Become a better student and a BETTER NURSE

Davis Advantage offers a personalized, interactive learning platform with proven results to help you succeed in your course.

94%
of students said Advantage improved their test scores.

"My grades have improved; my understanding about topics is much clearer; and overall, it has been the total package for what a nursing student needs to succeed."

— Hannah, Student, Judson University

Your journey to success BEGINS HERE!

Redeem your access code on the inside front cover of your text to access the tools you need to succeed in your course. Need a code? Visit FADavis.com to purchase access.

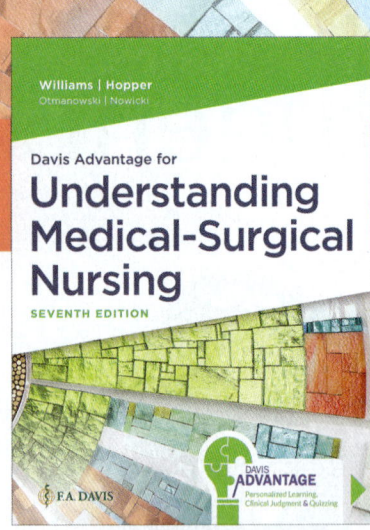

TEXT

STEP #1
Build a solid foundation.

Gerontological Issues
Age-Related Renal Changes
These changes typically occur in the renal system as people age:
- Decreased filtration efficiency of the kidneys affects the body's ability to eliminate drugs
- Decreased renal function slows the excretion of certain medications, so they remain in the body longer

Consequently, dehydration, common in older adults, and changes in renal function are a serious consideration for individuals in this age group who need medication therapy. The risk of adverse medication reactions, such as toxicity and overdose, increases. It can be important to monitor kidney function (such as serum creatinine and blood urea nitrogen [BUN] levels) in an older adult receiving medication therapy.

Gerontological Issues boxes prepare you to provide quality care to older adults.

Be Safe! boxes help you remember concepts essential to safe care.

BE SAFE!
AVOID FAILURE TO RESCUE! After an uncircumcised male is catheterized, the foreskin must be properly repositioned over the glans penis. It cannot be left retracted, as this can cause injury. If left retracted, subsequent swelling may make it impossible to pull the foreskin over the glans penis later. This can cause ischemia of the glans penis, a medical emergency. The HCP must be notified immediately. An emergency circumcision may be needed if the foreskin cannot be properly positioned. Always ensure that the foreskin is positioned properly after catheterization or perineal care.

Critical Thinking Exercises throughout each chapter help connect what you read to what you will see and do in the clinical setting, and include suggested answers at the end of the chapter to check your understanding.

CRITICAL THINKING
Mrs. Bohke is a 64-year-old female patient admitted to the hospital with a diagnosis of pneumonia. During her stay, she tells the nurse she has trouble getting to the bathroom in time and often dribbles before she can get there.

1. What type of urinary incontinence does Mrs. Bohke have?
2. When caring for a patient with incontinence, is it helpful to decrease fluid intake? Why or why not?

Suggested answers are a the end of the chapter.

Evidence-Based Practice

Clinical Question
What is the cumulative impact of social determinants of health on mortality in U.S. adults with CKD and diabetes?

Evidence
This study analyzed data from the 2005 through 2014 National Health and Nutrition Examination Surveys for 1,376 adults who had diabetes and CKD to look at the effect that social determinants of health had on mortality. Social determinates of health relate to socioeconomic; psychosocial; neighborhood environment; and political, cultural, and economic factors that people experience during their lifetime. This analysis looked at family income to poverty ratio, food insecurity, and depression. It was found that these social determinants had a cumulative effect on mortality that increased by 41% for each additional social determinant. Depression was independently associated with mortality (Ozieh et al, 2021).

Implications for Nursing Practice
An awareness of social determinants of health, and screening for them as well as for depression in CKD patients, to plan interventions or make referrals (e.g., for Meals on Wheels or mental health services) may help reduce mortality for CKD patients.

Reference: Ozieh, M. N., Garacci, E., Walker, R. J., Palatnik, A., & Egede, L. (2021). The cumulative impact of social determinants of health factors on mortality in adults with diabetes and chronic kidney disease. *BMC Nephrology, 22*(1), 76. https://doi.org/10.1186/s12882-021-02277-2

Evidence-Based Practice boxes feature an in-depth look at research that supports the best care and describe how that knowledge applies in practice.

CLINICAL JUDGMENT

Mrs. Wood, age 42, returns to the surgical unit after a hysterectomy. Her postoperative vital signs and data collection findings are normal. Mrs. Wood rates her pain level at 9 out of 10, and the nurse notes that she moans occasionally, repeatedly moves her legs, and pulls at her covers near her abdominal incision. She is drowsy but repeatedly says it hurts. In the PACU, a PCA pump was started. The last dose of medication was delivered 45 minutes ago. Her family is at her bedside trying to talk to her about her experience.

1. What nonverbal pain cues do you find Mrs. Wood is displaying?
2. How do you document Mrs. Wood's pain?
3. What action do you take to relieve Mrs. Wood's pain?
4. When will you next monitor Mrs. Wood's pain level?
5. If Mrs. Wood indicates that her pain remains unrelieved with the PCA pump, what action will you take?
6. Which team members do you collaborate with?
7. What action do you take to support the needs of the patient and family?

Suggested answers are at the end of the chapter.

Clinical Judgment case studies and questions help you practice and think about what you are learning, and then apply the learning to clinical decision-making.

CUE RECOGNITION 12.3

The surgeon's orders for a patient who had a colectomy are NPO with IV fluids and an NG tube to low intermittent suction to be irrigated prn. The patient reports stomach pressure and nausea with a need to vomit. What action do you take?

Suggested answers are at the end of the chapter.

Cue Recognition exercises provide practice in identifying actions to take when presented with patient cues or data.

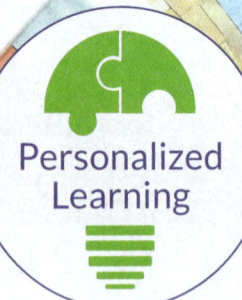
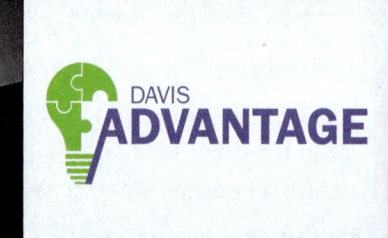

LEARN

STEP #2
Make the connections to key topics.

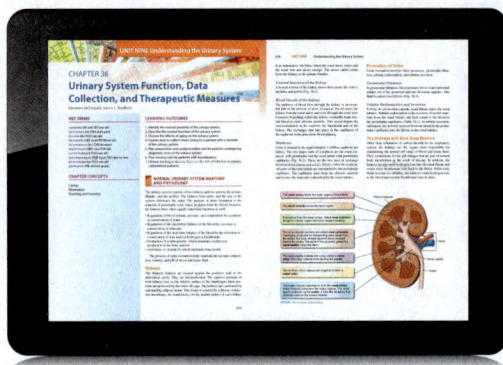
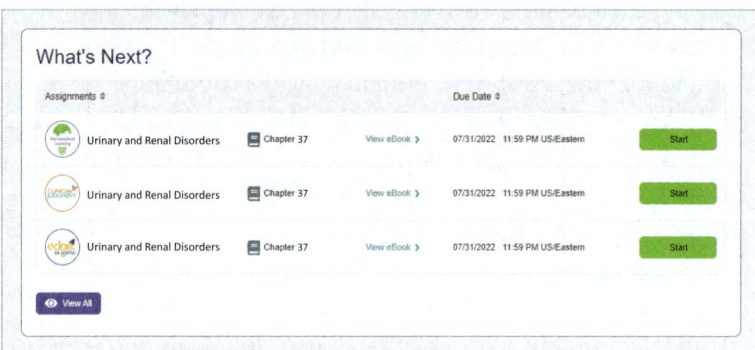

Assignments in Davis Advantage correspond to key topics in your book. Begin by reading from your printed text or click the eBook button to be taken to the **FREE, integrated eBook.**

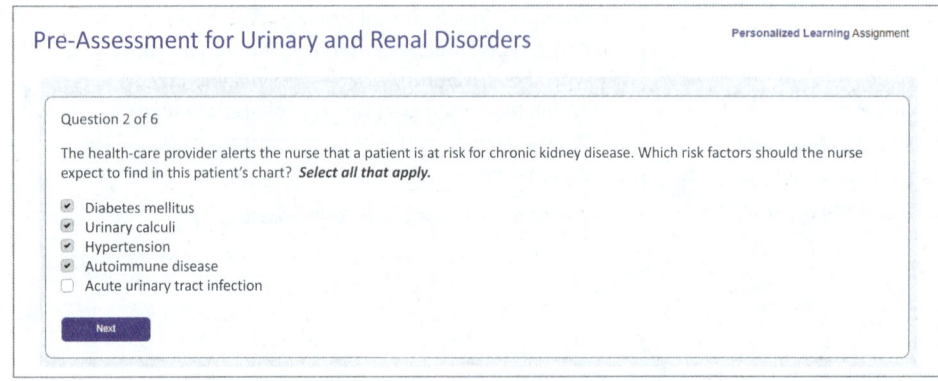

Following your reading, take the **Pre-Assessment** quiz to evaluate your understanding of the content. Questions feature single answer, multiple-choice, and select-all-that-apply formats.

You'll receive **immediate feedback** that identifies your strengths and weaknesses using a thumbs up, thumbs down approach. *Thumbs up* indicates competency, while *thumbs down* signals an area of weakness that requires further study.

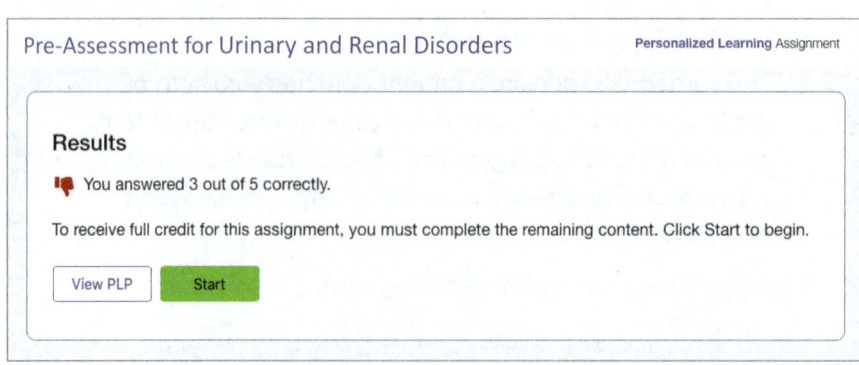

Online content subject to change upon publication.

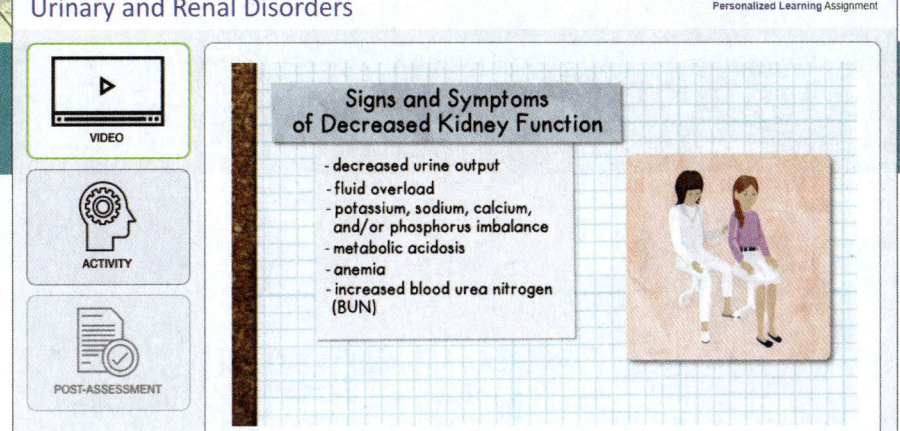

After working through the video and activity, a **Post-Assessment** quiz tests your mastery.

Animated mini-lecture videos make key concepts easier to understand, while **interactive learning activities** allow you to expand your knowledge and make the connections to important topics.

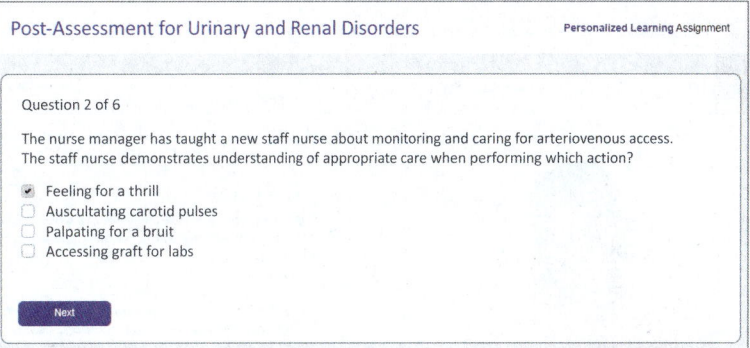

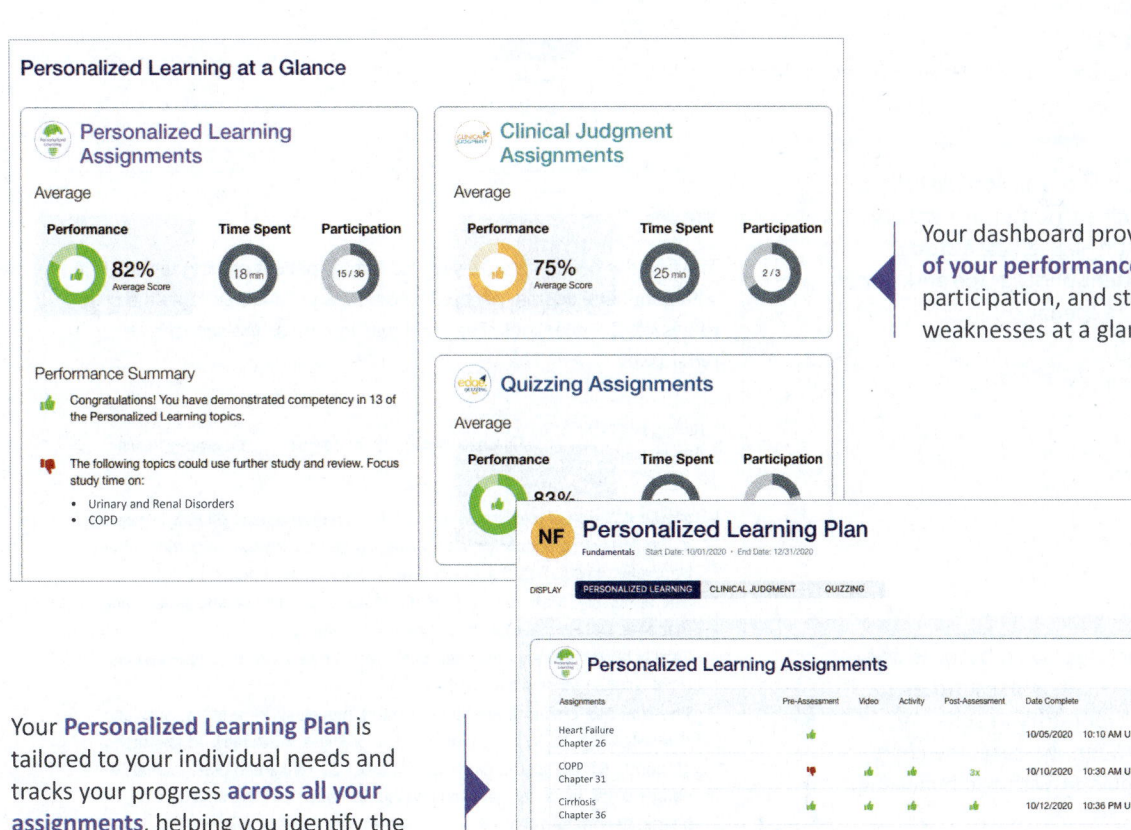

Your dashboard provides **snapshots of your performance**, time spent, participation, and strengths and weaknesses at a glance.

Your **Personalized Learning Plan** is tailored to your individual needs and tracks your progress **across all your assignments**, helping you identify the exact areas that require additional study.

Online content subject to change upon publication.

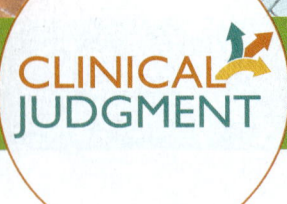

CLINICAL JUDGMENT

APPLY

STEP #3
Develop critical-thinking skills & prepare for the Next Gen NCLEX.®

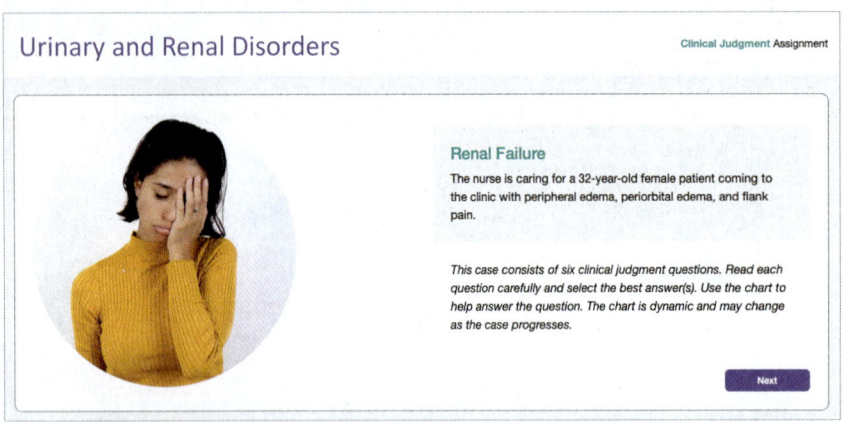

Urinary and Renal Disorders — Clinical Judgment Assignment

Renal Failure
The nurse is caring for a 32-year-old female patient coming to the clinic with peripheral edema, periorbital edema, and flank pain.

This case consists of six clinical judgment questions. Read each question carefully and select the best answer(s). Use the chart to help answer the question. The chart is dynamic and may change as the case progresses.

Real-world cases mirror the complex clinical challenges you will encounter in a variety of healthcare settings. Each **case study** begins with a patient photograph and a brief introduction to the scenario.

Scenario

The nurse is caring for a 32-year-old female patient coming to the clinic with peripheral edema, periorbital edema, and flank pain. Use the chart to answer the questions. *The chart may update as the scenario progresses.*

| History and Physical Assessment | Nurses' Notes | Vital Signs | Laboratory Results |

Medical/Surgical history: Systemic lupus erythematosus (SLE) x 12 years, controlled with glucocorticoids, diabetes mellitus x 2 years, recurring urinary tract infections (UTIs). Surgical history includes C-sections x 2.
Social history: Married with 2 healthy children. Works full time as an office manager. Denies use of alcohol, drugs, or tobacco.
Family history: Mother also had SLE, died at age 55 from complications of renal failure. Father is alive and healthy.
Physical Assessment: Alert and oriented, moves all extremities, grips and pushes strong, PERRLA. Lungs with fine crackles, bilaterally, no shortness of breath. S1, S2 heart sounds with murmur. 3+ radial and pedal pulses. 4+ edema of the lower legs, ankles and feet, 2+ edema of the fingers and hands, periorbital edema present. Pain with percussion of the costovertebral angle.
Medications: Prednisone 5 to 10 mg daily, titrated to symptoms; metformin

The Patient Chart displays tabs for History & Physical Assessment, Nurses' Notes, Vital Signs, and Laboratory Results. As you progress through the case, the chart expands and populates with additional data.

Urinary and Renal Disorders
Clinical Judgment Assignment

Scenario
The nurse is caring for a 32-year-old female patient coming to the clinic with peripheral edema, periorbital edema, and flank pain. Use the chart to answer the questions. *The chart may update as the scenario progresses.*

Tabs: History and Physical Assessment | Nurses' Notes | Vital Signs | Laboratory Results

Medical/Surgical history: Systemic lupus erythematosus (SLE) x 12 years, controlled with glucocorticoids, diabetes mellitus x 2 years, recurring urinary tract infections (UTIs). Surgical history includes C-sections x 2.
Social history: Married with 2 healthy children. Works full time as an office manager. Denies use of alcohol, drugs, or tobacco.
Family history: Mother also had SLE, died at age 55 from complications of renal failure. Father is alive and healthy.
Physical Assessment: Alert and oriented, moves all extremities, grips and pushes strong, PERRLA. Lungs with fine crackles, bilaterally, no shortness of breath. S1, S2 heart sounds with murmur. 3+ radial and pedal pulses. 4+ edema of the lower legs, ankles and feet, 2+ edema of the fingers and hands, periorbital edema present. Pain with percussion of the costovertebral angle.
Medications: Prednisone 5 to 10 mg daily, titrated to symptoms; metformin

Question 1 of 6
The nurse reviews the patient's record. *Select to highlight the areas that are the most concerning at this time.*

Physical Assessment: Alert and oriented, moves all extremities, grips and pushes strong, PERRLA. Lungs with fine crackles, bilaterally, no shortness of breath. S1, S2 heart sounds with murmur. 3+ radial and pedal pulses. 4+ edema of the lower legs, ankles and feet, 2+ edema of the fingers and hands, periorbital edema present. Pain of the costovertebral angle.
Vital Signs:
Temp 99.2° F (37.3° C)
HR 101 bpm; regular
RR 18 breaths/min
SpO₂ 95% on room air
BP 187/99 mm Hg (MAP 128)

Next

Complex questions that mirror the format of the Next Gen NCLEX® require careful analysis, synthesis of the data, and multi-step thinking.

Results

 You answered 0 out of 6 questions correctly.

Review the questions, answers and rationales below to improve your understanding. Identify which questions you answered correctly (indicated by a green check mark) and incorrectly (identified by a red x). Remember, you must choose all correct options and only the correct options to get a question correct. Expand the questions to review your individual answer choices, the correct answers (indicated by green shading), and complete rationales.

[Show All Details ▼] [Return to Assignments]

 Question 1 of 6 — Hide ▲

The nurse reviews the patient's record. *Select to highlight the areas that are the most concerning at this time.*

Physical Assessment: Alert and oriented, moves all extremities, grips and pushes strong, PERRLA. Lungs with fine crackles, bilaterally, no shortness of breath. **S1, S2 heart sounds with murmur.** 3+ radial and pedal pulses. **4+ edema of the lower legs, ankles and feet**, 2+ edema of the fingers and hands, periorbital edema present. **Pain of the costovertebral angle.**
Vital Signs:
Temp 99.2° F (37.3° C)
HR 101 bpm; regular
RR 18 breaths/min
SpO₂ 95% on room air
BP 187/99 mm Hg (MAP 128)

Rationale
The greatest concern at this time is hypertension, the severe lower extremity edema, and the risk for inflammation or infection in the kidneys. Pain of the costovertebral angle and a low-grade fever is indicative of inflammation or infection and requires further exploration. Neurological assessment is within normal limits. Although there are crackles in the lungs, the patient is not in distress and the SpO₂ on room air is normal, so it is not a priority concern. There is a murmur present, which is an abnormal finding but not a priority concern. Other findings are normal.

Clinical Judgment Cognitive Skill: Recognize Cues   Page Reference: p. 1447

 Test-Taking Tip — Even though a finding is abnormal (such as the mild edema of the hands and crackles in the lungs), that does not mean that it is concerning. Often the body compensates for other concerning events, and if compensatory, it is a welcomed assessment change.

Immediate feedback with **detailed rationales** encourages you to consider what data is important and how to prioritize the information, resulting in safe and effective nursing care.

Test-taking tips provide important context and strategies for how to consider the structure of each question type when answering.

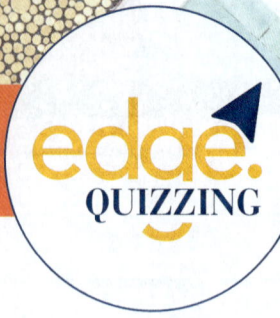

ASSESS

STEP #4
Improve comprehension & retention.

High-quality questions, including more difficult question types like **select-all-that-apply**, assess your understanding and challenge you to think at a higher cognitive level.

PLUS! Brand-new Next Gen NCLEX® stand-alone questions provide you with even more practice answering the new item types and help build your confidence.

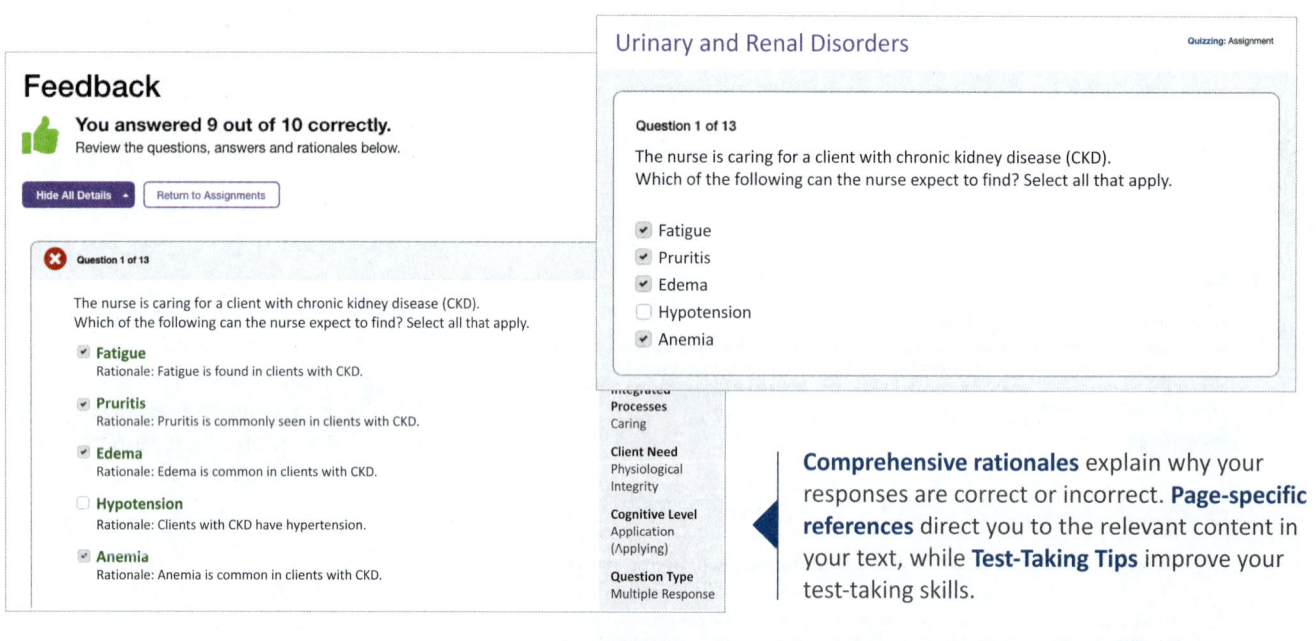

Comprehensive rationales explain why your responses are correct or incorrect. **Page-specific references** direct you to the relevant content in your text, while **Test-Taking Tips** improve your test-taking skills.

Create your own **practice quizzes** to focus on topic areas where you are struggling, or use as a study tool to review for an upcoming exam.

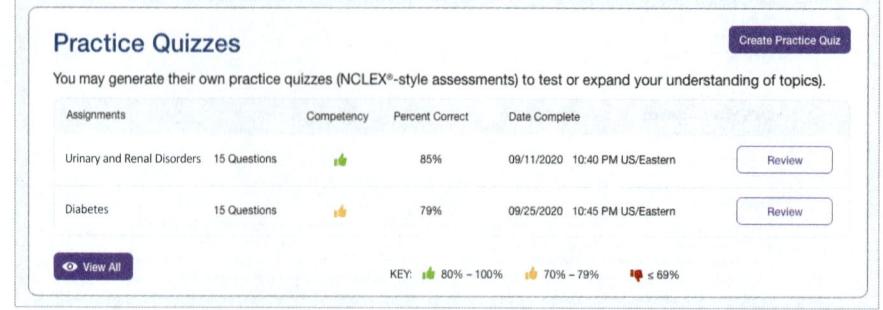

GET STARTED TODAY!
Use the access code on the inside front cover to unlock
Davis Advantage for **Understanding Medical-Surgical Nursing**

STUDY SMARTER | NOT HARDER

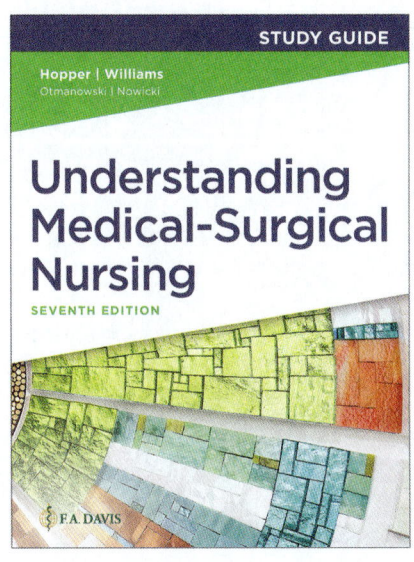

The perfect companion to the text!

Currently in nursing school.
"This workbook is a great review for each chapter!"

—David B.

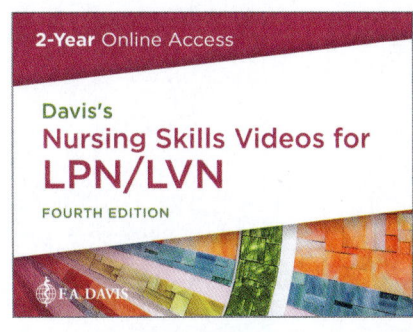

Real Nurses. Real People. Real Skills.

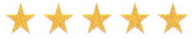

Five Stars
"Two thumbs up. Great product."

—Rebeccah T.

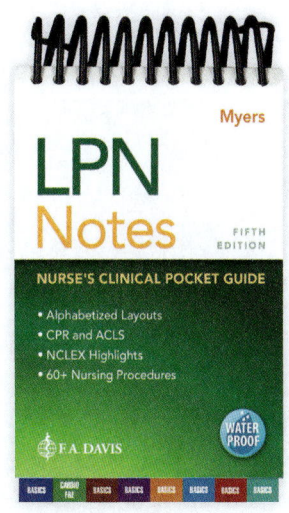

#1 LPN pocket guide for class & clinical.

Great. "A must-have during and after Nursing school. Wish I would've gotten this book sooner."

—Mary R.

SAVE 20% + FREE SHIPPING

Use Code: **DAVIS20**

ORDER TODAY!

at FADavis.com

Promotion subject to change without notice. Offer valid for individual purchases from FADavis.com in the U.S. only.

Brief Contents

UNIT ONE: Understanding Health-Care Issues, 1
1. Critical Thinking, Clinical Judgment, and the Nursing Process, 1
2. Evidence-Based Practice, 9
3. Issues in Nursing Practice, 15
4. Cultural Influences on Nursing Care, 31
5. Complementary and Alternative Modalities, 41

UNIT TWO: Understanding Health and Illness, 50
6. Nursing Care of Patients With Fluid, Electrolyte, and Acid–Base Imbalances, 50
7. Nursing Care of Patients Receiving Intravenous Therapy, 69
8. Nursing Care of Patients With Infections, 83
9. Nursing Care of Patients in Shock, 105
10. Nursing Care of Patients in Pain, 118
11. Nursing Care of Patients With Cancer, 140
12. Nursing Care of Patients Having Surgery, 164
13. Nursing Care of Patients With Emergent Conditions and Disaster/Bioterrorism Response, 192

UNIT THREE: Understanding Influences on Health and Illness, 211
14. Developmental Considerations and Chronic Illness in the Nursing Care of Adults, 211
15. Nursing Care of Older Adult Patients, 222
16. Patient Care Settings, 235
17. Nursing Care of Patients at the End of Life, 247

UNIT FOUR: Understanding the Immune System, 263
18. Immune System Function, Data Collection, and Therapeutic Measures, 263
19. Nursing Care of Patients With Immune Disorders, 277
20. Nursing Care of Patients With HIV and AIDS, 297

UNIT FIVE: Understanding the Cardiovascular System, 317
21. Cardiovascular System Function, Data Collection, and Therapeutic Measures, 317
22. Nursing Care of Patients With Hypertension, 342
23. Nursing Care of Patients With Valvular, Inflammatory, and Infectious Cardiac or Venous Disorders, 353
24. Nursing Care of Patients With Occlusive Cardiovascular Disorders, 377
25. Nursing Care of Patients With Cardiac Arrhythmias, 404
26. Nursing Care of Patients With Heart Failure, 425

UNIT SIX: Understanding the Hematologic and Lymphatic Systems, 448
27. Hematologic and Lymphatic System Function, Data Collection, and Therapeutic Measures, 448
28. Nursing Care of Patients With Hematologic and Lymphatic Disorders, 462

UNIT SEVEN: Understanding the Respiratory System, 486
29. Respiratory System Function, Data Collection, and Therapeutic Measures, 486
30. Nursing Care of Patients With Upper Respiratory Tract Disorders, 518
31. Nursing Care of Patients With Lower Respiratory Tract Disorders, 533

UNIT EIGHT: Understanding the Gastrointestinal, Hepatic, and Pancreatic Systems, 572
32. Gastrointestinal, Hepatobiliary, and Pancreatic Systems Function, Data Collection, and Therapeutic Measures, 572
33. Nursing Care of Patients With Upper Gastrointestinal Disorders, 598
34. Nursing Care of Patients With Lower Gastrointestinal Disorders, 618
35. Nursing Care of Patients With Liver, Pancreatic, and Gallbladder Disorders, 649

UNIT NINE: Understanding the Urinary System, 675
36. Urinary System Function, Data Collection, and Therapeutic Measures, 675
37. Nursing Care of Patients With Disorders of the Urinary System, 695

UNIT TEN: Understanding the Endocrine System, 723

38 Endocrine System Function and Data Collection, 723
39 Nursing Care of Patients With Disorders of the Endocrine System, 739
40 Nursing Care of Patients With Disorders of the Endocrine Pancreas, 765

UNIT ELEVEN: Understanding the Genitourinary and Reproductive Systems, 790

41 Genitourinary and Reproductive Systems Function and Data Collection, 790
42 Nursing Care of Women With Reproductive System Disorders, 815
43 Nursing Care of Male Patients With Genitourinary Disorders, 848
44 Nursing Care of Patients With Sexually Transmitted Infections, 869

UNIT TWELVE: Understanding the Musculoskeletal System, 884

45 Musculoskeletal Function and Data Collection, 884
46 Nursing Care of Patients With Musculoskeletal and Connective Tissue Disorders, 899

UNIT THIRTEEN: Understanding the Neurologic System, 929

47 Neurologic System Function, Data Collection, and Therapeutic Measures, 929
48 Nursing Care of Patients With Central Nervous System Disorders, 951

49 Nursing Care of Patients With Cerebrovascular Disorders, 1000
50 Nursing Care of Patients With Peripheral Nervous System Disorders, 1020

UNIT FOURTEEN: Understanding the Sensory System, 1038

51 Sensory System Function, Data Collection, and Therapeutic Measures: Vision and Hearing, 1038
52 Nursing Care of Patients With Sensory Disorders: Vision and Hearing, 1060

UNIT FIFTEEN: Understanding the Integumentary System, 1091

53 Integumentary System Function, Data Collection, and Therapeutic Measures, 1091
54 Nursing Care of Patients With Skin Disorders, 1107
55 Nursing Care of Patients With Burns, 1138

UNIT SIXTEEN: Understanding Mental Health Care, 1155

56 Mental Health Function, Data Collection, and Therapeutic Measures, 1155
57 Nursing Care of Patients With Mental Health Disorders, 1169

Davis Advantage for Understanding Medical-Surgical Nursing

SEVENTH EDITION

Linda S. Williams, MSN, RN
Professor Emeritus
Jackson College
Jackson, Michigan

Paula D. Hopper, MSN, RN
Professor Emeritus
Jackson College
Jackson, Michigan

Associate Editors

Jennifer Otmanowski, PhD, RN, CNE, CHSE
Professor
Baker College – Jackson
Jackson, Michigan

Lazette V. Nowicki, DNP, MSN, BS, RN
Professor, Nursing
American River College
Sacramento, California

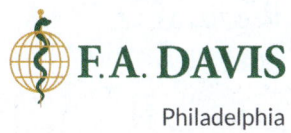

F.A. DAVIS
Philadelphia

F.A. Davis Company
1915 Arch Street
Philadelphia, PA 19103
www.fadavis.com

Copyright © 2023 by F.A. Davis Company

Copyright © 2023, 2019, 2015, 2011, 2007, 2003, 1999 by F.A. Davis Company. All rights reserved. This product is protected by copyright. No part of it may be reproduced, stored in a retrieval system, or transmitted in any form or by any means, electronic, mechanical, photocopying, recording, or otherwise, without written permission from the publisher.

Printed in the United States of America
Last digit indicates print number: 10 9 8 7 6 5 4 3 2 1

Publisher, Nursing: Terri Wood Allen
Senior Content Project Manager: Elizabeth Hart
Art and Design Manager: Carolyn O'Brien
Digital Project Managers: Elaine Finefrock & Jillian O'Hara

As new scientific information becomes available through basic and clinical research, recommended treatments and drug therapies undergo changes. The author(s) and publisher have done everything possible to make this book accurate, up to date, and in accord with accepted standards at the time of publication. The author(s), editors, and publisher are not responsible for errors or omissions or for consequences from application of the book, and make no warranty, expressed or implied, in regard to the contents of the book. Any practice described in this book should be applied by the reader in accordance with professional standards of care used in regard to the unique circumstances that may apply in each situation. The reader is advised always to check product information (package inserts) for changes and new information regarding dose and contraindications before administering any drug. Caution is especially urged when using new or infrequently ordered drugs.

ISBN: 978-1-7196-4458-7

Library of Congress Cataloging-in-Publication Data
Names: Williams, Linda S. (Linda Sue), 1954– editor. | Hopper, Paula D., editor |
  Otmanowski, Jennifer, editor. | Nowicki, Lazette V., editor.
Title: Davis advantage for understanding medical-surgical nursing /
  [editors], Linda S. Williams, Paula D. Hopper ; associate editors,
  Jennifer Otmanowski, Lazette V. Nowicki.
Other titles: Understanding medical-surgical nursing
Description: Seventh edition. | Philadelphia, PA : F.A. Davis Company, [2023] |
  Includes bibliographical references and index.
Identifiers: LCCN 2022002507 (print) | LCCN 2022002508 (ebook) |
  ISBN 9781719644587 (paperback) | ISBN 9781719644600 (ebook)
Subjects: MESH: Medical-Surgical Nursing | Nursing Process |
  Evidence-Based Nursing
Classification: LCC RT41 (print) | LCC RT41 (ebook) | NLM WY 150 |
  DDC 610.73—dc23/eng/20220422
LC record available at https://lccn.loc.gov/2022002507
LC ebook record available at https://lccn.loc.gov/2022002508

Authorization to photocopy items for internal or personal use, or the internal or personal use of specific clients, is granted by F.A. Davis Company for users registered with the Copyright Clearance Center (CCC) Transactional Reporting Service, provided that the fee of $.25 per copy is paid directly to CCC, 222 Rosewood Drive, Danvers, MA 01923. For those organizations that have been granted a photocopy license by CCC, a separate system of payment has been arranged. The fee code for users of the Transactional Reporting Service is: 978-1-7196-4458-7/22 0 + $.25.

Dedication

For practical and vocational nursing students: you are valuable members of the health-care team. We trust this text will help you learn to think like nurses and develop clinical judgment skills to become safe practitioners.

In memory of my father, Richard, who was so proud of every edition of this textbook.
—Linda

And for my grandchildren, Theo and Arthur, who light up my life.
—Paula

Acknowledgments

Many people helped us make this book a reality. First and foremost are the students, who provide us with the inspiration to undertake this project. We hope that students everywhere continue to find this text worth reading.

The F.A. Davis Company is an exceptional publishing partner. We feel fortunate to have had their continued enthusiasm and confidence in our book. The staff at F.A. Davis has guided us through this project for seven editions to help us create a student-friendly book that truly promotes understanding of medical-surgical nursing and the development of clinical judgment to provide safe, patient-centered care. Terri Allen and Elizabeth Hart as well as many others have been extremely patient and kind as we worked hard to provide a quality textbook.

Contributors from across the United States, including many well-known experts in their fields, brought expertise and diversity to the content. Their hard work is much appreciated. We are thankful to Gay Alcenius, PharmD, for her expertise in updating all of the medication information and to Sheria Robinson-Lane for her expertise in cultural issues.

We are especially excited to introduce two new associate editors, Jennifer Otmanowski and Lazette Nowicki. They have brought new voices and ideas to the project, and we are thankful for their expertise.

We wish to thank everyone who played a role, however large or small, in helping us to provide a tool to help students realize their dreams of becoming LPNs/LVNs. We hope this book will help educate nurses who can provide safe and expert care because we have helped them to learn to think critically and demonstrate sound clinical judgment.

Linda and Paula

Preface

Welcome to the Seventh Edition of *Davis Advantage for Understanding Medical-Surgical Nursing*! The material has been completely reviewed and updated. New evidence-based guidelines have been used wherever possible.

We continue to work hard to provide a text written at an understandable level, with features that help students understand, apply, and safely practice the challenging content required to succeed as practical/vocational nurses. We are thankful to the many faculty and students who tell us they find the book very readable and enjoyable. We welcome and value your comments on this edition.

We believe that students must have excellent thinking skills to supplement basic knowledge in order to make good, safe clinical judgments. To this end, we emphasize understanding and application over memorization and provide opportunities to practice critical thinking and clinical judgment throughout the text, study guide, and online resources. We hope you find this approach helps you to not only learn but understand and apply this information to your practice.

Content and Features

We have retained our most popular features from the first six editions and added new ones based on reader input and current practice.

New to the Seventh Edition are the following:

- **Expanded concept list** at beginning of each chapter.
- Up-to-the-minute information on **current issues** such as pandemics, COVID-19, and the opioid crisis.
- Discussion of **Social Determinants of Health** and **Healthy People 2030**.
- **Practice Analysis Tips** based on the NCSBN practice (job) analysis, which alert students to the skills that will be tested on the NCLEX-PN.
- **Cue Recognition** exercises, which provide practice in identifying actions to take when presented with patient cues or data; suggested answers are available at the end of the chapter.
- New **Clinical Judgment** and updated **Critical Thinking** case studies throughout each chapter. These exercises help students practice and think about what they are learning and then apply the learning to clinical decision making. **Suggested Answers** to case studies are available at the end of the chapter. Research supports the importance of immediate feedback to reinforce learning, so we feel strongly that students should have access to answers while they are studying. Because there can be many answers to some of the questions, we have provided sample answers to help stimulate students' thinking.

Based on feedback, we have retained, updated, and expanded the following:

- **Be Safe!, Nursing Care Tips,** and **Learning Tips** highlight important concepts to help make learning easier.
- Boxed presentations of **Cultural Considerations, Evidence-Based Practice, Gerontological Issues, Home Health Hints,** and **Nutrition Notes.** Boxes have been updated where needed.
- **Nursing Care Plans** with updated priority nursing diagnoses and gerontological considerations.
- **Patient Perspectives** that provide real patient experiences to bring life to theoretical material.
- **Pronunciation Guides** for new words at the beginning of each chapter.
- **Word Building** footnotes throughout the chapters.
- **Key Points** are now included at the end of chapters for quick and easy chapter review.
- **Glossary** that is comprehensive and updated in the back of the text.
- **Web links** in the text to help students do further research on topics of interest.

To Students: How to Use This Book

Learning Outcomes are provided for each chapter. Review them before reading, and then go back and check to be sure you understand each outcome after you complete your reading.

You will find a list of key terms and their pronunciations at the beginning of each chapter. These words appear in bold at either their first use or most relevant use in a chapter, and they also appear in the glossary at the end of the book. By learning the meanings of these words as you encounter them, you increase your understanding of the material. Many of these words are also broken down into component parts where they are used, so you can see how the parts of each word make up the whole.

Following the key terms is a list of concepts covered in the chapter. At the end of each chapter, consider what you have learned about each concept, how it relates to the other concepts, and what you already know about that concept.

You also will find learning tips to increase your understanding and retention of the material. You may want to develop your own memory techniques in addition to those provided. (If you think of a good one, send it to us at F.A. Davis, and you may find it in the next edition!) Many of the learning tips have been developed and used in our own classrooms. We find them to be helpful in fostering understanding of complex concepts or as memory aids. However, we want to stress that memorization is not the primary focus of the text but rather a foundation for understanding and thinking about more complex information. Understanding an application will serve you far better than memorization when dealing with new situations.

Each chapter includes brief critical thinking and clinical judgment case studies designed to help you apply material that has been presented. A series of questions related to the case will help you integrate the material with what you already know. Critical thinking questions emphasize WHY cues or events are important and what they mean. Clinical judgment questions focus on what you must DO to help or rescue the patient. Suggested answers are provided at the end of the chapter.

Generic medication names are a must for you to know for the NCLEX-PN. We provide both the generic and trade names for medications at their first mention in a chapter, and then only the generic name, to help you prepare for both the NCLEX-PN and nursing practice.

The following are included in the back of the text for easy reference:

- Common Diagnostic Tests (Appendix A)
- Normal Adult Reference Laboratory Values (Appendix B)
- Glossary
- Common Prefixes and Suffixes to help learn word-building techniques

The Teaching and Learning Package

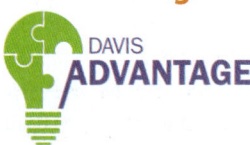

How students learn is evolving. In this digital age, we consume information in new ways. The possibilities to interact and connect with content in new, dynamic ways are enhancing student understanding and retention of complex concepts.

In order to meet the needs of today's learners, how faculty teach is also evolving. Classroom (traditional or online) time is valuable for active learning. This approach makes students responsible for the key concepts, allowing faculty to focus on clinical application. Relying on the textbook alone to support an active classroom leaves a gap. *Davis Advantage* is designed to fill that gap and help students and faculty succeed in core courses and across the LPN/LVN curriculum. It is comprised of the following:

- A **Strong Core Textbook** that provides the foundation of knowledge that today's nursing students need to pass the NCLEX® and enter practice prepared for success.
- An **Online Solution** that provides resources for each step of the learning cycle: learn, apply, assess.
  - **Personalized Learning** assignments are the core of the product and are designed to prepare students for classroom (live or online) discussion. They provide directed learning based on needs. After completing text reading assignments, students take a pre-assessment for each *topic*. Their results feed into their *Personalized Learning Plan*. If students do not pass the pre-assessment, they are required to complete further work within the topic: watch an animated mini-lecture, work through an activity, and take the post-assessment. The personalized learning content is designed to connect students with the foundational information about a given topic or concept. It provides the gateway to help make the content accessible to all students and complements different learning styles.
  - **Clinical Judgment** assignments are case-based and build off key Personalized Learning topics. These cases help students develop clinical judgment skills through exploratory learning. Students link their knowledge base (developed through the text and personalized learning) to new data and patient situations. Cases include dynamic charts that expand as the case progresses and use complex question types that require students to analyze data, synthesize conclusions, and make judgments. Each case ends with comprehensive feedback, which provides detailed rationales for the correct and incorrect answers.
  - **Quizzing** assignments (included for every topic) build off Personalized Learning Topics and help assess students' understanding of the broader scope and increased depth of that topic. The quizzes use NCLEX-style questions, including Next Generation NCLEX question types, to assess understanding and synthesis of content. Quiz results include comprehensive feedback for correct and incorrect answers to help students understand why their answer choices were right or wrong.
- **Online Instructor Resources** are aimed at creating a dynamic learning experience that relies heavily on interactive participation and is tailored to students' needs. Results from the post-assessments are available to faculty, in aggregate or by student, and inform a **Personalized Teaching Plan** that faculty can use to deliver a targeted classroom experience. Faculty will know students' strengths and weaknesses *before* they come to class and can spend class time focusing on where students are struggling. Suggested in-class activities are provided to help create an interactive, hands-on learning environment that helps students connect more deeply with the content. NCLEX-style questions from the **Instructor Test Bank** and **PowerPoint** slides that correspond to the textbook chapters are referenced in the Personalized Teaching Plans.

Davis Advantage is included with this text and is available for all titles across the LPN/LVN curriculum with *Davis Advantage LPN/LVN*.

Additional Online Resources for Students

An abundance of additional student resources come with this edition of *Davis Advantage for Understanding Medical-Surgical Nursing* in the form of digital assets found on ***Davis Advantage***:

- **References.** Comprehensive reference lists and bibliographies provide sources for content discussed in the chapter as well as for additional reading material. Web sites are included in the references for some chapters to aid in expanding information resources.

- **Audio Case Studies With Questions.** Students should listen to the chapter topic case scenarios on Davis Advantage and follow up with the critical thinking questions for thought and discussion that are available in the Study Guide chapters.
- **Procedures.** Selected LPN/LVN skills are provided for review.
- **Patient Teaching Guidelines.** Sample guidelines for disorders discussed throughout the text are printable for students to use in patient care settings while reinforcing teaching for patients.
- An **eBook** of the text is perfect for studying on the go!

Study Guide

A Study Guide is available to provide additional practice with the material. Each chapter includes questions to accompany the audio case studies, vocabulary practice, objective exercises, a case study with critical thinking and clinical judgment practice, communication (SBAR, ISBARR, CUS tools) practice, and other critical thinking and prioritization practice exercises. Expanded review questions written in NCLEX-PN style include hot spot questions. Study Guide answers are posted to the Instructor Resources on www.fadavis.com.

Additional Online Resources for Instructors

The online resources for instructors, available at FADavis.com, include guidance on how to utilize the text and *Davis Advantage* online resources throughout programs of different lengths, whether you teach traditionally or in a concept-based nursing program.

- **NCLEX-Style test bank** revised and updated for the 7th edition.
- **PowerPoint presentations** with newly added Practice Analysis Tips and interactive exercises, including concept-based case studies in select chapters, communication tools practice exercises, and other objective exercises. We want you to have the tools to promote an active, engaged classroom that learns by thinking and discussing as well as by lecture.
- **Digital image collection.** Many images are already included in the PowerPoint slides, but they are included here as well.
- **Study Guide Answer Key,** which allows instructors the option of providing answers to students for self-study or assigning the Study Guide exercises for grading.
- An **eBook** of the text.

LPN/LVN Connections

F.A. Davis is pleased to offer **LPN/LVN Connections,** a consistent and recognizable approach to design and content that will make it easier for students and instructors to use multiple F.A. Davis textbooks throughout the LPN/LVN curriculum. We have increased continuity whenever possible, without erasing the authors' autonomy or changing legacy content that has been popular in past editions. This makes it easier for instructors and students to move through the textbooks and ancillary products while recognizing shared themes and featured content.

Textbook Design, Style, and Pedagogy

All textbook chapters include:

- Numbered learning outcomes
- Key terms with phonetic pronunciations listed on the chapter opener and boldfaced where first defined in the chapter
- Chapter concepts
- Bulleted key points
- Chapter references, located online
- A reading level evaluation is performed during the manuscript development to ensure readability.
- Word-building footnotes help students build understanding of root terminology.
- A uniform, space-saving internal design features special heads and colors that are shared across titles for features with similar content to increase recognition.
- For consistent and current terminology and laboratory values across titles, the authors followed *Davis's Comprehensive Handbook of Laboratory & Diagnostic Tests With Nursing Implications* by Van Leeuwen and Bladh.

Standardized Student and Faculty Resources

For students:

- *Davis Advantage* online resources for students
- Study Guide with perforated pages so that students can hand in assignments if requested (Answer Key provided to instructors online to distribute if desired)

For instructors:

- *Davis Advantage* online resources for instructors
- **Davis Advantage LPN/LVN Curriculum Plan**, which includes implementation recommendations and engaging teaching strategies for programs of different lengths, whether you teach traditionally or in a concept-based nursing program
- NCLEX-style test bank
- PowerPoint presentations
- Digital image collection

F.A. Davis LPN/LVN Advisory Board

The authors and publisher extend a special thank you to the F.A. Davis LPN/LVN Advisory Board, whose members have provided guidance through their experience and expertise:

Deborah D. Brabham, PhD, RN, CNE
Professor of Nursing
Florida State College at Jacksonville
Jacksonville, Florida

Jennifer Briggs, MS, RN
Clinical Instructor, Practical Nursing
Adjunct Instructor, ADRN
Idaho State University
Pocatello, Idaho

Charlene Cowley, MS, RN, CPNP
Pediatric Nursing Instructor
Pima Community College – Desert Vista Campus
Tucson, Arizona

Shelley Eckvahl, MSN, RN
Professor, Nursing
Chaffey College
Chino Hills, California

Deana I. Elkins, MSN, RN
SCC Nursing Instructor
Southeastern Community College
Whiteville, North Carolina

Cynthia Hotaling, MSN, RN
Professor, LPN and ADN Programs
Owens Community College
Findlay, Ohio

Dawn Johnson, DNP, RN, Ed
Nurse Residency Coordinator & Nurse Educator
Renown Medical
Reno, Nevada

T. Camille Killough, PhD, RN
Instructor of Practical Nursing
Pearl River Community College
Poplarville, Mississippi

Jennifer Leer, MSN, RN, CCRN, SANE-P
Director, LPN and ADN Programs
West Virginia Junior College
Bridgeport, West Virginia

Chun Hee McMahon, RN, CHPN
Instructor, Vocational Nursing Program
Clovis Adult Education
Clovis, California

Paula K. Mundell, MSN, RN
Coordinator, Nursing Program
Delaware Technical Community College
Dover, Delaware

John H. Nagelschmidt, MSN, RN
Director, Practical Nursing
Assabet Valley Regional Technical School
Marlborough, Massachusetts

Deloris Paul, MSN, RN
Assistant Professor
Facilitator, Practical Nursing Program
Santa Fe College
Gainesville, Florida

Judith Pelletier, MSN, RN, CNE
Director, Division of Nurse Education
Upper Cape Cod Regional Technical School
Bourne, Massachusetts

Helen Rice, MSN, BSN, RN
LVN Program Director
Sacramento City College
Sacramento, California

Linda Rogers-Antuono, MSN/ED, RN
Nursing Faculty
Charlotte Technical College
Port Charlotte, Florida

Andrea D. Ruff, MS, RN
Coordinator of Healthcare Occupations
Cayuga-Onondaga BOCES
Auburn, New York

Ellen Santos, MSN, RN, CNE
Director of Practical Nursing, Retired
Assabet Valley Regional Tech
Marlborough, Massachusetts

Louise Schwabenbauer, MSN, RN, Med
Professor of Nursing
Practical Nursing Program Lead
Lord Fairfax Community College
Middletown, Virginia

Rosette Strandberg, MSN, Ed, RN
Director/Professor, Vocational Nursing Program
Santa Barbara City College
Santa Barbara, California

Amy Szoka, PhD, RN
Chair, School of Nursing
Daytona State College
Daytona Beach, Florida

Patricia Taylor, MSN-Ed, RN
Practical Nursing Coordinator
Kapi'olani Community College
University of Hawaii
Honolulu, Hawaii

Donna M. Theodore MSN, MA, RN, LMHC
Nurse Administrator/Director
Diman Regional Technical Institute
School of Practical Nursing
Fall River, Massachusetts

Loretta Vobr, MS, RN
LPN Instructor
Northwest Technical College
Bemidji, Minnesota

Dorothy L. Withers, MSN, RN
LPN Program Director and Director of Education
Prism Career Institute
Cherry Hill, New Jersey

Contributors

Gay Alcenius, PharmD, BCCCP
Clinical Pharmacy Manager
Henry Ford Allegiance Health
Jackson, Michigan
Medication Tables

Kathy Berchem, DNP, RN, APRN
Professor of Nursing
Lake Superior State University
Sault Ste. Marie, Michigan
Chapter 26: Nursing Care of Patients With Heart Failure

Christina Bode, MS, RND
Registered Dietician
San Diego, California
Nutrition Notes

Janice L. Bradford, MS
Associate Professor
Jackson College
Jackson, Michigan
Anatomy & Physiology

Michelle Corona, MS, BSN, RN
Assistant Professor
SUNY Morrisville
Norwich, New York
Chapter 44: Nursing Care of Patients With Sexually Transmitted Infections

Michele A. Dickson, DNP, MS, RN, CNE
Course Lead MSNED
Western Governor's University
Salt Lake City, Utah
Chapter 21: Cardiovascular System Function, Data Collection, and Therapeutic Measures
Chapter 25: Nursing Care of Patients With Cardiac Arrhythmias

Rebecca Ericson, MSN, RN
Perinatal Safety Specialist
Henry Ford Allegiance
Adjunct Instructor
Baker College
Jackson, Michigan
Chapter 41: Genitourinary and Reproductive Systems Function and Data Collection

Marge Gingrich, MSN, RN, CRNP
Adult Nurse Practitioner, Professor of Nursing
Harrisburg Area Community College
Harrisburg, Pennsylvania
Chapter 6: Nursing Care of Patients With Fluid, Electrolyte, and Acid–Base Imbalances

Kristy Gorman, MS, RN, OCN
Clinical Nurse
Baltimore County Public Schools and University of Maryland Medical Center
Baltimore, Maryland
Chapter 2: Evidence-Based Practice
Chapter 16: Patient Care Settings
Chapter 18: Immune System Function, Data Collection, and Therapeutic Measures
Chapter 19: Nursing Care of Patients With Immune Disorders

Debra Hadfield, DNP, MSN, RN, CNE
Director of Nursing
Baker College of Jackson
Jackson, Michigan
Chapter 43: Nursing Care of Male Patients With Genitourinary Disorders

Lynette P. Harvey, MS, BSN, RN
PhD Student and Teaching Assistant
Sinclair School of Nursing
University of Missouri
Columbia, Missouri
Chapter 5: Complementary and Alternative Modalities
Chapter 48: Nursing Care of Patients With Central Nervous System Disorders

Sarah Holda, MSN, RN, NP-C
Nurse Practitioner/Associate Professor of Nursing
Jackson College
Jackson, Michigan
Chapter 42: Nursing Care of Women With Reproductive System Disorders

Alene Homan, MEd, BSN, RN, CSN, CPN
Nurse Educator, Practical Nursing Program
Clearfield County Career and Technology Center
Clearfield, Pennsylvania
Chapter 38: Endocrine System Function and Data Collection
Chapter 39: Nursing Care of Patients With Disorders or the Endocrine System

Raja Issa, DNP, RN, CPHQ, CPPS, HACP, CJCP, NE-BC
Nursing Supervisor CVC-5 Moderate Care & CVC5-ICU
Michigan Medicine
Adjunct Clinical Instructor
University of Michigan School of Nursing
Ann Arbor, Michigan
Chapter 13: Nursing Care of Patients With Emergent Conditions and Disaster/Bioterrorism Response

Charlotte Kostelyk, MSN, RN, CNE
Assistant Professor of Nursing
Lake Superior State University
Sault Ste. Marie, Michigan
Chapter 23: Nursing Care of Patients With Valvular, Inflammatory, and Infectious Cardiac or Venous Disorders

Marina Martinez-Kratz, MS, RN, CNE
Professor of Nursing
Jackson College
Jackson, Michigan
Chapter 56: Mental Health Function, Data Collection, and Therapeutic Measures
Chapter 57: Nursing Care of Patients With Mental Health Disorders

Margaret J. McCormick, MS, RN, CNE
Clinical Associate Professor
Towson University
Towson, Maryland
Chapter 27: Hematologic and Lymphatic System Function, Data Collection, and Therapeutic Measures
Chapter 28: Nursing Care of Patients With Hematologic and Lymphatic Disorders

Maureen McDonald, MS, RN
Clinical Adjunct Faculty, Nursing
Laboure College
Milton, Massachusetts
Professor of Nursing, Retired
Massasoit Community College
Brockton, Massachusetts
Chapter 24: Nursing Care of Patients With Occlusive Cardiovascular Disorders
Chapter 36: Urinary System Function, Data Collection, and Therapeutic Measures
Chapter 37: Nursing Care of Patients With Disorders of the Urinary System

Amanda Miller, MSN, RN
Hospice Quality Assurance Nurse
Jerome, Michigan
Chapter 17: Nursing Care of Patients at the End of Life
Chapter 22: Nursing Care of Patients With Hypertension

John Nagelschmidt, MSN, RN
Director, Practical Nursing
Assabet Valley Regional Technical School
Marlborough, Massachusetts
Chapter 12: Nursing Care of Patients Having Surgery

Lisa Price, MSN, RN, CHSE
Associate Professor
Ivy Tech Community College
Kokomo, Indiana
Chapter 35: Nursing Care of Patients With Liver, Pancreatic, and Gallbladder Disorders

Sheria G. Robinson-Lane, PhD, RN
Assistant Professor
University of Michigan School of Nursing
Ann Arbor, Michigan
Cultural Connections
Chapter 4: Cultural Influences on Nursing Care
Chapter 10: Nursing Care of Patients in Pain

Linda Rogers-Antuono, MSN/ED, RN
Nursing Faculty
Charlotte Technical College
Port Charlotte, Florida
Chapter 34: Nursing Care of Patients With Lower Gastrointestinal Disorders

James Shannon, JD, MHSA, RN, CPHQ
Health Facilities Evaluator Nurse
California Department of Public Health
Santa Rosa, California
Chapter 3: Issues in Nursing Practice

Mary Anne Pietraniec Shannon, PhD, RN, GCNS-BC
Professor of Nursing
Sault College
Sault Saint Marie, Ontario, Canada
Chapter 15: Nursing Care of Older Adult Patients

Stephanie Skonos, RDN
Registered Dietitian
Center for Family Health
Jackson, Michigan
Nutrition Notes

Susan Sutton, MSN, RN
Instructor, Professional Nursing Program
Riverside College of Professional Nursing
Newport News, Virginia
Chapter 45: Musculoskeletal Function and Data Collection
Chapter 46: Nursing Care of Patients With Musculoskeletal and Connective Tissue Disorders

Heather Thornton, DNP, RN, CNE
Nursing Faculty
Baker College School of Nursing
Owosso, Michigan
Chapter 47: Neurologic System Function, Data Collection, and Therapeutic Measures

Gladdi Tomlinson, MSN, RN
Professor of Nursing
Harrisburg Area Community College
Harrisburg, Pennsylvania
Chapter 7: Nursing Care of Patients Receiving Intravenous Therapy

Rita Bolek Trofino, DNP, MNED, RN
Associate Dean, School of Health Sciences
Nursing Department Chair
Associate Professor
Saint Francis University
Loretto, Pennsylvania
Chapter 53: Integumentary System Function, Data Collection, and Therapeutic Measures
Chapter 54: Nursing Care of Patients With Skin Disorders
Chapter 55: Nursing Care of Patients With Burns

Kelli Verdecchia, MSN, RN
Assistant Professor, Chair
Lake Superior State University
Sault Sainte Marie, Michigan
Chapter 8: Nursing Care of Patients With Infections

Patrice Wade-Olsen, DNP, RN, AGPCWP-BC
Nurse Practitioner
Corktown Health Center
Detroit, Michigan
Chapter 20: Nursing Care of Patients With HIV and AIDS

Sara Wilk, DNP, MSN-ED, CCRN, CCRN-K Pediatrics, CHSE
Professor/Nursing Faculty
Baker College School of Nursing
Cadillac, Michigan
Chapter 49: Nursing Care of Patients with Cerebrovascular Disorders

Janet M. Yontas, MSN, RN
Nurse Educator
Career Technology Center, Practical Nursing–Lackawanna County
Scranton, Pennsylvania
Chapter 11: Nursing Care of Patients With Cancer

Contributors to Previous Editions

We would like to acknowledge and thank the following individuals for their contributions to previous editions. All contributions have helped to make *Davis Advantage for Understanding Medical-Surgical Nursing* what it has evolved into today.

Betty Ackley, MSN, EdS, RN

Nancy Ahern, PhD, RN

Cynthia Barrere, PhD, RN

Terri Blevins, BSN, MSEd

Michelle Block, MS, RN

Lucy L. Colo, MSN, RN

Colleen Delaney, PhD, RN, AHN-BC

Sharon Gordon, MSN, RN, CNOR(E)

Karen P. Hall, RN-C, MSHSA, NE-BC

Donna D. Ignatavicius, MS, RN, CNE, CNEcl, ANEF

Michelle Johnson, MSN, RN, CNE

Cindy Leffel, PhD, MSN, RN-BC

Carroll A. Lutz, MA, RN

Diane Mayo, MSN, RN

Erin Mazur, MSN, RN, FNP-BC

Kelly McManigle, MSN, RN

Kelly Ann Morris, DNP, RN

Sharon M. Nowak, MSN, EdD (ABD), RN

Lynn D. Phillips, MSN, RN, CRNI

Deb Richardson, MS, RN, CNS

John Sturtevant, MSN, RN

Deborah L. Weaver, PhD, RN

Patricia Williams, MSN, RN

Bruce K. Wilson, PhD, RN, CNS

Reviewers

Mindy Kay Barna, EdD, MSN, RN
Associate Dean of Health Professions, Assistant Professor
College of Saint Mary
Omaha, Nebraska

Caitlin F. Capodilupo, RN, BSN, MSN, DNP
Tenured Faculty, Lead Instructor (Medical Surgical Nursing), ADN Program Leader
Bay de Noc Community College
Escanaba, Michigan

James Chiles, MSN-Ed
Nursing Professor
San Jacinto Community College
Houston, Texas

Laure Frank, LPN
Assistant Professor
Santa Fe College
Gainesville, Florida

Louise S. Frantz, MHA, Ed, BSN, RN
Program Coordinator Practical Nursing
Penn State Berks
Reading, Pennsylvania

Lori Gehan, MSN, RN, CDP
Academic Department Head
Diman Regional School of Practical Nursing
Fall River, Massachusetts

Victoria Haynes, PhD, DNP, APRN, FNP-C
Tenured Professor of Nursing
Coordinator of Diversity & Cultural Competency
MidAmerica Nazarene University
Olathe, Kansas

Amanda Huber, DNP, APRN, FNP-C
Assistant Professor
Galen College of Nursing
Louisville, Kentucky

Lynn Lagasse, MSN, RN, CNE
Assistant Clinical Professor of Nursing
Keene State College
Keene, New Hampshire

Kimberly McClure, MSN, RN
Faculty, Level Coordinator
Victoria College
Victoria, Texas

Catherine R. Ratliff, PhD, GNP-BC, CWOCN, CFCN, FAAN
Nurse Practitioner, Clinical Associate Professor
University of Virginia
Charlottesville, Virginia

Mary L. Schreiber, MSN, RN, CMSRN
Nursing Education Consultant
RMS Consulting LLC
Ehrhardt, South Carolina

Melissa S. Smiley, MSN, RN
Nursing Faculty
Wayne Community College
Goldsboro, North Carolina

Rhonda Stangl, DNP, RN
Nurse Educator
Lake Area Technical College
Watertown, South Dakota

Hiba Wehbe-Alamah, PhD, RN, FNP-BC, CTN-A, FAAN
Professor and Interim Director of Graduate Nursing Affairs
University of Michigan-Flint
Flint, Michigan

Contents

UNIT ONE: Understanding Health-Care Issues, 1

1. Critical Thinking, Clinical Judgment, and the Nursing Process, 1
   What Are Critical Thinking and Clinical Judgment?, 2
   Critical Thinking Attitudes, 3
   The Nursing Process and Clinical Judgment, 3
   A Word about Vigilance, 5
   Communication With the Health-Care Team, 5
   Prioritizing Care, 6
   Collaboration, 7
   Nursing Knowledge Base, 7
   What Is on the NCLEX-PN®?, 7

2. Evidence-Based Practice, 9
   Reasons for Using EBP, 10
   Identifying Nursing Evidence, 10
   The EBP Process, 10
   Who Should Provide Evidence-Based Nursing Care?, 13
   EBP, Quality, and Safety: They Belong Together!, 13

3. Issues in Nursing Practice, 15
   Health-Care Delivery, 15
   Economic Issues, 16
   Nursing and the Health-Care Team, 17
   Compassion, 17
   Leadership in Nursing Practice, 17
   Ethics and Values, 20
   Legal Concepts, 26

4. Cultural Influences on Nursing Care, 31
   Concepts Related to Culture, 32
   Concepts Related to Spirituality, 32
   Health-Care Values, Beliefs, and Practices, 33
   Characteristics of Cultural Diversity, 34
   Space, 34
   Racial and Ethnic Groups in the United States, 37
   Culturally Responsive Care, 38

5. Complementary and Alternative Modalities, 41
   Complementary or Alternative: What's the Difference?, 41
   Introduction of New Systems Into Traditional Western Health Care, 42
   Complementary and Alternative Modalities, 43
   Safety and Effectiveness of Alternative Modalities, 47
   Role of the Licensed Practical Nurse/Licensed Vocational Nurse, 47

UNIT TWO: Understanding Health and Illness, 50

6. Nursing Care of Patients With Fluid, Electrolyte, and Acid–Base Imbalances, 50
   Fluid Balance, 50
   Fluid Imbalances, 52
   Electrolyte Imbalances, 57
   Acid–Base Balance, 65
   Acid–Base Imbalances, 65

7. Nursing Care of Patients Receiving Intravenous Therapy, 69
   Indications for Intravenous Therapy, 70
   Types of Intravenous Infusions, 70
   Methods of Infusion, 72
   Types of Fluids, 73
   Intravenous Access, 74
   Nursing Process for the Patient Receiving Intravenous Therapy, 75
   Complications of IV Therapy, 76
   Central Venous Access Devices, 76
   Other Therapies, 80

8. Nursing Care of Patients With Infections, 83
   The Infection Process, 83
   The Human Body's Defense Mechanisms, 88
   Infectious Disease, 89
   Infection Control in the Community, 91
   Infection Control in Health-Care Agencies, 92
   Antibiotic-Resistant Infections, 97
   Therapeutic Measures for Infectious Diseases, 97
   Nursing Process for the Patient With an Infection, 101

9. Nursing Care of Patients in Shock, 105
   Pathophysiology of Shock, 105
   Complications From Shock, 106
   Classification of Shock, 107
   Therapeutic Measures for Shock, 111
   Nursing Process for the Patient in Shock, 111

10. Nursing Care of Patients in Pain, 118
    The Pain Puzzle, 118
    Definitions of Pain, 119
    Risks of Uncontrolled Pain, 119
    Pain and Culture, 119
    Who's the Boss in Pain Management?, 120
    Myths and Barriers to Effective Pain Management, 121
    Opioid Addiction, 121
    Mechanisms of Pain Transmission, 122
    Options for Treatment of Pain, 123
    Nursing Process for the Patient Experiencing Pain, 131

11. Nursing Care of Patients With Cancer, 140
    Review of Anatomy and Physiology of Normal Cells, 140
    Introduction to Cancer Concepts, 142
    Nursing Process for the Patient With Cancer, 156
    Survivorship, 161
    Hospice Care of the Patient With Cancer, 161
    Oncological Emergencies, 162

12. Nursing Care of Patients Having Surgery, 164
    Surgery, 164
    Types and Phases of Surgery, 164

xxv

Preoperative Phase, 166
Intraoperative Phase, 174
Postoperative Phase, 178

13   Nursing Care of Patients With Emergent Conditions and Disaster/Bioterrorism Response, 192
Emergent Conditions, 192
Primary Survey, 192
Secondary Survey, 193
Shock, 194
Major Trauma, 194
Burns, 199
Hypothermia, 200
Frostbite, 201
Hyperthermia, 201
Poisoning and Drug Overdose, 202
Near-Drowning, 204
Psychiatric Emergencies, 204
Disaster Response, 204
Bioterrorism Agents, 205

UNIT THREE: Understanding Influences on Health and Illness, 211

14   Developmental Considerations and Chronic Illness in the Nursing Care of Adults, 211
Health, Wellness, and Illness, 211
The Nurse's Role in Supporting and Promoting Wellness, 212
Developmental Stages, 212
Chronic Illness, 215

15   Nursing Care of Older Adult Patients, 222
What Is Aging?, 222
Physiological Changes, 223
Cognitive and Psychological Changes in the Older Patient, 230
Health Promotion, 231

16   Patient Care Settings, 235
LPN/LVN Employment Settings, 235
Acute Care, 235
Medical Office Nursing, 236
Correctional Nursing, 236
Long-Term Care Services, 236
Home Health Care, 240

17   Nursing Care of Patients at the End of Life, 247
A Good Death, 247
Identifying Symptoms of Impending Death, 248
Advance Directives, Living Wills, and Durable Medical Power of Attorney, 248
End-of-Life Choices, 249
Communicating With Patients and Their Loved Ones, 251
Compassion Fatigue, 253
The Dying Process, 253
Care at the Time of Death and Afterward, 259
Grief, 260
Nursing Process for the Grieving Family, 260
The Nurse and Loss, 261

UNIT FOUR: Understanding the Immune System, 263

18   Immune System Function, Data Collection, and Therapeutic Measures, 263
Normal Immune System Anatomy and Physiology, 263
Antibody Responses, 265
Types of Immunity, 266
Aging and the Immune System, 268
Microbiota and the Immune System, 268
Immune System Data Collection, 268
Diagnostic Tests for the Immune System, 271
Therapeutic Measures for the Immune System, 275

19   Nursing Care of Patients With Immune Disorders, 277
Hypersensitivity Reactions, 277
Autoimmune Disorders, 288
Immune Deficiencies, 294

20   Nursing Care of Patients With HIV and AIDS, 297
History and Incidence, 299
Pathophysiology, 299
Prevention, 300
HIV Signs and Symptoms, 302
Complications, 302
Diagnosis, 304
Therapeutic Measures, 306
Resources, 315

UNIT FIVE: Understanding the Cardiovascular System, 317

21   Cardiovascular System Function, Data Collection, and Therapeutic Measures, 317
Normal Cardiovascular System Anatomy and Physiology, 317
Cardiovascular Disease, 323
Cardiovascular System Data Collection, 323
Diagnostic Tests for the Cardiovascular System, 330
Therapeutic Measures for the Cardiovascular System, 337

22   Nursing Care of Patients With Hypertension, 342
Pathophysiology, 342
Signs and Symptoms, 343
Diagnosis, 343
Social Determinants of Health, 343
Risk Factors, 344
Therapeutic Measures for Hypertension, 345
Complications, 345
Special Considerations, 349
Hypertensive Urgency, 349
Hypertensive Emergency, 349
Nursing Process for the Patient With Hypertension, 349

23   Nursing Care of Patients With Valvular, Inflammatory, and Infectious Cardiac or Venous Disorders, 353
Cardiac Valvular Disorders, 353
Inflammatory and Infectious Cardiac Disorders, 362
Venous Disorders, 370

24 Nursing Care of Patients With Occlusive Cardiovascular Disorders, 377
Atherosclerosis, 377
Coronary Artery Disease, 379
Acute Coronary Syndrome, 384
Peripheral Vascular System, 393
Lymphatic System, 400

25 Nursing Care of Patients With Cardiac Arrhythmias, 404
Cardiac Conduction System, 404
Electrocardiogram, 404
Components of a Cardiac Cycle, 405
Interpretation of Cardiac Rhythms, 407
Normal Sinus Rhythm, 409
Arrhythmias, 409
Cardiac Pacemakers, 418
Defibrillation, 420
Cardioversion, 420
Other Methods to Correct Arrhythmias, 421
Nursing Process for the Patient With Arrhythmias, 421

26 Nursing Care of Patients With Heart Failure, 425
Overview of Heart Failure, 425
Compensatory Mechanisms to Maintain Cardiac Output, 427
Pulmonary Edema (Acute Heart Failure), 428
Chronic Heart Failure, 429
Cardiac Transplantation, 441

UNIT SIX: Understanding the Hematologic and Lymphatic Systems, 448

27 Hematologic and Lymphatic System Function, Data Collection, and Therapeutic Measures, 448
Normal Hematologic and Lymphatic System Anatomy and Physiology, 448
Hematologic and Lymphatic Systems Data Collection, 454
Diagnostic Tests for the Hematologic and Lymphatic Systems, 456
Therapeutic Measures for the Hematologic and Lymphatic Systems, 458

28 Nursing Care of Patients With Hematologic and Lymphatic Disorders, 462
Hematologic Disorders, 462
Disorders of Red Blood Cells, 462
Hemorrhagic Disorders, 471
Disorders of White Blood Cells, 475
Multiple Myeloma, 478
Lymphatic Disorders, 480
Splenic Disorders, 482

UNIT SEVEN: Understanding the Respiratory System, 486

29 Respiratory System Function, Data Collection, and Therapeutic Measures, 486
Normal Respiratory System Anatomy and Physiology, 486
Respiratory System Data Collection, 492
Diagnostic Tests for the Respiratory System, 495
Therapeutic Measures for the Respiratory System, 499

30 Nursing Care of Patients With Upper Respiratory Tract Disorders, 518
Disorders of the Nose and Sinuses, 518
Infectious Disorders, 522
Malignant Disorders, 527

31 Nursing Care of Patients With Lower Respiratory Tract Disorders, 533
Infectious Disorders, 533
Restrictive Disorders, 543
Obstructive Disorders, 545
Pulmonary Vascular Disorders, 557
Chest Trauma, 559
Respiratory Failure, 562
Lung Cancer, 563
Thoracic Surgery, 566

UNIT EIGHT: Understanding the Gastrointestinal, Hepatic, and Pancreatic Systems, 572

32 Gastrointestinal, Hepatobiliary, and Pancreatic Systems Function, Data Collection, and Therapeutic Measures, 572
Normal Gastrointestinal, Hepatobiliary, and Pancreatic Systems Anatomy and Physiology, 572
Gastrointestinal, Hepatobiliary, and Pancreatic Systems Data Collection, 577
Diagnostic Tests for the Gastrointestinal, Hepatobiliary, and Pancreatic Systems, 583
Therapeutic Measures for the Gastrointestinal, Hepatobiliary, and Pancreatic Systems, 591

33 Nursing Care of Patients With Upper Gastrointestinal Disorders, 598
Anorexia, 598
Nausea and Vomiting, 598
Obesity, 599
Oral Health and Dental Care, 602
Oral Inflammatory Disorders, 603
Oral Cancer, 603
Esophageal Cancer, 603
Hiatal Hernia, 604
Gastroesophageal Reflux Disease, 605
Mallory-Weiss Tear, 606
Esophageal Varices, 607
Gastritis, 607
Peptic Ulcer Disease, 608
Gastric Bleeding, 611
Gastric Cancer, 612
Gastric Surgery, 613

34 Nursing Care of Patients With Lower Gastrointestinal Disorders, 618
Problems of Elimination, 618
Inflammatory and Infectious Disorders, 623

Inflammatory Bowel Disease, 626
Irritable Bowel Syndrome, 630
Abdominal Hernias, 633
Absorption Disorders, 634
Intestinal Obstruction, 635
Anorectal Problems, 637
Lower Gastrointestinal Bleeding, 638
Colorectal Cancer, 639
Ostomy and Continent Ostomy Management, 642

35 Nursing Care of Patients With Liver, Pancreatic, and Gallbladder Disorders, 649
Disorders of the Liver, 649
Disorders of the Pancreas, 662
Disorders of the Gallbladder, 668

UNIT NINE: Understanding the Urinary System, 675

36 Urinary System Function, Data Collection, and Therapeutic Measures, 675
Normal Urinary System Anatomy and Physiology, 675
Urinary System Data Collection, 679
Diagnostic Tests for the Urinary System, 683
Therapeutic Measures for the Urinary System, 690

37 Nursing Care of Patients With Disorders of the Urinary System, 695
Urinary Tract Infections, 695
Urological Obstructions, 699
Tumors of the Renal System, 702
Renal System Trauma, 705
Polycystic Kidney Disease, 705
Chronic Renal Diseases, 706
Glomerulonephritis, 707
Acute Kidney Injury or Chronic Kidney Disease, 708

UNIT TEN: Understanding the Endocrine System, 723

38 Endocrine System Function and Data Collection, 723
Normal Endocrine System Anatomy and Physiology, 723
Endocrine System Data Collection, 728
Diagnostic Tests for the Endocrine System, 729

39 Nursing Care of Patients With Disorders of the Endocrine System, 739
Pituitary Disorders, 740
Disorders of the Thyroid Gland, 745
Disorders of the Parathyroid Glands, 754
Disorders of the Adrenal Glands, 756

40 Nursing Care of Patients With Disorders of the Endocrine Pancreas, 765
Diabetes Mellitus, 765
Reactive Hypoglycemia, 786

UNIT ELEVEN: Understanding the Genitourinary and Reproductive Systems, 790

41 Genitourinary and Reproductive Systems Function and Data Collection, 790
Normal Genitourinary and Reproductive Systems Anatomy and Physiology, 790
Female Reproductive System Data Collection, 796
Male Reproductive System Data Collection, 805
Transgender Population Data Collection, 812

42 Nursing Care of Women With Reproductive System Disorders, 815
Breast Disorders, 816
Menstrual Disorders, 822
Irritations and Inflammations of the Vagina and Vulva, 825
Toxic Shock Syndrome, 826
Disorders Related to the Development of the Genital Organs, 828
Displacement Disorders, 829
Fertility Disorders, 831
Reproductive Life Planning, 833
Pregnancy Termination, 837
Tumors of the Reproductive System, 839
Gynecological Surgery, 843

43 Nursing Care of Male Patients With Genitourinary Disorders, 848
Prostate Disorders, 848
Penile Disorders, 859
Testicular Disorders, 860
Sexual Functioning, 861

44 Nursing Care of Patients With Sexually Transmitted Infections, 869
Disorders and Syndromes Related to Sexually Transmitted Infections, 870
Sexually Transmitted Infections, 871
Nursing Process for Sexually Transmitted Infections, 879

UNIT TWELVE: Understanding the Musculoskeletal System, 884

45 Musculoskeletal Function and Data Collection, 884
Musculoskeletal System Anatomy and Physiology, 884
Musculoskeletal System Tissues and Their Functions, 884
Role of the Nervous System, 886
Aging and the Musculoskeletal System, 887
Musculoskeletal System Data Collection, 887
Diagnostic Tests for the Musculoskeletal System, 890

46 Nursing Care of Patients With Musculoskeletal and Connective Tissue Disorders, 899
Bone and Soft Tissue Disorders, 899
Connective Tissue Disorders, 913
Musculoskeletal Surgery, 921

UNIT THIRTEEN: Understanding the Neurologic System, 929

47 Neurologic System Function, Data Collection, and Therapeutic Measures, 929
Normal Neurologic System Anatomy and Physiology, 929
Neurologic System Data Collection, 938
Diagnostic Tests for the Neurologic System, 945
Therapeutic Measures for the Neurologic System, 946

48 Nursing Care of Patients With Central Nervous System Disorders, 951
Central Nervous System Infections, 951
Increased Intracranial Pressure, 954
Headaches, 957
Seizure Disorders, 959
Traumatic Brain Injury, 963
Brain Tumors, 967
Intracranial Surgery, 969
Spinal Disorders, 971
Spinal Cord Injuries, 974
Neurodegenerative and Neurocognitive Disorders, 983

49 Nursing Care of Patients With Cerebrovascular Disorders, 1000
Transient Ischemic Attack, 1000
Stroke, 1000
Cerebral Aneurysm, Subarachnoid Hemorrhage, and Intracranial Hemorrhage, 1010
Nursing Process for the Patient With a Cerebrovascular Disorder, 1012

50 Nursing Care of Patients With Peripheral Nervous System Disorders, 1020
Neuromuscular Disorders, 1020
Cranial Nerve Disorders, 1031

UNIT FOURTEEN: Understanding the Sensory System, 1038

51 Sensory System Function, Data Collection, and Therapeutic Measures: Vision and Hearing, 1038
Vision, 1038
Hearing, 1048

52 Nursing Care of Patients With Sensory Disorders: Vision and Hearing, 1060
Vision Disorders, 1060
Hearing Disorders, 1075

UNIT FIFTEEN: Understanding the Integumentary System, 1091

53 Integumentary System Function, Data Collection, and Therapeutic Measures, 1091
Normal Integumentary System Anatomy and Physiology, 1091
Integumentary System Data Collection, 1094
Diagnostic Tests for the Integumentary System, 1100
Therapeutic Measures for the Integumentary System, 1100

54 Nursing Care of Patients With Skin Disorders, 1107
Pressure Injuries, 1107
Inflammatory Skin Disorders, 1118
Infectious Skin Disorders, 1121
Parasitic Skin Disorders, 1128
Skin Lesions, 1130
Dermatological Surgery, 1134

55 Nursing Care of Patients With Burns, 1138
Pathophysiology and Signs and Symptoms, 1138
Etiology, 1140
Complications, 1141
Diagnostic Tests, 1141
Therapeutic Measures, 1142
Nursing Process for a Patient With a Burn Injury, 1146

UNIT SIXTEEN: Understanding Mental Health Care, 1155

56 Mental Health Function, Data Collection, and Therapeutic Measures, 1155
Review of Neurologic Anatomy and Physiology, 1155
Mental Health and Mental Illness, 1155
Nursing Data Collection Related to Mental Health, 1158
Diagnostic Tests, 1158
Coping and Ego Defense Mechanisms, 1158
Therapeutic Measures, 1161

57 Nursing Care of Patients With Mental Health Disorders, 1169
Anxiety Disorders, Obsessive-Compulsive and Related Disorders, and Trauma- and Stressor-Related Disorders, 1169
Mood Disorders, 1176
Schizophrenia, 1179
Personality Disorders, 1182
Autism Spectrum Disorders, 1183
Eating Disorders, 1185
Substance Use Disorders, 1186
Mental Illness and the Older Adult, 1190

Appendix A Diagnostic Tests, 1194

Appendix B Normal Adult Reference Common Laboratory Values, 1198

Glossary, 1203

Photo & Illustration Credits, 1217

Index, 1219

Prefixes, Suffixes, and Combining Forms, IBC

References (online at Davis Advantage)

UNIT ONE Understanding Health-Care Issues

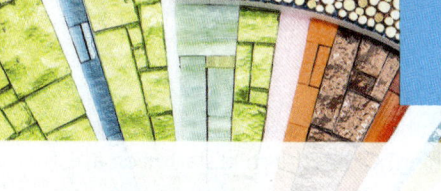

CHAPTER 1
Critical Thinking, Clinical Judgment, and the Nursing Process

Paula D. Hopper

KEY TERMS

clinical judgment (KLIN-ih-kull JUDJ-ment)
collaboration (koh-LAB-uh-RAY-shun)
critical thinking (KRIT-ih-kull THING-king)
cue (kyoo)
evaluation (e-VAL-yoo-AY-shun)
intervention (in-ter-VEN-shun)
nursing process (NER-sing PRAH-sess)
vigilance (VIJ-eh-lents)

CHAPTER CONCEPTS

Clinical judgment
Collaboration
Communication
Safety

LEARNING OUTCOMES

1. Explain the difference between critical thinking and clinical judgment.
2. Discuss why critical thinking and clinical judgment are essential in nursing.
3. Compare the nursing process to the clinical judgment process.
4. Describe attitudes of good critical thinkers.
5. Define vigilance.
6. Prioritize patient care activities based on the Maslow hierarchy of human needs.
7. Discuss the importance of collaboration in nursing practice.
8. Use the SBAR mnemonic to communicate a patient problem.

What do nurses do? What will you do as a nurse? Certainly, you will give injections and baths and change dressings. But your most important role will be to THINK like a nurse and make good decisions. What if a nurse gives an injection perfectly according to the book, but then the patient's blood pressure drops to an unsafe level because the medication was inappropriate for the patient? Even though the provider ordered it, the nurse must collect data and make a judgment about whether each dose is safe to give. What if the nurse provides expert tracheostomy care, but the patient hemorrhages during the procedure? Would a better chart review and careful thinking have uncovered this risk? Would better thinking have prevented these problems from occurring? Likely so.

Why is good thinking so important in the nursing profession? A study by Kavanaugh and Szweda (2017) found that only 23% of new nurses are ready to practice safely. Many new nurses are "unable to recognize a change in a patient's condition or identify the urgency of a situation" (Kavanaugh & Szweda, 2017). If a nurse is unable to recognize a change in condition and its urgency, a failure to rescue (FTR) can result. If a change is missed, then communication with the health-care team and subsequent **intervention** will be delayed or omitted. This places patients at serious risk of poor outcomes, including death. Many factors contribute to FTR events. Poor staffing, inadequate resources, and other systems limitations can play a role in addition to poor clinical judgment. Your job is to learn to think and make good decisions so you can recognize changes early and manage other limitations in order to have the best patient outcomes possible.

Let's look at an example. A new nurse notes a patient's blood pressure is 116/74 and thinks, "Great. That's perfect." But because two nurses called in sick, and the pharmacy missed sending some medications, the new nurse doesn't have time to review the chart before administering a routine dose of blood pressure medication. Otherwise, they would have found that the patient's blood pressure was 188/100 earlier in the day, and the patient received an extra dose of blood pressure medication. The patient's blood pressure continues to drop, but the nurse fails to recheck the blood pressure. The patient has a stroke as a result. This is an FTR. The system put the patient at risk by not having adequate staffing resources and by having disorganized pharmacy delivery. The nurse put the patient at risk by neglecting to review the chart, recheck the blood pressure, and recognize a change. These factors created the perfect storm to endanger the patient's life.

In this chapter, we talk about ways to critically think and make good clinical judgments. Then we provide opportunities to practice these skills throughout the book. You will learn why factors such as choosing priorities; using the **nursing process;** and establishing good communication, active listening, and **collaboration** go hand in hand with thinking skills when providing safe patient care.

Another important reason to learn good thinking skills is that you will need them to pass the NCLEX-PN®. The National Council of State Boards of Nursing (www.NCSBN.org) is the body that creates the NCLEX-PN®. They continuously study what nurses are doing in practice, to be sure the licensure examination focuses on the right topics. As patients become more complex, nurses must learn to think about the complexities at a whole new level. Soon, the NCLEX-PN® will focus more on clinical judgment to help ensure that new nurses are able to think and make good decisions that keep patients safer.

WHAT ARE CRITICAL THINKING AND CLINICAL JUDGMENT?

Critical Thinking

Halpern (2013) says that "**critical thinking** is the use of those cognitive [knowledge] skills or strategies that increase the probability of a desirable outcome" (p. 4). Critical thinking can help you understand the "what and why" of patient data and care needs.

SAMPLE CRITICAL THINKING EXERCISE

Your neighbor shows you her child's rash and asks your opinion. As a nursing student, you have learned how to collect data about alterations in skin integrity. What do you need to **THINK** about as you respond to your neighbor?

SUGGESTED ANSWERS

You can start by asking questions such as the following:
Where is the rash? How widespread is it? Is it getting worse?
How does it feel? Is it itchy or painful? Is it bothering the child?
What does it look like? How would you describe it?
Does anything make it better or worse? Was the child exposed to something? Or has the child started on a new medication?
How long has it been present?
Should you avoid touching it because it might be contagious? Does it look infected?

You will find Critical Thinking Exercises throughout the text. Suggested answers are provided at the end of each chapter.

As you can see from the exercise, one part of thinking critically is asking good questions. When collecting data, you can use the What's Up mnemonic to help you remember what to ask (Box 1.1).

Critical thinking also requires a good knowledge base so that your thinking and decisions are based on facts. You must collect appropriate data to have a solid base for decision making. Our goal is to provide you with this foundation of evidence-based, solid medical-surgical knowledge.

Clinical Judgment

Nursing **clinical judgment** can be defined as "the observed outcome of critical thinking and decision making" (Betts et al, 2019). This process uses nursing knowledge to collect appropriate data, identify a patient problem, and determine the best plan of action. Clinical judgment is based on good critical thinking. It determines what the nurse DOES after thinking about a problem.

LEARNING TIP

An easy way to remember the difference between critical thinking and clinical judgment is that critical thinking asks **why** (Why is this happening? Why is it important?) and clinical judgment is the **do**. What should you *do* after thinking through a problem?

Box 1.1

WHAT'S UP? Guide to Symptom Data Collection

W—Where is it?
H—How does it feel? Describe the quality (e.g., is it dull, sharp, stabbing?).
A—Aggravating and alleviating factors. What makes it worse? What makes it better?
T—Timing. When did it start? How long does it last?
S—Severity. How bad is it? This can often be rated on a scale of 0 to 10.
U—Useful other data. What other symptoms are present that might be related?
P—Patient's perception of the problem. The patient often has an idea about what the problem is or what the cause is but may not believe that their thoughts are important to share unless specifically asked.

SAMPLE CLINICAL JUDGMENT EXERCISE

Let's return to your neighbor's child. You have asked good questions and examined the rash. Now, what should you **DO**?

SUGGESTED ANSWERS

Because licensed practical nurses (LPNs) and licensed vocational nurses (LVNs) do not diagnose, you might encourage the mom to wash the area, to call a provider, or to check it again later. You will use your judgment to determine the best action.

You will find Clinical Judgment Exercises throughout the text. Suggested answers are provided at the end of each chapter.

CRITICAL THINKING ATTITUDES

It is important for nurses to possess attitudes that promote good thinking. The Foundation for Critical Thinking (2019) identifies eight attitudes associated with good critical thinking: (1) intellectual humility, (2) intellectual courage, (3) intellectual empathy, (4) intellectual autonomy, (5) intellectual integrity, (6) intellectual perseverance, (7) faith in reason, and (8) fair-mindedness. We explore three of these attitudes. For more information, go to www.criticalthinking.org.

Intellectual Humility

Have you ever known people who think they know it all? They do not have intellectual humility. People with intellectual humility have the ability to say, "I'm not sure about that. I need more information." Certainly, we want our patients to think we are smart and that we know what we are doing. However, patients and health providers also respect nurses who can say, "I don't know, but I'll find out." It is unsafe to care for patients when you are unsure of what you need to do.

Intellectual Autonomy

Did your parents ever say, "Just because everyone is doing it doesn't make it okay"? You may see some nurses cutting corners or doing things that you do not think are safe. If you have intellectual autonomy, you will think about what you observe and determine for yourself what is safe. And if you see unsafe practices, you will speak up appropriately.

Intellectual Integrity

A person with intellectual integrity values the truth. Consider the health-care team member who gossips about a patient over lunch. You know talking about patients in a negative way and in a public setting is wrong, but you don't want to rock the boat. If you have intellectual integrity, you will speak up—but you need to think carefully how to do so! Instead of saying, "You shouldn't do that," you could say, "I am not comfortable talking about a patient."

BE SAFE!

Avoid Failure to Communicate! Use the acronym CUS to speak up when you know something is not right.
C—I am **C**oncerned!
U—I am **U**ncomfortable!
S—This is a **S**afety issue!

From Agency for Healthcare Research and Quality, TeamSTEPPS, www.AHRQ.gov/teamstepps

THE NURSING PROCESS AND CLINICAL JUDGMENT

You studied the nursing process in your nursing fundamentals course. Now let's look at how the nursing process fits in with good thinking (Fig. 1.1).

Take a minute to study Figure 1.1. The clinical judgment model simply expands on the nursing process to better explain the type of thinking that is required for good decision making. Let's look at the steps in Table 1.1.

Cue recognition is so essential to providing safe care that you will find practice cue recognition opportunities (Cue Recognition) throughout the book to help you develop this skill.

SAMPLE CUE RECOGNITION

Let's go back to your neighbor with the child who has a rash. What if she calls you over to her house in a panic, and you see that her child is having severe difficulty breathing?
   Answer: *Sit her up and call 911!*

You will find Cue Recognition Exercises throughout the text. Suggested answers are provided at the end of each chapter.

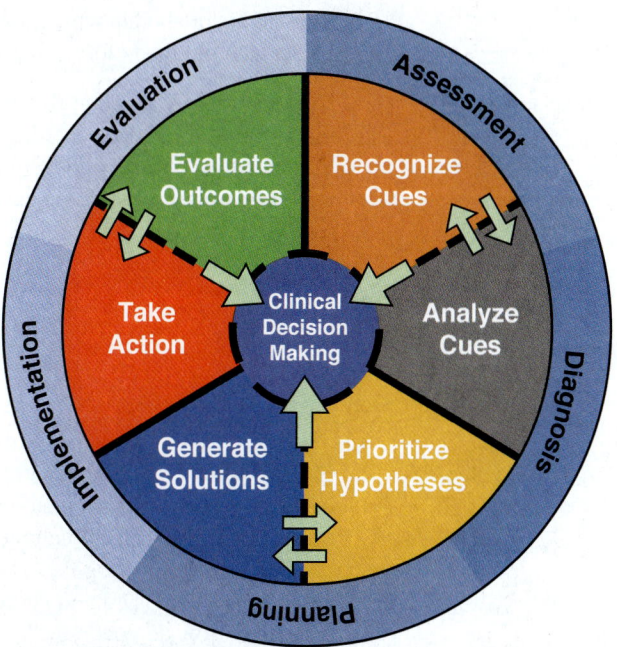

FIGURE 1.1 The nursing process and clinical judgment model.

Table 1.1
Clinical Judgment Process

Clinical Judgment	Explanation	Example
Identify and analyze cues	**Cues** are simply relevant bits of data that you have collected. They might include normal or abnormal findings in your patient, the setting you are working in, resource availability, and/or how much time you have. Once you have all the information you need, you must decide which data bits are the most relevant. Are there abnormal findings? Do you have to hurry? Do you have the equipment you need? If you go back to giving a perfect injection, how does the situation change if the medication is unavailable? Or if your patient is emaciated with little muscle mass? All this information must be analyzed before giving the injection.	Mr. Frank is in pain and asks for pain medication. His analgesic is not due for another 40 minutes. As a good critical thinker, you can use intellectual empathy as well as your knowledge base about pain to decide what data you need. You decide to use a pain-rating scale on which the patient rates pain from 0 (no pain) to 10 (the greatest pain possible). You find these cues: • Pain is in back, rates it at an 8 on scale • Pain worse since he's been confined to the hospital bed • History of spinal compression fractures Your empathetic attitude tells you that waiting for 40 minutes for pain relief is not acceptable.
Prioritize hypotheses	Once you have all your information and have decided which cues are relevant, you develop hypotheses. These may be in the form of nursing diagnoses, or you may simply have a list of possible problems. Now you must determine which problems are most urgent. (See later in the chapter for prioritization guidelines.)	• Mr. Frank is in pain. • Current analgesics are not sufficient to control pain.
Generate solutions	What is your goal? Once you determine an appropriate outcome, you can think about what to do for each priority problem. You pull together your knowledge base (yay nursing school!), your best thinking skills, and your resources to determine next steps. You might collaborate with a colleague or gather information before you proceed.	The goal? Pain relief! Possible solutions: • Wait 40 minutes and administer analgesic (does not help meet goal). • Give the analgesic early (against policy). • Use nondrug pain-relieving interventions, such as music and distraction. • Consult with RN or provider.
Take action	Next, carry out your plan. But as you know, things don't always go according to a plan. You will be continually collecting data and may need to think fast if you encounter a surprise.	You decide a 40-minute wait is not appropriate and giving the analgesic early does not follow orders. So, you help Mr. Frank reposition, turn on a television show he likes for distraction, and find the RN for a consultation. The RN contacts the provider for a new analgesic. You administer the first dose, being sure to evaluate his vital signs first and explain the drug's effects and side effects to Mr. Frank. The RN also informs Mr. Frank that the provider has ordered a consultation with the pain clinic.
Evaluate outcomes	Finally, you evaluate the outcome. **Evaluation** of the effectiveness of an intervention is an important part of clinical judgment. What results were you looking for? Did things go according to plan? Did you get results you expected? How do you know?	As you recheck Mr. Frank 30 minutes later, he rates his pain level at 2 on the 10-point scale. He smiles and thanks you for your attentiveness to his needs. You think back to the desired outcome, compare it with the current data collected, and determine that your interventions were successful.

Table 1.1
Clinical Judgment Process—cont'd

Clinical Judgment	Explanation	Example
Repeat	At any point in the cycle, if you encounter a problem or change, you can go back a step or two and try again. It would be great to go through the steps of the nursing process and say "Done!" but we are never truly finished with the nursing process or with clinical judgment. We need to continually refine our thinking and our plans in order to provide the best, safest nursing care.	Be sure to check back with Mr. Frank routinely—make sure his pain remains controlled. Discuss with him how often the medication can be given, and ask him to let you know if the pain returns. And teach him the value of distraction, relaxation, and other nondrug measures. (See Chapter 10.)

> **LEARNING TIP**
>
> Each time you exit a patient's room, do a mini-thinking assessment. Ask yourself, "Did I ask the right questions? Was my thinking clear and logical? Is there anything I could have done better?" This 1-minute metacognition exercise will help you develop as a great thinker.

A WORD ABOUT VIGILANCE

You can also use effective thinking in patient care by anticipating what might go wrong, watching carefully for signs that the problem might be occurring, and preventing it or notifying the registered nurse (RN) or health-care provider (HCP) in time to intervene. Nurses save many lives each year by anticipating and preventing problems. The state of awareness that enables you to anticipate problems is called **vigilance**. An example would be knowing the signs and symptoms of low blood glucose (because of your excellent knowledge base) and watching for them carefully (being vigilant) in a patient taking medication for diabetes. If early symptoms occur, you can intervene before the problem becomes severe. You could also teach the patient and family about low blood glucose and how to prevent it, further reducing the risk.

> **NURSING CARE TIP**
>
> As you review your patient care assignment at the start of each shift, ask yourself, "What is the worst thing that could happen to each patient today? What cues will tell me this is happening?" Then plan ahead to be vigilant for these cues and do all you can to prevent these occurrences. It's also a good idea to alert the nursing assistant what to watch for and inform you if cues occur.

COMMUNICATION WITH THE HEALTH-CARE TEAM

So far, we have established that you need a good knowledge base, good thinking skills, and effective clinical judgment to be a nurse. You also need to be a good communicator. You must be able to communicate patient data and care needs to the health-care team. One way to communicate effectively is to use the Situation-Background-Assessment/Analysis-Recommendation (SBAR) acronym. You learned this in your nursing fundamentals course. Let's review doing an SBAR with the RN, whom you need to communicate with about Mr. Frank's pain. If you collect good data and communicate it well, you will get the best recommendations for your patient.

Without SBAR, it might sound like, "Mr. Frank's pain is at an 8 out of 10, and his analgesic isn't due for another 40 minutes." Sounds pretty good, right? Now let's look at SBAR.

S—"Mr. Frank is in a lot of pain. He says it's an 8 out of 10."
B—"He has a history of spinal compression fractures. He looks very uncomfortable. I repositioned him in bed, and he is trying distraction, but it isn't helping much."
A—"I am concerned that 40 minutes is too long for him to wait and that his analgesic isn't adequate for him."
R—"I'd like to get an order for additional pain medication. What else do you recommend?"

Using SBAR, you helped focus the RN's attention on the situation, gave some good relevant data, and shared your thoughts. It was concise and is more likely than the first example to result in a good outcome for your patient.

Active Listening

Half of good communication involves being a good listener. No doubt you have had someone pretend to listen to you and then find that they didn't hear a word you said! We need to really listen to our patients. Active listening is much more than simply hearing words. You need to block out all distractions and really focus on what your patient is saying. You learned in your nursing fundamentals course to verify what you hear with responses such as "Let me clarify what I hear you saying," or "I hear you saying that your pain makes you feel sad." Clarification helps ensure that you and the patient don't have different perspectives on what has been said. You can also use follow-up questions such as "Can you tell me more?" or "What else are you concerned about?" to gather more information.

Using active listening with colleagues and providers can also help improve patient care. If you don't understand what a physician is explaining, never hesitate to say "I don't understand" or "Can you please explain that another way?" or even "Can you spell that please?" Carrying out orders that you don't fully understand can add to the nursing error statistics and harm your patients. Even when you do understand, *always* repeat orders back to the provider to verify that you heard correctly.

PRIORITIZING CARE

Once you know what problems need to be addressed, you must decide which problem or intervention should be taken care of first. Because care should always be *patient-centered*, with the patient at the center of the health-care team, such decisions should involve the patient as well as the RN and LPN/LVN. The Maslow hierarchy of human needs can be used as a basis for determining priorities (Fig. 1.2). According to Maslow, humans must meet their most basic needs, at the bottom of the triangle, first. They then move up the hierarchy to higher-level needs.

Physiological needs are the most basic. For example, a person who is having difficulty breathing is not worried about love or self-esteem; they just want to be able to breathe. Once physiological needs are met, the patient can concentrate on meeting safety and security needs. Love, belonging, and self-esteem needs are next; self-actualization needs are generally the last priority when planning care. Needs can occur simultaneously on different levels and must be addressed in a holistic manner, with prioritization guiding the care provided.

If several physiological needs are present, life-threatening needs are ranked first, health-threatening needs are second, and health-promoting needs, although important, are last.

You studied additional ways to prioritize care in your nursing fundamentals course. This is a good time to review them.

> **LEARNING TIP**
> If you are stuck wondering which physiological need should take priority, ask yourself, "Which problem is most threatening to my patient's life?"

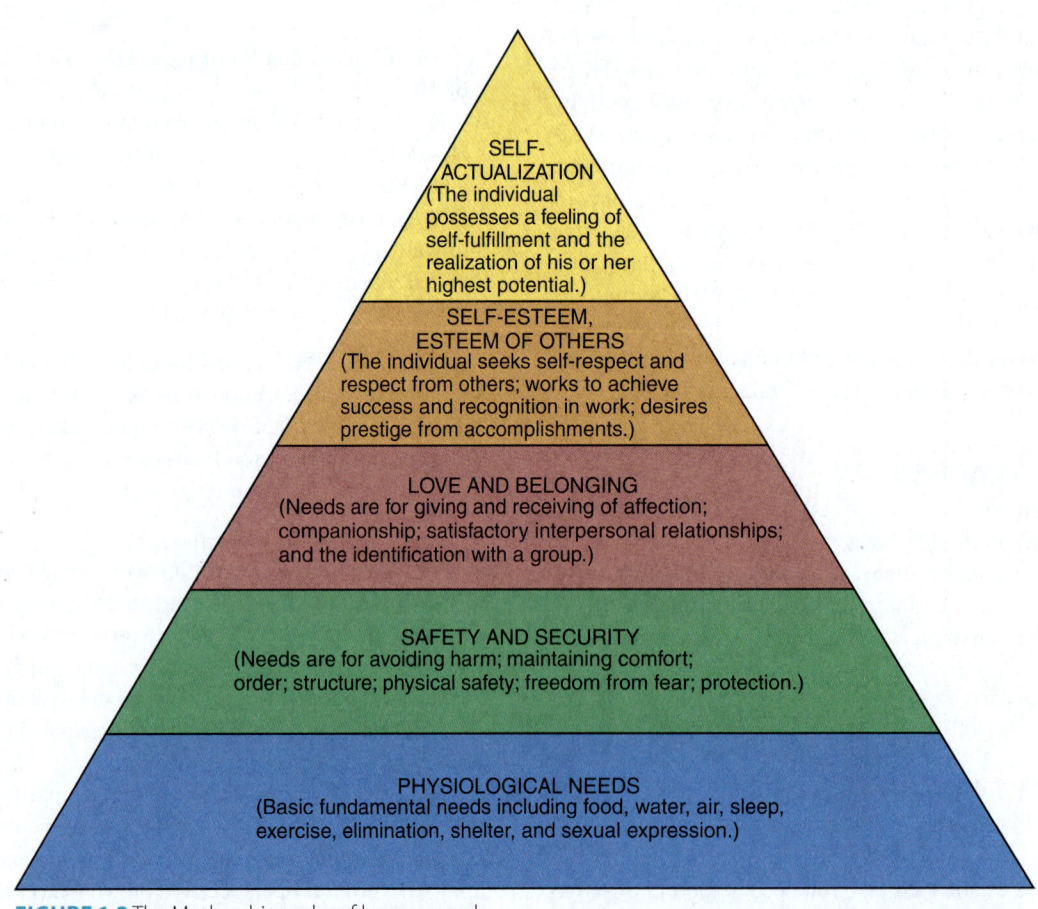

FIGURE 1.2 The Maslow hierarchy of human needs.

> **CRITICAL THINKING**
> **The Maslow Hierarchy of Human Needs:** Based on the Maslow hierarchy of human needs, list the following nursing diagnoses in order from highest (1) to lowest (5) priority. Give rationales for your decisions.
> ____ *Deficient Knowledge*
> ____ *Constipation*
> ____ *Disabled Family Coping*
> ____ *Readiness for Enhanced Self-Concept*
> ____ *Ineffective Airway Clearance*
> *Suggested answers are at the end of the chapter.*

COLLABORATION

Have you ever heard that two heads are better than one? It's almost always helpful to have another opinion, especially in complex situations. Fortunately, in most clinical settings, you can always find a partner for collaboration. It might be another nurse, a physician, a physical therapist, a dietary aide, or any of the multiple workers in your setting. ALWAYS include your patient in your collaboration efforts. Remember, the patient is the most important member of the health-care team. Sometimes, you might be part of a care team meeting, where various team members meet to discuss patient care. Because you, as the nurse, often have the most direct relationship with the patient, it will be your responsibility to think about who can be most helpful and to consult with others or request a team meeting. This approach results in improved patient outcomes.

NURSING KNOWLEDGE BASE

In addition to good thinking skills, nurses must have a solid knowledge base to safely care for patients. You would not drive a car without first learning the basics of how a car works and the rules of the road. In the same way, you must understand the human body in health and illness before you can understand how to take care of an ill patient. This is the reason you are going to school and studying this book.

Information is found in many places; some information is reliable, and some is questionable. For example, health information found on a Web site may have been put there by a major university or other reputable source, or it may have been put there by a patient or by someone who wants to sell you a product. The latter sources may be biased, or the information may simply be untrue. Therefore, you must select your information sources carefully.

The best knowledge on which to base your practice comes from research. When nursing care is based on good, well-designed research studies, it is called *evidence-based practice*. You will learn more about evidence-based practice in Chapter 2.

WHAT IS ON THE NCLEX-PN®?

That's the million-dollar question, right? But guess what! The NCSBN tells us what's on it! Every 3 years, NCSBN conducts a Practice Analysis (PA) for LPN/LVNs that tells them (1) what new LPN/LVNs do, and therefore, (2) what they should be tested on. They survey thousands of LPN/LVNs and educators and employers of LPN/LVNs. Access this information on the NCBSN Web site. Keep a copy of the Practice Analysis Average Frequency and Importance Ratings in your study area, and make sure you are studying the items to know what you will be expected to do as an LPN/LVN. You will also find PA tips throughout this book to remind you what is on the Practice Analysis. Following are some sample tips. You can see the importance of studying the information in this chapter!

> **PRACTICE ANALYSIS TIP**
> **Linking NCLEX-PN® to Practice**
> • Organize and prioritize client care based on client needs.
> • Participate in client data collection.
> • Use data from various credible sources in making clinical decisions.
> • Involve client in care decision making.
> • Recognize and report change in client condition.

Read each Practice Analysis Tip carefully and be sure to study the content—because it WILL be on NCLEX—and you will be prepared to safely care for your patients!

Key Points

- Only 23% of new nurses are ready to practice safely. Many new nurses are "unable to recognize a change in a patient's condition or identify the urgency of a situation" (Kavanaugh & Szweda, 2017). If a nurse is unable to recognize a change in condition and its urgency, an FTR can result.
- Critical thinking in nursing uses good thinking skills to improve patient care outcomes. Critical thinking can help you understand the "what and why" of patient data and care needs.

- Clinical judgment is the decision making nurses engage in every day. It must be based on good critical thinking. It determines what the nurse DOES after thinking about a problem.
- Good thinking requires attitudes such as intellectual humility, intellectual autonomy, and intellectual integrity.
- The clinical judgment process works well with the nursing process. Identifying and analyzing cues is part of good data collection. Prioritizing hypotheses might include problem statements in the form of nursing

diagnoses. Generating solutions is part of the planning process. Taking action and evaluating outcomes are analogous to intervention and evaluation.
- Nurses must be vigilant in anticipating and recognizing potential problems and then intervening before it's too late. Think ahead with each patient: "Based on my patient's diagnosis and current data collection, what could go wrong today?" Monitor closely for signs that a problem could be developing, and intervene to prevent the occurrence.
- Use the SBAR acronym to communicate effectively with the health-care team. S = What is the situation? B = What background is essential so the listener understands the situation? A = What is my assessment or analysis of the situation? R = What are my recommendations?
- Be an active listener with patients and the health-care team. Pay close attention to what is being said, and ask clarifying questions.
- Use Maslow's hierarchy to prioritize patient care. Physiological needs come first, then safety and security; love and belonging; self-esteem; and finally, self-actualization. If several physiological needs are present, manage life-threatening needs first, then health-threatening, and finally, health-promoting.
- Collaboration with others will lead to better outcomes. Remember, the patient is also on the health-care team. Patient-centered care means you always include the patient in planning and decision making.
- Become familiar with the NCSBN Practice Analysis for LPN/LVNs in order to be prepared for practice and also for the NCLEX-PN®.

SUGGESTED ANSWERS TO CHAPTER EXERCISES
Critical Thinking & Clinical Judgment
The Maslow Hierarchy of Human Needs
1. *Ineffective Airway Clearance:* physiological need that can be life-threatening
2. *Constipation:* physiological need that can be health-threatening
3. *Deficient Knowledge:* safety and security need
4. *Disabled Family Coping:* love and belonging need
5. *Readiness for Enhanced Self-Concept:* self-esteem need

Additional Resources

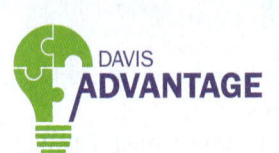

Go to Davis Advantage to complete your learning: strengthen understanding, apply your knowledge, and prepare for the Next Gen NCLEX®.

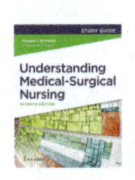

A Study Guide is also available.

CHAPTER 2
Evidence-Based Practice

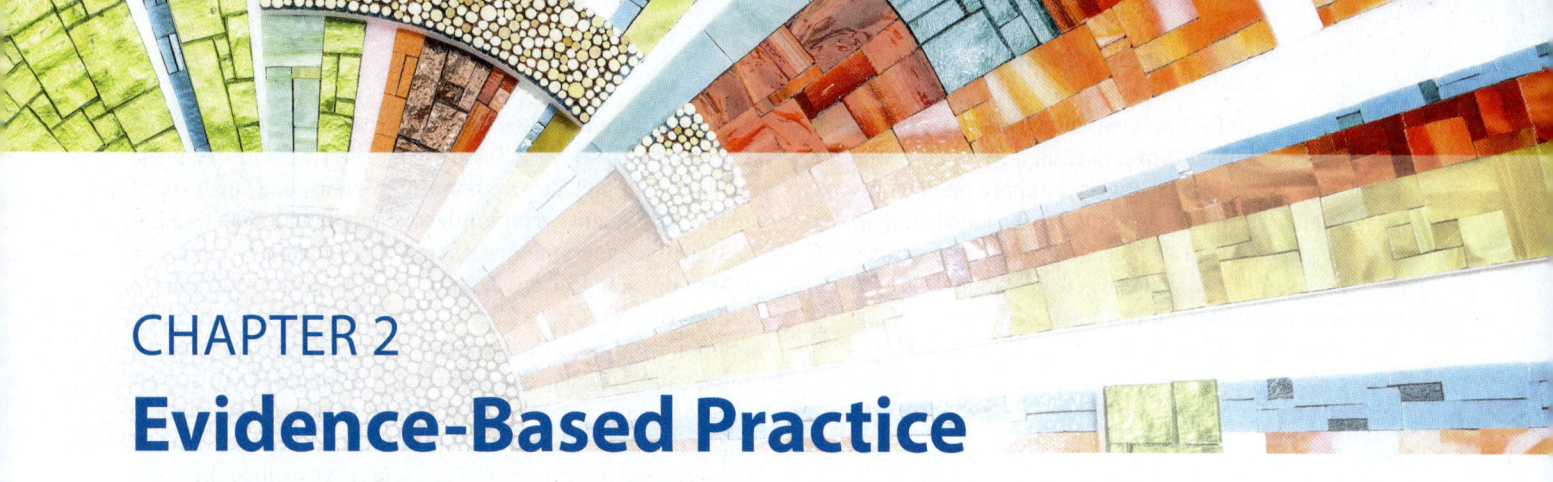

Kristy Gorman, Betty Ackley

KEY TERMS

evidence-based practice (EH-va-dense based PRAK-tis)
evidence-informed practice (EH-va-dense in-FORMD PRAK-tis)
randomized controlled trial (RAN-duh-mysd cun-TROLLD TRY-ul)
research (RE-surch)
systematic review (SIS-tem-AT-ik re-VIEW)

CHAPTER CONCEPTS

Caring
Evidence-based practice
Health-care technology
Quality improvement
Safety

LEARNING OUTCOMES

1. Define evidence-based practice (EBP) and evidence-informed practice (EIP).
2. Discuss benefits of using EBP.
3. Explain how to identify nursing evidence that should be put into practice.
4. Describe the EBP process.
5. List the six steps of EBP.
6. Identify who should give evidence-based nursing care, including when and where care should be given.
7. Describe how the Quality and Safety Education for Nurses (QSEN) project can promote safe patient care.

Amanda, a licensed practical nurse (LPN), is caring for patients in a long-term care facility. One of the patients, Mr. Samuel, suffers from dementia. He has difficulty carrying out activities of daily living. Upon inspection, his gums look red, and his tongue looks gray; he also has halitosis. He currently receives oral swabbing twice daily. Let's explore with Amanda what the evidence says should be done for oral care for Mr. Samuel.

Evidence-based practice (EBP) is a systematic process that uses current evidence to make decisions about patient care. Sackett and colleagues (1996) define evidence-based medicine as the "conscientious, explicit and judicious use of current best evidence in making decisions about the care of individual patients" and "integrating individual clinical expertise with the best available external clinical evidence from systematic research" (p. 71). This EBP definition has been adapted to other disciplines, including nursing.

A newer term also used to discuss the use of evidence in practice is **evidence-informed practice** (EIP). Peters, Hopkins, and Barnett (2016) adapted the work of Sackett and colleagues to define EIP as "conscientious, explicit and judicious use of best currently available evidence, integrated with clients' values and professional expertise, in making decisions about the care of individuals" (p. 145). EIP stresses consideration of patient factors along with the use of evidence for shared decision making between the health-care provider (HCP) and the patient.

EBP involves much more than simply evaluating **research** (scientific study, investigation, or experimentation) to determine which results apply to nursing care. Other factors include the context of care and the patient's preference for interventions and care. Because clinical reality can be very different from a research setting, it could be unrealistic or even unsafe to apply findings from a controlled laboratory research study to an actual clinical situation. Similarly, it could be unsafe to apply research results obtained on people of one age or medical diagnosis to those of another age or with multiple diagnoses.

REASONS FOR USING EBP

The use of EBP allows nurses to give patients the best care possible with improved patient outcomes. The reasons given for nursing care used to be, "This is how it was taught in nursing school," "This is what they told us in orientation," or "That's the way it is done here." Today, the rationale behind the best nursing care is, "Nursing care is based on evidence and how it applies to an individual patient in a specific setting." EBP is considered the gold standard of health care.

Evidence-based outcome measurement is built into the EBP process to measure and confirm the value of a change in nursing practice. For example, nurses measure the number of new pressure injuries and new urinary tract infections in health-care settings. These measured outcomes show nurses that they are giving the best care possible, based on the best evidence available at the time.

IDENTIFYING NURSING EVIDENCE

How do you identify nursing evidence that should be put into practice? It depends in part on the strength of the evidence. Evidence ranges from strong to weak, and levels can be assigned to rate its strength and quality. The rating scale used to label the quality of evidence ranges from Level I to Level VII (Table 2.1). Level I is the strongest evidence. It includes **systematic reviews** and analysis of many high-quality, **randomized controlled trials** (studies designed to determine the effects of a variable by randomly assigning subjects to experimental, placebo, or control groups). Level VII evidence is the weakest. It includes expert opinions and published clinical articles that are not based in research. Evidence from many disciplines, such as gerontology and social work, is used to develop EBP nursing care guidelines. Two of the best-known sources for Level I evidence are the Cochrane Database of Systematic Reviews for medical evidence and the Joanna Briggs Institute's evidence-based resources for nursing practice.

> **PRACTICE ANALYSIS TIP**
> Linking NCLEX-PN® to Practice
> The LPN/LVN will:
> • Apply EBP when providing care.
> • Use data from various credible sources in making clinical decisions.

THE EBP PROCESS

Evidence that guides nursing care can be used in two ways. It depends on whether the evidence is a dependent or an independent nursing intervention. Dependent nursing interventions are those that are delegated by an HCP. In the case

Table 2.1
Levels of Evidence

Level	Type of Evidence
Level I	*Systematic reviews:* Evidence from a systematic review of all relevant randomized clinical trials or evidence-based clinical practice guidelines that are developed from systematic reviews of randomized controlled trials. Three or more randomized controlled trials of good quality that have similar results also have been considered Level I evidence.
Level II	*Randomized controlled trials:* Evidence obtained from at least one well-designed randomized controlled trial. These are true experimental studies in which as many factors as possible that could falsely change the results are controlled.
Level III	*Quasi-experimental studies:* Evidence obtained from well-designed controlled trials without randomization.
Level IV	*Evidence from well-designed case-control or cohort studies*
Level V	*Systematic review of qualitative or descriptive studies*
Level VI	*Qualitative or a single descriptive study*
Level VII	*Expert opinion:* Evidence from the opinion of authorities and/or reports of expert committees or from nursing journal articles that are opinion based, not research based.

of dependent interventions, any change in practice must undergo committee review, such as by the policy and procedure committee, to determine whether it is appropriate for adoption. If the intervention is independent, however, you can implement an evidence-based change based on personal knowledge of the value of the intervention, as long as the change is safe and cannot harm the patient. An example of an independent intervention is reality orientation. Excellent research shows that the use of reality orientation can improve thinking ability in patients with dementia and delirium. You can implement this intervention independently because it does not require an order. Other independent intervention examples include the use of hand massage or music therapy.

A simplified version of the EBP process is discussed next and shown in Figure 2.1. The acronym **ASKMME!** is designed to help you remember the six essential steps: **A**sk, **S**earch, thin**K**, **M**easure, **M**ake it happen, and **E**valuate (Ackley et al, 2008).

Step 1: Ask the Burning Question

EBP begins with questioning the status quo, trying to solve a problem, or learning about new evidence that should be used in nursing practice. The initial question nurses often ask is, "Why do we do it that way?" or "How could we do this better?" Questioning the existing way of doing things is part of critical thinking. It helps ensure that the patient receives the best care possible. As a student nurse, you can do this as well.

A framework can be used to form the components of a researchable clinical question. Using a framework is a time saver that identifies keywords for the search. It narrows the focus for the search and produces more relevant findings. PICO(T) (Population, Intervention, Comparison, Outcome, Time) is an example of a method to form the question and identify keywords for the database search (Fineout-Overholt & Johnson, 2005). These types of frameworks can be filled in on database sites to get you started with your search (Box 2.1).

For Mr. Samuel, in the case study at the start of the chapter, Amanda was motivated to find the best way to give oral care. Amanda took her clinical question to the policy and procedure committee. Together, they began the evidence-based process to find best practices for giving oral care to patients at their agency.

Step 2: Search for and Collect the Most Relevant and Best Evidence Available

A thorough search of the literature in the subject area must be conducted. To find the best available evidence, you must search multiple databases for systematic reviews, research studies, and journal articles. One well-known database for nursing literature is the Cumulative Index to Nursing and Allied Health Literature (CINAHL). CINAHL is available through college and hospital libraries. Evidence-based care sheets are available on CINAHL. These sheets summarize current best practice on a specific topic. For

Step 6 Evaluate the practice change.
Step 5 Make it happen.
Step 4 Measure outcomes before and after change.
Step 3 Think critically.
Step 2 Search for and collect the most relevant and best evidence available.
Step 1 Ask the burning question.

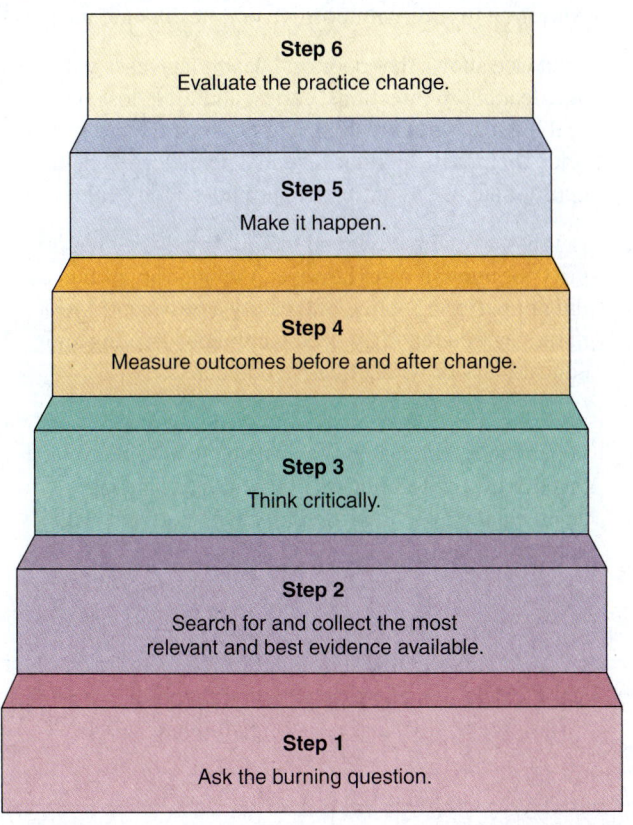

FIGURE 2.1 The six steps of the evidence-based practice process.

Box 2.1

Evidence-Based Practice Question Framework: PICO(T)

PICO(T) is a mnemonic to describe the five elements of a good searchable and answerable question. Let's explore how Amanda would use keywords to formulate a searchable clinical question.

P = Population/Problem: How would Amanda describe the problem among a group of patients?
Patients with dementia
I = Intervention: What main intervention is Amanda considering?
Suction toothbrushes
C = Comparison: Is there an alternative to compare with the intervention?
Foam swabs
O = Outcome: What does Amanda hope to accomplish, measure, improve, or affect?
Decreased periodontal disease
(T) = Time: Length of time for the intervention or to achieve the outcome
Time is not relevant for Amanda's question. It is not always required, which is why it appears in parentheses in PICO(T).

Amanda's PICO(T) question would be: *"In patients with dementia, how do suction toothbrushes as compared to foam swabs affect periodontal disease?"*

nursing evidence-based resources, visit the Joanna Briggs Institute Web site (https://jbi.global/ebp). For biomedical literature, which includes nursing, the comprehensive PubMed/Medline database can be accessed at https://pubmed.ncbi.nlm.nih.gov. Cochrane Reviews are available at www.cochranelibrary.com.

Amanda worked with a medical librarian and other members of her agency's policy and procedure committee to conduct an EBP search on oral care. They then summarized the research articles they found in this area (examples in Table 2.2).

Step 3: Think Critically

Always appraise the evidence you find for validity, relevance to the situation, and applicability. First, evaluate the quality of the evidence you find. It is helpful to determine the level of the evidence to make sure you have the best information available (see Table 2.1). For example, if you locate a systematic review, meta-analysis, or meta-aggregation, you have found a source of preappraised evidence using a prescribed step-by-step search of the best available evidence. Next, using critical thinking, evaluate the evidence as it applies to the individual patient or patient population, the clinical expertise of the nurse(s) involved, the values surrounding the situation, and agency policies that affect making a change in practice.

Amanda found research articles on the value of oral care, and the results were exciting. When the research was analyzed, it became obvious that patients with dementia were at greater risk for periodontal disease. Often, oral bacteria are noticeable as a coating on the tongue. In addition, Amanda discovered that increased severity of periodontal disease correlated with decreased health and quality of life. Mr. Samuels had trouble swallowing, so it was important that suction be readily available when oral care was given to prevent aspiration. Amanda discovered that various

Table 2.2
Summary of Research Findings for Patient Oral Care

Study	Key Findings
Castillo, Dora, Smith, Daniel, & Rosenfeld, Peri. (2020). Implementing and evaluating the impact of a nurse-led oral care initiative. *Journal of Nursing Care Quality, 35,* 123–129. https://doi.org/10.1097/NCQ.0000000000000426	This study focused on evaluating a multidisciplinary oral health initiative. The Oral Care Council, which included RNs, patient care technicians, and other oral health champions, focused on integrating practice standards, evaluating new products, and providing ongoing education to staff with positive oral health outcomes.
Coll, P. P., Lindsay, A., Meng, J., Gopalakrishna, A., Raghavendra, S., Bysani, P., & O'Brien, D. (2020). The prevention of infections in older adults: Oral health. *Journal of the American Geriatric Society, 68,* 411–416. https://doi.org/10.1111/jgs.16154	Evidence shows that poor oral health increases with age, leading to infections, caries, and tooth loss. Daily oral hygiene with brushing and flossing, the use of fluoride toothpaste, regular biannual dental care, and the appropriate use of antibiotics promotes oral health.
Dagnew, Z. A., Abraham, I. A., Beraki, G. G., Tesfamariam, E. H., Mittler, S., & Tesfamichael, Y. Z. (2020). Nurses' attitude towards oral care and their practicing level for hospitalized patients in Orotta National Referral Hospital, Asmara-Eritrea: A cross-sectional study. *BMC Nursing, 19*(63). https://doi.org/10.1186/s12912-020-00457-3	In this study, nurses agreed that oral care is a high priority for nursing care; however, the majority of nurses did not perform routine oral cavity assessment. Most nurses agreed that they need continuous training and education to provide effective oral care.
Manchery, N., Subbiah, G., Nagappan, N., & Premnath, P. (2020). Are oral health education for carers effective in the oral hygiene management of elderly with dementia? A systematic review. *Dental Research Journal, 17*(1), 1–9. https://doi.org/10.4103/1735-3327.276232	Four studies included in this systematic review revealed that caregiver education on oral health techniques is an efficient way to improve oral health for those with dementia.
Pitchika, V., Pink, C., Völzke, H., Welk, A., Kocher, T., & Holtfreter, B. (2019). Long-term impact of powered toothbrush on oral health: 11-year cohort study. *Journal of Clinical Periodontology, 46*(7), 713–722. https://doi.org/10.1111/jcpe.13126	The effects of long-term use of powered toothbrushes were examined. They showed powered toothbrushes are effective in improving periodontal health, reducing caries progression, and promoting tooth retention.

suction toothbrushes are available for patients who have difficulty swallowing. Amanda felt a renewed sense of purpose when she realized that small changes to oral care could have a positive impact on the well-being of patients such as Mr. Samuel.

Step 4: Measure Outcomes Before and After Change

Next, determine the patient outcomes that are likely to occur as a result of a change in nursing care. Usually, a small pilot study is done before any widespread change in practice to determine whether the change will be as effective as intended when implemented across the agency.

The committee members decided to implement a biannual evaluation of periodontal disease in patients.

Step 5: Make It Happen

Institute the desired change in nursing practice based on evidence through education and by setting up quality systems to ensure that the desired change is happening.

The policy and procedure committee developed an evidence-based procedure guideline for oral care of all patients, with separate policies for those with dementia. The new policy and procedure were introduced and became a care requirement for patients at the agency. A quality audit was done at intervals to ensure the appropriate oral care was being given.

Step 6: Evaluate the Practice Change

Evaluation is the process used to determine whether the change made a significant difference. What were the results of the initial small study? Was the change in practice effective in improving patient outcomes? If it made a difference, was it worth the extra cost or time it required?

Wow! Because of Amanda's concern about oral care, a policy change was made that, upon evaluation, showed a positive impact on the oral health for every patient.

WHO SHOULD PROVIDE EVIDENCE-BASED NURSING CARE?

All nursing care should be based on use of appropriate evidence, including care provided by assistive personnel (AP). A good way to ensure that evidence-based care is provided by AP is to explain why the care should be given at the time that the care is delegated.

Amanda asks a nursing assistant to provide oral care for each patient that includes brushing the teeth and tongue with a power suction toothbrush with fluoride toothpaste after meals, using mouthwash, and daily flossing. Along with the request, Amanda explains that research studies have shown that brushing both the teeth and the tongue decreases the bacteria that are responsible for periodontal disease. She also explains that preventing periodontal disease improves comfort, health, and quality of life. With this new knowledge, the nursing assistant understood the importance of giving effective oral care.

EBP, QUALITY, AND SAFETY: THEY BELONG TOGETHER!

EBP is critical thinking at its finest, working to determine the best care for the patient based on the evidence. The evidence provides core information to direct safe, quality-driven, excellent patient care. Multiple quality initiatives are currently having a positive impact on health care. Insurance companies, businesses, patients, and the government are demanding quality care. All quality initiatives require data collection, which is greatly facilitated by an EBP framework within the health-care agency. Some quality initiatives, such as those of The Joint Commission, are required for health-care agencies to receive accreditation. Others are voluntary but desirable for the agency's well-being. All quality initiatives should begin with a literature search to determine the most effective interventions.

Quality and Safety Education for Nurses Project

The Quality and Safety Education for Nurses (QSEN) project focuses on nursing education that promotes the continual improvement of quality and safety in patient care. The goal is for future nurses to develop the knowledge, skills, attitudes, and desire to continually improve the quality and safety of patient care. Information on the QSEN project can be found at qsen.org.

Teaching strategies for nursing students involve the following six areas of focus, which are supported throughout the book:

1. *Evidence-based practice:* Look for Evidence-Based Practice boxes throughout this book.
2. *Safety:* Many interventions are available to keep your patients safe (see Chapter 3, Safe Practice section). Look for Be Safe! boxes throughout the chapters for safety tips.
3. *Teamwork and collaboration:* These are important aspects of providing safe, quality care. You have learned about the members of the health-care team with whom you will work and collaborate. For example, you may discuss ways to increase social interaction for a newly admitted patient with the activity director or talk with the pharmacist if you have a question about a patient's medication to ensure it is given safely.
4. *Patient-centered care:* When collaborating on the development of nursing care plans, it is important to individualize interventions to provide patient-centered care. Nursing interventions should meet the patient's needs and preferred schedules rather than those of the institution or caregiver. You will find Nursing Care Plans throughout the chapters, but always remember that no plan fits all patients. Always evaluate each suggested intervention to see whether it fits with your patient's needs and then individualize it.
5. *Quality improvement:* Quality improvement (QI) is an ongoing process to improve patient care (see Fig. 3.2 in Chapter 3). You might participate in a QI project by collecting data, which is one aspect of this type of initiative.

6. *Informatics:* The use of technology is promoting safer patient care. Examples include electronic health records (EHRs), medication dispensing systems, medication barcoding systems, and computerized resources.

> **PRACTICE ANALYSIS TIP**
> **Linking NCLEX-PN® to Practice**
> The LPN/LVN will participate in quality improvement (QI) activities (e.g., collecting data, serving on QI committee).

> **CUE RECOGNITION 2.1**
> After a meal, you observe that a patient has reddened gums, dry oral mucous membranes, and a film on the teeth. What action do you take?
>
> *Suggested answers are at the end of the chapter.*

The author acknowledges the contribution to this chapter by Betty Ackley.

Key Points

- Evidence-based practice is a systematic process that employs current evidence to make decisions about patient care. Using evidence-based practice increases your ability to give the best nursing care possible by applying high-quality evidence to each patient in your specific setting.
- There are six steps in the evidence-based process: (1) Ask the burning question (using a framework such as PICO(T), (2) search for and collect the best evidence available, (3) think critically, (4) measure outcomes before and after change, (5) make it happen, and (6) evaluate the practice change.
- All nursing staff should provide evidence-based nursing care and understand why the care should be given in a certain way.
- Knowledge of QSEN promotes continual improvement of quality and safety in patient care based on evidence.

> **SUGGESTED ANSWERS FOR CHAPTER EXERCISES**
> **Cue Recognition**
> **2.1:** Develop an after-meal oral care schedule for the patient that uses a saliva substitute before meals, a power suction toothbrush, fluoride toothpaste, mouthwash, and daily flossing. Educate nursing assistants on the health benefits and improved quality of life with excellent oral hygiene.

Additional Resources

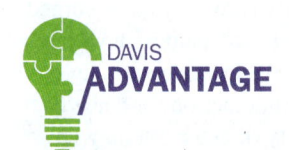

DAVIS ADVANTAGE — Go to Davis Advantage to complete your learning: strengthen understanding, apply your knowledge, and prepare for the Next Gen NCLEX®.

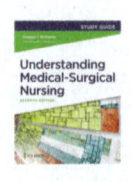

A Study Guide is also available.

CHAPTER 3
Issues in Nursing Practice

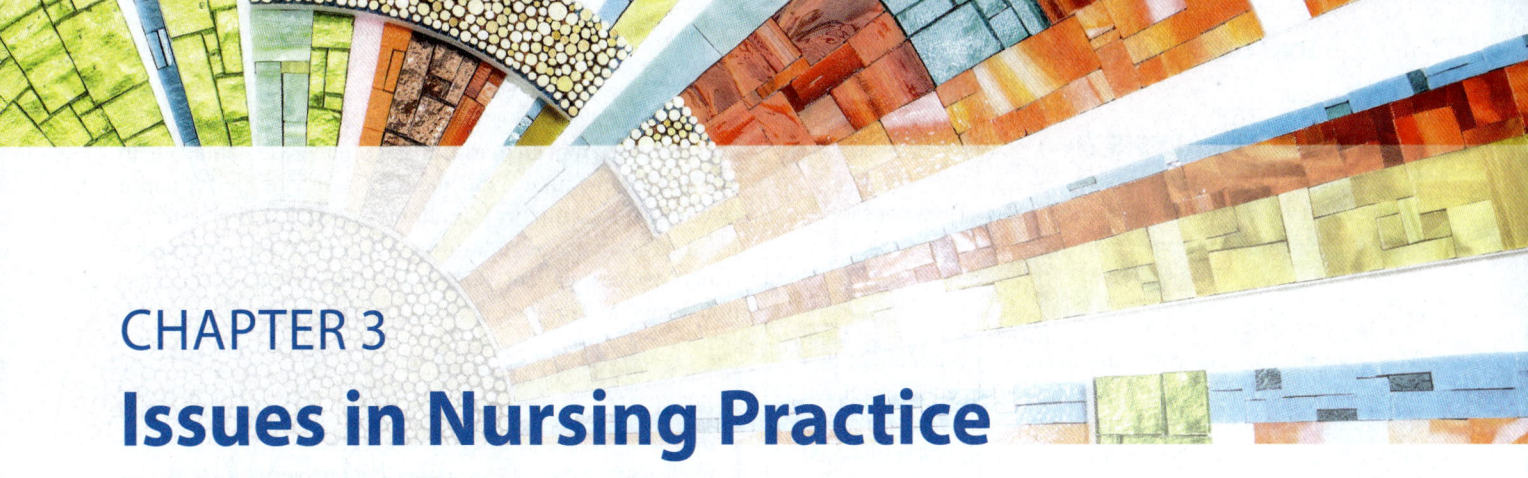

Linda S. Williams, James Shannon

KEY TERMS

administrative law (ad-MIN-i-STRAY-tiv law)
autocratic leadership (AW-tuh-KRAT-ik LEE-der-ship)
autonomy (aw-TAH-nuh-mee)
beneficence (buh-NEF-i-sens)
civil law (SIH-vil law)
confidentiality (KON-fi-den-she-AL-i-tee)
criminal law (KRIM-i-nuhl law)
delegation (DEL-a-GAY-shun)
democratic leadership (DEM-ah-KRAT-ik LEE-der-ship)
deontology (DEE-on-TOL-o-jee)
ethics (ETH-iks)
fidelity (FAH-del-eh-tee)
human trafficking (HUE-men TRA-fik-ing)
informatics (IN-for-MAT-iks)
justice (JUS-tis)
laissez-faire leadership (leh-say-FAIR LEE-der-ship)
leadership (LEE-der-ship)
liability (LY-uh-BIL-i-tee)
limitation of liability (LIM-i-TAY-shun of LY-uh-BIL-i-tee)
maleficence (ma-LEF-i-sens)
malpractice (mal-PRAK-tis)
moral distress (MOR-al di-STRES)
negligence (NEG-li-jens)
nonmaleficence (NON-ma-LEF-i-sens)
paternalism (puh-TER-nuhl-izm)
respondeat superior (ri-SPON-dee-et sue-PEER-ee-or)
summons (SUH-muns)
therapeutic privilege (THER-uh-PU-tik PRIV-uh-lej)
torts (TORTS)
utilitarian (yoo-TIL-ih-TAR-ee-en)
values (VAL-yooz)
veracity (ver-AH-sit-tee)

CHAPTER CONCEPTS

Collaboration
Communication
Health policy
Leadership and management
Professionalism
Quality improvement
Safety

LEARNING OUTCOMES

1. Identify factors influencing changes in the health-care delivery system.
2. Describe safe health-care practices.
3. Explain the significance of hospital-acquired conditions.
4. Describe four leadership styles.
5. Discuss the licensed practical nurse/licensed vocational nurse's role in leadership and delegation.
6. Describe the importance of ethics in health care.
7. Discuss moral distress and its effect on nursing care.
8. List the steps of the ethical decision-making model.
9. Identify where the regulation of nursing practice is defined.
10. Explain mandatory reporting for health-care professionals.
11. Describe human trafficking indicators to report.
12. Describe the Health Insurance Portability and Accountability Act of 1996.
13. Describe guidelines for professional use of social media.
14. Discuss how to provide quality care and limit liability.

HEALTH-CARE DELIVERY

Factors Influencing Health-Care Change

Health-care delivery is influenced by constant evolution that will impact your career. Ever-evolving evidence results in practice changes (see Chapter 2). Other factors that influence practice change include an aging and increasingly culturally diverse population; newly emerging viruses; multidrug-resistant infectious organisms; increased public awareness of issues such as human trafficking; electronic health records (EHRs); mobile health with digital apps, smartphones, tablets, and remote patient monitoring; robotics; and telehealth (smartphones, online video conferencing such as Zoom), which grew in use as a result of the 2020 pandemic. Nursing **informatics,** the study and use of information technology within nursing practice, is increasing as an area of expertise for nurses. Change makes learning an ongoing need. We hope that you are flexible and embrace change throughout your career!

> **PRACTICE ANALYSIS TIP**
> Linking NCLEX-PN® to Practice
> The LPN/LVN will use information technology in client care.

Safe Practice

Medication errors that can result in harm or death are of primary concern. The Institute for Safe Medication Practices has guidelines and recommendations to reduce medication errors that include resources on error-prone abbreviations, confused drug names, do-not-crush oral medications, high-alert medications in long-term care, and lookalike drug names distinguished by tall man letters (see www.ismp.org/tools). They also advocate to weigh patients only in kilograms to prevent mix-ups in pounds and kilograms for medication doses calculated in kilograms.

> **CUE RECOGNITION 3.1**
> You are preparing a medication, and its dose is labeled in milligrams per kilogram (mg/kg). The patient's weight is recorded in pounds. What action do you take for safety?
> *Suggested answers are at the end of the chapter.*

Distractions during medication administration can increase errors, so always stay focused and avoid interruptions during this time. Promote a culture of safety. Ask your coworkers to avoid interrupting others during medication administration. Ways to reduce distractions include outlining a designated area with bright tape that should not be entered during medication preparation and administration, a separate medication preparation room, or use of a colorful vest or sash that says, "Do Not Disturb Me While I Give Meds." Reducing errors requires everyone to be engaged and vigilant during patient care.

To promote safe tubing connections, a global initiative was developed for product redesign to prevent misconnections of medical tubing that have resulted in harm and death (www.stayconnected.org). For example, an enteral tubing connector, ENFit, has been designed that is *not* compatible with other types of tubing connections. This new design prevents feeding misconnections with other tubes such as IV central lines.

Preventing adverse events is of concern to organizations that promote safe health-care practices. The Joint Commission updates its National Patient Safety Goals annually (www.jointcommission.org). Clinical judgment is required to use them at the right time and in the right circumstances to provide safe care. The Joint Commission also identifies sentinel events, also called *never-events*, because they should never occur. These events result in death, severe temporary harm, or permanent harm. Analysis and corrective action are required after an event to protect patients by preventing future incidents.

The National Quality Forum seeks to improve health and safety for all Americans by setting standards and measurements of care. It identified a set of serious reportable events (SREs) that are harmful and often preventable to help prevent patient injury and measure safe care performance (www.qualityforum.org). Examples of SREs with resulting harm or death are assault of patient or staff, burns, contaminated devices, patient elopement (disappearance), medication errors, MRI injury, or wrong surgical procedure.

> **BE SAFE!**
> **BE VIGILANT!** Did you know that a medication is specifically made for only *one* type of administration route? It cannot be safely given by another route. For example, an IV medication cannot safely be given through a nasogastric (NG) or percutaneous endoscopy gastrostomy (PEG) tube. Avoid using a parenteral syringe to prepare an oral medication, as the medication is then sometimes mistakenly given intravenously. Instead, always use an oral medication syringe for an oral medication to prevent errors! (Yes, they are different types of syringes, so become familiar with each type and request that your institution stock both types for safety.) Serious effects, including death, can occur because the medication dosages or medication makeup is specific to its designated route. Request a medication order for an alternate route, if needed, to obtain the proper medication form for administration. Help keep your patients safe!

ECONOMIC ISSUES

Hospital-Acquired Conditions and Present-on-Admission Reporting

In 2008, the Centers for Medicare & Medicaid Services (CMS) implemented a payment policy change called the Hospital-Acquired Conditions (HACs) and Present on Admission (POA) Indicator Reporting. Box 3.1 shows the 14 categories of HACs. At discharge, if certain conditions were not POA, hospitals do not receive additional payment for those conditions. For example, if a patient was admitted with a stroke (primary diagnosis) and developed a pressure injury that was not POA (secondary diagnosis) and was preventable, the hospital would receive payment only for the primary diagnosis of stroke. The hospital must absorb the cost of care for the pressure injury.

With this requirement, nurses must carefully collect data and document patient conditions that are POA, using photos of these alterations or charts that detail them to show that they did not occur during the hospitalization. Screening tools such as the Braden Skin Scale can be used to identify complication risks to guide nursing interventions. Providing safe, quality care and educating patients to prevent complications, such as the need to do leg exercises, turn every 2 hours, or ambulate, are essential to prevent these conditions. Documenting interventions provided or the patient's refusal to participate (if applicable) are essential to help ensure payment for secondary diagnoses.

Box 3.1
Categories of Hospital-Acquired Conditions

The Centers for Medicare & Medicaid Services identified the following 14 categories of hospital-acquired conditions as those that increase health-care costs or that could have been prevented by using evidence-based guidelines:
- Foreign Object Retained After Surgery
- Air Embolism
- Blood Incompatibility
- Stage III and IV Pressure Ulcers
- Fall and Trauma Injuries (Burns, Crushing Injuries, Dislocations, Fractures, Intracranial Injuries, Other Injuries)
- Manifestations of Poor Glycemic Control (Diabetic Ketoacidosis, Nonketotic Hyperosmolar Coma, Hypoglycemic Coma, Secondary Diabetes With Ketoacidosis, Secondary Diabetes With Hyperosmolarity)
- Catheter-Associated Urinary Tract Infection
- Vascular Catheter-Associated Infection
- Surgical Site Infection, Mediastinitis After Coronary Artery Bypass Graft
- Surgical Site Infection After Bariatric Surgery for Obesity (Laparoscopic Gastric Bypass, Gastroenterostomy, Laparoscopic Gastric Restrictive Surgery)
- Surgical Site Infection After Certain Orthopedic Procedures (Spine, Neck, Shoulder, Elbow)
- Surgical Site Infection After Cardiac Implantable Electronic Device
- Deep Vein Thrombosis/Pulmonary Embolism (Total Knee Replacement, Hip Replacement)
- Iatrogenic Pneumothorax With Venous Catheterization

From Centers for Medicare & Medicaid Services. (Last modified February 11, 2020). Hospital-acquired conditions. www.cms.gov/Medicare/Medicare-Fee-for-Service-Payment/HospitalAcqCond/Hospital-Acquired_Conditions

NURSING AND THE HEALTH-CARE TEAM

Nursing is an integral part of the health-care network. Nurses practice as *licensed practical nurses* (LPNs) or *licensed vocational nurses* (LVNs), *registered nurses* (RNs), or RNs with advanced education and practice skills, which include *nurse practitioners* (NPs), *clinical nurse specialists* (CNSs), *certified nurse midwives* (CNMs), *certified registered nurse anesthetists* (CRNAs), and *doctors of nursing practice* (DNPs). *Student nurses* are enrolled in a nursing program and work under supervision of nursing faculty or RN preceptors in the clinical setting. *Unlicensed assistive personnel (AP)* such as *certified nursing assistants* (CNAs) work under supervision of registered or licensed nurses to provide bedside care and assistance with activities of daily living.

Collaborative Care

Nurses work in collaboration with the other members of the health-care team. For example, nurses might participate in multidisciplinary care conferences, request and make referrals (e.g., to chaplain, case manager, dietitian, social worker), or consult with health-care providers (HCPs) or pharmacists. Everyone plays a vital role in providing safe patient care. Excellent communication among team members is essential to providing quality patient-centered care.

> **PRACTICE ANALYSIS TIP**
> **Linking NCLEX-PN® to Practice**
> The LPN/LVN will participate as a member of an interdisciplinary team.

COMPASSION

Empathy is the ability to understand someone else's feelings. Compassion is putting empathy into action. A compassionate nurse understands how a patient is feeling and has the willingness to relieve their suffering, promote healing, or find a solution to their situation. While being a compassionate person may seem like a nice attribute for a nurse to have, it is actually an essential quality. Patients expect their nurse to be compassionate, and research has shown that compassion toward patients improves quality of care, motivates self-care, and decreases health-care costs (Trzeciak & Mazzarelli, 2019). Compassion also has benefits for the nurse. Patients view compassionate health-care workers as more competent, and acting compassionately can help you retain satisfaction in your career as a nurse (Kraft-Todd et al, 2017; Jazaieri, 2018). With all the demands on a nurse's time, how can you act compassionately? Surprisingly, it takes very little time to show compassion. Trzeciak and Mazzarelli (2019) found that demonstrating compassion takes an average of 40 seconds. Getting to know the patient, being kind and attentive, offering support, saying good morning, listening, smiling, holding the patient's hand, and respecting the patient's privacy are all small things that patients identify as compassionate gestures (Durkin, Gurbutt, & Carson, 2018). There will also be times during your career when there are no treatment options and compassion is all that you can give. While the demands on a busy nurse are many, never forget to let your compassion shine through!

LEADERSHIP IN NURSING PRACTICE

A leader seeks to influence, motivate, and enable others to achieve goals. **Leadership** skills are necessary for the LPN/LVN to effectively guide patient care and achieve patient care goals.

Effective leaders in a health-care setting must be knowledgeable about management and supervisory processes. They must use critical thinking and be able to make decisions. They should be role models and provide inspiration to others. A positive attitude and the use of humor are valuable assets of good leaders. Ultimately, leaders must earn the respect of their coworkers to be successful. To prepare for a leadership role, learning and applying the following principles of leadership, supervision, and management are helpful.

Leadership Styles

There are three traditional leadership styles: (1) autocratic, (2) democratic, and (3) laissez-faire. A fourth style, called *coaching,* is also used in health-care settings.

Autocratic (Authoritarian) Leadership

An autocratic leader leads with a high degree of control and gives little or no control to others. In **autocratic leadership,** the leader determines the goals and plans for achieving the goals. Others are told what to do without invitation to provide input. The group usually achieves high-quality outcomes under this style of leadership. This is an efficient leadership style for emergency situations when decisions must be made quickly, such as when evacuating a building or responding to a cardiac arrest.

Democratic (Participative) Leadership

A democratic leader has a moderate degree of control. Others are given some control and freedom. In **democratic leadership,** participation is encouraged in determining goals and plans for achieving the goals (Fig. 3.1). Decisions are made within the group. The leader assists the group by steering and teaching rather than dominating. The leader shares responsibility with the group. The group usually achieves high-quality outcomes and is more creative under this style of leadership than under autocratic or laissez-faire leadership. Democratic leadership is an efficient leadership style for most situations. With this type of leadership, group members have increased satisfaction and motivation to achieve goals as active participants.

Laissez-Faire (Delegative) Leadership

A laissez-faire leader exerts no control over the group. The group, therefore, is given complete freedom for decision making. With **laissez-faire leadership,** no one is responsible for determining goals and plans for achieving the goals. This can produce a feeling of chaos. Often, little is accomplished under this leadership style.

Coaching Leadership

By emphasizing active listening, clear communication, support, and accountability, coaching leaders work with others to develop problem-solving skills that facilitate effective communication, prioritization, critical thinking, and enhanced clinical judgment. This leadership style helps direct-care employees feel more empowered, valued, and respected.

Management Functions

The five major components in the management process are (1) planning, (2) organizing, (3) directing, (4) coordinating, and (5) controlling.

Planning

In the first step of the management process, a plan must be developed to ensure that desired patient care outcomes are achieved. To formulate the plan, desired outcomes or problems are identified and data about them are collected. Alternatives or solutions are considered using the collected data and input from others. A decision is then made about the best option or course of action. The leader should ensure that the choice is realistic and can be implemented. Involving others in the planning and decision-making process from beginning to end can increase acceptance at the time of implementation.

Organizing

Providing a framework for goals and the activities that accomplish them is the initial step in organization. Policies and procedures provide this framework and offer guidance to those carrying out tasks designed to accomplish the organization's goals.

Directing

Making assignments is the primary function of directing. One person, usually the nurse in charge or the team leader, makes the assignments for patient care. The nurse practice act in each state defines who can make assignments and delegate care. Communication is important in directing. Assignments must be clearly and specifically stated. The person making assignments must be sure that each assignment is correctly understood and should seek out the receiving person for clarification. Effective directing can be accomplished by providing verbal and written assignment information, making requests rather than giving orders, and giving instructions.

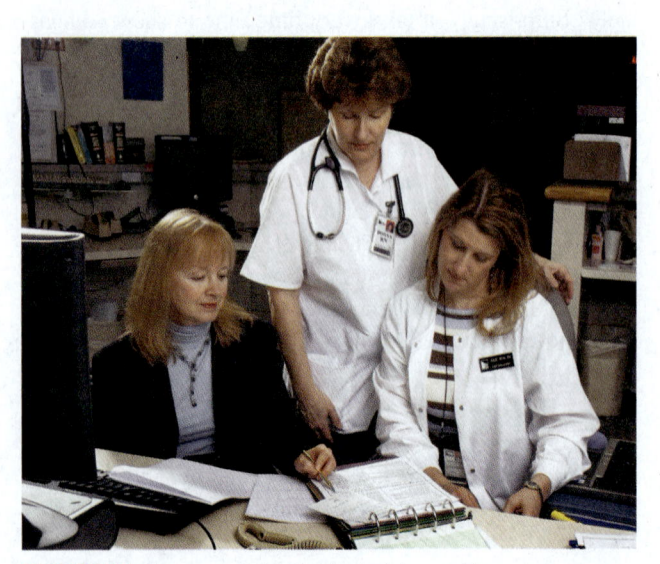

FIGURE 3.1 Group participation in decision making.

Coordinating

Coordination is the process of arranging services for a patient or looking at a situation to ensure that it is being handled most effectively for the organization. In a long-term care facility, for example, the nurse might want to review skin data collection to check for consistent, uniform care throughout the facility. If a concern is found, problem-solving techniques can be used.

Controlling

The final phase of the management process is controlling to evaluate the accomplishment of the organization's goals. Continuous quality improvement (CQI) is linked with controlling. If the organization's efficiency or ability to reach its goals is impaired, the use of the CQI model can facilitate correction of the concern (Fig. 3.2).

Leadership and Delegation for the LPN/LVN

LPNs/LVNs are managers of care for the patients to whom they are assigned while under the supervision of an RN, an HCP, or a dentist, as specified by each state nurse practice act. Beyond this application of a leader and manager role for the LPN/LVN, state nurse practice acts specify if the LPN/LVN can assume other leader or manager roles or can delegate.

The LPN/LVN might function as a team leader or charge nurse, usually in the long-term care setting, requiring some use of **delegation** to AP. When the LPN/LVN acts as a team leader or charge nurse, an RN delegates the authority to provide supervision and delegation of tasks. Team leaders are responsible for the coordination and delivery of care to each of the patients assigned to the team. They collect patient data to plan appropriate care and contribute to the nursing care plan. Team leaders receive information from team members and communicate patients' needs to appropriate individuals. Because team leaders guide patient care provided by the team, they must be knowledgeable about safety policies, patients' rights, and the accountability of being a team leader.

All patients are entitled to quality care and treatment with dignity and respect. The team leader is accountable for all care provided by the team. Supervision involves initial direction for the task, then monitoring of the task and outcome at intervals. At the end of the team's work shift, leaders are responsible for transferring patient care to the oncoming team in a way that prevents communication breakdowns that can harm patients. They must report hand-off communication of patient condition, status, and needs to the oncoming team leader (Fig. 3.3).

> **PRACTICE ANALYSIS TIP**
> **Linking NCLEX-PN® to Practice**
> The LPN/LVN will provide and receive report.

Delegation is the act of empowering another person to act. RNs delegate to LPNs/LVNs and AP. LPNs/LVNs in certain circumstances delegate to AP. When delegation occurs, care responsibility is transferred to the delegatee, but accountability for care remains with the delegator.

Within the leadership role, the LPN/LVN must decide when delegation would most benefit the situation and the patient. All nurses must follow their state nurse practice act and scope of practice when making any decisions regarding delegation. Consult the nurse practice act for your state, charge nurse, and team leader when deciding whether

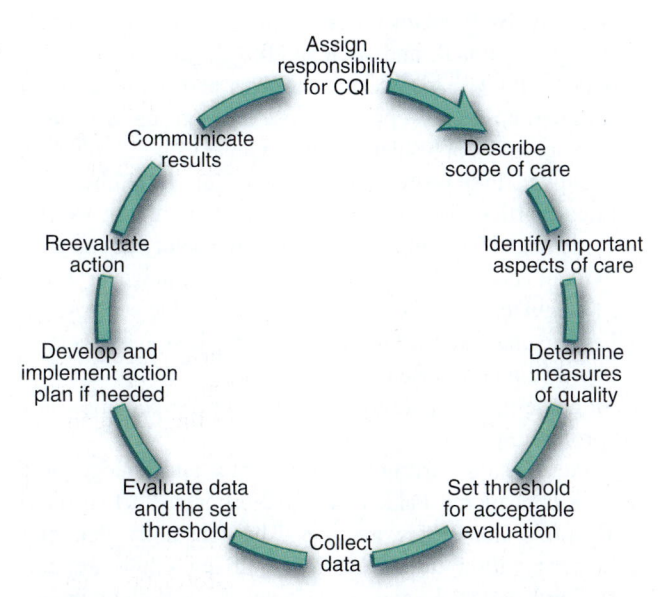

FIGURE 3.2 A continuous quality improvement (CQI) model.

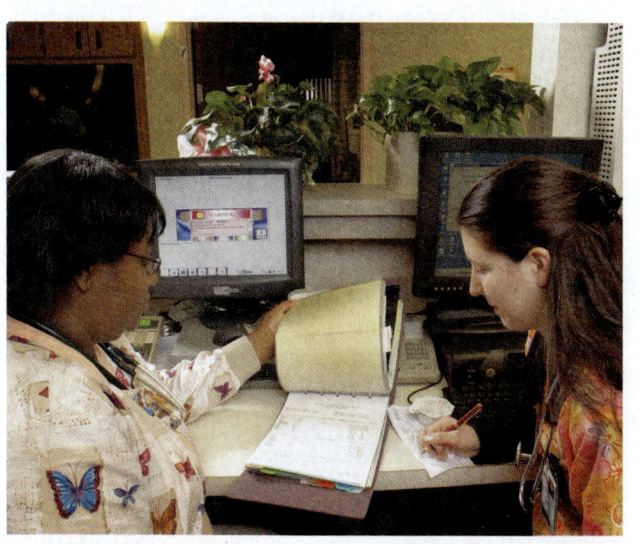

FIGURE 3.3 Hand-off communication of the patient's status by a team leader when transferring the patient's care to another team leader.

delegation is appropriate. Consider these important questions to determine when delegation is most beneficial:

- Does my state nurse practice act allow for delegation in this situation?
- Does the person to whom I am delegating have the knowledge and education to perform this skill, and is it documented for me to make the decisions regarding delegation?
- Would it benefit the patient if I delegated this skill to the support person?

Delegation Process

Delegation is a complex process encompassing the decision to delegate, what to delegate, and to whom:

1. Know your state nurse practice act rules for delegation. The LPN/LVN scope of practice usually does not provide legal authority for an LPN/LVN to delegate. However, some state board rules allow LPNs/LVNs to delegate tasks that are within the LPN/LVN's scope of practice as long as the RN has given the LPN/LVN authority to delegate the tasks.
2. Identify the skills of the person to whom you might delegate to determine whether they have the knowledge and ability to carry out the task. When deciding to delegate to a team member, consider if there is potential for harm to the patient during the task, whether it is a complex task that will require problem-solving, how predictable the outcome is, and how much interaction with the patient is needed. Match the skills and talents of the team member to the task being delegated.
3. Clear communication is essential to safe delegation. It is important to know and understand each other's methods of communicating so that miscommunications do not occur. Verify that the person who has been delegated a task clearly understands the task to be completed. Then check back to verify the task was completed and the outcome.
4. Use the National Council of State Boards of Nursing's five rights of delegation. Following these rights provides a framework for your decision-making process and comfort in knowing you used them to make good choices.

Delegation requires trust. You should be comfortable with which tasks can be delegated and the team member to whom you are delegating the tasks. When you first begin your career, the process of delegating can seem difficult. As with any skill, it takes practice to feel confident in carrying out the process.

> **NURSING CARE TIP**
> Nursing judgment can never be delegated.

> **PRACTICE ANALYSIS TIP**
> Linking NCLEX-PN® to Practice
> The LPN/LVN will monitor activities of assistive personnel.

ETHICS AND VALUES

The study and practice of ethics is grounded in philosophy and dates to the time of Hippocrates. **Ethics** is a systematic approach not only to understanding an ethical dilemma but also to examining the best outcome for each situation (Butts & Rich, 2019). *Bioethics* is a branch of ethics that studies moral values in the biomedical sciences. It has come to be most closely associated with health care. Today more than ever, nurses are confronted with situations and variables that can contribute to clinical ethical dilemmas. Therefore, it is necessary to understand how to identify, process, and address ethical dilemmas.

Although the terms *ethics* and *morals* are often used interchangeably, morals refer more specifically to personally derived values, beliefs, and behaviors. We tend to think of these behaviors as "right and wrong" or "good and bad" (Butts & Rich, 2019).

Values are unwritten standards, ideals, or concepts that give meaning to a person's life. They often serve as a guide for making decisions and setting priorities in daily life. Values can change throughout life on the basis of individual experiences and events. People make decisions based on their values; that is often how they solve conflicts that occur in everyday life. For example, a nurse who values both her career and her family might be forced to decide between going to work or staying home with a sick child. A patient who values both his personal health and family may have to decide between filling a prescription or buying necessary items for his family.

We may live by many types of values, including personal, group, professional, and societal. Just as individuals have personal values that govern their lives and actions, so do groups. Group values represent those of the group as a whole but may or may not be identical to personal values. Examples of groups include professional groups, clubs, churches, and political parties. Society also observes overarching values. As a member of a group, organization, or society/country, an individual accepts the values of that culture; however, he or she recognizes that those values may not be the same as his or her personal values. The values of a profession are usually outlined in a code of ethics. This code is a comprehensive set of guidelines that outlines the behavioral expectations for the profession.

Ethical issues surround us constantly and change over time. Kangasniemi, Pakkanen, and Korhonen (2015) found that professional ethics are shaped by constantly changing influences within the profession. Nursing ethics are not static, and ethical issues are particularly prevalent in our professional lives for several reasons. Advances in technology and therapeutics can prolong or save a life. Yet, questions arise: Who should receive treatment? How long should treatment continue? Should a patient receive a treatment because it is available or because it will be effective? How many health-care resources should be utilized for the treatment of terminal illnesses? Does quantity or length of life matter more than quality of life? Nurses contribute to deciding how and when resources are allocated. All nursing actions can potentially influence patient outcomes, so nurses must be prepared to consider the ethics behind their action(s) or inaction(s) (Milliken, 2018).

Not all bioethical issues make headline news. In fact, many ethical dilemmas are regular occurrences in the clinical setting. Nurses are involved every day in decision making based on traditional ethical principles: autonomy, beneficence, **maleficence**, and justice. Have you experienced an indication for ethical decision making? Here are some examples: You are asked to consistently work on a unit that is understaffed; a patient asks you to keep his prognosis from his spouse; you observe a reportable patient safety event and consider not reporting it to leadership because others were around, too, and you do not have time; you overhear a coworker on break, sharing patient health information with another employee without clinical reasons.

An ethical dilemma is a situation in which a person must choose between two options that will affect the outcome of the case. Although each option can be justified as "good," both have pros and cons. Therefore, when one option must be selected or implemented, it creates uncertainty in the outcome of the case (Butts & Rich, 2019).

Decision making in the clinical setting is a complex process involving many members of the health-care team. As a result of carrying out orders, nurses must handle consequences that arise from clinical problems. In addition, there is no one-size-fits-all solution for ethical problems. Even if dilemmas share a common thread, each has individual influences that make it unique.

When patients appear competent, their choices are usually respected. However, other intervening factors make decision making difficult. Disagreement is pervasive in the decision-making process, including disagreement between an HCP and a family, nurses and other HCPs, or family members.

Nurses are integral to resolving disagreements affecting patient care or outcomes. This role causes nurses to experience moral distress. **Moral distress** can be defined generally as distress one experiences when he or she identifies the correct action but cannot carry it out because of institutional constraints (Jameton, 1984). Moral distress can lead to job burnout, so finding ways to address moral distress is important. Stephens (2019) suggests that developing personal resilience helps nurses minimize moral distress in the workplace. Nurses can build resilience by looking within and identifying "personal protective factors," or coping skills that help defend against the effects of stress (Stephens, 2019). According to Stephens, one's *personal resiliency* is the ability "to navigate stressful situations or perceived adverse events to effectively cope and reach a higher level of well-being" (Stephens, 2019).

A basic mastery of several elements enhances your ability to perform competently when ethical issues arise, and good decision making is paramount. Understand your own personal ethics. Explore your personal values and how these values influence your nursing practice. As nurses, we must continuously acquire knowledge relevant to ethical scenarios we encounter. A standardized, evidence-based process for examining ethical dilemmas can build your understanding of ethics and develop a sound foundation on which you can competently resolve ethical concerns in the clinical environment.

Ethical Obligations and Nursing

As a nurse, you are an invaluable member of the health-care team, contributing to patient care according to your educational preparation and assigned responsibilities. You are guided by the law and the standards of the profession as well as by a professional code of ethics. In addition to practicing within the law, nurses are obliged to act ethically when using their license, and if the law is considered unethical or has serious limitations, a basic moral obligation of the nurse is to make an effort to change that law. Nurses may act individually, through representation, or through the political activism of professional organizations.

Nursing Code of Ethics

Some of the major ethical obligations of nursing practice are addressed in a nursing code of ethics. A code of ethics has several purposes and serves to provide (1) guidance for appropriate decision making based on current laws and professional standards; (2) a method for professional self-evaluation and reflection; and (3) a way to hold the profession accountable. The National Association of Licensed Practical Nurses has practice standards for ethical practice and conduct. NAPNES, the National Association for Practical Nurse Education and Service, also has standards of practice for LPNs/LVNs.

A code of conduct, ethics, or the like serves as a general guideline for professional practice. Although not documents of legal significance, codes generally harmonize with law. Codes are self-regulatory tools that are not enforced within the legal system. Ethical codes are occasionally updated to reflect current practice requirements, duties, and obligations of licensed practice.

> **PRACTICE ANALYSIS TIP**
> **Linking NCLEX-PN® to Practice**
> The LPN/LVN will practice in a manner consistent with code of ethics for nurses.

Building Blocks of Ethics

An understanding of basic concepts, presented here in the form of ethical principles and ethical theories, helps specifically target the ethical components of the problem. Principles and theories offer frameworks for ethical problem-solving and ethical decision making. Knowledge about ethics can help us to systematically look at an issue and determine the best course of action.

Ethical Principles

Ethical principles act as guidelines or standards. They provide a framework for moral conduct as well as how to approach ethical dilemmas. Ethical principles can be found in many professional codes of conduct. They are key components of ethical decision making. The ethical principles widely used in health-care delivery include autonomy, beneficence, nonmaleficence, fidelity, veracity, and justice. Given the prominence of these ethical principles in the bioethical literature, a basic understanding of them is necessary.

AUTONOMY. According to ethicists (as well as behaviorists, social scientists, and psychologists), what makes human beings different from nonhumans is that people have dignity based on their ability to choose freely what they will do with their lives. **Autonomy** is the right of self-determination, independence, and freedom founded on the notion that humans have value, worth, and moral dignity. Autonomy concerns the ability of all people to make self-interested health-care decisions. While a nurse may not agree with a patient or power of attorney's decision making, the nurse should respect the right of personal autonomy as well as the decision made. **Paternalism** occurs when a nurse tries to prevent autonomous decision making or decides the patient's course of action without regard for the patient's best interests. Autonomy can be harmonized with a professional nurse's beliefs and pursuits. *Advocacy* occurs when patients are not capable of making their own decisions and therefore lack autonomy. In this case, the nurse may work to advocate for the patient's best interests if the patient's interest is otherwise unstated or unwritten.

> **PRACTICE ANALYSIS TIP**
> Linking NCLEX-PN® to Practice
> The LPN/LVN will promote client self-advocacy.

Autonomy has limitations, which typically arise when one's individual autonomy interferes with the rights, health, or well-being of oneself or others. Federal legislation known as the Patient Self-Determination Act guarantees a patient's right to make certain health-care decision. One's health-care decision making may be limited. If a patient is no longer capable of self-care upon discharge, a request to live independently will not be granted. Therefore, the principle of autonomy cannot always be upheld.

BENEFICENCE. The principle of **beneficence** proposes that actions taken and treatments provided will benefit a person and promote welfare (Butts & Rich, 2019). The provision of good care means giving competent care as well as care that respects the patient's beliefs, feelings, and wishes, as well as those of the patient's family and significant others. Deciding what is good and beneficial for someone else can be a common problem when applying this ethical principle. As a tip, review the patient record and speak to the patient's close family and/or health-care decision maker. Ethical decision making can take time and requires balancing of benefits against risks.

NONMALEFICENCE. **Nonmaleficence** is one of the oldest obligations in health care, dating back to the Hippocratic Oath (400 BC). Nonmaleficence is the obligation to "do no harm" (Butts & Rich, 2019). It is common to hear beneficence and nonmaleficence talked about as "two sides of the same coin."

Licensed nurses are required to do no harm to their patients either *intentionally* or *unintentionally*. In current health-care practice, the principle of nonmaleficence may be intentionally violated to produce a greater good in the patient's long-term treatment. For example, a patient might undergo a painful and debilitating or disfiguring surgery to remove a cancerous growth, thereby avoiding death and prolonging life.

By extension, the principle of nonmaleficence also requires a nurse to protect from harm those who are considered vulnerable. Vulnerable groups include children, older adults, and those who are mentally incompetent or are too weak or debilitated to protect themselves.

FIDELITY. **Fidelity** is the obligation to be faithful to commitments made to self and others. In health care, fidelity includes faithfulness or loyalty to agreements and responsibilities accepted as part of the practice of nursing. It also means not promising the patient an outcome outside of the health-care team's control. Fidelity underpins the concept of accountability, although conflicts in fidelity may arise due to obligations owed to different individuals or groups. For example, nurses exhibiting fidelity demonstrate the highest quality care to all patients while employing care consistent with institutional policies and procedures. Nurses may experience an ethical dilemma when a hospital's staffing practice does not follow hospital policy and prevents nurses from meeting all patient needs throughout a shift.

Maintaining patient privacy and **confidentiality** is related to fidelity (Fig. 3.4). Privacy and confidentiality may or may not be an explicit promise. Nurses are obligated to discuss a patient's care only to facilitate care or ensure safety. Nurses may share information when a business purpose for sharing information exists. Some disclosures may be nonclinical, for example:

- When given specific instructions by the patient to share information.
- When a grave possibility of harm to the patient or another exists.
- When legally mandated to do so, under court order or regulatory mandate.

• WORD • BUILDING •
nonmaleficence: non—not + maleficentia—evil doing

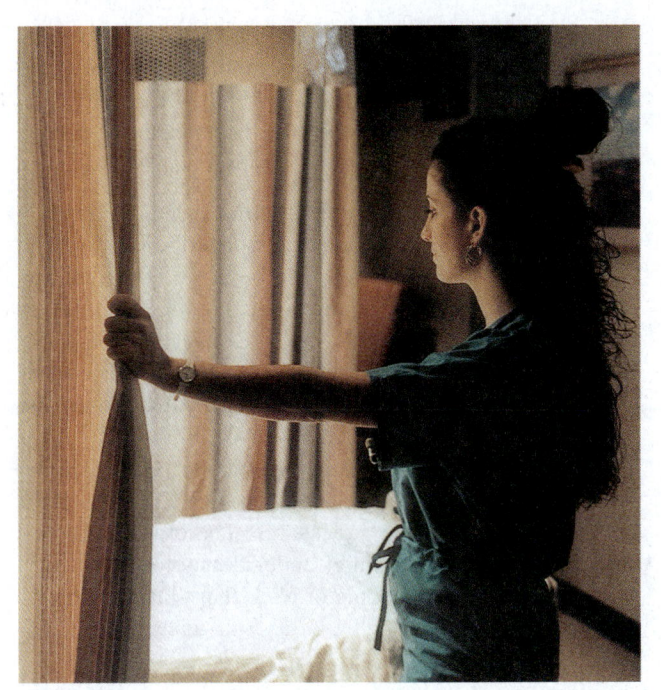

FIGURE 3.4 Maintaining privacy is a patient right and conveys caring to the patient.

Maintaining confidentiality also applies to communication of information posted on the unit, as evidenced by a patient census list, surgical or therapy schedules (e.g., operating room, physical therapy), computer storage of and access to patient information, and use of fax machines and e-mail to transmit patient information. Faculty members in the course of making student assignments, accrediting agencies, risk managers, quality assurance personnel, insurance companies, next of kin, and researchers all may access patient health information. However, each is obligated to maintain patient confidentiality.

> **PRACTICE ANALYSIS TIP**
> Linking NCLEX-PN® to Practice
> The LPN/LVN will provide for privacy needs; maintain client confidentiality.

VERACITY. **Veracity** is the virtue of truthfulness. Within health care, it requires licensed nurses to tell the truth and not intentionally deceive or mislead patients. As with other rights and obligations, there are limitations to this virtue. The primary limitation occurs when the truth would seriously harm a patient's ability to recover or when the truth can produce greater illness. This is known as **therapeutic privilege**. It is exercised by licensed nurses in cases when (1) they are trying to protect patients from heartbreaking news, as in the initial stages of treatment; (2) they do not know the facts, making it better not to answer rather than instill false hope; and (3) they state what is true rather than state what is not true (Butts & Rich, 2019).

Another difficult situation can be created in relation to diagnostic information. Although giving diagnostic information is generally the responsibility of the HCP or RN, LPNs/LVNs sometimes find themselves in situations in which they must deal with patients' questions. If LPNs/LVNs feel uncomfortable about reinforcing explanations given by the HCP or the RN, they might avoid answering patients' questions directly. However, patients do have a right to know this information. The LPN/LVN should inform the HCP or RN of the patient's request for information and follow the agency policy on patient information sharing.

JUSTICE. **Justice** is based on fairness and equality (Butts & Rich, 2019). Concerns for justice can focus on how we treat individuals and groups in society (psychologically, socially, legally, and politically). They can also focus on how we equitably distribute material resources, such as health care (distributive justice) and burdens (taxes), and the appropriate compensation to those who have been harmed. When a patient makes an appointment for 0900 at an outpatient clinic, the patient expects to be seen by the provider at the designated time, pending an emergency. Unequal, unjust treatment results when a provider sees a walk-in patient with no emergent condition instead of a patient who scheduled an appointment at 0900 and delays other scheduled appointments. Distributing resources justly is not easy. Just behavior requires one to understand benefits and burdens associated with a decision. Benefits and burdens may be tangible or intangible, monetary or nonmonetary. For example, one benefit may be participating in cutting-edge medication research, but the associated burden may be the risk of receiving a placebo instead of the medication being researched.

> **Evidence-Based Practice**
>
> **Clinical Question**
> What are nurses' perspectives of patient advocacy?
>
> **Evidence**
> A systematic review sought to identify nurses' attitudes and perceptions of patient advocacy (Saleh et al, 2020). Twenty-one studies showed nurses hold consistent positive attitudes for patient advocacy and that patient advocacy is a process with four elements: client situation, nurse, advocacy, and interventions and advocacy consequences.
>
> **Implications for Nursing Practice**
> To provide quality nursing care, nurses must be trained for the role of advocating for patients. A wide range of advocacy actions for nurses was identified, including establishing trust, empowering the patient, educating patients and families, providing respectful and dignified care, protecting patients, defending patient rights and choice, telling the truth, and assisting with end of life transition.
>
> *Reference:* Saleh, U. Aboshayga, A., O'Conner, T., Saleh, M., Patton, D., & Ampang, A. (2020). Nurses' perspective of patient advocacy: A systematic mixed studies review. *International Journal of Nursing & Clinical Practice, 7,* 317. https://doi.org/10.15344/2394-4978/2020/317

USE OF PRINCIPLES. One of the most serious limitations of ethical principles is the lack of built-in priority when faced with an ethical dilemma. Autonomy is not prioritized over justice, nor beneficence over nonmaleficence. Yet, each principle helps to categorize the perspectives shared during an ethical dilemma. Applying ethical principles enables discussion from a professional perspective, as opposed to discussion of one individual's viewpoint or feeling. Approach clinical concerns by applying ethical principles. This strategy can neutralize power struggles by those who simply want to win an argument and promote care that serves the patient's best interests.

> **LEARNING TIP**
> The following is an example of an ethical dilemma: A nurse supports a patient's refusal of surgery, while the surgeon asserts the patient must have surgery to avoid loss of limb. The nurse's approach is from the perspective of the patient's autonomy (self-determination), and the surgeon's approach is from the perspective of beneficence (to act in a way that benefits the patient). Here, you can see the issue is not a conflict between individuals but an issue arising out of the ethical conflict. Understanding ethical principles and variability does not resolve conflicts but makes conflicts less personal and drives just decision making and patient-centered outcomes.

Ethical Theories

Unlike ethical principles, ethical theories provide a robust framework for analyzing ethical dilemmas. Theories explain variables, guide inquiry, and create a foundation for ethical decision making. We describe only two major bioethical theories—utilitarianism and deontology—in this section, though other theoretical approaches to ethical decision making exist. One may combine several theories to address one ethical dilemma. In addition, this section explores the relationship of theology and religion to bioethics in medicine.

UTILITARIANISM. Utilitarian theory states that actions should be judged "right" or "wrong" purely on the utility of the action's outcome. Therefore, the relative utility of an outcome is the most important element to consider when making a decision. The right actions are morally preferred if they produce more happiness or greater benefits than unhappiness or burdens. In utilitarianism, each person's happiness is equally important. This approach can be used by institutions and organizations under the guise of cost-benefit ratios. A skilled nursing facility responsible for the care of 100 patients is less concerned with an individual patient who, unfortunately, is caught in the bureaucracy of the facility's functioning. Not all health-care facilities operate on this theory, but, generally, rules, policies, and procedures are developed with the majority's interests in mind.

The utilitarian theory is not without criticism. One criticism centers on the belief that an individual's needs are sacrificed for the good of the majority. Another criticism is based on the belief that it is difficult to predict outcomes, especially when human nature is involved.

DEONTOLOGY. Deontology is an ethical theory based on duty. Under this theory, the moral worth of an action (the result) should not be judged solely on the consequences of the action but on whether the action itself is right or wrong. For example, HCPs might project that ethically sound personnel should never lie even if the lie produces a positive outcome. Therefore, to be ethically sound, one must tell the truth always. Another rule might be to never use people to achieve an outcome. This ethical dilemma presents in medical research. An individual has the right to voluntarily participate in research. Therefore, no matter how good our intentions are, under deontological theory, one should not "use" people or trick them into participating in research.

THEOLOGICAL PERSPECTIVES. Theological perspectives on ethics derive from the many religious traditions represented in our culture. Religious teachings are key concepts for ethical decision making for some people. In fact, many consider these teachings a divine source of values and morals. Some examples include religion-based opposition to blood transfusions, abortion, and euthanasia. One complication of theologically derived ethics is that personal interpretation may vary according to religious teaching. As a nurse, you must collect data on religion in a patient's life to effectively analyze the patient's ethical framework(s) and needs.

Ethical Decision Making

A variety of models and frameworks are available for ethical decision making. In its simplest form, ethical decision making is a problem-solving process. The eight steps described here take nursing students through a set of strategies to help them understand ethical decision making in an organized and systemic manner.

Sample Ethical Dilemma

The Smith family was in an automobile accident out of state. Mrs. Smith is in critical condition with a head injury. Mr. Smith died in the emergency department, and their 12-year-old daughter, Melissa, is in critical condition. Mrs. Smith is still able to speak and asks you how her husband and daughter are doing. What action should you take?

STEP 1: IDENTIFY THE ETHICAL DILEMMA. The initial step is to identify the ethical dilemma. What is it in this case? You must separate the ethical and nonethical aspects of the case. Ethical dilemmas are different from clinical problems, which may have clearer interventions and rationales. Our sample case is an ethical dilemma because there is no obvious right answer. Do you tell the mother now or later that her spouse is dead and her child is critically injured?

STEP 2: IDENTIFY THE STAKEHOLDERS AND THEIR VALUES. The values, beliefs, and traditions of all participants are important. Each influences the decision-making process. The patient is at the center of the process, so patient autonomy is important to the steps of the process.

In our sample case, who are the stakeholders? Obviously, the patient (mother) and family members (daughter, others) are stakeholders, as are the health-care team members.

STEP 3: GATHER AND VERIFY THE INFORMATION. Examine all facets of the dilemma. Besides knowing who is involved, explore the context of the dilemma. How did the situation arise? Does objective data support one decision over another? The medical record, relevant law, facility policies and procedures, and other clinical resources or personnel can shed light on and add context to a dilemma. Therefore, it is necessary to comprehensively examine as much relevant information as is available, which is best gathered and facilitated by a health-care team.

In our sample case, what do you know? The objective data tell you the following: (1) The spouse is dead; (2) the daughter, who is 12 years old, is in critical condition; (3) the family is from out of state; and (4) it is found that the mother experienced head trauma, and although she is asking about her spouse and daughter, her vital signs are unstable and her condition is also critical. In addition to the objective information, you must gather information on processes that control patient communication. What comes to mind? What policies direct how health-care workers share medical information? What resources or departments should be called to assist in this case?

STEP 4: EXAMINE POSSIBLE ACTIONS AND FORECAST THE CONSEQUENCES OF EACH ACTION. Develop a comprehensive set of all possible actions, then forecast the potential consequences of each action, positive or negative. This allows you to weigh the benefit (positive) or risk (negative) of each action.

In our sample case, what are all the possible actions or alternatives to resolve the dilemma? If you consider the extremes, the choices appear clear: You either tell Mrs. Smith about her husband and child or you do not. If you tell Mrs. Smith that her husband is dead and her child is in critical condition, what are the positive and negative consequences of this action? Would this improve her autonomy or, moreover, her clinical outcome? Conversely, if you do not tell Mrs. Smith about her spouse and child, what are the consequences? There may be other tactful options, too. For example, you could calm Mrs. Smith by saying that her husband and daughter are both still being evaluated, or you could call a manager or chaplain to assist the staff in telling her the truth. Partial truths may seem unacceptable at first glance but should be added to a list of possible actions. Can you think of any more actions appropriate for this scenario? What would be the consequences for these actions?

STEP 5: DETERMINE THE ETHICAL FOUNDATION FOR EACH ACTION. Each action should be based on ethical values, principles, or theories. In addition, the code of ethics can lend support as an ethical rationale. One strategy that is proposed for an incompetent or unconscious patient is the *standard of best interest*. This standard involves determination of the best outcome for the patient, given the information known about the patient and the context of the situation. Typically, family members together with HCPs make this determination. However, this information may be memorialized on an advance directive or living will.

In our sample case, if you revisit the actions proposed in the previous section, you can see that telling the truth supports veracity but may violate the principle of beneficence and support maleficence. In contrast, by not telling the truth, you violate the principle of veracity but uphold beneficence, possibly nonmaleficence. Lastly, if you entertain the idea of telling only part of the truth, once again you are violating veracity, but the difference is that you are striving to meet the principle of beneficence. You realize that by telling the whole truth, Mrs. Smith's condition can worsen from the stress of the situation.

STEP 6: DETERMINE WHICH ACTION IS BEST, WITH THE MOST COMPELLING ETHICAL SUPPORT. Each action is judged on the basis of its risks and benefits and supporting rationale. The actions should then be ranked in priority order. Strong ethical support for the first priority is required, as is a reasonable potential for the action to be implemented. A team of health-care members is best suited to make judgment and priority decisions.

In our sample case, what do you think is the best outcome? Everyone must examine the actions and their respective consequences and supporting ethical principles before making a final decision.

Utilitarians and deontologists might disagree about the best outcome or how to best achieve that outcome. Do not assume, though, that people of different theoretical positions cannot achieve consensus. Although their rationales may differ, the final solutions sought may be identical.

STEP 7: IMPLEMENT THE ACTION. The selected action needs to be implemented in a logical way. Responsibilities for carrying out the plan can be assigned, especially if there are multiple steps in the process. In addition, a well-implemented plan can ensure that the plan is fully operationalized and increases the potential for success.

In our sample case, each person must implement a plan based on the stakeholders, the chosen action, and the underlying ethical principles. How would you implement your action? What resources would you need? Which members of the health-care team would you collaborate with?

STEP 8: EVALUATE THE OUTCOME. The evaluative process is most effective when the details of the care are still fresh. The resolution of an ethical dilemma, whether it has been successful or not, provides us with knowledge and experience to address the next ethical dilemma. Although each dilemma is unique in many ways, similarities between cases can provide insight into the best way to approach the decision-making process when a comparable case arises.

In our sample case, the outcome can be evaluated only after an action is implemented.

> **CRITICAL THINKING**
>
> **Ethical Decisions.** Identify a health-care-related ethical dilemma you have encountered as a student. How did you solve the dilemma? What evidence-based resources did you use?
>
> Apply the ethical decision-making steps to your ethical dilemma. How are your decision-making process and proposed actions different when using the steps?

LEGAL CONCEPTS

Regulation of Nursing Practice

Nursing is a licensed health-care profession that is regulated by individual states. Nurses must be licensed by their state to practice nursing. State licensure improves the quality of health-care services and protects the health, safety, and well-being of the residents of that state. Each state has a *board of nursing*. The board establishes requirements for nurses to be licensed and to practice in that state. To maintain licensure, continuing education requirements vary by state.

Each state has laws that define the scope of a nurse's practice in that state. In most cases, these laws are contained in a *nurse practice act*. If a nurse violates the nurse practice act, their license can be sanctioned—that is, suspended or revoked. Unprofessional conduct, incompetence, conviction of a crime, or misuse of controlled substances are examples of circumstances that can result in sanctions against a nurse's license.

> **PRACTICE ANALYSIS TIP**
> **Linking NCLEX-PN® to Practice**
> The LPN/LVN will provide care within the legal scope of practice.

> **BE SAFE!**
> - **BE VIGILANT!** Do not go into work after drinking alcohol, even the night before your shift. It takes time to metabolize alcohol from your system. Most, if not all, organizations have a zero-tolerance policy for alcohol. Many factors affect alcohol metabolism rates. Men metabolize alcohol faster than do women, especially petite women. A woman's menses may increase the time required to metabolize alcohol.
> - If you use a prescription medication, ensure you have a current prescription for a current condition. If you use controlled substances, even if legally prescribed, you cannot work when under their influence if the substance affects your ability to work safely.

Required Reporting to the Licensing Board

When you submit your application for state licensure, you must be honest and report any prior conviction for misdemeanors or felonies. Most states require a criminal background check for licensure, so they will know about it.

After you receive your license, address changes must be reported to the licensing board within 30 days. This ensures that you can always be contacted. Failure to do so can be a violation of state law. Failure to notify the licensing board could also result in missing important communications, such as license renewal mailings. Any conviction (occurring anywhere, not just in your own state) must also be reported to your state board within 30 days. If in doubt, report! They *will* find out. If you haven't reported a conviction, you could be sanctioned not only for the conviction but also for not reporting.

Mandatory Reporting

A state's mandated reporting laws require licensed nurses to report known or suspected abuse of a person to state authorities. In their profession, nurses interact with vulnerable populations. These populations need additional eyes and ears looking out for their best interests. Whereas state laws protect all patient populations, older adults, children, and those with mental or developmental disabilities are the most vulnerable. Be sure to learn how your state's laws will affect your practice if you are obligated to report known or suspected abuse. Know how and when to notify the authorities.

Generally, *abuse* is defined as willful behavior that causes harm to an intended recipient. Abuse takes several forms: physical, sexual, verbal, emotional, financial/economic, or neglect. It can occur to anyone, of any age, and in any setting. Although neglect and abuse are related, the intent of neglect differs from the intent of abuse. Abuse occurs when the nurse acts with a desire to harm, whereas neglect occurs when a nurse's inaction produces harm regardless of the nurse's intent. For example, neglect potentially occurs when a nurse decides to place two adult briefs on a patient with heavy urination patterns to minimize the frequency of necessary changes. The nurse may try to rationalize the intervention as a benefit to the patient, but the neglectful behavior does not satisfy the needs of the patient and has the potential to cause harm, including skin breakdown, pain, and discomfort. Neglect produces harm unintentionally. Abuse is intentional. Abuse can be done in person and through use of technology. Older adults are especially vulnerable to financial abuse as well as physical abuse and neglect. In long-term care, the risk of abuse is higher for residents who have dementia and direct unwelcome behaviors toward others. Other residents may harm this person as payback for past behaviors. Licensed nurses must be aware of potential for abuse to ensure safety of all residents.

> **PRACTICE ANALYSIS TIP**
> Linking NCLEX-PN® to Practice
> The LPN/LVN will follow regulation/policy for reporting specific issues (e.g., abuse, neglect, gunshot wound, communicable disease).

Human Trafficking and the Nurse's Role

Human trafficking refers to the act of recruiting, harboring, transporting, providing, or obtaining a person for labor or as a sex worker though the use of force, fraud, or coercion (which does not apply if the victim is a minor, as trafficking is child abuse) (US Department of State, 2015). Human trafficking is a worldwide problem. Some state boards of nursing are increasing awareness of the issue to help rescue victims. Nurses are being required, when seeking licensure, to obtain education on how to identify victims of human trafficking (Michigan Department of Licensing and Regulatory Affairs, 2017).

Human trafficking victims utilize the health-care system to access emergency, inpatient hospital, or community-based services (Michigan Department of Licensing and Regulatory Affairs, 2017). The US Department of Health and Human Services (n.d.) indicates that victims of human trafficking often lack access to quality health care for early treatment of health issues. Therefore, a victim may appear with late-stage issues that have gone untreated or have become chronic in nature. Victims seeking care often do not have identification or money. They are accompanied by someone in control, who will not leave them alone and who answers for them.

When providing care, licensed nurses have an opportunity to identify physical and psychological symptoms commonly seen in victims of human trafficking. Severe physical symptoms can include dizzy spells; headaches; fatigue; and back, abdominal, or stomach pain. Memory loss, depression, and anxiety are common psychological symptoms among human trafficking victims (Simkhada et al, 2018). Behaviors exhibited by human trafficking victims can resemble behaviors of sufferers of chronic abuse and neglect. Bruises, scars, and signs of physical abuse and torture, including malnutrition, should be noted. If you suspect a patient is a victim of human trafficking, discuss your suspicion with your clinical team (Box 3.2). After the suspicion is confirmed by the team, it must be reported to the appropriate authorities (Box 3.3).

Health Insurance Portability and Accountability Act

The Health Insurance Portability and Accountability Act of 1996 (HIPAA) ensures privacy of a patient's protected health information (PHI). All health-care workers and students must follow HIPAA. This act prohibits illegal sharing of a patient's medical or billing information.

> **Box 3.2**
> **Indicators of Human Trafficking**
>
> **Behaviors**
> Afraid, shy, or submissive
> Coached dialogue
> Sudden or dramatic change in behavior
>
> **Circumstances**
> Child involved with commercial sex acts
> Controlled by someone who makes all decisions, will not leave the person alone, and speaks for the person
> Evidence of poor housing conditions
> Kept away from family, friends, school, public organizations, and church
> Lack of personal possessions and adequate clothing
> Movements restricted
>
> **Signs and Symptoms**
> Abuse signs: mental, physical, sexual, torture
> Bruises (old and new)
> Confusion or disorientation
> Exhaustion
> Malnourishment and/or dehydration
> Minimal or no medical history
> Poor hygiene

> **Box 3.3**
> **Reporting Suspected Human Trafficking**
>
> **US Department of Homeland Security: Blue Campaign**
> The US Department of Homeland Security is the voice of the federal government efforts to combat human trafficking. Blue is a color code used internationally for human trafficking awareness: www.dhs.gov/blue-campaign, www.facebook.com/bluecampaign, Twitter: #BlueCampaign.
>
> The Blue Campaign recommends safety first: Do not confront a suspected trafficker or alert a suspected trafficking victim. Report it!
>
> To report suspected human trafficking, contact:
> - Your local law enforcement
> - The US Department of Homeland Security Tip Line: 1-866-347-2423
> - The National Human Trafficking Resource Center Hotline: 1-888-373-7888
> - Text HELP or INFO to BeFree (233733)

From US Department of Homeland Security. Blue Campaign: Indicators of human trafficking. Retrieved October 10, 2020, from www.dhs.gov/blue-campaign/indicators-human-trafficking

Nurses must be sensitive to all patient information that is learned during nursing care. HIPAA violations occur when PHI is shared without prior patient consent. An individual can be fined and/or sentenced up to 10 years in prison for

HIPAA violations. They can also be sued individually and face possible employment termination. Some states, such as California, have enacted laws ensuring the integrity of PHI. These state laws work in conjunction with HIPAA to deter unauthorized disclosure. If your agency reports an incident of unauthorized disclosure under federal or state law, a state agency may visit your organization to investigate. Review your employer's HIPAA compliance policies. Follow them. Review a patient's medical record (including your own) only when you have a business need to do so.

Social Media and Protecting Privacy

With the pervasive nature of social media, health-care agencies have increased oversight of employees' social media activity by monitoring for unauthorized disclosures of PHI. HIPAA as well as state law can be violated by uploading photos to social media that were taken on a personal device in a patient care setting. Examples of social media include Facebook, Instagram, Snapchat, and Reddit. Patient confidentiality and privacy must always be maintained. Use PHI only for intended purposes related to patient care. Nurses must afford dignity to patients and protect PHI in the virtual world. For information and examples about appropriate professional social media use, see the National Council of State Boards of Nursing's guide at www.ncsbn.org.

Nursing Liability and the Law

Nurses are expected to practice in accordance with the law. There are laws that establish **liability,** or responsibility for wrongful clinical decisions. Three subcategories of the law apply to nursing: civil law, criminal law, and administrative law. **Criminal laws** regulate human behavior within society. **Civil laws** protect individual and personal property rights. **Administrative laws** license and regulate the practice of nursing.

Criminal and Civil Law

Criminal laws establish rules for social behavior and define the punishment for breaking those rules. Criminal laws relate to wrongs against society. Their violation can result in imprisonment and/or monetary fines. Violation of criminal laws can also produce civil liability. For example, a nurse acts maliciously in causing the injury or death of a patient. This nurse can be found criminally liable for the malicious act (being against societal norms) and civilly liable for the extent of injury and damages caused by the action. Examples of criminal actions include assault, battery, murder, and rape. Civil laws generally concern disputes among individuals. Actions that violate civil law do not commonly rise to violations of criminal law. Nevertheless, liability for violating a civil law may entail stiff penalties, which are imposed to deter similar behavior in the future.

A nurse's civil liability can arise from negligent patient care. Civil law provides a means for patients and families to recover from injuries that occur after receiving negligent care. Recovery in civil law requires the injured party to show causation between the licensed professional's action and the patient's injury. To show causation, the patient must demonstrate how the licensed professional's action or omission caused the injury. An injury can be physical, emotional, or financial in nature. Lawsuits involving personal injuries are called **torts.**

The process of a civil lawsuit begins with the filing of a complaint in a court by a *plaintiff.* Court systems have their own rules. They require the plaintiff to serve a copy of the complaint on the *defendant,* or the party defending the complaint. A **summons** acts as a notice of a lawsuit and should be attached to the complaint. Nurses served with a summons and/or complaint that arises from work-related duties should notify their employers immediately. An employer may choose to answer the summons. If the employer does not answer the summons, the nurse must seek legal counsel to answer it within the required time frame. Failure to answer the summons and complaint is harmful to a nurse's personal and professional life.

An employer may be liable for the acts or omissions of a nurse it employs. This theory of liability is called *respondeat superior.* Nurses must appreciate how their behavior can create civil liability for employers. Always practice in accordance with agency policies and procedures.

Malpractice is a form of professional negligence. **Negligence** is a civil law claim that is presented when one's failure to exercise due care results in an injury to another. **Malpractice** arises when the resulting injury occurs as a result of the clinician–patient relationship. A nurse commits malpractice when the nurse fails to practice consistently within professional standards and the patient is injured as a result. For example, a nurse commits malpractice if the patient is injured because of a rough transfer performed inconsistently with organizational policy (e.g., to use lift sheets) and/or professional standards of practice. Professional standards of nursing practice are determined at the local and regional levels based on health-care services and care and equipment offered. Standards vary by state. Licensed nurses are expected to use their knowledge gained through school and experience wisely when interacting with patients and families.

Limitation of Liability

HCPs should strive to limit liability in practice. **Limitation of liability** reduces the actual and/or monetary responsibility for an undesired outcome. Prevention is the best way to limit liability. You can do this in the following ways: ensure patient rights, follow your employer's organizational policies, use current nursing practice standards, document accurately, and pursue continuing education.

Patient Rights

All patients are entitled to quality care that provides dignity, respect, and involvement in care planning and decision making. Ensure patient-centered outcomes. Question care directives that appear in conflict with patient rights. Rights are defined as something due an individual through legal guarantees or moral and ethical principles. Narrowly, the United States affords certain rights to patients who receive care at facilities reimbursed by the federal government through federal and state health insurance programs. Individual states may also enact laws that narrowly define rights for patients receiving care in that state. For example, Title 22 of the California Code of Regulations includes a bill of rights for patients at certain health-care facilities operating under state licensure. Generally, patient rights promote a patient's individuality and decision-making capacity. Patient rights also prevent patients from experiencing abuse and unauthorized disclosure of PHI. Be aware of patient rights as you practice. Be courteous to your patient. Knock before entering a patient's room. Introduce yourself to promote a patient's right to privacy and limit liability in practice.

> **PRACTICE ANALYSIS TIP**
> Linking NCLEX-PN® to Practice
> The LPN/LVN will advocate for client rights and needs.

Appropriate Documentation

The medical record is a legal record in which nurses must document all patient care. Documentation must be clear, honest, and accurate. Always document according to agency policy. Failure to do so can create potential embarrassment and liability for you and your employer. Your written record is all that remains to describe the care you provided. If it is not documented, it is not done.

Malpractice Insurance

Individual malpractice insurance may not be essential. Often, an employer's corporate insurance covers the costs of civil liability arising from a nurse's care. If curious, ask your employer whether or how the employer's insurance provides coverage for malpractice complaints against persons with your position/title. Employer-provided liability insurance is not personal liability insurance. Its coverage may not cover the cost of defending actions brought by a state licensing agency against an individual nurse. LPNs/LVNs may opt to carry their own personal liability insurance. A cost-benefit analysis prior to purchase is recommended.

Quality of Care and the Survey Process

State agencies are charged by federal law with overseeing the quality of care and services in long-term care and skilled nursing facilities. Annually, state agencies enter these facilities with a team of experienced evaluators. They assess the quality of care and review its environment and services during surveys. These surveys are stressful on facility staff and the surveyors. Surveyors appreciate honesty and candidness. The survey process helps to ensure skilled nursing facilities effectively assess and meet residents' needs in the normal course of business.

Acute care hospitals practice under different quality oversight rules than skilled nursing facilities. Acute care organizations may secure accreditation from a private organization, such as The Joint Commission, to improve operations and quality of services. Accreditation is helpful because it can shield an acute care organization from more frequent, on-site visits by state agencies and their critical eye.

State surveys and accreditation surveys review facility processes only. They are not intended to review an individual nurse's clinical practice methods.

Key Points

- Evidence that is always evolving results in practice changes, as do other influences, such as an aging and culturally changing population; newly emerging viruses and pandemics; multidrug-resistant infectious organisms; public awareness campaigns on identifying human trafficking; electronic health records (EHRs); mobile health with digital apps, smartphones, tablets, and remote patient monitoring; robotics; and telehealth.
- The Institute for Safe Medication Practices has guidelines and recommendations to reduce medication errors that include resources on error-prone abbreviations, confused drug names, do-not-crush oral medications, high-alert medications in long-term care, and look-alike drug names distinguished by tall man letters.
- The Institute for Safe Medication Practices advocates to weigh patients only in kilograms to prevent mix-ups in pounds and kilograms for medication doses that are calculated in kilograms.
- Safe health-care practices include following The Joint Commission's National Patient Safety Goals; preventing medication errors; preventing misconnections of tubing that can result in harm or death; preventing harmful, sentinel events (The Joint Commission) and serious reportable events (National Quality Forum); and improving the safety of health information technology.
- The CMS has identified 14 preventable conditions that often occur while a patient is hospitalized. If patients develop one or more of these secondary conditions while hospitalized, the CMS will not reimburse the hospital for the costs incurred in treating them. Therefore, it is essential for nurses to carefully assess and document any conditions *present on admission* to show that they did not occur during hospitalization.
- A leader seeks to influence, motivate, and enable others to achieve goals. The four leadership styles are autocratic, democratic, laissez-faire, and coaching.

- LPNs/LVNs are leaders and managers of care for the patients to whom they are assigned, under the supervision of an RN, HCP, or dentist, as specified by each state's nursing practice act.
- Delegation is the act of empowering another person to act without relinquishing responsibility for the delegated task. LPNs/LVNs delegate to assistive personnel.
- Ethical decision making is an informed, logical eight-step problem-solving process.
- Each state has laws that define the scope of a nurse's practice in that state, usually contained in the nurse practice act.
- Prevention is the best way to limit liability, and you can do this by ensuring that patients' rights are protected, following your employer's policies, using current nursing practice standards, documenting accurately, and pursuing continuing education.
- A state's mandated reporting laws often require licensed nurses and HCPs to report known or suspected abuse, neglect, communicable disease, and gunshot wounds to state authorities.
- Human trafficking is the act of recruiting, harboring, transporting, providing, or obtaining a person for labor or as a sex worker using force, fraud, or coercion. You should know how to identify victims of human trafficking and assist in reporting it to authorities.
- HIPAA can be violated when health-care workers place protected information on social media. It is safest to keep one's professional and personal life separate when using social media.

SUGGESTED ANSWERS TO CHAPTER EXERCISES
Cue Recognition
3.1: Weigh patient with a scale calibrated in kilograms, and document the kilogram weight.

Additional Resources

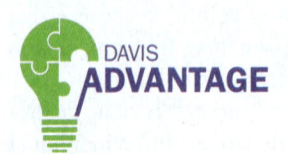

Go to Davis Advantage to complete your learning: strengthen understanding, apply your knowledge, and prepare for the Next Gen NCLEX®.

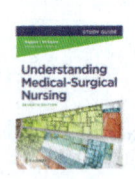

A Study Guide is also available.

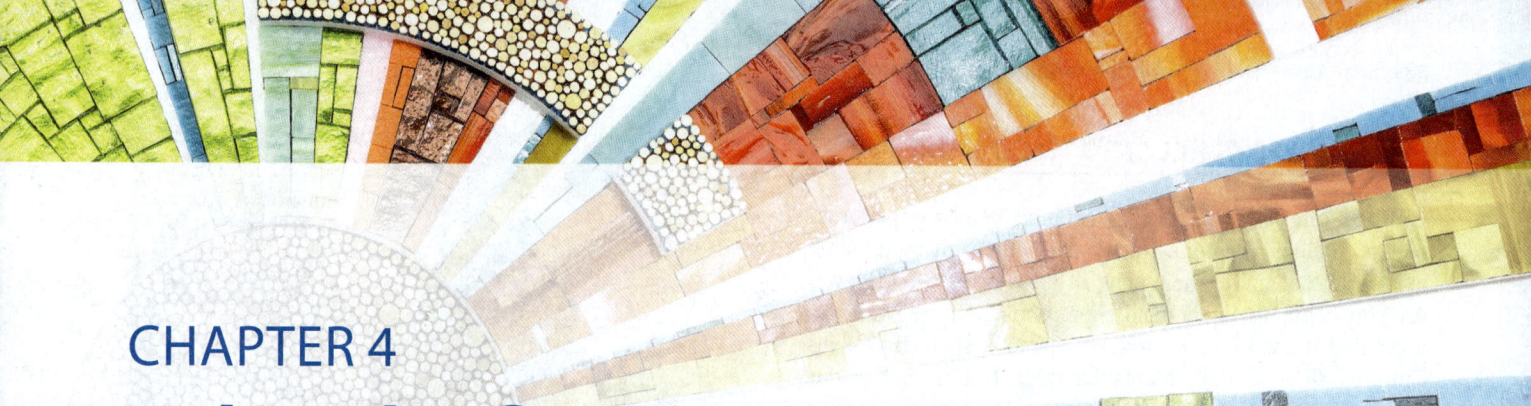

CHAPTER 4
Cultural Influences on Nursing Care

Sheria G. Robinson-Lane, Bobbi M. Martin

KEY TERMS

belief (bee-LEEF)
cultural (KUL-chur-uhl)
cultural awareness (KUL-chur-uhl a-WEAR-ness)
cultural competence (KUL-chur-uhl KOM-pe-tents)
cultural diversity (KUL-chur-uhl dih-VER-sih-tee)
cultural humility (KUL-chur-uhl hew-MIL-ih-tee)
cultural sensitivity (KUL-chur-uhl SEN-sih-TIV-ih-tee)
culture (KUL-chur)
customs (KUS-tums)
ethnic (ETH-nik)
ethnocentrism (ETH-noh-SEN-trizm)
practice (PRAK-tis)
spiritual (SPEER-ih-choo-al)
spirituality (SPEER-ih-choo-AL-it-ee)
stereotype (STER-ee-oh-TYPE)
traditions (tra-DISH-uns)
values (VAL-yooz)
worldview (WERLD-vyoo)

CHAPTER CONCEPTS

Caring
Communication
Family
Grief and loss
Self
Spirituality

LEARNING OUTCOMES

1. Define common concepts related to culture and spirituality.
2. Describe attributes of culturally diverse patients and their families and how they affect nursing care.
3. Identify data you should collect from culturally diverse patients and their families.
4. Apply a holistic approach to patient care that respects cultural and spiritual characteristics and attributes.

Can you think of examples of **cultural** practices you have seen or experienced that were different from your own? The images that likely come to mind depict people who look and dress very differently than you do, speak another language, eat different foods, and even have different religious beliefs. Everyone belongs to a *cultural group,* or social group in which people share learned patterns of behaviors, **beliefs,** and **values** that allow them to navigate through life (Robinson, 2013). The family is the first cultural group in which we take part. The people who raise us teach us what to believe, what to value, how to approach problem-solving, and ultimately how to survive in the world. Our cultural group expands as we enter new social relationships with others and develop new ways of behaving. These social relationships are formed and maintained by geography, shared histories, **customs, traditions,** and identities.

The United States is particularly diverse, made up of people who speak at least one of 350 different languages, have varying religious beliefs (or none at all), and of course have different stories about how their families came to be in the United States and where they find themselves now (U.S. Census Bureau, 2015). In health care, we find that culture often affects health outcomes, including how patients and families communicate health needs and how they respond to care. More than ever, nurses must develop cultural awareness, particularly self-awareness, and recognize the patient as a full partner in providing compassionate care based on respect for the patient's preferences, values, and needs. A foundational principle of Healthy People 2030 is the achievement of health, well-being, and health equity for all citizens (US Department of Health and Human Services, 2020). This chapter provides the basics of *culturally responsive care* and its effect on health promotion and wellness.

CONCEPTS RELATED TO CULTURE

Culture refers to socially transmitted behavior patterns, beliefs, values, customs, arts, and other characteristics of people that guide their view of the world (**worldview**). As you begin to understand more about culture, keep in mind that it encompasses several characteristics (Box 4.1). Culture influences daily habits that affect health, such as the foods we select as part of our diet, how we dress, how we raise children, and how we cope with stress. As you learn more about cultural groups, you will be challenged to look at differences and similarities across cultures.

Over the years, many different terms have been used to describe the ways to learn about culture and deliver appropriate care. For example, you may have heard the terms cultural sensitivity, cultural awareness, and cultural competence which are all similar but have different meanings. **Cultural sensitivity** is the awareness that cultural similarities and differences exist and are not right or wrong. **Cultural awareness** focuses on history and ancestry and emphasizes an appreciation for and attention to a culture's arts, music, crafts, celebrations, foods, and traditional clothing. **Cultural competence** refers to the development of skills and knowledge necessary to deliver effective care to diverse patients and families. **Cultural humility** is the idea that learning

Box 4.1
Characteristics of Culture

- Culture is learned. Learning occurs through life experiences shared with other members of the culture.
- Culture is taught. Cultural values, beliefs, and traditions are passed down from generation to generation, either formally (e.g., in schools) or informally (e.g., in families).
- Culture is shared by its members. Cultural norms are shared through teachings and social interactions.
- Culture is dynamic and adaptive. Cultural customs, beliefs, and practices are not static but change over time and at different rates. Cultural change occurs with adaptation in response to the environment.
- Culture is complex. Cultural assumptions and habits are unconscious, which may make them difficult for members of the culture to explain to others.
- Culture is diverse. Culture demonstrates the variety that exists between groups and among members of a particular group.
- Culture exists at many levels. Culture exists at material (e.g., art, dress, and things made and used) and nonmaterial (e.g., language, customs, beliefs, and practices) levels.
- Culture has common beliefs and practices. Members of cultural groups often share the same beliefs, traditions, customs, and practices.
- Culture is all encompassing. Culture can affect all of the ways its members think and act.
- Cultural beliefs and values often provide identity and a shared sense of community for members.
- Culture shapes spirituality. Spirituality gives meaning and purpose to our existence.

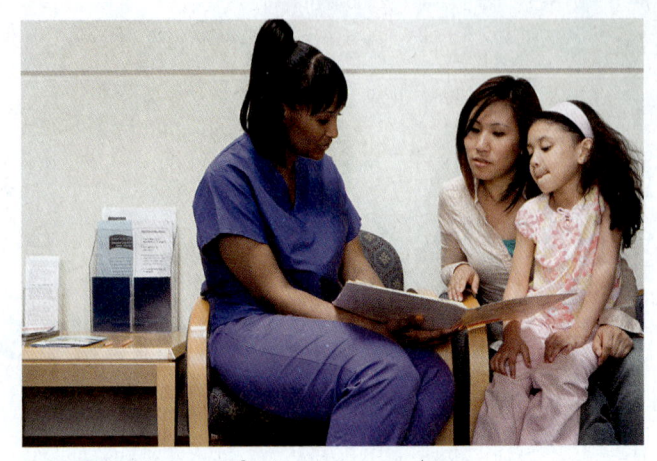

FIGURE 4.1 Nurse reinforcing patient teaching.

about culture with the intention to improve care and services is a lifelong process that also requires self-reflection of ones' own cultural beliefs and identities.

Although you may have knowledge about another culture, barriers such as ethnocentrism and stereotyping can keep you from appreciating cultural differences. **Ethnocentrism** is the tendency for people to think that their own culture's ways of thinking, acting, and believing are the only right and natural ways and that beliefs that differ greatly from those of their own culture are strange or bizarre and therefore wrong. This may result in racist attitudes and lead to individual and systemic discrimination when caring for people of different cultures. In addition to guarding against ethnocentrism, you must be careful not to stereotype your patient. A **stereotype** is an opinion or belief about a group of people that is attributed to an individual. Ethnocentrism and stereotypes are often a part of *racism*, or the belief that race determines specific traits and capabilities of individuals and that one race is superior.

Understanding the patient's cultural perspective helps the nurse to have cultural humility. If you have specific cultural knowledge, you can improve therapeutic interventions by partnering with patients and their families. To do so, it is important to develop a personal, open style of communication and be receptive to learning from patients from cultures other than your own. This is where cultural humility comes in: you are humble enough to recognize that it is unlikely that you will become an expert in someone else' culture, you understand that you will likely make some mistakes in the learning process, and yet you still commit to keep learning and working to deliver care that is responsive to the needs of the community that you are serving (Fig. 4.1).

CONCEPTS RELATED TO SPIRITUALITY

Spirituality, simply defined, is the essential connections that provide meaning and purpose in life (Dunn & Robinson-Lane, 2020). For some people, these essential connections include a belief in God or a higher power. Although religion and spirituality are distinct, they often overlap. Religion is more straightforward than spirituality and focuses on specific beliefs and practices that align with particular religious or philosophical ideas. Health-related behaviors such as diet, medical treatment choices, and communication about health can be linked to specific religious beliefs. For example, many people of the Jehovah's Witness faith do not believe in the use of blood transfusions as part of medical care and may refuse a treatment or procedure that would require a transfusion (Crookston, 2021). Identifying and documenting a patient's religious and **spiritual** practices should be a care priority during the initial data collection.

Knowing how to integrate spirituality into nursing care can be challenging. Exploring spirituality with patients may help them find hope and meaning during times of illness and crisis. Good starting points for being sensitive to the spiritual needs of patients include

- Being aware of your own spirituality and where your own sense of meaning, purpose, and value come from.
- Listening for cues and being attentive to patients raising issues of what their illness means.
- Promoting patient-centered care rather than task-centered care.

Growing evidence indicates that addressing spirituality improves a patient's comfort level emotionally and physically. It also has a positive effect on a patient's response to illness and treatments. Conversely, neglecting to deal with spiritual issues may expose a patient to additional suffering. Spiritual care may be influenced by many factors, including the nurse's own culture, religious affiliation, and clinical experience.

When people are in advanced illness, and particularly at end of life, they may begin to talk more about spiritual concerns with conversations about God and the afterlife. They may pose rhetorical questions such as "Why is this happening to me?" or "What have I done to deserve this?" Being responsive and sensitive to these signals may enable therapeutic communications. If a patient does not signal a desire to discuss spiritual matters, a sensitive and individualized approach is needed. Ask questions such as "How has this illness affected you?" or "What types of things have helped you to cope with great stress or big life changes in the past?" The discussion should result in a dialogue about how the patient can be supported in addressing their identified needs. It is also important for the nurse to pay attention to and document patient or family engagement in spiritual practices such as prayer, song, blessed oils, meditation, journaling, self-reflection, and even social engagement. Nurses can follow up after these activities to verify whether the patient finds them helpful in stress relief.

HEALTH-CARE VALUES, BELIEFS, AND PRACTICES

Cultural values, beliefs, and **practices** about the nature of disease and the human body are central in the delivery of health services, treatments, and preventive interventions. A *value* can be defined as a principle or standard that has meaning or worth to an individual. Values help shape people's beliefs and practices. Do you know what your values are regarding health and illness? "Cleanliness" is an example of a value. A *belief* is something that a person accepts as true (e.g., "I believe that germs cause illness and disease"). A *practice* is a set of behaviors that a person follows (e.g., washing hands before eating). As we discussed previously, values, beliefs, and practices are often culturally rooted.

There are three major health belief systems in the United States: scientific (Western medicine or biomedical), spiritual, and holistic. You are already familiar with the scientific health system, which dominates health care in Western societies. Belief or faith in God(s) or supernatural forces dominates the spiritual system, which is considered by many to be an alternative health-care system. The holistic belief system focuses on the need for balance and harmony of the body and spirit with nature. Folk remedies, or traditional medications or treatments that are not prescribed by a doctor, may be part of the holistic belief system.

Health care typically focuses on health promotion, illness prevention, and acute illness care while considering traditional, religious, and biomedical (scientific) beliefs. In addition, individual responsibility for health, self-medicating practices, views toward mental illness, response to pain, and the sick role are shaped by one's culture. Most societies combine aspects of biomedical health care with spiritual and holistic care practices. There are many examples of folk remedies for curing or treating specific illnesses. Think for a minute about such practices that you may use. What do you do for a cold? Does chicken noodle soup or a special tea come to mind? Many times, folk remedies are handed down from family members and may have their roots in religious beliefs. As you will see in Chapter 5, many people use complementary therapies such as acupressure or herbal remedies in addition to traditional Western therapies.

Generally, folk practices are not harmful and can be added to the patient's plan of care. However, some therapies may conflict with prescription medications or cause a toxic effect. For example, garlic supplements can cause very low blood pressure when combined with antihypertensive medications and interact with multiple other medications. It is essential to inquire about the full range of therapies being used by your patients, such as foods, teas, herbal remedies, nonfood substances, over-the-counter medications, vitamins, drops, supplements, medications prescribed by others, and medications borrowed from others.

If patients sense that you do not accept their beliefs and practices, they are less likely to share information or adhere to prescribed treatment. Your goal is to encourage practices that could be helpful and discourage those that may be harmful. Before encouraging or discouraging such practices, you must discuss them with the appropriate health-care team member.

It is important to note that mental illness, or behavioral health, may be seen by some cultures as unimportant compared with physical illness. In some instances, what is perceived as a mental illness in one society may not be considered a mental illness in another. Among some cultures, having a mental illness or an emotional difficulty is considered a taboo, a sign of weakness or a lack of faith. As a result, patients and families may not seek treatment or available support.

CHARACTERISTICS OF CULTURAL DIVERSITY

Primary and secondary characteristics of diversity affect how people view their culture. Primary characteristics of **cultural diversity** include nationality, race, skin color, gender identity, age, spirituality, and religious affiliation. Secondary characteristics include socioeconomic status, education, occupation, military experience, political beliefs, length of time away from one's country of origin, urban versus rural residence, marital status, parental status, physical characteristics, sexual orientation, and gender roles.

Culturally responsive care should consider eight cultural phenomena that may vary but can be seen in all cultural groups:

1. Communication styles
2. Space
3. Time orientation
4. Social organization
5. Environmental control/health beliefs
6. Choice of health-care providers (HCPs)
7. Biological variations
8. Death and dying issues

Communication Styles

Communication occurs both verbally and nonverbally. Verbal communication includes spoken language, dialects, and voice volume. Dialects include variations in grammar, word meanings, and pronunciation of spoken language. Nonverbal communication includes the use and degree of eye contact, the perception of time, and physical closeness when talking with peers and perceived superiors. In some cultures, people are expected to maintain eye contact without staring; this shows that they are listening and can be trusted. In other cultures, eye contact is a sign of disrespect, and it is believed that people should not maintain eye contact with superiors such as teachers and those in positions of higher status.

Nursing Data Collection and Strategies

Ask the following questions of your patients:

- What name do they prefer to be called?
- What language do they speak at home?

Be sure to do the following:

- Take cues from the patient regarding greetings and voice volume.
- Avoid appearing rushed.
- Speak slowly and clearly. Do not speak loudly or with exaggerated mouthing.
- Ask the patient to restate what they heard.
- Explain why you are asking specific questions.
- Provide written instructions in the patient's preferred language.
- Obtain an interpreter if needed, and avoid using family, particularly children, to interpret.

Although it may seem logical that a patient's best advocate is his or her family, it is risky to rely on family members to interpret medical or health information for the following reasons:

- Family members may not be proficient in medical terminology.
- They may unintentionally or intentionally omit or alter important information.
- Using family members to interpret may raise privacy issues protected by the Health Insurance Portability and Accountability Act of 1996 (HIPAA).
- If children are used, they may not be emotionally mature enough to handle the information being conveyed.

Patient Perspective

Amahle

Within a year after moving to the United States from South Africa, I gave birth to a daughter. My baby did not develop like my other child. During one of the baby's checkups, I was told through the interpreter that my baby needed to go to therapy. For many months, I took her to therapy with little improvement. I was very worried. I went back to the doctor to find out what was wrong and was told she had cerebral palsy. All this time, I worried over my baby and did not understand that she had cerebral palsy.

Interpreters vary in their abilities and their understanding of medical issues. It is important for doctors and nurses to take the time to make sure both the patient and the interpreter understand the information.

PRACTICE ANALYSIS TIP

Linking NCLEX-PN® to Practice
The LPN/LVN identifies and addresses barriers to communication.

SPACE

Space refers to one's "personal space." Are you aware of your comfort zone? In other words, how close can someone get to you before you feel less safe and secure? Most people have such a comfort zone. Personal space tends to be different when speaking with close friends versus strangers. It also differs across cultures. For example, people from some cultures stand close together when talking. This might make those from cultures who prefer more personal space uncomfortable. The need for space is important for the patient's privacy, autonomy, security, and self-identity. Understanding what space means for your patients supports patient-centered care.

Nursing Data Collection and Strategies
Ask your patients whether they are comfortable. Be sure to do the following:

- Make sure your patients are comfortable before you interview them.
- Maintain appropriate physical distance (observe for cues).
- Make sure that the patient's physical environment is arranged to ensure safety, security, and familiarity.

Time Orientation
Time orientation can vary among people from different cultures. The perception of time has two dimensions. The first dimension is related to clock time versus social time. For example, some cultures have a flexible orientation to time and events. An event scheduled for 1400 may not begin until 1430 or when most of the participants arrive.

The second dimension of time relates to whether the culture is predominantly concerned with the past, present, or future. Past-oriented cultures maintain traditions. Present-oriented cultures accept the day as it comes, with little regard for the past; the future is unpredictable. Future-oriented cultures anticipate a bigger and better future and place a high value on change. Some people balance all three views.

Understanding patients' time orientation can help you prepare them for the timing of appointments, tests, and treatments. In addition, learning about their usual routines allows you to incorporate these routines as much as possible into their daily care.

Nursing Data Collection and Strategies
Ask the following questions of your patients:

- Are there any routines that you prefer to follow?
- What time do you usually eat your meals? Take a shower or bath?

Be sure to do the following:

- Have a clock in the patient's room.
- Check for orientation and reorient to time as appropriate.
- Give time options when appropriate (e.g., "Would you like to take a walk now or in an hour?")

Social Organization
Family organization includes the perceived head of the household, gender roles, and roles of older and extended family members. The household may be patriarchal (male-dominated), matriarchal (female-dominated), or egalitarian (shared equally between men and women). An awareness of the family dominance pattern is important for determining which family members should be included when health-care decisions must be made. Confidentiality concerns can complicate this issue. Be sure to follow your institution's policies when communicating with family members. You may need to obtain the patient's permission before planning care with family members.

In some cultures, specific roles are outlined for men and women. Men may be expected to protect and provide for the family, manage finances, and deal with the outside world. Women may be expected to maintain the home environment and care for children. You must accept that not all societies have or even desire a family structure where roles are equal.

Roles for older adults and extended family vary among cultures. In some cultures, older adults are seen as wise, deferred to for making decisions, and held in high esteem. Their children are expected to provide for them when they are no longer able to care for themselves. In other cultures, although older people may be loved by family members, they may not be treated with the same regard. They may be cared for outside the home when self-care becomes a concern.

The extended family is very important in some cultures. A single household may include several generations living together out of desire rather than out of necessity. The extended family may include both blood-related and non-blood-related persons who are given family status. In other cultures, each generation lives in a separate home or living space.

Cultural Data Collection
Ask the following questions of your patients:

- Is there someone in particular whom you like to discuss decisions with?
- Are there particular responsibilities that you usually have at home?
- Who lives in your household? How are they related?

Be sure to do the following:

- Observe how the family is interacting.
- Let family members decide where they want to stand or sit for comfort.

Environmental Control
Environmental control consists of three major concepts: perception of one's ability to control what happens to them and their health, beliefs about health and illness, and beliefs in alternative health-care therapies such as folk medicine. For example, if a patient does not believe he or she has independent control of health, the patient may not be receptive to nursing interventions that require self-confidence, such as self-administration of insulin. Or, if a patient or family believes that an illness is due to a spiritual cause rather than a mental health disorder, he or she may not understand the need to take antipsychotics or antidepressants to treat the condition. In addition, many people put great faith in folk medicine healing practices. Nurses

should consider the patient's cultural values and beliefs, especially if they are different from their own.

Today, many patients and families are interested in complementary and alternative therapies, which are often more readily available and are becoming increasingly covered by health insurance. It is not unusual for patients to use alternative therapies and religious practices such as prayer in combination with the traditional medications and treatments we would see used in modern medicine.

Cultural Data Collection
Ask the following questions of your patients:

- What does being healthy look like to you?
- What do you do to keep well?
- When you feel sick, what is the first thing you do to get better?
- How do you deal with pain? What do you usually take for pain?
- How would I know if you were sad or grieving?
- Can you think of any beliefs or regular practices that I should know about to plan your care?

Be sure to do the following:

- Never stereotype on the basis of what you know about different cultures; always ask for specific information from each patient and family.
- Collect cultural data on all your patients.
- Ask what patients have done to date for their illness, including any home remedies, alternative therapies, or prescribed treatments/medications.
- Ask about religious beliefs and practices.

Choice of Health-Care Providers
HCP choices are made on the basis of the patient's perceived health status and previous use of traditional, religious, and biomedical HCPs. While a nurse practitioner or physician might be some patient's first choice in HCPs, other patients may prefer traditional healers.

It is also important to respect differences in gender relationships when providing care. Some people may be especially modest because of their culture or religion, seeking out same-gender nurses and HCPs for intimate care. Respect all patients' modesty by providing privacy, and support the assigning of same-gender care providers when requested if possible.

Cultural Data Collection
Ask the following questions of your patients:

- Do you have any natural practitioners or other care providers, besides physicians and nurses, that you see to help you to manage pain, an illness, or just overall health promotion?
- Do you object to male or female HCPs providing physical care for you?

Be aware of alternative care providers who may visit the patient in the health-care facility.

Biological Variations
Biological variations are ways in which people are different from one another physiologically and genetically. These differences can make individuals more susceptible to certain illnesses and diseases. They may also influence the effectiveness of different medications. Biological variations can include differences in (1) body build and structure, (2) skin color, (3) susceptibility to certain diseases, and (4) nutrition. For example, darker skin color combined with cooler climates can increase the likelihood of vitamin D deficiency.

Biological variations can also include differences in nutritional practices, such as the personal meaning of food, food choices and rituals, food taboos, and how food and food substances are used for health promotion and wellness. Cultural beliefs may influence what people eat or avoid. For example, many people avoid pork and pork products because of their religious beliefs. In addition to being important for survival, food offers security and acceptance, plays a significant role in socialization, and can serve as an expression of love.

Culturally responsive dietary counseling, such as adapting preparation practices and including ethnic food choices, can reduce health risks. Whenever possible, determine a patient's current dietary practices. Counseling about food group requirements or dietary restrictions must respect an individual's cultural background. Most cultures have their own nutritional practices for health promotion and disease prevention. For many, a balance of different types of foods is important for maintaining health and preventing illness. A thorough history and collection of data related to dietary practices can be an important diagnostic tool to guide health promotion.

Cultural Data Collection
Ask the following questions of your patients:

- What sorts of foods do you typically eat?
- Are there any foods or beverages that you try to avoid?
- Are you satisfied with your weight?
- Are you active? What is your normal exercise routine?
- Do you wear sunscreen or protect your skin from the sun in another way?
- Do you have any drug or food allergies?
- What do you eat when you are ill?
- Do certain foods cause you to become ill or upset your stomach? What are the foods, and how do they affect you?

Be sure to do the following:

- Teach about biological variations that may pertain to your patient.
- Determine and respect a patient's typical eating pattern whenever possible.
- Support the patient's choice to avoid particular foods by ensuring appropriate notifications are made to interdisciplinary team members (i.e., dietary department).
- Teach good nutrition habits, accounting for patient preferences. Refer to a dietitian if appropriate.

Death and Dying and End-of-Life Issues

Death rituals of cultural groups are the least likely to change over time. To avoid cultural taboos, become knowledgeable about rituals surrounding death and bereavement. In some cultures, the body should be buried whole. Therefore, an amputated limb may be buried in the amputee's future gravesite, and organ donation would probably not be acceptable. Cremation may be preferred in some cultures; in others burial is the preferred practice. Views on autopsy vary. Some cultural groups have elaborate ceremonies that last for days in commemoration of the dead. In some cultures, these rituals appear celebratory, and, in a sense, they are a celebration of the person's life rather than a mourning of the person's death. If you are uncertain, find out from the family if there is anything that the health-care team can do to facilitate cultural practices during the end-of-life phase.

The expression of grief in response to death varies among cultural and ethnic groups. For example, in some cultures, loved ones are expected to suffer the grief of death in silence, with little display of emotion. In other cultures, loved ones display elaborate emotions to show that they cared for the deceased. These variations in the grieving process may cause confusion, in that you may perceive some people as overreacting and others as not caring. You must accept that culturally diverse behaviors are associated with the grieving process. Bereavement support strategies include being physically present; assisting families in hospitals, nursing homes, or other care facilities to find a space to grieve and connect with one another privately when possible; openly acknowledging the family's right to grieve as they need to; helping the family express their feelings; and collaborating with other staff and spiritual leaders as appropriate.

End-of-life decisions such as advance directives, resuscitation status, and organ transplantation should involve collaboration with the registered nurse or HCP.

Cultural Data Collection

Ask the following questions of your patients:

- What are the usual burial or cremation practices in your family?
- What are your feelings about autopsy?

Be sure to do the following:

- Observe expressions of grief. Support the family in their expression of grief.
- Observe for differences in the expression of grief among family members.
- Offer to obtain a religious counselor/spiritual leader if the family wishes.

RACIAL AND ETHNIC GROUPS IN THE UNITED STATES

While race refers to how humans are generally categorized according to distinctive physical characteristics and common ancestry, ethnicity includes shared cultural traditions. Race and ethnicity are different concepts, but they cannot exist without one another. According to the US Census Bureau (2020), the primary racial categories in the United States are American Indian/Alaskan Native, Asian, Black, Native Hawaiian or other Pacific Islander, and White. Persons of any of these racial groups, though most often they are Black or White, may also identify with one of the two major ethnic groups Hispanic/Latino or Middle Eastern/North African. These groups of course do not represent all of the **ethnic** groups in North America; however, they represent those with the largest population percentages in the United States. Questions about race and ethnicity are typically asked during the initial visit or admission. Patients, or their family/representative, should be asked to identify the patient's race(s) and ethnicity during this first interaction. Your documentation system should have options to select multiple identities; if this is not the case, be sure to clarify race and ethnicity data within the narrative documentation.

Gerontological Issues

Aging and Cultural Diversity

Within specific age groups, people often have shared histories and experiences that are unique from those of other generations. For example, adults ages 65 and older who were raised in the United States would have experienced living in a segregated world where people of different races and ethnicities did not attend school together, worship together, or even receive health care in the same places. These experiences can affect the ways in which some older adults communicate and their expectations around care. To provide culturally responsive care, remember that older adults need to be assessed within their personal cultural context. Negotiation and explanation may be necessary when patients and families have preferences for same race/ethnicity providers that cannot be met.

CRITICAL THINKING & CLINICAL JUDGMENT

Ms. Kapahu is an older adult woman from a culture that is different from your own. She has had diabetes and hypertension (high blood pressure) for many years. She is admitted to the hospital for gangrene of her left foot. When you enter her room, you find Ms. Kapahu anxious and crying. As you approach her bed, she reaches out and takes your hand and holds it while you talk. When asked about her foot, she tells you that she has been applying a poultice to draw out the infection, but it has not worked yet. She adds that she has been praying for God to heal her foot. As you are collecting history information about her diabetes, Ms. Kapahu admits that her doctor advised her to follow a diabetic diet and to lose weight, but she doesn't like the foods on the diet. She quickly changes the subject to talk about her son and her grandchildren.

Critical Thinking (The Why)
1. What does your interaction with Ms. Kapahu tell you about her time orientation?
2. What do you know about her spirituality and social organization?
3. Do you have any clues about Ms. Kapahu's personal space needs?
4. Whom might you involve in discussions with Ms. Kapahu about her health?
5. How might you learn more about the unique health practices Ms. Kapahu uses to address her health concerns?

Clinical Judgement (The Do)
6. How can you use therapeutic communication to talk with Ms. Kapahu about her diet?

Suggested answers are at the end of the chapter.

CULTURALLY RESPONSIVE CARE

Culturally responsive care recognizes the value that patients and families bring to the care team as experts in their own culture-related health needs. By acknowledging the diverse beliefs and values that patients and families have and integrating cultural practices into care, when possible, more meaningful connections can be developed between nurses, patients, and families. In the event that an important cultural practice cannot be accommodated within the health-care setting, it is important that an explanation be provided.

The US Department of Health and Human Services Office of Minority Health (2018) has developed National Standards for Culturally and Linguistically Appropriate Services, or CLAS Standards. These 15 standards are guided by the primary idea that improved health-care quality and equity can be achieved when organizations are responsive to diverse cultural needs of the communities they serve (Box 4.2).

When culturally responsive care does not take place, *health disparities* can occur. Health disparities are preventable differences in disease burden, injury, or opportunities to achieve optimal health. As first-line care providers, nurses are best positioned to help ensure that patients receive optimal care that integrates the patients' beliefs, values, and traditions as much as possible. Nurses play a critical role as front-line care providers. They are often the first and last person with whom patients and families interact on the health-care team. Nurses who practice cultural humility and prioritize culturally responsive care practices can significantly improve the quality of life and overall health of the patients they serve.

Rarely do practicing nurses have the luxury to collect comprehensive data on each patient at the first encounter. The essentials for culturally responsive care are obtained as needed over time. As you meet patients from other cultures, continue to learn about these new cultures. Astute observations, openness to diversity, and willingness to learn from patients are essential for effective cross-cultural competence in clinical practice. Culturally responsive care is not a luxury; it is a necessity.

Box 4.2

National Standards for Culturally and Linguistically Appropriate Services (CLAS)

1. Provide care that recognizes the health beliefs and practices, preferred languages, health knowledge, and communication needs of the community.
2. Organization policies, practices, and resources should be incorporating concepts of CLAS and health equity.
3. The workforce and organizational leadership should be diverse and responsive to the population in the service area.
4. Education and training around CLAS policies and procedures should be ongoing.
5. Language assistance should be available free of charge and in a timely manner for any with limited English proficiency or other communication needs.
6. All patients/clients should be aware of the availability of language assistance services.
7. Language assistance services should be provided by trained and competent individuals, avoiding use of family and particularly minors as translators.
8. Provide print and multimedia materials and signage in the languages commonly used within the service area.
9. Culturally and linguistically appropriate goals should be imbedded into the organization's strategic plan.
10. Organization quality improvement evaluations should include CLAS measures and outcomes.
11. Patient demographic data should be monitored to evaluate any differences in health outcomes.
12. Collect data on community needs to identify service gaps.
13. Engage the community as partners in the development of polices, practices, and services to ensure cultural and linguistic appropriateness.
14. Ensure that complaint and grievance processes allow for appropriate solving of conflicts.
15. Communicate the organization's progress in implementing and sustaining CLAS standards to everyone.

U.S. Department of Health and Human Services. (n.d.) National Class Standards. https://thinkculturalhealth.hhs.gov/clas

---

LEARNING TIP
Take a trip to BALI:
Be aware of your own cultural heritage.
Appreciate that your patient is unique and influenced but not defined by their culture.
Learn about your patient's cultural groups.
Incorporate your patient's cultural values, beliefs, and practices into their plan of care.

Home Health Hints

The effects of a patient's cultural beliefs and practices related to health care are more evident when care is provided in the home. The nurse must adapt care to the patient's environment rather than the patient adapting to the nurse's hospital environment. The nurse is a guest in the patient's home and should respect the patient's unique cultural practices with these strategies:

- When scheduling a home visit, it is important to find out the primary language spoken in the home. The agency is required to inform the patient of his or her rights regarding care in a manner that the patient can understand. Check with your supervisor regarding the process for obtaining a translator.
- If you have a personal smartphone, you can download a language translator to assist with communication if approved by your agency.
- For some patients, their church is a source of spiritual support as well as physical support such as meals and transportation. Those who cannot attend church in person may be able to attend online.

Key Points

- Concepts related to culture include cultural humility and awareness. Cultural humility is the idea that learning about culture with the intention to improve care and services is a lifelong process that requires self-reflection of your own cultural beliefs and identities while learning about others. Cultural awareness focuses on history and ancestry and emphasizes an appreciation for and attention to a culture's arts, music, crafts, celebrations, foods, and traditional clothing. Cultural competence refers to the development of skills and knowledge necessary to deliver effective care to diverse patients and families.
- To provide culturally competent care, you need to know how the patients you encounter define health and illness, which may be based in a scientific, spiritual, or holistic approach.
- Responses to pain and the sick role can vary among cultures. In some cultures, people openly express pain, while in others people are expected to suffer in silence. In some cultures, the sick role is readily accepted, while in others people minimize illness.
- In order to provide culturally responsive care to a diverse population, take into account these eight things: communication styles, space preferences, time orientation, social organization, environmental control/health beliefs, choice of HCPs, biological variations, and death/dying issues. Nurses should collect data pertinent to each of these topics when caring for culturally diverse patients and their families.
- Some tips in providing culturally responsive care include the following: Consider each of your patients as unique, influenced by, but not defined by, their culture. Do not let your own biases about people and groups stand in the way of providing good care. Learn as much as possible about the cultural groups in your community.

SUGGESTED ANSWERS TO CHAPTER EXERCISES

Critical Thinking & Clinical Judgment

Ms. Kapahu

1. Ms. Kapahu may present as oriented. Her seeming lack of concern about her diabetes may reflect hesitance to worry about a future that is not yet here.
2. Family is important. She prays for healing.
3. Ms. Kapahu draws you close and holds your hand. This is a sign that she may not need a lot of personal space. Of course, you should ask her before you assume this.
4. Involving family members, both younger and older, might be helpful with Ms. Kapahu's permission. Because prayer is important to her, ask whether there is a minister or other religious person whom she might want to include in discussions and decision making. Contact the dietitian to suggest foods that fit Ms. Kapahu's preferences while she is in the hospital and to work with Ms. Kapahu to design a diabetes meal plan to be used at home that includes food she likes.
5. Ms. Kapahu is the expert on her own cultural practices. Do a thorough cultural data collection to learn whether any practices interfere with her health care. Work with the RN to develop an appropriate teaching plan. Remember to include any cultural practices she already uses if they are safe and don't interfere with her care.
6. Avoid putting Ms. Kapahu on the defensive about her diet. Try using open-ended questions such as "What kinds of food do you like to eat?"

Additional Resources

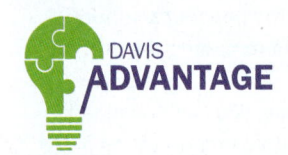

Go to Davis Advantage to complete your learning: strengthen understanding, apply your knowledge, and prepare for the Next Gen NCLEX®.

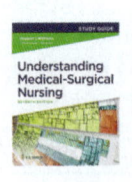

A Study Guide is also available.

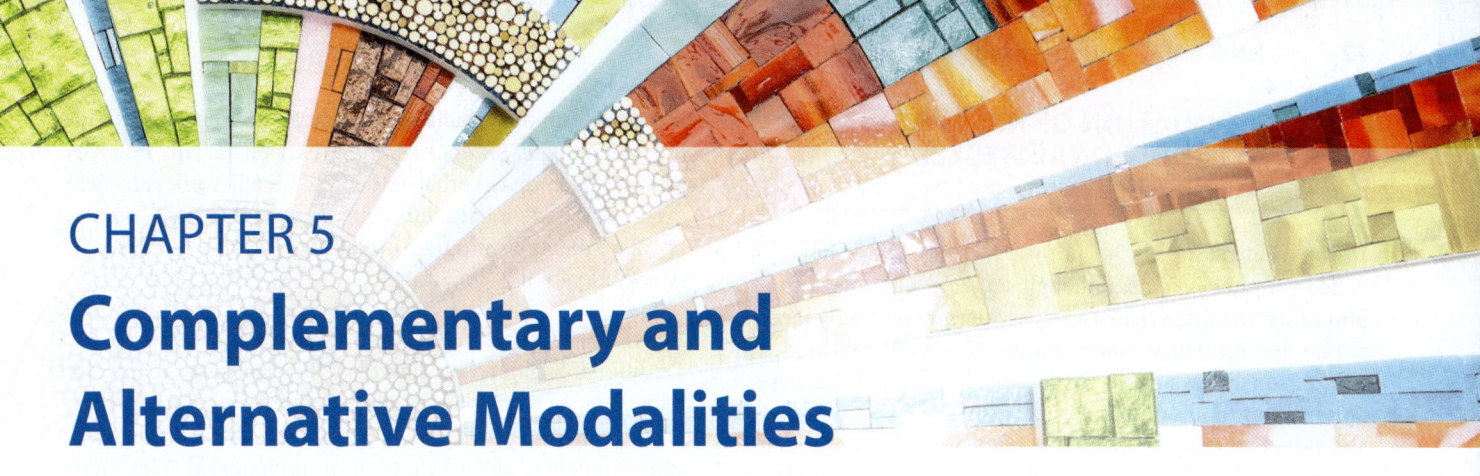

CHAPTER 5
Complementary and Alternative Modalities

Lynette Harvey

KEY TERMS

acupuncture (AK-yoo-PUNGK-chur)
allopathic (AL-oh-PATH-ik)
alternative modality (all-TERN-ah-tiv mo-DAL-ih-tee)
Ayurvedic (EYE-yur-VAY-dik)
chiropractic (ky-roh-PRAK-tik)
complementary modality (comp-la-MEN-ta-ree mo-DAL-ih-tee)
homeopathy (HO-mee-AH-pa-thee)
naturopathy (NAY-chur-AH-pa-thee)
osteopathic (AHS-tee-ah-PATH-ik)

CHAPTER CONCEPTS

Collaboration
Evidence-based practice
Health promotion

LEARNING OUTCOMES

1. Explain the difference between complementary and alternative modalities.
2. Describe systems of health care that have contributed to the development of new modalities.
3. Identify how selected modalities are classified.
4. Identify safety issues associated with complementary and alternative modalities.
5. Describe the role of the licensed practical nurse/licensed vocational nurse in assisting a patient with complementary and alternative modalities.

Health care in the 21st century requires that nurses recognize the shift toward the inclusion of complementary and alternative approaches in care. Nurses at all levels and in every area of practice are using new methods to care for those who are ill and enhance the health of those who are well.

Holistic nursing was a precursor to many of the now popular complementary and alternative modalities. It was introduced in the 1970s and has been growing ever since. *Holistic nursing* is simply defined as caring for the whole person—body, mind, and spirit—in a constantly changing environment.

COMPLEMENTARY OR ALTERNATIVE: WHAT'S THE DIFFERENCE?

The words *complementary* and *alternative* are sometimes used interchangeably, but they are not the same. A **complementary modality** refers to a therapy used *in addition* to a conventional modality. For example, a nurse might suggest guided imagery or relaxation techniques for pain control in addition to prescribed drug therapy. An **alternative modality** refers to a therapy used *instead* of a conventional modality. An example is using acupuncture instead of analgesics for pain. The terms *therapy, modality,* and *medicine* can be used interchangeably. For consistency, this chapter uses the term *modality*.

Myths and misinformation that exist about complementary and alternative modalities can be confusing for the patient. A good resource for current accurate information about complementary and alternative modalities is the National Center for Complementary and Integrative Health (NCCIH) at https://nccih.nih.gov.

INTRODUCTION OF NEW SYSTEMS INTO TRADITIONAL WESTERN HEALTH CARE

In the United States, the primary system of medicine is called simply *medicine,* although some people refer to it as **allopathic** medicine. American providers increasingly incorporate and introduce other schools of thought and philosophies, most frequently Ayurvedic, traditional Chinese, chiropractic, homeopathic, naturopathic, American Indian, and osteopathic medicine. Most of these systems use complementary and alternative modalities, sometimes referred to as complementary and alternative medicine (CAM).

Many adults in the United States use some form of complementary and alternative modalities. It is essential to ask your patients about CAM use so you can incorporate these modalities when appropriate and safe to do so.

> ### Gerontological Issues
> **Alternative Modalities**
> Many older adults use some form of CAM but may not report the use of these therapies to their health-care providers. Alternative modalities are commonly used to treat arthritis, back pain, memory issues, heart disease, allergies, and diabetes. Be sure to ask specifically about complementary and alternative modalities at every visit.

Allopathic/Western Medicine

The most common name for allopathic medicine is *Western medicine.* Other commonly used terms are *conventional medicine* and *mainstream medicine.* Allopathy is a method of treating disease with remedies that produce effects different from those caused by the disease itself. For example, when a patient has a bacterial infection, a Western medical practitioner prescribes an antibiotic to eliminate the invading pathogen.

Practitioners of Western medicine are medical doctors, nurses, and allied health personnel. This system of medicine uses scientific investigations to determine the validity of a diagnosis and the effectiveness of treatment; it is called *evidence-based medicine* (see Chapter 2). In scientific investigations, results can be verified and reproduced through various types of studies and statistical analyses. Practitioners use a variety of therapies, including drugs, surgery, and radiation therapy. Western medicine practitioners have made most of the significant advances and developments in modern medicine.

Ayurvedic Medicine

Ayurveda is the ancient Hindu system of medicine that originated in India. Ayurveda maintains that illness is the result of falling out of balance with nature. Diagnosis is based on three metabolic body types called *doshas*. An **Ayurvedic** doctor determines which *dosha* type is most appropriate for the patient: *vata, pitta,* or *kapha.* Treatment usually involves prescribing a diet, herbal remedies, breath work, physical exercise, yoga, meditation, massage, and a rejuvenation or detoxification program (National Ayurvedic Medical Association, n.d.).

Traditional Chinese Medicine

Traditional Chinese medicine is thousands of years old. It involves such practices as acupuncture, acupressure, herbs, massage, and qi gong. Chinese medicine involves diagnosis and treatment of disturbances of qi (pronounced "chee"), or vital energy.

Acupuncture is used commonly in the United States, most often for pain. To treat patients with acupuncture, practitioners insert one or more needles along the meridians (pathways) where qi flows (Fig. 5.1). Many acupuncturists prescribe herbal remedies as well. Find more information on the integration of acupuncture into Western medicine at https://nccih.nih.gov/health/acupuncture/.

Chiropractic Medicine

Chiropractic medicine is based on the belief that illness is a result of neuromusculoskeletal dysfunction. The main treatment modality of chiropractors is manual adjustment and manipulation of the vertebral column and the limbs. The goal is to remove interference with nerve function so the body can heal itself. In addition, chiropractors sometimes provide exercise and nutritional counseling. Chiropractors do not perform surgery or prescribe drugs. Learn more about chiropractic medicine at https://nccih.nih.gov/health/chiropractic/.

Homeopathic Medicine

Homeopathy was developed by Samuel Hahnemann in Germany in the early 19th century. Homeopathy is based on Hahnemann's principle that "like cures like," meaning that tiny doses of a substance that create the symptoms of disease in a healthy person will relieve those symptoms in a sick person.

Although schools and courses do exist for training homeopaths, no diploma or certificate from any school or program is a license to practice homeopathy in the United States. Medical doctors and doctors of osteopathy are granted national certificates of competency by the Council for Homeopathic Certification to practice homeopathy. There is very little current evidence that homeopathy is safe or effective. Learn more at https://nccih.nih.gov/health/homeopathy.

• WORD • BUILDING •
allopathic: allos—other + pathic—disease or suffering
Ayurvedic: ayu—life + veda—knowledge or science
acupuncture: acus—needle + punctura—puncture
chiropractic: cheir—hand + pracktos—to do
homeopathy: homeo—like + pathos—disease

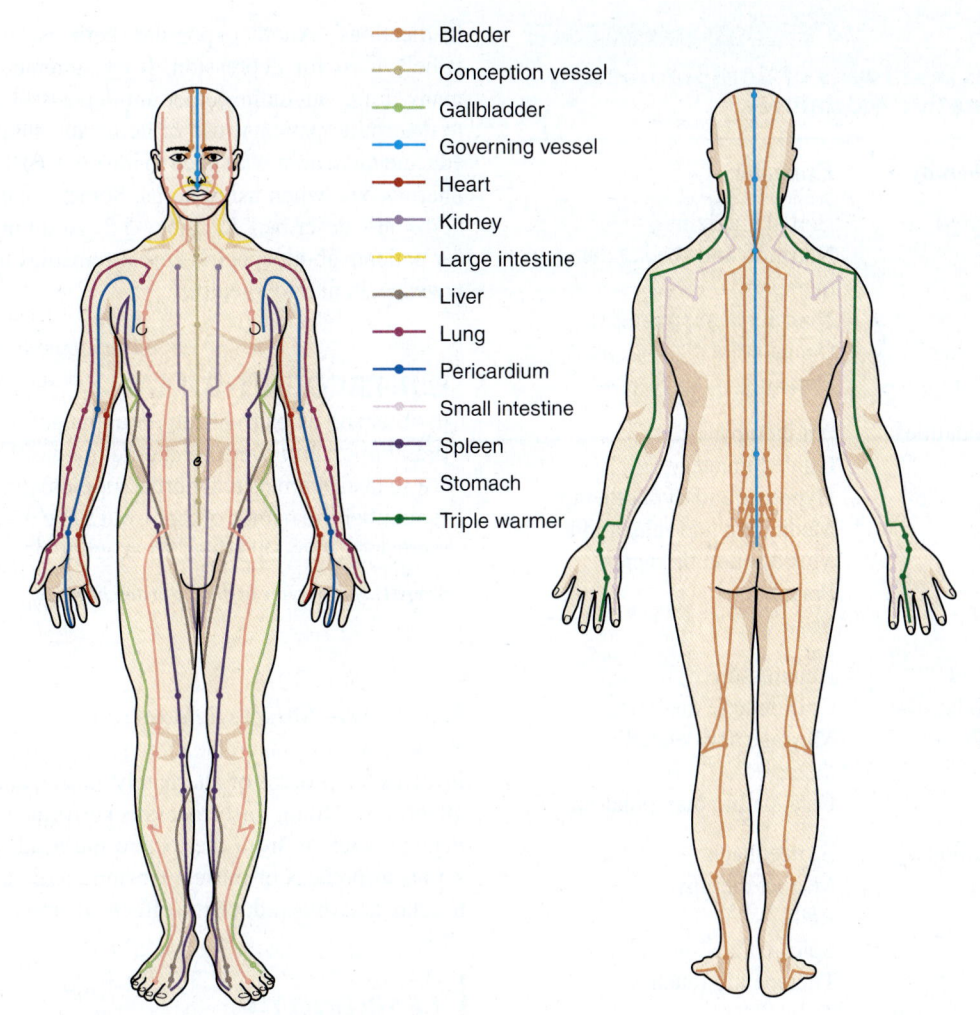

FIGURE 5.1 Qi meridians are used in the Chinese medicine techniques of acupressure and acupuncture.

Legend:
- Bladder
- Conception vessel
- Gallbladder
- Governing vessel
- Heart
- Kidney
- Large intestine
- Liver
- Lung
- Pericardium
- Small intestine
- Spleen
- Stomach
- Triple warmer

Naturopathic Medicine

Naturopathy primarily uses natural therapies such as nutrition, herbs, hydrotherapy (water-based therapy), counseling, and homeopathy to treat disease, promote healing, and prevent illness. Naturopathic physicians have a Doctor of Naturopathy (ND) degree and can be licensed in some states. For more information about naturopathy, visit https://nccih.nih.gov/health/naturopathy.

American Indian Medicine

American Indian medical practices vary from tribe to tribe. In general, American Indian medicine is a community-based system that uses "healers" or facilitators to guide health. These healers use stories, humor, music, tobacco, and various ceremonies to assist the patient with healing. Traditional healing encourages the patient to take initiative to heal themselves, but the healer guides the patient in healing (Redvers & Blondin, 2020). Learn more at the Association of American Indian Physicians Web site at www.aaip.org or www.nlm.nih.gov/nativevoices.

Osteopathic Medicine

Osteopathic medicine emphasizes the interrelationship of the body's nerves, muscles, bones, and organs. The osteopathic philosophy involves treating the whole person, recognizes the body's ability to heal itself, and stresses the importance of diet, exercise, and fitness with a focus on prevention. Osteopathic physicians are fully licensed in all states and often work closely with traditional Western medicine providers. For more information about osteopathy, visit the American Osteopathic Association Web site at https://osteopathic.org.

COMPLEMENTARY AND ALTERNATIVE MODALITIES

Discussion of all complementary and alternative modalities is beyond the scope of this text. Table 5.1 summarizes

• WORD • BUILDING •
naturopathy: naturo—nature + pathy—disease
osteopathic: osteo—bone + pathy—disease

Table 5.1
Categories and Types of Complementary and Alternative Modalities

Category of Therapy	Examples
Biologically based modalities	Herbal medicine Nutrition and special diet therapies Nutritional supplements Cannabidiol Detoxing
Mind–body modalities	Art therapy Guided imagery Hypnosis and hypnotherapy Meditation and relaxation Music/sound therapies Prayer Yoga
Manipulative and body-based modalities	Acupressure Chiropractic medicine Massage and related therapies Osteopathic manipulation
Energetic modalities	Biofeedback Magnet therapy Reiki Spiritual healing Therapeutic touch
Miscellaneous therapies	Heat/cold Aromatherapy Chanting Kinesiology Light therapy Animal-assisted therapy (companion animals, therapy animals, emotional support animals, assistance dogs)

the most commonly used modalities. It is important to have appropriate training and skills before using complementary and alternative modalities with patients.

Herbal Therapy

Herbal remedies are not foods. They have potent medicinal effects and should be taken under the supervision of a health-care provider (HCP). They can interact with prescribed medications and even complicate surgery. This can be problematic because many patients do not tell their doctors or nurses about their herb use. For example, the common herbs garlic, ginkgo, and ginseng can each increase the risk of bleeding when taken with anticoagulant or antiplatelet medications. Another popular herb is St. John's wort, widely used for depression. It can interact adversely with many drugs, including other antidepressant agents. Be sure to determine patients' use of herbs and supplements and to educate them about the need to inform HCPs, including their pharmacists, when using herbs. Some of the more common herbs are described in Table 5.2. Additional information for patients about specific herbal remedies may be found at www.nccih.nih.gov/health.

> **CUE RECOGNITION 5.1**
> In obtaining a health history, your patient names his prescription and over-the-counter medications, and states, "I also take vitamins and herbal supplements. I don't remember the names of them, but since they are not medicines, it's no big deal." What action do you take?
>
> *Suggested answers are at the end of the chapter.*

Relaxation Therapies
Progressive Muscle Relaxation

Progressive muscle relaxation is a simple technique that involves the process of alternately tensing and relaxing muscle groups. Often, this process is performed in a systematic manner, such as from the toes to the head. When our conscious awareness of muscle tension increases, we can learn to relax and thus reduce the effects of stress.

> **LEARNING TIP**
> Try progressive muscle relaxation next time you are anxious during a nursing examination.

Guided Imagery

Guided imagery involves using mental images to promote physical healing or changes in attitudes or behavior. Practitioners lead patients through visualization exercises or offer instruction in using imagery as a self-help tool. Guided imagery is used to alleviate stress, treat stress-related conditions such as insomnia and high blood pressure, and boost the immune system.

A common guided imagery technique begins with progressive muscle relaxation. Guided imagery works best when all the senses are used. The exercise in Box 5.1 is very basic but gives an idea of how the technique works. When used for healing, many more steps are involved. Find more on guided imagery at https://nccih.nih.gov; type "guided imagery" into the search window.

> **PRACTICE ANALYSIS TIP**
> **Linking NCLEX-PN® to Practice**
> The LPN/LVN will provide measures to promote sleep/rest.

Table 5.2
Common Herbs and Their Intended Uses

Herb	Purported Uses
Aloe vera	Used for skin lesions, acts as an astringent and may increase collagen production.
Bee pollen	No consistent evidence to support improvements in allergy symptoms, lowering of cholesterol, improvements in metabolism, or increase in stamina.
Black cohosh	May ease menopausal symptoms.
Capsaicin	When applied as a cream, may ease tenderness and pain of osteoarthritis, fibromyalgia, diabetic neuropathy, and healed shingles. Do not use on open wounds.
Chamomile	May be helpful for general anxiety disorder.
Echinacea	May reduce the chance of getting a cold, has not been shown to shorten the length of a cold.
Ephedra (ma huang)	A sympathomimetic agent used as a stimulant or weight loss supplement; banned by the Food and Drug Administration in 2004 because of deadly side effects, but patients may still obtain it outside the United States.
Feverfew	May help treat migraine headaches.
Garlic	May have a small effect on blood cholesterol. May reduce blood pressure. May reduce the incidence of colon cancer. May remove risk of platelet aggregation and bleeding.
Ginger	May reduce nausea and vomiting.
Ginkgo biloba	No consistent evidence to support improvements in memory and cognitive function in Alzheimer disease. Should be used with caution in patients taking anticoagulants.
Ginseng	May help balance blood glucose levels, improve short-term memory in healthy individuals, and reduce blood pressure in people with diabetes and hypertension.
Kava	May be effective for anxiety.
Red yeast rice	May reduce cholesterol and triglycerides.
St. John's wort	May help mild to moderate depression; may be effective against viral infections, including HIV and herpes. Interacts with many medications.

Warning: Herbs may have many side effects and may interact with many prescribed and over-the-counter medications. Urge patients to consult health-care providers before self-prescribing.

Biofeedback

Biofeedback is a technique that is used especially for conditions that are aggravated by stress, such as asthma, migraines, insomnia, and high blood pressure. Biofeedback is a way of monitoring and controlling tiny metabolic changes in one's body with the aid of sensitive machines that provide feedback (see "Patient Perspective").

Massage Therapy

Massage is the use of touch to achieve therapeutic results. It can include pressure, friction, and kneading of the body. Massage can be used to relax muscles, reduce anxiety, increase circulation, and reduce pain. Massage also provides a caring form of touch. Patients today are often not touched except during technical procedures. Try giving your patient a back massage to help them relax for sleep. You can learn basic massage techniques in nursing school. You may also choose to obtain formal massage therapy education to practice more advanced techniques.

> **BE SAFE!**
> **BE VIGILANT!** Be aware of the patient's health issues before giving a deep, firm massage. For example, do not use firm massage on a patient taking an anticoagulant or with a low platelet level. Tissue injury could cause bleeding. Check with the HCP before providing massage for any patient.

Box 5.1
Guided Imagery

Assist your patient to progress through the following steps:
- Assume a comfortable position in a quiet environment.
- Close your eyes and keep them closed until the exercise is completed.
- Breathe in and out deeply to the count of four, repeating this step four times.
- When relaxed, think of a peaceful place and prepare to take an imaginary journey there.
- Picture what this place looks like and how comfortable you feel being there.
- Listen to all the sounds; feel the gentle, clean air; and smell the pleasant aromas.
- Continue to breathe deeply and appreciate the feeling of being in this special place.
- Feel the sense of deep relaxation and peace of this place.
- As you continue to breathe deeply, slowly and gently bring your consciousness back to the setting in this room.
- Slowly and gently open your eyes, stretch, and think about how relaxed you feel.

Patient Perspective
Polly

I'm scared to death of flying. The minute I get on an airplane, I feel jittery, my heart races, and I can't calm down until we're safely back on the ground. Several years ago, I decided to try biofeedback therapy to overcome this fear.

My therapist immediately put me at ease and assured me I wasn't a crazy person to be afraid to fly. She listened to my fears and responses throughout all our sessions. At each practice session, she put a temperature sensor on my finger (my hands were usually pretty cold). In her calm, soft voice, she guided me through a relaxation exercise using imagery and progressive muscle relaxation. By the time we were finished, my hands would be several degrees warmer than when we started! This showed that my vessels were dilating, a sign that my sympathetic nervous system was slowing down its activity, so I felt calmer. The sensor gave me feedback that told me when my relaxation was working well. We did this every week for a couple of months until I got good at warming my hands and relaxing.

Now when I fly, I close my eyes, imagine a peaceful scene, and use my relaxation techniques. I still don't like flying much, but at least I feel a bit calmer!

Heat and Cold

Local application of heat or cold provides additional skin stimulation. A warm compress can soothe sore muscles and dilate vessels in a localized area, bringing healing circulation. People who suffer from arthritis or other chronic pain understand how warm water can ease their discomfort. Relaxing in water feels good for three reasons: warmth, water movement causing massage, and buoyancy. In addition, exercising in water (aqua therapy) can facilitate freer motion for patients who have limited mobility. Through research, we now know that warm water also stimulates the release of endorphins, the body's naturally occurring pain killers.

Ice or a cold gel pack can help numb an area. Cold can also cause dilated vessels to constrict, yielding relief from pain and throbbing of overstimulated nerve endings. Ice can be helpful on an acute injury and for some types of headaches. Heat or cold application may be contraindicated with certain health conditions and has the potential to make some health impairments worse, so an order from the HCP may be required.

Animal-Assisted Therapy and Animal-Assisted Activities

Animal-assisted therapy (AAT) and animal-assisted activities (AAA) are alternative modalities that use animals to assist humans in daily activities, stressful encounters, or rehabilitation (IAHAIO, 2020). These modalities strive to improve physical, emotional, or social health. The animals used vary depending on the therapy or activity. Common examples of AAA are the use of a visitation dog in an assisted living home or the use of a support animal to comfort someone after a trauma. AAT is a structured therapeutic treatment with animals by a trained professional. Examples of AAT include use of horses in physical therapy or dogs in speech therapy (Fig. 5.2).

Detoxing or Cleansing

Detoxing or cleansing is used to eliminate toxins from the body and/or aid in weight loss. Detoxing ranges from consuming only juice or certain foods for a period of time, using a commercial detox regimen, or using laxatives. Evidence is lacking in support for detoxing's effects on weight loss or the removal of toxins from the body. Detoxing has been associated with electrolyte imbalances, protein deficits, vitamin deficiencies, lactic acidosis, and even death.

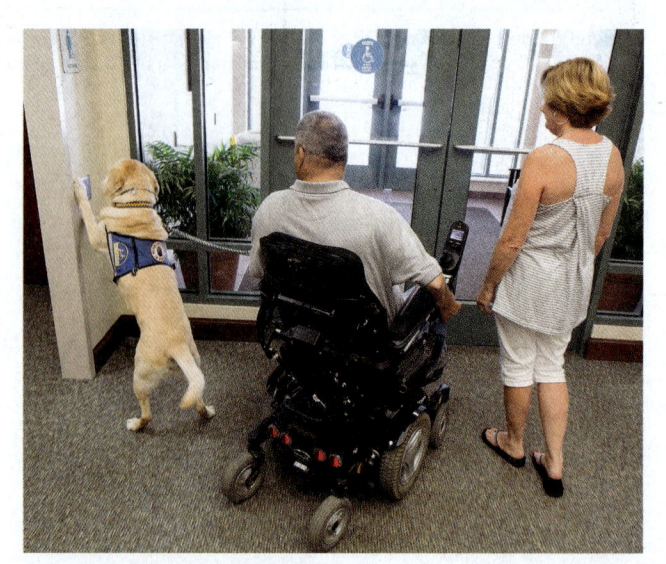

FIGURE 5.2 Animal-assisted activity.

Cannabis

Cannabidiol (CBD) and tetrahydrocannabinol (THC) are naturally found compounds in Cannabis plants (marijuana and hemp). THC is the compound in marijuana that causes the psychoactive "high," whereas CBD is the ingredient found in hemp and does not produce the same psychoactive high. These ingredients are available in oils, gels, gummies, capsules, and many other products. The laws that govern these substances vary significantly among states, and some states allow the use of both recreational and medical products.

CBD is thought to offer relief from many conditions, such as seizures, inflammation, pain, mental disorders, inflammatory bowel disease, nausea, migraines, depression, and anxiety. THC may offer relief from many of the same ailments, including pain, muscle spasticity, glaucoma, insomnia, low appetite, nausea, and anxiety. Side effects of THC include coordination problems, slower reaction times, and memory loss. Side effects of CBD include changes in appetite, weight loss, and fatigue. While CBD does not cause a euphoric high, the substance will still show up on drug screens, which can cause employment and legal concerns. Patients should be made aware that smoking cannabis is harmful to the lungs in many of the same ways tobacco smoking is harmful. In addition, no amount of cannabis is approved for use during pregnancy.

SAFETY AND EFFECTIVENESS OF ALTERNATIVE MODALITIES

Safety generally means that the benefits outweigh the risks of a treatment or modality. If a patient is interested in using complementary and alternative modalities, first counsel the patient to talk with the HCP. The patient also should ask the practitioner of the therapy about its safety and effectiveness. The patient should tell the HCP and alternative practitioners about all modalities they are using. This information may be important to consider in the safety of their overall treatment plan. The patient should be as informed as possible and continue gathering information even after a practitioner or therapy has been selected (Box 5.2).

Box 5.2
Questions Patients Should Ask Before Starting a Complementary or Alternative Modality

1. What will this modality do for me?
2. What are its advantages and disadvantages?
3. What are its risks and side effects?
4. How much will it cost? Will my insurance cover the cost?
5. How long will it take? How many treatments will I need?
6. How will it interact with my other therapies and medications?
7. What research has been done on this modality?

ROLE OF THE LICENSED PRACTICAL NURSE/LICENSED VOCATIONAL NURSE

Patients may ask you about the use of a complementary or alternative modality. Because the safety and effectiveness of many therapies are still unknown, advising patients presents a challenge. Collaborate with the HCP when discussing therapies with patients.

The following steps are suggestions for helping to advise patients regarding the use of these kinds of modalities. You should advise the patient to

1. Discuss use of the modality with the HCP before trying it.
2. Take a close look at the background, qualifications, and competence of the proposed practitioner. Check credentials with a state or local agency with authority over the area of practice in which the patient is interested. Is the practitioner licensed or certified? By whom?
3. Visit the practitioner's office, clinic, or hospital, and evaluate the conditions of the setting.

Evidence-Based Practice

Clinical Question
How are complementary and alternative modalities used by nurses to improve health outcomes?

Evidence
The following are examples of how complementary and alternative modalities have been used by nurses to enhance health outcomes in various patient populations:
- A meta-analysis by Hu et al (2018) showed that AATs are effective in reducing behavior and mental issues in patients with dementia.
- In a meta-analysis by Thomas et al (2019) found improvements in urinary incontinence after acupuncture therapies in patients who suffered from urinary incontinence after a stroke.
- A meta-analysis by Rusch et al (2019) found that mindful meditation is effective in improving sleep in those who suffer from insomnia.

Implications for Nursing Practice
Complementary and alternative modalities such as music, acupuncture, AAT, and meditation can improve health outcomes in diverse patient populations. Before incorporating complementary and alternative modalities into practice, check your state's nurse practice act for regulations. Discuss these therapies with the patient and the HCP before using them, and work within your institution's policies and procedures. Ask your patients if they use any complementary or alternative modalities and what their responses have been. Try to eliminate preconceived ideas you might have and avoid judgment. Your patients will feel more comfortable if they feel you understand the treatment and why they decided to use it.

4. Talk with others who have used this practitioner or modality.
5. Consider the costs. Are the treatments covered by insurance, or will the patient have to pay?

CRITICAL THINKING & CLINICAL JUDGMENT

Mr. Jones asks whether he should stop his chemotherapy and try magnet therapy for his prostate cancer.

Critical Thinking (The Why)
1. What are concerns about the patient stopping chemotherapy and starting magnet therapy?

Clinical Judgment (The Do)
2. How can you respond to Mr. Jones?
3. What other health-care team members might you collaborate with in helping Mr. Jones?

Suggested answers are at the end of the chapter.

> **Home Health Hints**
> - When taking a health history, ask the patient or caregiver about the use of complementary and alternative modalities because these may influence the effects or side effects of some prescription medications. Document and discuss concerns regarding potential interactions with the registered nurse or HCP.
> - If a pet in the home makes the HCP feel unsafe, ask the patient to secure the pet prior to the nurse's arrival. Securing pets during nursing procedures can help promote infection control.
> - To avoid secondhand exposure, ask your patient not to smoke cannabis while you are in the home.

Key Points

- A complementary modality refers to a therapy used in addition to a conventional modality, such as relaxation techniques to help control pain in addition to drug therapy.
- An alternative modality refers to a therapy used *instead* of a conventional modality, such as using acupuncture instead of analgesics for pain.
- The most frequently seen new systems include Ayurvedic, traditional Chinese, chiropractic, homeopathic, naturopathic, American Indian, and osteopathic medicine.
- Categories of complementary and alternative modalities include biologically based modalities, such as herbal medicines, CBD, and diet therapies; mind-body modalities, such as art and music therapies; manipulative and body-based modalities, such as chiropractic and massage; and miscellaneous therapies such as AAT.
- The patient should ask the practitioner of the therapy about its safety and effectiveness. The patient should tell the HCP and alternative practitioners about all modalities they are using.
- The role of the LPN/LVN in assisting patients with complementary and alternative medicine includes advising them to ask questions such as "Is the practitioner licensed or certified? By whom?" In addition, encourage the patient to discuss use of the modality with the HCP.

SUGGESTED ANSWERS TO CHAPTER EXERCISES

Cue Recognition
5.1: Inform your patient that it is important that you know his vitamins and herbal supplements because many of these remedies react with other medications.

Critical Thinking & Clinical Judgment
Mr. Jones
1. As with all medical treatments, it is important to support the established therapy the HCP has prescribed. If Mr. Jones stops chemotherapy and uses a therapy that has not been proven effective against cancer, his cancer may exacerbate.
2. A good response might be the following: "Mr. Jones, chemotherapy is an established medical treatment for your condition. There is a lot of evidence for its effectiveness in the medical literature. If you want to supplement your therapy, there may be some other treatments you can add. I suggest that you discuss your feelings about seeking some additional treatments with your oncologist."
3. Collaborate with the registered nurse as well as the oncologists; perhaps there are some complementary modalities Mr. Jones could try.

Additional Resources

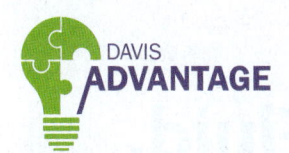

Go to Davis Advantage to complete your learning: strengthen understanding, apply your knowledge, and prepare for the Next Gen NCLEX®.

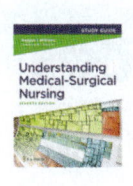

A Study Guide is also available.

UNIT TWO Understanding Health and Illness

CHAPTER 6
Nursing Care of Patients With Fluid, Electrolyte, and Acid–Base Imbalances

Marge Gingrich, Bruce K. Wilson

KEY TERMS

acidosis (as-ih-DOH-sis)
alkalosis (al-kah-LOH-sis)
anion (AN-eye-on)
antidiuretic (AN-ty-DY-yuh-RET-ik)
arrhythmia (uh-RITH-mee-ah)
cation (KAT-eye-on)
dehydration (DEE-hy-DRAY-shun)
diffusion (dih-FEW-shun)
edema (eh-DEE-mah)
electrolytes (ee-LEK-troh-lites)
extracellular (EX-trah-SELL-yoo-lar)
filtration (fill-TRAY-shun)
hydrostatic (HY-droh-STAT-ik)
hypercalcemia (HY-per-kal-SEE-mee-ah)
hyperkalemia (HY-per-kuh-LEE-mee-ah)
hypermagnesemia (HY-per-MAG-nuh-SEE-mee-ah)
hypernatremia (HY-per-nuh-TREE-mee-ah)
hypertonic (HY-per-TAH-nik)
hypervolemia (HY-per-voh-LEE-mee-ah)
hypocalcemia (HY-poh-kal-SEE-mee-ah)
hypokalemia (HY-poh-kuh-LEE-mee-ah)
hypomagnesemia (HY-poh-MAG-nuh-SEE-mee-ah)
hyponatremia (HY-poh-nuh-TREE-mee-ah)
hypotonic (HY-poh-TAH-nik)
hypovolemia (HY-poh-voh-LEE-mee-ah)
interstitial (IN-tur-STISH-uhl)
intracellular (IN-trah-SELL-yoo-ler)
intracranial (IN-trah-KRAY-nee-uhl)
intravascular (IN-trah-VAS-kyoo-ler)
isotonic (EYE-so-TAWN-ik)
osmolarity (OZ-moh-LAR-it-ee)
osmosis (ahs-MOH-sis)
osteoporosis (AHS-tee-oh-por-OH-sis)
semipermeable (SEM-ee-PER-mee-uh-bul)
transcellular (trans-SELL-yoo-lar)

CHAPTER CONCEPTS

Acid base
Fluid and electrolytes

LEARNING OUTCOMES

1. Identify the purposes of fluids and electrolytes in the body.
2. List the signs and symptoms of common fluid imbalances.
3. Predict patients who are at the highest risk for dehydration and fluid excess.
4. Identify data to collect in patients with fluid and electrolyte imbalances.
5. Describe therapeutic measures for patients with fluid and electrolyte imbalances.
6. Identify the education needs of patients with fluid imbalances.
7. Categorize common causes, signs and symptoms, and treatments for sodium, potassium, calcium, and magnesium imbalances.
8. Identify foods that have high sodium, potassium, and calcium contents.
9. Give examples of common causes of acidosis and alkalosis.
10. Compare how arterial blood gases change for each type of acid–base imbalance.

Have you ever wondered why you get thirsty? The body is continually changing. Water supports these changes. Approximately 60% of a young adult's body weight is water. Older people are less than 50% water. Infants are between 70% and 80% water.

In addition to water, body fluids contain dissolved solid substances, called *solutes*. Some solutes are electrolytes; some are nonelectrolytes. **Electrolytes** are chemicals that can conduct electricity when dissolved in water. Examples of electrolytes are sodium, potassium, calcium, magnesium, acids, and bases; these are discussed in this chapter. Nonelectrolytes do not conduct electricity; examples include glucose and urea.

FLUID BALANCE

Fluids are located in various compartments within the body. Fluid inside the cells is referred to as **intracellular** fluid (ICF). Fluid outside the cells is called **extracellular** fluid (ECF). ECF can be divided into three types: interstitial fluid, intravascular fluid, and transcellular fluid (Fig. 6.1).

• WORD • BUILDING •
electrolyte: electro—electricity + lyte—dissolve
intracellular: intra—within + cellular—cell
extracellular: extra—outside of + cellular—cell

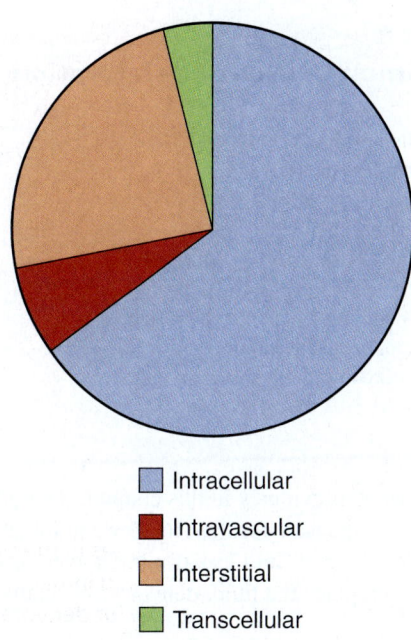

FIGURE 6.1 Normal distribution of total body water.

- Intracellular
- Intravascular
- Interstitial
- Transcellular

Interstitial fluid is the water that surrounds the body's cells and includes lymph. **Intravascular** fluid, or blood plasma, exists within arteries, veins, and capillaries. Fluids and electrolytes move between the interstitial fluid and the intravascular fluid. **Transcellular** fluids are those in specific compartments of the body, such as cerebrospinal fluid, digestive juices, and synovial fluid in joints.

Control of Fluid Balance

The primary control of water in the body is through pressure sensors in the vascular system that stimulate or inhibit the release of **antidiuretic** hormone (ADH) from the pituitary gland. A diuretic is a substance that causes the kidneys to excrete more fluid. ADH works in just the opposite way. ADH causes the kidneys to retain fluid. If fluid pressures within the vascular system decrease, more ADH is released, and water is retained. If fluid pressures increase, less ADH is released, and the kidneys eliminate more water.

Movement of Fluids and Electrolytes in the Body

Fluids and electrolytes move in the body by active and passive transport systems. Active transport depends on the presence of adequate cellular adenosine triphosphate (ATP) for energy. The most common examples of active transport are sodium-potassium pumps. These pumps are located in the cell membranes. They cause sodium to move out of the cells and potassium to move into the cells when needed.

In passive transport, no energy is expended specifically to move the substances. General body movements aid passive transport. The three passive transport systems are diffusion, filtration, and osmosis.

> **PRACTICE ANALYSIS TIP**
> **Linking NCLEX-PN® to Practice**
> The LPN/LVN provides care for a client with a fluid and electrolyte imbalance.

Diffusion is the movement of a substance from an area of higher concentration to an area of lower concentration. If you put a teabag in a cup of hot water, the movement of the molecules eventually causes the tea to be dispersed throughout the hot water. Like the tea fills the cup, the water molecules in the body move from high concentration to low concentration by diffusion. This passive movement of substances helps to maintain fluid and electrolyte balance.

Filtration is the movement of both water and smaller molecules through a **semipermeable** membrane from an area of high pressure to an area of lower pressure. A semipermeable membrane works like a screen that keeps larger substances on one side and permits only smaller molecules to filter to the other side of the membrane. Filtration is promoted by hydrostatic pressure differences between areas. **Hydrostatic** pressure, sometimes called *water-pushing pressure,* is the force that water exerts. In the body, filtration is important for the movement of water, nutrients, and waste products in the capillaries. The capillaries serve as semipermeable membranes, allowing water and smaller substances to move from the vascular system to the interstitial fluid. Larger molecules and red blood cells remain inside the capillary walls.

Osmosis is the movement of water from an area of lower substance concentration across a semipermeable membrane to an area of higher concentration. The power to pull water toward an area of higher concentration is referred to as *osmotic pressure.* This process continues until the concentration is the same on both sides of the membrane. The term **osmolarity** refers to the concentration of the substances in body fluids. The normal osmolarity of blood is between 270 and 300 milliosmoles per liter (mOsm/L).

Another term for osmolarity is *tonicity.* Fluids or solutions can be classified as isotonic, hypotonic, or hypertonic. A fluid that has the same osmolarity as the blood is called **isotonic.** For example, a 0.9% (normal) saline solution is

• WORD • BUILDING •

interstitial: inter—between + stitial—tissue
intravascular: intra—within + vascular—blood vessel
transcellular: trans—across + cellular—cell
antidiuretic: anti—against + diuretic—urination
diffusion: diffuse—spread, scattered
filtration: filter—strain through
semipermeable: semi—half or part of + permeable—passing through
hydrostatic: hydro—water + static—standing
osmosis: osmo—impulse + osis—condition
isotonic: iso—equal + tonic—strength

isotonic to the blood; it is often used as a solution for IV therapy. A solution that has a lower osmolarity than blood is called **hypotonic.** When a hypotonic solution is given to a patient, the water in the solution leaves the blood and other ECF areas and enters the cells. **Hypertonic** solutions exert greater osmotic pressure than blood. When a hypertonic solution is given to a patient, water leaves the cells and enters the bloodstream and other ECF spaces.

Fluid Gains and Fluid Losses

Water is very important to the body for cellular metabolism, blood volume, body temperature regulation, and solute transport. Although people can survive without food for several weeks, they can survive only a few days without water. Thirst is the major indicator that a healthy adult needs more water.

Water is gained and lost from the body every day. In addition to liquid intake, some fluid is obtained from solid foods. When too much fluid is lost, the brain's thirst mechanism tells the individual that more fluid intake is needed. Older adults are more prone to fluid deficits because they have a diminished thirst reflex and their kidneys do not function as effectively. An adult loses as much as 2,500 mL of sensible and insensible fluid each day. Sensible losses are those of which the person is aware, such as urination. Insensible losses may occur without the person recognizing the loss. Perspiration and water lost through respiration and elimination of stool are examples of insensible losses.

FLUID IMBALANCES

Fluid imbalances are common in all clinical settings. Older adults are at the highest risk for life-threatening complications that can result from either fluid deficit, more commonly called **dehydration,** or fluid excess. Infants are at risk for fluid deficit because they take in and excrete a large proportion of their total body water each day.

Dehydration

Although there are several types of dehydration, only the most common type is discussed in this chapter. Dehydration occurs when there is not enough fluid in the body, especially in the blood (intravascular area).

Pathophysiology and Etiology

The most common form of dehydration results from loss of fluid from the body, resulting in decreased blood volume. This decrease is referred to as **hypovolemia.** Hypovolemia occurs when the patient is hemorrhaging or when fluids from other parts of the body are lost. For example, severe vomiting and diarrhea, severely draining wounds, and profuse diaphoresis (sweating) can cause dehydration (Box 6.1).

Hypovolemia can also occur when fluid from the intravascular space moves into the interstitial fluid space. This process is called *third spacing.* Examples of conditions in which third spacing is common include burns, liver cirrhosis, and extensive trauma.

Box 6.1

Common Causes of Dehydration

Diarrhea
Diuretic therapy
Draining abscess or fistula
Fever
Gastrointestinal suction
Hemorrhage
Ileostomy
Long-term nothing-by-mouth (NPO) status
Profuse diaphoresis (sweating)
Systemic infection
Vomiting

As described previously in this chapter, the body initially attempts to compensate for fluid loss by a number of mechanisms. If the cause of fluid loss is not resolved or the patient is not able to replace the fluid, dehydration occurs.

Prevention

You can help prevent dehydration by identifying patients who have the highest risk for developing this condition and intervening quickly to correct the cause. High-risk patients include older adults, infants, children, and any patient with one of the conditions listed in Box 6.1. Also see "Gerontological Issues: Dehydration."

Adequate hydration is another important intervention to help prevent dehydration. Encourage patients to drink adequate fluids. Adults need 30 mL/kg/day of fluids. If a patient is unable to take enough fluid by mouth, alternate routes may be necessary.

Gerontological Issues

Dehydration. As a person ages, total body water decreases from 60% to 50% of total body weight. This age-related decrease in total body water is secondary to an increase in body fat and a decrease in thirst sensation. These factors increase the risk of developing dehydration.

Manifestations of dehydration in an older adult are different from typical manifestations in a younger person. They may include confusion, lightheadedness, and syncope (loss of consciousness). These occur because a patient with hypovolemia has an inadequate circulatory volume and, therefore, inadequate oxygen supply to the brain. If unable to replace fluids orally, remember IV infusions should be given only at the rate prescribed by the health-care provider.

• WORD • BUILDING •

hypotonic: hypo—less than + tonic—strength
hypertonic: hyper—more than + tonic—strength
dehydration: de—down + hydration—water
hypovolemia: hypo—less than + vol—volume + emia—blood

Signs and Symptoms

Thirst is the initial symptom experienced by otherwise healthy adults in response to hypovolemia. As the percentage of water in the blood goes down, the percentage of other substances goes up, resulting in the thirst response. As the blood volume decreases, the heart pumps the remaining blood faster but not as powerfully. This results in a rapid, weak pulse; rapid, shallow respirations; and low blood pressure. The body pulls water into the vascular system from other areas. This results in decreased tear formation, dry skin, and dry mucous membranes.

A dehydrated person will have decreased *skin turgor*. Turgor is considered decreased if the skin is pinched and a small "tent" or wrinkle remains (called *tenting*). Skin turgor should be palpated over the sternum or at the inner thigh. Tenting may be less reliable in older adults due to changes in skin elasticity. A dehydrated person's temperature increases because the body is less able to cool itself through perspiration. Temperature may not appear elevated in an older person because an older adult's normal body temperature is often lower than that of a younger person.

Urine output decreases. The urine becomes more concentrated as water is conserved. Dehydration should be considered in any adult with a urine output of less than 30 mL per hour. The urine may appear darker because it is less diluted. The patient becomes constipated as the intestines absorb more water from the stool. A major method of evaluating dehydration is weight loss. A pint of water (16 oz or 473 mL) weighs approximately 0.45 kg/1 lb. Symptoms of dehydration in older persons may be atypical (see "Gerontological Issues: Dehydration").

> **LEARNING TIP**
> Do you remember your grandmother saying, "A pint's a pound the world around"? It's a great way to remember how much fluid loss is represented by each lost pound.

Complications

If dehydration is not treated, lack of sufficient blood volume causes organ function to decrease and eventually fail. The brain, kidneys, and heart must be adequately perfused with blood to function properly. The body protects these organs by decreasing blood flow to other areas. When these organs no longer receive their minimum requirements, death results.

> **LEARNING TIP**
> The magic fluid number is 30: Healthy adults should drink approximately 30 mL of fluid per kilogram of body weight per day. They should urinate at least 30 mL per hour. This is just a basic rule of thumb and varies depending on individual circumstances.

Diagnostic Tests

A patient with dehydration usually has an elevated blood urea nitrogen (BUN) level and elevated hematocrit. Both values increase because there is less water in proportion to the solid substances being measured. The specific gravity of the urine also increases as the kidneys attempt to conserve water, resulting in a more concentrated urine.

Therapeutic Measures

The goals of therapeutic measures are to replace fluids and resolve the cause of dehydration. In a patient with moderate or severe dehydration, IV therapy is used. Isotonic fluids that have the same osmolarity as blood, such as normal saline, are typically administered.

Nursing Process for the Patient Experiencing Dehydration

Nurses can play a major role in identifying and caring for patients who are dehydrated.

DATA COLLECTION. Monitor the patient for signs and symptoms of dehydration. All the classic signs and symptoms may not be present.

When observing an older patient for skin turgor (tenting), palpate the skin over the forehead or sternum. The skin over these areas usually retains elasticity and is therefore a more reliable indicator of skin turgor. Also check mucous membranes, which should be moist.

Weight is the most reliable indicator of fluid loss or gain. A loss of 0.45 to 0.9 kg (1–2 lb) or more per day suggests water loss rather than fat loss. The patient in the hospital setting should be weighed every day. The patient in the nursing home or home setting should be weighed at least three times a week if the patient is at risk for fluid imbalance. Weigh the patient before breakfast using the same scale each time. Remember that 1 kg = 2.2 lb, so when a patient has gained or lost 1 kg in a day, this can represent a significant fluid loss or gain.

> **PRACTICE ANALYSIS TIP**
> Linking NCLEX-PN® to Practice
> The LPN/LVN monitors client intake and output.

> **LEARNING TIP**
> Here is a handy way to remember symptoms of dehydration. "No spit, no sweat, no need to go? Fix it all with H_2O."

NURSING DIAGNOSES, PLANNING, AND IMPLEMENTATION.

Risk for Deficient Fluid Volume or Deficient Fluid Volume [Isotonic or Hypotonic/Hypertonic] related to fluid loss or inadequate fluid intake

EXPECTED OUTCOME: The patient will be adequately hydrated as evidenced by stable weight, moist mucous membranes, and elastic skin turgor.

Cultural Considerations

Muslims who celebrate Ramadan traditionally fast for 1 month from sunup to sundown. Although ill individuals are not required to fast, they may still wish to do so. Fasting may include not taking fluids and medications during daylight hours. For a Muslim who is ill and is fasting, the nurse may need to alter times for medication administration, including intramuscular medication. Special precautions may need to be taken to prevent dehydration (Chehovich, Demler, & Leppien, 2019).

- Monitor daily weights and input and output (I&O) *so problems can be detected and corrected early.*
- Collaborate with the patient and other members of the health-care team on the type and timing of fluid intake. *Planning with the patient increases the likelihood that the plan will be followed.*
- Offer fluids often to the confused patient *because they may not drink independently.*
- Correct the underlying cause of the fluid deficit, *so it does not recur.*
- Be careful not to overhydrate the patient, *so fluid excess does not occur.*

See Box 6.2 for best practices for maintaining oral hydration in older people.

EVALUATION. The patient who is adequately hydrated will have elastic skin turgor, moist mucous membranes, and stable weight.

Patient Education
Reinforce with the patient, family, and significant others the importance of reporting early signs and symptoms of dehydration to the health-care provider (HCP). Encourage family members to offer low-sugar fluids throughout the day. Fresh lemon squeezed in water can make water more appealing. Reinforce the need to replace fluids lost through perspiration with fever, vomiting, or diarrhea.

CRITICAL THINKING & CLINICAL JUDGMENT

Mrs. Levitt is a 92-year-old widow who has been living for 4 years in the nursing home where you work. Today, she mentions that her urine smells bad and that her heart feels like it is beating faster than usual. You check her urine and find that it is a dark amber color and has a strong odor. Her heart rate is 98 beats per minute, blood pressure 126/74 mm Hg, respiratory rate 20 per minute, and temperature 99.2°F (37.3°C).

Critical Thinking (The Why)
1. What do you suspect is happening?
2. What other data should you collect, and what results do you expect?

Critical Judgement (The Do)
3. Which interventions should you provide at this time?
4. How should you document your subjective and objective findings?
5. What other team members should you collaborate with in your plan for Mrs. Levitt?
6. What data should you collect to determine if she is improving?

Suggested answers are at the end of the chapter.

Fluid Excess

Fluid excess, sometimes called *overhydration,* is a condition in which a patient has too much fluid in the body. Most problems related to fluid excess result from too much fluid in the bloodstream or from dilution of electrolytes and red blood cells.

Pathophysiology and Etiology
The most common result of fluid excess is **hypervolemia,** in which there is excess fluid in the intravascular space. Healthy adult kidneys can compensate for mild to moderate hypervolemia. The kidneys increase urinary output to rid the body of the extra fluid. Sometimes, however, the kidneys cannot keep up with the excess fluid.

Conditions that can cause excessive fluid intake are poorly controlled IV therapy or excessive ingestion of water. It can also occur secondary to excessive sodium intake, adrenal gland dysfunction, or use of corticosteroid drugs. Conditions that can result in inadequate excretion of fluid include kidney failure, heart failure, and the syndrome of inappropriate ADH. These conditions are discussed elsewhere in this book.

Box 6.2
Maintaining Oral Hydration in Older Adults

Following are best practice recommendations for maintaining oral hydration in older people:
- A fluid intake sheet is the best method of monitoring daily fluid intake.
- Urine-specific gravity may be the simplest, most accurate method to determine patient hydration.
- Evidence of a dry, furrowed tongue, mucous membranes, sunken eyes, confusion, and upper body muscle weakness may indicate dehydration.
- Regular presentation of fluids to bedridden older adults can maintain adequate hydration.
- Medication administration is a good time to encourage fluids.

Source: From Oates, L. L., & Price, C. I. (2017). Clinical assessments and care interventions to promote oral hydration amongst older patients: A narrative systematic review. *BMC Nursing, 16*(1), 4. https://doi.org/10.1186/s12912-016-0195-x

• WORD • BUILDING •

hypervolemia: hyper—more than + vol—volume + emia—blood

Prevention

One of the best ways to prevent fluid excess is to avoid excessive fluid intake. Monitor the patient receiving IV therapy for signs and symptoms of fluid excess. In at-risk patients, an electronic controller should be used to control the rate of infusion.

Also monitor the amount of fluid used for irrigations. For example, when a patient's stomach is being irrigated (gastric lavage), be sure an excessive amount of fluid is not absorbed.

Signs and Symptoms

Vital sign changes seen in the patient with fluid excess are the opposite of those found in patients with dehydration. Blood pressure is elevated, pulse is bounding, and respirations are increased and labored. Neck veins may become distended. Pitting dependent **edema** (excess water in tissues) in the feet and legs may be present. The skin is pale and cool. The kidneys increase urine output. Urine appears diluted, almost like water. The patient rapidly gains weight. In severe fluid excess, the patient develops moist crackles in the lungs, dyspnea, and ascites (excess peritoneal fluid).

Complications

Acute fluid excess typically results in congestive heart failure. As the fluid builds up in the heart, the organ cannot properly function as a pump. The fluid then backs up into the lungs, causing a condition known as pulmonary edema. Other major organs of the body cannot receive adequate oxygen. Organ failure can lead to death.

> **BE SAFE!**
> **BE VIGILANT!** Observe patients with impaired renal function closely for signs of fluid retention and cardiovascular complications. Symptoms may include weight gain, edema, shortness of breath, hypertension, tachycardia, and crackles in the lungs. If the patient is in bed, fluid may collect in the sacral area. If you recognize symptoms of overload notify the charge nurse and/or primary HCP.

Diagnostic Tests

In the patient experiencing fluid excess, BUN and hematocrit levels tend to decrease because the extra fluid dilutes the blood. The plasma content of the blood is proportionately increased compared with the solid substances. The specific gravity of the urine also diminishes as the urinary output increases.

Therapeutic Measures

Once the patient's breathing has been supported, the goal of treatment is to rid the body of excessive fluid and resolve the underlying cause of the excess.

POSITIONING. To facilitate ease in breathing, the head of the patient's bed should be in semi-Fowler or high Fowler position (Fig. 6.2). These positions allow greater lung expansion and thus aid respiratory effort. Once the patient has been properly positioned, oxygen therapy may be necessary.

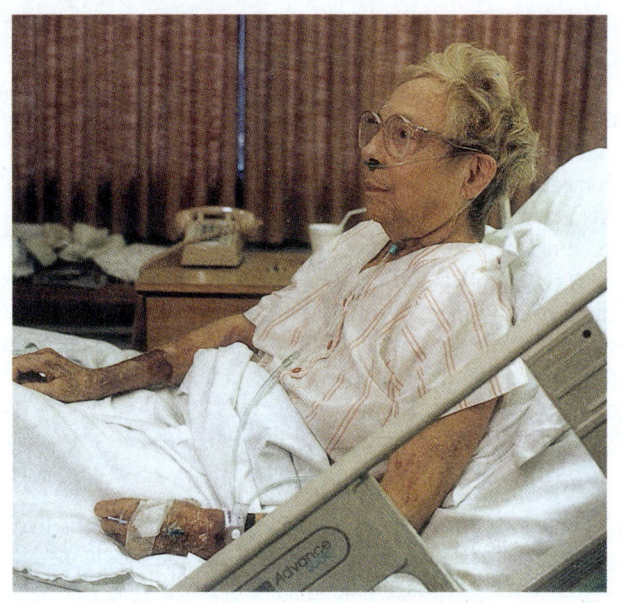

FIGURE 6.2 Patient in a high Fowler position with oxygen.

OXYGEN THERAPY. Oxygen therapy is used to ensure adequate perfusion of major organs and to minimize dyspnea. Monitor pulse oximetry and respiratory rate carefully.

DRUG THERAPY. Diuretics are commonly administered to rapidly rid the body of excess water. A diuretic is a drug that increases elimination of fluid by the kidneys. The drug of choice for fluid excess when the patient has adequately functioning kidneys is usually a loop diuretic, such as furosemide. Loop diuretics cause the kidneys to excrete sodium and water. Sodium (Na^+) and water tend to move together in the body. Potassium (K^+), another electrolyte, is also lost. This can lead to a potassium deficit, discussed later in this chapter.

Furosemide may be given by the oral, intramuscular, or IV route. The oral route is used most commonly for mild fluid excess. IV furosemide is administered for severe fluid excess. The patient should begin diuresis within 30 minutes after receiving IV furosemide. I&O, as well as daily weight, should be strictly monitored when a patient is receiving IV furosemide.

DIET THERAPY. Mild to moderate fluid restriction may be necessary along with a sodium-restricted diet. In collaboration with the dietitian, an HCP prescribes the specific restriction necessary, usually a 1 g to 2 g sodium restriction for severe excess. Different diuretics result in differing electrolyte elimination. Specific diet therapy depends on the medications the patient is receiving and the patient's underlying medical problems.

Nursing Process for the Patient Experiencing Fluid Excess

DATA COLLECTION. Observe a patient who is at high risk for fluid excess. Monitor fluid I&O carefully. If the patient is drinking adequate amounts of fluid (1,500 mL per day

• WORD • BUILDING •
edema: swelling

or more) but is voiding in small amounts, the fluid is being retained by the body.

Check for edema; if it is pitting, a finger pressed against the skin over a bony area such as the tibia leaves a temporary indentation. For patients in bed, check the sacrum for edema. For patients in the sitting position, check the feet and legs. Also auscultate lung sounds. Excess fluid accumulation in the lungs can cause crackles (see Chapter 29).

As mentioned earlier, weight is the most reliable indicator of fluid gain. Weigh at-risk patients daily. A gain of 0.45 to 0.9 kg (1 to 2 lb) or more per day indicates fluid retention, even though other signs and symptoms may not be present.

CUE RECOGNITION 6.1
You weigh your patient in the morning, and he weighs 1 kg more than yesterday. He has not had any changes in diet, medications, or fluid intake. What do you do?

Suggested answers are at the end of the chapter.

NURSING DIAGNOSES, PLANNING, AND IMPLEMENTATION.

Excess Fluid Volume related to excessive fluid intake or inadequate excretion of body fluid

EXPECTED OUTCOME: The patient will return to a normal hydration status as evidenced by return to weight that is normal for the patient, absence of edema, and clear lung sounds.

- Report increase in weight to the HCP. *Increased weight indicates fluid retention.*
- Implement fluid restriction as ordered *to reduce excess intake.* Work with the patient and registered nurse (RN) to determine how it should be implemented. For example, if a patient is on a 1,000 mL per day fluid restriction, you might plan for 150 mL with each meal, 450 mL to be given to the patient to use as they like during the day, and 100 mL to be used during the night. Be sure to include the patient in your planning. Remember to reserve enough fluid for swallowing medications. Post a sign in the patient's room so other caregivers know how much fluid the patient can have.
- Administer diuretics as ordered. Monitor patient response. Be sure to monitor potassium in patients receiving potassium-wasting loop or thiazide diuretics. *Diuretics promote diuresis.*
- Report urinary output below 30 mL per hour to the HCP or RN *because this may signify increasing renal complications.*

EVALUATION. If interventions have been effective, the patient will return to their normal weight with clear lung sounds and no edema. Many patients must remain on drug and diet therapy after hospital discharge to prevent the problem from recurring.

Table 6.1
Common Food Sources of Sodium

Food	Sodium Range (in milligrams)
1 cheeseburger, fast food restaurant	710–1,690
5 oz pork with barbecue sauce (packaged)	600–1,120
3 oz turkey breast luncheon meat (deli or prepackaged)	450–1,050
1 cup canned pasta with meat sauce	530–980
1 cup chicken noodle soup, canned prepared	100–940
3 oz chicken strips, restaurant, breaded	430–900
4 oz slice restaurant pizza, plain cheese, regular crust	510–760
1 corn dog, regular	350–620
3 oz chicken nuggets, frozen, breaded	200–570
1 oz slice American cheese, processed (prepackaged or deli)	330–460
1 cup lo mein	345–500
1 slice of white bread	80–230
1 oz potato chips, plain	50–200
1 package instant ramen noodles	1,340–1,760
1 burrito	985–1,420

Source: Adapted from Centers for Disease Control and Prevention. (2020). Sodium and food sources. https://www.cdc.gov/salt/food.htm

Patient Education
In collaboration with the dietitian, reinforce any fluid or sodium restrictions to prevent further problems ("Nutrition Notes"). Common foods that may have high sodium are listed in Table 6.1.

If a potassium-wasting diuretic is prescribed, encourage the patient to eat foods that are high in potassium (Table 6.2). The patient's serum potassium level must be periodically monitored by an HCP or home health nurse. If it becomes too low, an oral potassium supplement is needed.

Reinforce with the patient or caregiver common signs and symptoms of fluid excess that should be reported to the HCP. Of special importance is weight gain. A patient at high risk for fluid excess should be weighed at least three times a week in the home or nursing home at the same time each day and on the same scale. Weight gain should be reported.

Table 6.2
Food Sources of Potassium

Food	Potassium (mg)
Potato, baked, flesh and skin, 1 medium	941
White beans, canned, 1/2 cup	595
Sweet potato, baked in skin, 1 medium	542
Salmon, Atlantic, wild, cooked, 3 oz	534
Plain yogurt, low-fat, 8 oz	531
Tomato juice, canned, 1 cup	527
Orange juice, fresh, 1 cup	496
Banana, 1 medium	422

Source: Adapted from U.S. Department of Health and Human Services and U.S. Department of Agriculture. (2015). *2015–2020 Dietary guidelines for Americans* (8th ed.). Washington, DC: Author, Appendix 10, Food sources of potassium. https://health.gov/dietaryguidelines/2015/guidelines/appendix-10/#table-a10-1

Nutrition Notes

Reducing Sodium Intake. Americans consume excessive amounts of sodium, two to three times more than the adequate intake of 1,500 mg per day. The major sources of dietary sodium are prepackaged and prepared foods. For example, snack foods such as chips and crackers, baked goods, deli meats, hamburgers, burritos, pizza, soups, cheese, and processed meats are high in sodium. Patients should be taught to read labels for sodium content on all packaged foods (FDA, 2020).

Drinking water may contain significant amounts of sodium, particularly softened or mineral water. Because of the numerous hidden sources of sodium, patients on low-sodium diets will benefit from education by a registered dietitian.

The upper tolerable intake level (UL) for sodium is 2,300 mg daily. This is the amount contained in a teaspoon of salt. These recommendations may not apply to those losing large amounts of sweat daily or to those not used to exercising in a hot environment.

Specific definitions for reduced-sodium food products have been adopted. Note that serving size is an important variable:

- Salt or sodium free: Less than 5 mg sodium per serving
- Very low sodium: Less than 35 mg sodium per serving (per 100 g if main dish)
- Low sodium: Less than 140 mg sodium per serving (per 100 g if main dish)

ELECTROLYTE IMBALANCES

Natural minerals in food become electrolytes or ions in the body through digestion and metabolism. Electrolytes are usually measured in milliequivalents per liter (mEq/L) or in milligrams per deciliter (mg/dL).

CRITICAL THINKING & CLINICAL JUDGMENT

Mr. Peters is a 32-year-old man with a congenital heart problem. He is recovering from acute congestive heart failure and fluid excess. Today, his blood pressure is higher than usual, and his pulse is bounding. He is having trouble breathing and presses the call light for your assistance.

Critical Thinking (The Why)
1. What complications can occur if Mr. Peters's fluid imbalance is not corrected?

Clinical Judgement (The Do)
2. What should you do first when you discover Mr. Peters's condition?
3. What questions should you ask him?
4. What objective data should you collect?
5. What should you do with your findings?

Suggested answers are at the end of the chapter.

Electrolytes are either cations or anions. **Cations** carry a positive electrical charge. **Anions** carry a negative electrical charge. Although there are many electrolytes in the body, this chapter discusses the most important ones. These include sodium (Na^+), potassium (K^+), calcium (Ca^{2+}), and magnesium (Mg^{2+}). These electrolytes are maintained in different concentrations inside the cell and outside the cell because of pumps in the cell wall (Fig. 6.3).

At times, a patient may experience problems because of too much or too little of an electrolyte. In general, if a patient experiences a deficit of an electrolyte, the electrolyte is replaced either orally or intravenously. If the patient experiences an excess of an electrolyte, treatment focuses on getting rid of the excess, often via the kidneys. The underlying cause of the imbalance must also be treated.

The most important aspects of nursing care are preventing and recognizing electrolyte imbalances. You must be vigilant in watching for signs of imbalance in high-risk patients. Serum electrolytes are measured on a regular basis. As a rule, patients should be checked for electrolyte imbalance with a change in their mental status (either increased irritability or decreased responsiveness) or muscle function. Patient education is another important nursing role.

• WORD • BUILDING •
cation: cat—descending + ion—carrying
anion: an—without + ion—carrying

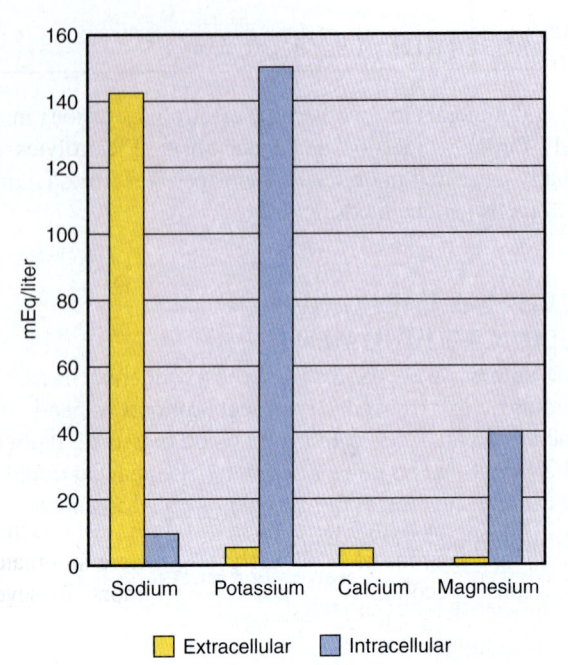

FIGURE 6.3 Extracellular and intracellular electrolytes.

Sodium Imbalances

The normal level of serum sodium is 135 to 145 mEq/L (135–145 mmol/L). Because sodium is the major cation in the blood, it helps maintain serum osmolarity. Therefore, sodium imbalances are often associated with fluid imbalances, described earlier in this chapter. Sodium is also important for cell function, especially in the central nervous system. The two sodium imbalances are **hyponatremia** (sodium deficit) and **hypernatremia** (sodium excess).

Hyponatremia

Hyponatremia occurs when the serum sodium level is less than 135 mEq/L.

PATHOPHYSIOLOGY AND ETIOLOGY. Many conditions can lead to an actual or relative decrease in sodium. In an actual decrease, the patient has inadequate intake of sodium or excessive sodium loss from the body. As the percentage of sodium in the ECF decreases, water is pulled by osmotic pressure into the cells. In a relative decrease, the sodium is not lost from the body; instead, it may leave the intravascular space and move into the interstitial tissues (third spacing), where it becomes trapped and useless. Another cause of a relative decrease occurs when the plasma volume increases (fluid excess), causing a dilutional effect. The percentage of sodium compared with the fluid is diminished.

PREVENTION. Additional sodium is commonly administered to patients at high risk for hyponatremia (Box 6.3), usually by the IV route. Individuals who have high fevers or who engage in strenuous exercise or physical labor, especially in the heat, need to replace both sodium and water. Hyponatremia is especially dangerous for the older patient.

Box 6.3

High-Risk Conditions for Hyponatremia

The following conditions place patients at high risk for hyponatremia:
- Nothing by mouth (NPO)
- Excessive diaphoresis (sweating)
- Diuretics
- Gastrointestinal suction
- Syndrome of inappropriate antidiuretic hormone
- Excessive ingestion of hypotonic fluids
- Freshwater near-drowning
- Decreased aldosterone

SIGNS AND SYMPTOMS. Unfortunately, the signs and symptoms of hyponatremia are vague and depend somewhat on whether a fluid imbalance accompanies the hyponatremia. The patient with sodium and fluid deficits has signs and symptoms of dehydration. The patient with a sodium deficit and relative fluid excess has signs and symptoms associated with fluid excess.

With more severe sodium deficit, the patient experiences mental status changes. These include disorientation, agitation, confusion, and personality changes. These changes occur because the low sodium and decrease in osmolarity cause more "water-pushing pressure." This causes water to collect in and around the brain (cerebral edema) and increase intracranial pressure. Weakness, elevated body temperature, tachycardia, nausea, vomiting, and diarrhea may also occur.

COMPLICATIONS. In severe hyponatremia, seizures, respiratory arrest, or coma can lead to death. The patient who also has fluid excess can develop pulmonary edema, another life-threatening complication.

LEARNING TIP

Hyponatremia Mnemonic: SALT LOSS
Stupor/coma
Anorexia, nausea, vomiting
Lethargy
Trouble concentrating, confusion
Limp muscles
Orthostatic hypotension
Seizures
Spasms of muscle

• WORD • BUILDING •

hyponatremia: hypo—less than + natr—sodium + emia—blood
hypernatremia: hyper—more than + natr—sodium + emia—blood

> **LEARNING TIP**
> Here is a handy way to remember the relationship between dehydration and confusion in the older adult: "You are not thinking if you are not drinking."

> **CUE RECOGNITION 6.2**
> A patient you are caring for has a sodium level of 124mEq/L and is becoming increasingly confused. What action do you take?
>
> *Suggested answers are at the end of the chapter.*

> **Evidence-Based Practice**
>
> **Clinical Question**
> Can improving hydration in nursing home patients decrease the number of urinary tract infections (UTIs)?
>
> **Evidence**
> The researchers were able to decrease the number of UTIs requiring antibiotics by 58% and the number of UTIs requiring hospitalization by 36% (Lean et al., 2019).
>
> **Implication for Nursing Practice**
> Researchers in four care homes developed a program of seven daily drink rounds. A brightly decorated cart was pushed around the facility to serve a variety of beverages and frozen ice treats at seven designated times throughout the day. The cart was brightly decorated with a theme such as sports or holidays. Staff training was provided, and staff were involved in choosing the seven times of the day that worked for their facility.
>
> *Reference:* Lean, K., Nawaz, R.F., Jawad, S., & Vincent, C. (2019). Reducing urinary tract infections in care homes by improving hydration. *BMJ Open Quality, 8*(3), e000563. https://doi.org/10.1136/bmjoq-2018-000563

DIAGNOSTIC TESTS. The primary diagnostic test is a serum sodium level, which in hyponatremia registers below 135 mEq/L. The serum osmolarity also decreases in patients with hyponatremia. Other laboratory results may be affected if the patient experiences an accompanying fluid imbalance. Serum chloride (Cl$^-$), an anion, is often depleted when sodium decreases because these two electrolytes commonly combine as NaCl (salt in solution, or saline).

THERAPEUTIC MEASURES. Therapeutic measures focus on resolving the cause of hyponatremia and replacing lost sodium. The HCP may order IV saline for patients who have hyponatremia without fluid excess.

For patients who have a fluid excess, a fluid restriction is often ordered. Diuretics that rid the body of fluid but do not cause sodium loss may also be used. For patients with cerebral edema, steroids may be prescribed to reduce intracranial swelling. I&O are strictly monitored. The patient is weighed daily. Implement interventions to keep patient safe if mental status is affected.

Hypernatremia

Hypernatremia occurs when the serum sodium level is above 145 mEq/L.

PATHOPHYSIOLOGY AND ETIOLOGY. A serum sodium increase may be an actual increase or a relative increase. In an actual increase, the patient receives too much sodium or is unable to excrete sodium, as in kidney failure. In a relative increase, the amount of sodium does not change, but the amount of fluid in the intravascular space decreases. Therefore, the percentage of sodium (solute) is increased in relationship to the amount of plasma.

In mild hypernatremia, most excitable tissues, such as muscle and neurons of the brain, become more stimulated. The patient becomes irritable and has tremors. In severe cases, these tissues fail to respond.

PREVENTION. Prevention of hypernatremia is not as simple as prevention of hyponatremia. Most patients have a sodium excess as a result of an acute or chronic illness. Patients with a potential for electrolyte imbalance must have their IV fluids carefully regulated.

SIGNS AND SYMPTOMS. Thirst is usually one of the first symptoms to appear. If you eat salty foods, such as potato chips, the amount of sodium in your body increases, and you become thirsty. Other signs and symptoms of hypernatremia are vague and nonspecific until severe excess is present. Like the patient with a sodium deficit, the patient experiencing sodium excess has mental status changes, such as agitation, confusion, and personality changes. However, this time the cause is too little fluid in the brain tissues. Seizures may also occur.

At first, muscle twitches and unusual contractions may be present. Later, skeletal muscle weakness occurs that can lead to respiratory failure if it affects the diaphragm. If fluid deficit or fluid excess accompanies the hypernatremic state, the patient also has signs and symptoms associated with these imbalances.

COMPLICATIONS. A patient with severe hypernatremia may become comatose or have respiratory arrest as skeletal muscles weaken.

DIAGNOSTIC TESTS. The most reliable diagnostic test is the serum sodium level. This indicates an increase above the normal level. Serum osmolarity may also increase. If the patient has a fluid imbalance, other laboratory values, such as BUN, hematocrit, and urine-specific gravity, are also affected (see earlier discussion).

• WORD • BUILDING •
intracranial: intra—within + cranial—cranium (skull)

THERAPEUTIC MEASURES. If a fluid imbalance accompanies hypernatremia, it is treated first. For example, fluid replacement without sodium in a patient with dehydration should correct a relative sodium excess. If the kidneys are not excreting adequate amounts of sodium, diuretics may help if the kidneys are functional. If the kidneys are not functioning properly, dialysis may be ordered (see Chapter 37). I&O and daily weights are strictly monitored.

The cause of hypernatremia is also treated in an attempt to prevent further episodes of this imbalance. For some patients, a sodium-restricted diet is prescribed.

Potassium Imbalances

Potassium is the most common electrolyte in the ICF compartment. Only a small amount, 3.5 to 5.3 mEq/L (3.5–5.3 mmol/L), is found in the bloodstream. Small changes in this laboratory value cause major changes in the body.

Potassium is especially important for cardiac muscle, skeletal muscle, and smooth muscle function. If the serum potassium level falls, the body attempts to compensate by moving potassium from the cells into the bloodstream.

The two potassium imbalances are **hypokalemia** (potassium deficit) and **hyperkalemia** (potassium excess). Hypokalemia is the most commonly occurring imbalance.

Hypokalemia

Hypokalemia occurs when the serum potassium level falls below 3.5 mEq/L.

PATHOPHYSIOLOGY AND ETIOLOGY. Most cases of hypokalemia result from inadequate intake of potassium or excessive loss of potassium through the kidneys. Hypokalemia most often occurs as a result of medications. Potassium-wasting diuretics (e.g., furosemide and hydrochlorothiazide) and corticosteroids (e.g., prednisone) are examples of drugs that cause increased excretion of potassium from the body. Potassium may also be lost through the gastrointestinal (GI) tract, which is rich in potassium and other electrolytes. Severe vomiting, diarrhea, and prolonged GI suction cause hypokalemia ("Patient Perspective"). Major surgery and hemorrhage can also lead to potassium deficit.

PREVENTION. Most patients having major surgery receive potassium supplements in their IV fluids to prevent hypokalemia. For patients receiving drugs known to cause hypokalemia, potassium supplements or foods high in potassium may prevent a deficit (see Table 6.2).

SIGNS AND SYMPTOMS. Many body systems are affected by a potassium imbalance. Muscle cramping or muscle fatigue can occur with either a deficit or an excess of potassium. Vital signs change because respiratory and cardiovascular systems need potassium to function properly. Diminished skeletal muscle activity results in shallow, ineffective respirations. The pulse is typically weak, irregular, and thready because the heart muscle is depleted of potassium. A major danger, irregular heartbeat (**arrhythmia**), can cause cardiac arrest. Orthostatic (postural) hypotension may be present.

> **Patient Perspective**
>
> **Patricia.** I take hydrochlorothiazide for my high blood pressure. Since it can make me lose potassium, I also take a potassium supplement. So, I thought I was all set. But recently I ate something that did not agree with me, and I had diarrhea for a couple of days. One morning as I was driving to work, I felt so weak it frightened me. I drove back home and asked my husband to drive me to work. I arrived safely, but as I walked down the hallway, I again felt so weak I had to sit down. I felt like I could not put one foot in front of the other. I kept thinking, "This is all in my head." I decided maybe I was dehydrated from the diarrhea, so I drank a bottle of Gatorade and a glass of orange juice. Slowly, I began to feel a bit better, and I made it through the day. After work, I had to take my daughter to the doctor, so I asked about my symptoms. I was sent to the lab, where I had my potassium level checked, and it was 3.1! Normal is 3.5 to 5.3 mEq/L. Mine must have been even lower before I drank the juice and Gatorade. I learned that I probably lost a lot of potassium because of the diarrhea. I also learned that low potassium made my muscles weak and could affect my heart function. Next time I have diarrhea, I will call my doctor.

The nervous system is usually affected as well. The patient experiences changes in mental status followed by lethargy. The motility of the GI system is slowed, causing nausea, vomiting, abdominal distention, and constipation. Vomiting may further increase potassium loss.

COMPLICATIONS. If not corrected, hypokalemia can result in death from arrhythmia, or respiratory failure and arrest. The patient must be treated promptly before these complications occur.

DIAGNOSTIC TESTS. The primary laboratory test is a serum potassium level. The patient's electrocardiogram (ECG) may show cardiac arrhythmias associated with potassium deficit. In addition to a decrease in the serum potassium level, the patient may have an acid–base imbalance known as metabolic **alkalosis**. This commonly accompanies hypokalemia. In metabolic alkalosis, the serum pH of the blood increases (more than 7.45) so that the blood is more alkaline than usual. Acid–base imbalances are discussed later in this chapter.

THERAPEUTIC MEASURES. The goal of treatment is to replace potassium in the body and resolve the underlying cause of the

• WORD • BUILDING •

hypokalemia: hypo—less than + kal—potassium + emia—blood
hyperkalemia: hyper—more than + kal—potassium + emia—blood
arrhythmia: dys—bad or disordered + rhythmia—measured motion
alkalosis: alkal—alkaline + osis—condition

imbalance. For mild to moderate hypokalemia, oral potassium supplements are given. For severe hypokalemia, IV potassium supplements are given. Because the kidneys eliminate excess potassium, potassium should be administered only after the patient has voided, to be sure the kidneys are functioning. Potassium is a potentially dangerous drug, especially when administered intravenously. In too high a concentration, it causes cardiac arrest. Only IV solutions that are premixed and carefully labeled should be used. Potassium is *never* given by IV push. The patient's laboratory values must be monitored carefully to prevent giving too much potassium.

Teach the patient about the side effects of oral potassium and precautions associated with potassium administration. Box 6.4 summarizes the precautions the patient should be aware of when taking oral potassium supplements.

LEARNING TIP
Six L's of Hypokalemia
Lethargy
Lethal cardiac arrhythmias
Leg cramps
Limp muscles
Low, shallow respirations
Less stool (constipation)

BE SAFE!
AVOID FAILURE TO RECOGNIZE! You can be alert for hypokalemia in patients who have several risk factors, such as having a nasogastric tube, taking a potassium-wasting diuretic, and being on NPO status (they are losing potassium without intaking more). Monitor the patient closely for weak pulses, decreased blood pressure, shallow respirations, muscle cramps, and weakness. Respond quickly if symptoms are present.

Hyperkalemia
Hyperkalemia is a condition in which the serum potassium level exceeds 5.3 mEq/L. It is rare in a person with healthy kidneys.

PATHOPHYSIOLOGY AND ETIOLOGY. Hyperkalemia may result from an actual increase in the amount of total body potassium or from the movement of intracellular potassium into the blood. Overuse of potassium-based salt substitutes or excessive intake of oral or IV potassium supplements can cause hyperkalemia. Use of potassium-sparing diuretics (e.g., spironolactone [Aldactone]) may contribute to hyperkalemia. Patients with kidney failure are at risk because the kidneys cannot excrete potassium.

Movement of potassium from cells into the blood and other ECF is common in massive tissue trauma and metabolic acidosis. Metabolic **acidosis** is an acid–base imbalance commonly seen with uncontrolled diabetes mellitus. Acid–base imbalances are discussed later in this chapter.

Box 6.4
Tips for Patients Taking Oral Potassium Supplements
- Do not substitute one potassium supplement for another.
- Take all forms of potassium with a full glass of water or juice.
- Dilute powders and liquids in water or juice exactly as directed.
- Do not crush extended-release potassium tablets, such as Slow-K or K-Dur tablets.
- Do not take potassium supplements if you take potassium-sparing diuretics such as spironolactone (Aldactone) or triamterene (Dyrenium).
- Tell your doctor if you use salt substitutes containing potassium.
- Take potassium supplements with meals.
- Report adverse effects, such as nausea, vomiting, diarrhea, and abdominal cramping, to the HCP.
- Have frequent laboratory testing for potassium levels as recommended by the HCP.

PREVENTION. For patients receiving potassium supplements, hyperkalemia can be prevented by monitoring serum electrolyte values and the patient's symptoms and adjusting the dose accordingly.

SIGNS AND SYMPTOMS. Most cases of hyperkalemia occur in patients who are hospitalized or undergoing therapeutic measures for a chronic condition. The classic manifestations are muscle twitches and cramps later followed by profound muscular weakness; increased GI motility (diarrhea); slow, irregular heart rate; weak pulse; and decreased blood pressure.

COMPLICATIONS. Cardiac arrhythmias and respiratory failure can occur in severe hyperkalemia, causing death.

DIAGNOSTIC TESTS. In addition to an elevated serum potassium level, electrocardiograph (ECG) changes are also associated with hyperkalemia. If the patient has metabolic acidosis, the serum pH falls below 7.35.

THERAPEUTIC MEASURES. For mild, chronic hyperkalemia, dietary limitation of potassium-rich foods may be helpful. Potassium supplements are discontinued. Potassium-wasting diuretics are given to patients with healthy kidneys. For patients with kidney problems, a cation exchange resin, such as sodium polystyrene sulfonate, may be administered either orally or rectally. This drug releases sodium and absorbs potassium for excretion through the stool and out of the body.

• WORD • BUILDING •
acidosis: acid—acidic + osis—condition

In cases in which cellular potassium has moved into the bloodstream, administration of glucose and insulin can facilitate the movement of potassium back into the cells. During treatment of moderate to severe hyperkalemia, the patient should be in the hospital on a cardiac monitor.

Calcium Imbalances

Calcium is a mineral that is primarily stored in bones and teeth. A small amount is found in ECF. The normal value for serum calcium is 8.2 to 10.2 mg/dL, or 2.1 to 2.6 mmol/L. Minimal changes in serum calcium levels can have major negative effects in the body.

Calcium is needed for the proper function of excitable tissues, especially cardiac muscle. The two calcium imbalances are **hypocalcemia** and **hypercalcemia.**

Hypocalcemia

Hypocalcemia occurs when the serum calcium level falls below 8.2 mg/dL, or 2.1 mmol/L.

PATHOPHYSIOLOGY AND ETIOLOGY. Although calcium deficit can be acute or chronic, most patients develop hypocalcemia slowly as a result of chronic disease or poor intake. Postmenopausal women are most at risk for hypocalcemia. As a woman ages, calcium intake typically declines. The parathyroid glands recognize this decrease and stimulate bone to release some of its stored calcium into the blood for replacement. The result is a condition known as **osteoporosis,** in which bones become porous and brittle and fracture easily. The woman who is postmenopausal has a decreased level of estrogens, a hormone that helps prevent bone loss in the younger woman. Immobility or decreased mobility also contributes to bone loss in many patients. The patients at highest risk for osteoporosis are thin, petite White women.

Hypocalcemia can also result from inadequate absorption of calcium from the intestines, as seen in patients with Crohn disease, a chronic inflammatory bowel disease. Insufficient intake of vitamin D prevents calcium absorption as well. Conditions that interfere with the production of parathyroid hormone, such as partial or complete surgical removal of the thyroid or parathyroid glands, can also cause hypocalcemia.

Finally, patients with hyperphosphatemia (usually those with kidney failure) often experience hypocalcemia. Calcium and phosphate have an inverse relationship. When one of these electrolytes increases, the other tends to decrease.

PREVENTION. In the United States, the typical daily calcium intake is less than 550 mg. The recommended dietary allowance (RDA) of calcium for adults ages 19 to 50 and men ages 51 and 70 is 1,000 mg; the RDA for women over age 50 and men over 70 is 1,200 mg.

Hypocalcemia can be prevented by consuming calcium-rich foods and taking calcium supplements. These supplements can be purchased over the counter in any pharmacy or grocery. At least half the recommended amount of calcium should come from foods. An inexpensive source of calcium for patients who do not require vitamin D supplementation is calcium carbonate (Tums), which has 240 mg of elemental calcium in each tablet. Caution patients not to routinely take high doses of calcium without checking with their HCP.

Vitamin D supplementation may be required in addition to calcium for patients whose sun exposure is limited. The sun's ultraviolet light causes the skin to manufacture vitamin D.

SIGNS AND SYMPTOMS. Chronic hypocalcemia is usually not diagnosed until the patient breaks a bone, usually a hip. Acute hypocalcemia can occur after surgery or in patients with acute pancreatitis. Signs include changes in heart rate, decreased blood pressure, mental status changes, hyperactive deep tendon reflexes, and increased GI motility, including diarrhea and abdominal cramping. Two classic signs that can be used to test for hypocalcemia are Trousseau sign and Chvostek sign.

To test for Trousseau sign, inflate a blood pressure cuff around the patient's upper arm for 1 to 4 minutes. In a patient with hypocalcemia, the hand and fingers become spastic and go into palmar flexion (Fig. 6.4). To test for Chvostek sign, tap the face just below and in front of the ear. Facial twitching on that side of the face indicates a positive test (Fig. 6.5). Trousseau sign is more specific for hypocalcemia than Chvostek sign.

> **LEARNING TIP**
> You can remember which sign is **CH**vostek sign because it causes spasm near the **CH**eek.

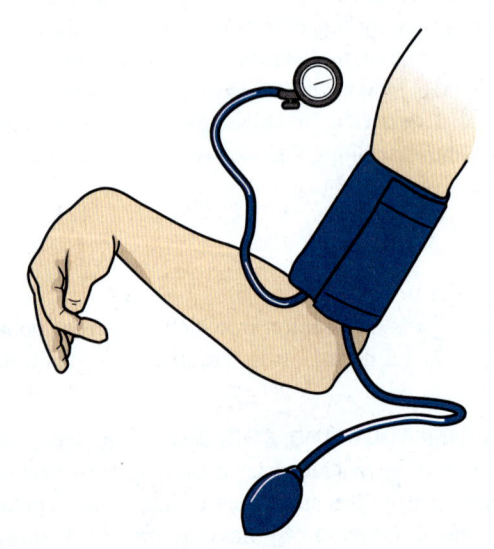

FIGURE 6.4 Trousseau sign.

• WORD • BUILDING •
hypocalcemia: hypo—less than + calc—calcium + emia—blood
hypercalcemia: hyper—more than + calc—calcium + emia—blood
osteoporosis: osteo—bone + porosis—porous

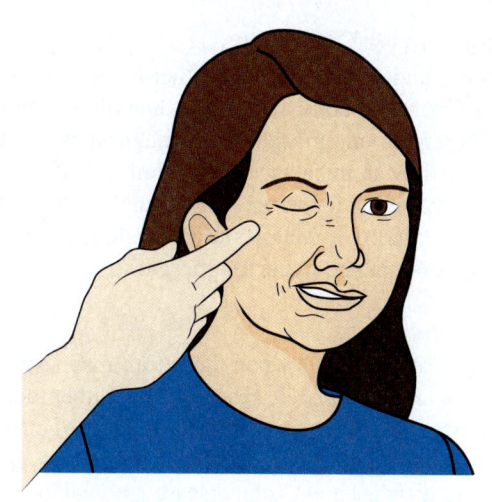

Chapter 6 Nursing Care of Patients With Fluid, Electrolyte, and Acid–Base Imbalances

FIGURE 6.5 Chvostek sign.

COMPLICATIONS. In severe hypocalcemia, neuromuscular irritability can lead to *tetany,* or continuous muscle contraction. The patient may have a sudden laryngospasm that will stop air from entering the lungs. Seizures, respiratory failure, or cardiac failure can occur and be fatal if not aggressively treated.

DIAGNOSTIC TESTS. The patient with hypocalcemia has a low serum calcium level and abnormal ECG. Parathyroid hormone level may increase as it attempts to stimulate bone to release calcium into the blood.

THERAPEUTIC MEASURES. In addition to treating the cause of hypocalcemia, calcium is replaced. For mild or chronic hypocalcemia, oral calcium supplements with or without vitamin D are given. Calcium supplements should be administered 1 to 2 hours after meals to increase intestinal absorption. Be sure to check compatibility when administering calcium with other medications.

For patients with acute or severe hypocalcemia, IV calcium gluconate or calcium chloride is given. When a patient has had thyroid or parathyroid surgery, there is a danger that parathyroid hormone will be decreased, causing serum calcium to drop. IV calcium must be readily available for emergency use if signs of hypocalcemia occur.

> **BE SAFE!**
> **ACT FAST!** Following thyroidectomy, if the patient becomes hypotensive and has a positive Chvostek sign, the nurse must collaborate with the HCP to correct the calcium imbalance and prevent serious complications for the patient.

For patients with hyperphosphatemia, usually those with kidney failure, aluminum hydroxide is used to bind the excess phosphate for elimination via the GI tract. As the phosphate decreases, the serum calcium level begins to normalize.

Diet therapy is an important part of treatment. Teach the patient, family, or other caregiver which foods are high in calcium (Table 6.3). Many foods today are fortified with calcium. Vitamin D foods are also encouraged, especially milk and other dairy products. For patients experiencing difficulty digesting dairy products and those who choose not to use dairy products, special attention must be paid to including other dietary calcium sources in the diet.

Hypercalcemia

Hypercalcemia occurs when the serum calcium is above 11 mg/dL, or 5.5 mEq/L.

PATHOPHYSIOLOGY AND ETIOLOGY. Chronic hypercalcemia can result from excessive intake of calcium or vitamin D, kidney failure, hyperparathyroidism, cancers, and overuse or prolonged use of thiazide diuretics, such as hydrochlorothiazide. Acute hypercalcemia can occur as an emergency in patients with invasive or metastatic cancers, especially cancers of the blood or bone.

Table 6.3
Food Sources of Calcium*

Food	Calcium (mg)
Fortified ready-to-eat cereals (various), 3/4 to 1 1/4 cup	137–1,000
Parmesan cheese, hard, 1.5 oz	503
Plain yogurt, nonfat, 8 oz	452
Almond milk (all flavors), 1 cup	451
Tofu, raw, regular, prepared with calcium sulfate, 1/2 cup	438
Soymilk (all flavors), 1 cup	340
Mustard spinach (tender, green), raw, 1 cup	315
Mozzarella cheese, part skim, 1.5 oz	304
Skim milk (nonfat), 1 cup	299
Cheddar cheese, 1.5 oz	287
Whole milk, 1 cup	276
White beans, 1 cup	179
Chia seeds, 1 tablespoon	126
Sardines canned with bones, 3 oz	325

*Both calcium content and bioavailability should be considered when selecting dietary sources of calcium.
Source: Adapted from U.S. Department of Health and Human Services and U.S. Department of Agriculture. (2015). *2015–2020 Dietary guidelines for Americans* (8th ed.). Washington, DC: Author, Appendix 11, Food sources of calcium. https://health.gov/dietaryguidelines/2015/guidelines/appendix-11/

> **CRITICAL THINKING & CLINICAL JUDGMENT**
>
> **Mrs. Wright** is a 77-year-old petite Caucasian woman who lives alone at home. She is on a fixed income and rarely eats calcium-rich foods. She recently fell and broke her hip. After surgery, she returned home under the care of a home health-care agency.
>
> **Critical Thinking (The Why)**
> 1. What factors made the patient at high risk for a fracture?
> 2. What would you expect her serum calcium level to have been before the fall?
>
> **Clinical Judgement (The Do)**
> 3. What patient teaching related to diet and calcium supplements should the home health nurse include during their home visits?
> 4. With whom should the nurse collaborate to assist Mrs. Wright?
>
> Suggested answers are at the end of the chapter.

PREVENTION. Although many causes of increased calcium cannot be prevented, a person receiving calcium supplements should be monitored carefully. Some patients believe that if two or three tablets a day are helpful, consuming twice as many will help even more. The result can be serum calcium excess. Educating the public about the proper amount of calcium needed each day and the danger of too much calcium is very important.

SIGNS AND SYMPTOMS. Patients who have mild hypercalcemia or a slowly progressing calcium increase may have no obvious signs and symptoms. However, acute hypercalcemia is associated with increased heart rate and blood pressure, skeletal muscle weakness, and decreased GI motility.

COMPLICATIONS. In some cases, the patient may experience kidney or urinary calculi (stones) resulting from excess calcium. In more severe cases of acute hypercalcemia, the patient may experience respiratory failure caused by profound muscle weakness or heart failure caused by arrhythmias.

THERAPEUTIC MEASURES. Patients with severe hypercalcemia should be hospitalized and placed on a cardiac monitor. Unless contraindicated by other conditions, the primary treatment is to give IV fluids and promote diuresis. Saline infusions are the most useful solutions to promote renal excretion of calcium.

The HCP also discontinues thiazide diuretics if the patient was receiving them and prescribes diuretics that promote calcium excretion, such as furosemide. Drugs such as pamidronate disodium (Aredia), zoledronic acid (Zometa), or calcitonin, which slow calcium movement from bones to the blood, may also be used.

If hypercalcemia is so severe that cardiac problems are present, hemodialysis, peritoneal dialysis, or ultrafiltration may be necessary to cleanse the blood of excess calcium. (See Chapter 37 for discussion of these procedures.)

Magnesium Imbalances

Magnesium and calcium work together for the proper functioning of excitable cells, such as cardiac muscle and nerve cells. Therefore, an imbalance of magnesium is usually accompanied by an imbalance of calcium.

The normal value for serum magnesium is 1.6–2.2 mg/dL (0.66–0.91 mmol/L). Magnesium imbalances are called **hypomagnesemia** and **hypermagnesemia.**

Hypomagnesemia

Hypomagnesemia occurs when the serum magnesium level falls below 1.6 mEq/L. It results from either decreased intake or excessive loss of magnesium. Causes of inadequate intake include malnutrition and starvation diets. Patients with severe diarrhea and Crohn disease are unable to absorb magnesium in the intestines.

One of the major causes of hypomagnesemia is alcoholism. Alcohol causes both decreased intake and increased renal excretion of magnesium. Certain drugs, such as loop and osmotic diuretics, aminoglycosides (e.g., gentamicin [Garamycin]), and some anticancer agents (e.g., cisplatin [Platinol]), can increase renal excretion of magnesium.

The signs and symptoms of hypomagnesemia are similar to those for hypocalcemia, including positive Trousseau and Chvostek signs, described earlier in this chapter.

The goal of management is to treat the underlying cause and replace magnesium in the body. Magnesium sulfate is administered intravenously. Oral replacement of magnesium oxide or magnesium-containing antacids can also be taken. If the serum calcium is also low, calcium replacement is prescribed. The patient is placed on a cardiac monitor because of magnesium's effect on the heart. Life-threatening arrhythmias can lead to cardiac failure and arrest.

Hypermagnesemia

Hypermagnesemia results when the serum magnesium level increases above 2.2 mEq/L. The most common cause of hypermagnesemia is increased intake coupled with decreased renal excretion caused by kidney failure.

Signs and symptoms are usually not apparent until the serum level is greater than 4 mEq/L. Then, the signs and symptoms include bradycardia and other arrhythmias, hypotension, lethargy or drowsiness, and skeletal muscle weakness. If not treated, the patient experiences coma, respiratory failure, or cardiac failure.

When kidneys are functioning properly, loop diuretics such as furosemide and IV fluids can increase magnesium excretion. For patients with kidney failure, dialysis may be the only option.

• **WORD** • **BUILDING** •

hypomagnesemia: hypo—less than + magnes—magnesium + emia—blood

hypermagnesemia: hyper—more than + magnes—magnesium + emia—blood

ACID–BASE BALANCE

The cells of the body function best when the body fluids and electrolytes are within a narrow range. Hydrogen (H^+) is another ion that must stay within its normal limits. The amount of hydrogen determines whether a fluid is an acid or base.

An *acid* is a substance that releases a hydrogen ion. The stronger the acid, the higher the number of hydrogen ions released. A common acid in the body is hydrochloric acid (HCl), which is found in the stomach. A *base* is a substance that binds hydrogen. A common base in the body is bicarbonate (HCO_3^-). *Alkali* is another word for "base."

Sources of Acids and Bases

Acids and bases are formed in the body as part of normal metabolic processes. Acids are formed as end products of glucose, fat, and protein metabolism. These are called fixed acids because they do not change once they are formed. Carbonic acid is a weak acid that can be formed when the carbon dioxide resulting from cellular metabolism combines with water. This acid can change to bicarbonate (a base) and hydrogen. It is, therefore, not a fixed acid.

The ECF maintains a delicate balance between acids and bases. The strength of the acids and bases can be measured by pH. The pH of a solution can vary from 0 to 14, with 7 being neutral, 0 to 6.99 being acid, and 7.01 to 14 being base, or alkaline. The normal serum pH level is 7.35 to 7.45, which is slightly alkaline. It must remain in this extremely narrow range to sustain life. An arterial pH lower than 6.9 or higher than 7.8 is usually fatal.

> **LEARNING TIP**
> The word *acid* has fewer letters and lower numbers (less than 7.35). *Alkaline* has more letters and higher numbers (greater than 7.45).

Control of Acid–Base Balance

The body has several ways in which it tries to compensate for changes in the serum pH. Three major mechanisms are used: cellular buffers, the lungs, and the kidneys.

Cellular buffers are the first to attempt a return of the pH to its normal range. Examples of cellular buffers are proteins, hemoglobin, bicarbonate, and phosphates. These buffers act as a type of sponge to "soak up" extra hydrogen ions if there are too many (too acidic) or release hydrogen ions if there are not enough (too alkaline).

The lungs are the second line of defense to restore normal pH. When the blood is too acidic (pH is decreased), the lungs "blow off" additional carbon dioxide through rapid, deep breathing. This reduces the carbon dioxide available to make carbonic acid in the body. If the blood is too alkaline (pH is increased), the lungs try to conserve carbon dioxide through shallow respirations.

The kidneys are the slowest to respond to changes in serum pH, taking as long as 24 to 48 hours to assist with compensation. The kidneys help in a number of ways, including regulating the amount of bicarbonate (base) kept in the body. If the serum pH lowers and becomes too acidic, the kidneys reabsorb additional bicarbonate rather than excreting it to help neutralize the acid. If the serum pH increases and becomes too alkaline, the kidneys excrete additional bicarbonate to get rid of the extra base. The kidneys also buffer pH by forming acids and ammonium (a base).

Acidosis or alkalosis that is corrected for by the body is referred to as *compensated*. The pH is returned to normal or near normal, but the gases that monitor acid–base balance (P_{CO_2} and HCO_3^-) are abnormal.

ACID–BASE IMBALANCES

Acid–base imbalances are caused by a number of acute and chronic illnesses or conditions. The primary treatment is to manage the underlying cause, which corrects the imbalance. The role of the nurse is to identify patients at risk and monitor laboratory test values for significant changes.

The laboratory tests used to evaluate acid–base balance are called arterial blood gases (ABGs). As the name implies, the blood sample analyzed must be from an artery rather than a vein. The femoral, brachial, and radial arteries are most often used. Table 6.4 lists ABG values and what they indicate.

The two broad types of acid–base imbalance are acidosis and alkalosis. Each of these imbalances can occur suddenly. This is called an *acute imbalance*. They can also develop over a long period, resulting in a *chronic imbalance*.

When the serum pH level falls below 7.35, the patient has acidosis because the blood becomes more acidic than normal. Too much acid or too little base in the body causes acidosis. Acidosis can be divided into two types: respiratory and metabolic. Respiratory acidosis is caused by problems occurring in the respiratory system. Metabolic acidosis is the result of problems in the rest of the body.

When the serum pH level increases above 7.45, the patient has alkalosis because the blood becomes more alkaline or basic. Alkalosis is caused by too little acid in the body or too much base. It can also be divided into two types: respiratory alkalosis and metabolic alkalosis.

See Figure 6.6 for details about respiratory and metabolic acid–base imbalances.

> **LEARNING TIP**
> Note the arrows in Table 6.4. In respiratory imbalances, the arrows are pointing in *opposite* directions. In metabolic imbalances, the arrows are pointing in the same or *equal* directions. So, simply remember "ROME": Respiratory Opposite, Metabolic Equal!

Table 6.4
Arterial Blood Gas Values and Changes in Acid–Base Imbalances

	pH	P_{CO_2}	HCO_3^-
Normal values	7.35–7.45	32–45 mm Hg	20–26 mEq/L
Respiratory acidosis	↓	↑	Normal
Respiratory acidosis with compensation	Nearly normal	↑	↑
Respiratory alkalosis	↑	↓	Normal
Respiratory alkalosis with compensation	Nearly normal	↓	↓
Metabolic acidosis	↓	Normal	↓
Metabolic acidosis with compensation	Nearly normal	↓	↓
Metabolic alkalosis	↑	Normal	↑
Metabolic alkalosis with compensation	Nearly normal	↑	↑

Acid-Base Imbalances

Acidosis
Too much acid or too little base

Respiratory
↓ pH ↑ CO_2
(Decreased ability of lungs to excrete CO_2)

Causes
- Decreased respiratory stimuli
- Anesthesia
- Drug overdose
- COPD, pneumonia
- Head injuries

Clinical Manifestations
- Headache
- Changes in LOC
- Hypoventilation
- Dyspnea
- Hyperkalemia

Body's Compensatory Mechanisms
Kidneys reabsorb more HCO_3 and excrete carbonic acid

Treatment
- Bronchodilators
- Noninvasive positive pressure ventilation
- Oxygen
- Smoking cessation

Metabolic
↓ pH ↓ HCO_3
(Decreased ability of kidneys to excrete acid or conserve base)

Causes
- DKA
- Severe diarrhea
- Renal failure
- Shock
- Intestinal suctioning

Clinical Manifestations
- Headache
- Decreased BP
- Hyperkalemia
- Warm, flushed skin
- Changes in LOC

Body's Compensatory Mechanisms
Deep, rapid breathing (Kussmaul's respirations) to rid body of CO_2

Treatment
- Sodium bicarbonate
- Treat underlying cause

Alkalosis
Too little acid or too much base

Respiratory
↑ pH ↓ CO_2
(Excessive excretion of carbonic acid)

Causes
- Hyperventilation (anxiety, fear)
- Mechanical ventilation
- Overactive thyroid

Clinical Manifestations
- Decreased LOC
- Deep, rapid breathing
- Tachycardia
- Hypokalemia
- Decreased BP

Body's Compensatory Mechanisms
Kidneys decrease the rate of HCO_3 reabsorption

Treatment
- Breathe into a paper bag
- Treat underlying cause

Metabolic
↑ pH ↑ HCO_3
(Excess HCO_3 or loss of acid)

Causes
- Overuse of antacids or baking soda
- Diuretics
- Vomiting
- Gastric suctioning

Clinical Manifestations
- Changes in LOC
- Nausea
- Vomiting
- Diarrhea
- Hypokalemia
- Tremors

Body's Compensatory Mechanisms
Slow, shallow respirations to increase CO_2 retention

Treatment
- Administer normal saline
- Supplemental potassium

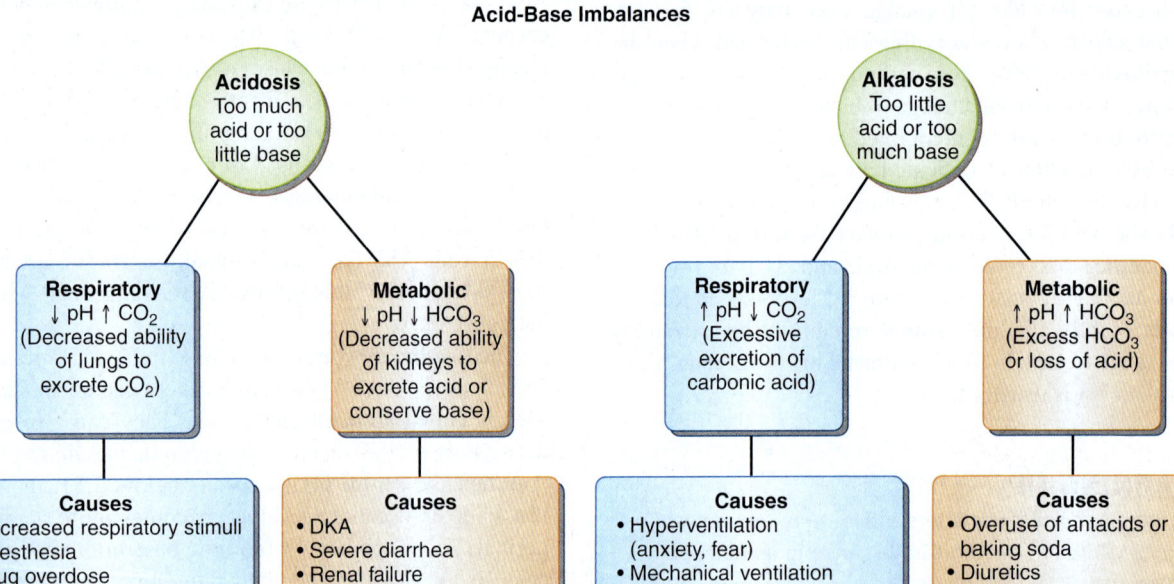

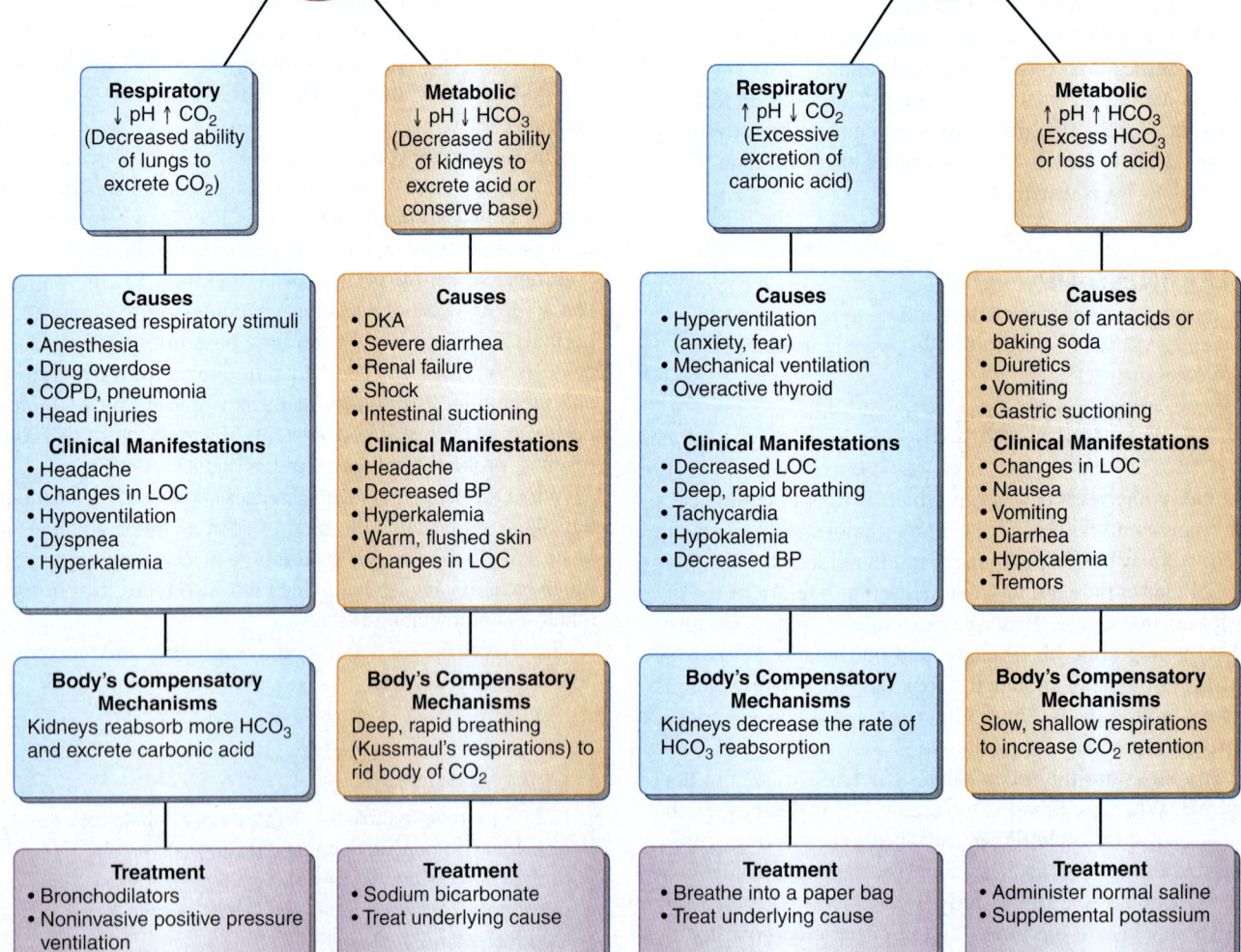

FIGURE 6.6 Mind map of acid–base imbalances.

Key Points

- Water is very important to the body for cellular metabolism, blood volume, body temperature regulation, and solute transport.
- Electrolytes are chemicals that can conduct electricity when dissolved in water. They carry either a positive electrical charge (cation) or a negative electrical charge (anion).
- Fluid deficit is the same as dehydration and occurs when there is not enough fluid in the body, especially in the blood.
- Fluid excess, also called overhydration, occurs when there is too much fluid in the bloodstream, causing dilution of electrolytes and red blood cells.
- Patients who are high risk for dehydration include older adults, infants, and children, as well as patients experiencing fluid loss through wounds, diseases, and suctioning. Patients at high risk for fluid volume excess are those receiving IV therapy, irrigations, and those with diseases that affect the kidneys or cause fluid retention.
- Data collection for patients with fluid and electrolyte imbalances includes comparing intake to output, monitoring rapid weight gain or loss, edema, lung sounds, and skin turgor, and reviewing electrolyte levels on laboratory reports.
- Therapeutic measures for patients with fluid and electrolyte imbalances include daily weights, strict intake and output, administering or withholding fluids as ordered, and determining and correcting the cause of the imbalances.
- Patient education for those with fluid imbalances includes identifying and reporting early signs and symptoms of dehydration or fluid excess to the HCP, reporting elevated temperature that can lead to fluid loss, recognizing foods high in sodium, using diuretics and potassium supplements correctly, and reporting any rapid weight gain.
- Electrolyte imbalances include either too much or too little of key electrolytes. In general, if a patient experiences a deficit of an electrolyte, the electrolyte is replaced either orally or intravenously. If the patient experiences an excess of an electrolyte, treatment focuses on getting rid of the excess, often via the kidneys. The underlying cause of the imbalance must also be treated.
- It is important to know the food sources of electrolytes to teach your patients with imbalances what to eat or what to avoid. Sodium is highest in processed and packaged foods such as frozen pizza, canned soups, and salad dressings. Potassium is found in sweet potatoes, baked potatoes, yogurt, milk, bananas, avocadoes, and orange juice. Foods highest in calcium include dairy products such as milk, cheese, and yogurt, as well as fortified cereals, soy, greens, and some fish, such as salmon and perch.
- Some common causes of acidosis include hypoventilation due to respiratory disease, drugs, or neurological problems that depress breathing. Other causes include end-stage renal disease and uncontrolled diabetes.
- Some common causes of alkalosis include hyperventilation due to anxiety or fear, mechanical ventilation, high altitudes, overuse of antacids or baking soda, as well as prolonged vomiting or gastric suction.
- The body strives to correct acidosis and alkalosis by making changes in respirations and the elimination of acids or bases. ABGs test for acidosis and alkalosis by measuring blood pH, carbon dioxide levels, and bicarbonate levels.

SUGGESTED ANSWERS TO CHAPTER EXERCISES

Cue Recognition

6.1: Consider that weight gain represents possible fluid retention. Check for signs of fluid overload such as edema, increased blood pressure, tachycardia, shortness of breath, or decrease in urine output.

6.2: As this level is dangerously low, the patient is at risk for changes in level of consciousness and possible seizures. Maintain a safe environment and protect the patient from injury.

Critical Thinking & Clinical Judgment

Mrs. Levitt

1. Mrs. Levitt is probably becoming dehydrated.
2. Check her weight and compare it with her previous weights. Dehydration is associated with weight loss. Monitor mental status for disorientation. Check skin turgor for tenting. Compare vital signs to usual vitals. Continue to monitor vital signs.
3. Encourage increased fluid intake. Notify the RN or HCP if Mrs. Levitt is unable to take in additional fluids or if the fluids do not normalize signs and symptoms.
4. Subjective: "My urine smells bad, and my heart is beating fast." Objective: Pt's urine is dark amber and smells strong. Weight 112# (baseline 116#); skin tenting present. VS: P 98 beats per minute, BP 126/74 mm Hg, RR 20 per minute, T 99.2. Fluids encouraged. RN notified.
5. Notify the RN but also the nursing assistant, who can help with encouraging fluids during and between meals as well as monitoring skin condition. Contact the dietary department to obtain beverages Mrs. Levitt prefers that do not contain caffeine.
6. Watch for her weight to return to normal, for her skin to feel more elastic, and for her urine to appear more dilute. Vital signs should also return to baseline.

SUGGESTED ANSWERS TO CHAPTER EXERCISES—Cont'd

Mr. Peters
1. If the fluid imbalance is not corrected, Mr. Peters could develop life-threatening pulmonary complications such as pleural effusions and/or pulmonary edema.
2. Raise the head of the bed to assist breathing.
3. Using the **WHAT'S UP?** format as a guide, ask the following questions: How are you feeling? Did anything aggravate your symptoms? When did your symptoms begin? On a scale of 0 to 10, how difficult is your breathing? Are you having any problems besides shortness of breath? What do you think might be happening? (If the patient is too dyspneic to answer, do not ask many questions.)
4. Check breath sounds for crackles, observe for dependent edema and ascites, observe for distended neck veins, observe skin for color and palpate temperature, check weight and compare with previous weight, and monitor I&O. Continue to monitor vital signs.
5. Notify the RN or HCP of your findings.

Mrs. Wright
1. The patient is at high risk for osteoporosis and, thus, fracture because she is an older, petite, Caucasian woman. In addition, she does not get much calcium in her diet.
2. Her serum calcium levels would be low or low-normal because the body will mobilize calcium in the bones to maintain serum calcium levels.
3. Teach her about consuming foods high in calcium, the need to be compliant with taking her calcium supplements, and to take the supplements 1 to 2 hours after meals for best absorption by the body.
4. She would benefit from physical therapy for ambulation and strengthening, occupational therapy for an evaluation of her home environment and possible assistive devices, and a dietitian for dietary counseling. Caution her to avoid taking more calcium than prescribed because that can also be harmful.

Additional Resources

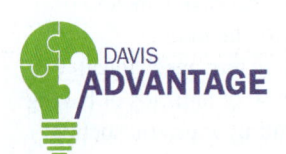

Go to Davis Advantage to complete your learning: strengthen understanding, apply your knowledge, and prepare for the Next Gen NCLEX®.

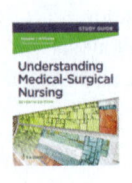

A Study Guide is also available.

CHAPTER 7
Nursing Care of Patients Receiving Intravenous Therapy

Gladdi Tomlinson

KEY TERMS

cannula (KAN-yoo-lah)
extravasation (eks-TRAH-vah-ZAY-shun)
hematoma (HEE-muh-TOH-mah)
hypodermoclysis (HY-poh-DUR-moh-CLY-sis)
infiltration (in-fil-TRAY-shun)
intravenous (IN-trah-VEE-nuss)
macrodrop (MACK-roh-DROP)
microdrop (MIKE-roh-DROP)
parenteral (pah-REN-ter-ul)
phlebitis (fleh-BY-tis)

CHAPTER CONCEPTS

Fluid and electrolyte balance
Nutrition
Safety

LEARNING OUTCOMES

1. Discuss how the practice of IV therapy is regulated.
2. List indications for IV therapy.
3. Plan nursing interventions to prevent IV therapy complications.
4. Identify common complications associated with IV therapy.
5. Calculate flow and drip rates for IV solutions.
6. Differentiate characteristics of isotonic, hypertonic, and hypotonic solutions.
7. Explain the differences between peripheral and central venous access devices.
8. Describe types of central venous access devices.
9. List indications for subcutaneous infusions (hypodermoclysis).

Intravenous (IV) therapy is the administration of fluids or medication via a needle or catheter (also called a **cannula**) directly into the bloodstream. Each state's nurse practice act governs the practice of IV therapy in that state. Some states' nurse practice acts now include IV therapy within the licensed practical nurse/licensed vocational nurse (LPN/LVN) role.

The Infusion Nurses Society (INS; www.ins1.org) is recognized as a global authority in infusion nursing and publishes standards of practice for infusion therapy. The INS (2021) standards of practice address the infusion-related scope of practice for LPNs and LVNs. The Institute for Healthcare Improvement (IHI, 2019; www.ihi.org; Jacob & Gaynes, 2019) provides information related to central line care. The National Institute for Occupational Safety and Health (NIOSH; www.cdc.gov/NIOSH) oversees workplace safety, including safety issues related to IV therapy. The American Society for Parenteral and Enteral Nutrition (ASPEN; www.nutritioncare.org) provides resources related to IV nutrition.

> **LEARNING TIP**
> National organizations provide guidelines, but you must look at your state nurse practice act to decide which of those guidelines applies to you!

• WORD • BUILDING •
intravenous: intra—within + venous—vein

69

INDICATIONS FOR INTRAVENOUS THERAPY

A variety of substances can be administered via IV therapy, including fluids, electrolytes, nutrients, blood products, and medications. Many medications are faster acting and more effective when given via the IV route. Fast action is especially important in an emergency. Medications can also be administered continuously via IV to maintain a therapeutic blood level. Patients with anemia or blood loss can receive lifesaving IV blood transfusions. Patients can receive life-sustaining fluids, electrolytes, and nutrition via IV when they are unable to eat or drink adequate amounts. Patients who cannot eat for an extended period can have their nutritional needs met with parenteral nutrition. The term **parenteral** refers to any medication route other than the digestive tract.

TYPES OF INTRAVENOUS INFUSIONS

There are four primary administration modes for IV medications: (1) continuous, (2) intermittent, (3) direct injection/IV push, and (4) patient-controlled analgesia.

Continuous Infusion

A continuous infusion is a large-volume infusion of solution or medications (typically 250–1,000 mL) administered over 2 to 24 hours. The HCP orders the infusion in milliliters (mL) to be delivered over a specific amount of time, such as 100 mL per hour or 1,000 mL over 8 hours. The infusion is kept running at the prescribed rate until ordered to be discontinued.

> **BE SAFE!**
> **BE VIGILANT!** Always verify that orders are complete and understandable. If you have any questions, contact the registered nurse, health-care provider, or pharmacist.

Continuous infusions are used when a medication must be highly diluted, a constant plasma concentration of a drug must be maintained, or a large volume of fluids and electrolytes must be administered. Rate control is important in the delivery of continuous infusions. It can be achieved by using an electronic infusion device (EID), mechanical controller, or roller clamp.

Intermittent Infusion

Some IV medications, such as antibiotics, need to be infused over a short period of time. For example, an antibiotic may be mixed with 50 to 100 mL of 5% dextrose or 0.9% sodium chloride solution and infused over 30 to 60 minutes. This is often done as an intermittent infusion. As with any IV therapy, health-care provider (HCP) orders must specify route, drug, dose, and amount to be infused over a specified time.

Primary Intermittent Infusion

Intermittent medications and solutions can be delivered using primary intermittent administration tubing that is connected and disconnected with each use. Access to the bloodstream can be provided by a short peripheral vascular access device, sometimes called a *saline lock*. With this device, an IV cannula is inserted and covered with a sterile needleless cap or valve that seals after each use.

> **BE SAFE!**
> **BE VIGILANT!** Each time a primary intermittent set is disconnected, the tip of the tubing must be kept sterile using a sterile end cap. To keep intermittent cannulas patent while not in use, flush peripheral intravenous (PIV) cannulas with saline, and flush central venous access devices (CVADs) with heparin (10 units/mL or 100 units/mL, based on agency policy.).

Piggyback (Secondary) Intermittent Infusion

If the patient already has a primary continuous IV infusing, the antibiotic (secondary) infusion can be "piggybacked" into the primary IV line. This is called an *intermittent infusion*, and the tubing is left attached to the primary administration set. For the intermittent infusion to work, it must hang higher than the primary infusion (Fig. 7.1). These can be infused using an EID, mechanical controller, or roller clamp.

> **PRACTICE ANALYSIS TIP**
> **Linking NCLEX-PN® to Practice**
> The LPN/LVN will administer intravenous piggyback (secondary) medications.

> **BE SAFE!**
> **BE VIGILANT!** The medication in the intermittent infusion tubing must be compatible with the solution that is in the primary intravenous tubing. Check with your pharmacy for compatibilities.

Needleless connectors provide connection to IV catheters (such as piggybacking into a primary IV line), administration sets, and syringes without a needle. They are important for avoiding needle stick injuries in nurses. Other terms used to describe such connectors are *injection cap*, *port*, or *injection valve*.

The hub or extension set of a peripheral cannula that is "capped off" with a needleless connector (saline lock, Fig. 7.2) is available for intermittent or emergency access.

• WORD • BUILDING •

parenteral: para—beside + enteral—intestines

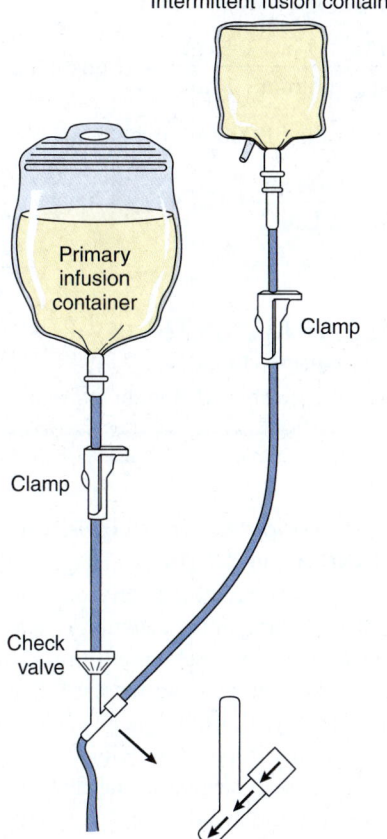

FIGURE 7.1 Gravity drip setup with intermittent infusion.

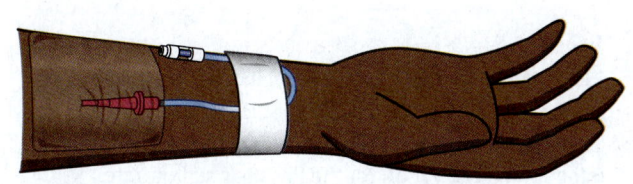

FIGURE 7.2 Peripheral IV with needleless connector attached to extension tubing.

In addition, because the needleless connector does not have to be removed to allow access, a sterile closed infusion system is maintained.

The patency (unobstructed flow) of an intermittent cannula must be maintained by flushing at periodic intervals based on institution flushing policy and procedure. Always check for patency of an intermittent device before administering a medication. Do this by first scrubbing the hub. Attach the syringe and draw back to check for backflow of blood. If blood is seen in the syringe, the catheter is patent. Once patency is confirmed, flush with normal saline (0.9% sodium chloride). To maintain patency of a cannula, flush the cannula after each use or at least every 12 hours if not in use or according to institution policy. In addition to ensuring patency, flushing with saline prevents mixing of incompatible medications and solutions. The INS recommends use of sodium chloride for maintaining peripheral intermittent devices. Heparin, an anticoagulant, is recommended for flushing CVADs. Remember that heparin is a medication and may be incompatible with other medications. Check your institution's policy for specific guidelines.

> **BE SAFE!**
> **BE VIGILANT!** "SCRUB THE HUB" with 70% alcohol or chlorhexadine and alcohol for 10 to 15 seconds using friction before each access to prevent infection!

Positive pressure must be maintained in the lumen of the cannula during the administration of the flush solution. This prevents a backflow of blood or solution into the cannula lumen, which could lead to an occlusion. Positive pressure maintains a closed infusion system within the needleless connector.

If resistance is met while a cannula is being flushed, a clot may be occluding the cannula. Do not exert pressure on the syringe plunger to restore patency. Doing so may dislodge the clot into the vascular system or rupture the cannula.

> **BE SAFE!**
> **BE VIGILANT!** Always check for cannula patency and follow manufacturer's guidelines for use before injecting any substance into the circulatory system. Forced flushing could cause a clot to dislodge from the cannula into the patient's circulatory system.

Direct Injection/Intravenous Push

An IV push, or direct injection medication, is injected slowly, between 1 and 10 minutes, via a syringe into an IV site or port. An IV push provides a rapid effect because it is delivered directly into the patient's bloodstream. IV push drugs can be dangerous if given incorrectly. A drug reference should always be checked to determine the safe amount of time over which the drug can be injected. IV push drugs are usually administered by registered nurses (RNs). They are not within the scope of practice of the LPN/LVN in some states. However, be aware of the drugs being given so you can assist in observing the patient for desired or adverse effects.

Patient-Controlled Analgesia

Patient-controlled analgesia (PCA) is used to deliver analgesic or pain medications. An EID or pump is used to deliver the analgesic drug. The EID is programmed to administer the prescribed amount to the patient when he or she presses a button. PCA administrations are usually done by RNs. They may not be within the scope of practice of the LPN/LVN. Verify with your state nurse practice act to determine whether PCA administration is within the LPN/LVN scope of practice. Again, be aware of the drugs being given so you can assist in observing the patient for desired or adverse effects.

> **BE SAFE!**
> **BE VIGILANT!** When administering medications through an IV line on a patient receiving PCA, remember to consider the PCA medication in the tubing when researching for incompatibilities.

METHODS OF INFUSION

Gravity Drip

Gravity can be used to administer a solution into a vein (see Fig. 7.1). The solution is positioned about 3 feet above the infusion site. If it is positioned too high above the patient, the infusion may run too fast. If positioned too low, it may run too slowly. Flow is controlled with a roller or screw clamp. A mechanical flow device can be added to achieve more accurate delivery of fluid.

Calculating Administration Rates

When using a gravity set, you must calculate the infusion rate and/or the drops (i.e., gtt, L. *guttae*) required per minute to deliver fluid at the ordered rate. Commercial parenteral administration sets vary in the number of drops delivering 1 mL of fluid. Sets typically deliver 10, 15, 20, or 60 drops per milliliter of fluid. Check the label on the administration set to determine how many drops per milliliter (known as the *drop factor*) are delivered by the set. Sets delivering 10, 15, or 20 drops per milliliter are called **macrodrop** sets. These are used for fluids that need to be infused more quickly. Sets delivering 60 drops per milliliter are called **microdrop** or minidrop sets. These are used for solutions that need to be infused more slowly.

To determine drops per minute for IV solution delivery, the nurse needs to know the amount of fluid to be given in a specified time interval and the drop factor of the administration set to be used. The formula for determining drops per minute is as follows:

$$\frac{mL}{hr \text{ or } hrs} \times \frac{1 \text{ hr}}{60 \text{ min}} \times \frac{gtt}{1 \text{ mL}} = gtt \text{ per minute}$$

> **LEARNING TIP**
> Always round to the nearest whole number when calculating drops per minute. You can't deliver a fraction of a drop!

The formula for determining milliliters per hour is as follows:

$$\frac{\text{Total \# of mL}}{\text{Total number of hrs}} = mL \text{ per hour}$$

SAMPLE PROBLEMS

Order: 125 mL of 5% dextrose and 0.45% sodium chloride per hour

Drop factor: 15 gtt/mL

$$\frac{125 \text{ mL}}{1 \text{ hr}} \times \frac{1 \text{ hr}}{60 \text{ min}} \times \frac{15 \text{ gt}}{1 \text{ mL}} = 31 \text{ gtt per minute}$$

Order: Normal saline 1,000 mL over 8 hours

$$\frac{1000 \text{ mL}}{8 \text{ hours}} = 125 \text{ mL per hour}$$

> **PRACTICE ANALYSIS TIP**
> **Linking NCLEX-PN® to Practice**
> The LPN/VN will calculate and monitor intravenous (IV) flow rate.

Factors Affecting Flow Rates of Gravity Infusions

CHANGE IN CANNULA POSITION. A change in the position of the cannula's tip can affect the infusion flow rate. If the *bevel* (the slanted opening of the cannula) is against the wall of the vein, the flow rate will decrease. If it is away from the wall of the vein, the flow rate can increase. Placement of a PIV in a joint area (wrist or elbow) can cause a kink in the cannula or change the tip position. Kinks may occur in the tubing. This can cause a change in the flow rate. Securing the cannula carefully and avoiding areas of joint flexion will minimize this problem. Remind patients to keep flexion to a minimum when an IV is placed near a joint.

> **BE SAFE!**
> **BE VIGILANT!** If the only useable vein is in an area of flexion (such as the wrist or antecubital space), secure the PIV appropriately. Remind patients to keep flexion to a minimum. Closely monitor the PIV site and flow rate.

HEIGHT OF THE SOLUTION. If an infusion is being administered by gravity, a change in the height of the infusion bag or bottle or a change in the level of the bed can increase or decrease the flow rate. The flow rate increases as the distance between the solution and the patient increases. A patient may inadvertently alter the flow rate greatly simply by standing up. The ideal height for a solution is 3 feet above the level of the patient's heart.

PATENCY OF THE CANNULA. A small clot or fibrin sheath can occlude the cannula lumen and decrease the flow rate or stop the flow completely. A fibrin sheath begins developing within the first 24 hours of the cannula insertion. Clot formation can result from irritation, vein wall injury from

• WORD • BUILDING •
macrodrop: macro—large + drop
microdrop: micro—small + drop

the insertion or tip position, increased venous pressure, or backup of blood into the cannula. Avoid use of a blood pressure cuff on the affected limb because of the resulting transient increase in venous pressure. A regular flush schedule helps maintain patency.

> **BE SAFE!**
> **BE VIGILANT!** Never exert pressure with a saline or heparin flush in an attempt to restore patency. Doing so could dislodge a clot into the vascular system or rupture the cannula.

Mechanical and Electronic Infusion Devices

Flow control devices, such as EIDs and mechanical controllers, regulate the rate of infusion and are used in all health care settings (Fig. 7.3). Mechanical controllers measure the amount of solution delivered and depend on gravity to deliver the infusion. EIDs, sometimes called *pumps*, use positive pressure to deliver the solution.

Pumps and controllers are used for infusing precise volumes and rates of solution. Institution policy often dictates use of controllers for very fast or slow rates and infusion of potent medications, such as heparin, concentrated morphine, and chemotherapy solutions. Some EIDs are portable and worn on the body. These are called ambulatory infusion devices. It is important to know the type of pump being used and follow the manufacturer's guidelines.

Filters

Filters can either be added to administration sets or built into the set during manufacturing. Various types of filters are available. The INS (2021) standards address the use of in-line filters to remove bacteria, fungi, particulate matter, air, and some endotoxins from IV fluids. In-line filters can also significantly reduce phlebitis in hospitalized patients. Check institution policy and manufacturers' guidelines for use of filters.

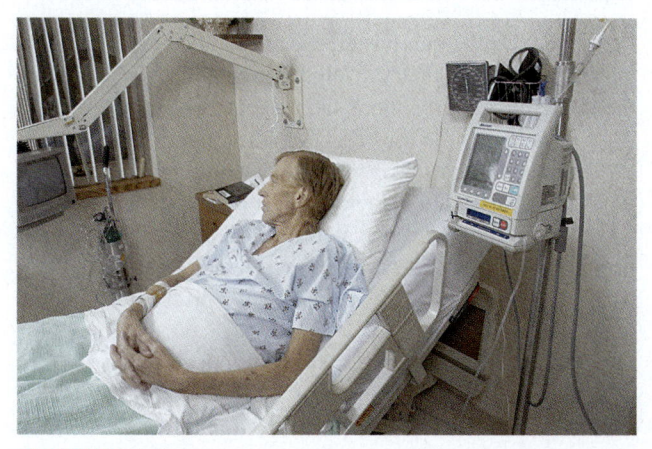

FIGURE 7.3 Infusion pump.

TYPES OF FLUIDS

There are three basic types of IV solutions: isotonic, hypotonic, and hypertonic (see Chapter 6). Fluids and electrolytes administered via the IV route pass directly into the plasma space of the extracellular fluid compartment. They are then absorbed based on the characteristics of the fluid and the hydration status of the patient. The most commonly infused fluids are dextrose and sodium solutions. These are called *crystalloid solutions.*

Crystalloid Solutions
Dextrose Solutions

Dextrose in water is available in many concentrations (2.5%, 5%, and 10%). It is typically used for continuous peripheral infusions. Concentrations above 10% must be infused via a central line into a large vein such as the subclavian vein.

Advantages of dextrose solutions include:

- They provide carbohydrates in a readily usable form for energy. This reduces breakdown of glycogen and catabolism of protein to help prevent negative nitrogen balance.
- They can be used to treat dehydration.
- They act as a means for medication administration.
- High concentrations can be used for treating hyperkalemia or hypoglycemia, or in combination with parenteral nutrition, because they supply a large number of calories.

Disadvantages of dextrose solutions include vein irritation, damage, and thrombosis. These issues can result when hypertonic dextrose solutions are administered in a peripheral vein.

Sodium Chloride Solutions

Sodium chloride solutions are available in concentrations of 0.25%, 0.33%, 0.45%, 0.9% (normal saline), 3%, and 5%. Sodium chloride 0.45% and 0.9% solutions are most common.

Advantages of sodium chloride solutions are as follows:

- They are useful for fluid replacement; treatment of shock, hyponatremia, and metabolic alkalosis; as a primer for blood transfusions; and during resuscitation after trauma. According to the American Association of Blood Banks, blood component administration sets can be primed only with 0.9% sodium chloride solution (Fung, Eder, Spitalnik, & Westhoff, 2017).
- They are useful to replace sodium and chloride in patients receiving nasogastric suctioning.
- Combination dextrose and sodium chloride solutions, such as 5% dextrose with 0.45% sodium chloride (often referred to as "D_5 and a half"), are commonly used for hydration and to check for kidney function before administration of potassium replacement therapy.

Disadvantages of sodium chloride solutions are as follows:

- They can cause circulatory overload if the prescribed rate is not monitored.
- If the patient is unable to excrete excess sodium (e.g., because of kidney disease or hormonal imbalance), hypernatremia can result.
- Acidosis can occur with continuous infusions.

Balanced Electrolyte Solutions

Electrolyte solutions replace lost fluids and electrolytes. A variety of balanced electrolyte solutions are available commercially. Maintenance electrolyte solutions, such as lactated Ringer solution, supply normal body electrolyte needs. Balanced solutions often contain lactate or acetate (yielding bicarbonate), which helps combat acidosis and provides a truly balanced solution. Potassium is an electrolyte commonly added to balanced solutions to replace potassium deficits. The patient must be monitored for signs and symptoms of potassium imbalance (see Chapter 6).

> **BE SAFE!**
> **BE VIGILANT!** Review institution guidelines for potassium administration before administration of any potassium-containing solution. An inappropriate rate or amount can cause a life-threatening cardiac arrhythmia!

Osmolarity of Intravenous Solutions

The osmolarity of an IV solution refers to its osmotic activity. As noted previously, IV fluids may be classified as isotonic, hypotonic, or hypertonic. (See Chapter 6 to review these concepts.) Isotonic fluids have the same ratio of solutes to water as body fluids. Hypertonic solutions have more solutes (i.e., are more concentrated) than body fluids. Hypotonic solutions have fewer solutes (i.e., are less concentrated) than body fluids. Water moves from areas of lesser concentration to areas of greater concentration. Therefore, hypotonic solutions send water into areas of greater concentration (cells). Hypertonic solutions pull water from cells.

Isotonic Solutions

Normal saline (0.9% sodium chloride) solution is an isotonic solution that has the same tonicity as body fluid. When administered to patients requiring water, it neither enters cells nor pulls water from cells; it therefore expands the extracellular fluid volume. A solution of 5% dextrose in water (D_5W) is also isotonic when infused. However, the dextrose is quickly metabolized, making the solution hypotonic. Lactated Ringer solution and 5% albumin are other examples of isotonic solutions. Isotonic solutions commonly treat dehydration, fluid loss, and hyponatremia.

> **BE SAFE!**
> **BE VIGILANT!** Since isotonic solutions expand the extracellular fluid volume, be vigilant for signs of fluid overload when infusing isotonic solutions. A good way to recognize early fluid overload is to monitor lung sounds for new onset or worsening of crackles.

Hypotonic Solutions

Hypotonic fluids are used when fluid is needed to enter the cells, as in the patient with cellular dehydration. They are also used as fluid maintenance therapy. Examples of hypotonic solutions are dextrose 2.5% water and 0.33% or 0.45% sodium chloride solution.

> **BE SAFE!**
> **BE VIGILANT!** Hypotonic solutions, because they leave the intravascular space and enter cells, can worsen hypotension, cause cardiovascular collapse, and increase intracranial pressure.

Hypertonic Solutions

Examples of hypertonic solutions include 5% dextrose in 0.9% sodium chloride, 3% sodium chloride, calcium chloride 10%, 5% dextrose in lactated Ringer solution, 10% dextrose in water, and albumin 25%. Hypertonic solutions are used to expand the plasma volume, for example, in a hypovolemic patient. They are also used to replace electrolytes.

> **BE SAFE!**
> **BE VIGILANT!** Monitor the patient receiving a hypertonic solution for circulatory overload. Monitor for and report elevation in blood pressure.

INTRAVENOUS ACCESS

IV therapy can be administered into the systemic circulation via the peripheral or central veins. Peripheral veins lie beneath the epidermis, dermis, and subcutaneous tissue of the skin. They usually provide easy access to the venous system.

Central veins are deeper and located closer to the heart. A CVAD is a special catheter with a tip that ends in a large vessel (i.e., superior vena cava) near the heart. This chapter primarily focuses on short peripheral catheters. The definitions of the various types of CVADs are discussed briefly at the end of the chapter.

See "Initiating Peripheral Intravenous Therapy" under Procedures in your online resources for a detailed explanation of how to initiate a peripheral IV cannula.

PRACTICE ANALYSIS TIP
Linking NCLEX-PN® to Practice
The LPN/VN will maintain and remove peripheral intravenous (IV) catheter.

NURSING PROCESS FOR THE PATIENT RECEIVING INTRAVENOUS THERAPY

IV therapy is a medical intervention. The nurse is responsible for appropriate assessment, monitoring, documentation, and reporting related to the therapeutic goals.

Data Collection
Some institutions require assessment of patients receiving IV therapy as often as every hour. The *INS Journal of Infusion Nursing* (2021) provides the INS infusion standards of practice for site assessment, including the following recommendations:

- Assess at least every 4 hours for patients not getting an irritant or vesicant who are alert and oriented.
- Assess every 1 to 2 hours for critically ill patients and adult patients who have cognitive sensory deficits, are receiving sedative medications or unable to notify the nurse of any problems, or have an IV placed in a joint area or external jugular vein.
- Assess every hour for pediatric or neonatal patients.
- Assess more frequently for any patient receiving vesicant medication.

Assessment should be systematic and thorough. It should include physiological and psychosocial data, critical laboratory values, allergies and environmental issues, and presence of adverse reactions or complications related to infusion therapy. Older adults are at increased risk for complications, making careful assessment essential ("Gerontological Issues").

The LPN/LVN collaborates with the RN to perform physical assessment. Daily weights and measurement of intake and output, help determine whether the patient is retaining too much fluid. Skin turgor, mucous membrane moisture, vital signs, and level of consciousness also indicate hydration status. New onset of fine crackles in the lungs can indicate fluid retention.

Inspect the insertion site for redness or swelling, evaluate the integrity of the dressing, and document your findings. Inspect the tubing to ensure tight connections and the absence of kinks or defects. Inspect the solution container and compare it with the HCP's order for type, amount, and rate. Report abnormal findings to the RN or HCP.

CLINICAL JUDGMENT
Mr. Rick, age 60, has a PIV with 0.9% saline infusing via gravity tubing. Blood is backed up in the IV tubing. When you open the clamp to increase the flow, nothing happens. What should you do?

Suggested answers are at the end of the chapter.

Gerontological Issues

Care of the Older Adult Receiving Intravenous Therapy.
When an older patient is receiving IV fluids, regularly monitor the patient for potential fluid volume excess. Symptoms of fluid volume excess include the following:

- Elevated blood pressure
- Increasing weight (a weight gain of 1 kg [2.2 lb] is equal to the retention of 1 L of body water)
- Peripheral edema
- Full bounding pulse
- Shallow, rapid respirations
- Jugular venous distention
- Increased urine output
- Development of moist crackles in the lungs
- Cyanosis (a late symptom of pulmonary edema)

If the above signs are present:

- Immediately notify the RN or turn down the IV to a minimum infusion rate (1 mL per minute); do not discontinue the IV because the HCP may want to order IV diuretics.
- Position the patient to maximize lung expansion.
- Check peripheral oxygen saturation with an oximeter.
- Apply oxygen by mask or nasal cannula if indicated and per institution guidelines.
- Closely monitor the patient's vital signs, level of consciousness, and oxygen saturation along with fluid output.
- Assist the HCP or RN with administration of diuretic medication such as furosemide if ordered.

Nursing Diagnoses, Planning, and Implementation
Priority nursing diagnoses for IV-related issues may include the following:

Risk for Fluid Volume Excess related to IV fluid administration

EXPECTED OUTCOME: The patient will have stable fluid balance as evidenced by stable vital signs, stable weight, and clear lung sounds (see "Gerontological Issues").

Impaired Physical Mobility related to placement and maintenance of IV cannula

EXPECTED OUTCOME: The patient will maintain mobility as evidenced by full range of motion and avoidance of complications related to immobility.

- Avoid insertion site close to joints if at all possible. *Joint areas are mobile, making it difficult to maintain an intact site.*
- If you must use a mobile site, such as the antecubital fossa or wrist area, immobilize the joint with an arm board or other immobilizer *to reduce cannula movement.* (Remember to get an order for this.)

- If site must be wrapped to protect from movement, be sure to leave insertion site visible or remove wrapping to view site according to agency policy. *The site must still be visualized for complications even if it is covered.*
- Assist patient with activities of daily living (ADLs). *The patient may have difficulty with ADLs if movement is limited.*

Risk for Infection related to broken skin or traumatized tissue

EXPECTED OUTCOME: The patient will be free from infection as evidenced by no redness, swelling, or purulence at IV insertion site; no fever; and normal white cell count.

- Monitor for signs of infection *so the IV can be removed and/or site rotated and infection treated quickly if it occurs.*
- Use good hand hygiene and strict aseptic techniques during cannula insertion and maintenance care *to prevent introduction of pathogens.*
- Change tubing and solutions regularly according to agency policy *to prevent growth of microorganisms.*
- Change or remove cannula when clinically indicated *to reduce prolonged risk.*

Evaluation

The RN is responsible for evaluation of outcomes and thus monitors the patient for evidence that the goals of therapy are being met and that complications are avoided. The LPN/LVN collects data that contribute to the evaluation. For example, if antibiotic therapy is administered, monitor for signs that the infection is resolving. If IV therapy is ordered to correct dehydration, monitor for improved fluid balance. Document all findings and report them to the RN.

> **BE SAFE!**
> **BE VIGILANT!** To prevent infection, the INS (2021) standards of practice state, "in addition to routine changes, the administration set (tubing) is changed whenever the peripheral catheter site is changed or when a new central vascular access device (CVAD) is placed." The INS also instructs clinicians to replace or remove any peripheral intravenous cannula placed in an emergency situation within 24 to 48 hours of the insertion or as soon as possible.

COMPLICATIONS OF IV THERAPY

Complications of infusion therapy fall into two categories: local and systemic. Any complication or unusual incident should be reported to the RN or HCP. A quality improvement report should be prepared according to institution policy.

The most common peripheral local complications are **hematoma, phlebitis,** or thrombophlebitis, **infiltration, extravasation,** and nerve injury (see Table 7.1). The INS (2021) lists the dorsal hand, radial wrist, and inner wrist as sites to avoid to prevent permanent nerve injury. Systemic complications can be serious. They include circulatory overload, septicemia, venous air embolism, and speed shock (a sudden reaction due to medication that is delivered too quickly). The nurse delivering infusion therapy must be knowledgeable in preventing, recognizing, and treating all complications of IV therapy (INS, 2021). See Table 7.1 for complications, prevention, and related care.

CRITICAL THINKING & CLINICAL JUDGMENT

Mrs. Gonzalez, age 47, has a PIV in the left forearm and is receiving 5% dextrose in water at 83 mL per hour via an EID. One hour after the infusion starts, she reports pain at the site. The site is cool to the touch and swollen, and the infusion rate is sluggish.

Critical Thinking (The Why)
1. What might be happening?

Clinical Judgment (The Do)
2. What additional data should you collect?
3. What action should you take?
4. How should you document your findings?
5. What other team members could be consulted to help in this situation?

Suggested answers are at the end of the chapter.

CUE RECOGNITION 7.1

You enter your patient's room to find the IV tubing disconnected from the bag of fluid and lying on the floor. The cannula is still in the patient's vein, and blood is backing up in the tubing. What should you do?

Suggested answers are at the end of the chapter.

CENTRAL VENOUS ACCESS DEVICES

The role of the LPN/LVN in CVAD care in most states is limited to assisting the RN with assessments. According to the 2020 NCLEX-PN Test Plan, the LPN can assist in maintaining a central venous catheter, assist in preparing the patient for insertion of the central line, and educate the patient on the reason for and care of a central venous device. It is important for you to be familiar with the different CVADs so you can recognize and report problems.

• WORD • BUILDING •
hematoma: hemat—blood + oma—tumor
phlebitis: phleb—vein + itis—inflammation
infiltration: in—inside + filtrate—to strain through + tion—condition
extravasation: extra—outside + vas—vessel + tion—condition

Table 7.1
Complications of Peripheral Intravenous Therapy

Complication	Signs and Symptoms	Prevention	Treatment
Local Complications of Intravenous (IV) Therapy			
Hematoma—bleeding around the cannula insertion site	• Ecchymoses • Swelling • Inability to advance cannula • Resistance during flushing	• Use indirect method of venipuncture (see procedure in online resources). • Choose smallest cannula appropriate. • Apply tourniquet just before venipuncture.	• Remove cannula. • Apply pressure with 2″ × 2″ gauze. • Elevate extremity. • Apply cold compress.
Thrombosis—a blood or fibrin clot in the cannula or vein	• Slowed or stopped infusion • Fever/malaise • Inability to flush or aspirate cannula	• Use an electronic infusion device (EID). • Choose microdrop sets with gravity flow if rate is less than 50 mL/hr. • Avoid use of flexion areas for insertion site.	• Discontinue cannula. • Apply cold compress to site. • Monitor for circulatory impairment. • Insert new cannula at another site.
Phlebitis—inflammation of the vein at or near the insertion site	• Redness/warmth at site • Local swelling • Pain • Palpable cord along vein • Sluggish infusion rate	• Use larger veins for hypertonic solutions. • Choose smallest cannula appropriate. • Use good hand hygiene. • Add buffer to irritating solutions. • Change solutions and containers every 24 hours. • Monitor peripheral IV (PIV) site per institution policy. • Remove cannula when clinically indicated.	• Discontinue cannula. • Apply cold compress initially; then warm. • Consult registered nurse (RN) or health-care provider (HCP) if severe.
Infiltration or extravasation—leaking of fluid or medication into the site around the cannula insertion (The term *extravasation* is used when a vesicant medication leaks and damages tissues.)	• Coolness of skin at site • Taut skin • Edema above or below site • Absent backflow of blood • Sluggish infusion rate • Pain or burning • Blisters (with extravasation)	• Place cannula in appropriate site. • Avoid antecubital fossa. • Stabilize cannula carefully. • Monitor PIV site per policy. • Instruct patient to notify RN immediately if any pain, burning, or swelling occurs.	• Discontinue cannula. • Apply cool/warm compress as indicated by solution type. • Elevate extremity. • Notify RN/HCP. • Follow agency infiltration/extravasation guidelines. • Have antidote available (if medication extravasates).
Local infection—infection at or near the insertion site	• Redness and swelling at site • Possible exudate • Elevated white blood cell and T lymphocytes	• Inspect all solutions for clarity. • Use sterile technique during venipuncture and site maintenance.	• Discontinue cannula. • Culture site and cannula. • Apply sterile dressing over site. • Notify RN/HCP. • Administer antibiotics if ordered.
Venous spasm—spasm in vein usually from irritation due to medication or cold fluids	• Sharp pain at site • Sluggish infusion	• Verify allergies. • Reduce infusion rate. • Dilute medications. • Keep IV solution at room temperature.	• Apply warm compress to site. • Restart infusion in new site if spasm continues. • Notify RN.

Continued

Table 7.1
Complications of Peripheral Intravenous Therapy—cont'd

Complication	Signs and Symptoms	Prevention	Treatment
Systemic Complications of Peripheral IV Therapy			
Septicemia—serious bloodstream infection	• Fever and chills • Profuse sweating • Nausea • Headache • Backache • Tachycardia/tachypnea • Hypotension • Altered mental status • Decreased urine output	• Use good hand hygiene. • Use aseptic techniques for insertion/maintenance of cannula, needleless connector, IV tubing, and solutions. • Carefully inspect fluids. • Cover infusion sites with appropriate dressings. • Follow standards of practice related to assessment and monitoring of PIV and hang time of infusions/IV tubing. • Use appropriate preparation solutions.	• Restart new IV system. • Obtain cultures. • Notify RN/HCP. • Initiate antimicrobial therapy as ordered. • Monitor patient closely.
Circulatory overload—too much fluid in circulatory system	• Rapid weight gain • Puffy eyelids • Edema • Increased blood pressure and pulse • Changes in input and output (I&O) • Rise in central venous pressure • Shortness of breath • Crackles in lungs • Cough • Distended neck veins	• Monitor infusion. • Maintain flow at prescribed rate. • Monitor I&O. • Know patient's cardiovascular history. • Do not "catch up" infusion if behind schedule. • Be alert that older patients are more prone to circulatory overload, and monitor closely.	• **CALL FOR HELP!** • Decrease IV flow rate. • Place patient in high Fowler position. • Keep patient warm. • Monitor vital signs. • Administer oxygen. • Use an EID with dose-error reduction system and anti-free-flow administration set. • Notify RN/HCP.
Venous air embolism—air in the venous system	• Lightheadedness • Dyspnea, cyanosis, tachypnea, expiratory wheezes, cough • Chest pain, hypotension • Changes in mental status	• Remove all air from administration sets. • Use Luer Lock connections. • Follow protocol for catheter removal. • Check for cracks in tubing/catheter hub.	• **CALL FOR HELP!** • Place patient in Trendelenburg position on left side. • Administer oxygen. • Monitor vital signs. • Notify RN/HCP.
Speed shock—sudden reaction due to medication that is injected too quickly	• Dizziness • Facial and neck flushing • Pounding headache • Tightness in chest • Hypotension • Irregular pulse • Progression of shock	• Use an EID. • Monitor infusion site and rate. • Give IV push medications over appropriate time.	• **CALL FOR HELP!** • Notify RN/HCP. • Stop infusion immediately. • Give antidote or resuscitation medications as ordered.

Source: Adapted from Gorski, L. A. (2018). *Phillips manual of IV therapeutics: Evidence-based practice for infusion therapy* (7th ed.). Philadelphia, PA: F.A. Davis.

Chapter 7 Nursing Care of Patients Receiving Intravenous Therapy 79

> **PRACTICE ANALYSIS TIP**
> Linking NCLEX-PN® to Practice
> The LPN/VN will maintain central venous catheter.

Central venous catheter tips terminate in the superior vena cava near the heart (Fig. 7.4). They are used when peripheral sites are inadequate. CVADs can be used to deliver all types of solutions, medications, or blood products when continuous infusion is required. They are also beneficial when irritant or vesicant medication must be given into a large vein. CVADs include tunneled and nontunneled catheters, peripherally inserted central catheters, and implanted ports. These devices can have one, two, or three lumens in the catheter or one or more port chambers. Each lumen of a multilumen device exits the site in a separate line, called a *tail*. Multilumen devices allow simultaneous administration of solutions while preventing mixing of incompatible solutions. Any CVAD will require special insertion site care according to agency policy.

> **BE SAFE!**
> **BE VIGILANT!** When utilizing more than one lumen concurrently on a multilumen device, monitor closely for fluid overload. Frequently auscultate lung sounds, palpate for lower extremity pitting edema, and monitor for weight increase. Report changes promptly.

Be careful not to confuse a central catheter with a dialysis catheter. Dialysis catheters should be used only for dialysis and not for IV therapy. Also, they should be accessed only by HCPs or specially trained dialysis nurses. If you are not sure what type of catheter your patient has, be sure to ask the RN or HCP.

Nontunneled Central Catheter

A nontunneled CVAD is inserted by an HCP into the jugular, subclavian, or femoral vein. After insertion, correct placement is determined by x-ray before the catheter is used. These short-term CVADs may remain in place up to several weeks. Nontunneled CVADs can be inserted at the bedside or in an outpatient setting. They are cost-effective for short-term use.

Tunneled Catheters

Tunneled catheters are used when venous access is needed for months to years. These catheters are typically composed of polymeric silicone with a Dacron polyester cuff. The cuff not only anchors the catheter in place subcutaneously but also provides a barrier to prevent bacteria from migrating to the tip of the catheter. The catheter tip is commonly placed in the superior vena cava (see Fig. 7.4C). The "tunnel" refers to the route of the catheter under the skin from the insertion site in the skin to the insertion in the vein.

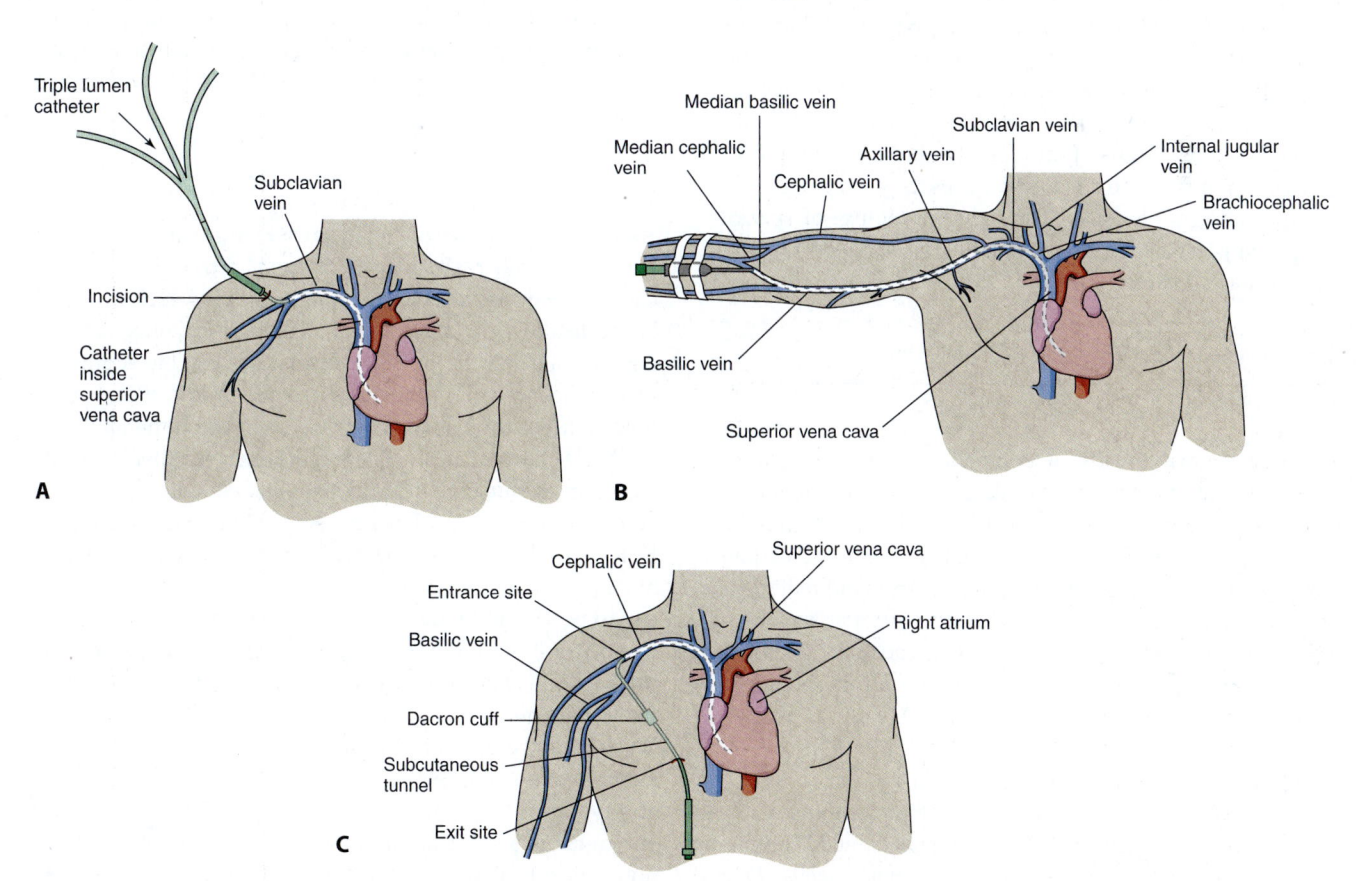

FIGURE 7.4 Central lines. (A) Triple-lumen subclavian catheter. (B) PICC line. (C) Tunneled catheter.

Peripherally Inserted Central Catheter

A peripherally inserted central catheter (PICC) is a long catheter that is inserted in the arm and terminates in the central vasculature (see Fig. 7.4B). A PICC can be tunneled or nontunneled. This device is used when therapy will last more than 2 weeks or the medication is too irritating for peripheral administration. Specially trained RNs can insert PICC lines, which can be left in place for long periods, minimizing the trauma of frequent IV insertions. Consult with the HCP for a PICC order if long-term therapy is anticipated.

It is important to follow the manufacturer's recommended guidelines for flushing the catheter and to be aware of your institution's PICC policy. A trained RN removes the PICC catheter when therapy is terminated. An LPN/LVN may assist the RN with this procedure if the state nurse practice act permits.

Ports

A port is a reservoir that is surgically implanted into a pocket created under the skin, usually in the upper chest. A catheter is attached to the reservoir and tunneled under the skin into a central vein, such as the superior vena cava. For this reason, a port is considered a central venous access device. An advantage of a port is that a dressing is not required when not in use. It can also be flushed and left unused for long periods. When the port is not in use, the patient can swim and shower without risk of contaminating the site.

Ports come in a variety of sizes and styles. They are now being placed in many areas of the body. Ports are suitable for long-term therapy. They can be used to administer all types of medications, including chemotherapeutic agents and antibiotics that are toxic to tissues. In addition, power injectable ports can be used for radiology imaging and procedures. Ports are usually accessed only by specially trained RNs. They require the use of special non-coring needles that are specifically designed for port access and infusions.

OTHER THERAPIES

Parenteral Nutrition

Parenteral nutrition (PN) is complete IV nutrition administered to patients who cannot take adequate nutrients via the enteral route (by mouth or tube feeding). PN may be used to promote nutrition for wound healing, help a patient achieve optimal weight before surgery, or avoid malnutrition from chronic disease or after surgery. Patients with ulcerative colitis, trauma, or cancer cachexia (wasting syndrome) are candidates for PN. Every effort should be made to return a patient on PN to enteral feedings as soon as possible.

PN provides and maintains the essential nutrients required by the body. Solutions contain carbohydrates, amino acids, lipid emulsions, electrolytes, trace elements, and vitamins in varied amounts according to the patient's needs. Due to the components in PN, compatibility issues must be considered. Therefore, medications should not be infused (piggybacked) directly into PN solutions. PN requires filtration and an EID for administration. A 0.22-micron filter is required for lipid-free PN. PN solutions with lipids must have a 1.2-micron filter. Patients receiving PN in the home setting may use an ambulatory infusion device to allow for more mobility.

Initial assessment includes the patient's height, weight, nutritional status, and current laboratory values. Because of high glucose concentration of PN, the patient is at risk for infection and blood glucose disturbances. Insulin therapy may be necessary during PN administration. Ongoing assessments include blood glucose levels according to institution policy and monitoring signs and symptoms of infection, hyperglycemia, and hypoglycemia. When starting PN therapy, the rate is increased gradually to the prescribed rate to prevent hyperglycemia.

When nutritional solutions contain concentrations exceeding 10% dextrose or 5% protein, they must be administered via a CVAD. When concentrations are less than 10% dextrose or 5% protein, they may be administered through a peripheral vein. This is referred to as peripheral parenteral nutrition (PPN). PPN is a short-term intervention because it does not provide adequate nutrition over an extended period. Some states allow LVN/LPNs to initiate PPN.

The entire health-care team must be involved in PN or PPN therapy. The pharmacist, dietitian, HCP, and nurse communicate as a team to discuss the assessment, plan, and outcome criteria. Many institutions have nutrition teams that assess the appropriateness of PN or PPN for individual patients.

Home Intravenous Therapy

As health-care costs continue to rise, a greater number of patients consider alternatives to hospitalization. Subacute care, skilled nursing care in long-term care facilities, and home health care are growing. Home IV therapy allows patients the benefit of early discharge and the ability to receive health care in the privacy and comfort of their own homes. Most patients requiring home infusion therapy have a CVAD rather than a PIV. Some home health-care agencies employ nurses to instruct patients and their families in administering home IV therapy (see "Home Health Hints"). Before discharge, the patient's insurance benefits for home health care should be verified.

Home IV antibiotic therapy is becoming the method of choice for long-term treatment of certain infections, including bacterial endocarditis, osteomyelitis, and septic arthritis. Other patients with various diseases may choose to receive PN, chemotherapy, or IV pain medications at home. The health team can assess patients and their families for their ability to manage home IV therapy. Cleanliness of the home environment and the ability to safely store equipment in the home must be determined before discharge.

> **Home Health Hints**
>
> Before discharge:
> - Coordinate discharge from the hospital with the home health-care agency so that no IV doses will be missed.
> - Provide home health-care agency contact information to the patient.
>
> At home:
> - Good hand washing is essential. To prevent cross-contamination, avoid visiting a patient with an infection prior to your patient receiving an infusion.
> - Instruct the patient to keep the IV site dry. If showering is permitted, instruct the patient to cover the IV with plastic and seal with tape on both ends to prevent water from entering site.
> - Assist the patient and caregiver to identify a safe place to store supplies. Note that some solutions or medications require refrigeration. Remind the patient to remove IV solution from the refrigerator 30 minutes prior to the arrival of the home health nurse.

Subcutaneous Infusion (Hypodermoclysis)

An alternative option for administration of medications or fluids is subcutaneous infusion, or **hypodermoclysis.** It is becoming a more common route in pediatrics, palliative care, home care, and hospice settings as well as for the elderly. Isotonic fluids, most commonly 0.9% sodium chloride or 5% dextrose in water, and limited medications can be administered via this route (Caccialanza, 2018; Gorski, 2018). Hypodermoclysis is recognized as a safe, low-risk, cost-effective route to treat dehydration and for use in patients with poor vein quality. Hypodermoclysis infusions were common in the 1950s, but complications and adverse reaction reports reduced the use of this infusion. Today, pharmacological companies are developing subcutaneous formulations of medications that will improve response, physiologic effect, and patient compliance. With new formulations, many medications are being evaluated for administration via the subcutaneous route.

To access the subcutaneous route, a needle or catheter is placed below the dermis and epidermis in the fatty tissue. Fluids may be administered by gravity or infusion pump, but the volume is limited based on the site. To reduce the risk of local edema, gravity is recommended because the infusion will slow down as pressure in the subcutaneous space increases; infusion rate of fluids is recommended not to exceed 62 mL/hr (1,500 mL total limit over 24 hr) (INS, 2021; Caccialanza et al, 2018). Two sites may be used for high volume solutions up to 1 liter per day per site (INS, 2021). However, when administering medications, the recommended rate should not exceed 5 mL/hr (Gorski, 2018; INS, 2021). Fluids and medications administered via this route will pass through the extracellular matrix to be absorbed by the capillaries and the lymphatic system. Locations for subcutaneous access include the abdomen, thighs, upper arms, chest, and scapular areas. To reduce the risk of infection, the needle and site should be changed every 24 hours. Some advantages are slow absorption rate, decreased severity of infection, and minimal training requirements.

Site assessment and monitoring are crucial to limit complications. Patient education should include reporting pain, redness, swelling, or leaking at the site (Smith, 2014). Patients and caregivers can be taught to obtain access and infuse the medications. Disadvantages include risk of edema, fluid overload, and infection and cellulitis. Drug choices are limited. (Caccialanza et al, 2018).

> **BE SAFE!**
> **BE VIGILANT!** When monitoring subcutaneous infusions, observe for edema at the infusion site. Edema could indicate that the infusion is exceeding the rate of absorption, and the rate must be decreased.

Key Points

- The Infusion Nurses Society is recognized as a global authority in infusion nursing and publishes standards of practice for infusion therapy and the infusion-related scope of practice for LPNs and LVNs. The Centers for Disease Control and Prevention (2020) provides guidelines for isolation precautions, hand hygiene, and prevention of intravascular catheter-related infections. The Institute for Healthcare Improvement provides information related to central line care. The National Institute for Occupational Safety and Health oversees safety issues related to IV therapy. The American Society for Parenteral and Enteral Nutrition provides resources related to IV nutrition.

- IV therapy is indicated when medications need to be fast-acting and at their most effective. Medications can be administered continuously via IV to maintain a therapeutic blood level or intermittently when a stable blood level is less critical. Patients with anemia or blood loss can receive lifesaving IV blood transfusions. Fluids, electrolytes, and nutrition are also administered via IV when patients are unable to eat or drink adequate amounts. Patients who are unable to eat for an extended

• WORD • BUILDING •

hypodermoclysis: hypo – under + dermo—skin + clysis—infusion of fluid

- period can have nutrition and fluids provided through IV parenteral nutrition.
- The most common peripheral local complications are hematoma, phlebitis, or thrombophlebitis, infiltration, extravasation, and nerve injury. Systemic complications can be serious. They include circulatory overload, septicemia, venous air embolism, and speed shock. The nurse delivering infusion therapy must be knowledgeable in preventing, recognizing, and treating all complications of IV therapy.
- To determine the correct IV flow rate, it is important for you to know the formula for determining milliliters per hour and drops per minute if you are using gravity flow.
- A fluid that has the same osmolarity as the blood is called *isotonic*. When given to patients requiring water, it neither enters cells nor pulls water from cells. Therefore, it expands the extracellular fluid volume. A solution with lower osmolarity than blood is called *hypotonic* and is used when fluid is needed to enter the cells, as in the patient with cellular dehydration. Hypertonic solutions exert greater osmotic pressure than blood and are used to expand the plasma volume, for example, in a hypovolemic patient. They also replace electrolytes.
- IV therapy can be administered into the systemic circulation via peripheral or central veins. Peripheral veins lie beneath the epidermis, dermis, and subcutaneous tissue of the skin. They usually provide easy access to the venous system. Central veins are larger and deeper and are located closer to the heart. A central venous access device (CVAD) is a special catheter with a tip that ends in a large vessel (i.e., superior vena cava) near the heart.
- CVADs include tunneled and nontunneled catheters, peripherally inserted central catheters, and implanted ports. These devices can have one to three lumens in the catheter or one or more port chambers. Each lumen of a multilumen device exits the site in a separate line, called a tail.
- Subcutaneous infusion (hypodermoclysis) is becoming a more common route in pediatrics, palliative care, and hospice settings, as well as for the elderly. Isotonic fluids and limited medications can be administered via this route. It is considered a safe, low-risk, cost-effective route to treat dehydration and for use in patients with poor vein quality.

SUGGESTED ANSWERS FOR CHAPTER EXERCISES

Cue Recognition
7.1: Because the IV is still in the patient's vein, there is serious risk of infection. There is a direct blood line from the floor to the patient's blood stream. Immediately clamp the tubing and call for the RN. The IV will need to be removed and restarted in another site.

Critical Thinking & Clinical Judgment
Mr. Rick
Your patient's IV line is likely clotted. If it has been so for a long time, it will not be salvageable. Do not flush it because doing so can dislodge the clot into the circulation. Discontinue the IV line and insert a new cannula.

Mrs. Gonzalez
1. The IV fluid may be leaking at the insertion site and flowing into the subcutaneous tissue, a problem known as *infiltration* or *extravasation*, depending on the type of drug infusing.
2. Consider whether the pain could be caused by the build-up of fluid under the skin. Compare the site with the opposite limb for size difference due to swelling caused by infiltration.
3. If the IV solution has infiltrated, stop the infusion, discontinue the cannula, and restart the cannula in a new site.
4. "Patient reports pain at IV site in right arm; area is cool to touch and edematous in 4.5 cm area around site. Flow rate sluggish. Infusion discontinued; IV restarted in left arm with 22-gauge cannula with good blood return. Infusing well with no signs of infiltration."
5. The registered nurse or IV therapy nurse would be good resources.

Additional Resources

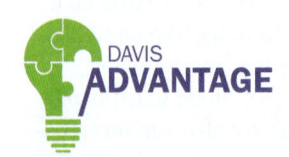

DAVIS ADVANTAGE Go to Davis Advantage to complete your learning: strengthen understanding, apply your knowledge, and prepare for the Next Gen NCLEX®.

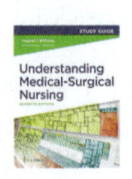

A Study Guide is also available.

CHAPTER 8
Nursing Care of Patients With Infections

Kelli Verdecchia

KEY TERMS

aerobic (air-OH-bik)
anaerobic (an-air-OH-bik)
antibodies (AN-ti-bah-dees)
antigens (AN-tih-jenz)
asepsis (ah-SEP-sis)
bacteria (bak-TEER-ee-ah)
clostridioides difficile (klos-TRID-e-OY-dees dih-fih-SEEL)
colonization (col-in-ih-ZAY-shun)
coronavirus disease (co-RONA-VY-rus diz-EZE)
dormant (DOOR-mant)
epidemic (eh-puh-DEH-mik)
fungi (FUNG-guy)
hand hygiene (HAND HY-jeen)
herd immunity (herd ih-MYOO-nih-tee)
host (HOHST)
morbidity (more-BIH-dih-tee)
mortality (more-TAH-lih-tee)
pandemic (pan-DEH-mik)
pathogen (PATH-o-jen)
personal protective equipment (PUR-sun-al pro-TEK-tiv i-KWIP-ment)
phagocytosis (fay-go-sy-TOH-sis)
protozoa (pro-tow-ZOH-ah)
reservoir (REZ-er-vwar)
rickettsia (rah-KET-see-ah)
sepsis (SEP-sis)
standard precautions (STAN-derd pre-KAW-shuns)
Staphylococcus aureus (staff-il-oh-KOK-us AW-ree-uhs)
trichinosis (TRIK-in-OH-sis)
vector (VEK-tur)
virulence (VEER-you-lence)
viruses (VY-rus-iz)

CHAPTER CONCEPT

Infection

LEARNING OUTCOMES

1. List the links in the chain of infection.
2. Explain how to interrupt the routes of transmission for infections.
3. Describe the body's defense mechanisms to fight infection.
4. Describe the principles of anti-infective medication administration.
5. Describe nursing care for a patient with an infection.

THE INFECTION PROCESS

A **pathogen** is an organism that can cause disease in a **host** (an infected person). **Colonization** occurs when pathogenic microbes are present in the body without causing symptoms or a detectable immune response. Infection occurs when a microbe multiplies within a host. Infection with only an immune response (increased antibody level for the microbe) and no symptoms is a *subclinical infection*.

To prevent infection, links in the chain of infection must be broken (Fig. 8.1). If an infection does occur, treatment focuses on breaking the chain of infection to prevent its spread to others.

Infectious Agents

Microorganisms that cause infection include bacteria, viruses, fungi, protozoa, helminths, and prions (Table 8.1). The organisms that occur naturally in or on a body part are known as *normal flora*. They are usually harmless (nonpathogenic). Normal flora are helpful to the human host. For example, intestinal flora (i.e., bacteria) assist in vitamin K production. This is a nutrient needed for normal blood clotting. However, if these same bacteria get into another area of the body, such as the blood, they may produce disease. They are then referred to as pathogens.

Bacteria

Bacteria are single-celled organisms. They may depend on a host, but they can also live and reproduce outside a host. Most bacteria have cell walls that are susceptible to antibiotic effects. However, bacteria can mutate to survive.

• WORD • BUILDING •
pathogen: pathos—suffering + genes—producer of

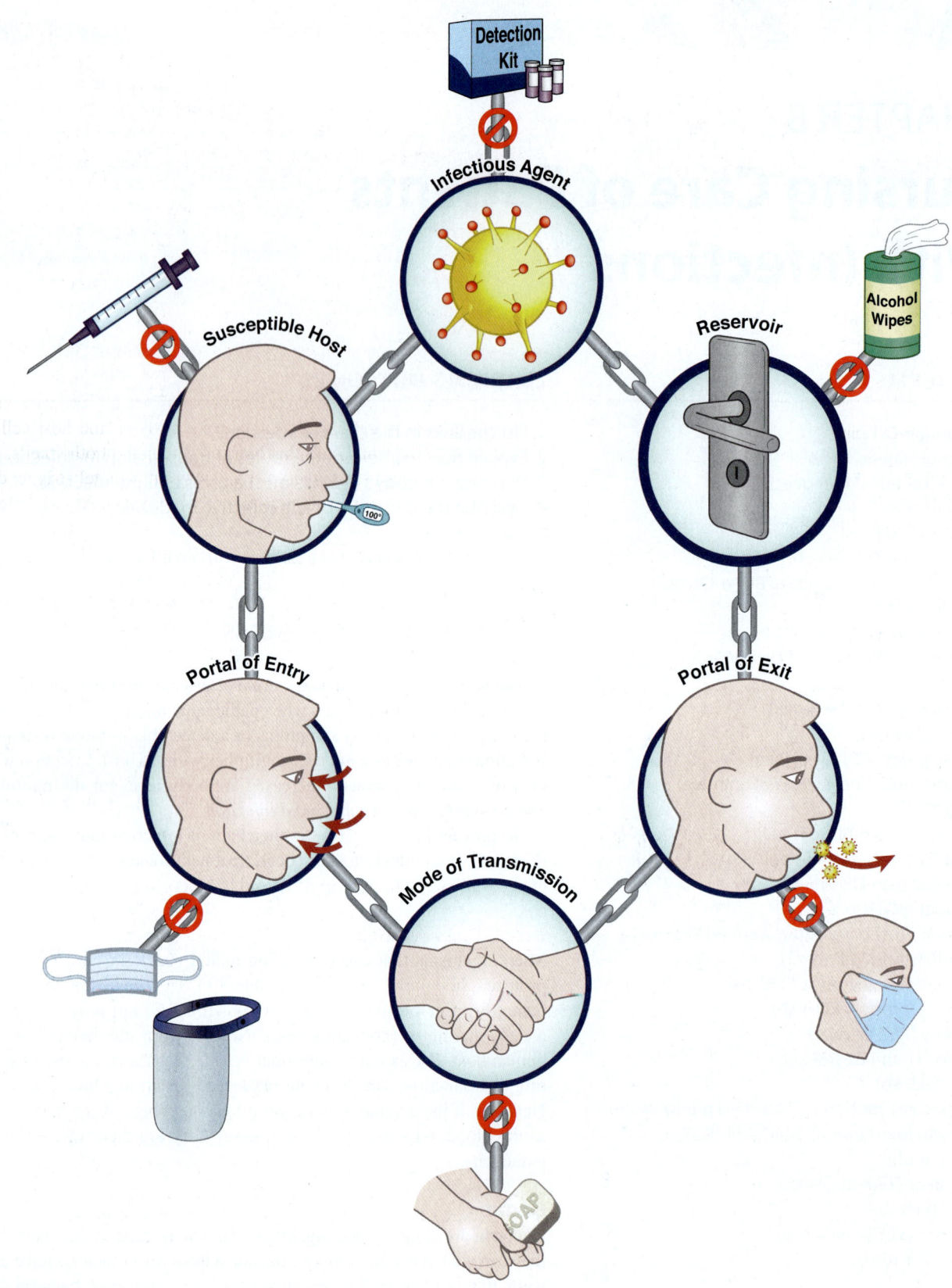

FIGURE 8.1 Breaking the chain of infection.

Bacteria are named according to their shape: spherical (coccus), rod (bacillus), and spiral (spirillum). They are classified according to their staining properties (e.g., Gram method, acid-fast staining). Bacteria respond to stains in one of three ways. Gram-positive bacteria stain purple. Gram-negative bacteria lose purple stain when exposed to alcohol but stain pink with a second dye. Acid-fast bacteria keep purple stain when an acid is applied.

Table 8.1
Common Infections

Microorganism	Type or Site of Infection
Gram-Positive Bacteria	
Staphylococcus aureus	Pneumonia, cellulitis, peritonitis, toxic shock
Staphylococcus epidermidis	Postoperative bone/joints, IV line–related phlebitis
Staphylococcus pneumoniae	Pneumonia, meningitis, otitis media, sinusitis, bacteremia
Gram-Negative Bacteria	
Escherichia coli	Urinary tract, pyelonephritis, bacteremia, gastroenteritis
Klebsiella pneumoniae	Pneumonia, wounds
Legionella pneumophila	Pneumonia
Neisseria gonorrhoeae	Gonorrhea
Pseudomonas aeruginosa	Wounds, urinary tract, pneumonia, IV lines
Salmonella enteritidis	Gastroenteritis, food poisoning
Viruses	
Epstein-Barr	Infectious mononucleosis
Hepatitis (A, B, C, D, E)	Liver
Herpes virus group	Cold sores/fever blisters, genital herpes
Human immunodeficiency virus (HIV)	Acquired immune deficiency syndrome (AIDS)
Influenza (A, B, C)	Bronchiolitis, pneumonia
Rubella	German measles
Rubeola	Measles
SARS-CoV-2	COVID-19
Varicella-zoster	Skin (chickenpox and shingles)
Fungi	
Candida albicans	Nailbed, thrush, vaginitis
Histoplasma capsulatum	Pneumonia
Protozoa	
Giardia lamblia	Gastroenteritis
Trichomonas vaginalis	Trichomoniasis
Dientamoeba fragilis	Diarrhea, fever
Entamoeba histolytica	Amoebic dysentery
Toxoplasma gondii	Toxoplasmosis
Plasmodium falciparum	Malaria

Bacterial growth depends on oxygen, nutrition, light, temperature, and humidity. **Aerobic** bacteria, such as those found on the skin, need oxygen to live. **Anaerobic** bacteria, such as bacteria in the gastrointestinal (GI) tract, live without oxygen. Most bacteria that inhabit humans grow best at a body temperature of 98.6°F (37°C).

Rod-shaped bacteria form spores that are thick walled. They are hard to kill. Spores remain in a resting state until favorable conditions exist to resume normal function. Prolonged exposure to high temperature destroys spores on surgical equipment. Bleach is used in patient rooms to kill spores from *Clostridioides difficile* (*C. difficile*; *C. diff*).

Rickettsiae are tiny bacteria that must be inside living cells to reproduce. Rickettsia **vectors** (living organisms that transmit disease) are infected fleas, ticks, mites, and lice. They bite humans and cause disease. These diseases include typhus, scrub typhus, and Rocky Mountain spotted fever.

Viruses
Viruses are organisms smaller than bacteria. They depend on host cells to live and reproduce (see Table 8.1). Invaded host cells make more of the virus material. The new viral particles are released either by destroying the host cell or forming small buds that break away to infect other cells.

When a virus enters a cell, it may immediately trigger disease or remain **dormant** (inactive) for years. An example of this is human herpesvirus 3 (varicella-zoster virus). It can cause disease quickly (e.g., chickenpox) or later erupt into the disease shingles. Antiviral drugs may decrease viral load (the number of viral cells in the patient's blood) and therefore viral symptoms. Antibiotics are not effective against viruses.

Fungi
Fungi include yeasts and molds. They can produce highly resistant spores (see Table 8.1). Normal flora of the mouth, skin, vagina, and intestinal tract include many fungi. Most fungi are not pathogenic, especially in healthy people. Serious fungal infections are rare, but if required, antifungal medications are available.

Protozoa
Protozoa are single-celled parasitic organisms that have flexible membranes and live in the soil (see Table 8.1). Protozoa infect humans through fecal–oral contamination, ingestion of food or water contaminated with cysts or spores, host-to-host contact, or the bite of a mosquito or other insect that has previously bitten an infected person.

Helminths
Helminths are wormlike parasitic animals. These include roundworms, flatworms, tapeworms, pinworms, hookworms, and flukes. Disease transmission occurs through skin penetration of larvae or ingestion of helminth eggs. **Trichinosis** (caused by the roundworm *Trichinella spiralis*) is a disease transmitted to humans by eating raw or undercooked meat of pigs or wild animals that contain *Trichinella* larvae.

Prions
Prions are transmissible pathogenic agents. They cause abnormal folding of normal cellular proteins known as prion proteins.

• **WORD • BUILDING •**
protozoa: proto—first + zoon—animal

Prion proteins are found mainly in the brain. They cause damage from the abnormal folding of prion proteins. Prion diseases have long incubation periods. They cause no inflammatory response but progress rapidly and are fatal. In humans, they include classic and variant Creutzfeldt-Jakob disease.

Reservoir

A **reservoir** is the place in the environment where infectious agents live, multiply, and reproduce. A reservoir can be animate (e.g., people, insects, animals, plants) or inanimate (e.g., water, soil, medical devices).

Portal of Exit

The portal of exit is the path by which the infectious agent leaves its reservoir.

Mode of Transmission

Once the causative agent exits the reservoir, a direct or indirect means of transfer to a susceptible host is needed.

> **NURSING CARE TIP**
> - Understanding the mode of transmission of a disease allows you to use the appropriate means of personal protection without using unnecessary supplies that increase costs.
> - Bundle interventions to conserve personal protective equipment and supplies and to reduce costs.

> **PRACTICE ANALYSIS TIP**
> Linking NCLEX-PN® to Practice
> The LPN/LVN will participate in providing cost-effective care.

Direct Transmission

Direct transmission occurs by direct contact or droplet spread. Direct contact occurs through touching, kissing, or sexual intercourse. Illnesses spread by this route include scabies, infectious mononucleosis, and sexually transmitted infections. **Personal protective equipment** (PPE) selection is guided by the task to be performed and the applicable precautions (standard precautions and/or transmission-based precautions; see the Infection Prevention and Control Guidelines discussion later). Contact precautions PPE includes gloves and gown.

Droplet spread occurs over short distances from spray during sneezing, coughing, or talking. **Coronavirus disease 2019 (COVID-19)**, influenza, and pertussis are spread in this way (Fig. 8.2). PPE for patients infected with COVID-19 includes fitted respirator mask (N95 respirator, powered air-purifying respirator or elastomeric respirator), eye protection, face shield, gloves, and gown (Fig. 8.3). Droplet PPE for patients with infectious non–COVID-19 conditions includes surgical mask, face shield or goggles, and gloves in addition to standard precaution requirements such as a gown (Fig. 8.4).

Indirect Transmission

Indirect transmission is either vehicle-borne, vectorborne, or airborne. Vehicles that can indirectly spread an infectious agent include biological products (e.g., blood, organs), soiled bedding, food, surgical instruments, toys, water, and wound dressings. Vehicle-borne illnesses include influenza, norovirus, and hepatitis. Rarely, SARS-CoV-2 can be transmitted in this way. Methods to avoid vehicle transmission include screening of biological products, meticulous **hand hygiene,** provisions for both clean water and food supplies, and cleaning of the patient environment and instruments per protocols.

Vectorborne transmission is the spread of infectious agents through a living source other than humans. Sources include fleas, mice, mosquitos, rats, and ticks. Diseases spread through vectors include Lyme disease, malaria, plague, and Zika virus disease. Vector transmission can be reduced with avoidance of infested areas, use of insect repellents, and rodent control.

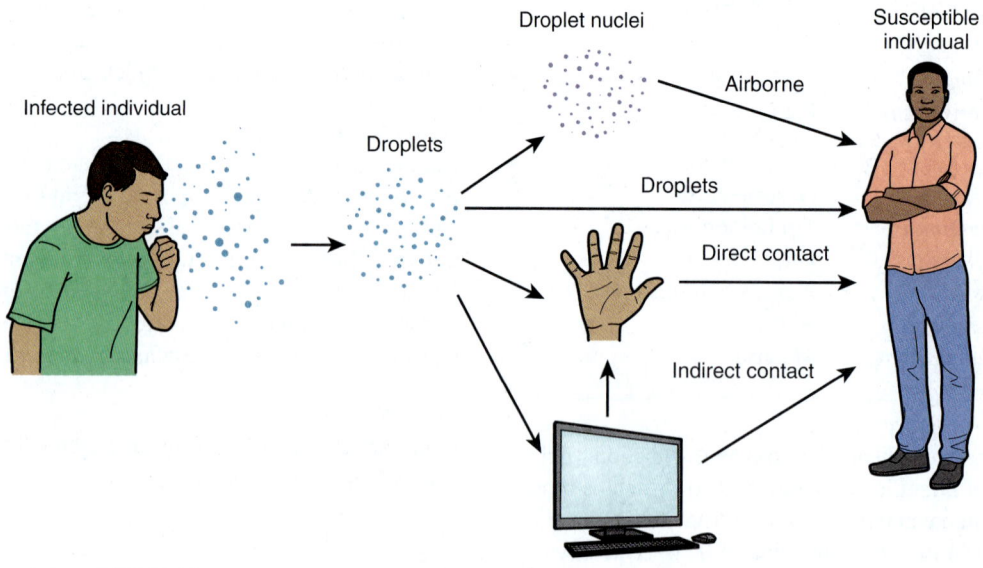

FIGURE 8.2 Transmission of COVID-19.

Chapter 8 Nursing Care of Patients With Infections 87

through the air in poorly ventilated enclosed spaces and from aerosol-generating medical procedures (World Health Organization, 2020). Airborne transmission is prevented with the use of a high-efficiency particulate air (HEPA) respirator that filters the tiniest particles more effectively than surgical masks. Fischer and colleagues (2020) noted the N95 mask is far superior to protect people nearby.

> **BE SAFE!**
> **BE VIGILANT!** If you provide care for patients with suspected or confirmed airborne diseases, you *must* have your own institution-provided fit-tested National Institute for Occupational Safety and Health–approved N95 or higher-level respirator to wear. Do not use other types of masks because they do not provide adequate protection. If you cannot obtain your own fit-tested mask, you should *never* enter the patient's room.

Multiple Modes of Transmission
Several diseases have multiple modes of transmission and require a variety of protective techniques. For example, chickenpox is transmitted by direct contact, indirect contact, and airborne transmission. Therefore, 90% of susceptible persons exposed to it develop the disease. It is thought that COVID-19 can also be transmitted in several ways, although direct contact is the most common mode. Airborne and indirect contact are much less common but have occurred.

Portal of Entry
To produce disease, organisms enter a susceptible host through the blood, genitourinary tract, GI tract, mucous membranes, skin (usually nonintact), placenta, or respiratory tract. The condition of the host, the **virulence** (ability to produce infection) of the organism, and other factors determine if the entry of the organism causes disease.

Susceptible Host
The body has many defense mechanisms to prevent infection. A breakdown in these defenses increases the possibility of infection. Factors that increase susceptibility to infection are burns, chronic disease, an immunocompromised state, invasive procedures, malnourishment, stress, and very young age or older age ("Gerontological Issues").

> ### Gerontological Issues
> **Infection and Older Adults.** Fever may not be a common sign of an infection for an older adult. Absence of fever can cause significant delay in providing appropriate treatment and care. Watch for atypical signs of infection in older adults:
> - Behavioral changes: pacing or irritability or new onset confusion
> - Infection symptoms that present like and are therefore masked by symptoms of existing chronic conditions

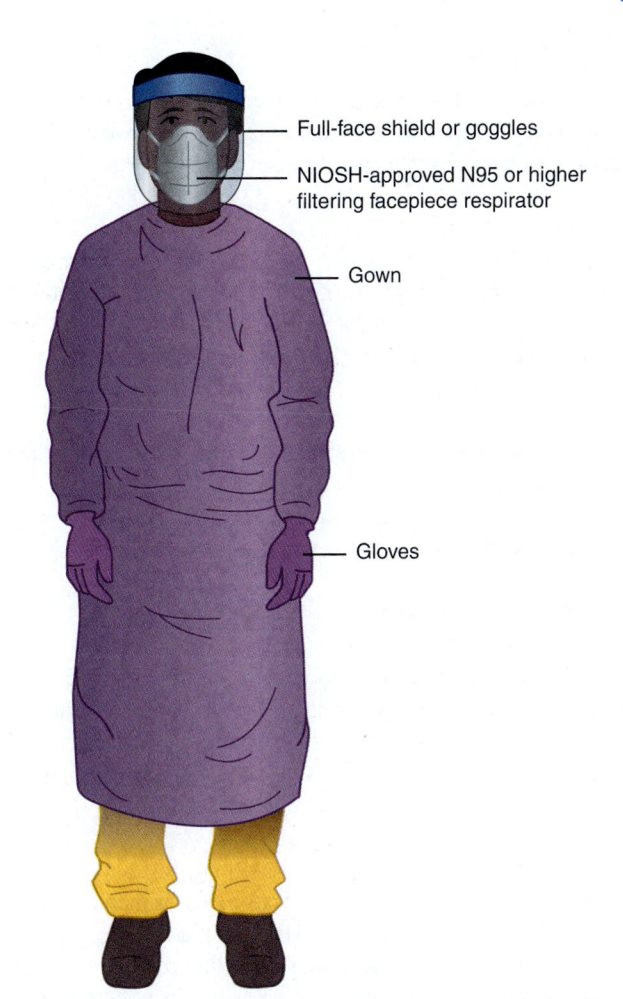

FIGURE 8.3 COVID-19 personal protective equipment for health-care workers.

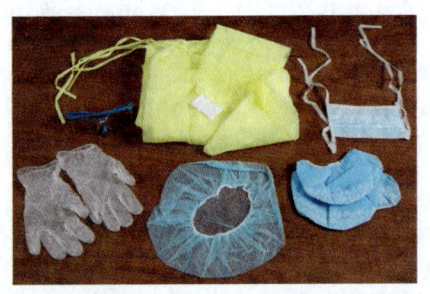

FIGURE 8.4 Personal protective equipment such as gloves, goggles, gown, surgical mask, shoe covers, and hair cover help prevent the spread of infection to health-care workers and patients.

Airborne transmission occurs by dust or droplet nuclei carrying an infectious agent through the air. It is different from droplet transmission (see Direct Transmission, discussed earlier). The floating particles are much smaller, remain suspended in the air longer, and travel farther distances. Airborne organisms can be inhaled or deposited on the mucous membrane of a susceptible host. *Mycobacterium tuberculosis* (TB), rubeola virus (measles), and varicella-zoster virus (chickenpox) are transmitted by airborne transmission. The severe acute respiratory syndrome coronavirus 2 (SARS-CoV-2) that causes COVID-19 can less commonly be transmitted

THE HUMAN BODY'S DEFENSE MECHANISMS

Skin and Mucous Membranes
Intact skin and mucous membranes are the body's first line of defense against infection. Preventing skin dryness and cracking with lotion keeps the skin intact, preventing an entry point for organisms. Oral mucous membranes have many layers which makes it difficult for organisms to enter the body. The skin has acidic (pH less than 7) properties to make some organisms unable to produce disease. Many bacteria prefer an alkaline (pH more than 7) environment for reproduction. The body also has an abundance of normal flora impairing the growth of pathogens both on the skin and in the GI tract.

Cilia
Cilia are hairlike structures lining the mucous membranes of the upper respiratory tract. They trap mucus, pus, dust, and foreign particles to prevent them from entering the lungs. Cilia push the trapped particles up to the pharynx with wave-like movements to be expectorated.

Gastric Acid
Gastric acid (pH 1 to 5) destroys most organisms that enter the stomach.

Antibodies
Antibodies, also called immunoglobulins, are proteins produced by plasma cells when foreign antigens of invading cells are detected (see Chapter 18). **Antigens** are markers on the surface of cells. They identify cells as being the body's own cells (autoantigens) or as being foreign cells (foreign antigens). Antibodies attach to specific foreign antigens on the surface of the invading organisms to identify them for destruction by neutrophils or macrophages.

Leukocytes and Macrophages
Leukocytes, or white blood cells (WBCs), are the primary cells that protect against infection and tissue damage. There are five types of leukocytes in order of abundance:

- Neutrophils are phagocytic cells that ingest and destroy bacteria and fungi.
- Lymphocyte functions include antigen recognition and antibody production.
- Monocytes become macrophages and mainly ingest and destroy tissue debris and large foreign particles.
- Eosinophils destroy parasites and respond in allergic reactions.
- Basophils are involved in inflammatory and allergic reactions.

After recognizing a foreign antigen, neutrophils and macrophages engulf and digest it. This is known as **phagocytosis**. The macrophages move the antigen fragments to their surface to be recognized by T lymphocytes to further stimulate action of the immune system.

Lysozymes
Lysozymes are bactericidal enzymes present in WBCs and most body fluids, such as tears, saliva, and sweat. These enzymes dissolve the walls of bacteria, destroying them.

Interferon
If an invading organism is a virus, WBCs and fibroblasts release interferon (a group of antiviral proteins). Interferon helps destroy infected cells, inhibits production of the virus within these cells, and may inhibit tumor cell growth.

Inflammatory Response
The inflammatory response occurs with any injury to the body. This response can be caused by pathogens, trauma, or other events causing injury to tissues. Infection may or may not be present.

Vascular Response
The first step of the inflammatory process is local vasodilation which increases blood flow to the injured area. Pathogenic organisms can trigger the first step of the inflammatory process. Increased blood flow creates redness and heat at the injury, bringing more plasma to the area to nourish tissue. Waste and debris are then carried away.

Inflammatory Exudate
The second step of the inflammatory process is increased permeability of the blood vessels. This lets plasma move out of the capillaries and into the tissues. Swelling can occur, which can cause pain from the pressure on nearby nerve endings.

Phagocytosis and Purulent Exudate
The final step of the inflammatory process is the destruction of pathogenic organisms and their toxins by leukocytes through phagocytosis. During this process, a purulent exudate (pus) may form that contains protein, cellular debris, and dead leukocytes.

Immune System
The immune system is the body's final line of defense against infection (see Chapter 18). The immune system is a finely tuned network of specialized parts. When this network breaks down, infection can result.

Risk Factors for Infection
Risk factors for infection include:

- Aging (e.g., decreasing immune function)
- Chronic disease
- Dysphagia (e.g., risk of aspiration pneumonia, malnutrition)
- Environment (e.g., hospitals, long-term care facilities)
- Immobility

• WORD • BUILDING •

phagocytosis: phagein—to eat + cytos—cell + osis—condition

- Immunocompromised
- Incontinence (e.g., voiding disturbances contribute to urinary tract infection [UTI])
- Instrumentation (e.g., central lines, endotracheal tubes, feeding tubes, IV lines, urinary catheters)
- Invasive procedures (e.g., cardiac catheterization, endoscopy, surgery)
- Malnutrition
- Medications (e.g., recent and/or multiple antibiotics, corticosteroids)

The older adult is most at risk for respiratory infections (e.g., influenza, coronavirus, pneumonia, TB), health-care-associated infection, hepatitis, methicillin-resistant *Staphylococcus aureus* (MRSA), sepsis, skin infection, and UTIs.

INFECTIOUS DISEASE

Localized Infection
Localized infection is caused by an increase of microbes in one area that triggers the inflammatory response. Signs and symptoms include pain, redness, swelling, and warmth at the site. Pain is most severe when the infection occurs in closed cavity areas. Redness and swelling are seen when surface structures are involved. Warmth may be felt at the site. Fever defined as 100.4°F (38°C) may occur to produce an antimicrobial effect (Centers for Disease Control and Prevention [CDC], 2018).

Sepsis
Sepsis is defined as "life-threatening organ dysfunction caused by dysregulated host response to infection" (Singer et al, 2016; see Chapter 9).

Laboratory Assessment
A Gram stain, using gentian violet, allows bacteria to be better seen under a microscope for identification. Gram-positive bacteria turn purple. Gram-negative bacteria become pink. A culture and sensitivity (C&S) identifies an illness-causing organism. It also determines the most effective antibiotic for treatment. Organisms in the culture specimen are grown on a laboratory plate within 24 to 48 hours. The organism is then exposed to several antibiotics to determine to which antibiotics the organism is sensitive.

A serum antibody test measures the reaction to a certain antigen. A positive result for this test does not always mean that an active infection is present. It can simply mean there has been an exposure to the antigen. Therefore, it is not as accurate as a culture.

A complete blood cell count with differential (CBC with diff) is usually obtained when an infection is suspected. The levels of the five leukocytes are measured. Elevations in specific leukocytes occur based on the type and severity of the pathogen.

Erythrocyte sedimentation rate (ESR, sed rate) is an early screening test for inflammation. It is not a definitive test for infection. During the inflammatory process, red blood cells (RBCs) become heavier. The ESR measures in millimeters per hour the speed at which the RBCs settle in a tube: the faster the settling (due to heavier RBCs), the greater the inflammation.

Other tests, such as x-rays, computed tomography (CT), and magnetic resonance imaging (MRI), are helpful in identifying abscesses (walled-off infections). Skin tests also diagnose infections. For example, the purified protein derivative (PPD) skin test screens for TB (see Chapter 31).

Pandemic
An **epidemic** occurs when there is a rapid rise in the number of those with a specific infection. A **pandemic** occurs when an infection affects large numbers of people and spreads across more than one continent or around the world. New infectious diseases, such as COVID-19, can result in a global pandemic because we have no immunity and no known cure. Those who are typically most vulnerable in a pandemic include the very young and the very old, the immunosuppressed, those with comorbidities, and those who live in institutions such as long-term care facilities. Health-care workers can be at high risk from exposure to those who are ill. Following transmission precautions and utilizing appropriate PPE is essential.

Immunity
Immunity is the ability of the body to protect itself from disease (see Chapter 18). There are several types of immunity:

- Natural immunity occurs in species and prevents one species from contracting illnesses found in another species.
- Innate immunity is genetic; hereditary immunity is that which a person is born with.
- Acquired immunity is obtained either actively or passively through exposure to an organism, from a vaccine, or from an injection of immunoglobulins (antibodies) or is passed from mother to baby. Visit www.cdc.gov/vaccines/schedules/easy-to-read.

Herd Immunity
Herd immunity to a specific disease occurs when a significant portion of the community becomes immune to the disease through infection or vaccination. Because the disease is less likely to spread among this population, herd immunity offers some protection to those who have not had the disease or been vaccinated. The percentage of immunity required to stop the uncontrolled spread of a disease varies with each disease.

Types of Infectious Diseases
Infectious disease examples are discussed next or in the chapters related to the body system they affect. For HIV, see Chapter 20; for respiratory diseases including COVID-19, see Chapter 31; for hepatitis, see Chapter 35.

• WORD • BUILDING •

pandemic: pan—all + demos—people

COVID-19

The novel severe acute respiratory syndrome coronavirus 2 (SARS-CoV-2) identified in 2019 created a pandemic because it was a new virus and no one had had previous exposure or immunity (Table 8.2). The disease this coronavirus caused was named COVID-19 (CO = corona, VI = virus, D = disease, 19 = 2019). Over time, variants of COVID-19, such as the Delta and Omicron, have evolved.

Ebola Virus Disease

In 1976, the Ebola virus was discovered near the Ebola River in the Democratic Republic of the Congo (see Table 8.2). Survivors of the disease develop antibodies that last about 10 years.

Infectious Mononucleosis

Infectious mononucleosis (IM) is usually caused by the Epstein-Barr virus (EBV), a herpes virus. EBV is spread through contact with saliva or mucus of an infected person. IM is mainly symptomatic in teens or young adults. Most adults by age 40 have developed antibodies to it. EBV remains inactive in the body for life. The incubation period for IM is 4 to 6 weeks. Symptoms include fever, severe sore throat, and generalized lymphadenopathy (enlarged lymph nodes in two different sites other than inguinal nodes) that last 1 to 4 weeks. The spleen enlarges 50% of the time. Occasionally, a rash develops, similar to the rash seen with measles. Signs and symptoms as well as diagnostic tests confirm IM. A positive mononucleosis test and EBV antibody tests confirm IM. No

Table 8.2
Viral Infections

Infection	Coronavirus Disease 2019 (COVID-19)	Ebola Virus Disease	Zika Virus Disease
Causative Organism	Severe acute respiratory syndrome coronavirus 2 (SARS-CoV-2)	Ebola virus (*Zaire ebolavirus*) Sudan virus (*Sudan ebolavirus*) Taï Forest virus (*Taï Forest ebolavirus*) Bundibugyo virus (*Bundibugyo ebolavirus*)	Zika virus is a member of the *Flaviviridae* family.
Transmission	Direct transmission person-to-person with close contact via respiratory droplets with: • Coughing • Sneezing • Talking Airborne possible in poorly ventilated enclosed spaces Indirect contact with contaminated surfaces and mouth, eyes, or nose	Direct contact via broken skin or mucous membranes with: • Infected blood, body fluids • Infected fruit bat or primate • Contaminated equipment (e.g., needles, syringes) • Semen from survivor	Day- and nighttime-active *Aedes* genus infected mosquito bite Sex with an infected partner Maternal–fetal
Prevention/ Isolation	Vaccine(s) Wear mask around those not living with you Hand hygiene frequently Stay 6 feet apart from others Avoid crowds Avoid unventilated indoor spaces Use tissue for coughs/sneezes, then throw in trash Disinfect frequently touched surfaces daily. Self-isolate if potential exposure or ill Use airborne, contact, droplet precautions	Vaccine: Ervebo Hand hygiene Avoid contact with infected blood, body fluids, objects, bats, primates, bodies of people who died of Ebola Wear specialized personal protective equipment Sterilize equipment Isolate patient Use contact and droplet precautions	Use Environmental Protection Agency–registered insect repellent Empty containers with stagnant water around the house Avoid unprotected sex and travel to areas of risk with Zika virus if pregnant Hand hygiene Disinfect household surfaces Wash contaminated clothing Avoid exposure to blood/bodily fluids Use standard precautions

Table 8.2
Viral Infections—cont'd

Infection	Coronavirus Disease 2019 (COVID-19)	Ebola Virus Disease	Zika Virus Disease
Symptoms	May appear 2–4 days after exposure to virus and include • Fever • Cough • Diarrhea • Fatigue • Headache • Loss of taste or smell • Muscle and body aches • Nausea, vomiting • Shortness of breath	Appear in 2–21 days (average 8–10 days) and include • Abdominal pain • Diarrhea • Fever • Headache • Muscle pain • Unexplained bruising/bleeding • Vomiting	Mild symptoms lasting several days to weeks include • Conjunctivitis • Fever • Headache • Muscle/joint pain • Rash
Diagnosis	Clinical examination: • New onset fever • Dyspnea, cough • New onset oxygen requirement • Close contact with known or suspected COVID-19 case Antigen test • Anterior nasal swab Polymer chain reaction (PCR) test • Nasal or throat swab	After onset of fever: • Antigen-capture enzyme-linked immunosorbent assay (ELISA) testing • Immunoglobulin M (IgM) ELISA • Polymerase chain reaction • Virus isolation	Symptomatic pregnant women who traveled to active transmission areas Dengue and Zika virus nucleic acid amplification test (NAAT) serum specimen Zika virus NAAT on urine specimen IgM for Dengue only
Complications	Acute respiratory distress syndrome (ARDS) Pneumonia Hypoxemia Sepsis Cardiomyopathy	Long-term joint and vision problems	Guillain-Barré syndrome Microcephaly birth defect Miscarriage Severe fetal brain defects
Treatment/Nursing Care	No cure Supportive care	No antiviral drug exists Supportive care Maintain blood pressure Maintain oxygenation IV fluids	Supportive care including acetaminophen Avoid NSAIDs Fluids and rest

Sources: Centers for Disease Control and Prevention (CDC). (Last reviewed October 25, 2021). Ebola (Ebola virus disease). www.cdc.gov/vhf/ebola/index.html; CDC. (Last reviewed December 9, 2019). Zika virus. www.cdc.gov/zika/hc-providers/testing-guidance.html; CDC. (Last updated February 16, 2021). Interim Clinical Guidance for Management of Patients with Confirmed Coronavirus Disease (COVID-19). www.cdc.gov/coronavirus/2019-ncov/hcp/clinical-guidance-management-patients.html; CDC. (Last updated October 25, 2021). Interim guidelines for collecting and handling of clinical specimens for COVID-19 testing. www.cdc.gov/coronavirus/2019-ncov/lab/guidelines-clinical-specimens.html; CDC. (Last updated February 22, 2021). Symptoms of COVID-19. www.cdc.gov/coronavirus/2019-ncov/symptoms-testing/symptoms.html; U.S. Food & Drug Administration. (2020). Ebola preparedness and response updates from FDA. www.fda.gov/emergency-preparedness-and-response/mcm-issues/ebola-preparedness-and-response-updates-fda.

specific treatment is needed. Antiviral drugs are not effective. Symptoms are treated with supportive care. Fatigue may last for months. Rest is important.

Zika Virus Disease

The Zika virus is named for the Zika Forest of Uganda where it was discovered in 1947 (see Table 8.2). Once infected, most people are protected from future infections of Zika virus.

INFECTION CONTROL IN THE COMMUNITY

Many levels of organizations work together to control communicable diseases. Global monitoring and virology surveillance supports crucial early identification of viruses that have a potential to create a pandemic. The World Health

Organization (WHO) and the Centers for Disease Control and Prevention (CDC) teach standards to prevent, monitor, and control disease outbreaks. Local health departments teach prevention and help control disease outbreaks. Immunization programs have helped to reduce communicable diseases.

> **NURSING CARE TIP**
>
> For infection control, teach the CDC coughing and sneezing instructions to patients and family members who have a cough, congestion, COVID-19, rhinorrhea, or respiratory secretions:
> - Cover your mouth and nose with a tissue when you cough or sneeze.
> - Put your used tissue immediately in the wastebasket.
> - If you do not have a tissue, cough or sneeze into your upper sleeve or elbow, not your hands.
> - Wash hands immediately with soap and water for 20 seconds; use a 60% to 95% alcohol-based hand cleaner if soap and water are not available.
> - Put on a facemask to protect others if asked.
>
> *Source:* Centers for Disease Control and Prevention. (2020). Coughing and sneezing. Retrieved from www.cdc.gov/healthywater/hygiene/etiquette/coughing_sneezing.html

INFECTION CONTROL IN HEALTH-CARE AGENCIES

A community-acquired infection is one a patient already has upon admission to a health-care facility. An infection that develops as a result of care provided in a health-care agency is called a health-care-associated infection (HAI). The host's condition plays a major role in whether an infection is acquired. Patients in the hospital are often debilitated, malnourished, or immunocompromised. Living in a long-term care facility rather than at home can increase infection risk. Multiple antibiotic therapy increases susceptibility to other types of infection. It also promotes resistance of pathogens to antibiotics. Therefore, risk of developing HAI is high.

Certain patient care areas tend to have an increased number of HAIs. These include burn, critical care, dialysis, neonatal, and oncology units. Patients in these units tend to undergo more invasive procedures and are more debilitated. Healthy People 2030 has two objectives for HAI: (1) reduce *C. diff* infections that people get in the hospital and (2) reduce MRSA bloodstream HAIs (Office of Disease Prevention and Health Promotion, 2020).

Several pathogens are commonly responsible for causing HAIs:

- *Escherichia coli* (*E. coli*) is the most common pathogen causing health-care-associated UTIs. *E. coli* normally lives in the healthy intestinal tract of humans. *E. coli* can be spread by the patient, by unwashed hands of a health-care worker, or through contaminated food and water.
- *Staphylococcus aureus* (known as staph) is the most common pathogen causing health-care-associated surgical wound infections. Staph usually lives in the nose and on the skin of healthy people.
- *Pseudomonas aeruginosa* is the most common pathogen in health-care-associated pneumonia. It is found in soil, around water, and in the health-care setting around sinks, water, irrigating solutions, and nebulizers on respiratory equipment.

Hand Hygiene

Proper hand hygiene is the single-most effective way to control and prevent the spread of infections. Hand hygiene removes the transient organisms that cause most HAIs. Most of these organisms are transmitted via the hands of health-care providers (HCPs). Hands must be cleansed before and after every patient contact to help prevent the direct transmission of organisms (Fig. 8.5). The use of gloves decreases the transmission of organisms. CDC guidelines require hand washing before and after glove use because hands may still become contaminated.

Hand hygiene is best performed with hand washing, but an alcohol-based hand rub containing at least 60% alcohol can be used if hand washing is not possible. Soap and water, however, are needed instead of a hand rub to remove *C. difficile*. For visibly soiled hands, wash with soap and water rather than using a hand rub. When using alcohol-based hand rubs, apply the specified amount of the hand rub to the palm of one hand. Rub both hands together, covering all surfaces, until

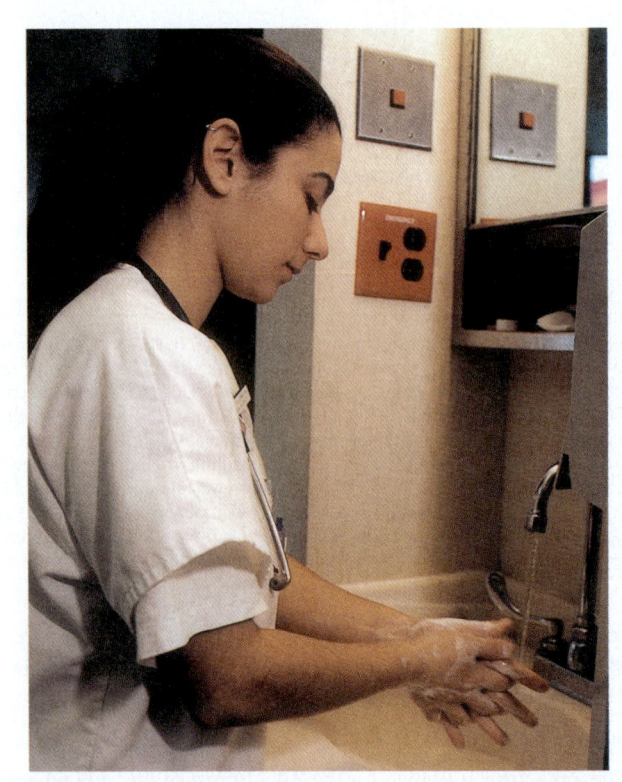

FIGURE 8.5 Frequent hand hygiene by health-care workers helps reduce the spread of microorganisms.

hands are completely dry to ensure the alcohol has evaporated. Do not wash off hand rub.

The CDC (2020b) describes proper hand washing. Wet your hands with warm—not hot—water, then soap and lather. Rub your hands together for at least 20 seconds (sing "Happy Birthday" twice), covering all surfaces. Interlace your fingers to cleanse between them. Rub your nails against your palms to clean under the nails. Then rinse your hands with fingertips pointed downward under running water. Dry your hands with clean paper towels/towels or air dry them. Use a paper towel to turn off the faucet.

The CDC has two campaigns to encourage excellent hand hygiene. The Clean Hands Count campaign is for improving HCP adherence and empowering patients to ask HCPs to use hand hygiene. A new community hand-washing campaign, Life Is Better with Clean Hands, encourages adults to incorporate hand washing into their daily routine.

> **BE SAFE!**
> **TAKE ACTION!** Did you know that patients may also transmit organisms with inadequate hand hygiene and that they are often never offered the opportunity to wash their hands? Research has shown that patient hand hygiene is a weak link in the prevention of HAIs. Offer and assist your patients with hand hygiene throughout the day! Teach them the importance of frequent hand hygiene before meals and after toileting, handling their own secretions, or leaving and returning to their room. If patients cannot get to a sink, place hand sanitizer or disinfecting wipes at the bedside.

Asepsis

Asepsis is freedom from organisms. Protect patients at risk of developing infections with aseptic techniques.

Medical Asepsis

Medical asepsis is referred to as *clean technique*. The goal is to reduce the number of pathogens or prevent the transmission of pathogens from one person to another. Frequent hand hygiene, use of PPE, patient rooms with special ventilation, disinfectants, and precautions as defined by the CDC help to achieve this goal. As part of medical asepsis, keep your own body, clothing, and shoes clean to prevent spread of infection to patients, yourself, and your family (Box 8.1).

You are responsible for using appropriate hand hygiene in the health-care setting. HCPs perform hand hygiene less than half of the time they should.

> **CUE RECOGNITION 8.1**
> A resident has neutropenia from chemotherapy treatments. What is the most important action for you to take to prevent infection?
>
> *Suggested answers are at the end of the chapter.*

> **Box 8.1**
> **Guidelines to Prevent the Spread of Infection to Patients, Self, and Family**
> - Bathe daily and *always* wear a clean uniform/clothing every day.
> - Keep your natural fingernail tips less than 1/4 inch long, and do not wear artificial nails. Studies have shown that long fingernails and artificial nails harbor harmful bacteria and have transmitted infections to patients that have sometimes resulted in death.
> - Avoid wearing rings and bracelets at work because they harbor organisms.
> - Use hand hygiene between each patient contact. The use of a 60% to 95% alcohol-based hand rub or hand washing is recognized as the single-most important action to take to prevent the spread of organisms.
> - Disinfect your stethoscope daily and in between patient use with alcohol wipes. Vancomycin-resistant enterococci have been cultured from stethoscopes in a hospital setting.
> - Follow prescribed isolation precautions for your protection as well as that of the patient.
> - Perform hand hygiene before going home to prevent transfer of bacteria to your home.
> - Remove your uniform in a contained area of your home to launder it, and bathe/shower when you come home from work. Doing so decreases the spread of antibiotic-resistant bacteria to your home and your family. Keep your nursing shoes clean and stored away from the rest of the family.

Surgical Asepsis

Surgical asepsis (sterile technique) refers to an item or area free of all microorganisms and spores. Surgical asepsis is used in surgery and to sterilize equipment. Items can be subjected to intense heat or chemical disinfectants to destroy all organisms. Use of pressurized steam sterilizers, called *autoclaves*, kills even the most powerful organisms. Some equipment cannot be exposed to moist heat and require gas sterilizers. After these items are sterilized, they are dated, packaged, and sealed. Once a package is opened or outdated, it is no longer sterile.

Ultraviolet Environmental Disinfection

Health-care agencies use ultraviolet (UV) light to disinfect patient care areas and rooms after traditional cleaning (Dong et al, 2020). Portable robots that emit UV-C light are placed into empty rooms with the doorways then blocked to prevent entry. All surfaces are disinfected with bouncing and reflecting light waves in minutes. To see a robot, visit www.xenex.com.

Infection Prevention and Control Guidelines

CDC guidelines for infection control and isolation precautions are used in policies at hospitals, long-term care facilities, and other health-care agencies. CDC and agency guidelines are continuously updated. Follow them for your patients' and your own protection. Current CDC guidelines for isolation precautions in hospitals and long-term care facilities include two tiers of precautions: standard precautions and transmission-based precautions (Table 8.3).

Table 8.3
Standard Precautions and Transmission-Based Precautions

Standard Precautions

Use standard precautions for all patient care as appropriate. Use standard precautions along with *all* transmission-based precautions as needed based on the patient's illness and anticipated contact with the patient and environment.

Hand hygiene	Use 60%–95% alcohol-based hand rub or wash hands with nonmicrobial soap, unless specifically contraindicated, before and after using gloves, between patients, and between procedures on the same patient.
Gloves	Wear gloves before contact with any body fluids or substances. Change gloves after each use.
Mask, eye protection, face shield	Use personal protective equipment for patient care if splashes or sprays of blood or body fluids are likely.
Gown	Wear gown to protect skin/prevent soiling of clothing for patient care if splashes or sprays of blood or body fluids are likely.
Occupational health and bloodborne pathogens	Dispose of sharps properly. Do not recap needles.
Patient care equipment	Clean reusable equipment before reuse. Dispose of single-use items properly.
Linen	Handle linen to avoid clothing contamination.
Patient placement	Use private room for infectious patients.

Transmission-Based Precautions

Airborne Precautions

Examples: *Mycobacterium tuberculosis* (TB), rubeola virus (measles), varicella-zoster virus (chickenpox), and SARS-CoV-2 (COVID-19) for aerosol generating procedures

Patient placement	Provide private room with regulated airflow. Keep door closed.
Personal protective equipment (PPE)	
Respiratory protection	Do not enter room if susceptible to measles or chickenpox unless no caregivers who are immune are available. If susceptible, wear a fit-tested (N95) disposable respirator or powered air-purifying respirator (PAPR). Do not enter room of patient with TB unless wearing a N95 disposable respirator or PAPR. Have patient with TB also wear surgical mask during times that care is performed. Offer visitors an N95 respirator per agency policy.
Standard precautions added as needed	Gloves, gown, goggles/face shield, foot covers.
Patient transport	Limit patient transport to essential purposes. Place surgical mask on patient.

Droplet Precautions

Examples: Adenovirus, coronavirus (COVID-19), diphtheria (pharyngeal), *Haemophilus influenzae* (epiglottitis, meningitis, pneumonia), influenza, mumps, mycoplasma pneumonia, *Neisseria meningitidis* (meningitis, pneumonia, pertussis, pneumonic plague, rubella, group A streptococcus)

Patient placement	Provide private room for patients with COVID-19. For other diseases requiring droplet precautions use a private room or separation greater than 3 feet between the infected patient and other patients, and close privacy curtain.

Table 8.3
Standard Precautions and Transmission-Based Precautions—cont'd

PPE	
Respiratory protection	Wear respirator mask upon entering patient area (N95 mask or PAPR for patients with COVID-19). Reinforce teaching on respiratory hygiene/cough etiquette.
Standard precautions added as needed	Gloves, gown, goggles/face shield, foot covers
Patient transport	Limit patient transport to essential purposes. Place appropriate type of mask on patient.
Contact Precautions Examples: Cellulitis, *Clostridioides difficile,* coronavirus (COVID-19), skin infections (cutaneous diphtheria, herpes simplex virus, impetigo, pediculosis, scabies), conjunctivitis, viral hemorrhagic infections (Ebola, Lassa, or Marburg), herpes zoster	
Patient placement	Provide private room or place with patient with same infection and no other infection.
PPE	Gloves, gown, and foot covers protect self and others from contaminated items.
Patient transport	Limit patient transport.
Patient care equipment	Dedicate the use of noncritical patient care equipment to a single patient.

Sources: Siegel, J. D., Rhinehart, E., Jackson, M., Chiarello, L., & Healthcare Infection Control Practices Advisory Committee. (2019). *Guideline for isolation precautions: Preventing transmission of infectious agents in healthcare settings.* (2007). Washington, DC: Centers for Disease Control and Prevention. www.cdc.gov/infectioncontrol/guidelines/isolation/index.html; Centers for Disease Control and Prevention (CDC). (Last reviewed August 30, 2018). Infection prevention and control recommendations for hospitalized patients under investigation (PUIs) for Ebola virus disease (EVD) in U.S. hospitals. www.cdc.gov/vhf/ebola/healthcare-us/hospitals/infection-control.html; CDC. (Updated September 10, 2021). Interim infection prevention and control recommendations for healthcare personnel during the coronavirus disease 2019 (COVID-19) pandemic. www.cdc.gov/coronavirus/2019-ncov/hcp/infection-control-recommendations.html.

Evidence-Based Practice

Clinical Question
What are barriers and facilitators to health-care workers' adherence to infection prevention and control (IPC) guidelines for respiratory infectious diseases?

Evidence
A qualitative evidence analysis of 20 studies from around the world looked at the experiences and perceptions of health-care workers in hospitals and primary and community care about factors that affect their ability to follow IPC guidelines (PPE, the isolation of these patients from others and meticulous cleaning routines) for respiratory infectious diseases. Barriers were identified as ever-changing local guidelines that did not reflect national or international guidelines; increased workloads; fatigue; lack of mandatory training on the IPC guidelines; lack of adequate isolation space; lack of high-quality, comfortable PPE; workplace culture; and personal value view. Facilitators included support by their management team, clear communication, reducing overcrowding, rapid identification of infected patients, limiting visitors, having easy access for hand hygiene, fear of self or family infection, and a responsibility to their patients.

Implications for Nursing Practice
To follow IPC guidelines effectively, all health-care staff need to be included and supported by their administration with clear communication for the education and implementation of IPC guidelines. Easy hand hygiene access, sufficient high-quality PPE, and adequate isolation space need to be available. A desire to provide good patient care is also important.

Reference: Houghton, C., Meskell, P., Delaney, H., Smalle, M., Glenton, C., Booth, A., Chan, X. H. S., Devane, D., & Biesty, L. M. (2020). Barriers and facilitators to healthcare workers' adherence with infection prevention and control (IPC) guidelines for respiratory infectious diseases: A rapid qualitative evidence synthesis. *Cochrane Database of Systematic Reviews, 4*(4), CD013582. https://doi.org/10.1002/14651858.CD013582.

Standard Precautions

Standard precautions are used in the care of all patients. These precautions require you to assume that all patients are infectious regardless of their diagnosis and to use PPE. Standard precautions apply to blood, secretions, excretions, open skin, mucous membranes, and all body fluids, excluding sweat. All patients with draining wounds or secretions of body fluids are considered infectious until an infection is confirmed or ruled out. Using PPE such as gloves, gowns, masks, goggles, and face shields along with meticulous hand hygiene helps prevent the spread of infection to health-care workers, other patients, and visitors. Surgical masks with a clear window help to improve the communication between the nurse and patients who are hearing impaired or cognitively impaired.

Transmission-Based Precautions

Transmission-based precautions are used for patients with specific infectious diseases that can be transmitted to others. They add an additional layer of protection to the standard precautions.

Prevention of Respiratory Tract Infections

Health-care-associated pneumonia has been linked with the highest infection mortality rate. Patients who are at highest risk for pneumonia are those with endotracheal, nasotracheal, or tracheostomy tubes. These invasive tubes bypass the normal defenses of the upper respiratory tract. Strategies to prevent infections such as ventilator-associated pneumonia (VAP) are "bundled" together so nurses remember to use these strategies.

Prevention of Genitourinary Tract Infections

The most common HAI is a catheter-associated UTI (CAUTI; CDC, 2020c). Patients with urinary catheters are at greatest risk. The urinary tract is sterile. Insertion of a catheter into the bladder may allow organisms to enter. Institutional policies on appropriate use of urinary catheters differ, so follow your agency's policy. Appropriate reasons for use of a urinary catheter may include urinary obstruction, a neurogenic bladder condition, shock, and palliative care.

Indwelling urinary catheters should be removed as soon as possible. For patients who need long-term catheterization, intermittent catheterization is preferred because it significantly reduces the risk of infection. Using strict aseptic technique while inserting and caring for the catheter in the health-care agency is imperative. The catheter tubing must be securely anchored to the patient's leg, according to agency protocol, to prevent moving in and out of the urethra. This movement can encourage organisms to enter the sterile urinary tract.

The closed urinary drainage system seal should never be opened. (If intermittent irrigation is ordered, sterile technique must be used to protect both ends of the system from contamination.) The drainage bag should always be positioned lower than the level of the bladder to prevent backflow of urine into the bladder, which could contaminate the sterile urinary tract. If an indwelling urinary catheter and a drainage system are used long term, the catheter and the entire system should be changed regularly using sterile technique. All long-term indwelling urinary catheters are considered colonized. Standards in home health care can differ from institutional care because patients are generally at lower risk of infection within their own environment.

The most crucial point at which bacteria may enter the patient is during insertion of the catheter. Excellent sterile technique is required. The urinary tract is highly vascular (many blood vessels close to the surface). Therefore, an infection can easily result in bacteremia (bacteria in the blood). This can progress to sepsis, a potentially life-threatening condition.

BE SAFE!
BE VIGILANT! Catheters should be used only when necessary because of the **morbidity** (sickness) and **mortality** (death) associated with infections that can develop. Continued need for an indwelling catheter should be monitored daily. The catheter should be discontinued as soon as possible.

CUE RECOGNITION 8.2
A patient is being transported in a wheelchair by a nursing assistant to the activity room with a urinary catheter bag hung on the arm of the wheelchair. What action do you take?

Suggested answers are at the end of the chapter.

Prevention of Surgical Wound Infections

The initial dressing for surgical wounds is applied in the operating room using sterile aseptic technique. Postoperative orders indicate when to change the dressing and any specific dressing supplies to use. Monitor the wound with each dressing change for signs of infection.

PRACTICE ANALYSIS TIP
Linking NCLEX-PN® to Practice
The LPN/LVN will apply principles of infection control (e.g., aseptic technique, isolation, sterile technique, universal/standard precautions).

CRITICAL THINKING
Risk of Infection: Of the following patients, who is at greatest risk of infection and why?
1. Mr. Ashland, age 55, had an ambulatory hernia repair. He has adult-onset diabetes.
2. Mrs. Burrows, age 72, is hospitalized with a fractured hip. She is thin and frail, has dementia, and has undergone placement of a urinary catheter.
3. Jackson Dunn, age 22, underwent an appendectomy in the hospital. Jackson is underweight.

Suggested answers are at the end of the chapter.

ANTIBIOTIC-RESISTANT INFECTIONS

Antibiotic-resistant infections are a worldwide health concern. Currently, there are 18 antibiotic-resistant organisms (CDC, 2020a). Resistant organisms are difficult or impossible to treat, can spread easily to others, and may result in death. It is up to each of us to help prevent antibiotic resistance. The CDC's Antibiotic Resistance Solutions Initiative aims to detect, respond to, contain, and prevent resistant infections within health-care settings.

> **LEARNING TIP**
> Do you know which type of organisms antibiotics kill? Bacteria, not viruses! (Remember the **b** in anti**b**iotics and **b**acteria.) Antibiotics are not effective against viral infections such as colds or the flu. Most upper respiratory infections do not require antibiotics. Taking antibiotics to treat viral infections increases the risk for antibiotic-resistant "superbugs" for everyone. Nurses play a vital role in educating people not to request antibiotics for a viral infection.

Methicillin-Resistant Staphylococcus aureus (MRSA)

MRSA is a serious, life-threatening antibiotic-resistant infection. It has resulted from long-term use of unnecessary antibiotics. People can be carriers of MRSA and spread it, even when they have no symptoms. MRSA occurs in health-care settings and nursing homes. Symptoms include painful warm red bumps, fever, and drainage. MRSA can also be seen in the community among those who are healthy, starting as a skin boil. Treatment includes draining skin boils or administering antibiotics such as vancomycin hydrochloride. Use contact precautions.

Vancomycin-Resistant Enterococci (VRE)

VRE infections are common. Although enterococci are normal flora in the GI and female genital tracts, VRE are a pathogenic strain. VRE are transmitted via direct or indirect contact. Patients at risk for VRE infections include those with indwelling urinary or central venous catheters, the immunocompromised or critically ill, those receiving multiple antibiotics or vancomycin therapy, surgical patients, and those with extended hospital stays. Preventive VRE measures focus on proper hand hygiene, education of HCPs, aggressive infection control methods, and restricting use of vancomycin. Use PPE and follow CDC and agency infection control policies. Treatment involves combination antibiotic therapy.

THERAPEUTIC MEASURES FOR INFECTIOUS DISEASES

When an infection-causing organism and the affected body system have been identified, the appropriate medication can be selected for treatment (Table 8.4).

Table 8.4 Medications Used to Treat Infections

Medication Class/Action

Bactericidal Antibiotics

Penicillin
Antibacterial agent that inhibits cell wall synthesis most effectively for gram-positive organisms.

Examples	Nursing Implications
amoxicillin (Amoxil) ampicillin (Omnipen) penicillin G ticarcillin (Ticar)	Monitor for allergic reaction or anaphylactic shock. *Teaching*: Hold medication and call HCP for allergy signs, oral white patches, or vaginal irritation.

Carbapenems
Antibacterial agent that inhibits cell wall synthesis for moderate to severe infection.

Examples	Nursing Implications
doripenem (Doribax) ertapenem (Invanz) imipenem/cilastatin (Primaxin) meropenem (Merrem)	Monitor for seizures. Ertapenem: Check for lidocaine (intramuscular diluent) allergy.

Continued

Table 8.4
Medications Used to Treat Infections—cont'd

Medication Class/Action

Cephalosporins
Antibacterial agent inhibits cell wall synthesis.
First generation: more effective against gram-positive organisms.
Second and third generation: more effective against gram-negative organisms.
Fourth generation: more gram-negative coverage.
Fifth generation: methicillin-resistant Staphylococcus aureus *coverage.*

Examples	Nursing Implications
First generation: cefazolin (Ancef) Second and third generation: cefaclor (Ceclor); ceftriaxone (Rocephin) Fourth generation: cefepime (Maxipime) Fifth generation: ceftaroline (Teflaro)	Use caution if penicillin allergy or renal or hepatic dysfunction. *Teaching:* Take on empty stomach.

Aminoglycosides
Gram-negative antibacterial agent that inhibits protein synthesis.

Examples	Nursing Implications
amikacin (Amikin) gentamicin (Garamycin) tobramycin (Nebcin)	Report elevated creatinine levels as nephrotoxic. Monitor peak/trough levels. *Teaching:* Report signs of allergy, tinnitus, vertigo, or hearing loss.

Fluoroquinolones
Antibacterial agent that inhibits bacterial DNA replication for variety of infections.

Examples	Nursing Implications
ciprofloxacin (Cipro) levofloxacin (Levaquin) moxifloxacin (Avelox) norfloxacin (Noroxin) ofloxacin (Floxin)	Boxed warning secondary to corrected QT interval prolongation, central nervous system (CNS) effects, peripheral neuropathy, tendon rupture, tendonitis. *Teaching:* Take on empty stomach with full glass of water. Do not take with antacids. Use sun protection of at least 30 and cover skin. Report joint or muscle pain, or tendon rupture immediately.

Nitroimidazoles
Inhibit nucleic acid synthesis in anaerobic bacteria and protozoa.

Example	Nursing Implications
metronidazole (Flagyl)	For sexually transmitted infection, treat partner also. *Teaching*: Take with or without food. Avoid alcohol; abstain for at least 48 hours after treatment to prevent severe flu-like reaction.

Glycopeptides
Inhibit the synthesis of cell walls in gram-positive cocci.

Examples	Nursing Implications
vancomycin (Vancocin HCL, Vancocin HCL Pulvules) Gram-positive skin and skin structure infections: dalbavancin (Dalvance) oritavancin (Orbactiv) telavancin (Vibativ)	Oral vancomycin given for *C. difficile* associated diarrhea. Review infusion recommendations specific to individual medication. Monitor medication levels and IV site. *Teaching:* Report sudden hearing or balance problems.

Table 8.4
Medications Used to Treat Infections—cont'd

Medication Class/Action

Bacteriostatic Antibiotics

Tetracyclines
Protein synthesis inhibitor for most gram-positive and gram-negative organisms.

Examples	Nursing Implications
tetracycline hydrochloride (Sumycin) doxycycline (Vibramycin) minocycline hydrochloride (Minocin)	*Teaching:* Do not take during pregnancy due to bone/teeth effects. Take on empty stomach. Do not take with antacids or dairy products. Use sun protection of at least 30 and cover skin.

Macrolides
Protein synthesis inhibitor for many gram-negative and gram-positive organisms.

Example	Nursing Implications
azithromycin (Zithromax)	*Teaching:* Take on empty stomach with a full glass of water. Do not take with antacids. Use sun protection of at least 30 and cover skin.
clarithromycin (Biaxin)	*Teaching:* Take with a full glass of water. Take time-release capsules with food.
erythromycin (E-Mycin, E.E.S.)	*Teaching:* Take orally on empty stomach with a full glass of water. Contact HCP if side effects such as gastric distress are intolerable.
For *C. difficile* only: fidaxomicin (Dificid)	*Teaching:* Take tablets with or without food.

Lincomycins
Inhibit protein synthesis within bacterial cell for serious bacterial infection.

Example	Nursing Implication
clindamycin (Cleocin)	*Teaching*: Report foul-odor diarrhea, fever, and abdominal pain indicating possible *C. difficile* infection.

Sulfonamides
Inhibit growth and multiplication for most gram-positive and many gram-negative organisms mainly in UTIs, Pneumocystis jiroveci pneumonia, and otitis media.

Example	Nursing Implications
trimethoprim sulfamethoxazole (Bactrim, Septra)	*Teaching:* Take on empty stomach with a full glass of water. Drink at least 1.5 liters daily and monitor output. Use sun protection of at least 30 and cover skin. Inform HCP for allergic reaction or bleeding.

Oxazolidinones
Synthetic protein synthesis inhibitor for complicated infections caused by gram-negative microorganisms.

Example	Nursing Implications
linezolid (Zyvox)	*Teaching:* Avoid tyramine (found in aged cheeses, smoked foods, draft beer, red wine, soy sauce, sauerkraut).

Continued

Table 8.4 Medications Used to Treat Infections—cont'd

Medication Class/Action

Antifungals

Amphotericin B
Interferes with the fungal cell wall structure for life-threatening fungal infections.

Examples	Nursing Implications
amphoteracin B (Fungizone)	May require premedication to prevent infusion reaction.
amphoteracin B lipid complex (Abelcet)	Monitor injection site and for signs of kidney damage.
amphotericin B liposome (Ambisome)	*Teaching:* Drink 1–2 liters of fluid daily to flush medication.

Triazoles
Inhibit cell membrane ergosterol synthesis for yeast or fungus infections.

Examples	Nursing Implications
fluconazole (Diflucan)	Monitor BUN and creatinine levels and liver function tests.
itraconazole (Sporanox)	*Teaching:*
posaconazole (Noxafil)	Notify HCP at the first sign of yellow skin, dark urine, or pale stools.
voriconazole (Vfend)	

Echinocandins
Disrupt fungal cell wall integrity for candidal infection.

Examples	Nursing Implication
anidulafungin (Eraxis)	Monitor liver function tests.
caspofungin (Cancidas)	
micafungin (Mycamine)	

Antivirals

Antiretrovirals
See Chapter 20

Anti-Influenza Virus
See Chapter 30

Anti-Hepatitis Virus
See Chapter 35

Anti-Herpes Virus and Cytomegalovirus
Inhibit viral DNA synthesis for viral infection.

Examples	Nursing Implications
acyclovir (Zovirax)	Use systemic preparations cautiously with CNS, hepatic, or renal disorders.
cidofovir (Vistide)	*Teaching:*
famciclovir (Famvir)	Maintain hydration with systemic preparations.
foscarnet (Foscavir)	
valacyclovir (Valcyte)	

The medication of choice must be able to destroy (or control) the identified pathogen:

- Antibiotics treat only bacterial infections, not viruses, fungi, helminths, or prions.
- Antiviral medications treat viral infections, but use is for symptom control rather than cure.
- Antifungal drugs are available for fungal infections, but cure may require extended use.

Antibiotics can be classified as either bactericidal or bacteriostatic. Bactericidal agents kill the bacteria. Bacteriostatic agents inhibit or retard bacterial growth. The final destruction of the bacteria is then completed by the infected host's immune system. Bacteriostatic agents may be less helpful for the patient who is immunocompromised.

> **BE SAFE!**
> **AVOID FAILURE TO RECOGNIZE!** When preparing to give an antibiotic, especially for the first time, ask what allergies a patient may have and report them to the HCP. Patients may have allergies to one antibiotic group that prevents the use of chemically similar drugs.

Many antibiotics are metabolized by the liver and excreted by the kidneys. Disorders of these organs may require lower doses. Antibiotic levels fluctuate depending on organ function, age, sex, health, and other factors. Antibiotic serum peak level (highest level occurring right after medication administration) and/or trough level (lowest level occurring just before a dose is due) are monitored per agency protocol to ensure nontoxic, therapeutic levels.

Antibiotic-Associated Diarrhea (AAD)

Antibiotic therapy may cause AAD because antibiotics upset the delicate balance of natural microbiota found in the intestine. Any antibiotic can cause AAD, but ampicillin, cephalosporins, and clindamycin are the most common. Antibiotics destroy both helpful bacteria and harmful bacteria. As a result, with fewer helpful bacteria, harmful bacteria increases. These harmful bacteria produce toxins that harm the intestinal wall, cause inflammation, and result in watery bowel movements. When AAD occurs, the antibiotic therapy may be stopped, which usually resolves the diarrhea. For severe diarrhea and colitis (colon inflammation), vancomycin (Vancocin) or fidaxomicin (Dificid) is given.

Clostridioides difficile

C. difficile is a gram-positive bacterium that can cause infection. It can be one of the most serious causes of AAD. It is sometimes found normally in the intestine. When normal gut microbiota has been destroyed, *C. difficile* can overgrow. This results in the release of toxins causing diarrhea of 20 or more stools daily, fever, bloating, and abdominal pain. *C. difficile* infection (CDI) often occurs after antibiotic therapy. It is seen in those who are hospitalized, in long-term care facilities as well as those in the community. Older adults are at greatest risk. *C. difficile* overgrowth can lead to pseudomembranous colitis, a serious and sometimes life-threatening condition with fever, diarrhea, and abdominal pain. The bacteria are transmitted by the fecal–oral route from touching feces-contaminated surfaces. Lidless toilets increase the risk of *C. difficile* environmental contamination by spraying organisms during flushing, so their use is discouraged. Hand washing is essential to reduce its spread, as alcohol-based rubs are not effective. To treat diarrhea caused by CDI, any antibiotic therapy is discontinued, and fidaxomicin (Dificid) or vancomycin (Vancocin) is given. Vaccines are in trials to prevent CDI.

Fecal Microbiota Transplantation

If CDI reoccurs, fecal microbiota transplantation can cure it, primarily when other treatments have failed. The purpose is to restore healthy bacteria in the intestine. Patients who have been gravely ill from recurrent CDI can be infection-free within days after the treatment. Donated feces from a screened healthy person is transplanted into the patient via oral capsules, colonoscopy, sigmoidoscopy, enema, nasogastric or nasoenteric tube, or esophagogastroduodenoscopy (EGD).

Nursing Care

Nurses are responsible for administering medications correctly and for teaching patients the importance of taking these medications properly (see "Patient Teaching Guide: Anti-infective Medications" in online resources). Follow these general guidelines before giving anti-infectives:

- Verify patient allergies and inform the HCP.
- Obtain ordered samples for culturing before starting ordered anti-infectives so culture accuracy is not affected.
- Monitor and report to HCP any side effects or signs of allergic response, especially anaphylactic reactions and peak and trough results.
- Observe and report to HCP any signs of superinfection (one that occurs as a result of antibiotic use). For example, oral thrush (white raised lesions on tongue) may develop because antibiotics disrupt the normal GI tract flora.

> **BE SAFE!**
> **BE VIGILANT!** Always review medication doses. Compare them with the normal dose of the medications before giving them to keep your patient safe and protect your nursing license. You are responsible for any medication you give, even if the dose was ordered incorrectly and you followed the order. If the dose is outside the normal range, do not give the medication. Contact your supervisor or pharmacist for consultation with the ordering HCP for clarification.

NURSING PROCESS FOR THE PATIENT WITH AN INFECTION

General Infections
Data Collection

Early detection of signs and symptoms can help provide early treatment to prevent major complications and reduce costs. Providing emotional support to the patient is also important ("Patient Perspective"). Patients who are prone to infection because of immunosuppression should take special precautions to prevent infection (see "Patient Teaching Guidelines: Prevention of Infection in Older, Frail, or Immunocompromised Patients" in online resources).

Patient Perspective

Jeff. It's back! I've been hospitalized four times with this same infection (cellulitis) in my leg. It feels like I've lost control of my life. My left leg is swollen, red, discolored, and very painful. I can tell when I'm infected. I feel weak and kind of spacey. I'm tired of going to the emergency room—waiting forever to get admitted, having an IV started and blood draws. With these infections, I've had a PICC [peripherally inserted central catheter] line twice. I've been sent home on IV antibiotics, sometimes for weeks at a time. I've learned how to hang my own IV antibiotics. My cellulitis is associated with chronic lymphedema, causing swelling in my legs. I'm working hard to keep the swelling down so the infection doesn't recur. Wish me luck and keep giving me psychosocial support during your nursing care.

CLINICAL JUDGMENT

Mr. Cheevers is admitted to the hospital for IV antibiotic therapy. He states that he has no allergies. One hour after the infusion begins, you happen to meet the nursing assistant coming down the hall with a blanket. He casually says, "Mr. Cheevers is very cold. I'm taking him a blanket. He is also restless and a bit short of breath."
1. What action do you take?
2. What health-care team members do you collaborate with?
3. What education do you provide to the nursing assistant after Mr. Cheevers is stable?

Suggested answers are at the end of the chapter.

Nursing Diagnoses, Planning, and Implementation

Risk for Infection related to external factors

EXPECTED OUTCOME: The patient will remain free from symptoms of an infection.

- Observe and report signs of infection such as redness, warmth, and fever promptly, especially for a neutropenic patient *who does not have a normal inflammatory response and in whom low-grade fever may be the only sign.*
- Monitor laboratory values of WBC counts and cultures *because they correlate to immune function for planning patient care.*
- Use standard and transmission-based precautions *to prevent the transmission of organisms.*
- Administer anti-infective medications as ordered *to treat infections.*

Evaluation
If interventions have been successful, the patient remains free from symptoms of an infection.

Deficient Knowledge related to infection and treatment

EXPECTED OUTCOME: The patient will describe therapy and carry out treatment.

- Explain infection and prevention *to control risk for infection.*
- Promote responsible use of antibiotics *to prevent resistant organisms.*
- Explain medications, side effects, and symptoms to report *to promote adherence to treatment and safe medication use.*

Evaluation
If interventions have been effective, the patient will state understanding of therapy and carry out treatment plan.

Respiratory Tract Infection
Data Collection
Symptoms of a respiratory tract infection may include a cough, nasal congestion, chest congestion, chest pain, or sore throat. The throat may be reddened or have white patches on the back. Lung sounds can include crackles, rhonchi, or wheezing. Ask if the cough is productive and, if so, the amount, frequency, and color of the sputum. A sputum culture identifies pathogenic organisms for appropriate treatment.

Nursing Diagnoses, Planning, and Implementation

Risk for Infection related to external factors

EXPECTED OUTCOME: The patient will remain free from symptoms of respiratory infection.

- Encourage fluids if not contraindicated, *as dehydration is associated with dry, sticky secretions that are difficult to cough up.*
- Encourage coughing and deep breathing *to keep airways clear and prevent atelectasis.*
- Provide pain relief *so patient will take deep breaths.*
- Provide oral care with toothbrush or suction-type toothbrush and fluoride toothpaste regularly *to remove plaque, as toothettes do not, which has been found to contribute to pneumonia development.*
- Use sterile water rather than tap water from faucet for oral care for immunocompromised patient *to prevent pneumonia.*
- Elevate head of bed 30 degrees or more when a tube feeding is infusing *to prevent aspiration pneumonia.*

Evaluation
If interventions have been effective, oxygen saturation will be 95% or greater, with report of decreased dyspnea. Respirations will not be labored, and the patient will be free of signs and symptoms of infection.

Gastrointestinal Tract Infection

Data Collection

Symptoms of GI tract infections may include anorexia, cramping, diarrhea, nausea, and vomiting. Signs of dehydration from fluid loss are reported. Stool cultures may be ordered.

Nursing Diagnoses, Planning, and Implementation

Risk for Infection related to external factors

EXPECTED OUTCOME: The patient will remain free from symptoms of GI tract infection.

- Encourage fluid intake *to replace fluid lost during fever, vomiting, and diarrhea.*
- Follow standard and transmission-based precautions *to prevent the spread of* C. difficile.
- Teach hand hygiene with antimicrobial soap and water *because alcohols, chlorhexidine, iodophors, and other antiseptic agents are not effective in destroying* C. difficile *spores.*

Evaluation

Patient will be free of infection and nausea, vomiting, diarrhea, cramping, anorexia, and dehydration if interventions have been successful.

Genitourinary Tract Infection

Data Collection

Symptoms of a UTI include voiding urgency, frequency, and burning, flank pain, change in urine color, foul urine odor, and confusion or change in mental status in older adults. Monitor frequency, amount, color, and odor of the urine. Urinalysis and urine cultures may be ordered.

Nursing Diagnoses, Planning, and Implementation

Risk for Infection related to external factors

EXPECTED OUTCOME: The patient will remain free from symptoms of UTI.

- Do not request a urinary catheter except for a justifiable reason *because patient is more likely to develop a CAUTI.*
- For urinary catheters: use sterile technique for insertion and avoid contamination when emptying the bag *to prevent HAI.*

Evaluation

If interventions have been effective, the patient will have normal urine output without symptoms of UTI.

Key Points

- The links in the chain of infection include a causative agent, a reservoir, a portal of exit, a mode of transmission, a portal of entry, and a susceptible host.
- To interrupt the route of direct transmission, use hand hygiene, aseptic technique, and personal protective equipment. Interrupt airborne transmission by using a high-efficiency particulate air (HEPA) respirator. Interrupt vehicle transmission by using hand hygiene, ensuring both clean water and food supplies are available, and cleaning the patient environment and instruments per protocols.
- The body's defense mechanisms include intact skin and mucous membranes, gastric acid, immunoglobulins in serum and body fluids, specialized blood cells, lysosomes, and interferon. The inflammatory response is the next defensive level. It can be caused by pathogens, trauma, or other events causing injury to tissue.
- Nurses are responsible for administering medications correctly and teaching patients the importance of taking these medications properly. Review patient allergies, obtain ordered samples for culture before starting ordered anti-infectives, monitor ordered peak and trough results, and monitor and report side effects or signs of allergic response.
- Health-care staff must be constantly vigilant to help prevent hospital-acquired infections (HAIs). Some of the more common HAIs include ventilator-associated pneumonia; urinary tract infections, especially with an indwelling catheter; and surgical wound infections.
- Antibiotic-resistant infections such as *C. difficile*, MRSA, and VRE are serious worldwide health concerns.
- Nurses plan and deliver care to prevent infection in those at risk and to care for patients with various types of infections.

SUGGESTED ANSWERS TO CHAPTER EXERCISES

Cue Recognition
8.1: Perform frequent hand hygiene to reduce microorganisms on your hands. Ensure that the patient and other health-care staff also perform hand hygiene.

8.2: Inform the nursing assistant that the urinary bag has been placed above the patient's bladder. Explain that the bag should always stay below the level of the bladder for both proper drainage and infection control. Assist the nursing assistant to reposition the bag properly. Ensure that the patient is monitored for signs of a bladder infection from the potential backflow of urine.

Critical Thinking & Clinical Judgment
Risk of Infection
1. Mr. Ashland has two risk factors: chronic disease and invasive procedure. The procedure was done outside of hospital, which reduces HAI risk.
2. Mrs. Burrows has multiple risk factors: older age, dementia (unable to participate in preventive care such as coughing and deep breathing), frailty, hospitalization, immobility (risk of pneumonia increased), injury, malnourishment, and an invasive procedure. This patient is at greatest risk.
3. Jackson has three risk factors: hospitalization, invasive procedure, and malnourishment.

Mr. Cheevers
1. Immediately, collect data from Mr. Cheevers, as he may be experiencing signs of allergic reaction to the medication. If allergy is suspected, the IV medication should be stopped.
2. Notify your supervisor and after immediate data collection, notify the HCP.
3. Later, the nursing assistant can be taught to report abnormal symptoms, as they may be a sign of an allergic response.

Additional Resources

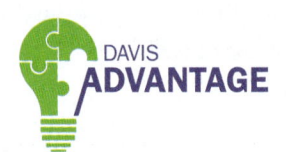

Go to Davis Advantage to complete your learning: strengthen understanding, apply your knowledge, and prepare for the Next Gen NCLEX®.

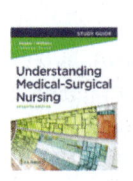

A Study Guide is also available.

CHAPTER 9
Nursing Care of Patients in Shock

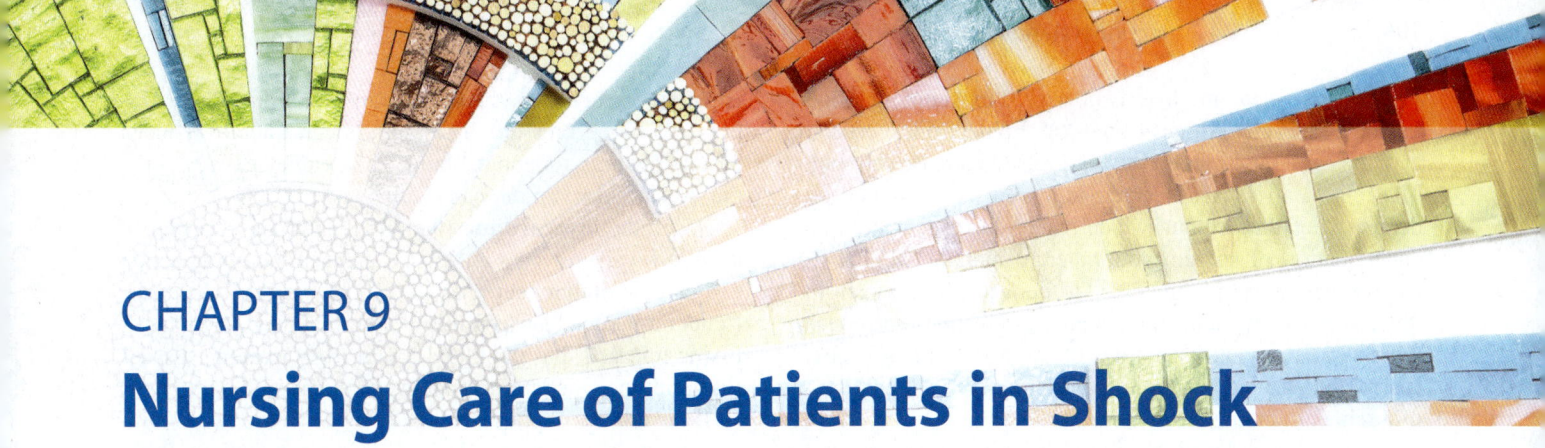

Linda S. Williams

KEY TERMS

acidosis (AS-ih-DOH-sis)
acute pulmonary hypertension (ah-KEWT PULL-muh-NAIR-ee HY-per-TEN-shun)
anaerobic (AN-air-ROH-bik)
anaphylaxis (AN-uh-fih-LAK-sis)
arrhythmia (uh-RITH-mee-ah)
bronchospasm (BRONG-koh-spazm)
capillary refill (KAP-ih-lar-ee REE-fil)
cardiac output (KAR-dee-ack OWT-put)
cardiogenic (KAR-dee-oh-JEN-ik)
cyanosis (SY-uh-NOH-sis)
distributive (dis-TRIB-yoo-tiv)
epinephrine (EP-ih-NEFF-rin)
hypoperfusion (HY-poh-per-FEW-shun)
hypotension (HY-poh-TEN-shun)
hypovolemic (HY-poh-voh-LEE-mik)
ischemia (is-KEY-mee-ah)
lactic acid (LAK-tik AS-id)
laryngeal edema (lah-RIN-jee-uhl eh-DEE-muh)
myocarditis (MY-oh-kar-DY-tis)
myocardium (MY-oh-KAR-dee-um)
neurogenic (NUR-roh-JEN-ik)
norepinephrine (NOR-ep-ih-NEFF-rin)
oliguria (ol-ih-GU-ree-ah)
perfusion (per-FEW-zhun)
pericardial tamponade (PER-ih-KAR-dee-uhl TAM-pon-AID)
sepsis (SEP-sis)
tachycardia (TAK-ih-KAR-dee-ah)
tachypnea (TAK-ip-NEE-ah)
tension pneumothorax (TEN-shun NEW-moh-THOR-raks)
toxemia (tock-SEE-mee-ah)
trauma (TRAW-mah)
urticaria (UR-tih-CARE-ee-ah)

CHAPTER CONCEPTS

Acid base
Fluid and electrolyte balance
Infection
Perfusion

LEARNING OUTCOMES

1. Explain the pathophysiology of shock and compensatory mechanisms.
2. Identify the etiology, signs, and symptoms for each of the four categories of shock.
3. Describe therapeutic measures for shock.
4. List data to collect when caring for patients in shock.
5. Plan nursing care for patients in shock.
6. Prioritize care for a patient in shock.
7. Identify findings that demonstrate a positive response to therapeutic measures for shock.

Shock is defined as inadequate cellular or tissue **perfusion** from a sudden drop in blood flow. When this happens, tissues do not receive enough oxygen to meet their metabolic needs. This imbalance in oxygen supply and demand leads to cellular and tissue hypoxia. **Hypoperfusion** of organs and cellular death can occur. It is important to identify patients at risk for shock. Monitor them for early signs and symptoms of shock, which can still be reversed to reduce injury to vital organs. Prolonged shock can lead to organ failure and death.

PATHOPHYSIOLOGY OF SHOCK

Blood pressure and tissue perfusion are maintained by three mechanisms: (1) adequate blood volume, (2) an effective cardiac pump, and (3) effective blood vessel tone. The body can compensate for a problem in one mechanism by making changes in one or both of the other mechanisms. Shock occurs when the compensatory mechanisms are unable to maintain blood pressure, resulting in poor tissue perfusion.

Metabolic and Hemodynamic Changes in Shock

When blood pressure falls, the sympathetic nervous system is activated and compensatory mechanisms begin. **Epinephrine** and **norepinephrine** are released from the adrenal medulla. This causes the heart to beat faster and stronger to increase **cardiac output.** Blood flow

• WORD • BUILDING •

hypoperfusion: hypo—low + perfuser—to pour over or through
epinephrine: epi—on + nephros—kidney

to the heart, brain, and liver is preserved by shunting blood from the intestines, kidneys, and skin. Epinephrine, cortisol, and glucagon raise blood glucose levels to increase cell fuel. The renin-angiotensin-aldosterone system is stimulated by decreased cardiac output, which results in vasoconstriction and retention of sodium and water to maintain fluid balance. Respiratory rate increases to deliver more oxygen to the tissues. Together, these compensatory responses produce the classic signs and symptoms of the first stage of shock: **tachycardia** (rapid heart rate), **tachypnea** (rapid breathing), **oliguria** (producing small amounts of urine), restlessness, anxiety, pallor, and cool, clammy skin. If blood pressure and oxygen delivery remain inadequate, signs and symptoms of progressive and then irreversible shock are seen (Table 9.1).

> **BE SAFE!**
> **TAKE ACTION!** Tachycardia is a compensatory mechanism that is usually the first sign of shock. Sustained tachycardia is a signal that the patient's condition is changing. Older patients cannot tolerate tachycardia for very long. Report tachycardia to the registered nurse (RN) or health-care provider (HCP). Then consider the cause of the tachycardia. For example, check a surgical patient who develops tachycardia for bleeding. Apply direct pressure to an area of hemorrhage. With internal hemorrhaging, there may not be visible bleeding. Vital sign changes may be the only cue.

When cells are deprived of oxygen, their energy production moves from efficient aerobic metabolism to less efficient **anaerobic** metabolism. The energy needs of the cell can only be met by anaerobic metabolism for a brief time. If the oxygen deficiency is prolonged, the body's metabolic rate and temperature fall.

Anaerobic metabolism produces lactate. **Lactic acid,** a by-product of lactate build-up, accumulates. If the lactic acid is not cleared from the bloodstream, it causes acidosis (an acid–base imbalance). **Acidosis** (blood pH below 7.35) is one of the classic signs of shock.

> **CRITICAL THINKING**
> **Shock**
> 1. What is the cause and compensatory purpose of each of the classic signs of shock: tachycardia, tachypnea, oliguria, pallor, and cool, clammy skin?
> 2. Why is anaerobic metabolism necessary and helpful if it produces the complication of metabolic acidosis?
>
> *Suggested answers are at the end of the chapter.*

Effect on Organs and Organ Systems

Why does prolonged shock cause extensive damage to organs? Inadequate blood flow results in tissue **ischemia** and injury throughout the body (Table 9.2). Early in shock, blood is shunted away from the kidneys to save fluid. This helps preserve blood pressure. The kidneys can tolerate reduced blood flow only for about 1 hour. Then kidney cells begin to die. Acute kidney injury can result.

When the **myocardium** (the middle and muscle layer of the heart wall) receives inadequate oxygen, pumping action and cardiac output decreases, and shock worsens. Acidosis, ischemia-induced **arrhythmias** (abnormal heart rhythm), or toxins released into the bloodstream from ischemic tissues further reduce the pumping ability of the heart.

If the brain is deprived of blood flow for more than 4 minutes, brain cells die from a lack of oxygen and glucose. Brain death can result from prolonged shock.

Organs of the gastrointestinal system can be injured early in shock. Inadequate circulation to the intestines injures the mucosa. Paralytic ileus (intestine paralysis) can occur. If gastrointestinal bacteria or endotoxins move from the bowel into the circulation, **toxemia** can result.

The liver can be injured by ischemia. If liver function is affected by this injury, elevated serum levels of ammonia, bilirubin, and liver enzymes and decreased production of plasma proteins can occur. The immune system is weakened by shock, leaving the body vulnerable to infection. If the liver has been damaged, it cannot assist the immune system in providing defense.

COMPLICATIONS FROM SHOCK

Acute respiratory distress syndrome (ARDS), disseminated intravascular coagulation (DIC), and multiple organ dysfunction syndrome (MODS; also referred to as multiple organ failure [MOF]) are three critical conditions that can follow prolonged shock. MODS is a major cause of death following shock. Inadequate perfusion of an organ leads to organ failure, which can cause the failure of other organs.

> **LEARNING TIP**
> To understand what disseminated intravascular coagulation (DIC) means, define each word:
> - *Disseminated:* scattered or widespread
> - *Intravascular:* intra = inside + vascular = vessel
> - *Coagulation:* clotting
>
> Together, these definitions tell you that DIC is scattered, widespread clotting inside the vessel!

• WORD • BUILDING •
tachycardia: tachy—fast + cardia—heart
tachypnea: tachy—fast + pnea—breathing
oliguria: olig—few + uria—urine
anaerobic: an—without + aerobic—presence of oxygen
acidosis: acid—sour + osis—condition
arrhythmia: a—without + rhythmia—rhythm

Table 9.1
Characteristics of Shock Stages

Characteristics	Stages		
	• Pre-shock (*compensated*) • Able to maintain blood pressure and tissue perfusion	• Shock (*progressive*) • Compensatory mechanisms start to fail	• End-organ dysfunction (*irreversible*) • No response to treatment • Multiorgan failure • Death is imminent
Heart rate	Tachycardia	Tachycardia Greater than 150 beats/min	Slowing
Pulses	Bounding	Weak, thready	Absent
Systolic blood pressure	Normal	Below 90 mm Hg In hypertensive patient, 25% below baseline	Below 60 mm Hg
Diastolic blood pressure	Normal	Decreased	Decreasing to 0
Respirations	Increased rate, deep	Tachypnea, crackles, shallow	Slowing, irregular, shallow
Temperature	Varies	Decreased, can rise in septic shock	Decreasing
Level of consciousness	Anxious, restless, irritable, alert, oriented, sense of impending doom	Confused, lethargic	Unconscious, comatose
Skin and mucous membranes	Cool, clammy, pale	Moist, cold, clammy, pale	Cyanotic, mottled, cold, clammy
Urine output	Normal	Decreasing to less than 20 mL/hr	15 mL/hr, decreasing to anuria
Bowel sounds	Normal	Decreasing	Absent

Hemorrhage may seem like an unlikely complication of a clotting problem. But when many clots form throughout the body in response to stressors, few clotting factors remain available to prevent hemorrhage. As a result, hemorrhage is a risk in DIC.

CLASSIFICATION OF SHOCK

The four types of shock discussed in this section are classified by their fluid and cardiovascular characteristics (Table 9.3). Undifferentiated shock is shock without a known cause. A combination of shock types may occur. The classic sign in all forms of shock is blood pressure too low to provide enough blood flow to the tissues for oxygenation.

Hypovolemic Shock

Hypovolemic shock results from circulating blood volume loss. This loss can be caused by dehydration; internal or external hemorrhage; fluid loss from burns, diarrhea, or vomiting; or loss of intravascular fluid into the interstitial space from sepsis or **trauma** (physical injury caused by an external force). Heat exhaustion or heatstroke can also cause hypovolemic shock from excessive water loss through sweating. Signs and symptoms include tachycardia; tachypnea; **hypotension;** restlessness; altered mental status; pale, cool, clammy skin; flat, nondistended jugular and peripheral veins; and decreased urine output.

> **NURSING CARE TIP**
> Research has shown that the Trendelenburg position (supine on 15- to 30-degree incline with feet higher than the head) is not helpful in improving cardiac output for patients in hypovolemic shock and can have profound negative effects on the lungs and brain.

Table 9.2
Effect of Shock on Organs and Organ Systems

Organ or Organ System	Effect
Lungs	Acute respiratory failure Acute respiratory distress syndrome (ARDS)
Renal system	Renal insufficiency Acute kidney injury
Heart	Arrhythmias Myocardial ischemia Myocardial infarction
Liver	Decreased production of plasma proteins Elevated serum levels of ammonia, bilirubin, and liver enzymes Impaired clotting
Immune system	Depletion of defense components
Gastrointestinal system	Absorption of endotoxins and bacteria Mucosal injury Pancreatitis Paralytic ileus
Central nervous system	Ischemic damage, necrosis, and brain death

CUE RECOGNITION 9.1
As you assist a patient who has returned from surgery, you notice a red stain on the sheet. You discover that the patient's jugular IV line has been dislodged. What action do you take?

Suggested answers are at the end of the chapter.

Cardiogenic Shock

Cardiogenic shock occurs when the heart fails as a pump and decreases cardiac output. It requires immediate treatment to prevent death. Signs and symptoms are like those of hypovolemic shock. Pulmonary edema may occur, which differentiates cardiogenic shock from other forms of shock. The main cause of cardiogenic shock is acute myocardial infarction. Other causes are arrhythmias, cardiomyopathy, cardiac trauma, endocarditis, heart valve defects, and **myocarditis** (inflammation of the heart muscle).

Distributive Shock

Distributive shock is caused by the loss of peripheral vascular resistance because of massive vasodilation. In hypovolemic shock, there is an actual loss of blood volume. But in distributive shock, there is no loss of fluid volume. Rather, the body's fluid distribution is altered within the body. There are three forms of distributive shock: anaphylactic, septic, and neurogenic.

Anaphylactic Shock

Anaphylactic shock is the most severe type of distributive shock. It occurs when the body has an extreme hypersensitivity reaction to an antigen (**anaphylaxis**) (Table 9.3; see Chapter 19). Death from anaphylactic shock can occur in minutes but is rare. Medical treatment must be sought immediately. Asthma or a delay in epinephrine injections increases the risk of death. For safety, patients are taught allergen avoidance techniques (Box 9.1).

Septic Shock

Sepsis is defined as "life-threatening organ dysfunction caused by dysregulated host response to infection" (Singer et al, 2016). In other words, the body's toxic response to an infection can lead to tissue damage, organ failure, and then death. Septic shock is defined as "a subset of sepsis with circulatory and cellular/metabolic dysfunction associated with a higher risk of mortality" (Singer et al, 2016). With septic shock, there is extreme hypoperfusion. It is a medical emergency. Early diagnosis and rapid treatment of sepsis are vital to increase survival rates and limit disability (Peltan et al, 2019). For every hour that sepsis remains untreated, mortality rises. One in three U.S. hospital deaths is due to sepsis (Centers for Disease Control and Prevention [CDC], 2020). The Surviving Sepsis Campaign, under the direction of the Society of Critical Care Medicine and the European Society of Intensive Care Medicine (www.sccm.org/SurvivingSepsisCampaign/Home), is a global initiative. Its goal is to reduce the sepsis mortality rate (see "Evidence-Based Practice"). A treatment bundle, Hour-1 Bundle, is used to guide initiation of quick treatment and ongoing management of sepsis to increase survival. Factors that increase sepsis risk include being older than 65, having a chronic illness, having a weakened immune system, having severe burns, or being critically ill (see "Gerontological Issues"). Infections of the lung (pneumonia), kidney, gastrointestinal tract, or skin are more commonly associated with sepsis. Sepsis is not contagious. Bacteria commonly cause sepsis, with *Escherichia coli, Staphylococcus aureus,* and some types of *Streptococcus* being the most frequent causes. Other infectious organisms that can also cause sepsis include viruses such as influenza or COVID-19. Educating the public

• WORD • BUILDING •

cardiogenic: kardia—heart + genesis—beginning
anaphylaxis: an—without + phylaxis—protection

Table 9.3
Categories of Shock

Category	Causes	Signs and Symptoms
Hypovolemic Shock	Any severe loss of body fluid, including dehydration; internal or external hemorrhage; fluid loss from burns, vomiting, or diarrhea; or loss of intravascular fluid into the interstitium	Tachycardia, tachypnea, hypotension, cyanosis, oliguria, flat and nondistended peripheral veins, altered mental status
Cardiogenic Shock	Myocardial infarction, traumatic cardiac injury, cardiomyopathy, endocarditis, myocarditis, arrhythmias, valvular disease	Arrhythmias, labored respirations, hypotension, cyanosis, oliguria, altered mental status, possibly distended jugular and peripheral veins, symptoms of heart failure
Obstructive Shock	Any block to the cardiovascular flow, such as pericardial tamponade, tension pneumothorax, intrathoracic tumor, massive pulmonary embolus, large systemic embolus	Tachycardia, tachypnea, hypotension, cyanosis, oliguria, altered mental status, possibly distended jugular veins
Distributive Shock	Any condition causing massive vasodilation of peripheral circulation, including the subcategories anaphylactic, septic, and neurogenic shock	*See below.*
• Anaphylactic shock	Reaction to an allergen, such as an insect sting, medication, peanuts, antibiotic, anesthetic, contrast dye, or blood product	• Tachycardia, tachypnea, wheezing, dyspnea, hypotension, cyanosis, oliguria, altered mental status • Can have **urticaria**, pruritus, angioedema, **laryngeal edema**, severe **bronchospasm** • If conscious, can be extremely apprehensive
• Septic shock	Loss of vascular autoregulatory control and loss of fluid into the interstitium caused by massive release of chemical mediators and endotoxins from pathogens	• *Early (warm) phase:* tachycardia; blood pressure, urine output, and capillary refill can be normal; skin warm and flushed; fever usually present; although temperature can be subnormal, fever may be absent in those who are older or immunosuppressed • *Late (cold) phase:* tachycardia; tachypnea; hypotension; oliguria; delayed capillary refill; cool, clammy skin; normal or subnormal temperature; mental status altered
• Neurogenic shock	Dysfunction or injury to the nervous system from spinal cord injury, general anesthesia, fever, metabolic disturbance, brain injury	• *Early phase:* hypotension; altered mental status; bradycardia; warm, dry skin • *Late phase:* tachycardia; tachypnea; cool, clammy skin

Box 9.1
Patient Education

Reinforce for patients who have severe allergies and a risk for anaphylaxis that they must have a prescribed epinephrine autoinjector available at all times for rapid onset, life-threatening reactions. After its use, medical treatment must be sought immediately before its effect wears off.

about sepsis, its signs and symptoms, and the need to seek urgent treatment and to ask, "Is this sepsis?" is vital to saving lives (Fig. 9.1).

Post-sepsis syndrome affects about half of sepsis survivors, with long-term physical and/or psychological effects. Others recover fully from sepsis with rehabilitation. Older adults are at higher risk for reduced cognitive and physical function following sepsis.

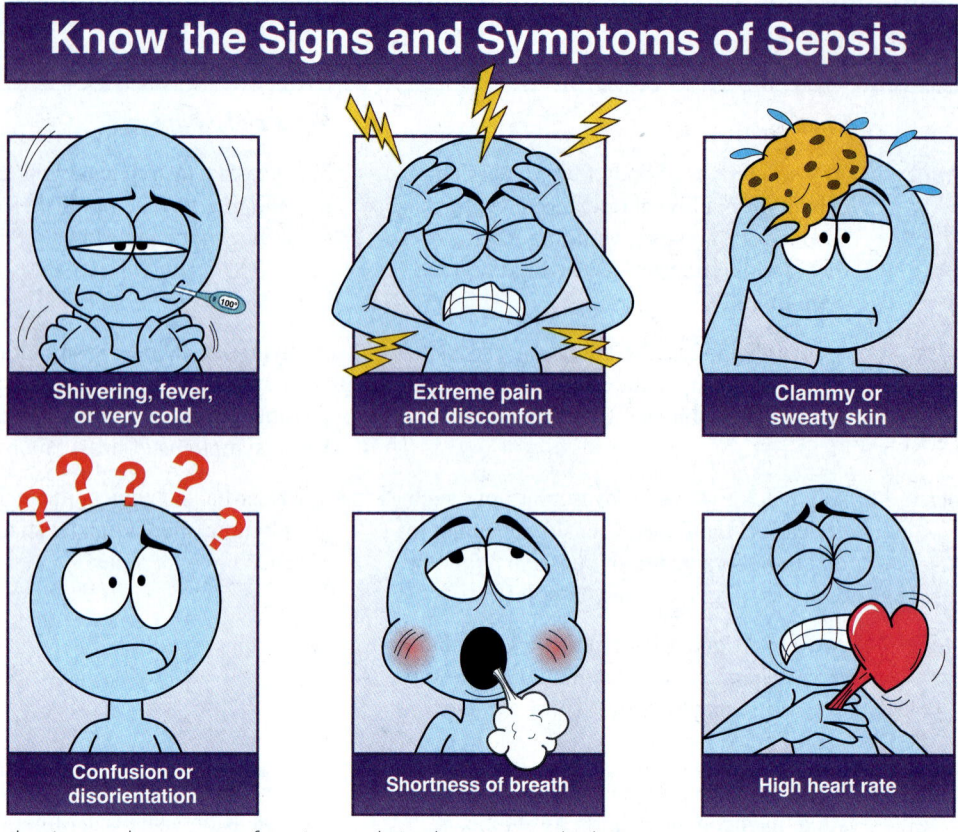

FIGURE 9.1 Know the signs and symptoms of sepsis to seek timely urgent medical care.

Evidence-Based Practice

Clinical Question
What are the best ways to manage sepsis and septic shock?

Evidence
The International Guidelines for Management of Sepsis and Septic Shock: 2021 provide updated evidence-based interventions. Nursing care interventions include the following:
- Use screening protocol for sepsis on acutely ill and high-risk patients with possible septic shock or high likelihood for sepsis.
- Report ordered laboratory results such as lactate level.
- Promptly obtain all ordered cultures (including two sets of blood cultures) prior to antimicrobial therapy so therapy is not delayed.
- Administer ordered IV antimicrobials (suggested as two gram-negative antimicrobials for multidrug resistant organisms; MRSA coverage antimicrobials with high risk of MRSA; antifungal therapy with high risk of fungal infection) immediately (within 1 hour) upon septic shock or highly suspected sepsis diagnosis, while cause of illness is sought.
- Administer and monitor ordered IV fluids (suggested at 30 mL/kg of IV balanced crystalloid fluid (rather than saline) for hypotension within first 3 hours of resuscitation).
- Administer ordered vasopressors (norepinephrine first choice; suggested peripherally until central venous access is available).
- Administer ordered IV corticosteroids when continued vasopressors are needed.
- Monitor arterial blood pressure invasively as soon as it is available to do so.
- Maintain ordered high flow nasal oxygen suggested for use in sepsis-induced hypoxemic respiratory failure.
- Use ordered prone positioning for mechanically ventilated patients with sepsis-related ARDS for more than 12 hours daily; veno-venous ECMO where available if mechanical ventilation fails.
- Implement ordered pharmacologic VTE prophylaxis.
- Maintain ordered glycemic control (arterial blood may be more accurate for point-of-care testing).
- Provide ordered enteral nutrition (early—within 72 hours—initiation).
- Assist with planning of care and the use of palliative care as appropriate.

Implications for Nursing Practice
Careful screening for sepsis and promptly carrying out ordered interventions included in the 2021 guidelines are vital to increasing patient survival rates from sepsis and septic shock.

Reference: Evans, L., Rhodes, A., Alhazzani, W., Antonelli, M., Coopersmith, C. M., French, C., Machado, F. R., Mcintyre, L., Ostermann, M., Prescott, H. C., Schorr, C., Simpson, S., Wiersinga, W. J., Alshamsi, F., Angus, D. C., Arabi, Y., Azevedo, L., Beale, R., Beilman, G., . . . Levy, M. (2021). Surviving sepsis campaign: international guidelines for management of sepsis and septic shock 2021. *Intensive Care Medicine, 47,* 1181–1247. https://doi.org/10.1007/s00134-021-06506-y

> **Gerontological Issues**
>
> **Sepsis**
> The older adult population has less ability to fight infections, placing them at higher risk for sepsis. Protect them with hand hygiene. Be vigilant and report abnormal signs and symptoms promptly.

Neurogenic Shock

Neurogenic shock occurs due to nervous system injury or dysfunction that causes extensive dilation of peripheral blood vessels. It is rare. Causes include spinal cord injury, general anesthesia, fever, metabolic disturbances, and brain contusions and concussions. Signs include hypotension and altered mental status and, during the early phases, bradycardia and warm, dry skin. As shock progresses, however, tachycardia and cool, clammy skin develops.

Obstructive Shock

Obstructive shock occurs when there is a blockage of blood flow to or from the heart. It is the rarest form of shock. **Pericardial tamponade** occurs when the pericardial sac fills with blood or fluid. This compresses the heart and limits its filling capacity. **Tension pneumothorax** compresses the heart because of an abnormal collection of air in the pleural space. **Acute pulmonary hypertension** is a sudden abnormally elevated pressure in the pulmonary artery. It increases resistance for the blood flowing out of the right side of the heart. All these conditions decrease cardiac output. This can lead to shock. A pulmonary embolism or tumor blocking blood flow can also lead to shock. Signs and symptoms of obstructive shock are similar to those of hypovolemic shock, except that jugular veins are usually distended.

THERAPEUTIC MEASURES FOR SHOCK

Because of the life-threatening nature of shock, immediate medical treatment is needed. The nature of the shock must be determined (Table 9.4) and interventions, including ventilatory and circulatory support, started. Life-threatening symptoms must be treated immediately (Table 9.5). If septic shock is identified, then current sepsis care guidelines are followed (visit www.survivingsepsis.org). Medications that are used in shock are listed in Table 9.6.

The order of interventions and testing is guided by the stability of the patient. Interventions include the following:

1. Airway management
2. Breathing and respiratory support
3. Cardiovascular support
4. Maintenance of circulatory volume
5. Control of bleeding if present
6. Monitoring of neurologic status
7. Treatment of life-threatening injuries
8. Determination and treatment of the cause of shock

Table 9.4
Data Collection for the Patient in Shock

Signs and Symptoms	Tachycardia, tachypnea, hypotension, cyanosis, mental status altered, oliguria
Laboratory Tests	Arterial blood gases, blood chemistries, blood typing and cross-match, cardiac isoenzymes, complete blood count, partial thromboplastin time, prothrombin time, serum lactate, serum osmolarity, urinalysis. Sepsis: C-reactive protein, endotoxins, procalcitonin
Imaging	Chest x-ray, computed tomography, echocardiogram, spinal x-ray
Monitoring	Arterial pressure, electrocardiogram, hemodynamic monitoring

NURSING PROCESS FOR THE PATIENT IN SHOCK

Data Collection

Recognizing and reporting patients at risk for shock is vital for increased patient survival. Being vigilant and screening patients for sepsis is important. Early detection and prevention of shock in patients at risk for shock are the desired goals. Rapid response teams can be helpful in providing quick assessment and care of patients at risk of developing shock.

For the patient in shock, assessment and data collection must be carried out quickly and should always start with ABCD: airway, breathing, circulation, and disability.

*A*irway is checked for patency and opened as necessary. A compromised airway must be treated immediately with the head-tilt/chin-lift method, an oral or nasal airway, or endotracheal intubation.

*B*reathing is checked for rate, depth, and symmetry of chest movement. The patient is observed for use of accessory muscles. Lung sounds are auscultated. Wheezing can be present in the patient with anaphylactic shock. Crackles can be found in the patient with cardiogenic shock or in the patient who has received too much intravenous fluid.

*C*irculation is monitored with blood pressure measurement. A narrowing pulse pressure can be present before a drop in systolic pressure. This indicates a decrease in cardiac stroke volume and peripheral vasoconstriction. Peripheral pulses are palpated. Tachycardia is the first sign of shock. However, patients on medications that block the sympathetic nervous system response will not exhibit tachycardia. The pulse is evaluated for quality; commonly, it is weak and thready in a patient with shock. As shock progresses, the peripheral pulses become

Table 9.5 Therapeutic Measures for Shock

Airway Management and Respiratory Support	Oxygen (nasal cannula, face mask, partial nonrebreather mask, assisted ventilations with bag-valve-mask, mechanical ventilator) SpO_2 over 95% Venous lactate less than 2 mmol/L
Cardiovascular Support	Vasopressor medication, if fluid resuscitation not effective Revascularization of heart in cardiogenic shock via angioplasty, with or without stent or fibrinolytic therapy Antiarrhythmics Positive inotropes
Adequate Circulatory Volume	Balanced crystalloid fluids (at least 30 mL/kg within first 3 hours for septic shock) Blood or blood products Hemoglobin greater than 10 g/dL Urine output greater than 30 mL/hr
Control of Bleeding	Pressure dressings Surgical intervention
Treatment of Life-Threatening Injuries	Medications Surgical intervention
Medications for Types of Shock	Sepsis/septic shock: antimicrobials (see discussion) immediately, within 1 hour of diagnosis Cardiogenic shock: diuretics, inotropics, nitrates, vasopressors Anaphylactic shock: epinephrine, diphenhydramine (Benadryl), methylprednisolone (Solu-Medrol)

Table 9.6 Medications Used for Shock

Medication Class/Action

Autonomic Nervous System Agents and Alpha- and Beta-Adrenergic Agents

Examples	Nursing Indicators
To strengthen myocardial contraction, increase systolic blood pressure, and increase cardiac output: epinephrine (Adrenalin) dopamine (Intropin) norepinephrine (Levophed) phenylephrine hydrochloride (Neo-Synephrine) vasopressin (V1) agent vasopressin (Pitressin)	Correct hypovolemia before giving medications Monitor vital signs often; vasopressor use should include arterial blood pressure monitoring; monitor intake and output Vasopressin usually added to norepinephrine or epinephrine for refractory shock
Examples *To bronchodilate:* epinephrine (Adrenalin)	**Nursing Indicators** First drug given in anaphylactic shock

Beta-Adrenergic Agent
Increases cardiac output in cardiogenic shock.

Examples	Nursing Indicators
dobutamine (Dobutrex)	Monitor vital signs often Monitor intake and output

Table 9.6
Medications Used for Shock—cont'd

Medication Class/Action

Antihistamine
Inhibits histamine release.
Examples
diphenhydramine (Benadryl)

Nursing Indicators
Monitor vital signs
May cause drowsiness

Anti-Inflammatory
Controls severe allergic reactions.
Examples
methylprednisolone (Solu-Medrol)
hydrocortisone (Solu-Cortef)
dexamethasone (Decadron)

Nursing Indicators
Monitor patient for elevated blood glucose, and signs and symptoms of infection

---

weaker or absent. A **capillary refill** greater than 3 seconds indicates inadequate arterial circulation. However, this is an unreliable indicator of shock in adults, especially older adults. Other observations for circulation include distended neck veins; skin that is cool, pale, and diaphoretic; presence of **cyanosis** (bluish color of skin and mucous membranes from decreased oxygen in the blood); mucous membranes that are pale and dry; and thirst. Rapidly scan the entire body for evidence of bleeding or other injuries.

> **LEARNING TIP**
> Gently squeeze and release your own nailbed. Do you see the lighter color change? Count the seconds until the color returns. That is your capillary refill time.

> **NURSING CARE TIP**
> A loss of peripheral pulses usually occurs in the patient whose systolic blood pressure has dropped below 80. If you can palpate a radial pulse on your patient, the systolic blood pressure is usually at least 80.

Disability is determined by the patient's level of consciousness. A decrease in level of consciousness indicates disability. This disability can range from lethargy to coma.

All four limbs are checked for circulation, sensation, and mobility (remember this as CSM). Bilateral responses are compared for equality. Circulation is assessed by palpating pulses for presence and quality. Sensation is determined by touching the patient's hands and feet and asking what the patient feels and if there is numbness or tingling. Mobility (motor ability) is determined by having the patient move all four limbs and wiggle fingers and toes. Have the patient push their feet against your hands and squeeze two of your fingers to determine strength.

A head-to-toe approach can follow the primary ABCD assessment. The presence, severity, and location of pain or nausea and vomiting are noted. Body temperature is measured. Bowel sounds are auscultated to determine whether they are normal, absent, hyperactive, or hypoactive. With an indwelling urinary catheter, the color, rate, and amount of urine output are noted.

> **PRACTICE ANALYSIS TIP**
> **Linking NCLEX-PN® to Practice**
> The LPN/LVN will:
> - Check and monitor client vital signs.
> - Recognize and report change in client condition.

> **NURSING CARE TIP**
> To determine whether a patient is alert and oriented, ask their name, current place, and the date. If the patient correctly answers all three questions, they are alert and oriented × 3 (person, place, time).

> **CRITICAL THINKING**
> **Mrs. Nabozny** takes a beta blocker. What sign of shock do you understand will not be present?
> *Suggested answers are at the end of the chapter.*

• WORD • BUILDING •

cyanosis: cyan—blue coloring + osis—condition

Nursing Diagnoses, Planning, Implementation, and Evaluation

See Table 9.7 for a shock summary. Also see "Nursing Care Plan for the Patient Experiencing Shock."

CRITICAL THINKING & CLINICAL JUDGMENT

Mr. Hall, who is 58 years old, had an acute myocardial infarction 2 days ago. He reports chest pain, rated 10 of 10, and shortness of breath. His blood pressure is 96/40, pulse 110, respiration rate 22, and Spo_2 89%. Crackles are heard in lung bases. The electrocardiogram shows an irregular and rapid heartbeat. He is restless and apprehensive.

Critical Thinking (The Why)
1. Would it be appropriate for IV fluids to be given to Mr. Hall now?
2. What signs and symptoms indicate that Mr. Hall is in cardiogenic shock?

Clinical Judgment (The Do)
3. What three priorities for Mr. Hall's nursing care do you and the RN discuss?
4. With what other members of the health-care team do you collaborate?

Suggested answers are at the end of the chapter.

Table 9.7 Shock Summary

Signs and Symptoms	Tachycardia Tachypnea Hypotension Mental status altered Cyanosis Oliguria
Diagnostic Tests	See Table 9.4
Therapeutic Measures	See Table 9.5
Complications	Acute respiratory distress syndrome (ARDS) Disseminated intravascular coagulation (DIC) Multiple organ dysfunction syndrome (MODS)
Priority Nursing Diagnoses	*Decreased Cardiac Output* *Risk for Ineffective Peripheral Tissue Perfusion*

Nursing Care Plan for the Patient Experiencing Shock

Nursing Diagnosis: *Decreased Cardiac Output* related to reduced circulating blood volume, structural damage, or decreased myocardial contractility as evidenced by abnormal vital signs and irregular cardiac rhythm
Expected Outcome: The patient will have adequate cardiac output as evidenced by vital signs and cardiac rhythm within normal limits.
Evaluation of Outcome: Are blood pressure, heart rate, and cardiac rhythm within normal limits? Are nailbeds and/or skin pink? Is skin warm, dry, and intact?

Intervention	Rationale	Evaluation
Monitor capillary refill, skin/nailbed color, heart rate, cardiac rhythm, peripheral pulses and report abnormalities.	*Inadequate perfusion is first evident in skin/nailbeds/mucous membranes and peripheral pulses. Changes in heart rate and cardiac rhythm need to be detected immediately for treatment.*	Is capillary refill less than 3 seconds? Are skin/nailbeds/mucous membranes their usual color? Is heart rate within normal limits? Is normal sinus rhythm present? Are peripheral pulses strong?
Administer cardiovascular medications and oxygen as ordered.	*Cardiac function can be supported with medications and oxygen.*	Is heart rate within normal limits? Is normal sinus rhythm present?
Provide comfort measures to alleviate pain and anxiety and maintain a normal body temperature.	*Pain, anxiety, and cold increase tissue demands for oxygen, which increases the heart's workload to supply it.*	Is patient free of pain and anxiety? Is body temperature within normal limits?
Geriatric		
Monitor perfusion by methods other than capillary refill, such as skin temperature.	*Capillary refill is frequently delayed in older adults. Blood flow warms the body.*	Is skin warm to the touch?

Nursing Care Plan for the Patient Experiencing Shock

Nursing Diagnosis: *Risk for Ineffective Peripheral Tissue Perfusion* related to hypovolemia or inadequate cardiac output or changes in circulatory volume or inadequate vascular tone, possibly evidenced by changes in skin color/temperature, tachycardia, hypotension, and oliguria.

Expected Outcome: The patient will display adequate tissue perfusion as evidenced by warm and dry skin, strong peripheral pulses, vital signs within normal parameters of baseline, breath sounds without adventitious sounds, and balanced intake and output.

Evaluation of Outcome: Is the patient's skin warm and dry? Are peripheral pulses present/strong? Are vital signs within the patient's normal range? Are lung sounds normal, intake/output balanced, edema absent, and pain/discomfort absent?

Intervention	Rationale	Evaluation
Maintain airway and provide oxygen as ordered.	*Ensures adequate oxygenation and tissue perfusion.*	Is SpO_2 over 95%? Are respirations between 12 and 20 per minute? Are signs of cyanosis absent?
Monitor vital signs and intake and output.	*Vital signs can indicate a change in status for prompt treatment. Urine output amount reflects renal function.*	Is heart rate between 60 and 100 beats per minute? Is heart rhythm regular? Are peripheral pulses strong? Is systolic blood pressure greater than 100 mm Hg? Is urinary output greater than 30 mL/hr?
Provide fluid replacement as ordered.	*Maintains fluid volume for tissue perfusion.*	Are vital signs within normal limits? Are mucous membranes moist? Is skin turgor less than 3 seconds?
Maintain body temperature with warmed IV fluids, room temperature, and blankets.	*Recovery is aided by a body temperature within normal limits.*	Is body temperature within normal limits?
Geriatric		
Change positions slowly.	*Age-related losses of cardiovascular reflexes can result in hypotension.*	Is systolic blood pressure greater than 100 mm Hg?

CUE RECOGNITION 9.2

A spouse is crying in the hallway that his wife, who is experiencing shock, is going to die. What action do you take?

Suggested answers are at the end of the chapter.

CLINICAL JUDGMENT

Mrs. Neal, age 45, arrived at the emergency department in severe hypovolemic shock. She sustained several bleeding lacerations and a ruptured spleen in a motor vehicle accident. Her shock is resolving after receiving several transfusions and surgical repair of her injuries. She has been admitted to your surgical unit for postoperative care.

1. What postoperative data do you collect first?
2. What do you do to promote patient-centered care for Mrs. Neal?
3. What data do you collect to detect postoperative complications in Mrs. Neal?
4. What family-centered care do you provide to Mrs. Neal's family, who is upset by her condition?
5. What documentation do you provide for your nursing care for Mrs. Neal?

Suggested answers are at the end of the chapter.

Key Points

- Shock is inadequate cellular or tissue perfusion from a sudden drop in blood flow. This results in an imbalance in oxygen supply and demand that leads to cellular and tissue hypoxia and potential death.
- Tissue perfusion and blood pressure are maintained by three mechanisms: adequate blood volume, an effective cardiac pump, and effective blood vessels. Shock occurs when the compensatory mechanisms for a problem in one mechanism fails to maintain blood pressure, leading to poor tissue perfusion.
- Hypovolemic shock results from a decrease in the circulating blood volume. It can be caused by dehydration; internal or external hemorrhage; fluid loss from burns, heat exhaustion, or heatstroke with sweating; vomiting or diarrhea; or loss of intravascular fluid into the interstitial space from sepsis or trauma.
- Cardiogenic shock occurs when the heart fails as a pump and decreases cardiac output. It requires immediate treatment to prevent death. Causes of cardiogenic shock include acute myocardial infarction, arrhythmias, cardiomyopathy, endocarditis, heart valve defects, myocarditis, or traumatic cardiac injury.
- Distributive shock, anaphylactic, neurogenic, septic, occurs when peripheral vascular resistance is lost because of excessive dilation of the venules and arterioles.
- Obstructive shock, which is rare, occurs with a blockage of blood flow outside of the heart. Causes include pericardial tamponade, tension pneumothorax or acute pulmonary hypertension.
- There are three stages of shock: Pre-shock (compensated), Shock (progressive), End Organ Dysfunction (irreversible).
- For the patient in shock, data collection must be carried out quickly and should always start with ABCD: airway, breathing, circulation, and disability.
- Therapeutic measures for shock include providing airway management and respiratory support, providing cardiovascular support, ensuring adequate circulatory volume, controlling bleeding, treating life-threatening injuries, and treating for the specific type of shock.
- The priority nursing diagnoses for patients in shock are *Decreased Cardiac Output* and *Risk for Ineffective Peripheral Tissue Perfusion*.
- Positive responses to therapeutic measures for shock include vital signs within normal limits, normal sinus rhythm, and intact peripheral circulation.
- Post-sepsis syndrome affects up to 50% of sepsis survivors with long-term physical and/or psychological effects.

SUGGESTED ANSWERS TO CHAPTER EXERCISES

Cue Recognition
9.1: Put on gloves and apply direct pressure with sterile gauze to the IV site while calling for immediate assistance.
9.2: Take him to a quiet place for privacy, provide tissues and a beverage, allow him to verbalize his feelings, and offer to contact the chaplain or social worker.

Critical Thinking & Clinical Judgment
Shock
1. Tachycardia is caused by decreased cardiac output and reduced tissue oxygenation. Its purpose is to increase cardiac output and oxygen delivery through more heartbeats to pump blood.

    Tachypnea is caused by decreased tissue oxygenation. Its purpose is to increase respirations so that more oxygen is available for delivery to tissues.

    Oliguria is caused by a reduced blood flow to the kidneys. Its purpose is to conserve fluid to help maintain normal blood pressure.

    Pallor results from reduced blood volume that shunts blood from the skin to vital organs.

    Cool, clammy skin is the result of decreased blood flow to the skin and the release of moisture (sweat) from the skin. Sweating cools the body in anticipation of the fight-or-flight response, which generates body heat when it occurs.

2. Anaerobic metabolism is the source of nutrition and energy for the cell that prevents cellular death when oxygen is not available. It is a *short-term* compensatory mechanism to help save the cell until oxygen becomes available again.

Mrs. Nabozny
Tachycardia will not be present. Beta blockers block the cardiac response of the sympathetic nervous system activated in shock.

Mr. Hall
1. No. Because Mr. Hall's lung sounds reveal crackles, indicating fluid in the lungs, he should not be given IV fluids. He already has too much fluid within his body for his heart to handle, and giving him more IV fluids could be life threatening. He should have an IV access for IV medications as needed.
2. Signs of cardiogenic shock include decreased blood pressure; increased heart and respiratory rates; cyanosis; decreased urine output; cool, pale nailbeds and/or skin; and decreased mental status.
3. Nursing priorities for Mr. Hall include adequate tissue perfusion, relief of chest pain and anxiety, and stabilization of cardiac rhythm and vital signs.
4. In addition to the RN, the HCP and case manager.

SUGGESTED ANSWERS TO CHAPTER EXERCISES—cont'd

Mrs. Neal

1. Data collection for respiratory and cardiovascular status, inspection of surgical wounds for bleeding, and noting mental status and the need for pain relief should be performed first. Then fluid balance should be monitored.
2. Develop a pain management plan to meet Mrs. Neal's patient-centered needs. Identify her normal coping techniques to support their appropriate use. Provide explanations and teaching as needed to keep her informed for decision making. Advocate for her needs, such as nutrition to help heal her wounds.
3. Pain rating to detect unrelieved *pain;* monitoring of dressings and vital signs for indications of *bleeding;* monitoring temperature and wounds for signs of *infection;* respiratory rate, presence of dyspnea, ease of breathing, lung sounds, and SpO_2 to detect *respiratory complications.*
4. Explain the cause of shock and all interventions, rationales, and desired outcomes. Keep the environment calm, provide for privacy, and answer questions in a matter-of-fact and reassuring manner. Encourage Mrs. Neal's family to visit to meet her psychosocial needs. Provide explanations to the family. Offer a chaplain and social worker referral.
5. *Airway:* breath sounds, ease of breathing, rate, depth, regularity of respirations, SpO_2. *Vital signs:* cardiac rate/rhythm, quality of pulses, skin color, blood pressure, body temperature. *Pain:* measures to relieve pain and evaluation of those measures. *Dressings:* drainage color and amount. *Fluid balance:* oral and IV intake, urine, and other output.

Additional Resources

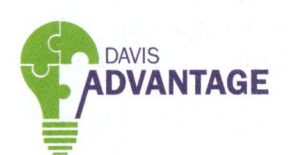

Go to Davis Advantage to complete your learning: strengthen understanding, apply your knowledge, and prepare for the Next Gen NCLEX®.

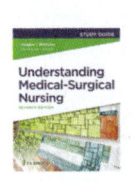

A Study Guide is also available.

CHAPTER 10
Nursing Care of Patients in Pain

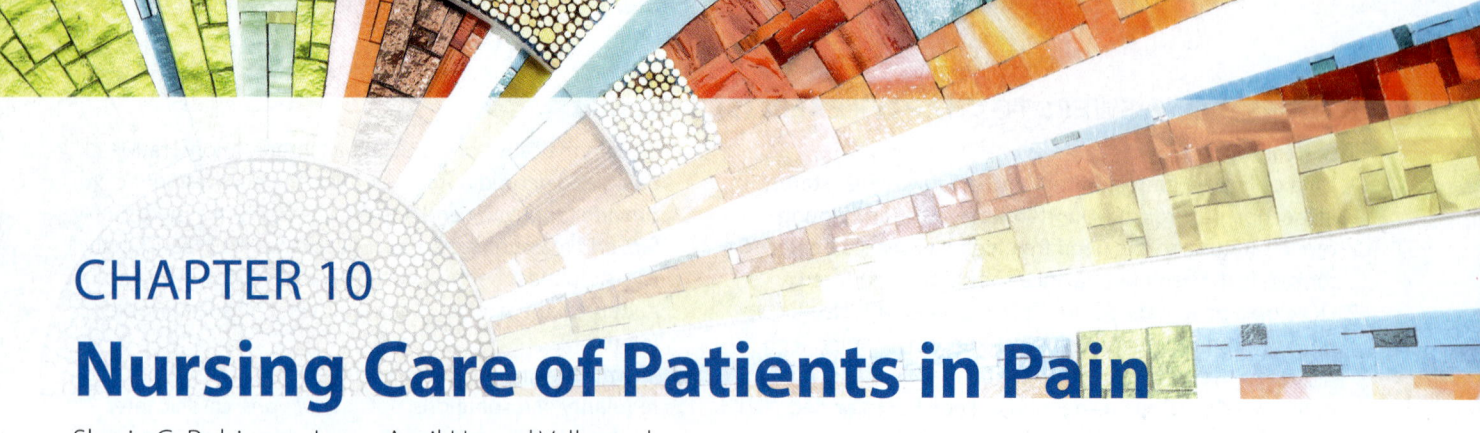

Sheria G. Robinson-Lane, April Hazard Vallerand

KEY TERMS

addiction (uh-DIK-shun)
adjuvant (ad-JOO-vant)
agonist (AG-un-ist)
analgesic (AN-uhl-JEE-zik)
antagonist (an-TAG-on-ist)
breakthrough (BRAYK-throo)
ceiling effect (SEE-ling eh-FEKT)
endorphins (en-DOOR-fins)
enkephalins (en-KEFF-eh-lins)
equianalgesic (EH-kwee-AN-uhl-JEE-zik)
hyperalgesia (HYPER-al-JEE-zee-ah)
malingerer (muh-LING-gur-er)
neuropathic (NEW-roh-PATH-ik)
nociception (NOH-sih-SEP-shun)
opioid (OH-pee-OYD)
patient-controlled analgesia (PAY-shunt kon-TROHLD AN-uhl-JEE-zee-ah)
physical dependence (FIZZ-ik-uhl dee-PEN-dense)
prostaglandins (PRAHS-tah-GLAND-ins)
pseudoaddiction (soo-doh-uh-DIK-shun)
psychological dependence (SY-ko-LAW-jik-al dee-PEN-dense)
somatic (so-MAT-ik)
suffering (SUH-fur-ing)
tolerance (TAH-ler-ens)
transdermal (trans-DER-mal)
visceral (VISS-er-uhl)

CHAPTER CONCEPTS

Addiction
Comfort
Safety

LEARNING OUTCOMES

1. Describe current definitions of pain.
2. Identify common myths and barriers to the effective management of pain.
3. Differentiate among addiction, physical dependence, and tolerance.
4. Explain current understanding about the basic physiology of the pain response.
5. Differentiate between nociceptive and neuropathic pain.
6. Collaborate in performing a pain assessment.
7. Describe the three classes of analgesics and their uses.
8. Identify commonly used pain medication treatment modalities and their appropriate use.
9. Recognize appropriate use of nonpharmacological pain management techniques.

THE PAIN PUZZLE

Pain is a complicated symptom of disease or injury. Although the cause of pain is not always apparent, the effects of poorly managed pain can be detrimental. In addition to causing physical discomfort, pain can also make us feel emotionally sad, angry, or spiritually empty. It can lead to social isolation, financial loss, and even death. Pain is an experience that can affect every aspect of a person's being and how they function in the environment. Pain management is the most common reason patients seek medical advice. Undiagnosed and untreated psychological concerns in individuals with pain are associated with increased health-care utilization and readmissions, decreased treatment adherence, and increased disability (U.S. Department of Health and Human Services, 2019). Nurses, however, can make a significant difference in pain management.

Nurses are often the first health professionals to whom patients report their pain symptoms. The nurse's response to the patient's complaint of pain or the nurse's own good observations of pain symptoms can set the tone for the health-care team's response to the patient's pain needs. Nurses may worry about overmedicating patients and may think that they are "doing good" (beneficence) or "doing no harm" (nonmaleficence) by withholding medication from a patient whom they believe is not in pain. But how can we know what pain is, and how can we really tell when others are experiencing pain?

DEFINITIONS OF PAIN

According to Margo McCaffery (1968), who was a nurse and well-known pain management expert, "Pain is whatever the experiencing person says it is, existing whenever the experiencing person says it does." This is a reminder to nurses that the patient's self-report of pain is the gold standard in pain assessment. The International Association for the Study of Pain (2020) describes pain in a bit more detail, as "an unpleasant sensory and emotional experience associated with, or resembling that associated with, actual or potential tissue damage." This definition was updated in 2020 to reflect the maladaptive nature of pain. It indicates that pain is a complex problem that is not just physical in nature or always a result of tissue injury.

Why does pain exist? Often, it is a protective mechanism or a warning. In the presence of an injury, pain may help prevent further injury. Consider the patient who has a fracture and holds it still to prevent further damage, or a child who touches a hot stove and pulls their hand away before a serious burn occurs. The immediate pain that often follows burns, surgery, or other trauma to the body is referred to as acute pain.

Acute pain prompts an inflammatory response in the body that subsides as healing takes place, usually within six months of the injury. This type of pain is often associated with short-term, objective, physical signs such as increased respiratory and heart rates, and elevated blood pressure. As acute pain continues, its physiological responses cannot be sustained without harm to the body. As the body adapts, vital signs return to normal. When acute pain persists beyond the anticipated time of healing, it is referred to as chronic pain.

Chronic pain is pain that lasts beyond the anticipated time of healing. Examples include neck pain that continues years after an accident, pain that accompanies diseases such as arthritis, and phantom limb pain. Because of the body's ability to adapt, patients with chronic pain may not appear to be in pain. Guard against labeling such a patient as a **malingerer** (someone who pretends to be in pain) or a drug seeker. When pain is not treated effectively or lasts longer than expected, suffering can occur. Healthy People 2030 has a goal to "reduce the proportion of adults with high impact chronic pain" (Office of Disease Prevention and Health Promotion, 2020). This goal includes not only pain reduction but also its impact on daily functioning, and it encompasses opioid alternatives and nonpharmacological interventions.

Suffering, or feelings of continuous distress, often accompanies pain, particularly chronic pain. It can diminish patient quality of life and motivation for self-care. In a paper examining the importance of treating suffering along with disease, del Giglio (2020) describes suffering as a complex concept that "can entail physical, psychological, and spiritual distress that prompts the sufferer to seek medical attention" (p. 215). Suffering can often be relieved if patients believe they can achieve comfort. In addition to medical treatment, many individuals find comfort from pain and related suffering through spiritual coping. Spiritual coping might include religious practices such as prayer, or non-religious practices such as self-reflection and connecting socially with others to affirm meaning and purpose in life (Dunn & Robinson-Lane, 2020). Nurses can encourage patients with persistent pain to continue to engage in spiritual practices that they find meaningful and with people who bring them joy. Further, a good assessment and individualized, culturally responsive approaches to care increase the likelihood of comfort.

RISKS OF UNCONTROLLED PAIN

How does untreated or undertreated pain affect the person? Complications can occur when pain is experienced. The body produces a stress response to pain that causes harmful substances to be released from injured tissue. Reactions include breakdown of tissue, increased metabolic rate, impaired immune function, and negative emotions. In addition, pain can prevent the patient from participating in self-care activities, such as walking, deep breathing, and coughing. Consider the patient who has had chest surgery and then has to cough and deep breathe. It hurts! Pain may make the patient want to avoid coughing, turning, or even moving. Retained pulmonary secretions and pneumonia can develop. If the patient is less active, return of bowel function is delayed, and an ileus (disruption of normal propulsive gastrointestinal activity) can result. When pain is well controlled, complications can be avoided, and patients can participate fully in recovery activities. This will speed discharge as well as allow patients to do things that are meaningful and important to them when they get home.

PAIN AND CULTURE

All individuals have learned patterns of behaviors, beliefs, and values that they share as members of particular social groups (Robinson, 2013). These cultural differences can affect responses to pain and expectations regarding treatment. As nurses, our beliefs, values, and experiences influence our perceptions of patients and can affect how we treat them. For example, if we are living and working with significant daily chronic pain ourselves, it may be hard to believe someone who reports severe pain but doesn't respond in the same way we would. While some patients may be dramatic and emotional when experiencing pain, others may tend to be stoic and quiet. It is important to evaluate a patient's pain care needs individually. Be culturally responsive to the needs of patients by taking the time to ask about treatment preferences and integrating these preferences into the plan of care as much as possible, reaching compromises as necessary, and providing explanations when care expectations cannot be met (Robinson-Lane & Booker, 2017). Also, be mindful of your patients' language, family engagement, and spirituality (see "Cultural Considerations"). Finally, pay careful attention to the ethical principles that influence patient care rather than making assumptions based on culture alone.

WHO'S THE BOSS IN PAIN MANAGEMENT?

The patient is at the center of the health-care team. The patient also knows best how pain feels and affects them. Providing accurate information and offering relevant choices in pain management help patients maintain autonomy. Just as risks, benefits, and alternatives to surgery and anesthesia are discussed with the patient, pain management options should be discussed while obtaining informed consent. It is important to learn as much as you can about pain and pain management so you can effectively advocate for and educate your patients.

The entire health-care team is responsible for pain management. All members must provide care in the most cost-effective manner possible while continuing to provide the best quality. Effective pain management helps to improve patient function and reduces costs by minimizing the side effects of opioids, preventing complications related to inadequate pain control, and reducing the length of hospital/nursing home stay or period of recovery.

Various regulatory bodies recognize the importance of good pain management. Many have incorporated a review of organizational pain management practices into accreditation and review processes. These standards support the importance of appropriate and effective management of pain. They address assessment and the safe pharmacological management of pain as well as patient and family teaching, postoperative pain, management of opioid-induced side effects, discharge planning, and process improvement. Examples of these guidelines are available through The Joint Commission Web site at www.jointcommission.org and the Centers for Medicare and Medicaid Services Web

Cultural Considerations

Pain experiences may differ among cultures and individuals of various geographical regions; family structures; and ethnic, racial, or religious groups. Remember that people within groups vary (see Chapter 4).

Cultural Expression	Data Collection	Intervention
Language	Listen for words or phrases the patient uses to describe discomfort, such as *achy, sore, fire, burning, shooting,* or *having a knot.* Observe use of nonverbal pain cues, such as moaning or crying, furrowed eyebrows, a clenched jaw, guarding or rubbing of body parts, and fetal positioning. Ask the patient about any nonverbal pain cues you see. Use standardized pain assessment scales.	Allow adequate time for the patient to respond to questions about pain. Use words the patient uses to discuss pain needs. Offer pain medications and interventions.
Family Engagement	Observe how involved the family is in the patient's care.	Teach the patient's family how to monitor the patient's discomfort and when to encourage pain medications or treatments. Engage the family to help with distraction and relaxation techniques.
Spirituality	Ask the patient whether they use religion or faith as a part of healing. Look for evidence of the patient's religious beliefs and spiritual practices. Clothing such as head coverings, jewelry, religious books or literature, clergy at the bedside, and patient engagement in prayer or meditation provide clues and insight.	Incorporate traditional healing methods as much as possible. Encourage the use of prayer, meditation, and relaxation as the patient desires. Offer and encourage pain medicines to promote healing. Support the patient's spiritual practices.
Treatment Preferences	Ask the patient how they usually treat pain at home. Ask the patient what they feel is needed to be comfortable.	Incorporate traditional home remedies, such as hot or cold packs and other practices, as permitted. Incorporate distraction and relaxation techniques. Administer medication promptly as requested.

site at www.cms.gov. For more information on pain management, visit these Web sites:

- Agency for Healthcare Research and Quality, www.ahrq.gov
- American Cancer Society, www.cancer.org
- American Chronic Pain Association, www.theacpa.org
- American Society for Pain Management Nursing, www.aspmn.org
- Centers for Disease Control and Prevention, www.cdc.gov
- GeriatricPain.org, www.geriatricpain.org

The care of patients with pain is challenging. However, with a systematic and holistic approach to data collection and treatment, good pain management can be achieved. In this chapter, the difficulties of pain management are discussed. Some of the tools needed to effectively deal with these challenges are presented. Common myths and barriers that continue to affect nursing practice are clarified first.

MYTHS AND BARRIERS TO EFFECTIVE PAIN MANAGEMENT

Many factors, including a nurse's personal experiences with pain, influence how patients with pain are treated. Why are some patients not believed when they report pain? Why do some nurses and other health-care team members insist that patients behave a certain way before they are believed? Common myths about pain can impair a nurse's ability to be objective. This may create barriers to effective treatment. Because there are few objective measures for pain, many nurses rely on assumptions rather than facts. Note the following myths:

Myth: A person who is laughing and talking is not in pain.
Fact: A person in pain is likely to use laughing and talking as a form of distraction. This can be effective in managing pain, especially when used with appropriate drug therapies. Patients may be more easily distracted when they have visitors and may ask for pain medication as soon as their family or significant other goes home.
Myth: Respiratory depression is common in patients receiving opioid pain medications.
Fact: Respiratory depression is uncommon in patients receiving opioid pain medications when medications are taken as prescribed. If patients are monitored carefully when they are at risk, such as with the first dose of an opioid or when a dose is increased, respiratory depression is preventable. A patient's respiratory status and level of sedation should be routinely monitored and recorded using a level-of-sedation scale.
Myth: Pain medication is more effective when given by injection.
Fact: Oral administration is the first choice if possible or whenever the IV route is not an option. The IV route has the most rapid onset of action and is the preferred route for postoperative administration. Intramuscular injections are not recommended because they are painful, have unreliable absorption from the muscle, and have a lag time to peak effect and rapid falloff compared with oral administration.

Myth: Teenagers are more likely than older patients to become addicted to opioids.
Fact: Addiction to opioids can occur in all age-groups. People with chronic pain who also have substance use disorders and/or mental health disorders have a higher risk for misuse of prescribed opioids.
Myth: Pain is a normal part of aging.
Fact: Although many older adults have medical conditions that cause pain, pain is not a normal or anticipated part of aging and should be treated proactively. Effective pain treatment for older people helps them to maintain their mobility longer and improve overall health.

CRITICAL THINKING

Mrs. Bao had an abdominal hysterectomy and is sitting up in bed the morning after surgery, putting on her makeup. On morning rounds, she is smiling but reports that her pain is at 6 on a scale of 0 to 10. **Mr. Brown** has just been transferred from the surgical intensive care unit the day after surgery for multiple injuries. He is moaning and reports his pain at 6 on a scale of 0 to 10. Which of these patients is really having as much pain as they say they are? How can you make this judgment?

Suggested answers are at the end of the chapter.

OPIOID ADDICTION

In 2018, nearly 47,000 Americans died of opioid overdose (Wilson et al, 2020). While the misuse of prescription medications like oxycodone and hydrocodone is decreasing, the use of illegally manufactured synthetic opioids such as fentanyl continues to rise (Centers for Disease Control and Prevention, 2021). Understandably, nurses often express concern about patients who need large amounts of opioid pain medication or know exactly when their next dose of pain medication is due. Nurses may worry that such patients are addicted or that they are "clock watchers." In truth, if a patient is watching the clock or asking for more medicine, the most likely reason is that they are in pain. Interestingly, patients are commonly taught to know the name, effects, and dosage of other medications, such as blood pressure medications and insulin; however, when they ask for a specific analgesic by name, concern that the patient is "drug seeking" is often raised.

Addiction is something that many patients fear—particularly today with increased media attention on opioid-related deaths. It is important to understand the differences between addiction, tolerance, and physical dependence. When talking with patients and their families about opioid medications, it is also important to verify that they understand these differences.

Tolerance is a normal biological adaptation to long-term use of a drug. The drug becomes less effective and the patient needs a larger dose to provide the same level of pain relief. **Physical dependence** is a normal physiological response that most people experience after a week or more of continuous opioid use. If an opioid is discontinued abruptly or an opioid antagonist such as naloxone (Narcan) is administered, the patient experiences withdrawal syndrome. Withdrawal symptoms can include headaches, sweating, tearing, runny nose, restlessness, irritability, tremors, dilated pupils, sleeplessness, nausea, vomiting, and diarrhea. These symptoms can be prevented by decreasing the dose slowly over several days rather than stopping it suddenly.

According to the American Society of Addiction Medicine (2019), **addiction** (also known as **psychological dependence**) is a chronic disease of the brain influenced by genetics, environment, and life experiences, which cause the compulsive pursuit of a substance or behavior to obtain reward or relief from craving. Addiction is characterized by poor control over drug use, craving, reduced recognition of problem behaviors, and continued use despite harm. Patients with uncontrolled pain who desire treatment are not addicts. Sadly, patients with a history of addiction are more likely to have poor pain control due to medication tolerance and health-care provider (HCP) bias. Careful assessment and monitoring of treatment are essential for *all* patients receiving treatment for pain—particularly patients who are prescribed opioid analgesics. Further, patients prescribed opioid analgesics to manage acute pain should also have a plan in place to wean down opioid doses as healing is anticipated.

Pseudoaddiction has been described in patients who are receiving opioid doses that are too low or spaced too far apart to relieve their pain. Behavioral characteristics resembling psychological dependence, such as clock-watching and repeatedly requesting pain medications, may develop in an attempt to get pain needs met. In contrast to the addicted patient, a patient with pseudoaddiction stops drug-seeking behaviors when the pain is reduced to a tolerable level.

CRITICAL THINKING & CLINICAL JUDGMENT

Lucy is hospitalized with pancreatitis and has severe abdominal pain. She has a history of IV drug abuse. She is receiving IV morphine every 3 hours. Two hours after her last dose, she puts on her call light and says she is in severe pain, which she rates as 15 on a 0 to 10 scale. You feel that you have given her enough morphine to kill a horse, yet she keeps requesting more.

Critical Thinking (The Why)
1. How is it possible for Lucy to be in pain when she is receiving so much morphine?

Clinical Judgment (The Do)
2. It's not time for more medication. What can you do?
3. You speak to the HCP, who prescribes acetaminophen (Tylenol) 1,000 mg for breakthrough pain (between morphine doses). When you take it to Lucy, she rolls her eyes and says, "You must be kidding me." How do you respond?
4. What communication with Lucy is important at this time?

Suggested answers are at the end of the chapter.

MECHANISMS OF PAIN TRANSMISSION

Pain is transmitted through four distinct processes:

1. *Transduction* represents the initiation of the stimulus and conversion of that stimulus into an electrical impulse at the time of the injury. Chemical neurotransmitters are released from damaged tissue including prostaglandins, bradykinin, serotonin, and substance P.
2. *Transmission* is the process of moving a painful message from the peripheral nerve endings through the dorsal root ganglion and the ascending tract of the spinal cord to the brain.
3. *Perception* is actually feeling pain. During perception, the hypothalamus activates, which controls emotional input and generates purposeful goal-directed behavior. Meanwhile, the cerebral cortex receives the pain message.
4. *Modulation* is the body's attempt to interrupt pain impulses by releasing endogenous (naturally occurring) opioids. **Endorphins** are endogenous chemicals that act like opioids, inhibiting pain impulses in the spinal cord and brain. Endorphins are the chemicals that stimulate the long-distance runner's "high." Unfortunately, they degrade too quickly to be considered effective analgesics. **Enkephalins** are one type of endorphin.

Pain Transmission: Nociceptive or Neuropathic?

Pain transmission can be nociceptive and neuropathic. **Nociception** refers to the body's normal reaction to noxious stimuli, such as tissue damage, with the release of pain-producing substances. Nociceptive pain may be somatic or visceral. **Somatic** pain is localized in the muscles or bones. Patients can often point to the exact location of pain and will describe it as throbbing or aching. Cancer patients may experience somatic pain when cancer spreads to bone or a tumor invades soft tissue. **Visceral** pain, or organ pain, is not well localized and is often described as cramping or pressure. Bowel obstructions and tumors in the lung can cause visceral pain symptoms. Pain may also be felt in parts of the body away from the pain source, such as low back/flank pain that often accompanies a bladder infection. This is called *referred pain* (Fig. 10.1).

Neuropathic pain is associated with injury to either the peripheral or central nervous system. Unlike nociceptive

• WORD • BUILDING •

pseudoaddiction: pseudo—false + addiction—psychological dependence
nociception: noci—pain + ception—reception
somatic: somato – body + ic – having to do with
neuropathic: neuro—nerves + pathy—disease, suffering

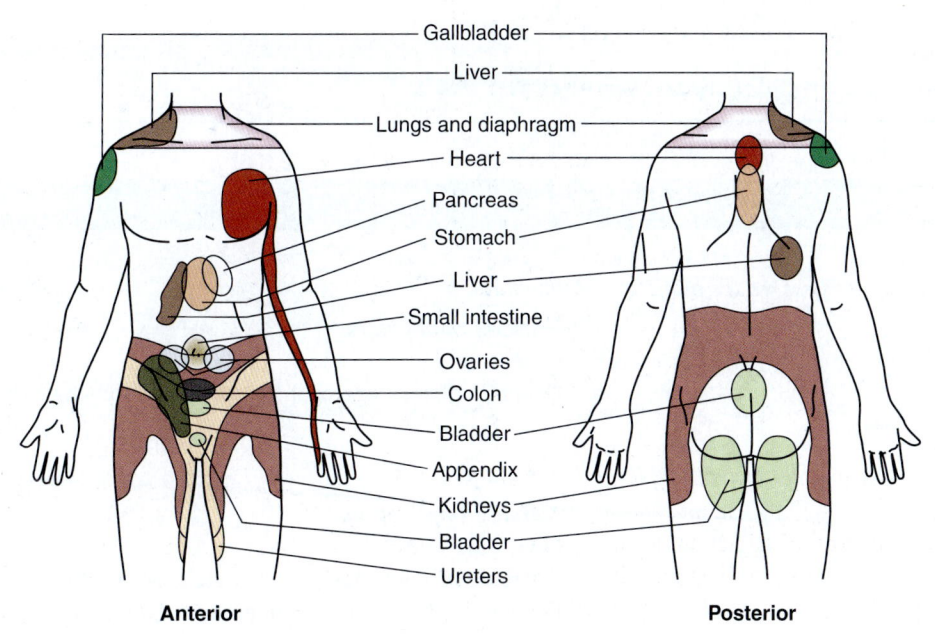

FIGURE 10.1 Sites of referred pain.

pain, neuropathic pain is poorly localized and may involve other areas along the nerve pathway. Neuropathic pain is common in cancer patients following chemotherapy or radiation therapy. It also occurs in patients who have fibromyalgia, diabetic neuropathy, and shingles. The pain is often described as numbing, tingling, sharp, shooting, or shocklike.

OPTIONS FOR TREATMENT OF PAIN

Medications that relieve pain are called **analgesics.** Analgesics make up a large piece of the pain management puzzle. They encompass three main classes of medications: opioids, nonopioids, and adjuvants. **Opioids** bind to opioid receptors in the brain, spinal cord, and other areas of the body, inhibiting the perception of pain. *Nonopioids* include NSAIDs and acetaminophen (Tylenol). **Adjuvants** are different from opioid and nonopioids in that they include categories of medications that were originally approved by the Food and Drug Administration (FDA) for purposes other than pain relief (e.g., depression). Some patients may require a combination of opioids, adjuvants, and NSAIDs to effectively manage their pain. Nurses should have a good understanding of these pharmacological treatment options.

Nonopioid Analgesics

Nonopioids are typically the first class of drugs used to treat mild pain (Table 10.1). They can be useful for acute and chronic pain from a variety of causes, such as surgery, trauma, arthritis, and cancer. These drugs are limited in their use because they have a ceiling effect to analgesia. A **ceiling effect** means that there is a dose beyond which there is no improvement in the analgesic effect, but there may be an increase in adverse effects. When used with opioids, the nonopioid dose must not exceed the maximum safe dose for a 24-hour period. For example, if a patient receiving two acetaminophen/hydrocodone (Norco) tablets every 4 hours continues to experience pain, the dose cannot be increased because of the potentially toxic effects of acetaminophen at that dosage. (See Table 10.1 for side effects and nursing implications.) Nonopioids do not produce tolerance or physical dependence.

Nonopioids work mainly peripherally at the site of injury, rather than in the central nervous system as opioids do. The exception in this class is acetaminophen, which is believed to act on the central nervous system. NSAIDs block the synthesis of **prostaglandins,** one of many chemicals needed for pain transmission. In general, it is helpful to include a nonopioid agent in any analgesic regimen, even if the pain is severe enough to require the addition of an opioid (see "Balanced Approach to Analgesia," later in this chapter).

Opioid Analgesics

Opioids are drugs that have actions similar to those of morphine. Opioids are classified by how they affect receptors in the nervous system. They may be full **agonists** (stimulators), partial agonists, mixed agonists, or **antagonists** (blockers). Full agonists have a complete response at the opioid receptor

• WORD • BUILDING •

analgesic: an—not + gesia—pain
antagonist: ant—against + agonist—stimulates receptor site

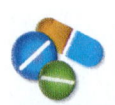

Table 10.1
Analgesic and Adjuvant Agents for Pain

Medication Class/Action

NONOPIOIDS

Salicylates
Peripherally acting analgesics; reduce pain, fever, inflammation.

Examples	*Nursing Implications*
aspirin	Give with food.
	Decrease platelet aggregation; watch for bruising or bleeding.

NSAIDs
Peripherally acting analgesics; reduce pain, fever, inflammation.

Examples	*Nursing Implications*
ibuprofen (Motrin)	Give with food.
ketorolac (Toradol)	Decrease platelet aggregation; watch for bleeding.
naproxen (Naprosyn, Aleve)	Do not give ketorolac for longer than 5 days.
	May cause constipation

COX-2 Inhibitors
Reduce pain and inflammation; no effect on platelet aggregation.

Examples	*Nursing Implications*
celecoxib (Celebrex)	Give with food.

Acetaminophen
Relieves pain and fever; no anti-inflammatory or antiplatelet effect.

Examples	*Nursing Implications*
acetaminophen (Tylenol, Ofirmev)	Maximum safe dose is 4 g per day; 3g for older adults and less for those who use alcohol.
	Be aware of other drugs that contain acetaminophen, such as cold remedies, to prevent accidental overdose.

Opioids and Opioid Combination Agents

Bind to opioid receptors in the central nervous system to alter perception of pain.

Examples	*Nursing Implications*
codeine (in Tylenol #2, #3, #4)*	May be combined with nonopioid (e.g., acetaminophen).
fentanyl (Sublimaze, Duragesic)	Monitor vital signs, level of sedation, and respiratory status.
hydromorphone (Dilaudid, Exalgo)	Avoid fentanyl patch in patient with fever; heat increases absorption.
methadone (Dolophine)	Encourage fluids and fiber to prevent constipation.
morphine (MS IR, MS Contin)	Codeine is contraindicated in pediatric patients.
oxycodone (Oxy IR, OxyContin, Xtampza ER)	Never crush extended-release tablets.
oxycodone/acetaminophen (Percocet, Endocet)	Tramadol lowers seizure threshold.
hydrocodone/acetaminophen (Norco, Lortab)	
tapentadol (Nucynta, Nucynta ER)	
tramadol (Ultram)	

Adjuvant Agents

Corticosteroids
Toxic to some cancer cells; reduce pain by decreasing inflammation.

Examples	*Nursing Implications*
prednisone	Administer with food. Monitor for increased blood glucose levels, insomnia, mood swings, and exacerbation of psychotic behaviors.
prednisolone	
methylprednisolone	
dexamethasone	

Table 10.1
Analgesic and Adjuvant Agents for Pain—cont'd

Medication Class/Action	
Benzodiazepines *Treat anxiety or muscle spasms associated with pain.* *Examples* midazolam (Versed) diazepam (Valium)	*Nursing Implications* Can cause sedation, which limits the amount of opioid that can be safely given at the same time. Increases risk of falls.
Tricyclic Antidepressants *Help relieve neuropathic pain.* *Examples* amitriptyline imipramine desipramine doxepin	*Nursing Implications* Often cause anticholinergic side effects (e.g., sedation, constipation, blurred vision, dry eyes, urinary retention).
Serotonin-Norepinephrine Reuptake Inhibitor *Effective for nerve pain and depression.* *Examples* duloxetine (Cymbalta)	*Nursing Implications* May take weeks before effect seen; teach patient to continue the medication even if it seems ineffective at first.
Anticonvulsants *Treat neuropathic pain.* *Examples* carbamazepine (Tegretol) gabapentin (Neurontin)	*Nursing Implications* Must be taken regularly to get full benefit.

*Tylenol #2 = Tylenol 300 mg + codeine 15 mg; Tylenol #3 = Tylenol 300 mg + codeine 30 mg; Tylenol #4 = Tylenol 300 mg + codeine 60 mg

---

site; a partial agonist has a lesser response. A mixed agonist or an antagonist activates one type of opioid receptor while blocking another.

Morphine, a full agonist, is often the drug of choice for treating severe pain. It is the standard against which all other analgesics are compared (see Table 10.2 for **equianalgesic** doses of medications). Morphine is long acting (4 to 5 hours) and available in many forms, including extended release, making it convenient and affordable for patients. It also has a slower onset than many other opioids. Other examples of opioids include controlled-release drugs such as oxycodone (OxyContin), hydromorphone (Exalgo ER), and tapentadol (Nucynta ER), which are effective for prolonged, continuous pain.

> **LEARNING TIP**
> Medication trade names often provide hints to their actions. Note the "ER," which means "extended release," and "Contin," which means "continuous."

> **BE SAFE!**
> **BE VIGILANT!** Never crush a controlled- or time-release tablet. Because the tablet is designed to deliver a dose of medication over time, crushing it could deliver the entire dose at once, resulting in overdose.

Opioids alone have no ceiling effect to analgesia. Doses can safely be increased to treat worsening pain if the patient's respiratory status and level of sedation are stable. However, inappropriate prescribing can lead to **hyperalgesia,** or increased sensitivity to pain. Patients with hyperalgesia have pain at the slightest touch, such as the moving of sheets, and require further medical intervention. Institutions must have policies and procedures in place related to opioids to prevent medication errors and reduce the risk of serious side effects. Other common opioid side effects include constipation, confusion, and fatigue; confusion or fatigue can increase a patient's

• WORD • BUILDING •

equianalgesic: equi—equal + analgesic—relieving pain

Table 10.2
Equianalgesic Chart

Drug	Parenteral Dose*	Oral Dose
Morphine	5 mg	15 mg
Codeine	60 mg	100 mg
Hydromorphone	1.5 mg	4 mg
Methadone	5 mg	10 mg
Meperidine	50 mg	150 mg
Oxycodone	Not applicable	10 mg

*IV, intramuscular, subcutaneous.

Note: Approximate doses of medications in milligrams to equal same amount of pain relief between drugs or same drug, different route. Consult pharmacist and health-care provider before changing drugs or routes.

risk for falls. See Table 10.1 for additional information and adverse effects of opioids.

Although opioids are important in pain management, they are also on a short list of "high-alert" drugs that can harm or even kill patients if they are not administered carefully (Institute for Safe Medication Practices, 2018). Institutions must have policies and procedures in place related to opioids to prevent medication errors and reduce the risk of serious side effects. It is especially important to be vigilant for side effects in patients unaccustomed to opioids. Such patients may be called "opioid-naïve." Opioids also have a high potential for abuse and misuse. Patients should be taught how to take their medications safely and keep medications safe in their homes.

CUE RECOGNITION 10.1
Thirty minutes after administering Joe's IV opioid for severe pain, you check on him and find him sleeping soundly. What do you do?

Suggested answers are at the end of the chapter.

NURSING CARE TIP
Be vigilant for side effects in patients unaccustomed to opioids, particularly constipation. Patients taking opioids for three days or more should be on bowel management programs that include a stimulant laxative such as senna (ExLax, Senokot). In cases of severe constipation, the HCP may prescribe a laxative specifically for opioid-induced constipation, such as naloxegol (Movantik) or methylnaltrexone (Relistor).

Opioids are added to nonopioids for pain that cannot be managed effectively by nonopioids alone. The use of a centrally acting opioid with a peripherally acting nonopioid can increase pain relief and reduce the amount of opioid needed.

Controlled-release opioids such as oxycodone (OxyContin) and morphine (MS Contin) are effective for prolonged, continuous pain. When a controlled-release form of medication is used, it is important to have an immediate-release medication available for **breakthrough** pain (transient pain that arises during generally effective pain control), such as oral morphine solution, oxycodone immediate-release (Oxy IR), or hydromorphone immediate-release (Dilaudid).

Meperidine (Demerol) was at one time a commonly used synthetic opioid but is no longer recommended in most cases. Meperidine is an opioid agonist; when broken down in the body, it produces a toxic metabolite called normeperidine. Normeperidine is a cerebral irritant that can cause adverse effects, ranging from dysphoria and irritable mood to seizures. Normeperidine has a long half-life even in healthy patients, so those with impaired kidney function are at increased risk. Meperidine use should be avoided in patients over age 65, patients with impaired kidney function, and patients taking a monoamine oxidase inhibitor (MAOI) antidepressant. In general, the use of meperidine should be limited to young, healthy patients who need an opioid for a short period and to those who have unusual reactions or allergic responses to other opioids. The effective dose of oral meperidine, three to four times the parenteral dose, is never recommended.

CRITICAL THINKING
Mrs. Zales, a 32-year-old woman, is admitted for a hysterectomy after being treated for painful endometriosis for 12 months. After her surgery, she has a patient-controlled analgesia (PCA) pump with hydromorphone, which is effective in relieving her pain. Forty-eight hours after surgery, the surgeon discontinues the PCA pump and orders oral hydrocodone with acetaminophen. It is ineffective, so an order is added for hydromorphone 2 mg orally every 3 to 4 hours, as needed. The nurse gives only one dose of the hydromorphone and then, thinking that her pain should be lessening, switches Mrs. Zales back to the hydrocodone with acetaminophen. By the next morning, Mrs. Zales is in severe pain. The on-call HCP orders intramuscular meperidine. Mrs. Zales's discharge is delayed until her pain can be controlled.

1. What do you think happened?
2. How could the delayed discharge have been avoided?
3. Who were the important team members in this scenario?

Suggested answers are at the end of the chapter.

Fentanyl can be given parenterally or intraspinally (Sublimaze) or by **transdermal** patch (Duragesic). Fentanyl is commonly used via IV with anesthesia for surgery. It also is used to relieve postoperative pain via IV, patient-controlled analgesia pump, or epidural (discussed later in this chapter). IV fentanyl has a short duration of action and must be given more often than other opioids to maintain an effective level of analgesia. The transdermal fentanyl patch is useful for a patient with stable chronic pain. The patch lasts 48 to 72 hours after application.

• WORD • BUILDING •
transdermal: trans—across + dermal—skin

CRITICAL THINKING & CLINICAL JUDGMENT

Mrs. Shepard is 92 years old and has undergone an open cholecystectomy. Her continuous epidural infusion of analgesic is discontinued at 1400 on her second postoperative day. The HCP orders oral hydrocodone/acetaminophen every 3 to 4 hours as needed for pain. At 1800, Mrs. Shepard refuses to get out of bed because her pain is 7 on a scale of 0 to 10. The nurse checks the medication administration record and notes that she has not yet received a dose of hydrocodone/acetaminophen.

Critical Thinking (The Why)
1. Why is Mrs. Shepard in so much pain?
2. Each analgesic tablet contains 5 mg of hydrocodone and 325 mg of acetaminophen. The maximum daily dose of acetaminophen is 3 g for an older adult. If she takes one tablet every 3 hours, is her dose safe?

Clinical Judgment (The Do)
3. What complications can occur as a result of her pain? How can you manage them?
4. What can you do to relieve her pain now and better prevent it in the future?

Suggested answers are at the end of the chapter.

Opioid Antagonists

Naloxone (Narcan) is a pure opioid antagonist that reverses, or antagonizes, the effect of opioids. It is often used in emergency departments and by emergency response personnel and others who have regular contact with people who abuse or misuse opioids or street drugs like heroin. Naloxone treats the effects of opioid overdose, such as sedation and respiratory depression. Caution must be used when giving naloxone to a patient who is receiving opioids for pain control. If too much naloxone is given too fast, not only can it reverse the unwanted effects—such as respiratory depression and sedation—but the pain may return as well.

Some antagonists are shorter acting than the opioid that is being used. If the antagonist is given because of respiratory depression, the dose may need to be repeated because its effect may wear off before the opioid wears off.

BE SAFE!
BE VIGILANT! Although respiratory depression is not a common side effect, it is a life-threatening one, and respiratory rate should be monitored, especially when beginning opioid use or with dose increases. Always check the respiratory rate before administering an opioid and report any respiratory rate that is lower than 12 per minute or lower than normal for that patient. An additional sign of opioid overdose is pinpoint (very small) pupils. Also be sure to ask about alcohol use before administering an opioid. Combining opioids and alcohol increases risk of respiratory depression, coma, and death.

Some analgesics are classified as combined agonists and antagonists or partial agonists. These drugs bind with some opioid receptors and block others. The most common drugs in this class are butorphanol, nalbuphine (Nubain), and buprenorphine (Buprenex).

How does this information translate into nursing practice? Consider a patient who receives sustained-release morphine every 12 hours to control metastatic bone pain, but the patient develops breakthrough pain between doses. You observe that butorphanol has been ordered for pain by another HCP and administer the medication. The butorphanol will antagonize, or counteract, some of the effects of the morphine, and the patient may experience acute pain. It is important to be informed about the actions of all drugs administered and to be aware of possible drug interactions that can interfere with patient care.

Analgesic Adjuvants

Adjuvants are classes of medications given in addition to other medications. Analgesic adjuvants can potentiate the effects of opioids or nonopioids, produce analgesic activity themselves, or counteract the unwanted effects of other analgesics. Some adjuvants are called *off-label* medications because they are used in a way not specifically approved by the FDA; that is, they were not initially developed to treat pain but may have pain-relieving properties for certain conditions. Although the use of adjuvants is common, nurses must be mindful of the side effects of these medications, which often affect the central nervous system. Examples of adjuvants are corticosteroids, benzodiazepines, antidepressants, and anticonvulsants (see Table 10.1).

Balanced Approach to Analgesia

A balanced analgesia approach should be used, combining analgesics and adjuvants from different classes to minimize adverse effects of opioids, such as nausea and vomiting or sedation, while maximizing pain relief. For example, giving an opioid and a nonopioid together can provide pain relief at lower doses than the patient would require with just one of the medications. Because these drugs have different mechanisms of action and different adverse effects, it is possible to safely use them together. Reducing doses in this manner may eliminate the need for additional sedating medications such as antiemetics and antihistamines to treat side effects.

Scheduling Options

Analgesics of any kind can be administered either as needed or on a scheduled basis. Intermittent, unpredictable pain may be best treated with as-needed doses. Pain that is predictable can be more effectively treated, or prevented, with scheduled doses of medication. Around-the-clock dosing is an effective way to schedule doses evenly over a 24-hour period to prevent pain from becoming unbearable. It is important to use around-the-clock dosing after surgery or trauma, with chronic pain, or in any other circumstance in which preventing pain will allow the patient to participate in daily or recovery activities.

Patient-Controlled Analgesia

Patient-controlled analgesia (PCA) involves an opioid on an IV controller. The patient has a button on a cord that can be pushed to receive a dose of IV medication. The registered nurse (RN) programs the pump to the dose and dosing interval ordered by the HCP. A "lockout" mechanism prevents the patient from receiving the medication more often than ordered. PCA is an excellent option after surgery because it gives the patient some control over pain management. Teach the patient and family that only the patient should push the button, never the nurse or a family member. If the patient is too sedated to push the button, a dose of opioid is not likely needed and could even be dangerous.

> **PRACTICE ANALYSIS TIP**
> **Linking NCLEX-PN® to Practice**
> The LPN/LVN will maintain pain control devices (e.g., epidural, patient-controlled analgesia, peripheral nerve catheter).

> **CRITICAL THINKING & CLINICAL JUDGMENT**
> **Ms. Jackson** had abdominal surgery 2 days ago. She has been receiving morphine via an IV patient-controlled analgesia pump at an average of 2.5 mg per hour for the past 6 hours. She rates her pain at 3 on a scale of 0 to 10. She is to be discharged today. Her HCP has ordered codeine 30 mg with acetaminophen (Tylenol with codeine No. 3), one or two tablets every 4 hours as needed for pain at home.
>
> **Critical Thinking (The Why)**
> 1. Will Ms. Jackson be comfortable at home? Why or why not? (Check the equianalgesic chart.)
>
> **Clinical Judgment (The Do)**
> 2. What should you do?
>
> *Suggested answers are at the end of the chapter.*

Other Interventions

Other pain treatments include topical local anesthetics, such as lidocaine/prilocaine cream (EMLA, or eutectic mixture of local anesthetics). These decrease the pain of procedures such as venipuncture and lumbar puncture. A lidocaine patch may be effective for patients with post-shingles or other nerve pain. In patients with osteoporosis, drugs that promote calcium uptake by the bones can aid in pain relief. These may include hormonal agents and medications that decrease calcium reabsorption from bone.

Placebos

Use of placebos involves the administration of an inactive substitute such as normal saline in place of an active medication. In the past, placebos were sometimes given to determine whether a patient's pain was "real." This is unethical and inappropriate unless the patient has given written consent. The use of placebos is a denial of the patient's report of pain. If a placebo is ordered for a patient, discuss concerns with the HCP and nurse supervisor. Placebos are only to be used in drug studies (clinical trials) to compare a new drug with an inactive substance. In this situation, patients are informed that they may be receiving a placebo.

Routes for Medication Administration

Analgesics can be administered by almost any route. The oral route is desired in most instances because it is easy and painless for the patient and can be used at home. See Table 10.3 for a comparison of the various routes.

Nonpharmacological Therapies

Nonpharmacological treatments are usually classified as cognitive-behavioral interventions or physical agents. The goals of these two groups of treatments differ. Cognitive-behavioral interventions can help patients understand and cope with pain and take an active part in its assessment and control. The goals of physical agents may include providing comfort, correcting physical dysfunction, or altering physiological responses. Nonpharmacological therapies should be used in conjunction with drug therapies. They are not expected to relieve pain on their own.

Cognitive-Behavioral Interventions

Cognitive-behavioral interventions include educational information, relaxation exercises, guided imagery, distraction (e.g., music, television), and biofeedback. These treatments require extra time for detailed instruction and demonstration. These methods will not help the patient if the patient does not find the chosen intervention acceptable. Educating patients about what to expect and how they can participate in their own care has been shown to decrease patients' reports of postoperative pain and analgesic use.

Relaxation can be accomplished through a variety of methods. The patient may prefer a scripted relaxation exercise that can be practiced and used the same way each time or simply the use of a favorite piece of music that allows a state of muscle relaxation and freedom from anxiety. Guided imagery uses the patient's imagination to take the patient away from the pain to a relaxing place, such as a beach in Tahiti. The success of guided imagery does not mean that the pain is in any way imaginary. See Chapter 5 for more information on relaxation and imagery.

As noted earlier, distraction is commonly used by patients to focus their attention on something other than the pain. They may watch a funny television program or laugh with visitors when they are in pain. When the program is over or the visitors leave, the patient may focus on the pain again and ask for a dose of pain medication.

Biofeedback is sometimes used in chronic pain programs to teach patients to train their bodies to respond to different signals. Biofeedback has been very useful in patients with migraine headaches. When an aura (warning sign) occurs before a migraine headache, patients begin the breathing and relaxation exercises that can often prevent the headache.

Table 10.3
Routes for Analgesic Administration

Uses	Advantages	Disadvantages	Nursing Considerations
Oral Preferred route in most cases.	Convenient. Less expensive than other forms. Immediate- and controlled-release forms available.	Slower onset than IV form.	Can provide consistent blood levels when given around the clock. Controlled-release form recommended for long-term use in chronic pain.
Rectal May be used to provide local or systemic pain relief.	Can be used when patient cannot take oral medication.	May be difficult for patient or family to self-administer.	Some oral preparations can be given rectally. (Place in empty gel cap for ease of use.) Check with health-care provider or pharmacist.
Transdermal Patch Used for chronic pain.	Easy to apply. Delivers pain relief for several days without patch change.	May take up to 3 days before maximum effective drug level reached; delay in excreting once removed. Patient must be closely monitored; alternative routes may be needed when starting and stopping therapy.	May be less effective in smokers and very thin people. Absorption may be erratic. Absorption may be increased with fever. Avoid heat application over patch. Avoid touching medication when applying patch. Keep used patches away from pets and children.
Intramuscular Acute pain.	Rapid pain relief, although slower than IV.	Painful administration. Inconsistent absorption.	Use only if other routes cannot be used.
IV Preferred route for postoperative and chronic cancer pain in patients who cannot tolerate oral route.	Provides rapid relief. Continuous infusion to achieve steady drug level.	Difficult to use in home health-care setting. Requires training and special equipment.	Follow drug manufacturer's instructions for administration.
Patient-Controlled IV Allows patient some control over administration schedule.	Patient pushes a button to administer a dose of opioid.	Requires special training. Pump must be programmed correctly.	An hourly limit and lockout interval are programmed into the pump to keep the patient from receiving too much drug. Caution patient and family that only the patient should push the button.
Subcutaneous May be used if IV route is problematic. A peripheral nerve catheter may be placed to deliver an anesthetic agent during and after surgery.	Can deliver effective pain relief. Some opioids may be given as continuous infusion.	Injection may be painful.	May be effective for treatment of chronic cancer pain.

Table 10.3
Routes for Analgesic Administration—cont'd

Uses	Advantages	Disadvantages	Nursing Considerations
Intraspinal (Epidural or Subarachnoid)			
Catheter into epidural or subarachnoid space used for traumatic injuries or chronic pain unrelieved by other methods. May also be used for orthopedic, chest, and abdominal surgical procedures.	May be able to control pain with lower doses of opioid because relief is delivered closer to site of pain. Fewer systemic side effects.	Requires single or continuous injection in back. May be associated with intense itching. Motor function must be monitored, especially when local anesthetic is used.	Steroids may be given with opioid to reduce pain by treating inflammation. Local anesthetic may be paired with opioid to enhance pain relief. Avoid use of anticoagulant and antiplatelet agents (including aspirin) because of risk of epidural hematoma.

Physical Agents

Physical agents can contribute directly to the patient's comfort. Examples of physical agents include applications of heat or cold, massage, and exercise. Additional physical interventions, such as immobilization or transcutaneous electrical nerve stimulation (TENS), are also available.

APPLICATION OF HEAT. The application of heat to sore muscles and joints is effective for pain relief. Heat works to increase circulation, induce muscle relaxation, and decrease inflammation when applied to a painful area. Heat can be applied using dry or moist packs or wraps, or in a bath or whirlpool. Many patients like to add Epsom salts (magnesium sulfate) with essential oils like lavender and/or peppermint to hot baths for additional comfort. Heat is contraindicated in conditions that would be worsened by its use, such as in an area of trauma, because of the possibility of increased swelling caused by vasodilation. To prevent burns, heat should not be applied directly to the skin or over areas of decreased sensation.

APPLICATION OF COLD. Cold can reduce swelling, bleeding, and pain when used to treat a new injury. It can also reduce the pain of an injection when applied prior to the injection, along with pressure, or vibration above the injection site. Cold can be applied by a variety of methods, such as cold wraps and cold packs as well as localized ice massage. Patients often choose heat over cold if they have the choice, because cold can be uncomfortable. Cold may be better tolerated over a small area. Alternating heat and cold therapies is most effective if not contraindicated.

> **PRACTICE ANALYSIS TIP**
> **Linking NCLEX-PN® to Practice**
> The LPN/LVN will provide non-pharmacological measures for pain relief (e.g., imagery, massage, repositioning).

MASSAGE AND EXERCISE. Massage and exercise are used to stretch and regain muscle and tendon length and relax muscles. Massage pressure can be superficial or deep and may involve vibration. It is important to ensure that massage is acceptable and inoffensive to the patient. Immobilization is used after a variety of orthopedic procedures as well as fractures and other injuries worsened by movement. Acupressure is also beneficial for pain reduction (see "Evidence-Based Practice").

Physical agents are readily available and inexpensive and often require little preparation or instruction. Remember, it is important to use nonpharmacological treatments as an enhancement of appropriate drug treatments, not as a substitute.

> **Evidence-Based Practice**
>
> **Clinical Question**
> Are noninvasive, nonpharmacological interventions effective for chronic pain?
>
> **Evidence**
> A systematic review looked at 218 clinical trials of patients with chronic low back, neck, knee, hip, tension headache, and fibromyalgia pain. A variety of nonpharmacological interventions were found to be effective. "Exercise, multidisciplinary rehabilitation, acupuncture, cognitive behavioral therapy, and mind-body practices were most consistently associated with durable slight to moderate improvements in function and pain for specific chronic pain conditions" (Skelly et al, 2018).
>
> **Implications for Nursing Practice**
> Nurses can assist patients with chronic pain to access training in non-pharmacological therapies. These therapies are not intended to replace medication for pain relief, but may help patients reduce analgesic doses and improve quality of life.
>
> *Reference:* Skelly, A. C., Chou, R., Dettori, J. R., Turner, J. A., Friedly, J. L., Rundell, S.D., Fu, R., Brodt, E. D., Wasson, N., Winter, C., & Ferguson, A. J. R. (2018). Noninvasive nonpharmacological treatment for chronic pain: A systematic review. Comparative Effectiveness Review No. 209. AHRQ Publication No 18-EHC013-EF. Rockville, MD: Agency for Healthcare Research and Quality. Posted final reports are located on the Effective Health Care Program search page. https://doi.org/10.23970/AHRQEPCCER209

NURSING PROCESS FOR THE PATIENT EXPERIENCING PAIN

Data Collection
Accurate assessment of pain is essential to effective treatment. Without accurate data, it is not possible to intervene in a way that meets the patient's needs. Because of regulatory requirements, most organizations require detailed pain assessments of patients at admission, with any change in condition, and at least every 3 months thereafter while in care. Nurses should verbally assess all patients under their care at least once per shift for pain and provide appropriate intervention as needed. The WHAT'S UP? format, introduced in Chapter 1, can help you collect complete and effective data. The following sections provide some additional key points for collecting data and putting together more pieces of the pain puzzle.

Accept the Patient's Report of Pain
Pain is what the patient says it is, not what the health-care team believes it is. The patient can usually sense when a member of the health-care team distrusts the patient's report of pain and may compensate by either underreporting pain or anxiously overreporting it. Patients may try to hide their pain for fear of being thought of as complainers or drug seekers.

Patient Perspective

Terry

I have had chronic back pain for 10 years. It is very real, related to multiple herniated discs in my thoracic and lumbar spine, arthritis, and degenerative disc disease. Because I've been dealing with it for 10 years, I have adapted. I never look like I am in pain. Sometimes I limp or move around a lot to find a comfortable position, but I don't have that pained look on my face, and my blood pressure doesn't go up like some people. I have tried many, many medications over the years and have become quite educated in pain treatments. I have tried antidepressants and antiseizure medications (both are used for neuropathic pain), ice, heat, transcutaneous electrical nerve stimulation (TENS), relaxation, physical therapy, more physical therapy, exercises, more exercises, massage therapy, steroid injections, and nerve blocks. I had relief once for about a month following some injections, and I kept thinking something was wrong. "Wait, where's the pain? This doesn't feel right!" Sometimes I would like a big dose of morphine, but I know that opioids for chronic pain are a one-way street to dependence. I do have a prescription for hydrocodone/acetaminophen (Norco) that I take a couple of times a month when I feel desperate. I ration them because I am afraid of them.

My friend Joanne also has back pain, which started 20 years ago. When it started, she was writhing in pain. I am positive her blood pressure was sky high! She couldn't move because of muscle spasms. She was also diagnosed with a herniated disc, but she had surgery to fix it. She said the nerve pain relief was already evident in the recovery room. Of course, surgery causes pain, so opioids are needed for a short while. But once healing started for Joanne, no pain! She still has acute pain from time to time, when she experiences muscle spasms and can't move very easily for several days. She takes muscle relaxers and has to lay low until the spasms resolve.

Sometimes Joanne looks at me and says, "You don't look like you're in pain." At first this made me feel bad, like she is comparing her pain to mine. Then one day, I realized the difference—she experiences *acute* pain, and I have *chronic* pain. I've adapted. She is way more miserable than I am when she is in pain, but it is short-lived. My pain is not as severe, but after 10 years, it has worn me down.

When you are a nurse, please believe your patients when they say they are in pain, even if they don't look like they are. Maybe they've gotten used to it, but that doesn't mean they enjoy feeling pain. Do whatever you can to help them feel better.

Obtain a Pain History
Obtain information from the patient about the pain they are experiencing. Letting the patient describe the pain in their own words helps establish a trusting relationship between you and the patient. Determine effects the pain is having on the patient's quality of life. Does the pain prevent the patient from eating, sleeping, or participating in work or family activities? Are there adverse effects such as nausea and vomiting or constipation that need to be addressed? Also observe for emotional and/or spiritual distress. Ask the patient about how they have coped with pain previously and what treatments have been effective or ineffective in the past. In nonverbal or cognitively impaired patients, information may be obtained from family members and the medical record. A painful diagnosis, such as arthritis, typically is a predictor of pain. A thorough history is essential so you can individualize pain interventions to fit the patient's needs.

Use Pain Assessment Tools
Various tools are available to assist with accurate and complete pain assessment. You should become familiar with the tools used in your clinical practice setting and use them consistently. It is of utmost importance that all health-care personnel caring for a particular patient use the same pain rating scale, whether it is a numerical scale (e.g., 0 to 10) such as a visual analog scale (Fig. 10.2) or the Wong Baker FACES Pain Scale (Fig. 10.3). There should also be consistent scales in place for nonverbal/cognitively impaired patients, such as the Pain Assessment in Advanced Dementia (PAINAD) Scale (Fig. 10.4; Warden, Hurley, & Volicer, 2003).

Whatever scale is used, it must be one that has been validated with research. The Wong Baker FACES Pain Scale was initially developed for use in children but can also be useful with adults. The PAINAD Scale was developed for patients with advanced dementia but is an effective tool for patients with other cognitive and communicative barriers. Longer questionnaires are useful in meeting regulatory requirements for the completion of comprehensive pain assessments (Fig. 10.5). These longer assessments are most often completed at admission and with any significant change in the patient's condition. A scale should also be used to monitor the patient's level of sedation after opioid administration (Fig. 10.6). Any unexpected increase in the patient's level of sedation should be reported promptly to the RN or HCP. Finally, keeping a pain diary helps patients to document pain ratings, interventions, and responses, which can help with the treatment plan. Cellular apps may facilitate journaling.

> **PRACTICE ANALYSIS TIP**
> Linking NCLEX-PN® to Practice
> The LPN/LVN will evaluate pain using standardized rating scales.

Assist with a Complete Physical Assessment

Collaborate with the RN to perform a thorough physical assessment. This is necessary to determine the effect of the pain and pain treatments on the body. It helps identify all pain sites and any medication side effects. It also helps prioritize the seemingly overwhelming task of helping the patient achieve acceptable pain relief and quality of life. As discussed previously, the patient with acute pain may exhibit objective signs such as grimacing and moaning or elevated pulse, respiratory rate, and blood pressure. For patients with cognitive impairments, these indicators can be particularly important; however, these signs cannot be relied on to "prove" that a patient is in pain. The only reliable source of pain assessment is the patient's self-report.

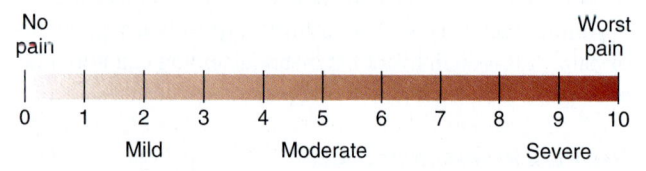

FIGURE 10.2 Analog pain scale.

> ### Gerontological Issues
> **Pain in Older Adults**
> Older adults frequently have unmet pain needs. Some believe that pain is an anticipated part of aging and may be hesitant to take strong medications such as opioids for pain. NSAIDs are often contraindicated for older adults due to medication interactions and gastrointestinal side effects; however, patients should be evaluated for medication needs on an individual basis. Patients in long-term care facilities, particularly patients with chronic pain and cognitive deficits, should have medications scheduled around the clock to ensure regular administration and effective pain control. Consider isolation, restlessness, confusion, aggression, and changes in appetite as possible signs of pain. Pulling at dressings, tugging at IV sites, and calling out can also be signs of discomfort. For patients at the end of life, a furrowed brow or restlessness may be signs of pain. Any change in the patient's usual behavior should be considered a possible sign of discomfort. A trial dose of pain medication can help to determine if the patient's behavior is because of pain. Remember to take more time when collecting data from older patients because they may need more time to process what you are asking. Consider using the Pain Assessment in Advanced Dementia (PAINAD) Scale when assessing confused patients.
>
> Opioid analgesic doses may need to be decreased by 25% to 50% initially because they tend to work longer and stronger in the older patient. The rule of thumb in starting opioid analgesics in older adults is to start low (in initial dosing) and go slow (in dose increases).

Nursing Diagnoses, Planning, and Implementation

See the "Nursing Care Plan for the Patient in Pain." Some additional principles to consider during planning and implementation follow.

Set Goals With Patients and Caregivers

Establish a pain control goal during the planning phase. Ask the patient to determine an acceptable level of pain if complete freedom from pain is not possible. Patients with

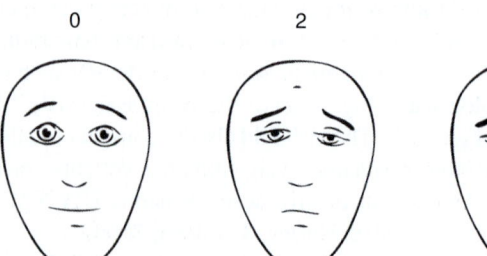

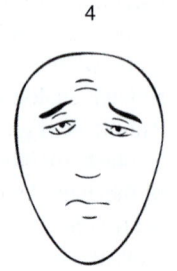

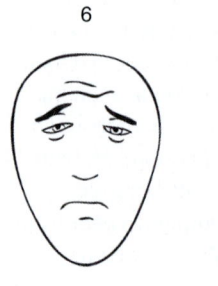

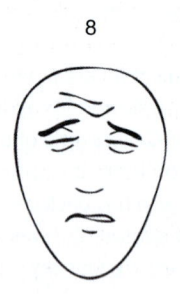

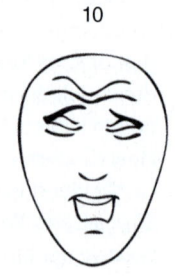

FIGURE 10.3 FACES Pain Scale–Revised.

Pain Assessment in Advanced Dementia Scale (PAINAD)

Behavior	0	1	2	Score
Breathing independent of vocalization	Normal	• Occasional labored breathing • Short period of hyperventilation	• Noisy labored breathing • Long period of hyperventilation • Cheyne-Stokes respirations	
Negative vocalization	None	• Occasional moan or groan • Low-level speech with a negative or disapproving quality	• Repeated troubled calling out • Loud moaning or groaning • Crying	
Facial expression	Smiling or inexpressive	• Sad • Frightened • Frown	• Facial grimacing	
Body language	Relaxed	• Tense • Distressed pacing • Fidgeting	• Rigid • Fists clenched • Knees pulled up • Pulling or pushing away • Striking out	
Consolability	No need to console	• Distracted or reassured by voice or touch	• Unable to console, distract, or reassure	
			Total*	

* Total scores range from 0 to 10 (based on a scale of 0 to 2 for five items), with a higher score indicating more severe pain (0–"no pain" to 10–"severe pain")

FIGURE 10.4 The PAINAD Scale.

cognitive deficits should also have pain goals established that include behavioral indicators. Education is important when helping patients and caregivers set realistic pain control goals. Although a pain goal of 0 is desirable, it may not be possible or safe. Conversely, a patient who chooses a pain goal of 6 may be unable to get out of bed and do daily or recovery activities.

Patients should also identify activity goals. After surgery, goals may include the ability to ambulate and achieve restful sleep. For patients with chronic pain, the goals may be different. For example, a patient with terminal cancer may want to be able to eat dinner with her family in the evening. You can assist the patient in reaching that goal by teaching her to conserve energy during the day for the activity that is most important to her. Instructing both types of patients in optimal timing of pain medications and appropriate use of nonpharmacological treatments will also assist them in reaching their desired activity goals.

Giving patients pain management options can provide autonomy and may help prevent feelings of helplessness and hopelessness. It is the nurse's responsibility to engage the patient and family in the pain management plan.

Understand That Pain Affects the Whole Family

It is important to include the whole family in the pain management plan. Understanding family dynamics helps in implementing an effective plan. Cultural influences are also important to consider (see Chapter 4 and "Cultural Considerations"). It is difficult for family members to see loved ones in pain or heavily sedated. When they help with planning, they feel that they help make the patient more comfortable and recognize the important role they have in patient care.

Recognize That Pain Is Exhausting

Pain may keep the patient from sleeping well. This cycle of sleeplessness and pain must be interrupted to help the patient. Fatigue is a common problem for the patient with chronic pain and can complicate treatment. Although older adults do not require as much sleep as younger adults, all patients must get at least 6 to 7 hours of uninterrupted sleep to be relaxed enough to break the cycle. Controlled-release opioids may help maintain pain relief throughout the night. If controlled-release medications are not used, it may be necessary to wake a patient to administer pain medication so that the pain does not get out of control. The addition of a sedative or sleep aid may be needed to allow the patient to sleep. Aromatherapy such as lavender, ensuring patient is comfortable, and limiting caffeine intake after 1500 can increase productive sleep.

Use a Team Approach to Pain Management

The interdisciplinary pain management team includes the patient and family, the licensed practical nurse/licensed vocational nurse, the RN, the HCP, therapists, spiritual advisers, social workers, and pharmacists. Communication among

Pain Assessment Chart (For Admission and/or Follow-up)

1. Patient _____ 2. DX _____

Assessment on Admission

Date _____/_____/_____   Pain ☐   No Pain ☐   Date of Pain Onset _____/_____/_____

1. Location of Pain (indicate on drawing)

2. Description of Predominant Pain (in patient's words) _____
   _____
   _____

3. Intensity [Scale 0 (no pain) — 10 (most intense)] _____   Right   Left   Left   Right
   _____

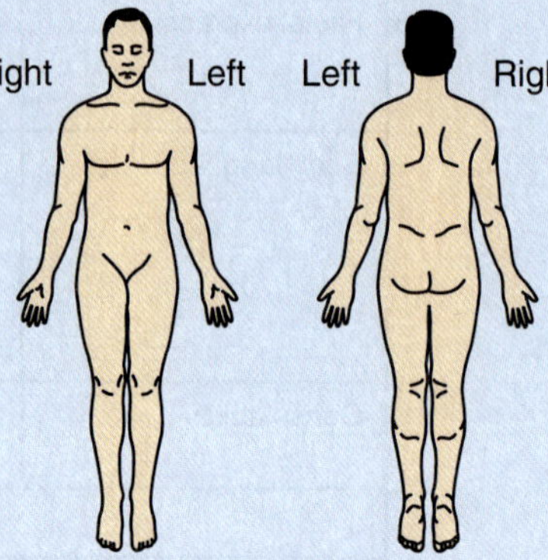

4. Duration and when occurs _____
   _____

5. Precipitating Factors _____
   _____

6. Alleviating Factors _____
   _____

7. Accompanying Symptoms

   GI: Nausea ☐   Emesis ☐   Constipation ☐   Anorexia ☐

   CNS: Drowsiness ☐   Confusion ☐   Hallucinations ☐

   Psychosocial: Mood _____   Anger _____

   Anxiety _____   Depression _____

   Relationships _____
   _____

8. Other Symptoms

   Sleep _____   Fatigue _____

   Activity _____   Other _____

9. Present Medications _____
   _____
   _____

   Doses and times medicated last 48 hours _____
   _____

10. Breakthrough Pain _____
    _____

Signature: _____

FIGURE 10.5 Pain assessment chart (modified).

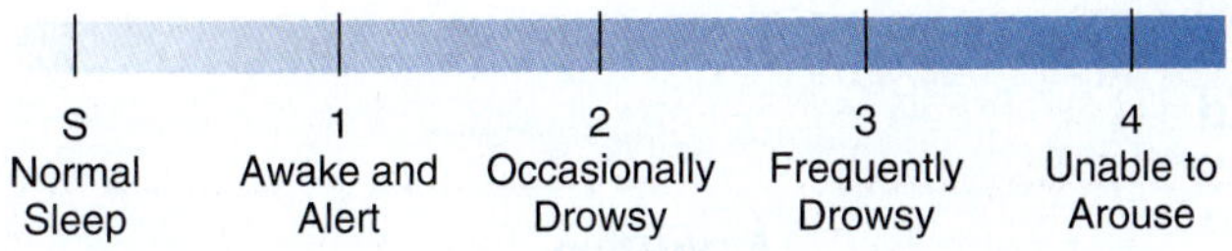

FIGURE 10.6 Level of sedation scale.

S — Normal Sleep
1 — Awake and Alert
2 — Occasionally Drowsy
3 — Frequently Drowsy
4 — Unable to Arouse

team members is essential. It is the important link that allows the team to be effective in creating a plan that works for the patient. As the nurse, you play a vital role in ensuring effective communication among team members, always remembering that the patient is at the center of the team.

Nursing Care Plan for the Patient in Pain

Nursing Diagnosis: *Pain (acute or chronic)*
Expected Outcomes: Pain will be at a level that is acceptable to the patient. The patient will be able to participate in activities that are important to him or her.
Evaluation of Outcomes: Is pain at a level that is acceptable to the patient? Is the patient able to participate in activities that he or she has identified as important?

Intervention	Rationale	Evaluation
Teach patient to use a pain rating scale. Use the same scales consistently.	A rating scale is the most reliable method for assessing pain severity.	Does patient understand the use of the scale and use it to report pain?
Have patient or caregiver keep a pain diary, documenting time of pain, interventions, and pre- and post-pain ratings.	A diary can show patterns of pain and pain relief, and help in planning care.	Does diary reveal patterns that help with planning?
Determine what is an acceptable pain level for the patient. Consider activities the patient should be able to perform.	Only the patient can decide what pain level is acceptable.	Is patient's pain at an acceptable level? Can they perform necessary activities of daily living with minimal pain?
Determine whether pain is nociceptive, neuropathic, or both.	Nociceptive and neuropathic pain may present differently and may require different interventions.	Has nociceptive versus neuropathic pain been identified? Are treatments appropriate?
Determine need for and offer emotional, spiritual, and social support for the experience of pain and suffering.	Pain, as well as disease processes, can be accompanied by feelings of powerlessness, distress, and isolation.	Does patient appear emotional, angry, or withdrawn? Does patient have difficulty making decisions? Does patient have a support system? Is patient–nurse relationship therapeutic?
Give analgesics before pain becomes severe. For persistent pain, give analgesics around the clock.	Pain can be more difficult to relieve when it becomes severe.	Is the analgesic schedule effective?
Combine opioid and nonopioid analgesics as ordered.	Balanced analgesia provides optimum pain relief with fewer side effects.	Is the analgesic combination effective?
Check for pain relief approximately 1 hour after administration of oral analgesics or 30 minutes after IV analgesics.	If pain is not relieved, additional measures will be needed.	Does patient report an acceptable level of relief?
Observe for adverse effects of pain medication.	Many pain medications cause nausea and fatigue. Both tend to subside after a few days.	Are adverse effects occurring? Can they be managed? Does medication regimen need to be adjusted?
If opioids and/or muscle relaxants are being used, monitor for respiratory depression and level of sedation at regular intervals.	Sedation and respiratory depression are risks if the patient is opioid-naïve or dose is increased. Sedation always precedes respiratory depression.	Is patient's respiratory rate greater than 8 per minute or above the parameter ordered by the HCP? What is patient's level of consciousness?

(nursing care plan continues on page 136)

Nursing Care Plan for the Patient in Pain—cont'd

Intervention	Rationale	Evaluation
Institute measures to prevent constipation: 8 to 10 glasses of noncaffeinated fluid daily (unless contraindicated), stimulant laxatives, and exercise as tolerated.	*Opioid-induced constipation is a problem of gastrointestinal motility; stimulant laxatives are most effective. Caffeine can exacerbate constipation.*	Is patient easily passing soft feces in the expected amount every 1 to 3 days?
Teach patient to incorporate nonpharmacological pain relief interventions, such as using hot or cold packs and initiating relaxation techniques when taking medication.	*Nonpharmacological interventions can help the patient feel in control and may help reduce the perception of pain.*	Does patient use nonpharmacological interventions effectively?
Determine whether patient is taking pain medications appropriately, and if not, determine the reasons. Discuss how interventions may be modified.	*Pain medications must be taken appropriately to be effective.*	Is patient able to manage the pain control regimen? Does patient have concerns about medications? Are adjustments necessary?

Patient Education

Patients, and in some instances their family members, must be informed about the medications they are taking for pain management. This allows them to take an active role in their care. Patients who are informed about the goals of pain management and who are confident that their providers believe them are more likely to report unrelieved pain so that they can receive prompt and effective treatment. Goals include a satisfactory comfort level with minimal side effects and complications of pain and its treatment as well as a reduced period of recovery.

The patient should be provided with information about a drug's effects, common adverse effects, frequency of the dose and duration of action, and potential drug-drug and drug-food interactions, if indicated. There are many special considerations for medications, such as controlled-release oral agents and transdermal patches. Care must be taken to include these considerations in the education plan for the patient taking these drugs at home. Drug-specific instructions are found in drug handbooks or databases. Education must be presented at a level that the patient can understand. Written information should be included when appropriate. Informed patients use their medications more effectively and safely.

Many patients are concerned about addiction when using opioids. Give accurate information on addiction risks and inform the patient of the importance of taking opioids exactly as directed. Also advise them on safe storage and disposal of opioids.

Evaluation

The final phase of the nursing process is evaluation. Once the plan of care has been implemented, evaluate whether the patient's goals have been met. What is the patient's pain rating? Has the patient's identified goal for an acceptable level of pain been met? How were the pain treatments tolerated? Was the patient able to participate in activities that they identified as important? The plan should be continuously updated based on the evaluation.

PRACTICE ANALYSIS TIP
Linking NCLEX-PN® to Practice
The LPN/LVN will evaluate client response to medication (e.g., adverse reactions, interactions, therapeutic effects).

CLINICAL JUDGMENT
Mr. Sebastian is a 75-year-old man diagnosed with lung cancer. He is anxious about leaving the hospital to return home following surgery. Home health care has been ordered for dressing changes and teaching about the medications he will need at home. While in the hospital, Mr. Sebastian has required 5 mg of IV morphine every 4 hours around the clock.
1. The morphine is available in syringes prefilled with morphine grains 1/6 per mL. How many milliliters should you administer while Mr. Sebastian is in the hospital?
2. What discharge instructions must be given to Mr. Sebastian and his wife before sending him home?
3. How might his pain be managed at home to prevent unnecessary readmissions?

Suggested answers are at the end of the chapter.

Home Health Hints
- Emotional or spiritual distress and fear related to dependence on family caregivers may alter the patient's perception or report of pain. Some patients may feel pain more intensely because of the influence of fear, and others may underreport if they are trying to protect family members.
- Weekly pill organizers are useful to manage administration of medications and for nurses to track usage.
- Opioids should be locked up and placed away from areas easily accessed by others.

Key Points

- The International Association for the Study of Pain (2020) describes pain in a bit more detail, as "an unpleasant sensory and emotional experience associated with, or resembling that associated with, actual or potential tissue damage." This definition indicates that pain is a complex problem that is not just physical in nature or always a result of tissue injury.
- Pain experiences may differ among cultures and individuals of various geographical regions. The nurse must assess for differences in language used, family engagement, spiritual practices, and treatment preferences based on each patient's unique background.
- While there are many common myths about pain, effective pain management helps to improve patient function and reduces costs by minimizing the side effects of opioids, preventing complications related to inadequate pain control, and reducing the length of hospital/nursing home stay or period of recovery.
- Tolerance is a normal biological adaptation to long-term use of a drug. The drug becomes less effective; therefore, a larger dose is required to provide the same level of pain relief. Physical dependence is a normal physiological response that most people experience after a week or more of continuous opioid use. Addiction is a disease of the brain that causes the compulsive pursuit of a substance or behavior to obtain reward or relief from craving.
- Pain is transmitted through four distinct processes: transduction, transmission, perception, and modulation.
- Nociceptive pain refers to the body's normal reaction to noxious stimuli, such as tissue damage, with the release of pain-producing substances. It may be localized in muscles or bones, or it may be organ pain.
- Neuropathic pain is poorly localized and may involve other areas along the nerve pathway. Neuropathic pain is common in cancer patients following chemotherapy or radiation therapy. It also occurs in patients who have fibromyalgia, diabetic neuropathy, and shingles.
- Analgesics make up the largest piece of the pain management puzzle. They encompass three main classes of medication: opioids, nonopioids, and adjuvants.
- Opioids bind to opioid receptors in the brain, spinal cord, and other areas of the body, inhibiting the perception of pain. Nonopioids include NSAIDs and acetaminophen. Adjuvants are different from opioid and nonopioids in that they include categories of medications that were originally approved by the FDA for purposes other than pain relief, such as depression.
- Nonopioids are typically the first class of drugs used to treat mild pain. They can be useful for acute and chronic pain from a variety of causes, such as surgery, trauma, arthritis, and cancer. These drugs are limited in their use because they have a ceiling effect to analgesia.
- Morphine, an opioid, is often the drug of choice for treating severe pain. It is the standard against which all other analgesics are compared. Opioids alone have no ceiling effect to analgesia. Although opioids are important in pain management, they are also on a short list of "high-alert" drugs that can harm or even kill patients if they are not administered carefully.
- Analgesic adjuvants can potentiate the effects of opioids or nonopioids, have analgesic activity themselves, or counteract the unwanted effects of other analgesics. Anticonvulsant and antidepressant medications are commonly used adjuvants.
- A balanced analgesia approach should be used, combining analgesics and adjuvants from different classes to minimize the adverse effects of opioids, such as nausea and vomiting or sedation, while maximizing pain relief.
- Nonpharmacological pain management techniques include cognitive-behavioral interventions (educational information, relaxation exercises, guided imagery, distraction, and biofeedback), as well as physical agents that can contribute directly to the patient's comfort. Examples of physical agents include applications of heat or cold, massage, and exercise. These techniques are intended to supplement, not replace medications for pain.
- The nurse should be familiar with a variety of pain assessment tools, such as a simple numeric scale, the Wong Baker FACES Pain Scale, and the PAINAD Scale.

SUGGESTED ANSWERS TO CHAPTER EXERCISES

Cue Recognition
10.1: Never assume that a sleeping patient is pain free or even safe. One option is to wake Joe and make sure his level of consciousness and pain levels are appropriate. You might also check his respirations as he sleeps. Suppressed respiratory rate could be a sign of too high of an opioid dose.

Critical Thinking & Clinical Judgment
Mrs. Bao and Mr. Brown
1. It is important to accept both patients' pain reports. Treatment should be based on what the patient says rather than what is observed. Each patient copes with their pain in a unique way, and the nurse cannot judge whether one is in more pain than the other.

Lucy
1. Remember, pain is whatever the experiencing person says it is, existing whenever the experiencing person says it does. You must assume that Lucy is in pain. She has pancreatitis, which is commonly very painful. She has a history of IV drug abuse and is likely tolerant to the effects of the morphine. She may be experiencing "end-of-dose failure," when pain medication

SUGGESTED ANSWERS TO CHAPTER EXERCISES—cont'd

does not last as long as expected. If her vital signs are within normal limits, it should be safe to treat her pain.
2. Contact the RN or HCP to explain the problem. Making Lucy wait another hour in pain is not appropriate.
3. Tylenol works differently from morphine and may offer minimal relief but is not an appropriate order for severe pain. Talk to the RN or supervisor and explain the situation.
4. Listen to Lucy and let her know that you understand she is in pain. Keep her updated at all times and assure her that you will continue to advocate for her until she achieves adequate pain relief. At the same time, be observant for visitors who might be bringing Lucy additional substances, including marijuana edibles (such as brownies) to help her control her pain. Additive effects of prescribed and nonprescribed medications can be deadly.

Mrs. Zales
1. Mrs. Zales may have been tolerant to opioids because of her need for medication for chronic pain during the past year. For this reason, she needed more medication than a nontolerant patient who does not usually use opioids. Intramuscular injections are not recommended because they are painful, absorption is not predictable, and there is a delay between injection and relief. A more rational approach to Mrs. Zales's pain management would have been regular pain assessment with around-the-clock treatment until the pain began to subside and a recommendation to the HCP to switch the meperidine to IV hydromorphone.
2. If her pain level had been better controlled, she might have been discharged on oral analgesics without the delay.
3. The most important team member here was Mrs. Zales—the patient should be the *center* of the team! If she had been listened to more carefully and her history considered, she might have been kept more comfortable.

Mrs. Shepard
1. Pain medication is most effective when given on a routine schedule around the clock to avoid breakthrough pain. Mrs. Shepard's epidural infusion should continue to relieve her pain for a time, up to several hours after it is discontinued, depending on the medication used. The oral medication is most effective when given at the time the epidural is stopped so that it is taking effect as the epidural effects wear off. See "Gerontological Issues" for special considerations for the older patient.
2. Pain prevents patients from moving freely. Postoperative complications such as retained pulmonary secretions and ileus can occur when patients are immobile. If you keep her pain controlled, she will be better able to move, cough and deep breathe, and get up to the bathroom, which will all reduce her risk of complications.
3. If she takes a dose every 3 hours, then she will receive eight doses in 24 hours: 325 mg × 8 = 2,600 mg, or 4 g, which is below the maximum safe dose of 3,000 mg for older adults. Recall that older adult patients metabolize and excrete medications more slowly than younger patients. Always be mindful of the total acetaminophen dosages consumed.
4. Give her a dose of hydrocodone/acetaminophen now. Or, call the HCP and ask for an IV analgesic order for faster action for her first post-PCA dose. Then consider administering it every 3 hours to prevent pain. Of course, check vital signs and ensure her safety before EVERY analgesic dose. Within 24 to 48 hours, you can begin to extend the time between doses, and then switch to acetaminophen alone. Remember to monitor her bowel function and administer a stimulant laxative as needed. Mrs. Shepard should be instructed about what her role will be whenever her pain management regimen is altered. Does she have to ask for the pain medication, or will it be brought to her? Patient and family education are vital to success in management of a patient's pain.

Ms. Jackson
1. Using an equianalgesic conversion, we can determine that Ms. Jackson is unlikely to have good pain relief based on her requirement with the PCA pump. Her current pain level of 3 shows that the morphine has been effective. Remember that the PCA pump keeps a history of what the patient uses, which is the best indicator of what the patient needs. Ms. Jackson has used 15 mg of morphine during the past 6 hours. An equianalgesic dose of codeine would be almost 200 mg of codeine, but only 30 to 60 mg has been ordered. In addition, if Ms. Jackson takes enough Tylenol with codeine No. 3 to get 200 mg of codeine, she will receive a dangerous dose of both the codeine and the acetaminophen.
2. The HCP needs to be contacted for different analgesic orders.

Mr. Sebastian
1. $\dfrac{5\text{ mg}}{60\text{ mg}} \cdot \dfrac{1\text{ grain}}{\text{grains }1/6} \cdot \dfrac{1\text{ mL}}{} = 0.5\text{ mL}$
2. Home instruction regarding around-the-clock administration of pain medication is indicated, as is education about effects and side effects to report. He will also need to implement measures to prevent constipation. Also, information about what to do and whom to contact if pain becomes unmanageable is necessary to help prevent readmission to the hospital.
3. A long-acting oral medication may be an option for Mr. Sebastian, along with an immediate-release preparation for breakthrough pain. Make sure to check an equianalgesic chart to be sure the oral dose ordered by the HCP is adequate.

Additional Resources

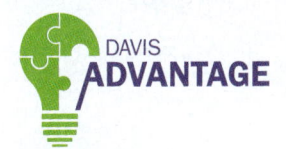

Go to Davis Advantage to complete your learning: strengthen understanding, apply your knowledge, and prepare for the Next Gen NCLEX®.

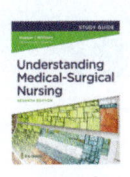

A Study Guide is also available.

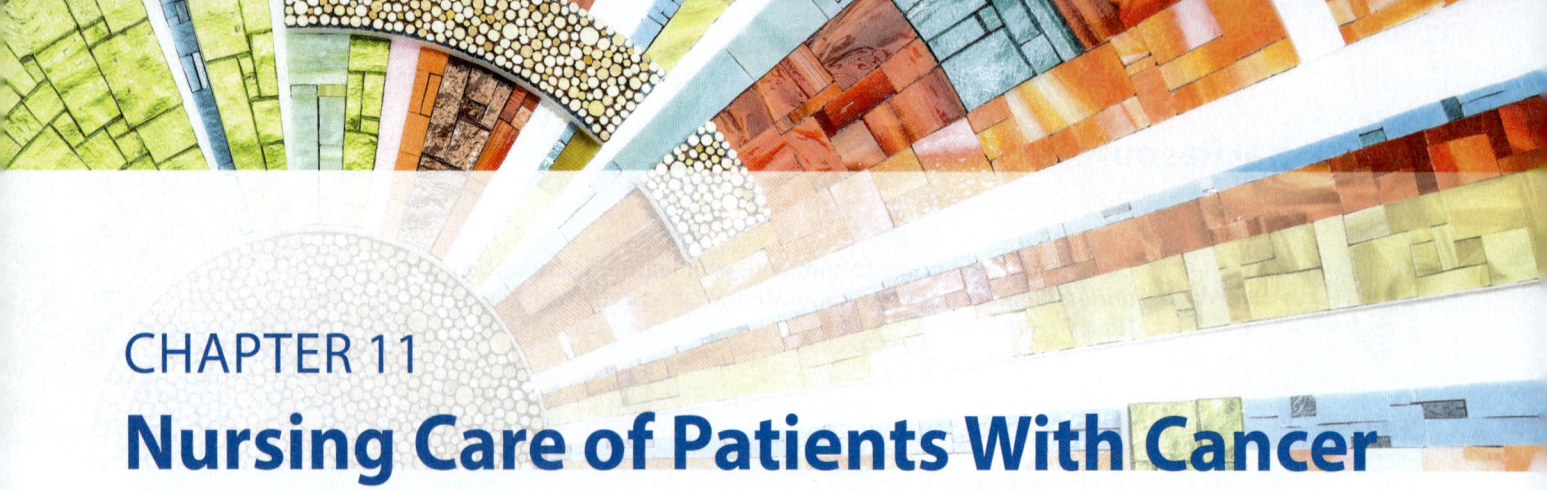

CHAPTER 11
Nursing Care of Patients With Cancer

Janet Yontas, Janice L. Bradford

KEY TERMS

alopecia (AL-oh-PEE-shah)
anemia (uh-NEE-mee-ah)
anorexia (AN-oh-REK-see-ah)
benign (bee-NINE)
biopsy (BY-op-see)
cancer (KAN-sir)
carcinogen (kar-SIN-oh-jen)
chemotherapy (KEE-moh-THAIR-uh-pee)
contact inhibition (kon-takt in-huh-BIH-shun)
cytotoxic (SY-toh-TOK-sik)
desquamation (dee-skwa-MAY-shun)
in situ (in SY-too)
leukopenia (LOO-koh-PEE-nee-ah)
malignant (muh-LIG-nunt)
metastasis (muh-TAS-tuh-sis)
mucositis (MYOO-koh-SY-tis)
nadir (NAY-dur)
neoplasm (NEE-oh-PLAZ-uhm)
neutropenia (noo-troh-PEE-nee-ah)
oncology (on-CAW-luh-gee)
oncovirus (ON-koh-VY-rus)
palliation (pal-ee-AY-shun)
radiation therapy (RAY-dee-AY-shun THAIR-uh-pee)
stomatitis (STOH-mah-TY-tis)
thrombocytopenia (THROM-boh-SY-toh-PEE-nee-ah)
tumor (TOO-mer)
vesicant (VES-ih-kent)
xerostomia (ZEE-roh-STOH-mee-ah)

CHAPTER CONCEPTS

Caring
Health promotion
Nutrition
Patient-centered care
Safety
Self

LEARNING OUTCOMES

1. Explain the structures and functions of the normal cell.
2. Describe changes that occur in a cell when it becomes malignant.
3. Identify common actions and side effects of chemotherapeutic agents.
4. Discuss the plan of care for the patient receiving chemotherapy and/or radiation therapy.
5. Identify data to collect when caring for a patient with cancer.
6. Recognize common oncological emergencies and related nursing care.
7. Discuss how you will know if your nursing interventions have been effective.
8. Discuss the role of hospice in providing care for patients with terminal illness.

REVIEW OF ANATOMY AND PHYSIOLOGY OF NORMAL CELLS

Cells are the smallest living structural and functional subunits of the body. Although human cells vary in size, shape, and certain metabolic activities, they have many characteristics in common.

Cell Structure

Human cells have a plasma membrane, cytoplasm (cytosol, organelles), and a nucleus (Fig. 11.1). Organelles are specific in structure and function. Variations in the relative amounts of organelles and cell features allow great diversity in cells and, therefore, in tissues.

Nucleus

The nucleus of a cell is its control center, containing the individual's unique deoxyribonucleic acid (DNA) sequence (Fig. 11.2). Most cells have one central nucleus, although variations exist.

DNA coding regions are called *genes*. Most genes code for a protein. Not all genes in a particular cell are active, only those needed for the proteins required to carry out their specific functions. These proteins may be structural, such as the collagen of connective tissue, or functional, such as the hemoglobin of red blood cells (RBCs). Important functional proteins are the enzymes that catalyze the specific reactions characteristic of each type of cell.

Chapter 11 Nursing Care of Patients With Cancer   141

Plasma membrane: The boundary of the cell

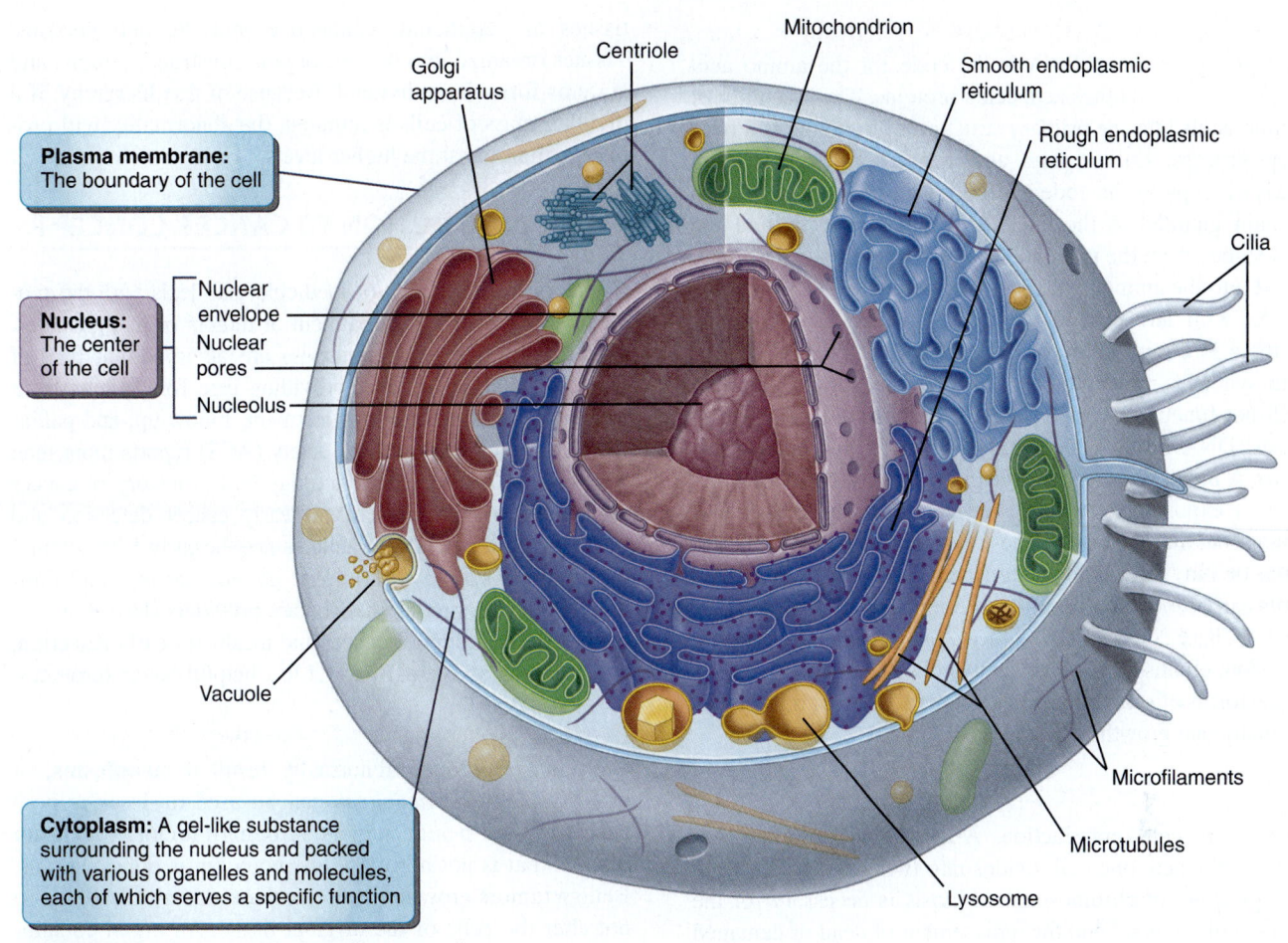

Nucleus: The center of the cell
- Nuclear envelope
- Nuclear pores
- Nucleolus

Golgi apparatus
Centriole
Mitochondrion
Smooth endoplasmic reticulum
Rough endoplasmic reticulum
Cilia
Vacuole
Microfilaments
Microtubules
Lysosome

Cytoplasm: A gel-like substance surrounding the nucleus and packed with various organelles and molecules, each of which serves a specific function

FIGURE 11.1 Schematic of a typical human cell.

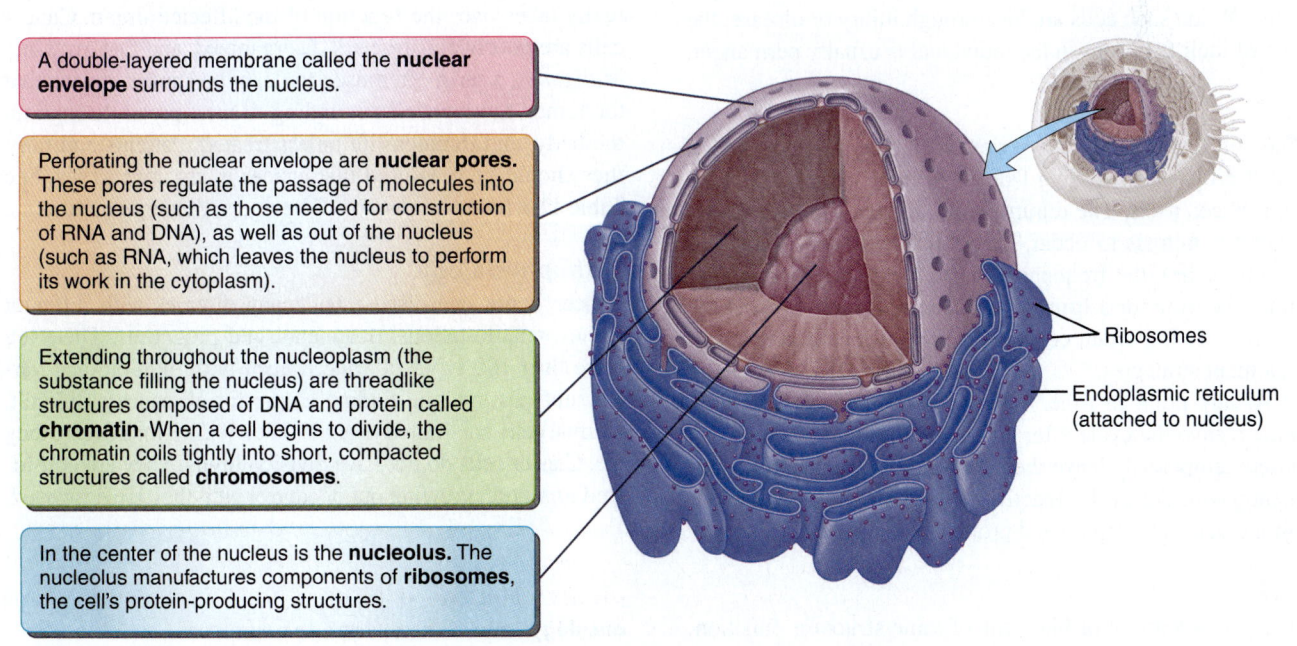

A double-layered membrane called the **nuclear envelope** surrounds the nucleus.

Perforating the nuclear envelope are **nuclear pores.** These pores regulate the passage of molecules into the nucleus (such as those needed for construction of RNA and DNA), as well as out of the nucleus (such as RNA, which leaves the nucleus to perform its work in the cytoplasm).

Extending throughout the nucleoplasm (the substance filling the nucleus) are threadlike structures composed of DNA and protein called **chromatin.** When a cell begins to divide, the chromatin coils tightly into short, compacted structures called **chromosomes.**

In the center of the nucleus is the **nucleolus.** The nucleolus manufactures components of **ribosomes,** the cell's protein-producing structures.

Ribosomes
Endoplasmic reticulum (attached to nucleus)

FIGURE 11.2 The nucleus.

Genetic Code and Protein Synthesis

The genetic code of DNA is the code for the amino acid sequences that synthesize a cell's proteins. The assembly of amino acids into the primary structure of a protein is a two-step process: transcription and translation. Transcription makes a copy of the code needed for a protein so DNA can remain guarded in the nucleus. Translation occurs at the ribosome where the nucleotide code of nucleic acids is translated into the amino acid code of protein (Fig. 11.3).

As with any complex process, mistakes are possible. If there is a mistake in the DNA code, the process of protein synthesis may continue. However, the resulting protein will not function normally; this is the basis for genetic diseases. DNA mistakes acquired during life are called *mutations*. A mutation is any change in the DNA code. Ultraviolet rays or exposure to certain chemicals may cause structural changes in the DNA code. These changes can kill the affected cells or may irreversibly alter their function. Such altered cells can become **malignant** and can no longer function normally. These cells actively replicate the mutated DNA during division, creating a mass of faulty cells. This process causes some forms of **cancer,** which is a general term for many types of malignant growths.

Mitosis

Mitosis is cell reproduction. After its 46 chromosomes have replicated, one cell divides into two cells, each with a complete set of chromosomes. Mitosis is necessary for the growth of the body and the replacement of dead or damaged cells. Not all cells are capable of mitosis. Of those that are capable, the rate of division varies widely by tissue type. Some cells are capable of only a limited number of divisions. Once that limit has been reached and the cells die, they are not replaced. Shortly after birth, almost all neurons lose their ability to divide, and muscle cells have limited mitotic capability. When such cells are lost through injury or disease, the loss of their functions in the individual is usually permanent.

Cell Cycle

The cell cycle involves a series of changes through which a cell progresses, starting from the time it develops until it reproduces itself. The duration of the cell's life, the time it takes for mitosis to occur, the growth ratio (percentage of cycling cells), the frequency of cell loss, and the doubling time (the time for a **tumor**—an abnormal mass—to double its size) are important concepts related to tumor growth and treatment strategies.

At any point in time, some cells are actively dividing, others leave the cycle after a certain point and die, and still others temporarily leave the cycle and remain inactive until reentry into the cycle. Inactive cells continue to synthesize ribonucleic acid (RNA) and protein (Fig. 11.4).

Cells and Tissues

A tissue is a group of like cells of same structure, function, and intercellular substance. The four categories of human tissues are epithelial, connective, muscle, and nervous. Tissues organize into organs, organs construct systems, and systems form the individual. Because of this hierarchy, if a dividing mass of cells is mutated, the abnormality will produce symptoms at the higher levels.

INTRODUCTION TO CANCER CONCEPTS

Oncology is the branch of medicine that deals with the prevention, diagnosis, and treatment of tumors or malignancies. Oncology nurses (cancer nurses) are an important part of the medical-surgical team, providing care for patients from prevention and detection to treatment, follow-up, and palliation. The American Cancer Society (ACS) reports more than 16.9 million Americans alive today have a history of cancer (ACS, 2020a). The benefits of early cancer detection and treatment have been documented since the early 19th century. Today, microscopic technology, genetic testing, and continued research provide health-care providers (HCPs) with a better understanding of cancer and means for early detection, interventions, and care. Box 11.1 lists helpful cancer resources.

Benign Tumors

Cells that reproduce abnormally result in **neoplasms,** or tumors. The term *neoplasm* can be used to describe both cancerous and benign tumors. A **benign** tumor is a cluster of cells that is not normal to the body but is noncancerous. Benign tumors grow more slowly than cancer cells. They do not alter the cells of the original tissue. An organ containing a benign tumor usually continues to function normally. A neoplastic growth is difficult to detect until it contains about 500 cells and is about 1 cm in diameter.

Cancer

Cancer is a group of cells that grows out of control and eventually takes over the function of the affected organ. Cancer cells are poorly constructed, disorganized, and fast growing. *Malignant,* a term often used to describe cancer, means that the tumor can invade surrounding tissue, spread throughout the body, and threaten life unless treated. Patients and families should be reassured that cancer is not contagious. See Table 11.1 for a comparison of benign and malignant tumors.

Pathophysiology

Cancer is not one disease but many diseases with different causes, manifestations, treatments, and prognoses. There are more than 100 types of cancer, each with multiple and varied subtypes, making finding a cure for all cancers difficult. Normal cells are limited to about 50 to 60 divisions before they die. Cancer cells do not have division limits. They are considered immortal, growing out of control until they are destroyed.

• WORD • BUILDING •
oncology: onco—mass + logy—word, reason
neoplasm: neo—new + plasm—form

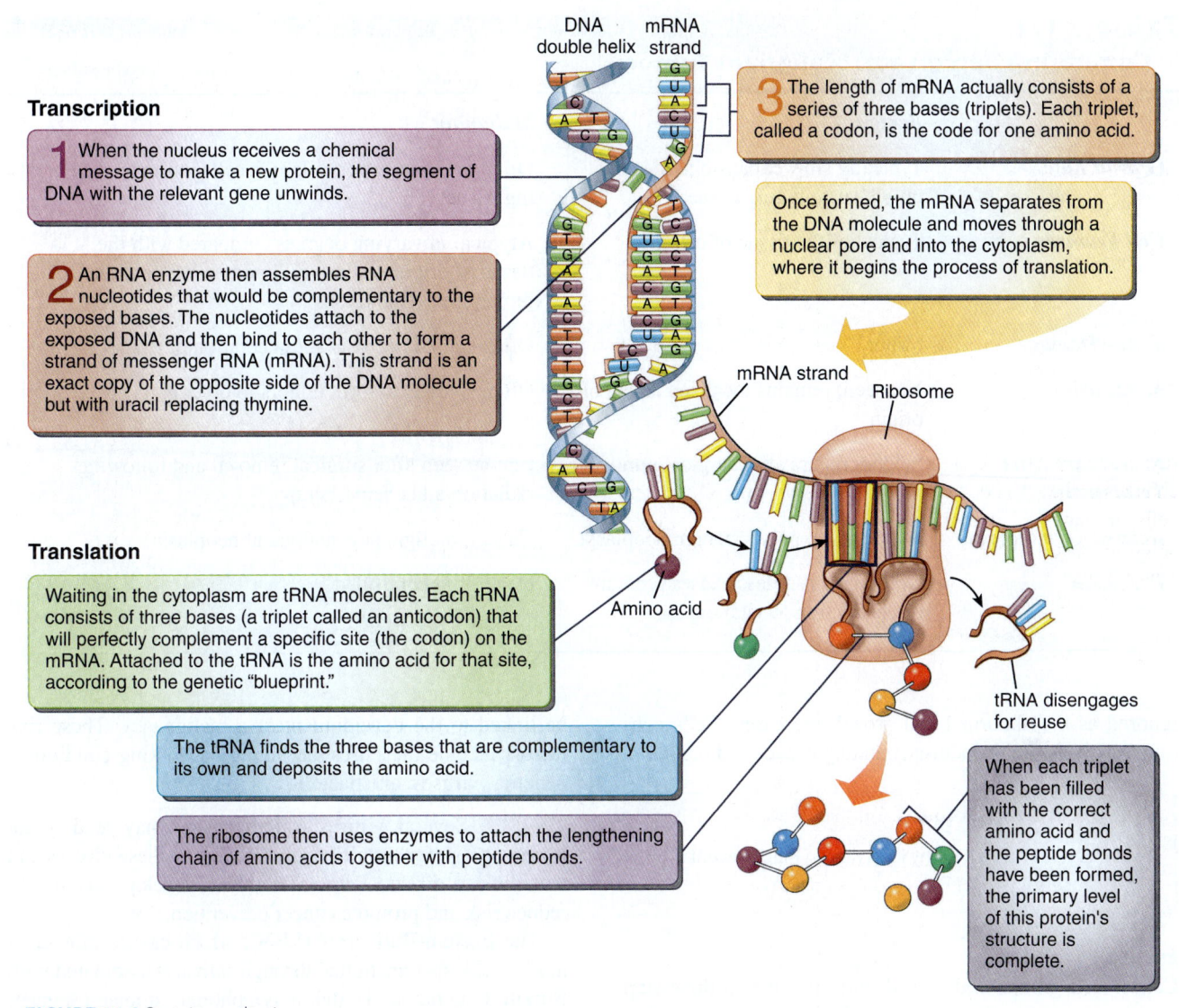

Chapter 11 Nursing Care of Patients With Cancer 143

Transcription

1 When the nucleus receives a chemical message to make a new protein, the segment of DNA with the relevant gene unwinds.

2 An RNA enzyme then assembles RNA nucleotides that would be complementary to the exposed bases. The nucleotides attach to the exposed DNA and then bind to each other to form a strand of messenger RNA (mRNA). This strand is an exact copy of the opposite side of the DNA molecule but with uracil replacing thymine.

3 The length of mRNA actually consists of a series of three bases (triplets). Each triplet, called a codon, is the code for one amino acid.

Once formed, the mRNA separates from the DNA molecule and moves through a nuclear pore and into the cytoplasm, where it begins the process of translation.

Translation

Waiting in the cytoplasm are tRNA molecules. Each tRNA consists of three bases (a triplet called an anticodon) that will perfectly complement a specific site (the codon) on the mRNA. Attached to the tRNA is the amino acid for that site, according to the genetic "blueprint."

The tRNA finds the three bases that are complementary to its own and deposits the amino acid.

The ribosome then uses enzymes to attach the lengthening chain of amino acids together with peptide bonds.

When each triplet has been filled with the correct amino acid and the peptide bonds have been formed, the primary level of this protein's structure is complete.

FIGURE 11.3 Protein synthesis.

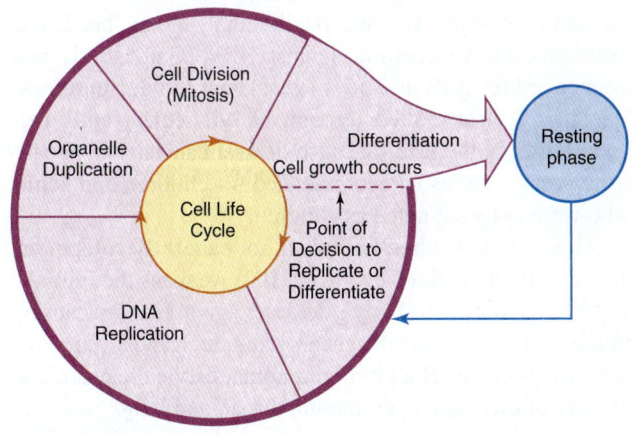

FIGURE 11.4 Cell cycle.

Box 11.1

Cancer Resources

American Cancer Society: 800-227-2345; www.cancer.org
CancerCare: 800-813-HOPE (4673); www.cancercare.org
National Cancer Institute: 800-4-CANCER (422-6237); www.cancer.gov
Oncology Nursing Society: 866-257-4ONS (4667); www.ons.org
Centers for Disease Control and Prevention: 1-800-CDC-INFO (800-232-4636); www.cdc.gov/cancer
American Society of Clinical Oncology (ASCO): 1-888-651-3038; www.cancer.net
OncoLink: www.oncolink.org

The progression from a normal cell to a malignant cell follows a pattern of mutation (change), defective division, abnormal growth cycles, and defective cell communication. Cell mutation occurs when an alteration affects the chromosomes, causing the new cell to differ from its parent cell. The malignant cell's enzymes destroy the glue-like substance found between normal cells disrupting the transfer of information and communication.

Cancer cells also lack **contact inhibition.** Growth-regulating signals in the cells' surrounding environment are

Table 11.1

Comparing Benign and Malignant Tumors

	Benign	*Malignant*
Growth Rate	Typically slow expansion: does not invade surrounding tissue	Often rapid growth; malignant cells infiltrate surrounding tissue
Cell Features	Typical of the tissue of origin	Atypical in varying degrees compared with the tissue of origin; altered cell membrane; contain tumor-specific antigens
Tissue Damage	Minor	Often causes necrosis and ulceration of tissue
Metastasis	Not seen; remains localized at site of origin	Often spreads to form tumors in other parts of the body
Recurrence After Treatment	Seldom recurs after surgical removal	Can be seen after surgical removal and following radiation and chemotherapy
Related Terminology	Hyperplasia, polyp, benign neoplasia	Cancer, malignancy, malignant neoplasia
Prognosis	Not injurious unless causes pressure or obstruction to vital organs	Death if uncontrolled

ignored as the abnormal cell growth increases. Cells continue to divide and invade surrounding tissues and organs.

> **NURSING CARE TIP**
> Teach families that a healthy lifestyle can help prevent some cancers.

Etiology

Cancer cell growth and reproduction involves a three-step process: initiation, promotion, and progression. The first step, *initiation,* results from alteration in the genetic structure of the cell (DNA). This occurs either spontaneously or following exposure to a **carcinogen** (a substance or agent that increases the risk of cancer). The cellular change primes the cell to become cancerous.

Promotion occurs after repeated exposure to carcinogens causes initiated cells to mutate. During the promotion step, a tumor forms from mutated cell reproduction. During *progression,* further genetic mutations occur, leading to growth and metastasis. Scientists are using this understanding of cancer cell growth to develop treatments to harm cancer cells at various stages of formation.

A healthy immune system can often destroy cancer cells before they replicate and become a tumor. It is important to remember that any substance that weakens or alters the immune system puts the individual at risk for cell mutation with the potential to develop into cancer.

Risk Factors

Researchers have determined that it is not known what causes cancer; however, there are many factors that may be linked to the development of a malignancy. These risk factors include diet, lifestyle, living or working conditions, genetics, viruses, and bacteria.

VIRUSES. Several viruses (**oncoviruses**) may lead to an increased risk for certain cancers. Studying these viruses and their link to disease helps researchers develop vaccines to reduce risk and promote cancer prevention.

The Epstein-Barr virus (EBV), which causes infectious mononucleosis transmitted through saliva, is associated with Burkitt lymphoma, Hodgkin lymphoma, stomach cancer, and nasopharyngeal cancer. Human papillomavirus (HPV) has strains that can lead to cancer in both men and women, including cervical, vaginal, penile, anal, throat, head, and neck cancers. Vaccination against HPV (Gardasil) is recommended for girls and boys age 11 to 12 to decrease risk. Hepatitis B, transmitted through blood, semen, and other body fluids, is the leading cause of liver cancer. The hepatitis B vaccine series is recommended for children and adults who were not vaccinated as children.

Although not directly linked to cancer development, human immunodeficiency virus (HIV) weakens the immune system and lowers the body's defenses against cancer-causing viruses. HIV-associated cancers include Kaposi sarcoma, non-Hodgkin and Hodgkin lymphoma, cervical cancer, and cancers of the anus, liver, mouth, throat, and lung.

BACTERIA. *Helicobacter pylori* (*H. pylori*) can irritate the stomach lining, causing changes that may lead to stomach

• WORD • BUILDING •
carcinogen: karkinos—cancer, crab + genesis—birth
oncovirus: onco—mass + virus

cancer. Chlamydia trachomatis may increase risk for cervical cancer. Prompt detection and treatment of these infections may decrease cancer risk.

RADIATION. An increased incidence of cancer occurs in persons exposed to prolonged or large amounts of radiation. Ionizing radiation involving ultraviolet rays (e.g., sunlight; x-rays; and alpha, beta, and gamma rays) plays a major role in promoting leukemia and skin cancers, primarily melanomas. A common type of cancer in adults is skin cancer; it is also considered the most preventable. Exposure to ultraviolet radiation (sunlight) and indoor tanning increases the risk of skin cancer. Wearing protective clothing and sunscreen can greatly reduce the risk of skin cancer (Fig. 11.5).

> **LEARNING TIP**
> Remember the ACS Slip, Slap, Slop, Wrap campaign: Slip on a shirt, slap on a hat, slop on the sunscreen, and wrap the sunglasses (ACS, 2020c).

Persons exposed to radioactive materials in large doses (e.g., a radiation leak or an atomic bomb) are at risk for leukemia and breast, bone, lung, and thyroid cancer. Controlled **radiation therapy** is used to treat cancer patients by destroying rapidly dividing cancer cells, but radiation can also damage normal cells. The decision to use radiation is made after careful evaluation of the tumor's location and vulnerability to other treatments.

> **Cultural Considerations**
> Although cancer rates and cancer deaths have decreased in the United States, some groups of people experience health disparities related to access to care. Black women are more likely than White women to die of breast cancer. Black men have a higher risk of dying from prostate cancer, and Hispanic/Latino and Black women have higher rates of cervical cancer. Generally, people who have low health literacy, lack health insurance, and have low income are less likely to be screened for cancer (National Cancer Institute, 2020), so the cancer may be quite advanced before it is discovered, leading to higher mortality rates.

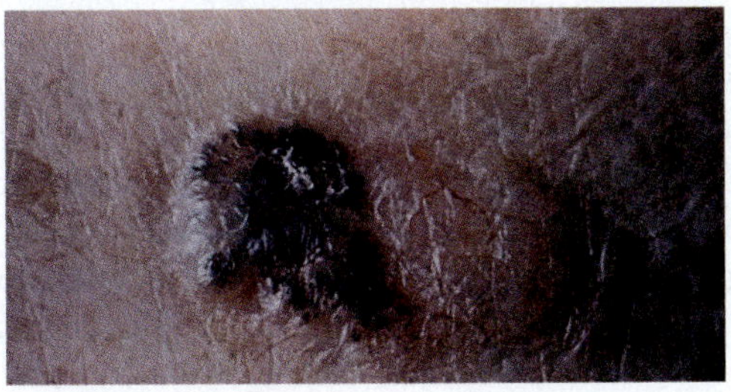

FIGURE 11.5 Melanoma.

CHEMICALS. Chemicals are present in air, water, soil, food, medications, and tobacco smoke. Length of time and degree of exposure to chemical carcinogens may trigger malignant tumor development, increasing the risk for cancer development.

Smoking accounts for 30% of all cancer deaths in the United States and 80% of all lung cancer deaths (ACS, 2020a). Other tobacco exposure, such as to cigars, smokeless tobacco, and secondhand smoke, also increases cancer risk. Scientists continue to study the effects of e-cigarettes (vaping) on cancer risk when used over a long period of time. E-cigarettes can contain harmful substances, including cancer-causing chemicals. Alcohol use, even a few drinks per week, has been associated with mouth, esophagus, liver, breast, colon, and stomach cancers. Alcohol and tobacco combined increase risk for the development of cancers of the mouth and esophagus. Lung cancer has the highest cancer mortality rate in both men and women and is mostly preventable. Cigarette smoking is the main cause of lung cancer, along with air pollution and exposure to radon and other chemicals.

Occupational exposures are associated with some cancers, such as bladder, liver, kidney, lung, and skin. Dyes in clothing and hair dye may increase cancer risk. Older buildings and homes should be monitored for asbestos, as this has been proven to cause lung cancer. Federal and state employee protection regulations have significantly reduced risk of occupational exposures.

GENETICS. Genetic mutations have been associated with 5% to 10% of all cancers, such as breast, ovarian, colorectal, and prostate (National Cancer Institute, 2020). People with chromosomal abnormalities such as Down syndrome have a higher risk of developing leukemia. Genetic predisposition is a factor for some early-onset cancers. The highest incidence of cancer in women is in the breast. Women with a family history of breast cancer have a greater risk than those with no family history. Commercial testing for the oncogene linked with breast cancer is available and marketed for women at high risk, especially those in the Ashkenazi Jewish population (CDC, 2019). Testing is done through genetic counseling programs. See Figure 11.6 for estimated new cancer cases and deaths for 2020. Although the genetic mutations are not the only factor for developing cancer, the study of genetics has led researchers to new treatments.

LIFESTYLE. Lifestyle is a modifiable risk factor for cancer. People who eat high-fat, low-fiber diets are at a higher risk for development of colon cancer. A diet high in fats has been associated with prostate cancer in men. Consumption of large amounts of salt-preserved, smoked, and charbroiled foods has been linked with esophageal and stomach cancers. A diet low in vitamins A, C, and E is associated with cancers of the lungs, esophagus, mouth, larynx, cervix, and breast. The Mediterranean diet, which includes a large variety of plant foods, fish, and olive oil, has been shown to contribute to the prevention of breast cancer.

HORMONES. Hormonal agents that disturb the body's balance can also promote cancer. Long-term use of the female

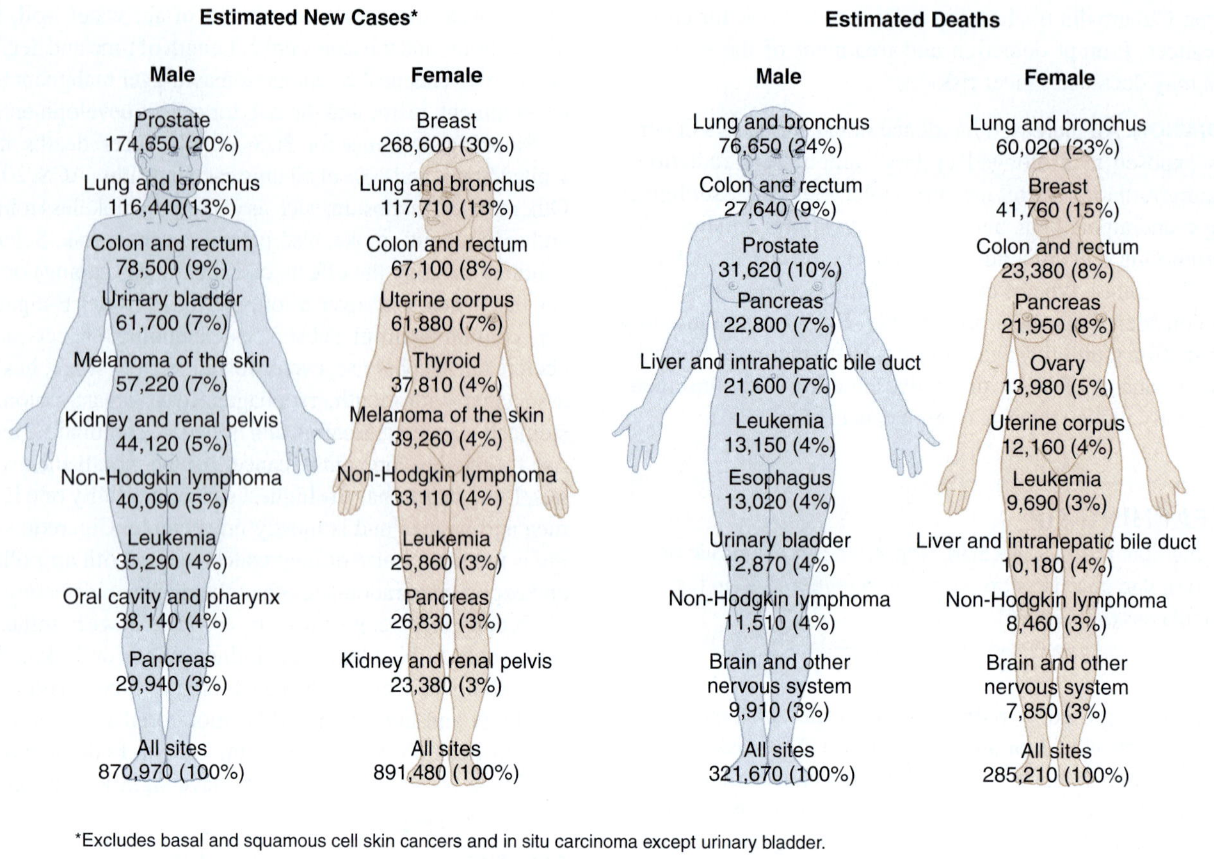

Estimated New Cases*

Male
- Prostate 174,650 (20%)
- Lung and bronchus 116,440 (13%)
- Colon and rectum 78,500 (9%)
- Urinary bladder 61,700 (7%)
- Melanoma of the skin 57,220 (7%)
- Kidney and renal pelvis 44,120 (5%)
- Non-Hodgkin lymphoma 40,090 (5%)
- Leukemia 35,290 (4%)
- Oral cavity and pharynx 38,140 (4%)
- Pancreas 29,940 (3%)
- All sites 870,970 (100%)

Female
- Breast 268,600 (30%)
- Lung and bronchus 117,710 (13%)
- Colon and rectum 67,100 (8%)
- Uterine corpus 61,880 (7%)
- Thyroid 37,810 (4%)
- Melanoma of the skin 39,260 (4%)
- Non-Hodgkin lymphoma 33,110 (4%)
- Leukemia 25,860 (3%)
- Pancreas 26,830 (3%)
- Kidney and renal pelvis 23,380 (3%)
- All sites 891,480 (100%)

Estimated Deaths

Male
- Lung and bronchus 76,650 (24%)
- Colon and rectum 27,640 (9%)
- Prostate 31,620 (10%)
- Pancreas 22,800 (7%)
- Liver and intrahepatic bile duct 21,600 (7%)
- Leukemia 13,150 (4%)
- Esophagus 13,020 (4%)
- Urinary bladder 12,870 (4%)
- Non-Hodgkin lymphoma 11,510 (4%)
- Brain and other nervous system 9,910 (3%)
- All sites 321,670 (100%)

Female
- Lung and bronchus 60,020 (23%)
- Breast 41,760 (15%)
- Colon and rectum 23,380 (8%)
- Pancreas 21,950 (8%)
- Ovary 13,980 (5%)
- Uterine corpus 12,160 (4%)
- Leukemia 9,690 (3%)
- Liver and intrahepatic bile duct 10,180 (4%)
- Non-Hodgkin lymphoma 8,460 (3%)
- Brain and other nervous system 7,850 (3%)
- All sites 285,210 (100%)

*Excludes basal and squamous cell skin cancers and in situ carcinoma except urinary bladder.

FIGURE 11.6 Leading new cancer cases and deaths: 2020 estimates.

hormone estrogen is associated with certain cancers of the breast, uterus, ovaries, cervix, and vagina. It has been found that children born of mothers who took diethylstilbestrol (DES) during pregnancy have an increased incidence of reproductive cancers. DES is a synthetic hormone with estrogen-like properties that was used in the past to prevent miscarriage. Tumors of the breast and uterus are tested for estrogen or progesterone receptiveness, meaning that the hormone is promoting their growth. Treatment varies depending on test results.

IMMUNE FACTORS. A healthy immune system destroys mutant cells quickly on formation. An individual with impaired immunity is more susceptible to cancer formation when exposed to small amounts of carcinogens compared to someone with a healthy immune system. Immune system suppression allows malignant cells to develop in large numbers.

Altered immunity is noted in persons with chronic illness and stress. An increased risk of cancer may follow a traumatic, stressful period in life, such as the loss of a mate or a job. Failure to decrease stress productively contributes to a higher incidence of chronic illnesses. Thus, a cycle of stress, illness, and increased cancer risk develops. People infected with HIV and patients on immunosuppressive medications after organ transplant have compromised immune systems and an increased risk for certain viruses that lead to cancer. People on medication that reduces immune function are also at risk.

AGE. Cancer affects all age-groups, but older adults have the highest incidence. In the United States, 80% of cancers are diagnosed in people 55 years and older (ACS, 2020a). Men have a higher incidence of cancer than women. Cancer in people older than 55 is thought to occur from a combination of exposure to carcinogens, body weight, and weakening of the body's immune system.

Acute lymphocytic leukemia, sarcomas, and cancers of the central nervous system and brain are common cancers found in children ages 0 to 14. Causes of childhood cancer are not understood; therefore, prevention is difficult. Adolescent and young adult cancers accounted for approximately 89,500 new cancers and 9,270 deaths in 2020. Common cancers include leukemia, thyroid, melanoma, cervical, and testicular (ACS, 2020a). Vaccines and teaching about screening play an important role in decreasing cancer risk and statistics for this age group.

Cancer Classification

Cancers are identified by the tissue affected, speed of cell growth, cell appearance, and location. Neoplasms occurring in the epithelial cells are called *carcinomas*. Carcinoma is the most common type of cancer. It arises from cells of the skin, gastrointestinal (GI) system, and lungs. *Sarcomas* are cancer cells affecting connective tissue, including fat, the sheath that contains nerves, cartilage, muscle, and bone. *Leukemia* is the term used to describe the abnormal growth of white blood cells (WBCs). Cancers involving cells of the lymphatic system, lymph nodes, and spleen are called *lymphomas*. See Table 11.2 for cancer types based on origin.

Metastasis (Spread of Cancer)

Neoplastic cells that remain in one area are considered localized, or **in situ,** cancers. These tumors may be difficult to detect on clinical examination and are identified through microscopic cell exam. In situ tumors are often removed surgically and may require no further treatment.

Metastasis is the term used to describe the spread of the tumor from the primary site into separate and distant areas (Fig. 11.7). Metastasis occurs mainly because cancer cells break away more easily than normal cells. Cancer cells can survive for a time independently from other cells. There are three steps in the formation of a metastasis: Cancer cells (1) invade blood or lymph vessels, (2) move by mechanical means, and (3) lodge and grow in a new location.

Table 11.2 Tumor Descriptions

Tumor Type	Character	Origin
Fibroma	Benign	Connective tissue
Lipoma	Benign	Fat tissue
Carcinoma	Cancerous	Tissue of the skin, glands, and digestive, urinary, and respiratory tract linings
Leukemia	Cancerous	Blood, plasma cells, and bone marrow
Lymphoma	Cancerous	Lymph tissue
Melanoma	Cancerous	Skin cells
Sarcoma	Cancerous	Connective tissue, including bone and muscle

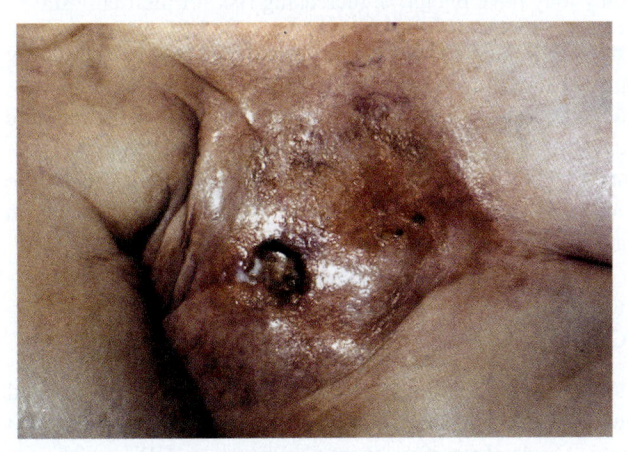

FIGURE 11.7 Invasive metastasis to skin area following mastectomy for breast cancer.

Metastatic tumors carry the cell characteristics of the original or primary tumor site. Under a microscope, the metastatic cancer has the same type of cancer cells as the original tumor. For example, breast cancer that spreads to the lung or brain is metastatic breast cancer, not primary lung or breast cancer. Common sites of metastasis are the lungs, liver, bones, and brain.

Mortality Rates

Cancer survival rates have improved with the recognition of risk factors and improvements in early detection and treatment. A 5-year period is used to monitor cancer patients' progress following diagnosis and treatment. Survival statistics are based on those who live 5 years in remission. Remission is considered to have occurred when all signs and symptoms of cancer have disappeared, even though there may still be cancer in the body.

Early Detection and Prevention

Nurses play an important role in preventing and detecting cancer by educating patients about risk factors, self-examination, genetic testing, and cancer screening programs. Early diagnosis and treatment are important factors in fighting cancer.

> **LEARNING TIP**
> CAUTION mnemonic:
> **C**hange in bowel or bladder habits
> **A** sore that does not heal
> **U**nusual bleeding
> **T**hickening or lump
> **I**ndigestion or difficulty swallowing
> **O**bvious change in mole
> **N**agging cough or hoarseness

BREAST CANCER SCREENING. The ACS recommends mammography (a special x-ray of breast tissue used to detect a mass too small for palpation) every year for women after age 40. After age 55, women can switch to mammograms every other year or continue yearly. Screening should continue as long as the woman is in good health and has a life expectancy of 10 years or more. Women of any age should discuss individual risk factors and recommended screenings such as genetic testing, mammogram, magnetic resonance imaging (MRI), or ultrasound with their HCP. Although considered optional, girls starting at puberty should perform self-breast examinations to recognize how their breasts normally look and feel and report changes to the HCP. A breast self-examination procedure can be found in Chapter 41. See breast changes with breast cancer, Figure 11.8.

CERVICAL CANCER SCREENING. Initial Papanicolaou (Pap) testing for cervical cancer is recommended to begin with a

• WORD • BUILDING •

in situ: in—in + situ—position
metastasis: meta—beyond + stasis—stand

Lump — Skin dimpling

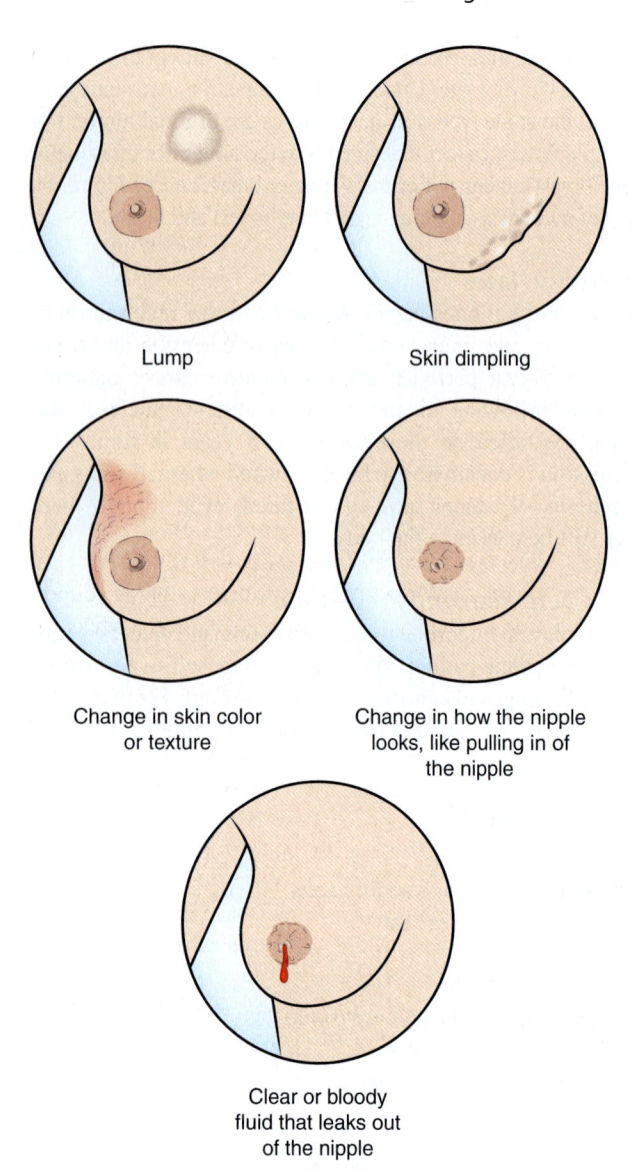

Change in skin color or texture — Change in how the nipple looks, like pulling in of the nipple

Clear or bloody fluid that leaks out of the nipple

FIGURE 11.8 Breast changes with breast cancer.

baseline screening no earlier than age 21. If normal, proceed to the preferred recommended schedule for women ages 25 to 65 of the Pap test with an HPV test every 5 years. However, it is acceptable to have just the Pap test every 3 years in this age-group. After age 65, a woman who has had three normal Pap tests in a row within the past 10 years needs no further screening. Women with a history of cervical precancer should be tested for at least 25 years after diagnosis regardless of age. Some women choose not to be screened even with access to health care. Barriers to screening include fear of health-care personnel and testing procedures as well as lack of knowledge. As a nurse, you can promote screening by developing a trusting relationship and providing information to your female patients.

COLON CANCER SCREENING. The ACS (2020b) recommends one of the following options to screen for colorectal cancer, beginning at age 45:

- Tests that find polyps and cancer
  - Flexible sigmoidoscopy every 5 years
  - Colonoscopy every 10 years
  - Double-contrast barium enema every 5 years
  - Colonography (virtual colonoscopy using computed tomography [CT]) every 5 years
- Tests that mainly find cancer
  - Fecal occult blood test every year
  - Fecal immunochemical test every year
  - Stool DNA test every 3 years

If any of the tests are positive, follow-up with an HCP is necessary for further testing.

PROSTATE CANCER SCREENING. The ACS currently recommends that men discuss the benefits of PSA testing and digital rectal examinations with their HCP starting at age 50 (ACS, 2020b).

LUNG CANCER SCREENING. The ACS currently recommends yearly lung cancer screening with a low-dose CT scan (LDCT) for high-risk people who meet the following conditions:

- Age 55 to 74 and in good health
- Currently smoke or quit smoking in the past 15 years
- Have at least a 30 pack-year smoking history (ACS, 2020b). (A pack-year is useful for determining lifelong tobacco exposure and is determined by multiplying the number of *packs* of cigarettes smoked per day by the number of *years* the person has smoked.)

The ACS considers testicular self-examinations to be optional for men. ACS guidelines encourage everyone to be familiar with their bodies and to report changes to their HCPs. Offer men and women instruction in breast and testicular self-examinations.

GENETIC TESTING. Genetic testing identifies persons at risk for certain cancers. This technology poses legal and ethical questions concerning confidentiality and insurance cost. The cooperation of family members is important because genetic testing is done after a member has been diagnosed with cancer. The family may experience various emotions about the increased risk for themselves as well as guilt over the role they may have played in increasing risk for their children.

HEALTHY LIFESTYLE. Practicing healthy lifestyles, including proper diet and exercise, helps strengthen the immune system and reduce cancer risk. Smoking is the most preventable cause of death from lung cancer. Smoking cessation and lifestyle programs are the subject of ongoing campaigns by the ACS and Healthy People 2030 (Office of Disease Prevention and Health Promotion, 2020).

Significant research about cancer risk and nutrition is underway. Visit www.cancer.org and "Nutrition Notes: Reducing Cancer Risk" for additional dietary recommendations.

VACCINES. Preventive vaccines target viruses associated with certain cancers. Recombinant HPV vaccine (Gardasil and Gardasil-9), for example, prevents HPV, which is responsible for various cancers. Hepatitis B vaccine protects

Nutrition Notes

Reducing Cancer Risk

The ACS estimates that at least 18% of cancers and 16% of cancer deaths in the United States could be prevented by following ACS diet and exercise recommendations. Excess body weight is responsible for about 11% of cancers in women and about 5% of cancers in men in the United States. The ACS recommends that Americans

- Achieve and maintain a healthy weight.
- Eat a healthy diet, with an emphasis on plant foods.
- Limit processed foods (cookies, deli meats, packaged snacks, most breakfast cereals).
- Read food labels to be aware of portion sizes and calories.
- Choose whole, unprocessed fruits and vegetables.
- Limit intake of sugar-sweetened beverages.
- Limit processed and red meats; choose fish, poultry, or beans.
- Eat a variety of at least 2 1/2 cups of fruit and vegetables each day.
- Choose whole grains instead of refined grain products.
- Limit alcohol intake to one drink for women and two for men per day (12 oz beer, 5 oz wine, or 1.5 oz distilled spirits).
- Spend 150 to 300 minutes per week in moderate-intensity physical activity (walking, dancing or biking) or 75 to 150 minutes per week in vigorous-intensity activity (jogging, running or swimming).
- Limit sedentary activity such as sitting or watching TV.

Source: American Cancer Society. (2020). ACS guidelines for nutrition and physical activity. www.cancer.org/healthy/eat-healthy-get-active/acs-guidelines-nutrition-physical-activity-cancer-prevention/guidelines.html

Patient Perspective

Nikki

When I was 27 years old, I went for a routine check-up. The doctor found a lump in my right breast. I had noticed it 6 months before, but I didn't think it was anything. When the doctor told me it was cancer, my reaction was, "Why me? I have such a healthy lifestyle!" I discussed treatments with my doctor, and he said I needed surgery, chemotherapy, and radiation. But because I was so young, I didn't want to lose my breast or my hair. The doctor said there was a new medicine that wouldn't make me lose my hair, but it wasn't covered by insurance.

The doctor put a port in my chest for chemo. It was so painful, I cried. After two chemo treatments, I had surgery. They were able to remove all the cancer and still leave most of my breast. When I was in the hospital, all the young medical students had to look at my breasts. After a while, I stopped feeling embarrassed.

Fortunately, my father was able to help me pay for the medicine I needed. When I went for chemotherapy, everyone was together in a group. All the older people looked at me because I was always the youngest patient. They had all lost their hair and had hats on. I lost about 20% of my hair, but I was the only one who could tell. I had four more chemo treatments and 30 radiation treatments. I started on tamoxifen to prevent the cancer from returning.

About 9 months later, when I was 28, I moved to Japan. I knew I wanted to have a baby someday, but I wasn't too worried at that time. Even the doctor wasn't sure whether I could have a baby. I met my husband, an American, when I was in Japan. I worried about telling him about the cancer because I knew he wanted children someday. But he said it was okay and that we could adopt if I couldn't have a baby. After we married, I stopped taking tamoxifen and had to wait 6 months to try to get pregnant. Then, it only took 2 months to get pregnant! I now have a healthy baby, and I feel very lucky and happy.

I worried that I wouldn't be able to breastfeed my baby, and it turns out I can only feed him from my left breast. Now when my breast is full of milk, I am very lopsided! I have to put in a pad on the right side when I go out. My left breast makes more than enough milk for my baby. I am not sure how long I will breastfeed before I have to go back on the tamoxifen, but for now I am happy that everything is working just fine.

Nothing is more important to me than staying healthy and for my husband and baby to be healthy, too. Now I have a good life and healthy body, and I can take care of my family. To stay healthy, I am careful to eat lots of fruits and vegetables and avoid unhealthy fats. I try to exercise a lot.

---

against the infection that increases susceptibility to liver cancer. Therapeutic vaccines are currently being researched and tested for various cancers. These vaccines stimulate the patient's immune system to destroy cancer cells. Currently, the only therapeutic cancer vaccines approved by the U.S. Food and Drug Administration are intravesical Bacillus Calmette-Guérin (BCG) Live (TheraCys; Sanofi Pasteur), which was approved by the FDA in 1990 for intravesical use in the treatment and prevention of urothelial carcinoma in situ of the urinary bladder; sipuleucel-T (Provenge) for the treatment of advanced prostate cancer; and talimogene laherparepvec, or T-VEC (IMLYGIC) for metastatic melanoma that cannot be surgically removed.

Diagnosis of Cancer

A cancer diagnosis is a frightening experience (see "Patient Perspective"). Often, people try to ignore symptoms because they are frightened of the disease. A physical examination along with careful and thorough assessment by the HCP of the patient's current status, medical and surgical histories, and family history is completed. It is important for the nurse to develop a trusting relationship with the patient. The most conclusive information is obtained through tissue biopsy.

For detailed explanations of the following tests, see Appendix A.

BIOPSY. Accurate identification of a cancer can be made only by **biopsy**. A biopsy can be done via an endoscopic procedure, surgical incision, or a small needle inserted into the site. Microscopic examination of a sample of tissue or aspirated body fluid can confirm the presence of abnormal or cancerous cells. A biopsy is typically done in an HCP office or as outpatient surgery.

RADIOLOGICAL PROCEDURES. X-ray examination is a valuable diagnostic tool in detecting cancer of bones and hollow organs. Chest x-ray examination is one diagnostic test used in detecting lung cancer. Mammography is a reliable and noninvasive low-radiation x-ray procedure to detect breast masses.

Contrast media x-ray studies are used to detect abnormalities that might not show up with regular x-rays. Barium is given orally for visualization of the esophagus and stomach. It can also be given rectally as a barium enema for visualization of the colon. IV injection of contrast media is used for visualizing vessels, the urinary tract, or fallopian tubes.

CT scans are important in the diagnosis and staging of malignancies. They can detect minor variations in tissue thickness. The use of a contrast medium enhances the accuracy of an abdominal CT scan. CT scans are also used to improve the accuracy of inserting a fine needle for biopsy. Be sure to ask the patient about a history of allergic reaction to dyes and for kidney function. Dyes are excreted by the kidneys.

NUCLEAR IMAGING PROCEDURES. Nuclear medicine imaging involves camera imaging of organs or tissues containing radioactive media. Radioactive compounds are given intravenously or by mouth. These studies are highly sensitive. They detect sites of abnormal cell growth months before changes are seen on an x-ray.

Positron emission tomography (PET) scanning provides information about cellular function. Patients are given biochemical compounds. Images are made of the tissue through gamma-camera tomography. PET scans have been useful in brain imaging as well as the detection of the spread of cancers of the lung, ovaries, colon, rectum, and breast.

ULTRASOUND PROCEDURES. Ultrasonography helps detect tumors of the pelvis, abdomen, heart, and breast. Ultrasound also may be used to distinguish between benign and malignant breast tumors.

MAGNETIC RESONANCE IMAGING. MRI is valuable in locating and staging malignant tumors in the central nervous system, spine, head, breast, and musculoskeletal system.

ENDOSCOPIC PROCEDURES. An endoscopic examination allows the direct visualization of a body cavity or opening. Endoscopy enables the surgeon to biopsy tissue. It is used to detect lesions of the throat, esophagus, stomach, colon, and lungs.

LABORATORY TESTS. For normal values for the following laboratory tests, see Appendix B. Blood, serum, and urine tests are important in establishing baseline values and general health status. An elevated WBC count is expected if the patient has evidence of infection; however, an increase in WBCs without infection raises suspicion of leukemia. Fifty percent of patients with liver cancer have increased levels of bilirubin, alkaline phosphatase, and glutamic-oxaloacetic transaminase.

Bone marrow aspiration is done to learn the number, size, and shape of RBCs, WBCs, and platelets. It is a major tool for diagnosis of leukemia. (See Chapter 27 for a description of this test and related nursing care.) Tumor markers, also called biochemical markers, are proteins, antigens, genes, hormones, and enzymes produced and secreted by tumor cells. Tumor markers help confirm a diagnosis of cancer, detect cancer origin, monitor the effect of cancer therapy, and determine cancer remission. Some examples of tumor markers are shown in Table 11.3.

CYTOLOGICAL STUDY. Cytology is the study of the formation, structure, and function of cells. Cytological diagnosis of cancer is obtained mainly through smears of cells shed from a mucous membrane (e.g., cervical, anal, oral). Test results are based on the degree of cell abnormality. Slight cellular changes are considered normal, with a possible link to abnormal cells seen in infection. Significant cellular changes reflect a higher probability of precancerous or cancerous activity.

Staging and Grading

Tumor staging helps to describe the extent of cancer. It provides valuable information for the development of a treatment plan. The most common system used for staging is the tumor-node-metastasis (TNM) system. This staging system classifies solid tumors by size and degree of spread (Table 11.4). For example, a breast cancer staged as T3 N2

Table 11.3
Tumor Markers and Associated Cancers

Tumor Marker	Associated Cancer
Alpha-fetoprotein (AFP)	Hepatocellular cancer
Cancer antigen (CA) 15-3	Breast cancer (useful in monitoring patient response to therapy for metastatic breast cancer)
CA 125	Ovarian, cervical, liver, and pancreatic cancers
CA 19-9	Colorectal, pancreatic, and hepatobiliary cancers (used to aid diagnosis and evaluation)
Carcinoembryonic antigen (CEA)	Colon and rectal cancers
Prostatic acid phosphatase (PAP)	Prostate cancer
Prostate-specific antigen (PSA)	Prostate cancer

Table 11.4
Tumor-Node-Metastasis System for Cancer Staging

Primary Tumor (T)	
TX	Primary tumor cannot be evaluated
T0	No evidence of primary tumor
Tis	Carcinoma in situ (early cancer that has not spread to neighboring tissue)
T1, T2, T3, T4	Size and/or extent of the primary tumor
Regional Lymph Nodes (N)	
NX	Regional lymph nodes cannot be evaluated
N0	No regional lymph node involvement
N1, N2, N3	Involvement of regional lymph nodes (number and/or extent of spread)
Distant Metastasis (M)	
M0	No distant metastasis
M1	Distant metastasis

Source: Data from American College of Surgeons. (Accessed December 9, 2021.) Cancer staging system. https://www.facs.org/quality-programs/cancer/ajcc/cancer-staging

M0 is a large breast cancer that has spread to regional lymph nodes, with no distant metastasis.

The TNM ratings correspond with one of five stages. However, ratings may differ based on the type of cancer. In this classification system, stages range from stage 0 (tumor in situ, no invasion of other tissues) to stage IV (distant metastasis to other sites). In general, a lower stage number means the cancer is less advanced and offers a better outcome. A higher number means a more serious situation exists, but treatment is possible. A rating system has also been established to define the cell types of tumors. Tumors are classified according to the percentage of cells that are differentiated (mature). If the tissue of a neoplastic tumor closely resembles normal tissue, it is called *well differentiated*. A *poorly differentiated* tumor is a malignant neoplasm that contains some normal cells, but most of the cells are abnormal. The better defined or differentiated the tumor, the easier it is to treat. For more information on staging systems, visit www.cancerstaging.org.

Treatment for Cancer

There are many types of treatment for cancer, including surgery, radiation therapy, chemotherapy (discussed here), immunotherapy, hormone therapy, targeted therapy (discussed in Chapter 42), and stem cell transplants (discussed in Chapter 28)

SURGERY. Surgery can be curative when it is possible to remove the entire tumor. Skin cancers and well-defined tumors without metastasis can be removed without any additional intervention. For some tumors, as much of the tumor as possible is removed (debulking). Follow-up chemotherapy or radiation is used to treat the remaining tumor cells.

Colon polyps are often removed to prevent malignancies from developing, especially if the polyps are considered premalignant. An extreme example of prophylactic surgery is a woman who elects to have a mastectomy (surgical removal of the breast) because of a high incidence of breast cancer in her family or positive genetic testing.

Surgery also may be done for **palliation** (symptom control). Surgical removal of tissue to reduce the size of the tumor mass is helpful, especially if the tumor is compressing nerves or blocking the passage of body fluids. Goals of palliative surgery are to increase comfort and quality of life.

Reconstructive surgery can be done for cosmetic enhancement or for return of function of a body part. Facial reconstruction is important for a patient's self-image after removal of head or neck tumors. Women can elect to have breast reconstruction after mastectomy.

Patients with a limited understanding of cancer may fear that tissues will not heal postoperatively. Nurses should encourage patients to express their fears. Smokers should be encouraged to enroll in cessation programs, as smoking decreases healing. Provide information about wound care, including dressing changes and drainage tubes, to increase the patient's understanding and sense of control. Visual aids of the tumor site and surgical procedures are valuable teaching tools. Include family members or caretakers in teaching when possible.

Patients who are undernourished are poor surgical candidates. They require intervention such as enteral or parenteral nutrition before and after surgery. Patients with cancer also are at increased risk for postoperative deep venous thrombosis (DVT). Preoperative teaching includes importance of leg movement, early ambulation, antiembolism stockings, sequential compression devices (SCDs), and recognizing symptoms of DVT, such as calf redness, warmth, or pain.

RADIATION. Radiation may be used as a curative treatment if the cancer is localized. It can also be used in cancer control and palliation. Radiation destroys cancer cells by affecting cell structure and the cell environment. The decision to use radiation is commonly based on cancer site and size. Treatments use special equipment to send radiation to break up the cancer cells locally, causing little systemic effect; however, side effects can occur in the area being treated because of damage to normal cells. Radiation can be delivered in three ways: external radiation, internal radiation (brachytherapy), or systemic radiation.

Radiation can be used before surgery to decrease the size of a large tumor. This makes surgical intervention more effective and less dangerous. It can also be used after surgery as adjuvant treatment. Palliative radiation is used to reduce the size of a large cancerous lesion and consequently reduce pressure and pain. Radioisotopes can be inserted into or near cancerous tissue (brachytherapy) during or after surgery to help destroy cancerous cells without removing the organ. Less skin damage occurs with brachytherapy.

Nursing Care of the Patient Receiving Radiation Treatment. Symptoms of tissue reaction to radiation can be expected about 10 to 14 days after treatment starts. Symptoms can continue for up to 2 to 4 weeks after treatment ends. Typical reactions and appropriate nursing interventions depend on the part of the body receiving the radiation. For example, radiation to the abdominal area may cause gastrointestinal symptoms. Some patients experience changes in the way food tastes. Other common side effects and interventions include the following:

- *Fatigue:* Encourage the patient to nap often and prioritize activities. Reassure the patient that the feeling will go away after the treatments are completed. See Evidence-Based Practice.
- *Skin reactions:* These can vary from mild redness to moist **desquamation** (peeling skin) similar to a second-degree burn. Skin surfaces that are warm and moist, such as the groin, perineum, and axillae, are especially vulnerable. Prophylactic skin care includes keeping skin dry; keeping it free from irritants, such as powder, lotions, deodorants, and restrictive clothing; and protecting it from exposure to direct sunlight for up to a year after radiation treatments. Irradiated skin can be fragile during treatment. It is important to wash these areas gently with mild soap and water, rinse well, and pat dry. The skin may have markings or tattoos to delineate the treatment field. Take care not to wash off the markings.
- *Bone marrow depression:* Low blood cell counts occur with both radiation and chemotherapy because they can attack all rapidly dividing cells, not just cancer cells. Weekly blood cell counts are done to detect low levels of WBCs, RBCs, and platelets. Transfusions of whole blood, platelets, or other blood components may be needed. See Table 11.5 for medications that can be used to stimulate production of blood cells.

> **PRACTICE ANALYSIS TIP**
> **Linking NCLEX-PN® to Practice**
> The LPN/LVN will monitor and provide for client nutritional needs.

> **CUE RECOGNITION 11.1**
> You receive a call in the Oncology Clinic from a patient complaining of bleeding when brushing teeth. She received radiation and chemotherapy 7 days ago. What do you do?
> *Suggested answers appear at the end of the chapter.*

Safety Considerations. Radiation may be administered externally or internally. External radiation is given by a trained medical specialist in a designated area of a hospital or clinic. Patients receiving external radiation therapy do not emit radiation, so they do not require safety precautions before or after treatment.

Internal radiation is administered to patients admitted to a health-care facility. Safety guidelines must be followed when caring for a patient with internal radioactive materials implanted into tissue or body cavities or administered orally or intravenously, because the patient will be radioactive. Nursing responsibilities include knowledge about the following:

- Radiation source being used
- Method of administration
- Start of treatment
- Length of treatment
- Prescribed nursing precautions

Personnel involved with radiation therapy must follow three limitations to protect themselves: *time, distance,* and *shielding.* These factors depend on the type of radiation used. *Time* involves the time spent administering care. *Distance* involves the amount of space between the radioisotope and the nurse. *Shielding* involves the use of a barrier such as a lead apron.

You must work efficiently when caring for patients who are receiving radioisotopes that are releasing gamma rays. Exposure to radiation is proportionate to the time spent and the distance from the radiation source. For example, you will receive less exposure standing at the foot of the bed of a patient with radioisotopes inserted into the head than at the head of the bed (Fig. 11.9). Principles of time and distance are used to protect the nurse, visitors, and other personnel.

It is important to teach the patient and family members the reason nursing focuses on providing only essential care. Speedy encounters and visitor restrictions are better accepted and less likely to promote feelings of isolation when patients and family understand the reasons.

Drainage from the site of a radioactive colloid injection is considered radioactive. The HCP must be informed immediately if it occurs. Dressings contaminated with radioactive seepage must be removed with long-handled forceps. Radioactive materials must never be touched with unprotected hands; shielding is required to prevent exposure to radiation. Contamination from radioisotope applicators or interstitial implants cannot occur when the capsule it is contained in is intact; contamination occurs when the capsule is broken.

> **BE SAFE!**
> **BE VIGILANT!** Remember to use the principles of time, distance, and shielding to protect yourself from radiation exposure.

• WORD • BUILDING •

desquamation: de—down, from + squamation—epidermis

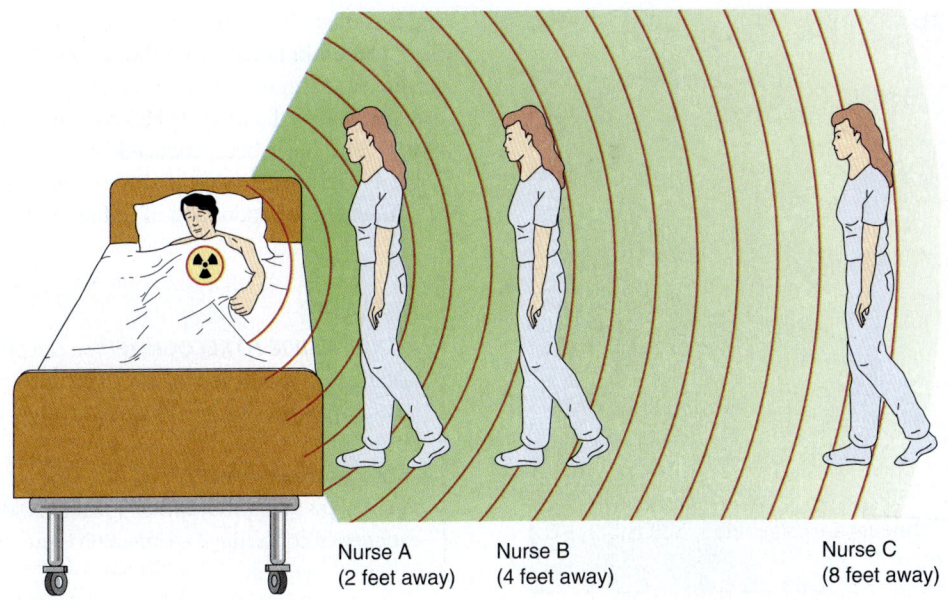

FIGURE 11.9 Radiation distancing. Nurse B receives less radiation than Nurse A, and Nurse C receives less radiation than Nurse B.

CHEMOTHERAPY. **Chemotherapy** is chemical therapy that uses **cytotoxic** medications to treat cancer. Cytotoxic medications can be used for cure, control, or palliation of cancerous tumors. They are classified according to how they affect cell activity. Some chemotherapy medications act on the cell DNA, some inhibit cell division or decrease hormone levels, and some prevent the growth and spread of cancer by blocking the growth of blood vessels. New chemotherapy medications are being developed all of the time. When working with a patient receiving chemotherapy, the licensed practical nurse/licensed vocational nurse (LPN/LVN) should refer to a drug manual or online resource for information on the patient's specific medications.

The effects of chemotherapy are systemic unless used topically for skin lesions. Chemotherapy is used preoperatively to shrink tumors and postoperatively to treat residual tumors. Tumor type and genetics influence the effectiveness of chemotherapy. Age is also a consideration; treatment should be based on physiological age rather than chronological age, taking into account the patient's comorbidities and functional status. Just because a patient might be 70 years old does not mean their body is the same as that of other 70-year-old patients.

Combination Chemotherapy. In this type of therapy, two or more antineoplastic agents are used together. This can expose a larger number of cells at different points in the cell cycle to chemotherapy. Combining medications also allows for smaller doses of each medication, which decreases the side effects of individual medications and the possibility of the tumor becoming resistant to the therapy.

For medications to be combined for chemotherapy, several criteria must be met. Each drug must be effective when used alone to treat the cancer. Each must have a different toxicity that would limit its use. For example, if three medications that are all toxic to the heart (cardiotoxic) are given, the patient is more likely to develop cardiotoxicity. Patients are still monitored for toxic effects from the treatment as well as for improvement in their status.

Routes of Administration. Chemotherapy can be given by oral, intramuscular, IV, or topical route. The dosage is determined by the size of the patient and the toxicities of the drug. IV administration of cytotoxic therapies requires specialized training and knowledge of antineoplastic medications.

Vesicant medications are given only by the IV route into a large vein. These medications cause blistering of tissue that eventually leads to necrosis if they infiltrate (leak out of the blood vessel and into soft tissue; Fig. 11.10). Skin grafts may be needed if tissue damage is extensive.

> **BE SAFE!**
> **AVOID FAILURE TO COMMUNICATE! ACT FAST!** If you recognize an extravasation by an IV vesicant, it is necessary to follow protocol. STOP infusion. Leave catheter in place. Notify RN and HCP. You can prevent serious infusion complications.

Oral Chemotherapy Agents. The number of oral chemotherapy agents has increased in the past several years. Be aware that oral agents can be just as potent as chemotherapy administered via the IV route. To keep family members safe, patients sharing a restroom with others should be instructed

• **WORD** • **BUILDING** •
chemotherapy: chemo—chemistry + therapy—treatment
cytotoxic: cyto—cell + toxic—poison
vesicant: vesicate—to blister

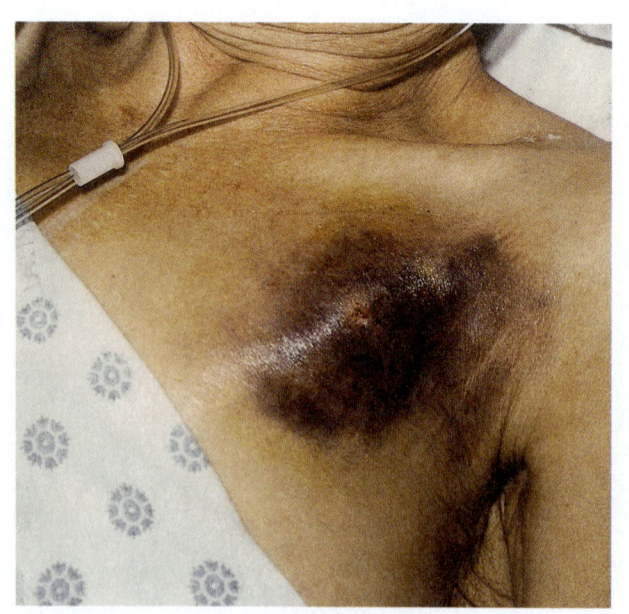

FIGURE 11.10 Necrosis of skin tissue resulting from administration of a vesicant chemotherapy drug.

to put the toilet lid down prior to flushing and to always flush twice. Nursing considerations for oral chemotherapy include safe storage and handling as well as monitoring for side effects. Some oral agents must be given concurrently with another treatment, such as radiation, so timing is important.

> **BE SAFE!**
> **BE VIGILANT!** Oral chemotherapy pills should not be stored with other oral medications. They should never be crushed or broken. The nurse giving the pills should wear chemotherapy safety gloves.

Side Effects. Toxicities in patients receiving chemotherapy vary with the medications given; however, some general side effects are common to chemotherapeutic medications because they affect all rapidly growing cells. Fast-growing epithelial cells, such as those of the hair, blood, skin, and GI tract, are usually the most affected by both chemotherapy and radiation. Typical side effects and interventions are listed next according to the body system they affect.

Hematologic System. Chemotherapy is toxic to bone marrow, which is where blood cells are produced. The number of blood cells (especially WBCs) drops after approximately 7 to 14 days of chemotherapy, depending on the medications. This period when the cell counts are lowest is called the **nadir**. This is when patients are most at risk for complications. Patients may develop low WBC counts (**leukopenia**), increasing their susceptibility to infection and sepsis. Sometimes this is called **neutropenia** because neutrophils are the most plentiful white cells. A reduction in platelets (**thrombocytopenia**) increases the risk of bruising and bleeding. It can require platelet transfusions. Increased risk of **anemia** occurs with the reduction of RBCs and may require blood transfusions. Special glycoproteins called colony stimulating factors can be given to patients whose white blood cells have been reduced by the chemotherapy (see Table 11.5). Erythropoietin-stimulating agents may be given to stimulate the production of red blood cells.

> **BE SAFE!**
> **AVOID FAILURE TO RECOGNIZE!** You can prevent infection leading to sepsis in your at-risk patients by monitoring laboratory values such as WBC count for elevations and observing for temperature 100.4 F° (38.0 C°) or above, chills, dysuria, or urinary frequency. Instruct patient to report signs and symptoms of infection. Older adults may experience confusion if an infection is present.

Gastrointestinal System. Because the lining of the GI tract is made up of rapidly dividing cells, it is susceptible to the toxicity of chemotherapy medications. **Stomatitis** (inflammation of the mouth) and **mucositis** (inflammation of mucous membranes, especially of the mouth and throat) can be painful for the patient and affect their ability to take in nutrients. Oral cryotherapy (ice water or ice chips swished around the mouth for 30 minutes) can be used preventively prior to the infusion of some chemotherapy medications. Urge the patient to avoid irritants such as smoking, alcohol, acidic food or drinks, extremely hot or cold foods and drinks, and commercial mouthwash. Advise the patient to perform mouth care before meals and every 3 to 4 hours. Rinsing with saline or with a solution of one-half teaspoon of salt and one teaspoon of baking soda in a quart of water is recommended. Mouthwashes containing lidocaine hydrochloride 2% viscous have an anesthetic effect on the mouth and throat and may be prescribed by the HCP.

Xerostomia (dry mouth) can also occur. Saliva substitute is available over the counter. It is especially helpful at night when patients describe a choking sensation from extreme dryness. Nausea, vomiting, and anorexia are common and bothersome problems. Encourage the patient to take prescribed medication for nausea and vomiting. **Anorexia** can be eased by providing small amounts of high-carbohydrate, high-protein foods and avoiding foods high in fiber. See "Treating Problems Related to Nutrition" for more interventions.

• **WORD** • **BUILDING** •
leukopenia: leuko—white cells + penia—lack
neutropenia: neutron—neutrophils + penia—lack
thrombocytopenia: thrombo—clot + cyte—cell + penia—lack
anemia: an—not + emia—blood
stomatitis: stoma—mouth + itis—inflammation
mucositis: muco—mucous (membrane) + itis—inflammation
xerostomia: xero—dry + stoma—mouth
anorexia: an—not + orexis—appetite

Table 11.5
Colony-Stimulating Factors

Medication Class/Action

Granulocyte–Colony-Stimulating Factor (G-CSF)
Stimulates proliferation of stem cells into granulocytes (neutrophils).

Examples	*Nursing Implications*
filgrastim (Neupogen)	Monitor complete blood count (CBC).
filgrastim-aafi (Nivestym)	Teach subcutaneous administration if drug will be given at home.
filgrastim-sndz (Zarxio)	
pegfilgrastim (Neulasta)	
pegfilgrastim-apgf (Nyvepria)	
pegfilgrastim-bmez (Ziextenzo)	
pegfilgrastim-jmdb (Fulphila)	
pegfilgrastim-cbqv (Udenyca)	

Erythropoietin
Stimulates proliferation of stem cells into red blood cells.

Examples	*Nursing Implications*
epoetin alfa (Epogen, Procrit)	Black-box warning for heart disease risk. Monitor blood pressure and hematocrit.
epoetin alfa-epbx (Retacrit)	Teach subcutaneous administration if drug will be given at home.
darbepoetin alfa (Aranesp)	Darbepoetin alfa (Aranesp) is long acting.

Note: Because these drugs are proteins, they all require refrigeration, and you cannot shake them. Many thousands of dollars have been lost because a drug was not returned to the refrigerator when it was not used. Be sure to check package instructions.

Hair. **Alopecia,** or hair loss, is common with many, but not all, chemotherapeutic medications (Fig. 11.11). This is a temporary condition. Growth of new hair usually starts when the chemotherapeutic medication is stopped. Alopecia involves the entire body, including eyebrows, eyelashes, and axillary and pubic hair. Hair that regrows may be a different color or texture than original hair. It is not uncommon for individuals who had straight hair to regrow curly hair.

> **NURSING TIP**
> Recognize your patient's self-image concerns. Suggest or support wig shopping before loss of hair so the patient may match their original hair.

Reproductive System. The effects of chemotherapy or radiation can cause temporary or permanent changes in the reproductive system. Chemotherapy can damage sperm and ova. Issues concerning fertility should be discussed with the patient before treatment. Measures such as freezing ova and using a sperm bank can provide options for patients and their partner. Patients should also talk to their HCPs before engaging in intercourse during chemotherapy and use protection against pregnancy.

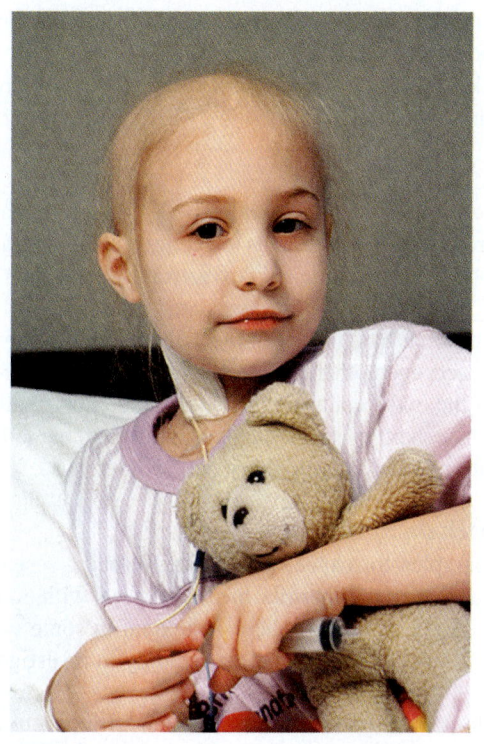

FIGURE 11.11 Chemotherapy-associated hair loss.

> **BE SAFE!**
> **AVOID FAILURE TO COMMUNICATE!** Some Web sites promote icing the scalp to cause vasoconstriction and reduce the amount of chemotherapy agent affecting hair loss. Encourage the patient to ask their HCP if scalp cooling is appropriate with the type of cancer they have before trying this therapy.

Neurologic System. Medications may affect the neurologic system. An adverse reaction to vincristine (Oncovin) is neurotoxicity. This can result in tingling or numbness in the extremities. In severe cases, it can cause foot drop from muscle weakness.

Other Systems. Less common complications include renal toxicities, such as pain and burning on urination, and hematuria. Doxorubicin (Adriamycin) has been associated with permanent heart damage. Bleomycin (Blenoxane) can cause pulmonary fibrosis. Severe toxic side effects can be controlled by carefully limiting the amount of each medication given and constantly monitoring the patient for complications.

> **LEARNING TIP**
> When assessing patients with possible side effects of chemotherapy and radiation, use the mnemonic BITES:
> **B**—Bleeding suggests low platelet count.
> **I**—Infection suggests low WBC count and a risk for infection.
> **T**—Tiredness suggests anemia.
> **E**—Emesis places the patient at risk for altered nutrition and fluid and electrolyte imbalance.
> **S**—Skin changes may be evidence of radiation reaction or skin breakdown.

Cytoprotective Agents. Cytoprotective agents protect healthy cells from some side effects of certain chemotherapeutic medications. For example, dexrazoxane (Zinecard) helps prevent cardiac damage associated with doxorubicin. Amifostine (Ethyol) helps protect the kidneys from platinum-based chemotherapy. It also protects normal cells in parts of the body against damage from radiation treatments. Mesna (Mesnex) protects the bladder against chemotherapy medications such as cyclophosphamide (Cytoxan).

Research on New Cancer Therapies

New therapies for cancer are constantly being researched. For example, hyperthermia has been used with radiation and chemotherapy. It has been beneficial in some types of cancer. However, it is typically used only in investigational studies.

Biological response modifiers (such as interferons) are medications used to stimulate the immune system. These medications are used commonly for specific types of cancer. They have produced some beneficial results. They are also being used in many investigational studies. Visit www.cancer.gov for information on current clinical trials.

NURSING PROCESS FOR THE PATIENT WITH CANCER

Data Collection

Thorough assessment of the patient with cancer will help the health-care team build a plan of care relevant to the patient's needs.

The nurse should monitor laboratory studies. Potential for bleeding exists when the platelet count is 50,000/mm^3 or less; risk for spontaneous bleeding occurs when the count is less than 20,000/mm^3. Monitor the WBC count for risk of infection and the RBC count for anemia.

Monitor the patient's weight. Note reports of nausea, changes in taste, vomiting, and diarrhea related to either the disease or treatment. Monitor the oral mucosa for lesions or inflammation. Also watch for signs of dehydration. The National Cancer Institute recommends that all cancer patients be screened for the need for nutritional support.

Psychosocial issues related to cancer are as varied as the persons afflicted with the disease. Help the patient explore perceptions about quality of life. Culture and age affect cancer perceptions. Determine the patient's ability to cope. Discuss coping strategies that have been effective in the past. Determine what information the patient has received and understands about their disease and prognosis.

Ask about the roles of the patient and caregiver in the family. Be aware of whether the caregiver can be at home or must work outside the home while also caring for the patient. Isolation can be either self-imposed or imposed by friends and family as issues surrounding terminal illness are confronted. It can be very distressing to see a loved one decline from cancer; often people say they are "afraid of saying or doing the wrong thing," so they "just stay away." Listen for cues from patients expressing self-blame, anger, or depression. It is important to recognize signs of depression and suicidal tendencies.

Ask about fatigue and anxiety in a patient being treated for cancer. A decline in sexual desire is not uncommon during cancer treatment. Determine whether the patient is feeling anxiety about sexual intercourse, including fears concerning contracting cancer from the patient and fears that sexual intercourse will make the cancer worse.

Allow the patient to share feelings about any actual or perceived change in appearance due to surgery, radiation, or chemotherapy.

Nursing Diagnoses, Planning, and Implementation

See the "Nursing Care Plan for the Patient With Cancer" for top nursing care priorities. Additional nursing diagnoses are presented next. Remember to collect supporting data before assuming a nursing diagnosis applies to that patient.

Nursing Care Plan for the Patient With Cancer

Nursing Diagnosis: Ineffective Coping related to the diagnosis and treatment of cancer as evidenced by behaviors such as denial, isolation, anxiety, and depression
Expected Outcomes: The patient will cope effectively as evidenced by identifying stressors related to illness and treatment; communicating needs, concerns, and fears; and use of appropriate resources to support coping.
Evaluation of Outcomes: Is the patient able to identify stressors and communicate concerns? Does the patient effectively draw on past coping mechanism? Does the patient have and appropriately use support systems?

Intervention	Rationale	Evaluation
Ask about effective coping mechanisms used in the past and currently available to the patient.	Coping mechanisms that worked in the past may be helpful again. The nurse can support appropriate choices.	Is patient able to identify and draw on past coping mechanisms?
Assist the patient to identify their meaning of quality of life.	Once identified, the nurse can assist patient to achieve quality-of-life goals.	Is patient able to identify the meaning of quality of life? Are there ways you can assist the patient to reach quality-of-life goals?
Ask about feelings of hopelessness and whether they have had thoughts of suicide.	A patient who feels hopeless may be at risk for suicide.	Is patient at risk? Are suicide precautions necessary?
Use active listening skills to encourage patient to express feelings and fears.	Patient must identify fears to be able to cope effectively with them.	Does patient identify fears and concerns?
Explore outlets that promote feelings of personal achievement.	Personal achievement promotes self-esteem.	Does patient have creative outlets that promote feelings of achievement? Can you assist in implementing these activities?
Consider the use of humor.	Humor can be both distracting and therapeutic.	Does patient use humor? Does it provide temporary distraction from concerns?

Nursing Diagnosis: Risk for Infection related to diminished immunity and bone marrow suppression as a result of chemotherapy or radiation
Expected Outcomes: The patient will be free and safe from infection as evidenced by being afebrile and stating self-care measures to protect from infection. Signs and symptoms of infection are identified and treated early.
Evaluation of Outcomes: Are signs and symptoms of infection absent? If present, are they reported quickly? Can the patient identify self-care measures for preventing infection?

Intervention	Rationale	Evaluation
Monitor body temperature every 4 hours.	Elevated body temperature is an early sign of infection.	Is body temperature within normal limits?
Monitor white blood cell (WBC) count daily.	For the neutropenic patient, the WBC count will not be elevated. Neutropenia is a risk factor for infection.	Is the WBC count 5,000 to 10,000/mm^3?
Monitor for signs of inflammation or drainage at potential infection sites, such as old aspiration sites, venipuncture sites, oral and rectal mucosae, perineal area, axillae, incisions, pierced earlobes, under breasts, and between toes.	Intact skin is the first line of defense against invading microorganisms.	Are there any sites that need special care to maintain skin integrity?

Continued

Nursing Care Plan for the Patient With Cancer—cont'd

Intervention	Rationale	Evaluation
Watch for signs of respiratory infection, such as sore throat, cough, shortness of breath, and sputum production.	*Hospital-acquired pneumonia has high morbidity and mortality rates.*	Are signs of respiratory infection present?
Monitor for signs of urinary tract infection (UTI) including burning, pain, urgency, and blood in urine.	*Genitourinary tract is the most common site for hospital-acquired infection.*	Are signs of UTI present?
Promote good hand washing technique before interaction with patient.	*Appropriate hand hygiene can reduce the transmission of antimicrobial organisms.*	Are you careful with your hand washing? Have you also instructed the patient, family, nursing assistants, and medical team about careful hand washing?
Limit visitors to only healthy adults.	*Viral infection in an immunosuppressed patient has a high mortality rate.*	Are patient and family aware of visiting restrictions and rationale? Is there a sign on the door reminding visitors?
Keep fresh flowers and potted plants out of the patient's room.	*Aspergillus is a fungus found in soil and water and can cause pneumonia.*	Is the room free from potential sources of infection?
Teach patient to ask health-care provider about avoiding unwashed fruits and vegetables (see "Nutrition Notes: Treating Problems Related to Nutrition").	*Unwashed fruits and vegetables can carry pathogens.*	Are patient and family aware of the risks of eating unwashed fruits and vegetables?
Teach administration of G-CSF (granulocyte–colony-stimulating factor) and GM-CSF (granulocyte macrophage–colony-stimulating factor) as ordered.	*These medications help the body produce more WBCs. Patient may need to administer it subcutaneously at home.*	Does patient or caregiver demonstrate correct administration? Is WBC count improving?

Evidence-Based Practice

Clinical Question
Does exercise help cancer-related fatigue?

Evidence
In a meta-analysis comparing exercise to non-exercise interventions for cancer-related fatigue, researchers found that exercise was effective at reducing cancer-related fatigue. There were no significant differences between types of cancer, and aerobic exercise had a more positive effect than a combination of aerobic and resistant exercises.

Implication for Nursing Practice
Encourage patients to participate in aerobic exercise such as walking, swimming, running, and cycling throughout their cancer treatment to reduce fatigue. Patients should check with their HCP before beginning an exercise program.

Reference: Kessels, E., Husson, O., & van der Feltz-Cornelis, C. M. (2018). The effect of exercise on cancer-related fatigue in cancer survivors: a systematic review and meta-analysis. *Neuropsychiatric disease and treatment, 14*, 479–494. https://doi.org/10.2147/NDT.S150464

Ineffective Protection related to thrombocytopenia associated with chemotherapy and radiation

EXPECTED OUTCOME: The patient will be free of bleeding as evidenced by stable blood counts and the absence of bruising, petechiae, or frank bleeding.

- Monitor platelet counts. *A platelet count of less than 50,000 indicates potential for bleeding.*
- Test all urine and stool for occult blood *to detect the presence of blood.*
- Observe for bruising, petechiae, bleeding gums, tarry stools, and black or coffee-ground appearing emesis. *These are signs of bleeding.*
- Avoid giving intramuscular, subcutaneous, or rectal medications. *Medications given via invasive routes can cause bleeding.*
- Apply pressure for at least 5 minutes to venipuncture or injection sites. *Pressure for a longer time is needed at sites of invasive procedures to stop bleeding.*
- Remind patient to avoid trauma to rectal tissue by avoiding rectal temperatures and enemas and using

soft toilet tissue. Teach importance of avoiding anal intercourse. *Trauma to rectal tissue can cause bleeding.*
- Reinforce to patient that they not take salicylates or NSAID medications *because they can interfere with platelet function and cause bleeding in GI tract.*
- Advise the patient to use an electric razor *to decrease risk for trauma and bleeding.*
- Remind patient to avoid forcefully blowing his or her nose or inserting objects into the nose *to reduce trauma to nasal mucosa to prevent spontaneous bleeding.*
- Reinforce teaching regarding the patient to monitoring for bleeding with intercourse *because of the risk of trauma to tissues.*
- Reinforce instructions for self-administration of oprelvekin (Neumega) as ordered, and observe patient's return demonstration. *Oprelvekin stimulates production of platelets.*
- Reinforce teaching about gentle mouth care, including not flossing, using a soft toothbrush, and wearing properly fitting dentures *to help prevent trauma and bleeding.*

Nutrition Notes

Treating Problems Related to Nutrition

Early Satiety and Anorexia
- Present meals in a calm, comfortable environment, offering assistance as necessary.
- Offer, every 2 hours, nutrient-dense foods that are high in protein and calories.
- Postpone liquids until after eating to prevent early satiety including liquid supplements.
- Encourage physical activity, which may stimulate appetite.
- Arrange for assistance in preparing meals when at home.

Changes in Taste and Smell
- Recommend oral hygiene before meals.
- Cook in glass containers in a microwave oven.
- Use plastic utensils for eating and paper for drinking (for metallic taste in mouth).
- Provide tart foods to stimulate saliva such as citrus, tomatoes, and plain yogurt.
- Serve food cold or at room temperature.
- Offer lemon drops, chewing gum, or mints.
- Provide eggs, fish, and poultry instead of red meats. Sweet sauces and marinades may improve the palatability of meats.
- Offer high-protein vegetarian meals if meats are not tolerated.

Local Oral Effects
- *Mucositis:* Offer soft, bland, moist foods; cream sauces, gravies, and dressings for lubrication; cold foods (such as ice chips) for soothing and numbing; and straws for liquids. Avoid hot items, salty or spicy foods, acidic juices, raw vegetables, sharp and crunchy foods. If an anesthetic mouthwash is prescribed, the mouth may be numb; caution the patient to chew carefully to avoid biting the lips, tongue, or cheeks.
- *Dry mouth:* Offer frequent sips of water or artificial saliva. Hard candy, chewing gum, popsicles, or ice chips may stimulate saliva production. Moisten food with sauce, gravy, or salad dressing. Perform oral hygiene after meals. Provide lip balm.
- *Dysphagia:* Have a speech pathologist, in consultation with the dietitian, evaluate the patient to determine the appropriate position for eating and the appropriate diet order. Liquids may be modified in viscosity to enable the patient to safely swallow and reduce risk for aspiration.

Nausea and Vomiting
- Administer antiemetics on a regular prophylactic schedule.
- Rinse mouth before and after eating. Offer lemon or peppermint hard candies.
- Provide small frequent meals every 2 to 3 hours.
- Provide foods that are bland and avoid spicy and greasy foods.
- Offer liquids between, instead of with, meals to reduce stomach volume. Offer low-fat meals to improve stomach emptying.
- Remove covers from food containers away from the bedside if strong odors disturb the patient's appetite.
- Instruct the patient to chew thoroughly, eat slowly, and rest afterward, sitting upright or reclining with the head raised for 1 hour after eating.
- Offer meals when patient feels better.
- Avoid serving favorite foods when the patient is nauseous to avoid an association between these foods and vomiting.

Diarrhea
- Suggest a low-fiber diet; per patient's tolerance. Provide fluids at room temperature. Avoid sugar alcohols in sugar-free items, which may cause diarrhea.
- Offer lactose-free milk or milk alternatives.
- Consult a dietitian about pre- and probiotic foods to repopulate the intestine.

Altered Immune Response
- Observe strict procedures for food safety and sanitation to avoid bacterial exposure in foods
- Keep foods within safe temperatures (cold: under 40°F, hot: over 140°F).
- Do not eat foods outside their expiration dates.
- Avoid deli meats, undercooked and raw meat, fish, poultry, or eggs. Cook all meats, fish, and poultry to well done.
- Avoid unpasteurized soft cheeses and beverages.
- Provide individually packaged foods, avoiding leftovers.
- Avoid salad bars and buffets when eating out.
- Wash fruits and vegetables before eating.

Source: National Cancer Institute. (2020). Nutrition in cancer care (PDQ)—Health professional version. www.cancer.gov/about-cancer/treatment/side-effects/appetite-loss/nutrition-hp-pdq

Disturbed Body Image related to cancer and its treatment (e.g., surgical procedures such as mastectomy, ostomy, or loss of hair from chemotherapy)

EXPECTED OUTCOME: The patient to accept changes in body image as evidenced by willingness to participate in care and adjust to changes in lifestyle.

- Allow the patient to discuss feelings of anger or depression and acknowledge that these feelings are normal when adjusting to body changes. *A patient may be better able to cope with body changes if he or she can talk about feelings and understand that they are normal and expected.*
- Encourage the patient to select a wig before hair loss *so the patient can find one resembling his or her own hair color and style.*
- Provide education and urge the patient to care for the ostomy site or surgical wound when ready *to promote independence.*
- Provide information about resources such as Reach to Recovery and Look Good Feel Better support groups. *Support groups provide a forum for patients to share their experiences with others undergoing similar changes.*
- Provide information about community assistance and financial aid for programs or services. *Social workers can help with community resources that can provide equipment or supplies for the patient.*

Additional nursing diagnoses that might be appropriate include *Self-Care Deficit* related to weakness and fatigue, *Ineffective Sexuality Pattern* related to change in body functions, Imbalanced Nutrition: Less Than Body Requires, Social Isolation and *Grieving* related to diagnosis and potential disease outcome. Grieving and end-of-life care are covered in depth in Chapter 17.

> **NURSING TIP**
> It is important to remember the patient caregiver is often a nonmedical person and may need to be assessed for caregiver stress.

Caregiver Role Strain related to needs of patient and anticipated outcomes

EXPECTED OUTCOME: The caregiver will be prepared to provide care effectively as evidenced by (1) identification of resources available to assist in providing care for the patient and (2) maintenance of the caregiver's physical and emotional health.

- Observe the caregiver's ability to provide care for the patient. *The nurse needs to know if the caregiver will be able to handle the care needs.*
- Observe the quality of the relationship between the patient and caregiver. *The quality of the relationship impacts the care delivered.*
- Watch for signs of depression in the caregiver and intervene to help with coping. *The caregiver can develop a weakened immune system secondary to stress and depression.*
- Actively listen to the caregiver's concerns. *Doing so can assist the nurse in determining the caregiver's ability to cope and can help in planning care.*
- Assist the caregiver to identify available supports. *Assistance can provide a break and decrease the risk of exhaustion and depression in the caregiver.*
- Consult the multidisciplinary team to provide the services needed at time of discharge. *Preparing the caregiver for discharge needs/care with the proper resources will help the caregiver feel empowered to deliver the care.*
- Arrange for respite for the caregiver or encourage the caregiver to utilize this service. *Respite care can provide a break for the caregiver.*
- Instruct the caregiver in the resources available in the community. *Support groups can help the caregiver by providing an outlet for sharing concerns and finding support.*
- Assist the caregiver with ways to decrease stress. *Encouraging caregivers to take time to care for themselves will leave them with the energy they need to continue providing care.*
- Teach appropriate caregiving skills as needed and have the caregiver demonstrate the skill in return to verify competency. *The caregiver may not be aware of how to bathe a patient or how to provide basic or advanced care.*

Evaluation

If the interventions have been effective, the patient will have no unusual bleeding or bruising. The patient and family will be knowledgeable about risk factors for bleeding and about signs of bleeding to report promptly. Caregivers will know how to provide care for the patient. They will make use of resources in the community to assist with patient care. Finally, the patient will adjust to changes in lifestyle and body image.

The patient will be able to openly discuss concerns regarding body changes and be able to maintain control of his or her body. The patient will know about community resources and support groups to assist with needs related to body image.

> **PRACTICE ANALYSIS TIP**
> **Linking NCLEX-PN® to Practice**
> The LPN/LVN will identify community resources for clients

> **CRITICAL THINKING & CRITICAL JUDGMENT**
> **Mrs. Morales** is admitted to your unit after a simple mastectomy for breast cancer. The tumor was staged as a T2, N0, M0. A bone scan was negative for metastasis. She is scheduled for four chemotherapy treatments, 3 weeks apart. The medications prescribed are high doses of doxorubicin (Adriamycin) and cyclophosphamide (Cytoxan). A central line (portacath) is inserted for chemotherapy.

Critical Thinking (The Why)
1. What does the staging of Mrs. Morales's tumor mean?
2. What major side effects of her medications should you look for?

Critical Judgement (The Do)
3. What special precautions should be taken knowing that Mrs. Morales is receiving a vesicant?
4. What nursing diagnoses are appropriate for Mrs. Morales?

Mr. Rodriguez presents to the outpatient oncology clinic for his third treatment for Hodgkin lymphoma. He is scheduled to receive doxorubicin (Adriamycin), bleomycin (Bleo 15k), and Vinblastine (Velban) through his portacath. He tells you he has no appetite, has not been eating, and has been very nauseated. He is only able to drink orange juice and sometimes likes his wife's spaghetti sauce. He has not taken his oral antiemetic prior to coming today as ordered because his throat hurts. He is exhausted. His mucous membranes are dry and cracked.

Critical Thinking (The Why)
1. Why are Mr. Rodriguez's mucous membranes dry and cracked?
2. What other data would be important to collect?
3. What orders do you anticipate from the HCP?

Critical Judgement (The Do)
4. What recommendations can you make to the HCP about Mr. Rodriguez's oral antiemetic?
5. What teaching can you provide Mr. Rodriguez to decrease his chemotherapy side effects and improve his nutrition? (Hint: see Nutrition Notes)
6. With whom can you collaborate to manage Mr. Rodriguez's symptoms and side effects?

Suggested answers are at the end of the chapter.

SURVIVORSHIP

Millions of people around the world are no longer dying from cancer. Many are either disease-free or continuing treatments to reduce the risk of recurrence or treat a chronic form of cancer. The need for medical and psychosocial interventions is ongoing as cancer survivors and their caregivers continue to deal with the emotional and physical effects of their disease and treatments. Continued monitoring of the patient's needs and creation of a survivorship plan are essential to maintaining a positive outcome. You can help your patients and families find local survivorship programs for needed assistance and counseling.

HOSPICE CARE OF THE PATIENT WITH CANCER

Hospice care is considered the model for quality compassionate care for patients and families facing a life-limiting illness. Hospice provides expert medical care, pain management, and emotional and spiritual support based on the patient and family's needs and wishes. Patients diagnosed with a terminal illness and a potential life expectancy of fewer than 6 months are eligible for hospice care. The hospice approach includes an interdisciplinary team working together to develop a plan of care that meets the patient's individual needs for management of pain and symptoms. Hospice care is offered as an inpatient or outpatient service. It may also be provided in nursing homes and assisted living facilities (see "Home Health Hints").

Inpatient services are used for symptom control and respite care for the family. Family and pets may be allowed to stay with the patient. Hospice care assists the family in crisis and continues 13 months and beyond if needed after the patient dies, with follow-up counseling, listening, nurturing, and referrals.

Outpatient care is given in the home with hospice staff educating family members in the care of the patient. Hospice staff also offers supportive care in pain management, psychosocial issues, bereavement, and symptom control as well as assistance during crisis. Hospice benefits are provided regardless of the ability to pay. They are covered by Medicare, Medicaid, and other insurances. In the home setting, a patient can maintain normal life patterns with familiar surroundings for as long as possible (Fig. 11.12). Refer to the National Hospice and Palliative Care Organization (NHPCO.org) and Chapter 17 for more information.

Home Health Hints

- The home health-care or hospice nurse helps manage cancer pain in the home. Oral, transdermal, or intravenous analgesics are preferred. For moderate to severe pain, doses should be given around the clock with as-needed doses for breakthrough pain. The nurse is in contact with the interdisciplinary team to update plan of care as necessary.
- The nurse should anticipate constipation from opioid administration and treat prophylactically.
- Some patients are fearful of taking prescribed pain medications. Explain the importance of taking the medications as ordered. Explain that it is easier to maintain pain relief than to reverse severe pain.
- Home health-care nurses are in key positions for making timely referrals for hospice care. Eligible patients are those who have a life expectancy of 6 months or less and who have a desire for supportive palliative care rather than curative treatments.
- Teach patients and caregivers to dispose of used transdermal patches immediately by folding the sticky sides of each patch together and taking back to the pharmacy or flushing down the toilet. Do not throw in the trash.

ONCOLOGICAL EMERGENCIES

Superior Vena Cava Syndrome
Superior vena cava syndrome (SVCS) occurs in patients with lung cancer or cancers of the mediastinum when the tumor or enlarged lymph nodes block circulation in the superior vena cava. This results in edema of the head, neck, and arms. Symptoms include shortness of breath, cough, chest pain, facial redness, and swollen neck veins. Radiation therapy can be used to shrink the tumor and allow circulation to resume naturally. Nursing interventions for the patient with SVCS include removing rings and restrictive clothing, avoiding taking blood pressures and venipunctures in the arms, and elevating the head of the bed to decrease feelings of dyspnea.

Spinal Cord Compression
Spinal cord compression occurs when a malignant growth presses on the spinal cord. This is a painful problem and requires pain management while radiation is given to relieve the symptoms. Patients may develop some motor loss when this occurs. A myelogram or bone scan may be used for diagnosis. Nursing care includes providing a safe environment, assisting with activity, and watching for changes in neurologic status as well as changes in the location or intensity of pain. Patients at risk include those with cancers that spread to the bone and spinal cord, such as lung, breast, and prostate cancer.

Hypercalcemia
In hypercalcemia, the serum calcium level exceeds 11 mg/dL. Hypercalcemia can result from the release of calcium into the blood from bone deterioration or from ectopic secretion of parathyroid hormone by a tumor. It is common in patients with bone metastasis, especially metastasis from breast cancer. It can be treated with IV medication and hydration to lower the calcium level. Nursing care includes maintaining safety and monitoring intake and output, pain control, and changes in pulse rate and rhythm.

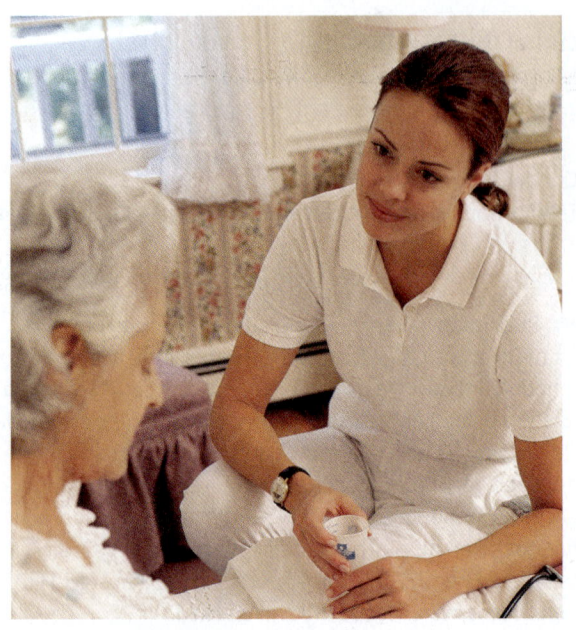

FIGURE 11.12 Hospice nurse and patient.

> **CUE RECOGNITION 11.2**
> You are caring for a patient who has lung cancer. You enter the room and the patient is suddenly short of breath and coughing. He has bulging neck veins. What do you do?
> *Suggested answers are at the end of the chapter.*

Key Points

- Human cells have a plasma membrane, cytoplasm (cytosol, organelles), and a nucleus. Organelles are specific in structure and function. Variations in the relative amounts of organelles and cell features allow great diversity in cells and, therefore, in tissues.
- Cancer refers to a group of cells that grows out of control and eventually takes over the function of the affected organ. Cancer cells are poorly constructed, disorganized, and fast growing. Often the tumor invades surrounding tissue, spreads throughout the body, and threatens life unless treated.
- Risk factors for developing cancer include exposure to oncoviruses, radiation, chemicals, and irritants. Other risk factors are a person's genetics, hormone levels, diet, physical activity level, and immune factors.
- Chemotherapy agents vary in their mechanisms of action.
- Cytoprotective agents protect healthy cells from some side effects of certain chemotherapeutic drugs.
- Data collection for cancer patients includes monitoring laboratory studies for adequate platelet count, monitoring WBC count for signs of infection, and monitoring red blood cell count for anemia. In addition, monitor the patient's weight and any complaints of nausea, changes in taste, vomiting, and diarrhea. Monitor for mouth lesions or inflammation. Also watch for signs of dehydration.
- Ask about the patient's psychosocial issues, including perceptions about quality of life and the individual's ability to cope, including which coping strategies have been effective in the past. Determine what information the patient has received and understands about the disease and prognosis.
- The plan of care for patients with cancer who are receiving chemotherapy and/or radiation therapy will focus on the nursing diagnoses of ineffective coping, acute or chronic pain, risk for infection, and ineffective protection due to low platelet count.

- Hospice care is considered the model for quality compassionate care for patients and families facing a life-limiting illness. Hospice provides expert medical care, pain management, and emotional and spiritual support based on the patient and family's needs and wishes.

- Oncological emergencies include superior vena cava syndrome due to the pressure of a growing tumor on the vena cava, spinal cord compression due to the pressure of a growing tumor on the spinal cord, and hypercalcemia due to bone deterioration or a parathyroid tumor. The nurse must take quick and decisive action in each of these situations.

SUGGESTED ANSWERS TO CHAPTER EXERCISES

Cue Recognition
11.1: Obtain platelet count and monitor for other signs of bleeding.
11.2: Remove restrictive clothing and elevate head of bed, provide oxygen, and prepare for tracheostomy if necessary.

Critical Thinking & Clinical Judgment
Mrs. Morales
1. Mrs. Morales's tumor is beginning to invade surrounding tissue. There is no lymph node involvement and no metastasis.
2. Doxorubicin (Adriamycin) is commonly associated with red urine. It also poses a risk for cardiac toxicity. Cyclophosphamide (Cytoxan) can cause blood in the urine and a risk for hemorrhagic cystitis. Therefore, the patient should take plenty of fluids and void often (every 2 hours). Both medications can cause nausea, vomiting, and alopecia. Both are vesicants.
3. Because the medications are vesicants, it is important to inject them into a large vein. It is also important to make sure that the catheter does not become dislodged during the infusion and no infiltration is present.
4. Many diagnoses are appropriate, including *Acute Pain* related to surgical incision, *Disturbed Body Image* related to alopecia and loss of a breast, *Imbalanced Nutrition: Less Than Body Requirements* related to nausea and vomiting, *Risk for Injury* related to medication side effects, and *Deficient Knowledge* about cancer treatment and management of side effects. A thorough nursing assessment is needed to determine actual diagnoses.

Mr. Rodriguez
1. Mr. Rodriguez is exhibiting signs of dehydration. He also may have an infection.
2. Check for further signs and symptoms of dehydration as well as look in Mr. Rodriguez's mouth and take his temperature.
3. Anticipate HCP orders for possible dehydration and mucositis. The HCP may order a complete blood count to rule out infection, a chemistry panel to rule out electrolyte imbalance, and IV fluids for rehydration. The HCP may order a prescription mouthwash for oropharynx lesions.
4. Ask the HCP for an alternative route, instead of by mouth, for the antiemetic.
5. Teach Mr. Rodriguez the signs and symptoms of mucositis and to use anesthetic mouthwash. Offer bland, moist foods, small frequent meals. Avoid acidic juices or spicy foods. Rinse mouth before or after eating.
6. RN, caregiver, dietitian, pharmacist

Additional Resources

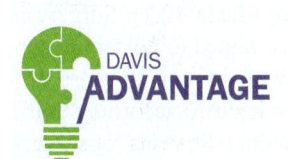

Go to Davis Advantage to complete your learning: strengthen understanding, apply your knowledge, and prepare for the Next Gen NCLEX®.

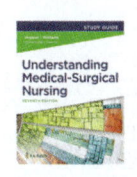

A Study Guide is also available.

CHAPTER 12
Nursing Care of Patients Having Surgery

John H. Nagelschmidt

KEY TERMS

adjunct (AD-junkt)
anesthesia (AN-es-THEE-zee-uh)
anesthesiologist (an-es-THEE-zee-ol-la-just)
aseptic (ay-SEP-tik)
atelectasis (AT-e-LEK-tah-sis)
débridement (da-breed-MAHNT)
dehiscence (dee-HIS-ents)
evisceration (ee-VIS-sir-ay-shun)
hematoma (HEE-muh-TOH-mah)
hypothermia (HY-poh-THUR-mee-ah)
induction (in-DUK-shun)
intraoperative (IN-trah-OP-pruh-tiv)
perioperative (PER-ee-OP-pruh-tiv)
postoperative (post-OP-pruh-tiv)
prehabilitation (pre-hah-BILL-ah-TAY-shun)
preoperative (pre-OP-pruh-tiv)
purulent (PURE-u-lent)
sanguineous (san-GWIN-ee-us)
serosanguineous (SEER-oh-san-GWIN-ee-us)
serous (SEER-us)
surgeon (SURJ-un)
surgery (SURJ-a-ree)

CHAPTER CONCEPTS

Caring
Comfort
Professionalism
Safety
Stress and coping
Teaching and learning
Tissue integrity

LEARNING OUTCOMES

1. Describe factors that influence surgical outcomes and reduce surgical risk factors.
2. Identify the role of the licensed practical nurse/licensed vocational nurse (LPN/LVN) in each perioperative phase.
3. Explain the role of the LPN/LVN in obtaining informed patient consent.
4. Assist in developing a teaching plan to enhance learning for the older preoperative patient.
5. Identify nursing interventions used for common postoperative patient needs.
6. Describe how to evaluate effectiveness of nursing interventions.
7. List signs and symptoms of common postoperative complications.
8. List the criteria for ambulatory discharge.
9. Describe the role of the home health-care nurse in caring for postoperative patients.

SURGERY

Surgery is the use of instruments during an operation to treat injuries, diseases, and deformities. Surgical procedures are named according to (1) the involved body organ, part, or location and (2) the suffix that describes what is done during the procedure (Table 12.1). Surgery is performed by **surgeons** and other physicians trained to do certain surgical procedures. Advanced practice nurses with training may also perform minor surgical procedures. Surgery is scheduled according to the urgency required for a successful patient outcome. Reasons for surgery appear in Table 12.2.

TYPES AND PHASES OF SURGERY

Laser, scope, and robotic technologies reduce the invasiveness of surgical procedures. Minimally invasive surgery is less damaging to tissues than traditional open incision surgery. This allows a faster and less painful recovery. Laser surgery uses a laser instead of a scalpel to cut tissue. It is often used for eye surgery. Minimally invasive surgery (called keyhole surgery) uses an endoscope for laparoscopic surgery (abdominal and pelvic cavity) and thoracoscopic surgery (chest and thoracic cavity). The endoscope is a flexible tube with an attached

Table 12.1
Surgical Procedure Suffixes

Suffix	Meaning	Word-Building Examples
-ectomy	Removal by cutting	crani (skull) + ectomy + craniectomy appen (appendix) + ectomy + appendectomy
-orrhaphy	Suture of or repair	colo (colon) + orrhaphy + colorrhaphy herni (hernia) + orrhaphy + herniorrhaphy
-oscopy	Looking into	colon (intestine) + oscopy + colonoscopy gastr (stomach) + oscopy + gastroscopy
-ostomy	Formation of a permanent artificial opening	ureter + ostomy + ureterostomy colo (colon) + ostomy + colostomy
-otomy	Incision or cutting into	oust (bone) + otomy + osteotomy thoro (thorax) + otomy + thoracotomy
-plasty	Formation or repair	oto (ear) + plasty + otoplasty mamm (breast) + plasty + mammoplasty

Table 12.2
Surgery Urgency Level and Purpose

Type	Definition	Examples
Urgency Level		
Emergency	Immediate surgery needed to save life or limb without delay	Ruptured aortic aneurysm or appendix, traumatic limb amputation, loss of extremity pulse from emboli
Urgent	Surgery needed within 24–30 hours	Fracture repair, infected gallbladder
Elective	Planned/scheduled, with no time requirements	Joint replacement, hernia repair, skin lesion removal
Optional	Surgery requested by patient	Cosmetic surgery
Purposes of Surgery		
Aesthetic	Requested by patient for improvement	Blepharoplasty, breast augmentation
Diagnostic	To obtain tissue samples, make an incision, or use a scope to make a diagnosis	Biopsy
Exploratory	Confirmation or measurement of extent of condition	Exploratory laparotomy
Preventive	Removal of tissue before it causes a problem	Mole or polyp removal to prevent cancer
Curative	Removal of diseased or abnormal tissue	Inflamed appendix, tumor, benign cyst, hernia
Reconstructive	Correction of defects of body parts	Scar repair, total knee replacement, face lift, mammoplasty
Palliative	Alleviation of symptoms when disease cannot be cured	Debulking (removal of as much of tumor as possible) to relieve pain or pressure, colostomy for incurable bowel obstruction, insertion of gastrostomy tube to provide tube feedings for swallowing problem, rhizotomy (cuts nerve root to relieve pain)

light, camera, and suction. It is inserted through a small incision and projects an image on a screen for the surgeon to watch. Additional incisions are made for insertion of other necessary instruments. Robotic-assisted surgery uses a robot with several moving arms that the surgeon controls. As the surgeon moves the controls, two of the robotic arms (inside the patient's body) translate the surgeon's movements to cut, suction, or suture.

There are three phases in the surgical process: **preoperative, intraoperative,** and **postoperative. Perioperative** refers to all three phases. It includes the time before, during, and after surgery. Each perioperative surgical phase has a defined time frame. Specific events related to surgery occur in each phase (Table 12.3).

PREOPERATIVE PHASE

Your primary role as a licensed practical nurse/licensed vocational nurse (LPN/LVN) in the *preoperative* phase is to:

- Assist in data collection and contribute to the patient's plan of care.
- Reinforce teaching and instructions given to the patient and family by the surgeon and registered nurse (RN).
- Provide emotional and psychological support for patients and families.

Other health-care team members also assist in preparing the patient for surgery. The surgeon obtains a medical history, performs a physical examination, and orders diagnostic testing. RNs perform a preoperative assessment, provide explanations and instructions, and offer patients and families emotional and psychological support to ease anxiety. They also develop a plan of care and verify the patient's name, surgical site (along with the patient), allergies, and related information when the patient arrives in the surgical area.

Factors Influencing Surgical Outcomes

When preparing a patient for surgery, the focus is to identify and implement actions that reduce surgical risk factors. **Prehabilitation** is planned preoperative functional, physical, and lifestyle preparation to help the patient achieve the best possible surgical and recovery outcome (Durrand et al, 2019). Its focus may be on controlling anxiety, preventing deconditioning after surgery through exercise preoperatively, providing nutritional support and weight loss counseling, or avoiding smoking, alcohol, or recreational drug use.

AGE. Surgery can potentially promote quality of life for anyone. For healthy older patients, age alone does not create greater surgical risk. They may take longer to recover from anesthetic agents due to aging changes that slow drug metabolism and elimination time frames. Older adults may have decreased ability to compensate for the stress of surgery due to declining physiological reserve (extra capacity of a body system or organ to carry out its function under stress). Perioperative nursing interventions focus on reducing complications.

CHRONIC DISEASE. Chronic diseases can increase the patient's surgical risk. A medical clearance for surgery may be needed from the patient's health-care provider (HCP).

EMOTIONAL RESPONSES. The word *surgery* causes a common anxious emotional reaction in patients and their families. *Anxiety* is a feeling of apprehension or uneasiness resulting from the uncertainties and risks associated with surgery. The thought of bleeding, disfigurement, mutilation, or a scar may cause great anxiety for some patients. *Fear* is a feeling of dread from a source known to the patient. Allow the patient to discuss concerns and assist them in coping with their feelings. If patient fears are extreme, such as a fear of dying during surgery, inform the surgeon. When fear is excessive, the surgeon might reschedule the surgery until the patient is better able to cope.

Surgical patients may experience various fears related to **anesthesia** (a reversible loss of sensation). These fears include feeling a loss of control, never waking up, and intraoperative awareness under general anesthesia (becoming conscious during surgery often without feeling pain). These concerns should be discussed with the patient by the anesthesia provider.

It is normal for patients to be concerned about pain. Analgesics are administered during and after surgery. Complementary techniques such as guided imagery, focused breathing, and music can also help reduce pain. A pain management plan should be discussed with the patient by the surgeon and anesthesia provider before surgery.

NUTRITION. Patients should be well nourished to heal and recover from surgery. Higher levels of protein (for tissue repair and healing), vitamin C (for collagen formation), and zinc (for tissue growth, skin integrity, and cell-mediated immunity) are required. Patients who are obese may have more delayed healing and wound *dehiscence* (opening of the incision). Patients with diabetes or who are emaciated may experience infection or delayed wound healing.

The Enhanced Recovery After Surgery (ERAS) Society guidelines (see https://erassociety.org) are an approach to surgical patient care that begins presurgery to ensure the best possible outcomes postsurgery. Screening for and correcting nutritional deficiencies before surgery lessens the impact of the metabolic stress of surgery so patients recover sooner.

Table 12.3
Perioperative Surgical Phases

Preoperative	Begins with decision for surgery and ends with transfer to the operating room
Intraoperative	Begins with transfer to operating room and ends with admission to perianesthesia care unit (PACU)
Postoperative	Begins with admission to PACU and continues until recovery complete

SMOKING AND ALCOHOL AND/OR DRUG ABUSE. Smoking thickens and increases the amount of lung secretions. It reduces the action of cilia that remove the secretions. Patients are encouraged to avoid smoking for at least 24 hours before surgery. If they have a chronic lung disorder, smoking avoidance should be for 4 weeks before surgery. Not smoking increases the action of the lungs' defense mechanisms, makes more hemoglobin available to carry oxygen, and improves wound healing.

Long-term alcohol and/or drug abuse may cause nutritional deficiencies and liver damage. This damage can create bleeding problems, fluid volume imbalances, and medication metabolism alterations. In addition, alcohol and drugs that are abused can interact with medications and should be avoided before surgery for safety.

Preadmission Surgical Patient Assessment

Surgical patients have a preoperative assessment. Nonemergent patients may have an assessment up to 30 days before their procedure. They have either an interview with the **anesthesiologist** or a preadmission telephone or face-to-face interview with an RN under the direction of the anesthesia provider. The interview process includes a health history, identification of risk factors, patient and family teaching, discharge planning, and necessary referrals to social workers, support groups, and educational programs. Self or family problems with anesthesia or malignant hyperthermia are identified (Box 12.1).

Preoperative diagnostic testing is based on the patient's age, medical history, data collection findings, and agency protocols (Table 12.4). A urine or serum pregnancy test is checked for female patients of childbearing age to prevent embryonic and fetal exposure to anesthetics and surgical risks. Health information and diagnostic testing results are reviewed by anesthesia providers. Abnormal test results are reported to the surgeon for intervention.

Federal law requires providers to ask patients before surgery if they have a signed advance directive (e.g., healthcare durable power of attorney or living will) for inclusion in their medical record (see Chapter 17). Providers must offer written information on advance directives to patients who do not have these documents.

Preoperative Teaching
Preoperative Routines

Preoperative teaching for common surgical routines includes:

- Date and time of admission and surgery
- Length of stay
- Clothing to wear and items to bring or leave at home (e.g., valuables and jewelry)
- Recovery after surgery
- Family information (e.g., waiting area and communication)
- Discharge (e.g., released to responsible adult after outpatient surgery; planned transfer to a rehabilitation facility)

Preoperative Instructions and Preparation

Special preps are explained to the patient. Bathing or skin preps to reduce skin bacterial counts before surgery to reduce surgical site infections may be ordered (World Health Organization, 2016). Nasal cultures for *Staphylococcus aureus* screening and treatment may be done. Enemas are prescribed before abdominal or intestinal surgery to empty the bowel. This reduces fecal contamination intraoperatively. It also prevents distension or straining postoperatively.

To prevent potential pulmonary aspiration, the American Society of Anesthesiologists (2017) practice guidelines recommend fasting time frames for solid and liquid intake before anesthesia (visit www.asahq.org/standards-and-guidelines). Medications to take the morning of surgery are explained. Patients may brush their teeth or rinse their mouth without swallowing. Surgery may be canceled if the patient has not stopped eating or drinking as specified.

Instructions for postoperative care are given before surgery. This allows the patient to be alert during teaching sessions and have time for practice of exercises and self-care. Patients are informed that active participation in postoperative care helps their recovery. Patients are shown how to report pain level using a pain rating scale (see Chapter 10). Pain relief methods are described that include oral, parenteral, or epidural analgesics or patient-controlled analgesia (PCA). Anticipated dressings, casts, tubes, and special equipment are also described. If needed, crutches are fitted and their use is demonstrated to the patient. If able, patients should perform a return demonstration so the nurse can evaluate it for correct performance.

Postoperative exercises that decrease complications are taught with return demonstrations performed. They include deep breathing and coughing, use of incentive spirometry, leg exercises, turning, and how to get out of bed.

Deep breathing expands and ventilates the lungs to prevent **atelectasis.** Atelectasis is the collapse of alveoli in one or more areas of the lung from hypoventilation or mucous obstruction. It reduces the lung's capacity to oxygenate the body. To deep breathe, instruct the patient to sit up, exhale fully, take in a deep breath through the nose, hold the breath and count to three, and then exhale completely through the mouth. This should be repeated hourly while awake, in sets of five, for 24 to 48 hours postoperatively.

Coughing moves secretions to prevent pneumonia. Give pain medication before asking the patient to cough. Reassure patient that coughing should not harm the incision. Reinforce teaching on coughing effectively if not contraindicated by the patient's condition (such as hernia repair, eye surgery, and head injury). Instruct the patient to sit up and lean forward; splint the incision using hands, a pillow, or a blanket if desired for comfort; inhale and exhale deeply three times through mouth; take in a deep breath and cough out

• WORD • BUILDING •

atelectasis: ateles—imperfect + ektasis—expansion

Box 12.1

Malignant Hyperthermia

Malignant hyperthermia is a potentially fatal hereditary muscular disease. It can be triggered by some types of general anesthetic agents and/or succinylcholine. A history of anesthetic problems in the patient or family members indicates the potential for this condition. Precautions can be taken. A muscle biopsy diagnoses this problem. Surgery can be safely done with planning. The anesthesia provider will carefully choose the anesthetic agents.

In malignant hyperthermia, metabolism in the muscles is increased. This produces a very high fever and muscle rigidity. In addition, tachycardia, tachypnea, hypertension, arrhythmias, hyperkalemia, metabolic and respiratory acidosis, and cyanosis occur. Malignant hyperthermia is life threatening. Immediate treatment is required to prevent death. Surgery is stopped. Anesthesia is discontinued immediately. Oxygen at 100% is given. The patient is cooled with ice and infusions of iced solutions. Dantrolene sodium (Dantrium) is a muscle relaxant that relieves the muscle spasms. It is the most effective medication for malignant hyperthermia. Dantrolene sodium is kept readily available in the operating room. It is given according to the treatment protocol of the Malignant Hyperthermia Association of the United States (www.mhaus.org).

Table 12.4 Preoperative Diagnostic Tests

Diagnostic Test	Purpose
Chest x-ray	Detect pulmonary and cardiac abnormalities
Electrocardiogram	Detect abnormalities in the conduction system of the heart
Oxygen saturation	Obtain baseline level and detect abnormality
Serum Tests	
Arterial blood gases	Obtain baseline levels and detect pH and oxygenation abnormalities
Bleeding time	Detect prolonged bleeding problem
Blood urea nitrogen	Detect kidney problem
Creatinine	Detect kidney problem
Complete blood cell count	Detect anemia, infection, clotting problem
Electrolytes	Detect potassium, sodium, chloride imbalances
Fasting blood glucose	Detect abnormalities, monitor diabetes control
Pregnancy	Detect early, unknown pregnancy
Partial thromboplastin time	Detect clotting problem
Prothrombin time/International normalized ratio	Detect clotting problem, monitor warfarin therapy
Type and cross-match	Identify blood type to match blood for possible transfusion
Urine Tests	
Pregnancy	Detect early, unknown pregnancy
Urinalysis	Detect abnormalities, infection

the breath forcefully with three short coughs using diaphragmatic muscles; then take in a quick deep breath through the mouth, cough deeply, and deep breathe. Several sets of coughing are performed hourly while the patient is awake, often in conjunction with deep breathing and incentive spirometry use.

Older adults perform deep breathing and coughing exercises better if you also perform the exercises with them. For example, say the following: "Let's take a deep breath in through the nose. Hold it and count to three. Slowly blow it out completely through the mouth. When you blow the air out, shape your lips like they are going to whistle."

Incentive spirometry may be ordered to prevent atelectasis (Chapter 29). It increases the volume of air inhaled, alveoli expansion, and venous return. Keep the spirometer within the patient's reach for self-use. Also, offer it to the patient as ordered to ensure that it is being used.

Leg exercises and foot circles should be done hourly while awake, if not contraindicated. Leg exercises improve circulation and prevent emboli formation. Instruct patients on these steps:

- For leg raises, lie down, raise leg, and flex the knee.
- Move the foot from plantar flexion to dorsiflexion, extend leg, and lower it to the bed.
- Do sets of five for each leg.
- For foot circles, raise a leg slightly off the bed with toes pointed (dorsiflexion).
- Draw a circle in the air with the great toe.
- Rotate to the right four times and then to the left four times.
- Repeat this five times and then repeat with the other foot.

Reinforce teaching that turning from side to side in bed is easier if the leg that is to be on top is bent. Then, place a pillow between the legs to support the top leg. Unless contraindicated, have patients use the bed's side rail to pull themselves over to the side. To promote comfort, have patients deep breathe while turning rather than holding their breath.

To make it easier to get out of bed and to reduce strain on the incision, instruct patients to:

- Turn on side without pillows between knees.
- Place hands flat against the bed.
- Push up while swinging legs out of bed into a sitting position.
- Sit for a few minutes after changing position to avoid dizziness and falling.
- Deep breathe while sitting to expand lungs.

> **PRACTICE ANALYSIS TIP**
> **Linking NCLEX-PN® to Practice**
> The LPN/LVN will reinforce client education about procedures and treatments.

Nursing Process for Preoperative Patients
Data Collection

HEALTH HISTORY. Patient data are collected on admission (Table 12.5). Ensure patients are wearing their contact lenses, glasses, or hearing aids to ensure accurate communication. Note the patient's emotional reaction to surgery (previously discussed).

All prescription, over-the-counter medications, herbal remedies, and recreational drugs are reviewed. The patient might have been told to stop anticoagulants, such as warfarin (Coumadin), or NSAIDs, including aspirin, several days before surgery. This is done to avoid bleeding problems during surgery. Contact the surgeon for clarification if needed. Herbal medicines can interfere with other medications. They can also increase bleeding times. Patients may be told to stop specific herbal medications 1 to 2 weeks before surgery. Patients on chronic oral steroid therapy cannot abruptly stop. This is true even when they are taking nothing by mouth (nil per os; NPO). Circulatory collapse can develop if steroids are stopped abruptly. The surgeon should order a parenteral route for the steroids. Ensure parenteral steroid therapy is continued while the patient is NPO. Patients with diabetes who take insulin are given insulin instructions (e.g., take an adjusted insulin dose or hold insulin on the day of surgery). After admission, blood glucose monitoring is done every 4 hours or as ordered to ensure blood glucose levels are maintained within a desired range.

Patients should be asked about their use of alcohol and recreational drugs (e.g., cannabis, cocaine, and opioids). These drugs can interact with anesthesia and medications and can cause withdrawal symptoms when stopped abruptly. To obtain honest, accurate information, tell patients of this potential interaction. Information and questions should be stated in a nonjudgmental, open-ended format. For example, ask, "How much alcohol do you drink daily or weekly?" instead of "Do you drink alcohol?" The first question requires more than a yes/no response and allows the patient who does not drink alcohol to indicate none. The patient who does drink alcohol can state an amount. The need for further questioning is eliminated. More accurate responses are given, as this approach is viewed more positively by the patient who drinks alcohol. Another example would be to ask the patient, "What role do drugs or alcohol play in your life?"

PHYSICAL ASSESSMENT. A physical assessment of body systems is performed. This information establishes the patient's baseline and identifies risk factors for surgery. Report a cough, cold, or fever to the surgeon. Surgery might be delayed until the acute infection is gone. Document dentures, bridges, capped teeth, and loose teeth. They can become dislodged during endotracheal (ET) intubation (insertion of breathing tube; see Fig. 29.27 in Chapter 29) or use of other airway adjuncts for general anesthesia.

Table 12.5
Nursing Data Collection of the Preoperative Patient

Subjective Data	Health History Questions
Demographic information	Name, age, marital status, occupation, roles?
Condition for which surgery is scheduled	Why are you having surgery?
Medical history	Any allergies, acute or chronic conditions, current medications, pain, or prior hospitalizations?
Surgical history	Any reactions or problems with anesthesia? Previous surgeries?
Tobacco use	How much do you smoke? Pack-year history (number of packs per day × number of years)?
Alcohol use	How often do you drink alcohol? How much?
Drug use	Do you use recreational or street drugs?
Coping techniques	How do you usually cope with stressful situations? Support systems?
Family history	Hereditary conditions, diabetes, cardiovascular or anesthesia problems?
Female patients	Date of last menses and obstetrical information?
Objective Data	**Physical Data Collection Findings**
Height and weight	
Vital signs, oxygen saturation	
Emotional status	Anxious, calm, tearful
Cardiovascular	Angina, cardiac rhythm, edema, heart failure, hypertension, jugular vein distention, mitral valve prolapse, myocardial infarction, peripheral pulses, valvular heart disease
Gastrointestinal	Abdominal distention, bowel sounds, date of last bowel movement, firmness, ostomy
Musculoskeletal	Crepitation, deformities, decreased range of motion, gait, prostheses, weakness
Neurologic	Ability to follow instructions
Respiratory	Infection (cough, breath sounds); barrel chest, chronic obstructive pulmonary disease; respiratory pattern, and effort
Skin	Bruises, color, dryness, lesions, mucous membrane status, turgor, warmth

Nursing Diagnoses, Planning, and Implementation

Anxiety or *Fear related to pain or unfamiliar situation of undergoing a surgical procedure*

EXPECTED OUTCOME: The patient will state reduced anxiety or fear prior to surgery.

- Inform the patient about procedures and surgical routines, *which helps reduce anxiety and fear.*
- Allow the patient to express their concerns *to allow inaccurate information to be corrected.*
- Ask if the patient would like a referral to a chaplain or social worker *to discuss anxiety and fear.*

Deficient Knowledge related to inadequate information with surgical routines and procedures

EXPECTED OUTCOME: The patient will demonstrate understanding of surgical information and routines before surgery.

- Identify knowledge deficiencies with patient and patient's family or caregivers *to provide appropriate information.*
- Ask the patient's preferred learning method, and use a variety of teaching methods (e.g., discussion, written materials and instructions, models, and videos) and individualize explanations *to allow for different learning styles and aging-related changes.* (See "Gerontological Issues: Considerations for Older Patient Teaching Sessions.")
- Reinforce preoperative information and new information as *teaching is caring in action and empowers patient to be a participant in own care.*
- Document teaching reinforcement and patient's understanding and continued learning needs *as evidence of teaching and the patient's level of understanding.*

> **PRACTICE ANALYSIS TIP**
> Linking NCLEX-PN® to Practice
> The LPN/LVN will identify barriers to learning.

Gerontological Issues
Considerations for Older Patient Teaching Sessions
Environmental Considerations
- Comfortable and safe: anxiety free, quiet, appropriate temperature
- Well lit: small, intense lighting with nonglare, soft white light (not fluorescent)
- Private: no distractions, no background noise

Presentation Considerations
- Identify readiness to learn.
- Plan learning based upon current knowledge.
- Use past experience and relate to new learning.
- Use simple, understandable words and avoid medical terminology.
- Use legible audiovisual materials (e.g., large print, black print on white nonglare paper).
- If using color, remember that older adults see red, orange, and yellow best; blue, violet, and green are more difficult to see.
- Remain aware of energy level of patient for learning.
- Answer questions as they occur.

Presenter Considerations
- Have a positive attitude and belief in self-care promotion for older adults.
- Earn trust by being a professional, credible, positive role model.
- Ensure that glasses and hearing aids are in use.
- Sit in front of patient for best visibility.
- Speak slowly in a low tone.
- Use touch appropriately to convey caring.
- Provide most important information first with one idea at a time.
- Provide instruction using multiple senses (vision and hearing) and memory aids such as pictures or diagrams.
- Allow patient increased response time.
- Provide repetition and obtain feedback to ensure comprehension.
- Provide positive reinforcement.

Evaluation
The goal to decrease anxiety is achieved if the patient states and demonstrates that anxiety is relieved. The goal for increasing knowledge is met if the patient is able to correctly state or accurately demonstrate the information presented.

Preoperative Consent

Before performing surgery, the surgeon must obtain written informed consent. It gives legal permission for the surgery. Consent has two purposes: One is to protect the patient from unauthorized procedures; the other is to protect the surgeon, anesthesia provider, agency, and agency employees from claims of performing unauthorized procedures. Informed consent is needed for all invasive procedures including anesthesia, surgery, and blood administration. Consent is typically valid for 30 days after signing and can be withdrawn at any time, even after signing.

Informed consent involves three elements:

1. The surgeon must explain in terms the patient understands about the diagnosis, the proposed treatment and who will perform it, the likely outcome, possible risks and complications of treatment, alternative treatments, and the prognosis without treatment. If the patient has questions before signing the consent, the surgeon must be contacted to provide further explanation to the patient. It is not within the nurse's scope of practice to provide this information.
2. The consent must be signed before analgesics or sedatives are given. Patients must demonstrate to a witness that they are informed and understand the surgery.
3. Consent must be given voluntarily. Persuasion or threats must never be used to influence the patient.

It may be your role to obtain and witness the patient's or authorized person's signature on the consent form. As the patient's advocate, ensure that the person signing the consent form understands its meaning. Ensure that the patient has no further questions to be directed to the surgeon and that the consent is being signed voluntarily. If the patient is unable to read, the entire consent must be read to the patient before it is signed.

Patients cannot give consent if they are unconscious, mentally incompetent, or minors. They also cannot give consent if they have received analgesics or any medications that alter central nervous system function within time frames specified by agency policy. Consent may be obtained in any of these cases in person or by phone from parents, next of kin, or legal guardians, as specified by law. A court order can also be obtained in a medical emergency. If time does not permit obtaining consent, the surgeon documents the need for treatment in the medical record as necessary to save the patient's life or avoid serious harm, according to state law and institutional policy.

> **NURSING CARE TIP**
> Your signature as a witness on a consent form indicates that you *observed* the *informed* patient or patient's authorized representative voluntarily sign the consent form. It does not mean that you informed the patient about the surgical procedure. That is the responsibility of the surgeon.

> **PRACTICE ANALYSIS TIP**
> **Linking NCLEX-PN® to Practice**
> The LPN/LVN will participate in client consent process.

> **CUE RECOGNITION 12.1**
> A 35-year-old man is being taken to the operating room. You hear him say to the transport technician that he does not want to have an operation. What action do you take?
>
> *Suggested answers are at the end of the chapter.*

Preparation for Surgery
Preoperative Preparation Checklist
A preoperative checklist that may include the following is completed by the nurse before the patient is transported to surgery:

- An identification band is placed on the patient. A hospital gown is given to the patient to wear. Underwear may need to be removed for access to the surgical site.
- Vital signs are taken and recorded as baseline information of the patient's status.
- Makeup, nail polish, and artificial nails (if applicable) are removed to allow assessment of natural color and pulse oximetry for oxygenation status during and after surgery.
- Removal of hairpins, wigs, and jewelry prevents loss or injury. Rings, such as wedding rings, are taped in place if the patient does not want to take them off (and if allowed by policy), except if the ring is on the operative side (arm or chest surgery), because edema may occur from the surgical procedure.
- Dentures, contact lenses, and prostheses are removed to prevent injury. Some patients are concerned about body image and do not want family members to see them without dentures, wigs, or makeup. These items can be removed after the family goes to the waiting room and reapplied before the family sees the patient postoperatively.
- Glasses and hearing aids go with patients to surgery if they are unable to communicate without them. Label them with the patient's name and document where they go.
- All orders, diagnostic test results, consents, and history and physical (required in medical record) are reviewed for completion and documented on the checklist.
- Patient valuables and their disposition (given to a family member or locked up per institutional policy by the nurse) are documented.
- Antiembolism devices are applied if ordered.
- Patients are asked to void before sedating preoperative medications are given, unless a urinary catheter is present, to prevent injury to the bladder during surgery.

Preoperative Medications
Preoperative medications are given at the time ordered or on call to surgery (i.e., surgery calls to instruct that it is time to give the medications; Table 12.6). If sedatives or analgesics are given, the bed rails are raised for safety per policy, and the patient is instructed not to get up alone.

Transfer to Surgery Department
When the surgery department is ready, the patient is transported to the surgical holding area on a stretcher or in their own bed (Fig. 12.1). The patient's inhaler medications for those with asthma and glasses or hearing aids to aid communication are taken with the patient. Family members can accompany the patient during transfer. During surgery, the family waits in the surgical waiting area, which is a communication center. The family is updated by cell phone or is given a beeper.

Post-Transfer to Surgery Department
After the patient goes to the surgery department, prepare the patient's room and necessary equipment to be ready when the patient returns from the perianesthesia care unit (PACU; Table 12.7).

Patient Arrival in Surgery Department
The holding area nurse greets the patient and completes a comprehensive surgical checklist (visit www.aorn.org/surgicalchecklist). Items verified include the patient's name, age, allergies, surgeon performing the surgery, and items on the preoperative checklist, including informed consent, surgical procedure (correct site, especially right or left when applicable), and medical history. Next, the nurse answers the patient's questions to alleviate anxiety. The operative site is confirmed by the patient and marked usually by the person most informed about the patient and procedure (surgeon). This helps ensure that the correct surgery will be done on the patient. Prophylactic antibiotics are typically given 60 to 120 minutes before the incision is made. This time frame has been shown to reduce surgical site infections (de Jonge et al, 2017).

Table 12.6 Preoperative Medications

Medication Class/Action	
Analgesic/Antipyretic *Relieves mild to moderate pain and reduces fever*	
Examples acetaminophen (OFIRMEV)	*Nursing Implications* Given intravenously as 15-minute infusion. Antipyretic effect may mask fever.
Antianxiety and Sedative Hypnotics *Sedation; anxiety reduction*	
Examples diazepam (Valium) lorazepam (Ativan) midazolam (Versed)	*Nursing Implications* Contraindicated for acute narrow-angle glaucoma. Monitor respirations.
Antiemetics *Control nausea and vomiting*	
Examples metoclopramide (Reglan) ondansetron (Zofran) prochlorperazine (Compazine) promethazine hydrochloride (Phenergan)	*Nursing Implications* Redness, pain, or burning at the site of injection. Increased drowsiness with opioids.
Antibiotics *Prevention of surgical infection*	
Examples Variety of antibiotics used	*Nursing Implications* Usually given within 60 to 120 minutes of incision time as prescribed for best outcome.
Opioids *Bind to opioid receptors in the central nervous system to alter perception of pain and enhance postoperative pain relief*	
Examples fentanyl (Sublimaze) hydromorphone hydrochloride (Dilaudid) morphine sulfate	*Nursing Implications* Monitor vital signs, level of sedation, and respiratory status.

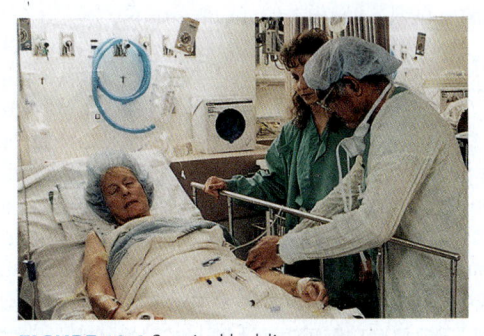

FIGURE 12.1 Surgical holding area.

The patient is introduced to the anesthesiologist and certified registered nurse anesthetist who verify patient information and explain the type of anesthesia to be used. IV fluids are started.

Before entering the operating room (OR), the patient should be reminded what to expect:

- "If the room feels cool, you can request extra blankets."
- "There is a lot of equipment in the room, including a table and large, bright overhead lights."
- "Several health-care team members will introduce themselves to you. You can ask questions or voice concerns to anyone present."
- "Your surgeon will greet you."
- "A safety checklist will be performed."

Preoperative Warming

Prewarming the patient's skin with a forced-air warming device for 30 minutes before anesthesia is helpful. It helps maintain normal body temperature (normothermia) and

Table 12.7
Postoperative Patient Hospital Room Preparation

Preparation	Rationale
Bed With Wheels Locked	
Ensure bed linens are clean and changed if used by patient before surgery.	Reduces contamination of surgical wound.
Place disposable, absorbent, waterproof pads on bottom sheet if drainage is expected.	Protects linen from wetness and soiling so a patient in pain does not have to be disturbed for linen change.
Apply lift sheet on bed of patient needing assistance with repositioning.	Makes lifting and turning easier for patient and nurse.
Have warm blankets available.	Patient may be cold.
Fanfold top cover to end of bed or to side of bed away from patient transfer side.	Readies bed to receive patient on transfer and allows covers to be easily pulled up over patient.
Obtain extra pillows as needed for positioning, elevating extremities, and splinting during coughing.	Pillows help maintain position when patient is turned, splint an incision during coughing, or elevate operative extremities for comfort and swelling reduction.
Equipment	
Have vital sign equipment available.	Promotes ability to promptly obtain vital signs.
Have IV pole/controller pump available.	Surgical patients have IV infusions postoperatively.
Have oxygen set up as needed.	After tracheostomy, patients wear humidified oxygen mask.
Prepare suction setup for tracheostomy, nasogastric tube, or drains as ordered.	Suction may be ordered related to surgical procedures: *Sterile suction:* tracheostomy *Nasogastric tube:* thoracic, abdominal, gastrointestinal surgery *T-tube:* cholecystectomy
Place emesis basin at bedside.	Nausea or vomiting may occur, especially after movement during transfer.
Place tissues and washcloths in room.	Promotes comfort (e.g., washing face or a cool cloth on forehead).
Have urinal or bedpan available in room.	Patients may be unable to get out of bed for first voiding.
Obtain special equipment as indicated by the surgical procedure.	Institutional policy and surgeon orders may require specialized equipment: *Jaw surgery:* suction, wire cutters, tracheostomy tray *Tracheostomy:* suction, extra tracheostomy set, tracheostomy care supplies

reduce intraoperative **hypothermia.** Associated complications of hypothermia can be prevented, including surgical wound infections (Zheng et al, 2020). Patients should be normothermic (body temperature within normal range) before transfer to surgery.

INTRAOPERATIVE PHASE

The next phase of the perioperative period is the *intraoperative* phase. It begins when the patient is transferred to the operating table (Fig. 12.2 and Fig. 12.3). Surgery can be done in a hospital or ambulatory (outpatient) surgical center. In addition, surgery is performed in HCP offices, cardiac catheterization laboratories, radiology centers, emergency rooms, and specialized units that perform endoscopy procedures.

The OR is designed to enhance **aseptic** (elimination of microorganisms) technique. Clean and contaminated areas are separated. Special ventilation systems control dust. They prevent air from flowing into the OR from hallways. The temperature and humidity in the OR are controlled to discourage bacterial growth. The OR temperature is recommended to be 68°F to 75°F (20°C to 24°C) to reduce patient hypothermia. Everyone entering the OR wears hospital-laundered surgical scrubs, shoe covers, caps, masks, and goggles to protect the

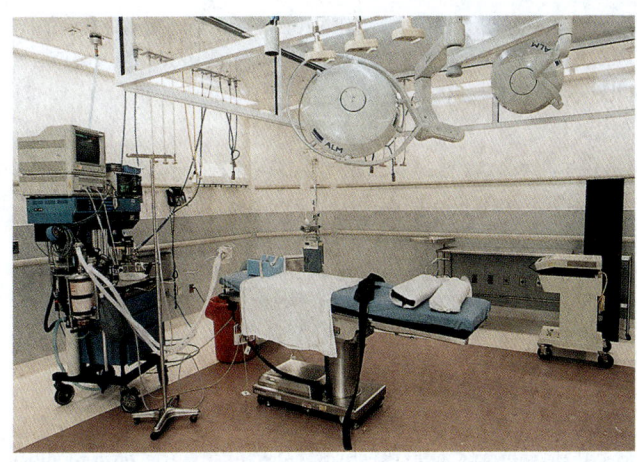

FIGURE 12.2 Operating room. Anesthesia equipment is on the left.

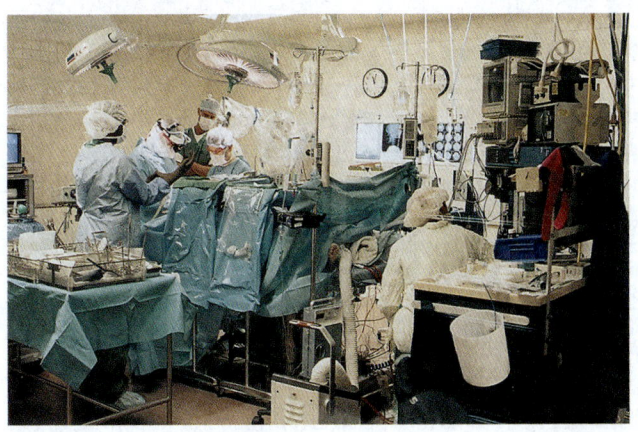

FIGURE 12.3 Operating room in use. Anesthesia equipment is on the right.

patient and staff from infection. Traffic in and out of the OR is limited. Strong disinfectants are used to clean the OR after each surgical case.

Prior to surgery, surgical team members (Box 12.2) must perform a sterile surgical hand scrub. This practice reduces the number of microorganisms on their hands and arms. Jewelry (e.g., watches, rings, bracelets) is removed. Fingernails are kept short and clean. Artificial nails and nail polish are not recommended, as they may harbor microorganisms ("Evidence-Based Practice"). Sterile gloves are worn by the surgical team to keep the surgical field sterile.

A surgical case cart contains sterile instruments specifically for the patient's case. The LPN/LVN may assist with maintaining the sterile surgical field.

A nursing plan of care focusing on safety is prepared before the patient arrives in surgery. It is developed with the patient's preadmission assessment data. Nursing diagnoses may include *Risk for Injury, Risk for Perioperative Positioning Injury,* and *Risk for Perioperative Hypothermia.*

The LPN/LVN may help position the patient onto the operating table. A safety strap is carefully applied. A time-out is taken to verify all patient and surgical information to prevent mistakes. All members of the OR team stop, listen to

Box 12.2

Surgical Health-Care Team Members and Roles

Members of the surgical health-care team and their roles are as follows:

- *Surgeon:* Medical doctor, doctor of osteopathy, oral surgeon, or podiatrist
- *Surgical (first) assistant:* Another physician, a specially trained RN (such as a nurse practitioner or clinical nurse specialist), or a physician's assistant who assists the surgeon
- *Anesthesiologist:* Physician who specializes in administering anesthesia and supervises certified registered nurse anesthetists (CRNAs) in the operating room
- *CRNA:* A certified RN with a master or doctorate degree in nurse anesthesia
- *RN:* Circulates in the operating room; roles include being the patient's advocate, planning care, protecting patient safety, monitoring patient positioning, checking vital signs and patient assessment, reducing patient's anxiety, monitoring sterility during surgery, preparing skin before incision, managing equipment (e.g., making sponge counts), documenting the procedure, and aiding health team communications
- *Surgical (second assistant) technician:* Assists surgeon (may be an RN, LPN/LVN, or surgical technologist)

Evidence-Based Practice

Clinical Question
What is the microbial growth on the nails of nurses who wear fingernail polish?

Evidence
A comparison of microbial cultures on unpolished fingernails, nails with one-day-old nail polish, and nails with four-day-old nail polish was conducted. Nails of 83 nurses in the study were cultured immediately after their shift ended. They were directed to perform routine hand washing during their shift. The one-day-old nail polish exhibited fewer gram-positive and gram-negative microorganisms than the unpolished nail. The four-day-old polish showed more microorganisms than the one-day-old polish.

Implications for Nursing Practice
Nurses should follow their agency policy regarding use of nail polish. Microbial growth increases the longer nail polish is in place.

Reference: Blackburn, L., Acree, K., Bartley, J., DiGiannantoni, E., Renner, E., & Sinnott, L. T. (2020). Microbial growth on the nails of direct patient care nurses wearing nail polish. *Oncology Nursing Forum, 47*(2), 155–164. https://doi.org/10.1188/20.onf.155-164

the information of the time out, and agree before the surgery begins. Then monitoring equipment is applied. Readings are recorded. The anesthesia provider begins anesthesia and directs when to position the patient. Positioning is done carefully to prevent pressure points that can cause tissue or nerve damage. Tubes that are needed, such as a nasogastric (NG) tube or urinary catheter, are inserted.

Patient allergies (e.g., to skin prep solutions) are rechecked. If the patient requires body hair removal, hair is removed with electric clippers. Shaving is avoided, as it can cause microabrasions that become colonized by microorganisms. Then the skin is cleaned with a skin prep solution such as povidone-iodine. A large area around the operative site is scrubbed, which allows the incision to be extended as needed. The scrub is completed in a circular motion from inner to outer edge. This technique allows for microbes to be mechanically moved away from the incision site. Allergic reaction to the antimicrobial solution can cause skin redness and blistering wherever the solution was used. After the skin is scrubbed, a sterile drape is applied. The incisional area is left exposed.

Anesthesia

The type of anesthesia and the anesthetic agents are ordered by the anesthesia provider with input from the patient and surgeon. There are two types of anesthesia: general and local (regional). General anesthesia causes the patient to lose consciousness, sensation, and reflexes. It acts directly on the central nervous system. Local anesthesia blocks nerve impulses along the nerve where it is injected, resulting in the loss of sensation to a region of the body. There is no loss of consciousness.

General Anesthesia

General anesthesia is given by IV or inhalation. It is used if the surgical procedure will take a long time and there is a need for muscle relaxation. It is also used when patients are anxious or do not want local anesthesia. In addition, it can be used for patients who are unable to cooperate, as with head injury, muscle disorders, or impaired cognitive function.

IV AGENTS. To begin most general anesthesia, the patient is induced (meaning "to cause anesthesia"). A short-acting IV agent is used to provide rapid, smooth **induction** (the period from when the anesthetic is first given until full anesthesia is reached). These agents last only a few minutes and are used along with inhalation agents. After induction, the patient is intubated with an endotracheal (ET) tube. This is used to provide anesthesia and mechanical ventilation.

INHALATION AGENTS. Inhalation agents maintain anesthesia during the surgery. These agents are delivered, controlled, and excreted via mechanical ventilation.

COMPLICATIONS. Side effects of general anesthesia are usually brief. They include nausea and vomiting, confusion (longer duration in older adult), sore throat, and shivering, likely from the body cooling. Serious complications occur rarely and include respiratory distress, malignant hyperthermia, and, more commonly in older adults, delirium (temporary) and cognitive dysfunction (e.g., long-term memory loss; difficulty learning, thinking, and concentrating). Inhalation agents and the ET tube can be irritating to the respiratory tract. Complications from them that can occur include laryngospasm (sudden violent contraction of the vocal cords), laryngeal edema, or injury to the vocal cords. When the ET tube is removed, closely monitor the patient's airway. Be prepared to provide respiratory support. Assist with reintubation if needed.

ADJUNCT AGENTS. An **adjunct** agent is a medication used with the primary anesthetic agents. These medications include opioids to control pain, muscle relaxers to avoid movement of muscles during surgery, antiemetics to control nausea or vomiting, and sedatives to supplement anesthesia. Side effects related to a specific medication, such as itching with opioids, can occur.

Local or Regional Anesthesia

Local or regional anesthesia is selected for the patient who wants to be awake, is not anxious, can tolerate the local agent, and is not required by the surgical procedure to be unconscious or to have relaxed muscles.

A local agent can be placed directly on the surgical area or injected into the tissue where the incision is to be made to numb a small area (common in dental procedures). A regional block is done by injecting the local agent along a nerve that carries impulses in the region where anesthesia is desired. There are several types of regional blocks. A nerve block is the injection of a local agent into a nerve at a specific point. A Bier block is done by placing a tourniquet (cuff) on an extremity to remove the blood; the local agent is then injected into the extremity. A field block is a series of injections surrounding the surgical area.

SPINAL AND EPIDURAL BLOCKS. Injection of a local agent into the subarachnoid space produces spinal block (Fig. 12.4). Epidural block occurs when the local agent is injected into the epidural space. Spinal and epidural blocks are used mainly for lower extremity, lower abdominal surgery, and childbirth. Both motor and sensory function are blocked. The patient must be carefully monitored for complications. Hypotension results from sympathetic blockade. The blockage causes vasodilation and reduces venous return to the heart. Cardiac output is reduced. Respiratory depression results if the block travels too far upward. As the block wears off, patients feel as if their legs are heavy and numb. This is normal. Reassurance should be offered to the patient that this type of feeling does not last after the block wears off. For safety, patients will remain in bed until full sensation returns.

COMPLICATIONS. Back pain, urinary retention, hematoma, nerve damage, or postdural puncture headache can occur with regional anesthesia. Headache may occur from leakage of cerebrospinal fluid (CSF) out of the needle puncture hole in the dura. Pressure is then reduced on the spinal cord and brain. This causes a low-pressure headache, which can be severe. The headache can worsen with standing or sitting.

• **WORD** • **BUILDING** •
induction: inductio—to lead in

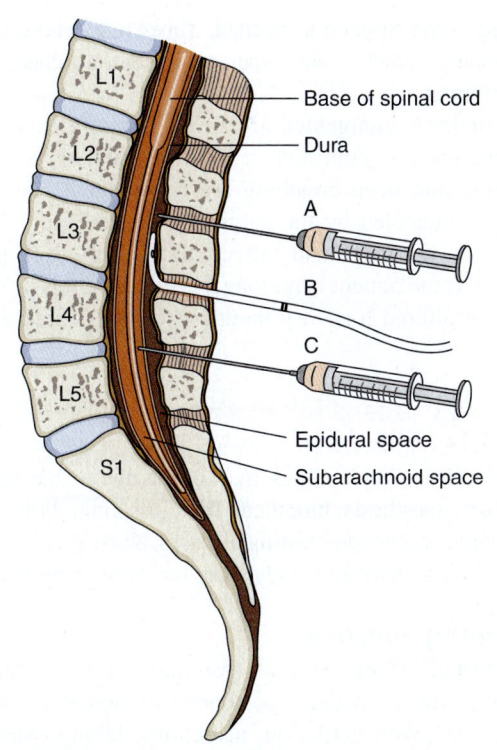

FIGURE 12.4 Injection of spinal anesthesia. (A) Epidural anesthesia. (B) Epidural catheter. (C) Spinal anesthesia.

Nausea, dizziness, tinnitus, and vision disturbances may be present. The headache usually will resolve in 7 to 10 days. If symptomatic and conservative treatment is not effective, an autologous epidural blood patch can be used. This sterile procedure is done by the anesthesiologist. To create an epidural blood patch, approximately 15 mL to 20 mL of the patient's blood is injected into the epidural space one interspace below the previous puncture site.

Procedural Sedation and Analgesia

Procedural sedation and analgesia is purposeful, minimal sedation. It does not cause the complete loss of consciousness. The patient may fall asleep but then arouse easily and respond. Patients remain in control of their own airway. They are comfortable and respond purposefully. Medications such as propofol (Diprivan), ketamine (Ketalar), midazolam (Versed), and opioids (fentanyl or morphine) are given to produce sedation. Selection of patients who are eligible for this sedation is based on the procedure, the patient's general health, and patient or physician preference. Examples of short procedures for which this type of sedation is used are dental procedures, endoscopy, cardioversion, and closed fracture reduction. Procedural sedation can be administered by anesthesia providers or ordered by an HCP and given by a specially trained RN.

The patient does not eat for 6 hours before the procedure. Clear liquids are allowed up to 2 hours before the procedure. A signed informed consent is obtained. Then an IV is started. Patients are placed on continuous electrocardiogram (ECG) and oxygen saturation monitors. Capnography waveforms may also be monitored. Vital signs are obtained every 5 minutes. Changes are announced to the surgeon. Oxygen may be given by nasal cannula or mask. Emergency equipment (e.g., airway suction, defibrillator, medications) is on standby.

After the procedure, the patient awakens quickly and remembers nothing or little about the procedure. The patient is monitored about every 15 minutes for response to the procedure and medications. Rare side effects include drowsiness, headache, and nausea. The patient is ready for discharge when vital signs return to baseline and are stable, oral fluids are retained, the patient can safely ambulate (if applicable), and voiding has occurred (if applicable). Written and oral discharge teaching must be given to both the patient and the responsible adult to whom the patient is being discharged. The responsible adult and the patient must sign the instructions. These state that an adult must drive the patient home and provide a safe environment. They also state that the patient must not and will not drive or operate heavy machinery or sign legal documents for 24 hours.

> **LEARNING TIP**
> In comparison with general anesthesia, procedural sedation and analgesia:
> - Is less invasive.
> - Requires less medication.
> - Causes less depression of the cardiovascular and respiratory systems.
> - Allows the patient to return more quickly to a wakeful state.

Transfer From Surgery

When surgery is completed and anesthesia stopped, the patient is stabilized for transfer. The patient is normothermic upon transfer from surgery. After local anesthesia, the patient may return directly to a nursing unit. After general and spinal anesthesia, the patient goes to the PACU (Fig. 12.5) or an intensive care unit (ICU).

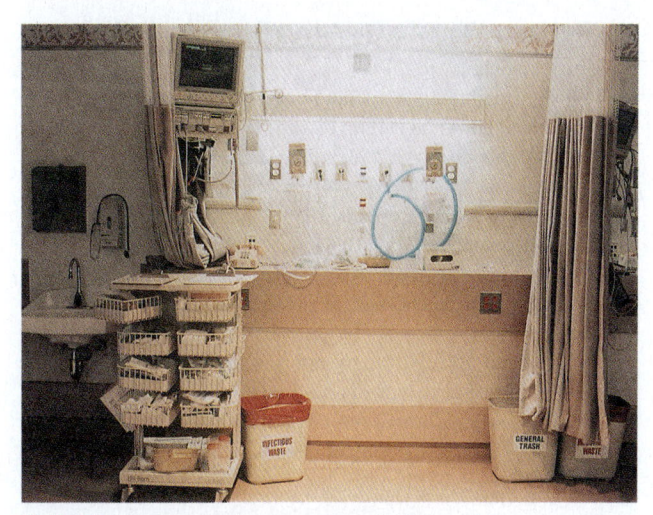

FIGURE 12.5 Perianesthesia care unit (PACU).

Patient safety is an important concern. The patient is never left alone. Ensuring a patent airway and preventing falls and injury from uncontrolled movements are priorities. The anesthesia provider and OR nurses transfer the patient to the PACU. They monitor the patient until the perianesthesia nurse can receive the hand-off report and assume care of the patient. This promotes safe recovery from anesthesia. The family is updated on the patient's status by the surgeon.

POSTOPERATIVE PHASE

The *postoperative* phase is the final perioperative phase. It begins when the patient is admitted to the PACU or directly to a nursing unit. It ends with the patient's postoperative evaluation in the surgeon's office.

Admission to the Perianesthesia Care Unit

Responsibilities of perianesthesia nurses are listed in Box 12.3. When patients are admitted to the PACU, an admission assessment is done. Hand hygiene between patients is essential.

Oxygen by nasal cannula, mask, or mechanical ventilation is given after general anesthesia. IV fluid infusion is maintained. Continuous monitoring of ECG, exhaled end-tidal carbon dioxide ($EtCO_2$), and pulse oximetry is done. Vital signs are obtained every 5 to 15 minutes. If the patient's temperature is normal, the temperature is monitored hourly and at PACU discharge. Passive methods to maintain temperature are continued. Room temperature is kept at or above 75°F (24°C). A head covering and warm blankets are used. If shivering due to hypothermia occurs, the temperature is retaken. For hypothermia, active warming, usually with a forced-air warming system, is used. Body temperature is monitored every 15 minutes until normal. The patient must be normothermic before PACU discharge.

The surgical site incision or dressing is monitored. Drainage amount, color, and **hematoma** formation are documented and reported to the surgeon as needed. Tubes (e.g., chest, drains, NG, urinary catheter) and other equipment are checked for proper function.

IV or PCA analgesics are given for pain as needed. Antiemetics are administered for nausea or vomiting. Coughing and deep breathing are encouraged unless they are contraindicated by the surgical procedure (e.g., hernia repair; ear, eye, jaw, and intracranial surgery; and plastic surgery). If the patient is no longer NPO, ice chips or sips of water are offered for a dry mouth when the patient is fully awake.

Nursing Process for Postoperative Patients in PACU

Postoperative complications may occur due to the surgical procedure, anesthesia, blood and fluid loss, immobility, unrelieved pain, or other preexisting diseases. Nursing care focuses on preventing, detecting, and caring for these complications.

Respiratory Function

DATA COLLECTION. Normal respiratory function can be altered in the immediate postoperative period by airway obstruction, hypoventilation, secretions, laryngospasm, or decreased swallowing and cough reflexes. Respiratory function monitoring includes respiratory rate, depth, ease, and pattern. Breath sounds, chest symmetry, accessory muscle use, and sputum are also monitored.

NURSING DIAGNOSES, PLANNING, AND IMPLEMENTATION

Ineffective Airway Clearance related to general anesthesia

EXPECTED OUTCOME: The patient will have a patent airway at all times.

- Ensure that the patient maintains a patent airway, as *airway obstruction may result when relaxed muscles allow the tongue to block the pharynx in patients with a decreased level of consciousness.*
- Use jaw-thrust method to manually open the patient's airway *if patient has snoring respirations and has not completely emerged from anesthesia.*

Ineffective Breathing Pattern related to anesthesia, analgesic medications, or pain

EXPECTED OUTCOME: The patient will maintain normal $EtCO_2$ and oxygen saturation (SaO_2) levels at all times.

- Maintain oxygen therapy as ordered *to prevent hypoventilation and hypoxemia, which can be an effect of anesthesia medications, analgesics, or decreased level of consciousness.*

Box 12.3

Perianesthesia Nursing Responsibilities

- Airway maintenance
- Vital signs including temperature, oxygen saturation (SaO_2), and exhaled end-tidal carbon dioxide ($EtCO_2$)
- Body systems assessment including surgical site
- Patient safety
- Monitoring anesthetic effects
- Pain management
- Accurate intake and output
- Identifying perianesthesia care unit discharge readiness
- Documentation
- Bedside hand-off report to receiving nurse (includes name, allergies, procedure, type of anesthesia, status, complications, oxygen, dressing/drains/equipment, medications, postoperative orders, pertinent history, family, opportunity to ask questions)

• WORD • BUILDING •

hematoma: heimatos—blood + oma—tumor

- Encourage deep breathing *to expand the lungs, expel anesthetic agents, and decrease alveolar collapse.*
- Report respiratory depression or abnormal EtCO$_2$ to the anesthesiologist *to obtain prompt treatment.*

Risk for Aspiration related to decreased level of consciousness, depressed gag reflex, and facial, neck, or oral surgery

EXPECTED OUTCOME: The patient will have clear lung sounds with no signs of acute aspiration (coughing, wheezing, fever, respiratory distress, cyanosis, chest pain) at all times.

- Position the patient onto side, *to protect the airway until fully awake, then elevate the head of bed 30 degrees,* unless contraindicated.
- Use suction equipment as needed *to clear secretions or emesis.*

EVALUATION. The goal for ineffective airway clearance and aspiration risk is achieved if the patient's airway remains patent and lung sounds remain clear. The goal for ineffective breathing pattern is met if the patient's respiratory rate is within normal limits, no dyspnea is reported, and arterial blood gases are within normal limits.

Cardiovascular Function

DATA COLLECTION. Alterations in cardiovascular function can include hypotension, arrhythmias, and hypertension. Hypotension can be the result of blood and fluid volume loss, cardiac abnormalities, or a side effect of anesthesia or pain medication. Shock can result from the significant blood and fluid volume loss or from sepsis (see Chapter 9). Arrhythmias can occur from hypoxia, altered potassium or magnesium levels, hypothermia, pain, stress, or cardiac disease (see Chapter 25). New-onset hypertension can develop from pain, a full bladder, or respiratory distress.

Cardiovascular function data collection includes heart rate, blood pressure, ECG, and skin temperature, color, and moistness. Vital signs are compared with baseline readings to determine patient status. Tachycardia; hypotension; pale skin color; cool, clammy skin; and decreased urine output indicate hypovolemic shock. This requires reporting and prompt treatment by the surgeon or anesthesia provider.

NURSING DIAGNOSES, PLANNING, AND IMPLEMENTATION

Risk for Deficient Fluid Volume related to blood and fluid loss or NPO status

EXPECTED OUTCOME: The patient will maintain blood pressure, pulse, and urine output within normal limits at all times.

- Monitor dressings, incisions, and drains for color and amount of drainage *to detect fluid loss.*
- Monitor intake and output *to detect imbalances.*
- Maintain IV fluids at ordered rate *to replace lost fluids but avoid fluid overload.*

EVALUATION. The goal for risk for deficient fluid volume is met if vital signs and urine output are within normal limits.

NURSING CARE TIP

Tachycardia is a compensatory mechanism designed to provide adequate delivery of oxygen in times of altered function. It is usually the earliest warning sign that an abnormality is occurring. It should be an indicator to evaluate the patient. Ask yourself what this patient is likely to be experiencing that is compromising oxygenation. Considering the cause allows you to begin prompt intervention.

Patient Condition	Possible Causes of Compromised Oxygenation
Postoperative	Hemorrhage, pain, respiratory depression
Myocardial infarction	Arrhythmia, cardiogenic shock, pain
Trauma	Hemorrhage, respiratory distress, severe pain

Pain

DATA COLLECTION. If the patient is awake, ask the patient to rate the presence of pain using a pain scale. Document the location and character of the pain. If the patient is not fully awake, monitor vital signs and nonverbal indications of pain. Nonverbal indications of pain can include abnormal vital signs, grimacing, moaning, restlessness, rubbing, or pulling at specific areas or equipment.

NURSING DIAGNOSES, PLANNING, AND IMPLEMENTATION

Acute Pain related to tissue damage (incision)

See "Nursing Care Plan for the Postoperative Patient."

Neurologic Function

Until its effects wear off, anesthesia can alter neurologic function. Patients may arrive in the PACU awake, arousable, or sleeping. Patients who are sleeping should become more alert during their stay in the PACU. As they emerge from anesthesia, they may become agitated or behave irrationally for a short time; this is called *emergence delirium*. During this time, it is important to prevent injury by providing safety measures such as side rails and restraints—following restraint protocols—and to protect IV lines and keep an ET tube in place. Once resolved, patients return to a calm state and have no recollection of the episode. Movement, sensations, and perceptions may also be altered by anesthesia. Movement is the first function to return after spinal anesthesia.

Patients who are confused may be agitated or frightened when they awaken. Review the patient's cognitive history. It is helpful to know how caregivers, family, and friends communicate with a patient. If possible, have a familiar relative or caregiver in the PACU with a patient who is confused. They can keep the patient calm and help with communication. Watch for nonverbal pain cues. Know that postoperative patients will have pain and require pain relief interventions, *even if they cannot report it*!

Neurological data collection includes level of consciousness; orientation to person, place, time, and event; pupil size and reaction to light; and motor and sensory function. Abnormalities are reported to the anesthesia provider.

Family Visitation
Family visitation in the PACU has been shown to help patients and their families. Allowing family visitation varies by agency. Patients and families should be educated about the expectations for family visitation. During visitation, confidentiality of all patients in PACU must be ensured per the Health Insurance Portability and Accountability Act of 1996 (HIPAA). For example, some patients may not want their surgical procedure revealed to any family members.

Discharge From the PACU
The length of stay in the PACU for a stable patient is about 1 hour. A postanesthesia recovery scale is used to score the patient's readiness to be discharged. The scale rates categories such as respiration, oxygen saturation, level of consciousness, activity, and circulation. The anesthesiologist discharges the patient for transfer to a nursing unit or home when discharge criteria are met (Box 12.4). The patient may be transferred to the ICU. This is done if the patient is unstable and/or frequent or invasive monitoring is needed.

Transfer to the Nursing Unit
The perianesthesia nurse provides a hand-off report to the unit nurse when the patient is transferred to the nursing unit. The patient is moved into a bed on the nursing unit unless the patient is being transferred in a bed, as may be done with major orthopedic procedures. Assistance is given to prevent dislodging of IVs, tubes, and drains. The following safety interventions are performed per agency policy to help prevent falls:

- The bed is placed in its lowest position with wheels locked, the side rails raised, and the call button within patient's reach.
- Instructions are given for the patient to call for assistance with ambulation.
- Assistance by one or two health-care workers is given to help the patient getting out of bed. The patient should be encouraged to sit on the side of bed prior to standing to prevent weakness or dizziness, especially when getting up for the first time postoperatively (Fig. 12.6).

Nursing Process for Postoperative Patients
A head-to-toe patient assessment is performed after transfer to the nursing unit. Respiratory status, vital signs (including temperature), level of consciousness, surgical site, dressings, and pain level are noted. IV site, patency, and IV solution and infusion rate are monitored. Chest tubes and NG are hooked to suction or clamped as ordered. Drains and catheters are positioned to promote proper functioning.

Interventions to promote recovery are implemented. They include monitoring for complications (e.g., respiratory depression, hemorrhage, and shock) and providing postoperative care. Complications can place the patient at *Risk for*

Box 12.4
Discharge Criteria for Perianesthesia Care Unit or Ambulatory Surgery
- Vital signs stable with temperature normal
- Respiratory function not depressed
- Oxygen saturation above 90%
- Patient awake or at baseline level of consciousness
- Drainage or bleeding not excessive

Additional Criteria for Ambulatory Surgery
- No nausea or vomiting/tolerating PO intake
- No IV opioids within last 30 minutes
- Voided if required by surgical procedure or ordered
- Is ambulatory or has baseline mobility
- Understands discharge instructions
- Provides means of contact for follow-up telephone assessment
- Released to responsible adult

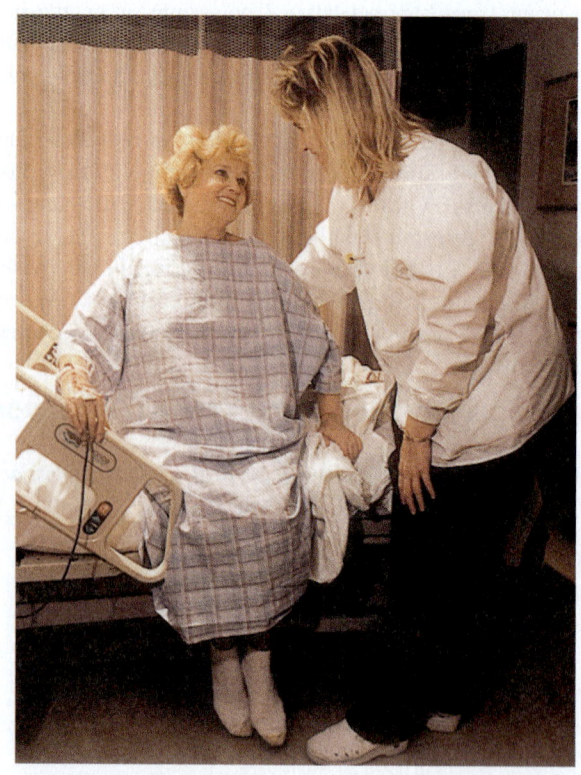

FIGURE 12.6 Postoperative patient sitting before standing.

Chapter 12 Nursing Care of Patients Having Surgery 181

> **BE SAFE!**
> **BE VIGILANT!!!** New nurses often focus only on postoperative comfort when receiving a patient from surgery or PACU. In addition to ensuring comfort, view the patient's surgical dressings and wounds and underneath the patient *upon* accepting care to identify and correct any problems such as bleeding quickly. *Always* perform a *line reconciliation* to identify every tube or catheter attached to a patient and verify its correct use and attachment to prevent harmful misconnections. Follow each tube or catheter from the patient to the point of origin *upon* accepting care during the hand-off report (e.g., feeding tubes, IV lines, peritoneal dialysis catheters, urinary catheters, wound drains).

Delayed Surgical Recovery. Other interventions reinforce teaching to patients and their significant others and assist with necessary referrals, including home health care.

Respiratory Function

DATA COLLECTION. Regular monitoring of the patient's respiratory system is performed. This includes rate, depth, effort, and breath sounds. Cough strength (if not contraindicated by the type of surgery, such as hernia repair or eye, ear, intracranial, jaw, or plastic surgery) is also noted. Postoperative patients are at risk for developing atelectasis, which can lead to pneumonia. They may have a weak cough from being drowsy from anesthesia or analgesics. Listen for fine crackles in the lung bases. If present, encourage the patient to deep breathe or cough. Listen again to see if the crackles have cleared. If the

---

Nursing Care Plan for the Postoperative Patient

Nursing Diagnosis: Ineffective Airway Clearance related to ineffective cough and secretion retention
Expected Outcomes: The patient will maintain a patent airway at all times. Breath sounds remain clear at all times.
Evaluation of Outcome: Is the patient able to clear own secretions? Are breath sounds clear?

Intervention	Rationale	Evaluation
Monitor breath sounds.	Abnormal breath sounds such as crackles or wheezes can indicate retained secretions.	Are breath sounds clear?
Encourage deep breathing and coughing hourly, use of incentive spirometer as ordered while awake, turning every 2 hours and early ambulation as able.	Lung expansion and coughing help prevent mucous plugs that block bronchioles.	Does patient perform deep breathing and coughing and use incentive spirometer?
Geriatric		
Ensure adequate hydration.	Older adults are prone to dehydration, making secretions thicker and more difficult to clear.	Does patient have balanced intake and output?

Nursing Diagnosis: Acute Pain related to tissue damage from surgery, muscle spasms, nausea, or vomiting
Expected Outcome: The patient will report that pain management relieves pain satisfactorily within 30 minutes of report of pain or when the patient awakens.
Evaluation of Outcome: Does the patient report satisfactory pain relief?

Intervention	Rationale	Evaluation
Monitor pain using a patient appropriate pain rating scale (self-report: 0 to 10; noncommunicative: pictogram; see Chapter 10).	Self-report is the most reliable indicator of pain unless patient is unable to report pain.	Is patient using the pain scale?
Provide ordered analgesics, PCA, or antiemetics as needed and monitor patient response.	Analgesics and antiemetics decrease pain, increase comfort, and promote willingness to deep breathe especially if incision is near the diaphragm.	Is patient's pain and/or nausea and vomiting reduced after receiving medication?
Position patient comfortably, assist to empty full bladder, and make environment soothing: comfortable room temperature, dim lights, quiet, offer to play preferred music.	Incisions, drains, tubing, equipment, and bedrest can cause discomfort, which positioning can relieve. Attention to environmental factors can help relieve pain.	Does patient report position and environment are comfortable?

(nursing care plan continues on page 182)

Nursing Care Plan for the Postoperative Patient—cont'd

Geriatric

Intervention	Rationale	Evaluation
Monitor patient who is cognitively impaired or nonverbal cognitively impaired at the beginning of a shift and then frequently, using an appropriate pain rating tool (see "Gerontological Issues") and observe nonverbal pain cues (e.g., grimacing, moaning, restlessness).	*Cognitively impaired patients are vulnerable to undertreatment of pain and deserve excellence in pain relief management. Using an appropriate pain rating tool and noting nonverbal cues can aid in pain treatment.*	Does patient exhibit signs of reduced or no pain per pain scale?
When monitoring pain, speak clearly and slowly so older patient can hear and understand.	*If older patient cannot hear or misunderstands, pain may not be reported accurately. Appropriate intervention would not be provided.*	Is patient able to report pain and relief accurately using pain rating scale?

Nursing Diagnosis: *Risk for Surgical Site Infection* related to contamination, immunosuppression, invasive procedure
Expected Outcome: The patient will remain free from infection at all times.
Evaluation of Outcome: Does the patient remain free from infection?

Intervention	Rationale	Evaluation
Observe incision and surrounding skin color and temperature for signs and symptoms of infection; report, if present.	*Fever and redness, warmth, and swelling at surgical site indicate infection.*	Are signs and symptoms of infection present?
Monitor dressings and note drainage color, amount, and consistency.	*Surgical wound drainage initially is* **sanguineous** *(red). It changes to serosanguineous (pink) and then serous (pale yellow) after a few hours to days.*	Is drainage color and amount as expected and not bright red or large amounts or purulent?
Maintain sterile technique for dressing changes.	*Sterile technique reduces infection development.*	Is incision free of signs and symptoms of infection?

Geriatric

Intervention	Rationale	Evaluation
Monitor for and report low-grade temperature or new-onset confusion.	*Older adults may exhibit a low-grade temperature or new-onset confusion as indicators of infection requiring treatment.*	Does patient have low-grade temperature or new-onset confusion to report?

---

patient's airway is compromised, take immediate action to support the airway. Notify the surgeon, anesthesia provider, or rapid response team if the condition is urgent.

NURSING DIAGNOSES, PLANNING, AND IMPLEMENTATION. See "Nursing Care Plan for the Postoperative Patient."

Circulatory Function

DATA COLLECTION. Monitor the patient's circulatory status to detect and prevent hemorrhage, shock, and venous thromboembolism. Vital signs, SaO_2, and skin temperature, color, and moistness are also monitored (per institutional policy). Report abnormal findings. Check the incision or dressing for drainage or hematoma formation. Drainage may leak down the patient's side and pool underneath the patient. Turn the patient if able or, while wearing gloves, slide hands underneath the patient to check for bleeding. Report signs of hemorrhage or shock (see Chapter 9) promptly.

Observe the lower extremities of surgical patients. Check peripheral pulses and capillary refill. Tenderness or pain in the calf may be the first indication of a deep vein thrombosis (DVT). Leg swelling, warmth, and redness as well as fever may also be present. Bilateral calf and thigh measurements are taken daily if DVT is suspected or diagnosed. DVT diagnosis is based on D-dimer lab test result and ultrasound.

NURSING DIAGNOSES, PLANNING, AND IMPLEMENTATION. See "Nursing Process for Postoperative Patients in Perianesthesia Care Unit: *Risk for Deficient Fluid Volume*."

Risk for Thrombosis related to surgery, dehydration, and impaired physical mobility

EXPECTED OUTCOME: The patient will not develop a thrombosis.

- Avoid pressure under the knee from pillows, rolled blankets, or prolonged bending of the knee, and elevate legs *to help prevent venous stasis.*
- Avoid pressure on the heels by elevating the ankles on rolled blankets or pillows *to help prevent heel breakdown.*
- Apply antiembolism compression stockings (TED hose) or sequential compression device as ordered *to help prevent stasis of blood* (see Chapter 21 Learning Tip on selecting appropriate compression stocking). *Thigh-length stockings are more effective than knee-length stockings in reducing the risk of thrombophlebitis.*
- Encourage leg exercises hourly while patient is awake *to prevent venous stasis and thrombosis.*
- Assist with early postoperative ambulation as ordered *to prevent thrombosis.*
- Administer anticoagulants as ordered *to reduce clot formation.*

EVALUATION. The goal for risk for thrombosis is met if tissue blood flow remains uncompromised by a thrombus.

> **PRACTICE ANALYSIS TIP**
> Linking NCLEX-PN® to Practice
> The LPN/LVN will apply and check proper use of compression stockings and/or sequential compression device.

Postoperative Pain

Pain is common after surgery. Each patient's pain experience varies. Incisional pain and painful muscle spasms can occur. Nausea and vomiting, ambulation, coughing, deep breathing, and anxiety can increase postoperative pain. Because unrelieved pain has negative physiological effects, pain relief should be provided as ordered to all surgical patients. It impairs deep breathing and coughing. Early ambulation is made more difficult. Increased complications, length of stay, and health-care costs can occur. Pain should not be ignored or undertreated, as it can lead to chronic pain and disability (Manworren et al, 2018), yet it has been found that it often is.

Increasing evidence shows that complementary and alternative therapies for pain management are effective (Bakker et al, 2020). These approaches allow lower doses of opioids to be used and result in fewer side effects. Opioid and nonopioid medications treat pain along various pathways, which provides better relief. Acetaminophen to reduce pain or the use of NSAIDs to reduce inflammation and pain should be considered. Nurses must make pain relief a priority and stay informed of advances in pain management. Being able to advocate for proper pain management reduces patient suffering and promotes recovery (see Chapter 10).

DATA COLLECTION. Monitor nonverbal indications of pain for patients who are not fully awake ("Gerontological Issues: Postoperative Pain"). Nonverbal indicators of pain may include grimacing, moaning, posturing, restlessness, and rubbing or pulling at specific body areas or equipment. Ask patients who are awake about the location of the pain, to rate the presence of pain, and to describe the pain quality, such as sharp, aching, throbbing, or burning. Document this data for use in developing a pain management plan of care.

NURSING DIAGNOSES, PLANNING, AND IMPLEMENTATION. See "Nursing Care Plan for the Postoperative Patient."

> **Gerontological Issues**
>
> **Postoperative Pain**
> Pain is not a normal part of aging. Careful identification of older patients' unique aging changes, chronic diseases, and pain relief needs is required to appropriately treat their postoperative pain. Cognitively impaired and nonverbal cognitively impaired adults are at risk for undertreatment of their postoperative pain. Make these patients a priority to observe, and provide pain relief at the start of your shift and then throughout it. Pain rating scales are available that work well for either of these types of adults with cognitive impairment to rate their pain (see Chapter 10). For the cognitively impaired adult these tools include Faces Pain Scale–Revised (FPS-R) and Iowa Pain Thermometer (IPT). For the nonverbal cognitively impaired adult, there is the Pain Assessment in Advanced Dementia (PAINAD).

Urinary Function

DATA COLLECTION. Monitor the patient's urinary status. The sympathetic nervous system is stimulated by the surgical experience. Fluid is saved by reducing urine output. Initially, urine output may be reduced and concentrated. Then it should gradually increase and become less concentrated and lighter in color. If present, ensure that the urinary catheter is functioning properly. Note the amount, color, and consistency of the urine. If no catheter is present, monitor for the patient's first postoperative voiding within 6 to 8 hours of their last preoperative voiding or last catheterization. Patients having urinary or gynecological procedures may have a surgeon's order to monitor that they void within 4 to 6 hours. If the patient does not void by the set time, the bladder should be palpated for distention and a bladder scan may be ordered to determine the amount of urine in the bladder.

Restlessness can be a sign of a full bladder. A distended bladder requires intervention to promote voiding and prevent increased pressure on the surgical site. Straight catheterization may be needed if the patient is unable to void. Inserting an indwelling urinary catheter is the last option because of the risk of infection and delirium in older patients. Epidural anesthesia and opioids may cause urinary retention. Evidence also suggests that age, obesity, chronic urologic conditions, and the type of surgery performed can predict postoperative urinary retention (Abdul-Muhsin et al, 2020). After outpatient surgery, patients may be required to void before discharge.

CLINICAL JUDGMENT

Mrs. Wood, age 42, returns to the surgical unit after a hysterectomy. Her postoperative vital signs and data collection findings are normal. Mrs. Wood rates her pain level at 9 out of 10, and the nurse notes that she moans occasionally, repeatedly moves her legs, and pulls at her covers near her abdominal incision. She is drowsy but repeatedly says it hurts. In the PACU, a PCA pump was started. The last dose of medication was delivered 45 minutes ago. Her family is at her bedside trying to talk to her about her experience.

1. What nonverbal pain cues do you find Mrs. Wood is displaying?
2. How do you document Mrs. Wood's pain?
3. What action do you take to relieve Mrs. Wood's pain?
4. When will you next monitor Mrs. Wood's pain level?
5. If Mrs. Wood indicates that her pain remains unrelieved with the PCA pump, what action will you take?
6. Which team members do you collaborate with?
7. What action do you take to support the needs of the patient and family?

Suggested answers are at the end of the chapter.

CLINICAL JUDGMENT

Mrs. Owens returned from a bowel resection 2 days ago. She is receiving 1,000 mL of 0.9% normal saline solution over 10 hours on an IV controller pump.

1. You verify that the IV controller pump is set at what rate?
2. How many milliliters do you record as Mrs. Owens's total intake for the last 12 hours?
   - Intake for 12 hours:
   - 8 oz coffee
   - 4 oz orange juice
   - 6 oz tomato soup
   - 3/4 cup gelatin
   - 2 cups of water
   - 1,200 mL of 0.9% normal saline solution IV
   - Output for 12 hours:
   - 1,700 mL of urine

Suggested answers are at the end of the chapter.

NURSING DIAGNOSES, PLANNING, AND IMPLEMENTATION

Risk for Urinary Retention related to surgery, pain, anesthesia, and altered positioning

EXPECTED OUTCOME: The patient will regularly and completely empty bladder.

- Measure and record output and urine characteristics of postoperative patient, especially for those having urological surgery, older patients, or those with an IV or urinary catheter *to detect urinary elimination problems such as output of less than 30 mL per hour.*
- Recognize that the patient who is voiding small amounts frequently (30 to 50 mL every 20 to 30 minutes) or who dribbles may have retention overflow and may not be fully emptying the bladder. This pattern may require a postvoid bladder scan to determine residual urine volume and need for catheterization *to empty the bladder and prevent complications.*
- Assist patient to the bathroom or bedside commode and provide privacy after safety is ensured, and allow male patients to stand or sit to urinate *to promote voiding.*
- Use techniques to stimulate voiding for patient who is unable to void to prevent need for catheterizing (e.g., running water, pouring warm water over a female patient's perineum, or drinking a hot beverage) *because catheterization increases the risk of infection.*
- Have patient place feet solidly on the floor to relax the pelvic muscles *to aid voiding.*
- Notify the surgeon if a patient is uncomfortable, has a distended bladder, or has not voided within the specified time frame *to obtain treatment orders.*

EVALUATION. The goal for urinary retention is met if the patient is able to void within specified time frame without pain or complications.

CLINICAL JUDGMENT

Mr. McDonald is a 48-year-old Black male who had a laparoscopic appendectomy at 1300. The hand-off report you received at 1900 included vital signs within normal parameters, pain of 3 out of 10, declined need for analgesic, due to void by 2200, voided 30 mL at 1830 and 20 mL at 1900, has not been out of bed, and tolerated light dinner well. You make your 1930 rounds and find Mr. McDonald alert but drowsy with vital signs unchanged, three bandaged laparoscopic incisions on his right lower abdomen dry with wound edges approximated, abdomen soft, bowel sounds present in all four quadrants, and slight bladder distention. He reports his pain level at 2 out of 10. He is repositioning his feet frequently and rubbing his hands during your data collection and states, "Nothing really hurts, I'm just restless. It must be the unfamiliar bed."

1. What additional data do you collect?
2. What actions do you take to alleviate Mr. McDonald's symptoms?
3. If Mr. McDonald does not empty his bladder on his own, what other data do you collect?
4. You find that Mr. McDonald's bladder contains 800 mL of urine after techniques to promote voiding are not effective, and you notify the surgeon. Develop your ISBARR (communication tool).

Suggested answers are at the end of the chapter.

Surgical Wound Care

An incision is a wound made by the surgeon with a sharp instrument such as a scalpel. A puncture wound is a small opening made to insert a tube or drain. Incisions are closed with sutures, staples (Fig. 12.7), surgical adhesives, or adhesive strips. As the wound heals, sutures or staples may be removed in 7 to 10 days.

> **PRACTICE ANALYSIS TIP**
> **Linking NCLEX-PN® to Practice**
> The LPN/LVN will remove wound sutures or staples.

Wounds can be clean or dirty. Clean wounds are surgical wounds that are not infected. Dirty (contaminated) wounds include accidental wounds or surgical incisions exposed to unsterile conditions. Infected wounds and dirty wounds contain microorganisms from trauma, ruptured organs, or contamination. Necrotic and infected tissue is removed before infected wounds are closed. This is known as **débridement.**

WOUND HEALING. Wound healing occurs in phases (Table 12.8). Wounds can heal by first (primary) intention, second (secondary) intention, and third (tertiary) intention (Fig. 12.8). In first-intention healing, the edges of the wound are approximated with staples or sutures. This usually results in minimal scarring. For second-intention healing, the wound is usually left open. It heals by granulation. Scarring is usually extensive with prolonged healing. For healing by third intention, an infected wound is left open until there is no evidence of infection. Then the wound is surgically closed.

WOUND COMPLICATIONS. Wound problems can include hematoma, infection, dehiscence, and evisceration. A hematoma occurs from bleeding in the wound and into the tissue around the wound. A clot forms from the bleeding. If the clot is large with swelling, the clot may need to be removed by the surgeon.

Infected wounds may be warm, reddened, or tender and have **purulent** drainage (pus). The drainage may have a foul odor. Increased inflammation may put visible tension on the incision and sutures. A fever and elevated white blood cell count may be present. Antibiotics can be used to treat the infection.

Dehiscence and evisceration are serious wound complications (Fig. 12.9). Wound **dehiscence** is the sudden bursting open of a wound's edges. It may be preceded by an increase in serosanguineous drainage. **Evisceration** is the viscera spilling out of the abdomen. The most relevant preoperative factor in wound dehiscence is the presence of infection, and the common postoperative risk factors include abdominal distention, excessive coughing, vomiting, and constipation (Chun et al, 2018). Increasing age, hypoalbuminemia, emergency surgery, cancer, and steroids have been shown to raise the risk of dehiscence (Rosen & Manna, 2020). To help prevent dehiscence and evisceration, support the wound during coughing and other activities that pull on the incision. Applying an abdominal binder can help reduce risk. If evisceration occurs, the patient may report that "something let loose" or "gave way," or "my gown is all wet." Pain and vomiting may occur. See "Be Safe!" for nursing actions to take.

> **BE SAFE!**
> **ACT FAST!** If dehiscence or evisceration occurs:
> - Position the patient in low Fowler position with knees flexed.
> - Cover the wound with sterile dressings or clean towels moistened with warm sterile normal saline. Apply very gentle pressure.
> - Notify the surgeon immediately of this surgical emergency.
> - Remain with the patient. Keep the patient still and calm.
> - Monitor vital signs and for evidence of shock (e.g., tachycardia, tachypnea, hypotension). Note dyspnea. Report abnormal findings to surgeon immediately.
> - Infuse IV fluids as ordered.
> - Prepare the patient for immediate surgery for cleaning and closure of the wound.

For dehisced surgical incisions that resist healing, vacuum-assisted closure (VAC) aids in healing the incision and other wounds (see Chapter 54).

> **CUE RECOGNITION 12.2**
> You hear a patient who is 2 days post-op after a colectomy cry out, "Oh no! I split open." You find the patient sitting on the bedside holding their wet abdomen with visible intestines protruding. What action do you take?
>
> *Suggested answers are at the end of the chapter.*

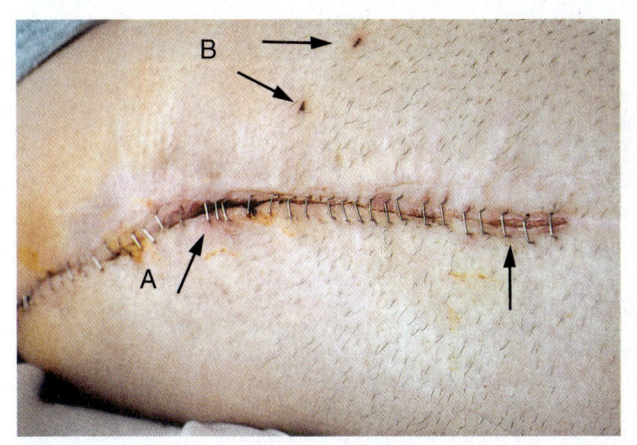

FIGURE 12.7 A stapled incision. (A) Note wound edges not approximated at arrows. (B) Arrows indicate puncture sites where drains were inserted.

• WORD • BUILDING •

evisceration: e—out + viscera—body organs

Table 12.8
Wound Healing Phases

Phase	Time Frame	Wound Healing	Patient Effect
I	Incision to second postoperative day	Inflammatory response	Fever, malaise
II	Third to 14th postoperative day	Granulation tissue forms	Feeling better
III	Third to sixth postoperative week	Collagen deposited	Raised scar formed
IV	Months to 1 year	Wound contracts and heals	Flat, thin scar

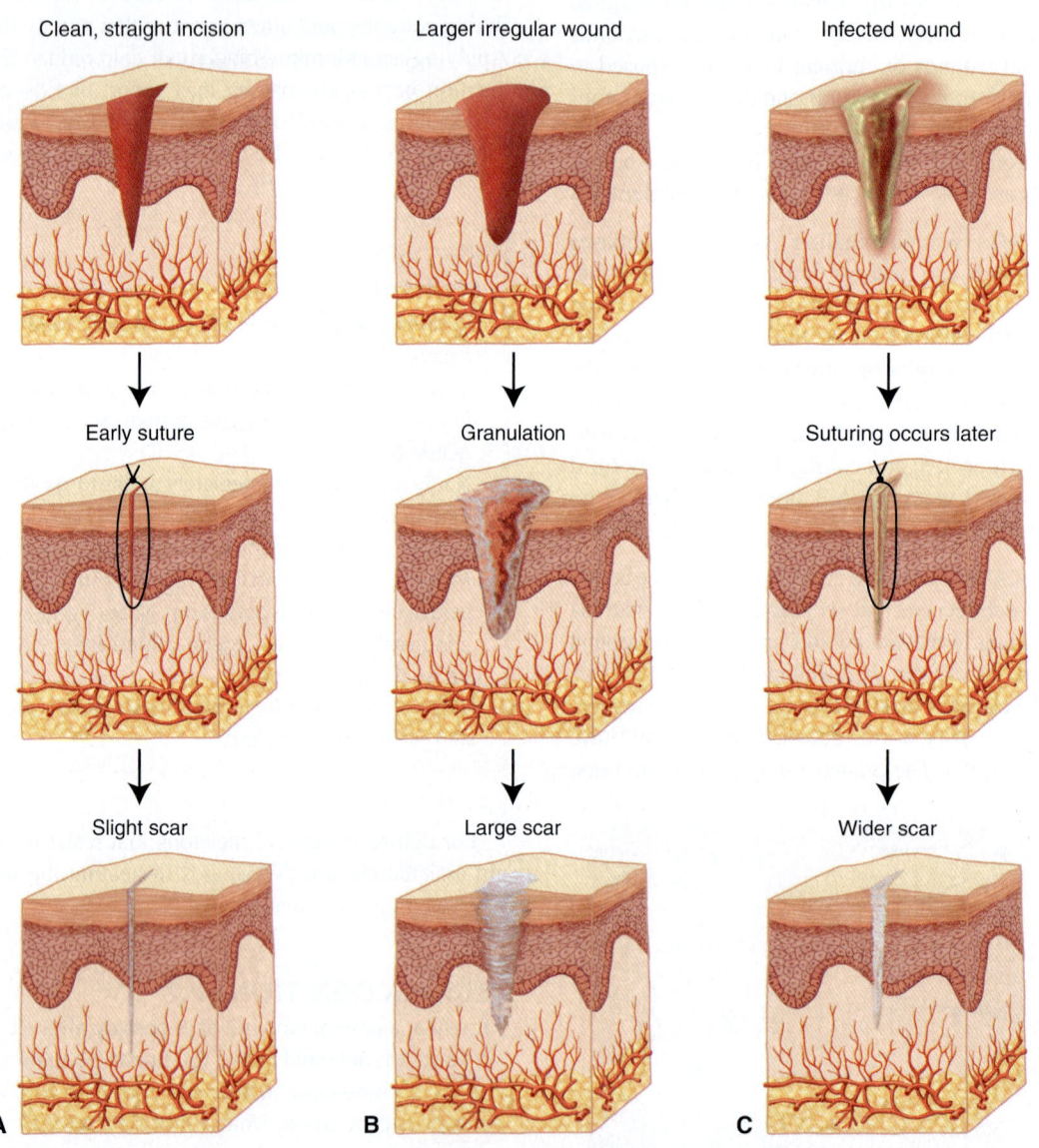

FIGURE 12.8 Wound healing. (A) Primary intention. Wound healing occurs in a clean wound, such as a surgical wound, for which edges are approximated, typically with staples or sutures. Healing occurs quickly with slight scarring. (B) Secondary intention. Large irregular or infected wounds are left open to allow healing to occur from the inside out. Pressure injuries or chronic wounds are often treated this way. Large scarring occurs with lengthy healing time. (C) Tertiary intention. Infected or contaminated wound is left open for a brief time period until wound is clean. Granulation tissue fills in for some wound healing, and then edges are approximated and closed surgically. Wider scarring occurs.

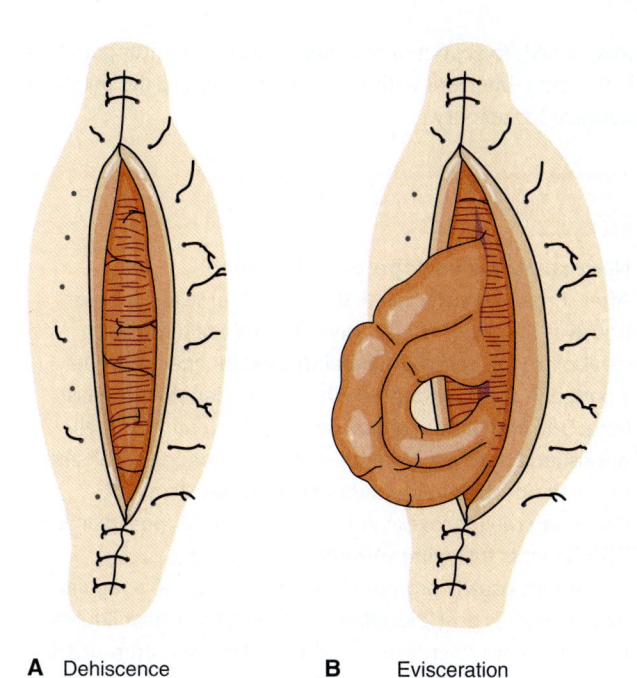

Chapter 12 Nursing Care of Patients Having Surgery

A Dehiscence   **B** Evisceration

FIGURE 12.9 (A) Wound dehiscence. (B) Wound evisceration.

DATA COLLECTION

Dressings. Dressings protect the wound, absorb drainage, prevent contamination from body fluids, and provide comfort. They can also apply pressure to reduce swelling or bleeding as in a pressure dressing. The initial dressing is applied in surgery. It can be removed as soon as 24 hours postoperatively by the surgeon or surgical physician assistant. If drainage appears on the initial dressing, reinforce it with another dressing. Follow the surgeon's dressing prescription and/or institution policy. Some dressings can remain in place until they are saturated or there are signs of infection.

After the initial dressing is removed, if the wound is dry and the edges intact (approximated), the surgeon can order the wound to be left uncovered. This allows easy observation of the wound and avoidance of applying tape to the skin. Draining wounds are dressed with several layers. They are changed as needed. When the old dressing is removed, it should be done carefully to prevent dislodging of tubes or drains. The condition of the wound is documented with each dressing change. It is normal for the incision to be puffy and red from the inflammatory response. The surrounding skin should be the patient's normal color and skin temperature without increased warmth. Correctly apply tape by gently laying it over the dressing and applying even pressure on each side of the wound. Pressure should not be applied on top of the wound by pulling on the tape from one side of the wound to the other side.

Drains. Drains may be inserted near the surgical area to prevent accumulation of fluid that could lead to infection or delayed healing. Drains may work by gravity (passive) or negative pressure (active; suction). Penrose drains are passive, soft, flat drains. Moderate, pink, **serosanguineous** (consisting of blood and **serous** fluid) drainage is expected from a Penrose drain. These drains may require frequent dressing changes. Active drains use suction to remove drainage. They include the Jackson-Pratt and Hemovac drains. These drains are closed systems. They may require periodic emptying. Be careful to keep them sterile when emptying them. Drain use is controversial as complications such as infection can occur.

Output is recorded when drainage is emptied. The amount of drainage expected varies with the type of surgery. Be alert for excessive amounts to report. Specialized drainage systems allow the transfusion of drainage containing blood back to the patient (autotransfusion). This maintains hemoglobin levels without the risks associated with blood transfusions (Chapter 27).

> **PRACTICE ANALYSIS TIP**
> **Linking NCLEX-PN® to Practice**
> The LPN/LVN will:
> - Provide care for client drainage device (e.g., wound drain).
> - Assist with client wound drainage device removal.

NURSING DIAGNOSES, PLANNING, AND IMPLEMENTATION

Risk for Surgical Site Infection related to contamination, immunosuppression, invasive procedure

See "Nursing Care Plan for the Postoperative Patient."

Gastrointestinal Function

Nutritional intake and bowel function can be affected by preoperative preps (NPO, bowel prep) surgery and anesthesia. After abdominal surgery, peristalsis, bowel sounds, and flatus usually stop (paralytic ileus). This may last for 24 to 72 hours. Flatus, bowel movements, and an appetite signal the return of gastrointestinal (GI) function. Interventions to shorten time of ileus include the following:

- Alvimopan (Entereg), which is a gut motility stimulator that promotes postsurgical bowel recovery after partial small or large bowel resections
- Early ambulation as ordered
- Chewing gum
- Early feeding as ordered
- Avoidance of NG tubes, as complications and delayed feeding can occur

DATA COLLECTION. After abdominal surgery, monitor for the return of flatus and appetite, first bowel movement, nausea or vomiting, or signs of paralytic ileus. Paralytic ileus signs are distention, bloating, and cramps. Document the abdomen as being soft or firm and flat or distended. Measure the patient's abdominal girth if distention occurs. Report abnormal findings to the surgeon.

• WORD • BUILDING •

serosanguineous: sero—whey + sanguineous—bloody

Traditionally, after GI surgery, bowel sounds were monitored by the nurse. The patient was kept NPO until flatus and bowel sounds returned. It is now known that bowel sounds are not correlated with bowel motility and the patient's ability to safely drink and eat postoperatively. In fact, patients can be hydrated and fed early, which promotes healing and faster recovery. Follow your institutions' policy if monitoring bowel sounds is required.

CUE RECOGNITION 12.3

The surgeon's orders for a patient who had a colectomy are NPO with IV fluids and an NG tube to low intermittent suction to be irrigated prn. The patient reports stomach pressure and nausea with a need to vomit. What action do you take?

Suggested answers are at the end of the chapter.

NURSING DIAGNOSES, PLANNING, AND IMPLEMENTATION

Imbalanced Nutrition: Less Than Body Requirements related to NPO, pain, and nausea

EXPECTED OUTCOME: The patient will resume normal dietary intake and maintain weight within normal limits.

- Maintain IV fluids, enteral feedings, or parenteral nutrition *until the patient resumes oral intake* ("Nutrition Notes: Nourishing the Postoperative Patient").
- Give antiemetics promptly as ordered *to control nausea and vomiting.*

Risk for Constipation related to decreased peristalsis, immobility, altered diet, and opioid side effect

EXPECTED OUTCOME: The patient will return to normal bowel elimination patterns within 3 to 4 days postoperatively.

- Monitor elimination and document *to detect problems.*
- Encourage early ambulation and exercise *to promote restoration of GI function.*
- Provide stool softeners or laxatives as ordered *to prevent constipation.*

EVALUATION. The goal for imbalanced nutrition is met if the patient is able to maintain the baseline weight and resume a normal dietary intake. The goal for constipation is met if the patient is free from discomfort and establishes a regular bowel elimination pattern.

Mobility

DATA COLLECTION. It is important for the patient to move as much as possible to prevent complications, promote healing, and regain their preoperative level of function. Pain, incisions, tubes, drains, dressings, and other equipment may make movement difficult. Determine the patient's ability to move in bed, to get out of bed, and to walk. Monitor pain levels that may interfere with movement. Observe the patient's tolerance for activity.

Nutrition Notes

Nourishing the Postoperative Patient

After surgery, 5% glucose in 0.45% normal saline intravenously is commonly prescribed. This is done to prevent catabolism (muscle protein being used for energy) while a patient is fasting. However, this prevention does not last long. One liter of this solution contains 170 calories. Well-nourished adults may tolerate not eating for up to 2 weeks, but malnourished adults should be fed early to avoid impacting their recovery. Advocate for a nutritional plan for your patients following surgery.

Patients usually progress from clear liquids to a regular diet as soon as possible. Offer water first, then clear liquids to see patient's tolerance. If "diet as tolerated" is prescribed, the patient should be asked, "What sounds good to eat?" Offering a full dinner when the patient doesn't feel well may "turn off" the appetite.

After GI surgery, if specific amounts of intake are prescribed, those limits should be strictly implemented to preserve the suture lines. After oral and throat surgery, no red liquids are given. This is so vomitus is not mistaken for blood.

NURSING DIAGNOSES, PLANNING, AND IMPLEMENTATION

Impaired Bed Mobility related to environmental constraints, insufficient muscle strength, and pain

EXPECTED OUTCOME: The patient will resume normal physical activity.

- Assist or turn patient at least every 2 hours with pillows for support, alternating from supine to side to side if not contraindicated, *to prevent complications and increase circulation and promote lung expansion.*
- If ambulation is not possible, encourage hourly exercises (e.g., deep breathing, range of motion of all joints, and active or passive isometric exercises of the abdominal, gluteal, and leg muscles) while awake *to prevent complications.*
- To prepare the patient to get out of bed, raise the head of the bed slowly, and if dizziness or feeling faint is reported, lower the head of the bed (and monitor orthostatic vital signs if the problem continues) *to let the circulatory system adjust to the position change slowly.*
- Allow patient to sit on the side of bed prior to standing and pedal the feet to "wake up" the muscles controlling the arteries *to prepare for ambulation* (see Fig. 12.6).
- Ensure patient wears nonslip footwear *to ambulate safely.*
- If a patient tolerates sitting, assist the patient to ambulate *to promote healing and reduce complications.* To rise, the patient should keep eyes forward and move slowly

until feeling adjusted to being up. Usually, the patient ambulates a short distance the first time and increases the distance as tolerated. One or two health-care workers should assist the patient and use a gait (walking) belt for safety. Walkers with wheels and seats also may be used for support and for resting if the patient becomes dizzy or tired. If the patient feels faint or dizzy or if vital signs change, help the patient back to bed. A wheelchair may be needed for safe transport back to the room.

EVALUATION. The goal for impaired physical mobility is met if the patient can increase ambulation and resume normal activities.

Postoperative Patient Discharge

Discharge planning begins during preadmission testing. It is ongoing after admission. This ensures a timely discharge.

Ambulatory Surgery

DISCHARGE CRITERIA. Usually, a patient is a candidate for discharge 1 hour after surgery if the PACU discharge scoring system or clinical discharge criteria are met (see Box 12.4). Clinical discharge criteria include stable vital signs, no bleeding, no nausea or vomiting, and controlled pain that is not severe. For certain surgical procedures (e.g., urological, gynecological, or hernia surgery), the patient may be required to void before discharge. The patient should also be able to sit up without dizziness. Patients meeting discharge criteria are discharged by the surgeon. They are released to a responsible adult. Patients are not allowed to drive themselves home because of the effects of anesthesia and medications.

DISCHARGE INSTRUCTIONS. Patients and their families are given written discharge instructions. The caregiver of an older patient should participate in the discharge instruction session. This promotes understanding for care and reporting of complications. The instruction form is signed by the patient or an authorized representative to indicate understanding. Ensure prescriptions have been ordered and a copy of the instructions sent with the patient. Encourage the patient to rest for 24 to 48 hours. Instruct the patient to avoid operating machinery, driving, drinking alcoholic beverages, and making major decisions for 24 hours. The effects of surgery and anesthesia can alter energy levels and thinking ability. The surgeon will order fluid, dietary, activity, or work restrictions.

Patients are taught wound care, medication information (including side effects), and complications to report to the surgeon. Phone numbers for the surgeon, surgical facility, and emergency care are provided. Patients are encouraged to call on the day of discharge to make a follow-up appointment with the surgeon to ensure appropriate scheduling. A follow-up phone call is usually made by a nurse to the patient the next day to check the patient's status and answer any patient or caregiver questions.

Inpatient Surgery

DISCHARGE CRITERIA. The surgeon determines the patient's readiness for discharge from the hospital. Before discharge, complete data collection of the patient is performed and documented.

DISCHARGE INSTRUCTIONS. Patients and families are taught wound care, medication information, and signs and symptoms of complications to report to the surgeon. The surgeon orders fluid, dietary, activity, or work restrictions and the date for a follow-up office visit. A copy of the signed written instructions is given to the patient. Prescriptions are usually sent electronically to the pharmacy for pick-up. If further teaching or reinforcement is needed, a referral to a home health-care nurse can be requested through the case manager.

> **PRACTICE ANALYSIS TIP**
> Linking NCLEX-PN® to Practice
> The LPN/LVN will:
> - Participate in client discharge or transfer.
> - Follow up with client after discharge.

> **Home Health Hints**
> A referral for home health care is made when the patient who had surgery needs skilled nursing care at home after discharge. (See Chapter 16 for examples of skilled care.) When the patient returns home, the home health-care nurse can provide the following guidance to caregivers for setting up the living area, bathroom, and equipment the patient will use:
> - It is helpful if the bedroom can be on the same floor as the bathroom and kitchen.
> - Lift sheets made of folded twin sheets are needed as well as extra pillows for positioning and splinting.
> - A bedside stand or TV tray table can be used for personal care items.
> - A bedside commode can be placed near the bed if the patient cannot walk to the bathroom. A bedpan or urinal may be needed.
> - A handheld shower is convenient and allows the patient more independence in bathing.
> - Installation of grab bars and tub chairs as well as skid-proofing of a shower or tub are important safety measures to help prevent falls. Physical or occupational therapy can make specific recommendations.
> - For the patient prescribed anticoagulants and/or compression stockings, their importance and instructions for correctly using them to prevent DVT should be reinforced.
> - Nutritional status should be monitored and reported to the RN to aid wound healing.
> - The patient and caregivers should be instructed on hand hygiene before and after personal care and wound care to prevent infection.
> - Medication regime, prescribed pain medication, pain management, and potential side effects to report should be discussed.

Key Points

- There are three defined phases in the surgical process: preoperative, intraoperative, and postoperative. Perioperative includes all the phases before, during, and after surgery.
- Factors that can influence surgical outcomes include alcohol and/or drug abuse, chronic disease, emotional responses, nutrition, and smoking.
- The primary role of the LPN/LVN in the preoperative phase is to assist in data collection, contribute to the patient's plan of care, reinforce teaching and instructions given to the patient and family by the surgeon and RN, and provide emotional and psychological support for patients and families.
- Nonemergent surgical patients have a preoperative assessment that includes an interview with the anesthesiologist or a preadmission telephone or face-to-face interview with the preadmission RNs. This includes a health history, identification of risk factors, patient and family teaching, discharge planning, and necessary referrals to social workers, support groups, and educational programs. Personal or family problems with anesthesia or malignant hyperthermia are also identified.
- It may be your role to obtain and witness the patient's or authorized person's signature on the consent form. As the patient's advocate, ensure that the person signing the consent form understands its meaning. Ensure that the patient has no further questions to be directed to the surgeon and that the consent form is being signed voluntarily. If the patient is unable to read, read the entire consent form to the patient before it is signed.
- When presenting preoperative information to older patients, sit in front of patients and speak slowly in a low tone. Ensure patient's glasses and hearing aids are worn. Allow for increased response time. Use memory aids (pictures or diagrams). Cover most important information first and present one idea at a time. Review important content. Obtain feedback. Provide positive reinforcement.
- Interventions to promote recovery are implemented in the postoperative phase. In addition to monitoring for respiratory depression, hemorrhage, and shock and providing postoperative care, the nurse reinforces teaching to patients and their family/caregivers and assists with necessary referrals, including home health care.
- Surgical incision complications can include hematoma, infection, dehiscence, or evisceration.
- Clinical discharge criteria for ambulatory surgery include stable vital signs, no bleeding, no nausea or vomiting with oral intake, and controlled pain that is not severe. For certain urological, gynecological, or hernia surgeries, the patient may need to void before discharge. The patient should also be able to sit up without dizziness and ambulate safely (if appropriate).
- Patients meeting ambulatory surgery discharge criteria are discharged to a responsible adult. Patients are not allowed to drive home because of effects of anesthesia and medications.
- Nursing interventions are evaluated as being effective if the patient's collected data is within normal parameters and complications do not develop.
- A referral for home health care is made when the patient who had surgery needs skilled nursing care at home after discharge.

SUGGESTED ANSWERS TO CHAPTER EXERCISES

Cue Recognition

12.1: Direct the technician to return the patient to his room, identify whether the patient is withdrawing his consent for surgery, and notify the surgeon.

12.2: Assist the patient to immediately lie down, and instruct them to lie still and not cough. Cover the dehisced and eviscerated wound with sterile normal saline–moistened dressings as the HCP is notified of this surgical emergency. Remain with the patient for safety and emotional support.

12.3: Confirm the NG tube is connected to a working wall suction and is patent (not compressed, kinked, or clogged). Confirm NG tube placement by checking pH of tube aspirate following agency policy, irrigate NG tube per orders, and administer antiemetic medication if needed.

Clinical Judgment & Critical Thinking
Mrs. Wood

1. Moaning occasionally, moving legs restlessly, and pulling covers near abdominal incision are nonverbal pain cues.
2. Document pain levels by actual observations: occasional moaning, restless leg movements, and pulling of covers near abdominal incision. Also use the patient's statement: "It hurts." Because Mrs. Wood is too drowsy to use the pain scale, other data are used. When Mrs. Wood is more awake, explanation of the pain scale should be reinforced and used.
3. Encourage patient to use PCA button if there is pain. Reinforce teaching on the PCA pump as able. Administer additional multimodality medications as ordered. Also, consider other pain relief measures, such as patient

SUGGESTED ANSWERS TO CHAPTER EXERCISES—cont'd

warmth and positioning as well as environmental issues such as bright lighting, room temperature, and noise.

4. After the PCA pump is pushed by the patient, monitor pain level in at least 30 minutes to determine pain relief. If Mrs. Wood is asleep, she should not be awakened unless it is necessary. Nonverbal cues should be observed. Count respirations and document. After Mrs. Wood is more alert, PCA monitoring is done hourly or per agency policy.
5. Document pain rating level such as on a scale of 0 to 10. Collaborate with the surgeon for report of inadequate pain relief.
6. Collaborate with the surgeon, pharmacist, and clergy to offer support to family and with nursing team members and case manager for discharge planning.
7. Introduce yourself to the family and explain that you will answer their questions about the patient's general status within limits of patient HIPAA rights so that the patient who is in pain may rest. Explain PCA function and that only the patient is to push the button. Explain that you are monitoring the patient's pain and your goal is for the patient to report pain is relieved within 30 minutes. As the patient's advocate, encourage family to either sit quietly at the bedside while the patient is sleeping or in the waiting room if they would be more comfortable, and assure them that you will let them know when the patient awakens. Ask if they would like to speak with clergy. Offer or direct them to beverages and snacks.

Mrs. Owens

1. 100 mL per hour. IV pumps are always set to deliver the number of milliliters per hour. Divide the total volume of 1,000 mL by the total time of 10 hours = 100 mL per hour.
2. Intake = 2,400 mL

   To calculate this, remember these conversions:
   30 mL = 1 oz; 1 cup = 8 oz

   Calculations:
   8 oz cup of coffee = 8×30 = 240 mL
   4 oz orange juice = 4×30 = 120 mL
   6 oz tomato soup = 6×30 = 180 mL
   3/4 cup gelatin = $3/4 \times 8 \times 30$ = 180 mL
   2 cups of water = $2 \times 8 \times 30$ = 480 mL
   1,200 mL of 0.9 normal saline IV

   The patient's output does not affect the intake total, so it is not used for this calculation.

Mr. McDonald

1. Review I&O and voiding record.
2. Run water audibly at sink, offer a hot beverage, assist to sit or stand to attempt voiding.
3. Bladder volume obtained with a bladder scan per policy.
4. Sample ISBARR: **I**: This is Dylan LVN. **S**: I am calling about Mr. McDonald in 612. **B**: He had a laparoscopic appendectomy at 1300 today. **A**: He is very restless. I am not sure why. His vital signs remain normal, pain is 2 on a scale of 0 to 10, he declined analgesics, voided 30 mL at 1830 and 20 mL at 1900, was due to void by 2200, and his bladder scan volume is 800 mL. **R**: Techniques to assist voiding were unsuccessful. I think a straight catheterization is needed based on the 800 mL bladder scan results. **R**: To restate your order: Straight catheterize one time now. Check residual bladder volume after each voiding for 12 hours and call if greater than 100 mL.

Additional Resources

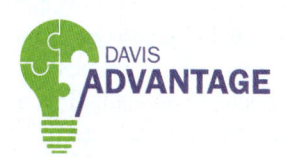

Go to Davis Advantage to complete your learning: strengthen understanding, apply your knowledge, and prepare for the Next Gen NCLEX®.

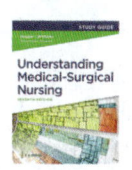

A Study Guide is also available.

CHAPTER 13
Nursing Care of Patients With Emergent Conditions and Disaster/Bioterrorism Response

Raja Issa

KEY TERMS

abrasion (ah-BRAY-zhun)
amputation (am-pew-TAY-shun)
anthrax (AN-thraks)
asphyxia (as-FIX-ee-ah)
bioterrorism (BY-oh-TARE-UR-is-um)
botulism (BOTCH-uh-liz-um)
cardiac tamponade (KAR-dee-yak TAM-pon-AYD)
flail chest (FLAYL CHEST)
gastric lavage (GAS-trik la-VAHJ)
laceration (las-ur-AY-shun)
plague (PLAYG)
shock (SHAWK)
tachycardia (TAK-ih-KAR-dee-yah)
tachypnea (TAK-ip-NEE-ah)
tetanus (TET-nus)
triage (TREE-ahj)

CHAPTER CONCEPTS

Cognition
Comfort
Fluid and electrolytes
Health-care systems
Infection
Intracranial regulation
Oxygenation
Perfusion
Stress and coping
Thermoregulation
Tissue integrity

LEARNING OUTCOMES

1. Explain the components of the primary survey.
2. Plan nursing interventions for a trauma victim.
3. Identify the symptoms and care for an inhalation injury.
4. Describe the stages of hypothermia.
5. Describe the stages of hyperthermia.
6. Explain the priorities of care for poison overdose.
7. Describe the role of the LPN/LVN in disaster response.
8. Discuss bioterrorist agents and subsequent care if exposed or infected.

EMERGENT CONDITIONS

Upon arrival in the emergency department (ED), most patients are **triaged** by a registered nurse (RN; Fig. 13.1). The ability to recognize an emergent condition is essential in nursing to prioritize life-saving care. This chapter presents common emergent conditions with application of the nursing process.

PRIMARY SURVEY

An initial assessment is conducted to identify the patient's general status and recognize life-threatening conditions to determine priorities of care in critically ill or injured patients. To quickly determine if the patient is alert, an assessment tool such as the AVPU scale can be used: alert (A), responds to verbal stimuli (V), responds to an applied painful stimulus (P), or is unresponsive to all stimuli (U). Then using an organized approach following an A, B, C type format, an assessment is conducted (U.S. National Library of Medicine, 2020).

A—Airway

If the patient is alert or responsive, have the patient open their mouth to inspect the airway. If the patient is not alert or unable to open their mouth, the jaw-thrust maneuver rather than the chin-lift maneuver must be used (Fig. 13.2). The neck should not be hyperextended, flexed, or rotated until a spinal injury is ruled out. The airway should be checked for obstruction caused by the tongue, loose or missing teeth, blood, emesis, edema, or foreign objects. If the airway is partially or completely obstructed, intervention is needed to keep it patent and open.

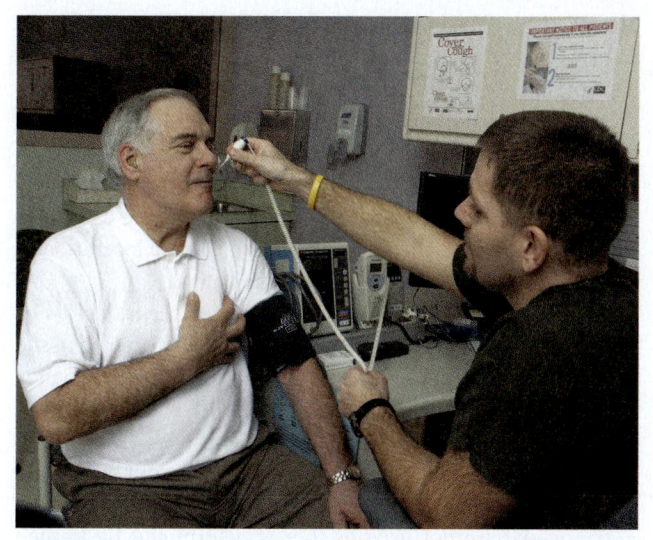

FIGURE 13.1 Triage nurse evaluating patient who has just arrived in the emergency department.

These interventions include foreign object removal, oropharyngeal suctioning, oropharyngeal or nasopharyngeal airway insertion, supraglottic airway insertion (laryngeal mask airway), retroglottic airway insertion (laryngeal tube airway), endotracheal intubation, cricothyroidotomy (needle or surgical). These airway interventions are performed by specially trained emergency personnel or health-care providers (HCPs).

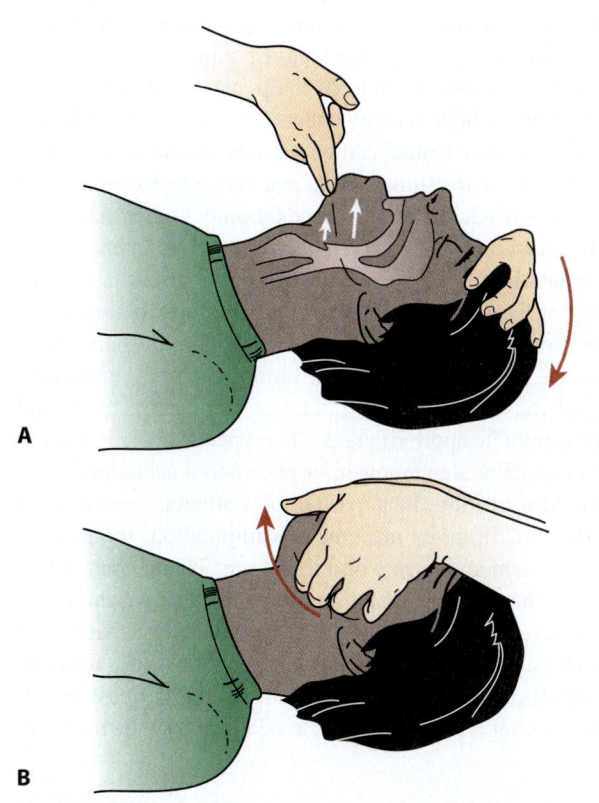

FIGURE 13.2 (A) Chin-lift maneuver is used to open the airway. (B) Jaw-thrust maneuver is used to open the airway if the patient might have a head or neck injury.

B—Breathing

After the airway is opened, the patient is checked for spontaneous breathing and respiratory rate and depth, the rise and fall of the chest for symmetry, the use of accessory muscles, and any open chest wounds. Breath sounds are auscultated bilaterally. If spontaneous respirations are present and the patient is alert, potential interventions include patient positioning, supplemental oxygen as indicated, or bilevel continuous positive airway pressure (BiPAP). If respirations are absent or abnormal, the patient can be ventilated with a mouth-to-face mask or a bag-valve face mask. For an unconscious patient, endotracheal intubation is the preferred method of establishing and maintaining an airway (see Fig. 29.27). This protects the lungs from aspiration.

C—Circulation

A central pulse (carotid or femoral) is palpated for quality and rate. The skin is checked for warmth, color, and moisture. External bleeding is controlled by external pressure. If bleeding of the extremities is not controllable by direct pressure, elevation or possibly applying a tourniquet as a last resort is considered. Life-threatening conditions like internal bleeding, shock, or burns are noted as they can compromise circulation. Large-gauge intravenous (IV) cannulas (16- or 18-gauge) are inserted for fluid resuscitation. If a pulse can be palpated, vital signs are taken and recorded. If the patient does not have a pulse, cardiac compressions are started.

D—Disability/Central Nervous System

A brief neurologic assessment is conducted using the Glasgow Coma Scale (GCS) to detect any central nervous system injury. GCS scoring quantifies the level of impaired consciousness based on three components: best motor response + best verbal response + eye-opening = GCS score (see "Nursing Process for the Patient Experiencing Trauma").

E—Exposure

To allow for a complete visual assessment, clothing must be removed. Respect the patient's dignity as this is done. Keep the patient covered to reduce heat loss and prevent shivering. Look for injuries, any uncontrolled bleeding, other signs of illness, and medical alert jewelry.

SECONDARY SURVEY

For victims of severe trauma, a secondary survey is conducted. This identifies areas of injury or medical problems that are not life-threatening but do require treatment. Major body areas that can sustain serious injury are quickly examined to detect additional injuries (Table 13.1). These include the head, spine, chest, abdomen, and musculoskeletal system. Each major body area is inspected and palpated. Deformity, bruising, open wounds, bleeding, and pain are noted.

Table 13.1 Components of the Secondary Survey

Head	Inspect for lacerations, bleeding from orifices. Check pupil size and response to light. Are pupils equal in size?
Chest	Auscultate for breath sounds in all lung fields. Inspect for lacerations, wounds, and foreign bodies.
Abdomen	Auscultate for bowel sounds in all four quadrants. Palpate for areas of tenderness and rigidity. Inspect for lacerations, wounds, and foreign bodies. Inspect for ecchymosis (bruising).
Extremities	Inspect for lacerations, wounds, and foreign bodies. Inspect for injuries and deformities. Note areas of tenderness. Palpate for pulses. Evaluate temperature and capillary refill and compare the left to the right extremities.

SHOCK

Shock is a condition of progressively decreasing blood pressure (see Chapter 9). It results in inadequate tissue perfusion. There are four types of shock. Hypovolemic shock signs and symptoms are caused by a decrease in the circulating blood volume. Cardiogenic shock signs and symptoms result from cardiac failure. Obstructive shock is caused by a blockage of blood flow in the cardiovascular circuit outside the heart. Distributive shock is caused by excessive dilation of the venules and arterioles.

Anaphylactic shock is a form of distributive shock. **Anaphylaxis** is the response to a severe allergic reaction that can progress to anaphylactic shock (see Chapters 9, 19). Signs of severe anaphylaxis include respiratory distress with wheezing, stridor and cyanosis due to airway constriction and fluid, hypotension due to vasodilation, and decreased level of consciousness due to decreased oxygenation. Immediate treatment with epinephrine is needed. Antihistamines, steroids, and oxygen may also be given.

MAJOR TRAUMA

Mechanism of Injury

It is important to determine the mechanism of injury for a victim of major trauma ("Gerontological Issues: Injuries Caused by Falls Versus Battery or Assault"). Injuries are classified as either penetrating or blunt. Penetrating (open) injuries can be caused by a sharp object (e.g., broken glass or a knife) or by projectiles traveling at high speed (e.g., bullets or fragments from an explosion). In blunt (closed) injuries, the skin surface is intact. An injury from blunt trauma may extend beyond the point of impact to surrounding and underlying structures. For example, a blow to the chest can cause rib fractures. These fractures could then cause a laceration or hematoma (collection of blood) of the spleen.

Damage caused by a gunshot wound and the trajectory of the bullet depends on the projectile mass, the type of tissue struck, the striking velocity, and the range. Entrance wounds are round or oval. They can be surrounded by a rim of abrasion. Powder burns are visible if the firearm was discharged at close range. Documentation of these wounds should include a clear description of their appearance. The words *entry* or *exit* are not used as that is determined by trained experts. Patients with gunshot wounds near the level of the diaphragm are evaluated for both abdominal and thoracic injuries.

Surface Trauma

Surface trauma includes closed wounds (skin intact) and open wounds (skin open). Closed wounds include contusions (bruising) and hematomas. Open wounds include abrasions, punctures, lacerations, avulsions, and amputations.

Abrasions are a scraping away of the epidermal and dermal layers of the skin. They bleed very little but can be extremely painful because of inflamed nerve endings. Dirt can become ground into abrasions. This increases the risk of infection, especially for large areas of skin.

Puncture wounds result from sharp, narrow objects such as knives, nails, or high-velocity bullets. They can often be deceptive. The entrance wound can be small with little or no bleeding. It is difficult to estimate the extent of damage to underlying organs as a result. Puncture wounds usually do not bleed profusely unless they are located in the chest or abdomen.

Lacerations are open wounds resulting from snagging or tearing of tissue. Skin can be partly or completely torn away. Lacerations vary in depth and can be irregular in shape. They can cause significant bleeding if blood vessels are involved.

Avulsions involve a full-thickness skin loss. The wound edges cannot be approximated. This type of injury is usually seen in machine, lawnmower, or power-tool accidents.

An **amputation** is a partial or complete severing of a body part. In cases of complete amputation, the arteries usually spasm and retract into the tissue. This results in less bleeding than does a partial amputation, in which the lacerated arteries continue to bleed. If the patient has sustained an amputation, bleeding is controlled with direct pressure and elevation. A tourniquet is applied only as a last resort. If a tourniquet is needed, it should be made of wide material,

• WORD • BUILDING •

anaphylaxis: an—without + phylaxis—protection

such as a blood pressure cuff. The wide material is less damaging to nerves and blood vessels. A dressing is applied to the amputated extremity, which is referred to as the stump. The stump is covered with sterile saline–moistened gauze followed by dry gauze. This is held in place with an elastic bandage for pressure. Amputated parts are sent with the patient for possible reattachment.

At the ED, it is very important and time sensitive to rinse the amputated part with saline solution and wrap it in sterile gauze before placing it in a patient-identified sealed plastic bag. The bag is then placed on ice (do not allow the amputated part to freeze or be submerged in liquid). The goal is to keep the body part cool without causing further damage with ice.

Gerontological Issues

Injuries Caused by Falls Versus Battery or Assault
Older adults are at high risk for falls. A fall can cause bruises, abrasions, cuts, or fractures. After a fall, patients must be evaluated for the reason for the fall and rule out abuse or neglect. Arrhythmias, neurologic, or syncope issues can cause falls.

Injuries related to falls have a predictable injury pattern related to the history and report of the fall. When an older adult attempts to break a fall, there is bruising of the hands and knees. Additional bruising or injuries to the front of the body, arms, and head could be caused by hitting something during the fall. Skin tears on the arms are common with a fall. If someone sees the older adult starting to fall, they may try to steady the person by grabbing the arms, which results in tearing the skin. Ask questions to be sure that the report of the fall incident is consistent with presenting injuries and the injuries are consistent with mechanism of injury.

Any unexplained bruises, burns, abrasions, cuts, fractures, evidence of old injuries or bruises, burns, and cuts that are in different healing stages are suggestive of abuse. The pattern of an injury can also suggest abuse: for example, cigarette burns in areas covered with clothing; bruises or friction burns in a ring around the neck, ankles, or wrists; welts, burns, or bruises in the outline of a hand or belt buckle; multiple similar injuries in an area, such as whip marks across the buttocks or back of the legs; defensive injury pattern of bruising; and trauma to the hands and forearms.

Abuse or the suspicion of abuse must be reported by health-care professionals to a designated state agency for investigation. It is not the nurse's responsibility to prove that there has been abuse or neglect, only to report it.

When a patient is impaled by an object, it is vital that the object is *not* removed unless it is obstructing the airway. Removing an impaled object can cause additional trauma. It can also cause uncontrollable internal bleeding. Impaled objects should never be cut off, broken off, or shortened unless transportation to the ED is otherwise impossible. A bulky dressing is applied around the object to stabilize it and reduce motion.

Tetanus

Tetanus is a disease caused by the bacillus *Clostridium tetani*. Its spores enter the body through an opening in the skin or a wound. The spores produce toxins. The toxins affect the central nervous system by blocking inhibitor impulses. This causes muscle contraction and spasm. The first sign of tetanus may be jaw muscle spasms (lockjaw). Other signs include abdominal rigidity, difficulty swallowing and breathing, painful muscle stiffness, and seizures. Tetanus can cause death in a small percentage of cases. Emergency treatment includes hospitalization, airway maintenance, human tetanus immune globulin (intramuscular), muscle spasm control, wound care, and tetanus toxoid booster. After pediatric tetanus vaccinations are completed, adults 19 and older need one booster shot of the tetanus/diphtheria (Td) vaccine every 10 years as part of their routine vaccine schedule in the absence of an open wound. If a deep cut or a burn occurs, especially if dirty, a booster may be needed earlier.

LEARNING TIP
For any injury, but especially head trauma, it is essential to ask if the patient is taking "blood thinners" such as apixaban (Eliquis), aspirin, heparin, rivaroxaban (Xarelto), or warfarin (Coumadin). Anticoagulants put the patient at higher risk for dangerous bleeding after an injury. There are reversal agents for some of these medications, but not all of them.

Head Trauma

Sharp blows to the head can cause shifting of intracranial contents. This leads to brain tissue contusion. The pathophysiology of head trauma can be divided into two phases. The first phase is the initial injury that cannot be reversed. The second phase involves intracerebral bleeding and edema from the initial injury. This causes increased intracranial pressure (ICP). Management of head trauma is directed at the second phase. It involves decreasing ICP. Early and late signs and symptoms of ICP are listed in Box 13.1.

Spinal Trauma

Spinal cord injury most often results from motor vehicle crashes, sports injuries, falls, and assaults. The cervical spine is especially vulnerable to traumatic injury. All trauma patients should be treated as though they have a spinal cord injury until proven otherwise. Moving a patient with a vertebral injury can displace the injured bones. This can damage the spinal cord. Patients should be moved only by trained

Box 13.1

Signs and Symptoms of Increased Intracranial Pressure

Early Signs and Symptoms
- Headache
- Nausea and vomiting
- Amnesia
- Changes in speech
- Altered level of consciousness or drowsiness

Late Signs and Symptoms
- Dilated nonreactive pupils
- Unresponsiveness
- Abnormal posturing
- Widening pulse pressure
- Decreased pulse rate
- Changes in respiratory pattern

---

professionals. Stabilizing the neck and back with a cervical collar and backboard is essential until a spinal cord injury is ruled out (Fig. 13.3).

> **BE SAFE!**
> **AVOID FAILURE TO RESCUE!** Do not move a patient with suspected vertebral or spinal cord injury. Paramedics, emergency medical technicians, or health-care providers should guide movement of the patient to prevent further injury to the spinal cord.

Chest Trauma

Chest trauma can cause damage to the heart and lungs that can be life-threatening. These injuries include pericardial tamponade, hemothorax, tension pneumothorax, and **flail chest** (condition of chest wall caused by two or more fractures on each affected rib, resulting in a segment of rib that is not attached on either end). Potentially life-threatening injuries can also occur, including pulmonary and myocardial contusion, aortic and tracheobronchial disruption, and diaphragmatic rupture.

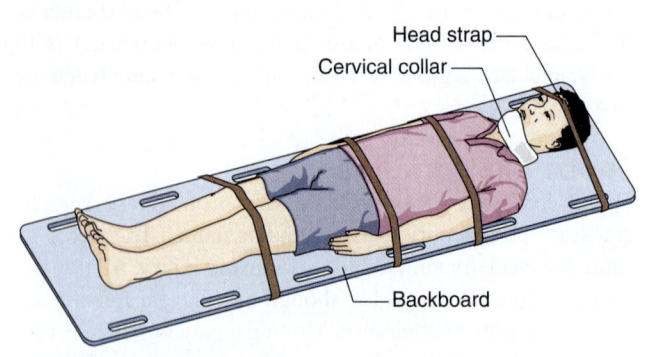

FIGURE 13.3 Immobilization of a patient suspected of having a spinal cord injury using a backboard and cervical collar.

Chest trauma can lacerate lung tissue. Air or blood leaking into the intrapleural space collapses the lung. This results in a pneumothorax (air) or hemothorax (blood). Ineffective ventilation occurs. In a tension pneumothorax, air is trapped in the pleural space during exhalation. This puts pressure on the unaffected lung. The heart, great blood vessels, and trachea shift toward the unaffected side of the chest. Blood flow to and from the heart is greatly reduced. This decreases cardiac output. An uncorrected tension pneumothorax is fatal.

Chest trauma can injure the heart and great blood vessels. It can reduce the amount of circulating blood volume. The heart can be bruised (myocardial contusion) or sustain direct trauma. **Cardiac tamponade** results when blood or fluid accumulates in the pericardial sac. This increases pressure around the heart, preventing its chambers from filling and contracting effectively. A patient with cardiac tamponade will have hypotension, **tachycardia** (rapid heart rate over 100 beats per minute), and jugular vein distention. It requires immediate intervention. Pressure must be reduced in the pericardial sac. This will restore normal filling and contraction of the heart chambers. Cardiac output will then increase.

Abdominal Trauma

The organs of the abdomen are vulnerable to injury. This is because of limited bony protection. Injury to organs such as the spleen and liver, which have a rich blood supply, can result in rapid loss of blood volume and hypovolemic shock. Abdominal organs can be injured from severe blunt or penetrating trauma. If hypotension is present, intra-abdominal hemorrhage may be the cause. If the urinary bladder ruptures, urine leaks into the abdomen and blood may be visible at the urinary meatus and perineum. Penetrating trauma can cause lacerations to abdominal organs. This results in rapid blood loss and hypovolemic shock.

Orthopedic Trauma

Fractured bones can result in blood loss, compromised circulation, infection, and immobility. Unstable pelvic fractures can cause injury to the genitourinary system or disrupt pelvic veins. Fractures of large bones, such as the femur and tibia, can cause significant blood loss. Joint dislocations can cause neurovascular compromise by applying pressure on nerves and blood vessels. Delayed fracture reduction (realignment or setting) can cause avascular necrosis. This leads to death of the affected tissue and bone.

> **LEARNING TIP**
> If a limb is fractured, splint it as it lies to prevent damage to blood vessels and nerves. Collect neurovascular data prior to and after splinting the limb. If the distal circulation is severely compromised, the patient needs immediate medical intervention.

• WORD • BUILDING •
tachycardia: tachy—fast + cardia—heart condition

Nursing Process for the Patient Experiencing Trauma

Data Collection

The mechanism of injury is identified to determine the potential extent of the injury. Loss of consciousness immediately after an injury indicates that a concussion has occurred. The Glasgow Coma Scale (GCS) is used to rate a patient's level of consciousness (see Chapter 47). The highest score is 15. It indicates that the patient is alert and needs only observation. Scores lower than 13 can indicate the need for immediate treatment. Morbidity and mortality are highest for patients with GCS scores of 8 or lower. Pupil size and reaction are monitored and recorded. Dilated or nonreactive pupils indicate increased ICP. This requires immediate intervention. Movement of extremities are also observed and documented. Posturing and differences between limb movement on the right and left side can indicate increased ICP.

Spinal nerves in the spinal cord transmit sensory impulses to the brain. They also send motor impulses to the body. The higher a traumatic injury is on the spinal column, the more extensive the loss of muscle and sensory function (Table 13.2). Identify the patient's level of muscle control and ability to feel each limb. A spinal cord injury at the C5 level or above interferes with diaphragm function and respiratory effort. Respirations must be carefully observed.

Major chest injuries can cause dramatic symptoms. These include classic signs of shock with restlessness, dyspnea, and cyanosis. Monitor the patient's breathing pattern and respirations. Observe the rise and fall of the chest to identify symmetrical chest movement. Any bruising on the chest or upper abdomen is noted. Seat belts and restraint systems can cause significant bruising in high-impact crashes.

Vital signs are taken to detect shock. The shape of the abdomen is observed for distention from intra-abdominal hemorrhage. Skin color, bruising, open wounds, and penetrating trauma are noted. The abdomen is auscultated for bowel sounds. The perineum is inspected for blood from the urethra.

Injured extremities are inspected. Skin integrity, protruding bone, or deformity is noted. Skin color and capillary refill time are noted. Pulses distal to the injury are palpated. This identifies the quality of circulation distal to the injury. Motor function and sensation are checked to determine nerve injury. Respiratory function is monitored to detect a pulmonary embolism from a long bone fracture.

Nursing Diagnoses, Planning, and Implementation

Acute Pain related to tissue trauma

EXPECTED OUTCOME: The patient will experience relief within 30 minutes after measures are provided to relieve pain as evidenced by verbal and nonverbal expressions of pain relief.

- For the affected area, rest it, apply ice and compression, and elevate it as ordered *to decrease swelling and relieve pain.*
- Have patient rate pain using a pain rating scale *to obtain pain data.*
- Provide analgesics as ordered *to relieve pain.*

Ineffective Breathing Pattern related to spinal neck injury or unstable chest wall segment or lung collapse

EXPECTED OUTCOME: The patient will maintain an effective respiratory rate and ABGs within normal parameters.

- If signs of respiratory distress are present, use the jaw-thrust or chin-lift maneuver, along with suction and airway adjuncts as needed, *to maintain patency of the airway.*
- Maintain chest tube drainage system when present *to help re-expand the lung.*

Risk for Bleeding related to trauma

EXPECTED OUTCOME: Patient's bleeding will be controlled to maintain vital signs within normal range for the individual.

- Apply direct pressure to external bleeding site, along with elevation if bleeding site is a limb *to stop the flow of blood and allow normal coagulation to occur.*
- When direct pressure and elevation do not control hemorrhage, pressure-point control should be attempted *to stop the bleeding* (Fig. 13.4). The chosen artery for pressure-point control must be proximal to the injury site and must be over a bony structure.

Risk for Ineffective Cerebral Tissue Perfusion related to cerebral edema

EXPECTED OUTCOME: The patient will maintain adequate cerebral homeostasis without cerebral edema as evidenced by a GCS score of 14 or greater.

Table 13.2
Correlating Spinal Injury With Impairment of Motor Function

Injury Level	Impairment
S3 to S5 or above	Patient unable to tighten anus.
L4 to L5 or above	Patient unable to flex foot and extend toes.
L2 to L4 or above	Patient unable to extend and flex legs.
C5 to C7 or above	Patient unable to extend and flex arms.

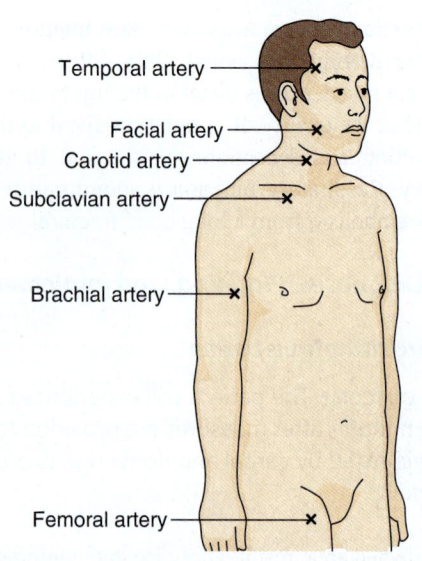

FIGURE 13.4 Arterial pressure points to control bleeding.

- Monitor neurologic checks and GCS score, and report changes *for intervention.*
- Elevate the head of the patient's bed 30 to 45 degrees, as possible, *to reduce ICP.*
- Maintain the patient's head position at midline *to ensure unobstructed venous drainage to help reduce ICP.*
- If the patient is agitated, provide calming measures *because agitation increases ICP.*

Risk for Aspiration related to neck injury

EXPECTED OUTCOME: The patient will maintain clear lung sounds at all times.

- Suction the oropharynx and nasopharynx as needed *to clear secretions and prevent aspiration of secretions into the airway.*
- If the patient vomits, log roll the patient onto one side and use suction as needed *to prevent aspiration of emesis.*

Impaired Physical Mobility related to neck injury or bone injury

EXPECTED OUTCOME: The patient will maintain movement of extremities that was usual for the patient prior to the injury.

- Maintain neck immobility during initial treatment of a patient with head or neck trauma *to prevent serious spinal injury until trauma damage is identified.*
- Monitor skin color, temperature, distal pulses, capillary refill, movement, and sensation of the extremity *to detect abnormalities.*
- Immobilize the joints above and below the affected area using a folded towel or a pillow *to provide comfort and protection until the patient is evaluated by an HCP.*
- Remove all jewelry before application of a splint *to prevent constriction from swelling.*

Decreased Cardiac Output related to compression of heart and great vessels

EXPECTED OUTCOME: The patient will maintain vital signs within normal ranges.

- Monitor the patient's vital signs and oxygen saturation and report if unstable *because the patient may need immediate treatment or surgical intervention in the operating room.*

Deficient Fluid Volume related to hemorrhage or abdominal organ injury

EXPECTED OUTCOME: The patient will maintain vital signs within baseline ranges.

- Monitor for signs of shock *to detect hypovolemic shock.*
- Monitor IV fluids or blood products administered via 18- or 16-gauge IV cannulas as ordered *to restore circulating volume.*
- Assist with ultrasound, if performed, *to detect intra-abdominal hemorrhage.*

Risk for Infection related to tissue trauma

EXPECTED OUTCOME: The patient's wounds will remain free of infection.

- Irrigate open wounds with sterile saline *to thoroughly remove dirt and debris and to clean exposed tissue to prevent infection.*
- Cover abdominal wounds with a sterile dressing, or sterile saline–soaked dressing when organs are exposed *to prevent infection and tissue necrosis.*
- With open wounds, give tetanus immunization if booster is needed as ordered *to prevent tetanus infection.*

Evaluation

If interventions have been effective, a patient with trauma reports an acceptable pain level. A patient with head or spinal injury maintains a normal sinus rhythm, and pattern of breathing; clear lung sounds; intactness of mobility; and GCS score of 14 to 15. A patient with hemorrhage has the bleeding controlled. A patient with chest trauma maintains an open airway and an effective breathing pattern. A patient with abdominal trauma has effective circulating volume as evidenced by vital signs within baseline parameters. A patient with altered tissue integrity has wounds that heal without infection. A patient with orthopedic trauma has strong and palpable pulses, normal blood pressure, normal skin color, skin that is warm and dry, capillary refill time of less than 3 seconds, pain controlled to a satisfactory level, and normal motor function and sensation in the extremity.

Chapter 13 Nursing Care of Patients With Emergent Conditions and Disaster/Bioterrorism Response

CRITICAL THINKING & CLINICAL JUDGMENT

Mrs. Aniston, 84, was brought to the ED for an unwitnessed descent (fall) and altered mental status after her son found her on the floor acting strangely. She is alert to person and place but does not recognize her son or remember what happened. She has bruises on her forehead and abrasions on her bilateral arms. She has a cervical collar on to protect her neck. Her son reports that she was diagnosed three weeks ago with atrial fibrillation and was started on warfarin. She has a history of dementia, type 2 diabetes, diabetic peripheral neuropathy, falls, and hypertension.

Critical Thinking (The Why)
1. What risk factors does Mrs. Aniston have for falls?
2. What is your priority concern for Mrs. Aniston?
3. In reviewing the mechanism of Mrs. Aniston's injury, what other injuries should be considered?

Clinical Judgment (The Do)
4. Upon Mrs. Aniston's arrival in the emergency department, what actions do you take?
5. When turned to the right side so that her back can be examined, Mrs. Aniston starts screaming with a sudden increase in her heart rate. What action do you take?

Suggested answers are at the end of the chapter.

Evidence-Based Practice

Clinical Question
What is the family perception of family presence during resuscitation?

Evidence
A systematic review analyzed 12 reviews from 1994–2017 that looked at the perspective of the family regarding family presence during resuscitation. Findings included that families viewed being present as a basic right; those that had been present reported benefits to the patient and health-care team; had a positive experience during resuscitation; and families want to have the option to be present.

Implications for Nursing Practice
Establishing policies and educating nurses and HCPs on family perceptions can decrease implementation barriers, provide consistency, and meet the needs of families.

Reference: Toronto, C. E., & LaRocco, S. A. (2019). Family perception of and experience with family presence during cardiopulmonary resuscitation: An integrative review. *Journal of Clinical Nursing, 28*(1–2), 32–46. org/10.1111/jocn.14649

BURNS

Skin function becomes impaired with a burn injury (see Chapter 55). Burns can lead to fluid and electrolyte losses, infection, and ineffective temperature regulation. The more extensive the burn injury, the greater the potential for complications and mortality, especially for those over age 60.

Data collection for the patient with burns begins with the ABCDE of the primary survey as well as F for "fluid resuscitation." The mechanism and time of the injury are noted. The presence of noxious chemicals or inhalation of smoke in an enclosed space is reported. The greatest threat to life in a patient with a major burn injury is smoke or heat inhalation because it causes edema in the respiratory passages. Lung injury from a burn is diagnosed with a bronchoscopy. Continuous monitoring of respiratory status is essential for burns or soot on the face, singed nasal hairs, a hoarse voice, coughing, or restlessness.

Burns of the face can swell rapidly and compromise the airway. The head of the bed is elevated to 30 degrees to reduce edema. Oxygen is administered regardless of the SPO_2 value, which will not be accurate in the presence of carbon monoxide. Equipment for endotracheal intubation should be readily available. Large fluid losses occur in burn injuries. An IV infusion with large-bore cannulas is started. The patient's weight and the percentage of the body burned guide fluid resuscitation needs. The patient is kept warm, as a burn victim cannot maintain body heat. IV opioids are administered for pain.

Burn depth is described as superficial, partial thickness, or full thickness. Small partial-thickness burns are cleaned with sterile saline solution. They are then covered with a 1/8-inch layer of an anti-infective cream such as silver sulfadiazine (Silvadene, Flamazine) and dry, bulky, fluffed dressings. Major full-thickness burns are covered with dry, sterile dressings or linen. Patients with major burns are transferred to a specialized burn unit.

CUE RECOGNITION 13.1
A patient with a burn is to have silver sulfadiazine applied to the burn during the dressing change. What action do you take?

Suggested answers are at the end of the chapter.

Gerontological Issues

Preventing Burns
Explain to older adults to avoid wearing loose clothing that can catch on fire when cooking over open flames or with heating equipment, such as wood stoves or electric heaters. Also include not to use a heating pad with ointments on the skin, such as methylsalicylate/menthol (Bengay), as it can cause severe burns.

LEARNING TIP
Over-the-counter ointments, lotions, butter, and antiseptics are never used on a major burn. They can retain heat (causing further tissue injury), promote infection, and increase pain.

CRITICAL THINKING & CLINICAL JUDGMENT

Mr. Smith is a 28-year-old man who was welding close to a natural gas line. The flame of the welder caused the gas line to explode, throwing Mr. Smith 50 feet. He landed on his back. He is brought to the emergency department by paramedics. Mr. Smith is awake, alert, and oriented. He has soot around his mouth and nose. During transport, an 18 gauge IV was started and a liter of lactated Ringers (LR) was administered. He sustained full thickness burns to his neck, upper chest, and both forearms. He reports pain from his burns as well as thoracic back and hip pain. His pulse rate is 100 beats per minute, blood pressure is 160/90 mm Hg, and respiratory rate is 20 per minute and his SPO_2 is 95% on room air. A urinary catheter is in place.

Critical Thinking (The Why)
1. What is the priority of care for Mr. Smith?
2. Does Mr. Smith have risk factors for respiratory burns? Why?
3. Does Mr. Smith require oxygen administration? Why?
4. Why is it critical to initiate fluid resuscitation on Mr. Smith?

Clinical Judgment (The Do)
5. Mr. Smith continues to report hip and back pain. In reviewing his mechanism of injury, what action do you take to identify other injuries Mr. Smith may have?
6. What action do you take for the urinary catheter?
7. What type of dressings do you apply on Mr. Smith's full-thickness burns?
8. With what members of the health care team do you collaborate?

Suggested answers are at the end of the chapter.

CUE RECOGNITION 13.2

You observe that a patient with severe burns is wearing a neck chain and a wedding ring. What action do you take?

Suggested answers are at the end of the chapter.

HYPOTHERMIA

Normally, the body maintains its temperature in a narrow range on either side of 98.6°F (37°C), which allows chemical reactions to work most efficiently. Heat loss is inversely proportional to body size and body fat. Fat insulates because it has fewer blood vessels that can vasodilate to cause heat loss. Hypothermia occurs when the core body temperature falls below 95°F (35°C). When this happens, the body is less able to regulate its temperature and generate body heat. A progressive loss of body heat then occurs.

Nursing Process for the Patient With Hypothermia

Data Collection

The defining characteristics of decreasing body temperature are listed in Table 13.3. In cases of mild hypothermia (core temperature between 90°F and 95°F [32.2°C and 35°C]), the patient is usually alert and shivering. More severe hypothermia occurs between 85°F and 89.6°F (29.4°C and 32°C). The patient's level of consciousness begins to markedly decrease at 89.6°F (32°C). There is less interest in fighting the cold environment. The profoundly hypothermic patient has a core temperature of less than 80.6°F (27°C) and usually appears dead, with no obtainable vital signs. Determination of death is made only after aggressive core rewarming above 90°F (32.2°C).

Nursing Diagnoses, Planning, and Implementation

Initial treatment of the patient who is hypothermic consists of rewarming the patient, stabilizing vital functions, and

Table 13.3
Defining Characteristics for Hypothermia

Core Body Temperature	Defining Characteristics
Below 95°F (35°C)	• Alert but apathetic or irritable • Vigorous shivering • Skin cold to touch • Lack of coordination • Slurred speech • Hypoglycemia from shivering • Vital signs decrease
Below 91.4°F (33°C)	• Cardiac arrhythmias • Cyanosis
Below 89.6°F (32°C)	• Shivering stops, muscles activity declines, then muscles rigid • Lethargic, disoriented, hallucinating • Dilated pupils • Hypotension
Below 82.4°F (28°C)	• Hypoventilation (3 to 4 breaths per minute) • Bradycardia, ventricular fibrillation possible • Absent deep tendon reflexes
Below 80.6°F (27°C)	• No vital signs detectable • Fixed, dilated pupils • Ventricular fibrillation to cardiac standstill

Nursing Care Plan for the Patient With Hypothermia

Nursing Diagnosis: *Hypothermia* related to exposure to cold environment
Expected Outcomes: The patient's body temperature and vital signs will be within normal ranges.
Evaluation of Outcomes: Is the patient's body temperature greater than 95°F (35°C)? Is the patient alert and oriented? Is patient in normal sinus rhythm?

Intervention	Rationale	Evaluation
Monitor and report defining characteristics of hypothermia (Table 13.3).	*Defining characteristics guide treatment and show response to treatment.*	Is body temperature greater than 95°F (35°C) and other defining characteristics absent?
Institute rewarming passively or actively as ordered.	*Rewarming is necessary to return body temperature to desirable range.*	Is body core temperature rising to normal range?

preventing further heat loss (see the "Nursing Care Plan for the Patient With Hypothermia"). The patient is removed from the cold environment. All wet clothing is removed to prevent further heat loss. The patient's core body temperature guides treatment. If body temperature is above 82.4°F (28°C), passive rewarming is preferred. The room temperature is set to 70°F to 75°F (21.1°C to 23.9°C). The patient is wrapped in warm, dry blankets. Heat loss from the person's head is reduced by covering the head with warm towels.

If core body temperature is below 82.4°F (28°C), active rewarming is needed. A heating blanket (carbon-fiber) and radiant heat lights are used. Warm, humidified oxygen is administered. Warm IV fluids are given. Body temperature is constantly monitored using a rectal probe. Heated **gastric lavage**, heated peritoneal lavage, or cardiopulmonary bypass can be used for profound hypothermia. Cardiac drugs are given sparingly. As the body warms, peripheral vasodilation occurs. Drugs that were trapped in the peripheral circulation are suddenly released during rewarming. This creates a bolus effect of the drug that can cause fatal arrhythmias.

Evaluation

Desired outcome criteria for the patient with hypothermia is a core body temperature higher than 95°F (35°C), being alert and oriented, no cardiac arrhythmias, vital signs within normal ranges, and normal acid–base balance.

FROSTBITE

The extremities are vulnerable to cold injury. *Frostnip* occurs when exposed parts of the body become very cold but not frozen. This condition usually is not painful. The skin becomes pale and blanched. Contact with a warm object such as someone's hand can be all that is needed to rewarm the part. During rewarming, the affected part might tingle and become red.

Frostbite occurs when body parts become frozen. The extremities are at increased risk because blood shunts away from them to maintain core body temperature and thrombus can form. The affected tissue feels hard and frozen. Most frostbitten parts are white, yellow-white, or blue-white. When rewarmed, the skin appears deep red, hot, and dry to touch. The severity of a cold injury is determined by the duration of the exposure, the temperature to which the body part was exposed, and the wind velocity during exposure.

Interventions for frostbite protect the affected area from further damage. The frostbitten area is handled very gently and never rubbed. It is loosely covered with a dry, sterile dressing. The patient is not allowed to stand or walk on a frostbitten foot. The affected extremity is elevated to heart level. This minimizes edema and promotes blood flow. Analgesics are administered as the rewarming process can be very painful. Aspirin or non-steroidal medication should be administered to prevent the risk of thrombus formation (McIntosh et al, 2019).

HYPERTHERMIA

The body's thermoregulation mechanisms usually work very well. This allows people to tolerate significant changes in temperature. To decrease body heat, sweating and dilation of blood vessels in the skin occur. When blood vessels dilate, blood comes to the skin surface. This increases radiation of heat from the body. If these mechanisms become overwhelmed, the consequences can be disastrous and irreversible. Those at greatest risk for heat illnesses include children, older adults, and those with cardiac disease.

Hyperthermia results when thermoregulation breaks down. This can be due to excess heat generation, an inability to dissipate heat, overwhelming environmental heat, or a combination of these factors. With a fever, the thermal set point is elevated; however, in a heat illness, the thermal set point remains normal. Hyperthermia occurs when heat builds up and cannot be lost. Antipyretics are of no use in hyperthermia and can contribute to complications.

> **BE SAFE!**
> **ACT FAST!** Recognize that older adults are vulnerable to hyperthermia. They do not readily perspire. In times of extreme summer temperatures, older people who live alone should be checked to make sure they are not experiencing hyperthermia. If they do not have fans or air-conditioning, they should be taken to a cooler environment.

Nursing Process for the Patient With Hyperthermia

Data Collection

Illness from heat exposure can take three forms: heat cramps, heat exhaustion, and heatstroke (Box 13.2). As heat illness progresses, circulating blood volume decreases, causing dehydration. Adequate fluid intake is crucial to prevent heat illness.

HEAT CRAMPS. Heat cramps are the mildest form of heat illness. They involve painful muscle spasms, usually in the legs or abdomen, that occur after strenuous exercise. Large amounts of salt and water can be lost as a result of excessive sweating. This causes stressed muscles to spasm. With adequate rest and fluid replacement, the body adjusts the distribution of electrolytes and cramps disappear.

HEAT EXHAUSTION. Heat exhaustion occurs when so much water and electrolytes have been lost through heavy sweating that hypovolemia occurs. Sodium and water loss cause dehydration. Heat exhaustion is a manifestation of the strain placed on the cardiovascular system as it tries to maintain normothermia. The body temperature is normal or slightly elevated, from 100.4°F to 102.2°F (38°C to 39°C).

> **Box 13.2**
> **Defining Characteristics for Environmental Hyperthermia**
>
> **Early Signs**
> - Core body temperature 100.4°F to 102.2°F (38°C to 39°C)
> - Diaphoresis
> - Cool, clammy skin
> - Alert, irritable, poor judgment
> - Dizzy, weak, headache
> - Vomiting, diarrhea
> - Pulse rate greater than 100
>
> **Late Signs**
> - Increasing body core temperature of 106°F (41.1°C) or higher
> - Inability to sweat
> - Hot, dry, flushed skin
> - Altered mental status
> - Seizures or coma possible
> - Hypotension

HEATSTROKE. If symptoms of heat exhaustion are not treated, heatstroke can develop. Altered mental status and an inability to sweat are key symptoms in heatstroke. The body temperature rises rapidly to 106°F (41.1°C) or higher, and level of consciousness decreases. If heatstroke is not treated, death results. Patients with heatstroke are treated in the intensive care unit. Late complications can appear suddenly. They require immediate management. Complications include seizures, cerebral ischemia, acute kidney injury, late cardiac decompensation, and GI bleeding. Prognosis varies with the length of time under heat stress and the patient's prior health status.

Nursing Diagnoses, Planning, and Implementation

Hyperthermia related to exposure to hot environment

EXPECTED OUTCOME: The patient will maintain body temperature within normal ranges.

- Remove the patient from the hot environment and remove layers of clothing *to allow the patient to cool more rapidly.*
- Mist-spray tepid water over the patient while maintaining a strong continual breeze from electric fans *because evaporative cooling is the most efficient method of cooling.*

Deficient Fluid Volume related to hypovolemia

EXPECTED OUTCOME: The patient will maintain blood pressure within normal range.

- Give the patient who is fully alert oral fluids as ordered *to replace lost fluids and electrolytes.*
- If the patient is hypotensive, maintain IV fluids as ordered *to restore fluid volume.*

Evaluation

Interventions have been successful if the patient who is hyperthermic has a core body temperature that is below 101°F (38.3°C); is alert and oriented; has warm, dry skin; and vital signs within normal range.

> **PRACTICE ANALYSIS TIP**
> **Linking NCLEX-PN® to Practice**
> The LPN/LVN will provide cooling/warming measures to restore normal body temperature.

POISONING AND DRUG OVERDOSE

Poisons enter the body by ingestion, inhalation, injection, absorption, or venomous bites. Poisons act by changing cellular metabolism, causing damage to structures, or disturbing body functions. Many toxins and poisons alter the patient's mental status. This can make it difficult to obtain an accurate history.

Nursing Process for the Patient With Ingested Poisoning

Data Collection
After an ingested poisoning has occurred, the poison must be identified. The method of exposure is established. This allows the removal or interruption of the toxin. Most ingested poisons are drugs. About one-third of poisonings are caused by cleaners, soaps, insecticides, acids, or alkalis. Many household plants are poisonous if they are ingested. Some plants cause local irritation of the skin. Others can affect the circulatory system, GI tract, or central nervous system.

Empty medication bottles, scattered pills, or chemicals are examined by emergency medical personnel at the scene. This helps identify the poisonous substance. The patient's physical appearance also can give clues to the type of substance ingested. IV needle tracks, burns, erythema, and flushed skin may help identify the poison.

Nursing Diagnoses, Planning, and Implementation

Risk for Injury related to absorption of poisoning agent

EXPECTED OUTCOME: The patient will maintain vital signs within normal ranges and be free of injury.

- Administer naloxone (Narcan) as ordered *to treat an opioid overdose. Naloxone is available over-the-counter without a prescription in many states.*
- Contact the nationwide 24/7 poison control hotline at 1-800-222-1222 or use the webPOISONCONTROL® online or app tool at www.triage.webpoisoncontrol.org *to get quick specific recommendations based on age, substance, and amount.*
- The nationwide 24/7 poison control hotline number (1-800-222-1222) should be kept near every home telephone and in cell phones. Text "POISON" to 797979 to save the contact number in a smartphone.

Evaluation
Interventions have been successful if the patient is awake and has vital signs within normal ranges and remains free from injury.

NURSING CARE TIP
- Syrup of ipecac is *not* recommended for at-home treatment of accidental overdose. Evidence shows that its use does not improve patient outcomes. For example, giving it to a person who has swallowed a caustic chemical can result in greater tissue damage from vomiting the caustic chemical. Also, after being given syrup of ipecac, a person who was poisoned may vomit the necessary antidote that was administered.
- Gastric decontamination, activated charcoal, and gastric lavage are no longer routinely recommended except in severe cases such as when the patient has ingested a large quantity of a drug or is unconscious.

Inhaled Poisons
Inhaled poisons include carbon monoxide, chlorine, natural gas, pesticides, and other gases. Carbon monoxide is odorless. It can produce profound hypoxia by combining with hemoglobin molecules. This displaces oxygen in red blood cells. The patient's carboxyhemoglobin level is monitored to guide therapy. Inhalation of chlorine is irritating to the respiratory system. It can produce airway obstruction and pulmonary edema.

When an inhalation injury from a poison occurs, the patient must be moved into fresh air and away from the toxin. Supplemental oxygen is given as ordered. Prolonged inhalation of a poison can cause lung damage. Respiratory status must be closely monitored to detect complications.

Injected Poisons
Injected poisons pose problems because they are difficult to remove or dilute. Usually, they result from drug overdose. However, they can also result from the bites and stings of insects or animals. Local swelling and tissue destruction can occur at the injection site. Any jewelry the patient is wearing is removed because swelling can occur and impair circulation. A cold pack is applied to decrease local pain and swelling around the injection site. The identity of the injected drug or toxin must be established so that adverse effects can be anticipated and managed.

Insect Stings or Bites
Insect stings or bites cause anaphylaxis in only a small percentage of people. Symptoms in most people are limited to localized pain, swelling, heat, and redness. Treatment involves applying ice to and elevating the affected part. Cellulitis can occur hours later and requires medical treatment.

When a patient has sustained a bee or wasp sting, examine the area for the stinger and remove it by gently scraping it off the skin. Tweezers or forceps are not used to remove the stinger. Squeezing the stinger can inject more venom into the patient. Placing ice over the injury site can help slow the rate of toxin absorption.

Snakebites
Only a small percentage of snakebites are caused by poisonous snakes. The most prevalent poisonous snakes are the coral snake and the pit vipers, which include rattlesnakes, copperheads, and cottonmouth moccasins. Envenomation occurs when the snake's hollow fangs puncture the skin and inject stored venom. A poisonous snakebite leaves two painful small puncture wounds with surrounding discoloration and swelling that occurs within 5 to 10 minutes after the bite. Envenomation by any pit viper snake produces burning pain at the site of the injury.

Evidence-based interventions are focused on decreasing the circulation of venom throughout the patient's system. This is done by keeping the patient calm and immobilizing the affected body part until antivenin can be given under the direction of an experienced toxicologist. An affected extremity should be positioned below the level of the heart. The site of the bite is cleaned with soap and water. It should not be irrigated or flushed. The wound is covered with a loose, clean dressing. A tourniquet or ice should not be used.

NEAR-DROWNING

Drowning is death from **asphyxia** (insufficient oxygen intake) after submersion in water. *Near-drowning* is submersion with at least temporary survival of the victim. When submersion occurs, conscious victims hold their breath until reflex inspiratory efforts override breath holding. As water is aspirated, laryngospasm occurs. In wet drowning, the laryngospasm is less prolonged. Fluid enters the lungs after the vocal cords relax. In dry drowning, cold water causes laryngospasm and vagal stimulation. This produces severe hypoxia. Most successfully resuscitated victims experience dry drowning. Risk factors for drowning include inability to swim, diving accidents, use of alcohol and drugs before swimming, exhaustion, and hypothermia. Factors that influence the outcome of near-drowning include the temperature of the water, length of time submerged, cleanliness of the water, and age of the victim. The younger the patient, the better the chance of survival.

After submersion, acute respiratory failure can occur. Symptoms of impaired gas exchange (known as secondary near-drowning) can be delayed as long as 72 hours after the incident. Contaminants in the water can irritate the pulmonary system and cause inflammatory reactions and impaired surfactant functioning. Metabolic acidosis is usually present. Hypoxemia and hypothermia predispose the patient to arrhythmias. Neurologic damage and cerebral edema can occur.

Aggressive resuscitative efforts are used for victims of cold-water drowning when submersion time is 1 hour or less. Hypothermia can decrease the metabolic needs of the brain. This can contribute to neurologic recovery even after prolonged submersion. Resuscitation should not be stopped until the core body temperature is at least greater than 90°F (32°C). Supportive respiratory care is provided; this may include mechanical ventilation.

Nursing Process for the Near-Drowning Patient

Data Collection

Conduct ABCDE of the primary survey. Take vital signs. Observe respiratory rate and pattern, dyspnea, or signs of airway obstruction to report. Note skin color or cyanosis. The patient's level of consciousness may be altered from anoxia. Most near-drowning victims have mild dyspnea, a deathlike appearance with blue or gray skin color, apnea or **tachypnea** (breathing over 20 respirations per minute), hypotension, slow heart rate (possibly less than 10 beats per minute), cold skin temperature, dilated pupils, hypothermia, and vomiting.

Nursing Diagnoses, Planning, and Implementation

Risk for Ineffective Cerebral Tissue Perfusion related to severe anoxia

EXPECTED OUTCOME: The patient will maintain level of consciousness and vital signs within normal range, with clear breath sounds that are equal bilaterally.

- Give supplemental oxygen as ordered *to increase tissue oxygenation.*
- Ensure that adjunct airway equipment is available *because endotracheal intubation and insertion of a nasogastric tube to decompress the stomach may be needed.*

Evaluation

Interventions have been successful if the patient has normal respiratory rate and pattern, has normal vital signs, and is alert and oriented.

PSYCHIATRIC EMERGENCIES

A psychiatric emergency occurs when a person no longer has the coping skills to maintain the usual level of functioning. The patient's moods, thoughts, or actions can be so disordered that the patient could harm self or others if the situation is not quickly controlled. If acute psychiatric episodes are not managed, they can result in life-threatening, suicidal, violent, or psychologically damaging behavior (see Chapter 57).

DISASTER RESPONSE

A *disaster* is defined as any event that overwhelms existing personnel, facilities, equipment, and the capabilities of a responding agency, institution, or community. Potential sources of disaster include internal events such as fires and explosions; external events such as floods, storms, fires, earthquakes, and tornadoes; and created events such as motor vehicle accidents, plane crashes, and acts of terrorism. In 2003, a campaign to educate the American people on preparing for emergencies and disasters was launched at www.ready.gov. In addition to more information about disasters, you can complete courses and training at www.fema.gov.

External disasters involve a community-wide response of several agencies. These include first responders (i.e., emergency medical system [EMS] providers, fire departments,

• WORD • BUILDING •

tachypnea: tachy—fast + pnea—breathing

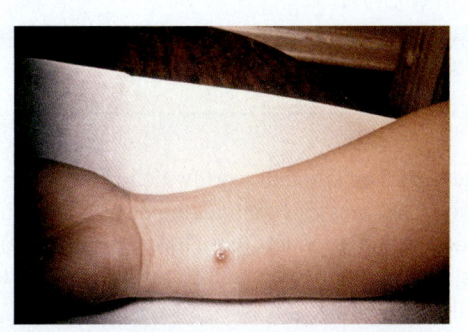

FIGURE 13.5 Cutaneous anthrax on right forearm in early stage of infection.

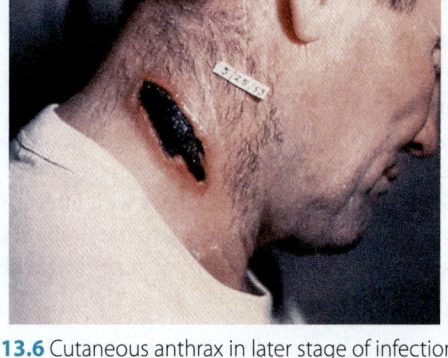

FIGURE 13.6 Cutaneous anthrax in later stage of infection.

law enforcement) and hospitals. These agencies coordinate communication, search, rescue, transportation, and treatment of multiple victims. Each agency and hospital involved in responding to a disaster follows a disaster plan. It outlines the role and responsibilities of the agency and its staff. It identifies procedures to follow when interacting with the casualties, families, media, or other agencies. Community-wide disaster drills are conducted regularly to evaluate and rework plans.

Hospitals serve as the major treatment area for injured victims of a disaster (casualties). When a disaster occurs, the hospital activates its disaster plan. There are external and internal disaster plans. External plans respond to events occurring outside the hospital. Internal disaster plans are specific to an institution. They cover internal water, power, sewer, or computer issues that could cause harm. Specific duties for all staff and each department are outlined. You should be familiar with your agency's disaster plan. Know your role and responsibilities during a disaster.

In a disaster, each nursing unit calls available off-duty staff to report to work. Units prepare for the influx of casualties by discharging noncritical patients. Each nursing unit is designated to receive specific types of casualties such as burns, major trauma, medical, mental health, or pediatric. The ED serves as the triage (to assign priorities) and stabilization area for casualties. A hospital disaster plan may assign one or more staff from other areas to work in the ED. These staff members assist in decontamination, first aid, critical care, burn treatment, family room, or transportation. During a disaster, decision making and prioritization of patient care are guided by the personnel and resources available. Patients who are seriously injured but have the greatest chance of full recovery are treated first.

Long-Term Care Facilities

Long-term care facilities have disaster plans in place to respond to various types of disasters and ensure continuity of essential functions. These plans may be linked to a community-wide disaster plan and those of other agencies to ensure smooth implementation of the plan. The CDC provides planning guidelines to assist long-term care facilities in being prepared for disasters (www.cdc.gov/cpr/readiness/healthcare/longtermcare.htm). The plan should prepare the facility to be self-sufficient for a minimum of 96 hours during a disaster. Review your facility's disaster plan to know what your role in a disaster is. Participate in training or drills to ensure familiarity with protocols that you may need to implement. It is essential for you to keep vulnerable older adults and those with disabilities safe in a disaster.

> **PRACTICE ANALYSIS TIP**
> **Linking NCLEX-PN® to Practice**
> The LPN/LVN will participate in preparation for internal and external disasters (e.g., fire, natural disaster).

BIOTERRORISM AGENTS

The Centers for Disease Control and Prevention (CDC) evaluates bacteria, viruses, and toxins on their risk for use in a **bioterrorism** attack (visit www.cdc.gov). Early recognition of a bioterrorism attack is vital. It allows for rapid implementation of preventive interventions, treatment, and public communication. Some of the agents a nurse may encounter are **anthrax, botulism,** and **plague** (Table 13.4).

Table 13.4
Potential Bioterrorism Agents

Anthrax
A disease caused by the spore-forming bacterium *Bacillus anthracis*. The organism is found worldwide in soil. Animals become infected by grazing in contaminated areas. Under natural conditions, humans can contract the disease, which most often occurs after close contact with infected animals or contaminated animal products (e.g., hides, meat, wool). The spores activate upon exposure to the tissues or blood of an animal or infected human. Person-to-person transmitted anthrax is not known to occur. A vaccine is available.

Type & Transmission	Incubation	Signs & Symptoms	Diagnosis	Treatment & Nursing Care

Cutaneous (skin) can occur when people handle contaminated animal products and spores enter a cut or scrape on their skin; it is the most common type.	1 to 7 days (up to 12 days)	• Group of small blisters or bumps that may itch
		• Painless skin sore (ulcer) with black center that appears after the small blisters or bumps
		• Swelling around sore
		• Sore most often on face, neck, arms, or hands (See Figs. 13.5 & 13.6.)
			• Chest x-ray
			• CT scan
			• *Culture:*
			  • Peripheral blood
			  • Pleural fluid
			  • Cerebrospinal fluid
			  • Fluid under eschar
			  • Pleural & Lung Biopsy
				• Antibiotics:
				  • ciprofloxacin
				  • doxycycline
				  • a quinolone

Inhalation (lung) can occur when a person inhales aerosolized spores during the industrial processing of contaminated materials, such as wool, hides, or hair.	1 to 6 days (can also develop within a week or take as long as 2 months)	• Fever and chills
		• Chest discomfort
		• Confusion or dizziness
		• Cough
		• Shortness of breath
		• Headache
		• Nausea, vomiting, or stomach pains
		• Sweats (often drenching)
		• Extreme tiredness, body aches
			See above. Diagnosis is the same for all types of anthrax.	• Antibiotics:
				  • ciprofloxacin
				  • doxycycline
				• Antitoxins
				• Antibodies
				• Aggressive care: maintenance of fluid, electrolytes, and acid-base balance, and drainage of pleural effusions

Gastrointestinal (digestive) can occur when a person eats raw or undercooked meat from infected animals.	1 to 7 days	• Fever and chills
		• Swelling of neck or neck glands
		• Sore throat, painful swallowing
		• Hoarseness
		• Headache
		• Nausea and vomiting (bloody vomiting)
		• Diarrhea (bloody)
		• Red face and eyes
		• Stomach pain
		• Swelling of abdomen (stomach)
		• Fainting
			See above. Diagnosis is the same for all types of anthrax.	• Antibiotics:
				  • ciprofloxacin
				  • doxycycline
				• Antitoxins
				• Antibodies
				• Aggressive care: maintenance of fluid, electrolytes, and acid-base balance

Table 13.4
Potential Bioterrorism Agents—cont'd

Botulism

An illness caused by the most potent lethal toxin known, botulinum toxin. This neurotoxin is produced by *Clostridium botulinum*, an anaerobic, spore-forming bacterium. The toxin is colorless, odorless, and likely tasteless. Botulinum toxin blocks neurotransmission. It binds to the presynaptic nerve terminal at the neuromuscular junction which prevents the release of acetylcholine. Skeletal muscle weakness results. Person-to-person transmitted botulism is not known to occur. Natural forms of the disease are foodborne botulism, wound botulism, and infant botulism.

Botulinum toxin has been developed as a biological weapon. An aerosol attack is considered the most likely use of botulinum toxin for bioterrorism. A bioterrorism attack is considered in any outbreak of botulism. It is especially considered when a cluster of cases occurs, when an outbreak has a common geographical location but there is no common dietary exposure (suggestive of possible aerosol exposure), when there is an outbreak of an unusual botulinum toxin type, or when multiple simultaneous outbreaks occur. A careful patient dietary and travel history is taken to help identify the source. Patients are asked if they know of others with similar symptoms.

Type & Transmission	Incubation	Signs & Symptoms	Diagnosis	Treatment & Nursing Care
Inhalation botulism from biological weapon.	Unknown	• Classic triad of botulism: (1) afebrile, (2) symmetrical descending flaccid paralysis with prominent bulbar palsies (impairment of cranial nerves IX, X, XI, XII) (3) clear mentation • Difficulty seeing, speaking, swallowing • Anticholinergic symptoms: dry mouth, ileus, constipation, nausea, vomiting, urine retention, mydriasis • Dizziness • Sore throat	• Based on clinical presentation	• For aerosol exposure: wash clothes; shower; 0.1% hypochlorite bleach solution for surfaces • Immediately: Trivalent equine antitoxin • Intensive care, mechanical ventilation, parenteral nutrition • Frequent monitoring of gag and cough reflexes, swallowing, oxygen saturation, vital capacity, inspiratory force • Airway intubation for secretion control or impending respiratory failure
Foodborne botulism from ingestion of improperly processed foodstuffs containing preformed toxin produced by *C. botulinum*.	12 to 72 hours (range is 2 hours to 8 days)	See above. Signs & Symptoms are the same for all types of botulism.	• Based on clinical presentation • Foodborne: Toxin assay of blood, gastric aspirate, emesis, and stool for confirmation	See above. Treatment & Nursing Care is the same for all types of botulism.
Wound botulism from production of botulinum toxin by *C. botulinum* organisms in wounds.	10 days	See above. Signs & Symptoms are the same for all types of botulism.	• Based on clinical presentation	See above. Treatment & Nursing Care is the same for all types of botulism.

Continued

Table 13.4
Potential Bioterrorism Agents—cont'd

Plague

Plague is caused by the gram-negative coccobacillus *Yersinia pestis*. Under natural conditions, plague is transmitted to humans by the bite of an infectious flea. It can also be transmitted by direct contact with infectious body fluids or tissues of an infected animal or by inhaling infectious droplets. Plague has a long history of use and development as a biological weapon. After a biological attack, primary pneumonic plague would most likely occur. Pneumonic plague is the most serious form of the disease and is the only form of plague that can be spread from person-to-person (by infectious droplets).

Type & Transmission	Incubation	Signs & Symptoms	Diagnosis	Treatment & Nursing Care

Pneumonic plague from inhaling infectious droplets. It may also develop from untreated bubonic or septicemic plague after the bacteria spreads to the lungs. The pneumonia may cause respiratory failure and shock.	1 to 6 days	• Fever
		• Headache
		• Weakness
		• Rapidly developing pneumonia with shortness of breath, chest pain, cough, and sometimes bloody or watery mucous
			During a confirmed outbreak of pneumonic plague after a biological attack, a diagnosis can be made based on symptoms. Leukocytes elevated. Neutrophils increased. Platelets normal or low. International normalized ratio (INR), prothrombin time (PT), and partial thromboplastin time (PTT) increased. Liver function tests elevated. Abnormal renal function tests with systemic disease. Culture of blood and sputum.	• For pneumonic plague, use droplet precautions as patients are contagious.
				• Antibiotics
				  • gentamicin
				  • streptomycin
				  • levofloxacin
				  • ciprofloxacin
				  • doxycycline
				  • moxifloxacin
				  • chloramphenicol

Bubonic plague from the bite of an infected flea.		• Sudden onset of fever • Headache • Chills • Weakness • One or more swollen, tender and painful lymph nodes (called buboes)	See above. Diagnosis is the same for all types of plague.	See above. Treatment & Nursing Care is the same for all types of plague.
Septicemic plague results from bites of infected fleas or from handling an infected animal. It can occur as the first symptom of plague or may develop from untreated bubonic plague.		• Fever • Chills • Extreme weakness • Abdominal pain • Shock • Possible bleeding into skin, other organs • Skin, other tissues may turn black and die, especially fingers, toes, nose	See above. Diagnosis is the same for all types of plague.	See above. Treatment & Nursing Care is the same for all types of plague.

Key Points

- When a patient first arrives in the emergency department (ED), a primary survey is done. The patient's alertness is determined. Then the patient's airway, breathing, circulation status, and any disability are assessed. The patient's area of distress is exposed (clothing removed) for inspection.
- For victims of severe trauma, a secondary survey is conducted to identify areas of injury or medical problems that are not life threatening but do require treatment.
- When planning care for a victim of spinal, neck, or chest trauma, focus on managing pain, establishing effective breathing patterns, and airway clearance.
- With hemorrhage or an abdominal organ injury, hypovolemia will be of great concern.
- When an inhalation injury from a poison occurs, the patient must be moved into fresh air and away from the toxin. Inhaled poisons include carbon monoxide, chlorine, natural gas, pesticides, and other gases. Supplemental oxygen is given as ordered. Respiratory status must be closely monitored to detect complications.
- In mild hypothermia, the patient is usually alert and shivering and appears clumsy, apathetic, or irritable. Respiratory rate, heart rate, and cardiac output decrease. When more severe hypothermia occurs, shivering stops and muscle activity decreases. Eventually, as the body temperature continues to drop, all muscle activity stops. Muscles become rigid and the patient becomes lethargic.
- Hyperthermia from heat exposure can take three forms: heat cramps, heat exhaustion, and heatstroke. As the illness progresses, circulating blood volume decreases, causing dehydration. Adequate fluid intake is crucial to prevent heat illness.
- After an ingested poisoning has occurred, the poison must be identified and the method of exposure established. Most ingested poisons are drugs. About one-third of poisonings are caused by cleaners, soaps, insecticides, acids, or alkalis.
- During a disaster situation, nursing units prepare for the influx of casualties by discharging noncritical patients. Each nursing unit is designated to receive specific types of casualties: major trauma, burns, medical, pediatric, or psychiatric issues. The ED serves as the triage and stabilization area for casualties.
- The Centers for Disease Control and Prevention evaluates bacteria, viruses, and toxins on their risk for use in a bioterrorism attack. Early recognition of a bioterrorism attack is vital. It allows for rapid implementation of preventive interventions, treatment, and public communication. Bioterrorism agents include anthrax, botulism, and plague.

The author acknowledges contributions to this chapter by Patricia Williams.

SUGGESTED ANSWERS TO CHAPTER EXERCISES

Cue Recognition

13.1: Check allergies to sulfa medications before applying the silver sulfadiazine. Note that the name of the medication contains "sulfa." A patient allergic to sulfa drugs should not be given this sulfa medication!

13.2: Remove the jewelry including the wedding ring immediately before edema formation occurs to prevent them from compromising circulation.

Critical Thinking & Clinical Judgment

Mrs. Aniston
1. Dementia, diabetic peripheral neuropathy, and a history of falls are risk factors for falling.
2. Intracerebral bleeding due to possible head trauma and use of warfarin.
3. Closed head injury; Spinal trauma; Other fractures.
4. Assist health-care team with initial data collection during the primary and secondary survey in order to recognize life-threatening conditions and determine priorities of care.
5. Mrs. Aniston had an unwitnessed fall. She could have sustained fractures of the pelvis or back. Gently return her to a supine position. Collect data regarding her pain and other symptoms. Notify the HCP. Offer analgesic as prescribed. Provide emotional support.

Mr. Smith
1. The airway is the priority because edema from inhalation burns can occlude the airway.
2. Mr. Smith may have experienced respiratory burns as evidenced by the soot near his mouth and nose. He should be closely monitored. Monitoring should include respiratory rate and pattern and the patient's ability to speak without having a hoarse voice. Abnormal breathing sounds such as wheezing indicate partial upper airway occlusion and require immediate treatment.
3. Yes. Oxygen must be administered regardless of SPO_2 value. Pulse oximetry cannot differentiate between oxygen-bound hemoglobin and carboxyhemoglobin, so the reading could be inaccurate in the presence of carbon monoxide.
4. Patients with burns tend to develop third-spacing of fluid and are at an increased risk for shock and hypothermia. Therefore, it is critical to administer isotonic fluids (preferably lactated Ringer's) to replace the fluid loss. Continually monitor the patient for signs and symptoms of hypovolemia.
5. Since Mr. Smith was involved in an explosive incident and thrown 50 feet, he could have fractures of the pelvis or back or internal organ injuries. You collect data on his symptoms to share with the HCP to assist in identifying

SUGGESTED ANSWERS TO CHAPTER EXERCISES—cont'd

other injuries. Until his complete status is known, keep him immobile. Be alert for any change in his status and report it promptly.
6. Monitor hourly urine output. Urine output is the gold standard for monitoring fluid resuscitation for burns.
7. Full-thickness burns are covered with dry dressings. Because the skin can no longer provide protection, wet dressings would provide a medium for bacterial invasion. They could also decrease body temperature because the skin can no longer maintain thermoregulation.
8. The emergency department health-care provider, registered nurse, respiratory therapist, social worker, case manager, and clergy.

Additional Resources

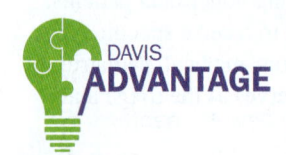

Go to Davis Advantage to complete your learning: strengthen understanding, apply your knowledge, and prepare for the Next Gen NCLEX®.

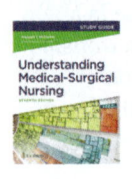

A Study Guide is also available.

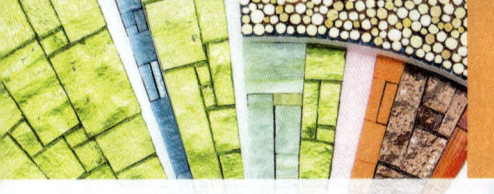

UNIT THREE Understanding Influences on Health and Illness

CHAPTER 14
Developmental Considerations and Chronic Illness in the Nursing Care of Adults

Linda S. Williams

KEY TERMS

chronic illness (KR-ON-ik ILL-ness)
developmental stage (de-VEL-up-MEN-tal STAYJ)
health (HELTH)
hopelessness (HOHP-less-ness)
illness (IL-ness)
immunosenescence (IM-u-no-sen-ESS-ents)
powerlessness (POW-er-less-ness)
reminiscence therapy (reh-meh-NISS-ents THER-a-pee)
respite care (RESS-pit CARE)
spirituality (SPEER-ih-chu-AL-ih-tee)

CHAPTER CONCEPTS

Caring
Family
Growth and development
Health promotion
Safety
Self
Reproduction and sexuality

LEARNING OUTCOMES

1. Explain the nurse's role in promoting wellness.
2. List Erikson's eight stages of psychosocial development.
3. Identify the effects of chronic illness.
4. Describe special needs that caregivers have.
5. Explain health promotion methods.
6. Plan nursing interventions for a patient who is chronically ill.

HEALTH, WELLNESS, AND ILLNESS

Have you ever known someone with a seemingly small health problem who considered themselves unwell or disabled? Or perhaps a person with major health problems who views themselves as well? Many factors play a role in a person's perception of **health.** These include the ability to perform activities of daily living (ADLs) and desired tasks, fulfilment of life roles (e.g., student, parent, employee), and quality of life. *Wellness* is a term describing movement toward a higher level of functioning. Even though a person has a disabling illness, they may still achieve a higher level of wellness.

The concept of **illness** is one of imbalance or disharmony with the environment. Physical causes of illness are most easily recognized, such as a fall that breaks a bone. But illness can also result from a psychological, sociological, cultural, or spiritual imbalance. After the loss of a spouse, for example, one may experience loneliness, depression, and a loss of balance in the social and psychological aspects of life. A hospitalization or long-term care stay may increase disharmony if cultural beliefs and practices are not understood or upheld by health-care providers (HCPs). A person faced with a terminal diagnosis may lose hope and direction in life, causing anxiety and despair.

Rather than being exclusive concepts, health and illness are dynamic and ever-changing states of being. A health crisis such as a myocardial infarction overwhelms a patient's ability to maintain a normal level of wellness. Two months later, however, the patient could be enjoying a higher level of wellness than before the myocardial infarction if they begin to follow a healthy lifestyle.

THE NURSE'S ROLE IN SUPPORTING AND PROMOTING WELLNESS

The goal of nursing care is to help patients achieve their highest possible level of wellness. To do this, the nurse must consider the patient's strengths and resources. Working together, the patient, family, nurses, and other members of the healthcare team develop a plan of care. The plan includes wellness goals and interventions to accomplish those goals. The plan of care focuses on six main areas:

- Mobilizing resources
- Providing a safe and adaptable environment
- Helping the patient learn about their health problem and treatment and promoting self-management of the illness
- Performing and teaching the patient to perform healthcare procedures
- Anticipating problems and recognizing potential cues for crises
- Evaluating the plan and progress toward the goals with the patient and family

Nurses assume a variety of roles in promoting the health of their patients, such as advocate, caregiver, consultant, and educator.

> **NURSING CARE TIP**
> Displaying photos, provided by family, in a patient's room, showing the patient at various ages when healthy and active, enables caregivers to appreciate the patient in wellness roles.

DEVELOPMENTAL STAGES

There are many theories of **developmental stages.** Erik Erikson's theory (1980, 1993), which describes eight stages of psychosocial development, is discussed in this chapter (Table 14.1). The developmental stages of life focus on the balance a person must achieve for high-level wellness within that stage. Each stage must be completed before accomplishing the next. The first five stages relate to the child and adolescent. The last three stages, discussed here, are young adulthood, middle adulthood, and late adulthood.

> **PRACTICE ANALYSIS TIP**
> Linking NCLEX-PN® to Practice
> The LPN/LVN will provide care that meets the needs of the adult client ages 18 through 64 years.

The Young Adult

Erikson's sixth psychosocial developmental stage, from ages 18 to 40, addresses intimacy versus isolation. The young adult's task is to develop warm, affectionate relationships with a spouse, family, and friends created through fondness, understanding, caring, and love. The inability to do so results in isolation from others. Physically, growth is usually complete by age 20. Socially, young adults begin to move away from their parents to start their own families. The young adult begins to develop a place in society through school, work, and social activities. In this stage, intimacy or closeness develops with partners and friends. Having a pet, marrying, and having children shows the desire for intimacy. Challenges to intimacy are tasks that must be overcome in this stage.

Table 14.1
Erikson's Stages of Psychosocial Development

Stage	Age Range	Developmental Task
Infancy	Birth to 18 months	Trust versus Mistrust
Toddler	18 months to 3 years	Autonomy versus Shame and doubt
Preschool	3 to 5 years	Initiative versus Guilt
School age	5 to 12 years	Industry versus Inferiority
Adolescence	12 to 18 years	Identity versus Role confusion
Young adulthood	18 to 40 years	Intimacy versus Isolation
Middle adulthood	40 to 65 years	Generativity versus Stagnation
Late adulthood	65 through death	Integrity versus Despair

Erikson, E. H. (1980). *Identity and the life cycle.* New York: W.W. Norton & Company.

Common Health Concerns

The lifestyle choices of young adults may place their health at risk. Establishing lifelong positive health practices helps prevent long-term health complications. Health promotion for this age-group focuses on risk prevention through teaching. The importance of diet and exercise, sunscreen use to avoid increased risk of skin cancer, and avoiding tobacco use to prevent lung disease and cancer in later life should be explained.

In the early part of young adulthood, the individual is in the workforce or is preparing for a career with a college or vocational education. Being a novice in the work world and accepting new independence, freedom, and responsibilities can introduce stressors into the young adult's life. Overeating; engaging in violence; and alcohol, drug, or tobacco use are risky lifestyle choices and poor coping mechanisms for stress. Young adults should be aware of their individual stressors and develop positive coping mechanisms such as exercise, music, and meditation.

Young adults may be sexually active with multiple partners. This puts them at risk for sexually transmitted infections. Safer sex guidelines and information on birth control should be available for the young adult.

The Middle-Aged Adult

In the middle adult years, ages 40 to 65, the psychological developmental stage is developing generativity versus self-absorption. Generativity includes a sense of productivity and creativity and is demonstrated by concern and support for others, along with a vision for future generations. The inability to develop generativity may be displayed as preoccupation with personal needs or self-absorption.

Physically, middle-aged adults may notice signs of intolerance for physical exercise if they have not maintained a healthy lifestyle. Traditionally, their children are adolescents or young adults who need assistance with entering adulthood and launching their own careers and families; however, people are having children later in life, so this is not always the case. The term *empty nest* is used to describe the middle-aged couple's home after their children have left.

Today's middle-aged adults have been labeled the *sandwich generation*. People in this age-group often care for their children and their aging parents at the same time. Middle-aged adults look back over their lives and compare accomplishments versus unrealized goals. Midlife crisis may occur when a desire to change work, social, or family situations results. Planning for retirement occurs by developing interests outside of work. Preparing for financial security is another important task during this stage.

Common Health Concerns

The need for immunizations continues into adulthood (visit www.cdc.gov). Unhealthy lifestyle choices often lead to serious health consequences during middle adulthood. These choices may include a diet high in saturated fat, overeating, use of alcohol or drugs, a sedentary lifestyle, or smoking. Chronic bronchitis, emphysema, hypertension, heart disease, and lung cancer are major health concerns. Cardiovascular disease and cancer cause most deaths in this age-group. However, middle adulthood is not too late for lifestyle changes to positively affect health. Helping adults in this age-group recognize the benefits of positive lifestyle choices and empowering them to make changes is a major nursing goal.

> ### CRITICAL THINKING
> **Mr. Crowley**, age 54, calls his HCP's office for the fourth time this month to request medication for severe indigestion. He has refused to have diagnostic tests because he "can't fit them" into his schedule. Mr. Crowley travels for work and eats fast-food daily. His wife quit her job to supervise their 15-year-old son, who was not going to school every day. Their twin daughters are both in college.
> 1. What might be causing Mr. Crowley to experience health problems?
> 2. What is affecting the developmental tasks Mr. Crowley needs to perform?
>
> *Suggested answers are at the end of the chapter.*

The Older Adult

The final psychological developmental stage affects adults from age 65 until death. Advances in living conditions and health care and increased knowledge of age-related changes to the immune system (**immunosenescence**) have allowed more people to live productive, fulfilling lives into their 80s, 90s, and 100s. Older adults are likely to be found gardening, hiking, exercising, and socializing (Fig. 14.1). Some may continue to work beyond retirement age or begin a second career after retiring.

Developmental work for older adults focuses on integrity versus despair. In this stage, older adults look back to see what they have done with their lives. *Integrity* refers to accepting responsibility for one's life thus far and reflecting on it in a positive way. Reaching this stage is a sign of maturity. Failing to reach this stage is an indication of unsuccessful completion of previous stages, causing feelings of despair that life has been lived in vain and also a fear of death. **Reminiscence therapy** may be one way to assist the older adult through this stage.

Aging is associated with role changes and transitions. Some roles, such as employee or spouse, are lost because of retirement or illness, or death of a spouse, causing sadness or depression. New roles may arise, such as grandparent, volunteer, or widow/widower. With retirement, household roles may need to change. If an older adult becomes ill and dependent and needs to be cared for by an adult child, the parent–child role may be reversed.

Life events such as decreased physical ability, illness, retirement, or death of a spouse are challenges that older adults face.

• WORD • BUILDING •

immunosenescence: immuno—immune + senescere—to grow old

reminiscence: re—backward + minisc—mind + ens—action

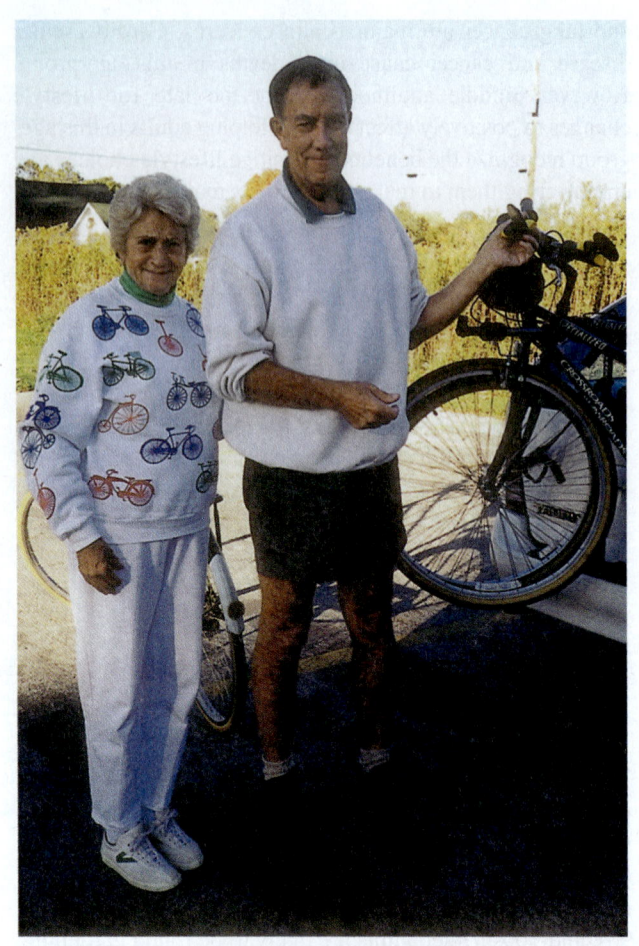

FIGURE 14.1 Socialization helps older adults maintain integrity.

The older adult's ability to cope with these stressors is essential for healthy aging and maintaining a sense of control. Coping with aging is influenced by the individual's cultural beliefs and the community's value of older adults. Sometimes the greatest loss for older adults is their lack of connection with the world and a lack of being part of a greater purpose. However, being alone is not the same as being lonely. For some older adults, being by oneself allows for reflection to better understand one's situation. Older adults who feel unwanted or unloved are more likely to develop anxiety and depression and fail to thrive.

> **PRACTICE ANALYSIS TIP**
> **Linking NCLEX-PN® to Practice**
> The LPN/LVN will:
> - Recognize stressors that affect client care.
> - Participate in reminiscence therapy.
> - Assist client with expected life transition (e.g., retirement).

Common Health Concerns

The focus of care for the older adult is assistance in meeting physical, psychological, cultural, sociological, and spiritual needs. Promoting self-care and encouraging the use of community services for seniors is important. Most older adults continue to live in their own residences. Impairment in mobility and the ability to carry out instrumental activities of daily living (IADLs) threaten their independence. IADLs include shopping for groceries, preparing meals, and cleaning and maintaining a home. Asking or paying others to perform tasks that they formerly could do themselves is a significant loss for many older adults. The loss of a spouse, death of friends, or lack of social contacts can isolate an older adult. Isolation can lead to depression and a feeling of **hopelessness.** The accumulation of losses can overwhelm an older adult's coping mechanisms. Hopelessness is related to a high rate of suicide, especially for older men. Suicide is the ultimate expression of hopelessness.

Older adults may need encouragement to remain active. Many cities have transportation services for older adults. Senior centers offer programs such as bowling leagues, dances, trips, and tax assistance. Older adults can also continue to work as volunteers for schools, nursing facilities, parks, museums, zoos, and youth groups. Colleges and universities may offer discounts for older adults.

Chronic diseases can limit an older person's ability to be independent in performing ADLs and IADLs. Hypertension and heart disease are common in this age-group. Managing these conditions helps keep the older adult active.

One of the most difficult tasks for the nurse who is interacting with an older adult is distinguishing normal age-related changes from pathological changes. Changes in mobility and chronic pain may limit an older person's activity and active lifestyle. Pain is not a normal part of aging and should always be investigated.

> **CRITICAL THINKING & CLINICAL JUDGMENT**
> **Mr. Klein,** age 82, visits his HCP. He reports left hip pain. The HCP replies, "It can be common to experience pain as you get older." Mr. Klein thinks a minute and says, "But my right hip doesn't hurt, and it's as old as my left hip!"
>
> **Critical Thinking (The Why)**
> 1. What is occurring in this situation?
>
> **Clinical Judgment (The Do)**
> 2. What actions do you take to provide patient-centered care and improve the quality of life for Mr. Klein?
>
> *Suggested answers are at the end of the chapter.*

Falls are a serious concern for older adults. They result from multiple factors (Chapter 15) and can indicate the decline of the musculoskeletal system at the subcellular level that occurs with aging. Falls increase dependence and can be predictors of poor outcomes. Healthy People 2030 has set objectives to reduce the rate of emergency department visits due to falls among older adults and to reduce fall-related deaths among older adults (Office of Disease Prevention and Health Promotion, 2020). Fall prevention includes fall risk assessments and in-home safety assessments to alter the home environment for safety.

Vision and hearing loss can affect physical and psychological health in the older adult. Sensory input is needed to protect oneself from accidents, social isolation, and limitations in self-care. Visual impairments (e.g., cataracts, glaucoma, macular degeneration, or decreased peripheral vision) can limit driving ability as well as isolate the older adult. Decreased hearing is also common in older adults. Social stigmas related to memory changes such as forgetfulness and dementia are a serious concern for many older adults. Older adults experiencing depression often believe they have memory changes and attempt to hide their symptoms rather than seek treatment for their depression.

CHRONIC ILLNESS

A **chronic illness** is defined as an illness that is long lasting or that recurs and is never completely cured. It usually interferes with the person's ability to perform ADLs. The degree of disability a person has depends not only on the condition and its severity but also on the individual effects for that person. For example, both John F. Kennedy and Franklin D. Roosevelt would have been eligible for disability benefits because of their chronic illnesses, but both were able to serve as president.

When caring for those with chronic illnesses, the goal of nursing care is to maintain and, when able, improve the patient's quality of life. A chronic illness also affects the family dynamics of the patient's family. Therefore, when planning patient care, the family's needs must also be considered.

Fostering hope is a primary foundation of care planning for people who are chronically ill. Whenever there is life, there is potential for growth in areas such as developmental tasks, health promotion, knowledge, and spirituality. Individuals have psychological developmental tasks to perform even as they cope with illness or prepare for a peaceful death.

The Chronic Disease Self-Management Program (CDSMP) is an effective self-management education program for people with chronic health problems that was developed by Stanford University and is now offered by the Self-Management Resource Center (www.selfmanagementresource.com). Healthy People 2030 supports the use of these interactive community-based programs to teach those with chronic illnesses, such as arthritis, ways to cope with and manage their condition. Program participants have increased their ability to perform ADLs and IADLs and have fewer concerns, anxiety, frustration, depression, and pain and more confidence in managing their condition. Providing information about these local programs is a way to provide support to your patients.

Incidence of Chronic Illness

Incidences of chronic illness are rising for three reasons. First, people are living longer, and fewer people are dying from acute diseases. This is in part due to antibiotics, better hygiene, exercise, nutrition, new treatments, and vaccinations. Second, medical advances have reduced mortality from some chronic illnesses. In turn, people are living longer with these illnesses. Third, today's technologically advanced and modern lifestyle contributes to the development of some chronic illnesses. Examples include a sedentary lifestyle; exposure to air and water pollution, chemicals, and carcinogens; substance abuse; and stress.

Types of Chronic Illnesses

Chronic illnesses have different causes (Box 14.1). One chronic illness can lead to development of other illnesses (e.g., hypertension can cause chronic kidney disease). Chronic illness can begin at any age. With age, there is an increasing likelihood of developing one or more chronic illnesses, such as arthritis, hypertension, or sensory losses.

> **CRITICAL THINKING & CLINICAL JUDGMENT**
>
> **Mrs. Lucia,** age 87, lives alone and one day has a dizzy spell. Her daughter takes her to the emergency department, where her blood pressure reading is 170/88. She is diagnosed with hypertension. Mrs. Lucia is started on metoprolol (Lopressor) 50 mg bid. She is discharged to her home with instructions on taking her medication, following a low-sodium diet, and home safety.
>
> **Critical Thinking (The Why)**
> 1. Why might Mrs. Lucia have an increased risk of falling?
>
> **Clinical Judgment (The Do)**
> 2. What patient-centered nursing interventions do you implement to promote Mrs. Lucia's independence and safety?
> 3. With what health team members do you collaborate?
>
> *Suggested answers are at the end of the chapter.*

Gerontological Influence

As people live longer, spouses or older relatives are increasingly being called on to care for chronically ill family members. Children of older adults who themselves are reaching their 60s and may have chronic illnesses of their own are being expected to care for their frail parents. A family in

---

Box 14.1

Examples of Chronic Illnesses by Cause

Genetic
- Cystic fibrosis
- Huntington disease
- Sickle cell anemia

Congenital
- Heart defects
- Malabsorption syndromes
- Spina bifida

Acquired
- AIDS
- Diabetes mellitus
- Emphysema
- Multiple sclerosis

this situation is at great risk for ineffective coping or further development of health problems. Assessment of all older members of the family is essential to ensure that all their health and coping needs are being met.

Older adults are concerned about becoming dependent on others. They may become depressed and give up hope if they feel that they are a burden to others. Establishing short-term goals or self-care activities that allow them to participate or have small successes is an important nursing action that can increase self-esteem. The nursing diagnosis *Frail Elderly Syndrome* may apply to older chronically ill patients.

Barriers to care can exist for a chronically ill older patient. These include not understanding medications; being on special diets that require knowledge to follow, are difficult to prepare or obtain, or exceed a modest food budget; needing treatments that require complex care; and being unfamiliar with supportive services in the community. Share information with older patients and their families about meal programs or respite care. Provide a resource person they can contact with questions.

Effects of Chronic Illness

To cope with a chronic illness and resulting functional limitations, lifelong routines and habits may need to be changed. Treatment needs, such as going to therapy sessions, performing peritoneal dialysis exchanges, or monitoring blood glucose, can interrupt daily life and require adaptation into the daily routine.

Chronic Sorrow

Chronic sorrow is felt by those affected by a chronic illness as well as their significant others and caregivers. This intermittently occurring sadness occurs in response to losses caused by a chronic illness. When chronic sadness occurs, nursing care should be focused on active listening. Understanding the loss allows nurses to offer comfort, information, and support. To provide patient-centered care, a patient-identified social network care map can be helpful to the health-care team in promoting self-care management (Young et al, 2019). The nursing diagnosis *Chronic Sorrow* may apply to those with chronic illnesses.

Spiritual Distress

Patients with chronic illness can experience spiritual distress when faced with the limitations of their illness. Maintaining a patient's quality of life includes assisting with spiritual needs. Several factors may make you uncomfortable in caring for a patient's spiritual needs. These include a lack of training, a lack of understanding of your own spiritual needs and beliefs, and not recognizing or believing that this is your role. Examine your own spiritual needs, and then define a personal spiritual view. Doing this can help you develop insight into others' spiritual needs and resources. It will help you gain insight into issues surrounding your patients' spiritual needs, which may help you become more comfortable with addressing these needs.

Spirituality helps many patients cope with chronic illness. It gives them a sense of wholeness, hope, and peace during uncertain times. Spirituality empowers patients to handle their condition. It is a source of inner strength. A meditation room for quiet reflection or prayer, chaplain visits, or worship services can be used to support spirituality in the hospital or long-term care facility.

Accreditation agencies require that the spiritual needs of patients are addressed and documented by nurses. Nursing diagnoses related to spiritual needs include *Spiritual Distress, Readiness for Enhanced Spiritual Well-Being,* and *Impaired Religiosity.*

> **NURSING CARE TIP**
> Spirituality is feeling connected to a higher power. It should not be considered in only religious terms. Everyone has spiritual needs that involve hope, peace, and wholeness. Spiritual care goes beyond asking a patient's religion. It involves identifying the patient's perceptions of spirituality and ways to meet the person's spiritual needs.

> **CUE RECOGNITION 14.1**
> A new resident whom you are caring for states, "I am so sad that I can no longer go to church." What action do you take?
>
> *Suggested answers are at the end of the chapter.*

Powerlessness

A chronic illness can be unpredictable. This leaves the patient vulnerable during the phases of a chronic illness: the diagnosis, the instability phase, an acute illness or crisis, remissions, and a terminal phase. Treatments that the patient undergoes may be painful, frightening, and invasive. A patient who does not understand what is happening can feel overwhelmed and alone. These feelings contribute to a sense of **powerlessness** because the patient cannot control the outcome (Fig. 14.2). This lack of control throughout an illness influences the patient's reactions to the illness. The nursing diagnosis *Powerlessness* may apply to chronically ill patients.

Coping With the Impact of Chronic Illness

Patients can be helped to feel more in control of their illness if you remember to include them in their care. Listen to their feelings, values, and goals. Explain all procedures before they occur. Avoid using complex medical language when talking with patients to increase their understanding and feeling of being included in their care. Developing a positive attitude toward dealing with the illness can help patients cope. This can be accomplished if patients gain knowledge, use a problem-solving approach, become motivated to continue adapting to the illness, and have resilience ("Evidence-Based Practice").

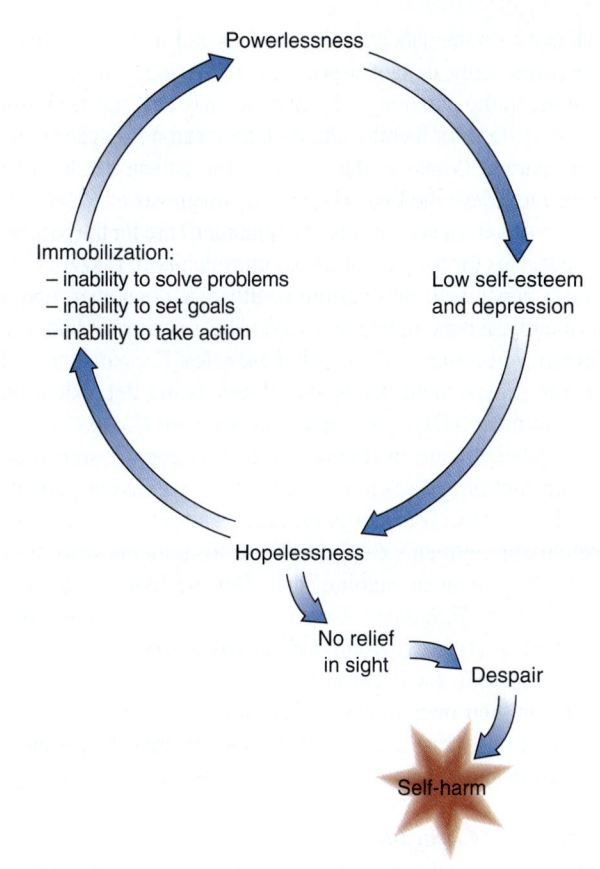

FIGURE 14.2 Powerlessness–hopelessness cycle.

Having a variety of coping techniques can be useful. Ask patients about their perception of the illness and coping techniques that were previously used successfully. New coping resources may need to be added to help patients effectively deal with the chronic illness. Make referrals to social workers in long-term care, or provide community support service information to patients and families living in the community. To promote effective coping, help patients learn to be comfortable with the newly defined person they are to become. The nursing diagnoses *Ineffective Coping and Disabled Family Coping* may apply to those dealing with chronic illness.

Hope

Before coping resources can be used, hope must be established in the patient. False hope is not beneficial and should be replaced with realistic hope. Providing the patient with accurate knowledge regarding their fears helps do this. Hope should not be directed toward a cure that may not be possible but rather at living a quality life within the patient's functional capacity. Over the course of the illness, hope must be maintained for both the patient and the family. Periodically identify whether the patient is maintaining hope. Studies have shown that patients adapt better when hope is high. The nursing diagnoses *Readiness for Enhanced Hope* or *Hopelessness* may apply to chronically ill patients.

Encouraging patients to live each moment to the fullest helps them experience the joy of being alive. Using humor aids patients in being lighthearted and hopeful. Simple things, such as a cool breeze, the warm sun on the skin through a facility window, the clean scent of the air after it rains, or the scent of pine trees, inspire hope and allow individuals to appreciate the beauty of nature. Family members can be encouraged to foster hope in the patient. Doing so can make them feel hopeful as well. During times of acute illness, it is beneficial for the patient to maintain as much control as possible and be informed if any loss of control related to treatments is temporary. This prevents a continual feeling of loss of power. The use of music or inspirational reading material can reduce stress and help the patient find meaning in life. This in turn fosters hope. Hopeful patients are empowered and do not feel powerless.

Sexuality

Chronic illness can affect a patient's sexuality, which includes femininity and masculinity as well as sexual activity. Changes in the physical body affect the way patients view themselves and are viewed by others. Patients with a negative body image perception may withdraw and become depressed. When interacting with patients, be aware of your facial expressions, nonverbal cues such as appearing hurried or keeping a distance, use of or lack of touch, and amount of time spent with the patient. When patients believe they have lost their femininity or masculinity, their self-worth decreases. Interventions to enhance sexuality should be used. One example is obtaining a wig for patients undergoing chemotherapy.

Sexual intimacy can include touching, hugging, or sharing time together. Provide patients with the opportunity to

---

Evidence-Based Practice

Clinical Question
What lifestyle behavioral factors affect multimorbidity resilience?

Evidence
Data for 6,771 Canadian adults 65 or older who had two or more chronic illnesses was reviewed to identify lifestyle behavioral factors associated with multimorbidity resilience. For those who identified cardiovascular/metabolic and osteo-related illness clusters, having a non-obese body mass, not smoking, getting satisfactory quality of sleep, having a good appetite, and not skipping meals are associated with multimorbidity resilience.

Implications for Nursing Practice
Reinforcing teaching about healthy lifestyle choices and including interventions in the plan of care that support achievement of these choices, such as weight loss, smoking cessation, promoting sleep and proper nutrition, promotes resilience during a chronic illness.

Reference: Wister, A., Cosco, T., Mitchell, B., & Fyffe, I. (2020). Health behaviors and multimorbidity resilience among older adults using the Canadian Longitudinal Study on Aging. *International Psychogeriatrics, 32*(1), 119–133. https://doi.org/10.1017/S1041610219000486

CRITICAL THINKING

Mr. Webb, age 90, lives in his own home with his wife of 65 years. He is in good health except for limited vision and is very active physically as he continues to golf with friends whom he still beats on the golf course even with limited vision. Mr. Webb's wife is in the early stages of Alzheimer disease. She cannot perform ADLs, so he has assumed the caregiver role. They complement each other's limitations because she has good vision and is helpful when she is not confused. Over time, Mr. Webb's wife's health declines, and she enters a long-term care facility. Mr. Webb remains in his home alone, which concerns his family. They eventually convince him to move into senior housing. He is very reluctant to leave his home and does not actively participate in moving and selling his home. Mr. Webb rarely leaves his new apartment, sleeps 14 hours a day, and eats one daily meal. He tries to visit his wife by taking a bus but finds it difficult because of his limited vision, so he rarely sees her. Three months later, Mr. Webb develops pneumonia and dies.

1. Why do you think Mr. Webb behaved the way he did after he moved?
2. What patient-centered interventions could have been used to empower Mr. Webb?
3. Why might Mr. Webb have developed pneumonia and died?

Suggested answers are at the end of the chapter.

discuss sexuality questions. Be professional and confidential. Sexuality counselors can help chronically ill patients cope with their sexuality needs.

Because sexuality is a part of a person's lifelong identity, ensure older patients' sexuality is addressed in their plans of care. Patients in long-term care facilities should be given private time with their significant other as appropriate. Grooming methods can increase a patient's self-esteem and sexual identity. Women may want to get their hair and nails done; men can be shaved or get a haircut. Older patients' sexuality needs should be met just as younger patients' needs are. The nursing diagnoses of *Disturbed Body Image, Sexual Dysfunction,* or *Ineffective Sexuality Pattern* may apply.

Roles

Chronically ill patients usually are faced with altering their accustomed roles in life, such as spouse, grandparent, parent, provider, homemaker, employee, and friend. Not only must the patient deal with these role alterations, but the family must adapt to them as well. Family members may have to take on new roles to compensate for roles the patient can no longer perform. The nursing diagnosis of *Ineffective Role Performance* should be included in the plan of care for the patient and family.

The patient is faced with giving up aspects of old roles at the same time that new roles related to being chronically ill need to be assumed. Grieving accompanies the loss of old roles. If a patient can no longer participate in social activities, grief work can help the patient accept the loss and maintain dignity. Sometimes, only certain aspects of a role may change. For example, in the parenting role, patients may still function as a support system for a child, although they can no longer be the disciplinarian. Whatever the role loss, the patient needs to be allowed to grieve the loss. The nursing diagnosis of *Readiness for Enhanced Grieving* may help in planning care for the patient.

New roles for the patient who is chronically ill may include being a dependent, an ongoing health-care consumer, and a chronically ill person. Patients need to be given understanding while they become familiar with these roles. For patients used to being independent before the illness, being dependent on others to meet ADLs can impact self-esteem. Navigating the complex health-care and financial reimbursement systems can be overwhelming. Patient care navigators can assist patients with these tasks. Transportation needs and waiting times for medical appointments can be difficult for patients who must deal with them on an ongoing basis. *Deficient Knowledge* and *Readiness for Enhanced Knowledge* are nursing diagnoses helpful for fostering learning for these new roles.

As patients live with chronic illness over time, they become experts on their own illness. Today, patients are being viewed as partners in their health care. Being sensitive to patients' knowledge and respecting it increases patients' self-esteem.

Family and Caregivers

Families are affected by the chronic illness of a family member in many ways. Most chronic illness care is provided in the home so that families can become involved in the management of the illness. Family members may have to take on new family roles or assume the role of caregiver. Decreased socialization, lost income, and increased medical expenses can increase family stress and tension.

Families must learn to cope with the stress of illness and its often-unpredictable course. Most families develop ways to cope with the patient's illness. They may become closer as a family unit. Families often deal with the illness on a day-by-day basis. They may take a passive approach to letting problems work themselves out. During times of exacerbation or crisis, however, the family may need coping assistance (Box 14.2).

Patients are often concerned about being a burden to their families. It is important to determine both the family's and the patient's feelings about the care required for the patient. The family's ability to provide this care adequately must also be considered in care planning. If the family lacks the desire, skills, or resources to adequately care for the patient, alternative care options, such as home health care, adult foster care, or long-term care, must be explored.

Box 14.2

Caregiver Resources

AARP: Family Caregiving, www.aarp.org/caregiving
Eldercare Locator, https://eldercare.acl.gov
Family Caregiver Alliance, www.caregiver.org

Patients' caregivers often have certain ideas about the care that the patient should receive. Caregiver input into the patient's plan of care should be sought so that everyone has a clear understanding of the goals and expectations for the patient's care.

Caregivers can experience depression, role strain, guilt, powerlessness, and grieving related to caregiving. Awareness of these potential feelings helps nurses detect indications that caregivers need help in dealing with them. Chronic care coaches are available to provide caregivers with insight, encouragement, and support for caring for someone who is chronically ill. Nursing diagnoses for caregivers include *Risk for Caregiver Role Strain* and *Caregiver Role Strain*.

RESPITE CARE. When caregivers are required to provide 24-hour care for a patient, they can experience burnout, fatigue, and stress. If extreme, this may lead to patient abuse. Patients may not be able to be left alone, even briefly, because of wandering behaviors, confusion, or safety issues. Caregivers might find it impossible to get a normal night's sleep and suffer from sleep deprivation because of the patient's wandering or around-the-clock treatment needs. It is essential for caregivers to have periodic relief from caregiving to reduce the stress of constant responsibility. Everyone requires private time for reflection or pursuing favorite hobbies and interests. Caregivers may need a night or weekend away simply to sleep soundly and be refreshed. **Respite care** is designed to provide caregivers with a much-needed break from caregiving by providing someone else to assume the caregiver role. Be familiar with your community's respite care services, and share that information with caregivers.

CUE RECOGNITION 14.2
During a home care visit, the caregiver begins to cry and says, "I can't do this anymore!" What action do you take?

Suggested answers are at the end of the chapter.

CLINICAL JUDGMENT
Mrs. Bow, age 68, is caring for her husband, who has Alzheimer disease. He wanders at night and has been found outside in his pajamas in freezing winter weather. He tries to cook and burns the pans. He cannot express his needs. He disrobes frequently and is incontinent. Mrs. Bow quit her job to care for him. She no longer goes to lunch weekly with her friends. Her children live out of town. She places a chair and tin cans in front of the home's doors as an alarm in case her husband opens the doors while she tries to sleep.
1. What data do you identify that indicates that Mrs. Bow is experiencing caregiver role strain?
2. What additional data do you collect for Mrs. Bow?
3. What nursing diagnoses do you suggest to the RN to include in Mrs. Bow's plan of care?
4. What nursing interventions do you plan to implement in collaboration with the RN to assist Mrs. Bow?
5. With what health team members do you collaborate?

Suggested answers are at the end of the chapter.

FINANCES. Managing a chronic illness can be expensive. Income can be lost if the patient is unable to work or caregivers are forced to stay home. Insurance may not cover all

Home Health Hints
Patient-Centered Care
- Medicare requires that the home health-care (HHC) patient participates in the development of the plan of care. The patient has the right to be informed in advance about the care to be furnished and of any changes in care. Involve the patient in care planning by asking about care preferences and assisting the patient to set realistic and meaningful goals. Praise the effort the patient is making toward meeting their goals.
- Asking about displayed photos or mementos can increase a patient's self-concept.
- Reminiscing with the patient can reveal how they have coped with challenges in the past.
- Using appropriate humor can relieve stress and humanize care. However, humor can be irritating if the patient is distraught, anxious, or angry.

Resources
- Caregivers of bed-confined patients can use a portable monitor to hear the patient.
- Occupational and physical therapists can recommend adaptive equipment for ADLs to increase patient independence.
- The HHC social worker should be informed of any patient financial concerns.

Education
These patients and their families have tremendous educational needs if they are to learn to cope successfully with a long-term illness. The following are primary tasks that chronically ill patients and their families/caregivers will need to perform:
- Be willing and able to carry out the medical regimen.
- Reorder time for treatments, medication schedules, and pacing of activities.
- Understand and control symptoms. Know when symptoms should be reported to the HCP.
- Prevent and manage crises.
- Adjust to positive or negative changes in the disease over the course of time.
- Compensate for symptoms and limitations to be treated as normally as possible by others.
- Prevent social isolation related to physical limitations or altered body image.

Explain individualized interventions to deal with these tasks during educational sessions. Have the patient or family teach back instructions in their own words to evaluate understanding. Provide dignity and show respect to all patients ("Patient Perspective"). Unique approaches can positively assist chronically ill patients and their families on their long-term journey.

of the patient's expenses. Family savings can quickly be used up and place a strain on families. Financial difficulties can lead to the nursing diagnoses *Disabled Family Coping*. Social work referrals can be made to assist with financial aid.

Health Promotion

Health promotion is possible and necessary at all ages and levels of disability. Patients with chronic illness make daily lifestyle choices that affect their health. For example, the patient with chronic lung disease makes the choice to smoke or to quit smoking, and a patient with degenerative joint disease chooses whether to maintain an ideal weight to reduce wear and tear on the joints. Providing patients with the knowledge to make informed decisions empowers them to take control of their lives and reach their greatest potential.

Nursing Care

Because of the nature of chronic illness, nurses should understand the unique needs of patients and their families experiencing chronic illness. These needs differ from those of patients experiencing acute care. In-depth knowledge is needed by the patient. Recognize that the wishes of the patient must be respected. Patients have the right to establish their own goals along with the health-care team. Today, patients participate in their own daily bedside rounds with their health-care team. This is true patient-centered care! Most chronic illness care occurs in the home and community ("Home Health Hints"). Family members and caregivers must be included in the plan of care to offer support to the patient.

Patient Perspective

Mr. Lyman
A note to my nurse:
- Be polite!
- Don't call me "sweetie" or "honey." My name is Mr. Lyman. If I want you to call me by my first name, I'll tell you.
- Don't give me a huge glass of water; give me a small glass and don't fill it full. Otherwise, when I drink it, it spills all down the front of me.
- When you leave my meal tray, make sure I can reach it. Then when you take it away, don't leave a bunch of stuff on my table. There is not much room on those little tables.
- Ask how I like my blankets. Don't just fix them the way you do for anyone else.
- Make sure my call light is where I can reach it.
- Make sure my overhead light is working and that I can reach it.
- Keep a wastebasket where I can reach it.
- Ask whether I need anything before you leave the room.
- Try to talk quietly in the hallway instead of being so loud.
- Thank you for preserving my dignity and showing me respect. I appreciate it!

Key Points

- Erickson's eight developmental stages of life focus on the balance a person must achieve for high-level wellness within that stage before accomplishing the next stage: young adulthood, ages 18 to 40, intimacy versus isolation; middle adulthood, ages 40 to 65, generativity versus self-absorption; and late adulthood, age 65 through death, integrity versus despair.
- A chronic illness is long-lasting or recurs and is never completely cured. It usually interferes with the person's ability to perform ADLs.
- Caregivers of people with chronic illnesses can experience depression, role strain, guilt, powerlessness, and grieving related to caregiving. Awareness of these potential feelings helps nurses detect indications that caregivers need help in dealing with them.
- It is essential for caregivers to have periodic relief (respite care) from caregiving to reduce the stress of always having to be responsible.
- Health promotion is possible and necessary at all ages or levels of disability. Providing patients with the knowledge to make informed decisions empowers them to take control of their lives and reach their greatest potential.
- Most chronic illness care occurs in the home and community so family members and caregivers must be included in the plan of care.
- A major focus of nursing care for the chronically ill is teaching. These patients and their families have tremendous educational needs if they are to learn to cope successfully with a long-term illness.

SUGGESTED ANSWERS TO CHAPTER EXERCISES

Cue Recognition

14.1: Inform resident of transportation options to her church and worship options at the long-term care facility.

14.2: Allow caregiver to express feelings, collect data, collaborate with the health-care team, arrange support resources such as respite care.

SUGGESTED ANSWERS TO CHAPTER EXERCISES—cont'd

Critical Thinking & Clinical Judgment

Mr. Crowley
1. Mr. Crowley's physical health is being affected by poor diet choices and stress.
2. It is easy to recognize the psychological stress related to parenting skills when a child is in trouble. Decreased family income with increased family expenses (two children in college) can cause financial strains. With family problems and health problems, Mr. Crowley may be questioning why things are happening to him and his family, causing him spiritual distress.

Mr. Klein
1. Stereotypical misconceptions about older adults are occurring. They can lead to the belief that pain is part of the aging process. Therefore, Mr. Klein's issue may not be diagnosed and treated appropriately.
2. Gathering data to assist with the diagnosis of the cause of the pain and possible treatment would improve Mr. Klein's quality of life. Taking him seriously would also convey that Mr. Klein is a valued member of society and would increase his self-esteem.

Mrs. Lucia
1. Falls could be caused by changes due to aging; things in the environment, such as throw rugs, clutter, or electrical cords in walking paths; lack of hand grips in the bathroom; or lack of nonskid mats in the shower or tub. Poor vision and altered depth perception can result in missing a stair step or obstacles. Weakness or orthostatic hypotension can cause an unsteady gait or a fall.
2. Explain home safety to the patient and family. Discuss with Mrs. Lucia the benefit of using a cane or a walker if she is unsteady. Because Mrs. Lucia lives alone, a referral for a wearable emergency alert system could be beneficial. When activated, the transmitter alerts an answering service to contact designated individuals to check on the patient. Discussing medication safety is also important. Patients who take medications that lower blood pressure must be aware of the potential for orthostatic hypotension (drop in blood pressure with position changes), which can cause dizziness or lightheadedness and result in a fall.
3. Physical therapist for walking aids; social worker for emergency alert system information.

Mr. Webb
1. Mr. Webb lost control of his world and felt powerless. His environment, both home and outdoors, was shrinking. He had to give up his daily routines and interactions with others. His purpose in life was gone when he was no longer caring for his wife, whom he no longer could visit. His visual limitations made his new environment unfamiliar and frightening.
2. Options to keep him safely in his home could have been explored with his input. He should have been thoroughly oriented to his new environment and asked what his goals were for his new situation. Hobbies and interests, like golfing, should have been encouraged. Visual support services could have been contacted for support ideas. Transportation could have been arranged to allow him to visit his wife and continue golfing.
3. He was depressed and slept from a lack of interests. His lungs were at risk for pneumonia because of his long periods of immobility. He lost hope and gave up on living, which decreased his ability to fight the pneumonia.

Mrs. Bow
1. Mrs. Bow is at risk for sleep deprivation, fatigue, stress, and burnout.
2. How she is able to meet her own ADLs: bathing, hours of sleep per night, nutrition and appetite, privacy and time alone to relax. IADLs: shopping for groceries, cooking, paying the bills. Financial concerns. Social support—nearby family members.
3. Nursing diagnoses include *Disturbed Sleep Pattern, Fatigue, Social Isolation, Risk for Caregiver Role Strain,* and *Deficient Knowledge.*
4. Beneficial nursing interventions would include teaching her about Alzheimer disease, recommending a chronic care coach, providing a respite care referral, using alarm devices for wandering, and teaching her stress management techniques.
5. Case manager, chaplain, social worker.

Additional Resources

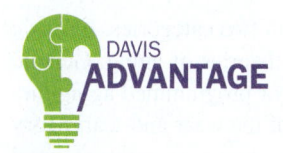

Go to Davis Advantage to complete your learning: strengthen understanding, apply your knowledge, and prepare for the Next Gen NCLEX®.

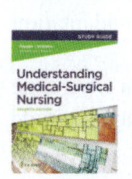

A Study Guide is also available.

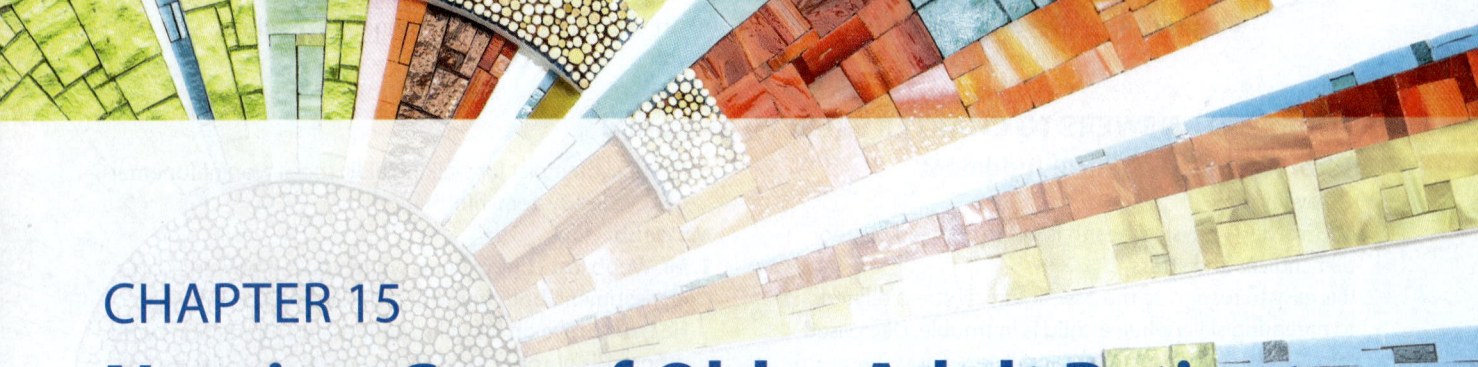

CHAPTER 15
Nursing Care of Older Adult Patients

MaryAnne Pietraniec-Shannon

KEY TERMS

activities of daily living (ack-TIH-vih-tees of DAY-lee LIH-ving)
aspiration (AS-pi-RAY-shun)
constipation (KON-sti-PAY-shun)
contractures (kon-TRAK-churs)
delirium (dih-LEER-ee-um)
dementia (dih-MENT-sha)
depression (dih-PRESH-shun)
edema (eh-DEE-muh)
expectorate (ek-SPEK-tuh-RAYT)
frailty (FRAYL-tee)
holistic (ho-LIS-tik)
homeostasis (HO-mee-oh-STAY-sis)
nocturia (nok-TOO-ree-ah)
osteoporosis (OS-tee-oh-puh-ROH-sis)
perception (per-SEP-shun)
pressure injury (PRESH-ur IN-jer-ee)
range of motion (RAYNJ of MOH-shun)
reality orientation (ree-AL-ih-tee OR-ee-en-TAY-shun)
sensory deprivation (SEN-suh-ree DEP-rih-VAY-shun)
sensory overload (SEN-suh-ree OH-ver-lohd)
urinary incontinence (YOOR-ih-NARE-ee in-KON-tih-nents)

CHAPTER CONCEPTS

Caring
Cognition
Safety
Self-care
Sensory perception
Stress and coping

LEARNING OUTCOMES

1. Define aging.
2. Describe basic physiological changes associated with advancing age.
3. Describe the psychological and cognitive changes associated with advancing age.
4. Plan nursing care for physiological and psychological changes associated with advancing age.
5. Identify nursing practices that promote safety for the older patient.

WHAT IS AGING?

In this chapter, *aging* is defined as a maturational process that creates the need for individual adaptation because of physical and psychological declines that occur throughout life. Even though aging truly begins at conception, the focus in this chapter is on the maturational process that is experienced after age 65 (older adult). People ages 85 and older are usually the frailest, although chronological age alone should never be the basis for determining health status. Functional age (health, independence, and functional abilities) should be used to determine individual care needs.

NURSING CARE TIP
Aging is a unique experience. Placing older adults into one category titled "old" overlooks this fact of aging. The concept of *functional age* recognizes that aging is individual, which promotes the need for individualized patient-centered care for the older adult.

Factors that contribute to aging fall within two categories. Intrinsic factors focus on genetic and physiological theories of aging. Genetic theories include the biological clock theory or programmed aging theory. Physiological theories include aspects of the wear-and-tear theory or stress adaptation theory. Extrinsic factors focus on environmental influences, such as pollutants, free-radical theory, and stress-adaptation theory.

Perception and attitude play key roles in how changes over time affect the individual. It is through the filter of perception and attitude that a person identifies, defines, and adapts to the changes that occur in body structure and function over time.

According to the 2019 profile of older Americans, 16% of the population consisted of older adults (Administration for Community Living, 2020a). Over the past 10 years, the population ages 65 and over increased 35% and is projected to reach 94.7 million in 2060 The fastest growing age-group continues to be adults 85 and older.

Approximately 70% of people turning age 65 can expect to use some form of long-term care during their lifetime (Administration for Community Living, 2020b). Adults who live in the United States and need elder care can choose from diverse settings such as home care, assisted living care, hospice care, adult day services, and residential aging communities (see Chapter 16). Regardless of care setting, it is quality nursing care that allows the older person the ability to function at the highest possible level.

> **PRACTICE ANALYSIS TIP**
> **Linking NCLEX-PN® to Practice**
> The LPN/LVN will provide care that meets the needs of the adult client ages 65 and over.

PHYSIOLOGICAL CHANGES

Over time, cells change and do not function as efficiently as in earlier years. Cellular decline in structure and function increases in severity and extent over time. Although the body works hard to maintain **homeostasis**, it is often unable to fully adapt to many of the declines that result from aging. Some cells that die cannot regenerate themselves. As a result, structures are altered. The body then tries to make the revised structure meet functional demands, which increases the **frailty** of the individual (Box 15.1).

Common Physiological Changes in Older Adults and Their Implications for Nursing Care

Key Changes in the Muscular System
Age-related changes in the muscular system include the following:

- Decreased elasticity of tendons and ligaments, resulting in restricted movements
- Decreased muscle mass, making muscles look smaller
- Slower muscle response, increasing response time
- Decreased muscle tone, making muscles flabbier
- Weakness from decreased muscle mass or tone

NURSING CARE. Changes in the muscular system impact movement, strength, and endurance. These changes can also increase the risk for injury. Because muscle response is slower, movement takes longer. This can impact the older person's confidence and ability to perform routine tasks. Collaborate with an occupational therapist for assistive devices.

> **Box 15.1**
> **Preventive Strategies to Slow the Onset of Elder Frailty**
> **F**ood intake maintenance
> **R**esistance exercises
> **A**therosclerosis prevention activities
> **I**solation avoidance
> **L**imit pain
> **T**ai Chi and other balance exercises
> **Y**early testosterone level checks for men
>
> Reprinted from Morley, J. E., Vellas, B., Abellan van Kan, G., Anker, S. D., Bauer, J. M., Bernabei, R., Cesari, M., Chumlea, W. C., Doehner, W., Evans, J., Fried, L. P., Guralnik, J. M., Katz, P. R., Malmstrom, T. K., McCarter, R. J., Gutierrez Robledo, L. M., Rockwood, K., von Haehling, S., Vandewoude, M. F., & Walston, J. (2013). Frailty consensus: A call to action, *Journal of the American Medical Directors Association, 14*(6), 392–397, with permission from Elsevier.

Key Changes in the Skeletal System
Age-related changes in the skeletal system include the following:

- Exaggerated bony prominences, increasing risk for skin breakdown
- Eroding cartilage, making joint movement painful
- Joint stiffening, decreasing flexibility
- **Osteoporosis,** thinning (decrease in density) and softening of the bone
- Water loss in the intervertebral discs of the spinal column and flexion of the spine associated with the influence of gravity over time, reducing height

NURSING CARE. Muscles and bones work together for movement, so age-related skeletal changes are most obvious when the older patient is moving. **Range of motion** (ROM) can be limited in the arms, legs, and neck of the older patient. **Contractures** of the fingers and hands can limit the person's ability to perform **activities of daily living** (ADLs). Assisting the patient with ROM exercises can prevent long-term disabilities from contractures (Fig. 15.1). Prescribed anti-inflammatory medications for arthritis can be administered so their action peaks when exercises are beginning. Older patients taking anti-inflammatory medicines should be taught to monitor for gastrointestinal (GI) upset or bleeding to report symptoms to their health-care provider (HCP). Performing ROM exercises in warm water can also help prevent pain.

Bone density is influenced by diet and weight-bearing exercise. Nutrition should be balanced and rich in calcium and vitamin D. Safe weight-bearing exercise programs should

• WORD • BUILDING •

homeostasis: homios—similar + stasis—standing
osteoporosis: osteon—bone + poros—a passage + osis—condition

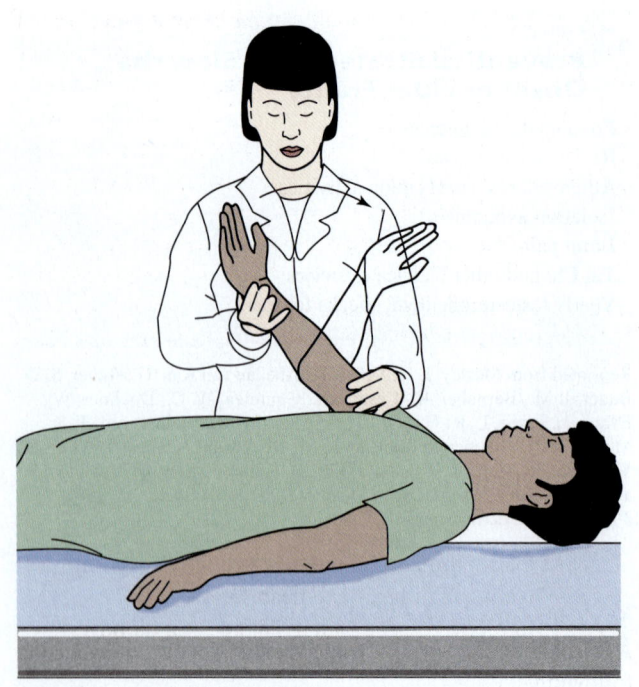

FIGURE 15.1 Nurse assists patient in range-of-motion exercises to prevent the development of contractures.

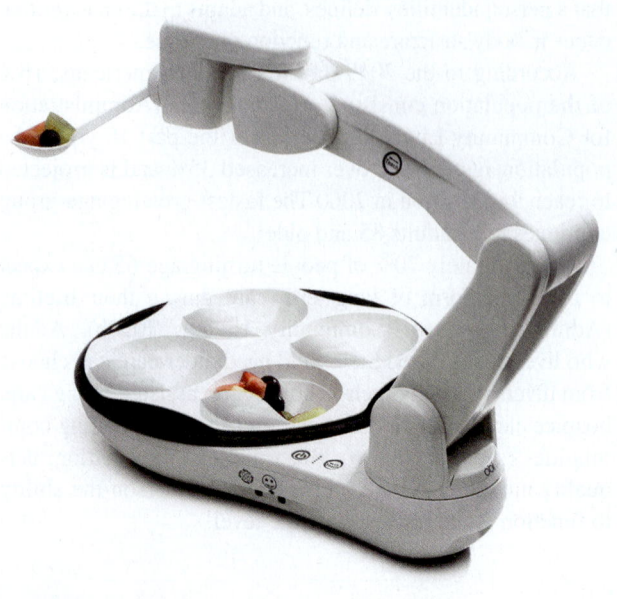

FIGURE 15.2 Obi robotic dining device.

> **PRACTICE ANALYSIS TIP**
> Linking NCLEX-PN® to Practice
> The LPN/LVN will assist with activities of daily living.

be encouraged. Tai-chi, an ancient Chinese gentle system of exercise and stretching, is helpful in promoting balance and flexibility for the older adult to prevent falls. The environment needs to be safe for walking. Sturdy assistive devices such as handrails, canes, or walkers should be used as needed. Supportive shoes with nonskid soles can keep patients safe when walking.

Decreasing density of bones can cause fractures that result in falls or falls that cause fractures. In both genders, severe pain, increased frailty, low level of activity, and one or more chronic diseases are linked to falling. Gender differences also exist for fall risk (Resnick et al, 2020). Women are more likely to fall if they have higher depression scores and incontinence. Men are more likely to fall if they have poor hearing and currently smoke (Gale et al, 2018). Consider gender in planning for frailty prevention and fall risk precautions.

Gerontological Issues

Technology can be used to improve quality of life and promote safety for the older adult.
- Intelligent assistive technology (IAT): Robotic devices such as the Obi robotic dining device provide assistance with eating (Fig. 15.2; https://meetobi.com). Robotic pets can decrease loneliness. Other IAT tools, such as wearable sensors, assist in gait assessment and fall prevention.
- Video games that appeal to the older adult can provide exercise, socialization, and diversion to reduce boredom and loneliness.

Key Changes in the Neurologic System

Age-related changes in the neurologic system include the following:

- Decreased blood flow to the brain, causing short-term memory loss
- Decreased number of brain cells; remaining cells are functional
- Decreased endorphins, increasing risk for depression
- Decreased equilibrium and motor coordination, resulting in fall risk
- Decreased hypothalamus function and regulation of body temperature, increasing risk of hyper/hypothermia
- Slower reaction times, increasing risk for injury
- Decreased sensitivity, increasing risk for injury

NURSING CARE. Changes in the nervous system of the older patient occur in both the peripheral and central systems. These changes have significant meaning for the older person. They impact safety. With normal aging, there is a slowed response to stimuli. There is a marked decrease in the speed of the psychomotor response to the stimuli. Stronger stimuli are needed to elicit a neurologic response. The older patient may be unable to recognize early signs of danger. To protect from accidental skin burns, the thermostat on water heaters should be lowered, and electrical heating devices (heating pads, electric blankets, and mattress pads) should not be used.

With aging, maintaining balance becomes a safety issue. Musculoskeletal changes can affect balance. Plan care to assist older patients to safely transfer, stand, and ambulate.

Fine tremors of the hand can be a normal finding with age. These movements tend to increase when the older patient is active, cold, excited, or hungry. Collaborate with an occupational therapist for assistive devices for ADLs to help reduce the unsteadiness.

Normal neurologic changes that arise with age usually occur on both sides of the body at the same time. One-sided weakness, sensory deficits, and performance problems should always be referred for further evaluation. Coarse tremors of the finger, forearm, head, eyelids, or tongue that occur when the body part is at rest can be a sign of a neurologic problem such as Parkinson disease. These tremors typically occur on one side of the body first. Patients with these tremors should always be referred to HCP for further evaluation.

Key Changes in the Integumentary System

Age-related changes in the integumentary system include the following:

- Thin skin layers, making the skin more fragile
- Decreased subcutaneous fat layer, resulting in less insulation and less protective cushioning
- Water loss, causing increased dryness of the skin
- Decreased sebaceous and sweat glands, resulting in skin dryness and decreased temperature regulation.
- Increased pigmentation, causing aging spots
- Decreased melanin, resulting in gray hair
- Thinning scalp hair, resulting in baldness
- Harder and drier nails, making them more brittle

NURSING CARE. The skin is the first line of defense against infection and injury. In the older adult, skin injuries take longer to heal. Healing times can be affected by the presence of multiple chronic diseases. These diseases include diabetes and circulatory disorders. The older person with limited mobility is at risk of developing **pressure injuries** (see Chapter 54). It is important to take time to check skin integrity daily, especially in high-risk areas of the body. To prevent accidental injury to the feet, instruct patients not to walk barefoot. Potential pressure points on the feet should be monitored. Referral to a podiatrist is made when there are concerns. People with neuropathy (decreased sensation) or diabetes should assess their feet daily to prevent injury.

> **BE SAFE!**
> **BE VIGILANT!** A person with severe foot neuropathy wore shoes for 8 hours without recognizing that a small toy was wedged in the toe of the shoe. Because he could not feel the irritation of the toy, he continued to walk. It was not until the end of the day when he removed that shoe that he saw a severe pressure injury on his toe that required hospitalization. Encourage patients to check their shoes thoroughly before putting them on to ensure there is nothing in the shoes that could cause injury!

Skin care for the older adult should be gently performed (Ronch et al, 2004). Visit the New York State Department of Health Web site for gentle bathing techniques at www.health.ny.gov/diseases/conditions/dementia/edge/interventions/gentle. These techniques include the towel bath, bag bath, and glove bath. These methods of bathing avoid the drying effects from using hot water and soap. Applying moisturizers regularly (except between toes); gently stimulating non-reddened, intact skin sites with massage; and avoiding use of heating pads that can cause burns are all helpful in protecting the skin. Nail care is also important for older people. Soaking nails in warm water helps soften nails for filing and promotes blood flow. Filing nails with an emery board is safer than cutting them.

Key Changes in the Cardiovascular System

Age-related changes in the cardiovascular system include the following:

- Increased arrhythmias (irregular heartbeats), resulting in poor oxygenation of heart and heart failure
- Decreased blood vessel elasticity, increasing blood pressure and cardiac workload
- Decreased cardiac output, causing less oxygen to body tissues
- Increased cardiac conduction time, possibly causing slower heart rate and making it unable to increase quickly
- Less efficient leg vein valves, creating fluid accumulation in tissues
- Atypical classic symptoms of cardiac emergencies, delaying recognition and treatment

NURSING CARE. Observe for early, subtle symptoms related to circulatory problems and report them to the HCP. Educate older patients on promotion of healthy circulation and prescribed medications. Monitoring fluid balance is important. Thirst may be decreased in the older adult. Oral fluids may need to be encouraged. Any IV fluids must be carefully monitored to prevent fluid overload. If leg **edema** is present, the legs should be elevated higher than the heart to promote blood return to the heart. Compression stockings should be worn for edema as ordered.

Changes in body position from lying to sitting to standing should occur gradually. Quickly changing body position can make the older patient feel weak and dizzy. Stand next to older patients as they dangle their legs over the side of the bed before rising to stand. For safety, use an ambulatory belt and a walker for unsteady older patients. Falls continue to be a leading cause of accidental death in older patients. A history of falls is a key predictor of future falls. Identify patients who are at risk of falling. Then implement interventions to prevent falls.

Key Changes in the Respiratory System

Age-related changes in the respiratory system include the following:

- Reduced emptying of the lungs, causing carbon dioxide (CO_2) retention

• WORD • BUILDING •
edema: oidema—swelling

- Decreased lung capacity, causing dyspnea with activity
- Decreased lung recoil strength or gag reflex, producing weaker cough and pulmonary **aspiration** risk

NURSING CARE. The respiratory system is less efficient with advancing age. Older patients have a decreased tolerance for activity. It can take longer for normal respiratory functioning to return when under stress. Help older patients pace their activities. Schedule rest periods to prevent overexertion. Rest periods should not outnumber activity sessions. This will help prevent the older adult from becoming immobile.

Cough, fatigue, and confusion can be early signs of inadequate oxygenation. Respiratory rates over 25 per minute can be an early indicator of a lower respiratory tract infection. Normally, the larger lower lobes of the lungs perform the oxygen (O_2) to CO_2 exchange. However, the older patient performs this exchange in the less efficient upper lobes of the lung. Because lung recoil strength is decreased, mucus is more difficult for the older patient to **expectorate** (cough up). A weaker cough or gag reflex causes greater potential for lung problems.

Lifelong habits and exposures can contribute to respiratory sensitivity for the older patient. These include smoking, second- or thirdhand smoke exposure, work-related respiratory pollutant exposure, or paints and glues used in hobbies. It is important to include coughing, deep breathing, and position changes in the plan of care to stimulate all lobes of the older patient's lungs. Encourage the older adult to receive recommended pneumococcal and flu vaccines. You can help prevent the spread of respiratory illnesses to older patients. Receive an annual flu shot, perform hand hygiene between patients, and do not work when ill. Your patients will appreciate it!

Key Changes in the Gastrointestinal System

Age-related changes in the GI system include the following:

- Altered taste and smell, affecting eating enjoyment
- Decreased saliva production, causing dry mouth and altered taste
- Delayed gastric emptying, reducing appetite
- Decreased peristalsis, causing constipation
- Declining liver enzymes, reducing medication metabolism and detoxification

NURSING CARE. Age-related structural and functional changes put the older patient at risk for poor nutrition and illness ("Nutrition Notes"). Ask family members to bring in the patient's favorite approved seasoning in shakers to help stimulate appetite. Dietitians can provide ideas to promote healthful eating. Offering a calm and comfortable environment helps food digestion.

Older people may wear dentures or partial plates. But tooth loss is not a normal part of aging. With proper dental care, teeth should last a lifetime. For those with dentures, a significant change in body weight can affect the fit and comfort of dentures. Ask the patient about denture fit and comfort regularly. When assisting the older patient with oral care, examine gum health and the oral cavity.

> **Nutrition Notes**
> **Older Adult Nutritional Needs**
> Changes in physiology and psychosocial conditions make older adults vulnerable to protein-calorie malnutrition. This negatively impacts their functional status. Decreased muscle mass, increased fat stores, and nutrient deficiencies can cause anemia, cognitive function impairment, immune dysfunction, osteoporosis, impaired wound healing, and weakness. These conditions can further impair the ability of individuals to shop, cook, and consume adequate calories and nutrients.
>
> Achlorhydria (low or absent gastric acid in the stomach) can occur as a result of age-related changes or from chronic ingestion of stomach acid-reducing medications such as protein pump inhibitors. In either case, protein digestion and absorption of iron and vitamin B_{12} can be impaired by the lack of gastric acid and intrinsic factor required for vitamin B_{12} absorption (see "Nutrition Notes" in Chapter 28). Malabsorption of iron and vitamin B_{12} can lead to anemia; however, sources of blood loss should also be considered. If a vitamin B_{12} deficiency is identified, fortified foods or supplements are recommended (Klemm, 2020).
>
> Decreased visual acuity and impaired dexterity can make shopping for food and preparing it difficult or even hazardous. Arthritis can affect jaw movements, so chewing can be problematic. Approximately 13% of U.S. residents ages 65 to 74 and 26% of adults over age 74 have lost all their teeth (edentulous) (Lauritano et al, 2019).
>
> Food, nutrient, and medication interactions can occur. A nutritional assessment by a registered dietitian should be done if alcohol consumption, polypharmacy (multiple medications), or a chronic illness is identified.
>
> Older adults should be offered the opportunity for toileting before eating. Providing enough time to eat is essential to accomplish the task of eating. If a patient needs help with eating, be sensitive to the patient's pace. Give the patient as much control when eating as possible. A robotic dining device can learn the patient's feeding preferences and pace to provide patient-centered feeding assistance (Fig. 15.2; https://meetobi.com). Adequate nutritional intake can be impaired by social isolation (Roberts et al, 2019). Therefore, encourage the patient to be out of bed and to eat with others, as much as possible. However, it is also important to respect the patient's right of refusal to eat in a designated social setting. Some patients might not eat as well when seated next to agitated or confused residents in a common dining hall.

Medications can cause taste disturbances or problems with dry mouth, which can affect the older patient's ability to eat. Some medications reduce bowel motility. **Constipation** may occur. Stress, anxiety, or a change in routine can also

- WORD - BUILDING -

expectorate: ex—out + pectus—breast

> ### Evidence-Based Practice
>
> **Clinical Question**
> Can a 1-year Mediterranean diet intervention alter the gut microbiota and reduce frailty?
>
> **Evidence**
> The gut microbiota of 612 non-frail or pre-frail participants from five European countries was analyzed before and after a 12-month long Mediterranean diet intervention for older adults. It was found that promoting a Mediterranean diet was associated with signs of lower frailty, such as improved cognitive function, hand strength, walking speed, and inflammatory markers. A higher intake of fiber, vitamin C, thiamine, copper, iron, and manganese from this diet likely contributed to this finding.
>
> **Implications for Nursing Practice**
> Planning care to overcome obstacles to maintaining a Mediterranean diet helps protect the older patient's microbiome from changes to it that relate to frailty and disease. These obstacles include limited fresh produce, high cost, poor dentition, reduced saliva production, dysphagia, or irritable bowel syndrome.
>
> *Reference:* Ghosh, T. S., Rampelli, S., Jeffery, I. B., Santoro, A., Neto, M., Capri, M., Giampieri, E., Jennings, A., Candela, M., Turroni, S., Zoetendal, E. G., Hermes, G., Elodie, C., Meunier, N., Brugere, C. M., Pujos-Guillot, E., Berendsen, A. M., De Groot, L., Feskins, E., . . . O'Toole, P. W. (2020). Mediterranean diet intervention alters the gut microbiome in older people reducing frailty and improving health status: The NU-AGE 1-year dietary intervention across five European countries. *Gut, 69*(7), 1218–1228. https://doi.org/10.1136/gutjnl-2019-319654

cause constipation. Obtain baseline information about bowel routines unique for each older patient. Ask what the patient expects when it comes to "regular bowel movements." Identify what has worked for bowel elimination in the past. Over-the-counter and prescribed enemas, suppositories, and medications are often misused in this age-group. When overused, these products can create an unhealthy dependency. Teach the older patient realistic expectations for bowel elimination. Discuss the intake of fiber and water and exercise to promote safe elimination.

Key Changes in the Endocrine-Metabolic System

Age-related changes in the endocrine-metabolic system include:

- Decreased pancreatic insulin release and impaired glucose tolerance, increasing potential for hyperglycemia
- Altered adrenal hormone production, decreased ability to respond to stress
- Slowing basal metabolic rate, requiring a 5% reduction in calorie consumption to maintain weight

NURSING CARE. Increased incidence of metabolic disease, such as diabetes, occurs with age. Encourage older adults to be screened for metabolic problems. With aging, there is also a notable decrease in the effectiveness and interaction of all hormones. It becomes more difficult for the older body to respond to stressful situations. Address the psychological needs of your older patients to help reduce stressors affecting their care.

Typical symptoms of hyperthyroidism or hypothyroidism are not seen in older patients. It is important *not to assume* that cold sensitivity, constipation, fatigue, fluid retention, forgetfulness, and skin changes are caused by "old age." These symptoms may actually be a result of an impaired thyroid gland. Blood tests can identify a thyroid problem.

Key Changes in the Genitourinary System

Age-related changes in the genitourinary system include the following:

- Benign prostate hypertrophy, causing difficult voiding
- Decreased bladder size and tone, increasing urinary frequency
- Decreased kidney filtration rate and tubular function, decreasing renal clearance of medications
- Weakened pelvic floor muscles, resulting in incontinence
- Increased incidents of urinary tract infections (UTIs), affecting mainly women
- Decreased urine concentrating ability, resulting in nocturia

NURSING CARE. Many older people have to urinate during the night (**nocturia**). Changes within the kidneys, medication effects, and heart failure can contribute to nocturia. Review patient medications and personal medication practices. For example, taking diuretics late in the day can cause nocturia and sleep disruption. Adjusting the diuretic schedule to earlier in the day can prevent this problem.

> ### NURSING CARE TIP
> With advancing age, older patients do not get the urge to void as early in the process as they did when younger. This aging change, accompanied with other normal aging changes in the urinary system (such as the pear-shaped bladder becoming funnel-shaped), contributes to the older patient's voiding urgency. If the patient is not assisted to void promptly upon making a request, incontinence can quickly result. This can create a fall risk if the patient attempts to get up alone and the floor is slippery. Provide safe patient-centered care by planning for and meeting the patient's voiding needs *promptly*.

> ### CUE RECOGNITION 15.1
> A patient, 77 years of age, who awakens from a nap calls for assistance to the bathroom. What action do you take?
>
> *Suggested answers are at the end of the chapter.*

• WORD • BUILDING •

nocturia: nocte—night + ouron—urine

Urinary incontinence is *not* a normal condition of aging. It is usually a treatable condition that requires evaluation. It is one of the main reasons older people enter long-term care facilities. In older men, urinary incontinence results from benign prostate hypertrophy (enlargement). In older women, it is likely due to a short urethra and weakened perineal muscles. Teaching pelvic floor muscle exercises is successful for some patients. All patients with urinary incontinence should be referred to a specialist.

Management of urinary incontinence is tailored to the need of the patient. Bladder training programs can be effective. They remind the older patient on a regular basis to toilet. Incontinence can result from problems that affect the toileting task itself. The toilet should be nearby, and pathways should be uncluttered. Clothing must be easy to remove. Velcro fasteners can replace buttons or zippers. Urinary briefs can help instill confidence in older patients who fear urine leakage so activity can be maintained. Ensure proper fit of the correct type of brief. Monitor for early signs of perineal skin breakdown.

Older patients may try to decrease urine leakage by severely limiting their fluid intake. This can result in dehydration and acid–base and electrolyte imbalances with confusion, diarrhea, vomiting, or weakness. Instead, a balanced fluid intake needs to be encouraged. Focus education on timing of liquid intake and beverage selection. Caffeine and alcoholic beverages promote urinary output and should be avoided.

UTIs are more common in older people and often more serious. Monitoring the patient's intake and output to ensure balanced hydration helps prevent UTIs.

> **CUE RECOGNITION 15.2**
> Two days ago, you cared for an 80-year-old patient who was alert and oriented × 4. Today, the patient is responding inappropriately to questions and searching for her dog. What action do you take?
>
> *Suggested answers are at the end of the chapter.*

Key Changes in the Immunological System
Age-related changes in the immune system include the following:

- Increased autoimmune response, increasing autoimmune diseases
- Declining immune response, increasing infection and cancer risk
- Decreased T cell number and function, leading to impaired ability to produce antibodies to fight disease

NURSING CARE. Older adults tend to have more chronic diseases, which can depress their immune responses and take them longer to recover from infections. They are also at higher risk for complications and death from influenza (flu) or COVID-19. It is important that older patients are taught ways to prevent illness, such as hand hygiene, exercising, maintaining a healthy lifestyle, healthy eating, age-appropriate immunizations, and stress reduction. Vaccines include an annual flu shot; COVID-19, pneumococcal 13 and/or 23 to prevent pneumonia; and zoster (Shingrix preferred) for age 50 and over to prevent shingles (see www.cdc.gov/vaccines/vpd/index.html). Shingles is a painful, contagious rash caused by the chickenpox virus (varicella-zoster). Those who are immunocompromised (such as those who take steroids) also need to take safety precautions when around others who are ill.

> **CLINICAL JUDGMENT**
> **Mr. Jones,** age 72, lives at home and is visited by a home health-care nurse. His home has wood floors with throw rugs. The bathroom is located in the hall outside his bedroom. Mr. Jones has nocturia and is occasionally incontinent from urgency to void. He takes bumetanide (Bumex) 1 mg orally daily.
> 1. What additional data do you obtain for Mr. Jones's urinary status and home environment?
> 2. What safety concerns do you identify in the home environment?
> 3. What nursing diagnoses do you suggest as you collaborate on Mr. Jones's nursing care plan?
> 4. What topics do you recommend for inclusion in Mr. Jones's teaching plan?
> 5. Mr. Jones is to take bumetanide 1 mg orally now. Bumetanide 0.5 mg tablets are available. How many tablets do you administer?
>
> *Suggested answers are at the end of the chapter.*

Key Changes in the Sensory System
Age-related changes in the sensory system include:

- Decreased visual acuity
- Decreased elasticity of the eardrum
- Decreased sense of smell
- Decreased taste perception
- Decreased touch sensation

NURSING CARE. Sensory changes associated with age often occur gradually. Early diagnosis and treatment help to minimize these changes. Sensory losses can affect the older person's psychological health. Disorientation, withdrawal, or social isolation may occur from **sensory deprivation.** On the other hand, overstimulation caused by **sensory overload** can create psychological and physical strain. This strain is difficult for an older patient to cope with. Be aware of the environment you provide for the older patient. As a patient advocate, identify and minimize overload situations.

Normal age-related changes affect the focus ability of the eye's lens (see Chapter 52). This can affect near and far vision (see Box 52.1). It is often difficult for adults after about the age of 40 to read fine print (presbyopia). Reading glasses or bifocal lenses assist with this. Help the older patient keep glasses clean and in good repair. When glasses are not being worn, keep them accessible and in a protective, labeled case. The older person has difficulty adjusting to changes between light and dark settings. Seeing in the dark is enhanced with the use of an amber or red nightlight. Red-hued lighting is more easily detected by the cones and rods in the older person's eye. Sensitivity to glare occurs and can create fall risks. Reduce sunlight glare. The glare from car headlights can impair night vision in older people, so many older people avoid driving at night.

Hearing loss is common in older adults (see Chapter 52). Although the severity of age-related hearing loss is variable, the stigma it carries is the same. Hearing aids are often not well accepted by older persons because they are visual signs of a loss. See Box 52.2 for interventions to assist the older patient with hearing difficulty. Wearing a mask, such as in an airborne pandemic or protective isolation, can make it more difficult to see facial expressions and lip read. When possible, wearing a transparent mask helps the hearing impaired communicate more easily with you, as your face will be visible. If the older patient has a hearing aid, always keep it accessible and clean, with working batteries (see Box 52.3 for hearing aid care).

The senses of taste and smell work closely together. Ill-fitting dentures, poor oral care and oral disease medications, and tobacco products can contribute to an alteration in the sense of taste. A medication review and daily mouth inspections can help identify sources of the taste alteration. In some cases, the loss of smell can result from allergies, nasal obstruction, or sinus problems. If damaged olfactory receptors are the primary cause for losing the sense of smell, little can be done. Loss of smell increases risk for consuming spoiled or toxic substances. Encourage patients to read all item labels and to review expiration dates to ensure the food or beverage is safe. Smoke alarms and natural gas/propane alarms in addition to carbon monoxide alarms should be used at home. Instruct patients to report any sudden loss in taste or smell sensation to the HCP because it can signal other significant health-care problems.

Decreased touch sensation can occur with age or disease and put older people at risk of injury. Burns can occur when hot water is not felt. The thermostat should be turned down on the hot water heater to less than 120°F (49°C). A thermometer can be used to test bath water temperature, which should be lukewarm at about 100°F (37.77°C). It is better to use a hot-water bottle than electrical heating devices, to prevent burns.

Key Changes in Sexuality
Age-related changes in sexuality include the following:

- Chronic illnesses that affect sexual functioning
- Functional sexual changes in older men (e.g., altered ability to obtain or maintain an erection and to ejaculate), causing psychological concerns
- Functional sexual changes in older women (e.g., decreased vaginal lubrication causing painful intercourse and reduced vaginal acidity), resulting in risk for vaginal infection and psychological concerns
- Increased nonintercourse intimacy behaviors, including various forms of touch
- Sexual problems caused by psychological factors, which are more common than physical ones in older patients
- Increased sexual arousal time, requiring more time for stimulation

NURSING CARE. The older patient's sexuality is an important aspect of **holistic** care. Sexuality is one of the basic physiological needs identified in Maslow's hierarchy of needs. This is true for everyone regardless of age. Become aware of your personal attitudes and values about sexuality, sex, and aging. Be respectful so that your personal beliefs and potential stereotypes do not interfere with the older patient's sexual identity. Privacy remains a common problem for patients in all health-care settings. Provide the patient with scheduled private time. Sexual enhancement treatments are becoming more available to older people, providing openness to discuss sexual expression with older patients. Many older patients have difficulty overcoming barriers to sexual expression. This can be due to certain chronic diseases, cultural or religious beliefs, fear of failure, fear of consequences, lack of a suitable partner, illness, or side effects of medications. It is important to address the older patient's sexual history sensitively, professionally, and completely (Box 15.2).

Box 15.2
Sexuality Data Collection

As with any nursing skill, practice will increase your comfort in collecting sexuality data from your older patient. Although older patients will respond to your questions, they are less apt to bring up this topic on their own. Establish rapport with the patient by collecting other data first and collecting sexual data at the end of your discussion. As you collect data, be aware of problems that were already identified that could impact sexuality (such as angina, dexterity, elimination, medication side effects, mobility, pain, and surgeries).

Naturally, you should use a professional approach and manner. These questions may lead to the discovery of other health issues. Tell the patient that you will be asking questions about sexuality. Start with questions that are likely to be more comfortable for the patient:

- Address roles first. For example: What concerns do you have or has your illness created in carrying out your roles with your spouse or sexual partner?
- Address relationship issues next. For example: What effect on your relationship with your spouse or sexual partner(s) has this symptom or illness had?
- Then address body image. For example: What effects have your (illness, surgery [mastectomy, ostomy, prostate], chronic illness, age-related changes) had on your self-concept of being a (man or woman)?
- Afterwards, you can address safer sex practices. For example: How many sexual partners do you have? What type of protection do you use (condoms, female condoms or dental dams)?
- Finally, address history of sexually transmitted infections. For example: Do you have any discharge or open sores (vaginal, penile)?

COGNITIVE AND PSYCHOLOGICAL CHANGES IN THE OLDER PATIENT

Cognition

Older patients can experience age-related changes that influence cognition. Cognition involves abilities related to intelligence, judgment, learning, memory, orientation, and problem-solving. Cognition focuses on intake, storage, processing, and retrieval of information. Older patients store information without much conscious effort. When remembering becomes difficult, the older person can begin to worry. This worry needs to be addressed. If it is not, the patient's concern can result in psychological problems and fear.

Sensory changes and diseases associated with age can alter and cause misinterpretation of patient data. For example, pain from chronic diseases can limit cognition as pain takes over the body and mind. Sleep deprivation caused by worry or fear can make it more difficult to perform ADLs. Medications that cause drowsiness can also impair cognition.

Long-term memory retrieval is easier than short-term memory retrieval for the older adult. Use written lists and visual cues to strengthen short-term memory skills.

Intelligence does not decline as one ages. Cognitive abilities tend to slow down with advancing age, but they are not lost. Most of the subtle declines that occur with information processing and retrieval do not interfere with the older patient's abilities in performing ADLs.

It is common knowledge that health, good nutrition and hydration, and adequate sleep are important for brain function. So is the use of technology with guidance, such as an Internet-connected tablet, which encourages curiosity and engagement. It can help older adults thrive.

Coping Abilities

People make choices in adapting to changes in functional ability over time. These choices impact how a person will work through the entire maturational process called *aging*. In addition to normal aging changes, many older patients cope with chronic diseases. They are also dealing with societal and cultural losses associated with aging. Role changes in employment status, society, and family can create a shift from independence to dependence. This dependence can have a strong psychological impact on patients and their families. With all these losses, an older person's confidence level can be affected. Nurses may need to encourage self-care behaviors.

Personality, attitude, past life experiences, and the desire to adapt to change are all intrinsic influencing factors. They help the older patient cope with changes brought on by aging. Extrinsic factors include financial status and family and caregiver support. It is helpful for older people to have the energy, desire, determination, and support of their caregivers. This allows them to better utilize their cognitive function in maintaining health.

Depression

There are times when the psychological impact of change is difficult to manage and loneliness, grief, or sadness can occur, disrupting the older person's ability to cognitively focus on health. **Depression** can result and can disable the older person's mind and body. Depression is the most common psychiatric problem among older adults (Gale et al, 2018). Mood disturbance increases the risk for suicide, physical health problems, and sleep issues.

Depression can result from many factors, such as physical changes in the brain, a medication or a condition affecting neurotransmitters, or psychological changes on an emotional level. Depression may be reversed with prompt identification and a referral for treatment.

Dementia

Unlike depression, **dementia** involves a more permanent progressive deterioration of mental function (see Chapter 48). There are various types of dementia, with Alzheimer disease being the main type. Dementia is characterized by confusion, forgetfulness, impaired judgment, and personality changes. Refer any patient with confusion for a mental status examination to help determine if the person has depression or dementia.

Help patients who have dementia maintain an optimum level of functioning. Provide an environment with physical and emotional safety. To help the patient who is confused, consider using **reality orientation.** Provide orienting information (e.g., clocks, calendars). Sensory overload should be avoided. Speak calmly and slowly. Provide nonthreatening therapeutic touch, if acceptable to the patient. Address the education and support needs of the patient's family. They will need to learn to cope with changes in the patient's behavior.

> **PRACTICE ANALYSIS TIP**
> Linking NCLEX-PN® to Practice
> The LPN/LVN will participate in reality orientation.

Delirium

Delirium reflects the patient's level of alertness and psychomotor activity. It is an acute, reversible state of disorientation and confusion characterized by difficulty focusing attention, inability to sleep, and hyperactivity from an underlying cause. Based on patient behaviors, delirium is classified as hypoactive, hyperactive, or mixed. It is commonly a complication of acute illness and treatments. It can occur in hospitalized patients at any age. However, it occurs most often in hospitalized older patients. It is usually documented as "confusion." The actual mechanism through which delirium occurs is not known. It is thought to occur from changes in brain neurotransmitters that control cognitive function, mood, and behavior. Unlike depression and dementia, delirium has a sudden onset and tends to worsen at night. The patient appears to be disturbed or frightened. It can last for a few hours or a few weeks.

Delirium is different from depression and dementia. It is a cognitive state that can be easily reversed once the cause is identified and treated. The nurse must not assume that the older patient's current mental status is their usual state. Know the risk factors for this condition: acute illness, alcohol or drug use, hip fracture, infection, metabolic disturbance, or surgery. Promptly report any changes in patient functioning to help prevent delirium.

Sleep and Rest Patterns

The need for sleep (7–9 hours daily) does not decrease with age. However, the sleeping pattern of older adults often changes from when they were younger. Lack of sleep leads to fatigue, irritability, reduced ability to make memories of yesterday's activities, increased sensitivity to pain, and increased likelihood of accidents. It is important to obtain a baseline sleep and rest history for the older patient. Ask about bedtime rituals, rest and nap patterns, sleep patterns, exercise patterns, dietary patterns, and stress level. Include caffeine, alcohol, and nicotine intake during the data collection.

Circulatory problems can disrupt normal sleep patterns for the older adult. Report disrupted sleep, as it might be the only sign of an impending health problem. Use interventions to reduce stimulation and calm the anxious older patient who is unable to sleep. These can include back rubs, foot rubs, a warm towel bath, warm milk, or a glass of wine, if allowed. Sleep medications should generally be avoided. They can affect the quality and depth of sleep for the older adult and cause side effects.

Medication Management

Medication management is one of the most difficult tasks for older adults and their caregivers. Older adults are susceptible to medication-induced illness and adverse side effects. This happens for a variety of reasons previously addressed in this chapter. The Beers Criteria identifies potentially inappropriate medications for older adults (American Geriatrics Society Beers Criteria® Update Expert Panel, 2019; also see www.healthinaging.org/tools-and-tips/tip-sheet-ten-medications-older-adults-should-avoid-or-use-caution). Be aware of what medications the older adult is taking. Monitor the effects of each medication. Ask patients about their recreational drug use (caffeine, alcohol, CBD, THC, other) during patient data collection. Although substances or drugs may be advertised as safe for such things as pain and anxiety, they can have side effects. These side effects affect the circulation, kidneys and liver systems, cognition, and balance.

Older adults often have more than one chronic illness. As a result, they take multiple medications. Polypharmacy can cause side effects that can be dangerous. Duplication of medications with similar actions can occur. HCPs need to be aware of all prescribed medicines. They also need to review all over-the-counter medicines and self-prescribed extracts, elixirs, herbal remedies, herbal teas, cultural healing substances, home remedies, and recreational drugs, including alcohol being used by the older adult.

Older patients must understand how to take their medications correctly. For example, an enteric-coated tablet or a time-released medication should not be crushed. Doing so would destroy the enteric protection designed to protect the stomach and intestines or release the medication too rapidly. Some older patients cut pills in half or skip medication doses to save money. When prescribed doses are not being taken as ordered, problems can result.

Be a patient advocate. Reinforce the importance of adhering to medication regimens. For each medication, explain its action, purpose, route, when to take it, how to take it, food-beverage-medicine combinations that are not safe, and any early or late side effects to report to the HCP. Older adults with a disability and with no or partial high school education tend to use medications inappropriately more often than those who have a college education. Review medications with the older patient and caregiver regularly so concerns can be promptly addressed. Visual and verbal reminders that have meaning for the older patient are helpful.

> **BE SAFE!**
>
> **AVOID FAILURE TO COMMUNICATE!** For medication safety:
> - Document a list of all the patient's medications (prescribed, over-the-counter, herbal, and traditional) upon admission. Question the patient and family about anything the patient calls "my medicines."
> - Ensure new medications are reviewed by a pharmacist.
> - During discharge teaching, review and provide a written list of new and prior medicines, dosages, and information on how to take the medicine to the patient and family/caregiver.

HEALTH PROMOTION

To promote health, first determine the present health status of the older patient. When gathering holistic health data, focus on the older patient's mind, body, and spirit. Use valid and reliable data collection tools designed specifically for older adults. This helps provide a true picture of the older patient's condition, needs, and strengths. Listening and observing are two key nursing skills required to accurately obtain information from older patients. Recognize that symptoms often differ between younger and older patients who have the same health conditions. For example, older patients can exhibit confusion rather than chest pain during a heart attack.

Health education is the most important health promotion tool for older patients. Educational efforts must first focus on erasing stereotypes about aging. Erroneous associations between aging and illness must be corrected. As an example, research shows that urinary incontinence is not a normal sign of aging and is treatable. Yet, many still think it is inevitable with old age and do not seek treatment. Provide evidence-based health information. Do this at the right time, in the right amount, and in the right way to empower the older patient. This will help them value a proactive approach for wellness in old age. Help the older patient with health screenings, immunization updates, safety program participation, and activity planning aimed at an optimal level of functioning and wellness (Table 15.1).

Table 15.1
Nursing Care Focus on Safety Alphabet for Older Patients

A is for ABILITIES	• Know your abilities. • Know your patient's abilities. • Base nursing actions on your abilities. • Seek out assistance when needed.
B is for BODY MECHANICS AND ALIGNMENT	• Use proper body mechanics. • Use appropriate assistive devices. • Ensure patient is in proper body alignment.
C is for COMFORT	• Ensure physical and emotional comfort during care. • Use pain scale during every data collection.
D is for DELIBERATE MOVEMENTS	• Plan ahead and communicate plans to patient. • Alert patient to planned movements by saying, "Moving on three. One, two, three." • Ensure patient assists with moves as able.
E is for ENVIRONMENT	• Always place nurse call light within reach. • Keep environment uncluttered and safe. • Ask patient's permission before moving items.
F is for FALLS	• Remember that falls are a primary concern for older patients. • Use interventions to prevent falls: assist patients with ambulation, use assistive devices, answer call lights promptly, provide accessible toileting facilities, use nightlights, avoid use of throw rugs.
G is for GIVING YOUR TIME	• Allow more time to perform actions. • Do not rush older patients. • Provide time for listening and observing, so concerns are addressed before becoming problems.
H is for HAND HYGIENE	• Use hand hygiene protocols and standard precautions to protect yourself and older patients. • Cleanse your stethoscope before and after each patient use.

Home Health Hints

Home Visits
- Wear layers of clothing to adjust layers as needed for comfort.
- Place cell phones and pagers on a silent mode, if possible, to avoid startling or confusing the older patient.
- Do not assume that the older patient will remember all the home health-care nurses. Each time you visit, state your name and why you are there. Wear a large-letter, photo nametag in clear view.
- To enhance the effectiveness of a visit, talk with the older patient in a quiet room. Invite the main caregiver to join at the appropriate time. This ensures privacy and fosters the person's ability to hear.

Lab Draws
- When drawing blood from an older patient, use the smallest needle possible. Anchor the vein securely before needle insertion.
- Do NOT use a taped bandage on the fragile skin of an older patient. After applying pressure to the needle site for 2 minutes, check the site for bleeding. Be vigilant if the patient has a history of taking anticoagulants. Firmly secure a cotton ball with a gauze wrap on the site.

Home Environment
- Evaluate the older patient's environment for safety hazards at each visit, and promote safety. Urge the patient and caregiver to avoid using scatter rugs and to declutter walkways to promote safe ambulation.
- It can be difficult for older adults to regulate their body temperature, so they should be asked at what temperature they are comfortable in their home. Typically, thermostats are kept at or above 75°F (24°C) during cold months. In addition, the older adult must have a way to keep cool during a heat wave.

- Assist patients in obtaining a medical alert device that can be worn around the neck and activated in case of falls or other emergencies.

Medications
- Assist patients and/or caregivers with obtaining and setting up a daily/weekly pill organizer. For patients who are forgetful, a pill dispenser with a timed audible or visual alarm and lockbox feature can be used to safely remind the patient of medication schedules.
- It is important for the home health-care nurse to evaluate the patient's ability to follow instructions. During visits, check the medication dispenser to ensure that the medication is being taken as prescribed and by the patient only. If there is a concern, inform the HCP.

Nutrition/Fluids
- Check the refrigerator for outdated food. Many older patients are on a limited budget and have been taught not to waste food. These factors, along with a decreased sense of smell and taste, can increase the risk of foodborne illness.
- If the older patient has dentures, ask if they are worn for eating. If not, ask why they are not worn (e.g., sores, improper fit from weight loss) and discuss solutions.
- Instruct the patient on adequate hydration to prevent dehydration and explain one of the first signs of dehydration is tachycardia or confusion.
- Encourage the uses of spices and herbs (parsley, oregano, lemon, garlic, and basil) instead of salt and sugar. Suggest keeping pared apples and segments of oranges in the refrigerator for snacks.
- If a Meals-on-Wheels program is available, ask whether the older patient would like to consider this type of assistance.
- Use a warming tray when feeding an older patient who takes a longer time to eat to keep food warm and tasty.
- When swallowing is difficult, freezing of liquids helps, so that they can be eaten with a spoon or as a popsicle. Eggnog, instant breakfast mixes, high-protein drinks, and milkshakes are thicker liquids that are easier to control when swallowing than non-thickened liquids are.

Elimination
- If an older person wears perineal pads or adult briefs, ask how many are used in a 24-hour period to evaluate the degree of incontinence. Have the patient keep a voiding diary to further determine the degree of incontinence.
- Suggest a bedside commode to help reduce the risk of falls and ease caregiver burden if an older patient is confused, on diuretics, or has a history of falling.
- If the older patient reports constipation, review patient's diet and make suggestions regarding fluid and fiber intake and physical activity. A mixture of equal parts of applesauce, bran, and prune juice is often helpful to prevent or relieve constipation. Discourage the use of mineral oil because it will interfere with vitamin absorption.

Rest
- If the older patient seems fatigued early in the day, ask about night-time sleeping patterns and things that disrupt sleep, such as nocturia or restless legs. Check medications for insomnia side effects and suggest dosing of these medications early in the day if appropriate. Napping is not recommended if the patient is having insomnia.

Infection
- Suggesting that limiting visitors or not allowing persons with colds or other illnesses to visit can be helpful in preventing illness in the older patient.
- One of the first signs of infection in the older patient is confusion.

Education
- When reinforcing teaching, it is important to acknowledge the patient's health literacy, knowledge, and life experiences. Older patients can tell you how they have successfully maintained their health over the years.
- Reinforcing teaching should occur *with* patients, not *to* them. The nurse is a visitor in the older adult's space/home, and patient's respect and dignity must always remain intact during home visits.
- Use open-ended scenarios to guide education, such as "What would you do if you fell and you were all alone?"
- When reinforcing teaching, include a return demonstration for any procedures.
- When auscultating lungs, ask the older patient to take deep breaths slowly in and out through the mouth. This can stimulate coughing, which is a perfect time to reinforce teaching for deep-breathing and coughing exercises.

Key Points

- Aging is defined as a maturational process that creates the need for individual adaptation because of physical and psychological declines that occur throughout life. Aging has many different components and is a unique process for each individual.
- Cellular decline in structure and function increases in severity and extent over time. Some cells that die cannot regenerate themselves. As a result, structures are altered. The body then tries to make the revised structure meet functional demands. These changes are cumulative over time, which impacts nursing care measures required to care for older patients.
- Normal aging cognition issues result from structural shrinkage of the brain over time, decreased blood flow

to the brain and all major organs/structures, decreased sensory acuity, and increased body response time. These expected changes due to advancing age are often impacted by other factors, such as genetics, diseases, medication use, sleep cycle dysfunction, and lifestyle behaviors, that complicate the cognitive functioning of older people.
- Confusion, depression, delirium, and dementia seen in some older adults are NOT a part of normal aging. These factors make older adult care more complex. For this reason, it is important for the nurse to collaborate with the older patient and the health-care team when planning care.
- To assist the older patient to reach an optimal level of functioning, plan health promotion strategies. Focus on interventions for these high-risk areas: medication management, fall prevention, and quality-of-life.

SUGGESTED ANSWERS TO CHAPTER EXERCISES

Cue Recognition

15.1: Promptly assist the patient or ask an immediately available nursing assistant to provide patient-centered care to preserve the patient's dignity and safety, knowing the patient physiologically does not have the ability to wait.

15.2: Ensure patient safety, check the patient's hydration status (documented intake and output trends), collect data for signs of dehydration, notify RN or HCP immediately for order to check electrolytes.

Critical Thinking & Clinical Judgment

Mr. Jones

1. Does he live alone? Does he have a history of falls? If so, does he use a device to signal for help? What type of nightlight is used? How far is it to the bathroom? Does he take his bumetanide (Bumex) early in the day? Does he void before going to bed? Does he anticipate needing to void 30 minutes after lying down?
2. Wood floors that are slippery when wet from incontinence are a safety hazard. Scatter rugs can slide or cause tripping. No nightlight is used, and the bathroom is in the hallway.
3. Nursing diagnoses include *Urge Urinary Incontinence* related to distance to bathroom; *Deficient Knowledge* related to safety, medication administration, and nocturia; and *Risk for Injury* related to slippery floors from incontinence, use of scatter rugs, and inadequate lighting.
4. A teaching plan should include the following:
   - *Safety:* Place urinal at bedside to prevent incontinence on the way to the bathroom. Consider a nightlight to improve vision and prevent falls. Use an easily cleaned floor covering that is secure and absorbent to avoid falls. Consider the need for using a device that can send a signal for help.
   - *Medication administration:* Take diuretics prior to 4 p.m. to avoid having to get up frequently while sleeping during the night.
   - *Nocturia:* Void before lying down. Anticipate the need to void after lying down by reclining in a chair for 30 minutes with legs elevated before going to bed, and then void on way to bed.
5. Two 0.5 mg tablets.

Additional Resources

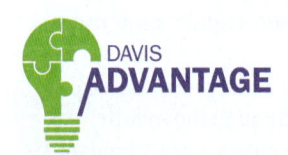

Go to Davis Advantage to complete your learning: strengthen understanding, apply your knowledge, and prepare for the Next Gen NCLEX®.

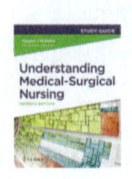

A Study Guide is also available.

CHAPTER 16
Patient Care Settings

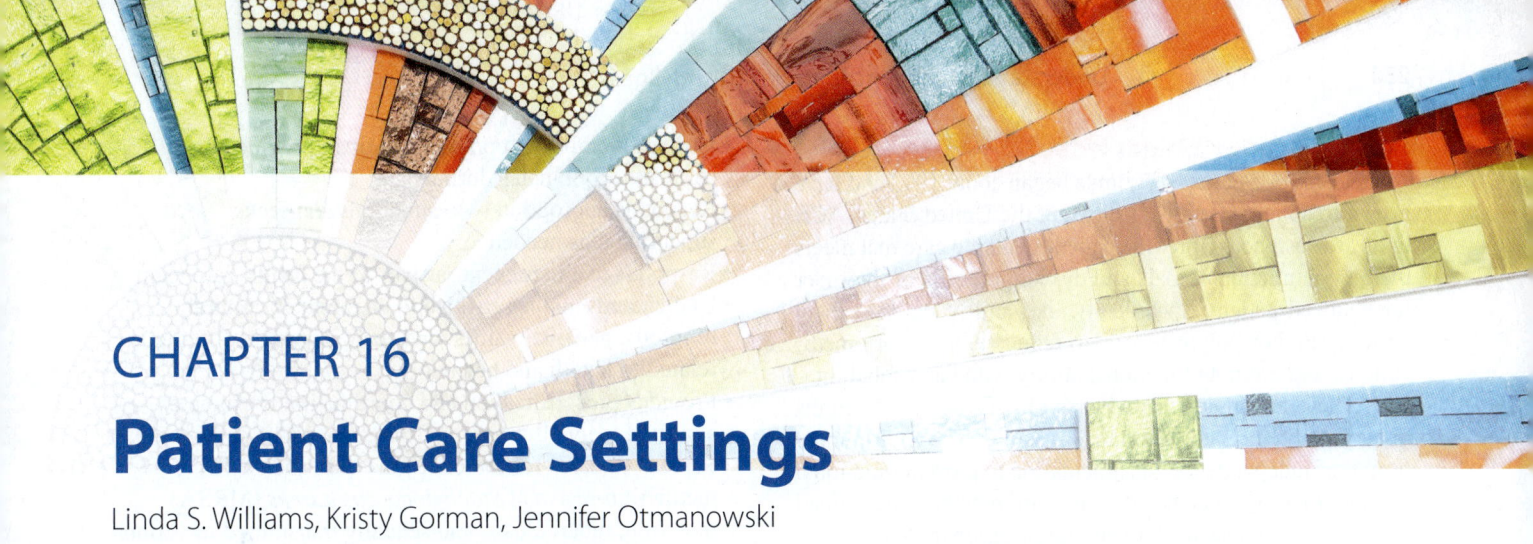

Linda S. Williams, Kristy Gorman, Jennifer Otmanowski

KEY TERMS

autonomous (aw-TAH-nah-mus)
collaborative (kuh-LAB-er-uh-tiv)
elopement (ih-LOPE-munt)
respite (RES-pit)
telenursing (TEL-a-nurs-ing)
trauma-informed care (TRAW-muh in-FORMD care)

CHAPTER CONCEPTS

Caring
Collaboration
Health-care system
Safety

LEARNING OUTCOMES

1. Describe acute care for elders units in hospitals.
2. Describe the role of the licensed practical nurse/licensed vocational nurse (LPN/LVN) in medical offices or clinics.
3. Describe the role of the LPN/LVN in correctional nursing.
4. Identify long-term care options.
5. Describe services offered in long-term care settings.
6. Describe the role of the LPN/LVN in long-term care settings.
7. Describe patient safety interventions in long-term care.
8. Describe home health-care eligibility.
9. Explain differences in hospital versus home health nursing care.
10. Explain the steps involved in making a home health-care visit.
11. Explain safety practices for the nurse while making home visits.
12. Identify home safety interventions for the patient.
13. Describe methods of infection control for the home health-care nurse.
14. Identify documentation required for a home visit with a patient.
15. Plan nursing interventions for the home health-care patient and caregiver.

LPN/LVN EMPLOYMENT SETTINGS

The need for licensed practical nurses/licensed vocational nurses (LPNs/LVNs) is expected to grow 9% between 2020 and 2030. This growth is much faster than the average for all occupations (Bureau of Labor Statistics, 2021). LPNs/LVNs may work in child day-care centers, clinics (urgent care or addiction), correctional health-care facilities, dentist offices, dialysis centers, home health care, hospices, hospitals, long-term care facilities, medical offices, occupational health departments such as in factories, rehabilitative facilities, or schools. The roles of the LPN/LVN in acute care and acute care for elder units, medical offices, correctional health-care facilities, long-term care, and home health care are discussed in this chapter.

ACUTE CARE

While hospital employment of LPNs/LVNs is declining, employment is growing in other settings. Employment of and types of roles for LPNs/LVNs vary by hospital. Some hospitals do not employ LPNs/LVNs. Others may, although the job title of LPN/LVN may not be used.

Acute Care for Elders Hospital Units

Acute care for elders (ACE) units began about 1993 and have grown to about 200 units throughout the United States. ACE units are designed to provide patient-centered care that meets the unique treatment goals and discharge needs of the older hospitalized patient. Specifically, they utilize daily medical review, monitor polypharmacy to reduce unnecessary medications, and promote functional ability with early rehabilitation. These actions reduce adverse effects, decrease lengths of stay, and reduce costs and readmissions. The environment promotes independence and ambulation to prevent functional decline. In ACE units, health-care team members are trained in geriatric care and work in an interdisciplinary team.

MEDICAL OFFICE NURSING

LPN/LVNs provide patient care in medical offices and work with patients of all ages. Following are the types of duties the LPN/LVN might perform:

- Greet, triage (assignment of degree of urgency to decide order of treatment of patients), and register patients.
- Escort patients to examination rooms.
- Follow the Health Insurance Portability and Accountability Act of 1996 (HIPAA).
- Obtain and document patients' vital signs, height, and weight.
- Obtain patients' medical and medication histories.
- Enter data into the electronic medical record.
- Contribute to the patient's plan of care and advocate for patients.
- Provide patient care (e.g., wound care, dressings).
- Administer immunizations and other medication injections.
- Monitor patients after medications or treatments.
- Reinforce teaching for health promotion and new medications.
- Answer questions regarding the patient's care.
- Document understanding of education.
- Obtain prior authorization of medications.
- Assist with renewal of prescriptions.
- Communicate health information to patients.

CORRECTIONAL NURSING

Local, regional, and state correctional facilities hire LPN/LVNs in growing numbers to care for inmates and handle worksite wellness programs for correctional staff. In this practice setting, the LPN/LVN:

- Works safely, effectively, and efficiently as a team member in conditions involving incarcerated patients.
- Follows health-care standards, procedures, and protocols when providing care.
- Demonstrates professionalism, effective interpersonal skills, and high-quality oral and written communication skills in providing health-care delivery to inmates.
- Utilizes therapeutic communication to provide empathetic assistance to inmates during care.
- Responds appropriately to situations and seeks supervision as needed.
- Responds to emergencies as part of the health-care team.
- Understands and is sensitive to an inmate's cultural, religious, personal values, and socioeconomic differences related to health and behaviors.
- Provides precertification and coordination for inmates admitted to and discharged from acute care facilities.
- Screens inmates for infectious diseases such as HIV, methicillin-resistant *Staphylococcus aureus* (MRSA) infection, tuberculosis, and sexually transmitted infections (STIs) and adheres to Centers for Disease Control and Prevention (CDC) guidelines.
- Screens inmates for mental health disorders and/or emergencies to make appropriate referral for acute and/or chronic mental health treatment.
- Utilizes the nursing process and nursing skills when implementing health-care provider (HCP) orders.
- Utilizes knowledge of medications (e.g., actions, interactions, uses, and side effects).
- Reinforces patient education on health promotion and chronic conditions.
- Maintains institutional health records and provides required reports.

LONG-TERM CARE SERVICES

Long-term care services describes both health- and non-health-care services to assist those who are disabled or frail with self-care. In 2016, more than 8.3 million people were served by about 65,600 regulated long-term care services providers (Harris-Kojetin et al, 2019). Long-term care services can be provided in the home, via home health care (discussed later in this chapter) or hospice (see Chapter 17). Services can also be provided in community settings (e.g., adult day-care services), residential care settings (e.g., independent living, skilled nursing and memory care, adult foster care, assisted living facilities), and institutions (e.g., nursing homes) (Table 16.1). Some institutions specialize in care for people with chronic illnesses and physical impairments, such as those requiring mechanical ventilators. However, most long-term care is provided in the home setting.

Types of Long-Term Care Services

Long-term care services include daily personal care; dental care; physical, occupational, and speech therapies; pharmacist medication monitoring; podiatry; skilled nursing; IV therapy; intensive services such as dialysis; mechanical ventilator and tracheostomy care; and palliative or hospice care. Support services involve social workers, mental health professionals, and counselors.

Most long-term care that is provided is not medical or nursing care. It is primarily assistance with activities of daily living (ADLs) and instrumental activities of daily living

Table 16.1
Long-Term Care Service Settings

Community

Adult day-care service	Provide patient-centered assistance, supervision, socialization, and health care to older adults, adults with disabilities, and those with dementia during the day so that caregivers can work or receive respite. Services are provided by an interdisciplinary staff, including aides, nurses, social workers, and therapists (occupational, physical, and speech). Services may include assistance with activities of daily living (ADLs), meals, therapies, and transportation.

Residential

Adult foster care	Private residences in which the owner lives with the residents to offer personal care, meals, supervision, and sometimes other supportive services. The number of residents allowed by each state varies.
Continuing care retirement community	Residential care setting offering independent living, assisted living (assistance with ADLs, meals, medication assistance and supervision), skilled nursing, and memory care on site. Residents entering independent living pay an entrance fee and then a monthly fee for the various levels of care based on needs.
Residential care community (semiassisted/assisted living)	Residential care setting that combines housing, ADL assistance, supervision, support services, and limited health-care for older adults. Residents are independent. Medication assistance and other treatments may be provided. Residents may have a kitchen to prepare meals and/or group meals may be provided.

Institution

Nursing home	Provides the most comprehensive range of services, including housing, ADL assistance, nursing care, and 24-hour supervision. Short-term rehabilitation is also offered for physical, occupational, or speech therapy. *Skilled care:* Licensed nurses or therapists are required to perform medical care 24 hours a day, such as IV therapy, complex wound care, monitoring health status, tube feedings, or short-term rehabilitation services. A health-care provider order is required. *Intermediate care:* ADL assistance and some (but not constant) nursing care is provided. *Custodial care:* Supervision and ADL assistance is provided. Nursing care is not required. This type of care is often provided for those with dementia. *Green House Project/Small House model:* This model for institutional long-term care represents a culture change toward long-term care in institutions that promotes natural living. Care is provided in a home environment in small houses on a campus with up to 12 residents per home. A great room, kitchen with dining, and outdoor access are open to everyone. Each resident has a bedroom and bathroom. A care team provides all patient-centered care and prepares meals. A nurse is available 24 hours a day. Up to an additional 30 minutes of direct care is given daily with this model. Residents are nurtured and thrive as their individual needs are met.

(IADLs). ADL services include bathing, dressing, feeding, incontinence care, toileting, transferring (to or from bed or chair), and supervision for safety. IADL services include food preparation, grocery shopping, money and bill management, housekeeping, laundry, pet care, and transportation.

Dementia Care

The physical environment is a key component in safe, patient-centered care for those with Alzheimer disease or dementia. Six in 10 people with dementia will wander (Alzheimer's Association, 2020). There are positive benefits to wandering, such as exercise, more energy, improved appetite, pain control, and reduction of boredom and anxiety. However, there are negative effects, such as fatigue, risk of falls, and risk for **elopement** (leaving a facility unsupervised when unable to protect oneself). A long-term memory care unit should use a variety of strategies to manage wandering behavior while giving a person with dementia a sense of freedom and independence (Neubauer et al, 2018).

Innovative thinking in the design of long-term memory care units stimulates the senses, reduces agitation, improves eating, and encourages safe wandering. Innovations include curvy or figure-8 hallways with seating areas and refreshment stations. Such elements encourage wandering, without agitating dead ends. Themed units provide sensory stimulation and use of color to help the resident recognize where he or she lives. Sensors also provide knowledge of the resident's location. The addition of fish tanks in dining areas can be calming and promote eating. Murals of peaceful rivers can discourage residents from going through a door. Memory stations can engage residents with activities during wandering. In addition, multisensory areas allow residents to use self-selected sensory stimulating items (e.g., aromas, sounds, textures) and interact with items used in the past by the resident for work or tasks. Encouraging residents' self-care ability (e.g., combing their own hair and brushing their teeth) reduces their anxiety and enhances their well-being.

Residents' moods may improve and become more receptive to care when personal items are in their environment. The Green House Project model, or Small House model, of institutional long-term care (discussed in Table 16.1) has shown that providing residents with an activity that reminds them of what they loved to do in the past makes them feel more comfortable and confident (Boumans et al, 2019).

Role of the LPN/LVN in Long-Term Care Services

Licensed nursing hours per resident per day are higher in long-term care facilities than in residential care communities and adult day-care services centers (Harris-Kojetin et al, 2019). The LPN/LVN is responsible for patient safety and direct bedside care in nursing homes under the supervision of a registered nurse (RN). General LPN/LVN duties in long-term care facilities include administering medication; supervising, educating, and mentoring nursing assistants; nursing care; contributing to the plan of care; communicating with the HCP; making rounds; ensuring patient comfort; documentation; and reporting concerns to the supervising RN.

Common resident care tasks for the LPN/LVN include but are not limited to:

- Collecting the resident's history
- Monitoring vital signs and resident health status
- Monitoring fluid intake and output
- Monitoring nutritional intake
- Monitoring residents to prevent and detect pressure injury (see Chapter 54)
- Documenting resident information
- Giving medication (oral and injection) prescribed by the HCP
- Monitoring for adverse effects of medications
- Monitoring intravenous lines
- Assisting with ADLs
- Providing wound care, tube feedings, enemas, and insertion of urinary catheters
- Providing emotional support
- Reinforcing teaching to residents and families
- Assisting with end-of-life care

> **PRACTICE ANALYSIS TIP**
> Linking NCLEX-PN® to Practice
> The LPN/LVN will:
> - Evaluate client response to medication (e.g., adverse reactions, interactions, therapeutic effects).
> - Identify signs and symptoms related to acute or chronic illness.

> **CUE RECOGNITION 16.1**
> You assisted a long-term care resident to transfer safely from the bed to wheelchair. You are called to another room to assist the resident with obtaining a drink of water. What action do you take as you exit or enter a residents' room to promote infection control?
>
> *Suggested answers are at the end of the chapter.*

Medicare and Medicaid Participation Requirements

Health and safety standards must be met for long-term care facilities to participate in Medicare or Medicaid. In 2016, revisions were made to the requirements for long-term care facilities in response to advances in knowledge and evidence-based practice to improve the quality of care and life of residents. Visit www.CMS.gov for current standards; see Table 16.2 for examples.

Patient Safety and Wellness in Long-Term Care Facilities

Activity and Exercise

For older adults to maintain health and independence in long-term facilities, activities and exercise should be promoted by the nursing staff in collaboration with activity directors. Strength, balance, and stretching exercises can assist residents in maintaining a normal weight, preventing falls, and improving freedom of movement. A recent study in nursing home residents with dementia found that physical activity interventions positively affect cognitive, physical, and mood outcomes (Henskens et al, 2018).

Fall Prevention

It is important to prevent residents from falling. In 2018, more than 88 older adults died from falls each day (Centers for Disease Control and Prevention [CDC], 2020). The National Council of Aging (2020) recommends exercise to strengthen leg muscles and improve balance and flexibility as well as keeping the environment clutter-free and well lit. In addition, the CDC's STEADI (Stopping Elderly Accidents, Deaths & Injuries) initiative (2020) recommends fall prevention education; identification of vitamin D and calcium intake; annual vision checks and hearing tests; measurement of orthostatic blood pressure; a medication review for side effects or interactions; obtaining adequate sleep; use of assistive walking devices; wearing nonskid, rubber-soled low-heeled shoes; and not walking in socks only because they can be slippery.

Table 16.2
Medicare and Medicaid Long-Term Care Facilities Reform Examples

Person-centered care	Develop and implement a baseline person-centered care plan for each resident within 48 hours of the person's admission. At discharge, planning must include resident's discharge goals to prepare residents to be active participants in their post-discharge care, transition, and prevention of readmission.
Quality of care	Focus on care and services so residents achieve their highest possible physical, mental, and psychosocial well-being.
Quality of life	Updated focus on special care issues that are based on an assessment of a resident and the person-centered plan of care and preferences. These include accidents, dialysis, incontinence, elimination ostomies, mobility, assisted nutrition and hydration, pain management, pharmacy (e.g., unnecessary medications, medication errors, antipsychotic medications, immunizations), restraints and bed rails, skin integrity, and **trauma-informed care** (e.g., special care to avoid traumatization triggers for trauma survivors, such as those of abuse, Holocaust survivors, veterans, or victims of large-scale disasters).
Alignment with U.S. Department of Health and Human Services Initiatives	Reduce avoidable hospitalizations and unnecessary hospital readmissions. Reduce incidences of health-care-acquired infections. Improve behavioral health care. Safeguard nursing home residents from the use of unnecessary antipsychotic medications.

Source: Adapted from U.S. Department of Health and Human Services. (2016). Medicare and Medicaid programs; reform of requirements for long-term care facilities. *Federal Register, 81*(192) (October 4, 2016). www.gpo.gov/fdsys/pkg/FR-2016-10-04/pdf/2016-23503.pdf; and LongTermCare.gov. (2020). https://acl.gov/ltc

As part of a fall prevention program, facilities can use a standardized fall risk assessment tool, such as the Morse Fall Scale, the Johns Hopkins Fall Risk Assessment Tool (JHFRAT), or St. Thomas's Risk Assessment Tool in Falling Elderly Inpatients (STRATIFY). These scales can be used upon admission, after a fall, and when there is a change in the resident's status or medications to quickly identify a risk of falling. To help prevent falls within the long-term care environment, closely monitor residents with cognitive impairment, balance problems, or incontinence. Ensure the environment is modified for safety by removing rugs or obstacles, installing grab bars and bathmats in the shower, checking on residents every 2 hours or more frequently for those at greater risk of falling, and encouraging residents to participate in activities outside of their rooms throughout the day to be more visible.

> **CUE RECOGNITION 16.2**
> You are caring for an older patient who has a history of falls within the past month. The patient is to go to the physical therapy room for an exercise session now. What action do you take?
>
> *Suggested answers are at the end of the chapter.*

Lighting
Older adults require additional light for vision due to changes within the pupil and lens of the eye. They benefit from amber motion sensor nightlights and tunable lighting. Tunable lighting is lighting that can be adjusted to the desired intensity and color at various times of the day (e.g., brighter in morning and reduced over 24 hours) to promote normal circadian rhythms. This newer researched lighting has been shown to reduce falls, improve sleep with reduced need for psychotropic or sleep medication, and decrease agitation. Advocating for new technology such as this lighting at your agency promotes patient-centered care.

Restraints
The Centers for Medicare and Medicaid Services (CMS, 2020b) defines *physical restraints* as "any manual method or physical or mechanical device, material, or equipment attached to or near your body so that you can't remove the restraint easily." *Chemical restraint* is the use of medication to restrict the freedom of movement to sedate the resident or control his or her behavior. Federal law says restraints may not be used as discipline, as punishment, or for the convenience of staff and can be used only when the resident's behavior could cause harm to self or others. When used, the medical record must include an order for the restraint, a defined plan for the use, and the length of time it will be used. A new order for the restraint may be required every 24 hours. Restraint use is controversial and done as a last resort. The resident must be frequently monitored, as restraint use can result in injury or death of the resident. A long-term care facility must have a plan in place to reduce restraint use (e.g., gradually increasing the time for ambulation and muscle strengthening activities). Restraint use regulations can vary by state.

Infection Prevention

Long-term care facility residents are at the greatest risk of morbidity and mortality due to health-care-associated infections. Residents living within a confined environment are at a higher risk of cross-infection. Hand hygiene, personal protective equipment use (such as wearing a mask during an airborne pandemic), adhering to standard precautions and transmission precautions, and cleaning and disinfecting surfaces are examples that can help reduce the spread of some infections.

HOME HEALTH CARE

Ask a patient in a hospital where he or she would choose to be, and chances are the answer will be "home." The number of home health-care patients is growing as a result of the aging population in the United States as well as many older adults' desire to age in place. Home health care provides an affordable and convenient option for providing care in the community. Technological advances such as telehealth allow home health-care agencies to provide high-quality complex care. The LPN/LVN is a valuable member of the home health-care team.

Home Health-Care Eligibility

The home health-care patient must require skilled services that can be provided only by nurses, physical therapists, occupational therapists, and speech therapists (Box 16.1). Home health-care aides are also available for patients who are receiving skilled care (care that cannot be provided by the patient alone and requires intervention of a qualified nurse or therapist). Depending on the patient's health insurance, a patient who is receiving home health care may be required to be homebound. For example, Medicare has very specific guidelines for determining homebound status. If the nurse suspects a patient is not homebound, the nurse should alert the RN. Alternative options to home health care can be arranged to help the patient receive the care that they need. These options can include going to a clinic to have a blood pressure reading done, attending an outpatient physical therapy or occupational program, or having skilled needs (such as dressing changes) completed in an ambulatory surgery facility or wound care clinic.

Home health-care services usually are ordered after discharge from the hospital when there is a need for skilled care in the home. It is not uncommon, however, for an HCP's office to request home health-care services after seeing a patient in the office. For example, a patient who is having difficulty controlling blood glucose levels could benefit from having a nurse visit to see how the patient uses a glucometer, observe what types of food are being purchased, monitor the glucose level, and teach the patient diabetic management. These types of home health-care visits are usually short-term with the goal of facilitating independent care by the patient and/or family.

Home health care may be provided to residents in an assisted living facility. Because these facilities are not skilled nursing facilities, the facility staff is not trained to perform skilled nursing tasks. Home health-care nurses need to understand the facility's policies when visiting a patient in assisted living. They must maintain communication with the facility staff regarding health-care instructions for the patient.

Collaborative Home Health Care

Home health care is **collaborative.** Teamwork is facilitated through team meetings and written communication (Fig. 16.1). Home health care is patient-centered, and the patient should be involved in the plan of care as well as in setting their own goals.

Based on recommendations from the home health-care RN case manager or hospital case manager, the HCP may order a social worker to evaluate community resources to

Box 16.1

Skilled Activities for the Home Health-Care Nurse

According to the Medicare Benefit Policy Manual (CMS, 2020a), to be considered as skilled nursing services, the services must require the skills of an RN, or an LPN/LVN under the supervision of a RN, and they must be reasonable and necessary to the treatment of the patient's illness or injury, as discussed, and must be intermittent. Examples of skilled nursing care include the following:
- Blood draws
- Wound care
- IV medication administration
- Monitoring a patient's status following a change in medications or condition
- New feeding tube management
- New ostomy management
- Patient and family education
- Urinary catheter insertion and maintenance

If a family member is able to perform a skill part of the time, the nurse can teach that person how to perform the skill. The nurse can still complete skilled visits to monitor the patient's progress and provide care when family members are not available.

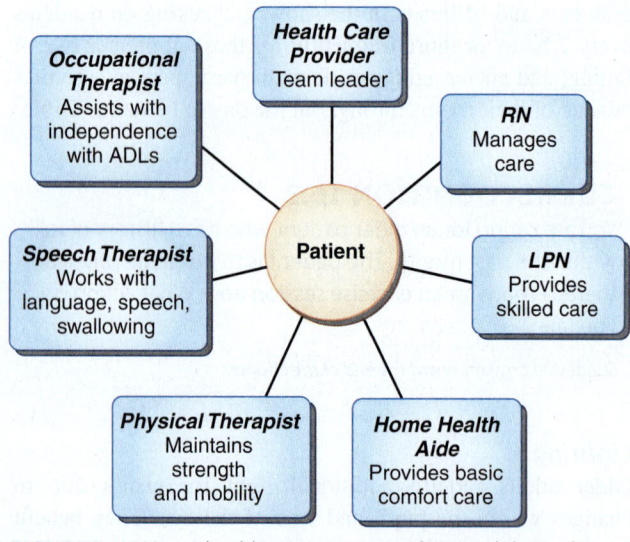

FIGURE 16.1 Home health-care team members and their roles.

- Occupational Therapist: Assists with independence with ADLs
- Health Care Provider: Team leader
- RN: Manages care
- LPN: Provides skilled care
- Home Health Aide: Provides basic comfort care
- Physical Therapist: Maintains strength and mobility
- Speech Therapist: Works with language, speech, swallowing
- Patient (center)

assist the patient. Social services can create a link between the patient and resources available within the community.

> **PRACTICE ANALYSIS TIP**
> **Linking NCLEX-PN® to Practice**
> The LPN/LVN will identify signs and symptoms related to acute or chronic illness.

CRITICAL THINKING & CLINICAL JUDGMENT

Mr. Perez, 75, needs a dressing change for the diabetic ulcer on the bottom of his right foot. When you take vital signs, you notice that his temperature is 100.4°F (38°C), one degree higher than yesterday's temperature. Other vital signs are within his normal range. After opening the box with his supplies, you note that there are no more blue pads to put under his foot while you change the dressing. You proceed with the dressing change, wash your hands, and document the wound care noting that the old dressing on the right foot was soiled with purulent drainage.

Critical Thinking (The Why)
1. Which cues are concerning and will require you to take action?

Clinical Judgment (The Do)
2. What did you use instead of a blue pad to complete the dressing change?
3. What additional data do you collect?
4. Which members of the health-care team do you collaborate with?

Suggested answers are at the end of the chapter.

Transition From Hospital-Based Nursing to Home Health-Care

Patients who enter the hospital are leaving behind the comfort of their own homes. They may be scared and isolated, trying to adjust not only to an illness but also to a new environment. The opposite is true for home health-care nursing. In the patient's home, the nurse is the visitor and the surroundings are unfamiliar. This can be a difficult adjustment for a nurse. As confidence in being a home health-care nurse grows, so does the comfort level with entering someone else's home. The nurse should recognize and consider cultural issues. The nurse should remain nonjudgmental about the home environment to maintain communication with the patient and caregiver. Patients may be less likely to share information with the nurse if they feel judged. If the home environment poses a health or safety risk, it may be necessary to inform the RN.

When working in the hospital, the nurse has many staff and supply resources available. These resources are not always easily available when working in a patient's home. As such, the nurse must have a mastery of nursing skills. Home health-care nursing requires an ability to adapt and remain flexible because, unlike the hospital environment, the home environment is unknown. Consequently, it is necessary to evaluate both the patient and the home setting. Home health-care nurses must evaluate the patient's case based not only on the referral diagnosis but also on what may be occurring within the home that is contributing to the diagnosis. The home health-care nurse needs good data collection skills and the ability to recognize changes in patient condition.

> **CUE RECOGNITION 16.3**
> Your patient reports falling yesterday and reports that she is lightheaded. Orthostatic blood pressures indicate a decrease in blood pressure with standing. What action do you take?
>
> *Suggested answers are at the end of the chapter.*

Families play an important role in the care of patients in the home. It is not surprising to walk into a home and find several anxious family members with a list of questions. Family members may be very involved in visits. Initially, their presence may be intimidating. When preparing for a visit, take the time to learn about an unfamiliar diagnosis or medication so you can answer their questions. In addition, be prepared for the unexpected. Carry extra common supplies, such as various sizes of urinary catheters, sterile dressing gauze, different types of tape, and alcohol wipes. Being prepared will help develop a trusting relationship with patients and families.

Visiting the patient in their home provides you with a good opportunity to look for cues indicating caregiver stress. A caregiver who is impatient with the patient or is leaving a patient in soiled clothing may be experiencing caregiver stress or burnout. You can provide information and encouragement to the caregiver to attend caregiver support groups or make a referral to a program that provides **respite** care. Provide a listening ear to the caregiver and allow them to express their challenges and frustrations with caregiving. Educating the caregiver on how to care for their loved one can also help and is a very rewarding part of home care. Be sure to keep the case manager updated. A referral to a social worker may be indicated.

Because of the **autonomous,** or independent, nature of home health care, most agencies require at least 1 year of medical-surgical nursing experience to ensure that the nurse has the basic knowledge needed to work in home health care. Home health-care agencies also hire nurses for specialty areas such as cardiac, wound care, or pediatrics. See Box 16.2 for a review of liability issues.

The Role of the LPN/LVN in Home Health Care

The LPN/LVN's role in home health care is varied and complex. Skilled nursing care is similar to care performed in the hospital setting, only the setting is different (Fig. 16.2). The

• WORD • BUILDING •

Autonomous: autos -self + nomos - law

Box 16.2
Liability Issues to Consider When Working in Home Health Care

When starting in home health care, review your state nurse practice act and scope of practice (visit www.NCSBN.org). When in patients' homes, they might ask you to perform a skill or request something that is outside your scope of practice. It is important that you explain to them that it is outside your scope of practice but that you will notify your agency immediately about their request. For example, if a patient asks you whether it is okay to change a medication dose, you should understand that, as an LPN/LVN, you cannot prescribe medications. If you changed the medication dose, you would be altering the prescribed dose and thus practicing outside your scope of practice because only an HCP can prescribe medications.

Always discuss your concerns with your supervisor and review your agency's guidelines, policies, and procedures. Know what you can and cannot do before you start, and never be afraid to question something that you feel or know violates your nurse practice act. Remember: It is your license, so protect it by following your nurse practice act!

LPN/LVN works under the supervision of a home health-care RN or RN case manager. The LPN/LVN role involves collecting patient data, providing compassionate patient care, educating patients and caregivers, and documenting visits.

Here is one LPN's personal testimonial:

> *Being a licensed practical nurse in a home health-care setting requires many skills such as organization, excellent critical thinking skills, dedication, and the flexibility to adjust to patient and staffing needs. Being a home health-care nurse allows you to focus on one patient at a time, to see patients in their homes, and to see the challenges they face day-to-day. It gives you the ability to change lives and make a difference in someone's life.*

Steps in the Home Health-Care Visit
Preparing for the Visit

The typical day of a home health-care nurse consists of six to seven home visits. These visits typically last 30 to 45 minutes. Most agencies try to arrange visits in the same geographical location for convenience. Agencies usually provide mileage reimbursement, so mileage is recorded from house to house.

The day before your visits, develop a plan of action for how your visits will be structured. Sometimes, you will need to be at a certain place at a particular time, so factor this into your planning. Each patient must be contacted. Give the patient a 1- to 2-hour window for your arrival time. Remember, you cannot always anticipate what is going to happen during a visit. It is better to give your patients a time range as opposed to an exact time. If you are unsure how to locate your patient's home, ask for directions when you arrange the visit time. A global positioning system (GPS) or mapping application can help you arrive at your patient's home in a timely manner, improving patient satisfaction.

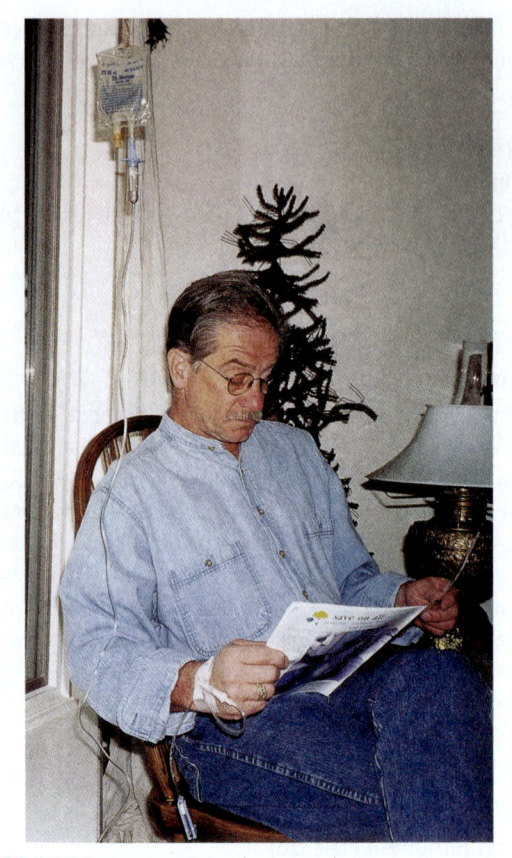

FIGURE 16.2 Patient receiving home IV therapy.

Many agencies utilize electronic documentation. You will likely be issued a laptop or tablet that allows you access to the patient's history and documentation from previous home health-care visits. You can review the patient's diagnosis, pertinent medical information, and the reason for home health care prior to the visit. When in the home, it is important to compare vital sign and other data from the previous nurse's documentation to the data you collect. This information will help you identify and address any changes in the patient's condition. You will collect data about the patient as well as the home environment each time you visit.

CUE RECOGNITION 16.4
You are visiting a 74-year-old man with a history of heart failure who is recovering from a knee replacement. Today the patient has edema bilateral ankles. You note from the chart that his physical therapist visited this morning and documented an increase in shortness of breath that made therapy difficult. What action do you take?

Suggested answers are at the end of the chapter.

Safety Considerations

A home health-care nurses' travels can take them to areas that may be unsafe. It is important to be vigilant about personal safety. Box 16.3 lists tips on how to protect yourself before, during, and after a home health-care visit.

Box 16.3
Safety Guidelines for Home Health-Care Nurses

In general, providing home health care is a safe occupation. Most communities recognize the importance of the role of home health-care nurses and are receptive to visits made to members of the community. However, it is still important to understand how you can protect yourself in case an unsafe situation arises.

Here are some tips for maintaining safety when completing a home health-care visit:
- Keep your gas tank filled.
- Complete recommended maintenance on your car and have the tires checked regularly.
- Always carry a cell phone charger.
- Keep your laptop or tablet with you at all times—it contains patient information and, if stolen, could result in a HIPAA violation.
- If lost in an unknown area, go to a familiar place and contact the patient for directions.
- If possible, park on the street or road in front of the house. This prevents someone from blocking you in the driveway.
- When entering a home, be aware of where the exit doors are and of any windows that will allow safe evacuation from the home.
- Be aware of your outside surroundings. When leaving the home, have your supplies packed up and keys out, ready to open the car door.
- If you need to complete a visit at night, request an escort. Some communities will have a police officer accompany you to and from the home. Discuss this option with your supervisor.
- Call your agency if you are concerned about your safety. Never complete a visit if you feel concerned for your safety.

Patient safety in the home is also important. Observe things in the home that can pose a hazard to the patient and educate the patient about injury prevention at home. Physical or occupational therapy can help the patient build strength, use assistive devices effectively, and maintain safety. (See "Gerontological Issues" for patient safety considerations in the home of older patients.)

Gerontological Issues
Safety
Older adults make up a significant proportion of home health-care patients. Many items in older patients' homes are potential safety hazards that should be addressed. Following are examples:
- Electrical cords
- Lighting
- Overcrowded spaces
- Pets
- Scatter/throw rugs
- Steps used to enter home
- Lack of sturdy grab bars and a tub mat in the bathroom

BE SAFE!
AVOID FAILURE TO RECOGNIZE! Be aware of the following signs of elder abuse: Caregiver refuses to let the older adult be seen alone by the HCP, patient has unexplained injuries, caregiver displays controlling behavior and/or prevents older adult from seeing friends and family members, utilities are turned off, or there is no food in the house.

Evidence-Based Practice
Clinical Question
How do failed communication attempts between home health-care nurses and physicians affect hospital readmission?

Evidence
Participants were Medicare recipients with a diagnosis of heart failure who were receiving home care. Researchers tracked communication attempts where the nurse and the HCP failed to connect with each other, such as calls in which messages were left or the nurse communicated only with the office staff. Among high-risk patients, communication failures increase the chance that the patient will be readmitted to the hospital.

Implications for Nursing Practice
Excellent communication skills and the ability to collaborate with physicians is essential for home health-care nurses. Nurses should be persistent in their attempts to reach physicians when their patient has a change in condition.

Reference: Pesko, M. F., Gerber, L. M., Peng, T. R., & Press, M. J. (2018). Home health care: Nurse-physician communication patient severity, hospital readmission. *Health Research and Educational Trust, 52*(2), 1008–1024. https://doi.org/10.1111/1475-6773.12667

Infection Control
Maintaining asepsis in the patient's home may be a challenge. In the hospital, everything is readily available for infection control. However, in the home, the nurse is responsible for inventorying and bringing supplies provided by the home health-care agency. All equipment should be cleaned prior to going back in the nursing bag. The nursing bag should be placed on a barrier on a hard chair, never on the kitchen table.

It is always important to have extras of basic equipment, including the following:

- Personal protective equipment (e.g., disposable gowns, masks, goggles, shoe covers), N95 mask kept in a plastic box with air holes to avoid being crushed
- Latex-free gloves
- Biohazard bags
- Disposable underpads (which can be used to provide a clean field or barrier for supplies and for the equipment bag)
- Antibacterial soap and paper towels
- Hand sanitizer and sanitizing wipes
- Disinfecting spray to clean equipment and your bag after each visit

- Alcohol wipes
- A small chemical spill kit

An important infection control measure is hand hygiene. Always wash your hands with soap and water before and after completing patient care and before reaching into your nursing bag. If water is not available, use hand sanitizer. Do not wash your hands in the patient's kitchen sink. Always ask to use the bathroom for washing your hands, and never use the patient's hand towel.

> **CLINICAL JUDGMENT**
>
> **Mrs. Ortiz** was referred to your home health-care agency after an appointment with her HCP. During that visit, Mrs. Ortiz was diagnosed as being anemic with dizziness, fatigue, and alterations in her blood pressure. The HCP requested home health-care nurse visits for Mrs. Ortiz to evaluate her safety and recommend appropriate safety devices.
>
> 1. What hazards in the home do you look for?
> 2. What safety devices do you request for Mrs. Ortiz?
> 3. What referrals and collaborations with other disciplines do you discuss with the RN case manager?
>
> *Suggested answers are at the end of the chapter.*

Documentation

Because of reimbursement guidelines, the nurse must document specific things during the home visit. Home health-care agencies receive their income based on a prospective pay system (rate determined by patient care needs), not per-visit payments. On admission, the RN fills out information that is entered into a computer system. This information is called the Outcome and Assessment Information Set, or OASIS (CMS, 2019). This tool is used to generate information about the home health-care agency and patient outcomes. Home health-care outcomes generated from OASIS are publicly reported via Home Health Compare (www.medicare.gov/homehealthcompare/search.html). OASIS allows the RN to implement an evidence-based plan of care, helping to eliminate potential complications, improve outcomes, and prevent unnecessary rehospitalizations. The LPN/LVN should be familiar with the general function of OASIS and its relevance to creating a plan of care.

For home health-care agencies to be reimbursed, they need to demonstrate that a skill was completed. Documenting information is based on the patient's plan of care and the corresponding skill that was completed at the visit. For example, the HCP orders skilled nursing observation and medication management for a patient. In documenting the visit for this order, the nurse needs to state that this skill was completed. Documentation of the skill might include the following:

- The patient's response to medication (e.g., vital signs, level of consciousness, or other potential side effects)
- The patient's current understanding of medication regimen and the action the nurse took to improve that understanding
- The patient's response to education and any areas in which they may need more assistance

The following items are typically included in home health-care agency documentation:

- Nurse's arrival and departure times
- Vital signs
- Data collection findings
- A description of any procedures performed
- A narrative note, including patient education provided
- The patient's signature verifying that the nurse was present

A folder with information is also kept at the patient's residence. It usually consists of relevant patient information and a communication form that all staff members complete at each visit. This documentation is important to ensure continuity of care.

Patient Education

A primary responsibility of nurses in home health care is educating patients or caregivers about the patient's illness and ways to effectively manage that illness at home. Education is provided with the intention of improving health outcomes and decreasing the need for hospitalization. Handouts are available from the home health-care agency as well as other sources to help reinforce the verbal instructions the nurse provides. When reinforcing teaching given to the patient or caregiver for a procedure, always have them do a return demonstration before evaluating them as competent to perform the procedure.

> **LEARNING TIP**
>
> An easy way to make sure you always have the handouts you need is to organize them into a three-ringed binder. The information can be organized on the basis of diagnoses or alphabetically. Have plenty of handouts when making a visit. Many times, family members who do not live with the patient request copies so that they can have a copy at their own home.

Nursing Process for the Home Health-Care Patient

Data Collection

Monitor and document patient and family adjustment to change and illness. Perform a complete patient evaluation during each visit. Monitor the home environment for potential safety hazards and the need for devices to assist with care.

Nursing Diagnoses, Planning, and Implementation

Ineffective Health Self-Management related to deficient knowledge, complexity of medical needs, and limited access to social support

EXPECTED OUTCOME: The patient will demonstrate the changes in lifestyle needed to maintain health.

- Include the patient in the development of short- and long-term health goals *to promote patient cooperation.*

- Recognize cues that health status has changed *to report them and collaborate with other members of the home health-care team as needed.*
- Look for cues to patient's ability to take medications correctly *to provide assistance as needed.*
- Look for cues that psychosocial needs are not being met *to make referral to friendly visitor programs and support groups as needed.*
- Instruct patient regarding diet and help patient set short-term goals related to making healthy dietary choices, including home delivered meals if needed *to promote health.*
- Reinforce correct use of assistive devices such a cane and walker *to promote safety.*
- Instruct patient on recommended amounts of physical activity and help patient set physical activity goals such as walking 10 times around dining room table *to prevent immobility.*
- Encourage participation in home exercise program provided by physical therapy *to support collaboration.*
- Talk with RN about referral for physical therapy if patient is experiencing falls *to promote safety.*

Other Forms of Home Health-Care Nursing

Telenursing

Technology makes it possible to provide care in the home to patients in remote or rural areas or after office hours or when home visits are not possible. **Telenursing,** a branch of telehealth, uses information technology and telecommunication (telephone, fax, e-mail, and video/audio conferencing) to provide nursing care. The nurse interacts with the patient via equipment set up in the patient's home. Because the nurse can see the patient, data collection can be obtained, including visualizing wounds. The nurse then plans care and educates the patient. Other patients may have remote monitoring of their weight and vital signs, alerting the nurse in the home care office to changes in the patient's condition.

Private-Duty Nursing

This chapter has focused on home health care that is covered under the Medicare and Medicaid systems or private insurance. Additional types of home health-care agency employment are available for nurses, including private-duty nursing and hospice nursing (see Chapter 17).

Private-duty nursing consists of scheduled care to assist patients with personal and homemaking needs as well as helping patients fill weekly medication dispensers. These services have been called *home companion services, homemaker services,* and *private-duty care.* They generally are not covered by insurance. Nurses may enjoy this type of work because of the long-term relationships that are formed with the patient and family.

Key Points

- ACE units are designed to meet the unique needs of hospitalized older adults and to provide care that meets the treatment goals and discharge needs of the older patient. Specifically, ACE unit staff utilize daily medical review, monitor polypharmacy to reduce unnecessary medications, and promote functional ability with early rehabilitation.
- LPNs/LVNs provide patient care in medical offices and work with patients of all ages. Their duties may include greeting and triaging patients; obtaining and documenting patients' vital signs, height, and weight; obtaining patients' medical and medication histories; contributing to the plan of care for the patient; providing patient care; and administering immunizations and other medication injections.
- Local, regional, and state correctional facilities hire LPNs/LVNs to care for inmates and handle worksite wellness programs for correctional staff.
- Long-term care services can be provided in the home, via home health care or hospice. Services can also be provided in community settings and residential care settings, which include independent living, skilled nursing and memory care, adult foster care, assisted living facilities, and nursing homes.
- Long-term care services include daily personal care; dental care; physical, occupational, and speech therapies; pharmacist medication monitoring; podiatry; skilled nursing; IV therapy; intensive services such as dialysis; mechanical ventilator and tracheostomy care; and palliative or hospice care. Support services involve social workers, mental health professionals, and counselors.
- The LPN/LVN is responsible for patient safety and direct bedside care in nursing homes under the supervision of an RN. General duties in long-term care facilities include administering medication; supervising, educating, and mentoring nursing assistants; providing nursing care; contributing to the plan of care; communicating with the HCP; making rounds on residents; ensuring patient comfort; documenting; and reporting concerns to the supervising RN.
- The home health-care patient must require skilled services that can be provided only by nurses, physical therapists, occupational therapists, and speech therapists. Home health-care aides are also available for patients who are receiving skilled care. Medicare has very specific guidelines for determining homebound status and requires that the patient be homebound to receive home health care.
- Home health-care nursing requires an ability to adapt and remain flexible because, unlike the hospital environment, the home environment is unknown.
- The LPN/LVN role in home health care involves understanding and following infection control procedures, collecting patient data, providing patient care, educating patients and caregivers, and documenting visits.

- The LPN/LVN must be alert to things in the home that can pose a hazard to the patient and teach the patient how to prevent injuries in the home.
- During a home visit, the nurse is responsible for bringing supplies provided by the home health-care agency. It is always important to have extras of basic equipment.
- Because of reimbursement guidelines, the nurse must document specific things during the home visit. Home health-care agencies receive their income on the basis of a prospective pay system (predetermined rate), not per-visit payments.
- The home health-care team collaborates. Physical or occupational therapy can help the patient build strength, learn how to use assistive devices, and maintain safety.

The author acknowledges the contributions to this chapter by Anna Ricks, LPN, for the "Medical Office Nursing" section and MaryAnne Pietraniec-Shannon, RN, PhD, and Linda Rogers-Antuono RN, MSN/Ed. for the "Correctional Nursing" section.

SUGGESTED ANSWERS TO CHAPTER EXERCISES

Cue Recognition
16.1: Perform hand hygiene upon entry to and exit from each room.
16.2: Ensure your patient is wearing nonskid, rubber-soled low-heeled shoes.
16.3: Collect head-to-toe patient data, noting any injuries and including a review of the patient's medications to see if the patient is taking them correctly.
16.4: Observe for further cues of heart failure exacerbation and notify the RN.

Critical Thinking & Clinical Judgment
Mr. Perez
1. The increase in the patient's temperature and the purulent drainage may indicate infection.
2. A paper towel, paper napkin, or clean towel provided by the patient could be used under the patient's foot and as a barrier for wound care supplies.
3. Collect data about the patient's blood sugar, today and over the last couple of days. An elevated blood sugar may indicate the patient has an infection. In addition, collect data to look for other signs and symptoms of infection. If the wound is infected, the patient may have chills and increased pain, redness, and/or swelling in the area of the wound.
4. The RN and/or HCP should be notified of the patient's signs and symptoms. The HCP may order a wound culture, an antibiotic, or a change in the type of wound dressing.

Mrs. Ortiz
1. Important observations include scatter/throw rugs, overcrowded spaces, sharp edges along furniture, inadequate lighting, and stairs. Instruct the patient to keep frequently used kitchen appliances and foods on shelves that are easy to reach. Assist the patient with setting up a "command center" in the living room so that favorite items are kept in proximity and the patient does not have to get up too frequently.
2. Because anemia can cause extreme fatigue, it is important for Mrs. Ortiz to have safety devices in the home to prevent falls. Equipment to consider includes a bath bench for the shower so she can sit while bathing, a detachable shower head, handrails in the shower and hallways, a bedside commode, an over-the-toilet seat, a reacher device to assist with obtaining objects at a distance, and a medical alert device that can be worn at all times.
3. A physical therapist or occupational therapist can determine what adaptive equipment would be most beneficial for the patient and teach safe use of it. The patient may benefit from a home health aide to provide safety with bathing.

Additional Resources

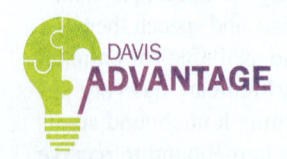

DAVIS ADVANTAGE Go to Davis Advantage to complete your learning: strengthen understanding, apply your knowledge, and prepare for the Next Gen NCLEX®.

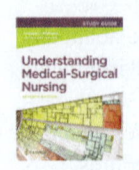

A Study Guide is also available.

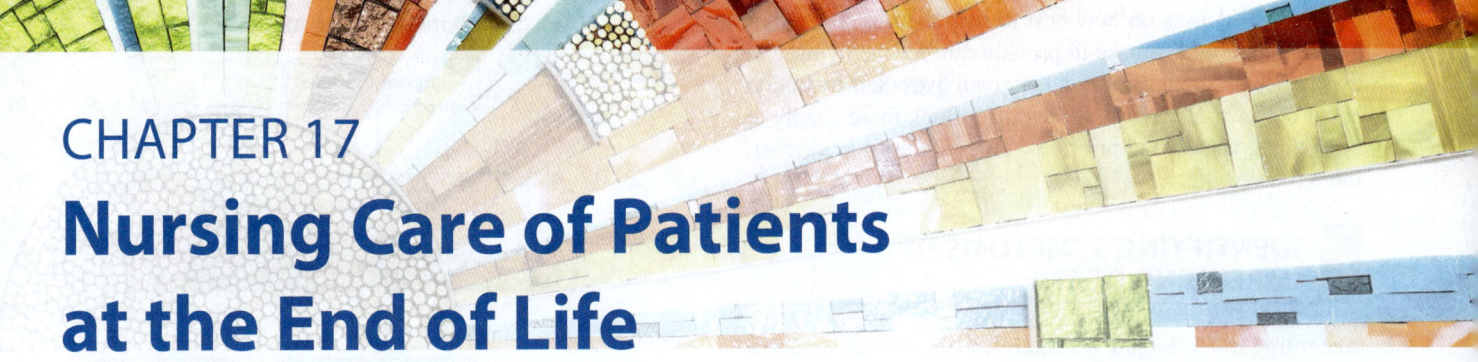

CHAPTER 17
Nursing Care of Patients at the End of Life

Amanda J. Miller, Betsy Murphy

KEY TERMS

advance medical directive (ad-VANTS MED-ih-kuhl dur-EK-tiv)
advocate (AD-vuh-ket)
artificial feeding (ART-ih-FISH-uhl FEE-ding)
artificial hydration (ART-ih-FISH-uhl hy-DRAY-shun)
do not resuscitate (DNR) (DOO not re-SUSS-ih-TATE)
durable power of attorney (DUR-uh-buhl POW-ur OV uh-TUR-nee)
hospice (HOS-pis)
living will (LIH-ving WIL)
palliative (PAL-ee-uh-tiv)
postmortem care (pohst-MOR-tum CARE)

CHAPTER CONCEPTS

Collaboration
Comfort
Communication
Grief and loss
Growth and development

LEARNING OUTCOMES

1. Identify characteristics of the patient who is approaching the end of life.
2. List legal documents for patients with life-limiting illness.
3. Explain choices that are available to patients at the end of life.
4. Demonstrate empathetic communication with dying patients and their families.
5. Describe physical changes that may occur during the dying process.
6. Specify nursing interventions for patients at the end of life.
7. Describe postmortem care.
8. Plan nursing interventions for the grieving patient and family.
9. Explain compassion fatigue.
10. Discuss the role of the licensed practical nurse/licensed vocational nurse in hospice care.

A GOOD DEATH

Despite our best efforts, there will come a time when our patients die. Death is the expected end to life. In the 21st century, most Americans die from acute and chronic illnesses such as cancer, heart disease, stroke, and dementia. We have the technology to prolong life, but sometimes this longer life can carry profound disability and reduced quality of life. Our patients sometimes tell us that this is not what they intended for the last phase of life. What is the role of the nurse with patients nearing the end of life? Two priorities are to (1) identify patients nearing the end of life and (2) help them define and communicate their end-of-life goals to ensure that their wishes are understood and followed.

Perhaps the most important role for nurses is to validate our patients' needs and concerns as they move through the series of changes leading to a good death. Dying is, after all, the final phase of our growth and development. The developmental tasks associated with this phase involve reflecting on life accomplishments and saying "goodbye," "I'm sorry," and "I love you." The goal of having a "good death" is a valid one.

Multiple studies have focused on identifying the needs of terminally ill patients and their families. According to the National Institute on Aging, "People who are dying need care in four areas—physical comfort, mental and emotional needs, spiritual issues, and practical tasks" (2017). These needs may be met with collaboration between the patient, physician, nurse, and caregivers. This partnership helps facilitate patients' desires and focuses on how best to help them achieve their goals. Nurses who choose to provide care for the dying will experience personal growth in their own lives. Self-reflection about our own mortality can help us to look more deeply at our beliefs, values, and priorities. This can result in a richer, more focused life.

IDENTIFYING SYMPTOMS OF IMPENDING DEATH

According to Cross and Warraich (2019), most Americans say that they want to die at home, and this is now the most common setting where death takes place. "Home" for many patients means the place where they are most comfortable, surrounded by caregivers who understand their needs and provide attentive care. Home can be where they live independently or with others, such as a continuing care retirement community, assisted living facility, or nursing home. Nurses who are working in long-term care and assisted living facilities will find themselves in a position to support these patients and their families in planning for a good death. Because many patients die within months of admission to long-term care facilities, their preferences should be identified soon after admission. Without proper documentation available, patients who become ill are routinely transported to the hospital, possibly receiving unwanted treatments.

What are common signs and symptoms in patients nearing the end of their lives? Some patients exhibit rapid decline in their condition despite aggressive treatment. They may also have accompanying weight loss, increased dependency in activities of daily living, increased hospitalizations, mental status changes, and increased sleep. Knowing these symptoms can help to identify patients who are dying. Another symptom of decline is aspiration, a risk associated with recurrent pneumonia. Decreased respiratory muscle strength, lack of lung elasticity, and poor immune response make meaningful recovery unlikely. Older patients with poor renal and cardiac function are also at high risk for dying. For some older patients with chronic illness, many aggressive treatments such as IV fluids or chemotherapy offer little benefit.

For most patients and their families, the transition from treating an illness to allowing the patient to die comfortably is a gradual process. Figure 17.1 shows the evolving relationship between treatments intended to cure and treatments intended to comfort as the patient approaches the end of life. As curative therapies are reduced, comfort care, also known as **palliative** measures, is increased. This chapter explores some of the choices people need to make at the end of life and the interventions you can use to help patients during this time.

ADVANCE DIRECTIVES, LIVING WILLS, AND DURABLE MEDICAL POWER OF ATTORNEY

The Patient Self-Determination Act, which took effect in 1991, ensures that every patient has the right to accept or refuse any medical treatment that is offered. The act also requires health-care professionals to ask patients entering a hospital if they have prepared **advance medical directives.** These directives include the patient's advance set of instructions for health-care wishes (sometimes called a **living will**). In preparing advance medical directives, patients are exercising their right to make their wishes known regarding specific medical treatments if they become unable to express their decisions. Check individual state policy to confirm what is legal within that state.

A **durable power of attorney** (DPOA) for health care specifies a person who (1) will speak for a patient when that patient cannot speak and (2) will honor the patient's instructions. Many states provide standard forms to use and may require the patient to have both a DPOA for health care and an advance directive to ensure the patient's wishes are followed. An attorney, although not required, may be helpful in preparing these documents.

The nurse may encourage patients not only to fill out the necessary forms but also to discuss their wishes with all caregivers. Patients are often reluctant to complete these documents ahead of time, as they may be overwhelmed or concerned that they may change their minds about treatments in the future. It is helpful to talk about advance care planning as a *process* that may require collaboration with other team members, such as a social worker, to complete. Patients can change their minds at any time about treatment and write a new advance directive. If no advance directive is on record or a DPOA has not been chosen, the state law where the patient resides will dictate their proxy decision maker.

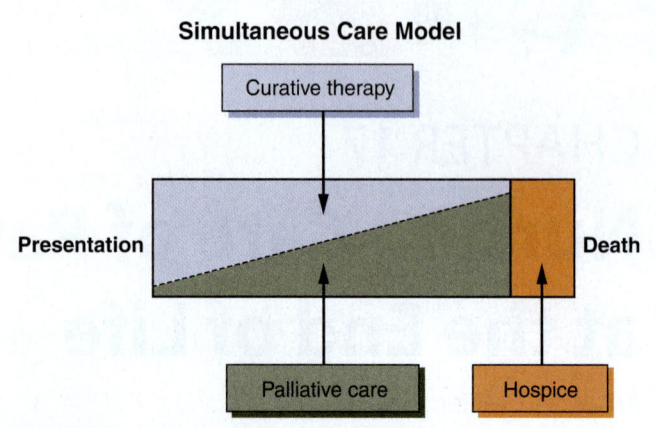

FIGURE 17.1 The simultaneous care model.

> **PRACTICE ANALYSIS TIP**
> Linking NCLEX-PN® to Practice
> The LPN/LVN will:
> - Provide information about advance directives.
> - Provide end-of-life care and education to clients.

END-OF-LIFE CHOICES

Cardiopulmonary Resuscitation

During the 1960s, cardiopulmonary resuscitation (CPR) was developed to rescue people who suffered a cardiac or respiratory arrest. Today, CPR has become standard in many health-care facilities. All patients receive CPR unless they have documentation in place that opposes receiving CPR.

Patients often have the misperception that CPR can save most lives. In reality, very few lives are saved by CPR. The overall rate of survival that leads to hospital discharge for someone who experiences cardiac arrest is about 10.6% (Ouellette et al, 2018). One reason for the low survival rate is that CPR must begin within 3 to 5 minutes of collapse. The most successful cases are those in which CPR and an automatic external defibrillator (AED) are used within 3 to 5 minutes of collapse. A helpful way of presenting the CPR option to patients and families is to provide them accurate information about outcomes. They should understand that after CPR, their underlying health condition will still be present, and they will likely be further debilitated. Reassure patients that they will receive appropriate comfort care as they die a natural death.

Do Not Resuscitate Orders

A "No Code," or **do not resuscitate (DNR)** order, is written in collaboration with the patient, family, and health-care provider (HCP), usually after it has been determined that the patient will not benefit from CPR. The patient will still have choices regarding all other treatments. A DNR order simply means that CPR will not be done, and the patient will be allowed to die a natural death. Mostafa and El-Din (2019) suggest that CPR is not an effective treatment for those who are nearing the end of life.

An advance directive or hospital DNR order does not cover patients' wishes in the home or nursing home. A durable DNR (also called an out-of-hospital or prehospital DNR) is a document for emergency medical services workers to follow. The form may be called Physician Orders for Life-Sustaining Treatment (POLST), Medical Orders for Life-Sustaining Treatment (MOLST), Medical Orders for Scope of Treatment (MOST), or Physician Orders for Scope of Treatment (POST). This document is signed by both the patient or the patient's decision maker and the patient's HCP. Emergency medical services workers are trained to look for such a document, often in a bright color and hanging on the patient's refrigerator. Document names may vary by state.

Some patients fear that if they choose a DNR status, a treatment that may benefit them might be withheld. It is important to tell patients that DNR does not mean *do not treat*. Patients who have a DNR order will still receive treatments such as oxygen and medications to manage their symptoms and will be given psychosocial support to ensure a comfortable death. Furthermore, a patient can choose which treatment options they would like, if any, and still remain a DNR. This may include defibrillation or medication administration. A gentler way of discussing these choices may be to ask patients and families if they prefer to allow a natural death. All DNR orders and discussions with the patient and their caregivers should be documented on the patient's chart ("Patient Perspective").

> **LEARNING TIP**
> A Full Code order means that, if the patient's heart stops, everything possible will be done to save the patient, including CPR. Often, the patient will require artificial ventilation following CPR. A No Code/Full Therapeutic Support order means that everything possible will be done up to but not including CPR or ventilator. A No Code/Comfort Care Only order means that only medications and treatments that keep the patient comfortable will be provided.

Patient Perspective

Anna

My mom, Anna, was diagnosed with cardiomyopathy and congestive heart failure when she was just 60 years old. At that time, she was still working and had recently remarried. She thought she had many years left in life. She did not have an advance directive—why would she?

Two years later, as her disease progressed, she decided she did not ever want to "live on machines." So, with the help of her doctor and our family, she wrote her living will and made her new husband her durable power of attorney for health care, with me as his backup person. Because she was still functioning well, with lots of medications and occasional hospitalizations, she chose a do not resuscitate (DNR) status, but with full therapeutic, aggressive interventions. She even took a tour of Europe during this time in her life, knowing she would not be able to do it later.

By age 67, she had a lot less energy to do things, and her heart failure really cramped her lifestyle. But she still enjoyed life, and her goal was to see my son, who was her oldest grandson, graduate from high school. She considered a heart transplant, but her doctor told her she was too old to qualify. She did have a new kind of valve surgery that was supposed to make her feel better, but it didn't help much.

Three months after my son's graduation, my mom was hospitalized several times with progressively worse outcomes. She weighed barely 100 pounds and could not eat much. She was only 70 years old and still looked and acted so young! Finally, she was in a semicoma in the hospital, and our family had to make the difficult decision to withdraw all therapeutic support. She was now a DNR, with comfort measures only. We were confident this would be what she wanted because we had talked about it with her. She was alert enough to let us know that she wanted to die at home.

She was discharged home with hospice care and died within a week. I moved in for her final days to help out. Between her husband, me, and her hospice team (which was a godsend), as well as frequent visits from family and her minister, she was well cared for. We kept her comfortable with lots of attention and morphine. She was alert and able to converse some of the time. She ate what and when she wanted, which amounted to one-quarter of a cheese and tomato sandwich one day, but she enjoyed it! She could finally enjoy a glass of grapefruit juice, which she had been unable to have for years because it interacted with one of her heart medications.

At the end, she died with me holding her left hand and her husband holding her right. We were telling her we loved her. It was a good death.

CLINICAL JUDGMENT

Mrs. Hung has written an advance directive, specifying her health-care wishes should she become incapacitated. Because she has advanced disease, she tells you she would not want to be resuscitated if she has a cardiac arrest. She is currently hospitalized but will be discharged to her home in a few days.

1. What documents does Mrs. Hung need to have in place to ensure she will not receive unwanted resuscitation?
2. What health-care team members should you collaborate with in helping Mrs. Hung through this process?

Suggested answers are at the end of the chapter.

Artificial Feeding and Hydration

Healthy patients who are unable to eat while recovering from an acute illness may benefit from **artificial feeding** or **artificial hydration** (also called clinically assisted nutrition and hydration [CANH]). For example, a patient may benefit from receiving parenteral nutrition (see Chapter 7) or tube feeding to prevent weight loss while receiving chemotherapy or radiation, as both treatments are known to cause weight loss.

Other patients may be unable to eat or drink as a result of a chronic illness with multiple medical problems, or failure to thrive. Failure to thrive is defined as "a syndrome of weight loss, decreased appetite and poor nutrition, and inactivity, often accompanied by dehydration, depressive symptoms, impaired immune function, and low cholesterol" (Agarwal, 2020). Such patients will not likely benefit from CANH.

If the patient is able to swallow, they should be allowed to eat and drink when, what, and how much they choose. However, research has shown that CANH increases the risk of aspiration, pressure ulcers, edema, heart failure, infections, hospital admissions, and discomfort in terminally ill patients (Carter, 2020). Once the body reaches a point of cachexia, it can no longer break down nutrients like before. In addition, some studies suggest that dehydration can benefit the terminal patient by releasing increased naturally occurring endorphins, providing analgesia and a heightened state of well-being (Suchner et al, 2019). Other benefits may include fewer secretions with less shortness of breath, reduced swelling, and less urination, resulting in reduced risk of skin breakdown.

Providing families with evidence-based information as part of advance care planning can help families make the best possible decisions for their loved ones. See the nursing diagnosis *Impaired Oral Mucous Membrane Integrity* in the "Nursing Care Plan for the Patient at the End of Life" later in this chapter for suggestions to increase comfort in the patient unable to drink.

The issue of feeding at the end of life is emotionally difficult for some families. Bringing favorite foods may be one way family and friends show love and communicate caring. The following are three ways you can support families in making decisions about feeding:

- Identify goals of care and evaluate whether artificial feeding will help meet those goals.
- Weigh the benefits and burdens of feeding.
- Help the family find alternative ways (besides feeding) to communicate love, such as skin care, mouth care, or reading to their loved one.

Hospitalization

Patients may go to the hospital at the end of life to manage illness or symptoms, to relieve family caregivers, or sometimes even to feel safe. However, there are also burdens associated with hospitalization for older adult patients approaching the end of life, and they may decline more rapidly in a hospital setting. When removed from predictable routines and known caregivers, the older patient often suffers from confusion, decreased appetite, increased risk of infection, and withdrawal (Allers et al, 2019). Frail patients with poor immunity risk often develop infections. They may enter the hospital with one infection and be discharged with another infection. Patients in nursing facilities who are approaching the end of life may benefit from having a "do not hospitalize" order. This will keep them in an environment that feels safe and preserves their chosen quality of life. Having hospice care established (see next section) in nursing facilities reduces the chances of unwanted hospital and intensive care unit admissions.

Hospice Care

Hospice service, or end-of-life care, is covered as a benefit under most insurance coverages and Medicare. Hospice can be provided in various settings, including the patient's home, assisted living facilities, hospitals, and nursing homes when there is a signed contract between the hospice organization and the facility (see "Home Health Hints"). There are free-standing hospice facilities, but these often require an out-of-pocket expense to the patient for room and board, unless the patient qualifies for a grant or receives other financial assistance to help with these costs. According to Cross and colleagues (2020), home hospice care ranges from $153.72 to $194.50 per day to an inpatient cost of $1,021.25 per day.

To qualify for hospice care, a patient must have an estimated prognosis of 6 months or less, assuming the illness runs the typical course. Patients can receive hospice care longer than 6 months if their health continues to decline. Some indicators of a 6-month or less prognosis (regardless of diagnosis) are 10% unintentional loss of weight in 6 months, mental status decline, increased weakness, frequent hospital admissions, and recurrent infections. The goal of hospice care is holistic: to manage symptoms such as pain and nausea, to provide emotional and spiritual counseling for the patient and family, and to support the patient in achieving their goals of care. Each patient is assigned a multidisciplinary hospice team to assist with care (Table 17.1). In addition, medications, medical supplies, and medical equipment are covered by the hospice benefit if they are related to the terminal diagnosis.

Hospice care does not provide 24-hour in-home health care, but a nurse is available for home visits 24 hours a day. Nurses and other team members also make regular visits to support and teach the patient and family. In times of medical crisis or caregiver fatigue, many insurance providers and home hospice agencies provide short-term inpatient hospice services or respite care.

CUE RECOGNITION 17.1

You are passing medications to your residents when a family member runs out of a room in a panic, yelling, "He's not breathing! Help!" What do you do?

Suggested answers are at the end of the chapter.

CUE RECOGNITION 17.2

A resident is transferred from the hospital to the long-term care facility where you work. The resident has a gastrostomy tube for artificial feeding. The resident pulls the tube out. What do you do?

Suggested answers are at the end of the chapter.

COMMUNICATING WITH PATIENTS AND THEIR LOVED ONES

Terminal illness is often a team experience that affects not only the patient but also their loved ones. The team includes the patient and may include blood relatives, friends,

Home Health Hints

- Encourage discussion regarding advance directives with the patient and family/caregiver early in the care process. Decisions regarding resuscitation and the use of technology to prolong life are more difficult when the patient is in crisis.
- Allow time during your visit to sit with the patient and caregiver. Sitting quietly lets the patient and caregiver know you are there to meet both physical and emotional needs.
- Encourage family involvement with care. Caregivers need reassurance that they are not going to hurt the patient; take the time to teach them how to assist the patient with basic care, including administration of medications.
- Prepare the caregiver on signs of impending death. Offer resources such as books, handouts, and reputable Web sites.
- When the patient is no longer conscious, encourage the family to continue to spend time at the bedside sharing thoughts and happy memories with the patient. It is theorized that the last sensation to be lost is hearing.

Table 17.1
The Hospice Team

Team Member	Role
Medical director—a physician or other health-care provider (HCP)	Works with the patient's primary HCP, offering suggestions to improve care. Directs team activities and often makes visits to the patient's home.
Nurse	Makes routine home visits, assessing patient needs and implementing a plan of care. Nurses are available 24 hours per day to make visits as needed.
Social worker	Provides emotional counseling and long-term planning, assists patients with insurance issues, assists with completing an advance directive, and helps identify community resources.
Chaplain or minister	Provides spiritual counseling or coordinates care of spiritual issues with the patient's chosen spiritual counsellor. May participate in funeral or memorial service.
Home health-care aide	Provides personal care, linen changes, and may assist with feeding the patient.
Volunteers	Support caregivers by staying with the patient while they leave the home. May also read to patient, run errands, etc.
Bereavement counselor/team	Provides counseling for family and significant others for 13 months after the patient's death.

significant others, or partners. The primary role of the nurse is to facilitate a comfortable death that honors the patient's choices. The nurse is the patient's **advocate,** ensuring their wishes are communicated to loved ones and other members of the health-care team. In addition, the nurse is often the professional caregiver and educator of the nonprofessional caregivers and family members.

Good communication requires active listening and honest answers. The nurse can help to identify patient choices and allow verbalization of fears. Nonverbal communication can be expressed through eye contact, body language, and tone of voice.

Take time to identify your own communication barriers that may affect your ability to talk with families. Do you have fears about your own mortality or lack personal experience with death? Do you fear being blamed for decisions or disagree with decisions that were made? These barriers will affect your ability to support patients and families in crisis. Practice attentive listening with patients and families. Allow them to talk. Don't change the subject. Know that you do not need to have all the answers. Your role can be to help them reflect on what they are communicating and to clarify their goals so you can advocate for them.

Set the stage by sitting down to show you are not in a hurry (Fig. 17.2). Maintain eye contact, encourage patients to speak, repeat what they say to gain clarification, and reflect on its meaning. Some things to say to facilitate good communication include the following:

- "Tell me more about. . . ."
- Repeat back what you hear: "I hear you saying. . . ."
- "How can I help?"

From the patient's perspective, many factors influence the content and quality of communication with you. Trust is paramount between the nurse and the patient/caregiver. Fears may interfere with their hearing what they are being told about the illness. It may be helpful to ask what they heard the HCP tell them about the illness and prognosis. If they ask questions, answer honestly; dishonesty destroys trust and credibility (see "Evidence-Based Practice"). To successfully work with dying patients and families, you must demonstrate empathy, unconditional positive regard, trustworthiness, and clinical judgment. You are part of an interdisciplinary team (see Table 17.1). Each discipline has expertise and can lend support to patients and their loved ones using evidence-based information to make appropriate decisions.

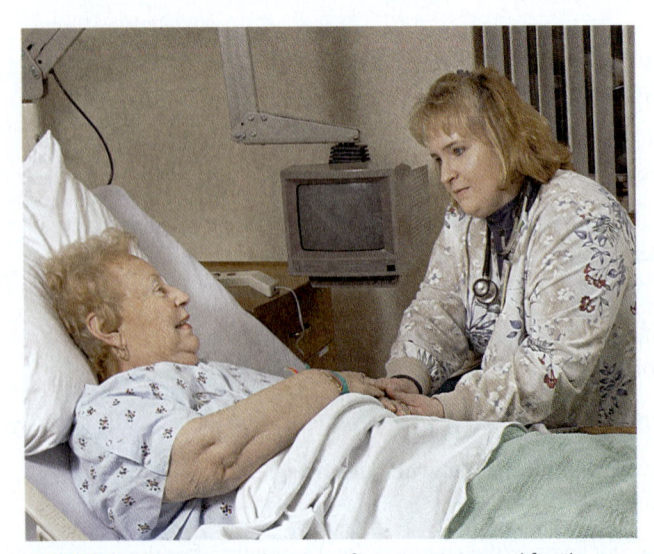

FIGURE 17.2 Nurses can be a comfort to patients and family members.

Evidence-Based Practice

Clinical Question
Do patients with a terminal diagnosis understand their prognosis? Do health-care professionals benefit from end-of life communication training?

Evidence
Multiple studies have suggested that an alarming number of patients at the end of life do not understand their prognosis or options, which leads to futile aggressive care, increased pain, and decreased quality of life (Trevino et al, 2019). According to Abernethy and colleagues (2020), in a study of nearly 600 patients with advanced cancer, only 17.6% of the 71% who wanted to know their prognosis reported being told. In other words, if a patient at the end of life wants to know their prognosis, what keeps them from receiving this accurate and often life-changing information from their medical team? Abernethy and colleagues state that this is related to dread of disclosing "bad news" or destroying the patient's hope, balancing sensitivity and honesty, and fear of damaging the rapport with the patient. We need to remember that although these discussions are often difficult, focus needs to be placed on meeting the patient's needs, not our own. Medical teams have a responsibility to their patients to have end-of-life conversations that are effective and comprehensive (Pfeifer & Head, 2018). The earlier patients know about their disease and prognosis, the sooner they are able to make decisions about the end of their life. This leads to fewer unnecessary treatments, earlier pain intervention, and decreased symptom burden (Trevino et al, 2019). End-of-life communication training may increase health-care professionals' ability to deliver prognoses to patients that are accurate and honest, while being culturally, racially, and socioeconomically sensitive (Loh et al, 2019).

Implications for Nursing Practice
It is important that all patients understand their disease status and prognosis. This may begin with health-care professionals' ability to effectively communicate with those facing end-of-life issues. Successful communication between health-care professionals and patients may help patients understand their conditions more clearly and increase their participation in end-of-life decision making.

> **References:** Abernethy, E., Campbell, G., & Pentz, R. D. (2019). Why many oncologists fail to share accurate prognoses: They care deeply for their patients. *Cancer, 126*(6), 1163–1165. https://doi.org/10.1002/cncr.32635
> Loh, K., Mohile, S. G., Lund, J. L., Epstein, R., Lei, L., Culakova, E., McHugh, C., Wells, M., Gilmore, N., Mohamed, M. R., Kamen, C., Aarne, V., Conlin, A., Bearden, J., Onitilo, A., Wittink, M., Dale, W., Hurria, A., & Duberstein, P. (2019). Beliefs about advanced cancer curability in older patients, their caregivers, and oncologists. *The Oncologist, 24*(6). https://doi.org/10.1634/theoncologist.2018-0890
> Pfeifer, M., & Head, B. A. (2018). Which critical communication skills are essential for interdisciplinary end-of-life discussions? *AMA Journal of Ethics, 20*(8), E724–731. https://doi.org/10.1001/amajethics.2018.724
> Trevino, K. M., Prigerson, H. G., Shen, M., Tancredi, D. J., Xing, G., Hoerger, M., Epstein, R. M., & Duberstein, P. R. (2019). Association between advanced cancer patient-caregiver agreement regarding prognosis and hospice enrollment. *Cancer, 125*(18), 3259–3265. https://doi.org/10.1002/cncr.32188

COMPASSION FATIGUE

Compassion fatigue can occur when caring for a loved one who is terminally ill. It is defined as "emotional, physical, and spiritual distress in those providing care to another" who is "experiencing significant emotional or physical pain and suffering" (Compassion Fatigue Awareness Project, 2020). Loved ones who care for the patient do so with the best intentions to help provide the person with a good death. Often, caregivers do not realize that caring for another human at the end of life is a 24-hour per day, 7-day per week undertaking. The patient's cognition and physical body will undergo frequent changes and demands. The patient may have restlessness and agitation, or pain levels may quickly fluctuate. Without proper support, providing care in these circumstances can become emotionally and physically straining on the caregiver. Remember, the caregiver is already grieving the anticipated loss of the patient; this combined with lack of sleep, frequent demands of the patient, and the need for self-care can be exhausting.

As the nurse, it is important to educate the caregiver on the importance of self-care, including adequate sleep, nutrition, exercise, and allowing time to grieve the patient. Offer to contact other professionals who may provide support to the caregiver, such as a social worker, chaplain, or volunteers. Validate the caregiver's efforts and diligence in providing comfort to their loved one.

THE DYING PROCESS

This section discusses the expected changes in the days and hours before death. Assessing patients, planning and implementing treatments, and evaluating responses to interventions are all important. Nursing interventions are summarized in the "Nursing Care Plan for the Patient at the End of Life."

Educating family caregivers about what to expect is essential. Caregivers who anticipate the expected changes and understand the rationale behind the interventions are more successful in their caregiving and have fewer regrets or concerns after the death. The "Nursing Care Plan for the Patient at the End of Life" includes specific communications that may help caregivers understand what is happening and how they can help.

Eating and Drinking

As the body moves toward death, patients lose desire for food and fluids. They are conserving energy and often do not feel hunger. The swallowing reflex is impaired, so patients fear choking and may hold their mouth tightly closed when food or fluids are offered. This is normal, and the resulting dehydration will increase comfort due to endorphin production.

Changes in Breathing

Research suggests that as many as 70% of dying patients report shortness of breath during end-of-life care (Huffman & Harmer, 2020). Patients who are not alert must rely on their caregivers to identify their distress. Signs of distress are tachypnea (respiratory rate greater than 24 per minute), facial grimacing, gasping, and use of accessory muscles to breathe. Untreated dyspnea can lead to fear and agitation, resulting in worsening shortness of breath. Dyspnea can be effectively managed without aggressive treatment (see "Nursing Care Plan for the Patient at the End of Life"). Some patients also have episodes of apnea or Cheyne-Stokes respirations (Chapter 29) in the days or hours before they die.

Oral Secretions

Saliva that the patient is now unable to swallow may collect in the back of the throat, causing a sound sometimes called a *death rattle*. This can be disconcerting for the family (see "Nursing Care Plan for the Patient at the End of Life").

Temperature Changes

As the body loses its ability to control temperature, the patient may become diaphoretic or feel cold all the time. Some patients have experienced fevers as high as 105°F (40.5°C). As death approaches, the feet and legs may become cool, cyanotic, and mottled. This occurs autonomically as the body tries to preserve the vital organs by bringing the blood back to the core of the body, thus decreasing warmth in the periphery. It is often an indicator that death will occur within hours. It is important to continue to keep the patient comfortable and calm (see "Nursing Care Plan for the Patient at the End of Life").

Bowel and Bladder Changes

Most patients become incontinent of bowel and bladder during the dying process. Urine output will decrease as dehydration occurs. Urine often darkens in color and has a strong odor. At the time of death, there may be a release of urine or stool as the pelvic muscles relax.

Sleeping
In the final weeks of life, patients may sleep most of the time. They also begin to emotionally detach from families as part of their preparation to leave. Although the family may sense the patient beginning to distance from their surroundings, it is part of the natural dying process.

Mental Status Changes
As patients go through the process of dying, they often become confused. Some patients will say things like, "I have to catch a train" or "I need my passport." This metaphorical communication is their way of notifying loved ones and caregivers that they are getting ready to die.

Terminal Restlessness
Terminal restlessness is a syndrome observed in a significant number of patients during the final days of life. The patient may be unable to concentrate or relax and may show nonpurposeful motor activities such as picking at bed sheets. The patient may hallucinate or try to climb out of bed. Some physical causes may be reversible, so it is important to assess whether dyspnea, pain, urinary retention, or fecal impaction may be the cause.

Restlessness may also be caused by medications. As kidney and liver functions decline, medication levels rise in the body and cause toxicity. Consult with the HCP and pharmacist to determine if all the medications the patient is receiving are beneficial or necessary. Table 17.2 reviews medications that may be helpful at the end of life.

Unconsciousness
Most patients are unconscious for hours or days before they die. Before they lose consciousness, their ability to see may be diminished. Hearing is the final sense to be lost. It is important for you to remember as you are caring for the patient and conversing with the family that your patient likely hears everything you are saying. Encourage the family to continue talking to the patient.

CRITICAL THINKING & CLINICAL JUDGMENT
Mr. Johnson is in the final hours of his life and has become increasingly short of breath throughout the day. With each inspiration, his respirations are moist and noisy. His family is extremely upset with his gurgling breathing. Currently, his respiratory rate is 30 per minute, and you notice he is using his accessory muscles to breathe.

Critical Thinking (The Why)
1. What is the cause of his noisy breathing?

Clinical Judgment (The How)
2. What can be done to help Mr. Johnson be more comfortable?
3. How can you help ease the family's anxiety?

Suggested answers are at the end of the chapter.

Nursing Care Plan for the Patient at the End of Life

Nursing Diagnosis: *Impaired Gas Exchange* related to dying heart and lungs as evidenced by dyspnea, apneic pauses, irregular breathing patterns, increase in oropharyngeal secretions, and change in respiratory rate
Expected Outcomes: The patient will not be in distress and will appear comfortable.
Evaluation of Outcomes: Is the patient's breathing relaxed and is the patient calm?

Intervention	Rationale	Evaluation
Monitor respiratory rate and effort.	Increased rate and effort indicate distress.	Is the patient in distress? Are further interventions needed?
Administer diuretics or antibiotics as ordered.	Diuretics or antibiotics may be given to treat causes of dyspnea and promote comfort, not to prolong life.	Do diuretics or antibiotics reduce dyspnea?
Plan activities to conserve energy.	Spacing rest with activity helps reduce oxygen consumption.	Can the patient tolerate spaced activities?
Place the patient in a recliner with pillows to 45 degrees.	An upright position allows lung expansion.	Does positioning reduce dyspnea?
Offer alternative comfort measures, such as massage for muscle relaxation.	Relaxation may reduce anxiety and resulting dyspnea.	Are alternative measures effective?

Nursing Care Plan for the Patient at the End of Life—cont'd

Intervention	Rationale	Evaluation
Administer oxygen as ordered.	Oxygenation reduces dyspnea.	Does oxygen relieve dyspnea?
Place a fan in the room if the patient desires.	The feeling of a breeze may reduce subjective feelings of dyspnea.	Does the patient report increased comfort or appear more comfortable with a fan on?
Administer low-dose morphine as ordered.	Morphine causes peripheral vasodilation, which can reduce pulmonary edema. It can also slow breathing and reduce anxiety.	Are respirations less labored after morphine administration?

Nursing Diagnosis: Ineffective Airway Clearance related to excessive secretions and inability to swallow as evidenced by gurgling sound ("death rattle")
Expected Outcome: The patient's airway will be free of secretions.
Evaluation of Outcome: Is the patient's breathing quiet and unlabored?

Intervention	Rationale	Evaluation
Adjust the patient's head to allow secretions to move down the throat.	This can help the patient swallow the secretions and decrease frightening noise.	Is breathing quieter?
Place a humidifier in the room.	Humidified air can liquefy secretions and help the patient cough.	Is the patient able to cough up secretions?
If secretions are copious, administer hyoscyamine (Levsin) as ordered.	Anticholinergic medications can dry secretions.	Do medications help dry secretions?
Administer low-dose morphine as ordered.	Morphine has an anticholinergic action that can help dry secretions.	Does morphine help quiet breathing and help the patient stay calm?
Suction patient as needed.	If secretions are copious, suctioning may be needed.	Is suctioning needed? Is it effective?
Explain to the family that, because the patient is unresponsive, a small amount of secretions is unlikely to be disturbing to the patient. The noisy breathing can often be reduced by repositioning the patient's head.	The informed family is able to cooperate and assist with keeping the patient comfortable.	Do the patient and family understand reasons for care and feel secure that the patient is receiving the best possible care?

Nursing Diagnosis: Imbalanced Nutrition: Less Than Body Requirements related to inability to swallow and lack of appetite as evidenced by refusing food and weight loss
Expected Outcomes: The patient will state satisfaction with the amount and types of food offered. The patient will not aspirate food or fluid.
Evaluation of Outcomes: Does the patient appear content with foods and fluids offered? Does the patient swallow without aspirating?

Intervention	Rationale	Evaluation
Let the patient choose when, how much, what to eat. Do not force the patient to eat if they do not wish to.	The goal is no longer providing adequate nutrition but keeping the patient comfortable.	Is the patient receiving the foods and fluids they want?
Sit the patient upright to eat or drink.	This can help the patient swallow and prevent aspiration.	Does the patient swallow effectively?

(nursing care plan continues on page 256)

Nursing Care Plan for the Patient at the End of Life—cont'd

Explain to family, as needed, that the patient is afraid to swallow now because swallowing is impaired and it causes the patient to choke. As the patient becomes dehydrated, the patient's comfort will increase as the body produces naturally occurring anesthesia.	*The informed patient and family are able to cooperate and assist with keeping the patient comfortable.*	Do the patient and family understand the reasons for care and feel secure that the patient is receiving the best possible care?

Nursing Diagnosis: *Impaired Oral Mucous Membrane Integrity* related to dehydration, not eating, and medication side effects
Expected Outcome: The patient's mucous membranes will be clean and moist.
Evaluation of Outcome: Are the patient's mucous membranes clean and moist? Does the patient indicate that the mouth is comfortable?

Intervention	Rationale	Evaluation
If the patient is alert, offer ice chips or sips of water.	*These keep mucous membranes moist.*	Does the patient indicate their mouth feels comfortable?
Provide frequent mouth care with sponge-tipped Toothettes.	*This can keep mucous membranes moist when the patient is not able to drink adequate fluids.*	Is the mouth clean and moist?
Apply lip balm or lanolin to lips.	*Lip balm and lanolin keep the mouth and lips from becoming dry and crusty.*	Are lips smooth and moist?

Nursing Diagnosis: *Impaired Comfort* (pain, terminal restlessness) related to disease process, dying process, and medications
Expected Outcome: The patient will acknowledge that they are comfortable or, if unable to speak, will appear calm and peaceful, not restless or agitated.
Evaluation of Outcome: Is the patient comfortable, calm, and peaceful?

Intervention	Rationale	Evaluation
Determine reversible causes of agitation (e.g., pain or other discomfort, urine retention or fecal impaction, medications that are no longer beneficial).	*Often, agitation is a sign of discomfort. Identifying and removing the cause of the discomfort can help calm the patient.*	Can causes be identified? Are they removed?
Reposition the patient in bed at least every 2 hours and as needed.	*Repositioning frequently can promote comfort and relieve pressure on bony prominences. When other medical interventions are discontinued, the patient still needs to be repositioned regularly to prevent uncomfortable complications.*	Does repositioning promote comfort?
Discuss with the HCP discontinuing all uncomfortable procedures such as blood draws and finger sticks for blood glucose, and discontinuing all nonessential medications.	*Many procedures are not beneficial to the patient at the end of life. Nonessential medications are difficult to swallow for some patients and are often ineffective at the end of life. They should be discontinued.*	Are any uncomfortable procedures and nonessential medications still being administered that are not absolutely necessary?
If the cause of the agitation cannot be determined, try medication for pain, dyspnea, or anxiety as ordered.	*Medication may need to be administered based on objective observations if the patient is unable to communicate.*	Does medication promote comfort?

Nursing Care Plan for the Patient at the End of Life—cont'd

Intervention	Rationale	Evaluation
Keep the patient safe with one-on-one monitoring.	A fall would increase the patient's discomfort.	Is patient safety maintained?
Keep the perineal area clean and dry, frequently checking adult briefs.	A wet brief is not comfortable. Unchanged briefs can also lead to skin breakdown, another source of discomfort.	Is the patient clean and dry with intact skin?
Teach the patient and family that restlessness can have many causes. It can be a sign of pain, bowel or bladder problems, or a medication issue. Tell them you will work with the HCP to improve the situation.	The informed patient and family are able to cooperate and assist with keeping the patient comfortable.	Do the patient and family understand the reasons for care and feel secure that the patient is receiving the best possible care?

Nursing Diagnosis: Hypothermia or Hyperthermia related to dysregulation of central nervous system
Expected Outcomes: The patient's temperature will be maintained as close to normal as possible, and discomfort from temperature extremes will be managed.
Evaluation of Outcomes: Is temperature within normal limits? If unable to control temperature, does the patient appear comfortable?

Intervention	Rationale	Evaluation
Administer acetaminophen suppository as ordered.	Acetaminophen is an antipyretic. It is given by suppository if the patient cannot swallow.	Does acetaminophen reduce fever?
Keep the patient clean and dry. Change gown and bed linens as needed.	A fever can cause diaphoresis (excessive sweating), and lying in damp sheets can be uncomfortable and cause skin breakdown.	Is the patient kept dry and comfortable?
If the patient is cold, add blankets as needed. Do not use an electric blanket or heating pad.	Blankets warm the patient without risking burns from electric heating devices.	Are blankets helpful?

Nursing Diagnosis: Acute Confusion related to neurologic changes
Expected Outcomes: The family will voice understanding that confusion is not uncommon and will show appropriate responses if it occurs.
Evaluation of Outcomes: Does the family respond appropriately to the patient during times of confusion?

Intervention	Rationale	Evaluation
Assure families that some confusion is common.	If family is prepared, confusion will be less disturbing.	Is the family informed? Do family members verbalize understanding of what to expect?
Teach the family to not correct the patient but instead encourage the patient to talk about what is happening.	Sometimes patients talk about their fears in metaphor. Allowing them to express their fears promotes relaxation and decrease loneliness.	Is the patient less distressed after speaking?
Keep a dim light on in the room (but enough light to avoid shadows), and remind the patient gently of who is present.	Being able to see clearly helps keep the patient oriented if the patient awakens during the night.	Is the light on? Is the patient able to orient on awakening?

(nursing care plan continues on page 258)

Nursing Care Plan for the Patient at the End of Life—cont'd

Intervention	Rationale	Evaluation
Explain to the family that many patients don't make sense at times. It is as if "they are in two worlds at the same time." Patient will be less distressed if the family lets the patient talk about what the patient is experiencing.	Family members will be less distressed if they understand what is happening.	Does the family respond appropriately to the patient's confused statements?

Nursing Diagnosis: *Fear* related to threat of death
Expected Outcome: The patient will be treated as still present and respected, and not as though the patient is already gone.
Evaluation of Outcome: Is communication respectful toward the patient?

Intervention	Rationale	Evaluation
When providing care, always speak as if the patient can hear you. When conversing with family members in the room, remember that the patient also can hear what you are saying.	Patients may be able to hear even when they appear to be nonresponsive. Always assume the patient can hear you.	Are caregivers and family members sensitive to the patient's presence when communicating?
When giving care, explain softly to the patient what you are doing and why.	Knowing what is happening can reduce anxiety and increase cooperation.	Does the patient appear calm? Does the patient respond to your explanations?
Explain to the family that it is believed that hearing is the last sense to go in the dying patient. This can be a good time to say the things they have not been able to say.	Continued communication can be comforting to both patient and family.	Is communication appropriate?

Nursing Diagnosis: *Grieving* related to impending death
Expected Outcome: The patient and family will be able to openly communicate their feelings to each other and say goodbye.
Evaluation of Outcome: Are the patient and family able to communicate effectively and say goodbye to each other?

Intervention	Rationale	Evaluation
Encourage the family to be present with the patient. Just sit quietly and hold the patient's hand for a period of time if they wish.	This can help the patient feel less alone. Many patients fear dying alone.	Is someone present with the patient as much as possible?
Show appropriate concern.	This promotes trust and empowers family members to ask for what they need.	Is the family communicating openly with the HCPs?
Provide a quiet environment where loved ones can say goodbye in a way that reflects their culture and values.	These interactions serve as valuable memories after the death and provide a feeling that all participants did what they needed to do for their loved one.	Do family members appear satisfied with their participation in the process?
Consult a minister or religious counselor of the family's choice.	A minister often has special skills and training in communicating with people during difficult times. Talking about an afterlife may also be comforting to the patient and family.	Does the family appear to benefit from the presence of a minister or religious counselor?
Ask about the family's cultural and religious beliefs, and allow time for prayers and ceremonies.	Providing a culturally familiar environment can reduce patient's and family's anxieties and give them more control over the process.	Do the family members feel free to carry out cultural and religious beliefs?

Table 17.2
Medications to Increase Comfort at the End of Life

Medication Class/Action

Opioids
Bind to opioid receptors to reduce pain and dyspnea.

Examples	*Nursing Implications*
morphine (MS, MS-IR, MS Contin, Roxanol) hydromorphone (Dilaudid) fentanyl (Duragesic, Sublimaze, Actiq, Fentora)	For pain and dyspnea. Longer-acting agents must be given routinely to be effective. Give short-acting analgesia for 24 to 72 hours until longer-acting agents take effect. Do not cut patches before application. Wear gloves when applying or removing the patch because the drug may be absorbed during handling. Do not apply heat over a patch. Heat increases drug absorption and may cause overdoses. Used patches may still contain drug. Dispose of used patches to prevent accidental exposure to others, especially children and pets.

Anxiolytics
Depress the central nervous system to reduce anxiety.

Examples	*Nursing Implications*
lorazepam (Ativan) alprazolam (Xanax) diazepam (Valium)	Not first-line drugs for treating dyspnea. Effective for dyspnea caused by anxiety.

Neuroleptics
Reduce severe agitation and terminal restlessness.

Examples	*Nursing Implications*
haloperidol (Haldol)	Useful in treating anxiety or agitation when lorazepam is ineffective.

Anticholinergics
Treat excessive pharyngeal secretions.

Examples	*Nursing Implications*
hyoscyamine (Levsin) atropine drops scopolamine (Transderm-Scop) glycopyrrolate (Robinul)	Place a scopolamine patch behind the ear.

CARE AT THE TIME OF DEATH AND AFTERWARD

Death has occurred when you observe the absence of heartbeat and respirations. The skin becomes pale and waxen, the eyes may remain open, and pupils are fixed. Telling the family that the patient has died should be done with sensitivity, with consideration of the family's cultural and religious preferences. Provide small amounts of information according to the family's level of understanding. Be sure to check and adhere to the policies in your health-care setting and state regarding death pronouncement and organ donation. Document the absence of pulse and lung sounds. Your goal now is to provide a personal closure experience for the family and caregivers.

After death has been pronounced, you will provide **postmortem care.** First, remove the tubes, medical supplies, and equipment. Bathing and dressing the patient and making him or her look presentable for the family shows respect. Some cultures dictate specific care of the body after death and who should provide that care. Ask the family their preferences and follow them as long as they are within agency policy. Allow loved ones to assist with this process if they choose to do so. Work toward providing a clean, peaceful impression of the deceased. Position the body in proper alignment, insert dentures, place dressings on leaking wounds, and use briefs as needed. Allow loved ones time with the body. Do not remove the body from the room until the family is ready. Covering or uncovering the face at removal should be done according to the family's preference. Additional activities, such as contacting the HCP or funeral home, should be carried out according to agency policy.

> **PRACTICE ANALYSIS TIP**
> Linking NCLEX-PN® to Practice
> The LPN/LVN will assist in providing postmortem care.

GRIEF

Grief is the emotional response to a loss. Loss is a daily experience in everyone's life. People express grief in their own way based on their coping skills, life experiences, and cultural norms. In end-of-life care, grief is a process that begins before the patient's death and continues through a series of tasks that the survivors move through to resolve grief. Feelings associated with grief may include anger, frustration, regret, guilt, sadness, and many others. Although each person is different, the process commonly includes three general stages (Table 17.3).

Interventions for the grieving patient are addressed in the "Nursing Care Plan for the Patient at the End of Life."

NURSING PROCESS FOR THE GRIEVING FAMILY

Data Collection
Some things to consider when assessing grief include the following:

- Where is the family in the grief process?
- Is the stress of grieving exacerbating medical conditions?
- What support systems are available to the family?
- What interventions might facilitate their grief process?

Nursing Diagnoses, Planning, and Implementation
Although many nursing diagnoses may be appropriate, the priority diagnosis is simply *Grieving*.

> **Grieving related to impending death or loss of a loved one**
>
> **EXPECTED OUTCOME:** Family members will be able to express feelings of anger, guilt, or sadness. They will be able to think about the future and perform activities of daily living as needed.

- Simply be present. *Sitting with the bereaved, without having to have all the answers, is very powerful. If you don't know what to say, just be silent.*
- Actively listen and let the bereaved talk about the loved one and their feelings about the loss. Ask open-ended questions to encourage them to continue talking. *One of the greatest needs of the bereaved is to trust someone enough to share their pain.*
- Help family members identify their support systems (e.g., religious or spiritual affiliation, friends, family) and encourage them to use them. *Support systems can help in practical ways (e.g., meals, transportation) as well as lend emotional support.*
- Consider acknowledging the event by attending the memorial service or sending a card. *This simple act of caring is very important to families.*

Table 17.3
Stages of Grief

Stage	Tasks	Characteristics
Stage 1 Shock and disbelief	Acknowledge the reality of the loss. Recognize the loss.	Has difficulty with feelings of numbness, emotional outbursts, poor daily functioning, and avoidance.
Stage 2 Experiencing the loss	Work through the pain by expressing and experiencing the feelings.	Anger, bargaining, depression. May feel guilt over not preventing the death or not providing enough care. May feel angry at a loved one who has "left them behind." May experience insomnia, loss of appetite, apathy, lack of interest in daily life.
Stage 3 Reintegration	Adjust to an environment without the deceased.	Finds hope in the future, participates in social events, and feels more energetic.

Evaluation

Healing takes time. If interventions have been effective, family members will have the support to function effectively while they grieve.

THE NURSE AND LOSS

Working with dying patients triggers awareness of your own losses and fears about death and mortality. Adapting to the care of the dying requires that you explore and experience your personal feelings toward death. Unresolved losses from your past can resurface and affect your ability to care for dying patients. You may find that you continue to think about patients who have died long after the event. Portoghese and colleagues (2020) recognize that staff working within a palliative care environment may be exposed to patient suffering, and this takes its toll on the nurse. Unresolved grief can lead to symptoms that resemble burnout, such as insomnia, headaches, and fatigue. If you find yourself distancing and withdrawing from your dying patients, it is an indicator that you need to attend to caring for yourself. Some nurses may find counseling helpful to effectively process losses from the past and learn healthy ways to process future losses. Both formal and informal support systems should be in place to support staff through multiple losses. Informal support can be one-on-one sharing of experiences with coworkers, peers, pastoral counselors, and HCPs. Understanding and acknowledging your limitations, asking for help, and getting regular exercise and relaxation are important components. Some nurses find journal writing a helpful process; writing down feelings may allow you to release them. Formal support systems can be established in many ways:

- Preplanned gatherings where nurses can express feelings in a safe environment
- Post-clinical debriefings after difficult deaths to alleviate anxiety and promote learning
- Ceremonies such as memorial services in facilities to allow both staff and residents to recognize and honor the loss of patients

In addition, many employers offer free employee assistance programs that provide counseling.

Key Points

- The Patient Self-Determination Act ensures that every patient has the right to accept or refuse any medical treatment offered. The act also requires health-care practitioners to ask patients entering a hospital if they have prepared advance medical directives. A helpful way of presenting the DNR option to patients and families is to help them to understand that, after receiving CPR, their medical condition will not improve and that it is likely that they will be more debilitated. Reassure patients that they will receive aggressive comfort care as they are dying a natural death.
- Symptoms of impending death include a rapid decline in condition, weight loss, difficulty swallowing and aspiration, increased dependence, increased hospitalizations, mental status changes, and increased sleep.
- Patients who are losing weight because of a life-limiting illness with multiple medical problems will probably not benefit from artificial feeding.
- The primary role of the nurse in communicating with dying patients and their loved ones is to facilitate a comfortable death that honors the choices of the patient and loved ones. The nurse, therefore, becomes the advocate, ensuring that patient wishes are communicated to other members of the health-care team.
- Good communication requires that you take time to listen, answer questions honestly, help identify choices, and allow verbalization of fears. Physical changes to expect during the dying process include diminished appetite, dyspnea/apnea, changes in ability to regulate body temperature, incontinence of bowel and bladder, decreased urine output, sleeping most of the time, mental status changes, terminal restlessness, and unconsciousness.
- Part of the nurse's role is to support the family caregivers. *Compassion fatigue* can occur when caring for a loved one who is terminally ill. It is defined as "emotional, physical, and spiritual distress in those providing care to another" who are "experiencing significant emotional or physical pain and suffering." It is important to educate caregivers on self-care and assist with locating resources to allow caregivers to do so.
- The dying process may involve changes in eating and drinking, changes in breathing, inability to swallow oral secretions, temperature changes, bowel and bladder incontinence, increased sleeping, mental status changes, restlessness, and unconsciousness.
- During postmortem care. you will remove tubes, medical supplies, and equipment. Bathe and dress the patient and make them look presentable for the family. Some cultures dictate specific care of the body after death and who should provide that care. Position the body in proper alignment, insert dentures, place dressings on leaking wounds, and use briefs as needed. Allow the family time with the body. Do not remove the body from the room until the family is ready.
- Working with dying patients may trigger awareness of your own losses and fears about death and mortality. Adapting to the care of the dying requires that you explore and experience your personal feelings toward death. Unresolved losses from your past can resurface and affect your ability to care for dying patients.

- Hospice care can help a family take care of a patient at home, but hospice nurses do not routinely provide 24-hour in-home health care. Rather, a nurse is on call for in-home visits 24 hours a day. Nurses and other team members make regular visits to support and teach the patient and family. In times of medical crisis, short-term inpatient hospice services or respite care may be provided under some hospice benefits.

SUGGESTED ANSWERS TO CHAPTER EXERCISES

Cue Recognition

17.1: Check your assignment quickly to determine whether the patient has a DNR order. If so, go with the family member into the room and do a calm, respectful assessment to determine whether the patient has a heartbeat or is breathing. If not, gently tell the person that the resident has died, and remind them that the patient had chosen a DNR status. Notify the RN. If the patient does NOT have a DNR order, call for help and begin CPR.

17.2: Check the resident's advance directive. The resident may have a directive in place about artificial feeding. Communicate with the family or patient advocate as needed. Have this information ready before notifying the HCP.

Critical Thinking & Clinical Judgment

Mrs. Hung

1. Mrs. Hung will need a DNR order in the hospital setting. When she goes home, she will need an out-of-hospital or prehospital, durable DNR (whatever the form is called, such as MOLST, MOST, POST, or POLST, in her state of residence). In addition, her family members should be aware of her wishes.
2. Her HCP, hospital social worker, or case manager can be helpful. She may also wish to speak with the chaplain or her spiritual advisor.

Mr. Johnson

1. Mr. Johnson's noisy breathing may be caused by saliva collecting in the back of the throat or by pulmonary edema.
2. Mr. Johnson may benefit from oxygen, positioning, and suctioning oral secretions. Low-dose morphine will decrease his respiratory rate and improve his oxygenation. Morphine also has a drying effect on secretions. If morphine is unsuccessful, the addition of an anticholinergic medication may be helpful.
3. The "death rattle" can be distressing for loved ones. Explain to the family what is happening, and how the care you are providing will help.

Additional Resources

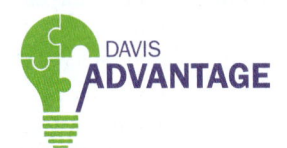

Go to Davis Advantage to complete your learning: strengthen understanding, apply your knowledge, and prepare for the Next Gen NCLEX®.

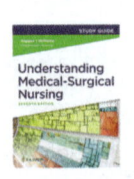

A Study Guide is also available.

UNIT FOUR Understanding the Immune System

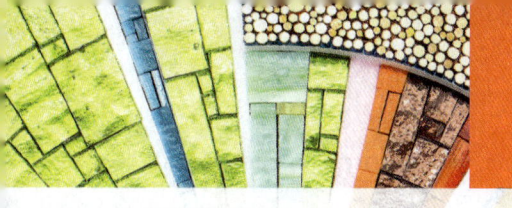

CHAPTER 18

Immune System Function, Data Collection, and Therapeutic Measures

Kristy Gorman, Janice L. Bradford

KEY TERMS

active immunity (AK-tiv ih-MYOO-nih-tee)
anaphylactic (AN-uh-fih-LAK-tik)
antibody (AN-tih-bah-dee)
antigen (AN-tih-jen)
autoimmune (AW-toe-ih-mewn)
cell-mediated immunity (SELL MEE-dee-ay-ted ih-MYOO-nih-tee)
humoral immunity (HYOO-mur-uhl ih-MYOO-nih-tee)
immunosenescence (ih-MEWN-oh-sen-ESS-ents)
lymphocyte (LIM-fuh-site)
microbiota (MY-kro-by-OTT-a)
neutrophil (NEW-troh-fil)
passive immunity (PASS-iv ih-MYOO-nih-tee)
white blood cells (WYTE BLUHD SELLS)

CHAPTER CONCEPTS

Immunity
Safety
Self-care
Teaching and learning

LEARNING OUTCOMES

1. Identify the type of immunity that is obtained with a vaccine.
2. Describe the two mechanisms of immunity.
3. Discuss the function of each class of immunoglobulin and how each behaves in a particular immune response.
4. Describe how aging affects the immune system.
5. Explain subjective data that are collected when caring for a patient with a disorder of the immune system.
6. Explain objective data that are collected when caring for a patient with a disorder of the immune system.
7. Describe nursing care for patients undergoing diagnostic tests for the immune system.
8. Discuss common therapeutic measures used for disorders of the immune system.

NORMAL IMMUNE SYSTEM ANATOMY AND PHYSIOLOGY

Immunity is the ability to destroy pathogens or other foreign material and to prevent further cases of infectious disease. Immunity is typically the body's response to foreign microorganisms such as bacteria, viruses, and fungi. However, immune responses can be directed toward other cells or substances that are identified by the body, correctly or incorrectly, as foreign. Mutated cells are considered foreign and are usually destroyed by the immune system after mutation but before they become malignant. Unfortunately, transplanted organs are usually perceived as foreign and, therefore, rejected. Occasionally, the immune system mistakenly reacts to self (**autoimmune** disease) or to a substance that should be tolerated (allergic reaction).

The immune system consists of lymphoid organs and tissues, **lymphocytes** and other **white blood cells** (WBCs), and many chemicals that activate our own cells for the destruction of foreign antigens (Fig. 18.1). The lymphatic system includes lymphatic vessels that return lymph (tissue fluid) to the circulatory system; lymph nodes, nodules, and the spleen, where macrophages phagocytize (engulf and destroy) pathogens and where thymus-derived lymphocytes (T cells)

• WORD • BUILDING •
lymphocyte: lympho—lymph + kytos—cell

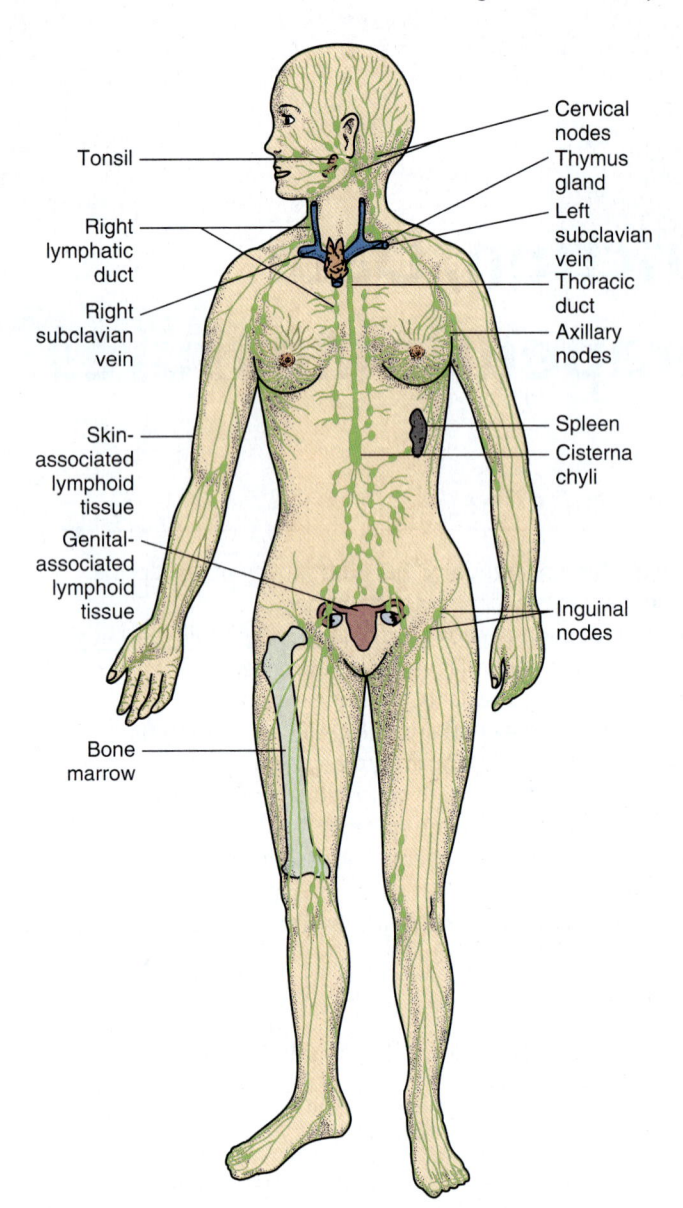

FIGURE 18.1 Immune system organs, lymph vessels, and major lymph nodes.

and bone marrow–derived lymphocytes (B cells) carry out immune functions; and red bone marrow and the thymus (which functions primarily in childhood and atrophies with age). Lymph flows from vessels through lymph nodes, where pathogens are percolated out and destroyed. Lymph nodes are especially concentrated in the cervical, axillary, and inguinal areas. Lymph nodules, lacking encapsulation, are found under the surface of mucous membranes (e.g., tonsils).

Antigens

Antigens are chemical markers that identify cells or molecules. Human cells have their own antigens—thousands of markers that identify the cell as "self." These are the major histocompatibility complex antigens, also called human leukocyte antigens, which are genetically determined. Major histocompatibility complex antigens are tolerated by the body's immune system, whereas foreign antigens will be destroyed in one of several ways.

Lymphocytes

There are three types of lymphocytes: natural killer (NK) cells, T cells, and B cells, each with different functions.

Natural Killer Cells

Natural killer (NK) cells patrol the body and produce a quick attack. They destroy a variety of foreign cells, including altered self-cells (tumors) and infected cells. After binding with an abnormal cell, NK cells release perforins and granzymes, which cause cytolysis (destruction of cell). Cell fragments are then phagocytized by WBCs.

T Cells and B Cells

T cells and B cells are involved in specific immune responses; that is, each cell is programmed to respond to one kind of foreign antigen. Both T cells and B cells arise in the red bone marrow. T cells then migrate to the thymus, where the thymic hormones bring about their maturation. From the thymus, T cells migrate to the lymph nodes and nodules and to the spleen. B cells mature in the bone marrow and migrate directly to lymphatic tissue. When activated during an immune response, T cells perform a direct attack, whereas B cells differentiate into plasma cells that release antibodies for an indirect approach.

Antibodies

Antibodies are glycoproteins produced by plasma cells in response to foreign antigens. They are also called immunoglobulins (Ig). Antibodies do not themselves destroy foreign antigens but rather become attached to such antigens to label them for destruction. Each antibody is specific for only one antigen. B cells (which become plasma cells) can produce millions of different antibodies. There are five classes of human antibodies, designated by letter names: IgG, IgA, IgM, IgD, and IgE (Fig. 18.2). Their functions are summarized in Table 18.1.

Mechanisms of Immunity

The two mechanisms of immunity are *cell-mediated immunity,* which involves T cells, and *humoral immunity,* which involves mainly B cells but is assisted by T cells. Although the mechanisms are different, invasion by a pathogen often triggers both.

Cell-Mediated Immunity

Cell-mediated immunity is effective against intracellular pathogens (infected host cells), malignant cells, and grafts of foreign tissue. A T-cell response results in cytotoxic T cells,

• WORD • BUILDING •

antigen: anti—against + gennan—to produce

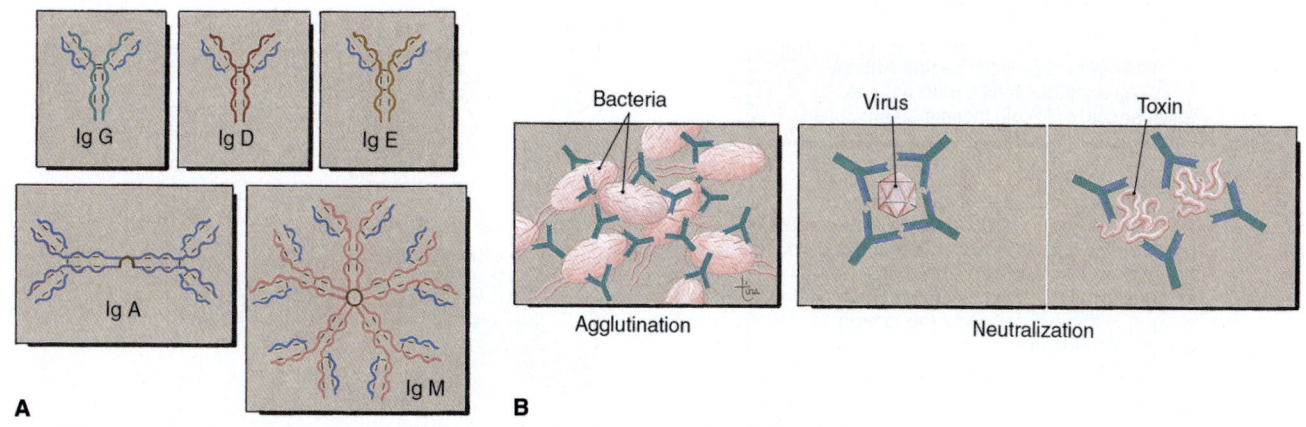

FIGURE 18.2 Antibodies. (A) Structure of the five classes of antibodies. (B) Antibody activity.

Table 18.1
Classes of Antibodies

Immunoglobulin (Ig)	Location	Function
IgG	Blood, extracellulwar fluid, lymph	Provides long-term immunity after vaccine or illness recovery Crosses the placenta to provide passive immunity in newborns
IgA	External secretions (e.g., tears, saliva)	Found in secretions of all mucous membranes Provides passive immunity for breastfed infants
IgM	Blood, lymph	Produced first during an infection (IgG production follows)
IgD	B cells	Antigen-specific receptors on B lymphocytes
IgE	Mast cells or basophils	Important in allergic reactions Mast cells release histamine

Source: From Scanlon, V., & Sanders, T. (2019). *Understanding human structure and function* (8th ed.). Philadelphia, PA: F.A. Davis.

which attack altered cells; helper T cells, which assist; and memory T cells, which retain knowledge of the pathogen in the event of future encounters with the same (Fig. 18.3).

Humoral Immunity

Humoral immunity involves antibody production. It is also called *antibody-mediated immunity*. It is effective against extracellular pathogens, which are often bacteria but can also be viral or fungal infections (Fig. 18.4).

Although B cells are stationary, the antibodies produced by plasma cells circulate throughout the body and bond to the antigen, forming an antigen–antibody complex. This bonding immobilizes the pathogen; also, the antigen is now labeled for phagocytosis by macrophages or **neutrophils**. The antigen–antibody complex also activates the *complement cascade*.

Complement is a group of more than 30 plasma proteins that circulate in the blood until activated by either the presence of pathogen or by an antigen–antibody complex. The activation of complement results in a protein cascade that lyses (causes disintegration of) the cell. Other complement proteins bind to foreign antigens, serving as labels to attract macrophages.

ANTIBODY RESPONSES

The first exposure to a foreign antigen stimulates antibody production. However, the antibodies are produced too slowly to prevent the disease. With time, the person accumulates antibodies and memory cells specific for that pathogen. On second exposure, the memory cells begin rapid production of large amounts of antibody, often enough to prevent a second occurrence of the illness (Fig. 18.5). This is the basis for the protection given by vaccines. A vaccine contains an antigen that is not pathogenic. The vaccine stimulates formation of antibodies and memory cells.

• WORD • BUILDING •

neutrophil: neutro—neuter + philein—to love

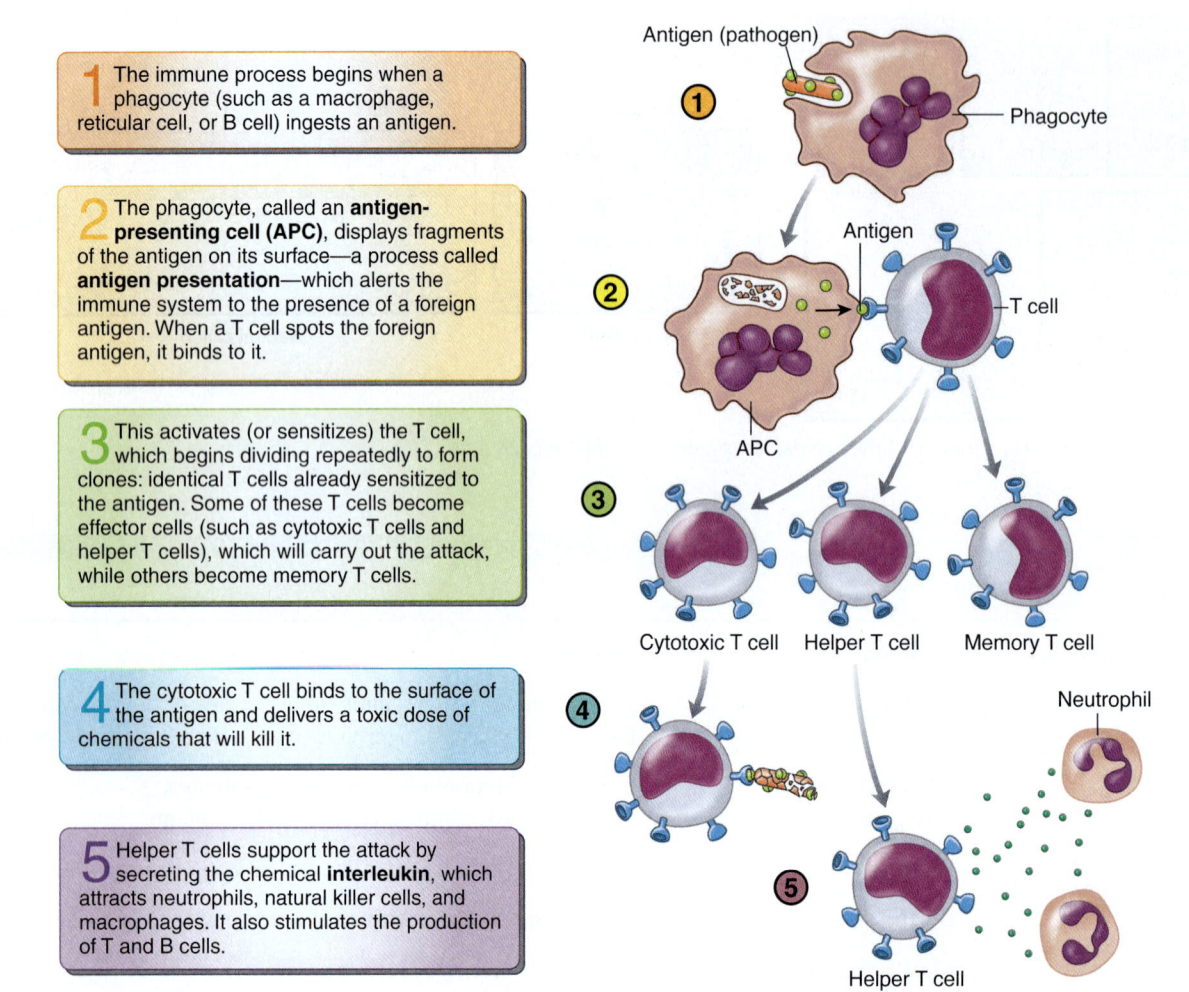

1. The immune process begins when a phagocyte (such as a macrophage, reticular cell, or B cell) ingests an antigen.

2. The phagocyte, called an **antigen-presenting cell (APC)**, displays fragments of the antigen on its surface—a process called **antigen presentation**—which alerts the immune system to the presence of a foreign antigen. When a T cell spots the foreign antigen, it binds to it.

3. This activates (or sensitizes) the T cell, which begins dividing repeatedly to form clones: identical T cells already sensitized to the antigen. Some of these T cells become effector cells (such as cytotoxic T cells and helper T cells), which will carry out the attack, while others become memory T cells.

4. The cytotoxic T cell binds to the surface of the antigen and delivers a toxic dose of chemicals that will kill it.

5. Helper T cells support the attack by secreting the chemical **interleukin**, which attracts neutrophils, natural killer cells, and macrophages. It also stimulates the production of T and B cells.

FIGURE 18.3 Cellular immunity.

Antibodies may also neutralize viruses; that is, they attach to a virus and render it unable to enter a cell (see Fig. 18.2). Viruses cannot reproduce outside of living cells. Those coated with antibodies are phagocytized by macrophages. Interferon, another defense against viruses, is a chemical produced by cells infected with viruses. Although it does not help the infected cell, interferon protects surrounding cells by enabling them to resist viral replication.

Antibodies are also involved in allergic responses. During an allergic response, the immune system responds to foreign but harmless antigens (an allergen), such as plant pollen. IgE antibodies on mast cells bind to an allergen, causing release of histamine and other chemicals that contribute to inflammation. **Anaphylactic** shock is an allergic reaction, but massive in response. It is characterized by loss of plasma from capillaries (an effect of histamine) and a sudden drop in the intravascular blood volume and blood pressure.

TYPES OF IMMUNITY

Two categories of immunity are passive immunity and active immunity. In **passive immunity,** antibodies are not produced by the person but are obtained from another source. One form of *naturally* acquired passive immunity includes placental transmission of antibodies from mother to fetus and transmission of antibodies in breast milk. *Artificially* acquired passive immunity involves injection of preformed antibodies; this may help prevent disease after exposure to a pathogen such as the hepatitis B virus. Passive immunity is always temporary, in that antibodies from another source eventually break down.

Active immunity means that the person produces his or her own antibodies. An example of *naturally* acquired active immunity occurs when a person recovers from an infection and then has antibodies and memory cells specific for that pathogen. *Artificially* acquired active immunity occurs as the result of a vaccine that stimulates production of antibodies and memory cells. The duration of active immunity depends on the disease or vaccine; some confer lifelong immunity, but others do not due to antibody loss over various time frames.

• WORD • BUILDING •
anaphylactic: ana—up + phylaxis—protection

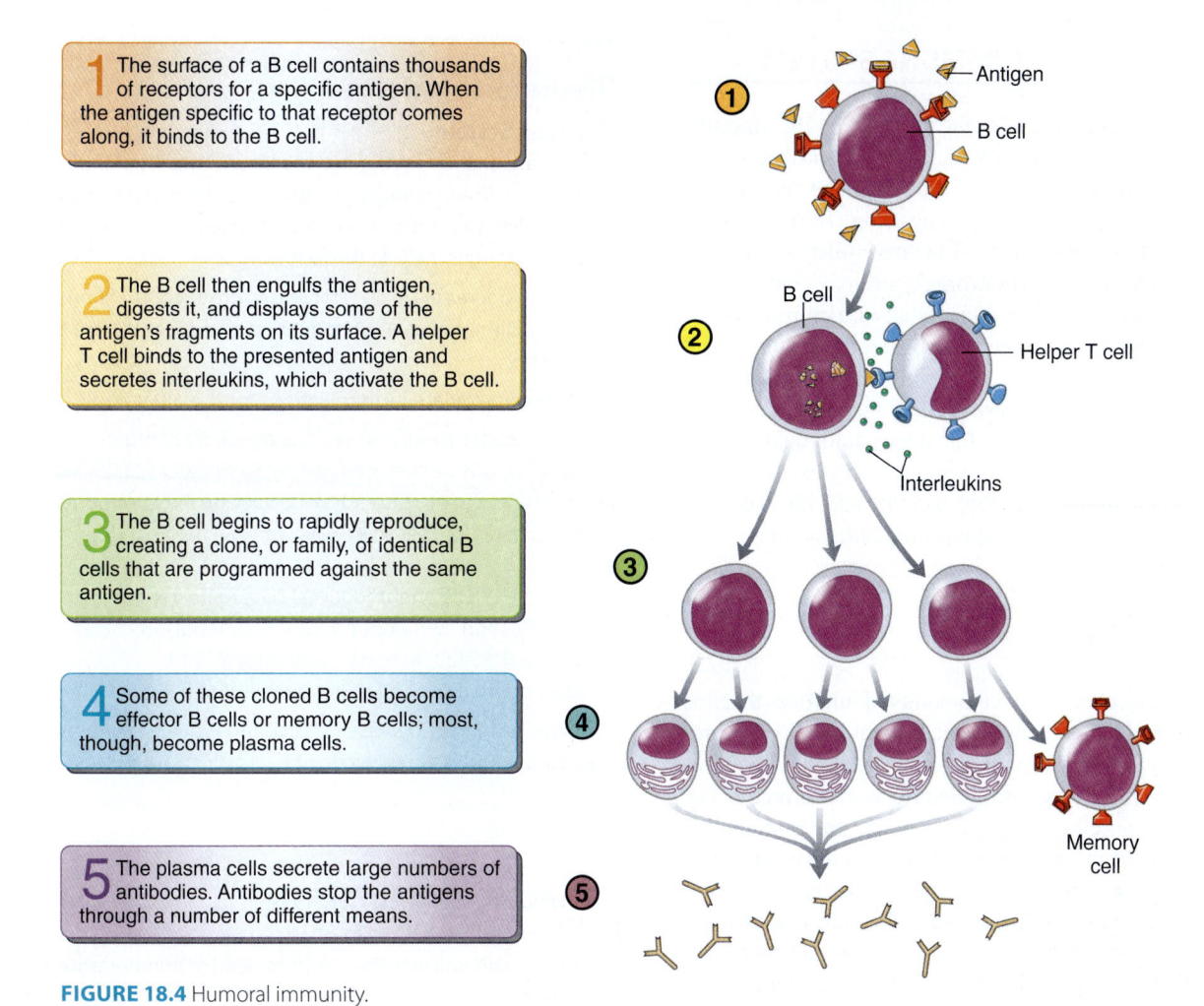

Chapter 18 Immune System Function, Data Collection, and Therapeutic Measures   267

1. The surface of a B cell contains thousands of receptors for a specific antigen. When the antigen specific to that receptor comes along, it binds to the B cell.

2. The B cell then engulfs the antigen, digests it, and displays some of the antigen's fragments on its surface. A helper T cell binds to the presented antigen and secretes interleukins, which activate the B cell.

3. The B cell begins to rapidly reproduce, creating a clone, or family, of identical B cells that are programmed against the same antigen.

4. Some of these cloned B cells become effector B cells or memory B cells; most, though, become plasma cells.

5. The plasma cells secrete large numbers of antibodies. Antibodies stop the antigens through a number of different means.

FIGURE 18.4 Humoral immunity.

Primary and secondary antibody responses

FIGURE 18.5 Antibody responses to a first and then subsequent exposure to a pathogen.

AGING AND THE IMMUNE SYSTEM

Immunosenescence refers to the decline in the immune system especially seen in older adults. The production of new immune cells, the efficiency of the immune system, and response to vaccines decrease with age (Fig. 18.6). Lifetime influences such as environmental factors, lifestyle, medications, and repeated exposures to organisms may contribute to immunosenescence. As such, older adults are more susceptible to infections and autoimmune disorders ("Gerontological Issues"). Incidence of cancer is also higher; malignant cells that might once have been destroyed by the immune system live and proliferate. Mortality for older adults increases. A healthy lifestyle of avoiding alcohol, avoiding excessive sun exposure, maintaining a normal weight, and not smoking can help promote immune health for the older adult.

MICROBIOTA AND THE IMMUNE SYSTEM

Microbiota is a collection or community of microbes that live in or on the body. See www.gutmicrobiotaforhealth.com for more information. Ongoing research suggests that microbes are essential for our immune system to work correctly. The term *microbiome* refers to the genes within the microbes of the microbiota. Microbes affect metabolic pathways that provide the body nutrients. Some microbes can cause disease with their overgrowth, but most microbes are essential for health. Lack of diversity and disruption of the microbiota are being studied as contributing factors in the development of some diseases (e.g., anorexia nervosa, cardiovascular disease, depression, irritable bowel syndrome, and immune disorders such as lupus and rheumatoid arthritis). Research findings may lead to new treatments for these diseases.

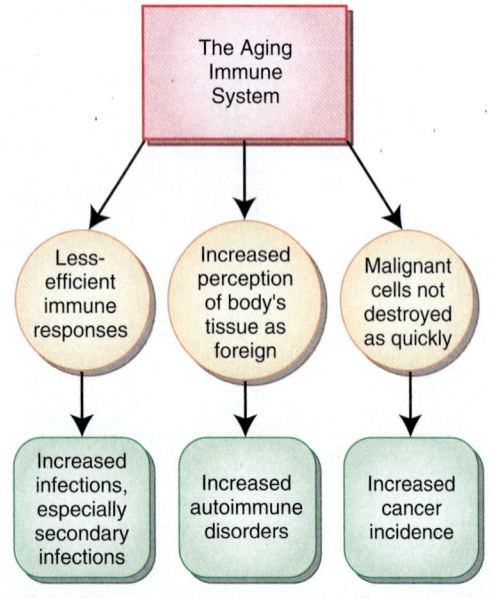

FIGURE 18.6 This concept map shows the effects the aging process has on the immune system.

Gerontological Issues

Immune System

Significant changes occur in the immune system of the older adult. These changes are known as *immunosenescence*, which refers to a decline in immune system function. Some specific changes include the following:

- Thymus decreases in size, increases production of immature T cells, and has a subsequent decline in response to antigens.

    Age-appropriate immunizations for the older adult:

- Herpes zoster (shingles) vaccine at age 50 or older (Shingrix; CDC recommended) or 60 or older (Zostavax)
- Influenza vaccine (plus H1N1 flu vaccine if recommended) yearly, mid-October to mid-November, before influenza season
- Thirteen-valent pneumococcal conjugate vaccine (PCV13), then 23-valent pneumococcal polysaccharide vaccine (PPSV23) at least 1 year after PCV13
- Tetanus and diphtheria booster every 10 years

    See Centers for Disease Control and Prevention immunization schedules at www.cdc.gov.

PRACTICE ANALYSIS TIP
Linking NCLEX-PN® to Practice
The LPN/LVN will identify clients in need of immunizations (required and voluntary).

IMMUNE SYSTEM DATA COLLECTION

Disorders of the immune system can affect every system in the body, so it is important to collect head-to-toe data as well as a patient history (Table 18.2).

Subjective Data

Data are collected regarding the patient's health history and current health condition using the **WHAT'S UP?** format (see Chapter 1). A family history is also obtained. Some diseases tend to be associated with a certain gender or ethnicity. For instance, systemic lupus erythematosus (SLE; see Chapter 19), an autoimmune disorder, affects more women than men. Ninety percent of people living with lupus are women. Black, Asian American, Hispanic/Latino, American Indian, and Pacific Islander women are affected more than White individuals (Lupus Foundation of America, 2021, https://www.lupus.org/resources/lupus-facts-and-statistics).

• WORD • BUILDING •

immunosenescence: immunis—exempt from + senescere—to grow old

Table 18.2
Subjective Data Collection for the Immune System

Questions to Ask During the Health History	Rationale/Significance
Demographic Data	
Where were you born?	Determines ethnic and cultural background influences.
What is your ethnic or cultural background?	Some immune disorders are associated with certain cultural/ethnic groups.
Where have and do you currently live?	Shows ethnic, cultural, and environmental exposures and influences.
What is your occupation? Have you been exposed to hazardous chemicals, fumes, or radiation?	Chemicals can produce local reactions (skin) or systemic immune reactions, and some can lead to bone marrow suppression.
What risky behaviors do you engage in?	Intravenous drug use, unprotected sex, or multiple partners increase risk for contracting HIV.
Allergies	
Do you have allergies to medications? Latex? Foods? Stinging insects? Environmental allergens?	Medication side effects are often inaccurately considered to be allergies by patients, which requires education.
If yes, have you had a recent exposure to any of these? Describe the reaction.	Recent exposure may provide cause for current symptoms.
What allergies do immediate relatives have?	If immediate family members have allergies, the patient may also be predisposed to the reaction.
Medications, Herbs	
What prescription or over-the-counter medications or herbal preparations do you take?	Corticosteroids and immunosuppressants suppress immune responses; anti-infectives and antineoplastics depress the bone marrow and white blood cells.
Medical Conditions	
What conditions have you been diagnosed with?	May provide insight into patient's current condition or symptoms.
Surgeries	
What surgeries have you had?	If any immune organs have been removed, this may reduce immune function.
Coping	
What do you do to cope with stress?	Identifying patient coping behaviors allows incorporation into the plan of care.
Who or what are your support systems?	Support systems can buffer stress that affects immune function.

Many atopic (allergic) disorders, such as allergic rhinitis (see Chapter 19) and asthma (see Chapter 31), and autoimmune disorders, such as ankylosing spondylitis (see Chapter 19), are thought either to be familial or to have a genetic predisposition in certain ethnic or cultural groups. For example, four genes have been identified that are strongly associated with SLE and 10 others identified as risk factors. It is suggested that different genes may affect how the disease presents in individual patients. As an example, certain genetic mutations have been associated with lupus nephritis.

Ask about allergies. If the patient indicates a latex allergy, ask whether they have a latex detection service dog. Anaphylactic reactions can be caused by exposure to airborne latex or by direct contact. Latex may be found in gloves and other medical products. Some fruits and nuts are latex-reactive foods (such as avocado, banana, chestnut, kiwi, apple, carrot, celery, papaya, potatoes, tomatoes, melons). Be aware of this potentially life-threatening allergy and know your agency's latex allergy protocol.

A surgical history can give clues to a patient's health status. For example, with thymus removal (thymectomy), T-cell production may be altered. This affects the cell-mediated immune response. If the spleen is removed (splenectomy), lymphocyte and plasma cell production may be altered. This affects the humoral immune response.

> **PRACTICE ANALYSIS TIP**
> **Linking NCLEX-PN® to Practice**
> The LPN/LVN will identify client allergies and intervene as appropriate.

Objective Data

Physical data collection begins by observing the patient's general appearance, facial expression, hearing, vision, posture, gait, skin, and nailbeds. Rashes should be examined for size, shape, location, texture, drainage, and pruritus (itching). Additional objective data are collected (Table 18.3). Lymph nodes are not normally palpable by the health-care provider (HCP; see Fig. 18.1). When they are enlarged, the following characteristics are noted: location, size, shape, tenderness, temperature, consistency, mobility, symmetry, pulsation, and whether red streaks, redness, or edema are

Table 18.3
Objective Data Collection for the Immune System

Abnormal Findings	Possible Causes
Heart Sounds	
Pericardial friction rub	Rheumatoid arthritis or systemic lupus erythematosus (SLE) from inflammation of connective tissue surrounding the heart (pericardium).
Lung Sounds	
Crackles with a dry cough	Pneumocystis jiroveci pneumonia
Pleural effusion with tachypnea, diminished sounds; pleural friction rub	Rheumatoid arthritis, SLE
Wheezing	Allergic reaction
Lymph Nodes	
Painful, enlarged lymph nodes	Inflammation, infection
Enlarged, painless, firm, fixed lymph nodes	Cancer
Gastrointestinal	
Diarrhea or diarrhea alternating with constipation	Irritable bowel syndrome
Musculoskeletal	
Swollen, painful joints and limited joint range of motion	Rheumatoid arthritis
Decreased strength and coordination	Multiple sclerosis
Strength and endurance loss during repetitive movements	Myasthenia gravis
Neurologic	
Confusion, lethargy	Later stages of SLE or AIDS
Muscle weakness and coordination abnormalities	Multiple sclerosis or myasthenia gravis
Renal	
Urine output less than 30 mL/hour, protein in urine, edema	SLE or serum sickness
Hematuria, flank pain, oliguria	Glomerulonephritis, transfusion reaction
Skin	
Rash, erythema (redness), urticaria, pruritus, pustules	Allergic reaction
"Butterfly rash" (red rash over bridge of nose and cheek bones)	SLE (most typical rash)
Onycholysis (nail detaches from nailbed)	Hashimoto thyroiditis
Painless purple lesions	Kaposi sarcoma, associated with HIV/AIDS
Pale, edematous mucous membranes, rhinorrhea, "allergic shiners" (dark circles under eyes)	Allergic rhinitis
Pale conjunctiva	Anemia
Periorbital edema	Hypothyroidism

present. An enlarged spleen may be palpable by the HCP in the left upper quadrant of the abdomen. Enlargement occurs with overproduction or excessive destruction of red blood cells.

> **LEARNING TIP**
> A normally functioning immune system is required to trigger an inflammatory response and production of the signs of inflammation or infection (e.g., fever, redness, pain, swelling, and warmth). If the immune system is suppressed or functioning abnormally, this normal inflammatory response may not occur. The patient may have only a low-grade fever with none of the other signs of inflammation or infection.
> Recognize patients who have suppressed immune systems so that low-grade fevers are reported to the HCP for prompt treatment. This may be the only sign of a life-threatening infection that develops.

> **CUE RECOGNITION 18.1**
> You are caring for a patient who received chemotherapy one week ago via a central line. When you check vital signs, the patient has a temperature of 100.4°F (38°C) but has no chills or sweating. What action do you take?
> *Suggested answers are at the end of the chapter.*

> **CLINICAL JUDGMENT**
> **Mrs. Sims** is scheduled for a lymph node biopsy and reports for preadmission testing before surgery. As you prepare to draw blood specimens, you learn that Mrs. Sims is allergic to latex.
> 1. What do you do to promote patient-centered care during this laboratory draw?
> 2. What actions do you take after learning of the allergy?
> 3. What precautions do you take when drawing the blood specimen?
> 4. What health-care team members do you collaborate with?
>
> *Suggested answers are at the end of the chapter.*

DIAGNOSTIC TESTS FOR THE IMMUNE SYSTEM

Table 18.4 describes the most common blood tests for patients with allergic, autoimmune, or immune disorders. Table 18.5 presents common noninvasive and invasive procedures for immune disorders. Chest x-ray, magnetic resonance imaging (MRI), and computed tomography (CT) scans might also be used.

Gene Testing

With human genome mapping data, scientists can test for numerous diseases, predisposition to diseases, and enzyme deficiencies that can alter immune response.

Table 18.4
Laboratory Tests for the Immune System

Test/Definition	Normal Value	Significance of Abnormal Findings
Red Blood Cell (RBC) Count—Number of RBCs per 1 mm of blood.	Adult male: $4.21–5.81 \times 10^6$ cells/microL Adult female: $3.61–5.11 \times 10^6$ cells/microL	Decreased in all forms of anemia, such as pernicious anemia that develops from the autoimmune form of gastritis or idiopathic autoimmune hemolytic anemia.
Differential—Each of these tests (MCV, MCH, MCHC, RDW) provides information about RBC size, shape, color, and intracellular structure.	See below.	Can help determine the cause of anemia. Pernicious anemia can develop because of the autoimmune form of gastritis.
• MCV	Adult male: 77–97 fL Adult female: 78–98 fL Older adult male: 79–103 fL Older adult female: 78–102 fL	
• MCH	Adult: 26–34 pg/cell Older adult: 27–35 pg/cell	
• MCHC	32–36 g/dL	

Continued

Table 18.4
Laboratory Tests for the Immune System—cont'd

Test/Definition	Normal Value	Significance of Abnormal Findings
• RDWCV	11.6–14.8	
• RDWSD	38–48	
White Blood Cell (WBC) Count—Number of WBCs per 1 mm of blood.	Adult: 4.5–11.1 × 10^3/microL^3	Increased with immunosuppression and infection.
Differential—Percentage of each type of WBCs in 100 cell count. Absolute count is the actual number of specific types of WBCs present.	See below.	Eosinophils elevate with type I hypersensitivity reactions such as allergic rhinitis or anaphylaxis.
	% Absolute/microL^3	
• Neutrophils	40–75 2.7–6.5	
• Lymphocytes	12–44 1.5–3.7	
• Monocytes	4–9 0.2–0.4	
• Eosinophils	0–5.5 0.05–0.5	
• Basophils	0–1 0–0.1	
Erythrocyte Sedimentation Rate (ESR)—A nonspecific test for generalized inflammation. Measures the RBC descent (in millimeters) in test tube after being in normal saline solution for 1 hour (Westergren method).	*Male under 50:* 0–15 mm/hr *Female under 50:* 0–25 mm/hr *Male 50 and over:* 0–20 mm/hr *Female 50 and over:* 0–30 mm/hr	False negative may result if steroids or NSAIDs are taken when test is performed.
Rheumatoid Factor (RF)—An abnormal protein found in serum when IgM reacts with an abnormal IgG; found in 80% of patients with rheumatoid arthritis and other autoimmune disorders.	Less than 14 IU/mL (60 years and older may be elevated)	Increased in rheumatoid arthritis, SLE, leukemia, tuberculosis, older age, scleroderma, and infectious mononucleosis.
Antinuclear Antibody (ANA)/Anti-ds DNA (ANA subset)—Measures autoantibodies that attack the cell's nucleus.	*Negative:* Less than 5 IU *Indeterminate:* 5–9 IU *Positive:* 9 IU	Presence strongly associated with SLE. Also indicates leukemia, scleroderma, rheumatoid arthritis, and myasthenia gravis; many medications influence levels.
Complement—Specific serum proteins that help mediate inflammation. Measures amount of each component in the complement system.	See below.	Deficiencies of specific complement proteins are seen in SLE.
• Total	CH50 31–60 units/mL	
• C3	83–177 mg/dL	
• C4	12–36 mg/dL	

Table 18.4
Laboratory Tests for the Immune System—cont'd

Test/Definition	Normal Value	Significance of Abnormal Findings
C-Reactive Protein (CRP)—An abnormal protein found in plasma during acute inflammatory processes; more sensitive than sedimentation rate.	Less than 10 mg/L	Increased in rheumatoid arthritis, cancer, and SLE. Suppressed by aspirin and steroids.
Antigen/Antibody Combination Immunoassay—Detects both HIV-1 and HIV-2 antibodies and HIV-1 p24 antigen.	Negative	Shows established infection with HIV-1 or HIV-2 and acute infection for HIV-1. If positive, antibody immunoassay test is done to differentiate between HIV-1 and HIV-2 antibodies.
Antibody Differentiation Immunoassay—Differentiates between HIV-1 and HIV-2 antibodies.	Negative	Identifies infection with HIV-1 or HIV-2.
Nucleic Acid Test—Confirmation test for HIV-1 if antigen/antibody combination immunoassay is positive but antibody differentiation immunoassay is nonreactive or inconclusive.		Positive HIV-1 indicates acute HIV-1 infection.
Immunoglobulin Assay or Electrophoresis—Antibodies are made up of immunoglobulins, of which there are five different classes.	See below.	See below.
• IgG	650–1600 (mg/dL)	Increased in all types of infections, liver disease, rheumatoid arthritis, multiple myeloma, and dermatological disorders. Decreased in agammaglobulinemia, lymphoid aplasia, and Bence-Jones proteinuria.
• IgM	50–300 (mg/dL)	Increased in malaria, infectious mononucleosis, SLE, and rheumatoid arthritis. Decreased in lymphoid aplasia and chronic lymphoblastic leukemia.
• IgA	40–350 (mg/dL)	Increased during exercise and obstructive jaundice. Decreased in familial inheritance, immunosuppressive therapy, and benzene exposure.
• IgE	Less than 160 units/L	Increased in allergic reactions and allergic infections.
• IgD	Less than 15 (mg/dL)	Decreased in agammaglobulinemia.
Radioallergosorbent Test (RAST)—Patient serum is mixed with a specific allergen, incubated with radiolabeled anti-IgE antibodies, and then the total amount of the specific IgE antibodies is measured.		A viable alternative to skin testing if the patient does not have multiple allergies.

Continued

Table 18.4
Laboratory Tests for the Immune System—cont'd

Test/Definition	Normal Value	Significance of Abnormal Findings
CD4 Count—CD4-helper T lymphocytes are counted.	*Percentage:* 28%–51% *Count:* 332–1642 cells/microL	Increased in allergy-proven patients. Decreased in patient with cancer, AIDS, and immunosuppression. Guides antiretroviral therapy.
CD8 Count—CD8-suppressor T lymphocytes are counted.	*Percentage:* 12%–38% *Count:* 170–811 cells/microL	Increased in viral infections. Decreased in SLE.

AIDS = acquired immune deficiency syndrome; HIV = human immunodeficiency virus; Ig = immunoglobulin; IU = international units; MCH = mean corpuscular hemoglobin; MCHC = mean corpuscular hemoglobin concentration; MCV = mean corpuscular volume; NSAIDs = nonsteroidal anti-inflammatory drugs; RDW = red blood cell distribution width; SLE = systemic lupus erythematosus.

Table 18.5
Diagnostic Procedures for the Immune System

Procedure	Definition/Normal Finding (if applicable)	Significance of Abnormal Findings	Nursing Management (if applicable)
Noninvasive			
Gene Testing	A sample of DNA, which can be taken as an oral or nasal swab, is examined and mapped for a variety of genetic disorders.	Abnormal findings may confirm a diagnosis or indicate patient may develop symptoms or pass on a disorder to children.	Identify patient support systems and need for counseling referral.
Invasive			
Biopsy (of a Specific Organ)	Biopsy tissue examined microscopically to confirm a diagnosis, determine a prognosis, or evaluate treatment. Specimen obtained through needle aspiration, incision, excision, or gavage, with or without endoscopy, fluoroscopy, stereotaxic, or needle localization.	Cancers, lymphomas, leukemias, and transplant rejections.	Ensure informed consent has been obtained. Monitor vital signs and site for bleeding, as organs are very vascular with a higher risk for bleeding after the biopsy.
Skin Testing	Done if immune system is intact. Testing is done for *Candida*, tetanus, tuberculosis (purified protein derivative [PPD] test), or specific allergens such as medications, food, or environmental factors.	If erythema (redness) or induration (firmness) occurs at the site within a prescribed time frame, test is positive. Indicates patient has been exposed to an organism, has an active infection, or has developed antibodies that stimulate an immune response.	Ask if patients have any allergies and the type of reaction or symptoms that occur.

THERAPEUTIC MEASURES FOR THE IMMUNE SYSTEM

Allergies

For patients with allergies, medical identification jewelry or other readily available identification is essential. Allergies must always be verified before giving any medications or foods. All allergies must be taken very seriously.

Food allergies create significant management problems. A food allergen can be contained within other food, such as baked goods. Food can be contaminated with an allergen from a previous batch of food made with the same equipment. Food allergies have become the most common cause of anaphylaxis in the community setting. Death from anaphylactic shock can result ("Nutrition Notes"). Occasionally, a food allergen may enter the body by inhalation or contact with skin or mucous membranes rather than eating.

Treatment for allergen exposure includes an epinephrine auto-injector (e.g., AUVI-Q, EpiPen) and antihistamines such as diphenhydramine (Benadryl). An epinephrine auto-injector must always be carried when exposure to known allergens is possible. It must be checked routinely for discoloration or cloudiness and a past-due expiration date, all of which require replacement. The patient should also be instructed to obtain emergency medical care immediately after using the epinephrine auto-injector because the effect is brief (less than 15 minutes) and relapse can occur (Mustafa, 2018).

> **Nutrition Notes**
>
> **Food Allergies**
> The Academy of Nutrition and Dietetics (2020) reports that more than 16 foods cause allergic reactions. The Food Allergen Labeling and Consumer Protection Act of 2004 requires food labeling for eight foods that are responsible for 90% of all food allergies: eggs, milk, fish, peanuts, tree nuts, crustacean shellfish, wheat, and soybeans (U.S. Food and Drug Administration, 2018). If a food allergy is suspected, an in-depth medical history and physical examination should be conducted, along with other testing (e.g., skin testing).
>
> Maternal diet should not be restricted during pregnancy or breastfeeding as an attempt at preventing the development of food allergies in infants. Infants should be fed peanut-containing foods after successful feeding of other foods at age 4 to 6 months per guidelines based on allergy risk to decrease peanut allergy development (McCarthy, 2020).

> **CUE RECOGNITION 18.2**
> A patient who has a peanut allergy reports a "lump" in his throat and difficulty swallowing while eating breakfast. What action do you take?
>
> *Suggested answers are at the end of the chapter.*

Immunotherapy

Allergen immunotherapy, such as subcutaneous immunotherapy (SCIT) and sublingual immunotherapy (SLIT), aims to desensitize a patient with anaphylactic reactions or chronic allergic symptoms. SCIT involves preparing an extract of the allergen and injecting small amounts of it as a vaccine. The concentration of the allergen in the vaccine is increased over time until the desired hyposensitivity is reached. Anaphylactic reactions can occur during treatment. The HCP and emergency equipment should be readily available if a reaction occurs. The patient and family should be taught how to respond if a reaction occurs after discharge.

SLIT is the use of tablets or drops containing specific allergen extracts. These are placed under the tongue and swallowed. Studies have shown SLIT to be effective in dust mite allergy–related asthma as well as in demonstrating long-lasting symptom control for certain allergens. SLIT has significantly lower anaphylactic event occurrence when compared with SCIT.

Medications

Medications are one of the primary treatment options for immune disorders. General medication categories used include antibiotics, antihistamines, antivirals, corticosteroids, decongestants, epinephrine, histamine (H_2) blockers, hormone therapy, immunosuppressants, interferon, leukotriene antagonists, and mast cell stabilizers (see Chapter 19).

Surgical Management

In some cases, splenectomy is needed to control symptoms of an immune disorder. A significant side effect of this surgery is the reduced ability of the immune system to fight infections.

Monoclonal Antibodies

Monoclonal antibodies can be produced against various antigens. A monoclonal antibody is made by cloning one specific antibody and then growing unlimited amounts of it in tissue cultures. These antibodies have many uses, such as therapy for transplant rejections and cancer.

Recombinant DNA Technology

Recombinant deoxyribonucleic acid (DNA) technology combines genes from one organism with genes from another. This therapy is used to replace an abnormal or missing gene with the goal of producing a normal gene. The normal gene can then be injected into a patient to cure a disorder if the patient's body then reproduces the normal genes. T-lymphocyte-directed gene transfer and injection of stem cells into abnormal areas to produce normal cells have been performed successfully. For more information, visit www.genome.gov or www.ncbi.nlm.nih.gov/guide.

Key Points

- Artificially acquired active immunity occurs as the result of a vaccine that stimulates production of antibodies and memory cells.
- The two mechanisms of immunity are cell-mediated immunity, which involves T cells, and humoral immunity, which involves mainly B cells but is assisted by T cells.
- Classes of immunoglobulin include IgG, IgA, IgM, IgD, and IgE. Each function differently in the body to contribute to the immune response.
- The efficiency of the immune system decreases with age. As such, older adults are more susceptible to infections and autoimmune disorders.
- Subjective data are collected regarding the patient's health history and current health. A family history is also obtained. Many allergic disorders, such as allergic rhinitis and asthma, and autoimmune disorders, such as ankylosing spondylitis, are thought either to be familial or to have a genetic predisposition in certain ethnic or cultural groups.
- Objective data collection begins by observing the patient's general appearance, facial expression, hearing, vision, posture, gait, skin, lymph node enlargement, and nailbeds. Rashes are examined for size, shape, location, texture, drainage, and pruritus.
- Education provided for patients undergoing diagnostic tests for the immune system includes the rationale for the test, preparation for the test, what to expect during the test, and care after the test. Informed consent is obtained for invasive procedures.
- General medication categories used to treat immune disorders include antibiotics, antihistamines, antivirals, corticosteroids, decongestants, epinephrine, histamine (H_2) blockers, hormone therapy, immunosuppressants, interferon, leukotriene antagonists, and mast cell stabilizers.

SUGGESTED ANSWERS TO CHAPTER EXERCISES

Cue Recognition
18.1: Check the central line insertion site for redness or swelling and notify the HCP immediately of findings. Prepare to obtain blood and urine for cultures as ordered to rule out infection.
18.2: Quickly identify if a food allergen has been consumed while calling for assistance. Immediately administer an injection of epinephrine as prescribed. Maintain airway. Notify HCP.

Critical Thinking & Clinical Judgment
Mrs. Sims
1. Review the patient's history and allergies to prevent complications. Explain the procedure and allow the patient to ask questions or verbalize concerns.
2. Follow the agency's latex allergy protocol, enter this data into the patient's medical record, notify surgery scheduling so latex precaution protocols can be planned for surgery, and ensure that the patient's HCP is informed.
3. Following the agency's protocol, wear nonlatex gloves and use nonlatex equipment to draw the specimens.
4. HCP, anesthesia provider, surgical team, dietitian.

Additional Resources

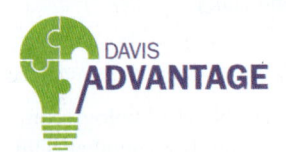

Go to Davis Advantage to complete your learning: strengthen understanding, apply your knowledge, and prepare for the Next Gen NCLEX®.

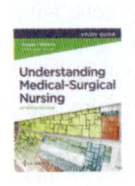

A Study Guide is also available.

CHAPTER 19
Nursing Care of Patients With Immune Disorders

Kristy Gorman

KEY TERMS

anaphylaxis (AN-uh-fih-LAK-sis)
angioedema (AN-gee-oh-eh-DEE-mah)
ankylosing spondylitis (ANG-kih-LOH-sing SPON-da-LY-tis)
histamine (HISS-tah-mean)
urticaria (UR-tih-CARE-ee-ah)

CHAPTER CONCEPTS

Caring
Clinical judgment
Collaboration
Immunity
Teaching and learning

LEARNING OUTCOMES

1. Explain the immunological mechanism for the four types of hypersensitivities.
2. Explain the pathophysiology of disorders of the immune system.
3. Identify the etiologies, signs, and symptoms of immune system disorders.
4. Plan nursing care for patients undergoing tests for immune system disorders.
5. Describe current medical treatment for immune system disorders.
6. List data collected when caring for patients with disorders of the immune system.
7. Explain factors that alter or influence the self-recognition portion of the immune system.
8. Plan nursing care for patients with disorders of the immune system.
9. Evaluate effectiveness of nursing interventions for disorders of the immune system.

Disorders of the immune system can be divided into three categories: hypersensitivity reactions (e.g., anaphylaxis), autoimmune disorders (e.g., systemic lupus erythematosus), and immune deficiencies (e.g., AIDS; see Chapter 20).

HYPERSENSITIVITY REACTIONS

The immune system is an adaptive system that protects the body. However, sometimes this system can cause injury to the body because of its exaggerated response, known as a hypersensitivity reaction. In 1963, Gell and Coombs developed a system of classifying hypersensitivity reactions as types I, II, III, and IV, according to the way the tissue is injured.

Type I Hypersensitivity Reactions

Type I hypersensitivity reactions involve the release of **histamine** and other mediators from mast cells and basophils. The reaction may lead to urticaria, eczema, angioedema, conjunctivitis, allergic rhinitis, asthma, gastroenteritis, and anaphylaxis. Symptoms may range from mild to severe and life threatening. An anaphylactic reaction is an immediate reaction that occurs on exposure to a specific antigen after a prior exposure (sensitization; Fig. 19.1). During the initial exposure, the immune system overreacts to the antigen and makes immunoglobulin E (IgE)

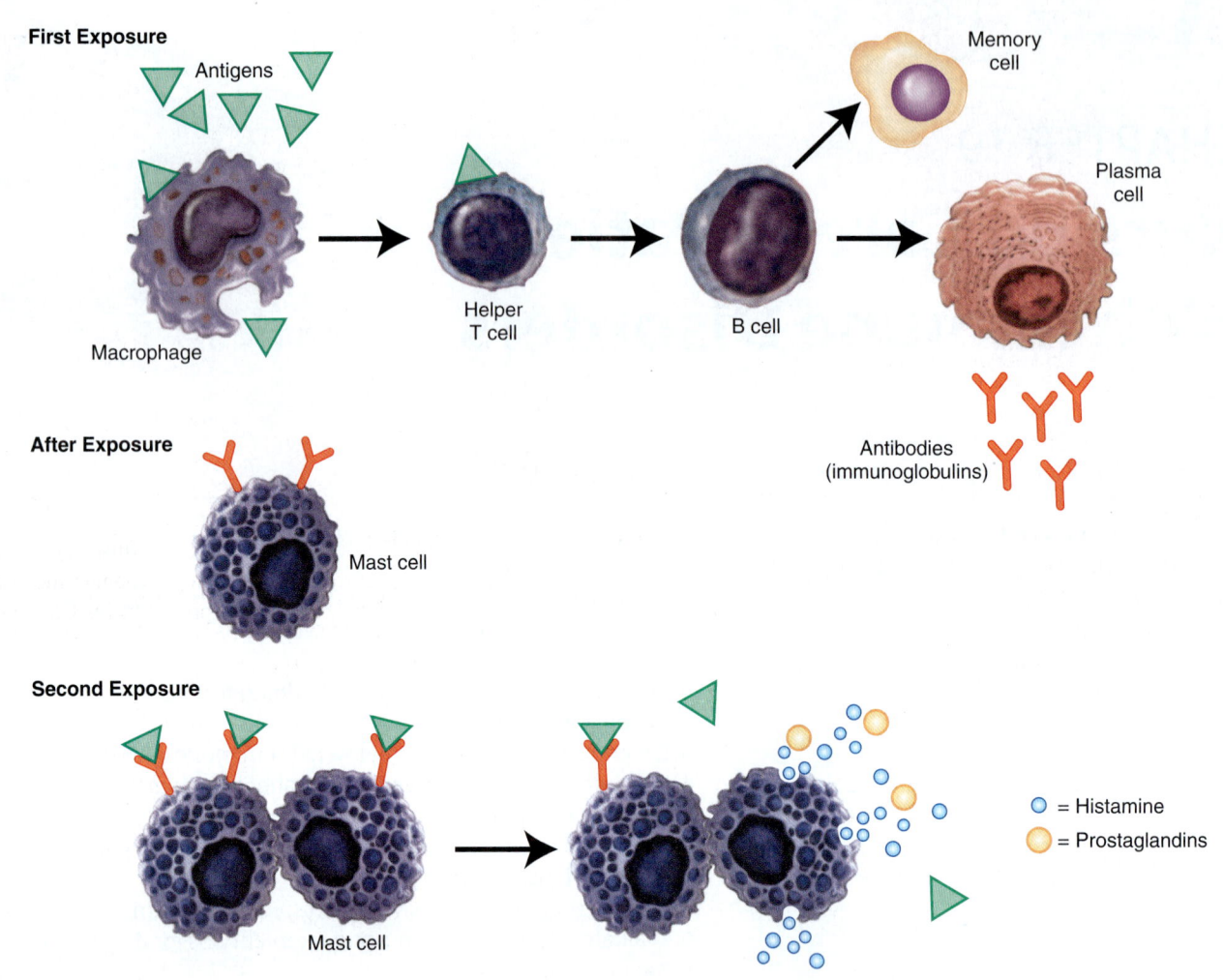

FIGURE 19.1 Type I hypersensitivity.

antibodies that attach to mast cells throughout the body. When a subsequent exposure occurs, the antigen causes IgE to trigger mast cells to release their contents. When histamine is released, vasodilatation, bronchoconstriction, mucus secretion, and vascular permeability occur. If the exposure is localized, the reaction is mild and remains local. However, if the exposure is systemic, the reaction is massive and widespread.

Allergic Rhinitis

Allergic rhinitis is the most common form of allergy. When symptoms occur throughout the year, it is called *perennial allergic rhinitis*. If the symptoms occur seasonally, it is called *hay fever*. The causative antigens are environmental and airborne.

PATHOPHYSIOLOGY. Allergic rhinitis is the result of an antigen–antibody reaction. Ciliary action decreases and mucous secretions increase. Vasodilation and local tissue edema occur.

SIGNS AND SYMPTOMS. Signs and symptoms vary in intensity. They include sneezing, nasal itching, profuse watery rhinorrhea (runny nose), and itchy red eyes. The nasal mucosa is pale, cyanotic, and edematous. Frequently there are dark circles under the eyes, called *allergic shiners*, caused by venous congestion in the maxillary sinuses.

COMPLICATIONS. Sinusitis, nasal polyps, asthma, and chronic bronchitis can occur with repeated episodes of allergic rhinitis.

DIAGNOSTIC TESTS. Skin testing may be performed to identify the specific offending allergens to allow avoidance of the allergen. However, skin testing does not always identify the allergen. The in-vitro allergy test, or radioallergosorbent test (RAST), which identifies IgE antibodies, is an alternative to skin testing for some patients.

THERAPEUTIC MEASURES. Initial treatment involves eliminating the offending environmental stimuli. Antihistamines and nasal decongestants may be prescribed to relieve symptoms. If the symptoms are severe, corticosteroids may also be given via inhalation or nasal spray. Nasal corticosteroids should be used cautiously in the older adult because these medications can be drying to the nares. Intranasal saline irrigation can be an inexpensive and effective way to reduce nasal congestion.

Rhinophototherapy uses bilateral intranasal light waves to reduce the hyperimmune response seen in this disorder. The treatment is usually done three times a week for 3 weeks and relieves symptoms such as sneezing, itching, and runny nose.

Immunotherapy, known as allergy shots, is reserved for patients with severe or debilitating symptoms (see Chapter 18).

This therapy continues until the patient no longer has symptoms when exposed to the environmental antigen.

Atopic Dermatitis (Eczema)

Atopic dermatitis, often called *eczema*, is a familial, chronic inflammatory skin response.

PATHOPHYSIOLOGY. Two theories exist regarding the pathophysiology of atopic dermatitis. One theory suggests the allergic response is mediated by IgE antibodies, because it is commonly found in patients with allergic rhinitis or allergic asthma. Another theory suggests atopic dermatitis is a defect in epithelial cells that damages the skin's protective barrier.

SIGNS AND SYMPTOMS. Initially, the patient experiences pruritus, edema, and extremely dry skin. This is followed by red, weeping lesions that break open, crust over, and scale off. The skin eventually thickens in the affected areas (lichenification).

DIAGNOSTIC TESTS. A diagnosis of atopic dermatitis is based on clinical examination and exclusion of other diseases with similar symptoms. Serum IgE levels will be elevated in patients with atopic dermatitis and tend to correlate with the severity of the disease. If an infection is present, culture and sensitivity tests may be ordered to determine the infecting organism and treatment.

THERAPEUTIC MEASURES. The focus of treatment for eczema is to reduce the itchy, dry, inflamed skin. Antipruritics (cortisone, antihistamines) are vital in reducing the itch-scratch cycle that predisposes the patient to skin infections. Diluted household bleach in lukewarm water baths, up to three times weekly, can kill bacteria on the skin to prevent infection, which also contributes to itching. Cool soaks can also relieve itching. The use of soaps for sensitive skin and oatmeal bath products helps prevent dryness (see "Home Health Hints"). Fragrance-free moisturizers, emollients (baby oil, petroleum jelly), or oil-in-water lubricants should be applied after baths to prevent further dryness Topical corticosteroids or topical calcineurin inhibitors such as tacrolimus (Prograf) and pimecrolimus (Elidel), if corticosteroids are not effective, are used to reduce the inflammatory response. If skin lesions become infected, topical or systemic antibiotics can be prescribed. For long-term prevention of symptoms, it is important to identify and eliminate hypersensitivity triggers while controlling environmental temperature and humidity to prevent extreme skin dryness.

Anaphylaxis

Anaphylaxis is a severe systemic type I hypersensitivity reaction. Some causes of anaphylaxis are antibiotics such as cephalosporins, penicillin, and sulfonamides; anticonvulsants such as phenytoin (Dilantin); NSAIDs such as aspirin; foods such as eggs, nuts, shellfish, and wheat; latex rubber; food additives such as monosodium glutamate (MSG) and bisulfites; and venom from insect bites or stings.

PATHOPHYSIOLOGY. IgE antibodies produced from previous antigen sensitization are attached to mast cells throughout the body. With this hypersensitivity reaction, an antigen is introduced at a systemic level. This causes widespread release of histamine and other chemical mediators contained within the mast cells. The most profound complications of an anaphylactic reaction are respiratory and cardiac arrest. Immediate treatment is needed to prevent death.

SIGNS AND SYMPTOMS. Anaphylaxis produces sudden and life-threatening signs and symptoms (Table 19.1). Generalized smooth muscle spasms occur, causing bronchial narrowing and creating stridor, wheezing, dyspnea, and laryngeal edema, which can lead to respiratory arrest. Cramping, diarrhea, nausea, and vomiting also result from these spasms. Capillary permeability increases, allowing fluid to shift from the blood vessels to the interstitium. This causes hypotension, tachycardia, and an increase in respiratory symptoms. While the blood volume in the blood vessels decreases from fluid shifting, the vessels are dilating, resulting in a further decrease in circulating blood volume. The dilation also causes diffuse erythema (redness) and warmth of the skin. Neurologic changes include apprehension, drowsiness, headache, profound restlessness, and possible seizures.

DIAGNOSTIC TESTS. The patient's history, signs, and symptoms establish the diagnosis. Arterial blood gases may reveal hypoxemia, hypercarbia, and acidosis. Electrocardiogram (ECG) monitoring may show cardiac arrhythmias. After the patient's recovery, allergen testing may be considered for future prevention.

THERAPEUTIC MEASURES. Epinephrine is given IM immediately. IV access is a priority for administration of vasopressor drugs and fluids to increase blood pressure. Oxygen therapy is started. If respiratory symptoms are severe, a tracheostomy or endotracheal intubation may be needed, with mechanical ventilation. Antihistamines and corticosteroids may also be given.

CRITICAL THINKING & CLINICAL JUDGMENT

Mrs. Barnes, a 32-year-old woman, was brought into the emergency department after having been stung multiple times by bees while gardening. She has numerous red welts over her body that she says are itchy. She is very anxious. Her temperature is 99.2°F (37.22°C), blood pressure is 102/58 mm Hg, pulse is 102 bpm, and respiratory rate is 26 breaths per minute.

Critical Thinking (The Why)

1. What might be the cause of Mrs. Barnes's symptoms?

Clinical Judgment (The Do)

2. What additional data do you collect?
3. What actions do you take to care for Mrs. Barnes?
4. What are you most vigilant about monitoring?
5. With which members of the health-care team do you collaborate?

Suggested answers are at the end of the chapter.

• WORD • BUILDING •

anaphylaxis: ana—up + phylaxis—protection

Table 19.1 Anaphylaxis Summary

Signs and Symptoms	Generalized smooth-muscle spasms: • Bronchial narrowing, leading to stridor, wheezing, dyspnea, laryngeal edema • Abdominal cramping and diarrhea • Nausea and vomiting Increased capillary permeability (allowing fluid to shift from blood vessels to the interstitium): • Hypotension • Tachycardia • Increased respiratory symptoms Dilation of blood vessels: • Further decreasing circulating volume • Diffuse erythema (redness) • Increased skin temperature Apprehension Drowsiness Profound restlessness Headache Possible seizures
Diagnostic Tests	Testing to guide treatment: • Arterial blood gases • Electrocardiogram monitoring History and physical examination After recovery, allergen testing for prevention
Therapeutic Measures	Oxygen IV access Epinephrine IM Vasopressor drugs IV (dopamine) Antihistamines (oral, IV, injection) Corticosteroids (oral, IV, injection) If severe respiratory compromise: • Tracheostomy or endotracheal intubation • Mechanical ventilation
Complications	Respiratory and cardiac arrest
Priority Nursing Diagnoses	*Impaired Gas Exchange* *Anxiety*

Urticaria

Urticaria (hives) is a type I hypersensitivity reaction. The causes of urticaria are numerous. In addition to various medicines and foods, chemicals, cold, and stress can also cause urticaria. Many patients with chronic conditions, such as systemic lupus erythematosus, lymphoma, hyperthyroidism, or cancer, are susceptible to urticaria.

PATHOPHYSIOLOGY. Urticaria is triggered by the antigen-stimulated reaction of IgE antibodies, which causes the release of mast cell contents, especially histamine.

SIGNS AND SYMPTOMS. The lesions of urticaria are raised, pruritic, nontender, and erythematous wheals on the skin. They tend to be concentrated on the trunk of the body and proximal extremities.

DIAGNOSTIC TESTS. Diagnosis is based on physical examination and history.

THERAPEUTIC MEASURES. Treatment depends on the degree of symptoms. In the most severe cases, epinephrine may be given to quickly resolve the urticaria. Corticosteroids may be given orally, topically, or via IV to reduce inflammation. Antihistamines and histamine (H_2) blockers are given to block the release of histamine. The use of corticosteroids and antihistamines together resolves the reaction more quickly. Patients suffering with the chronic form of urticaria might require IgE monoclonal antibody therapy, such as omalizumab (Xolair). Studies have found that acupuncture as an adjunctive measure may relieve symptoms (Qin et al, 2020; Shi et al, 2019).

Angioedema

Angioedema is a type I hypersensitivity reaction. There are several types of angioedema with varying causes. The most common type occurs from an allergic reaction while other types occur from angiotensin-converting enzyme (ACE) inhibitors or an unknown cause (idiopathic). In addition, there are hereditary (HAE; rare) or acquired (AAE; rarer) forms with subtypes caused by C1 esterase inhibitor (C1-INH; blood protein) deficiency or dysfunction. Triggers for HAE include anxiety, infection, physical stimuli (e.g., cold, physical activity, surgery), or trauma. Visit the U.S. Hereditary Angioedema Association (www.haea.org).

PATHOPHYSIOLOGY. Angioedema (swelling) results from temporary vascular permeability that occurs within the submucosal and subcutaneous layers.

SIGNS AND SYMPTOMS. Localized swelling of the skin, mucosa, or submucosa occurs. Angioedema can happen with or without urticaria (hives). Depending on the type of angioedema, it can affect any part of the body or primarily the face, eyes, and lips. Depending on the location and extensiveness of the edema, these eruptions are usually nonpruritic and painless. However, it can be life threatening if the upper airway is involved. It is always an emergency, and medical care must be sought if obstruction of the airway is developing.

• WORD • BUILDING •

angioedema: angeion—vessel + oidema—swelling

DIAGNOSTIC TESTS. A comprehensive history and physical examination confirm the diagnosis. Skin testing can determine if there is a specific causative antigen.

THERAPEUTIC MEASURES. The most basic treatment involves avoiding the antigen or allergen desensitization. Cinryze, a C1-INH, is for routine prophylaxis against angioedema attacks. Acute symptoms may be relieved with antihistamines, corticosteroids, or other medications. Berinert, also a C1-INH, treats angioedema of the abdomen, face, or throat. Haegarda is a human plasma–derived, concentrate prepared from donors. Ecallantide (Kalbitor), a plasma kallikrein inhibitor, and icatibant (Firazyr), a selective bradykinin B2 receptor antagonist, help control symptoms. Infusion of fresh frozen plasma reverses the angioedema symptoms associated with ACE inhibitor–induced angioedema, which tends to resist standard treatments. Androgens, antifibrinolytics, and immunosuppressive therapy are useful in the long-term treatment of some acquired types of angioedema.

Nursing Process for the Patient With a Type I Hypersensitivity Disorder

DATA COLLECTION. Gather data about the patient's signs and symptoms. Immediately report to the health-care provider (HCP) any sudden dyspnea, anxiety, restlessness, or chest or back pain. Identify allergies and reactions. Observe the patient's skin and take photos to document lesions or rashes. Include signs of infection, such as redness, warmth, and drainage. Identify the patient's knowledge of the disease process, causes, treatment plan, and self-care to develop an educational plan.

NURSING DIAGNOSES, PLANNING, AND IMPLEMENTATION

Impaired Gas Exchange related to laryngeal edema

EXPECTED OUTCOME: The patient will maintain clear lung fields and remain free of signs of respiratory distress at all times.

- Monitor respiratory rate, depth, use of accessory muscles, nasal flaring, abdominal breathing, restlessness, changes in mentation, level of consciousness, changes in voice, or dysphagia *to identify respiratory problems for early intervention.*
- Position the patient in a high-Fowler or semi-Fowler position *to improve ventilation and decrease upper airway edema.*

Anxiety related to dyspnea or pruritus

EXPECTED OUTCOME: The patient will state that anxiety is controlled.

- Stay with the patient and speak calmly *to reduce anxiety or frustration.*
- Encourage patient to visualize absence of anxiety, itching, or dyspnea *to decrease anxiety.*

Deficient Knowledge related to lack of knowledge of condition, prevention, and treatment regimen

EXPECTED OUTCOME: The patient or caregiver will state understanding and follow the mutually agreed-on plan of care.

- Identify the patient's knowledge of the disease and barriers to implementing the plan of care *to develop an education plan.*
- Explain to the patient the benefit of using medical identification for allergies *so prompt medical attention can be given if the patient is unable to give this information.*
- Reinforce education on methods to avoid allergens, such as wearing a mask when mowing the lawn or working outdoors, having heating ducts cleaned, covering heat registers with filters, and frequent home vacuuming and dusting, *to promote an understanding of preventive methods and prevent allergen exposure and anaphylaxis.*
- Reinforce education to obtain an epinephrine auto-injector and how to use it to provide *prompt treatment if the antigen is environmental* (e.g., food or insect sting).
- For atopic dermatitis, reinforce education on signs and symptoms of infection, use of humidification during the winter months *to prevent dryness*, wearing cotton clothing *to minimize irritation*, and cool soaks *to decrease pruritus.*
- For urticaria, reinforce education for stress management and relaxation techniques *to relieve urticaria* and to follow therapeutic regimen, including prescribed medications and their correct usage, *to reduce symptoms.*

Risk for Impaired Skin Integrity related to effects of allergic reaction

See "Nursing Care Plan for the Patient With Contact Dermatitis."

EVALUATION. If interventions have been effective, there will be no signs of respiratory distress, and lung fields will be clear. The patient's facial expressions, gestures, and posture will reflect no anxiety. The skin will remain intact. If there are lesions, they will be smaller and healing. The patient will express knowledge of the disorder and the treatment plan.

> **CUE RECOGNITION 19.1**
> A patient with a diagnosis of angioedema states that her throat is feeling tingly. What action do you take?
> *Suggested answers are at the end of the chapter.*

Type II Hypersensitivity Reactions

A type II hypersensitivity reaction involves the destruction of a cell or substance that has an antigen attached to its cell membrane, which has been sensed by either immunoglobulin G (IgG) or immunoglobulin M (IgM) as being a foreign antigen (Fig. 19.2). When an antigen is sensed as foreign, an antibody attaches to the antigen on the cell membrane, causing lysis of the cell or accelerated phagocytosis

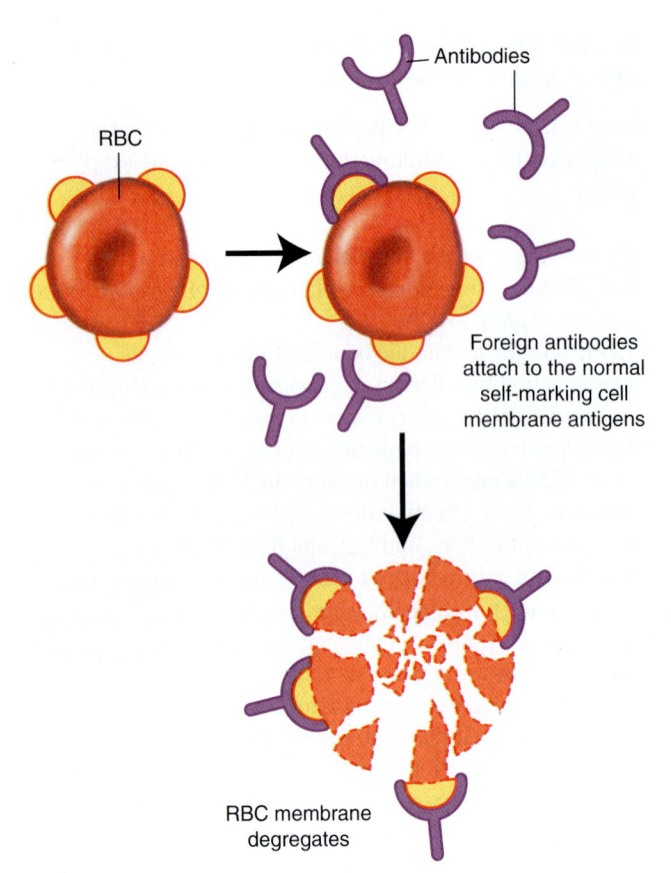

FIGURE 19.2 Type II hypersensitivity.

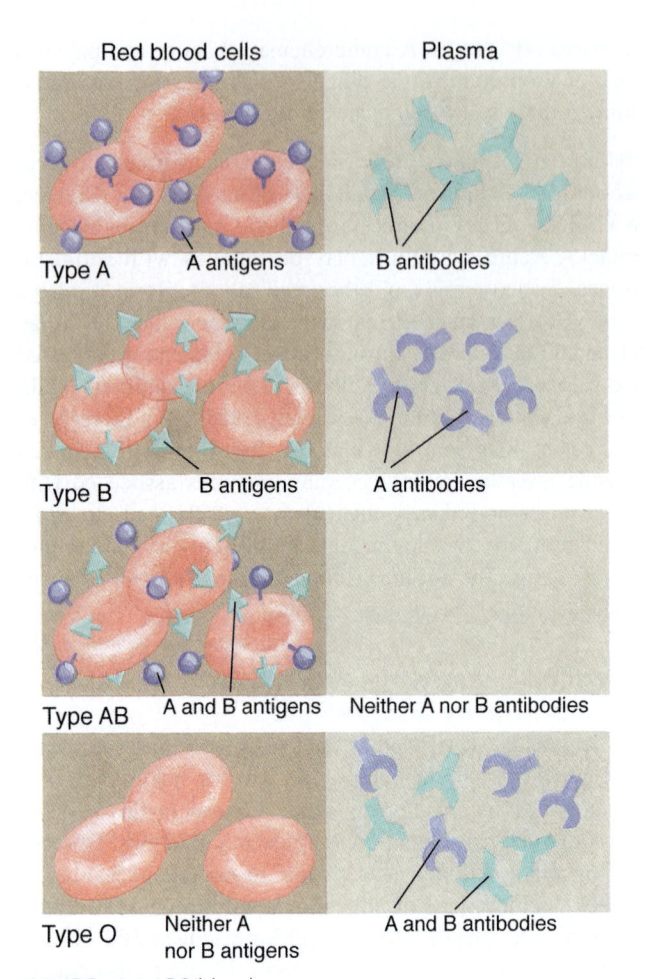

FIGURE 19.3 ABO blood types.

(engulfing and ingestion). When a cell is foreign, such as a bacterium, this process is beneficial. However, if the antigen on the surface of a red blood cell (RBC) is sensed as foreign because it is from a different ABO blood type, then the RBC is destroyed.

Hemolytic Transfusion Reaction

PATHOPHYSIOLOGY. A hemolytic transfusion reaction is a rare type II hypersensitivity reaction that can be due to ABO or Rh incompatibility. ABO and Rh [Rhesus] are human blood group systems. The antigens found on RBCs may be ABO or Rh incompatible. If they are, the recipient's antibodies attach to the foreign antigens on the transfused RBCs surface, causing rapid lysis (destruction) of the RBC. The rapid RBC lysis results in a massive amount of cellular debris that blocks blood vessels throughout the body. This leads to ischemia and necrosis of tissue and organs. It can be life threatening.

ETIOLOGY. The ABO blood group system types are A, B, AB, and O (Fig. 19.3). The donor's and recipient's ABO and Rh blood types must be matched for compatibility for a transfusion. Antibodies are continually made naturally for A or B antigens that a person does not have. People with blood type O are *universal donors* because they do not have A or B antigens to be sensed as foreign by the recipient's anti-A or anti-B antibodies. Consequently, they themselves can receive only type O blood because a donor's A or B antigen would be recognized as foreign and attacked. People with type AB blood are *universal recipients* because they do not make anti-A or anti-B antibodies. Those with blood types other than AB cannot receive AB blood because they have either A or B antibodies that would attack the A or B antigens. Antibodies may form for other types of RBC antigens due to prior sensitization, most often from previous blood transfusion or pregnancy.

Rh antigens are present on the RBC surface in people who are Rh$^+$. A person who is Rh$^+$ typically has the D antigen, which is the strongest antigen of the 50 possible antigens. A person who is Rh$^-$ does not have the D antigen. Rh anti-D antibodies are present in those who are Rh$^-$ only after a sensitizing event. Those who are Rh$^+$ can receive Rh$^-$ blood. Those who are Rh$^-$ cannot receive Rh$^+$ blood. When maternal and fetal Rh antigens are different, the mother becomes sensitized by the fetal Rh type and develops antibodies that can affect future fetuses. For example, an Rh$_0$(D)-negative pregnant woman becomes sensitized by an Rh$_0$(D)-positive fetus. As a result, the blood cells of future Rh$_0$(D)-positive fetuses can be destroyed by maternal anti-Rh$_0$(D) antibodies crossing the placenta.

SIGNS AND SYMPTOMS. See Table 19.2 for signs and symptoms of a hemolytic transfusion.

Table 19.2
Hemolytic Transfusion Reaction Summary

Signs and Symptoms	Low back or chest pain Hypotension Fever rising more than 1.8°F (1°C) Chills Tachycardia Tachypnea, wheezing, dyspnea Urticaria Anxiety Headache Nausea
Diagnostic Tests	Direct Coombs test
Therapeutic Measures	Depends on severity of reaction and organs affected Antihistamines Corticosteroids Epinephrine Diuretics, to assist kidneys
Complications	If severe: shock, acute kidney injury
Priority Nursing Diagnosis	*Risk for Injury*

DIAGNOSTIC TESTS. The direct Coombs test confirms the reaction. In the laboratory, a small amount of the patient's RBCs is washed to remove any unattached antibodies. Antihuman globulin is added to see if agglutination (clumping) of the RBCs results. If agglutination occurs, an immune reaction, such as a hemolytic transfusion reaction, is taking place.

THERAPEUTIC MEASURES. If a reaction occurs, medications are given to treat the reaction and symptoms (Table 19.3).

To prevent production of anti-$Rh_0(D)$ antibodies, an $Rh_0(D)$ immune globulin (RhoGAM) injection is given to $Rh_0(D)$-negative patients who were accidentally given $Rh_0(D)$-positive blood or exposed to $Rh_0(D)$-positive fetal blood by delivery, miscarriage, abortion, amniocentesis, or intra-abdominal trauma. When antibodies do not form, a hemolytic reaction can be prevented.

NURSING CARE AND EDUCATION. Prevention of hemolytic reactions is crucial. Following strict institutional guidelines for blood transfusion administration helps ensure the patient's safety. After blood is released from the hospital blood bank, two nurses, designated per institutional policy, double-check specified data. At the bedside, transfusion guidelines include double-checking the patient's name and identification number in the medical record, unit of blood, and patient's identification bracelet as well as checking the patient's blood type in the medical record, on the unit of blood, and on the paperwork with the unit of blood.

Follow agency policy for vital sign monitoring during a blood transfusion. Minimally, vital signs are taken before the start of the blood transfusion, 15 minutes into the transfusion, and when the transfusion is completed. It takes only a small amount of blood to trigger a hemolytic transfusion reaction, so it is critical to stay with the patient at the bedside during the first 15 minutes of any blood transfusion.

If symptoms of a reaction are noted, the blood transfusion is immediately stopped. Follow the agency policy for a suspected transfusion reaction. Start a normal saline infusion with new tubing to keep the vein patent. Immediately notify the HCP and blood bank of the patient's symptoms. Stay with the patient for reassurance and monitoring of symptoms and vital signs. Return the unused blood and blood tubing to the blood bank for testing. A series of blood and urine specimens will be collected and sent to the laboratory for analysis. Follow the HCP's orders to treat the patient's symptoms.

Encourage the patient if having future elective surgery to discuss autologous (self-) blood donation options with the HCP to avoid another transfusion reaction. Explain to the patient the importance of informing future HCPs about the hemolytic transfusion reaction so specific blood tests are performed for less common antibodies if blood typing occurs again.

> **PRACTICE ANALYSIS TIP**
> **Linking NCLEX-PN® to Practice**
> The LPN/LVN will:
> - Verify the identity of client.
> - Use precautions to prevent injury and/or complications associated with a procedure or diagnosis.

> **BE SAFE!**
> ***AVOID FAILURE TO RECOGNIZE!*** Every unit of blood, even of the same blood type, is unique and can trigger a blood transfusion reaction. Careful monitoring with every transfusion is necessary.

Type III Hypersensitivity Reactions

A type III hypersensitivity reaction involves immune complexes formed by antigens and antibodies, usually of the IgG type (Fig. 19.4). The patient is sensitized with an initial exposure to the antigen, and a reaction occurs with a later exposure. The reaction is localized and evolves over several hours. Symptoms range from a red, edematous skin lesion to hemorrhage and necrosis. The process involves formation of antigen–antibody complexes in the blood vessels as the antigen is absorbed through the vessel wall. Neutrophils are attracted to the area and release enzymes that ultimately lead to blood vessel damage.

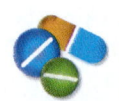

Table 19.3
Medications Used in Hemolytic Transfusion Reactions

Medication Class/Action

Antihistamines
Block histamine at histamine$_1$ receptors, thereby preventing or reversing the effects of histamine (capillary permeability, itching, and bronchospasms).

Examples
diphenhydramine (Benadryl)

Nursing Implications
Teach:
- Take with or without food.
- Avoid alcohol, central nervous system depressants, and over-the-counter antihistamines.
- Avoid prolonged exposure to sunlight.
- Use caution with activities requiring mental alertness.

Corticosteroids
Hormones with marked anti-inflammatory effects due to inhibition of prostaglandin synthesis and accumulation of macrophages and leukocytes at site.

Examples
dexamethasone (Decadron)
hydrocortisone (Solu-Cortef)
methylprednisolone (Solu-Medrol)
prednisolone (Delta-Cortef)
prednisone (Deltasone)

Nursing Implications
Teach:
- Take orally with food.
- ***Never*** stop taking suddenly.

Monitor:
- Weight
- Edema, shortness of breath, jugular vein distention for heart failure development
- Blood glucose level
- Gastrointestinal bleeding

Sympathomimetics
Marked stimulation of alpha, beta$_1$, and beta$_2$ receptors, causing vasoconstriction, bronchodilation, and cardiac stimulation.

Examples
epinephrine (Adrenalin, EpiPen)

Nursing Implications
Educate patient to avoid exposing drug to heat or light.

Serum Sickness

Serum sickness is a rare type III immune-mediated hypersensitivity reaction in which antigen–antibody complexes form due to exposure to nonhuman proteins. This exposure to nonhuman antigens is typically through medications such as antivenoms, rabies vaccinations, and immune modulating agents (rituximab). The complexes lodge in small vessels, leading to inflammation, tissue damage, and necrosis. Signs and symptoms can occur 7 days to 3 weeks after antigen exposure once antibodies have formed. Arthralgia, edema, fever, lymphadenopathy, muscle soreness, nausea, rash, and urticaria may occur. Leukocytosis or leukopenia may occur. Sedimentation rate and C-reactive protein elevate due to inflammation. IgG and IgM increase substantially, while the complement assay decreases as it is tied up in the complexes.

Once the exposure to the antigen ends or is reduced, serum sickness is self-limiting within about 10 days. It has an excellent prognosis. The treatment focuses on symptoms. Antipyretics may be given for fever, and analgesics and anti-inflammatories for arthralgia. For more severe symptoms, antihistamines and corticosteroids may be given. Collect data to identify a causative agent. Inform the patient about the agent so it can be avoided and discussed with the HCP. Provide supportive care for symptoms, including pain management, as ordered. Document patient response to prescribed medications and the treatment plan.

Type IV Hypersensitivity Reactions

A type IV hypersensitivity reaction, also called a *delayed* reaction, occurs when a sensitized T lymphocyte comes in contact with the particular antigen to which it is sensitized (Fig. 19.5). The resulting necrosis is caused by the actions of macrophages and the various T lymphocytes involved in the cell-mediated immune response.

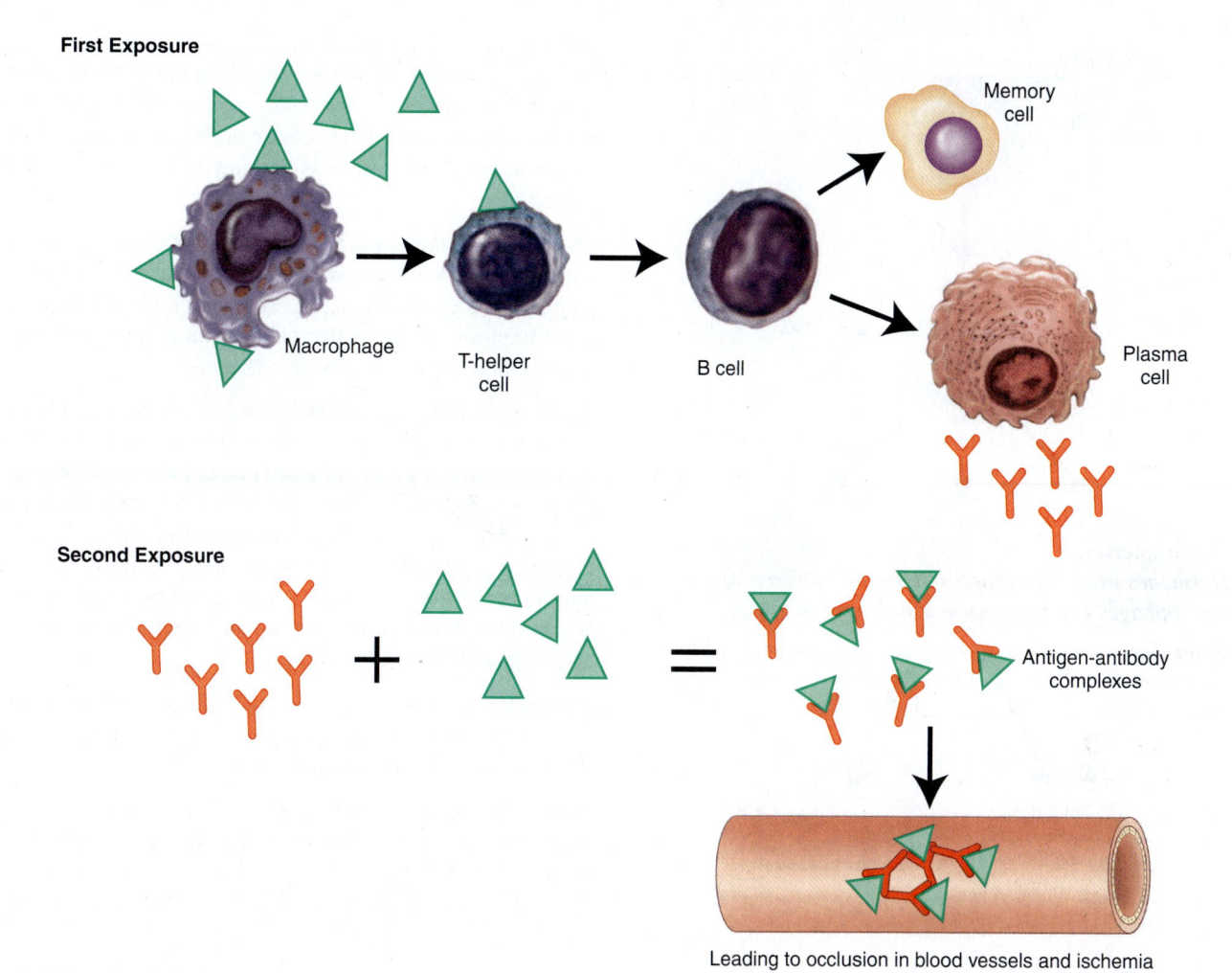

FIGURE 19.4 Type III hypersensitivity.

Contact Dermatitis

PATHOPHYSIOLOGY. When a substance or chemical comes in contact with the skin, it is absorbed and binds with special skin proteins called *haptens*. With the first contact, there is no reaction or symptoms, but within 7 to 10 days, T memory cells are formed. On subsequent exposures, the T memory cells quickly become activated T cells, which secrete chemicals that may cause symptoms.

ETIOLOGY. Poison ivy and poison oak are the most common irritants that cause this reaction. Latex, which is produced from rubber trees, may cause contact dermatitis and can also trigger a type I anaphylactic reaction. Anaphylactic reactions to latex can be fatal. A latex allergy is a serious concern for those who work in health care due to regular exposure to latex in the health-care setting. Implementation of standard precautions and the use of latex gloves began in 1987, resulting in increased exposure to latex. Latex-free gloves are available. For patients who are allergic to latex, special protocols are followed using latex-free gloves and equipment. Those who are allergic to latex can also be allergic to fruits and vegetables such as avocado, bananas, kiwi, and tomatoes. For more information on latex allergies, visit the American Academy of Allergy, Asthma, and Immunology at www.aaaai.org.

SIGNS AND SYMPTOMS. Within a few hours of exposure, the area of contact becomes red and pruritic, with fragile vesicles. Secondary infections may develop. (See "Atopic Dermatitis (Eczema).")

DIAGNOSTIC TESTS. Diagnosis is made through skin and lesion observation and patient history. Biopsy, culture, and patch testing of the skin may also be done.

THERAPEUTIC MEASURES. Oral or topical antihistamines and topical drying agents can be used to control skin symptoms. Topical corticosteroids may be used and are most effective if sparingly applied after a bath or shower. If symptoms are severe, systemic corticosteroids or topical immunomodulators, such as tacrolimus (Protopic) or pimecrolimus (Elidel), may be prescribed.

Special protocols are used for patients who are allergic to latex. Agencies may prepare special latex-free kits containing common supplies nurses use to care for patients. Ensure that latex allergy protocols are followed when a patient has a latex allergy to prevent development of life-threatening

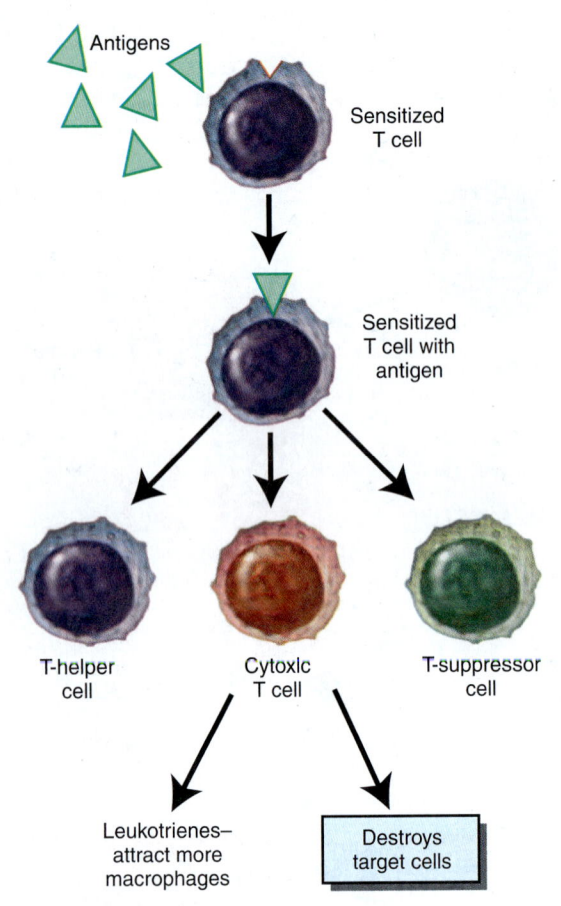

FIGURE 19.5 Type IV hypersensitivity.

anaphylaxis (see "Home Health Hints" at the end of the chapter).

> **NURSING CARE TIP**
> One of the causes of anaphylactic shock is a latex allergy reaction. Latex-free products limit latex exposure to reduce development of latex allergies.

NURSING PROCESS FOR THE PATIENT WITH CONTACT DERMATITIS

Data Collection. Observe symptoms and identify the causative agent. Determining patient understanding of the cause is important to prevent a recurrence of the condition. Ask if patient has medical alert identification for allergies.

Nursing Diagnoses, Planning, and Implementation. See "Nursing Care Plan for the Patient With Contact Dermatitis."

Transplant Rejection

PATHOPHYSIOLOGY AND ETIOLOGY. Transplanted living tissue is sensed as being foreign to the immune system. Therefore, lifelong immunosuppression is required to prevent transplant rejection, which can occur at any time. Lymphocytes become sensitized during an induction phase immediately after the tissue is transplanted. If immunosuppression is not effective, the sensitized lymphocytes invade the transplanted tissue and destroy it via the release of chemicals and macrophage activity. This results in varying degrees of transplant rejection.

SIGNS AND SYMPTOMS. Various signs and symptoms occur depending on the transplanted tissue or organ that is involved along with the severity of the rejection (Table 19.4). Signs and symptoms are reflective of the failing organ or tissue, such as heart failure for a rejected heart.

COMPLICATIONS. The rejected tissue or organ may be damaged from immunological reactions. It then may not function at full capacity. A total failure and loss of the transplanted tissue or organ can occur. The greatest cause of death following a transplant is infection. Immunosuppression therapy, which is needed to prevent tissue rejection after the transplant, is a major contributory factor for severe infection development. Because the immune system is suppressed, it may be unable to effectively fight an infection.

DIAGNOSTIC TESTS. Arteriography, biopsy, blood tests, scans, and ultrasonography are tests that may be performed to aid in diagnosing a transplant rejection.

THERAPEUTIC MEASURES. Depending on the type of transplant, the body's immunological system is prepared before surgery with medications, transfusions, or radiation to minimize the risk of rejection. After the transplant, lifelong

Table 19.4
Transplant Rejection Summary

Signs and Symptoms	Dependent on involved transplanted tissue or organ and degree of failure
Diagnostic Tests	Arteriography Biopsy Blood tests Scans Ultrasonography
Therapeutic Measures	Preventive preoperative preparation with medications, transfusions, or radiation to minimize the risk of rejection
Complications	Total failure and loss of transplanted organ or tissue Cause of death most commonly due to infection, with immunosuppression therapy a contributory factor
Priority Nursing Diagnoses	*Grieving* *Fear*

immunosuppression is needed, unless a newer option that also transplants the same organ donor's bone marrow is used. This option can reduce or eliminate the need for antirejection drugs. Improved specificity of immunosuppressants has reduced medication side effects while improving patient outcomes. If rejection occurs, medications may be used to attempt to reverse the rejection. Supportive care is provided based on the failing tissue or organ, such as hemodialysis if kidney rejection occurs.

NURSING CARE. Observing for signs of rejection is a priority after transplant. Educating the patient on signs and symptoms of transplant rejection to report is important before discharge. The patient often will be afraid of transplant rejection and should be allowed to discuss these fears. If rejection occurs, nursing care depends on the type of signs and symptoms occurring.

Education for prescribed medications is a must because the long-term success of a transplant depends on compliance with immunosuppressant therapy. Rejection can take place weeks, months, or years after a transplant (with decreasing risk). The patient and family need to be informed of specific signs and symptoms of rejection and when to notify the HCP.

Nursing Care Plan for the Patient With Contact Dermatitis

Nursing Diagnosis: *Impaired Skin Integrity* related to effects of allergic reaction and pruritus
Expected Outcome: The patient's skin will remain intact.
Evaluation of Outcome: Is the patient's skin intact or healing?

Intervention	Rationale	Evaluation
Identify and document skin status and lesions.	*Provides a basis for intervention planning and evaluation of healing.*	Are lesions present? Are lesions healing?
Encourage patient to wear clean, white cotton socks, underwear, gloves, or mittens over affected area, especially at bedtime.	*Cotton is breathable. White cloth is less irritating than those with dyes. Scratching decreases during sleep by covering affected area.*	Are symptoms of skin irritation reduced?
Encourage patient to keep fingernails short and use gentle rubbing or pressure instead of scratching.	*Use of gentle rubbing or pressure instead of scratching with longer nails causes less skin trauma.*	Does skin remain intact despite itchy sensation?
Explain that tepid baking soda baths, colloidal oatmeal baths (e.g., Aveeno), and cool washcloths or cool baths reduce itching.	*These items help dry the vesicle and minimize the pruritus.*	Is itching reduced?

Nursing Diagnosis: *Deficient Knowledge* related to lack of knowledge of methods to decrease inflammation and reduce episodes of inflammation
Expected Outcome: The patient or caregiver will follow the mutually agreed-on plan of care.
Evaluation of Outcome: Can the patient express knowledge of etiology, signs and symptoms, and treatment plan? Does the patient discuss any emotional, social, financial, or material blocks to attaining treatment goals?

Intervention	Rationale	Evaluation
Identify knowledge of disease and barriers to patient's ability to carry out plan of care and plan interventions to decrease barriers.	*Lack of knowledge and barriers can prevent patient from carrying out plan of care.*	Is knowledge level identified? Are barriers present? Are solutions to barriers planned?
Discuss methods of avoiding allergen with patient.	*Understanding prevention methods can help prevent allergen exposure.*	Does patient state methods to help prevent allergen exposure?
Teach patient to wash with a brown soap (e.g., Fels-Naptha) or, if unavailable, any soap when contact with the offending agent occurs.	*Washing with soap removes offending agent.*	Does patient state understanding of the need to wash off the agent with exposure?

AUTOIMMUNE DISORDERS

In autoimmune disorders, the immune system no longer recognizes the body's normal cells as self. Instead, antigens on these normal body cells are recognized as foreign material. The body then launches an immune response to destroy them.

Several factors either cause or influence this breakdown of self-recognition, including viral infections, smoking, alcohol, drugs, and cross-reactive antibodies. Some microbes stimulate production of antibodies that are so closely related to normal cell antigens that the antibodies also attack some normal cells. Hormones also may influence this breakdown of self-recognition.

Some autoimmune disorders are discussed next, whereas others are discussed in chapters related to the body system most affected (Table 19.5).

Pernicious Anemia

PATHOPHYSIOLOGY AND ETIOLOGY. In the most common form of pernicious anemia, the body's immune system develops antibodies that destroy the stomach parietal cells and disrupt intrinsic factor (protein that binds with B_{12} to carry it through the ileum for absorption) production. A vitamin B_{12} (cobalamin) deficiency results. This leads to insufficient and deformed RBCs with poor oxygen-carrying capacity. There tends to be a familial tendency toward the autoimmune form of pernicious anemia.

Causes of the acquired form of pernicious anemia (non-immune-related) include any type of gastric or small-bowel resections that impair absorption of vitamin B_{12} in the ileum coupled with no or inadequate vitamin B_{12} or intrinsic factor replacement.

SIGNS AND SYMPTOMS. The patient experiences increasing weakness, loss of appetite, glossitis (inflammation or infection of the tongue), and pallor. Irritability, confusion, and numbness or tingling in the extremities (peripheral neuropathy) occur because the nervous system is affected from the B_{12} deficiency.

DIAGNOSTIC TESTS. On microscopic examination of the patient's RBCs, macrocytic (enlarged cell) anemia is diagnosed. Macrocytic anemia and low cobalamin levels are indicators of pernicious anemia. To determine if the diagnosis is pernicious anemia, intrinsic factor and parietal cell antibodies are tested. Methylmalonic acid and homocysteine are elevated when cobalamin is low.

THERAPEUTIC MEASURES. Corticosteroids may correct the problem if it is immunologically caused. Otherwise, vitamin B_{12} therapy is needed, usually for life. Parenteral B_{12} therapy may be required, but if not, there are also oral and nasal gel or spray therapy options for mild cases.

NURSING CARE. Vitamin B_{12} is administered as ordered. Care related to fatigue and safety are important. Ambulation, frequent rest periods, and assistance with activities of daily living (ADLs), as indicated by the patient's activity tolerance, are helpful for the patient with anemia.

The patient and family require education regarding B_{12} replacement therapy. Patients should not miss injections, periodic vitamin B_{12} testing, or follow-up appointments.

Idiopathic Autoimmune Hemolytic Anemia

PATHOPHYSIOLOGY. In this disorder, the body produces autoantibodies for no known reason; the autoantibodies attach to RBCs and cause them to either lyse or agglutinate (clump). When lysis occurs, fragments of the destroyed RBCs circulate in the blood. If agglutination occurs, occlusions in the small blood vessels are followed by tissue ischemia.

SIGNS AND SYMPTOMS. Clinical manifestations vary from mild fatigue and pallor to severe hypotension, dyspnea, palpitations, headaches, and jaundice. Problems concentrating and thinking frequently occur.

DIAGNOSTIC TESTS. The RBC count, hemoglobin (Hgb) level, and hematocrit (Hct) level are low. Microscopic examination reveals fragmented RBCs. Lactate dehydrogenase and serum bilirubin levels are elevated because of RBC destruction and tissue ischemia. The direct antiglobulin test (also called the Coombs test) helps determine whether hemolytic anemia is caused by antibodies attached to RBCs.

THERAPEUTIC MEASURES. Supportive measures such as supplemental oxygen may be started. Folic acid may be prescribed to increase production of RBCs. IV immunoglobulin, immunosuppressant medications, and corticosteroids may be useful in obtaining remission. In more severe cases, blood transfusions and erythrocytapheresis (a process in which abnormal RBCs are removed and replaced with normal RBCs) may be instituted. For severe cases, a splenectomy may be performed to stop the destruction of RBCs.

NURSING CARE. The patient's signs and symptoms should be monitored and reported as needed. Frequent rest periods should be planned into the patient's daily routine to prevent fatigue. Blood products may be administered to replace

Table 19.5
Autoimmune Disorders

Disorder	Refer to
Immune thrombocytopenia	Chapter 28
Multiple sclerosis	Chapter 50
Myasthenia gravis	Chapter 50
Rheumatoid arthritis	Chapter 46
Ulcerative colitis	Chapter 34

RBCs. The patient and family are instructed on the medical regimen, and their understanding is verified.

Hashimoto Thyroiditis

PATHOPHYSIOLOGY. Autoantibodies for thyroid-stimulating hormone (TSH) form in Hashimoto thyroiditis (also known as *chronic lymphocytic thyroiditis*). However, instead of inactivating TSH, the autoantibodies bind with hormone receptors on the thyroid gland and stimulate the thyroid gland to secrete thyroid hormones. The thyroid gland enlarges as a result of this overstimulation (hyperthyroidism). It becomes infiltrated with lymphocytes and phagocytes, causing inflammation and further enlargement. Different autoantibodies then appear that destroy thyroid cells. This slows secretion activity, causing hypothyroidism.

ETIOLOGY. Although the exact cause is unknown, it may be viral, bacterial, or genetic. It occurs more in females, middle age, and people with Down syndrome and Turner syndrome.

SIGNS AND SYMPTOMS. Initial signs and symptoms are those of hyperthyroidism, such as restlessness, tremors, chest pain, increased appetite, diarrhea, moist skin, heat intolerance, and weight loss. These manifestations may go unrecognized and progress quickly into hypothyroidism. At this point, an enlarged thyroid gland (goiter) may be seen. Signs and symptoms may include fatigue, bradycardia, hypotension, dyspnea, anorexia, constipation, dry skin, weight gain, sensitivity to cold, facial puffiness, and a slowing of mental processes.

DIAGNOSTIC TESTS. Immunofluorescent assay, a test that detects antigens on cells using an antibody with a fluorescent tag, detects antithyroid antibodies. Serum TSH levels will be elevated, while triiodothyronine (T_3) and thyroxine (T_4) levels are low. A thyroid scan is also done.

THERAPEUTIC MEASURES. Thyroid hormone replacement therapy of thyroxine is the primary means of treatment. Lifelong thyroid hormone therapy is required.

NURSING CARE. If the patient has a goiter, a soft diet may be needed for comfort. Frequent rest periods may be needed while slowly increasing patient activity. Compression stockings may help prevent venous stasis during the low-energy, decreased-activity phase. Daily weights and monitoring of intake and output when cardiac status is compromised are important to detect abnormalities such as fluid retention. Because weight gain and facial puffiness alter patients' self-image, patients need an opportunity to verbalize their feelings to help them adjust to this disease process.

EDUCATION. Patients taking thyroid hormone replacement therapy should avoid foods excessively high in iodine. During the hyperthyroidism phase, a diet high in protein and carbohydrates encourages weight gain. Education regarding prescribed medications is needed. Cholestyramine, ferrous sulfate, sucralfate, iron-containing multivitamins, calcium carbonate, and all other antacids interfere with the absorption of levothyroxine from the gastrointestinal tract. Therefore, levothyroxine should be taken a minimum of 4 hours after taking these medications.

> **CUE RECOGNITION 19.2**
> Your patient with Hashimoto disease recently started taking a thyroid hormone replacement and asks if it is okay to eat seafood. What response do you give?
>
> *Suggested answers are at the end of the chapter.*

Systemic Lupus Erythematosus

Three types of lupus occur in adults. (A fourth type is neonatal, a rare form that is passed on from a mother who has lupus to her fetus.) Drug-induced lupus erythematosus (DILE) affects a low percentage of lupus patients and rarely affects major organs. Research has identified about 80 prescription medications that have caused DILE (Box 19.1). A small percentage of lupus patients have the type that affects only the skin, a condition called discoid lupus erythematosus (DLE). This form is not life threatening and does not affect any internal organs. Most patients with lupus have systemic lupus erythematosus (SLE). SLE can be life threatening because it is a progressive, systemic inflammatory disease that can cause major body organ and system failure. Although this definition seems similar to the definition of rheumatoid arthritis, one distinct difference exists: Patients with SLE typically have more body organ involvement earlier in their disease than do patients with rheumatoid arthritis.

PATHOPHYSIOLOGY. SLE is an autoimmune disease characterized by spontaneous remissions and exacerbations. In SLE, the body develops abnormal antibodies (antinuclear antibodies [ANAs]) against its own tissue, leading to the formation of immune complexes. These in turn activate the complement system, resulting in negative autoimmune effects on the patient's healthy connective tissue. Many of the manifestations result from recurring injuries to the patient's vascular system. The resulting immune complexes lodge in the blood and organs, leading to inflammation, damage, and possibly death.

Box 19.1

Medications Associated With Triggering Lupus Erythematosus*

- Adalimumab
- Chlorpromazine
- Diltiazem
- Etanercept
- Hydralazine
- Infliximab
- Isoniazid
- Methyldopa
- Minocycline
- Nitrofurantoin
- Phenytoin
- Procainamide
- Quinidine
- Rifampin

*Information is inconclusive and contradictory regarding some medications.

ETIOLOGY. The cause of SLE is unknown, but the disorder tends to occur in families. Identified chromosomal markers indicate a genetic link. Environmental factors may also play a critical role in the development of SLE. Infections, high stress levels, various hormones and medications (especially antibiotics such as sulfonamides and penicillin), and ultraviolet light have all been linked to triggering SLE. Exacerbation of symptoms, also called a *flare*, often occurs before the start of menstruation and during pregnancy, demonstrating the link hormones may have in triggering SLE. See Box 19.2 for a list of flare triggers.

People who are Black, Asian, Hispanic, or American Indian are more likely to develop SLE than are White individuals (Centers for Disease Control and Prevention, 2018). Women are most affected, typically between the ages of 15 and 44.

With improved therapy, the mortality rate for patients with SLE has improved greatly. The leading causes of death are kidney failure, heart failure, and central nervous system involvement.

SIGNS AND SYMPTOMS. Clinical manifestations vary from mild to severe (Table 19.6; "Evidence-Based Practice"). The classic feature of lupus is the characteristic reddened butterfly rash found over the bridge of the nose that extends to both cheeks, although less than half of patients develop the rash (Fig. 19.6). The rash is typically flat, is not painful or pruritic, and is photosensitive, worsening when exposed to ultraviolet light. Instead of the butterfly rash, some patients have discoid (coinlike) skin lesions on other parts of the body.

DIAGNOSTIC TESTS. Skin lesions can be biopsied and examined microscopically for signs of inflammation. Other tests include the erythrocyte sedimentation rate (ESR; to detect systemic inflammation) and ANA titers (to detect the presence of abnormal antibodies). Two subtypes of ANA, anti-double stranded DNA (anti-dsDNA) and anti-Smith (anti-Sm) antibodies, are found only in patients with SLE and can be useful in confirming a diagnosis of SLE. A blood test involving serine/arginine-rich (SR) proteins also may aid in diagnosis of SLE. Although no laboratory test can confirm a diagnosis of SLE, the results of immunological tests may support the diagnosis.

> ### Evidence-Based Practice
>
> **Clinical Question**
> What effect does SLE have on bone mineral density and risk for fracture?
>
> **Evidence**
> A meta-analysis was done by Xia and colleagues (2019) of 71 studies involving the frequency and risk factors of reduced bone mineral density (BMD) in patients with SLE. Risk factors such as multiorgan inflammation, corticosteroid therapy, postmenopausal status, and increasing age were found to affect BMD, leading to bone loss and fractures.
>
> **Implications for Nursing Practice**
> Because patients with SLE are at higher risk for fractures, stress the importance of BMD testing. To reduce fracture risk, reinforce the need for adequate dietary calcium intake and adherence to prescribed calcium supplementations.
>
> *Reference:* Xia, J., Luo, R., Guo, S., Yang, Y., Ge, S., Xu, G., & Zeng, R. (2019). Prevalence and risk factors of reduced bone mineral density in systemic lupus erythematosus patients: A meta-analysis. *BioMed Research International, 2019*, 3731648. https://doi.org/10.1155/2019/3731648

THERAPEUTIC MEASURES. Treatment of SLE focuses on decreasing inflammation and preventing life-threatening organ damage (Table 19.7). The human monoclonal antibody belimumab (Benlysta) is the only medication directed at one of the underlying processes of SLE, overstimulated B lymphocytes (which produce an antibody-mediated response known as a *humoral response*). This medication decreases the activity of these cells. This decreases the production of autoantibodies. Many of the drugs used for SLE have serious side effects. Patients receiving them are carefully monitored.

Research is ongoing regarding the possible cause of SLE. Researchers have found more than 100 genes that are associated with SLE or that, in combination, increase the risk for the development of lupus (Scofield, 2020). These genetic discoveries are enabling researchers to develop new methods of therapy, including gene therapy.

NURSING CARE. Prevention of exacerbations (flares) is important. Minimizing exposure to the sun and artificial ultraviolet light by wearing protective clothing and 70 SPF sunscreens will help those patients who are photosensitive. Fatigue during ADLs can be minimized using a daily

> ### Box 19.2
> **Common Systemic Lupus Erythematosus Flare Triggers**
>
> - Emotional crisis
> - Environmental sensitivities or allergies
> - Fluorescent and halogen lights
> - Hormones
> - Immunizations
> - Infection
> - Injury
> - Lack of rest, overwork
> - Pregnancy and after delivery (postpartum)
> - Certain prescription drugs, some over-the-counter drugs (cough syrup)
> - Stopping medications suddenly
> - Stress
> - Sunlight (reflected off water and snow; window glass does not fully protect)
> - Surgery

Table 19.6
Systemic Lupus Erythematosus Summary

Signs and Symptoms	Discoid: • Patchy, crusty, sharply defined skin plaques • Tend to occur on face or sun-exposed areas Drug-induced: • Pleuropericardial inflammation • Fever • Rash • Arthritis Systemic: • Early symptoms are vague, then fatigue, fever • Dermatological: Butterfly rash (face), photosensitivity, mucosal ulcers, alopecia, pain, pruritus, bruising • Musculoskeletal: Arthralgia, arthritis • Hematologic: Anemia, leukocytopenia, elevated erythrocyte sedimentation rate (ESR), thrombocytopenia, false-positive venereal disease research laboratory test • Cardiopulmonary: Pericarditis, myocarditis, myocardial infarction, vasculitis, pleurisy, valvular heart disease • Renal: Renal failure, urinary tract infections, fluid and electrolyte imbalances • Central nervous system: Cranial neuropathies, cognitive impairment, mental changes, seizures • Gastrointestinal: Anorexia, ascites, pancreatitis, intestinal vasculitis • Ophthalmological: Cataracts, conjunctivitis, dry eye, glaucoma, retinal pigmentation
Diagnostic Tests	Complete blood count Antinuclear antibody (ANA) Anti-Smith (a highly specific immunoglobulin for systemic lupus erythematosus [SLE]) Anti-nDNA positive in 60% to 80% of SLE patients Anti-Ro (SSA), an immunoglobulin, positive in 30% of SLE patients Anti-La (SSB), an immunoglobulin, positive in 15% of SLE patients Complement ESR and C-reactive protein (CRP) nonspecific 24-hour urine creatinine clearance If ruling out kidney involvement: • Urinalysis • Serum creatinine • Kidney biopsy
Therapeutic Measures	Symptom management NSAIDs Immunosuppressants Corticosteroids Antimalarials Immunoglobulin intravenously
Complications	Emboli Mesenteric or intestinal vasculitis leading to obstruction, perforation, or infarction Myocarditis Osteonecrosis Renal failure Sepsis Thrombocytopenia Vasculitis
Priority Nursing Diagnoses	*Acute Pain* *Disturbed Body Image* *Fatigue*

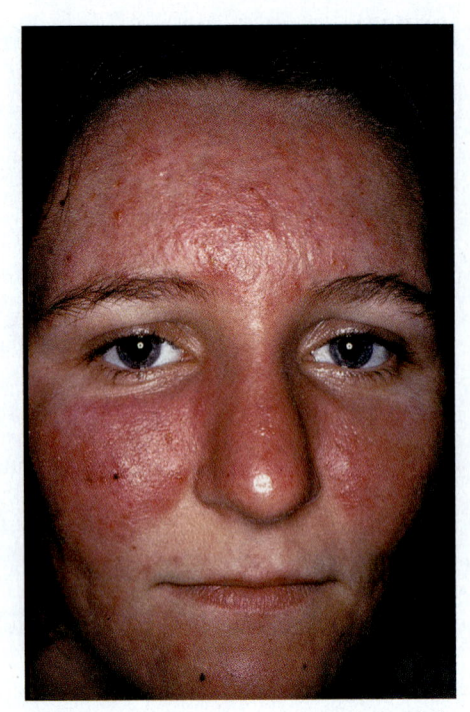

FIGURE 19.6 Lupus erythematosus: red papules and plaques in butterfly pattern on face.

personal schedule. The patient needs a minimum of 8 hours of sleep per night with naps as needed to combat fatigue. Because most patients with SLE develop transitory arthralgia (joint pain), maintaining fitness and joint range of motion through a regular fitness program while decreasing activity during flares is vital. Warm baths may help with morning stiffness, and application of heat and cold compresses, splints, assistive devices, and physical therapy may help soreness. Eating a well-balanced diet will also influence the level of fatigue and the corticosteroid-induced weight gain, which also can affect joint soreness. Patients should keep immunizations up to date.

Finally, but most important, the patient's psychological state and support systems need to be addressed. The period from the onset of symptoms to the diagnosing of lupus is usually costly in terms of time, money, and emotions. Patients may face anger, frustration, and confusion before the diagnosis. For many, there is a sense of relief at diagnosis that may quickly be replaced with feelings of anger, fear, depression, or grief. This is when empathy, support, hope, and, most important, education for the patient, family, and significant others are vital for acquiring successful long-term coping skills. In addition, local support groups and educational and self-management programs available through the Lupus Foundation of America (www.lupus.org) can provide patients with avenues for attaining more specific knowledge and skills for coping and taking control of their lives.

Explain the signs of bleeding and of cardiac and vascular problems, such as myocardial infarction and thrombophlebitis. Encourage medical alert identification usage. Provide smoking cessation information to patients who smoke. Because kidney disease is a major complication of SLE, patients must learn the signs of impending problems that need to be relayed to the HCP immediately. These include facial puffiness and "foamy" or "cola-colored" urine, which are indicative of proteinuria or hematuria, respectively. Explain that regular ophthalmic examinations are needed

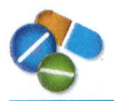

Table 19.7
Medications Used to Treat Systemic Lupus Erythematosus

Medication Class/Action

NSAIDs
Reduce inflammation.

Examples
ibuprofen (Motrin)
indomethacin (Indocin)
naproxen (Naprosyn)

Nursing Implications
Teach:
- Take with food and avoid alcohol.
- Protect self from ultraviolet light.
- Monitor for abnormal bleeding.

Antimalarials
Action is not clearly understood but can significantly help reduce inflammation and decrease platelet aggregation while lowering plasma lipid levels.

Examples
chloroquine (Aralen)
hydroxychloroquine sulfate (Plaquenil)

Nursing Implications
Obtain baseline physical assessment, including an ophthalmic examination.
Teach:
- Administer either before or after meals at the same time of day.
- That it may take weeks or months for effects to be noticed.

Table 19.7
Medications Used to Treat Systemic Lupus Erythematosus—cont'd

Medication Class/Action

Corticosteroids
Reduce inflammation and suppress immune response.

Examples	*Nursing Implications*
dexamethasone (Decadron) methylprednisolone (Solu-Medrol) hydrocortisone (Solu-Cortef) prednisone (Deltasone)	Monitor for weight gain, elevated blood sugar, decreased urine output, pulse irregularities, increased blood pressure, edema, and temperature. *Teach:* • Take with food or milk. • Do not miss doses. • ***Never*** stop taking suddenly. • Use methods to avoid infection.

Immunosuppressants
Target and damage auto-antibody-producing cells.

Examples	*Nursing Implications*
azathioprine (Imuran) cyclosporine (Sandimmune) methotrexate (Rheumatrex)	Monitor complete blood count, renal and liver function tests, abnormal bleeding, joint range of motion, edema, temperature, and erythema. *Teach:* • Take with food for gastrointestinal upset. • Protect from infection.

Human Monoclonal Antibody
Only drug aimed at one of the underlying processes of systemic lupus erythematosus: overstimulated B-lymphocytes.

Examples	*Nursing Implications*
belimumab (Benlysta)	May have serious side effects; careful monitoring is needed.

---

for early detection and treatment of the complications that antimalarial drugs and corticosteroids can produce, such as cataracts, glaucoma, retinal bleeding,

CLINICAL JUDGMENT
Mr. Sauceda is suffering from a flare of SLE. The HCP has ordered intramuscular Solu-Cortef 80 mg to be given every 8 hours. Solu-Cortef 125 mg per 2 mL is available. How many milliliters would you administer for each dose?

Suggested answers are at the end of the chapter.

CUE RECOGNITION 19.3
You are caring for a patient with SLE who has had multiple procedures and tests. You enter her room and find her very tired and reporting that her wrists are hurting very badly. What action do you take?

Suggested answers are at the end of the chapter.

Ankylosing Spondylitis
Ankylosing spondylitis is a chronic progressive inflammatory disease primarily of the spine and sacroiliac area. It can also affect the ribs and large limb joints.

PATHOPHYSIOLOGY. The inflammatory process begins in the lower region of the back and progresses upward. A specific histocompatibility antigen (antigen that identifies self), human leukocyte antigen (HLA) B27, is formed that stimulates an immune response. It can result in complete fusion of the spine as new bone is laid down to attempt to heal from the inflammation. This causes complete rigidity in the spine, a condition known as "bamboo spine."

• WORD • BUILDING •
ankylosing spondylitis: anayle—stiff joint + osing—condition + spondyl—vertebrae + itis—inflammation

ETIOLOGY. There is strong evidence of a familial tendency, but no other specific causes are known. Ankylosing spondylitis tends to afflict men more than women. It is usually diagnosed between the later teens and age 40.

SIGNS AND SYMPTOMS. Ankylosing spondylitis causes an insidious onset of lower back stiffness and pain, which is worse with immobility at night and in early morning. Activity eases the pain. As the disease progresses, the pain worsens and spasms of the back muscles occur. The normal curvature of the lower back (lordosis) flattens, and the curvature of the upper back (kyphosis) increases. Patients may also experience fatigue, anorexia, weight loss, iritis or uveitis, and occasionally heart and lung involvement.

DIAGNOSTIC TESTS. Spinal range of motion, deep breaths to identify rib involvement, and x-rays are used to diagnose this condition. Radiographs of the joints showing spinal changes and fusion (although these changes are a late finding) confirm a diagnosis of ankylosing spondylitis. There are no specific immunological tests to diagnose ankylosing spondylitis.

THERAPEUTIC MEASURES. Because there is no cure for ankylosing spondylitis, treatment consists of measures to minimize the symptoms. Analgesics and muscle relaxants for pain relief, anti-inflammatory agents to decrease joint inflammation, and physical therapy to maintain muscle strength and joint range of motion are used. Biological agents such as anti-tumor necrosis factor (TNF)-a, including etanercept adalimumab (Humira), certolizumab pegol (Cimzia), etanercept (Enbrel), Golimumab (Simponi), and infliximab (Remicade), reduce symptoms and help change the disease's progression. An interleukin-17 (IL-17) inhibitor, such as ixekizumab (Taltz) or secukinumab (Cosentyx), can also be helpful to prevent infection and inflammation. Surgery can be done to replace fused joints. For kyphosis, cervical or lumbar osteotomy can be performed. Physiotherapy and exercise are very beneficial in managing symptoms.

Klebsiella bacterium, found naturally in the gut, is found in high levels in the feces of patients with ankylosing spondylitis. It may be a trigger for the disease. This bacterium requires starch to grow, so it is being researched to see if reducing starch in the diet might reduce symptoms. For more information, visit the Spondylitis Association of America at www.spondylitis.org.

NURSING CARE. Nursing care focuses on administration and evaluation of response to prescribed medications as well as reinforcing patient education to help reduce pain and stiffness. Explain proper posture, range-of-motion exercises, and changing positions frequently. Also encourage patients to sleep on a mattress that is firm without a pillow or with a thin pillow. Pain management, rest periods, assistance with ADLs, and exercise promotion are provided.

CLINICAL JUDGMENT

Mr. Asfaw, a truck driver who was recently diagnosed with ankylosing spondylitis, verbalizes concern about how this diagnosis will affect his ability to work.

1. How would you answer his questions:
   a. "What is happening to me?"
   b. "Will I have to quit my job driving an interstate truck?"
   c. "Am I going to have really bad pain?"
   d. "Am I going to be dependent on someone?"
2. Mr. Asfaw plans to continue driving his truck and therefore has a need, upon discharge, for specific interventions that will help him maintain his independence. What rationale will you provide to Mr. Asfaw to reinforce education about the importance of using each of the following interventions?
   a. Perform range-of-motion exercises daily.
   b. Do not stay in one position too long. Stop and walk around often.
   c. Sleep on a firm mattress without a pillow or with a thin pillow.
   d. Maintain good posture, even when driving the truck.

Suggested answers are at the end of the chapter.

IMMUNE DEFICIENCIES

Immune deficiencies occur when one or more components of the immune system are either completely absent or deficient in quantities sufficient to elicit or sustain an adequate immune response to combat an infectious agent.

Hypogammaglobulinemia

PATHOPHYSIOLOGY AND ETIOLOGY. Hypogammaglobulinemia is either a hereditary congenital disorder or acquired after childhood from unknown causes. It is characterized by the absence or deficiency of one or more of the five classes of immunoglobulins (IgG, IgM, IgA, IgD, and IgE) from defective B-cell function. The lack of normal function of these antibodies makes the patient prone to infections. The congenital form of this disorder affects males. Patients usually have a normal life span.

SIGNS AND SYMPTOMS. Recurrent infections occur, especially from *Staphylococcus* and *Streptococcus* organisms.

DIAGNOSIS. Immunoelectrophoresis, which measures the level of each immunoglobulin, can be performed.

THERAPEUTIC MEASURES. Treatment is aimed at minimizing infections while increasing immune system function through subcutaneous injections or IV infusions of immunoglobulin. Immunoglobulin mainly contains IgG, so fresh frozen plasma is given to replace IgM. IgA cannot be replaced, increasing the risk for frequent pulmonary infections. Gene therapy can successfully stabilize infant immune systems with severe combined immunodeficiency but is less effective with older patients.

NURSING CARE AND EDUCATION. Monitor for infections. Any break in the skin must be cleansed immediately and monitored for infection development. Genetic counseling may be recommended. Education on signs and symptoms of various infections and seeking medical help promptly, avoiding crowds, the need for good nutrition, hydration, and hygiene is provided.

> **Home Health Hints**
>
> **Atopic Dermatitis**
> - If a skin rash develops, encourage the use of a mild laundry soap, such as Dreft.
>
> **Latex Allergy**
> - Always have latex-free gloves available.
> - Use latex-free silicone urinary catheters.
>
> **Post-Transplant**
> - Encourage patients who are taking immunosuppressant medications to avoid people who are contagious such as with exposure to COVID-19 or who are ill with COVID-19, a cold, or the flu to prevent becoming ill.

Key Points

- Type I hypersensitivity reactions involve the release of histamine and other mediators from mast cells and basophils. Examples of this type of reaction include allergic rhinitis, atopic dermatitis, anaphylaxis, urticaria, and angioedema.
- A type II hypersensitivity reaction involves the destruction of a cell or substance that has an antigen attached to its cell membrane, which is sensed by either immunoglobulin G (IgG) or immunoglobulin M (IgM) as being a foreign antigen. An example of this type of reaction is a hemolytic transfusion reaction.
- A type III hypersensitivity reaction involves immune complexes formed by antigens and antibodies, usually of the IgG type. This type of reaction is seen in serum sickness.
- A type IV hypersensitivity reaction, or delayed reaction, occurs when a sensitized T lymphocyte comes in contact with the particular antigen to which it is sensitized. This type of reaction is seen in contact dermatitis, including latex allergy and transplant rejection.
- Treatment may vary depending on the type of an allergic reaction. Immediate treatment is guided by symptoms. Patients should be taught what measures to take in case of an anaphylactic reaction (e.g., always carry an epinephrine auto-injector).
- In autoimmune disorders, the immune system no longer recognizes the body's normal cells as self. Instead, antigens on these normal body cells are recognized as foreign material. The body then launches an immune response to destroy them. Examples of this are ankylosing spondylitis, Hashimoto thyroiditis, idiopathic autoimmune hemolytic anemia, pernicious anemia, and SLE.
- Several factors, including viral infections, drugs, and cross-reactive antibodies, either cause or influence this breakdown of self-recognition. Some microbes stimulate production of antibodies that are so closely related to normal cell antigens that the antibodies also attack some normal cells. Hormones also may influence this breakdown of self-recognition.
- Immune deficiencies occur when one or more components of the immune system are either completely absent or deficient in quantities sufficient to elicit or sustain an adequate immune response to combat an infectious agent. An example of this is hypogammaglobulinemia.

> **SUGGESTED ANSWERS TO CHAPTER EXERCISES**
>
> **Cue Recognition**
> **19.1:** Immediately observe and maintain patency of the airway while calling for assistance for this emergency to ultimately prevent respiratory arrest.
> **19.2:** "Avoid eating excessive amounts of iodine-rich foods, such as fish and shellfish."
> **19.3:** Collect pain rating data and administer analgesics as ordered. Cluster nursing care to promote periods of rest.
>
> **Critical Thinking & Clinical Judgment**
> **Mrs. Barnes**
> 1. Mrs. Barnes is most likely having an anaphylactic reaction to the bee stings with accompanying urticaria or possibly angioedema.
> 2. Further data collection might include identification of any previous allergies to food, medications, and environmental stimuli and what reactions occur with these allergies.

SUGGESTED ANSWERS TO CHAPTER EXERCISES—cont'd

Thorough respiratory data collection is needed, noting any adventitious sounds, particularly wheezing. Note any dysphagia, changes in the voice, or hoarseness.
3. Therapeutic measures to implement include monitoring vital signs, staying with the patient, using semi-Fowler to high-Fowler position, giving oxygen at 2 to 3 L per minute, and ensuring a patent intravenous access. Notify the registered nurse and/or HCP right away. Anticipate administration of antihistamines, epinephrine, and fluids.
4. Mrs. Barnes's airway.
5. HCP, registered nurse, and respiratory therapist.

Mr. Sauceda
1. 28 mL per dose.

Mr. Asfaw
1. a. "Human leukocyte antigen B27 is formed, stimulating a chronic immune (inflammatory) response specifically in the spine, sacroiliac area, and large limb joints. This leads to thickening of the joints, joint pain, and stiffness."
   b. "No, you shouldn't have to quit your job, but you may need to alter how you travel."
   c. "No, you may not have severe pain with use of medication and exercise."
   d. "No, this disease may not affect your independence with proper treatment and rehabilitation."
2. a. "Range-of-motion exercises will help maintain joint mobility and a full range of motion and prevent contractures from forming."
   b. "Again, this frequent movement prevents stiffness and joint pain and contractures."
   c. "Sleeping on a firm mattress without a pillow or with a thin pillow keeps the spine in correct alignment, which in turn helps prevent progressive changes in spine alignment (kyphosis, scoliosis) that affects various major body systems (respiratory, etc.)."
   d. "Again, good posture will aid in preventing bone deformities."

Additional Resources

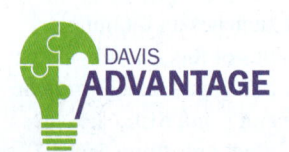

Go to Davis Advantage to complete your learning: strengthen understanding, apply your knowledge, and prepare for the Next Gen NCLEX®.

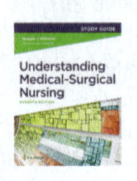

A Study Guide is also available.

CHAPTER 20
Nursing Care of Patients With HIV and AIDS

Patrice Wade-Olson

KEY TERMS

acquired immunodeficiency syndrome (uh-KWHY-erd im-yoo-noh-dee-FISH-en-see SIN-drohm)
cytomegalovirus (SY-tow-MEH-guh-low-vy-rus)
human immunodeficiency virus (HYOO-man im-yoo-noh-dee-FISH-en-see VY-rus)
personal protective equipment (PUR-sun-al pra-TEK-tiv ee-KWIP-ment)
pneumocystis pneumonia (new-moh-SIS-tis new-MOHN-yah)
undetectable viral load (un-dee-TECH-tah-bul VY-ruhl lohd)

CHAPTER CONCEPTS

Caring
Collaboration
Health promotion
Immunity
Nutrition

LEARNING OUTCOMES

1. Define HIV and AIDS.
2. Explain how HIV is transmitted.
3. Explain tests for diagnosing HIV.
4. Describe the prognosis for HIV and AIDS.
5. Develop an education plan for prevention of an HIV infection.
6. Identify prevention measures used to decrease infection and opportunistic diseases for patients with HIV.
7. Develop an education plan for a patient with HIV receiving antiretroviral therapy.
8. Plan nursing care for patients with HIV and AIDS related to medications, coinfection prevention, and maintenance of nutritional status.

Acquired immunodeficiency syndrome (AIDS) is the final stage of a **human immunodeficiency virus** (HIV) infection. AIDS can happen at any point during an HIV infection. The Centers for Disease Control and Prevention (CDC) identifies criteria for determining when HIV disease has developed into AIDS (Box 20.1).

In the United States, most people with HIV who are diagnosed early and receive treatment do not develop AIDS because antiretroviral medications suppress HIV replication. This improves immune function and reduces the risk of life-threatening opportunistic infections. The first antiretroviral (ARV) HIV drug was introduced in 1987. Highly active antiretroviral therapy (HAART) began in 1996. A newer term for HAART is antiretroviral therapy (ART). Both the latter terms refer to the use of a combination of at least two ARV medications that have different actions to suppress HIV replication.

> ### NURSING CARE TIP
> When caring for patients who are HIV positive or who have AIDS, it is important to be aware of and understand current information. Being informed helps you to provide competent, nonjudgmental care without fear (Table 20.1). Knowledge about HIV/AIDS and treatments is continually evolving.

Box 20.1

CDC AIDS-Defining Opportunistic Conditions in HIV Infection

AIDS is diagnosed when CD4 T-lymphocyte count below 200 cells/mm^3 or certain opportunistic infections or cancers develop:

- Candidiasis of mouth, vagina, esophagus, bronchi, trachea, or lung
- Cervical cancer, invasive
- Coccidioidomycosis
- Cryptococcosis
- Cryptosporidiosis
- Cystoisosporiasis
- Cytomegalovirus
- Encephalopathy attributed to HIV
- Herpes simplex virus
- Histoplasmosis
- Kaposi sarcoma
- Lymphoma
- *Mycobacterium avium* complex
- *Mycobacterium* tuberculosis
- *Pneumocystis* pneumonia (*Pneumocystis jiroveci*)
- Pneumonia
- Progressive multifocal leukoencephalopathy
- Salmonella septicemia
- Toxoplasmosis
- Wasting syndrome attributed to HIV

Source: Centers for Disease Control and Prevention. (2020). AIDS and opportunistic infections. Retrieved January 30, 2021, from www.cdc.gov/hiv/basics/livingwithhiv/opportunisticinfections.html.

Table 20.1

Staying Current: HIV/AIDS Information Resources

Association of Nurses in AIDS Care	www.nursesinaidscare.org (800) 260-6780
AVERT: AVERTing HIV and AIDS	www.avert.org
The Body: The Complete HIV/AIDS Resource	www.thebody.com
Centers for Disease Control and Prevention (CDC) National HIV, STD, and Hepatitis Testing	https://gettested.cdc.gov (800) CDC-INFO
CDC: HIV/AIDS	www.cdc.gov/hiv (800) CDC-INFO (888) 232-6348 (TTY)
CDC National Center for HIV/AIDS, Viral Hepatitis, STD, and TB Prevention	www.cdc.gov/nchhstp
HIV.gov (gateway to federal domestic HIV/AIDS resources)	www.hiv.gov
HIV Prevention Trials Network	www.hptn.org
NAM AIDSMaps	www.aidsmap.com
Prevention Access Campaign	www.preventionaccess.org
University of California, Los Angeles, National Clinician Consultation Center (Post-Exposure Prophylaxis hotline)	www.nccc.ucsf.edu (888) 448-4911
U.S. Department of Health and Human Services AIDSinfo (in English and Spanish)	www.aidsinfo.nih.gov (800) HIV-0440
U.S. National Library of Medicine	www.nlm.nih.gov (888) FIND-NLM
World Health Organization: HIV/AIDS information	www.who.int/hiv

HISTORY AND INCIDENCE

The HIV epidemic was first reported by the CDC in June 1981. Cases of HIV infection and AIDS increased rapidly through the 1980s. A decrease followed in the late 1990s. At the end of 2018, the CDC estimated that 1.2 million people were infected with HIV. Of these, an estimated 14% were not aware of being infected. In 2018, an estimated 39,968 people were newly infected with HIV. Of those infected in 2018, 24% were heterosexual, 42% were Black, and 19% were women (CDC, 2020a; CDC, 2020b). Although HIV or AIDS can occur in a person of any age, this chapter focuses on adults with HIV or AIDS.

PATHOPHYSIOLOGY

Infection with HIV kills immune cells. A weakened immune system allows infections and cancers to take over. AIDS is the final phase of this immunodeficiency.

Two strains of HIV have been identified: HIV-1 and HIV-2. HIV-1 is found around the world; it is more pathogenic. HIV-2 is found mainly in a small area in West Africa; it is less pathogenic. It is possible to become infected with both strains of HIV. Because of genetic differences, they require different types of diagnostic testing. They are transmitted in the same way, are incurable, and can progress to AIDS. Because HIV-1 is most common, reference to HIV in this chapter is to HIV-1, unless noted.

HIV is a retrovirus, which only has ribonucleic acid (RNA) for genetic material. HIV is attracted to immune cells with a surface-attaching site. This is the CD4 receptor. Cells with CD4 receptors include lymphocytes [called CD4 T lymphocytes, CD4+ T lymphocytes, T4 lymphocytes (or helper T lymphocytes)], and macrophages (found in the brain). HIV hides in these latent reservoirs for infection flare-ups, which makes finding a cure difficult. The CD4 T lymphocytes are the main targets of HIV. CD4 T lymphocytes coordinate all immune functions. Consequently, the destruction of these cells by HIV results in progressive impairment of the body's immune response. The study of macrophages and HIV has led to the discovery of how HIV enters these cells. Continued research to assess latent HIV reservoirs and macrophages and monocytes is needed to help discover a cure (Kruize & Kootstra, 2019).

The HIV replication process has seven steps: (1) The first is *binding* (attachment) to the CD4 receptor of the host cell (Fig. 20.1). Cellular chemokine receptor type 5 (CCR5) antagonist drugs act here to block HIV attachment. (2) Binding leads to fusion of the HIV envelope (membrane) and host cell membrane. Fusion inhibitor drugs act here. (3) After fusion, the HIV capsid (which encloses genetic material of the virus) is released into the host cell. HIV uses its enzyme *reverse transcriptase* to convert its RNA to HIV DNA. The new HIV DNA then enters the host cell's nucleus. Nonnucleoside reverse transcriptase inhibitors (NNRTIs) and nucleoside reverse transcriptase inhibitors (NRTIs) act here. Inhibitors of reverse transcriptase that act here were the first anti-HIV drugs developed. (4) HIV releases the enzyme *integrase*, which incorporates its HIV DNA into the host cell's DNA. Integrase inhibitors act here. (5) HIV then uses the machinery of the host cell to replicate long chains of HIV proteins for building more HIV. (6) Packaging of HIV RNA and HIV proteins within a viral envelope created from part of the cell membrane occurs next. (7) The immature, noninfectious HIV then buds from the host cell. It releases the enzyme *protease* to cut the HIV protein chains into their shorter functional forms. Mature, infectious HIV is then formed from these proteins. Protease inhibitors, which are potent antiviral medications, block this critical step.

HIV can persist in a latent (inactive) state for many years. The virus has no cure, as it lies dormant in a small number of cells called *viral reservoirs* even when at undetectable levels in the blood. However, HIV can be controlled with lifelong antiviral treatment. The goal of researchers is to use knowledge of the HIV life cycle to test potential vaccines in ongoing clinical trials and to develop a cure.

After a person has been infected with HIV, other immune system components form antibodies to fight HIV. These HIV antibodies typically become present within 3 months after infection. The time between infection and developing antibodies is called the window period. Testing for these antibodies can be done to diagnose HIV.

Progression of HIV Infection

The initial infection is followed by a relatively symptom-free period. This is called the *clinical latency stage*. The virus remains in the lymph nodes, liver, and spleen, and it reproduces. If the infection is untreated, CD4 T lymphocytes gradually decrease. B lymphocytes also become dysfunctional and dysregulated by HIV progression. B and T lymphocytes normally work together in a healthy immune system. The period from infection to the beginning of the symptomatic stage varies for each person. It averages 8 to 12 years. During this stage, the person is considered HIV-positive. In the early symptomatic stage of HIV disease, symptoms of the weakening immune system are seen. When CD4 counts drop below 200 cells/mm^3 or certain opportunistic infections or cancers occur, a diagnosis of AIDS is given (see Box 20.1).

> **LEARNING TIP**
> Being HIV positive means that the person has been infected with the HIV virus. It does not mean that the person has AIDS.

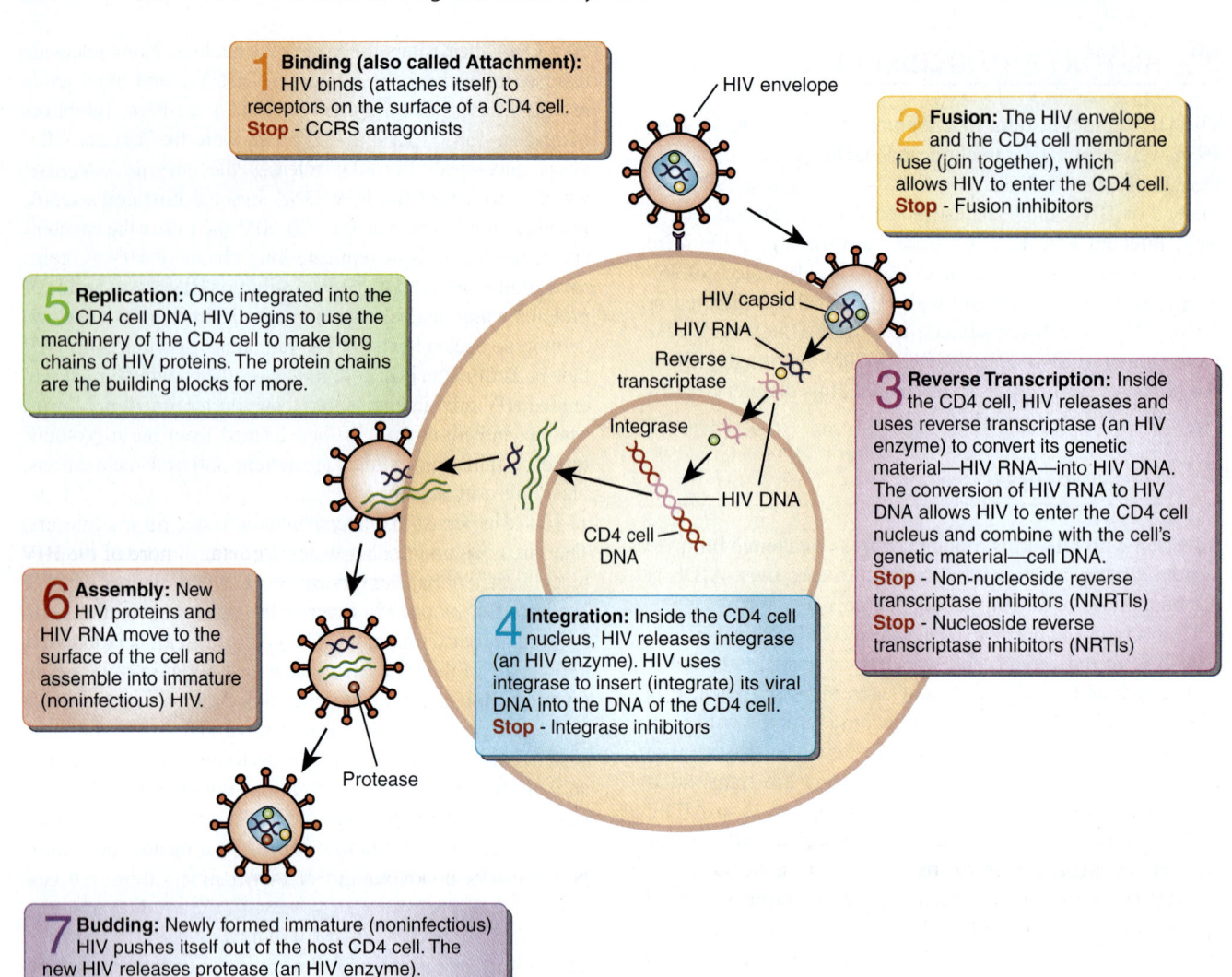

1 Binding (also called Attachment): HIV binds (attaches itself) to receptors on the surface of a CD4 cell.
Stop - CCR5 antagonists

2 Fusion: The HIV envelope and the CD4 cell membrane fuse (join together), which allows HIV to enter the CD4 cell.
Stop - Fusion inhibitors

3 Reverse Transcription: Inside the CD4 cell, HIV releases and uses reverse transcriptase (an HIV enzyme) to convert its genetic material—HIV RNA—into HIV DNA. The conversion of HIV RNA to HIV DNA allows HIV to enter the CD4 cell nucleus and combine with the cell's genetic material—cell DNA.
Stop - Non-nucleoside reverse transcriptase inhibitors (NNRTIs)
Stop - Nucleoside reverse transcriptase inhibitors (NRTIs)

4 Integration: Inside the CD4 cell nucleus, HIV releases integrase (an HIV enzyme). HIV uses integrase to insert (integrate) its viral DNA into the DNA of the CD4 cell.
Stop - Integrase inhibitors

5 Replication: Once integrated into the CD4 cell DNA, HIV begins to use the machinery of the CD4 cell to make long chains of HIV proteins. The protein chains are the building blocks for more.

6 Assembly: New HIV proteins and HIV RNA move to the surface of the cell and assemble into immature (noninfectious) HIV.

7 Budding: Newly formed immature (noninfectious) HIV pushes itself out of the host CD4 cell. The new HIV releases protease (an HIV enzyme). Protease acts to break up the long protein chains that form the immature virus. The smaller HIV proteins combine to form mature (infectious) HIV.
Stop - Protease inhibitors (PIs)

FIGURE 20.1 The HIV life cycle and the medication classes that stop HIV in various life cycle stages.

PREVENTION

Education and prevention are the best ways to manage HIV/AIDS. Education should begin with older school-age children and continue with adults of all ages ("Gerontological Issues"). *Ending the HIV Epidemic: A Plan for America (EHE)* is an initiative that seeks to reduce new HIV infections by 90% by 2030 using four science-based strategies: diagnose, treat, prevent, and respond (U.S. Department of Health and Human Services [HHS], 2020). Visit www.hiv.gov for more information. The Healthy People 2030 HIV objectives and targets support the indicators in the new EHE initiative. They include reducing the number of new HIV infections and new diagnoses, increasing knowledge of HIV status, increasing linkage to medical care, increasing viral suppression, and reducing perinatal transmission.

Mode of Transmission

HIV is a fragile virus. It is transmitted from person to person only through certain body fluids from a person infected with HIV. These fluids include blood, semen, preseminal fluid, vaginal secretions, rectal fluids, and breast milk. HIV can be transmitted to others within 2 to 4 weeks of initial infection and then, without treatment, throughout all stages of the HIV infection and AIDS (HHS, 2019). HIV is not spread casually. It does not live long outside of the body. HIV needs a portal of entry into the body. Entry portals include a tear in a mucous membrane or nonintact skin or direct injection into the bloodstream (via needle). Casual contact such as hugging, closed-mouth kissing, shaking hands, or sharing eating utensils, towels, or bathroom fixtures with an HIV-positive person does not transmit HIV. Transmission does not occur by air, water, food, or insects. Since 1985, donated

Gerontological Issues

Older Adults and HIV

In 2016, the Centers for Disease Control and Prevention (2019) reported that almost half of those living with HIV are age 50 or over. Older adults are often diagnosed with an HIV infection when AIDS is already present. Ask older adults about their sexual and drug use history. Explain preventive measures. Share information on products to reduce transmission of HIV and sexually transmitted infections (STIs). At-risk adults over age 50 are less likely than younger at-risk adults to use condoms during sex. They tend to think of condoms only as a birth control measure. They are also less likely to be tested for HIV.

Erectile dysfunction treatments have contributed to more older adults being sexually active. They may have multiple partners. Some are also contracting HIV through same-sex contact.

A decline in the older adult's immune system increases the risk for infection with HIV. Increased vaginal dryness and friability further increase an older woman's susceptibility to HIV infection. The rise in HIV infection among older adults is expected to continue due to a lack of preventative knowledge. With AIDS death rates dropping as a result of more effective treatments, the number of older adults living with HIV will increase.

Symptoms of HIV in older adults can be confused with commonly perceived problems of aging. These include fatigue, decreased endurance, and altered cognitive status. The brain effects of HIV can be mistaken for Alzheimer disease. Misinterpretation of symptoms can delay appropriate treatment.

---

blood has been tested for HIV antibodies. Donated organs are also tested. HIV infection is rare from blood transfusions or organ donation. Transmission within households from contact with HIV-infected blood or body secretions is also rare. Education for those living with someone infected with HIV is important (visit www.cdc.gov/hiv).

Pre-exposure Prophylaxis

Pre-exposure prophylaxis (PrEP) with an ARV is an effective way to prevent HIV transmission for those at high risk of contracting the virus (CDC, 2020c; Krakower et al, 2020). If PrEP is taken as directed, it is 99% effective at preventing HIV transmission. Emtricitabine/tenofovir disoproxil (Truvada) and emtricitabine/tenofovir alafenamide (Descovy) are PrEP medications. Emtricitabine/tenofovir alafenamide is currently approved for certain populations. Both medications should be taken once daily consistently.

Counseling

Early knowledge of one's HIV status helps reduce the spread of HIV. The U.S. Preventive Services Task Force (USPSTF, 2019) recommends routine testing for those ages 15 to 65, pregnant females, and individuals who have experienced sexual assault. Testing is done either confidentially or anonymously. Permission is needed to release one's test results to others. Post-test counseling is available to help the patient understand the test results, assist with informing sexual partners and drug needle sharers, reduce risk factors, and provide care options.

Sexual Transmission

HIV can be transmitted through sexual contact with infected body fluids and mucous membranes. Some types of sexual contact carry a higher rate of transmission. Vaginal and anal sex have high rates of transmission for both males and females. Anal sex has the highest risk, as it may result in tearing of the mucous membrane, which allows exposure to infected semen. Females have a greater risk of infection because the vagina has a greater area of mucous membranes than the penis and because semen contains more of the HIV virus than vaginal secretions do. Early initiation of ART leads to faster viral suppression and less risk of transmission. In 2017, the CDC (2020d) reported that when testing consistently does not detect the virus for at least 6 months, the individual cannot transmit the HIV virus to other people.

Safer Sex Practices

Abstaining from sexual intercourse is the only 100% way to prevent sexual exposure to HIV. A long-term, mutually monogamous sexual relationship is considered safest when both partners are known to be HIV negative. Limiting sexual partners, wearing latex gloves to protect hands during genital or anal contact, using latex condoms and dental dams (latex sheets) correctly and regularly as a barrier for the mouth and genitals or anus are other measures to reduce sexual exposure to HIV (Box 20.2; see "Patient Teaching Guidelines: Preventing HIV Transmission" in the online resources). People with HIV must legally disclose their HIV status to

---

Box 20.2

Patient Education

Condom Use to Prevent HIV Transmission

Condoms should be:
- New for each sex act.
- Made of latex (highly effective) because other materials have large pores that allow HIV to pass.
- Undamaged and used before expiration date.
- Applied before partner is touched. (Tip of condom is held while unrolling over erect penis, allowing room at tip for semen collection.)
- Used with adequate amounts of only water-soluble lubricant. (Petroleum or oil-based lubricants such as petroleum jelly, cooking oil, shortening, or lotions can damage latex condoms.)
- Replaced if broken. (If ejaculation occurs before replacement, immediate use of a spermicide can give some protection.)
- Withdrawn from partner by holding condom against base of erect penis to avoid semen leakage.

any intimate partner. Using safer sex techniques reduces the risk of HIV transmission.

Parenteral Transmission

The best way to prevent parenteral transmission of HIV is to avoid or stop injecting drugs. If a person who injects drugs is unable or unwilling to stop, it is recommended that a new sterile syringe and needle, obtained from pharmacies, is used each time along with new sterile water and new or disinfected preparation equipment. Alcohol swabs should be used to clean the injection site. Afterward, the syringe should be disposed of safely. Drug injection equipment should never be shared or reused. Syringe exchange program availability varies by location. These programs decrease the risk of transmission of HIV and other bloodborne pathogens. If injection equipment is reused, it should be boiled or cleansed with bleach. Sexual activity should be discouraged when judgment is impaired by drug use because protective measures may not be used during this impairment. PrEP with an ARV for non-HIV-infected people who inject drugs can reduce HIV infection.

Autologous (one's own) blood transfusion, when possible, is the safest type of blood transfusion to prevent HIV infection. Donated blood is screened for HIV. There is a very low chance of HIV transmission from donated blood that is infected but has not yet had time to develop antibodies.

Perinatal Transmission

Guidelines for HIV screening of pregnant women recommend that HIV counseling and testing be offered during routine prenatal care for all pregnant women and again in the third trimester for women at high risk (Panel on Treatment of HIV-Infected Pregnant Women and Prevention of Perinatal Transmission, 2019). All pregnant women who are HIV positive can reduce the risk of perinatal HIV transmission with ART during pregnancy, labor, and delivery. At the time of labor, pregnant women who have not been tested for HIV should be offered rapid HIV tests. Therapy should be started if infection with HIV is confirmed.

Health-Care Providers (HCPs) and HIV Prevention

Occupational HIV transmission is rare. Using standard precautions (see Chapter 8), appropriate hand hygiene, and safety devices to prevent needlesticks (e.g., needleless systems, protective covers, and *never* recapping used needles) reduce the risk of HIV exposure. It is essential to use these practices with all patients to protect yourself from exposure and transmission of HIV. If you are unsure of the appropriate **personal protective equipment** (e.g., gloves, gown, goggles, face shield) or isolation precautions to use for the situation, ask your instructor or the patient's nurse before providing care to a patient.

Know the occupational exposure protocol for the agency in which you are practicing. If exposure occurs, wash the exposure site with soap and water immediately. For mucous membrane exposure, flush the area with water. Then seek immediate medical care. The U.S. Public Health Service guidelines for occupational exposures can be viewed at www.jstor.org/stable/10.1086/672271. Visit www.cdc.gov/niosh/topics/bbp/guidelines.html for National Institute for Occupational Safety and Health guidelines.

CUE RECOGNITION 20.1

You are administering a subcutaneous insulin injection to Mr. Sims, who is HIV positive, when he suddenly moves, and the needle pierces your gloved finger. What action do you take?

Suggested answers are at the end of the chapter.

HIV SIGNS AND SYMPTOMS

Each patient's HIV infection response is different. In Stage 1, the patient may not have any symptoms but later may develop acute retroviral syndrome. Symptoms of this syndrome are extreme fatigue, headache, fever, lymphadenopathy (enlarged lymph nodes in two sites other than inguinal nodes), diarrhea, or a sore throat (Fig. 20.2 and Table 20.2). Symptoms can develop 2 to 4 weeks after transmission of HIV (CDC, 2020a). They can last a few days to weeks. The symptoms are usually mild and are not usually associated with being infected with HIV.

An extended asymptomatic phase, Stage 2, also known as chronic HIV infection, can then occur. If the HIV infection is untreated, this phase could last up to 10 to 15 years before progressing to a symptomatic state, which occurs when the virus has greatly impaired the immune system. The patient may have shortness of breath, fever, weight loss, fatigue, night sweats, persistent diarrhea, oral or vaginal candidiasis ulcers, dry skin, skin lesions, peripheral neuropathy, shingles (varicella zoster virus reactivation), seizures, or dementia. In the final stage of HIV infection, Stage 3, AIDS is diagnosed if the CD4 T-lymphocyte count is below 200 cells/mm^3 or opportunistic infections or cancers occur (see Box 20.1).

COMPLICATIONS

Complications from HIV and AIDS vary from patient to patient. With ART, fewer complications are seen than in the past. Some, such as Kaposi sarcoma (a connective tissue tumor), are rarely seen anymore.

AIDS Wasting Syndrome

AIDS wasting syndrome is defined by involuntary loss of more than 10% of baseline body weight plus chronic weakness or fever or chronic diarrhea for more than 30 days. Several factors contribute to this syndrome, including decreased appetite, oral lesions, altered metabolism, malabsorption, gastrointestinal (GI) infections, diarrhea, medication side effects, and cognitive impairment. The progressive weight loss impairs the function of all body systems from

CD4+ T-lymphocyte Count During HIV Disease and AIDS

HIV Infection Phases:
- 1–4 weeks: Seroconversion flu-like illness
- 2 months: Positive HIV antibody test
- Asymptomatic latency period
- AIDS
- Death

Infection after exposure to HIV

Early symptoms of HIV infection

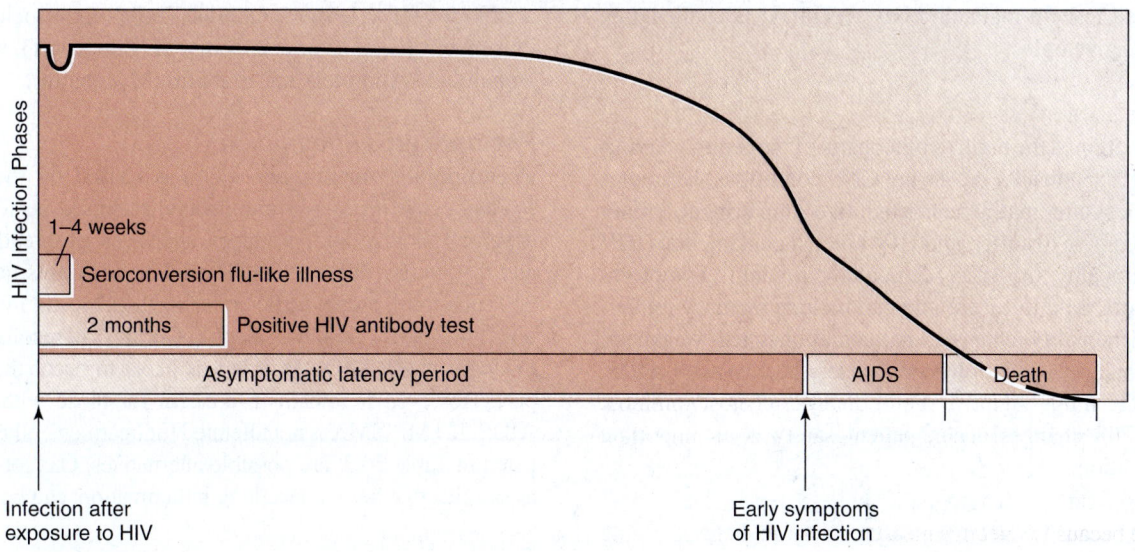

FIGURE 20.2 Typical phases of HIV infection, AIDS development, and CD4+ T-lymphocyte counts without treatment. Length of latency period varies but is usually many years. As CD4+ T-lymphocyte counts drop, symptoms, AIDS, opportunistic infections, and then death can result.

Table 20.2
HIV/AIDS Summary

Signs and Symptoms	Initially vary; none or acute retroviral syndrome Asymptomatic phase Immune system impairment (e.g., dyspnea, fever, weight loss, fatigue, night sweats, persistent diarrhea, oral or vaginal candidiasis ulcers, dry skin, skin lesions, peripheral neuropathy, shingles, or dementia) AIDS diagnosed when CD4 T-lymphocyte count is below 200 cells/mm^3 or opportunistic infections or cancer occur
Diagnostic Tests	Fourth-generation antigen/antibody combination immunoassay Antibody differentiation immunoassay HIV-1 nucleic acid test Complete blood cell count/lymphocyte count CD4 T-lymphocyte count Viral load testing Genotyping
Therapeutic Measures	Cellular chemokine receptor type 5 (CCR5) antagonists Fusion inhibitors Integrase inhibitors Nonnucleoside reverse transcriptase inhibitors (NNRTIs) Nucleoside reverse transcriptase inhibitors (NRTIs) Post attachment inhibitors Protease inhibitors
Complications	AIDS wasting syndrome Opportunistic infections or cancer AIDS dementia complex
Priority Nursing Diagnoses	*Ineffective Protection* *Deficient Knowledge*

malnourishment. Begin patient education when HIV is first diagnosed to help maintain body weight. It is challenging, but don't give up!

HIV-Associated Neurocognitive Disorder

HIV infection in the brain or other parts of the central nervous system (CNS) results in varying CNS conditions. Examples include asymptomatic neurocognitive impairment, minor neurocognitive disorder, and HIV-associated dementia (HIV encephalopathy or AIDS dementia complex). Symptoms range from mild to severe and can include memory impairment, personality changes, hallucinations, leg weakness, loss of balance, and slower responses. In advanced AIDS, with ART, minor cognitive motor disorder is most common. When CNS changes occur, patient safety is an important consideration.

Cancer and Opportunistic Infections

Why does a person with HIV or AIDS have increased risk for cancer and opportunistic infections? With an impaired immune system, cancer incidence rises because the abnormal cancer cells are not being destroyed. Opportunistic infections, so named because they take advantage of the opportunity to attack a weakened immune system, are not fought off as a healthy immune system would be able to do. Opportunistic infections can be viral, bacterial, mycobacterial, fungal, protozoal, or parasitic. Some opportunistic infections can be prevented with prophylactic treatments. Examples of opportunistic infections are discussed next.

Candida Albicans

Candida albicans is a fungus normally found in the GI tract. It does not cause infection in a person with a healthy immune system. In a person with AIDS, overgrowth of this fungus occurs, commonly affecting the mouth or esophagus. Signs and symptoms of candidiasis include oral or esophageal pain, dysphagia, and yellow-white plaques that look like cottage cheese in the mouth and throat. Nutrition can be affected by oral or esophageal candidiasis. Recurrent vaginal candidiasis, with severe itching and a white discharge, is common in women with AIDS.

Cytomegalovirus

Cytomegalovirus (CMV) infection can be serious. It can cause retinitis, which can result in blindness. Signs and symptoms include fever, fatigue, diarrhea, GI upset, and hepatitis.

Mycobacterium Avium Complex

Mycobacterium avium complex (MAC) is a serious nontuberculous mycobacterial infection. Occurrence rises when CD4 T-lymphocyte counts drop below 50 cells/mm^3. MAC is found in water, foods such as raw or partially cooked fish or shellfish, and soil. A prophylactic antibiotic may be given when CD4 T-lymphocyte counts fall below 50 cells/mm^3 if ARVs are not being taken. With infection, symptoms can include fever, night sweats, weight loss, fatigue, abdominal pain, and diarrhea. Treatment includes a combination of antibiotics for at least 12 months. These might include clarithromycin (Biaxin) or azithromycin (Zithromax), with ethambutol (Myambutol) and rifabutin (Mycobutin).

Pneumocystis Pneumonia

Pneumocystis pneumonia (PCP) is caused by the fungus *Pneumocystis jiroveci* in immunocompromised persons. PCP develops slowly and produces shortness of breath, fever, and dry cough. When CD4 T-lymphocyte counts fall below 200 cells/mm^3, prophylactic oral trimethoprim-sulfamethoxazole (TMP-SMX [Bactrim, Septra, Cotrim]) is recommended. Owing to TMP-SMX, PCP is less likely to occur than in the past. However, it remains a concern for those with HIV or AIDS. If TMP-SMX is not tolerated for treatment, other agents, listed in Table 20.3, are possible alternatives. Oxygen, as well as steroids that help reduce lung inflammation, can be used.

Tuberculosis

Tuberculosis is a bacterial infection caused by the mycobacterium tuberculosis. Symptoms include dyspnea, cough, chest pain, fever, night sweats, and weight loss. A Mantoux tuberculin skin test with tuberculin-purified protein derivative should be performed at least yearly in people with HIV infection. Induration of 5 mm or more is considered a positive result in patients with HIV infection (see Chapter 31) and would define the onset of AIDS.

DIAGNOSIS

HIV testing is recommended for people from 15 to 65 years of age at least once, during pregnancy, and after sexual assault (USPSTF, 2019). Those with increased risk outside of this age range should also be screened. Frequent screening should occur for those at higher risk.

Finger stick blood, oral fluid (e.g., OraQuick Rapid HIV test, which tests a swab done of the complete upper and lower outer gums), and serum specimens can be used for HIV testing. Urine can also be tested but is slightly less accurate and is rarely used. Results can be available in less than 20 minutes with the Alere DETERMINE fourth-generation HIV 1 and 2 antigen and antibody combination test or in 1 hour for immunoassay testing. Consumer-controlled test kits (home sample collection devices) can be purchased at drug stores. The blood sample for this testing is mailed to a laboratory as directed. The person then anonymously calls for the results and counseling and referral, if needed.

After infection with HIV, HIV antigen can be detected within 2 weeks of the exposure. Antibodies form within 3 weeks to 3 months, or even longer in some cases. Early-detection HIV tests are available to detect HIV infection as soon as 1 week after potential exposure.

• WORD • BUILDING •

Cytomegalovirus: cyto—cell + megalo—big + virus—poisonous secretion

Table 20.3
Treatment for AIDS-Related Conditions

Opportunistic Infection/Complication	Treatment
Candidiasis	Amphotericin B (Fungizone), fluconazole (Diflucan), isavuconazole (Cresemba), ketoconazole (Nizoral), nystatin (Nyamyc)
Cytomegalovirus retinitis	Ganciclovir (Cytovene)
Hepatitis B virus	Hepatitis B virus vaccine when HIV infection diagnosed, unless already infected with hepatitis B
Hepatitis C virus	Interferon, lamivudine, tenofovir for infection; pegylated interferon and ribavirin
Herpes simplex, herpes zoster, varicella zoster	Acyclovir (Zovirax), valacyclovir, famciclovir, foscarnet
Influenza	Annual influenza vaccine
Mycobacterium avium complex (MAC)	Azithromycin, clarithromycin, ethambutol
Pneumococcal pneumonia	Pneumococcal vaccine when HIV infection diagnosed
Pneumocystis pneumonia (PCP)	Trimethoprim-sulfamethoxazole (Bactrim, Septra, Cotrim), dapsone, atovaquone, pentamidine isethionate
Tuberculosis	Tuberculosis skin test; drug therapy per Centers for Disease Control and Prevention guidelines: pyrazinamide, isoniazid (Laniazid, Isotamine), ethambutol (Myambutol)
AIDS wasting syndrome	*Patient education:* Develop easy meal plan (e.g., favorite foods, meal programs, frozen dinners, cold food to control nausea). Eat frequent small, high-calorie and high-protein meals with snacks daily. Eat low-residue diet for diarrhea control. Use artificial saliva for dry mouth. Numb painful oral sores with ice, popsicles, or topical analgesic; avoid spicy foods. Control odors if they cause nausea. Use antiemetics, appetite stimulants, and/or testosterone. Use nutritional supplements. Use Supplemental Nutrition Assistance Program, community food pantries, or free meal programs as needed. Exercise to increase muscle mass. Rest or listen to music. Take medications prescribed to treat wasting.

HIV Antibody and Antigen Tests

In 2018, the CDC updated recommendations for HIV testing and diagnosis (CDC, 2018a, 2018b). It recommends testing with a U.S. Food and Drug Administration (FDA)-approved antigen/antibody combination (fourth-generation) immunoassay that detects both HIV-1 and HIV-2 antibodies and HIV-1 p24 antigen. Established infection with HIV-1 or HIV-2 and acute infection for HIV-1 is identified. If the test is positive, an antibody immunoassay test to differentiate between HIV-1 and HIV-2 antibodies should be done. If the combination immunoassay is positive, but the antibody differentiation immunoassay is nonreactive or inconclusive, an FDA-approved HIV-1 nucleic acid test should be done for confirmation. The updated algorithm allows earlier detection of HIV and fewer false positives for those within the "window period."

Complete Blood Cell Count/Lymphocyte Count

Patients with HIV are susceptible to leukopenia, lymphopenia, anemia, and thrombocytopenia due to the HIV infection and as a complication of ART. A complete blood cell count (CBC) with a lymphocyte count is obtained and repeated as needed.

CD4 T-Lymphocyte Count

The CD4 T-lymphocyte count is essential for initial evaluation of the status of the immune system and the need for ART. In healthy adults, CD4 levels range from 332 to 1,642 cells/mm^3. In people with HIV disease, CD4 levels drop. After ART begins, a rapid CD4 increase can occur during the first 3 months, with an increase of 50 to 150 cells/mm^3 in the first year. This is followed by an annual increase of 50 to 100 cells/mm^3 until stabilization occurs, which is considered a satisfactory response. CD4 T-lymphocyte counts should be performed before ART begins, 3 months after ART is begun, every 3 to 6 months for the first 2 years, and then annually for consistently suppressed viral load and a CD4 count at 300 to 500 cells/mm^3 (Panel on Antiretroviral Guidelines for Adults and Adolescents [Panel], 2019).

Viral Load Testing

Viral load testing measures the amount of HIV RNA in the plasma. It shows the risk of the disease progressing without treatment, the risk of opportunistic infections, and, most important, response to ART. ART usually produces a 50% decrease in total-body HIV levels within just a few days. Viral load testing should be performed before starting ART and then within 1 month afterward, continuing every 1 to 2 months until viral load is suppressed to less than 200 copies/mL, then every 3 to 4 months for the first 2 years. After 2 years, monitoring for consistently suppressed viral load is done every 6 months or for detectable viremia every 3 months (Panel, 2019). The goal of ART is to obtain and maintain an ultrasensitive, **undetectable viral load**. With ART, an optimal viral load would be less than 20 to 75 copies/mL or below the level of detection, which is under 20 copies/mL. Failure to respond to ART is considered a viral load above 200 copies/mL. Medication resistance testing is recommended for a viral load greater than 1,000 copies/mL.

Genotyping

Genotyping measures resistance to currently available ARV treatments. This guides HCPs in choosing treatment that will be most effective against each individual's virus.

General Tests

Standard serological testing for syphilis is recommended annually in patients who are HIV positive and sexually active. Hepatitis A, B, and C serologies and liver chemistry panels are done because of the high incidence of concurrent hepatitis coinfection in patients who are HIV positive. Coinfections can influence the course of either the patient's HIV infection or the coinfection. Coinfections can also affect HIV treatment options.

THERAPEUTIC MEASURES

The goal of HIV therapy is to suppress the virus to protect health and prevent or delay development of opportunistic diseases and an AIDS diagnosis. In 2019, the Federal Guidelines for the Use of Antiretroviral Agents in Adults and Adolescents Living with HIV was updated (Panel, 2019). It is recommended that all patients with HIV be started on ART, regardless of their CD4 T-lymphocyte count. To increase life expectancy and treatment cost effectiveness, prophylactic treatment for certain opportunistic infections is recommended. These include hepatitis A and hepatitis B, herpes simplex virus, and PCP (see Table 20.3). Other opportunistic infections are treated if they occur.

Antiretroviral Therapy

ARV medications inhibit reproduction of HIV but do not kill it. ARV medication classes have been developed to act on processes specific to HIV (see "Pathophysiology" section). Use of these medications in combination is referred to as *antiretroviral therapy*, or ART. Each ARV medication class affects HIV in a different stage of its life cycle. Initial treatment for most treatment-naive patients is three medications (two-medication regimen sometime used) in at least two classes of treatment categories are used in ART (Table 20.4). This makes medication therapy more effective and reduces drug resistance. Most people treated with ART achieve undetectable viral loads within 6 months or less. Having a durably undetectable viral load (viral load is undetectable for at least 6 months after first undetectable test result) prevents transmission of HIV. It allows CD4 T-lymphocyte counts to rise to protect health and promote quality of life.

The major cause of medication resistance is not taking medications as directed. *Adherence* is the term used to describe taking medications exactly as directed. Promoting adherence is important. Medication resistance can occur when a person with resistant HIV exposes someone else with HIV to resistant HIV with unprotected sex or shared injected drug use.

> ### NURSING CARE TIP
> Reinforce education to patients that it is essential to take every medication every day as ordered. Missing just 10% of doses (1 out of 10) decreases effectiveness to about 80%, depending on the drug. This means that, if a patient is taking three to seven pills each day, missing one to two pills a week will decrease the medication's effectiveness by 20%. When ART is interrupted, HIV can reemerge and multiply again to detectable levels in the blood.

Anti-HIV medications can have side effects. If they occur, the medication regimen can be changed or interventions used to help control side effects. Explain potential side effects. Encourage patients to report them immediately.

Table 20.4
Antiretroviral Medications for HIV Infection

Medication Class/Action

Nonnucleoside Reverse Transcriptase Inhibitors (NNRTIs)
Block reverse transcriptase enzyme activity to prevent conversion of HIV RNA to HIV DNA.

Examples	*Nursing Implications*
delavirdine mesylate (Rescriptor) efavirenz (Sustiva) etravirine (Intelence) nevirapine (Viramune, Viramune XR) rilpivirine (Edurant)	Monitor for rash (especially first month); Stevens-Johnson syndrome can occur, requiring discontinuation of the drug. Can be life threatening. *Education:* • Report rash immediately. • Monitor white blood cell count, liver tests, especially with history of hepatitis B or C.

Nucleoside/Nucleotide Reverse Transcriptase Inhibitors (NRTIs/NtRTIs)
Block reverse transcriptase enzyme by binding to the enzyme to prevent conversion of HIV RNA to HIV DNA.

Examples	*Nursing Implications*
abacavir sulfate (Ziagen)* abacavir sulfate/lamivudine (Epzicom) didanosine (Videx, Videx EC) emtricitabine (Emtriva) lamivudine (Epivir) lamivudine/zidovudine (Combivir) stavudine (Zerit, Zerit XR) tenofovir disoproxil fumarate (Viread)** abacavir sulfate/lamivudine/zidovudine (Trizivir) emtricitabine/tenofovir disoproxil fumarate (Truvada) zidovudine (Retrovir)	Monitor for peripheral neuropathy, bone marrow suppression, lactic acidosis, and kidney and liver function. *Report flu-like symptoms immediately as a life-threatening condition can develop. **Monitor for hepatomegaly with steatosis and for lactic acidosis, which can be fatal, especially in women. **Education: Take 2 hours before or 1 hour after didanosine.

Protease Inhibitors
Bind to active site of HIV protease enzyme (cuts reproduced HIV strands), interrupting formation of mature viral particles.

Examples	*Nursing Implications*
atazanavir sulfate (Reyataz) darunavir (Prezista) darunavir/cobicistat (Prezcobix) fosamprenavir calcium (Lexiva)* indinavir sulfate (Crixivan)** lopinavir/ritonavir (Kaletra) nelfinavir mesylate (Viracept) ritonavir (Norvir) saquinavir mesylate (Invirase) tipranavir (Aptivus)	Manage gastrointestinal symptoms. Monitor lab results. Watch for increased bleeding in patients with hemophilia. *Report rash. *Should not be given if patient is allergic to sulfa. **Education: Importance of hydration (at least 48 oz of liquids in 24 hours).

Fusion Inhibitors
Block HIV-1 fusion with the CD4 cell membrane to prevent cell entry.

Examples	*Nursing Implications*
enfuvirtide (Fuzeon)	*Education*: • Subcutaneous injection technique and injection site rotation. • If dizzy, do not drive.

Continued

Table 20.4
Antiretroviral Medications for HIV Infection—cont'd

Medication Class/Action

Cellular Chemokine Receptor Type 5 (CCR5) Antagonists
Block CCR5 receptor preventing HIV-1 entry into CD4 cells.

Examples	*Nursing Implications*
maraviroc (Celsentri, Selzentry)	Monitor for liver problems.

Post-Attachment Inhibitors
Blocks binding to CCR5 and CXCR4 coreceptors after HIV-1 binds to CD4 receptor. For adults with multidrug resistant HIV-1 infection failing current antiretroviral regimen.

Examples	*Nursing Implications*
ibalizumab (Trogarzo)	Monitor post intravenous infusion for side effects.

Integrase Inhibitors
Block HIV from combining with its genetic code so more copies of itself cannot be made.

Examples	*Nursing Implications*
bictegravir (in combination form only) dolutegravir (Tivicay) elvitegravir (in combination form only) raltegravir (Isentress, Isentress HD)	*Education*: Side effects to report.

Combination Agents
Multiclass combined single tablet regimens

Examples	*Nursing Implications*
bictegravir/tenofovir alafenamide/emtricitabine (Biktarvy) dolutegravir/lamivudine (Dovato) dolutegravir/abacavir/lamivudine (Triumeq) dolutegravir (Tivicay) or raltegravir (Isenstress) plus one of these: emtricitabine + tenofovir alafenamide (Descovy); emtricitabine + tenofovir disoproxil fumarate (Truvada); emtricitabine + tenofovir disoproxil fumarate; lamivudine + tenofovir disoproxil fumarate (Temixys, Cimduo)	See individual agents above. Patient adherence is key to efficacy. Combination medications increase patient adherence with fewer tablets to take.

Rashes (e.g., from TMP-SMX) or abdominal pain (e.g., from azidothymidine [AZT; Retrovir]) can be serious or life threatening.

When someone with a suppressed immune system (very low CD4 T-lymphocyte count) is started on ART, the person can experience immune reconstitution syndrome. The patient's immune system can be greatly improving, but the patient feels worse. When the patient's immune system was severely damaged, immune responses were too weak or absent to produce the signs of an existing infection. When immune function improves, the immune system begins to fight off the infections already present in the body, resulting in symptoms. This serious, sometimes fatal condition can occur a few weeks after ART starts. Educate the patient to report immediately any symptoms of opportunistic infections after starting therapy. This will allow for prompt diagnosis and treatment of the infection which can save the person's life.

Treatment as Prevention
Research has shown that ART that results in undetectable blood levels prevents transmission of HIV sexually. Those infected with HIV who take ART as prescribed and achieve and maintain an undetectable viral load have effectively no risk of sexually transmitting the virus to an HIV-negative partner (CDC, 2020d). It takes 1 to 6 months of ART to achieve undetectable viral loads plus 6 months of maintained undetectable viral levels after the first undetected test result (known as durably undetected) to effectively have no risk of transmitting HIV sexually (Eisinger et al, 2019).

The Undetectable = Untransmittable (U = U) Campaign (Prevention Access Campaign, 2020; see www.preventionaccess.org) was developed to promote this important information. It is giving hope to those with HIV that they can live healthy lives without fear of transmitting HIV. Many worldwide health organizations are publicly sharing this message to reduce the stigma associated with being HIV positive. This may encourage more people to be tested and treated to prevent the transmission of HIV.

Nursing Process for the Adult Patient With HIV/AIDS

People with HIV/AIDS continue to face discrimination, rejection, and isolation, even from relatives and friends. The Americans with Disabilities Act makes discrimination toward patients with HIV/AIDS illegal. Being knowledgeable about the transmission of HIV allows appropriate interaction with the patient. Take care to maintain confidentiality per HIPAA. Patients with HIV may choose not to share their diagnosis with family or friends.

Nursing Diagnoses, Planning, and Implementation

HIV/AIDS can affect every body system and aspect of a person's life. Nurses can positively influence a patient with HIV/AIDS with a nonjudgmental approach, empathy, and psychological support. All patients with HIV/AIDS will need protection from infections and education (see Patient Teaching Guidelines: Signs and Symptoms of Opportunistic Infections to Report" in your online resources). Other types of care and nursing diagnoses are individualized to a patient's symptoms. Examples are presented. See "Nursing Care Plan for the Patient With HIV/AIDS."

> **Deficient Knowledge related to inadequate information about the chronic, potentially life-threatening nature of HIV**
>
> **EXPECTED OUTCOME:** The patient will state understanding of HIV infection, treatment, and disease progression.

- Include the patient's family or caregivers with patient's permission in educational sessions and determine everyone's baseline knowledge *to develop an educational plan that allows the family to assist the patient.*
- Educate patient on HIV infection, symptoms, transmission and prevention, progression, health and safety precautions including food and water safety (see Table 20.5), and treatment *to empower patient to manage condition and reduce fear of transmitting HIV, which decreases social isolation.*
- Discuss medication regimens, including taking medications exactly as instructed and not missing doses; use of a memory aid such as an alarm watch; taking a

---

Nursing Care Plan for the Patient With HIV/AIDS

Nursing Diagnosis: *Ineffective Protection* related to deficient immunity
Expected Outcomes: The patient will remain free of infection. The patient and/or caregiver explains precautions to take to prevent infection.
Evaluation of Outcomes: Is the patient free of infection? Does the patient and/or caregiver explain precautions for preventing infection?

Intervention	Rationale	Evaluation
Identify patient's risk factors, such as CD4 T-lymphocyte counts, skin condition, and portals of entry for infections.	*Status of risk factors provides input for plan for care.*	Does patient have risk factors present?
Inform patient and caregiver of ways to avoid transmission of microorganisms, including excellent hand hygiene/bathing, washing toothbrush, not sharing grooming items, using clean dishes, and avoiding others when ill (Table 20.5).	*It is difficult for the weakened immune system to fight opportunistic infections.*	Does patient and caregiver state understanding of ways to prevent transmission?
Promote skin integrity with frequent turning, optimum mobilization, use of specialized mattress and chair pads, gentle washing/drying of skin, and application of emollients as needed to keep skin dry.	*Skin is the body's first line of defense.*	Does patient's skin remain intact and infection free?

Table 20.5
Patient Education: Preventing Opportunistic Infections

Environmental/Occupational	
To protect from:	*Consider risk and prevent exposure to infectious agents from:*
Tuberculosis	Health-care settings, correctional facilities, homeless shelters
Cytomegalovirus (CMV), cryptosporidiosis, hepatitis A, giardiasis	Child-care settings: Wash hands after diaper changing/body fluid contact.
Cryptosporidiosis, toxoplasmosis, salmonellosis, campylobacteriosis	Animal contact: Exposure possible from veterinary work, pet stores, farms.
Cryptosporidiosis, toxoplasmosis, histoplasmosis, coccidioidomycosis	Gardening/soil contact: Avoid gardening/houseplant care or bird-roosting site or soil, cleaning chicken coops. Wear gloves and mask, and wash hands after soil contact.

Food/Water Safety	
To prevent or protect from:	*General measures for home or restaurants:*
Foodborne and waterborne infections caused by bacterial, viral, protozoal, or parasitic pathogens	Food handlers must practice excellent hand hygiene. Discard food past expiration date and dented or swollen cans. Control insects and rodents to prevent food contamination. Disinfect kitchen counters and food preparation appliances (e.g., cutting boards, can openers). Avoid cross-contamination of foods with uncooked meat on food preparation surfaces. Do not thaw foods at room temperature, as freezing does not kill bacteria in foods. Maintain adequate refrigeration and cooking temperatures. *Foods to avoid:* Buffets and salad bars Cheese (e.g., soft cheeses, such as feta, brie, camembert, blue veined, queso fresco, which can harbor bacteria) Dairy (e.g., unpasteurized milk/dairy products and fruit juice, raw seed sprouts) Eggs (e.g., raw/undercooked eggs and foods with raw eggs, such as hollandaise sauce, Caesar dressing, mayonnaise, uncooked batters, ice cream, eggnog) Meat if not cooked until internal temperature is 180°F (82.2°C) for poultry or 165°F (73.8°C) for red meats with no trace of pink Seafood raw or undercooked
Cryptosporidiosis, giardiasis	Foods to avoid or cook until steaming hot: delicatessen foods, leftovers, meat spreads, ready-to-eat, and refrigerated pâtés.
Hepatitis A, campylobacteriosis, *Escherichia coli*, giardiasis, leptospirosis, norovirus, rotavirus, shigellosis	*Water safety:* Use safe water supply or, when unsure, boil water for 1 minute for drinking or making ice cubes. Drink bottled water purified from reverse osmosis, filtration through absolute 1-micrometer filter, or distillation (only safe methods) in areas where water sources are known not to be safe. (For information, visit www.bottledwater.org.) Bottled or canned carbonated soft drinks, commercially packaged unrefrigerated beverages, pasteurized beverages, and beers are safe. Avoid beverages made from tap water in public places in areas where water sources are known not to be safe. Avoid public drinking fountains and water directly from lakes or rivers.

Table 20.5

Patient Education: Preventing Opportunistic Infections—cont'd

Sexual Relations	
To protect from:	*General measures:*
Sexually transmitted infections, herpes simplex virus, CMV, human papillomavirus, resistant HIV strain	Always use latex (if no allergy) condom for every sex act.
Intestinal infections: amebiasis, hepatitis A, cryptosporidiosis, shigellosis, campylobacteriosis, giardiasis	Avoid oral–anal contact or use dental dams; use latex gloves for hand–anal contact; wash hands and genitals with warm soapy water after contact.
Hepatitis A and B	Get hepatitis A and hepatitis B vaccines.

Injection Drug Use	
To protect from:	*General measures:*
Hepatitis A, hepatitis B, hepatitis C, resistant HIV strain	Get hepatitis A and B vaccines. Stop using injection drugs and enter substance abuse treatment. If unable to stop, never reuse or share syringes, needles, water, or drug preparation equipment. If shared, use bleach and water to clean equipment. Use sterile syringes from pharmacies or community syringe exchange programs and dispose of safely. Use clean water and equipment and new alcohol swab.

Pet-Related Issues	
To protect from:	*General measures:*
Cryptosporidium, Salmonella, Campylobacter spp. infection	Avoid pet feces/diarrhea; seek veterinary treatment for pet's diarrheal illness. Counsel on pet contact risks but recognize emotional benefits of pets and do not suggest parting with pet. Immunize pets. For new pets, avoid those younger than 6 months old (and cats younger than 1 year old); obtain pets from known sanitary source; avoid strays; wash hands after handling pets.
Toxoplasmosis, *Bartonella* spp. infection, salmonellosis, campylobacteriosis	Cat ownership increases risk from litter box cleaning, scratches, bites, licking, and fleas. If cleaning litter box, wear gloves and wash hands well afterward. Keep cats indoors to avoid hunting infected prey.
Cryptococcus neoformans, Mycobacterium avium, Histoplasma capsulatum infection	Unhealthy birds can transmit infectious organisms.
Salmonellosis	Avoid reptiles, turtles, chicks, and ducklings.
Mycobacterium marinum infection	Wear gloves for cleaning aquariums.

Table 20.5
Patient Education: Preventing Opportunistic Infections—cont'd

Pet-Related Issues

To protect from:

Opportunistic pathogens, food-borne and waterborne infections

General measures:

Consult health-care providers on travel to developing countries.
Traveler's diarrhea prophylaxis is not recommended. Carry supply of antimicrobial agent to take for diarrhea.
Consider prophylaxis for other types of exposures.
Avoid raw fruits, vegetables, raw/undercooked seafood or meat, tap water, ice from tap water, unpasteurized milk/dairy products, and items from street vendors.
Safe items include steaming-hot foods, self-peeled fruits, bottled (especially carbonated) beverages, hot coffee/tea, beer, wine, and water boiled 1 minute.
Avoid soil/sand contact by wearing shoes, using beach towels.

Source: Panel on Opportunistic Infections in HIV-Infected Adults and Adolescents. (2020). *Guidelines for the prevention and treatment of opportunistic infections in HIV-infected adults and adolescents: Recommendations from the Centers for Disease Control and Prevention, the National Institutes of Health, and the HIV Medicine Association of the Infectious Diseases Society of America.* https://clinicalinfo.hiv.gov/sites/default/files/guidelines/documents/Adult_OI.pdf.

---

missed dose as soon as possible unless it is too close to the time of the next dose, as doses should not be doubled; medication side effects and promptly contacting the HCP for side effects or questions, *as understanding medication regimens is vital—missing doses could cause therapy failure because viral loads can then rise and resistance to treatment develop.*

Imbalanced Nutrition: Less Than Body Requirements related to anorexia, diarrhea, nutrient malabsorption, nausea or vomiting, oral sores, or side effects from medications

EXPECTED OUTCOME: The patient will maintain a normal BMI.

- Instruct patient to document weight weekly *to monitor effectiveness of interventions.*
- Provide interventions promoting adequate nutrition (See "Nutrition Notes: Nourishing the Patient with HIV or AIDS") *to maintain normal BMI.*
- Use antiemetics as ordered *to control nausea and vomiting.*
- Encourage exercise *to maintain muscle mass* ("Evidence-Based Practice") *and promote relaxation, sleep, and a sense of control and well-being.*

Impaired Oral Mucous Membrane Integrity

EXPECTED OUTCOME: The patient will maintain intact mucous membranes.

- Explain importance of daily mouth care using a soft toothbrush *to maintain oral health and prevent injury to mucous membranes.*
- Encourage patient who smokes to quit *to reduce risk of oral thrush.*
- Explain use of antifungal medication as prescribed *to treat oral or esophageal candidiasis.*
- Discuss use of a numbing agent, such as lidocaine viscous (Xylocaine Viscous) *to decrease pain during eating.*

Fatigue

EXPECTED OUTCOME: The patient will be able to perform desired tasks without injury.

- Identify potential causes of fatigue for patient such as infections, medications, anemia, dehydration, depression, or poor nutrition *to plan interventions.*
- Alternate periods of activity and rest *to manage fatigue.*
- Plan tasks that use more energy when patient will be most energetic *to protect the patient from injury.*

Risk for Situational Low Self-Esteem

EXPECTED OUTCOME: The patient will state feelings of positive self-esteem.

- Provide a climate of acceptance *to promote a trusting relationship.*
- Provide emotional and spiritual support *to improve the patient's self-esteem.*
- Encourage patient to express feelings, when ready, *to help identify positive aspects of self.*
- Administer tesamorelin (Egrifta), a synthetic growth hormone–releasing hormone, as prescribed *to treat acquired lipodystrophy (abnormal fat distribution).*

Evaluation

Patient goals are met if the patient remains free from infection; explains precautions for preventing infection; states understanding of HIV infection, treatment, and disease progression; maintains a normal BMI; maintains intact mucous membranes; performs desired tasks without injury; and states feelings of positive self-esteem. If the disease should progress, goals are met if the patient's needs are being met and the patient's dignity is maintained.

> **PRACTICE ANALYSIS TIP**
> **Linking NCLEX-PN® to Practice**
> The LPN/LVN will provide emotional support to client.

Nutrition Notes
Nourishing the Patient With HIV or AIDS

Nutrition has preventive and therapeutic functions for patients with HIV or AIDS. Those who are well nourished stay healthier. They are better able to resist opportunistic infections and tolerate the side effects of treatment. Anorexia, diarrhea, nutrient malabsorption, nausea or vomiting, oral sores, or side effects from medications can cause the loss of lean body mass (Total weight – Fat weight).

A dietitian should be consulted for the nutritional care of the patient with HIV or AIDS. Interventions to optimize nutrition include:

- Reviewing nutritional status for adequacy and identified concerns related to disease or treatment.
- Optimizing the diet with consideration to side effects of disease and treatment should include meeting calorie needs, adequate protein intake, nutrient dense foods, dietary fiber, and food safety.
- Consult dietitian for dietary changes to reduce diarrhea (e.g., low-residue diet, no dairy products, no spicy foods, no caffeine or alcohol).
- Seek resources from community health programs to optimize nutritional support (e.g., food pantries, Meals on Wheels).

Every effort should be made to provide nourishment orally (see "Nutrition Notes: Treating Problems Related to Nutrition," in Chapter 11). Helpful strategies include the following:

- Offering small, frequent meals
- Serving food cold or at room temperature
- Using a variety of seasonings
- Modifying texture to accommodate chewing difficulty or oral lesions
- Providing high calorie high protein nutritional supplements

Reference: Ellis, E. (Reviewed 2021, November). Nutrition Tips to Keep the Immune System Strong for People with HIV-AIDS. *Academy of Nutrition and Dietetics.* Retrieved December 9, 2021 from https://www.eatright.org/health/diseases-and-conditions/hiv-aids/nutrition-tips-to-keep-the-immune-system-strong-for-people-with-hiv-aids.

Evidence-Based Practice
Clinical Question

Does cardiovascular disease (CVD) have more negative health implications for people living with HIV as compared to people who are not living with HIV?

Evidence

A systematic review of 16 studies found that people living with HIV have a twofold increased risk of having an acute myocardial infarction (AMI) as compared to people with similar risks who did not have HIV. The authors also found that hypertension, tobacco use, and hyperlipidemia significantly increased the risk of AMI. Hypertension increased AMI risk by 20%, while hyperlipidemia increased the risk by 9% and tobacco use increased it by 9% as well.

Implications for Nursing Practice

Whole-person care is critical for persons living with HIV. It is not enough to focus only on medication adherence. Focusing on lifestyle modifications including exercise and diet, along with tobacco cessation, are very important to help lower CVD risk factors.

Reference: Rao, S., Galaviz, K., Gay, H., Wei, J., Armstrong, W., Rio, C., Narayah, V., & Ali, M. (2019). Factors as sociated with excess myocardial infarction risk in HIV-infected adults: A systematic review and meta-analysis. *Journal of Acquired Immunodeficiency Syndrome, 81*(2): 224–230. https://doi.org/10.1097/QAI.0000000000001996.

CLINICAL JUDGMENT

Chloe Rogers, age 19, is diagnosed as HIV positive. She is tearful and asks many questions.

1. How do you answer the following questions:
   a. "Am I going to die?"
   b. "How is AIDS diagnosed?"
   c. "Can my boyfriend get it?"
2. What food and water safety methods do you explain to her?
3. Later, Chloe loses weight and becomes malnourished. What interventions do you use to promote adequate nutrition for her?

Suggested answers are at the end of the chapter.

CUE RECOGNITION 20.2

You are assisting with skin care for Mrs. Dexter, a resident with HIV disease who takes ART. You notice a red rash on both of her inner arms and then collect data and photograph the rash for documentation. What action do you take?

Suggested answers are at the end of the chapter.

Patient Perspective

Aimee

As a productive, single mother of three, I never expected to hear the term HIV infected, but at 45 years of age, that diagnosis became my reality. In February 2016, I had viral symptoms that progressively manifested into AIDS, and my world turned upside down in a split second. I was immediately consumed with shame and fear, but most important, a small glimpse of hope. Within weeks of my diagnosis, my body responded as expected to treatment, and my psychological state healed at literally the same pace.

What I eventually discovered is that an 8-month-long sexual relationship was with an individual of high risk. He was diagnosed with HIV shortly after we ended our relationship and left "the call" up to the clinic that helped him. They never called. Almost 3 years later, I was on my deathbed. My HIV doctor confirmed that I would have died had it been 10 to 15 years earlier, before effective therapies became available.

What I would like for people to learn from my story is that everyone should be screened for HIV according to the guidelines. People with HIV disease, whose antiretroviral therapy is effective and who continue to take their medication as prescribed, not only can become undetectable (virus undetected in blood) but also are no longer able to transmit the virus sexually (U = U, Undetectable = Untransmittable). It's imperative that medical professionals treat people living with HIV as human beings. We are not contagious in every aspect of casual contact. We feel small nuanced stigma, and it's a human rights failure on every level when our treatment is handled in any other manner. With today's medical advancements in HIV treatment, I take one pill a day, my virus is undetectable, and I'm back to doing things that I love, like surfing and skateboarding. Life is good!

Data Collection

Ongoing monitoring is important for the patient with HIV/AIDS to detect problems early. Health history information is obtained (Box 20.3). A physical examination provides data on the effects of HIV/AIDS and ART. Monitoring the patient's pain, if present, is ongoing. Many patients with HIV do not have pain related to HIV. Signs and symptoms of opportunistic infections are noted. Oral or esophageal candidiasis is more common in the late stage of AIDS. The painful lesions interfere with swallowing and nutrition. Identify if the patient with AIDS smokes, as there is an increased incidence of oral thrush (candidiasis). Varied skin conditions can occur with HIV infection. Some medications can cause skin infections that can be life threatening. Identify and report skin rashes immediately.

Changes in self-esteem and self-concept occur from several of the effects of HIV infection. Patients often experience changes in their relationships with others and in day-to-day activities such as work. Major weight loss and abnormal fat distribution from protease inhibitors, a condition called *acquired lipodystrophy*, can cause dramatic changes in appearance that alter body image and reduce self-esteem.

> **LEARNING TIP**
>
> Key points to remember:
> - HIV and AIDS are disease labels, not people labels.
> - Each person reacts to an HIV or AIDS diagnosis differently.
> - It is not the HIV that ultimately causes death; it is an opportunistic infection or disease that the compromised immune system is unable to fight off, even with medical intervention.
> - With today's antiretroviral therapy, HIV has changed from being a life-ending infection to a chronically managed disease.
> - With ART, a person who achieves and then maintains an undetectable viral load for 6 months and continues to do so is effectively unable to transmit HIV sexually, thus reducing the fear and stigma of being HIV positive.

Box 20.3

Data Collection: Health History Information for HIV/AIDS

- Demographic data (e.g., gender identity, sexual orientation, age, marital status, occupation, residence, pets)
- Date of diagnosis of HIV or AIDS
- Height/weight (also weight loss)
- Allergies
- Current health status and concerns
- Immunizations
- Past medical history and surgeries
- Infections/cancers (see Box 20.1)
- Family history
- Medication history of antiretrovirals used with reason for discontinuing
- History of any gaps in ARV use
- Current prescribed medications, over-the-counter medications, supplements
- For females, gynecological history, last Pap test
- Sexually transmitted infections and treatments
- Social and sexual history, risk behaviors, safe sex practices
- Needlestick/blood exposure, injection drug use, blood transfusions/treatment for hemophilia
- Lifestyle (e.g., nutrition, exercise, sleep)
- Tobacco use
- Drug and alcohol use
- Occupational history

RESOURCES

Financial resources may need to be addressed so that food and medications can be obtained. Treatment can be expensive, and the patient may be unable to work. With ART, many people are able to continue working. The Ryan White Comprehensive AIDS Resources Emergency Act provides funding for some services and treatment-related needs. Knowledge of local resources and referrals to financial resources and support groups are very important.

If an HIV infection progresses, the patient may need more care from caregivers and home health care nurses ("Home Health Hints"). Support services should be identified, such as community AIDS organizations, Meals on Wheels, respite care services, community mental health services, and Internet support groups. When a patient is terminal, comfort care and emotional support for the family are essential. Hospice care can be helpful at this time.

Home Health Hints

- When providing patient care, perform hand hygiene and wash hands frequently; follow standard precautions.
- Observe caregivers for role strain. Respite care may be helpful to reduce caregiver stress.
- Educate the family of a patient with AIDS on which symptoms to report to the HCP or nurse immediately: fever; increased dyspnea; pain; change in sputum production; upper respiratory tract infection; pneumonia; respiratory distress syndrome; diarrhea five times a day or more for 5 days; uncontrolled weight loss greater than 10 pounds in the past month; persistent headaches; falling; seizures; mental status changes, including memory loss and personality changes; rashes and skin changes; difficulty swallowing; and problems with urination.
- To dispose of sharps (e.g., needles, lancets, razors), use a red biohazard container if provided. If not, use a rigid labeled container such as a tin can with a sealable lid. Add 1:10 bleach solution to disinfect the sharps. Tape the lid. Place in a bag and dispose of in the trash.
- Dispose of contaminated articles by sealing them in a plastic bag and placing in the trash.
- Educate patients with HIV/AIDS and their families on proper cleaning and disinfecting of the home to prevent infection:
  - Use disinfectant to (1) disinfect body fluid spill areas, (2) clean toilet seats and bathroom fixtures, and (3) clean inside the refrigerator to avoid mold growth.
- Flush body fluids, solid body waste, and contaminated solutions down toilet.
- Rinse clothing and then wash separately from other clothes with 1 cup of bleach if soiled with blood, urine, feces, or semen.
- Wash dishes and silverware in hot, soapy water, and rinse thoroughly or place in dishwasher. Patients with HIV/AIDS do not require separate sets of dishes or silverware.

Key Points

- AIDS is the late phase of a chronic immune function disorder. This disorder is caused by infection with HIV. AIDS develops after a long period of untreated HIV infection and can be fatal.
- HIV is transmitted from person to person through certain body fluids from a person infected with HIV. These fluids include blood, semen, preseminal fluid, vaginal secretions, rectal fluids, and breast milk. HIV can be transmitted to others within 2 to 4 weeks of initial infection and then without treatment throughout all phases of HIV infection and AIDS.
- Diagnostic tests for HIV include beginning with an FDA-approved fourth-generation antigen/antibody combination immunoassay that detects both HIV-1 and HIV-2 antibodies and HIV-1 p24 antigen. If the test is positive, an antibody immunoassay test to differentiate between HIV-1 and HIV-2 antibodies should be done. If the combination immunoassay is positive but the antibody differentiation immunoassay is nonreactive or inconclusive, an FDA-approved HIV-1 nucleic acid test should be done for confirmation.
- Additional diagnostic tests include complete blood count, CD4 T-lymphocyte count, viral load testing, genotyping, and standard serological testing for syphilis.
- With today's ART, HIV has changed from being a life-ending infection to a chronically managed disease.
- With ART, a person who achieves and then maintains an undetectable viral load for 6 months and continues to do so is effectively unable to transmit HIV sexually, thus reducing the fear and stigma of being HIV positive.
- It is recommended that all patients with HIV be started on ART, regardless of their CD4 T-lymphocyte count. To increase life expectancy and treatment cost effectiveness, prophylactic treatment for certain opportunistic infections is recommended. These include hepatitis A and hepatitis B, herpes simplex virus, and pneumocystis pneumonia. Other opportunistic infections are treated if they occur. Mycobacterium avium complex treatment is not recommended unless there is a delay in ART initiation.
- Research has shown that ART results in undetectable blood levels that prevents transmission of HIV sexually.

So, those infected with HIV who take ART as prescribed and achieve and maintain an undetectable viral load have effectively no risk of sexually transmitting the virus to an HIV-negative partner.

- Extensive education is required for patients to understand the chronic, potentially life-threatening nature of HIV. ART adherence is crucial to preventing drug resistance and reducing the risk of disease progression.

SUGGESTED ANSWERS TO CHAPTER EXERCISES

Cue Recognition

20.1: Wash the exposure site with soap and water immediately. Then notify your supervisor and seek immediate medical care following your agency exposure protocol.

20.2: Notify the HCP, as it could be a life-threatening side effect to ART.

Critical Thinking & Clinical Judgment

Chloe Rogers

1. a. "There is no cure for HIV/AIDS; however, medications are available that make an HIV infection a manageable chronic disease. Research continues in the search for a cure."
   b. "AIDS is diagnosed when CD4 T-lymphocyte counts are below 200 cells/mm^3 and/or an opportunistic infection or cancer, as defined by the CDC, is present in an HIV-infected person."
   c. "If you do not have durably undetectable viral loads, then your boyfriend could become infected through exposure to your blood and vaginal or rectal secretions. You can learn about transmission, preventive measures, and undetectable viral loads. Then you can discuss it with him. If you have had unprotected sex, he should be tested for HIV."

2. Food handlers must maintain good hand-washing and hygiene practices. Discard food that is past the expiration date and dented or swollen cans. Ensure adequate refrigeration and cooking of food. Control insects and rodents to prevent food contamination. Drink purified bottled water if you live in an area with unsafe drinking water. Use a safe water supply or boil water for 1 minute when unsure. Avoid unpasteurized milk, dairy products, and fruit juice, as well as raw seed sprouts. Avoid raw and undercooked eggs, meats, and seafood (see Table 20.5).

3. Eat three to four high-calorie, high-lean protein meals and snacks daily. Eat a low-residue diet if diarrhea is present. Develop an easy meal plan. Use antiemetics, if needed. Numb any painful oral sores. Request a referral for Supplemental Nutrition Assistance Program (SNAP)/free meal program if necessary. Engage in regular exercise.

Additional Resources

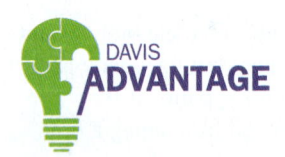

Go to Davis Advantage to complete your learning: strengthen understanding, apply your knowledge, and prepare for the Next Gen NCLEX®.

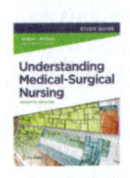

A Study Guide is also available.

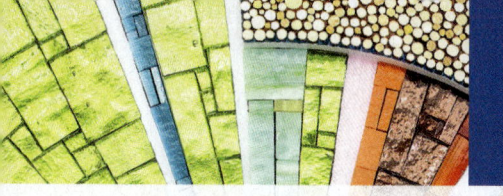

UNIT FIVE Understanding the Cardiovascular System

CHAPTER 21
Cardiovascular System Function, Data Collection, and Therapeutic Measures

Michele Dickson, Janice L. Bradford

KEY TERMS

arrhythmia (uh-RITH-mee-ah)
atherosclerosis (ATH-er-oh-skleh-ROH-sis)
bruit (brew-EE)
claudication (KLAW-dih-KAY-shun)
clubbing (KLUH-bing)
endothelium (EN-do-THEE-lee-um)
hyperkalemia (HY-per-kuh-LEE-mee-ah)
hypokalemia (HY-poh-kuh-LEE-mee-ah)
hypomagnesemia (HY-poh-MAG-neh-SEE-mee-ah)
ischemic (is-KEY-mik)
murmur (MUR-mur)
pericardial friction rub (PER-ih-KAR-dee-uhl FRIK-shun rub)
poikilothermy (POY-kih-loh-THER-mee)
point of maximum impulse (POYNT of MAKS-ih-muhm IM-puls)
preload (PREE-lohd)
pulse deficit (PULS DEF-ih-sit)
Starling's law (STAR-lings law)
sternotomy (stir-NAH-tuh-mee)
thrill (THRIL)

CHAPTER CONCEPTS

Caring
Perfusion
Teaching and learning

LEARNING OUTCOMES

1. Identify the normal anatomy of the cardiovascular system.
2. Explain the normal function of the cardiovascular system.
3. List data to collect when caring for a patient with a disorder of the cardiovascular system.
4. Identify tests commonly performed to diagnose disorders of the cardiovascular system.
5. Plan nursing care for patients undergoing diagnostic tests for cardiovascular disorders.
6. Describe current therapeutic measures for disorders of the cardiovascular system.
7. Describe preoperative and postoperative care for patients undergoing cardiac surgery.

NORMAL CARDIOVASCULAR SYSTEM ANATOMY AND PHYSIOLOGY

The cardiovascular system consists of the heart, blood, and vessels (including arteries, capillaries, and veins). Its function is to perfuse the organs and tissues with blood.

Heart

Cardiac Structure and Function

LOCATION OF THE HEART. The heart is located in the mediastinum within the thoracic cavity. It is enclosed by three membranes. The outermost is the fibrous pericardium, which forms a loose-fitting pericardial sac around the heart. The second, or middle, layer is the parietal pericardium, a serous membrane that lines the fibrous layer. The third and innermost layer, the visceral pericardium or epicardium, is a serous membrane on the surface of the heart muscle. Between the parietal and visceral layers is serous fluid, which prevents friction as the heart beats.

STRUCTURE OF THE HEART AND CORONARY BLOOD VESSELS. The walls of the four chambers of the heart are made of cardiac muscle (myocardium) and are lined with endocardium, smooth epithelial tissue that prevents abnormal clotting. The epithelium also covers the valves of the heart and continues into blood vessels, at which point it is called the **endothelium.** Coronary circulation provides oxygenated blood throughout the myocardium and returns deoxygenated blood to the right atrium via the coronary sinus. The two main coronary arteries

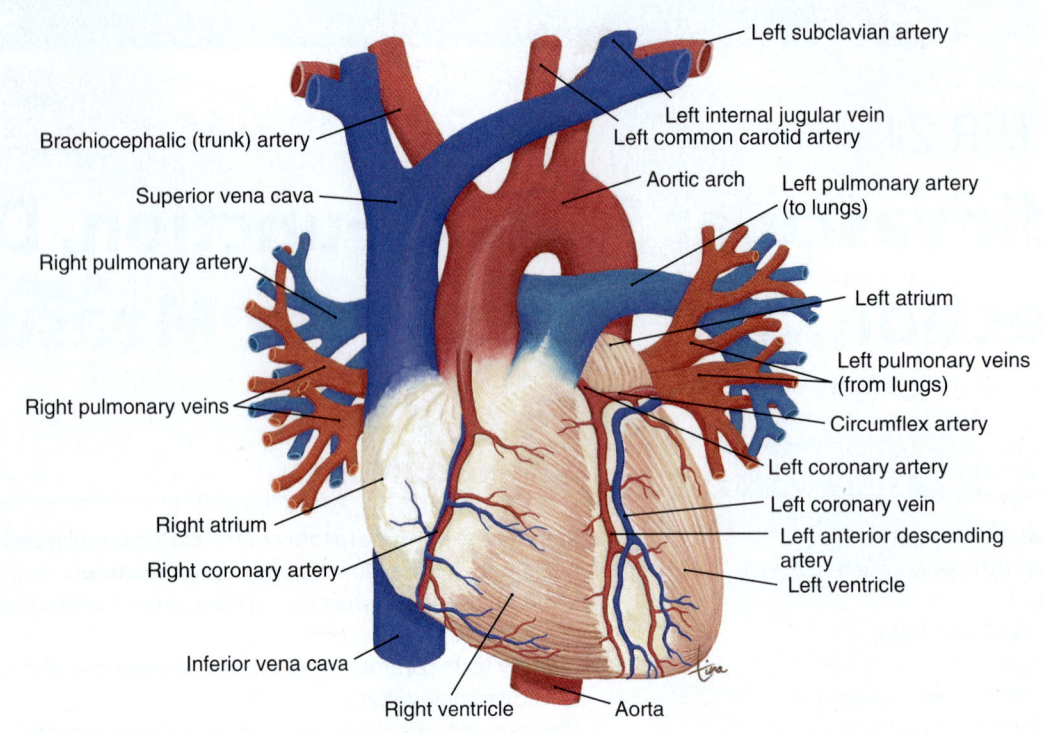

FIGURE 21.1 Anterior view of the heart and major blood vessels.

are the first branches of the ascending aorta, just outside the left ventricle (Fig. 21.1).

The superior chambers of the heart are the thin-walled right and left atria, separated by the interatrial septum. The lower chambers are the thicker-walled right and left ventricles, separated by the interventricular septum. Each septum is made of myocardium that forms a common wall between the two chambers.

CORONARY BLOOD FLOW. The right atrium receives deoxygenated blood from the coronary sinus, from the upper body by way of the superior vena cava, and from the lower body by way of the inferior vena cava (see Fig. 21.1). This blood flows from the right atrium through the tricuspid valve into the right ventricle. Backflow during ventricular systole (contraction and emptying) is prevented by the tricuspid, or right atrioventricular (AV) valve (Fig. 21.2). The right ventricle pumps blood through the pulmonary semilunar valve to the lungs by way of the pulmonary trunk and arteries. The pulmonary semilunar valve prevents backflow of blood into the right ventricle during ventricular diastole (relaxation and filling).

The left atrium receives oxygenated blood from the lungs by way of the four pulmonary veins. This blood flows through the mitral, or left AV valve (also called the *bicuspid valve*) into the left ventricle. The mitral valve prevents backflow of blood into the left atrium during ventricular systole. The left ventricle pumps blood through the aortic semilunar valve to the body by way of the aorta. The aortic valve prevents backflow of blood into the left ventricle during ventricular diastole.

The tricuspid and mitral valves consist of three and two cusps, respectively. These cusps, or flaps, are connective tissue covered by endocardium. They are anchored to the floor of the ventricle by the chordae tendineae and papillary muscles. The papillary muscles are columns of myocardium that contract along with the rest of the ventricular myocardium. This contraction pulls on the chordae tendineae and prevents hyperextension of the AV valves during ventricular systole (see Fig. 21.2).

Although each ventricle pumps the same amount of blood, the much thicker walls of the left ventricle pump with approximately five times the force of the right ventricle to distribute the blood throughout the body. This difference in force is reflected in the large difference between systemic and pulmonary blood pressure.

Cardiac Conduction Pathway and Cardiac Cycle

The cardiac conduction pathway is the pathway of electrical impulses that generates a heartbeat. The sinoatrial (SA) node in the wall of the right atrium is autorhythmic and depolarizes about 100 times per minute, initiating each heartbeat. (While at rest, parasympathetic fibers dominate and slow the SA node to about 75 beats per minute.) For this reason, the SA node is called the *pacemaker*, and a normal rhythm is called a *normal sinus rhythm*. From the SA node, impulses travel on a specific path (Fig. 21.3). If the SA node becomes nonfunctional, the AV node can initiate each heartbeat, but at a slower rate of 40 to 60 beats per minute. The *bundle of His* can generate the beat of the ventricles, but at the much slower rate of about 20 to 35 beats per minute.

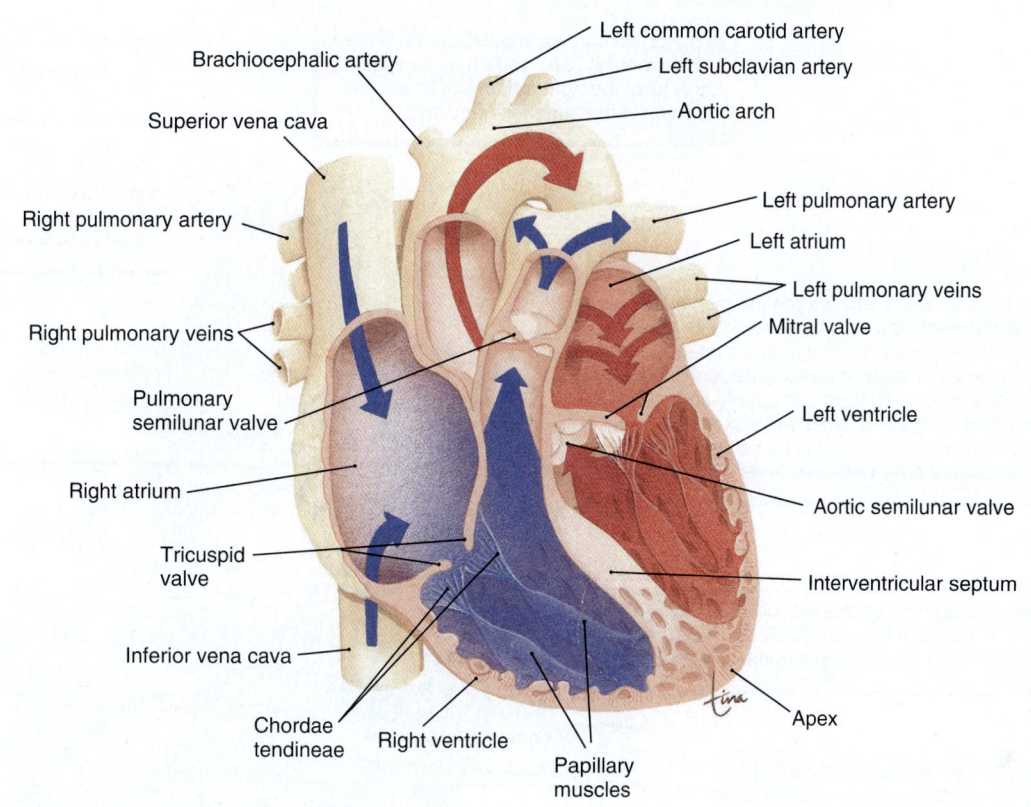

FIGURE 21.2 Frontal section of the heart showing internal structures and cardiac blood flow.

A cardiac cycle is the sequence of mechanical events that occurs during each heartbeat. Simply stated, the two atria contract simultaneously, followed by the simultaneous contraction of the two ventricles (a fraction of a second later). The contraction (emptying), or systole, of each set of chambers is followed by relaxation (filling), or diastole, of the same set of chambers.

The events of the cardiac cycle create the normal heart sounds. The first of the two major sounds (the "lub" of "lub-dub") is caused by closure of the AV valves during ventricular systole. The second sound is created by the closure of the aortic and pulmonary semilunar valves.

Cardiac Output

Cardiac output is the amount of blood ejected from the left ventricle in 1 minute (the right ventricle pumps a similar amount). It is determined by multiplying stroke volume by heart rate. Stroke volume is the amount of blood ejected by a ventricle in one contraction. It averages 60 to 80 mL/beat. With an average resting heart rate of 75 beats per minute, average resting cardiac output is 5 to 6 L (approximately the total blood volume of an individual that is pumped within 1 minute). Ejection fraction is a measure of ventricular efficiency. It is normally 55% to 70% of the total amount of blood within the left ventricle that is ejected with every heartbeat.

During exercise, venous return increases and stretches the ventricular myocardium, which in response contracts more forcefully. This is known as **Starling's law** of the heart, and the result is an increase in stroke volume. More blood is pumped with each beat. At the same time, the heart rate increases, causing cardiac output to increase by as much as four times the resting level (or more for athletes).

Regulation of Heart Rate

The heart generates its own electrical impulse, which begins at the SA node. The nervous system, however, can change the heart rate in response to environmental circumstances. In the brain, the medulla oblongata receives sensory input and alters heart function (Fig. 21.4).

Hormones and the Heart

The hormone epinephrine is secreted by the adrenal medulla in stressful situations. It is sympathomimetic in that it increases the heart rate and force of contraction and dilates the coronary vessels. This in turn increases cardiac output and systolic blood pressure.

Aldosterone is a hormone produced by the adrenal cortex. It is important for cardiac function because it helps regulate blood levels of sodium and potassium, both of which are needed for normal electrical activity of the myocardium.

The atria of the heart secrete a hormone of their own, called atrial natriuretic peptide or *atrial natriuretic hormone*. As its name suggests, atrial natriuretic peptide increases the excretion of sodium by the kidneys by inhibiting secretion of aldosterone by the adrenal cortex. Atrial natriuretic peptide is secreted when a higher blood pressure or greater blood volume stretches the walls of the atria. The loss of sodium is accompanied by the increased loss of water in urine. This decreases blood volume and, therefore, blood pressure as well.

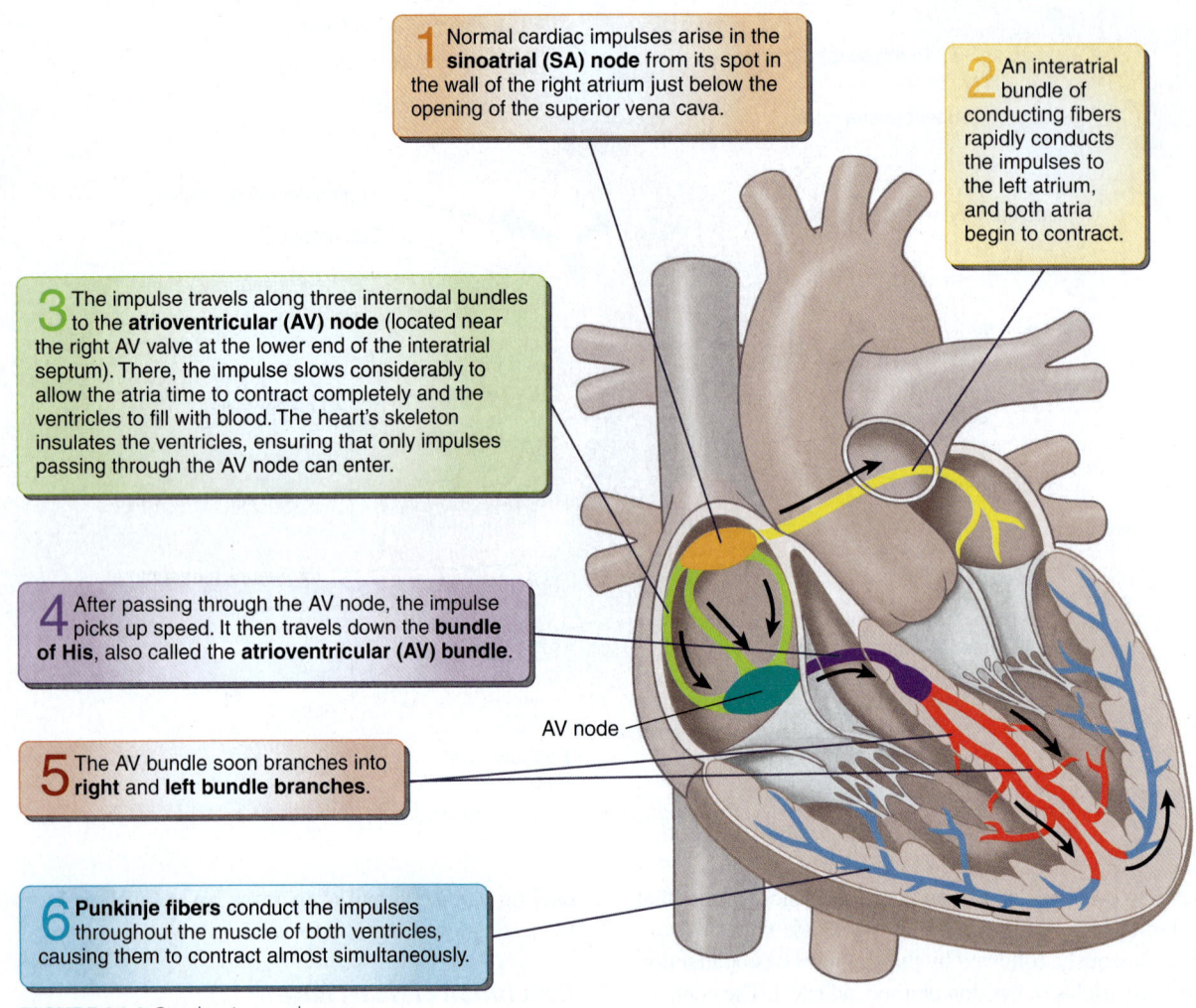

1 Normal cardiac impulses arise in the **sinoatrial (SA) node** from its spot in the wall of the right atrium just below the opening of the superior vena cava.

2 An interatrial bundle of conducting fibers rapidly conducts the impulses to the left atrium, and both atria begin to contract.

3 The impulse travels along three internodal bundles to the **atrioventricular (AV) node** (located near the right AV valve at the lower end of the interatrial septum). There, the impulse slows considerably to allow the atria time to contract completely and the ventricles to fill with blood. The heart's skeleton insulates the ventricles, ensuring that only impulses passing through the AV node can enter.

4 After passing through the AV node, the impulse picks up speed. It then travels down the **bundle of His**, also called the **atrioventricular (AV) bundle**.

AV node

5 The AV bundle soon branches into **right** and **left bundle branches**.

6 **Punkinje fibers** conduct the impulses throughout the muscle of both ventricles, causing them to contract almost simultaneously.

FIGURE 21.3 Conduction pathway.

Blood Vessels

Arteries and Veins

Arteries and arterioles carry blood from the heart to capillaries. Their walls are relatively thick and consist of three layers. Arteries carry blood under high pressure. The outer layer of fibrous connective tissue prevents rupture of the artery. The middle layer of smooth muscle and elastic connective tissue contributes to the maintenance of normal blood pressure, especially diastolic blood pressure, by changing the diameter of the artery. The diameter of arteries is regulated primarily by the sympathetic division of the autonomic nervous system. By use of the smooth muscle, the arteries can also alter where the greatest volume of blood is directed. The inner layer, or lining, of the artery is simple squamous epithelium, called *endothelium*, which is very smooth to prevent abnormal clotting.

Veins and venules carry blood from capillaries to the heart. Their walls are relatively thin because they have less smooth muscle than arteries. However, sympathetic impulses can bring about extensive constriction of veins. This becomes important in situations such as severe hemorrhage. The lining of veins is, like arteries, endothelium that prevents abnormal clotting; at intervals, it is folded into valves to prevent backflow of blood. Valves are most numerous in the veins of the extremities, especially the legs, where blood must return to the heart against the force of gravity.

Capillaries

Capillaries carry blood from arterioles to venules and form extensive networks in most tissues. The exceptions are cartilage, covering/lining epithelia, and the lens and cornea of the eye. Capillary walls are a continuation of the lining of arteries and veins. They are one-cell thick to permit the exchange of gases, nutrients, and waste products between the blood and tissues (Fig. 21.5). Blood flow through a capillary network is regulated by a precapillary sphincter, a smooth muscle fiber ring that contracts or relaxes in response to tissue needs. In an active tissue such as exercising skeletal muscle, for example, the rapid oxygen uptake and carbon dioxide production cause dilation of the precapillary sphincters to increase blood flow. At the same time, precapillary sphincters in less active tissues constrict to reduce blood flow. This is important because the body does not have enough blood to fill all the capillaries at once; the fixed volume must constantly be shunted or redirected to where it is needed most.

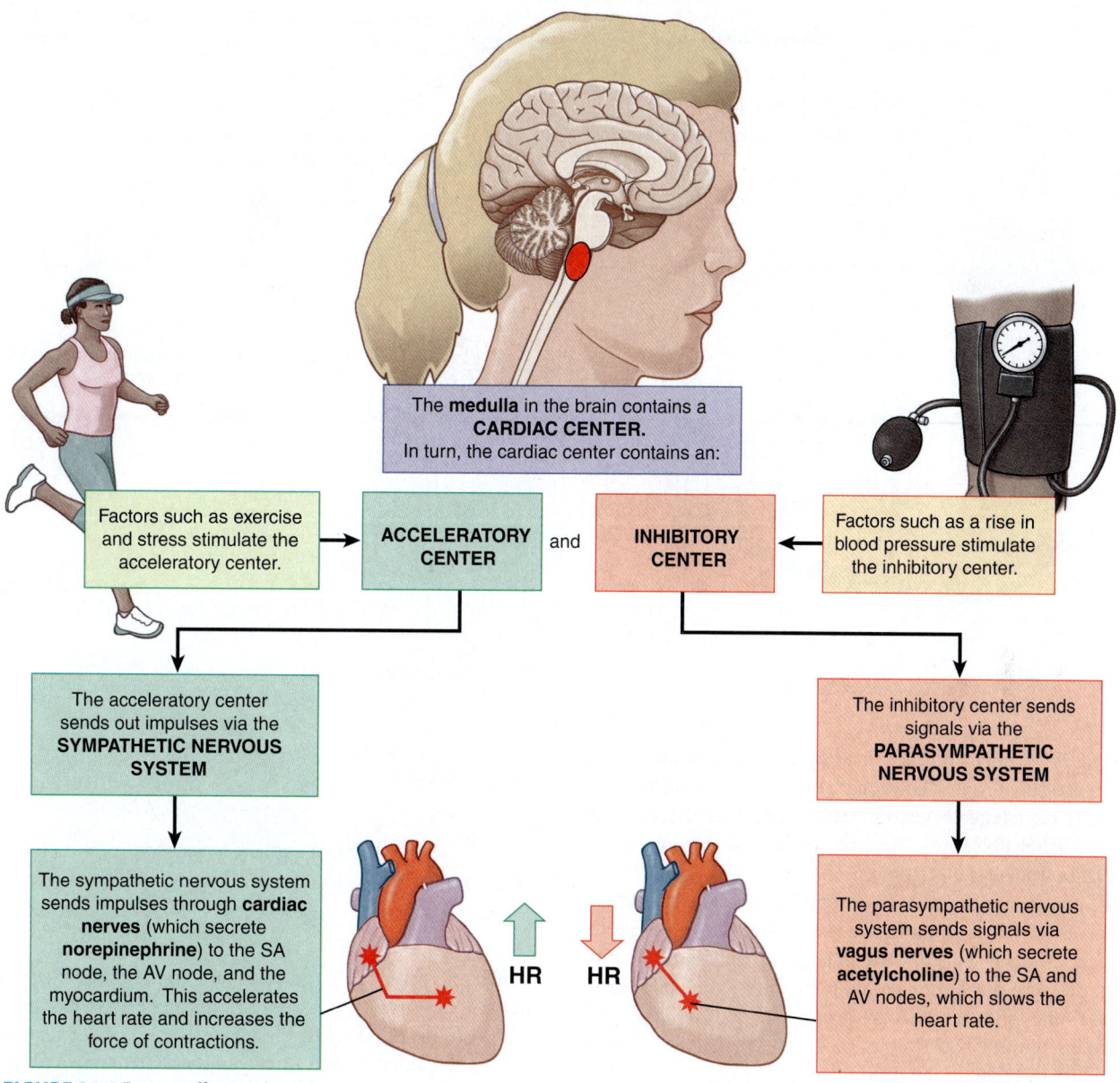

FIGURE 21.4 Factors affecting heart rate.

Exchange between blood and tissue fluids occurs primarily due to diffusion and/or filtration at the capillaries. Diffusion is important to gas exchange. Filtration is a vital mechanism for homeostasis of extracellular fluids. Some of this tissue fluid returns to the capillaries, and some is collected in lymph capillaries. Lymph is returned to the blood by lymph vessels. Should blood pressure within the capillaries increase, more tissue fluid than usual is formed, too much for the lymph vessels to collect. This may result in tissue swelling, called *edema*.

Blood Pressure

Blood pressure is the force of the blood against the walls of the blood vessels. It is measured in millimeters of mercury (mm Hg), systolic over diastolic. The normal average of systemic arterial pressure is 120/80 mm Hg. Blood pressure decreases in the arterioles and capillaries, and the systolic and diastolic pressures merge into one pressure. As blood enters the veins, blood pressure decreases further and approaches zero as it flows into the right ventricle. As mentioned previously, the blood pressure in the capillaries is of great importance. Normal blood pressure is high enough to permit filtration for nourishment of tissues but low enough to prevent rupture.

The arterioles (and veins during increased sympathetic stimulation) are usually in a state of slight constriction that helps to maintain normal blood pressure, especially diastolic pressure. This contributes to peripheral resistance; it is regulated by the vasomotor center in the medulla, which receives input via the glossopharyngeal and vagus nerves.

Blood pressure is also affected by many other factors. If heart rate and force increase, blood pressure increases within limits. If the heart is beating very fast, the ventricles are not

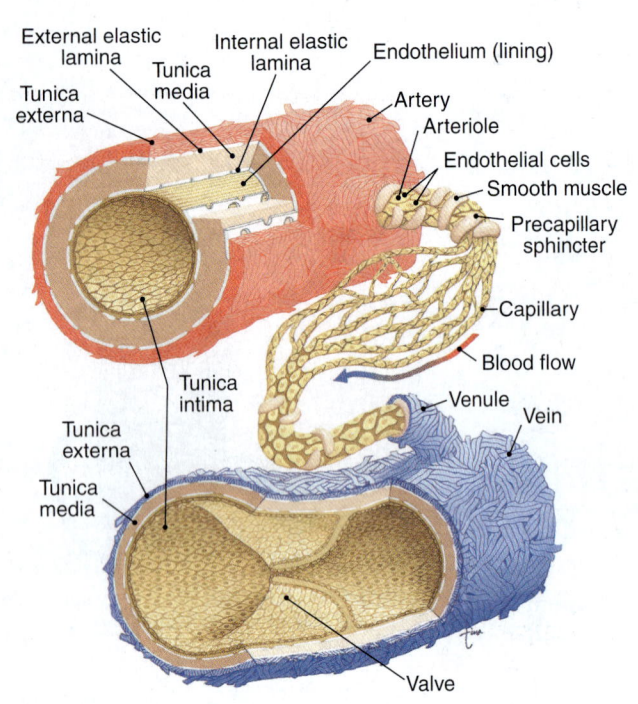

FIGURE 21.5 Structure of an artery, arteriole, capillary network, venule, and vein.

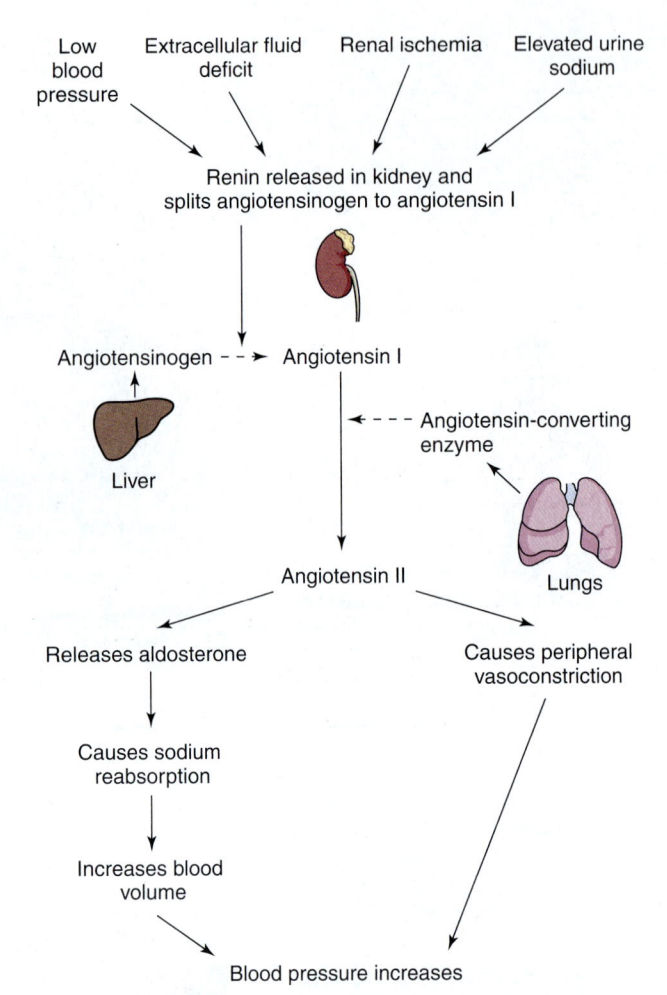

FIGURE 21.6 The renin-angiotensin-aldosterone mechanism.

filled before they contract, cardiac output decreases, and blood pressure drops. The strength of the heart's contractions depends on adequate venous return, which is the amount of blood that flows into the atria. Decreased venous return results in weaker contractions.

Venous return depends on several factors: constriction of the veins to reduce pooling, the skeletal muscle pumping to squeeze the deep veins of the legs, and the diaphragm's downward pressure during inhalation to compress the abdominal veins as the thoracic veins are decompressed. The valves in the veins prevent backflow of blood and thus contribute to the return of blood to the heart.

The elasticity of the large arteries also contributes to normal blood pressure. When the left ventricle contracts, the blood stretches the elastic walls of the large arteries, which absorb some of the force. When the left ventricle relaxes, the arterial walls recoil, exerting pressure on the blood. Normal elasticity, therefore, lowers systolic pressure, raises diastolic pressure, and maintains normal pulse pressure. Pulse pressure is the difference between the systolic and diastolic pressures. The usual ratio of systolic to diastolic to pulse pressure is 3:2:1.

Renin-Angiotensin-Aldosterone Mechanism

The kidneys are of great importance in the regulation of blood pressure. If blood flow through the kidneys decreases, renal filtration decreases and urinary output decreases to preserve blood volume. Decreased blood pressure stimulates the kidneys to secrete renin, which initiates the renin-angiotensin-aldosterone mechanism, raising blood pressure (Fig. 21.6).

Other hormones that affect blood pressure include those of the adrenal medulla (norepinephrine and epinephrine), which increase cardiac output and cause vasoconstriction in skin and viscera. Antidiuretic hormone is released from the posterior pituitary. It directly increases water reabsorption by the kidneys, thus increasing blood volume and blood pressure. Atrial natriuretic peptide is secreted by the atria of the heart. It inhibits aldosterone secretion and thereby increases renal excretion of sodium ions and water, which decreases blood volume and subsequently blood pressure.

Circuits of Circulation

The two circuits of circulation are pulmonary and systemic (see Fig. 21.2). Pulmonary circulation begins at the right ventricle, which pumps deoxygenated blood toward the lungs for gas exchange at the alveoli. Oxygenated blood returns to the left atrium by way of the pulmonary veins. Low pressure in the pulmonary capillaries prevents filtration in pulmonary capillaries. This keeps tissue fluid from accumulating in the alveoli of the lungs, which can otherwise result in pulmonary edema.

Systemic circulation begins in the left ventricle, pumping oxygenated blood into the aorta, the many branches of which eventually give rise to capillaries within the tissues. Deoxygenated blood returns to the right atrium by way of

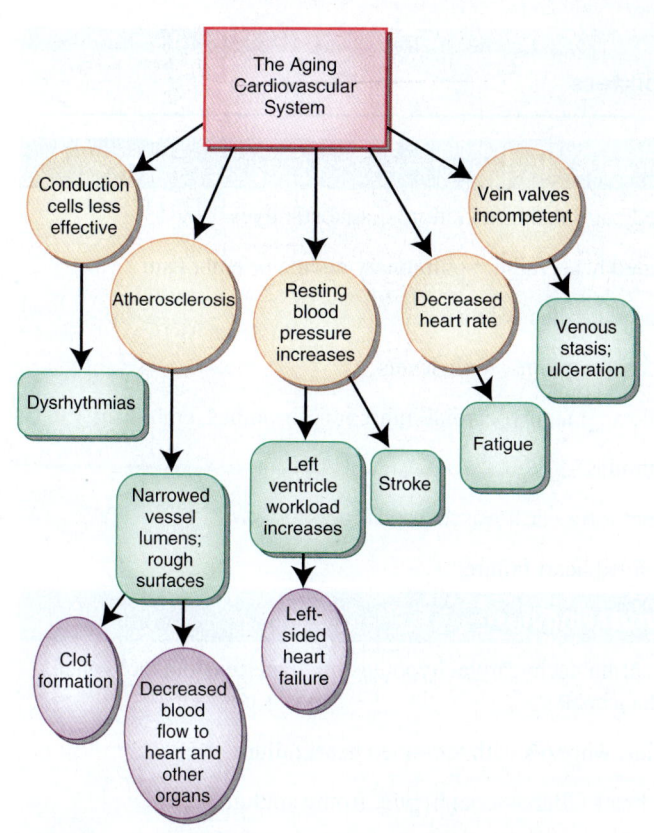

FIGURE 21.7 Aging and the cardiovascular system concept map.

the superior and inferior vena cava and the coronary sinus. The hepatic portal circulation is a special part of the systemic circulation in which blood from the capillaries of the digestive organs and spleen flows through the portal vein and into the sinusoids in the liver before returning to the heart. This pathway permits the liver to regulate the blood levels of nutrients such as glucose, amino acids, and iron and to remove potential toxins such as alcohol or medications from circulation.

Aging and the Cardiovascular System

The aging of blood vessels, especially arteries, is believed to begin in childhood, although the effects are not apparent until later in life (Fig. 21.7). **Atherosclerosis** is the deposition of lipids in the walls of arteries over a period of years. The deposited lipids can narrow the arteries' lumens and form rough surfaces that may stimulate intravascular clot formation. Atherosclerosis decreases blood flow to the affected organ. With age, the heart muscle becomes less efficient, and maximum cardiac output and heart rate both decrease, although resting levels may be more than sufficient. Valves may become thickened by fibrosis, leading to heart murmur.

CARDIOVASCULAR DISEASE

An estimated 121.5 million American adults have one or more types of cardiovascular disease (Benjamin et al, 2019).

Lifestyle and access to quality health care play leading roles in risk factors for cardiovascular disease. Many Americans lead a sedentary lifestyle and eat excess calories. Ways to improve cardiovascular health include not smoking, exercising, eating healthy, and maintaining normal blood pressure, blood glucose, total cholesterol levels, and weight. Culturally competent engagement in health promotion and disease prevention education is important to address and reduce heart disease risk in all racial and ethnic groups. In women, the greatest cause of death is cardiovascular disease. The movement Go Red for Women (www.goredforwomen.org) gives women encouragement and tools to prevent cardiovascular disease and live healthy.

CARDIOVASCULAR SYSTEM DATA COLLECTION

Data collection of the cardiovascular system includes a patient health history and physical examination ("Gerontological Issues: Atypical Symptoms"). If the patient is experiencing an acute problem, focus on the most serious signs and symptoms and physical data until the patient is stabilized (Table 21.1).

Gerontological Issues

Atypical Symptoms

Older adults commonly have signs and symptoms that are not typical of a myocardial infarction (MI). For example, the only symptom of MI in an older patient may be dyspnea. Chest pain, a typical symptom, may not be present. It is important for the older adult to have a complete assessment for this reason.

Health History

For cardiovascular problems, data collection focuses on the areas listed in Table 21.2. Patient allergies, medications, medical disorders, and surgeries are documented. Functional limitations that are related to cardiovascular problems, such as difficulty performing activities of daily living, walking, climbing stairs, or completing household tasks, are noted.

Physical Examination

The patient's general appearance is observed. Height, weight, and vital signs are recorded (Table 21.3).

• WORD • BUILDING •
atherosclerosis: athere—porridge + sklerosis—hardness

Table 21.1
Data Collection for Acute Cardiovascular Disorders

History	Significance
Allergies	For medication administration, diagnostic dyes
Dyspnea	Left-sided heart failure; pulmonary edema or embolism
Fatigue	Decreased cardiac output
Medications	Effect on symptoms; toxic levels
Pain: Description, location, radiation, or referred	Possible angina, myocardial infarction, thrombus, embolism
Palpitations, dizziness	Arrhythmias
Smoking history	Risk factor for cardiovascular disorders
Weight gain	Right-sided heart failure
Physical Examination	**Abnormal Findings**
Vital signs	Bradycardia, tachycardia, hypotension, hypertension, tachypnea, apnea, shock
Breath sounds	Crackles, wheezes with left-sided heart failure
Cough, sputum	Acute heart failure—cough, pink frothy sputum
Edema	Right-sided heart failure
Heart rhythm	Arrhythmias
Jugular vein distention	Right-sided heart failure

Table 21.2
Subjective Data Collection for the Cardiovascular System

Questions to Ask During Health History	Rationale/Significance
Pain: WHAT'S UP? Format	
Where is your pain? Does it radiate? Is it referred pain?	Chest pain may also *radiate* to adjacent areas such as the shoulders, neck, jaw, arms, or back. If pain is present in the shoulders, neck, jaw, arms, or back due to a cardiac problem but there is no chest pain, then it is *referred* pain. Vascular disorders cause extremity pain.
How does it feel? Discomfort, burning, aching, indigestion, squeezing, pressure, tightness, heaviness, numbness in chest area? Fullness, heaviness, sharpness, throbbing in legs?	Pain can be associated with angina or myocardial infarction. The quality of pain varies. Arterial pain is sharp or throbbing. Venous pain is a fullness or heaviness.
Aggravating/alleviating factors that increase/relieve your pain?	Activity may cause or increase angina. Rest or medications may relieve angina. Leg activity pain, intermittent claudication, results from decreased perfusion that is aggravated by activity. Rest pain, from severe arterial occlusion, increases when lying. Dangling reduces the pain as blood flow increases with gravity.

Table 21.2
Subjective Data Collection for the Cardiovascular System—cont'd

Timing of your pain: onset, duration, frequency?	Pain may be continuous, intermittent, acute, or chronic. Arterial occlusion causes acute pain.
Severity of pain?	Pain is rated, such as on a scale of 0 to 10.
Useful data for associated symptoms?	Accompanying symptoms and their characteristics guide diagnosis and treatment.
Perception of your problem?	Patient's insight to problem is helpful in planning care.
Dyspnea Are you short of breath? What increases or relieves your shortness of breath?	Dyspnea can be present with heart failure that reduces cardiac output, on exertion in angina pectoris, or from a pulmonary embolus resulting from thrombophlebitis, heart failure, or arrhythmias.
Palpitations Are you having palpitations or irregular heartbeats? Does your heart race, pound, or skip beats?	Palpitations can occur from arrhythmias resulting from ischemia, electrolyte imbalance, or stress. Dizziness can be associated with arrhythmias.
Fatigue Have you noticed a change in your energy level?	Fatigue occurs from reduced cardiac output resulting from heart failure.
Are you able to perform activities that you would like to?	Functional abilities can be limited from fatigue.
Edema Have you had swelling in your feet, legs, or hands? Are rings, shoes, or gloves tighter?	Right-sided heart failure can cause fluid accumulation in the tissues.
Have you gained weight?	Fluid retention causes weight gain.
Paresthesia Any numbness, tingling, or other abnormal sensations in your extremities?	Numbness and tingling, pins and needles, and crawling sensations are paresthesia.
Childhood Diseases Did you have rheumatic fever or scarlet fever?	These childhood illnesses can lead to heart disease.
Risk Factors What is your typical diet? Do you exercise, smoke? Any recent stressors?	Modifiable risk factors include diet, being sedentary, smoking, and stressors.
Family History Do your parents, siblings, or grandparents have cardiovascular disorders?	Many cardiac problems are hereditary.

Blood Pressure

Normal blood pressure is considered less than 120/80 mm Hg (see Chapter 22). Readings in both arms are done for comparison (Box 21.1). A difference in the readings is reported to the health-care provider (HCP). The arm with the higher reading is used for ongoing measurements. If necessary, blood pressure is suggested to be measured at the ankle, which reduces discomfort and ease in applying the cuff as compared to the thigh. The systolic reading at the ankle averages 17 mm Hg higher than in the arm with no difference in the diastolic reading (Sheppard, 2020).

ORTHOSTATIC BLOOD PRESSURE. Measurements are taken with the patient lying, sitting, and standing to detect abnormal

Table 21.3
Objective Data Collection for the Cardiovascular System

Abnormal Findings	Possible Causes
Vital Signs	
Bradycardia	Athletes, arrhythmias, medications (digitalis, beta blocker), myocardial infarction
Tachycardia	Arrhythmias, dehydration, shock
Hypotension	Dehydration, hemorrhage, medication, shock
Orthostatic hypotension	Deficient fluid volume, diuretics, analgesics, pain
Respiratory	
Breath sounds	Crackles, wheezes with left-sided heart failure
Dry cough	Airway irritation from heart failure, medication (ACE inhibitor)
Cardiovascular	
Edema	Right-sided heart failure, peripheral venous disease
Heart sounds—S_3; S_4	Left-sided heart failure, fluid volume overload, mitral valve regurgitation; hypertension, CAD, pulmonary stenosis
Jugular vein distention	Right-sided heart failure
Murmur	Valvular disease
Pericardial friction rub	Inflammation of pericardium
Skin	
Light skin: cyanosis; dark skin: grayish green; yellowish skin: whitish gray	Tissue hypoxia
Pallor	Anemia, insufficient arterial blood flow
Dependent rubor—lower extremities	Insufficient arterial blood flow
Brown discoloration, dependent purple	Venous blood flow problem
Cool temperature	Insufficient arterial blood flow
Warm temperature	Venous blood return problem, infection, thrombophlebitis
Increased capillary refill time	Anemia, decreased arterial blood flow
Clubbing	Chronic oxygen deficiency
Decreased hair distribution, thick, brittle nails, shiny, taut, dry—lower extremities	Insufficient arterial blood flow

variations with postural changes (Box 21.2). When the patient sits or stands, a drop in the systolic pressure of up to 15 mm Hg and either a drop or slight increase in the diastolic pressure of 3 to 10 mm Hg is normal. In response to the drop in blood pressure, the pulse increases 15 to 20 beats per minute to maintain cardiac output. Orthostatic hypotension (postural hypotension) is a drop in systolic blood pressure greater than 15 mm Hg, a drop or slight increase in diastolic blood pressure greater than 10 mm Hg, and an increase in heart rate greater than 20 beats per minute in response to the drop in blood pressure. It indicates a problem that should be investigated by the HCP. The patient often reports light-headedness or syncope because the drop in blood pressure decreases the amount of oxygen-rich blood traveling to the brain. Factors that may cause orthostatic hypotension include deficient fluid volume, diuretics, analgesics, or pain.

Box 21.1
Taking Accurate Blood Pressure Measurements

- Instruct the patient to avoid exercise, caffeine, and smoking for 30 minutes before the blood pressure (BP) measurement.
- Instruct the patient to void before taking the BP measurement.
- Use the auscultatory method with a properly calibrated and validated BP instrument.
- Seat the patient quietly for at least 5 minutes in a chair (not on an examination table) with feet on the floor and arm supported at heart level before the BP measurement.
- Use the appropriate-sized cuff so that the cuff bladder encircles at least 80% of arm when placed 1 inch above the antecubital fossa.
- Ask the patient to remain still and quiet during BP measurement, as motion alters reading.
- Determine the patient's baseline blood pressure by inflating cuff and noting the reading when the radial pulse is no longer felt. When taking BP, inflate the cuff to 20 numbers above the obtained baseline reading. (Overinflation may cause inaccurate reading.)
- During BP measurement, deflate the cuff slowly at rate of 2 mm Hg/second.
- Take at least two BP measurements and average them.
- Remember that systolic BP is the first of two or more sounds heard and that diastolic BP is the final sound before the disappearance of sounds.
- Provide patients, verbally and in writing, with their specific BP reading.

BE SAFE!
AVOID FAILURE TO RECOGNIZE! Anticipate orthostatic hypotension with position changes. A drop in blood pressure increases the risk of fainting and falling. Older adults are at increased risk for developing orthostatic hypotension, which could precipitate a fall. This is often due to a combination of age-related changes, immobility, chronic illness, and medications. Inform the patient to sit up and stand slowly before walking. Use fall precautions such as a walking belt or two-person assist for patients at risk of or with orthostatic hypotension.

PRACTICE ANALYSIS TIP
Linking NCLEX-PN® to Practice
The LPN/LVN will:
- Assist in and/or reinforce education to client about safety precautions.
- Use transfer assistive devices (e.g., gait/transfer belt).

Pulses

The apical pulse is auscultated for 1 minute to identify rate and regularity. Normal heart rate is 60 to 100 beats per minute. In athletic people, the heart rate is often slower, around

Box 21.2
Orthostatic Hypotension

To identify orthostatic hypotension:
1. Explain the procedure to the patient; determine whether the patient can safely stand.
2. Tell the patient not to exercise, eat, or smoke for 30 minutes before BP measurements.
3. Have the patient lie flat in bed for at least 5 minutes before BP measurements.
4. Use the correct size BP cuff.
5. Tell the patient not to talk during BP measurements.
6. Take the patient's lying BP and heart rate.
7. Assist the patient to a sitting position. Inform the patient to sit with legs uncrossed. Ask if dizzy or lightheaded with each position change. If yes, ensure safety from fainting or falling. A gait or walking belt should be used. With any position change, if the patient experiences additional symptoms with the dizziness and decreased BP and increased heart rate, assist the patient to lie down, take BP, and notify the HCP. Consider the possible cause of the orthostatic hypotension (e.g., hemorrhaging, dehydration, diuretics) to plan patient care.
8. Wait 3 minutes and then take the patient's sitting BP and heart rate. If the patient is dizzy or lightheaded, continue sitting position for 5 minutes if tolerated. Do not attempt to bring the patient to standing. Repeat sitting BP. If BP has increased and the patient is no longer dizzy, assist the patient to stand.
9. After the patient is standing, take BP and pulse immediately. Repeat in 3 minutes. If BP drops and the patient is dizzy or lightheaded, do not attempt to ambulate the patient.
10. Document all heart rate and BP measurements, including extremity used and patient position when reading was obtained (e.g., "right arm: lying 132/78 mm Hg, sitting 118/68 mm Hg, standing 110/60 mm Hg"). Also document patient tolerance, symptoms, and nursing interventions if symptomatic.
11. Report abnormal findings to HCP.

50 beats per minute, because the well-conditioned heart pumps more efficiently. Apical pulse is documented as regular or irregular. Compare the apical rate with the radial rate for equality. If there are fewer radial beats than apical beats, a **pulse deficit** exists and should be reported to the HCP.

Arterial pulses are palpated bilaterally for volume and pressure quality and compared for equality. A normal vessel feels soft and springy. A sclerotic vessel feels stiff. The quality of the pulses is described on a four-point scale as follows: 0 absent; 1+ weak, thready; 2+ normal; and 3+ bounding. An absent pulse is not palpable. A thready pulse is one that disappears when slight pressure is applied and returns when the pressure is removed. The normal pulse is easily palpable. The bounding pulse is strong and present even when slight pressure is applied. When the normal vessel is palpated, a tapping is felt. In an abnormal vessel with a bulging or narrowed wall, a vibration is felt, called a **thrill.** When auscultating an abnormal vessel, a humming is heard because of turbulent blood flow through the vessel. This is referred to as a **bruit**.

Respirations
The rate and ease of respirations are observed. Breath sounds are auscultated. Sputum characteristics such as amount, color, and consistency are noted. Pink, frothy sputum is an indicator of acute heart failure. A dry cough can occur from the irritation caused by the lung congestion resulting from heart failure.

> **CUE RECOGNITION 21.1**
> Mrs. Goldberg, a resident who is 77, stands up to ambulate and becomes unsteady and places her hand on her forehead as you walk by her in the hallway. What action do you take?
>
> Suggested answers are at the end of the chapter.

Inspection
During the health history, inspection begins by noting shortness of breath when the patient speaks or moves. The patient's oxygenation status is noted through skin, mucous membrane, lip, and nailbed color. For those with dark skin, oxygen deficiency appears as a whitish or gray color around the mouth and conjunctiva that are blue or gray. For those with yellowish skin, a grayish-greenish color is seen. For those with light skin, it appears as dark blue skin and mucous membranes, also referred to as *cyanosis*. Pallor may indicate anemia or lack of arterial blood flow. A dependent rubor (red) found in the lower extremities occurs from decreased arterial blood flow. Brown discoloration and purple skin when the lower extremity is dependent may be seen in the presence of venous blood flow problems. Decreased hair distribution; thick, brittle nails; and shiny, taut, dry skin on the lower extremities occurs from reduced arterial blood flow. Varicose veins, stasis ulcers, or scars around the ankles and signs of thrombophlebitis such as swelling, redness, or a hard, tender vein reveal venous blood return problems.

The patient's internal and external jugular neck veins are observed for distention in a 45- to 90-degree upright position. Normally, the veins are not visible in this position. Distention indicates an increase in the venous volume, often caused by right-sided heart failure.

Capillary refill time is normally 3 seconds or less and reflects arterial blood flow to the extremities. The patient's nailbed is briefly squeezed, causing blanching, and then released. The time it takes for the color to return to the nailbed after release of the squeezing pressure is the capillary refill time. Longer times indicate anemia or a decrease in arterial blood flow to the extremity.

Clubbing of the nailbeds occurs from oxygen deficiency over time. It is often caused by congenital heart defects or long-term use of tobacco. The distal ends of the fingers and toes swell and appear clublike. With clubbing, the normal 160-degree angle formed between the base of the nail and the skin is lost, causing the nail to be flat (Fig. 21.8). Later, the nail base elevates, the angle exceeds 180 degrees, and the nail feels spongy when squeezed. These findings should be reported to the HCP. To demonstrate how to check for this, touch your index fingers together at the nailbeds and first joint. Look at the space created between the nailbeds. Do you see a diamond? If so, that is normal. If no diamond is seen, it indicates the nailbeds are clubbed and therefore filling that space.

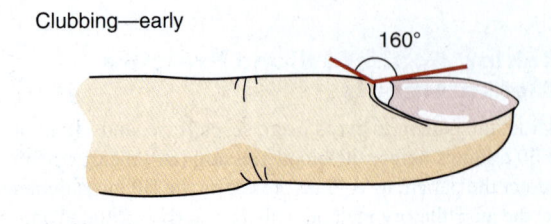

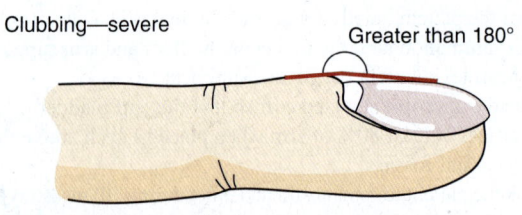

FIGURE 21.8 Clubbing of the fingers.

> **LEARNING TIP**
> Six Ps characterize peripheral vascular disease:
> - Pain
> - Paresthesia (decreased sensation)
> - Pallor
> - Pulselessness
> - Paralysis
> - Poikilothermia (assumes temperature of the environment)

Palpation
In addition to palpating the arteries, the thorax can be palpated at the **point of maximum impulse** (PMI). The PMI is palpated by placing the right hand over the apex of the heart. If palpable, a thrust is felt when the ventricle contracts. An enlarged heart may shift the PMI to the left of the midclavicular line.

The temperature of the extremities is palpated bilaterally for comparison. Palpation begins proximally and moves distally along the extremity. In areas of decreased arterial blood flow, the **ischemic** area feels cooler than the rest of the body because it is blood that warms the body. In the absence of sufficient arterial blood flow, the area becomes the temperature of the environment (**poikilothermy**). A warm or hot extremity indicates a venous return problem.

• WORD • BUILDING •
ischemic: ischein—hold back + haima—blood
poikilothermy: poikilos—varied + therme—heat

Chapter 21   Cardiovascular System Function, Data Collection, and Therapeutic Measures

Edema is palpated in the lower extremities or dependent areas such as the sacrum for the supine patient (Fig. 21.9). Edema can occur from right-sided heart failure, gravity, or altered venous blood return. Severity of the edema is identified by applying pressure for 5 seconds over the bone where the edema is. If the finger imprint or indentation remains, the edema is pitting. Measuring the leg circumference is an accurate method for monitoring the edema.

Auscultation

Normal heart sounds are produced by the closing of the heart valves. See the figure in the "Learning Tip" that follows for the areas to auscultate to best hear these sounds. Erb's point is where S_2 is best heard. In blood-flowing vessels, sound is transmitted in the direction of the blood flow. The first heart sound (S_1) is heard at the beginning of systole as "lub" when the tricuspid and mitral (AV) valves close (Fig. 21.10). The second heart sound (S_2) is heard at the start of diastole as "dub" when the aortic and pulmonic semilunar valves close. The diaphragm of the stethoscope is used to hear the high-pitched sounds of S_1 and S_2. Normally, no other sounds are heard between S_1 and S_2. With the bell of the stethoscope placed at the apex, a third heart sound (S_3) or a fourth heart sound (S_4) may be heard. Having patients lean forward or lie on their left side can make the heart sounds easier to hear by bringing the area of the heart where the sound may be heard closer to the chest wall. The S_3 heart sound is normal for younger adults. It sounds like a gallop and is a low-pitched sound heard early in diastole. In older adults, S_3 may be heard with left-sided heart failure, fluid volume overload, and mitral valve regurgitation. The S_4 heart sound is also a low-pitched sound, similar to a gallop but heard late in diastole. It occurs with hypertension, coronary artery disease (CAD), and pulmonary stenosis.

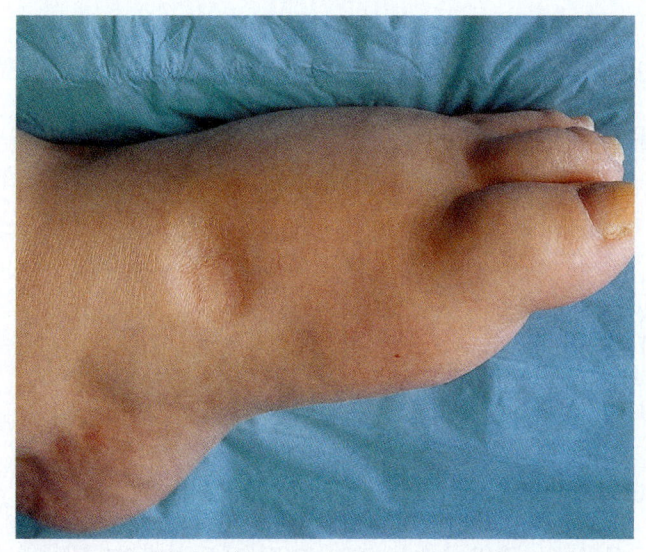

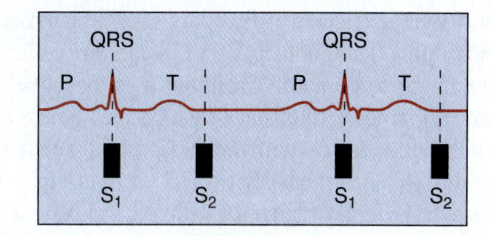

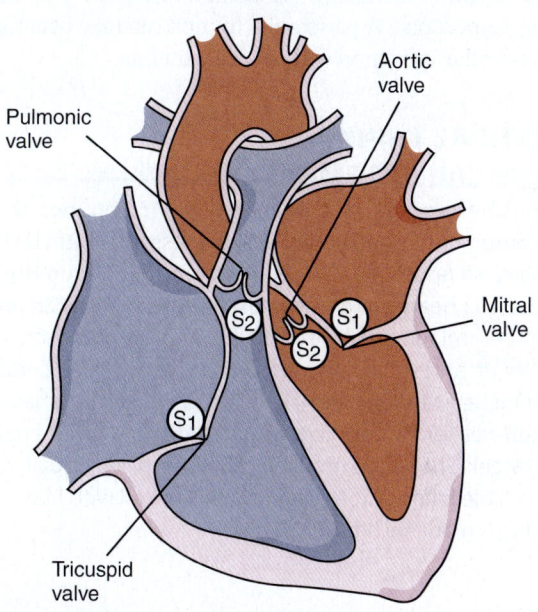

FIGURE 21.10 Heart sounds correlated with electrocardiogram: S_1 is heard at the beginning of systole, and S_2 is heard at the beginning of diastole.

> **LEARNING TIP**
> This sentence can help you remember the heart's auscultation points:
>
> | All | (aortic) |
> |---|---|
> | People | (pulmonic) |
> | Eat | (Erb's point) |
> | Three | (tricuspid) |
> | Meals | (mitral) |

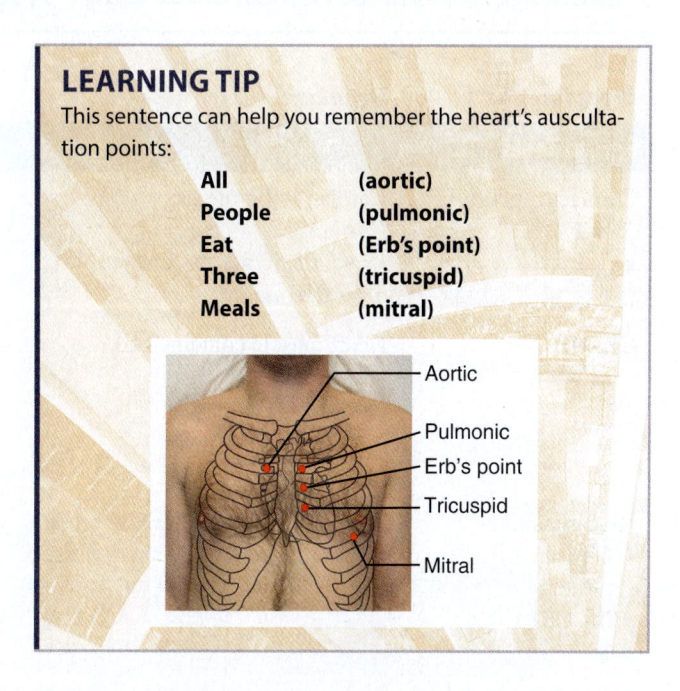

FIGURE 21.9 Pitting edema. Application of pressure over a bony area displaces the excess fluid, leaving an indentation or pit.

Murmurs are caused by a narrowed valve opening or a valve that does not close tightly. A **murmur** is a prolonged, swishing sound that ranges in intensity from faint to very loud.

A **pericardial friction rub** occurs from inflammation of the pericardium. The intensity of a rub can range from faint to loud enough to be audible without a stethoscope. A rub has a grating sound, like that of sandpaper being rubbed together, that occurs when the pericardial surfaces rub together during a heartbeat. (See the "Learning Tip" on pericardial friction rub in Chapter 23.) Having the patient sit and lean forward allows a rub to be heard more clearly. The rub is best heard to the left of the sternum using the diaphragm of the stethoscope. A pericardial friction rub may occur after a myocardial infarction (MI) or chest trauma.

CRITICAL THINKING & CLINICAL JUDGMENT

Mrs. Cheung, age 78, baseline weight 162 pounds, is admitted to the hospital with shortness of breath. Data collection findings are blood pressure 152/88 mm Hg, pulse 104 beats per minute, respirations breaths 26 per minute, and temperature 99.4°F (37.2°C). She has shortness of breath at rest that increases with activity, ankle edema, distant heart tones, pale nailbeds, and no pain. She has not eaten well for 2 weeks but has had a 6-pound weight gain in 1 week. She sleeps on three pillows, and her jugular veins are visible bilaterally. A diagnosis of acute MI with heart failure is made by her HCP.

Critical Thinking (The Why)
1. Why would Mrs. Cheung not be feeling chest pain with a diagnosis of acute MI?

Clinical Judgment (The Do)
2. How do you collect ankle edema data to provide complete and measurable data?
3. How do you document the date for the ankle edema?
4. How do you document the additional symptoms Mrs. Cheung has?
5. How do you document Mrs. Cheung's weight in kilograms?
6. What health-care team members do you collaborate with in caring for Mrs. Cheung?

Suggested answers are at the end of the chapter.

DIAGNOSTIC TESTS FOR THE CARDIOVASCULAR SYSTEM

Diagnostic test results are combined with the health history and physical data collection to diagnose disorders and plan care for the patient (Table 21.4 and Table 21.5). Additional tests can identify genetic and inflammation factors contributing to cardiovascular risk to develop a preventive plan of care for the patient.

Table 21.4
Laboratory Tests for the Cardiovascular System

Procedure	Definition	Significance of Abnormal Findings	Nursing Management
Serum Tests			
Cardiac troponin I or T	Cardiac cell proteins. Normal: I = <0.05 ng/mL T = <0.01 ng/mL	Elevated levels sensitive indicator of myocardial damage.	No special care.
CK-MB	Heart muscle contains MB isoenzyme. Normal = 0–5 ng/mL	Rises with acute MI in 4–6 hours, peaks in 15–20 hours, returns to baseline in 2–3 days.	Avoid IM injections. Obtain baseline CK before IV insertion to avoid elevating CK from damaging muscle cells.
High-sensitive C-reactive protein (hs-CRP)	CRP level can indicate low-grade inflammation in coronary vessels.	CAD risk: Low = <1 mg/L Average = 1–3 mg/L High = >3 mg/L (after repeated)	No special care.
Homocysteine	Amino acid in the blood. Normal = 4.6–11.2 micromol/L	Elevated levels linked with higher risk of CAD and PVD.	Encourage high-risk patients with CAD to have adequate intake of folic acid and vitamin B.

Table 21.4
Laboratory Tests for the Cardiovascular System—cont'd

Procedure	Definition	Significance of Abnormal Findings	Nursing Management
Lipoproteins: HDL, LDL, VLDL	HDL: Desirable = 60 mg/dL or higher Acceptable = 40–60 mg/dL Low = < 40 mg/dL LDL: Optimal = <100 mg/dL Near optimal = 100–129 mg/dL Borderline high = 130–159 mg/dL High = 160–189 mg/dL Very high = > 190 mg/dL VLDL: 2–30 mg/dL	Elevated LDL increases CAD risk. Elevated HDL cardio protective.	May be instructed to fast except for water 6–12 hours and avoid alcohol 24 hours before test.
Total Cholesterol: LDL + HDL	Desirable = <200 mg/dL Borderline = 200–239 mg/dL High = 240 mg/dL or higher	Elevation increases risk of CAD.	May be instructed to fast except for water 6–12 hours and avoid alcohol 24 hours before test.
Triglycerides	Normal = <150 mg/dL Borderline high = 150–199 mg/dL High = 200–499 mg/dL Very high = >500 mg/dL	Elevation increases risk of CAD.	May be instructed to fast except for water 6–12 hours and avoid alcohol 24 hours before test.

CAD = coronary artery disease; PVD = peripheral vascular disease.

Table 21.5
Diagnostic Procedures for the Cardiovascular System

Procedure	Definition	Significance of Abnormal Findings	Nursing Management
Noninvasive			
Chest x-ray film	Anterior-posterior and left lateral views of chest.	Heart enlargement, calcifications, fluid around heart	Ask females if pregnant. Remove metal items. Teaching: No discomfort.
Cardiac computed tomography scan and angiography	Evaluates heart and structures. Contrast agent may be given to visualize arteries.	Classification system used to report cardiac event risk	Kidney function checked if contrast used.
Cardiac magnetic resonance imaging (MRI) or magnetic resonance angiography (MRA)	MRI: Provides three-dimensional image of heart. MRA: Contrast agent given to visualize arteries.	Cardiac structural abnormalities, blood vessel abnormalities	Ask if has cardiac or orthopedic implant and its MR designation, or metallic items in body, or claustrophobia. Ask if history of reaction to contrast medium (reaction to iodine-based contrast dye is not the same as a shellfish allergy, as iodine is not an allergen [Long et al, 2019]). Give antianxiety medication as ordered. Teaching: Lie still in cylinder that makes loud, pounding sounds.

Continued

Table 21.5
Diagnostic Procedures for the Cardiovascular System—cont'd

Procedure	Definition	Significance of Abnormal Findings	Nursing Management
Electrocardiogram (ECG)	Electrodes on skin carry electrical activity of heart from various cardiac views.	Arrhythmias, enlarged heart chamber size, myocardial ischemia or infarction, electrolyte imbalances	Teaching: No discomfort.
Holter monitor	Recording of ECG for up to 24 hours to match abnormalities with symptoms recorded in patient's diary.	Arrhythmias, infrequent myocardial ischemia	Teaching: Keep accurate diary; push event button for symptoms. No showers or baths.
Event recorder	Worn for long time periods and can record three cardiac events.	Infrequent cardiac events	Teaching: Push event button for symptomatic event. Can bathe.
Echocardiogram	Sound waves bounce off heart to produce heart images and show blood flow.	CAD, heart enlargement, thickened cardiac walls or septum, pericardial effusion, valvular abnormalities	May be done at bedside. Patient lies on left side. Teaching: No discomfort, gel applied.
Strain echocardiogram	Comprehensive assessment of the function of the heart muscle.	Guides treatment in heart failure and cardiomyopathy; evaluates for cardiac surgery or transplant.	May eat before test.
Transesophageal echocardiogram	Probe with transducer on end inserted into esophagus.	See Echocardiogram.	Monitor vital signs and oxygen saturation. Suction continually during procedure. Check gag reflex before NPO status is discontinued. Teaching: NPO 6 hours before test. Sedation and local throat anesthetic given.
Exercise stress echocardiogram	Evaluates effects of exercise on heart and vascular circulation.	Arrhythmias, ischemia	Monitor vital signs and ECG before, during, and after test until stable. Teaching: Wear walking shoes and comfortable clothes.
Doppler ultrasound	Sound waves bounce off moving blood cells, producing color recordings.	Decreased blood flow occurs from peripheral vascular disease.	Teaching: Explain procedure.
Radioisotopes			
Single-photon emission computed tomography (SPECT-CT) thallium imaging	IV thallium-201 is injected, and gamma camera images evaluate viable myocardium at rest. Repeat in 3–4 or 24 hours to show myocardial perfusion and viability.	Shows viable myocardium and identifies ischemic heart disease via "cold spots" in which thallium is not taken up.	Check renal function and if had prior reaction to contrast medium. Ensure patent IV line. Apply cardiac monitor. Monitor vital signs at baseline, every 2 minutes and up to 1.5 hours after test. Teaching: No caffeine 12 hours or aminophylline 24 hours before test.

Table 21.5
Diagnostic Procedures for the Cardiovascular System—cont'd

Procedure	Definition	Significance of Abnormal Findings	Nursing Management
Adenosine, dipyridamole, or regadenoson SPECT-CT thallium imaging	Regadenoson most common of these vasodilators given to increase blood flow to coronary arteries.	Same as in thallium imaging.	Same as thallium in imaging.
Technetium pyrophosphate or technetium-99m (TC-99m) sestamibi imaging	The radioisotope is given IV. Scanned 1.5–2 hours later.	Areas of myocardial cell damage take up the radioisotope, which appears as hot spots.	Teaching: Same as thallium imaging.
Multiple-gated acquisition (MUGA) scan	TC-99m pertechnetate is given IV to be detected by a camera to evaluate pumping function of the ventricles.	Decreased cardiac output indicates heart muscle damage.	Teaching: Explain procedure. Takes 1–2 hours.
Positron emission tomography (PET)	Nitrogen-13 ammonia IV given and scanned to show cardiac perfusion. Then fluoro-18-deoxyglucose IV given and scanned for cardiac metabolic function. Exercise may be used.	In normal heart, scans match; in damaged heart, they differ.	Patient's blood glucose must be 60–140 mg/dL for accuracy. Teaching: Must lie still during scan. If exercise used, NPO and no tobacco use.
Invasive			
Angiography	Contrast medium injected into vessels to make them visible on x-rays. Cardiac: Coronary arteries via cardiac catheter. Peripheral: Peripheral arteries or veins.	Identifies vessel patency, injury, or aneurysm.	Precare: Identify prior reaction to contrast medium. Informed consent. NPO 4–18 hours before test. Teaching: Sedative and local anesthesia used; burning sensation from dye. Postcare: Monitor vital signs, injection site bleeding, peripheral pulses.
Cardiac catheterization	Catheter inserted into heart for diagnostic and therapeutic purposes. Contrast medium may be used.	Cardiac disease	Precare: Same as angiography. See Cardiac Catheterization section for sensory education and postcare.
Hemodynamic monitoring	Diagnoses and guides treatment with various continuous readings.	Blood pressure, central venous, cardiac, and pulmonary pressure abnormalities	Informed consent signed. Monitor insertion site for signs of infection.
Electrophysiological studies	Assesses heart's electrical system, with electrodes inserted into the right side of the heart.	Arrhythmias	Consent is obtained. Patient is NPO 6–8 hours before the test.

Laboratory Tests
Cardiac Biomarkers

Proteins and enzymes released into the blood by damaged cardiac cells are known as *cardiac biomarkers*. With other data, they help identify if a patient is having or has had a recent MI.

CARDIAC TROPONIN. Cardiac muscle contains the proteins troponin I and troponin T, which control the muscle fibers that contract or squeeze the heart muscle. These biomarkers are specific and sensitive for myocardial damage. Troponin testing is the preferred test, but it can be used along with less specific biomarker tests that were routinely used in the past such as creatine kinase, the isoenzyme CK-MB and myoglobin (protein that is a non-site-specific indicator of muscle damage). The high sensitivity troponin T assay, that the U.S. Food and Drug Administration (FDA) approved in 2017, provides earlier detection of myocardial injury. Normally, troponin levels are very low, so even a slight increase indicates some heart damage. High levels are indicative of MI. Levels elevate within 2 to 6 hours of damage, peak in about 15 to 20 hours, and remain elevated for up to 5 to 7 days.

CK-MB. Creatine kinase (CK) is an enzyme found in the brain, skeletal muscle, and heart muscle. The isoenzyme CK-MB found in heart muscle may be used if troponin is not available to help diagnose an MI. It rises within 4 to 6 hours after cardiac cells are damaged, peaks in 15 to 20 hours, and returns to normal in 24 to 36 hours.

High-Sensitive C-Reactive Protein
C-reactive protein is an acute-phase protein that increases with vascular inflammation. Elevated high-sensitive C-reactive protein (hs-CRP) levels reflect a higher risk for heart attack and vascular disease. Nurses can help patients understand and reduce cardiac and vascular risk factors.

Homocysteine
Homocysteine is an amino acid in the blood that may damage the lining of arteries and promote blood clots. Elevated levels are associated with increased cardiovascular disease risk. Folic acid, vitamin B_6, and vitamin B_{12} break down homocysteine. Green leafy vegetables and grains fortified with folic acid as well as vitamin B can help reduce homocysteine levels.

Lipids
Lipids include triglycerides, cholesterol, and phospholipids. Lipoproteins carry these lipids attached to proteins. Triglycerides are found in very low-density lipoproteins (VLDLs). Cholesterol is mainly found in low-density lipoproteins (LDLs). High-density lipoproteins (HDLs) are a mixture of one-half protein and one-half phospholipids and cholesterol.

A lipid profile can screen for increased risk of CAD. Patients may be asked to fast for 6 to 12 hours and avoid alcohol for 24 hours before the test. Water is not withheld. High levels of LDLs are linked to an increase in CAD because they circulate cholesterol in the arteries. HDLs play a protective role against CAD because they carry cholesterol to the liver to be metabolized. Triglycerides are a fat that can raise the risk of CAD. They are not a form of cholesterol but are included in a lipid panel. Controlling lipids and triglycerides is important in reducing CAD.

Magnesium
Magnesium, an electrolyte, is important to many functions in the body. Among these is control of the heartbeat and regulation of blood pressure. A normal magnesium level is 1.6 to 2.2 mg/dL. **Hypomagnesemia**, a low level of magnesium in the blood, can cause cardiac arrhythmias, hypertension, and tachycardia. Many things can contribute to low magnesium levels, including diuretic therapy, digitalis, some antibiotics, diabetes mellitus, and MI.

Potassium
A normal potassium level of 3.5 to 5.3 mEq/L is essential for normal cardiac function (see Chapter 6). **Hypokalemia** (low potassium level) can cause the pulse to become weak, irregular, and thready. **Hyperkalemia** (high potassium level) can result in muscle twitches and cramps followed by muscular weakness and a slow, irregular heart rate; weak pulse; and reduced blood pressure. An abnormal potassium level can be dangerous. Arrhythmias can occur, resulting in cardiac arrest.

Noninvasive Studies
Arterial Stiffness Index
Stiffness of the brachial artery is measured to determine arteriosclerosis and cardiovascular disease risk. The brachial artery correlates with the coronary arteries in regard to the extent of atherosclerosis. The arterial stiffness index test is done with a device that has a blood pressure cuff hooked to a computer that maps the waveforms during the blood pressure reading.

Chest Radiograph (X-Ray)
A chest x-ray uses radiation to reveal heart enlargement, calcifications, fluid around the heart, heart failure, and placement of pacemaker leads and pulmonary artery catheters. Fluoroscopy uses a luminescent x-ray screen to guide cardiac catheter or pacemaker lead placement. Visit www.radiologyinfo.org for test information.

Computed Tomography Angiography
Computed tomography angiography (CTA) views arteries to identify abnormalities. Coronary CT angiography (CCTA) views coronary arteries to identify CAD and risk for a cardiac event. An iodine contrast agent is used. For CCTA,

• WORD • BUILDING •

hypomagnesemia: hypo—low + magnes—magnesium + emia—in blood nitroglycerin is given to dilate the coronary arteries to identify narrowing. Also, a beta blocker may be given to slow the heart rate. Kidney function (i.e., glomerular filtration rate, creatinine) must be checked before these tests to help prevent contrast-induced acute kidney injury (see Chapter 36).

Coronary Magnetic Resonance Imaging

Two- or three-dimensional still or moving images of the beating heart are produced with magnetic resonance imaging (MRI). Cardiac MRI is useful for identifying ischemia and heart damage as well as other conditions affecting the heart. Before the test, determine if the patient has any cardiac or orthopedic implants and if they are designated MR safe (no hazard), MR conditional (able to carefully use MRI), or MR unsafe (unacceptable risk). Studies are showing that even people with non-MRI-conditional cardiac devices have been able to safely have MRIs following strict protocols ("Evidence-Based Practice"). See patient teaching guidelines for screening and preparation information for MRI on Davis Edge.

> ### Evidence-Based Practice
>
> **Clinical Question**
> Can an MRI be safely done for patients with non-MRI-conditional cardiac devices?
>
> **Evidence**
> From September 2015 to June 2019, 532 participants in the Patient Registry of Magnetic Resonance Imaging in Non-Approved DEvices underwent a total of 608 MRI examinations. An electrophysiology nurse monitored participants during the MRI. There were no complications. This demonstrated that MRI examinations can be performed safely in patients who have non-MRI-conditional devices, in pacemaker-dependent patients with implantable cardioverter defibrillators, and in patients with abandoned leads. This finding is helpful, as MRI results influence and guide patient treatment plans (Gupta et al, 2020).
>
> **Implications for Nursing Practice**
> It cannot be assumed that an implanted cardiac device prevents an MRI from being performed. Inform the HCP if the patient has an implanted cardiac device.
>
> References: Gupta, S. K., Ya'qoub, L., Wimmer, A. P., Fisher, S., & Saeed, I. M. (2020). Safety and clinical impact of MRI in patients with non–MRI-conditional cardiac devices. *Radiology: Cardiothoracic Imaging, 2*(5). https://doi.org/10.1148/ryct.2020200086

Electrocardiogram

The electrocardiogram (ECG) records electrical activity of the heart in various views. Abnormalities related to conduction, rate, rhythm, heart chamber enlargement, myocardial ischemia, MI, and electrolyte imbalances may be reflected on an ECG.

To obtain an ECG, electrodes are placed on the skin to transmit electrical impulses to the ECG machine for recording. The electrical impulses from the heart appear as waves on graph paper. One view of the heart using a combination of the electrodes to obtain the view is called a *lead*. The standard 12-lead ECG provides 12 views of the heart. In addition, 15- and 18-lead ECGs can be obtained.

SIGNAL-AVERAGED ECG. The signal-averaged ECG uses a computer to record electrical heart signals for 20 minutes to capture undetected low-level signals that are averaged. This test can identify whether a patient is at risk for ventricular **arrhythmias** (abnormal heart rhythms; also known as *dysrhythmias*).

HOLTER MONITORING (AMBULATORY ECG). A Holter monitor is worn by the patient and continuously records an ECG in one lead (view) for 24 to 48 hours as a patient goes about their daily activities. The patient records a diary of activities and symptoms and pushes the event button if symptoms occur. Symptoms are later correlated with the ECG recordings. The recordings are scanned by a computer and interpreted by an HCP. Arrhythmias or myocardial ischemia that occur infrequently can be detected.

Echocardiogram

An echocardiogram is an ultrasound that records the motion of the heart structures, including the valves and chambers, as well as the heart size, shape, and position. Three-dimensional images of the heart and four-dimensional (real-time) heart imaging are possible. Color Doppler (change in sound wave pitch as they bounce off blood cells) can record blood flow and blood pressure through the heart arteries and valves.

- The standard transthoracic echocardiogram transmits ultrasonic sound waves across the chest wall and through lung and rib tissue into the heart so that the returned echoes can be recorded. An ECG is recorded at the same time.
- A strain echocardiogram shows changes in the shape of the heart (deformation). It is used for heart failure, in cardiomyopathy, to guide treatment, or to evaluate cardiac surgery or transplant.
- An exercise stress echocardiogram shows exercise-induced cardiac ischemia to diagnose CAD. If the patient is unable to exercise, dobutamine (a cardiac inotrope and chronotrope) is given, as the heart rate responds to it as it does to exercise.
- A transesophageal echocardiogram (TEE) produces clear images using a transducer on a probe placed in the esophagus because lung and rib tissue does not have to be penetrated by the sound waves. Patients take nothing by mouth (NPO) for 6 hours before the test and receive a sedative. The patient's throat is anesthetized with a local anesthetic.

> ### BE SAFE!
> **BE VIGILANT!** Whenever a patient's throat is anesthetized for a procedure, the patient must not take anything by mouth (NPO) until the nurse has verified (by touching the back of the throat with a cotton tip swab) that the gag reflex has returned. The patient could aspirate or choke while drinking or eating if the gag reflex is not present.

Exercise Stress Test

The exercise stress test measures cardiac function or peripheral vascular disease during a defined exercise protocol. If the patient is unable to exercise, a coronary vasodilator such as adenosine or dipyridamole can be given to increase blood flow in healthy vessels and show unhealthy areas with reduced blood flow. Test instructions include an explanation of the test; not smoking, eating, or drinking for 2 to 4 hours before the test; and wearing comfortable walking shoes, a loose top, and, for women, a supportive bra.

Before the test, baseline vital signs are obtained. Then, while the patient exercises on a treadmill, on a stationary bicycle, or by climbing stairs, vital signs, oxygen saturation, skin temperature, physical appearance, chest pain, and ECG are monitored to help ensure patient safety. The test is completed when the patient reaches his or her peak heart rate (patient's age subtracted from 220), experiences chest pain or other symptoms, is unable to exercise further, or develops abnormal vital sign or ECG changes. Vital signs and ECG continue to be monitored after the test until they return to baseline.

For a peripheral vascular stress test, the patient walks for 5 minutes at 1.5 miles per hour on the treadmill. Pulse volume measurements are taken at baseline resting, during the test, and at final resting after the test. If intermittent **claudication** (pain in the legs with activity) occurs, the test is stopped.

Nuclear Radioisotope Imaging

For nuclear radioisotope imaging, small amounts of radioisotopes are given via IV route. The patient is then scanned with a gamma camera to produce a radionuclide image. Radiation exposure is small. These tests can provide information about organ function such as myocardial ischemia or infarction, cardiac blood flow, and ventricle size and motion. Examples include the following:

- Technetium (TC-99m) pyrophosphate shows hot spots in areas of ischemia or myocardial cell damage. Acute MI size and location can be detected, but old MIs cannot be detected.
- TC-99m sestamibi shows hot spots in areas of myocardial cell damage.
- TC-99m pertechnetate is used in a multiple-gated acquisition scan to follow the flow of radioactivity in the bloodstream to show ventricular function, wall motion, and the ejection fraction of the heart.
- Thallium-201 detects impaired myocardial perfusion and ischemia or MI through cold spot areas where the thallium was not absorbed. The patency of a coronary artery graft may also be assessed with this test. Exercise testing may be combined with thallium injection to detect blood flow changes with activity and after rest. If patients are unable to participate in exercise for the thallium stress test, coronary vasodilators can be given.

Positron Emission Tomography Scan

A cardiac positron emission tomography (PET)/CT myocardial perfusion scan shows blood flow to the heart muscle during stress and at rest. A small amount of radiation is used. CAD can be identified for treatment.

Tilt Table Test

The tilt table test is used to help diagnose the cause of syncope (fainting spells). Heart rate and blood pressure are monitored during a change in position from lying down to standing up.

Doppler Ultrasound

In a Doppler ultrasound test, sound waves bounce off moving blood cells in the peripheral blood vessels and return a sound frequency in relationship to the amount of blood flow. With decreased blood flow, the sounds are reduced. This test requires no patient preparation, takes about 20 minutes to complete, and is painless.

Invasive Studies

Angiography

Arteriography and venography are the two types of angiography (Fig. 21.11). Arteriography examines arteries. Venography studies veins. Angiography uses dye injected into the vascular system to visualize the vessels on radiographs. This test is used to assess blood clot formation, diagnose peripheral vascular disease, and test vessels for potential grafting use.

The patient must be asked about allergies, assessed for risk for contrast-induced acute kidney injury (see Chapter 36), give informed consent, be NPO for about 4 hours before the test, and be informed that the dye produces a hot, burning feeling when injected. After the procedure, vital signs, allergic reaction signs, hemorrhage at the injection site, and pulses are monitored for several hours.

Cardiac Catheterization

Cardiac catheterization allows the heart's right or left anatomy and physiology to be studied and therapeutic procedures to be done. As an invasive diagnostic procedure, it measures pressures in the heart chambers and great blood vessels, cardiac output, and oxygen saturation (see "Hemodynamic Monitoring"). The wrist, forearm, groin, or neck blood vessels

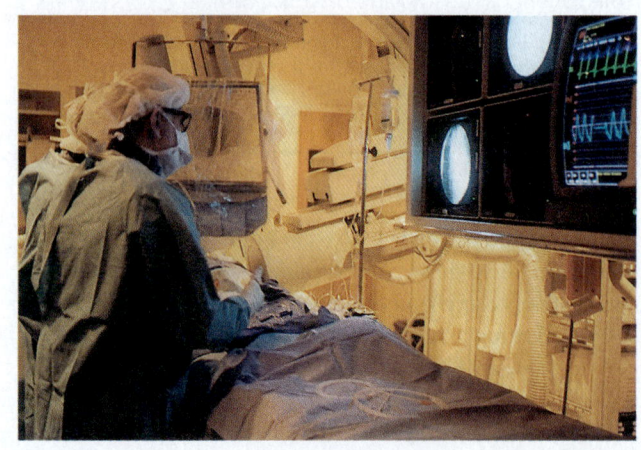

FIGURE 21.11 Coronary angiography and cardiac catheterization.

can be used as catheter insertion sites. The radial artery is growing in use to access the left side of the heart, while the femoral vein is typically used for the right side of the heart, although the brachial vein is becoming more popular. The arm bleeds less and has fewer complications and mobility restrictions than the groin. To guide the insertion of the catheter into the heart, fluoroscopy, which uses x-ray to produce real-time images of internal organs in motion on a video monitor, is used. Dye can be injected to visualize the heart chambers and vessels to diagnose CAD.

Prior to the procedure, an informed consent is obtained and a prior reaction to a contrast medium is noted and reported. The patient is NPO for about 8 hours before the test. IV hydration may be given before the procedure while the patient is NPO. Patient education includes informing the patient that they will be awake but sedated during the procedure; a local anesthetic, which may sting, will numb the catheter insertion site prior to insertion; a warm, flushing sensation may be felt when the dye is injected; the room will have a lot of equipment; a movable table will be used; vital signs and ECG are monitored constantly; and the procedure takes up to 2 to 3 hours.

After the procedure, the catheter is removed. Firm pressure must be applied to the insertion site to prevent hemorrhage, hematoma formation, or retroperitoneal bleeding, which are the most common complications. Methods used to control the bleeding include manual pressure for up to 15 to 30 minutes, devices to close the arterial puncture using sutures or an internal absorbable plug, and a mechanical clamp applied and monitored by skilled staff. Vital signs, the insertion site, and pedal pulses are monitored. If the wrist is used, sitting and ambulation are permitted. If the groin is used, the patient is on bedrest without moving or flexing the leg for a few hours to prevent bleeding. For comfort, modified positioning and use of a pillow may be used without complications as ordered. Patients can eat and are encouraged to drink fluids to help eliminate the dye from the body. If the patient is stable and no significant findings are found, the patient may be discharged by the HCP to a responsible adult.

Hemodynamic Monitoring

A catheter attached to a transducer and monitor, called an *arterial line*, can be inserted into the radial or femoral artery to measure continuous arterial blood pressure. A catheter inserted into the vena cava or the pulmonary artery can monitor pressure. Normal central venous pressure (CVP) is 1 to 6 mm Hg. CVP reflects **preload** (pressure stretching the ventricle of the heart from fluid returned to the heart). Normal right atrial pressure is 2 to 6 mm Hg. Normal cardiac output is 4 to 8 L/min. Normal pulmonary artery systolic/diastolic pressures are 20–30/0–10 mm Hg, and pulmonary artery wedge pressure is 4 to 12 mm Hg. Normal venous oxygen saturation (SvO_2) is 60% to 80%.

Electrophysiological Study

To study the heart's electrical system, one or more catheters with two to three electrodes are inserted via the femoral vein into the right side of the heart. The heart's electrical impulses are recorded, and cardiac pacing can be done. Arrhythmias can be triggered to help the HCP diagnose why they are occurring. A consent is obtained. The patient is NPO 6 to 8 hours before the test.

THERAPEUTIC MEASURES FOR THE CARDIOVASCULAR SYSTEM

Health Promotion and Lifestyle Changes

To reduce risk factors or promote recovery from cardiovascular disease, lifestyle changes are often needed. Long-standing habits are difficult to change. Refer patients to community support groups that can offer encouragement to promote a healthy lifestyle.

> **PRACTICE ANALYSIS TIP**
> Linking NCLEX-PN® to Practice
> The LPN/LVN will participate in client referral process.

Diet

A healthy, balanced diet is important to help reduce the risk for CAD. Weight loss, if needed, is encouraged. Eating at least five servings of fruits and vegetables daily, increasing fish intake, eating poultry without skin, and limiting saturated fats and sodium are parts of a healthy diet.

Exercise

A prescribed walking program helps promote blood flow by contracting the skeletal muscles and may reduce symptoms of peripheral vascular disease. Exercise is very important for optimum cardiac functioning.

Smoking Cessation

Smoking causes vasoconstriction that can last up to 1 hour after smoking one cigarette. For patients with cardiac or vascular disease, the reduced blood flow can exacerbate symptoms. Patients should be encouraged to stop smoking and be referred to cessation programs and support groups (see www.americanheart.org).

Antiembolism Devices

Antiembolism devices improve arterial blood flow and venous return to prevent the formation of blood clots. They are used for patients on bedrest, with peripheral vascular disease, or after surgery or trauma.

Compression Stockings

There are two types of compression stockings for two different types of medical issues. *Antiembolism stockings* (TED hose = thromboembolism deterrent) apply 8 to 18 mm Hg of compression to the leg to promote normal venous return to prevent stasis of fluid in immobile patients. *Medical graduated compression stockings* apply 15 to 20 mm Hg or higher of compression to the leg in ambulatory people with venous or lymphatic disorders. The greatest pressure is applied at the ankle and decreases going up the leg. Their uses include edema, post-thrombotic syndrome, post-venous procedures, venous stasis, and varicose veins which require higher compression than antiembolism stockings provide. Compression stockings may be knee or thigh length. All stockings must be applied correctly so as not to produce a tourniquet effect. For ease in application, turn the stocking inside out to the heel, put the foot portion on the patient's foot up to the heel, and pull the remaining stocking up over the leg. Knee-length stockings should be 1 to 2 inches below the bottom of the kneecap. They should not roll down, or they will cause rather than prevent stasis. Some patients may require assistance in applying the stockings if they have impaired manual dexterity. Devices are available that aid in applying the stockings.

> **LEARNING TIP**
> Selection of the appropriate compression stocking:
> - Antiembolism stockings: Immobile patients on bedrest to maintain normal venous return
> - Medical graduated compression stockings: Ambulatory patients with chronic venous or lymphatic disorders
> - Nonmedical uniform, nongraduated compression support hosiery: People with tired, aching legs or who are traveling

Intermittent Pneumatic Compression Devices

An intermittent pneumatic compression device consists of plastic inflatable stockings that are filled intermittently with air by an attached motor. This device simulates the contraction of the leg muscles, promoting fluid movement, which helps to prevent thrombosis development. The compartments in the stockings inflate to 35 to 55 mm Hg of pressure, beginning in the ankle compartment and progressing next to the calf compartment and finally the thigh compartment. Monitor the device for proper pressure inflation.

Oxygen

Supplemental oxygen is administered to patients with chest pain to help ensure that the heart receives sufficient oxygen to function. Oxygen may be delivered via a nasal cannula or facemask. Reinforce teaching on safety precautions for home use of oxygen, such as avoiding open flames and not smoking when oxygen is in use.

Medications

The primary cardiovascular drugs are antihypertensives, antiarrhythmics, antianginals, anticoagulants, cardiac glycosides, thrombolytics, and vasodilators. They are discussed in further detail where the disorders they are used to treat are discussed (see "Nutrition Notes").

> **Nutrition Notes**
> **CYP Enzymes and Certain Citrus Fruits**
> Cytochrome P450 (CYP450) is a superfamily of more than 50 enzymes found mainly in the liver but also in the gastrointestinal tract, lungs, placenta, and kidneys. The isoenzyme CYP3A4, found in the small intestine, plays a major role in metabolizing medications and regulating their oral bioavailability, a function that may have evolved to protect the body from toxins. Grapefruit, Seville oranges (often in orange marmalade), pomelos, and tangelos (cross between tangerine and grapefruit) appear to inhibit intestinal CYP3A4, which can then cause too much medication to be absorbed into the bloodstream (see www.fda.gov and search "grapefruit juice" for a video). Not all medications in the same medication class are affected by grapefruit in whole or juice form. For medication interactions with grapefruit, search "grapefruit" on https://medlineplus.gov. Consult a pharmacist for specific medication and grapefruit information.

Cardiac Surgery

As heart disease symptoms increase in severity and frequency or the disease process worsens, cardiac surgery may be used as treatment.

Preparation for Surgery

Baseline data collection is important for postoperative comparison and early discharge planning. In addition to an electrocardiogram, chest x-ray, complete blood cell count, coagulation studies, chemistry profile, and blood crossmatch, patients with chronic obstructive pulmonary disease may have baseline arterial blood gases and pulmonary function tests. Patients with carotid bruits may have carotid studies to determine the amount of occlusion in the carotid artery. If the occlusion is significant, a carotid endarterectomy, which removes the plaque on the lining of the blocked or diseased carotid artery, is performed, usually several weeks before cardiac surgery.

Medications that may increase bleeding or reduce fluid volume may be ordered to be held before surgery by the HCP. Medications that increase bleeding include aspirin, often stopped 3 to 7 days preoperatively; warfarin (Coumadin), often stopped 4 to 5 days preoperatively; and heparin, usually stopped 4 hours preoperatively. During surgery, fluid volume and blood pressure may be decreased by blood loss or medications. Therefore, diuretics, which could further reduce fluid volume and blood pressure, are withheld up to 2 days before surgery. The patient is NPO as specified before surgery. For this reason, patients with diabetes are instructed on management of their insulin or oral hypoglycemic agents for the morning of surgery. Blood glucose monitoring is done. The anesthesiologist assesses the patient before surgery and orders preoperative medications.

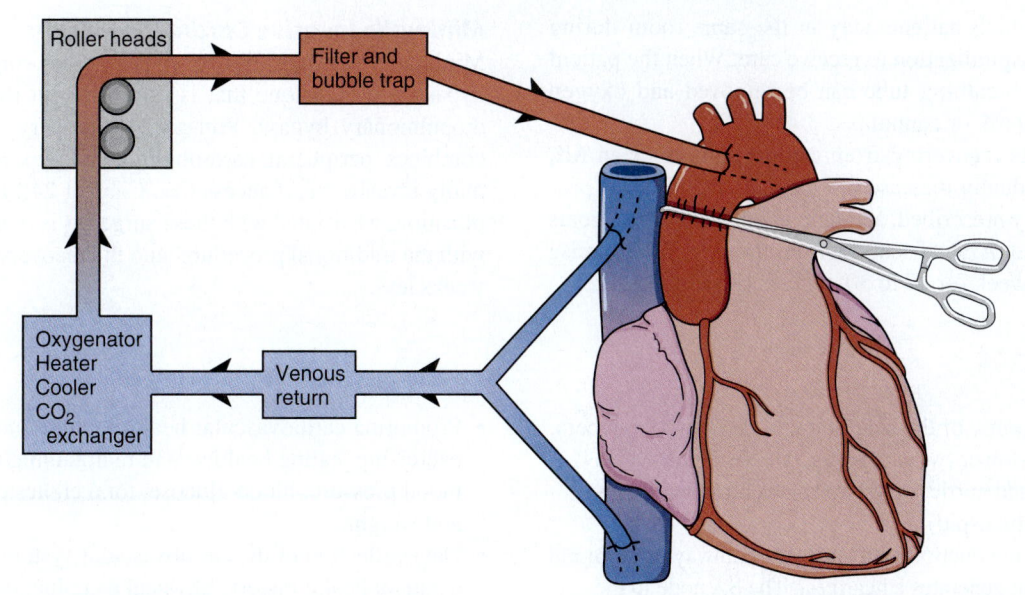

FIGURE 21.12 Cardiopulmonary bypass pump components.

Patients recover more quickly and have less postoperative stress with thorough preoperative education on pain management; coughing and deep breathing exercises; incision care; equipment, including the endotracheal tube and mechanical ventilator, and methods of communicating while intubated; chest tubes; IV lines; the urinary catheter; and equipment alarms. It should be emphasized to the patient and family that the patient will not be able to talk while the endotracheal tube is in place. In addition, a preoperative family tour of the patient's postoperative unit and the waiting area helps prepare them for the surgical experience. A referral to pastoral care, if desired, can be comforting to the patient and family.

Cardiopulmonary Bypass

Cardiac surgery may use a cardiopulmonary bypass pump in which blood is temporarily diverted away from the heart and lungs to the special pump (Fig. 21.12). This diversion allows for a bloodless and motionless surgical field while the function of the heart and lungs is maintained by the pump (Fig. 21.13).

Before going on the pump, the patient is anticoagulated with heparin until the partial thromboplastin time is five to six times greater than normal. Immediately before the patient comes off the pump, the effects of the heparin are reversed with protamine sulfate (antidote for heparin). Heparin is absorbed and stored in organs and tissue and can be sporadically released hours after surgery. As a result, the patient may have excessive bleeding. The risk of an air embolism is minimized by priming the pump with lactated Ringer's solution. This priming solution increases circulating volume, which then results in a shifting of fluid into the interstitial tissue causing edema formation. These fluid shifts can continue up to 6 hours after surgery and may cause hypotension.

General Procedure for Cardiac Surgery

After the patient is placed on cardiopulmonary bypass, a cardioplegic solution is infused into the aortic root along with iced saline to cause cardiac standstill. When the surgery is completed, the patient's blood is warmed in the cardiopulmonary bypass circuit, and the patient is slowly weaned from bypass. The heart starts beating again after it is warmed and defibrillated. Temporary pacing wires are attached to the heart before the cardiopulmonary bypass pump is discontinued, so an external temporary pacemaker can be used if bradycardia develops. Once the heart is beating, bypass is stopped. Mediastinal chest tubes are placed to drain remaining blood and fluid from the chest. The **sternotomy** (sternum cut in half) is closed with wires through the sternum and then dissolving sutures or staples for the layers of tissue and skin. While still under anesthesia and on the mechanical ventilator, the patient is transferred to a cardiac care unit. Cardiac universal beds (CUB) may

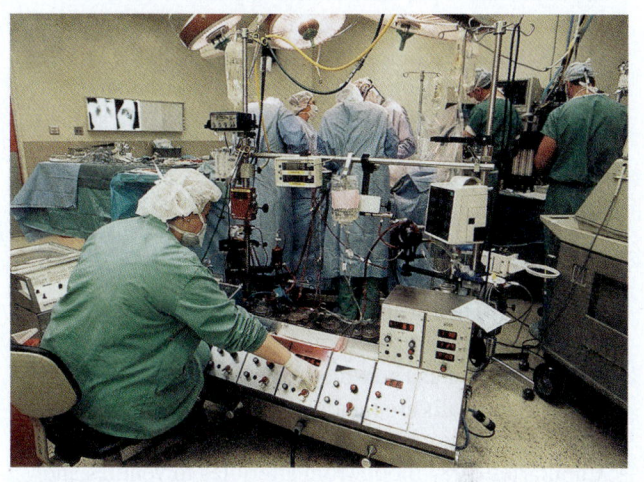

FIGURE 21.13 Cardiopulmonary bypass pump in use.

• WORD • BUILDING •

sternotomy: stern—sternum + otomy—incision into

be used, in which patients stay in the same room during their entire hospitalization to receive care. When the patient awakens, the breathing tube can be removed and oxygen delivered by mask or cannula.

For patients recovering from cardiac surgery or an MI, activity is gradually increased. A cardiac rehabilitation program is usually prescribed, and individualized exercise goals are determined. After discharge from the hospital, exercise three times a week for 20 to 30 minutes is encouraged.

Minimally Invasive Cardiac Surgery

Minimally invasive direct visualization coronary artery bypass is a technique that is done without the use of cardiopulmonary bypass. Port-access coronary artery bypass combines peripheral cardiopulmonary bypass with minimally invasive heart access (see Chapter 24). Risk for complications associated with these surgeries is much lower than with the traditional procedure, and the recovery time is often weeks less.

Key Points

- Normal anatomy of the heart: atria—upper two chambers, ventricles—lower two chambers, two semilunar valves (pulmonic and aortic), and two atrioventricular valves (mitral and bicuspid).
- The cardiac conduction pathway is the pathway of electrical impulses that generates a heartbeat. The SA node in the wall of the right atrium is autorhythmic and depolarizes about 100 times per minute, initiating each heartbeat.
- A cardiac cycle is the sequence of mechanical events that occurs during each heartbeat. Simply stated, the two atria contract simultaneously, followed by the simultaneous contraction of the two ventricles (a fraction of a second later).
- Cardiac output is the amount of blood ejected from the left ventricle in 1 minute (the right ventricle pumps a similar amount).
- Arteries and arterioles carry blood from the heart to capillaries. Their walls are relatively thick and consist of three layers.
- Veins and venules carry blood from capillaries to the heart. Their walls are relatively thin because they have less smooth muscle than arteries.
- Capillaries carry blood from arterioles to venules and form extensive networks in most tissues. They are one-cell thick to permit the exchange of gases, nutrients, and waste products between the blood and tissues.
- Atherosclerosis is the deposition of lipids in the walls of arteries over a period of years.
- Promoting cardiovascular health includes not smoking; exercising; eating healthy; and maintaining normal blood pressure, blood glucose, total cholesterol levels, and weight.
- Data collection of the cardiovascular system includes a patient health history, physical examination, and diagnostic tests.
- Blood tests done for cardiovascular disease can include cardiac troponin, CK-MB, hs-CRP, homocysteine levels, lipid profile, magnesium and potassium, triglycerides.
- Noninvasive diagnostic tests commonly performed to diagnose disorders of the cardiovascular system include arterial stiffness index, chest x-ray, cardiac or artery CTA, ECG, echocardiogram, MRI, magnetic resonance angiography, and cardiac PET scan.
- Invasive diagnostic tests include angiography, cardiac catheterization, electrophysiological study, and hemodynamic monitoring.
- Therapeutic measures for disorders of the cardiovascular system include health promotion and lifestyle changes, antiembolism devices, compression stockings, diet, exercise, medications, oxygen, and smoking cessation.
- Minimally invasive direct visualization coronary artery bypass is a technique that is done without the use of cardiopulmonary bypass. Port-access coronary artery bypass combines peripheral cardiopulmonary bypass with minimally invasive heart access.

SUGGESTED ANSWERS TO CHAPTER EXERCISES

Cue Recognition

21.1: Quickly assist Mrs. Goldberg to sit down to prevent a fall. Ask how she is feeling. Did you recognize that the cue of her hand on her forehead may mean she is feeling dizzy and at risk of falling? Lightheadedness or syncope may be reported due to a drop in blood pressure decreasing the amount of oxygen-rich blood traveling to the brain. Take orthostatic blood pressure readings and report abnormal data (see "Orthostatic Blood Pressure" section) to the HCP. Explain to the resident why it is important to change positions slowly. Encourage the resident to request assistance to ambulate. Use a walking belt during ambulation for safety.

Critical Thinking & Clinical Judgment

Mrs. Cheung

1. An older person may not experience typical MI symptoms. Chest pain is often not present in MI because of reduced nerve sensitivity with aging. Dyspnea is the classic symptom of MI in the older patient.
2. Inspect both legs to determine edematous areas. Determine location and severity of edema by pressing for 5 seconds over the medial malleolus and moving up the leg along the tibia until no edema is found. Palpate bilaterally. Measure leg circumference.

SUGGESTED ANSWERS TO CHAPTER EXERCISES—cont'd

3. Document location of edema and whether edema is nonpitting or pitting for both legs: "bilateral pitting ankle edema" along with the leg circumference measurement number.
4. Additional symptoms should be documented as follows: dyspnea at rest that increases with exertion, heart tones clear and distant, nailbeds pale, pain free, poor appetite for 2 weeks, 6-pound weight gain in 1 week, three-pillow orthopnea, bilateral jugular venous distention.
5. Unit analysis method:

$$\frac{162 \text{ pounds}}{} \times \frac{1 \text{ kilogram}}{2.2 \text{ pounds}} = 73.6 \text{ kilograms}$$

6. HCP, nurses, pharmacist, respiratory therapist, dietitian, and social worker or case manager.

Additional Resources

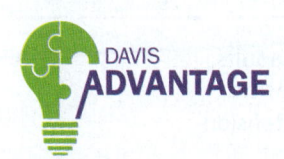

Go to Davis Advantage to complete your learning: strengthen understanding, apply your knowledge, and prepare for the Next Gen NCLEX®.

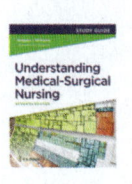

A Study Guide is also available.

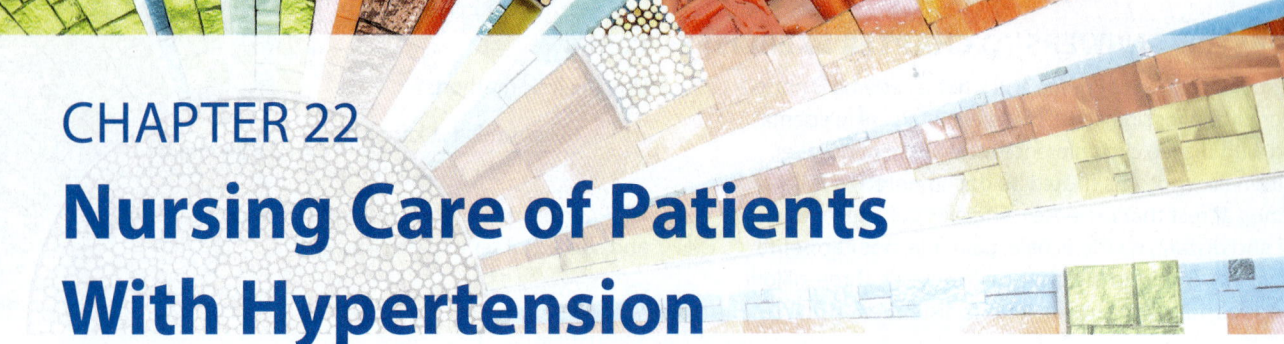

CHAPTER 22
Nursing Care of Patients With Hypertension

Amanda Miller

KEY TERMS

cardiac output (KAR-dee-yak OWT-put)
diastolic (dy-uh-STAH-lik)
hypertension (HY-per-TEN-shun)
hypertensive emergency (HY-per-TEN-siv ee-MUR-gen-see)
hypertensive urgency (HY-per-TEN-siv UR-gen-see)
hypertrophy (hy-PER-truh-fee)
peripheral vascular resistance (puh-RIF-uh-ruhl VAS-kyoo-lar ree-ZIS-tents)
plaque (PLAK)
primary hypertension (PRY-mer-ee HY-per-TEN-shun)
secondary hypertension (SEK-un-DAR-ee HY-per-TEN-shun)
systolic (sis-TOL-ik)
viscosity (vis-KAW-sih-tee)

CHAPTER CONCEPTS

Caring
Health promotion
Perfusion
Teaching and learning

LEARNING OUTCOMES

1. Define classifications of hypertension in adults.
2. Explain the pathophysiology of hypertension.
3. Identify causes and risk factors for hypertension.
4. List signs and symptoms of hypertension.
5. Describe therapeutic measures for hypertension.
6. Define hypertensive emergency.
7. List common complications of hypertension.
8. Plan nursing care for patients with hypertension.
9. Evaluate effectiveness of nursing interventions.

Consistent elevation in blood pressure results in **hypertension**, or high blood pressure (BP), which is a primary risk factor for cardiovascular disease (CVD) and stroke. In 2017, hypertension was the 13th leading cause of death, a 4.7% increase from 2016 (Kochanek et al, 2019). The American College of Cardiology (ACC) and the American Heart Association (AHA) redefined normal and abnormal BP for adults ages 18 and older (Table 22.1; Whelton et al, 2018). Other expert groups have slightly different definitions of hypertension categories that might be used for diagnosis and treatment by health-care providers (HCPs).

PATHOPHYSIOLOGY

BP is a measure of the pressure exerted by blood on the walls of the blood vessels. BP is determined by **cardiac output** (CO; the amount of blood that the heart pumps each minute), **peripheral vascular resistance** (PVR; the ability of the vessels to stretch), the **viscosity** (thickness) of the blood, and the amount of circulating blood volume. Decreased stretching ability of blood vessels, increased blood viscosity, and/or increased fluid volume may cause an increase in BP.

Factors that impair normal regulation of BP may lead to hypertension. Many of these factors are not well understood. Sympathetic nervous system overstimulation, which causes vasoconstriction, and alterations in baroreceptors and chemoreceptors may influence the development of hypertension. Specifically, baroreceptors may become

• WORD • BUILDING •

hypertension: hyper—excessive + tensio—tension
viscosity: viscous—sticky

Table 22.1
Categories of Blood Pressure (BP) in Adults*

BP Category	Systolic BP		Diastolic BP
Normal	<120 mm Hg	and	<80 mm Hg
Elevated	120–129 mm Hg	and	<80 mm Hg
Hypertension			
Stage 1	130–139 mm Hg	or	80–89 mm Hg
Stage 2	≥140 mm Hg	or	≥90 mm Hg

*Individuals with SBP and DBP in 2 categories should be designated to the higher BP category. BP indicates blood pressure (based on an average of ≥2 careful readings obtained on ≥2 occasions).

Reprinted with permission. *Hypertension*, 2018;71:e13-e115. ©2018 American Heart Association, Inc.

Table 22.2
Hypertension Summary

Signs and Symptoms	Often none Increased blood pressure Headache, bloody nose, severe anxiety, shortness of breath
Diagnosis	See Table 22.1
Therapeutic Measures	Lifestyle modification Medication
Complications	Heart failure Kidney disease Myocardial infarction Stroke
Priority Nursing Diagnoses	*Readiness for Enhanced Health Literacy* *Ineffective Health Self-Management* *Risk for Unstable Blood Pressure*

less sensitive from prolonged increases in vessel pressure and then fail to stimulate vasodilation through vessel stretching. Increases in hormones that cause sodium retention, such as aldosterone, lead to increased fluid retention. Changes in kidney function, altering the excretion of fluid, also results in excess fluid volume that may contribute to hypertension.

Types of Hypertension
Primary Hypertension
Primary hypertension (formally essential hypertension) is elevation of **systolic** and/or **diastolic** BP with no identifiable cause.

Secondary Hypertension
Secondary hypertension has a known cause. It occurs as the result of another disease process, such as a kidney abnormality or a tumor of the adrenal gland. When the cause of secondary hypertension is treated before permanent structural changes occur, BP usually returns to normal.

SIGNS AND SYMPTOMS

Hypertension often does not exhibit symptoms for many years. As a result, it is referred to as the "silent killer." Patients with hypertension are often first diagnosed when seeking health care for reasons unrelated to hypertension. In a small number of cases, a patient with hypertension may report a headache, bloody nose, severe anxiety, or shortness of breath (Table 22.2).

DIAGNOSIS

BP should be measured at least every year after the age of 3 (National Heart, Lung, and Blood Institute, 2020). Diagnosis of hypertension requires that at least two BP measurements are taken at different points in time, usually a week(s) apart, preferably by an ambulatory or home monitoring BP monitoring device. A patient's risk factors, presence of signs and symptoms, history of kidney or heart disease, and current use of medications are also considered.

> **CUE RECOGNITION 22.1**
> You observe the nursing assistant escort Mr. Haiken, a patient in the HCP's office, into an examination room and seat him on the table with his legs dangling. The nursing assistant immediately begins to take a BP reading as she talks with the patient. What action do you take?
>
> *Suggested answers are at the end of the chapter.*

SOCIAL DETERMINANTS OF HEALTH

Social determinants of health (SDOH) are categorized by Healthy People 2030 (health.gov) as economic stability, education access and quality, health-care access and quality, neighborhood and built environment, and social and community context. SDOH can influence the development and management of hypertension. Embracing healthy habits and obtaining and properly using antihypertensive medications can be more difficult for people in lower socioeconomic levels. Licensed practical nurses/licensed vocational

• WORD • BUILDING •
systolic: systole—concentration
diastolic: diastole—expansion

nurses (LPNs/LVNs) can provide education on hypertension, healthy lifestyles to prevent hypertension, and use of medication as well as information on resources for obtaining medications to manage hypertension.

RISK FACTORS

A combination of genetic (nonmodifiable) and environmental (modifiable) risk factors are thought to be responsible for the development of hypertension. Nonmodifiable risk factors—those that *cannot* be changed—include a family history of hypertension, age, and ethnicity. Modifiable risk factors—those that *can* be changed—include blood glucose level, activity level, smoking, salt and alcohol intake, and insufficient sleep (less than 5 hours per night). Managing these risk factors can help to decrease BP. Healthy People 2030 has an objective to increase the proportion of adults with hypertension whose BP is under control from the baseline 47.8% to 60.8%.

Nonmodifiable Risk Factors
Family History of Hypertension
Hypertension is more common among people with a family history of hypertension; people with a family history have almost twice the risk of developing hypertension as those with no family history and should have their BP monitored regularly.

Age
Genetics, environmental risk factors, and lifestyle habits affect how we age, resulting in wide variations of BP among older adults. With age, **plaque** builds up in the arteries. Blood vessels become stiffer and less elastic, causing the heart to work harder to force blood through them.

Race or Ethnicity
High BP is more common in non-Hispanic Black adults (54%) than in non-Hispanic White adults (46%), non-Hispanic Asian adults (39%), or Hispanic adults (36%) (Centers for Disease Control and Prevention [CDC], 2020). Hypertension among Black individuals is often caused by increased renin activity, resulting in greater sodium and fluid retention. This population may respond well to diuretics such as hydrochlorothiazide (HydroDIURIL) and furosemide (Lasix).

Modifiable Risk Factors
Lifestyle
Lifestyle modifications to reduce hypertension risk include access to health care, maintenance of a healthy weight, reduced sodium intake, adequate potassium intake, reduced alcohol consumption, regular physical activity, and compliance with medication regimen (Carey et al, 2018). They are used along with antihypertensive medications to control hypertension. A dietitian can help the patient develop a healthy low-sodium diet plan ("Nutrition Notes"; "Evidence-Based Practice").

Nutrition Notes
Reducing Blood Pressure With Diet
The Dietary Guidelines for Americans 2020–2025 recommend a sodium intake of 2,300 mg for healthy adults (www.dietaryguidelines.gov). Those with hypertension should reduce their sodium intake more. The average sodium intake of Americans is 3,393 mg per day. Examples of low-sodium dietary patterns include the Dietary Approaches to Stop Hypertension (DASH) dietary pattern, Healthy Mediterranean-Style Dietary Pattern, and Healthy Vegetarian Dietary Pattern (USDA, 2020). On a 2,000-calorie diet, a person following the DASH Eating Plan (www.nhlbi.nih.gov/health-topics/dash-eating-plan) would consume the following:

Food Group	Number of Servings	Example of One Serving
Grains	6–8	• 1 slice of bread • ½ cup cooked cereal or pasta
Vegetables	4–5	• 1 cup raw leafy • ½ cup cooked, nonstarchy
Fruits	4–5	• 1 medium fresh • ½ cup canned or frozen • ¼ cup dried
Dairy, low-fat or fat-free	2–3	• 8 ounces of milk • 1½ ounces of cheese
Meat (lean), poultry, or fish	6 or less	• 1 ounce cooked
Fats and oils, preferably monounsaturated (e.g., canola, olive, peanut)	2–3	• 1 teaspoon
Nuts, seeds, dry beans, peas	4–5 weekly	• ⅓ cup of nuts • 2 tablespoons of seeds • ½ cup cooked beans

---

Diabetes Mellitus
Many adults who have diabetes mellitus also have hypertension. Lifestyle modifications and adherence to therapy are crucial to prevent heart attacks, strokes, blindness, and kidney disease associated with high blood glucose and BP levels.

Evidence-Based Practice

Clinical Question
Does the Dietary Approaches to Stop Hypertension (DASH) diet affect high BP?

Evidence
A systematic review and meta-analysis of 30 random controlled trials revealed that the DASH diet led to significant reductions in both systolic and diastolic BP (Filippou et al, 2020).

Implications for Nursing Practice
Teach patients that the DASH diet is an effective way to help control BP. Even small decreases in BP can reduce cardiovascular disease and mortality.

Reference: Filippou, C. D., Tsioufis, C. P., Thomopoulos, C. G., Mihas, C. C., Dimitriadis, K. S., Sotiropoulou, L. I., Chrysochoou, C. A., Nihoyannopoulos, P. I., & Tousoulis, D. M. (2020). Dietary Approaches to Stop Hypertension (DASH) diet and blood pressure reduction in adults with and without hypertension: A systematic review and meta-analysis of randomized controlled trials. *Advances in Nutrition, 11*(5), 1150–1160. https://doi.org/10.1093/advances/nmaa041

CRITICAL THINKING

Ms. Diaz, age 54, visits a health-care clinic because she has a headache every morning. The nurse collects data on Ms. Diaz and finds that she is an office manager, smokes a pack of cigarettes a day, and eats fast food for lunch at her desk. She has two adult children, is recently divorced, and has two to three alcoholic drinks every evening. Ms. Diaz has been in good health and takes two aspirin tablets daily for her headaches.

1. What are Ms. Diaz's risk factors for hypertension?
2. What is the most significant patient information identified? Why?
3. Why is hypertension referred to as the "silent killer"?
4. Why should Ms. Diaz be told of the need for lifelong therapy if she is diagnosed with hypertension?

Suggested answers are at the end of the chapter.

THERAPEUTIC MEASURES FOR HYPERTENSION

The 2014 Evidence-Based Guideline for the Management of High Blood Pressure in Adults by the Eighth Joint National Committee (James et al, 2014) defines pharmacologic treatment thresholds and recommends drug therapy. Treatment begins with lifestyle modifications and then individualized consideration of antihypertensive medication therapy. See Table 22.3 for examples of medications used to treat hypertension. The treatment plan of lifestyle modifications and medications is effective if patients are motivated to accept the diagnosis of hypertension and include the lifelong treatment in their daily routine. Empathy and trust between patients and nurses can increase patient motivation. Remind them that although they may feel fine with treatment, the hypertension condition is still present. Inform patients not to stop taking their medications unless told to by their HCP.

Antihypertensive medications can have unpleasant side effects. The nurse should be proactive and inform patients about these side effects and to report them if they occur, so that medications can be adjusted as needed. As an example, erectile dysfunction can be a side effect. Men may be reluctant to discuss this side effect and instead choose to stop the medication.

BE SAFE!
BE VIGILANT! Explain to patients who take antihypertensive drugs to change positions slowly to prevent the effects of orthostatic hypotension and the risk of falling.

Gerontological Issues
Managing Antihypertensive Therapy
- Deficiencies in fluid volume are a common problem for older adults. Diuretics can worsen dehydration. Careful monitoring of fluid balance is important to prevent dehydration.
- Older adults may be more sensitive to medications and require lower dosages. Monitor them carefully for adverse effects.

BE SAFE!
AVOID FAILURE TO RECOGNIZE! Clonidine, an alpha-adrenergic agonist, and clonazepam, a benzodiazepine, have look-alike and sound-alike drug names. Be aware of drug names that look alike and sound alike to prevent errors involving these drugs.

COMPLICATIONS

Common complications of hypertension include coronary artery disease, atherosclerosis, myocardial infarction (MI), heart failure (HF), stroke, and kidney or eye damage. High BP levels may also increase the size of the left ventricle, referred to as **hypertrophy.** Over time, elevated BP damages the small vessels of the heart, brain, kidneys, and retina. The results are a progressive functional impairment of these organs, known as *target-organ disease.*

Table 22.3
Medications Used to Treat Hypertension

Medication Class/Action

Diuretics
Increase urine output by inhibiting sodium and water reabsorption by the kidney.

Examples	Nursing Implications
thiazide and thiazide-like diuretics loop diuretics potassium-sparing diuretics	Give with food to prevent gastrointestinal upset. Monitor intake and output (I&O) and weight to determine fluid loss. Monitor for improvement of edema in patients with heart failure and reduced blood pressure (BP) for hypertension. Electrolyte imbalances may occur quickly. *Teach:* Take early during the day to prevent excessive urination during sleeping hours. If sleep during the day, take early at night when awaken.

Thiazide and Thiazide-Like Diuretics
Increase urine output by promoting sodium, chloride, and water excretion; cause loss of potassium, sodium, and magnesium; calcium saved; no immediate effect; most effective in normal kidney function.

Examples	Nursing Implications
Thiazide: hydrochlorothiazide (HydroDIURIL) chlorothiazide (Diuril) *Thiazide-like:* chlorthalidone (Hygroton) indapamide (Lozol) metolazone (Zaroxolyn)	Hypercalcemia could be hazardous to patients on digoxin. Monitor potassium level for hypokalemia. Blood glucose can increase in those with diabetes. *Teach:* Wear sunscreen and protective clothing to prevent photosensitivity.

Loop Diuretics
Act on the ascending loop of Henle in the kidney to cause sodium and water loss; also cause loss of potassium, magnesium, and calcium.

Examples	Nursing Implications
bumetanide (Bumex) furosemide (Lasix) torsemide (Demadex)	Contraindicated if allergic to sulfonamides. Monitor potassium level for hypokalemia. *Teach:* Take with food or milk to prevent gastric upset. Wear sunscreen and protective clothing to prevent photosensitivity.

Potassium-Sparing Diuretics
Mild diuretic; can be used as combination therapy; promote sodium and water excretion and potassium retention by the kidney.

Examples	Nursing Implications
amiloride (Midamor) spironolactone (Aldactone)	Check potassium level for hyperkalemia before administration. Check BP before administration.

Sympatholytics (Beta Blockers)
Decrease sympathetic nervous system response, resulting in decreased BP, heart rate, contractility, cardiac output, and renin activity.

Examples	Nursing Implications
atenolol (Tenormin) metoprolol (Lopressor) metoprolol extended release (Toprol XL) nadolol (Corgard)	Check heart rate and BP before administration, as it causes bradycardia and orthostatic hypotension. Check daily I&O and weight. Monitor for bronchospasm.

Table 22.3
Medications Used to Treat Hypertension—cont'd

Medication Class/Action

propranolol (Inderal) propranolol long-acting (Inderal LA)	*Teach:* Rise slowly. Do not stop the medication abruptly to avoid rebound hypertension, angina, or arrhythmias.

Alpha-1 Blockers
Block effects of sympathetic nervous system on smooth muscle of blood vessels, resulting in vasodilation and decreased BP.

Examples	Nursing Implications
prazosin (Minipress) terazosin (Hytrin)	Check heart rate and BP before administration; it causes hypotension and tachycardia. *Teach:* Rise slowly.

Combined Alpha and Beta Blockers
Block alpha-adrenergic receptors, causing vasodilation and reduced BP; decrease sympathetic nervous system response, resulting in decreased heart rate and contractility.

Examples	Nursing Implications
carvedilol (Coreg) labetalol (Normodyne)	Check heart rate and BP before administration, as it causes bradycardia and hypotension. Check daily I&O and weight. Monitor edema, neck vein distention, and lung sounds. *Teach:* Rise slowly. Do not stop the medication abruptly to avoid rebound hypertension, angina, or arrhythmias.

Central-Acting Alpha-2 Agonists
Block effects of sympathetic nervous system centrally.

Examples	Nursing Implications
clonidine (Catapres) tablets or patch guanfacine hydrochloride (Tenex)	Check for decreased BP and edema. *Teach:* Rise slowly. Do not stop the medication abruptly to avoid rebound hypertension, angina, or arrhythmias. Suggest gum or hard candy for dry mouth.

Angiotensin-Converting Enzyme (ACE) Inhibitors
Block production of angiotensin II, a potent vasoconstrictor; reduces peripheral arterial resistance and BP.

Examples	Nursing Implications
benazepril hydrochloride (Lotensin) captopril (Capoten) enalapril maleate (Vasotec) fosinopril (Monopril) lisinopril (Prinivil, Zestril) moexipril (Univasc) perindopril (Aceon) quinapril (Accupril) ramipril (Altace) trandolapril (Mavik)	Monitor for edema with heart failure, decreased BP with hypertension, and new-onset cough. *Teach:* Rise slowly. Report new-onset cough. Wear sunscreen and protective clothing to prevent photosensitivity. Understand angioedema can occur anytime during therapy. Do not stop the medication abruptly to avoid rebound hypertension, angina, or arrhythmias.

Table 22.3 Medications Used to Treat Hypertension—cont'd

Medication Class/Action

Angiotensin II Receptor Blocker (ARB)
Blocks angiotensin II receptors, causing vasodilation and reduction in BP.

Examples	Nursing Implications
candesartan (Atacand) eprosartan (Teveten) irbesartan (Avapro) losartan (Cozaar) olmesartan (Benicar) telmisartan (Micardis) valsartan (Diovan)	Monitor for edema with heart failure and decreased BP with hypertension. Teach: Report new-onset cough. Wear sunscreen and protective clothing to prevent photosensitivity.

Aldosterone Receptor Antagonist
Blocks binding of aldosterone at receptor site to reduce sodium reabsorption and then BP.

Example	Nursing Implication
eplerenone (Inspra)	Monitor potassium for hyperkalemia before and during therapy.

Calcium Channel Blocker (CCB)
Prevents movement of extracellular calcium into the cell causing vasodilation.

Examples	Nursing Implications
amlodipine (Norvasc) diltiazem (Cardizem) felodipine (Plendil) isradipine (DynaCirc) nicardipine hydrochloride (Cardene, Cardene SR) nifedipine (Procardia) nisoldipine (Sular) verapamil (Calan SR, Isoptin SR)	Check BP (for hypotension), heart rate (for bradycardia), arrhythmias, and angina. Might increase blood levels of digoxin.

Direct Vasodilators
Relax smooth muscles of blood vessels, causing vasodilation and decreased BP.

Examples	Nursing Implications
hydralazine (Apresoline) minoxidil (Loniten)	Monitor BP for hypotension/hypertension and increasing heart rate. Treat headache with acetaminophen. Often given with diuretic to reduce edema resulting from water and sodium retention.

Combination Agents
See individual agent for action.

Examples	Nursing Implications
losartan (Cozaar) + hydrochlorothiazide (HydroDIURIL) = Hyzaar telmisartan (Micardis) + hydrochlorothiazide (HydroDIURIL) = Micardis HCT	See individual agent.

LEARNING TIP

Walking for 30 minutes is an effective way to lower BP, as is listening daily to 30 minutes of classical, Celtic, or raga type music while practicing slow abdominal breathing. Transcendental meditation also helps control high BP. Here are additional, important lifestyle modifications in an easy-to-remember mnemonic:

L—Limit salt, caffeine, and alcohol.
I—Include daily potassium and calcium.
F—Fight fat and cholesterol.
E—Exercise regularly (e.g., walking).
S—Stay on your BP regimen.
T—Try to quit smoking.
Y—Your medications are to be taken daily.
L—Lose weight.
E—End-stage complications will be avoided!

SPECIAL CONSIDERATIONS

BP should be controlled before the patient has an invasive procedure. Hypertensive patients are at greater risk for strokes, MI, HF, kidney disease, and pulmonary edema.

CLINICAL JUDGMENT

Mrs. Bell, 80 years old, is seen in her physician's office. She lives a sedentary lifestyle and lives independently in her own home with a bathroom down the hall from the bedroom. Mrs. Bell's son lives in the same city and visits her often. She has wood floors with throw rugs in the hall and a tile floor in the bathroom. She wears glasses and has a cataract. She has an unsteady gait and nocturia. She is 40 pounds overweight and has a 10-year history of hypertension for which she is taking hydrochlorothiazide (HydroDIURIL) and lisinopril (Zestril), when she remembers to take them.

1. What teaching methods do you use to help ensure that Mrs. Bell will understand and follow her treatment plan?
2. What patient safety needs do you identify?
3. What interventions do you contribute to the nursing care plan?
4. What patient-centered safety interventions do you contribute to the patient's and family's teaching plan?
5. With whom do you collaborate to assist Mrs. Bell to remember to take her medication?
6. Lisinopril 20 mg by mouth is ordered now because Mrs. Bell forgot to take her lisinopril. You have on hand lisinopril 10 mg tablets. How many tablets do you give?

Suggested answers are at the end of the chapter.

HYPERTENSIVE URGENCY

Acute **hypertensive urgency** occurs when the BP is as elevated as in a hypertensive emergency but without progression of target-organ dysfunction. A patient with hypertensive urgency may have severe headaches, nosebleeds, shortness of breath, and severe anxiety. Appropriate oral medication is implemented with a follow-up visit within several days.

HYPERTENSIVE EMERGENCY

Hypertensive emergency occurs with elevations in systolic BP higher than 180 mm Hg or diastolic BP higher than 120 mm Hg (Brathwaite & Reif, 2019). If there is a risk for or progression of target-organ dysfunction (such as MI, HF, dissecting aortic aneurysm) immediate BP treatment is required in an intensive care unit. Gradual reduction of BP is often desired to prevent decreased blood flow to the kidneys, heart, and/or brain. An IV medication such as nitroprusside (Nipride) may be given to reduce BP during the crisis. The nursing diagnosis *Risk for Unstable Blood Pressure* is applicable to the patient with hypertensive emergency.

CUE RECOGNITION 22.2

You obtain a BP reading of 188/96 on Mr. Slugay, a resident who has no history of hypertension. What action do you take?

Suggested answers are at the end of the chapter.

NURSING PROCESS FOR THE PATIENT WITH HYPERTENSION

Data Collection

Data collection for a patient with hypertension includes the patient's health history, BP measurements, medications, and physical assessment (Fig. 22.1). Determining what

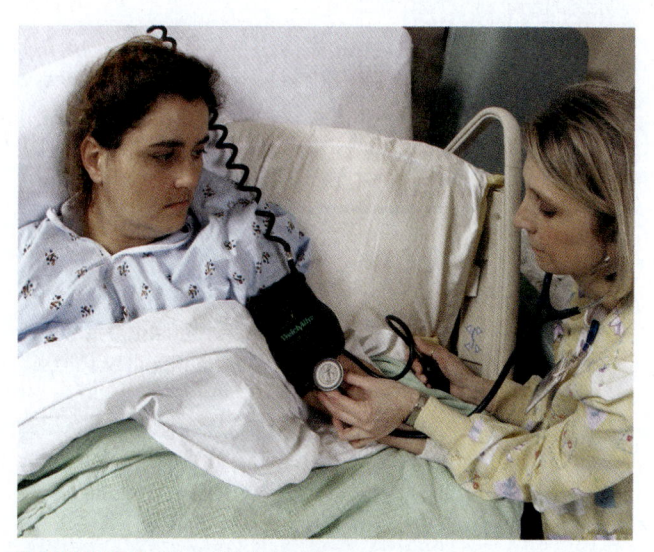

FIGURE 22.1 Nurse obtaining BP measurement. Correct cuff size is essential for accurate reading.

hypertensive patients and their families know about hypertension and associated risk factors is essential for planning patient and family education and subsequent lifelong lifestyle modification needs.

Nursing Diagnoses, Planning, Implementation, and Evaluation

See "Nursing Care Plan for the Patient With Hypertension."

Nursing Care Plan for the Patient With Hypertension

Nursing Diagnosis: *Readiness for Enhanced Health Literacy* related to desire to learn about hypertensive disease process and treatment regimen
Expected Outcome: The patient will verbalize understanding of hypertension and treatment regimen.
Evaluation of Outcome: Is the patient able to explain hypertension, including its risk factors, complications, and treatment regimen?

Intervention	Rationale	Evaluation
Verify patient's readiness and ability to learn and preferred method of learning.	*Patient must express the desire to understand the hypertension diagnosis and be able to receive information.*	Does patient verbalize readiness to learn about hypertension? Is patient able to retain information presented in the preferred learning method?
Provide patient with information concerning disease process, including risk factors, complications, and treatment regimen.	*Provides understanding for need to make changes in behavior and follow treatment regimen.*	Is patient able to accurately state information explained about hypertension?

Nursing Diagnosis: *Ineffective Health Self-Management* related to complexity of treatment, costs and side effects of medications, lack of symptoms, and need to alter long-term lifestyle habits
Expected Outcome: The patient will verbalize willingness to adhere to treatment.
Evaluation of Outcome: Is the patient able to state types of lifestyle changes that will be made? Does the patient identify and problem-solve barriers for therapy?

Intervention	Rationale	Evaluation
Develop plan for lifestyle modification needs and ways to overcome barriers to therapy. Make referrals as needed.	*Identified barriers can be overcome with planning and intervention: provide instructions at patient's learning level; simplify to a combination medication; make referrals to support groups, financial assistance, or prescription delivery service.*	Have barriers been eliminated? Can patient self-administer medications accurately?

Geriatric

Teach patient to take medications as prescribed and not to skip dosages.	*Older patients may skip dosages in order to save money or reduce side effects.*	Does patient take dosages as prescribed? Does patient express concern over cost or side effects?

Home Health Hints

Medications
- Discuss medication compliance with the patient. Count the number of remaining pills in the patient's pill bottles, as needed.
- Note on a calendar medication refills and medical appointment dates to remind the patient.
- Communicate with the HCP and pharmacist if medicines are reported to be too expensive for the patient.
- Reinforce teaching the patient or caregiver proper use of a home BP monitoring device and record results. Review at each visit.
- Reinforce teaching for the patient to monitor pulse and to call the nurse if it is below 60 beats per minute or parameters defined by the HCP. Many antihypertensive medicines can cause bradycardia.
- Reinforce teaching to take medication as prescribed even if patient feels fine and has no symptoms; report side effects if they occur.

- Reinforce teaching patient who is traveling to refill medicines ahead of time to make sure they do not run out. The HCP can write a prescription for the patient to have for emergency refills.

Nutrition
- Refer to a dietitian to review the DASH eating plan if appropriate (www.nhlbi.nih.gov/health-topics/dash-eating-plan).
- Reinforce teaching patient to read food labels for high salt content and avoid sweets to avoid weight gain.

Lifestyle
- Ask about cigarette smoking at every visit, and offer assistance to make a plan to quit (Quitline 1-800-QUIT-NOW).
- Encourage patient to put "No Smoking" signs on their entrance door to prevent second- and thirdhand smoke.
- If cleared by HCP, patient should work toward 150 minutes of moderate-intensity aerobic activity per week such as brisk walking, swimming, dancing, or biking.

Key Points

- The pressure exerted by blood on the walls of the blood vessels is measured as BP. BP is determined by CO, PVR, the viscosity of the blood, and the amount of circulating blood volume.
- Sympathetic nervous system overstimulation, which causes vasoconstriction, alterations in baroreceptors and chemoreceptors, or changes in kidney function that cause fluid retention, may each contribute to hypertension.
- Nonmodifiable risk factors for hypertension are those that *cannot* be changed and include a family history of hypertension, age, and ethnicity. Modifiable risk factors are those that *can* be changed and include blood glucose level, activity level, smoking, salt and alcohol intake, and insufficient sleep.
- Hypertension often causes no signs or symptoms other than elevated BP readings. As a result, hypertension is referred to as the "silent killer."
- Hypertension complications include coronary artery disease, atherosclerosis, myocardial infarction, heart failure, stroke, and kidney or eye damage. The severity and duration of the increase in BP determine the extent of the vascular changes causing organ damage.
- Hypertensive emergency occurs with elevations in systolic BP higher than 180 mm Hg or diastolic BP higher than 120 mm Hg. It can be asymptomatic and treated with oral antihypertensives or cause target-organ dysfunction, which requires immediate treatment in an ICU often with IV medication.
- Nursing diagnoses for patients with hypertension may include *Readiness for Enhanced Health Literacy*, *Ineffective Health Self-Management*, and *Risk for Unstable Blood Pressure*.
- Nursing interventions are effective if the patient can explain hypertension, including its risk factors, complications, and treatment regimen; how lifestyle changes will be made; how problem-solving for barriers to therapy will be made.

SUGGESTED ANSWERS TO CHAPTER EXERCISES

Cue Recognition

22.1: Speak with the nursing assistant when she leaves the room to review the appropriate techniques to use when measuring BP (see Box 21.1). Accompany the nursing assistant into the patient room, greet the patient, and assist the nursing assistant to repeat the BP reading using the appropriate techniques and providing feedback as necessary.

22.2: Ensure appropriate BP cuff size and measurement techniques are used. Repeat the BP reading. If it remains elevated, inform the HCP urgently.

Critical Thinking & Clinical Judgment

Ms. Diaz
1. Risk factors include gender; age; smoking; a diet high in fat, salt, and calories; consumption of two to three alcoholic drinks per evening; and possibly her morning headaches.
2. Morning headaches. Ms. Diaz may be experiencing an episode of hypertensive urgency and should be evaluated immediately by an HCP.
3. "Silent killer" refers to the fact that hypertension often has no signs or symptoms.
4. Lifelong therapy is required because hypertension has no cure and complications must be prevented.

Mrs. Bell
1. Identify patient's reading level and primary language. Provide patient with written instructions in large letters about medications. Include family members and enlist their support in reinforcing adhering to the treatment plan.
2. Patient is 80 years old, makes frequent trips to the bathroom related to diuretics, and has vision problems; throw rugs pose a fall/slip risk; and a side effect of lisinopril is fatigue.

SUGGESTED ANSWERS TO CHAPTER EXERCISES

3. Discuss with the HCP a combination medication to reduce the number of pills to be consumed. Order a bedside commode to reduce distance and urgency to get to the bathroom.
4. Encourage the placement of nightlights in the bedroom, hall, and bathroom. Explain that throw rugs increase the risk of falling and should be removed. Suggest the use of safety bars in the hall and bathroom for support or other walking aids as needed. If incontinence is a concern, suggest wearing an incontinence product. Suggest discussing with the HCP an exercise program for strengthening that will reduce fall risk.
5. Family, pharmacist, social worker.
6. Unit analysis method:

$$\frac{20 \text{ mg}}{} \cdot \frac{1 \text{ tablet}}{10 \text{ mg}} = 2 \text{ tablets}$$

Additional Resources

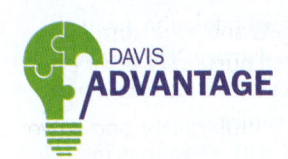

Go to Davis Advantage to complete your learning: strengthen understanding, apply your knowledge, and prepare for the Next Gen NCLEX®.

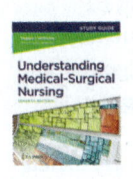

A Study Guide is also available.

CHAPTER 23
Nursing Care of Patients With Valvular, Inflammatory, and Infectious Cardiac or Venous Disorders

Charlotte Kostelyk

KEY TERMS

allograft (AL-oh-graft)
annuloplasty (AN-yoo-loh-PLAS-tee)
autograft (AW-toh-graft)
bioprosthesis (by-oh-prahs-THEE-sis)
cardiac tamponade (KAR-dee-yak TAM-pon-AYD)
cardiomegaly (KAR-dee-oh-MEG-ah-lee)
cardiomyopathy (KAR-dee-oh-my-AH-pah-thee)
chorea (core-REE-ah)
commissurotomy (KOM-ih-shur-AHT-oh-mee)
Dressler syndrome (DRESS-ler SIN-drohm)
emboli (EM-boh-ly)
heterograft (HET-er-oh-graft)
homograft (HOH-moh-graft)
infective endocarditis (in-FEK-tive EN-doh-kar-DY-tis)
insufficiency (IN-suh-FISH-en-see)
international normalized ratio (IN-ter-NASH-uh-nul NOR-muh-lized RAY-she-oh)
murmur (MUR-mur)
myectomy (my-EK-tuh-mee)
myocarditis (MY-oh-kar-DY-tis)
pericardial effusion (PER-ih-KAR-dee-uhl ee-FYOO-zhun)
pericardial friction rub (PER-ih-KAR-dee-uhl FRIK-shun RUB)
pericardiectomy (PER-ih-kar-dee-EK-tuh-mee)
pericardiocentesis (PER-ih-KAR-dee-oh-sen-TEE-sis)
pericarditis (PER-ih-kar-DY-tis)
petechiae (peh-TEE-kee-eye)
regurgitation (ree-GUR-jih-TAY-shun)
rheumatic fever (roo-MAT-ik FEE-vur)
stenosis (steh-NOH-sis)
streptococci (STREP-toh-KOK-eye)
thrombophlebitis (THROM-boh-fleh-BY-tis)
valvotomy (val-VAH-tuh-mee)
valvuloplasty (VAL-vyoo-loh-PLAS-tee)
xenograft (ZEE-no-graft)

CHAPTER CONCEPTS

Caring
Perfusion
Safety
Teaching and learning

LEARNING OUTCOMES

1. Explain the pathophysiology, etiology, signs and symptoms, diagnostic tests, therapeutic measures, and nursing care for each of the valvular disorders.
2. Compare and contrast commissurotomy, annuloplasty, and valve replacement.
3. Identify postoperative complications that can occur following any type of cardiac valve replacement.
4. Explain the pathophysiology, etiology, signs and symptoms, diagnostic tests, therapeutic measures, and nursing care for infective endocarditis, pericarditis, and myocarditis.
5. Explain the pathophysiology, etiology, signs and symptoms, complications, diagnostic tests, therapeutic measures, and nursing care for dilated, hypertrophic, and restrictive cardiomyopathy.
6. Explain the pathophysiology, etiology, signs and symptoms, prevention, complications, diagnostic tests, therapeutic measures, and nursing care for thrombophlebitis.

CARDIAC VALVULAR DISORDERS

Within the normal heart, blood flows in one direction because of the presence of heart valves. There are four valves in the heart: mitral, tricuspid, pulmonic, and aortic (see Fig. 21.2). The chordae tendineae and papillary muscles are attachment structures for both the mitral and tricuspid valves. They ensure that these valves close tightly.

Damage to the valves or their surrounding structures can result in abnormal valvular functioning (Fig. 23.1). The valves of the left side of the heart are more commonly affected. There are two major types of valvular dysfunction: **stenosis** and **insufficiency**. Forward blood flow is reduced if the valve is narrowed (*stenosed*) and does not open completely. If the valve does not close completely, blood backs up; this is referred to as **regurgitation** or *insufficiency*. Either type of valve damage increases the heart's workload and increases pressure in the

• WORD • BUILDING •
stenosis: stenos—narrow
insufficiency: in—not + sufficiens—sufficient
regurgitation: re—again + gurgitare—to flood

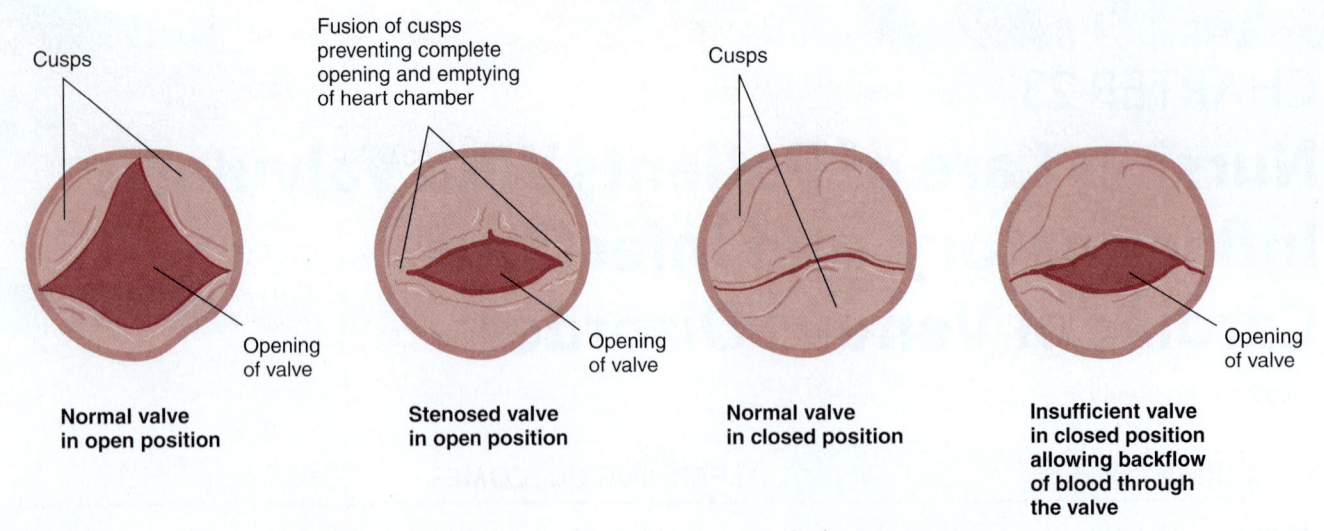

FIGURE 23.1 Openings of stenosed and insufficient valves compared with a normal valve.

affected heart chamber due to a backup of blood flow. These conditions may result from congenital defects, infections, or rheumatic fever. Valvular disorders are summarized in Table 23.1 and discussed in more detail in the following sections.

Rheumatic Fever

Rheumatic fever is an autoimmune reaction about 2 to 4 weeks after tonsillopharyngitis due to group A **streptococci**. Although rheumatic fever can occur at any age, it typically occurs between ages 5 and 15. Rheumatic fever and subsequent rheumatic heart disease and valvular damage can be prevented by detecting and treating streptococcal infections promptly with penicillin. This rare complication of untreated strep throat or scarlet fever is not commonly seen in the United States. Worldwide it is common in developing countries. A throat culture is used to diagnose a streptococcal infection. Predominant signs and symptoms include polyarthritis, subcutaneous nodules (painless), a painless rash, carditis with valvulitis, Sydenham **chorea** (brief, rapid, uncontrolled movements that occur 1 to 8 months after the infection) with unusual exhibition of emotions. Minor signs and symptoms include fever; arthralgia (joint pain); and red, hot, swollen joints and pneumonitis, a rare complication. Rheumatic heart disease may not be evident for years after rheumatic fever; however, when manifested, the valves are most affected.

Mitral Valve Prolapse
Pathophysiology and Etiology

During ventricular systole, as pressure in the left ventricle rises, the flaps of the mitral valve normally remain closed and stay within the atrioventricular junction. In mitral valve prolapse (MVP), however, one or both flaps bulge backward into the left atrium (like a parachute) during systole. This can happen when one flap is too large or if a defect occurs in the chordae tendineae that secure the valve to the heart wall. If the bulging flaps do not fit together, blood can leak backward into the left atrium (mitral regurgitation). Increased pressure on the papillary muscles results in ischemia (inadequate blood supply) within the muscle, causing further dysfunction of the mitral valve.

MVP results from changes in the valve structure (myxomatous degeneration), connective tissue disorders (*Ehler-Danlos syndrome*—a group of inherited connective tissue disorders affecting the skin, blood vessels, and joints with cardiac abnormalities being common such as MVP), or a hereditary trait or gene mutation. It is the most common form of valvular heart disease for both genders. Risk rises with age (Shah et al, 2020).

Signs and Symptoms

Most patients with MVP are asymptomatic and have a good prognosis (see Table 23.1). MVP severity ranges from having a **murmur** (caused by blood leaking backward) to chordae tendineae rupture with mitral regurgitation. The murmur is best heard at the heart apex. It begins in the middle of systole (*midsystolic*) and becomes more intense until the end of systole. Symptoms may include anxiety, atypical chest pain not related to exertion, arrhythmias causing palpitations, dizziness or syncope (fainting), fatigue, and dyspnea (shortness of breath), especially when lying flat or during activity.

Complications

Rare complications include mitral regurgitation, arrhythmias, heart failure (HF), emboli, or infective endocarditis (IE).

Diagnostic Tests

Auscultation for a murmur or a click caused by the stress on the chordae tendineae or valve leaflets when they prolapse is the first diagnostic step for MVP. A normal electrocardiogram (ECG) is common, although inverted (downward) T waves (indicating ischemia) may be seen (see Fig. 25.6). A two-dimensional echocardiogram with Doppler and a transesophageal echocardiography can show valve abnormalities

Table 23.1
Cardiac Valvular Disorders Summary

Valve Disorder	Signs and Symptoms	Diagnostic Tests	Complications	Therapeutic Measures	Priority Nursing Diagnoses
Mitral valve prolapse	None Murmur Atypical chest pain Palpitations Arrhythmias Dizziness Syncope Fatigue Dyspnea Anxiety	Echocardiogram Electrocardiogram (ECG) Cardiac catheterization	Emboli Infective endocarditis Mitral regurgitation Arrhythmias Heart failure (HF)	None Beta blockers Antiarrhythmics Aspirin or anticoagulants Valvuloplasty Valve replacement	*Decreased Activity Tolerance* *Decreased Cardiac Output*
Mitral stenosis	None Murmur Chest pain Palpitations Dizziness Syncope Fatigue Edema Exertional dyspnea Cough Hemoptysis Respiratory infections	ECG Chest x-ray Echocardiogram Doppler ultrasound Transesophageal endoscopy (TEE) Cardiac catheterization Magnetic resonance imaging (MRI)	Emboli HF	None Anticoagulants Antiarrhythmics Valvuloplasty Valve replacement	*Decreased Activity Tolerance* *Decreased Cardiac Output*
Mitral regurgitation	None Murmur Chest pain Palpitations Syncope Fatigue Exertional dyspnea Cough Hemoptysis Peripheral edema *Acute:* Pulmonary edema Shock	ECG Chest x-ray Echocardiogram Doppler ultrasound TEE Cardiac MRI Cardiac catheterization	Arrhythmias Emboli HF	None Angiotensin-converting enzyme (ACE) inhibitors Antiarrhythmics Anticoagulants Valvuloplasty Valve replacement	*Decreased Activity Tolerance* *Decreased Cardiac Output*
Aortic stenosis	None Angina Murmur Syncope Orthopnea Exertional dyspnea	ECG Chest x-ray Serial echocardiograms Stress (exercise) test Computed tomography (CT) scan	HF	Valve replacement: Surgical or transcatheter	*Decreased Activity Tolerance* *Decreased Cardiac Output*

Continued

Table 23.1
Cardiac Valvular Disorders Summary—cont'd

Valve Disorder	Signs and Symptoms	Diagnostic Tests	Complications	Therapeutic Measures	Priority Nursing Diagnoses
	Fatigue HF	MRI Cardiac catheterization			
Aortic regurgitation	None Forceful pulse Murmur Chest pain Palpitations Fatigue Exertional dyspnea Corrigan pulse Diaphoresis	ECG Chest x-ray Echocardiogram Cardiac catheterization	HF Life-threatening arrhythmia Symptoms of shock	Diuretics Vasodilators Valve replacement	Decreased Activity Tolerance Decreased Cardiac Output

and identify mitral regurgitation from MVP. For more severe cases, cardiac catheterization can show the bulging flaps of the mitral valve on a coronary angiogram (dye-injected X-ray).

Therapeutic Measures

MVP is a benign disorder. No treatment is needed unless symptoms become severe. A healthy lifestyle, including a heart-healthy diet, exercise, stress management, and avoidance of stimulants such as caffeine, can help prevent symptoms. Treatment depends on severity of symptoms and may include beta blockers to reduce the heart rate and perhaps relieve chest pain, aspirin or anticoagulants to help prevent formation of blood clots on the valve, and antiarrhythmics (also known as *antidysrhythmics*) for an arrhythmia. Surgical repair or replacement of the valve can be done for severe cases of MVP. (See surgical interventions discussion later in the chapter.)

> **CRITICAL THINKING & CLINICAL JUDGMENT**
>
> **Mr. Goldfarb,** age 51, presents with chest pain, increase in fatigue with exercise, weight gain, and job stress. He reports a history of MVP with surgical repair 3 years ago.
>
> **Critical Thinking (The Why)**
> 1. How does weight gain and stress affect cardiac health?
>
> **Clinical Judgment (The Do)**
> 2. What data do you collect for Mr. Goldfarb's medical and surgical history of MVP?
> 3. What patient-centered resources do you provide to help Mr. Goldfarb manage his MVP?
>
> *Suggested answers are at the end of the chapter.*

Mitral Stenosis

Pathophysiology and Etiology

Mitral stenosis (MS) results from thickening of the mitral valve flaps and shortening of the chordae tendineae, causing narrowing of the mitral valve opening. Older patients with MS usually have calcification and fibrosis of the mitral valve flaps. This obstructs blood flow from the left atrium into the left ventricle. The left atrium enlarges to hold the extra blood volume caused by the obstruction. Due to the increased blood volume, pressure rises in the left atrium; in turn, pressure rises in the pulmonary circulation and the right ventricle. The right ventricle dilates to handle the increased volume. Eventually, the right ventricle fails from excessive workload, reducing blood volume delivered to the left ventricle and decreasing cardiac output.

Rheumatic fever is the major cause of MS, which is seen in older adults who had rheumatic fever as children or in those in developing countries. Even though rheumatic fever is rare in developed nations, when it does occur, any resultant rheumatic heart disease may not appear for 5 to 10 years or longer after the rheumatic fever is resolved. This time frame depends on the severity of the rheumatic fever. Less common causes of MS include congenital defects of the mitral valve, systemic lupus erythematosus, and calcium deposits.

Signs and Symptoms

Patients can be asymptomatic with MS (see Table 23.1). A click or low-pitched murmur might be heard as a rumbling sound over the heart apex during diastole. The click or murmur is more pronounced right before systole. The most common symptoms, which are often unnoticed because they develop gradually as disease severity increases, are exertional dyspnea and intolerance to activity. Additional pulmonary symptoms include hemoptysis (bloody sputum), hoarseness, cough, and respiratory infections. Fatigue, dizziness, syncope, and more rarely chest pain result from decreased cardiac output. Palpitations from atrial flutter or atrial fibrillation caused by atrial enlargement may occur.

Complications
Stasis of blood in the left atrium could form a thrombus. A moving thrombus called an **emboli** could cause a stroke. If the right ventricle fails, symptoms of right-sided HF can occur (see Chapter 26).

Diagnostic Tests
Transthoracic two-dimensional color flow Doppler echocardiogram and Doppler ultrasound are the noninvasive gold standard tests for evaluation of valvular disease. They show the narrowed mitral valve opening and decreased motion of the valve. Exercise stress echocardiography can be helpful for severe symptoms. The ECG shows enlargement of the left atrium and right ventricle and changes in the P waveform (see Fig. 25.1). Atrial flutter or fibrillation may be seen (see Chapter 25). An incidental chest x-ray examination shows enlargement of the left atrium.

Therapeutic Measures
When the patient is asymptomatic, no treatment is needed. Anticoagulants might be given to prevent emboli from stasis of blood in the atrium. Atrial fibrillation, an irregular heart rhythm, or HF may develop and require treatment (see Chapter 26).

If invasive treatment is needed, percutaneous balloon **valvotomy** (a balloon dilates the stenosed heart valve) can be done in the cardiac catheterization lab (Fig. 23.2). Surgical treatment can include valvular repair (**valvuloplasty**), but mitral valve replacement is typically needed (Fig. 23.3).

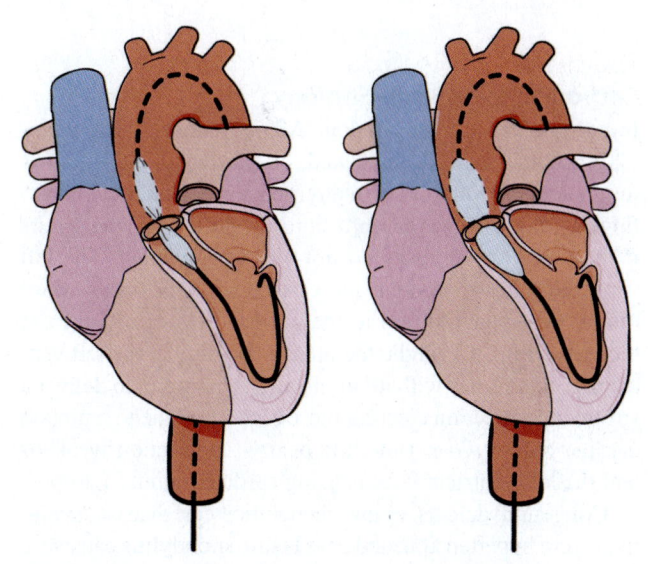

FIGURE 23.2 Percutaneous balloon valvuloplasty.

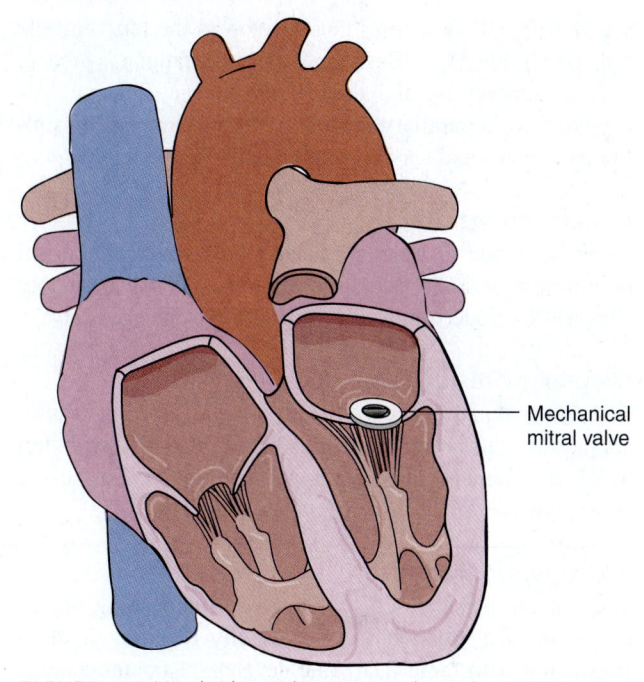

FIGURE 23.3 Mitral valve replacement with mechanical valve.

> **CUE RECOGNITION 23.1**
> A patient who has mitral valve stenosis is experiencing shortness of breath, oxygen saturation (SaO$_2$) 90%, hoarseness, palpitations, and dizziness. What action do you take?
>
> *Suggested answers are at the end of the chapter.*

Mitral Regurgitation
Pathophysiology and Etiology
Mitral regurgitation (MR), or insufficiency, is the incomplete closure of the mitral valve leaflets. It allows backflow of blood into the left atrium with each contraction of the left ventricle. This extra blood volume is added to the incoming blood from the lungs. With chronic MR, the increase in blood volume dilates and increases pressure in the left atrium. In response to the extra blood volume delivered by the left atrium, the left ventricle compensates by dilating. If the compensatory mechanism of dilation is inadequate, pressure rises in the pulmonary circulation and then in the right ventricle as blood volume backs up from the left atrium. The left ventricle and eventually the right ventricle may fail from this increased strain.

Causes of MR include rheumatic heart disease, endocarditis, rupture or dysfunction of the chordae tendineae or papillary muscle, MVP, hypertension, myocardial infarction (MI), cardiomyopathy, annulus calcification, aging, or congenital defects.

Signs and Symptoms
Patients with MR are usually asymptomatic initially. A murmur may be heard. It begins with S$_1$ (first heart sound) and continues during systole up to S$_2$ (second heart sound). With

severe MR, HF symptoms can develop as the left ventricle fails (see Table 23.1). Exertional dyspnea, fatigue, syncope, cough, hemoptysis, and edema may occur. If acute MR develops, as in papillary muscle rupture following MI, pulmonary edema and shock symptoms will be exhibited.

Complications
Palpitations due to atrial fibrillation may result as the left atrium enlarges. Pulmonary hypertension or HF may occur (see Chapter 26). Endocarditis is a risk due to the damaged valve.

Diagnostic Tests
Two-dimensional echocardiogram with Doppler or transesophageal echocardiogram (TEE) confirms MR with left atrial enlargement and regurgitation of blood. For severe symptoms, cardiovascular MRI may be useful.

Therapeutic Measures
Without the presence of symptoms and depending on the cause, medical treatment is not usually required. If atrial fibrillation with rapid heart rate develops, calcium channel blockers or beta blockers may be ordered. Anticoagulants are used to prevent thromboembolisms. When symptoms develop and surgery is needed, a mitral valve repair or percutaneous mitral valve repair is preferred over mitral valve replacement when possible.

Aortic Stenosis
Pathophysiology and Etiology
In aortic stenosis (AS), blood flow from the left ventricle into the aorta is obstructed through the stenosed aortic valve. The opening of the aortic valve may be narrowed from thickening, scarring, calcification, or fusing of the valve's flaps. To compensate for the difficulty in ejecting blood into the aorta, the left ventricle contracts more forcefully. In chronic AS, the left ventricle hypertrophies to maintain normal cardiac output. As narrowing increases, the compensatory mechanisms are unable to continue. The left ventricle fails to move blood forward, resulting in decreased cardiac output and HF.

The major causes of AS are congenital defects or rheumatic heart disease. Calcification of the aortic valve may be age related and occurs after age 60.

Signs and Symptoms
Many years may pass before signs or symptoms of AS are observed (see Table 23.1). Early symptoms include exertional angina, exertional dyspnea or activity intolerance, and exertional dizziness or syncope. Late end-stage symptoms are angina, syncope, and HF signs and symptoms. A systolic murmur can develop, beginning just after systole (S_1) with increasing intensity until midsystole, then decreasing and ending right before the second heart sound (S_2).

Complications
HF, pulmonary hypertension, life-threatening arrhythmias, sudden cardiac death, endocarditis, and emboli can occur.

Diagnostic Tests
Ultrasound may be used initially and shows thickness of aortic valve leaflets and their reduced motion. Then two-dimensional and Doppler echocardiogram shows thickening of the left ventricular wall, impaired movement of the aortic valve, and the severity of the disease. The ECG commonly shows enlargement of the left ventricle and left atrium.

Therapeutic Measures
Aortic valve replacement is the only effective treatment for AS. For those considered high risk for traditional open-heart surgery, a transcatheter aortic valve replacement (TAVR) can be done (see the section on heart valve replacement). Valvotomy is used only for those who are unable to have valve replacement.

If symptoms of HF are present, they are treated. Medications that reduce the contractility of the heart and, subsequently, cardiac output are avoided to prevent further HF.

> **CLINICAL JUDGMENT**
>
> **Mrs. Pryor,** age 48, has aortic stenosis and is admitted to the hospital with angina. She had an episode of syncope two days ago. She reports that she tires easily. Mrs. Pryor asks what aortic stenosis is.
>
> 1. What do you tell Mrs. Pryor?
> 2. How do you document this education?
> 3. If Mrs. Pryor experiences angina, whom do you collaborate with?
> 4. What interventions do you perform for the anginal episode?
> 5. What do you contribute to Mrs. Pryor's plan of care for safety?
> 6. What discharge education do you reinforce for the patient regarding digoxin on signs and symptoms indicating the medication should be held?
>
> *Suggested answers are at the end of the chapter.*

Aortic Regurgitation
Pathophysiology and Etiology
In chronic aortic regurgitation (AR), the aortic valve cusps may become scarred, thickened, or shortened. Chronic AR may slowly develop over many years or decades. A backflow of blood from the aorta into the left ventricle occurs if the aortic valve cusps do not close completely. The left ventricle's blood volume increases with this backflow of blood; this is in addition to the normal flow of blood from the left atrium. To handle the increased volume, the left ventricle compensates with dilation and hypertrophy to deliver a stronger contraction ejecting more blood volume to maintain cardiac output. Over time, the heart's contraction weakens and the left ventricle fails, causing cardiac output to drop.

Congenital defects, aging, rheumatic heart disease, syphilis, severe hypertension, and ankylosing spondylitis can cause AR. Acute causes include endocarditis or aortic dissection.

Signs and Symptoms

Symptoms may not become apparent for many years with chronic AR (see Table 23.1). Initially, the patient may report feeling a forceful heartbeat that is more pronounced when lying down. Palpitations and pounding in the head may also be experienced. Next, exertional dyspnea, fatigue, and worsening levels of dyspnea (e.g., orthopnea, paroxysmal nocturnal dyspnea) occur after years of progressive valvular dysfunction. A murmur is heard during diastolic after the second heart sound. The palpated pulse is forceful and then quickly collapses (Corrigan pulse). The diastolic blood pressure decreases to widen the pulse pressure. This compensates for an increase in systolic blood pressure. Later in the disease, atypical angina pectoris may occur. This often happens at rest or at night, along with diaphoresis, when a lower pulse rate results in delivery of less oxygen to the myocardium. Eventually, symptoms of HF develop if the left ventricle fails. In acute aortic dysfunction, profound symptoms of pulmonary distress, chest pain, and cardiogenic shock symptoms occur and require immediate treatment.

Diagnostic Tests

An echocardiogram, Doppler echocardiogram, or transesophageal echocardiogram detect an enlarged left ventricle and severity of the AR. Cardiovascular MRI can provide accurate disease severity assessment and effect on ventricular function.

Therapeutic Measures

Treatment with vasodilators or diuretics may be useful to reduce systolic blood pressure and, subsequently, cardiac workload or heart failure prior to surgery or for patients who cannot have surgery. Aortic valve replacement is typically the surgery that is required. Rarely, an aortic valve repair can be done.

Nursing Process for the Patient With a Cardiac Valvular Disorder

Data Collection

A history is obtained that includes information presented in Table 23.2. Vital signs are measured, heart sounds are auscultated to detect murmurs, and signs and symptoms of HF are noted and reported (see Chapter 26).

Table 23.2
Data Collection for Patients With Cardiac Valvular Disorders

Data Collection	Subjective Data Questions
Health History	Infections (rheumatic fever, endocarditis, streptococcal or staphylococcal, syphilis)? Congenital defects? Cardiac disease (myocardial infarction, cardiomyopathy)?
Respiratory	Dyspnea at rest, on exertion, when lying, or that awakens patient? How many pillows are you accustomed to sleeping on? Cough or hemoptysis?
Cardiovascular	Chest pain, qualities—when does it occur? Loss of consciousness? Edema? Palpitations, dizziness, fatigue, activity intolerance?
Medications	What medications are you taking?
Knowledge of Condition	What is the reason that you are here today? Have you ever been diagnosed with any type of heart disease?
Coping Skills	How do you normally cope with stressors? Support system? What, if anything, seems to help alleviate symptoms? Have there been any adaptations in lifestyle and/or environment?
	Objective Data
Respiratory	Crackles, wheezes, tachypnea, use of accessory muscles
Cardiovascular	Murmurs, extra heart sounds, arrhythmias, edema, jugular venous distention, Corrigan pulse, increased or decreased pulse pressure or blood pressure
Integumentary	Clubbing; cyanosis; diaphoresis; cold, clammy skin; pallor
Diagnostic Test Findings	Review test results.

Nursing Care Plan for the Patient With a Cardiac Valvular Disorder

Nursing Diagnosis: *Decreased Cardiac Output* related to cardiac valvular stenosis or insufficiency or heart failure
Expected Outcome: The patient will have adequate cardiac output as evidenced by vital signs within normal parameters for patient; strong pulses, warm extremities; lack of dyspnea and minimal fatigue.
Evaluation of Outcome: Are the patient's vital signs within normal parameters for the patient, pulses strong, extremities warm, without dyspnea or fatigue?

Intervention	Rationale	Evaluation
Monitor heart and lung sounds, vital signs, oxygen saturation, chest pain, skin temperature, capillary refill and peripheral edema.	Indicators of cardiac output decline are new onset of murmurs, hypotension, tachycardia, reduced SaO_2 chest pain, edema or crackles in the lungs.	Are vital signs, oxygen saturation, and heart and lung sounds within the patient's normal parameters? Is skin warm, capillary refill less than 3 seconds with no chest pain or peripheral edema?
Administer oxygen as ordered.	Supplemental oxygen increases oxygen to the heart by increasing the oxygen saturation in the blood.	Does oxygen saturation remain within normal patient parameters at rest and with activity?
Elevate head of bed 45 degrees.	Venous return to heart is reduced and chest expansion improved when head of bed is elevated, which increases the amount of oxygen coming into the lungs.	Is there use of accessory muscles of respiration? Does patient report shortness of breath?

Intervention	Rationale	Evaluation
Geriatric		
Review cardiac medications and presence of side effects, and teach patient side effects to report.	Toxic side effects are more common, owing to altered metabolism and excretion of medications in the older adult.	Are side effects present for medications patient is taking? Does patient understand side effects to report?

Nursing Diagnosis: *Decreased Activity Tolerance* related to decreased oxygen delivery from cardiac valvular stenosis or insufficiency and output
Expected Outcome: The patient will exhibit normal changes in vital signs and less fatigue in response to activity.
Evaluation of Outcome: Does the patient have normal changes in vital signs with activity? Does the patient report less fatigue with activity?

Intervention	Rationale	Evaluation
Assist as needed with activities of daily living (ADLs).	Conserve energy with ADL assistance.	Are all ADLs completed? Are vital signs within range during activity?
Geriatric		
Slow pace of care and allow patient extra time to perform activities.	Patients can often perform activities if allowed time to slowly perform them and rest at intervals.	Does blood pressure remain within normal patient parameters when changing position?
Ensure safety when mobilizing older patient.	Orthostatic hypertension is common in the older adult.	Does patient ambulate without feeling faint or unsteady?

Nursing Diagnoses, Planning, Implementation, and Evaluation

The major nursing diagnoses for all the valvular disorders are the same. They include those for HF as well, if symptoms of HF are present. See "Nursing Care Plan for the Patient With a Cardiac Valvular Disorder."

Patient Education

Education should include caregivers and focus on the understanding of the nature of the disorder, health maintenance including medications, prevention of complications, and early recognition of symptoms in order to seek medical care. Highest-risk patients are counseled according to the

AHA guidelines for prophylactic antibiotics to prevent IE (see "Prevention" under "Infective Endocarditis" later in this chapter).

For patients on warfarin (Coumadin), **international normalized ratio** (INR) should be regularly monitored (see "Learning Tip"), a consult with a dietitian and diet education is essential (see "Nutrition Notes"), and a medical ID should be used (see Patient Teaching Guidelines for this chapter on Davis Edge).

> **LEARNING TIP**
> - Before administering the anticoagulant warfarin, the patient's INR value must be compared with the desired therapeutic INR value to determine whether it is safe to give the warfarin.
> - An INR range of 2 to 3 is therapeutic for patients on warfarin who have a blood clot, tissue heart valve, or atrial fibrillation. For a mechanical heart valve, the therapeutic INR range is usually 2.5 to 3.5. Hold the warfarin until any value outside of therapeutic range is reported to the HCP for patient safety.
> - Check for bleeding or ecchymosis (excessive bruising) prior to warfarin administration and, if present, report these findings to the HCP for orders regarding warfarin administration.

> **Nutrition Notes**
> The most important role of vitamin K is its participation in blood clotting. Vitamin K is required for the activation of four (factor II or prothrombin, VII, and X) of the 13 proteins (factors) involved in the blood clotting process. These four proteins contain several glutamic acid residues that must be activated by an enzyme (gamma-glutamyl carboxylase). This enzyme requires vitamin K as a coenzyme.
>
> Foods sources of vitamin K include green leafy vegetables (collard greens, turnip greens, kale, broccoli), legumes, and some vegetable oils. Anticoagulants such as warfarin interfere with vitamin K function by preventing the conversion of vitamin K to its active coenzyme form. It is important to inform patients that, to maintain a therapeutic level of warfarin, they should eat a consistent amount of these types of foods on a day-to-day basis rather than increase or decrease the amounts. Inconsistent day-to-day intake can alter the effects of the warfarin and make it difficult to establish and maintain a therapeutic INR. A consultation with a dietitian can be helpful in developing a meal plan (National Institutes of Health, 2020).

Cardiac Valve Repairs

A **commissurotomy** repairs a stenosed valve, most commonly the mitral valve. It can be done via percutaneous (preferred), open with bypass, or rarely via closed surgical approach. The valve flaps that have adhered to each other—and thus closed the opening between them, known as the *commissure*—are separated during one of these approaches to enlarge the valve opening.

Annuloplasty is the repair or reconstruction of the valve flaps or annulus. Sutures or a prosthetic ring may be placed in the valve annulus to improve closure of the leaflets. The mitral valve is the most common valve repaired in this way. Similar procedures are used on the tricuspid valve.

Heart Valve Replacement

Valves used for cardiac valve replacement may be either mechanical or biological (tissue). Research is ongoing to develop tissue engineered heart valves. Tissue valves (**bioprosthesis**) come from **xenograft** (porcine [pig] and bovine [cow]; also known as a **heterograft**) or **allograft** (a human cadaveric or living donor; also known as a **homograft**); see "Cultural Considerations." Allografts are available in limited numbers because they rely on donors. An **autograft** (self-donor) in the Ross procedure uses the patient's own pulmonary valve to replace the removed aortic valve; an allograft (human donor) pulmonary valve then replaces the patient's pulmonary valve. Visit www.lifenethealth.org for more information on allografts.

> **Cultural Considerations**
> Religious groups such as Jewish, Muslim, Hindu, Buddhist, and Seventh Day Adventists may not consume pork or beef products depending on their beliefs. It is important that patients' and families' views about cardiac valve options such as porcine (pork-derived) and bovine (beef-derived) tissue valves are discussed in case they wish to avoid them (Koshy et al, 2020).

For mitral valve replacement, a left atriotomy is made after the patient is on cardiopulmonary bypass (CPB). For an aortic valve replacement, an incision is made above the right coronary artery in the aorta. Then, in either valvular procedure, the diseased valve is excised and the new valve sutured in place. The incision is closed. Surgery then continues as described in Chapter 21.

TAVR is a minimally invasive procedure that replaces the valve without removing the defective valve. A balloon catheter is introduced via the femoral artery. It is inserted through the diseased valve and inflated to open the stenosed valve leaflets. For

• WORD • BUILDING •

commissurotomy: commissura—joining together + tome—incision
annuloplasty: annulus—ring + plasty—formed

mitral valve valvoplasty, after the balloon catheter is inserted into the right atrium, it is threaded through a small hole pierced into the right atrial septum that emerges into the left atrium. The catheter is passed through the mitral valve. Inflating the balloon within the mitral valve opens the stenosed valve flaps. Complications may include arrhythmias, emboli, hemorrhage, and cardiac tamponade. A balloon valvuloplasty results in fewer complications than traditional open-heart surgery.

Complications of Valve Replacement

Tissue valves have a low incidence of thrombus formation. They do not require lifelong anticoagulant therapy. However, they do not last as long as mechanical valves because of degenerative changes and calcification. Mechanical valves are durable (lasting 20 to 30 years). However, they create turbulent blood flow, requiring lifelong anticoagulant therapy to prevent blood clots. Anemia from hemolysis of red blood cells as they come in contact with mechanical valve structures can occur. Also, IE can occur due to microorganisms growing on the valve leaflets or the sewing ring of mechanical valves. These growths can make valves incompetent or can break off to become emboli.

Nursing Process for the Preoperative Cardiac Surgery Patient

DATA COLLECTION. Baseline data collection is important for postoperative comparison and to begin discharge planning. Pain management, circulatory status, and results of diagnostic tests are all significant. Typing and crossmatching for units of blood as ordered is done.

NURSING DIAGNOSES, PLANNING, IMPLEMENTATION, AND EVALUATION. See the "Nursing Process for Preoperative Patients" in Chapter 12.

Nursing Process for the Postoperative Cardiac Surgery Patient

After cardiac surgery, the patient goes to a cardiac universal bed (CUB) unit or an intensive care unit (ICU) to be monitored for 1 to 2 days. In a CUB unit, the patient recovers in the same room until discharge, which avoids transfers to other units and increases continuity of care. In an ICU, as recovery progresses, the patient is transferred to a step-down or general surgical unit for continued cardiac monitoring.

DATA COLLECTION. The patient is accompanied to ICU/CUB by the anesthesiologist. The anesthesiologist gives the nurse a report of the procedure, complications, and hemodynamic and ventilatory management of the patient. The patient remains on a cardiac monitor and mechanical ventilator for up to 24 hours.

A head-to-toe assessment of the patient is performed. It includes dressings, tubes (chest tube, nasogastric tube, urinary catheter), and IV lines. Of importance are signs of awakening, pain, lung and heart sounds, and palpation of the entire chest and neck to detect crepitus (air in the subcutaneous tissue from opening the chest). Trends in cardiac output are monitored.

Body temperature is continuously monitored if warming measures such as a warming blanket are used. Warming is discontinued when the core body temperature nears 98.6°F (37°C). Warming should occur slowly to avoid peripheral vasodilation, which can result in shock. While being rewarmed, patients are monitored for shivering. Shivering may be felt as a fine vibration at the mandibular angle of the jaw. Shivering greatly increases cardiac oxygen needs. As ordered, paralyzing agents given with narcotics eliminate shivering. Complete blood count (CBC), electrolytes, coagulation studies, and arterial blood gases (ABGs) are monitored.

After the initial transfer assessment, vital signs, oxygen saturation, and cardiac pressures are monitored. They are recorded every 15 to 30 minutes, with decreasing frequency as the patient stabilizes. Intake and output are measured. A 12-lead ECG is done to detect perioperative MI. A chest x-ray is done to check central line and endotracheal tube placement and to detect a pneumothorax or hemothorax, diaphragm elevation, or mediastinal widening from bleeding.

Awakening with many questions, strange auditory and tactile sensations, and the inability to speak is frightening and frustrating to the patient. Give explanations regarding procedures in simple terms. Keeping eye contact with the patient and using touch appropriately can be soothing to the patient. Communicating with the intubated patient is done with simple closed-ended questions for yes and no answering, nonverbal gestures, communication boards, or magic slates. The family will need a great deal of support during this time.

After cardiac surgery, pain is monitored in relation to the patient's preoperative anginal or MI-associated pain. Chest pain after surgery can be frightening. Knowing that chest pain can occur from the surgical incision rather than from anginal or MI pain is comforting to the patient.

NURSING DIAGNOSES, PLANNING, IMPLEMENTATION, AND EVALUATION. Nursing diagnoses for postoperative care after cardiac surgery are discussed in the "Nursing Care Plan for the Postoperative Patient" in Chapter 12. After cardiac surgery, the patient will have a chest tube in place. Monitor the amount of drainage in the chest tube. Report amounts above 200 mL per hour to help prevent complications.

INFLAMMATORY AND INFECTIOUS CARDIAC DISORDERS

The layers of the heart are the endocardium, pericardium, and myocardium (Fig. 23.4). They can become inflamed or infected, leading to endocarditis, pericarditis, and myocarditis, respectively.

Infective Endocarditis

Infective endocarditis, or IE, is an infection of the endocardium that occurs primarily in hearts with artificial or damaged valves and in those who inject drugs. Men develop IE more often than women, as do older adults compared with younger adults.

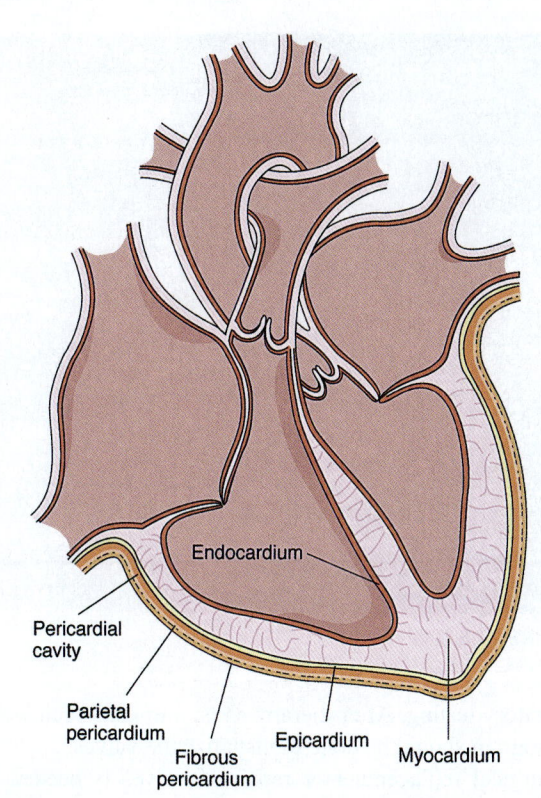

FIGURE 23.4 Layers of the heart.

Pathophysiology and Etiology

Cardiac defects result in turbulent blood flow that erodes the normally infection-resistant endocardium. IE begins when the invading organism (most commonly bacteria but possibly a fungi or other organism) attaches to eroded endocardium where platelets and fibrin deposits have formed a vegetative lesion. Then, more platelets and fibrin cover the multiplying organism. This covering protects the microbes, reducing the ability to destroy them. Damage to valve leaflets occurs as the vegetation grows. As blood flows through the heart, the vegetation may break off and become emboli.

Damaged valves from conditions such as MVP with regurgitation, rheumatic heart disease, congenital defects, and valve replacements are especially prone to bacterial invasion. The mitral valve is the valve most commonly infected, with the aortic valve second. HF may result from valve damage, especially of the aortic valve. Risk factors include compromised immune system, intravenous catheter, artificial heart valve, congenital or valvular heart disease, history of IE, IV drug use, and gingival gum disease.

Prevention

Dental disease may be a contributing factor to IE. Therefore, daily tooth brushing and flossing along with regular dental care is important. The AHA (2021) recommends antibiotic prophylaxis before certain dental procedures that manipulate oral tissue for the highest risk individuals who have a history of IE, a prosthetic heart valve or valve repair, a heart transplant with abnormal valve function, or certain congenital heart defects. It is not routinely recommended for any other medical procedures.

Signs and Symptoms

The onset of symptoms can be rapid or slow. Fever (99°F to 103°F [37.2°C to 39.4°C]) is a common sign (Table 23.3). Chills, anorexia, weight loss, aching muscles and joints, fatigue, dyspnea, cough, night sweats, and hematuria may occur. A new or different murmur is heard with valvular damage. Splinter hemorrhages may be seen in the distal nailbed (black or red-brown longitudinal short lines). **Petechiae** (tiny red or purple flat spots) resulting from microembolization of the vegetation may occur on mucous membranes, conjunctivae, or skin and may be seen in less than half of patients with IE (Fig. 23.5). Janeway lesions (small, painless red-blue lesions on palms and soles) are an acute finding. Osler nodes (small, painful nodes on fingers and toes) from cardiac emboli are a late finding (Fig. 23.6). Roth spots, which are hemorrhages in the retina that have a white center, can occur.

Complications

Vegetative emboli can be a major complication of IE. If organ embolization occurs, signs and symptoms vary based on the affected organ. For example, brain emboli may produce changes in level of consciousness or stroke. Kidney emboli cause pain in the flank area, hematuria, or renal failure. Pulmonary emboli result in sudden dyspnea, cough, and chest pain. Spleen emboli cause abdominal pain. Emboli in the small blood vessels can impair circulation in the extremities.

Heart structures can be damaged or destroyed by IE, leading to MI or arrhythmias. Stenosis (narrowing) or regurgitation (leakage) of a heart valve may also result. As the infection progresses and causes more damage to heart structures, HF may occur. Abscesses may also develop in the heart or other parts of the body.

Diagnostic Tests

Table 23.3 lists diagnostic tests for IE. Positive blood cultures identify the causative organism. Echocardiogram shows cardiac vegetation and effects. Cardiac CT scan or MRI may be used to identify other areas of infection.

Therapeutic Measures

Prompt diagnosis is followed with hospitalization and IV antibiotics. The specific pathogen will be identified by blood cultures. The length of therapy is dependent on the type of pathogen, often up to 6 weeks. A combination of two antibiotics may be used. Rest and supportive symptom care are also used. When afebrile without complications, the patient is discharged to continue IV antibiotic therapy at home. Monitoring is continued by the home health-care nurse and

• WORD • BUILDING •

petechiae: petecchia—skin spot

Table 23.3
Infective Endocarditis Summary

Signs and Symptoms	Dyspnea, cough Fatigue, weakness Fever, chills, aching muscles Heart murmur Janeway lesions, Osler nodes, Roth spots Nailbed splinter hemorrhages Petechiae Weight loss
Diagnostic Tests	Blood cultures Complete blood count Echocardiogram or transesophageal echocardiogram Chest x-ray Electrocardiogram
Therapeutic Measures	Antibiotic prophylaxis per criteria *Acute therapy:* Prolonged IV antimicrobial medications such as penicillin, vancomycin, amphotericin B Antipyretics Rest Valve replacement or repair
Complications	Emboli Heart failure Abscesses
Priority Nursing Diagnoses	*Decreased Cardiac Output* *Decreased Activity Tolerance*

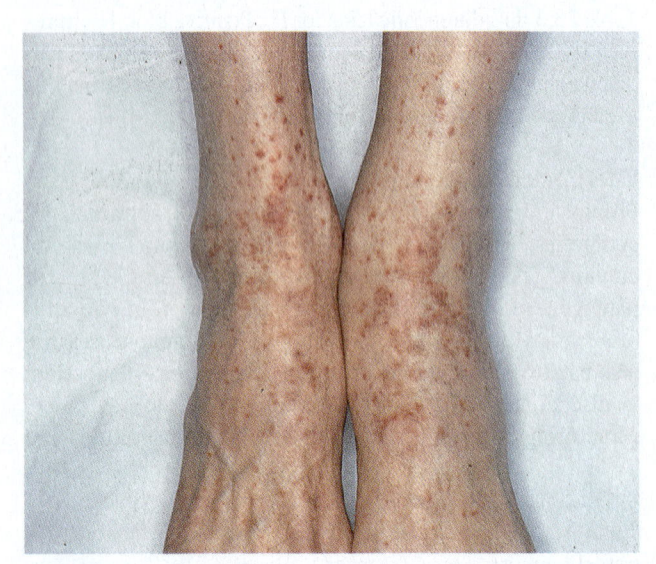

FIGURE 23.5 Petechiae.

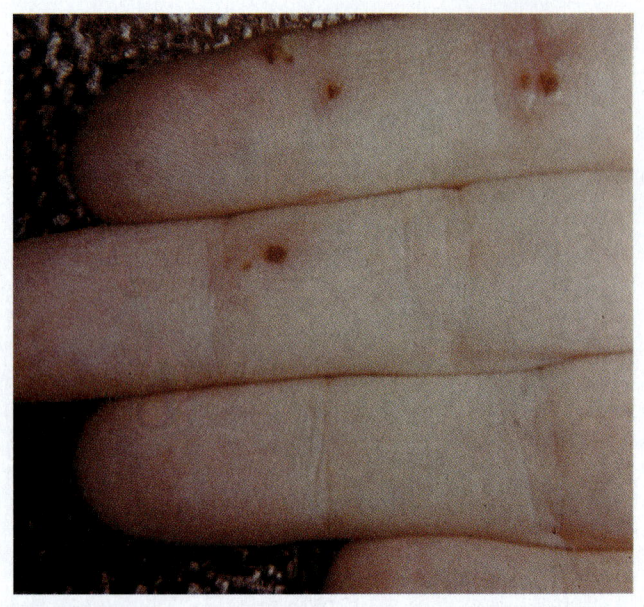

FIGURE 23.6 Osler nodes.

laboratory testing. After therapy ends, a transthoracic echocardiogram should be done to visualize the valves.

Surgical replacement or repair of valves is needed for severely damaged heart valves, prosthetic valve infection, multiple emboli from damaged valves, or HF. Surgery may be needed for infections that do not resolve.

Nursing Process for the Patient With Infectious Endocarditis

DATA COLLECTION. A patient history is obtained that includes risk factors for IE and recent infections or invasive procedures (Table 23.4). Vital signs are recorded, and heart sounds are auscultated for murmurs. Signs of HF and emboli are noted. The HCP should be notified immediately if circulatory impairment (e.g., cool or cold skin, increased capillary refill time, cyanosis, or absent peripheral pulses in an extremity) or symptoms of organ-related emboli are detected.

NURSING DIAGNOSES, PLANNING, AND IMPLEMENTATION. See the nursing diagnosis *Decreased Cardiac Output* under "Nursing Care Plan for the Patient With a Cardiac Valvular Disorder."

Decreased Diversional Activity Engagement *related to restricted mobility from prolonged intravenous (IV) therapy*

EXPECTED OUTCOME: The patient will state diversional activities are satisfying.

- Plan relaxing and fun activities for patient to do during IV therapy, using the patient's input *to increase patient self-esteem through increased patient control.*

EVALUATION. Interventions are successful if the patient's vital signs are within normal parameters for the patient, pulses are strong, extremities are warm, no dyspnea or fatigue are present, and the patient participates in diversional activities.

Table 23.4
Data Collection for Patients With Infective Endocarditis

Data Collection	Subjective Data Questions
Health History	Infections (rheumatic fever, scarlet fever, previous endocarditis, streptococcal or staphylococcal, syphilis)? Cardiac disease (valvular surgery, congenital)? Childbirth? Invasive procedures (surgery, dental, catheterization, IV therapy, cystoscopy, gynecological)? Injectable drug use?
Gastrointestinal	Malaise? Anorexia? Weight loss?
Respiratory	Dyspnea on exertion or orthopnea (when lying down)? Cough?
Cardiovascular	Palpitations, chest pain, fatigue, activity intolerance?
Musculoskeletal	Weakness, arthralgia, myalgia?
Medications	Steroids, immunosuppressants, prolonged antibiotic therapy? IV drug use?
Knowledge of Condition	What is your understanding of this condition?
	Objective Data
Body Temperature	Fever, diaphoresis
Respiratory	Crackles, tachypnea
Cardiovascular	Murmurs, tachycardia, arrhythmias, edema
Integumentary	Nailbed splinter hemorrhages; petechiae on lips, mouth, conjunctivae, feet, or antecubital area; paleness
Renal	Hematuria
Diagnostic Test Findings	Positive blood cultures, anemia, elevated white blood cell count, elevated erythrocyte sedimentation rate, electrocardiogram showing conduction problems, echocardiogram showing valvular dysfunction and vegetation, chest x-ray examination showing heart enlargement (cardiomegaly) and lung congestion

PATIENT EDUCATION. Education provides patients and families with the ability to provide IV antibiotics at home and maintain health to prevent future IE. Good hygiene, including brushing with a soft-bristle toothbrush (to prevent gum trauma) twice a day, flossing daily, and having biannual dental cleaning, is important. Good skin care includes bathing, proper hand-washing technique, avoiding nail biting, not popping pimples or lancing boils, and cleansing and applying antibiotic ointment to cuts. Recognition of symptoms (e.g., fever, chills, sweats), seeking prompt medical care, and a statement of patient's understanding along with printed material for home reference promote health maintenance.

CRITICAL THINKING & CLINICAL JUDGMENT

Mrs. Jones, age 28, is admitted to the hospital with a fever of 100°F (37°C), chills, fatigue, anorexia, and pain in her joints. A physical examination reveals splinter hemorrhages in the left index finger nailbed and petechiae on her chest. She is diagnosed with a heart murmur and infective endocarditis.

Critical Thinking (The Why)
1. Why is a heart murmur heard with endocarditis?
2. What do splinter hemorrhages look like?
3. What do petechiae indicate?

4. What type of medication would the nurse expect to be ordered to treat the infection?
5. Why does Mrs. Jones have chills if her temperature is elevated?
6. What signs and symptoms might occur if the complications of heart failure develop?

Clinical Judgment (The Do)

7. How would Mrs. Jones's data collection findings be documented?
8. What health-care team members will you collaborate with to care for this individual?
9. Acetaminophen (Tylenol) 650 mg every 6 hours for pain is ordered. It comes as 325 mg tablets. How many tablets would be given for each dose?

Suggested answers are at the end of the chapter.

Pericarditis

Pathophysiology and Etiology

Pericarditis is an acute or chronic (greater than 3 months) inflammation of the pericardium (the sac surrounding the heart for protection and to reduce friction). The inflammation creates a problem for the heart as it tries to expand and fill. As a result, ventricular filling is reduced, which then decreases cardiac output and blood pressure. Acute pericarditis usually resolves in less than 4 to 6 weeks but can persist up to 3 months or reoccur at any time. The cause may be unknown or due to infections (e.g., viruses, bacteria, fungi, or Lyme disease), **Dressler syndrome** (autoimmune response), medications, neoplastic disease, post–cardiac injury (e.g., after myocardial infraction, cardiac surgery, trauma), renal disease or uremia, or rheumatic disorders (e.g., systemic lupus erythematosus, rheumatoid arthritis).

There are several forms of chronic pericarditis. It is the result of fibrous scarring of the pericardium. The heart becomes surrounded by a thickened, stiff sac that limits the stretching ability of the heart's chambers for filling and may result in HF. Chronic constrictive pericarditis results from neoplastic disease and metastasis, radiation, or tuberculosis.

Signs and Symptoms

Chest pain is the most common symptom of acute pericarditis (Table 23.5). The pain is located substernally and over the heart. It may radiate to the clavicle, neck, and left scapula. Typically, the chest pain is an intense, sharp, creaky, grating pain that increases with deep inspiration, coughing, moving of the trunk, or lying flat. For some, the pain is not as intense and is instead a dull ache. The pain is often relieved by sitting up and leaning forward. Other symptoms depend on the cause of the pericarditis. They may include orthopnea, low-grade fever, fatigue, cough, and edema.

A **pericardial friction rub** is a grating, scratchy, high-pitched sound that is the result of friction from the inflamed pericardial and epicardial layers rubbing together as the heart fills and contracts. Depending on the severity of the pericarditis, the rub may be faint when auscultated or loud enough to be audible without auscultation. It may be heard intermittently or continuously. It is usually heard over the lower left sternal border of the chest during each heartbeat.

Chronic constrictive pericarditis produces dyspnea and signs and symptoms of right-sided HF. It may also cause atrial fibrillation.

Table 23.5 Pericarditis Summary

Signs and Symptoms	Chest pain Cough Dyspnea, orthopnea Edema Low-grade fever Palpitations Pericardial friction rub Weakness
Diagnostic Tests	Complete blood count Blood chemistry Chest x-ray Electrocardiogram Echocardiogram Magnetic resonance imaging Computed tomography scan
Therapeutic Measures	Treat underlying cause Anti-inflammatory medication Corticosteroids Pericardiocentesis Pericardial window Pericardiectomy
Complications	Pericardial effusion Cardiac tamponade
Priority Nursing Diagnoses	*Acute Pain* *Anxiety* *Decreased Cardiac Output*

> **LEARNING TIP**
> To simulate the sound of a pericardial friction rub, hold the diaphragm of a stethoscope against the palm of one hand; listen through the stethoscope as you rub the index finger of the opposite hand over the knuckles of the hand holding the diaphragm. This sound is similar to a pericardial friction rub.

Diagnostic Tests

Table 23.5 lists diagnostic tests for pericarditis. Initially, the ECG reveals new widespread ST segment elevation which resolves over time (see Fig. 25.8). Echocardiogram results will show a **pericardial effusion** (buildup of fluid in pericardial space) when present. Erythrocyte sedimentation rate and C-reactive protein (CRP) are elevated from inflammation and can be monitored to show therapy effects. A CT scan or MRI may show a thickened pericardium.

Therapeutic Measures
Mild acute cases may resolve without treatment. The cause is determined for appropriate treatment such as antibiotics for bacterial infections. NSAIDs or aspirin are given along with colchicine (Colsalide) to resolve inflammation and reduce pain. Corticosteroids are used if initial treatment is not effective. Hemodialysis is used to treat uremic pericarditis. If the patient is unstable, prompt intervention is required, such as an emergency pericardiocentesis.

Chronic effusive pericarditis can be treated with a pericardial window, which is a surgical opening to remove a portion of the outer pericardial layer, allowing continuous drainage of pericardial fluid into the pleural space. Chronic constrictive pericarditis is treated with **pericardiectomy**, which is the surgical removal of the entire tough, calcified pericardium, relieving constriction of the heart and allowing normal filling of the ventricles.

Complications
A pericardial effusion is the most common complication of pericarditis. A rapidly developing effusion, such as one occurring from trauma, can produce symptoms with smaller amounts of fluid than slowly developing effusions, such as pericarditis from tuberculosis, with larger amounts of fluid. The increasing fluid presses on nearby tissue, such as lung tissue producing dyspnea, cough, and tachypnea. The heartbeat sounds distant.

As the fluid accumulation grows, **cardiac tamponade**, another complication of pericarditis, can occur. Cardiac tamponade is a life-threatening compression of the heart by fluid accumulated in the pericardial sac. Cardiac output decreases. To compensate, the heart rate increases. Then, blood pressure falls as compensatory mechanisms fail. Symptoms of decreased cardiac output, such as restlessness, confusion, tachycardia, and tachypnea, occur. Jugular venous distention is present from increased venous pressure, and heart sounds are distant.

Cardiac tamponade requires emergency treatment with **pericardiocentesis**. The pericardium is punctured with a needle, and excess fluid in the pericardial sac is removed (Fig. 23.7). Fluid obtained during pericardiocentesis can be examined to diagnose the cause. Complications include bleeding, infection, pneumothorax, or heart damage from laceration of a coronary artery or the myocardium.

Nursing Care
Nursing care focuses on relieving the patient's pain and anxiety and maintaining normal cardiac function. Pain is rated and treated as ordered. Allowing the patient to assume a position of comfort by sitting up and leaning forward also

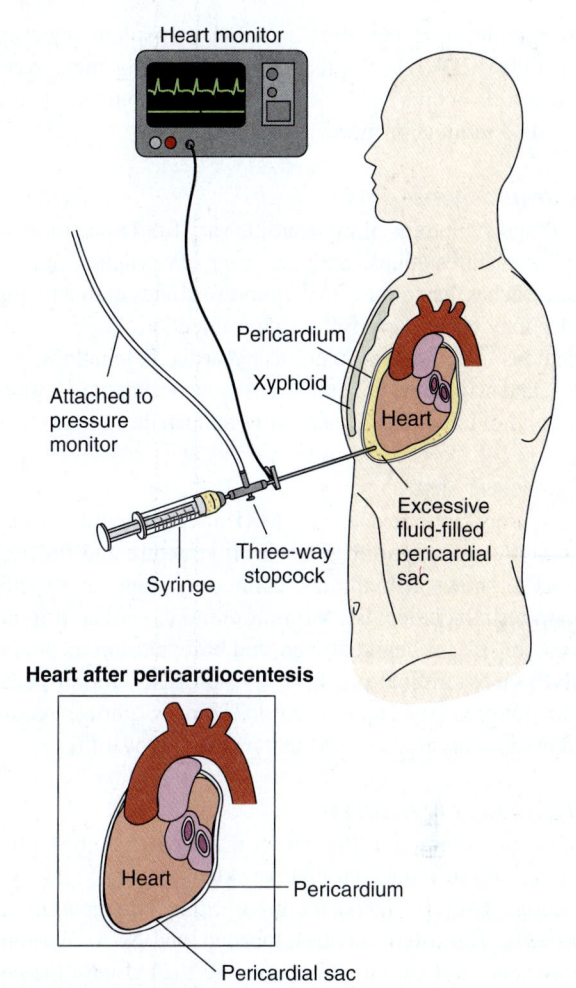

FIGURE 23.7 Pericardiocentesis.

relieves pain. Reinforcing teaching about pericarditis and its treatment relieves anxiety, giving a feeling of control by allowing the patient to make knowledgeable health-care decisions.

Myocarditis
Pathophysiology and Etiology
Myocarditis is inflammation of the myocardium. The amount of muscle destroyed with myocarditis determines the extent of damage to the heart and resultant heart failure. The heart may enlarge in response to the damaged muscle fibers. However, most cases of myocarditis are benign, with few signs or symptoms.

Myocarditis is a rare condition that most commonly develops after a viral infection, including COVID-19 in some cases. Other causes are bacteria, parasites, fungi, rickettsiae, or protozoa. Noninfectious causes may include

• WORD • BUILDING •

cardiac tamponade: kardia—heart + tamponade—plug
pericardiocentesis: peri—around + kardia—heart + centesis—puncture
myocarditis: myo—muscle + kardia—heart + itis—inflammation

autoimmune, cocaine abuse, cardiac transplant rejection, or (rarely) COVID-19 vaccination for young men. Acute myocarditis occurs for 3 months or less; chronic myocarditis lasts 3 months or more.

Signs and Symptoms
Signs and symptoms of myocarditis vary from none to severe cardiac manifestations. Fatigue, fever, pharyngitis, malaise, muscle aches, gastrointestinal discomfort, and enlarged lymph nodes may occur early from a viral infection. Cardiac manifestations such as chest pain, tachycardia, palpitations, dyspnea, and symptoms of heart failure may occur about 2 weeks after a viral infection. Occasionally, sudden death may occur.

Diagnostic Tests
Chest x-ray, echocardiogram, MRI or radionuclide ventriculography are helpful to show heart structure and function. An ECG shows arrhythmias, commonly sinus tachycardia. Blood tests include CBC with differential, cardiac troponin levels to look for heart damage, and brain natriuretic peptide (BNP) or N-terminal pro-BNP (NT-proBNP) for suspected heart failure. An endomyocardial biopsy during cardiac catheterization may be used to diagnose myocarditis.

Therapeutic Measures
Treatment is aimed at the cause, if known. Limiting physical activity to reduce cardiac workload during recovery is essential. Exercise increases myocardial inflammation and mortality. The use of alcohol, tobacco, and NSAIDs should be avoided. Symptoms of HF may be treated with medications such as angiotensin-converting enzyme (ACE) inhibitors, angiotensin II receptor blockers (ARBs), beta blockers, or diuretics to reduce the heart's workload. Severe myocarditis may require inotropic medications to vasodilate and strengthen contraction, ventricular assist device, or heart transplantation.

Nursing Care
Nursing care is aimed at maintaining normal cardiac function by monitoring vital signs and symptoms, and administering medications as ordered. Interventions to reduce fatigue include providing assistance as needed, allowing for frequent rest periods, and teaching energy conservation methods. Determining diversional activities with the patient when activity is restricted further reduces patient anxiety.

Cardiac Trauma
Two types of cardiac trauma can occur: nonpenetrating and penetrating. Nonpenetrating injuries, or contusions, occur from blunt trauma such as motor vehicle accidents or contact sports in which direct compression or force is applied to the upper torso. Contusions may vary from small bruises to hemorrhage.

There may be no external trauma indicating cardiac injury. The patient may be asymptomatic or exhibit signs and symptoms identical to an MI. In severe contusions, laboratory results may show elevated creatine kinase MB (CK-MB, an enzyme) or troponin I (a protein).

If bleeding into the pericardial sac occurs, cardiac tamponade can occur. If signs of shock are present, a pericardiocentesis must be performed. With its own pressure, the tamponade may seal the area of bleeding, so no cardiac decompensation occurs. In this case, only bedrest and observation are required. There are no long-term effects with most contusions. With severe contusions, however, scarring and necrosis of the myocardium may decrease cardiac output and increase the risk for cardiac rupture.

Penetrating traumas include an external injury to the chest, such as a stab or gunshot wound, or an internal injury, such as invasive lines that penetrate the cardiac muscle. Complications vary depending on the size, location, and cause of injury. Tamponade occurs from bleeding into the pericardial sac if the pericardium is sealed off by clot formation. A hemothorax develops if blood drains into the pleural space in the chest. A pneumothorax occurs if air collects in the pleural space. Signs and symptoms of hemorrhage and myocardial ischemia can be noted. Surgical repair may be indicated.

Cardiomyopathy
Cardiomyopathy is abnormality and enlargement of the heart muscle that leads to ineffective pumping of the blood. It is often a genetic condition. There are three types of cardiac structure and function abnormalities in cardiomyopathy: dilated, hypertrophic, and restrictive (Fig. 23.8). A consequence of each type of cardiomyopathy can be HF, myocardial ischemia, or MI due to reduced cardiac output. There is no cure.

Dilated Cardiomyopathy
In dilated cardiomyopathy, the size of the heart chambers increases and the walls of the heart become thin. Because the heart is weakened, cardiac output is reduced. Blood moves more slowly from the left ventricle, often resulting in blood clot formation. Dilated cardiomyopathy is the most frequent type of cardiomyopathy and one of the most frequent causes of HF. The left ventricle is most often affected. Dilated cardiomyopathy may be genetic (family testing may be recommended) or caused by infectious myocarditis, hypertension, heart valve disorders, MI, chronic alcohol or cocaine use, metals such as lead, elevated iron levels, HIV, thiamine or zinc deficiencies, cardiac infections, chemotherapy, or neuromuscular disorders.

Hypertrophic Cardiomyopathy
Hypertrophic cardiomyopathy is a hereditary disorder that is transmitted as an autosomal dominant trait (family testing with ECG and echocardiogram is recommended). Prognosis

---

• WORD • BUILDING •

cardiomyopathy: kardia—heart + myo—muscle + pathy—disease

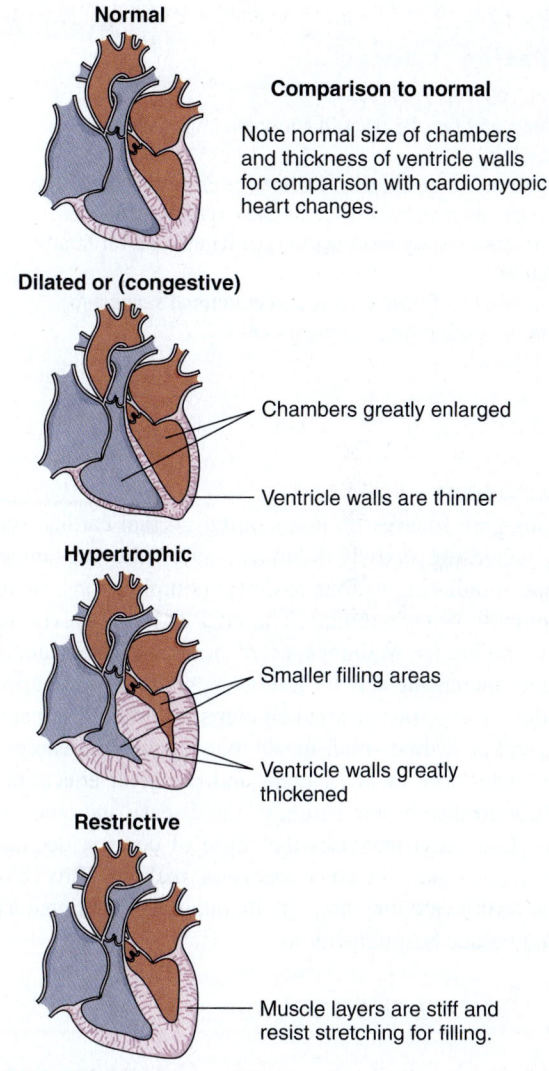

Chapter 23 Nursing Care of Patients With Valvular, Inflammatory, and Infectious Cardiac or Venous Disorders

FIGURE 23.8 Comparison of the normal heart structure with each type of cardiomyopic heart structure.

amyloid within the myocardial cells. This makes the muscle stiff and resistant to stretching for easy ventricular filling. Treating the underlying cause may help reduce heart damage.

Signs and Symptoms

Manifestations of cardiomyopathy depend on the type of abnormality, with varying degrees of HF (Table 23.6). Often there are no early symptoms, and it can occur abruptly. With dilated cardiomyopathy, left ventricular and then right-sided HF with a poor prognosis are seen. Dyspnea on exertion, orthopnea, extreme fatigue, and sometimes atrial fibrillation occur. With hypertrophic cardiomyopathy, if symptoms develop, middle to older age is the most common time. These symptoms can include exertional dyspnea, fatigue, chest pain, syncope, dizziness, and palpitations related to obstruction of cardiac output through the aortic valve. With restrictive cardiomyopathy, HF

Table 23.6 Cardiomyopathy Summary

Signs and Symptoms	Angina Arrhythmias Dyspnea Edema Fatigue Syncope
Diagnostic Tests	Brain natriuretic peptide (BNP) Electrocardiogram Chest x-ray Cardiac catheterization Cardiac magnetic resonance imaging Echocardiogram

Therapeutic Measures	Anticoagulants
	Antihypertensives
	Diuretics
	Corticosteroids
	Antiarrhythmics
	Dilated cardiomyopathy:
	   Vasodilators, cardiac glycosides, cardiac resynchronization, implantable cardioverter device, heart transplant
	Hypertrophic cardiomyopathy:
	   Beta blockers, calcium channel blockers, myectomy, septal ablation
	Restrictive cardiomyopathy:
	   Vasodilators, heart transplant

Complications	Heart failure
Priority Nursing Diagnoses	*Decreased Activity Tolerance* *Anxiety* *Decreased Cardiac Output*

and life span are very good, as symptoms often do not develop to restrict lifestyle. Thickening (hypertrophy) of the cardiac muscle wall, often of the upper ventricular septum and left ventricle during adolescence, occurs. The hypertrophy may occur asymmetrically. Hypertrophic cardiomyopathy causes the ventricular wall to be rigid. Therefore, it does not relax to allow normal ventricular filling. If the mitral valve is affected and, along with the enlarged septum, obstructs the outflow of blood through the aortic valve, it is known as *obstructive hypertrophic cardiomyopathy*. Occasionally, sudden death can occur, primarily in those who are young.

Restrictive Cardiomyopathy

Restrictive cardiomyopathy impairs ventricular stretch, limiting ventricular filling. Cardiac muscle stiffness is present with no ventricular dilation, although systolic emptying of the ventricle is normal. Restrictive cardiomyopathy is the rarest form of cardiomyopathy. It may be caused by infiltrative diseases such as amyloidosis that deposit the protein

symptoms result from the ventricles' inability to fill during diastole. Syncope, arrhythmias, and thrombi may occur.

Diagnostic Tests

Cardiomegaly is visible on a chest x-ray. Echocardiogram shows muscle thickness and chamber size to differentiate between the types of cardiomyopathy. Changes related to enlarged chamber size, tachycardia, and arrhythmias can be seen on the ECG. Cardiac catheterization and biopsy as well as cardiovascular MRI may be useful. An endomyocardial biopsy may be done for restrictive cardiomyopathy. Blood tests may be done to identify HF (BNP), infections, or elevated metal or iron levels. For those with hypertrophic cardiomyopathy, a stress (exercise) test may identify exertional problems due to obstruction.

Therapeutic Measures

Treatment for both dilated and restrictive cardiomyopathies is palliative, focusing on the underlying cause, if known, and managing HF (see Chapter 26). For dilated cardiomyopathy, treatment focuses on the symptoms of HF. ACE inhibitors, ARBs, beta blockers, diuretics, aldosterone antagonists, and digoxin (Lanoxin) may be given. Biventricular pacing and implantable defibrillators may be used. For severe HF, primarily in those with dilated cardiomyopathy, a heart transplant may be done. A ventricular assist device and extracorporeal membrane oxygenation (ECMO) may be used until a donor heart is found (see Chapter 26).

Therapy is not very useful for restrictive cardiomyopathy. Diuretics or nitrates may be used to relieve venous congestion that occurs because of HF. However, a fine balance is needed when using these drugs so that preload is not reduced too greatly, which would worsen symptoms. With atrial fibrillation, anticoagulants are given to prevent emboli formation. Antiarrhythmics or cardioversion is used for arrhythmias.

Treatment is not required for most people with hypertrophic cardiomyopathy, as symptoms do not usually develop. For obstructive hypertrophic cardiomyopathy, beta blockers and calcium channel blockers are given to slow the heart rate to allow more filling time and lessen the strength of the heart's contraction. An antiarrhythmic agent might be used. Adequate hydration is vital, helping to maintain cardiac output. Digoxin and vasodilators are avoided because they can increase the obstruction. Strenuous exercise and athletic sports are restricted to prevent sudden death. Lower levels of exercise may be allowed. For patients in whom medical therapy is not effective, dual chamber pacemakers, implantable automatic defibrillators, or invasive procedures are considered. For those without obstruction, fewer treatment options exist. Diuretics are used to reduce elevated pressures along with beta blockers and calcium channel blockers.

When medical therapy is not successful, surgery can be done for the hypertrophied muscle to remove part of the ventricular septum (**myectomy**). This allows greater outflow of blood. For those that are not candidates for surgery, a septal ablation delivers alcohol via a catheter to necrose and reduce septal heart wall thickness over time.

Box 23.1 Patient Education
Cardiomyopathy

Patients and families should know the importance of the following:
- Adherence to medication regimen to prevent heart failure
- Having emergency contact numbers readily available
- Cardiopulmonary resuscitation (CPR) training for family members
- Availability of hospice care and emotional support for families during the grieving process

---

Nursing Care

Nursing care focuses on maintaining normal cardiac function, increasing activity tolerance, and relieving anxiety. Careful monitoring is done to detect complications, such as HF, emboli, or arrhythmias. The HCP is immediately notified of problems. Maintenance of normal cardiac function includes increasing activity tolerance, planning rest periods, scheduling activities in small amounts, avoiding tiring activities, and providing small meals that require less energy to digest than large meals. Patient and caregiver education is vital due to the chronic nature of the disease and emotional needs. Education increases the sense of control, decreases anxiety, and aids informed decision making (Box 23.1). Home health care may assist in maintaining functional ability and reduce hospitalizations.

VENOUS DISORDERS

Venous Thromboembolism Disease

Venous thromboembolism (VTE) disease includes DVT and pulmonary emboli. **Thrombophlebitis** is the formation of a clot, followed by inflammation within a vein. It is the most common disorder of veins. It can occur in any superficial or deep vein but most often affects the legs, thighs, or pelvis. Deep vein thrombosis (DVT) is the most serious form because pulmonary emboli, which can be fatal, can result if the thrombus detaches (see Chapter 31). DVT occurs most often in patients who are immobile because of recent surgery or hospitalization.

Pathophysiology and Etiology

A venous thrombus is made up of platelets, red blood cells, white blood cells, and fibrin. Platelets attach to a vein wall. Then, a tail forms as more blood cells and fibrin collect. As the

---

• WORD • BUILDING •

cardiomegaly: kardia—heart + mega—large
myectomy: myo—muscle + ectomy—cutting out
thrombophlebitis: thromb—lump (clot) + phleb—vein + itis—inflammation

tail grows, it drifts in the blood flowing past it. The turbulence of blood flow can cause parts of the drifting thrombus to break off, becoming emboli that travel to the lungs.

Three factors are involved in the formation of a thrombus: stasis of blood flow, damage to the lining of the vein wall, and increased blood coagulation (Table 23.7). They are referred to collectively as *Virchow's triad*.

Prevention

Identification of risk factors for thrombosis (see Table 23.7) and patient education promote the use of interventions (discussed later) to prevent thrombosis ("Evidence-Based Practice"). See the Stop the Clot campaign at www.stoptheclot.org. Dehydration should be avoided to reduce thrombus risk.

Managing the risk of thrombosis in transgender adults undergoing hormone therapy is important. Hormone therapy can improve overall mental health and gender identity for transgender adults. However, it has been suggested that hormone treatment regimens should avoid ethinyl estradiol or progestin in order to reduce thrombosis risk in this population (Goldstein et al, 2019).

> **BE SAFE!**
> **TAKE ACTION!** For prevention of thrombophlebitis:
> - Explain and encourage leg exercises for immobilized patients.
> - Ambulate as early as possible.
> - Maintain balanced hydration.

> **Evidence-Based Practice**
>
> **Clinical Question**
> What interventions support vulnerable patient populations taking oral anticoagulants?
>
> **Evidence**
> A systematic review of 41 studies included 37 studies focused on older adults, with 20 focused on INR monitoring, 17 on education interventions, 2 on health literacy, and 2 on cultural and linguistical diversity (Yiu & Bajorek, 2019). Findings of the review showed that INR monitoring with point-of-care testing, pharmacist-led INR monitoring especially during transition periods, and telephone monitoring were effective for older adults. The review also revealed that there is a need for long-term follow-up, with regular reinforcement of information using multiple modes of conveying the information (written, verbal, and video), that is tailored to a patient's health literacy and culture. Patient understanding helps reduce adverse events and improve INR control.
>
> **Implications for Nursing Practice**
> Collect data on patient's understanding of his or her prescribed anticoagulant and reinforce teaching using written, verbal, and video information at regular intervals and at each encounter.
>
> *Reference:* Yiu, A., & Bajorek, B. (2019). Patient-focused interventions to support vulnerable people using oral anticoagulants: A narrative review. *Therapeutic Advances in Drug Safety, 10.* https://doi.org/10.1177/2042098619847423

Table 23.7
Predisposing Conditions for Thrombophlebitis (Virchow's Triad)

Condition	Example
Venous stasis	
• Reduction of blood flow	Shock, heart failure, myocardial infarction, atrial fibrillation
• Dilated veins	Vasodilators
• Decreased muscle contractions	Sitting for long periods (e.g., traveling) Immobility due to fractured hip, paralysis, anesthesia, surgery, obesity, advanced age
• Faulty valves	Varicose veins, venous insufficiency
Venous wall injury	Venipuncture, venous cannulation at same site for more than 48 hours, venous catheterization, surgery, trauma, burns, fractures, dislocation, IV medications (potassium, chemotherapy drugs, antibiotics, IV hypertonic solutions), IV contrast agents, diabetes, cerebrovascular disease
Increased coagulation of blood	Anemia, malignancy, antithrombin III deficiency, oral contraceptives, estrogen therapy, smoking, discontinuance of anticoagulant therapy, dehydration, malnutrition, polycythemia, leukocytosis, thrombocytosis, sepsis, pregnancy

IMMOBILITY. People traveling long distances (e.g., in cars, airplanes) or with sedentary jobs that require extended periods of sitting or standing should change positions, perform knee and ankle flexion exercises, or walk at regular intervals to prevent stasis of blood. Patients on bedrest should have legs elevated above the level of the heart, if possible, and turn every 2 hours to prevent pooling of blood. Postoperatively or during bedrest, active or passive range-of-motion exercises should be done to increase blood flow. Ambulation should begin as soon as the patient's condition allows. Pain should be controlled to facilitate movement. Deep-breathing aids improve blood flow in large thoracic veins. Smoking should be avoided, as nicotine causes vasoconstriction.

PROPHYLACTIC ANTIEMBOLISM DEVICES. Patients with peripheral venous disease, those on bedrest, and those who have had surgery or trauma may use antiembolism devices to improve blood flow. Knee- or thigh-length compression stockings apply pressure to the leg. They must be applied correctly to avoid a tourniquet effect. Older patients with decreased manual dexterity may need assistance. Stockings should be removed for skin inspection, cleansing, and moisturizing daily. Intermittent pneumatic compression (IPC) devices fill intermittently with air to move venous blood in the legs by simulating contraction of the leg muscles. They may be used in combination with compression stockings for greater effectiveness.

PROPHYLACTIC MEDICATION. Low molecular weight heparin (LMWH) can be given postoperatively to prevent thrombosis (Table 23.8). Anticoagulation monitoring is not required with LMWH because of the predictability of its dose-related response. Subcutaneous heparin may also be used postoperatively to prevent thrombosis. Platelet counts must be monitored with either LMWH or heparin to detect heparin-induced thrombocytopenia. Oral anticoagulants such as warfarin (Coumadin) can be used in the high-risk patient to prevent thrombosis.

IV THERAPY. Monitoring of IV sites is performed according to institutional policy to detect signs of thrombophlebitis. Venous cannula sites should be changed regularly per institutional guidelines to prevent thrombus formation.

Table 23.8
Anticoagulant Medications

Medication Class/Action

Coumarin
Inhibits liver synthesis of vitamin K dependent clotting factors: II, XII, IX, X.

Examples	*Nursing Implications*
warfarin (Coumadin)	Monitor international normalized ratio (INR) regularly and signs of bleeding. Teach patient to report bleeding.
	Acetaminophen (Tylenol) is given for analgesia instead of aspirin while on warfarin (can continue aspirin for heart disease).
	Antidote: Vitamin K.
	Teach:
	Maintain regular monitoring of INR, report signs of bleeding, and eat amounts that are consistent for foods that are high in vitamin K to maintain INR level (see "Nutrition Notes").

Direct Thrombin Inhibitors

Examples	*Nursing Implications*
dabigatran (Pradaxa)	Monitor for bleeding.

Heparin
Binds to antithrombin III, which then inhibits fibrin formation.

Examples	*Nursing Implications*
heparin sodium	Monitor heparin antifactor Xa or partial thromboplastin time: 1.5 to 2 times control.
	Do not give intramuscularly, as can cause pain and hematoma.
	Monitor for bleeding and decreased platelet count.
	Antidote: Protamine sulfate.
	Teach:
	Report bleeding.

Table 23.8
Anticoagulant Medications—cont'd

Medication Class/Action

Factor Xa Inhibitors
Bind with antithrombin III, inhibiting making of factor Xa and the formation of thrombin.

Examples	Nursing Implications
apixaban (Eliquis) dalteparin sodium (Fragmin) enoxaparin (Lovenox) fondaparinux (Arixtra) rivaroxaban (Xarelto) edoxaban (Savaysa)	Bleeding rare. Contraindicated with kidney disease due to increased bleeding risk. Compliance is key for efficacy. *Teach:* Give injection subcutaneously (with a prefilled syringe the air bubble is not to be removed).

Thrombolytics
Promote fibrinolysis to break down fibrin in blood clot.

Examples	Nursing Implications
reteplase; rPA (Retavase) tenecteplase; TNK (TNKase) tissue plasminogen activator; tPA (Alteplase)	Minimize blood draws for 24 hours. Monitor for bleeding. Avoid acetylsalicylic acid, NSAIDs.

Signs and Symptoms

Symptoms vary according to the size and location of a thrombus. In some cases, the thrombus becomes an embolus (Table 23.9).

SUPERFICIAL VEINS. Thrombophlebitis in a superficial vein may produce redness, warmth, swelling, and tenderness in the area. The vein feels like a firm cord. This effect is called *induration*. The saphenous vein is the most commonly affected vein in the leg. Varicosity of the vein is usually the cause. In the arm, IV therapy is the most common cause.

DEEP VEINS. Patients may have no symptoms with thrombophlebitis in the leg. With a DVT in a femoral vein, swelling, pain, warmth, venous distention, edema, and tenderness of the calf may be present in the affected leg. Obstruction of blood flow from the leg back to the heart causes the edema. An elevated temperature can be present. Cyanosis and edema may occur if the large veins (vena cava) are involved.

Complications

The most serious complication is pulmonary embolism (PE), a life-threatening emergency (see Chapter 31). Chronic venous insufficiency results from damage to the valves in the vein and can cause venous stasis. Signs and symptoms that may appear years after a thrombus include edema, pain, brownish discoloration and ulceration of the medial ankle, venous distention, and dependent cyanosis of the leg. Post-thrombotic syndrome (PTS) is a symptomatic chronic venous insufficiency after a DVT that occurs in about 50% of DVT patients within 2 years. It occurs from damage to the vein valves that normally prevent backflow of blood within the leg veins. PTS results in pain, swelling, and sometimes leg ulcers, which can

Table 23.9
Thrombophlebitis Summary

Signs and Symptoms	*Superficial veins:* Redness, warmth, swelling, tenderness, induration *Deep veins:* Swelling, pain, warmth, venous distention, edema and tenderness
Diagnostic Tests	D-dimer (small protein fragment in blood as a blood clot dissolves) Compression ultrasonography Contrast venography Magnetic resonance imaging or computed tomography
Therapeutic Measures	*Superficial veins:* Warm, moist heat; analgesics; NSAIDs; compression stockings *Deep veins:* Anticoagulants; warm, moist heat; leg extremity elevation above heart level; compression stockings; thrombolytic therapy; thrombectomy; early ambulation
Complications	Pulmonary embolism Chronic venous insufficiency Recurrent deep vein thrombosis
Priority Nursing Diagnoses	*Acute Pain* *Impaired Skin Integrity* *Anxiety*

reduce quality of life. Routine compression stockings use for those with acute DVTs is not recommended for preventing PTS. Compression use for those with extensive lower leg edema is suggested (Kavali & Vedantham, 2018).

Diagnostic Tests
Diagnostic tests guide treatment needs (see Table 23.9). Compression ultrasonography is a reliable, rapid bedside test to diagnosis a suspected DVT, allowing quick initiation of treatment.

Therapeutic Measures
The goals of treatment are to relieve pain and to prevent pulmonary emboli, thrombus enlargement, or development of another thrombus. Superficial thrombophlebitis is treated at home with warm, moist heat; analgesics; NSAIDs; and, for the leg, compression stockings and leg elevation for symptom relief. Determining if the patient will be able and willing to use compression therapy is important. Anticoagulants are not typically needed because the risk of PE is low. A proximal DVT may be treated at home if there is no PE. Mobilization has not shown an increase in risk for PE and DVT progression. Early mobilization in smaller studies has shown a decrease in pain and swelling when a DVT is present (Chatsis & Visintini, 2018).

Traditional medical care for DVTs involves a hospital stay. Interventions may include warm, moist heat; elevation of the leg above heart level for swelling; compression stockings; and anticoagulants. Additional classes of anticoagulants that do not require ongoing laboratory monitoring have provided options to the traditional anticoagulant therapy of heparin and warfarin (see Table 23.8). Usually, anticoagulants are prescribed for 3 months. Then, the patient is evaluated for further need for them.

Other approaches are venous thrombectomy to remove the clot to prevent pulmonary emboli or chronic venous insufficiency when the risk of pulmonary emboli is great or anticoagulant therapy cannot be used. Occasionally, a permanent or retrievable vena cava filter is placed into the vena cava through the femoral or right internal jugular vein. Once in place, it is opened and attached to the vein wall to trap clots traveling toward lungs without hindering blood flow.

Nursing Process for the Patient With Thrombophlebitis

DATA COLLECTION. A patient history is obtained that includes questions regarding recent IV therapy or use of contrast media, surgery, extremity trauma, childbirth, bedrest, recent long trips, cardiac disease, recent infections, and current medications that can put the patient at high risk of thrombus. Data are gathered for pain, fever, peripheral pulses, sensation, tenderness, redness, warmth, edema, and a firm, cordlike vein in the affected extremity. Daily extremity circumference measurements are taken and documented (bilateral thighs and calves for leg DVT) and recorded to monitor edema. Coagulation tests are monitored. Signs and symptoms of a pulmonary embolism must be immediately reported to the HCP (see Chapter 31).

NURSING DIAGNOSES, PLANNING, AND IMPLEMENTATION. For the patient identified as being at risk for blood clots, the nursing diagnosis *Risk for Thrombosis* applies. Interventions would include the preventive measures previously discussed. Educating the patient about the disease and its treatment is important to reduce anxiety about complications and to enhance adherence to treatment to prevent complications (see Patient Teaching Guidelines for this chapter on Davis Edge).

Acute Pain related to inflammation of vein

EXPECTED OUTCOME: The patient will report satisfactory pain relief within 30 minutes of pain report.

- Ask patient to rate pain with a pain rating scale (such as 0 to 10) *to provide consistency in pain reporting*.
- Provide analgesics and NSAIDs, as ordered, *to reduce pain*.
- Apply warm, moist compresses, as ordered, *as moist heat penetrates deeply to relieve pain*.

Impaired Skin Integrity related to venous stasis

EXPECTED OUTCOME: The patient's skin will remain intact.

- Observe skin for edema, skin color changes, and ulcers and measure both extremities' circumference at the same site in each extremity daily *to detect skin integrity impairment as edematous skin breaks down more easily*.
- Elevate feet above heart level when at rest *to decrease swelling*.
- Apply compression stockings after acute edema decreases, as ordered, *to maintain reduced swelling*.
- Reinforce teaching for patient to avoid crossing legs or wearing constricting clothes *to avoid impairing venous return*.

EVALUATION. Interventions are successful if the patient is pain-free and skin remains intact.

CUE RECOGNITION 23.2
A patient who is on bedrest reports tenderness in the calf. What action do you take?

Suggested answers are at the end of the chapter.

Home Health Hints
- Upon admission, measure a patient's midcalf circumference for baseline size. Reassess measurements at every visit. If a difference in sizes is detected, check for signs and symptoms of thrombophlebitis or deep vein thrombosis.
- Consider patient need for active and passive range-of-motion exercises. If necessary, consider involving occupational and physical therapists.

- Encourage the patient to move often because immobility can contribute to thrombophlebitis and other complications.
- If pressure is applied on the popliteal area or calf muscle when a patient with venous circulation problems is sitting in a recliner with the leg rest in the up position, use a small, flat pillow under the knees and lower legs to open the angle and relieve the pressure.
- Assist patients to develop energy-conserving techniques by being observant of their environment. Place frequently used items nearby. Put a carrying pouch on the front bar of a walker for carrying items. Place a chair for resting at the top and bottom of stairs.
- Reinforce teaching for patients to report the signs and symptoms of thrombophlebitis, pulmonary emboli, incisional infection, or pneumonia.

Key Points

- Damage to the valves or their surrounding structures can result in abnormal valvular functioning. The valves of the left side of the heart are more commonly affected. The two major types of valvular dysfunction are stenosis and insufficiency.
- Valvular diseases include rheumatic fever, mitral valve prolapse, mitral stenosis, mitral regurgitation, aortic stenosis, and aortic regurgitation.
- A commissurotomy repairs a stenosed valve, which is most commonly the mitral valve. The valve flaps that have adhered to each other are separated to enlarge the valve opening.
- Annuloplasty is the repair or reconstruction of valve flaps or annulus. Sutures or a prosthetic ring may be placed in the valve annulus to improve closure of the leaflets. The mitral valve is the most common valve repaired in this way.
- Valves used for cardiac valve replacement may be either mechanical or biological.
- Postoperative complications of valve replacements include the concern that tissue valves do not last as long as mechanical valves because of degenerative changes and calcification. Mechanical valves, while more durable, create turbulent blood flow, requiring lifelong anticoagulant therapy to prevent blood clots.
- Infective endocarditis is an infection of the endocardium that occurs primarily in hearts with artificial or damaged valves.
- Pericarditis is an acute or chronic inflammation of the pericardium that creates a problem for the heart as it tries to expand and fill. As a result, ventricular filling is reduced, which then decreases cardiac output and blood pressure.
- Myocarditis is inflammation of the myocardium. The amount of muscle destroyed with myocarditis determines the extent of damage to the heart. The heart may enlarge in response to the damaged muscle fibers; however, most cases of myocarditis are benign, with few signs or symptoms.
- Cardiomyopathy—dilated, hypertrophic, and restrictive—is abnormality and enlargement of the heart muscle that leads to ineffective pumping of the blood.
- Thrombophlebitis is the formation of a clot, followed by inflammation within a vein. It can occur in any superficial or deep vein in the body.

SUGGESTED ANSWERS TO CHAPTER EXERCISES

Cue Recognition

23.1: Place the patient on bedrest with the head of bed elevated, apply oxygen per agency protocol, obtain an ECG per orders to identify atrial fibrillation, notify HCP, provide emotional support.

23.2: Measure and document bilateral thighs and calves. Observe skin color and temperature. Note swelling and edema. Maintain bedrest. Notify the HCP of findings.

Critical Thinking & Clinical Judgment

Mr. Goldfarb
1. Weight gain and stress can increase blood pressure, which increases the risk for heart disease, stroke, and damage to other organs.
2. Symptoms, other medical conditions such as hypertension, medications, diet, lifestyle, and surgical complications.
3. Suggest referral to a cardiac rehabilitation program for education on mitral valve prolapse and when to seek medical assistance, managing medications, activity, and setting lifestyle goals. Referral to dietitian and social worker to support nutrition and stress management techniques.

Mrs. Pryor
1. "In aortic stenosis, the aortic valve is narrowed, making it more difficult for blood to leave the left ventricle and go into the aorta, resulting in less blood flow to the body." This is most likely why Mrs. Pryor is feeling tired.
2. Documentation: Subjective data—"What is aortic stenosis?" Objective data—Listened attentively during explanation of aortic stenosis and its effects. Expressed interest in learning more about diagnosis.
3. Respiratory therapist, HCP.

SUGGESTED ANSWERS TO CHAPTER EXERCISES—cont'd

4. Collect data: vital signs with oxygen saturation, pain (location, radiation, severity, characteristics), other signs or symptoms, and ECG. Give prescribed nitroglycerin or other medications or oxygen as needed.
5. Nursing interventions for safety should include fall precautions due to syncope and fatigue. Patient education should be based on Mrs. Pryor's need for safety at home, assistance with ADLs, and answering her questions and concerns.
6. Contact your physician if you experience a heart rate less than 60 bpm, fatigue, anorexia, nausea/vomiting, diarrhea, seeing halos around lights.

Mrs. Jones

1. A heart murmur is heard from damaged heart valves.
2. Splinter hemorrhages appear as black or red-brown lines in the distal nailbed.
3. Petechiae indicate that tiny pieces of a lesion on the endocardium or valves have broken off and become microemboli.
4. Expected medications include IV antibiotics.
5. Shivering is muscular work that raises the body's temperature. It is the body's attempt at developing an unfavorable environment for the pathogen. Removing blankets to decrease fever results in chills and shivering. This further increases body temperature and adds to cardiac workload from muscular activity during shivering. Therefore, Mrs. Jones should be kept covered to prevent chills.
6. For left-sided heart failure, crackles or wheezes may be auscultated and cough or dyspnea might be noted. In right-sided hear failure, peripheral edema or jugular venous distention may be present.
7. Subjective data may include statements such as "I have pain in my joints and am chilled" or "I am fatigued and have no appetite." Objective findings may include fever of 100°F (37°C), splinter hemorrhages in the nailbed, petechiae on chest.
8. HCP, occupational therapist for diversional activities, social worker, or case manager for home IV therapy planning.
9. Two tablets.

$$\frac{650 \text{ mg}}{} \times \frac{1 \text{ tablet}}{325 \text{ mg}} = 2 \text{ tablets}$$

Additional Resources

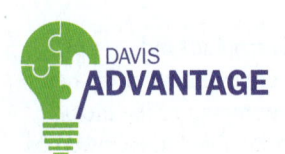

Go to Davis Advantage to complete your learning: strengthen understanding, apply your knowledge, and prepare for the Next Gen NCLEX®.

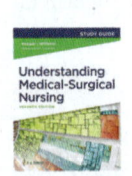

A Study Guide is also available.

CHAPTER 24
Nursing Care of Patients With Occlusive Cardiovascular Disorders

Maureen McDonald

KEY TERMS

acute coronary syndrome (ah-KYOOT KOR-uh-nare-ee sin-DROHM)
anastomosed (an-AST-tah-most)
aneurysm (AN-yur-izm)
angina pectoris (an-JY-nah PEK-tuh-ris)
arteriosclerosis (ar-TEER-ee-oh-skleh-ROH-sis)
atherosclerosis (ATH-er-oh-skleh-ROH-sis)
collateral circulation (kuh-LAH-tur-al SIR-kew-LAY-shun)
coronary artery disease (KOR-uh-nar-ee AR-ter-ee dih-ZEEZ)
embolism (EM-buh-lizm)
endarterectomy (en-DAR-ter-eck-toe-mee)
high-density lipoprotein (HY DEN-sih-tee LIH-poh-PROH-teen)
hyperlipidemia (HY-per-LIH-pih-DEE-mee-ah)
intermittent claudication (IN-tur-MIT-ent KLAW-dih-KAY-shun)
ischemia (is-KEY-me-ah)
low-density lipoprotein (LOH DEN-sih-tee LIH-poh-PROH-teen)
lymphangitis (lim-FAN-jee-EYE-tis)
myocardial infarction (MY-oh-KAR-dee-uhl in-FARK-shun)
peripheral arterial disease (puh-RIFF-uh-ruhl ar-TEER-ee-uhl dih-ZEEZ)
plaque (PLAK)
Raynaud disease (RAY-noh dih-ZEEZ)
thrombosis (throm-BOH-sis)
varicose veins (VAR-ih-kohz VAINS)
venous stasis ulcers (VEE-nus STAY-sis UL-sers)

CHAPTER CONCEPTS

Collaboration
Comfort
Health promotion
Nutrition
Oxygenation
Perfusion

LEARNING OUTCOMES

1. Explain the etiology, signs, symptoms, and therapeutic measures of coronary artery disease, angina pectoris, and myocardial infarction.
2. List data to collect for patients with coronary artery disease, angina pectoris, or myocardial infarction.
3. Describe therapeutic measures used to treat coronary artery disease, angina pectoris, and myocardial infarction.
4. Explain the etiology, signs, and symptoms for each of the peripheral vascular disorders.
5. Identify therapeutic measures used to treat peripheral vascular disorders.
6. Plan nursing care for patients with a peripheral vascular disorder.

Heart disease is the leading cause of death of adults in the United States with a fatality every 36 seconds (Centers for Disease Control and Prevention [CDC], 2018). After a heart attack, women are more likely than men to die or develop heart failure within 5 years (Ezekowitz et al, 2020).

ATHEROSCLEROSIS

Arteriosclerosis is the thickening, loss of elasticity, and calcification of arterial walls. It occurs with aging. **Atherosclerosis** is the formation of plaque in the arteries. Arteriosclerosis and atherosclerosis are both conditions that may begin in early childhood and progress without symptoms through adulthood. Atherosclerosis causes coronary heart disease (CHD), also known as **coronary artery disease** (CAD), discussed shortly.

Pathophysiology

Atherosclerosis is a multistep process that affects the inner lining of the artery (Fig. 24.1). Injury to the endothelial cells that line the walls of the arteries occurs, causing inflammation and immune response. Damage to the endothelium stimulates the growth of smooth muscle cells. These cells secrete collagen and fibrous proteins. Lipids, platelets, and other clotting factors accumulate. This buildup of fatty deposits that

• WORD • BUILDING •

arteriosclerosis: arterio—artery + sklerosis—hardness

378 UNIT FIVE Understanding the Cardiovascular System

Normal artery

Atherosclerotic artery

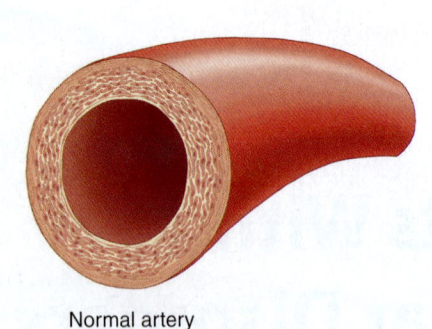

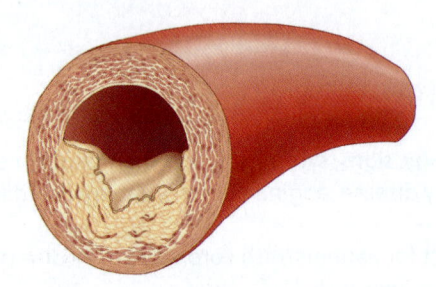

FIGURE 24.1 (Top) Cross section of normal coronary artery. (Bottom) Coronary artery with atherosclerosis narrowing the lumen.

adheres to the wall of the artery is known as **plaque**. It is composed of smooth muscle cells, fibrous proteins, and cholesterol-laden foam cells. The plaque develops a fibrous cap that calcifies. The plaque's fibrous cap can tear or rupture, and a blood clot forms on the plaque. The clot can completely block the coronary artery, or it may break loose and lodge within a smaller artery leading to the heart. The artery may also become stenosed (narrowed) by the plaque buildup causing partial or total occlusion of the artery, resulting in reduced blood flow. The area distal to the occlusion can become ischemic as a result.

Etiology

Risk factors for atherosclerosis can be divided into two categories: those that can be modified and those that cannot (Table 24.1). Patient education to prevent risk factors is important.

Diagnostic Tests

Total cholesterol levels above 200 mg/dL increase risk of CAD and **myocardial infarction** (MI; Table 24.2). Elevated **low-density lipoproteins** (LDLs) and low levels of **high-density lipoproteins** (HDLs) are associated with increased risk of CAD. A risk factor for premature CAD is a high level of Lp(a) cholesterol (a genetic variation of plasma LDL). An excellent predictor of MI risk is the LDL particle number. It is measured directly or indirectly as apolipoprotein B, the protein particle in each LDL. A high LDL particle number with a low LDL still creates a high risk for MI. (The amount of cholesterol contained in each LDL particle varies.) Apolipoprotein B particles in LDL-type cholesterol are able to infiltrate the arterial wall, rapidly causing damage. C-reactive protein (CRP) can indicate low-grade inflammation in blood vessels and an increased CAD risk. Elevated blood glucose levels can increase the risk for atherosclerosis. Radiological studies of the arteries can be performed to show narrowed or occluded vessels (see Chapter 21).

Table 24.1
Risk Factors for Atherosclerosis/Coronary Artery Disease

Risk Factors That Cannot Be Changed	
Age	Men have increased incidence after age 50. Women have increased incidence after menopause.
Ethnicity	Black Americans have a higher incidence of atherosclerosis.
Gender	Men have more risk factors and higher incidence of coronary artery disease (CAD).
Genetics	CAD risk factors such as hyperlipidemia can run in families.

Risk Factors That Can Be Changed or Controlled	
Diabetes mellitus	Increases the risk of hypertension, obesity, and elevated blood lipids.
Hypertension	Vasoconstriction increases myocardial oxygen demand.
Elevated serum cholesterol	Level above 200 mg/dL increases risk of developing CAD.
Elevated low-density lipoprotein (LDL) particle number or apolipoprotein B	Infiltrates arterial wall, rapidly causing damage.

Table 24.1
Risk Factors for Atherosclerosis/Coronary Artery Disease—cont'd

Elevated serum homocysteine	Increases CAD risk. Foods that contain folic acid (e.g., fruits, green leafy vegetables) reduce homocysteine level.
Excessive alcohol use	Raises blood pressure, increases triglycerides, and causes irregular heartbeats.
Obesity	Increases heart workload and risk of hypertension, diabetes, glucose intolerance, and hyperlipidemia.
Sedentary lifestyle	Increases obesity, hypertension, and hyperlipidemia.
Emotional stress	Increases heart workload and risk for hypertension.
Tobacco use, secondhand and thirdhand smoke	Causes vasoconstriction and increases myocardial oxygen demand. Decreases high-density lipoproteins (HDLs).

Table 24.2
Atherosclerosis Summary

Diagnostic Tests	Cholesterol Low-density lipoprotein (LDL) particle number Triglycerides Arteriogram
Therapeutic Measures	Low-fat, low-cholesterol diet Smoking cessation Exercise
Priority Nursing Diagnoses	*Acute Pain* *Deficient Knowledge*

Therapeutic Measures
A healthy lifestyle, preventing risk factors, medications, and regular physical examinations are helpful in controlling atherosclerosis.

Diet
Because plaque within arteries is primarily caused by fatty deposits, an adherence to a heart-healthy diet (Dietary Approaches to Stop Hypertension [DASH] eating plan) is beneficial (see Chapter 22, "Nutrition Notes").

Smoking
The risk of developing CAD is greater in cigarette smokers than in nonsmokers. Risk is proportionate to the number of cigarettes smoked. Smoking contributes to a loss of HDL. Smoking also causes vasoconstriction, which leads to angina pectoris and cardiac arrhythmias. The benefits of smoking cessation are dramatic and almost immediate. Education about the risks of smoking and effects of exposure to secondhand and thirdhand smoke should be presented to patients and their families. Thirdhand smoke is residual nicotine and toxic chemicals left on surfaces (e.g., skin, hair, clothing, bedding, carpets, floors, furniture, walls) by tobacco smoke. The American Cancer Society has many programs to help people quit smoking (visit www.cancer.org).

Exercise
Increased activity raises HDL levels. Increasing physical activity may also lower insulin resistance and facilitate weight loss. Over time, exercise also leads to the development of **collateral circulation**, which allows blood to flow around occluded sites. Before starting an exercise program, patients should consult their health-care provider (HCP).

Medications
Lowering lipid levels is the primary therapy for atherosclerosis. If dietary control is not effective, medication is also used (Table 24.3). It may take 4 to 6 weeks before lipid levels respond to medication therapy. For those with familial hypercholesterolemia, which is a genetic disorder that prevents the removal of LDL due to a chromosome 19 defect, injectable monoclonal antibodies agents such as alirocumab (Praluent) and evolocumab (Repatha) are used.

CORONARY ARTERY DISEASE

CAD is the obstruction of blood flow through the coronary arteries to the heart muscle cells, typically from atherosclerosis.

Prevention
Risk factors for CAD are listed in Table 24.1. Risk factors that can be modified should be changed (see therapeutic measures for atherosclerosis above). Low-dose aspirin may be recommended for certain patients by their HCP to prevent the formation of a thrombus. Million Hearts® 2022 is a national initiative to prevent 1 million heart attacks and strokes within

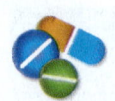

Table 24.3 Medications Used to Lower Lipid Levels

Medication Class/Action

Statins
First-line medications to reduce low-density lipoprotein (LDL) by reducing cholesterol synthesis.

Examples	Nursing Implications
atorvastatin (Lipitor) fluvastatin (Lescol XL) lovastatin (Mevacor) pravastatin (Pravachol) rosuvastatin (Crestor) simvastatin (Zocor)	Monitor liver function studies. Monitor for rhabdomyolysis (lethal breakdown of skeletal muscle). Teach: Take medication in evening when cholesterol synthesis is highest. Report muscle pain to health-care provider.

Fibrates
Reduce triglycerides.

Examples	Nursing Implications
clofibrate (Atromid-S) fenofibrate (TriCor) gemfibrozil (Lopid)	Teach: Take 30 minutes before morning and evening meal. May increase the effects of anticoagulants and hypoglycemia.

Niacin
Prevents conversion of fats into very low LDLs. Rarely used because of flushing.

Examples	Nursing Implications
niacin (nicotinic acid) extended-release niacin (Niaspan)	Teach: Take aspirin 30 minutes before taking medication to reduce flushing.

Cholesterol Absorption Inhibitor
Inhibits the absorption of cholesterol. Decreases LDLs and increases high-density lipoproteins (HDLs).

Examples	Nursing Implications
ezetimibe (Zetia)	Teach: Take with liquids and meals. Take other medications 1 hour before or 4 hours after.

Combination Agent
See each agent.

Examples	Nursing Implications
Vytorin = ezetimibe (Zetia) + simvastatin (Zocor)	See each agent.

---

5 years (https://millionhearts.hhs.gov). Evidence-based priorities to improve cardiovascular health for everyone focus on cholesterol management, self-measured blood pressure monitoring, hypertension control, tobacco cessation, and cardiac rehabilitation.

> **CUE RECOGNITION 24.1**
>
> A patient who has hypertension and had an episode of angina is tearful and frightened. The patient asks you how to prevent future pain episodes. What action do you take?
>
> *Suggested answers are at the end of the chapter.*

Angina Pectoris

Angina pectoris is chest pain due to **ischemia** resulting from a reduction in coronary artery blood flow and oxygen delivery to the myocardium. Angina is a symptom, not a disease.

Types of Angina

STABLE ANGINA. Stable angina occurs with moderate exertion in a pattern familiar to the patient. The pain is predictable and lasts a few minutes. It can usually be relieved by resting and use of prescribed nitroglycerin.

• WORD • BUILDING •
angina pectoris: angina—to choke + pectora—chest

Chapter 24   Nursing Care of Patients With Occlusive Cardiovascular Disorders

VASOSPASTIC ANGINA. This type of angina is caused by coronary artery spasms and is serious. The pattern of occurrence is often cyclical, with the pain happening about the same time each day. The pain lasts longer than stable angina, can occur with exercise or at rest, and often occurs at night.

MICROVASCULAR ANGINA. Spasms in the walls of the tiniest arteries of the heart reduce coronary blood flow and result in microvascular angina. Compared with other types of anginal pain, this pain is often more severe and lasts longer.

Signs and Symptoms

Patients (especially men) often describe anginal chest pain as discomfort, burning, fullness, heaviness, pressure, or squeezing (Fig. 24.2). The pain can radiate to adjacent areas such as one or both arms (left arm is common), shoulders, neck, jaw, or back. If pain is present in the shoulders, neck, jaw, arms, or back due to a cardiac problem but there is no chest pain, then it is *referred* pain. Patients may also describe heaviness in their arms or a feeling of impending doom. During the episode of pain, the patient may be pale, diaphoretic, or dyspneic.

Women might also experience chest pain, jaw pain, or heartburn with angina but often have atypical symptoms. These include shortness of breath, fatigue, nausea, or pain that is described as less severe. Atypical symptoms should not be ignored. Treatment should be sought immediately. (See the "Women and Heart Health" section.)

Diagnostic Tests

Common tests used to diagnose CAD or anginal causes include electrocardiogram (ECG), exercise stress test, echocardiography, chemical stress testing, cardiac computed tomography (CT) scan, cardiac magnetic resonance imaging (MRI)/magnetic resonance angiogram (MRA), radioisotope imaging, and coronary angiography.

Therapeutic Measures

Risk factors identified for the patient determine treatment to prevent anginal attacks with activity and MI. Weight reduction, a heart-healthy diet, smoking cessation, and reduction of emotional stress may help slow disease progression. Three major classes of medications—nitrates, beta blockers, and calcium channel blockers—and a newer medication, the antianginal ranolazine (Ranexa), are used alone or in combination for reducing angina (Table 24.4).

Nitroglycerine (NTG), a vasodilator, is the medication of choice for *acute* anginal attacks. For acute use, it is available sublingually (buccal, powder, spray, tablet) or intravenously in the hospital. When administered sublingually, NTG may relieve chest pain within 1 to 2 minutes (Box 24.1). Long-acting nitrates (oral or topical: ointment, transdermal patch) are used to *prevent* acute chest pain. To prevent development of nitrate tolerance, a common issue with nitrates, the ointment or patch is removed for a 10- to 12-hour nitrate-free period (removed at bedtime/reapplied in the morning for exertional angina; removed in the morning/reapplied at bedtime for nocturnal angina). Oral nitrates (non-extended-release capsules) are also scheduled to give the patient a nitrate-free period.

BE SAFE!
ACT FAST!
Sublingual Nitroglycerin
- If after one tablet and 5 minutes have elapsed, pain is unrelieved or worsens, especially with symptoms of an MI, call 911. Take two more doses, 5 minutes apart, if needed while waiting.
- For angina, take one NTG tablet. If the symptoms are not worsening but are not completely relieved, repeat a tablet every 5 minutes up to a total of three tablets. If pain is not relieved after three tablets, call 911.

BE SAFE!
AVOID FAILURE TO COMMUNICATE! Inform patients who take nitrates not to take medications for erectile dysfunction, such as sildenafil (Viagra), tadalafil (Cialis), or vardenafil (Levitra). These types of medications dilate blood vessels and may cause a significant drop in blood pressure if used with nitrates.

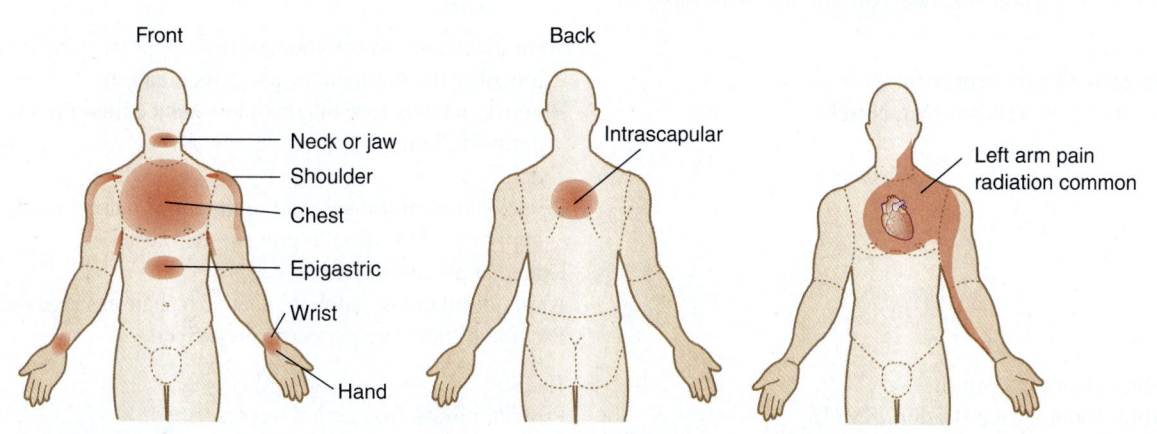

FIGURE 24.2 Common locations of anginal pain, which may vary in combination and intensity.

Table 24.4
Medications Used to Treat Angina Pectoris

Medication Class/Action

Antiplatelets
Inhibit platelet activation, adhesion, or procoagulant activity.

Examples	*Nursing Implications*
aspirin clopidogrel (Plavix) ticagrelor (Brilinta)	Enteric-coated aspirin beneficial for daily use. Monitor for bleeding.

Beta Blockers
Decrease heart rate, contractility, and BP to reduce cardiac workload and exertional angina. Decrease the risk of sudden death.

Examples	*Nursing Implications*
atenolol (Tenormin) metoprolol (Lopressor, Toprol XL)	If pulse is less than 60 bpm or systolic BP less than 90 mm Hg, consult HCP before administering medication. *Teach:* Explain need to rise slowly. Abrupt withdrawal may result in diaphoresis, palpitations, headache, and tremors.

Calcium Channel Blockers
Dilate peripheral arteries, decrease myocardial contractility, depress conduction system, and decrease workload of the heart. In vasospastic angina, reduce coronary artery spasm.

Examples	*Nursing Implications*
amlodipine (Norvasc) diltiazem (Cardizem, Dilacor XR) felodipine (Plendil) verapamil (Calan SR)	If pulse is less than 60 bpm or systolic BP less than 90 mm Hg, notify HCP before administering medication.

Nitrates
Vasodilate to increase blood flow to coronary arteries and reduce preload and afterload to reduce oxygen consumption of myocardium.

Nursing Implications:
Do not use any NTG with erectile dysfunction medication as it can cause a significant drop in blood pressure.
Document onset, location, type, radiation, and duration of pain.
Monitor blood pressure (BP) pre- and postadministration.

Examples	*Nursing Implications*
Fast Acting: nitroglycerin sublingual powder (GONITOR) nitroglycerin sublingual, buccal (Nitrostat, NitroQuick) nitroglycerin sublingual spray (Nitrolingual, Nitromist)	*Teach:* See Be Safe! Act Fast! and Box 24.1.
Long Acting: nitroglycerin (Transderm Nitro, Nitro-Bid) nitroglycerin patch (Nitro-Dur, Nitrek)	Wear gloves to protect yourself from hypotension from touching the ointment or patch medication. Remove patch before magnetic resonance imaging or defibrillation. *Teach:* Remove current transdermal ointment or patch before applying a new dose to prevent overdose. Rotate application sites. Apply ointment or patch to clean, dry, hairless area daily. Provide nitrate-free period as prescribed.
isosorbide dinitrate (Isordil) isosorbide mononitrate (Imdur, ISMO) nitroglycerin extended release (Nitro-Time)	*Teach:* Provide nitrate-free period as prescribed.

Table 24.4 Medications Used to Treat Angina Pectoris—cont'd

Medication Class/Action

Anti-Ischemic Agent
Antianginal agent used as combination therapy for those not responding to other antianginal medication.

Examples	*Nursing Implications*
ranolazine (Ranexa)	May not be as effective in women. Prolongs QT interval on electrocardiogram.

Statins
See Table 24.3.

Box 24.1
Key Points for Using Fast-Acting Nitroglycerin

- Carry nitroglycerin (NTG) at all times.
- Keep NTG tablets tightly sealed in the dark container to protect from heat, light, and moisture.
- Maintain a fresh supply of NTG tablets, replacing it as needed, or every 6 months for maximum effect.
- Use NTG before an activity known to cause chest pain.
- Tingling should be felt under the tongue when sublingual (SL) NTG tablets are used.
- Pour SL packet of powder under the tongue to dissolve without swallowing.
- Do not shake NTG aerosol canister before spraying it on or under the tongue, and close mouth immediately.
- NTG may cause lightheadedness. Sit or lie down when taking NTG, if possible. Rise slowly to prevent falls, especially with sublingual spray.
- NTG may cause a headache initially for 1 to 2 weeks. Aspirin may relieve it.

Beta blockers are initial therapy for exertional angina prevention. They decrease heart rate and contractility and lower blood pressure to reduce the workload of the heart. Beta blockers are not effective for coronary artery spasms, so they should not be used for vasospastic angina.

> **LEARNING TIP**
> To help you identify beta blockers, remember that their generic names end with *-olol*.

Calcium channel blockers dilate the coronary arteries and peripheral vessels, which increases the myocardial oxygen supply and reduces cardiac workload. They are ineffective in relieving acute anginal attacks. Antiplatelets are used to prevent cardiovascular events that would occur from blood clots and cause angina. Statins prevent and treat atherosclerosis since cholesterol and inflammation in artery walls are involved in atherosclerosis development (see Table 24.3).

Nursing Process for the Patient With Coronary Artery Disease and Angina

Data Collection

Record height, weight, allergies, over-the-counter and prescription medications, use of herbs, and typical diet. Identify the patient's nonmodifiable and modifiable risks for atherosclerosis and CAD. Obtain vital signs and oxygen saturation. Note dyspnea, labored respirations, diaphoresis, nausea, skin color, and temperature.

Note a history of chest pain, fatigue, or activity intolerance. Document the patient's description of anginal pain, factors making the pain worse or better, how long the patient has had angina, triggering activities, and how the pain has been relieved in the past (see Table 21.2).

Nursing Diagnoses, Planning, and Implementation

Acute Pain related to reduced perfusion of coronary arteries

EXPECTED OUTCOME: The patient will report an absence or acceptable level of pain within 30 minutes of reporting pain.

- Ask patient to rate pain with a scale (such as 0 to 10) *to provide consistent pain reporting.*
- Administer oxygen as prescribed *to increase oxygen availability to myocardium to ease pain.*
- Administer fast-acting NTG (sublingual) as prescribed *to provide pain relief.*
- Notify HCP if pain is unrelieved after three doses of NTG or as prescribed, or if vital signs change. *Chest pain unrelieved by nitrates (sublingual) may represent MI.*
- Remain with patient and provide emotional support. *A patient who has chest pain should never be left alone.*

Deficient Knowledge related to ineffective management of regimen for coronary artery disease

EXPECTED OUTCOME: The patient will report understanding of management of atherosclerosis and CAD.

- Identify patient's readiness to learn, desired learning needs, baseline knowledge and feelings about incorporating lifestyle changes into daily routine *to prioritize teaching topics.*
- Include significant other as appropriate *to support patient during learning.*
- Explain pathophysiology of atherosclerosis and CAD, control of risk factors, management of CAD symptoms and medications *to promote understanding and reduce complications.*
- Provide information about community resources *that can assist in making lifestyle changes.*
- Encourage questions and allow patient the opportunity to verbalize new information and skills *to enhance learning.*

Evaluation

Interventions are successful if the patient is pain-free, demonstrates increased understanding of atherosclerosis and CAD and their management, and states plans to modify risk factors of CAD.

CUE RECOGNITION 24.2

You are caring for a patient who reports chest pain. What action do you take?

Suggested answers are at the end of the chapter.

ACUTE CORONARY SYNDROME

Acute coronary syndrome (ACS) refers to conditions involving myocardial ischemia: unstable angina, non–ST-elevation MI (NSTEMI), and ST-elevation MI (STEMI). With unstable angina, the ischemia does not cause enough cardiac damage to release cardiac biomarkers. NSTEMI is caused by a partial coronary artery blockage. STEMI is usually caused by a complete blockage of a coronary artery. In a small percentage of patients with a STEMI, there is no obstruction (i.e., cocaine, embolism, myocarditis, spasm). (See Chapter 25 for ST-segment definition.) MI due to ischemia is discussed.

Silent Ischemia

Silent ischemia occurs without pain. It can carry great risk because the ischemia goes undetected. Older adults, women, and those with hypertension or diabetes most often have silent ischemia.

Sudden Cardiac Death

Sudden cardiac death is cardiac arrest triggered by lethal ventricular arrhythmias or asystole (see Chapter 25) from an abrupt occlusion of a coronary artery. Immediate treatment is required to attempt to prevent death.

Myocardial Infarction

The ability of the heart to contract, relax, and propel blood throughout the body requires healthy cardiac muscle. An acute MI due to ischemia results in the death of heart muscle cells from a sudden partial or complete blockage of a coronary artery. The extent of the cardiac damage varies depending on the location and amount of blockage in the coronary artery. Cellular death may be avoided with timely and effective reperfusion.

Pathophysiology

Ischemic injury evolves over several hours before complete necrosis and myocardial infarction take place. The ischemic process affects the subendocardial layer, which is most sensitive to hypoxia. This process leads to depressed myocardial contractility. The body's attempt to compensate for decreased cardiac function triggers the sympathetic nervous system to increase the heart rate. The change in heart rate increases myocardial oxygen demand, further depressing the myocardium.

Once necrosis takes place, the contractile function of the muscle is permanently lost. The heart has a zone of ischemia and injury around the necrotic area (Fig. 24.3). The zone of injury is next to the necrotic area. It is susceptible to becoming necrosed. If treatment is initiated within the first hour of symptoms of the MI and restores the blood supply from the blocked artery, the area of damage can be minimized. Around the injury zone is an area of ischemia and viable tissue. If the heart responds to treatment, this area can rebuild and develop collateral circulation.

The area affected by an MI depends on the coronary artery (Fig. 24.4). Being familiar with the anatomy of the heart and the area of the MI helps the nurse anticipate arrhythmias, conduction disturbances, and heart failure. All of these are the major complications of MIs (Table 24.5).

The left coronary artery supplies the anterior wall of the heart, which also includes most of the left ventricle. An occlusion in this area causes an anterior wall MI. When the left ventricle is affected, there can be severe loss of left ventricular function. This leads to severe changes in the hemodynamic status of the patient.

LEARNING TIP

To remember coronary artery occlusion and subsequent myocardial infarction location, personalize the locations with initials of places familiar to you.

Location	Coronary Artery	Resulting MI Location
Los **A**ngeles	**L**eft **a**nterior descending	**A**nterior
Cedar **P**oint	**C**ircumflex	**P**osterior
Rhode **I**sland	**R**ight	**I**nferior

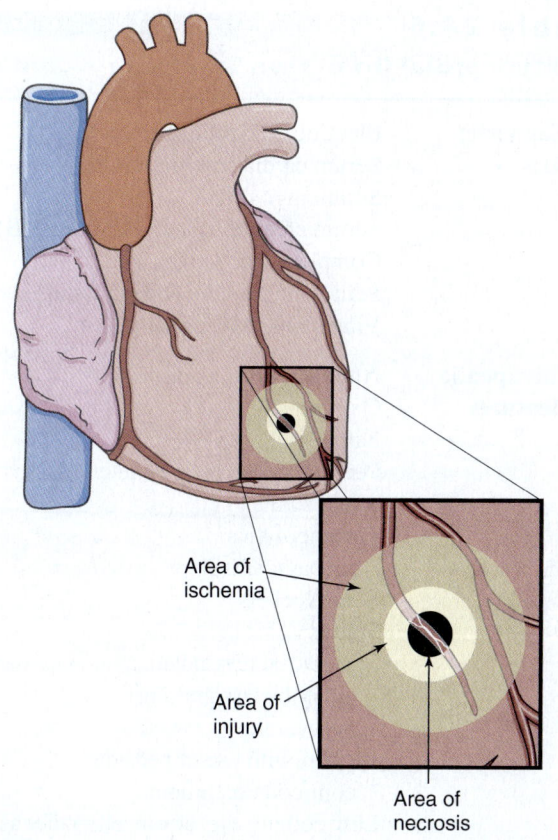

FIGURE 24.3 Myocardial infarction. Areas of ischemia, injury, and necrosis caused by a blockage in the left anterior coronary artery.

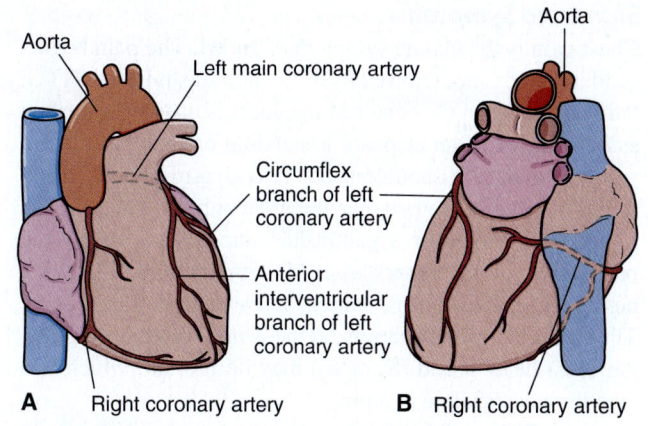

FIGURE 24.4 Coronary arteries. (A) Anterior view. (B) Posterior view.

The right coronary artery supplies the heart's inferior wall and parts of the atrioventricular node and the sinoatrial node. An occlusion of the right coronary artery leads to an inferior MI and abnormalities in cardiac conduction. Serious arrhythmias can occur early in an inferior MI that may be life-threatening.

The left circumflex coronary artery supplies the heart's lateral wall and part of the posterior wall. A blockage in this artery causes a lateral wall infarction of the left ventricle.

Table 24.5
Complications of Myocardial Infarction

Complication	Types or Symptoms	Interventions
Arrhythmias	Premature ventricular contractions, ventricular tachycardia, ventricular fibrillation, heart block	Continuous cardiac monitoring Protocol treatment of arrhythmias (see Chapter 25)
Cardiogenic shock	Decreased blood pressure; increased heart rate; diaphoresis; cold, clammy, gray skin	Immediate initiation of treatment to decrease infarct size, control pain and arrhythmias Intra-aortic balloon pump Thrombolytic therapy Dopamine, dobutamine
Heart failure/pulmonary edema	Dizziness, orthopnea, weight gain, edema, enlarged liver, jugular venous distention, crackles	Correct underlying cause Relieve symptoms Increase cardiac contractility Administer diuretics as ordered
Emboli	Dependent on location of emboli	Anticoagulants to prevent clots Supportive symptom treatment
Rupture of muscles or valves of the heart, septal rupture	Signs of cardiogenic shock, death	Immediate treatment of myocardial infarction to limit extent of damage
Pericarditis (inflammation of the pericardium)	Chest pain, increased with movement, deep inspiration, or cough; pericardial friction rub (fine grating sound)	Position upright, leaning forward Anti-inflammatory medications

Signs and Symptoms

Chest pain is the classic symptom of an MI. The pain begins suddenly and is not relieved by rest or administration of NTG. Pain occurring in the center of the chest is usually described as crushing, as if an elephant is standing on the chest. Chest pain can radiate to shoulders, one or both arms, hands, neck, throat, lower jaw, teeth, upper abdomen or back. The pain can imitate indigestion or a gallbladder attack with abdominal pain and vomiting. Other classic MI symptoms include shortness of breath, dizziness, nausea, and sweating (Table 24.6). The heart rate may be rapid and the heart's rhythm irregular. An extra heart sound (S_3 or S_4) may be present, which is a sign the myocardium is failing.

TIMELY SYMPTOM TREATMENT. Individuals, especially women, often deny or fail to recognize that an MI is occurring because they experience symptoms that are atypical or similar to other mild conditions such as indigestion ("Gerontological Issues"). Patients have reported that the symptoms of an MI they experienced were not what they expected. If people expect and do not experience the dramatic heart attack symptoms seen on television shows (which are usually not the same as those in real life), they are likely to delay seeking treatment. Waiting 2 to 24 hours before seeking medical care is common, yet the first hour after symptom onset is crucial for administering reperfusion treatments that restore blood flow, minimize tissue damage, and save lives. Individuals should not drive themselves or let someone drive them to the hospital when having chest pain. Calling for emergency medical services allows lifesaving treatment to begin. Individuals, especially women, need to be educated that "time is muscle." As time passes during an MI, more muscle is lost.

Women and Heart Health

Heart disease remains the leading cause of death in women in the United States (Office on Women's Health, 2019). Compared with men, women tend to have acute MIs at an older age, with a higher mortality rate and more complications, such as ventricular fibrillation and heart failure. This may be due to women waiting longer than men do before seeking help.

Women may have classic chest pain, but they are also likely to have other symptoms as well that men do not typically have. Atypical symptoms reported by women may

Table 24.6 Myocardial Infarction Summary

Signs and Symptoms	*Classic* Crushing, vicelike chest pain with radiation to arms, shoulder, hands, neck, throat, lower jaw, teeth, or back Shortness of breath Dizziness Nausea Sweating *Atypical* Absence of chest pain Fatigue Cramping in chest Anxiety Feeling of impending doom Falling *More Common in Women* Shortness of breath Fatigue Epigastric or abdominal pain Chest discomfort, pressure, or burning Arm, shoulder, neck, jaw, or back pain Discomfort/pain between shoulder blades Indigestion or gas pain Nausea or vomiting
Diagnostic Tests	Electrocardiogram (ECG) Serum cardiac troponin I or T Serum myoglobin Serum creatine kinase-MB (CK-MB) Complete blood count (CBC) Serum magnesium and potassium Vital signs, oxygen saturation
Therapeutic Measures	Antiplatelets (e.g., aspirin) Oxygen Nitrates Percutaneous coronary interventions and stents Thrombolytics Anticoagulants Beta blockers Statins Myocardial revascularization (coronary artery bypass grafting) Daily weight Bedrest with use of bedside commode/bathroom Low-sodium diet advanced to diet as tolerated; no caffeine Cardiac rehabilitation
Complications	Arrhythmias Heart failure Cardiogenic shock Valvular insufficiency
Priority Nursing Diagnoses	*Acute Pain* *Decreased Cardiac Output* *Fear*

Gerontological Issues

Myocardial Infarction

With age, the heart has decreased elasticity, which increases both resistance to its pumping action and the workload of the myocardium. Older adults should be taught never to neglect symptoms of shortness of breath, fatigue, fast or slow heartbeats, or chest discomfort. For older adults, the following is common with MI:

- When pain is not present, the only symptom may be a sudden onset of shortness of breath or fainting, restlessness, or a fall. Atypical presentation of MI symptoms is normal in older adults, especially those older than age 85.
- Because the older adult has had more time than younger people to develop collateral circulation, they often do not have as many complications with an MI.
- In the older adult, reperfusion therapies such as angioplasty and bypass surgery seem to be superior in improving quality of life without increasing mortality risk.

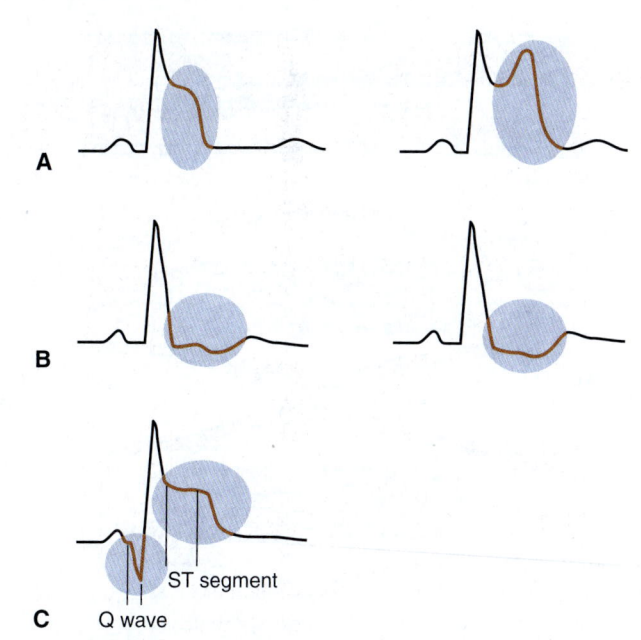

FIGURE 24.5 Electrocardiogram changes during STEMI myocardial infarction. (A) Injury: ST-segment elevation. (B) Ischemia: ST-segment inversion. (C) Necrosis: large Q-wave and ST-segment elevation.

include extreme fatigue, epigastric pain, lower jaw pain, indigestion, nausea and vomiting, dyspnea, shortness of breath, or cramping in the chest. Many women note prodromal symptoms a month before an acute MI. These symptoms include unusual fatigue, sleep disturbances, and shortness of breath.

Diagnostic Tests

Patients with a strong familial history of MI should be considered at risk until an MI is ruled out. Combined indicators of an MI are patient history, ECG changes, and elevated levels of highly sensitive cardiac troponin T (cTnT) or I (cTnI), and myoglobin and creatine kinase (CK)-MB if used (see Chapter 21). The ECG may show the area that is infarcted as well as ischemic areas of the heart. Myocardial damage can be seen as ST-elevation, the presence of a Q wave, or T-wave abnormalities (Fig. 24.5). Serial ECGs monitor changes indicating damage or ischemia. Magnesium and potassium levels are checked. Both are essential for normal cardiac function, especially for those on diuretic therapy.

Therapeutic Measures

Time until intervention is directly related to mortality (Box 24.2). Medical treatment should be sought within 5 minutes for unrelieved chest pain or other symptoms. The goal is to restore blood flow to the heart muscle within 90 minutes of the patient's arrival at the emergency department.

PERCUTANEOUS CORONARY INTERVENTION WITH STENTING. Coronary artery stenting with drug-eluting stents is the preferred percutaneous coronary intervention (PCI) for cardiac revascularization. A stent is an expandable metal mesh tube that is implanted during angiography at the site of the atherosclerotic blockage in the coronary artery (Fig. 24.6).

Box 24.2
Preventing Delays in Myocardial Infarction Treatment

- Understand symptoms, the "time is muscle" principle, and that a delay in calling for help results in untoward effects.
- Develop an action plan and rehearse it.
- Understand normal emotional responses of anxiety, denial, or embarrassment.
- Educate family to follow action plan.
- Establish protocols in workplaces for employees experiencing myocardial infarction.
- Establish emergency department policies that reduce delays, such as having equipment and medication readily available.

It provides support to the coronary artery wall at the area of stenosis to keep the artery open and the blood flowing through the artery. Drug-eluting stents, which are coated with immunosuppressant medication, are more effective in preventing the need for revascularization of the artery than is percutaneous transluminal cardiac angioplasty (PTCA). The drug is released over months to inhibit smooth muscle cell proliferation to reduce risk of restenosis. Antiplatelet medications are recommended after stent placement to help prevent clot formation. Complications associated with stent placement include **thrombosis** (formation of a blood clot inside a blood vessel), bleeding from anticoagulation, stent occlusion, or coronary artery dissection.

THROMBOLYTIC THERAPY. PCI, when available onsite, has greatly reduced the use of thrombolytics to dissolve a blood clot that is occluding a coronary artery. When used,

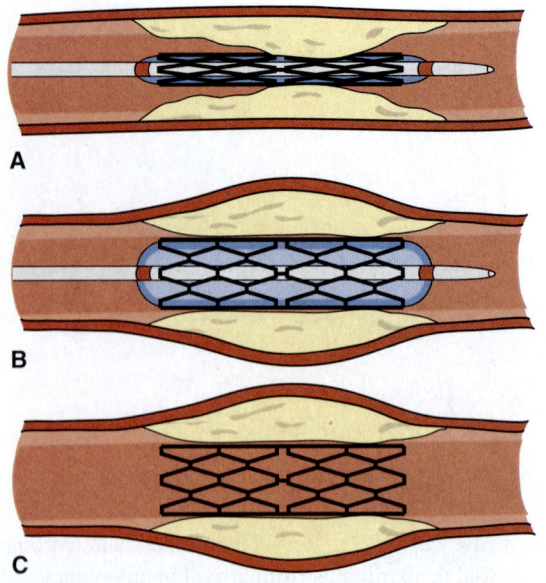

FIGURE 24.6 Insertion of a coronary artery stent: (A) A balloon catheter with a collapsed stent is advanced to the location of a coronary artery lesion. (B) The balloon is inflated, which expands the stent and compresses the lesion to increase the artery opening. (C) The balloon is then deflated and removed, leaving the expanded stent in place to prevent the artery from closing.

the thrombolytic medication must be started within a specified time range from the onset of symptoms, usually within 1 to 6 hours, before necrosis results. The goal is to give a thrombolytic within 30 minutes of arrival in the emergency department.

OXYGEN. Arterial blood gases (ABGs) guide the patient's oxygen needs. Routine oxygen was not found to be beneficial when oxygen levels were normal (Abuzaid et al, 2018).

MEDICATION. Table 24.7 summarizes pharmacological treatment of MI. Antiplatelet medication is given to reduce platelets from forming clots. Chewing one nonenteric aspirin (165–325 mg) is prescribed after diagnosis of acute coronary syndrome. For acute cardiac-related pain, NTG is given sublingually or by IV drip. NTG causes vasodilation, which supplies increased blood flow to the myocardium, thereby relieving ischemia and reducing the pain. Nitrates should not be given if the patient has taken a phosphodiesterase inhibitor for erectile dysfunction, as catastrophic hypotension may result (see "Be Safe!" earlier in the chapter). Morphine sulfate is given carefully for ischemic pain that is unrelieved by other therapy, as it may worsen patient outcomes. Dual antiplatelet therapy may be given long term after an MI.

Table 24.7
Medications Used to Treat Myocardial Infarction

Medication Class/Action

Anticoagulants
Heparin: Inhibits conversion of prothrombin to thrombin to prevent thrombus formation.

Examples	Nursing Implications
heparin sodium	Do not give if bleeding risk.
	Dose regulated by heparin antifactor Xa or activated partial thromboplastin time (aPTT Goal: 1.5 to 2.5 times control).
	Monitor for bleeding.

Low Molecular Weight Heparin (LMWH): Antithrombotic prophylaxis of ischemic complications in non-ST-elevation myocardial infarction with aspirin therapy.

Examples	Nursing Implications
dalteparin (Fragmin)	Do not remove prefilled syringe air bubble.
enoxaparin (Lovenox)	Rotate sites.
fondaparinux (Arixtra)	Give deep subcutaneously: Hold fold of skin while giving injection. Do not massage site.
	Teach: Monitor for bleeding.

Antiplatelets
Inhibit platelet activation, adhesion, or procoagulant activity.

Examples	Nursing Implications
aspirin	*Teach:*
clopidogrel (Plavix)	Chew aspirin when myocardial infarction (MI) suspected.
prasugrel (Effient)	Report bleeding or bruising.
ticagrelor (Brilinta)	
vorapaxar (Zontivity)	

Table 24.7
Medications Used to Treat Myocardial Infarction—cont'd

Medication Class/Action

Glycoprotein IIb/IIIa Inhibitors
Inhibit platelet aggregation during percutaneous coronary intervention.

Examples	Nursing Implications
abciximab (ReoPro)	Prevent injury due to bleeding risk.
bivalirudin (Angiomax)	Monitor vital signs and ECG.
eptifibatide (Integrilin)	Teach:
tirofiban (Aggrastat)	Report bleeding or bruising.

Thrombolytics
Dissolve blood clots in blood vessels.

Examples	Nursing Implications
alteplase; tissue plasminogen activator [t-PA] (Activase)	Most effective when given within 6 hours of acute coronary event. Goal is 30 minutes from arrival in emergency department.
reteplase; rPA (Retavase)	Baseline international normalized ratio (INR), activated partial thromboplastin time (aPTT), platelet count, and fibrinogen levels checked.
tenecteplase; TNK (TNKase)	Avoid venipunctures for 24 hours after administration.

Beta Blockers
See Table 24.4.

Nitrates
See Table 24.4.

Statins
See Table 24.3.

Additional Medications as Needed
Specific for medications given.

Examples	Nursing Implications
antiemetics	Control nausea, vomiting, anxiety, gastric upset, and straining/constipation.
anxiolytics	
antacids	
stool softeners	

Antiarrhythmics are given if atrial or ventricular arrhythmias occur (see Chapter 25).

ACTIVITY. Initially, patients are kept on bedrest to decrease myocardial oxygen demand. A bedside commode for bowel movements is usually ordered to reduce straining on a bedpan. Activity is advanced gradually when stable as tolerated.

DIET AND WEIGHT LOSS. Initially, a low-sodium, clear liquid diet is ordered as tolerated, which helps reduce the risk of vomiting. Then, small, easily digested, heart-healthy meals are served. Caffeine is restricted because it increases heart rate and causes vasoconstriction. Fluids may be restricted if the patient is in heart failure as well. If the patient is overweight, weight loss can reduce cardiac workload. A dietitian can help the patient and family to devise a weight-loss diet for the patient.

Coronary Artery Bypass Graft

During coronary artery bypass graft (CABG) surgery, the saphenous vein from the leg and/or an internal mammary artery from the chest wall is used to reroute blood around a segment of a coronary artery that is narrowed by atherosclerosis (Fig. 24.7). One or more vessels can be bypassed (see "Patient Perspective"). The surgery can be done either on cardiopulmonary bypass (arrested heart surgery) or off cardiopulmonary bypass (beating heart surgery). See Chapter 21.

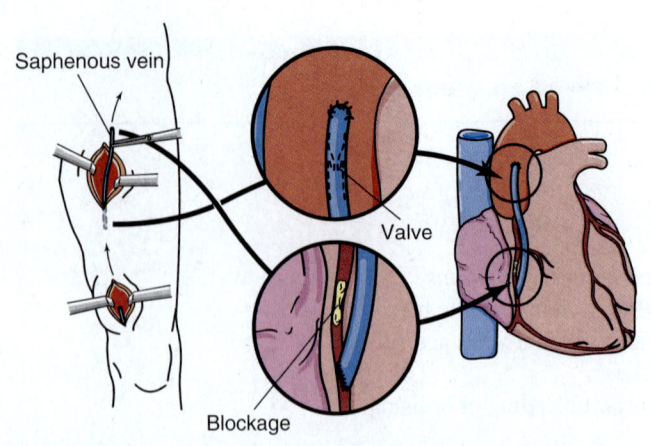

FIGURE 24.7 Myocardial reperfusion by coronary artery bypass graft surgery.

Patient Perspective
Keith
When I was 72, a heart catheterization showed significant coronary artery blockage, so I had five coronary artery bypass grafts performed. It was a long surgery. I felt disoriented for several days afterward, mostly while I was in the intensive care unit.

I was provided excellent care at home after discharge from the hospital. I had a capable visiting nurse, physical therapist, or occupational therapist almost every day. Physical therapy was difficult at first but shortly became routine and easy. I have had a strange sensation in my legs at the incision sites ever since surgery but no pain. I have not experienced depression, although I hear post-op depression is common.

My experience during cardiac rehab of three sessions per week for 12 weeks was outstanding. I enjoyed the association with others in the same situation. We even staged a graduation when we finished. I wore a tuxedo jacket with my gym shorts!

Since completing my rehab, I have maintained a minimum 40-minute exercise schedule three times per week. I am trying to be more conscious of my diet. I do this because I want to stay healthy for a long time.

CARDIOPULMONARY BYPASS: ON PUMP. Most bypasses are done while the heart is stopped with cardiopulmonary bypass (on pump) in use. While the median sternotomy is made, the vein graft is being removed from the body. The graft is flushed with a heparinized solution to check for leaks and then set aside for use during the surgery. After the patient is placed on cardiopulmonary bypass and the heart is stopped, one end of the graft is **anastomosed** (joined) to the coronary artery distal to the occlusion, and the proximal end of the graft is anastomosed, often to the ascending aorta.

CARDIOPULMONARY BYPASS: OFF PUMP. This surgery is done with the heart beating and does not use the cardiopulmonary bypass (off pump). A device is used to stabilize a vessel while the surgeon works on it. Either traditional median sternotomy or minimally invasive surgery can be used.

MINIMALLY INVASIVE SURGERY. Less-invasive approaches include the minimally invasive direct CABG (MIDCAB), which is done off pump, and totally endoscopic CABG (TECAB), which can be done on or off pump. MIDCAB is done through a small fifth intercostal incision. TECAB uses three or four chest holes for insertion of robotic arms and a camera that a surgeon views to control the robotic arms.

Nursing Process for the Patient Experiencing Myocardial Infarction

DATA COLLECTION. A thorough history is obtained to identify risk factors that may contribute to an MI. All patients admitted with chest pain are treated for a possible MI until it has been ruled out. Continuous cardiac monitoring and serial ECGs and laboratory values determine the degree of cardiac damage and detect life-threatening arrhythmias. Controlling ischemic pain immediately helps diminish anxiety and the negative physiological effects pain has on the body. Screening for depression, common after an MI, is important for appropriate therapy referrals.

NURSING CARE TIP
Surgical site infection following CABG (i.e., mediastinitis) is a "Never Event." This means that Medicare will not pay the hospital for care for this condition, as it *never* should have occurred. Use infection-control procedures at all times to prevent this surgical site infection.

NURSING DIAGNOSES, PLANNING, IMPLEMENTATION, AND EVALUATION. See "Nursing Care Plan for the Patient With Myocardial Infarction." Also see "Nursing Care Plan for the Patient Undergoing Surgery" in Chapter 12. Patients undergoing cardiac surgery will have a chest tube placed. Chest tube drainage is observed, and more than 200 mL/hr should be reported. Vital signs, peripheral pulses, electrolytes, ABGs, and ECGs are monitored. Acidosis, low calcium and magnesium levels, and abnormal potassium levels decrease cardiac contractility and cardiac output. Acute pain may be experienced due to sternotomy, leg incisions, or internal mammary artery resection. The patient should be taught sternal precautions: no pushing or pulling with arms; hug pillow with all movements; do not use arms to rise out of a chair; do not lift more than 5 to 10 pounds; do not raise elbows above shoulders; and bend elbows and lower head for grooming.

Patient Education
Education about the therapeutic regimen includes information about the disease, medications, diet, activity, and rehabilitation needs that may require lifestyle changes, such as smoking cessation, exercise, stress management, and weight

loss. Heart disease can affect all aspects of a patient's lifestyle, including family and job roles.

Patients recovering from cardiac disorders are often anxious about resuming sexual activity but are embarrassed to discuss it. This is an area that is often overlooked when caring for patients. Sexuality counseling should be offered to patients and their partners. Patients often have misconceptions that are unfounded but interfere with resuming sexual activity. If patients have angina, NTG can be taken prophylactically before sexual activity. After an MI, sexual activity can be resumed in 1 to 2 months or when the patient can climb two flights of stairs without symptoms, as approved by the HCP. Patients are given information to make an informed decision on when they are ready to resume this physical activity. Referral to a sexuality counselor for information on ways to cope with sexual issues in relation to the illness can be helpful to the patient.

Cardiac Rehabilitation and Exercise

Cardiac rehabilitation to improve cardiac function and quality of life begins when the patient's acute symptoms are relieved (see "Evidence-Based Practice"). Phase 1 of rehabilitation occurs in the hospital. Activities for each hospital day, such as types and amounts of self-care and activity, are specified in protocols. Phase 2 occurs 4 to 6 weeks after discharge in an outpatient program. It focuses on returning the patient to previous levels of activity and function. Phase 3 follows, during which patients are encouraged to maintain optimal physical fitness and continue healthy lifestyles that include exercising and losing weight to maintain an ideal body weight.

CRITICAL THINKING & CLINICAL JUDGMENT

Mr. Jones was transferred to the critical care unit after a quadruple coronary artery bypass graft. Preoperative vital signs were blood pressure 144/84 mm Hg, apical pulse 62 beats per minute (regular), respiratory rate 18 breaths per minute, and temperature 98.4°F (36.9°C). Postoperative data collection findings are blood pressure 100/56 mm Hg, apical pulse 115 beats per minute, respiratory rate 28 bpm (irregular and shallow), temperature 99.8°F (37.7°C), lung sounds diminished with crackles in bilateral bases, chest tube intact with 300 mL of red drainage over 1 hour, pedal pulses weak bilaterally, and chest and leg dressings dry and intact.

Critical Thinking (The Why)
1. Why might Mr. Jones's blood pressure be decreased?
2. Why might Mr. Jones's apical pulse be elevated?
3. Which data collection findings require action?

Clinical Judgment (The Do)
4. What priority action do you take?
5. With which health-care team members do you collaborate?
6. What patient education topics do you reinforce in sessions with the patient and family?

Suggested answers are at the end of the chapter.

Evidence-Based Practice: Clinical Question

What are the effects of eHealth-based interventions on patient adherence to components of cardiac rehabilitation?

Evidence

A systematic review including 105 studies was conducted on eHealth and its effect on patient adherence to components of cardiac rehabilitation. Most studies focused on medication adherence, and others looked at adherence to diet, physical activity, vital signs, weight, step counts, smoking, and fluid restriction. It was found that telemonitoring and Web-based applications for self-care behavior were more effective than telephone calls to promote patient adherence.

Implications for Nursing Practice

Nurses and health-care team members may find it beneficial to include telemonitoring and Web-based applications for self-care to encourage and support patients in reducing modifiable risk factors for cardiovascular disease.

References: Kebapci, A., Ozaynak, M., & Lareau, S. (2020). Effects of eHealth-based interventions on adherence to components of cardiac rehabilitation: A systematic review. *Journal of Cardiovascular Nursing, 35*(4), 74–85.

CRITICAL THINKING & CLINICAL JUDGMENT

Mrs. Sims, age 43, is admitted to the intensive care unit with a diagnosis of atypical chest pain that radiates to her left shoulder and down her left arm. She has a history of midsternal chest cramping. Her pain increases with activity and decreases with rest. She smokes 1.5 packs of cigarettes per day and is 50 pounds overweight. The cardiac monitor shows normal sinus rhythm without arrhythmias. She has nitroglycerin sublingual ordered as needed for chest pain.

One hour after admission, Mrs. Sims reports acute midsternal chest pain radiating to her left neck and lower jaw. The cardiac monitor shows sinus tachycardia of 108 bpm with occasional premature ventricular contractions. Her blood pressure is 100/70 mm Hg, respirations are 20 breaths per minute and unlabored, and skin is warm and dry.

Critical Thinking (The Why)
1. What is likely occurring with Mrs. Sims?
2. How is angina differentiated from an MI?
3. What are the indicators of an MI that will be checked for Mrs. Sims?
4. What medical interventions could be used for Mrs. Sims?

Clinical Judgment (The Do)
5. What priority actions do you take?
6. What do you remain vigilant about?
7. What psychosocial actions do you provide Mrs. Sims?
8. With which health-care team members do you collaborate?
9. What patient-centered education topics do you reinforce in educational sessions with Mrs. Sims and her family?

Suggested answers are at the end of the chapter.

Nursing Care Plan for the Patient With Myocardial Infarction

Nursing Diagnosis: *Acute Pain* related to decreased coronary blood flow causing myocardial ischemia
Expected Outcomes: The patient will report an absence or acceptable level of pain within 30 minutes of reporting pain.
Evaluation of Outcomes: Does the patient state that pain is reduced?

Intervention	Rationale	Evaluation
Monitor pain level with a pain rating scale and its characteristics.	*Identifies severity and type of pain.*	What is pain level, location, duration, intensity, and radiation?
Administer nitrates and analgesics as needed and prescribed.	*Relieves pain.*	Is pain relieved?
Assist with alternative pain relief measures (e.g., positioning, rest, relaxation techniques).	*These measures help decrease oxygen demand.*	Does patient express pain relief and decreased emotional stress?

Geriatric

Intervention	Rationale	Evaluation
Monitor and ensure that older patient's pain is relieved.	*Pain is not an expected part of the aging process as may be believed.*	Does patient report pain is relieved?

Nursing Diagnosis: *Decreased Cardiac Output* related to ischemia or infarction, changes in heart rate and rhythm, and decreased contractility
Expected Outcomes: The patient will maintain adequate cardiac output and tissue perfusion.
Evaluation of Outcomes: Does the patient have vital signs and urine output within normal limits (WNL)?

Intervention	Rationale	Evaluation
Monitor blood pressure, heart rate, electrocardiogram and urine output, and report abnormalities.	*These are indirect indicators of cardiac output.*	Are indicators WNL?
Monitor peripheral pulses, capillary refill, color, and temperature.	*These are indicators of adequate tissue perfusion.*	Does patient have strong peripheral pulses, capillary refill less than 3 seconds, pink nailbeds, and warm skin?
Administer cardiac medications as ordered by health-care provider.	*Helps improve cardiac output and tissue perfusion.*	Does patient show signs of improved contractility, increased cardiac output, and tissue perfusion?
Promote quiet environment and rest in semi-Fowler position.	*Decreases cardiac workload.*	Is patient relaxed?

Geriatric

Intervention	Rationale	Evaluation
Observe for atypical pain or no pain with dyspnea or fatigue.	*In acute myocardial infarction (MI), older adults may not have typical chest pain or may have a silent MI.*	Does patient have atypical symptoms of MI?
Monitor for medication side effects.	*Older patients may have more medication toxicity due to reduced renal and hepatic function.*	Does patient exhibit side effects of medications?

Nursing Care Plan for the Patient With Myocardial Infarction—cont'd

Nursing Diagnosis: ***Decreased Activity Tolerance*** related to imbalance between oxygen supply and demand, weakness, and fatigue
Expected Outcome: The patient will tolerate progressive activity as evidenced by heart rate, blood pressure, pulse oximetry, and respiratory rate WNL.
Evaluation of Outcome: Is the patient's heart rate, blood pressure, pulse oximetry, and respiratory rate WNL with progressive activity?

Intervention	Rationale	Evaluation
Obtain baseline vital signs and observe and stop activity and report abnormal responses, if heart rate over 120 beats per minute or 20 beats over resting rate, systolic blood pressure increases more than 20 mm Hg, chest pain, dizziness, skin color changes, diaphoresis, dyspnea, arrhythmias, excessive fatigue, and ST-segment changes on ECG occur.	*Observation allows detection of abnormal responses to stop activity.*	Are vital signs WNL and activity tolerated without symptoms?
Maintain progression of ordered activities as tolerated. *Initial activities:* Activities of daily living, dangling feet at bedside for 15 minutes, using commode with assistance. *Progressive activities:* Out of bed to chair for 30 to 60 minutes, partial bath, range-of-motion exercises.	*Patient should have increasing activity to condition the myocardium.*	Is patient able to progress activity?
Geriatric		
Slow the pace of care but allow independence.	*Allow patient extra time to complete activity to reduce cardiac demand and fatigue.*	Is patient able to complete care without symptoms or fatigue?
Request referral for cardiac rehabilitation.	*Older adults benefit comparably to younger persons from exercise programs.*	Does patient participate in cardiac rehabilitation?

PERIPHERAL VASCULAR SYSTEM

Peripheral vascular disease (PVD) may be either arterial or venous in origin. Understanding whether the origin of the problem is arterial or venous can prevent serious complications.

Arterial Thrombosis and Embolism

Pathophysiology

Acute arterial occlusions are often sudden and dramatic. They are most common in the lower extremity. A thrombus (blood clot) adheres to the artery wall. Acute arterial thrombi occur with injury to an arterial wall, sluggish flow, or plaque formation secondary to atherosclerotic changes. Other causes of arterial thrombosis are polycythemia, dehydration, and repeated arterial needlesticks. If a thrombus breaks off and travels, it becomes an **embolism** that occludes an arterial vessel that is too small to allow it to pass. Causes of an arterial embolism are arrhythmias, prosthetic heart valves, MI, and rheumatic heart disease.

Signs and Symptoms

Usually there is an abrupt onset of symptoms with acute arterial occlusion, unless collateral circulation has developed that is able to supply blood flow to the occluded area. Symptoms depend on the artery occluded, the tissue supplied by that artery, and whether collateral circulation is present. The clinical signs of acute arterial occlusion are known as the six Ps: **p**ain, **p**allor, **p**ulselessness, **p**aresthesia (numbness), **p**aralysis, and **p**oikilothermia (assumes the environmental temperature). There is decreased movement in the affected extremity. The extremity is pale, mottled, and without pulses distal to the occlusion. The extremity will feel cold because blood provides warmth.

Therapeutic Measures

Immediate treatment is necessary to save the affected limb. IV fluids and anticoagulant therapy, usually with IV unfractionated heparin (UFH), is started immediately to prevent further clotting. UFH has no effect on the existing clot. The patient remains on UFH therapy for several days. UFH levels are monitored with activated partial thromboplastin time (aPTT) or antifactor Xa. After 3 to 7 days, a low molecular weight heparin (LMWH) such as enoxaparin (Lovenox), dalteparin (Fragmin), or tinzaparin (Innohep) or an oral anticoagulant such as warfarin (Coumadin) is started. LMWH medications often require no laboratory monitoring. Warfarin takes 3 to 5 days to reach therapeutic levels. UFH is continued until a therapeutic warfarin level is reached, unless LMWH injections are used for bridging therapy. Warfarin levels are monitored by international normalized ratios (INRs). Daily adjustments in warfarin doses are made to reach therapeutic levels. Other types of anticoagulants may also be used.

For patients with severe occlusions, especially if the risk of limb loss is imminent, surgery is usually performed to save the extremity. During an emergency embolectomy or thrombectomy, the artery is cut open, the emboli or thrombus is removed, and the vessel is sutured closed. In milder cases, thrombolytic agents may be used to dissolve the clot.

Peripheral Arterial Disease

Peripheral arterial disease (PAD) is a disorder of the arterial circulation usually caused by chronic, progressive narrowing of arterial vessels that leads to obstruction or occlusion. PAD usually affects the lower extremities. Atherosclerosis is the leading cause of occlusive disease. PAD can be described as organic or functional. Organic disease is caused by structural changes from plaque or inflammation in the blood vessels. Functional disease is a short-term localized spasm in the blood vessel, as occurs in Raynaud disease.

Pathophysiology

The purpose of the arterial system is to deliver oxygen-rich blood to the vascular beds. Anything that impedes this flow causes an imbalance in supply and demand for oxygen. Decreased nutrition, cellular waste accumulation, and development of ischemia occur distal to the obstruction. With increased debris and sluggish flow, thrombosis and embolism can become major problems.

The body has several mechanisms that attempt to compensate for reduced blood flow, including peripheral vasodilation, anaerobic metabolism, and development of collateral circulation. However, these mechanisms are not intended to meet the ongoing blood supply needs of the body. It takes time for collateral circulation to develop. Blood vessels eventually reach their limit of dilation, and anaerobic metabolism is only a very short-term compensatory mechanism. Eventually, a lack of blood supply produces signs of ischemia. If not corrected, this results in ulceration, gangrene, and necrosis of the extremity; amputation of the limb may become necessary.

> ### CRITICAL THINKING & CLINICAL JUDGMENT
>
> **Mrs. Mehta** is a resident with severe rheumatoid arthritis that has limited her mobility for 7 months. She is returning to her room following physical therapy in a wheelchair when she suddenly reports severe pain in her left groin.
>
> **Critical Thinking (The Why)**
> 1. What might be possible causes of this sudden symptom?
>
> **Clinical Judgment (The Do)**
> 2. What priority action do you take?
> 3. What action do you take for abnormal findings?
> 4. How do you document Mrs. Mehta's signs and symptom?
>
> *Suggested answers are at the end of the chapter.*

Signs and Symptoms

Many people with PAD, especially women, may have no early symptoms. It is not until late in the course of PAD when diminished blood flow begins to produce changes within the extremities that symptoms occur. Pain in the calves associated with activity or exercise, a common symptom, is called **intermittent claudication**. When blood supply to the muscles is decreased, the muscles are unable to receive adequate oxygen. As ischemia increases, the muscle develops a cramping-type pain that usually subsides when activity is stopped. As PAD worsens, the pain is present even at rest, indicating severe arterial occlusion.

Skin color changes are associated with decreased blood supply. The extremity is pale when the leg is elevated. In a dependent position, it becomes reddish-purple or cyanotic. The extremity is cool to touch even in warm environments. There may be hair loss on the lower calf, ankle, and foot. Other findings include dry, flaky, scaly, pale, or mottled skin. Toenails may be thickened. As occlusion of the arteries progresses, arterial pulses become diminished or absent.

Diagnostic Tests

The ankle-brachial index (ABI) is used to compare blood pressures in the upper and lower extremities. Normally, blood pressure readings in the thigh and calf are higher than those in the upper extremities. With the presence of arterial disease, thigh and calf blood pressures are lower than the brachial blood pressure. Ankle blood pressure is normally equal to or greater than the brachial blood pressure. When an occlusion occurs in the lower extremities, the blood pressures between the upper and lower extremities become unequal. With arterial insufficiency, the ABI decreases following diagnostic treadmill exercise. A duplex ultrasound measures the velocity of the blood flow. MRI and CT scan can give definitive images of blood vessels and degrees of arterial closure. Plethysmography and angiography can also be used to evaluate arterial flow in lower extremities (see Chapter 21).

Therapeutic Measures

Conservative treatment is initiated with mild to moderate occlusive disease. Lifestyle modifications to promote vascular health include smoking cessation, exercise therapy, and statins. Cilostazol (Pletal), an antiplatelet medication, treats claudication to improve walking ability. Invasive intervention is considered for the patient who experiences pain at rest or who has leg ulcers that do not heal. This includes balloon angioplasty to dilate a narrowed peripheral vessel, stents to maintain patency of the artery, atherectomy to remove atherosclerotic lesions, or grafting to bypass the occluded area. (See the discussion of vascular surgery later in this chapter.) Statins and antiplatelets are prescribed post-procedure to prevent complications.

Raynaud Disease

Raynaud disease (also called syndrome or phenomenon) is a local overreaction by the blood vessels that results in vasospasm, primarily in the digits, when exposed to cold or emotional stress. The abnormal vasoconstriction in the small arteries in the digits reduces arterial blood flow. It also can affect the ears, lips, or nose. Primary Raynaud disease does not occur as a result of another disorder. Secondary Raynaud disease may be seen with collagen diseases such as rheumatoid arthritis, scleroderma, systemic lupus erythematosus, or endocrine disorders.

Women who live in cold climates are more often affected. With exposure to cold (e.g., opening the refrigerator/freezer, touching cold water) or emotional stress, the affected skin area exhibits obvious skin color changes that can vary. The affected area of skin may turn white and then blue, with reports of coldness and numbness. With warming, pain, tingling, and redness (hyperemia) occur. Normal blood flow returns in about 15 minutes.

Initial therapy goals are to improve quality of life and prevent tissue injury from ischemia. Education on avoiding cold, keeping warm, and managing emotional stress is essential for patients with Raynaud disease. To protect hands from cold, gloves should be worn when going outside, cleaning a refrigerator, or preparing cold foods. Patients are instructed in the importance of protecting the hands from injury and avoiding vasoconstrictors such as smoking, alcohol, caffeine, and emotional stress. Immersing the hands in warm water may decrease vasospasm. A calcium channel blocker may be prescribed if preventive measures do not effectively prevent vasoconstriction. Other medications such as nitrates may be used if initial therapy is not effective.

Thromboangiitis Obliterans (Buerger Disease)

Thromboangiitis obliterans, or Buerger disease, is a rare recurring inflammation and thrombosis of small and medium arteries and veins in the limbs. The cause is unknown but may be autoimmune. It is only known to be associated with tobacco (cigarettes, cigars, smokeless) or cannabis use. To stop its progression and risk for amputation, all use of tobacco and cannabis must be avoided. Periodontal disease may be a factor in the development of the disease. Symptoms include intermittent pain or claudication (pain with activity) in the legs and feet or arms and hands, tingling, numbness in the feet or hands, reddish or blue tinged feet or hands, pale fingers or toes with cold exposure, and vein inflammation under the skin if a blood clot occurs. Distal extremity ischemia can lead to ulceration, gangrene, and even amputation. There is no cure, so there is urgency in helping the patient cease smoking. Treatments such as intermittent pneumatic compression to increase blood flow for pain relief and vasodilators may be tried. The goal of nursing care for patients with Buerger disease is to reduce the complications of ulceration, gangrene, and amputation.

Nursing Process for the Patient With a Peripheral Arterial Disorder

DATA COLLECTION. Careful assessment of intermittent claudication (leg pain), extremity pulses, capillary refill, temperature, color, presence of edema, and activity intolerance helps identify patients at risk for complications. Absent pulses are reported immediately to prevent limb loss. Skin that is shiny and hairless points to chronic diminished blood flow to the extremity. A serum glucose and lipid panel identifies diabetes and **hyperlipidemia**, which are significant risk factors for PAD. Skin lesions and ulcerations are photographed for documentation.

NURSING DIAGNOSES, PLANNING, IMPLEMENTATION, AND EVALUATION. See "Nursing Care Plan for the Patient With a Peripheral Arterial Occlusive Disorder."

> **Readiness for Enhanced Health Literacy** *related to complications, medications, or postoperative care*
>
> **EXPECTED OUTCOME:** The patient and family will verbalize self-care measures to be implemented to control disease and prevent complications.

- Determine patient's and family's health literacy for the physiology of the disease and treatment and preventive techniques; then provide missing knowledge *to determine their ability to learn.*
- Reinforce teaching of healthy lifestyle and risk factor control for PAD (e.g., smoking cessation, healthy diet, walking programs, hyperlipidemia, and diabetes and hypertension control) *to promote circulation and decrease functional impairment and pain.*
- Explain daily foot care: Inspect feet for ingrown toenails, redness, sores, or blisters; wash feet with warm soap and water; dry with gentle patting; lubricate skin to prevent cracking; wear clean socks; do not walk barefoot; and inspect inside of footwear for foreign objects before inserting foot *to promptly identify and report problems.*

• WORD • BUILDING •

hyperlipidemia: hyper—above + lipos—fat + emia—blood

Nursing Care Plan for the Patient With a Peripheral Arterial Occlusive Disorder

Nursing Diagnosis: *Ineffective Peripheral Tissue Perfusion* related to interruption of arterial flow in arms and legs
Expected Outcome: The patient will show signs of increased arterial blood flow and tissue perfusion.
Evaluation of Outcome: Does the patient have strong peripheral pulses, capillary refill less than 3 seconds, warm skin, pink nailbeds, and absence of edema?

Intervention	Rationale	Evaluation
Check extremity peripheral pulses, capillary refill, color, temperature, and presence of edema, and skin status every 4 hours, and report abnormal findings.	These are indications of adequate tissue perfusion.	Are peripheral pulses strong, nailbeds pink, and capillary refill of 3 seconds or less with no edema noted?
Maintain extremities lower than heart, feet on floor in sitting position, or head of bed elevated on blocks.	Dependent position increases blood flow to the legs and feet.	Does patient have adequate tissue perfusion signs?
Avoid bending knees, pillows under knees, prolonged sitting, or crossing legs.	These activities impede blood flow to extremities.	Does patient exhibit understanding of ways to improve peripheral blood flow?

EVALUATION. Interventions are successful if the patient and family demonstrate health literacy of the disease and implement interventions to control disease and prevent complications.

Aneurysms

An **aneurysm** is a bulging, ballooning, or dilation at a weakened point of an arterial wall. The artery diameter is often increased by 50%. Atherosclerosis, hypertension, smoking, trauma, and congenital abnormalities are risk factors for an aneurysm. Heredity may also play a role. Aneurysms can occur in any artery in the body but are common in the abdominal aorta, which is the focus of the rest of this discussion.

An abdominal aortic aneurysm (AAA) is often silent if it is less than 4 cm. The incidence of AAA increases with age. Medicare covers a one-time screening ultrasound for those with a family history of AAA or men ages 65 to 75 with a smoking history of 100 or more cigarettes. Men older than age 50 are at the highest risk of death from rupture and bleeding of an AAA. The mortality rate is high with a ruptured aneurysm. Survival improves with elective repair.

Types of Aneurysms

The various types of aneurysms are shown in Figure 24.8. A fusiform aneurysm is the dilation of the entire circumference of the artery. A saccular aneurysm is one that bulges on only one side of the artery wall. A dissecting aneurysm occurs when a cavity is formed from a tear in the artery wall, usually the intimal (inner) layer. The layers of the artery wall separate as blood is pumped into the tear with each heartbeat, expanding the cavity, which then becomes prone to rupturing.

Signs and Symptoms

An AAA usually exhibits few if any symptoms until it enlarges (Table 24.8). Back or flank pain is the classic symptom; the pain is caused by the aneurysm pressing against nerves of the vertebrae. Depending on the location and size of the aneurysm, there may be reports of abdominal pain, a feeling of fullness, or nausea caused by pressure on the intestines. Changing positions may temporarily relieve the symptoms. Because the symptoms are vague, they are often not associated with an AAA. There may be a pulsating mass in the abdomen caused by an AAA that is discovered during routine physical or x-ray examination.

Severe, sudden back, flank, or abdominal pain and a pulsating abdominal mass can indicate that the aneurysm may be about to rupture. With rupture and bleeding, signs of shock may develop. Emergency surgery is required for a ruptured AAA to prevent death.

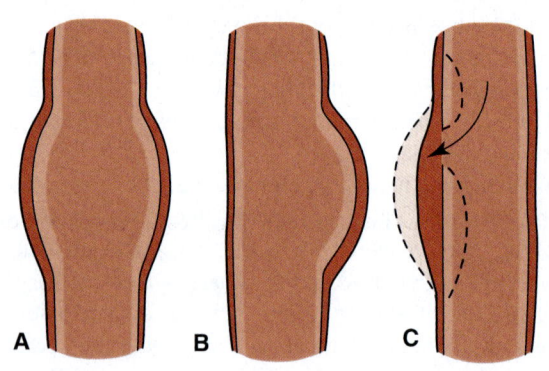

FIGURE 24.8 Types of aneurysms. (A) Fusiform: The entire circumference of the artery is dilated. (B) Saccular: One side of the artery is dilated. (C) Dissecting: A tear in the inner layer causes a cavity to form between the layers of the artery and fill with blood. The cavity expands with each heartbeat.

Diagnostic Tests

Abdominal ultrasound, CT scan, MRI, or aortography diagnose an AAA. Small aneurysms, less than 4 cm, are monitored for enlargement with ultrasound about every 6 to 12 months.

Table 24.8
Aneurysm Summary

Signs and Symptoms	Back pain Flank pain Abdominal fullness Nausea Pulsating mass in abdomen Severe sudden back pain with rupture
Diagnostic Tests	Ultrasound Computed tomography (CT) scan Aortography
Therapeutic Measures	Monitor growth of aneurysm Maintain normal blood pressure Surgical repair and graft
Complications	Rupture Hemorrhage Shock
Priority Nursing Diagnoses	*Acute Pain* *Risk for Deficient Fluid Volume* *Risk for Ineffective Peripheral Tissue Perfusion*

Therapeutic Measures

Medical treatment includes smoking cessation, gentle exercise such as walking and bike riding, avoiding lifting of heavy objects, blood pressure control to prevent arterial wall rupture, and beta blockers to slow AAA enlargement. Elective surgical repair (a bypass graft) is performed for pain, signs of circulatory compromise, or an aneurysm larger than 5.5 cm or rapidly enlarging.

An open surgical repair or an endovascular stent graft may be done to repair an AAA. Open repair is done under anesthesia. The dilated aorta section is removed and replaced with a synthetic graft that is sutured in place. Endovascular grafting involves the placement (through the femoral artery) of a stent graft at the site of the AAA. Dye is used to guide a balloon catheter that positions and opens the graft against the aorta wall. Blood flows through the stent graft to reduce pressure on the aneurysm, which will shrink over time. A fenestrated (perforated) endograft is used when the AAA is near other arteries, such as the renal arteries, to maintain their blood flow. Endovascular surgery requires less hospitalization time (2 to 3 days) and has a quicker recovery. Lifelong monitoring of the endograft is necessary.

Nursing Process for the Patient With an Abdominal Aortic Aneurysm

DATA COLLECTION. Careful monitoring of a patient with an AAA is necessary. Emotional stress may be a risk factor that should be addressed. Patient understanding must be determined so patients understand their medication regimen and the importance of taking antihypertensives as prescribed. The patient is cared for in the intensive care unit after surgery.

NURSING DIAGNOSES, PLANNING, IMPLEMENTATION, AND EVALUATION. See Chapter 12, "Nursing Care Plan for the Postoperative Patient."

Ineffective Peripheral Tissue Perfusion *related to aneurysm*

EXPECTED OUTCOME: The patient will have palpable peripheral pulses; adequate capillary refill; and normal color, temperature, motor, and sensory function of extremities.

- Monitor circulation, movement, and sensation in extremities every 1 to 4 hours *to detect reduced blood flow to minimize risk of ischemia and necrosis.*
- Measure abdominal girth every shift *to detect increasing girth indicating bleeding into abdomen.*
- Monitor complete blood count (CBC) as ordered *to detect insidious bleeding into abdomen or significant hematoma formation.*

EVALUATION. Interventions are successful if the patient does not develop postoperative complications and maintains normal neurovascular checks.

Varicose Veins

Varicose veins are elongated, tortuous, dilated veins. Primary varicosities are likely caused by a structural defect in the vessel wall. Along with the defect, the dilation of the vessel can lead to incompetent venous valves. Valves normally help prevent blood from refluxing. If reflux occurs, it can cause further dilation of the vessel and blood pooling in the lower extremities. Superficial veins are most often involved in primary varicosities. Secondary varicosities are caused by an acquired or congenital pathological condition of the deep venous system.

Etiology

Wall defects have been identified as a familial tendency. Any factor that contributes to increasing hydrostatic pressure within the leg, such as obesity, prolonged standing, or pregnancy, can promote venous dilation.

Signs and Symptoms

The appearance of telangiectasias (spider veins) indicates minor chronic venous disease. More advanced disease can cause dull pain, cramping, edema, and feelings of heaviness in the lower extremities, especially after prolonged standing. This can usually be relieved by walking or elevating the extremity. With secondary varicosities, pain and disfigurement can be more severe. Edema or ulceration can develop if venous return is severely compromised.

Therapeutic Measures

To help prevent varicose veins from prolonged standing during your nursing career, consider wearing compression stockings. The primary goals for varicose vein therapy are to improve circulation, relieve pain, and avoid complications. Conservative treatment is exercise, leg elevation, and compression therapy (e.g., compression stockings, intermittent pneumatic compression pump, or compression bandages) as prescribed. Injection sclerotherapy to collapse the vein and laser or light therapy can treat superficial varicosities. Minimally invasive ablation to seal the vein includes radiofrequency or laser ablation. These procedures can be done in the HCP's office with local anesthesia. Traditional vein stripping that is done in surgery is rare.

Venous Insufficiency

Venous insufficiency is a chronic condition. Damaged or aging valves within the veins interfere with blood return to the heart, causing pooling of blood in the lower extremities. Chronic venous insufficiency can lead to venous stasis ulcers.

Venous Stasis Ulcers

Venous stasis ulcers are the end result of chronic venous insufficiency. Dysfunctional valves in the venous system prevent or reduce venous blood return. As venous pressure increases, venous stasis occurs. Over time, the congestion and decreased venous circulation lead to changes in the lower extremities. There may be edema and a brownish discoloration of the leg and foot, with the surrounding skin hardened and leathery in appearance. The brown color occurs when veins rupture, releasing red blood cells into the tissues; the red blood cells then break down and stain the tissue brown.

Stasis ulcers develop from the increased pressure and rupture of small veins. Signs of skin breakdown are most commonly seen at the medial malleolus of the ankle. Stasis ulcers are a serious complication of venous insufficiency that are difficult to cure and can affect the patient's quality of life.

THERAPEUTIC MEASURES. The focus of treatment is to decrease edema and heal skin ulcerations. Compression with stockings or bandage wraps is necessary to decrease edema. Elevation of the legs and feet above the heart is important to assist with venous drainage of lower extremities. Patients are advised not to keep legs dependent and to avoid long periods of standing or sitting to prevent increased pressure and pain. The foot of the bed should be elevated 5 to 6 inches. In addition, patients should be encouraged to exercise and walk often during nonacute episodes. They should be informed not to cross their legs or wear constrictive clothing that decreases venous blood return to the heart.

Skin ulcers are cultured and treated with topical antibiotics if needed. Wound care can be chronic and challenging (see Chapter 54). An Unna boot is a gauze dressing coated with zinc oxide, calamine, and glycerine. It may be used to promote healing in severe ulcers. Zinc promotes wound healing and can be soothing. The Unna boot is applied snugly and provides compression therapy as well. It is changed every 2 to 7 days. Skin grafting may be necessary if ulcerations are severe or do not heal.

Nursing Process for the Patient With a Venous Disorder

DATA COLLECTION. Risk factors and knowledge of contributing factors for venous disorders are identified for teaching plans. Symptoms and concerns about body image are noted. Leg appearance, presence of edema, and ulcerations are observed. Patient-coping skills are identified to cope with the chronic ulcers that may impact quality of life.

NURSING DIAGNOSES, PLANNING, AND IMPLEMENTATION.

Acute Pain related to edema in extremities

EXPECTED OUTCOME: The patient will report an absence or acceptable level of pain within 30 minutes of reporting pain.

- Elevate legs above heart level and avoid long periods of sitting or standing *to reduce impaired venous return or pooling of fluid.*
- Utilize compression therapy as ordered *to reduce edema.*

Impaired Skin Integrity related to chronic venous congestion

EXPECTED OUTCOME: The patient will have intact skin.

- Note and document size, shape, and depth of wound *to evaluate healing of wound over time.*
- Provide a comprehensive plan for wound care including pressure relief, treatments, and nutrition as ordered *to ensure that quality wound care is provided.*
- Provide wound care as ordered *to aid in wound healing.*

Ineffective Health Self-Management related to deficient knowledge of venous disorder

EXPECTED OUTCOME: The patient will report understanding of how to manage venous disorder.

- Identify patient's understanding of the venous disorder *to determine baseline knowledge.*
- Explain venous disorder pathophysiology, signs and symptoms, prevention, and therapeutic regimen *to empower patient to manage disorder.*
- Explain that tight-fitting clothes at tops of legs or waist should not be worn *to prevent venous occlusion.*
- Explain how to control risk factors and prevent varicose veins (e.g., weight reduction, elevation of the extremities, walking, exercise, and compression therapy) *to assist blood flow return to the heart.*
- Document reinforcement of teaching and evaluation of patient knowledge *to communicate patient progress toward goal attainment.*

Also, see Chapter 12 for the "Nursing Care Plan for the Postoperative Patient."

EVALUATION. Interventions are successful if the patient reports pain is at an acceptable level and verbalizes an understanding of venous disease and prevention.

Vascular Surgery

Vascular impairments requiring surgery may be acute or chronic. They may involve arteries, veins, or lymphatic vessels.

When intermittent claudication becomes severe or disabling or when the limb is at risk for amputation, then surgical vascular grafting may be done.

Nursing Process for the Patient Undergoing Preoperative Vascular Surgery

DATA COLLECTION. Circulatory status and pain control needs are monitored. Laboratory test results, including CBC, INR, partial thromboplastin time (PTT), and bleeding time, are reviewed.

NURSING DIAGNOSES. The nursing diagnoses for preoperative vascular surgery may include the following:

- *Acute* or *Chronic Pain* related to ischemia of tissue distal to occlusion or aneurysm
- *Anxiety* related to unknown outcome, pain, powerlessness, or threat of death
- *Deficient Knowledge*, preoperative and postoperative procedures, related to unfamiliar process

See Chapter 12 for preoperative nursing process information.

Embolectomy and Thrombectomy

When an artery becomes completely occluded by an embolus or thrombus, it is considered a surgical emergency. Surgical removal to restore blood flow and oxygenation to the tissue distal to the occlusion is imperative to decrease ischemia and necrosis.

Vascular Bypasses and Grafts

Vascular bypass surgery involves the use of either autografts, such as the patient's own saphenous vein, or a synthetic graft material. The graft is anastomosed to the artery proximal to the occlusion and tunneled past the occlusion. The distal end of the graft is anastomosed to the artery (Fig. 24.9). The graft is assessed for hemostasis and function. The wound is then sutured closed.

Endarterectomy

Arteriosclerotic plaques are dissected from the lining of the arterial wall and removed in a procedure called an **endarterectomy**. To control blood flow, the artery is clamped on both sides of the occlusion. An incision is made into the artery. The plaque within the artery is removed with forceps. The artery is irrigated to remove further debris and then closed with sutures. Clamps are removed and the skin incision is closed. A drain may be placed to prevent hematoma formation.

Angioplasty

Minimally invasive techniques can also be used to open plaque-blocked arteries. These techniques include balloon or laser angioplasty. A flexible laser-tipped catheter is inserted into an artery and advanced to the site of the blockage. The laser sends out pulsating beams of light that vaporize the plaque. This procedure is used for patients with smaller occlusions in the distal superficial femoral, proximal popliteal, and common iliac arteries.

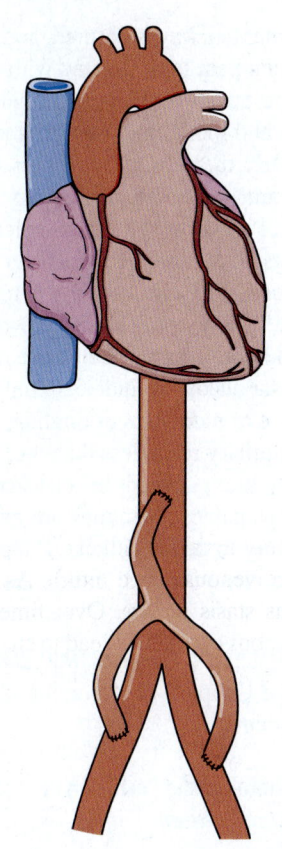

FIGURE 24.9 Aortofemoral bypass.

Stents

Stents are placed inside an artery to provide support to the artery walls to keep them open. See the PCI discussion earlier.

Complications of Vascular Surgery

Bleeding and hemorrhage can occur with any vascular surgery. If hemorrhage occurs, manual pressure is applied to the site of bleeding and the HCP is notified immediately. Drainage may cause swelling and hematoma formation. Drains can be placed to help prevent this. Extensive surgeries may result in significant blood loss, leading to fluid volume deficit or shock.

Reocclusion is possible with any vascular surgery. If thrombi or emboli develop and block blood flow, a surgical emergency results. Loss of a pedal pulse may signify reocclusion and must be immediately reported to the HCP. Blood flow needs to be reestablished within 4 to 6 hours to prevent risk of amputation of the extremity.

Nursing Process for the Patient After Vascular Surgery

DATA COLLECTION. Upon transfer postoperatively to either the intensive care or surgical unit, the patient is positioned comfortably. Head-to-toe data collection is obtained and

• WORD • BUILDING •

endarterectomy: end—inside + arter—artery + ectomy—excision

documented. A patent airway is ensured, and vital signs monitored. The patient's pain level is rated with a pain scale. All IVs and drains are traced to their source, labeled to prevent misidentification, and monitored. Measurement of intake and output is done hourly, then every 4 to 8 hours. CBC, INR, PTT, and electrolytes are monitored. Increasing abdominal girth measurements (for AAA repair) can indicate hemorrhage. Abnormal findings are reported immediately to the HCP.

Initially, neurovascular checks are ordered every 15 minutes for the first 2 hours, then every 30 minutes for 1 to 3 hours, and then hourly for aortic or extremity vascular surgery. Neurovascular checks include extremity movement and sensation, presence of numbness or tingling, pulses, temperature, color, and capillary refill (less than 3 seconds normally). Peripheral pulses are palpated or checked with Doppler ultrasound if not palpable. Then, they are compared with the unaffected extremity to detect deficits. If a pulse is absent or weak or the extremity is cool or dusky, the HCP is notified immediately.

NURSING DIAGNOSES, PLANNING, IMPLEMENTATION, AND EVALUATION. See Chapter 12, "Nursing Care Plan for the Postoperative Patient."

Ineffective Peripheral Tissue Perfusion related to emboli, vascular spasm, or reocclusion

EXPECTED OUTCOME: The patient will have palpable peripheral pulses; adequate capillary refill; and normal color, temperature, motor, and sensory function of extremities.

- Monitor circulation, movement, and sensation in extremities every 1 to 4 hours *to detect reduced blood flow to minimize risk of ischemia and necrosis.*
- Avoid constricting measures on affected extremity (e.g., knee gatch of bed, adhesive tape, tight dressings) *to prevent further decrease in blood flow to compromised extremity.*
- Assist the patient with early ambulation as prescribed *to reduce complications of immobility and increase blood flow to the extremities.*

EVALUATION. Interventions are successful if the patient does not develop postoperative complications and maintains normal neurovascular checks.

NURSING CARE TIP

Neurovascular checks refer to data collection of an extremity. (Note: Neurologic checks refer to data collection of the central nervous system.) The following are areas to examine on an extremity when doing neurovascular checks:

NEURO	VASCULAR
Movement	Pulses
Sensation	Capillary refill
Numbness	Color (nailbed or skin)
Tingling	Temperature

CLINICAL JUDGMENT

Mr. Janway, age 63, has just returned from surgery after an embolectomy of the right lower leg. He has a history of type 2 diabetes mellitus, hypertension, renal insufficiency, and an MI 3 months ago. He is 6 feet tall and weighs 316 pounds. His gait is impaired, and he uses a cane, although he has not been very active since his MI.

1. What priority data do you collection for Mr. Janway?
2. What additional data do you collect about Mr. Janway's medical history?
3. What priority nursing diagnoses and outcomes do you contribute to the plan of care for Mr. Janway?
4. What priority nursing interventions do you implement for each nursing diagnosis identified?
5. What priority equipment do you obtain to safely care for Mr. Janway?
6. Which health-care team members do you collaborate with for Mr. Janway's care?

Suggested answers are at the end of the chapter.

LYMPHATIC SYSTEM

The lymphatic system returns fluid from other tissues in the body to the bloodstream. It is a pumpless system with one-way valves that return the fluid to the heart. Any interruption in the flow of lymph results in edema.

Lymphangitis

Lymphangitis is inflammation of the lymphatic channels due to an infection. The infection can occur in the arms or legs. It is most commonly caused by *Streptococcus* bacteria but can also result from *Staphylococcus* bacteria and other organisms. It is a serious infection that can cause sepsis and death. Symptoms include painful red streaks in the extremity. Fever and chills may be present. Lymph nodes in the area of infection can be enlarged and painful. Therapy is initiated with an appropriate antimicrobial agent. Moist heat and elevation help reduce pain and swelling.

Nursing Process for the Patient With Lymphangitis

DATA COLLECTION. The affected area is monitored for size changes, edema, and skin breakdown to prevent complications. Pain level and fever occurrence are monitored. Abnormal changes are reported to the HCP.

NURSING DIAGNOSES, PLANNING, AND IMPLEMENTATION.

Acute Pain related to tissue damage and edema from infection

EXPECTED OUTCOME: The patient will report an absence or acceptable level of pain within 30 minutes of reporting pain.

- Monitor pain level with a pain rating scale *to identify severity of pain.*

- Administer analgesics as prescribed and recheck pain level in 30 minutes *to provide pain relief.*
- Position extremity *for comfort*, and elevate *to reduce edema, which can cause pressure and pain.*

Excess Fluid Volume related to congested lymph nodes from infection

EXPECTED OUTCOME: The patient will exhibit no evidence of edema.

- Apply moist heat on the extremity as ordered *to increase circulation and reduce edema.*
- Elevate extremity *to help improve circulation and prevent edema.*

EVALUATION. Interventions are successful if the patient reports pain is at an acceptable level and no edema is present.

Home Health Hints

Cardiac
- After open-heart surgery, many patients suffer from depression. Utilize a depression screening tool and follow up with the HCP as needed.
- Chest pain from esophageal reflux can mimic cardiovascular symptoms. Ask if the pain is related to consuming large meals, lying down, or bending over, or if it is relieved with antacids or food. Inform the HCP of these findings.
- Check the expiration date on the patient's nitroglycerine bottle and facilitate getting a new bottle if needed.
- Reinforce teaching for stress management techniques for the caregiver to use: deep-breathing exercises, reading a book, meditation, massage therapy, guided imagery, exercise, socializing with friends, and/or working on a favorite hobby.
- Refer to a social worker if caregiver is overwhelmed for services such as respite care or housekeeping services.

Vascular
- Monitor peripheral pulses and capillary refill. Report absent pulses or slow capillary refill to the HCP.
- Reinforce teaching for the patient to monitor extremities. Patients with peripheral vascular disorders are at a high risk for developing lower extremity wounds that are slow to heal.
- Reinforce teaching for the patient to stop and rest if pain develops in the lower extremities during exercise.

Key Points

- Arteriosclerosis (thickening, loss of elasticity, and calcification of arterial walls) and atherosclerosis (formation of plaque in the arteries) both begin in early childhood and progress without symptoms through adulthood. Atherosclerosis causes CAD.
- CAD is the obstruction of blood flow through the coronary arteries to the heart muscle cells, typically from atherosclerosis. This blood flow reduction can cause angina, MI, or sudden death if blood flow is not restored.
- Angina pectoris is chest pain due to ischemia resulting from a reduction in coronary artery blood flow and oxygen delivery to the heart muscle. Angina is a symptom, not a disease.
- Weight reduction, a heart-healthy diet, and emotional stress reduction may help slow CAD progression. Medications used for reducing angina include nitrates, beta blockers, calcium channel blockers, and ranolazine.
- Acute coronary syndrome involves ischemia of the myocardium. It includes unstable angina, NSTEMI, and STEMI.
- An MI results in the death of heart muscle cells from a sudden partial or complete blockage of a coronary artery, although a few MIs have non-occlusion causes. The extent of the cardiac damage varies depending on the location and amount of blockage in the coronary artery.
- PVD may be either arterial or venous in origin. It is important to understand whether the origin of the problem is arterial or venous to prevent serious complications from occurring.
- Arterial disorders include arterial thrombosis and embolism, peripheral artery disease, Raynaud disease, and thromboangiitis obliterans (Buerger disease).
- Monitoring of extremity pulses, capillary refill, temperature, color, and presence of edema helps identify patients at risk for complications from vascular disorders. Absent pulses are reported immediately to prevent limb loss.
- An aneurysm is a bulging, ballooning, or dilation at a weakened point of an arterial wall. Atherosclerosis, hypertension, smoking, trauma, congenital abnormalities or heredity are risk factors for an aneurysm.
- Varicose veins are elongated, tortuous, dilated veins that can lead to incompetent venous valves.
- In venous insufficiency, damaged or aging valves within the veins interfere with blood return to the heart, causing pooling of blood in the lower extremities. Chronic venous insufficiency can lead to venous stasis ulcers.
- Stasis ulcers are a serious complication of venous insufficiency that are difficult to cure and can affect the patient's quality of life. Stasis ulcers develop from the increased pressure and rupture of small veins often at the medial malleolus of the ankle.

SUGGESTED ANSWERS TO CHAPTER EXERCISES

Cue Recognition
24.1: Reinforce teaching to modify risk factors: Avoid smoking, eat a heart-healthy diet, maintain normal blood pressure and normal blood sugar, and reduce stress.
24.2: Ask the patient to rate the pain level from 0 to 10.

Critical Thinking & Clinical Judgment
Mr. Jones
1. Hemorrhage, decreased cardiac output, shock.
2. Pain, compensation for respiratory status, hemorrhage, reduced cardiac output, shock, elevated temperature.
3. Excessive chest tube drainage, abnormal vital signs, weak pedal pulses. Respiratory rate of 28 breaths per minute (irregular and shallow), lung sounds diminished with crackles in bilateral bases.
4. Notifies the HCP of data collection findings immediately due to excessive chest tube drainage and signs of heart failure and shock.
5. HCP for orders, pharmacist for medication orders, and respiratory therapist for pulmonary concerns.
6. Postoperative topics: Splinting incision, deep breathing, incentive spirometer, activity, wound care, signs of infection. Cardiac topics: Medications, lifestyle modifications—smoking cessation, heart-healthy eating pattern, physical activity, weight management, stress reduction, maintaining blood pressure, blood sugar, and cholesterol within prescribed parameters.

Mrs. Sims
1. Mrs. Sims is likely experiencing an anginal attack or an acute MI.
2. NTG usually stops chest pain associated with angina. Rest may also alleviate chest pain. Neither NTG nor rest will relieve the pain of an acute MI.
3. Patient history, ECG changes with or without ST-elevation (STEMI; NSTEMI), elevated highly sensitive troponin, and possibly myoglobin and CK-MB elevation.
4. Initial medical interventions may include NTG (sublingual or IV), antiplatelet and anticoagulant therapy. Then a cardiac catheterization is done to determine coronary artery disease and, if indicated, percutaneous coronary intervention (drug-eluting stenting) or a coronary artery bypass graft is performed.
5. Maintain patient on bedrest, obtain vital signs and ECG, administer NTG sublingual as prescribed, administer oxygen if prescribed, and notify HCP.
6. Continuously monitor chest pain level and relief obtained, ECG, and vital signs.
7. Remain at the bedside and offer Mrs. Sims reassurance that her condition and heart actions are being continually monitored to provide appropriate treatment. Ask if there is anything you can provide to assist her with coping after the acute pain episode is over, such as a significant other or clergy visit.
8. HCP, pharmacist, respiratory therapist, dietitian, clergy.
9. Educate Mrs. Sims about lifestyle risks of smoking and being overweight and offer referrals to tobacco cessation programs and a dietitian.

Mrs. Mehta
1. An injury during physical therapy or a thromboembolism within the left femoral artery.
2. Assist Mrs. Mehta safely to her bed. Monitor her left leg for color, temperature, capillary refill, and pulses (femoral, popliteal, dorsalis pedis, and posterior tibial). Compare findings with those of right leg.
3. Immediate interventions include protecting the patient's leg, preventing complications such as a pulmonary embolism with strict bedrest, and notifying the HCP.
4. This is a sample **SOAP** (Subjective, Objective, Analysis, Plan) charting to document findings: **S:** "I have severe pain in my left groin that just started. It is at 9 on a scale of 0 to 10"; **O:** Grimacing, moaning, and holding left upper leg. Left leg cool, color pale, nailbeds pale, capillary refill 8 seconds, unable to palpate pulses. Faint femoral and popliteal pulse, no dorsalis pedis or posterior tibial pulse heard with Doppler. Right leg warm, pink, capillary refill 3 seconds, with all pulses palpable; **A:** There is ineffective peripheral tissue perfusion; **P:** Notify HCP immediately.

Mr. Janway
1. Priority areas for data collection include respiratory status due to anesthesia, circulatory status of right leg and foot due to the embolectomy, vital signs, and pain level.
2. Mr. Janway's cardiac status, usual blood glucose values, medications, ambulation aids, gait, knowledge base regarding his various disease processes, and cause of his current diagnosis.
3. Priority nursing diagnoses include (1) *Acute Pain* related to surgery of right lower leg; (2) *Ineffective Peripheral Tissue Perfusion* related to embolectomy of right lower leg; and (3) *Risk for Injury* related to leg surgery, diabetes, and obesity. Outcomes include (1) verbalizes relief of pain; (2) maintains adequate tissue perfusion, as evidenced by palpable peripheral (pedal) pulses and warm, dry skin; and (3) remains free from injury.
4. Nursing interventions include the following: (1) Position (especially right leg) for comfort; keep the right leg slightly elevated; educate the patient regarding the need to ask for pain medication before pain is too severe; educate the patient regarding the need to take pain medication to minimize the negative physiological effects of pain; monitor pain on a pain scale; evaluate the effectiveness of medication using the same pain scale; report ineffective pain measures. (2) Check pedal pulses, surgical dressing, pedal sensation and movement, and color initially and every hour; report changes; check capillary refill; monitor for pain in extremities; monitor for edema in extremities; keep leg elevated slightly. (3) Ensure the nursing call light is within reach; consult physical therapy to aid with ambulation; use walking aids.
5. Gait belt for ambulation, a walker, a large recliner.
6. HCP, physical therapist, occupational therapist, dietitian, clergy.

Additional Resources

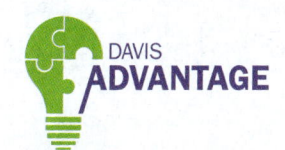

Go to Davis Advantage to complete your learning: strengthen understanding, apply your knowledge, and prepare for the Next Gen NCLEX®.

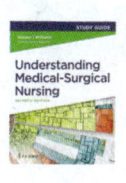

A Study Guide is also available.

CHAPTER 25
Nursing Care of Patients With Cardiac Arrhythmias

Michele Dickson

KEY TERMS

ablation (uh-BLAY-shun)
arrhythmia (uh-RITH-mee-ah)
atrial depolarization (AY-tree-uhl DEE-poh-lur-ih-ZAY-shun)
bigeminy (by-JEM-ih-nee)
bradycardia (BRAY-dih-KAR-dee-ah)
cardioversion (KAR-dee-oh-VER-zhun)
defibrillation (dee-FIB-ri-lay-shun)
dysrhythmia (dis-RITH-mee-ah)
electrocardiogram (ee-LEK-troh-KAR-dee-oh-GRAM)
fluoroscopy (fluh-RAHS-kuh-pee)
hyperkalemia (HY-per-kuh-LEE-mee-ah)
hypomagnesemia (HY-poh-MAG-nuh-ZEE-mee-ah)
isoelectric line (EYE-so-ee-LEK-trik LINE)
multifocal (MUHL-tee-FOH-kuhl)
quadrigeminy (kwa-drih-JEM-ih-nee)
sinoatrial node (SY-noh-AY-tree-al NOHD)
trigeminy (try-JEM-ih-nee)
unifocal (YOO-ni-FOH-kuhl)
ventricular repolarization (ven-TRIK-yoo-lar RE-pol-lahr-i-ZAY-shun)
ventricular tachycardia (ven-TRIK-yoo-lar TAK-ee-KAR-dee-ah)

CHAPTER CONCEPTS

Caring
Perfusion
Stress and coping
Teaching and learning

LEARNING OUTCOMES

1. Describe how electrical activity flows through the heart.
2. List the six steps used for arrhythmia interpretation.
3. Explain current medical treatments for cardiac arrhythmias.
4. Discuss cardiac pacemakers and implantable cardioverter defibrillators and their uses.
5. Plan nursing care for patients with an arrhythmia.
6. Plan nursing care for patients with an implanted device.

CARDIAC CONDUCTION SYSTEM

The heart's electrical conduction system initiates an impulse that stimulates the mechanical cells of the heart to contract (see Chapter 21, section "Cardiac Conduction Pathway and Cardiac Cycle"; Fig. 21.3). Electrical activity can be seen on a cardiac monitor or recorded on an **electrocardiogram** (ECG) tracing. Activity seen on an ECG is not *proof* that the mechanical cells of the heart have contracted in response to the electrical impulse seen. So how can you verify that the heart muscle contracts and perfusion occurs? With physical data collection! Obtain the patient's blood pressure and apical and peripheral pulses. These provide the evidence that cardiac contraction and perfusion occurred.

Cardiac Cycle

The electrical representation of the cardiac cycle (impulse that stimulates depolarization [contraction] and repolarization [relaxation] of the atria and ventricles) is a P wave, a QRS complex, and a T wave (Fig. 25.1).

ELECTROCARDIOGRAM

The electrical activity of the heart can be seen with either an ECG or continuous cardiac monitoring. An ECG shows electrical activity during the moment the ECG is obtained. Electrodes placed on the patient's skin allow various views of the heart's electrical activity to be seen. Each view of the heart is referred to as a *lead*. A 12-lead ECG provides 12 different views of the heart's electrical activity. An 18-lead ECG shows 18 views. For continuous monitoring, one lead or two leads are viewed. Continuous 12-lead monitoring can also be done. By learning the characteristics of a normal heart rhythm and rules for common **arrhythmias**, you will be able to report rhythm changes to your supervisor or the health-care provider (HCP).

• WORD • BUILDING •

arrhythmia: an—without or away + rhythm—rhythm + ia—condition

Chapter 25 Nursing Care of Patients With Cardiac Arrhythmias 405

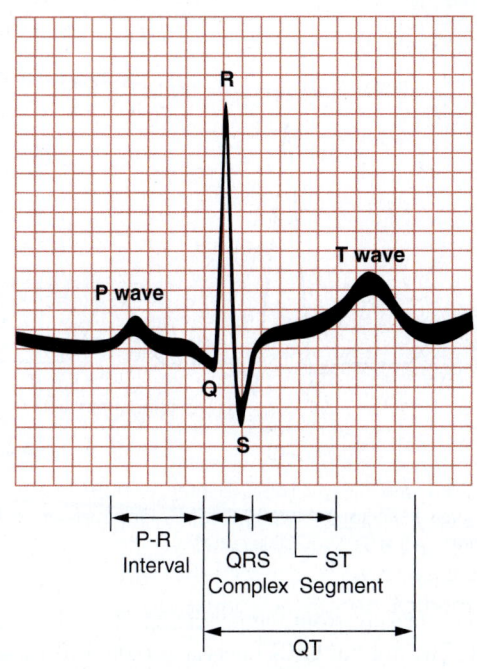

FIGURE 25.1 Components of the cardiac cycle.

Electrocardiogram Graph Paper

Intervals of each of the components of a cardiac cycle tracing are measured in seconds of time on the ECG graph paper. The graph paper is calibrated within a grid. Small squares are divided into heavy lined blocks of 25 that are five squares wide and five squares high (Fig. 25.2). Each small square is 0.04 seconds wide. One-half of a square is 0.02 seconds wide. Nothing smaller than one-half of a square is used. There are five small squares horizontally between two heavy, vertical black lines. The waveforms are measured horizontally from left to right on the graph paper. The height of the waveforms (amplitude) is measured vertically.

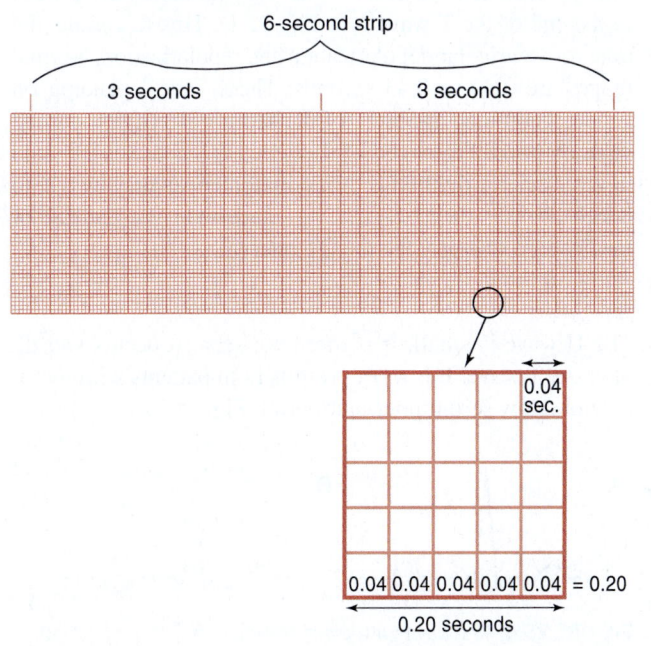

FIGURE 25.2 Electrocardiogram graph paper time intervals.

You have probably seen a heart monitor, perhaps on television, with a straight line displayed on it. This straight line is called the **isoelectric line** (baseline). It occurs when there is no electrical current (e.g., when the ECG machine is turned on but not attached to a person) or when the positive and negative electrical activity is equal if attached to a person. The ECG graph paper displays a straight line when there are no positive (upward) or negative (downward) electrical wave deflections present.

COMPONENTS OF A CARDIAC CYCLE

P Wave
The P wave is the first wave of the cardiac cycle. It represents **atrial depolarization.** When the SA node fires, the electrical impulse spreads from the right to left atrium. The normal P wave appears rounded. When compared with other waveforms, it looks like a small hill. Disorders that change atrial size cause alterations in P-wave shape and size.

PR Interval
The PR interval (PRI; duration) represents the time it takes for the electrical impulse to travel from the SA node to the AV node. The PRI starts at the beginning of the P wave and ends at the beginning of the QRS complex. To calculate the PRI, count the number of small squares horizontally that the interval covers. Then multiply by 0.04 to identify the length of the PRI (Fig. 25.3). The normal PRI is 0.12 to 0.20 seconds (three to five small horizontal squares).

> **LEARNING TIP**
> To remember the normal PR interval (PRI), use the *R* to recall normal respiratory rate and then add a decimal before each number. A normal respiratory rate is 12 to 20 breaths per minute, and a normal PRI is 0.12 to 0.20 seconds!

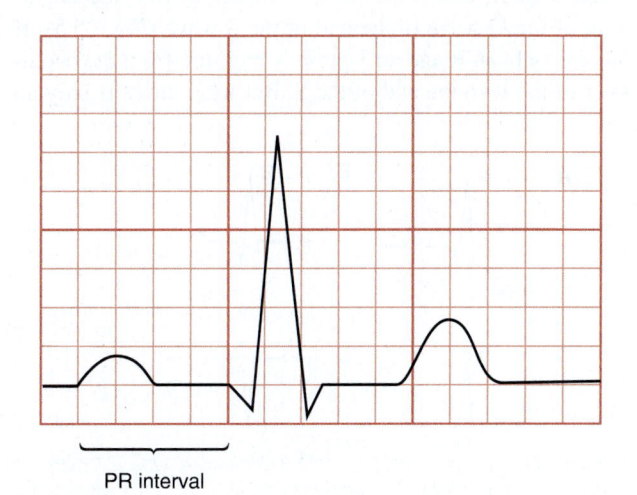

FIGURE 25.3 PR interval. This PR interval covers four squares. Each square is 0.04 seconds: 4 × 0.04 = 0.16 seconds.

LEARNING TIP
To make identification and measuring of waves easier:
- Identify the isoelectric line and place a straight-edged item exactly along the isoelectric line and let it lie below the line; note any positive waves that are above the isoelectric line. Then, lay the straight-edged item above the isoelectric line and note any negative waveforms that occur below the isoelectric line.
- Find a wave that begins on a vertical line, if possible, to make it visually easier to double check the caliper measurement (see Fig. 25.3).

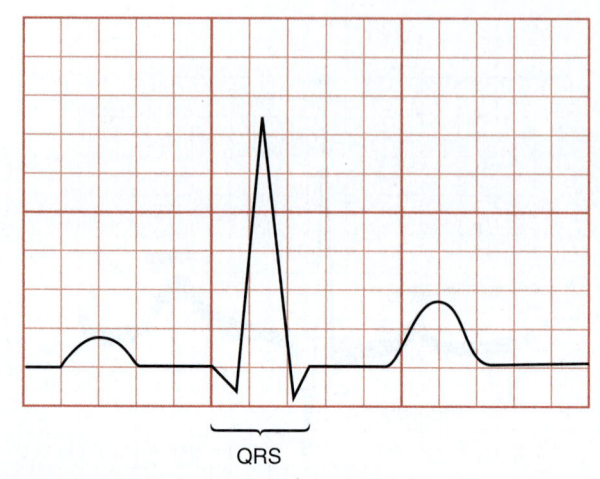

FIGURE 25.5 QRS interval. This QRS interval covers two and a half squares. Each square is 0.04 seconds. One-half square is 0.02 seconds: 2.5 × 0.04 = 0.10 seconds.

QRS Complex

The QRS complex represents ventricular depolarization. It is composed of three waves: Q, R, and S. The Q wave is the first downward deflection after the P wave. The R wave is the first upward deflection after the P wave. The S wave is the first negative deflection after the R wave (see Fig. 25.1). The S wave ends when it returns to the isoelectric line. (This is why locating the isoelectric line is helpful when first learning to identify waves.) It is very important to note that all three waves are not always present in every QRS complex. But even with absent waves, it is still referred to as the *QRS complex* and is considered normal (Fig. 25.4). The QRS complex is larger than the P wave because the ventricles are larger owing to more muscle mass. This makes the QRS complex look like the "mountain" when compared with other waveforms.

QRS Interval

The QRS interval represents the time it takes for the electrical impulse to travel from the AV node rapidly through the ventricles. To measure the QRS interval, count the number of squares from the wave that begins the QRS complex to the end of the wave that ends the QRS complex. For example, when a Q, R, and S are present, measure from the beginning of the Q wave to the end of the S wave (Fig. 25.5). If there is only an R and an S present, measure from the beginning of the R to the end of the S. But when there is only an R present, measure from the beginning of the R to the end of the R. The normal QRS interval is 0.06 to 0.10 seconds (1.5 to 2.5 boxes).

T Wave

The T wave represents **ventricular repolarization**, which is the resting state of the heart when the ventricles are filling with blood and preparing to receive the next impulse. The T wave is a rounded wave. In size comparison with the other waves, it is a "medium-sized hill." In most leads, the normal T wave is an upward (positive) deflection. It follows the QRS complex (remember, depolarization must occur first!). The T wave ends with a return to the isoelectric line. An inverted (downward) T wave can indicate cardiac ischemia (Fig. 25.6).

QT Interval

The QT interval measures the time from the start of the Q wave to the end of the T wave (see Fig. 25.1). This represents the time for ventricular depolarization and repolarization. Normal ranges are 0.34 to 0.43 seconds. These vary depending on gender, heart rate, and age. A QT chart for identifying normal values is used. Prolonged or shortened QT intervals can lead to ventricular arrhythmias. Abnormal intervals may be due to genetic causes, heart conditions, electrolyte imbalances, or medications that prolong the QT interval.

U Wave

The U wave is small. It is often not seen. It occurs shortly after the T wave. It is most prominent in patients with hypokalemia (low serum potassium level; Fig. 25.7).

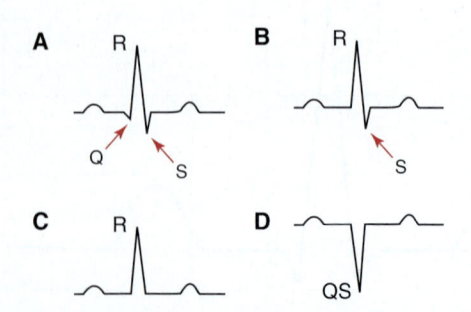

FIGURE 25.4 (A) QRS complex with a Q wave. (B) QRS complex without a Q wave. (C) QRS complex without a Q or an S wave. (D) QRS complex with no R wave. The wave present is called a QS because it is not known whether it is a Q or an S.

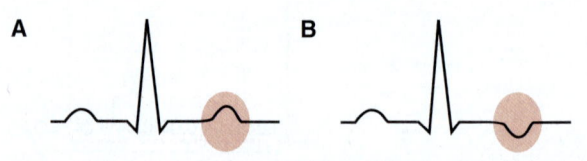

FIGURE 25.6 (A) T wave with positive deflection. (B) T wave with inverted, negative deflection, indicating ischemia.

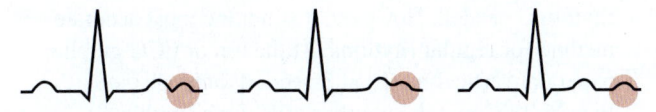

FIGURE 25.7 Various locations where U waves may appear.

ST Segment

The ST segment reflects the time from completion of a contraction (depolarization) to recovery (repolarization) of myocardial muscle for the next impulse. The ST segment starts at the end of the QRS complex. It ends at the beginning of the T wave (Fig. 25.8A). The ST segment is checked when patients experience chest pain. If a patient has nontransmural (occurring across the entire wall of an organ) ischemia, the ST segment can become inverted or depressed (Fig. 25.8B). With transmural ischemia, the ST segment can rise from the isoelectric line (Fig. 25.8C).

INTERPRETATION OF CARDIAC RHYTHMS

Six-Step Process for Arrhythmia Interpretation

An orderly, systematic method for interpreting ECG rhythms should be used. This will increase understanding of the items to examine and ensure nothing is overlooked. Six steps are used (Table 25.1). The findings of the first five steps identify the ECG rhythm according to the five rules for each arrhythmia. Then, the QT interval is measured in the sixth step. A 6-second ECG tracing is used when interpreting rhythms (see Fig. 25.2).

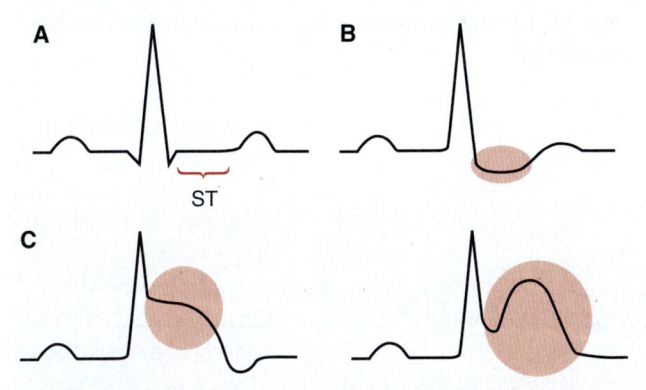

FIGURE 25.8 (A) ST segment. (B) ST segment inverted or depressed. (C) ST segment elevated.

Table 25.1
Six-Step Process for Arrhythmia Interpretation

After answering these questions with the patient's electrocardiogram (ECG) data, you can name the patient's arrhythmia.

Step	Questions
Step 1: Regularity of the rhythm	Is the rhythm regular? Irregular? Is there a pattern to the irregularity?
Step 2: Heart rate	What is the heart rate?
Step 3: P waves	Is there one P wave in front of every QRS complex? Is the atrial rate the same as the ventricular rate? Are the P waves smooth, rounded, and upright?
Step 4: PR interval	Is the PR interval normal and constant? Does the PR interval vary?
Step 5: QRS interval	Is the QRS duration normal and constant? Do the QRS complexes all look alike?
Step 6: QT interval	Is the QT interval normal?

Step 1. Regularity of the Rhythm

The regularity of the rhythm can be determined by looking at the R-to-R spacing on the ECG tracing (Fig. 25.9). The same spacing between each R to R, with a rare variation of no greater than two small squares, is seen in a normal rhythm. To determine the regularity of a rhythm, count the number of small squares between each R wave. They should normally be the same number. A caliper (a two-sided, movable metal instrument with sharp points) can also be used to measure the R-to-R spacing.

To use a caliper for measuring R waves, place one metal point on an R wave. Place the other point in the exact same location on the next R wave. Next, stabilize the caliper.

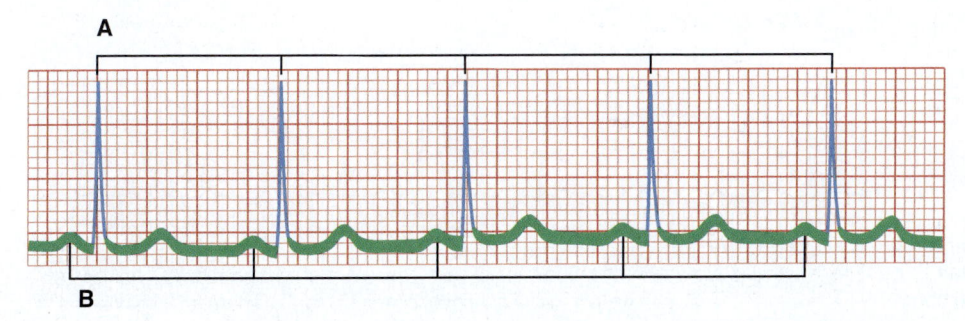

FIGURE 25.9 Normal cardiac waves are equal distances apart. (A) R-to-R waves. (B) P-to-P waves.

Without changing the distance between the caliper points, move the caliper from R wave to R wave across the ECG tracing (also known as an *ECG strip*) to see if R waves are regularly (evenly) spaced. If the distance is always the same, the rhythm is regular. If the distance varies, the rhythm is irregular. An irregular rhythm can be regularly irregular or irregularly irregular. *Regularly irregular* means it has a predictable pattern of irregularity. *Irregularly irregular* means it has no pattern to the occurrence of the irregularity.

> **LEARNING TIP**
> If a caliper is not available, a mark can be made on a piece of paper at the peak of one R wave and another mark made at the peak of the following R wave. Then the marks on the paper can be moved along the R-to-R intervals on the tracing (just as caliper points are) to determine the rhythm's regularity.

Step 2. Heart Rate
After rhythm regularity is determined, a 1-minute heart rate is calculated. One of the two following methods is used:

1. Count the number of small (0.04-second) squares between two R waves. Divide that number into 1,500. This gives the bpm, because 1,500 small squares equal 1 minute (Fig. 25.10). This method is used *only* for regular rhythms. It is very accurate. A *rate meter* is a visual paper copy of this mathematical calculation for an entire 6-second ECG tracing. You view it to calculate a 1-minute heart rate.
2. The 6-second method is used for irregular rhythms. It may also be used when a rapid estimate of a regular rhythm is needed. However, it is not the most accurate method for regular rhythms. At the top of ECG graph paper are vertical marks at 3-second intervals (see Fig. 25.2). Count the number of R waves within a 6-second strip (three vertical marks) and multiply the total by 10 (the number of 6-second time periods in a minute) to obtain the bpm (6 seconds × 10 = 60 seconds, or 1 minute; Fig. 25.11).

Step 3. P Waves
The P waves on the ECG tracing are examined to see whether (1) there is one P wave in front of every QRS, (2) the P waves are regularly occurring, and (3) the P waves all look alike (see Fig. 25.9). If all of the P waves meet these criteria, they are considered normal. If they do not, further examination of the tracing is necessary to determine the arrhythmia.

Step 4. PR Interval
All PRIs are measured to determine whether they are normal (0.12 to 0.20 seconds) and constant. If the PRI is found to vary, it is important to note whether there is a pattern to the variation.

Step 5. QRS Interval
The QRS complexes are measured to determine whether they are all within normal range (0.06 to 0.10 seconds). Abnormal QRS complexes require further examination.

Step 6. QT Interval
Finally, the QT interval is measured to ensure that it is not shortened or prolonged. Abnormal intervals can lead to arrhythmias. They should be reported to the HCP. A prolonged QT could become life threatening if it slows the heart rate enough.

FIGURE 25.10 Normal sinus rhythm, rhythm regular: Count the small squares between two of the R waves and divide into 1,500: 1,500/22 = 68 bpm.

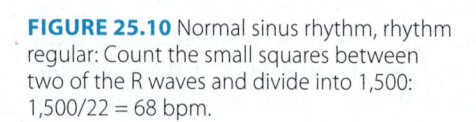

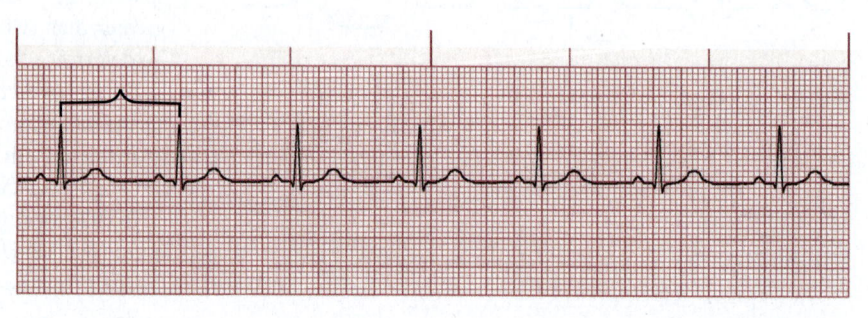

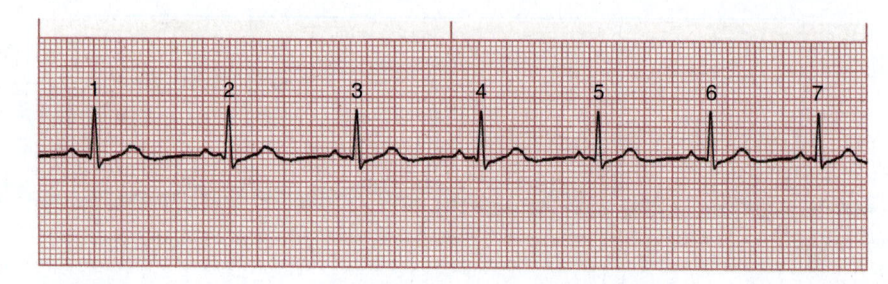

FIGURE 25.11 Rhythm irregular: Counting R waves in a 6-second strip. There are seven R waves in this 6-second strip. 7 × 10 = 70 bpm.

NORMAL SINUS RHYTHM

Normal sinus rhythm (NSR) is the heart's normal rhythm (see Fig. 25.10). It originates in the SA node. NSR has complete, regular cardiac cycles at 60 to 100 bpm.

Normal Sinus Rhythm Rules
1. Rhythm: Regular
2. Heart rate: 60 to 100 bpm
3. P waves: Rounded, upright, precede each QRS complex, alike
4. PRI: 0.12 to 0.20 seconds
5. QRS interval: 0.06 to 0.10 seconds

ARRHYTHMIAS

An arrhythmia, which is used interchangeably with the term **dysrhythmia**, is an abnormal rhythm of the heart. Several mechanisms can cause an arrhythmia. Examples of these mechanisms are disturbances in the formation of an impulse or in the conduction of the impulse. When impulse formation is disturbed, an impulse may arise from the atria, the AV node, or the ventricles instead of the SA node. This disturbance can result in an increased or decreased heart rate, early or late beats, or atrial or ventricular fibrillation. With a disturbance in conduction, the impulse becomes blocked within the electrical conduction system (as in heart blocks or right or left bundle branch block).

See the American Heart Association (AHA) Guidelines for Cardiopulmonary Resuscitation (CPR) and Emergency Cardiovascular Care (ECC) at www.heart.org. Systemic reviews and research trials have looked at safe performance of CPR during an airborne pandemic such as COVID-19 (Brown & Chan, 2020; Couper et al, 2020; Malysz et al, 2020).

> **PRACTICE ANALYSIS TIP**
> **Linking NCLEX-PN® to Practice**
> The LPN/LVN will:
> - Recognize and report basic abnormalities on a client cardiac monitor strip.
> - Respond and intervene to a client life-threatening situation (e.g., cardiopulmonary resuscitation).

Arrhythmias Originating in the Sinoatrial Node

Rhythms arising from the SA node are referred to as *sinus rhythms*. Disturbances in conduction from the SA node can cause irregular rhythms or abnormal heart rates. Arrhythmias arising from the SA node are rarely dangerous. People who cannot tolerate a rapid or slow heart rate, especially those with heart, lung, or kidney disease, may require treatment.

> **LEARNING TIP**
> The origin and the type of a problem are used to name an arrhythmia. Let's name a slow arrhythmia that originates in the **sinoatrial (SA) node**. The origin is sinus, and the type of problem (slow rate) is bradycardia. So, the arrhythmia's name is *sinus bradycardia*. The term *normal* is not used because there is an abnormality in the rate! What would a fast arrhythmia originating in the SA node be called? *Sinus tachycardia*, of course. It is easy to understand what is happening within an arrhythmia when you look at the name and what it conveys.

Sinus Bradycardia

Bradycardia is a rate slower than 60 bpm. It can be asymptomatic or symptomatic (usually when below 50 bpm). Sinus bradycardia has the same cardiac cycle components as NSR. The only difference between the two is a slower rate caused by fewer impulses originating from the SA node (Fig. 25.12). Look to the name "sinus bradycardia," which tells us that the impulse is coming from the sinus node (sinus) but at a slower rate than normal (bradycardia).

ETIOLOGY. Electrolyte imbalances, medications such as digoxin (Lanoxin), or myocardial infarction (MI) can cause bradycardia. Well-conditioned athletes, whose hearts work very efficiently, can also have slow heart rates.

SINUS BRADYCARDIA RULES
1. Rhythm: Regular
2. Heart rate: Less than 60 bpm
3. P waves: Rounded, upright, precede each QRS complex, alike
4. PRI: 0.12 to 0.20 seconds
5. QRS interval: 0.06 to 0.10 seconds

SIGNS AND SYMPTOMS. With symptomatic bradycardia, decreased blood pressure, respiratory distress, diminished or absent peripheral pulses, fatigue, or syncope can occur.

THERAPEUTIC MEASURES. Asymptomatic bradycardia does not require treatment. Observe the patient for symptom development. The underlying cause must be identified for correction. For the symptomatic patient, begin treatment while the cause is corrected. Treatment can include IV atropine or infusions of dopamine or epinephrine. Transcutaneous pacing is used if atropine is ineffective (Table 25.2). Transvenous pacing can also be considered.

Sinus Tachycardia

Tachycardia is defined as a heart rate greater than 100 bpm. It originates from the SA node. Sinus tachycardia has the same components as NSR except the rate is faster (Fig. 25.13).

• WORD • BUILDING •

dysrhythmia: dys—difficult or abnormal + rhythm—rhythm + ia—condition
bradycardia: bradys—slow + kardia—heart

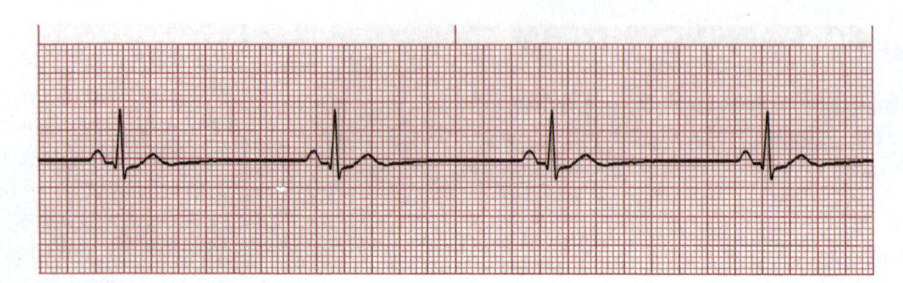

FIGURE 25.12 Sinus bradycardia. Heart rate is 38.

Table 25.2
Medications Used in Treatment of Arrhythmias

Medication Class/Action

Anticoagulant (Oral)
Increases clotting time.

Examples	*Nursing Implications*
Reduces risk of blood clots in atrial fibrillation (AF). warfarin (Coumadin)	Monitor international normalized ratio regularly. Monitor for bruising and bleeding. Acetaminophen (Tylenol) should be used rather than aspirin for analgesia during therapy. Reversal agent is vitamin K.
Reduces risk of blood clots in nonvalvular AF. apixaban (Eliquis) dabigatran (Pradaxa) edoxaban (Savaysa, Lixiana) rivaroxaban (Xarelto)	No regular monitoring needed. No specific reversal agent available. Dosage adjustment may be required with reduced kidney function.

Antiarrhythmics

Examples	*Nursing Implications*
In supraventricular tachycardia, slows conduction through AV node to restore normal sinus rhythm. adenosine (Adenocard)	Inform health-care provider (HCP) if female pregnant or nursing. Record rhythm strip during administration. Given via IV push fast (1–3 seconds), followed by normal saline flush fast.
Inhibits AF, atrial flutter, and ventricular arrhythmias. amiodarone (IV: Nexterone; oral: Cordarone, Pacerone) dronedarone (Multaq)	Contraindicated in atrioventricular (AV) block or pregnancy. Obtain baseline vital signs and electrocardiogram. Monitor for toxicity. Monitor for multiple medication interactions.

Anticholinergic
Increases heart rate to treat symptomatic bradycardia and asystole.

Examples	*Nursing Implications*
atropine sulfate	Contraindicated in angle-closure glaucoma.

Beta Blockers
Decrease myocardial contractility. Control rate in sinus tachycardia, premature atrial contraction, atrial flutter, AF, and premature ventricular contractions.

Examples	*Nursing Implications*
atenolol (Tenormin) esmolol (Brevibloc) metoprolol succinate (Lopressor, Toprol XL)	Check apical pulse and blood pressure (BP) before giving. If pulse is less than 60 bpm and BP less than 100 mm Hg systolic, notify HCP. Teach: Change positions slowly and do not stop drug abruptly.

Table 25.2
Medications Used in Treatment of Arrhythmias—cont'd

Medication Class/Action

Calcium Channel Blocker

Decreases myocardial contractility and depresses conduction system. Controls rate in sinus tachycardia, atrial flutter, and AF.

Examples	Nursing Implications
diltiazem (Cardizem) verapamil (Calan, Isoptin, Verelan)	IV route used for symptomatic arrhythmias. Monitor for bradycardia and hypotension.

Inotrope—Cardiac Glycoside (Positive Inotrope and Negative Chronotrope)

Slows heart rate. Maintains sinus rhythm for sinus tachycardia, atrial flutter, and AF.

Examples	Nursing Implications
digoxin (Lanoxicaps, Lanoxin)	Take apical pulse for 1 minute; if less than 60 bpm, notify HCP. Therapeutic digoxin levels: 0.5 to 2 mg/mL. Monitor drug level and electrolytes as hypokalemia, hypomagnesemia, and hypercalcemia increase toxicity.

Vasopressors

Examples	Nursing Implications
For cardiac stimulation, vasoconstriction, and bronchodilation. Treats asystole, ventricular tachycardia, ventricular fibrillation, and symptomatic bradycardia. epinephrine/adrenalin norepinephrine *Increases cardiac output and blood pressure; treats bradycardia.* dopamine	Contraindicated with nonselective beta blockers. Monitor blood pressure and heart rate.

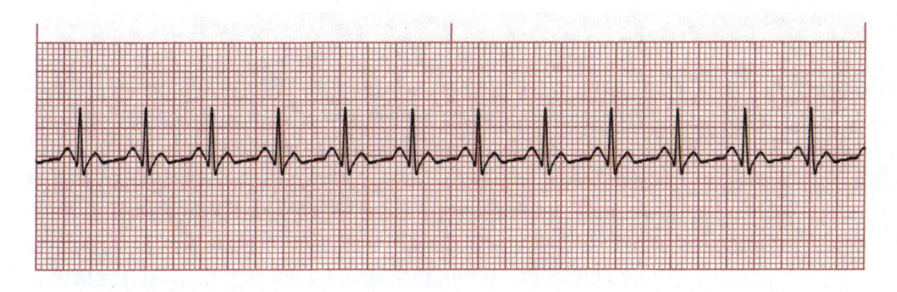

FIGURE 25.13 Sinus tachycardia. Heart rate is 125.

ETIOLOGY. Sinus tachycardia causes include physical activity; hemorrhage; shock; medications such as epinephrine, atropine, or nitrates; dehydration; fever; MI; electrolyte imbalance; fear; and anxiety. Tachycardia occurs as a compensatory mechanism for hypoxia. It helps produce additional cardiac output to deliver oxygen to tissues.

SINUS TACHYCARDIA RULES
1. Rhythm: Regular
2. Heart rate: 101 to 180 bpm
3. P waves: Rounded, upright, precede each QRS complex, alike
4. PRI: 0.12 to 0.20 seconds
5. QRS interval: 0.06 to 0.10 seconds

SIGNS AND SYMPTOMS. Sinus tachycardia can be asymptomatic. A very rapid rate (usually greater than 150 bpm) that is sustained for long periods may cause symptoms. The patient may have angina, dyspnea, syncope, or tachypnea. Older patients can become symptomatic more rapidly than younger patients (see "Gerontological Issues"). Patients with an MI may not tolerate a rapid heart rate. They can have more severe symptoms because cardiac workload is increased.

THERAPEUTIC MEASURES. If the patient is stable, obtain an ECG and treat the cause. Medications such as adenosine (Adenocard), beta blockers, and calcium channel blockers are considered to slow the heart rate (when equal to or greater than

> **Gerontological Issues**
>
> **Arrhythmia Risk**
> Factors that increase the risk of arrhythmias in older adults include:
>
> - Digitalis toxicity (most common)
> - Hypokalemia
> - Angina
> - Coronary insufficiency or cardiomyopathy (exercise, stress)
> - Sleep apnea
> - Hypothyroidism or hyperthyroidism
>
> Arrhythmias that occur most often in older adults include the following:
>
> - Atrial fibrillation (atria beating 400 to 700 times per minute)
> - Sick sinus syndrome (alternating episodes of bradycardia, normal sinus rhythm, tachycardia, and periods of long sinus pause)
> - Heart blocks (delayed or blocked impulses to the atria or ventricles)
>
> Some of the common age-related effects of arrhythmias include the following:
>
> - Bradycardia
> - Confusion
> - Dizziness
> - Dyspnea or shortness of breath
> - Fatigue
> - Hypotension
> - Palpitations
> - Syncope
> - Weakness
>
> Older adults have less ability to adapt to sudden changes or stressors. They may not be able to tolerate tachycardia for very long. Any new-onset tachycardia in an older patient should be reported promptly.

> **LEARNING TIP**
> Tachycardia is often the first sign of hemorrhage. It is a compensatory mechanism to maintain cardiac output. If a patient develops sudden tachycardia, consider whether hemorrhage could be the cause in postoperative patients, patients with gastrointestinal bleeding or cancer, or trauma patients. Consider both external and internal bleeding. Apply pressure to a bleeding site. Report the tachycardia and any bleeding promptly for treatment.

150 bpm; see Table 25.2). The treatment goal is to decrease the heart's workload and correct the cause. This usually resolves the tachycardia. For example, if the patient is hemorrhaging, immediate intervention is needed to stop bleeding and restore normal blood volume. Once normal blood volume is restored, the heart rate should return to normal.

Arrhythmias Originating in the Atria

As reviewed, all areas of the heart can initiate an impulse (see Chapter 21). If the atria begin to initiate impulses faster than the SA node, the primary pacemaker, the atria become the primary pacemaker. Atrial rhythms are usually faster than 100 bpm. They can exceed 200 bpm. When an impulse originates outside the SA node, the P waves produced look different (flatter, notched, or peaked) from the rounded P waves of the SA node. This is an indicator that the SA node is not controlling the heart rate. When the atrial impulses travel to the ventricles, they initiate a normal-shaped QRS complex after each P wave.

> **LEARNING TIP**
> If a QRS complex measures 0.06 to 0.10 seconds and an arrhythmia is present, the problem originated above the ventricles. This is known as a *supraventricular* (above the ventricle) *arrhythmia*. Ventricular-originating arrhythmias produce wide QRS complexes that are greater than 0.10 seconds.

Premature Atrial Contractions

The term *premature* refers to an "early" beat. When the atria fire an impulse before the SA node fires, a premature beat results. If the underlying rhythm is NSR, the distance between R waves is the same except where the early beat occurs. When looking at the ECG strip, a shortened R-to-R interval is seen where the premature beat occurs. The R wave preceding the premature atrial contraction (PAC) and the PAC's R wave are close together, followed by a pause, with the next beat being regular (Fig. 25.14).

ETIOLOGY. Causes of PACs include enlarged atria in valvular disorders, atrial fibrillation onset, cigarette smoking, electrolyte imbalances, heart failure, hypoxia, medications (such as digoxin), myocardial ischemia, and stress.

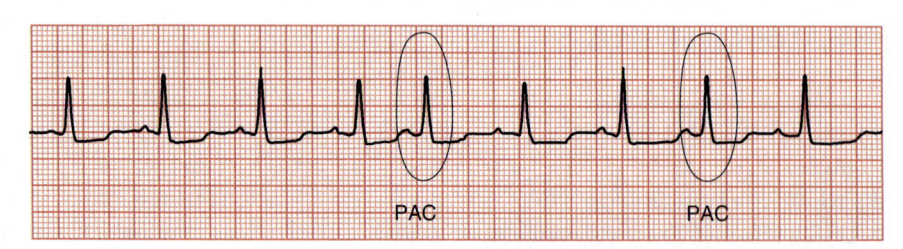

FIGURE 25.14 Premature atrial contractions.

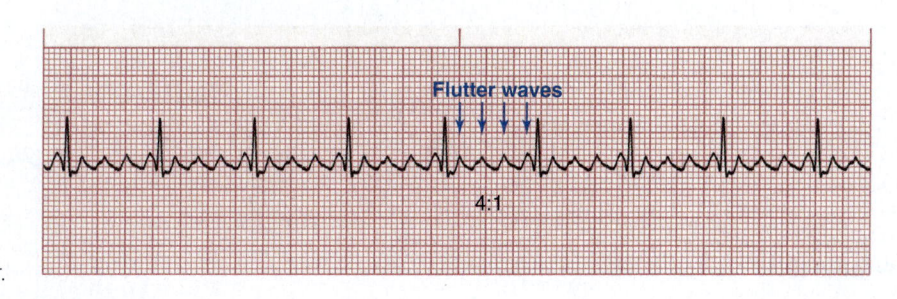

FIGURE 25.15 Atrial flutter.

PREMATURE ATRIAL CONTRACTIONS RULES
1. Rhythm: Premature beat interrupts the underlying rhythm
2. Heart rate: Depends on the underlying rhythm; if NSR, 60 to 100 bpm
3. P waves: Early beat is abnormally shaped
4. PRI: Normal if underlying rhythm normal; premature beat can have shortened or prolonged PRI
5. QRS interval: 0.06 to 0.10 seconds (indicates normal conduction to ventricles)

SIGNS AND SYMPTOMS. PACs can occur in healthy individuals as well as those with a diseased heart. No symptoms are usually present. If several PACs occur in succession, the patient may report feeling palpitations.

THERAPEUTIC MEASURES. PACs are usually not serious. Often, no treatment is required other than correcting a cause. Frequent PACs indicate atrial irritability, which could worsen into other atrial arrhythmias. Beta blockers can be given for frequent PACs to slow the heart rate (see Table 25.2).

Atrial Flutter
In atrial flutter, the atria contract, or flutter, at a rate of 250 to 350 bpm. The very rapid P waves appear as *flutter*, or F waves, on the ECG. They appear in a sawtooth pattern. Some of the impulses travel through the AV node and reach the ventricles. This results in normal QRS complexes on the ECG. There can be from two to four F waves between QRS complexes. If impulses pass through the AV node at a consistent rate, the rhythm will be regular (Fig. 25.15). The classic characteristics of atrial flutter are more than one P wave before a QRS complex, a sawtooth pattern of P waves, and an atrial rate of 250 to 350 bpm.

ETIOLOGY. Causes of atrial flutter include heart failure, hypertension, rheumatic or ischemic heart diseases, pericarditis, pulmonary embolism, and postoperative coronary artery bypass surgery. Many medications can also cause this arrhythmia.

ATRIAL FLUTTER RULES
1. Rhythm: Atrial rhythm regular; ventricular rhythm regular or irregular depending on consistency of AV conduction of impulses
2. Heart rate: Ventricular rate varies
3. P waves: Flutter or F waves with sawtooth pattern
4. PRI: None measurable
5. QRS interval: 0.06 to 0.10 seconds

SIGNS AND SYMPTOMS. The presence of symptoms in atrial flutter depends on the ventricular rate. If the ventricular rate is normal, usually no symptoms are present. If the rate is rapid, the patient may experience palpitations, angina, or dyspnea.

THERAPEUTIC MEASURES. The ventricular rate and adequacy of cardiac output guide treatment. The goal is to control the ventricular rate with conversion to NSR. For an unstable patient with a rapid ventricular rate, synchronized **cardioversion** (electrical shock) is used. Medications such as calcium channel blockers can be used to control the ventricular rate (see Table 25.2). Antiarrhythmic medications are used to convert atrial flutter. To terminate the atrial flutter in symptomatic patients, catheter **ablation** (usually in the right atrium) may be done.

Atrial Fibrillation
In atrial fibrillation (AF), the atrial rate is extremely rapid and chaotic. An atrial rate of 350 to 600 bpm can occur. However, the AV node blocks most of the impulses. Consequently, the ventricular rate is much lower than the atrial rate. There are no definable P waves. The atria are fibrillating, or quivering, rather than beating effectively. No P waves can be seen or measured. A wavy pattern is produced on the ECG. Because the atrial rate is so irregular and only a few of the atrial impulses are allowed to pass through the AV node, the R waves are irregular. The ventricular rate varies from normal to rapid.

AF can be self-limiting, persistent, or permanent; permanent AF doubles the risk of death. Stroke risk is increased with AF because of the risk of thrombus formation in the atria from blood stasis caused by poor emptying of blood from the quivering atria (Fig. 25.16).

ETIOLOGY. AF increases with age (65 and above), especially in those with heart disease. Causes include cardiac surgery, emphysema, heart failure, heart valve disease, hypertension, hyperthyroidism, MI, sleep apnea, and certain medications. Sometimes the cause is unknown.

• **WORD • BUILDING** •
ablation: ab—away from + lat—carry

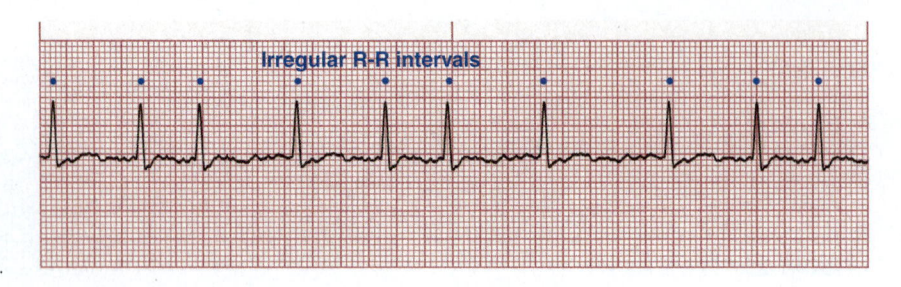

FIGURE 25.16 Atrial fibrillation.

ATRIAL FIBRILLATION RULES
1. Rhythm: Irregularly irregular
2. Heart rate: Atrial rate not measurable; ventricular rate under 100 bpm is controlled response; greater than 100 bpm is rapid ventricular response
3. P waves: No identifiable P waves
4. PRI: None can be measured because no P waves are seen
5. QRS interval: 0.06 to 0.10 seconds

> **LEARNING TIP**
> Atrial fibrillation is easy to identify based on two classic characteristics on an ECG: lack of identifiable P waves and an irregularly irregular rhythm (R waves).

SIGNS AND SYMPTOMS. With AF, most patients feel the irregular rhythm. Many describe it as palpitations, a racing heart, or a skipping heartbeat. They may feel shortness of breath, dizziness, or chest discomfort. A patient's radial pulse may be faint because of a decreased stroke volume (volume of blood ejected with each contraction). If the ventricular rhythm is rapid and sustained, the patient can go into left-sided heart failure.

THERAPEUTIC MEASURES. The focus of AF treatment is to control rate, prevent thromboembolism, and restore normal rhythm. If the patient is unstable, synchronized cardioversion is done immediately to try to return the heart to NSR. For the patient who is stable, medications to control the ventricular rate are used. These include beta blockers, calcium channel blockers, or sometimes digoxin (see Table 25.2). Anticoagulant therapy may be given to reduce thrombi and stroke risk. Pharmacological or electrical cardioversion can be used to attempt to convert the rhythm to NSR. This should be done after sufficient anticoagulation (3 to 4 weeks) to stabilize or resolve any existing blood clots in the atria. This prevents clots from being dislodged and causing a stroke. Rhythm control medications such as sodium or potassium channel blockers are used to restore and maintain NSR. If known, the underlying cause of AF is treated. For patients with AF who do not respond to medications or electrical cardioversion, other therapies can be used.

Catheter Ablation. To stop impulses coming from the pulmonary veins (most AF impulses arise from pulmonary veins) or AV node, catheter ablation may be used. Intracardiac echocardiography maps the area of the heart requiring treatment. Then, released energy, such as cryothermy or radiofrequency energy, creates lesions either on all four pulmonary veins or near the AV node. The lesions heal and scar. This blocks those pathways for future impulses. Postprocedural care is similar to postangioplasty or postcardiac catheterization care (see Chapter 21).

Surgery. The maze procedure creates multiple lines of scar tissue (a maze-like pattern) with cryothermy or radiofrequency energy to block reentry of the electrical impulses traveling to the AV node.

Third-Degree Atrioventricular Block

In third-degree AV block, SA node impulses are blocked and do not reach the ventricles to stimulate them to contract (Fig. 25.17). This is also known as *complete heart block* (CHB) or *third-degree heart block*. The *escape* pacemakers for the heart (junctional [AV node] or ventricular)

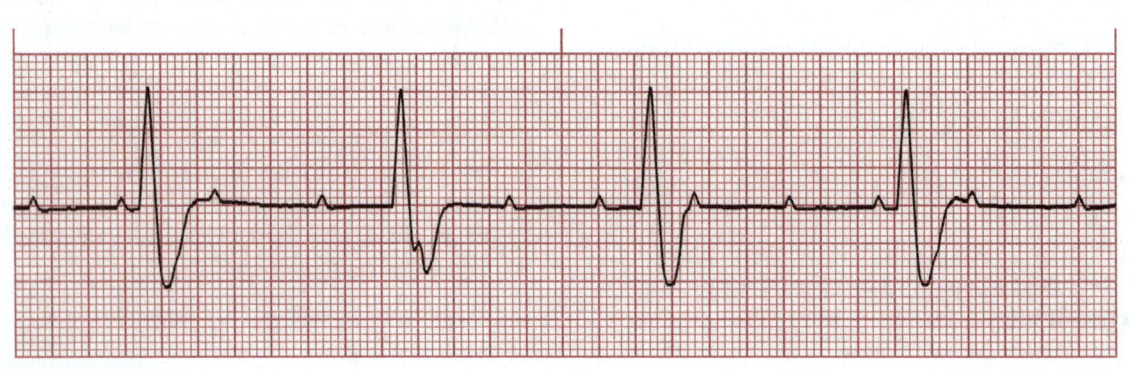

FIGURE 25.17 Third-degree atrioventricular block.

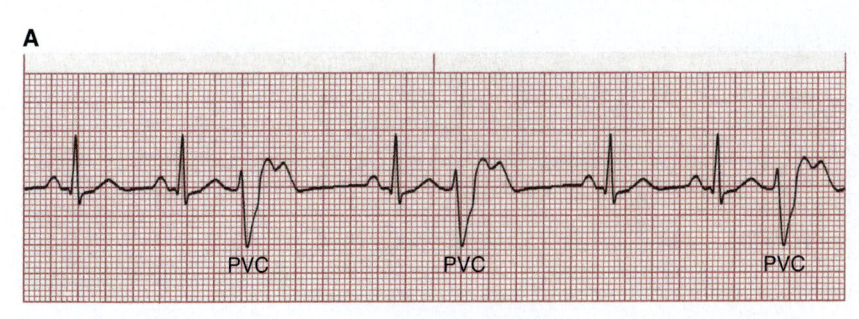

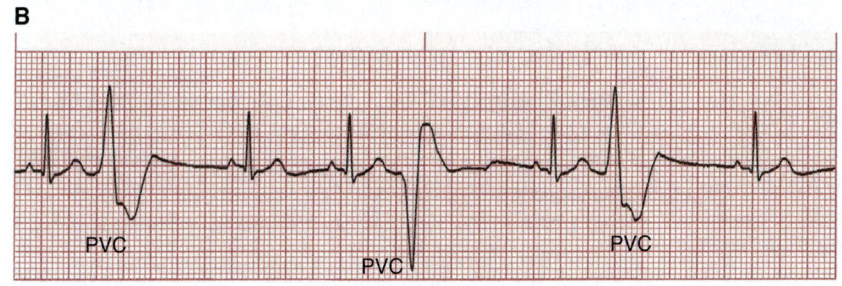

FIGURE 25.18 Premature ventricular contractions. (A) Unifocal PVCs arise from one foci (area) and look the same. (B) Multifocal PVCs arise from different foci and may look different.

must produce electrical impulses to cause the ventricles to contract, or else cardiac arrest will occur. Depending on the origin of the escape beat, the QRS complex will be either narrow (junctional) or wide (ventricular) on the ECG. Normal P waves march across the ECG strip at a constant P-to-P interval without any relationship to the regularly occurring but slower QRS complexes on the ECG.

ETIOLOGY. Cardiac ischemia or infarction, **hyperkalemia** (elevated serum potassium), infection, antiarrhythmic medications, or digoxin toxicity are some common causes of CHB.

SIGNS AND SYMPTOMS. Typically, severe symptoms are seen. These include confusion, dyspnea, severe chest pain, hypotension, or syncope. With narrow QRS complex escape rhythms, fewer symptoms occur. They include dizziness, chest pain, and fatigue.

THIRD-DEGREE ATRIOVENTRICULAR BLOCK RULES
1. Rhythm: P-to-P interval regular; R-to-R interval regular; atria and ventricles controlled by separate electrical impulses from foci that are firing regularly
2. Heart rate: Atrial 60 to 100 bpm; ventricular rate slower: 40 to 60 bpm is junctional foci; 20 to 35 bpm is ventricular foci
3. P waves: Rounded, upright, alike; more P waves than QRS complexes; may occur within a QRS complex or upon a T wave
4. PRI: No P waves conducted to the ventricles, so no relationship to the QRS complexes; therefore, there is no actual PRI (may appear as if the PRI varies)
5. QRS interval: 0.06 to 0.10 seconds (junctional origin); greater than 0.10 (ventricular origin)

THERAPEUTIC MEASURES. CHB is a medical emergency. Treatment is based on the level of the block in the heart. Atropine is considered. If the patient is symptomatic, transcutaneous pacing is needed immediately. Depending on the cause, a permanent pacemaker may be required for the rest of the patient's life. A temporary pacemaker may be used until the permanent pacemaker can be implanted. If medication toxicity is the cause, the CHB may be gone after the toxicity is resolved. A temporary pacemaker may be needed until this occurs.

CUE RECOGNITION 25.1

You are caring for a patient who displays complete heart block with a wide QRS complex escape rhythm on the continuous ECG and reports dyspnea and severe chest pain. What action do you take?

Suggested answers are at the end of the chapter.

Ventricular Arrhythmias

Premature ventricular contractions (PVCs) originate in the ventricles from an ectopic focus (a site other than the SA node). The irritable ventricles fire prematurely, before the SA node does. When the ventricles fire first, the impulses are not conducted normally through the electrical pathway. This results in a wide (greater than 0.10 seconds), bizarre QRS complex (Fig. 25.18).

PVCs can occur in different shapes. **Unifocal** (one focus) PVCs all look the same. This is because they come from the same irritable ventricular area. **Multifocal** (multiple foci) PVCs do not all look the same because they are originating from several irritable areas in the ventricle.

There can be several repetitive cycles or patterns of PVCs:

- **Bigeminy** occurs every other beat (a normal beat and then a PVC; Fig. 25.19).

• WORD • BUILDING •
hyperkalemia: hyper—above + kalium—potassium + emia—blood

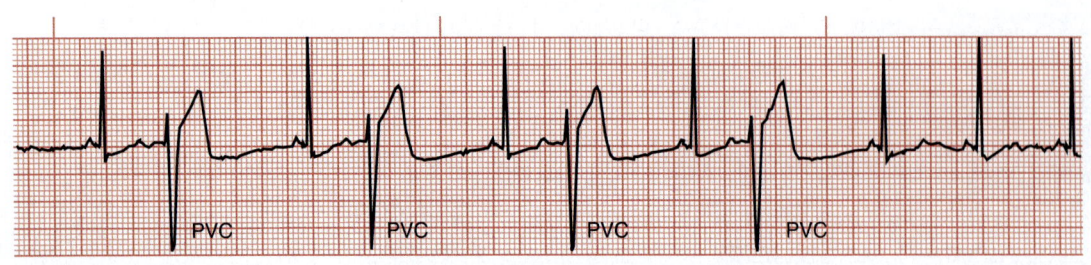

FIGURE 25.19 Bigeminal premature ventricular contractions.

- **Trigeminy** occurs every third beat (two normal beats and then a PVC).
- **Quadrigeminy** occurs every fourth beat (three normal beats and then a PVC).
- When two PVCs occur together, they are referred to as a *couplet* (pair).
- If three or more PVCs occur in a row, it is referred to as a *run* of PVCs, or ventricular tachycardia.

ETIOLOGY. Anxiety, use of caffeine or alcohol, cardiomyopathy, hypokalemia, ischemia, and MI are common causes of PVCs.

PREMATURE VENTRICULAR CONTRACTION RULES
1. Rhythm: Depends on the underlying rhythm; PVC usually interrupts rhythm
2. Heart rate: Depends on underlying rhythm
3. P waves: Absent before the PVC QRS complex
4. PRI: None for PVC
5. QRS interval: In a PVC, is greater than 0.10 seconds; T wave is in the opposite direction of QRS complex (i.e., QRS upright, T downward; or QRS downward, T upright)

SIGNS AND SYMPTOMS. PVCs may be felt by the patient. They are described as a skipped beat or palpitations. With frequent PVCs, cardiac output can be decreased. This leads to fatigue, dizziness, or more severe arrhythmias.

THERAPEUTIC MEASURES. Treatment depends on the type and number of PVCs and whether symptoms are produced. Occasional PVCs do not usually require treatment. However, if the PVCs are more than six per minute, regularly occurring, multifocal, falling on the T wave (known as *R-on-T phenomenon*, which can trigger life-threatening arrhythmias), or caused by an acute MI, they can be dangerous. Typically, a beta blocker or sometimes a calcium channel blocker is used to treat PVC symptoms (see Table 25.2). Antiarrhythmic medications can be used if these are ineffective.

CLINICAL JUDGMENT

Mrs. Zhang, age 74, is 4 days postmyocardial infarction without complications. You assist her back to bed after she ambulates at 1400 hours. Her oxygen is on at 2 L/min via nasal cannula. Her vital signs are blood pressure 126/78 mm Hg, apical pulse 82 bpm, and respiratory rate 18 breaths per minute. She has no pain and says she feels good after walking. The cardiac monitor shows normal sinus rhythm. Five minutes later, you see that the monitor shows sinus rhythm with premature ventricular contractions of less than six per minute. Her vital signs are now blood pressure 132/84 mm Hg, apical pulse 92 bpm (regularly irregular), and respiratory rate 22 breaths per minute. She reports no pain but says, "I can feel my heart skipping. It takes my breath away."

1. What do you do first?
2. What do you do regarding the arrhythmia?
3. As you collect data, what symptoms do you look for?
4. What do you do if symptoms are present?
5. What causes do you consider for this arrhythmia?
6. With which health-care team members do you collaborate?
7. How do you document your findings?
8. What do you remain vigilant for?

Suggested answers are at the end of the chapter.

Ventricular Tachycardia

The occurrence of three or more PVCs in a row is referred to as **ventricular tachycardia** (VT; Fig. 25.20). VT results from the continuous firing of an ectopic ventricular focus. During VT, the ventricles rather than the SA node become the pacemaker of the heart. The pathway of the ventricular impulses is different from the normal conduction pathway, so it produces a wide (greater than 0.10 seconds), bizarre QRS complex.

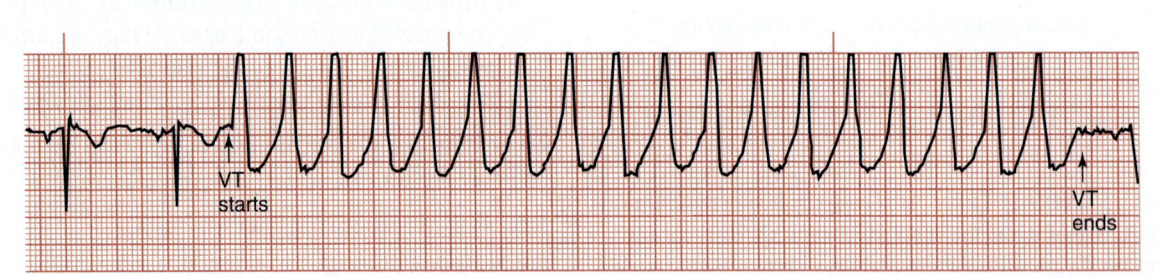

FIGURE 25.20 Ventricular tachycardia.

ETIOLOGY. Myocardial irritability, MI, and cardiomyopathy are common causes of VT. Respiratory acidosis, hypokalemia, digoxin toxicity, cardiac catheters, and pacing wires can also produce VT.

VENTRICULAR TACHYCARDIA RULES
1. Rhythm: Usually regular, may have some irregularity
2. Heart rate: 150 to 250 ventricular bpm; slow VT is below 150 bpm
3. P waves: Absent
4. PRI: None
5. QRS interval: Greater than 0.10 seconds

SIGNS AND SYMPTOMS. Patients are aware of a sudden onset of rapid heart rate. They can experience dyspnea, palpitations, and lightheadedness. Angina commonly occurs. The seriousness of VT is determined by the duration of the arrhythmia. Sustained VT compromises cardiac output. It can become pulseless VT, a life-threatening rhythm.

Evidence-Based Practice

Clinical Question
What is the best method for bystander CPR on an adult?

Evidence
A systematic review of 42 studies that included 32 randomized control trials identified interventions associated with improved quality of bystander CPR such as telephone-dispatcher assisted CPR with instructions, compression-only CPR, or heel of the hand only when the rescuer is tiring. Compression-only CPR had better CPR quality than conventional CPR because compression-only CPR provided more chest compressions, less hands-off time, and less time to first compression. Devices providing real-time feedback and mobile devices containing CPR applications or software were found to be beneficial, although they could cause a delay in CPR onset (Chen et al, 2019).

Implications for Nursing Practice
Encourage patients and their families to become certified in basic life support to be able to respond to an emergency.

Reference: Chen, K., Ko, Y., Hsieh, M., Chiang, W., Ma, M., & Lin, S. (2019). Interventions to improve quality of bystander cardiopulmonary resuscitation: A systematic review. *PloS One, 14*(2), e0211792. https://doi.org/10.1371/journal.pone.0211792

THERAPEUTIC MEASURES. For a patient who is stable, antiarrhythmic medications are used. If the patient is pulseless or not breathing, cardiopulmonary resuscitation (CPR) and immediate **defibrillation** are required (see "Evidence-Based Practice"). Advanced cardiac life support (ACLS) protocols for pulseless VT treatment are used. Medications may include epinephrine and amiodarone (see Table 25.2).

CRITICAL THINKING & CLINICAL JUDGMENT

Mrs. Parker, age 76, is admitted to the long-term care unit where you are working. She has been transferred from the hospital after treatment for a recent MI and several episodes of ventricular tachycardia (VT). At 1600 hours, you find her unresponsive, with no palpable pulses and with shallow respirations. Vital signs are blood pressure 60/20 mm Hg, apical pulse 160 bpm, and respiratory rate 6 breaths per minute.

Critical Thinking (The Why)
1. Why are there no palpable pulses?
2. What is happening to the heart when VT is occurring?

Clinical Judgment (The Do)
1. What action do you take?
2. How do you document your findings?

Suggested answers are at the end of the chapter.

Ventricular Fibrillation
Ventricular fibrillation (VF) occurs when many ectopic ventricular foci fire at the same time. Ventricular activity is chaotic. There are no discernible waves (Fig. 25.21). The ventricle quivers. It is unable to initiate a contraction. There is a complete loss of cardiac output. If this rhythm is not corrected immediately, death occurs.

ETIOLOGY. Hyperkalemia, **hypomagnesemia** (low serum magnesium), electrocution, coronary artery disease, and MI are all possible causes of VF. Placement of intracardiac catheters and cardiac pacing wires can also lead to ventricular irritability and then VF.

VENTRICULAR FIBRILLATION RULES
1. Rhythm: Chaotic and extremely irregular
2. Heart rate: Not measurable
3. P waves: None
4. PRI: None
5. QRS complex: None

SIGNS AND SYMPTOMS. Patients experiencing VF lose consciousness immediately. There are no heart sounds, peripheral pulses, or blood pressure readings. These are all indicative of circulatory collapse. Respiratory arrest, cyanosis, and pupil dilation occur.

THERAPEUTIC MEASURES. Immediate defibrillation is the best treatment for terminating VF. Each minute that passes without defibrillation reduces survival. CPR is started until the defibrillator is available. Automatic external defibrillators provide quick access to easily used technology for defibrillation (see "Defibrillation" section). Endotracheal intubation

• WORD • BUILDING •

hypomagnesemia: hypo—below + magnes—magnesium + emia—blood

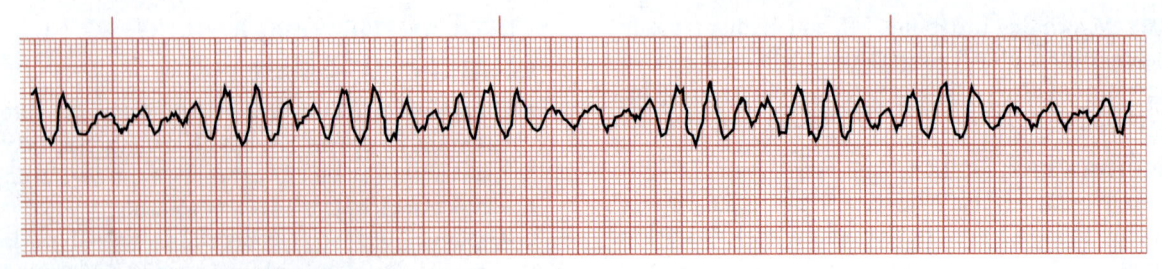

FIGURE 25.21 Ventricular fibrillation.

with oxygen supports respiratory function. Medications are given according to ACLS protocols. They include epinephrine and amiodarone (see Table 25.2).

Asystole
Asystole (the silent heart) is the absence of electrical activity within the cardiac muscle. It is referred to as *cardiac arrest*. A flat or straight line appears on an ECG strip (Fig. 25.22).

ETIOLOGY. Hyperkalemia, VF, or a loss of a majority of functional cardiac muscle due to an MI are common causes of asystole. VF usually precedes asystole. VF must be reversed immediately to help prevent progression to asystole.

ASYSTOLE RULES
1. Rhythm: None
2. Heart rate: None
3. P waves: None
4. PRI: None
5. QRS interval: None

SIGNS AND SYMPTOMS. Patients in asystole are unconscious and unresponsive. There are no heart sounds, peripheral pulses, blood pressure readings, or respirations.

THERAPEUTIC MEASURES. CPR is started immediately. Endotracheal intubation and oxygen support respiration. Epinephrine is administered per ACLS protocols (see Table 25.2). Reversible causes are treated.

CARDIAC PACEMAKERS

Pacemakers are used to generate an electrical impulse when there is a problem with the heart's conduction system.

Temporary Pacemaker
Temporary pacemakers treat bradycardia or tachycardia (overdrive pacing) that does not respond to medications or synchronized cardioversion. They may also be used after an MI to allow the heart time to heal. The temporary pacemaker becomes the electrical conduction system. It stimulates the atria and ventricles to contract, which maintains cardiac output. Temporary pacemakers can be inserted during valve or open-heart surgery (epicardial). They can also be used in the cardiac catheterization laboratory or critical care unit (CCU; transvenous) for emergency treatment. They are kept in place until surgery can be scheduled to implant a permanent pacemaker. Transcutaneous pacemakers are used in emergency situations. They are quick and easy to apply. Impulses are delivered from the external generator via electrodes on the skin to the heart. The electrodes are placed on the chest and back.

Permanent Pacemaker
Permanent pacemakers are used for symptomatic bradycardia and third-degree AV block (complete dissociation between atrial and ventricular activity). Permanent pacemaker implantation is a procedure in which **fluoroscopy**, a screen that shows an image similar to a radiograph, is used. The pacemaker generator is implanted subcutaneously. It is attached to leads (insulated conducting wires) that are inserted via a vein into the heart. The lead then delivers an impulse directly to the heart wall. A single-lead pacemaker paces either the right atrium or right ventricle into which it is placed. Dual-chamber pacemakers have two leads (Fig. 25.23). One is in the right atrium, and the other is in the right ventricle. This allows pacing of both chambers. Activity-responsive pacemakers provide a rate range (e.g., 60 to 115 bpm). They allow rate changes in response to a person's activity level. This provides the patient with greater flexibility for increasing cardiac output when needed, such as during exercise.

Leadless Pacemaker
The leadless permanent pacemaker was approved in 2016 (visit www.medtronic.com). It is inserted via a leg vein, so no chest incision is needed for implantation into the right ventricle, without leads. Everything is contained within the

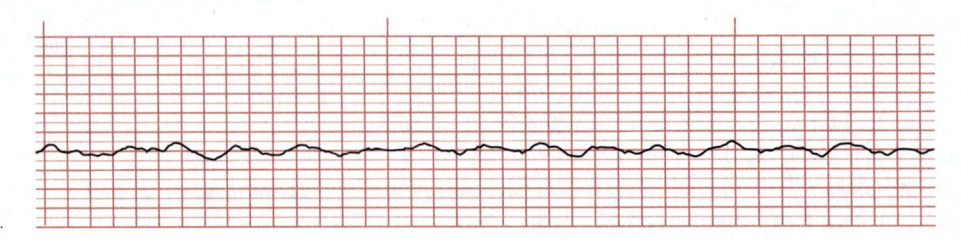

FIGURE 25.22 Asystole.

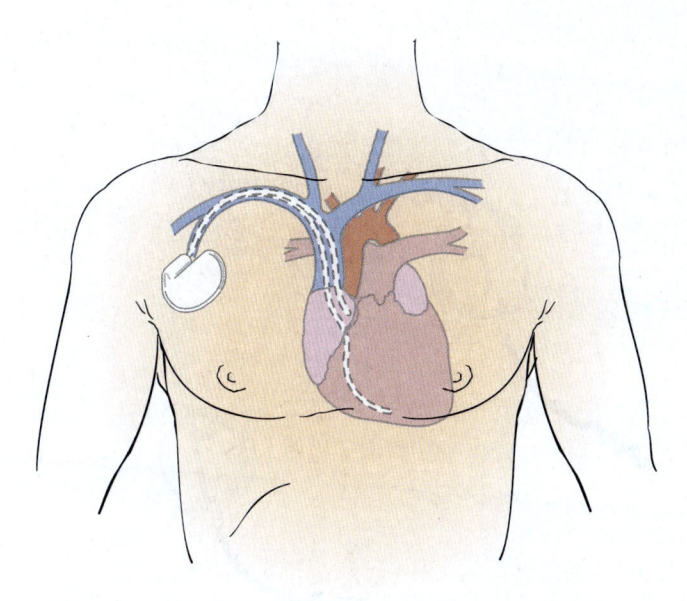

FIGURE 25.23 Dual-chamber permanent pacemaker.

pacemaker, which is about the size of a vitamin capsule. The battery lasts about 8 to 12 years. Few complications occur with this type of pacemaker.

Pacemaker Activity

When a patient is in a paced rhythm, a small spike (vertical line) is seen on the ECG at the start of the paced beat. This spike is the electrical stimulus. It can precede the P wave, QRS complex, or both depending on what is being paced (Fig. 25.24). Patients may have 100% paced beats, a mixture of their own beats and paced beats, or 100% their own beats. Pacemakers should not fire during a patients' own beat to prevent complications.

Problems that can occur with pacemakers include the following:

- Failure to sense a patient's own beat
- Failure to pace because of a malfunction of the pulse generator
- Failure to capture, which is the heart's lack of depolarization (turn patient onto left side)

Nursing Care for Patients With Pacemakers

Patients' heart rhythm, apical pulse, and incision are monitored after implantation of a pacemaker. Irregular heart rhythms or a rate slower than the pacemaker's set rate can indicate pacemaker malfunction. Any change in heart rhythm, reports of chest pain, or changes in vital signs are reported to the HCP immediately. The patient may have outpatient surgery or remain in the hospital overnight.

Pacemaker teaching before discharge includes the following:

- Care for an incision as instructed (e.g., dressing removal, keeping it clean and dry, resuming showers).
- Maintain ordered activity restrictions (e.g., limit raising arm on pacemaker side, driving, returning to work).

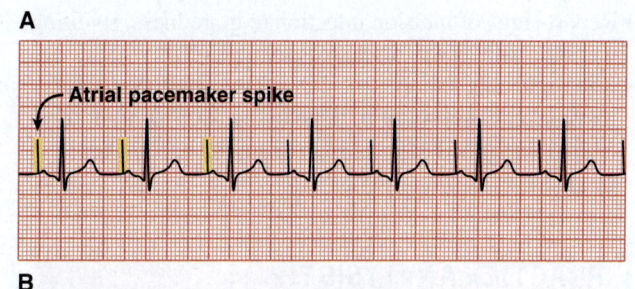

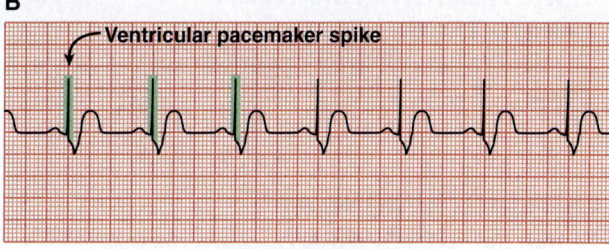

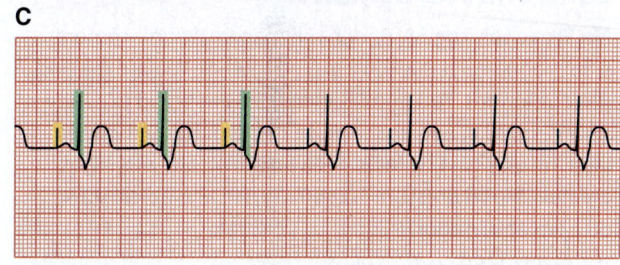

FIGURE 25.24 ECG tracings. (A) Atrial-only pacemaker (yellow spike before P wave). (B) Ventricular-only pacemaker (green spike before QRS). (C) Dual-chamber pacemaker that paces both atrial and ventricular chambers (yellow spike before P and green spike before QRS).

- Be aware of other devices:
  - Safe devices: microwaves, most cell phones if not held too closely to the cardiac device, Bluetooth headset, most common household devices.
  - Caution to be used with devices: antitheft systems, some cell phones with more magnets, security metal detectors (avoid having a hand wand passed over the pacemaker), MP3 player headphones, extracorporeal shock-wave lithotripsy.
  - Devices with possible risk: strong electromagnetic fields (magnetic resonance imaging with a cardiac device requires evaluation to determine if it is safe; newer pacing systems and cardiac devices are designed for use with MRI, such as the complete Revo MRI SureScan pacing system), welders above 130 amps, radio towers, or touching running car engines (information is available on the pacemaker manufacturer and AHA Web sites regarding various devices).
  - If you become lightheaded or dizzy near an electromagnetic device, move away from it.
- Carry a pacemaker identification card to show to HCPs, airport security, or other security staff. Pacemaker metal may set off alarms, but the device is not harmed if one walks normally through the security device.
- Report chest pain, dizziness, fainting, irregular heartbeats, palpitations, muscle twitching, or hiccups to the HCP.

- Report signs of incision infection (e.g., redness, swelling, warmth, pain, fever, discharge) to the HCP.
- Keep scheduled appointments with the HCP. Periodic pacemaker checks will be done by the HCP or remotely from home. The HCP can reprogram the pacemaker if needed.

> **PRACTICE ANALYSIS TIP**
> **Linking NCLEX-PN® to Practice**
> The LPN/LVN will assist in the care of a client with a pacing device.

> **CRITICAL THINKING & CLINICAL JUDGEMENT**
>
> **Mr. Treacher,** age 58, underwent pacemaker placement 6 days ago and has a 100% paced rhythm. You are making patient rounds. You find his vital signs are blood pressure 138/72 mm Hg and apical pulse 72 bpm. Thirty minutes later, he says that he feels weak and tired. His vital signs are now blood pressure 100/60 mm Hg and apical pulse 60 bpm and irregular.
>
> **Critical Thinking (The Why)**
> 1. What might be happening to Mr. Treacher?
>
> **Clinical Judgment (The Do)**
> 2. What action do you take first?
> 3. What actions do you take next?
> 4. What interventions do you anticipate?
>
> *Suggested answers are at the end of the chapter.*

DEFIBRILLATION

Defibrillation is a lifesaving procedure used for pulseless VT or VF. It delivers an electrical shock to attempt to reset the heart's rhythm. Self-adhesive pads (saline or with conductive jelly) are placed on the patient's chest. They prevent electrical burns and promote conduction of the electrical charge. The defibrillator is charged, then the paddles are pressed firmly and evenly against the chest wall to prevent burns or electrical arcing (Fig. 25.25). For safety, the person who is defibrillating must announce "Clear." The phrase "One. I'm clear. Two. You're clear. Three. All clear" is suggested. No one, including the person defibrillating, should touch the bed or patient during this time to avoid being shocked. ACLS protocols specify guidelines for resuscitation.

After successful defibrillation, the patient is checked for a pulse and adequate tissue perfusion. The patient is treated in the CCU after successful resuscitation.

Emotional support for an alert patient who experiences cardiac arrest and defibrillation is an important aspect of nursing care. This can be an extremely frightening event for the patient. It is important to explain to the patient what

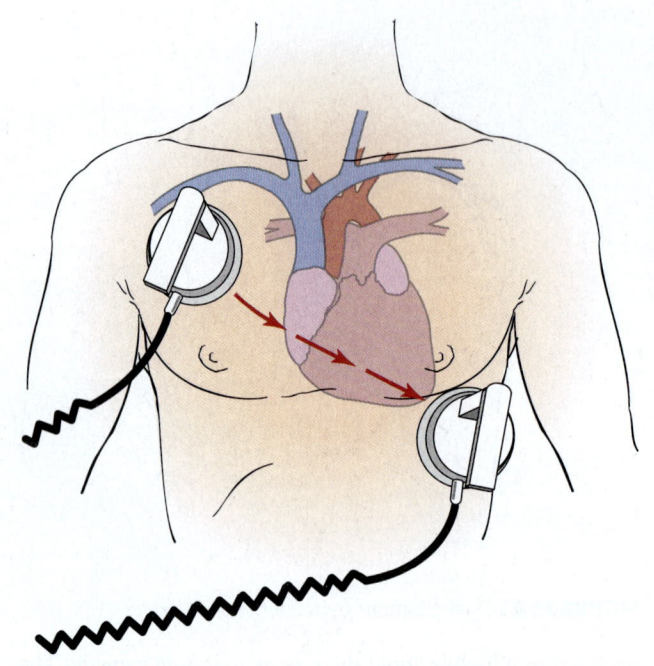

FIGURE 25.25 Placement of defibrillator paddles on chest.

happened. Then listen and allow them to express concerns. The patient is reassured that continuous cardiac monitoring will be done in the CCU. Families also require emotional support during resuscitation of a loved one. They may be present during the resuscitation per agency policy.

CARDIOVERSION

Cardioversion is performed with a defibrillator set in the synchronized mode. In the synchronized mode, a mark is highlighted on the patient's R waves. The R wave must be recognized for a shock to be delivered. When the discharge button is pressed, the shock is released when the machine senses it is safe to do so. The number of joules delivered with each shock usually ranges from 25 to 50. The procedure for delivering the shock safely is the same as for defibrillation.

Synchronized cardioversion is used for VT with a pulse. Elective synchronized cardioversion is used for arrhythmias that are not responsive to medication therapy. These include AF, atrial flutter, and supraventricular tachycardia. The patient is given a sedative and monitored by anesthesia professionals during the procedure.

If cardioversion is successful, there should be a return to NSR. If the rhythm does not immediately convert, additional cardioversion attempts can be made by the HCP. After the procedure, the patient is monitored for skin burns, rhythm disturbances and changes in the ST segment, vital sign changes and hypotension, and respiratory problems.

• WORD • BUILDING •

defibrillation: de—from + fibrillation—quivering fibers

Chapter 25 Nursing Care of Patients With Cardiac Arrhythmias

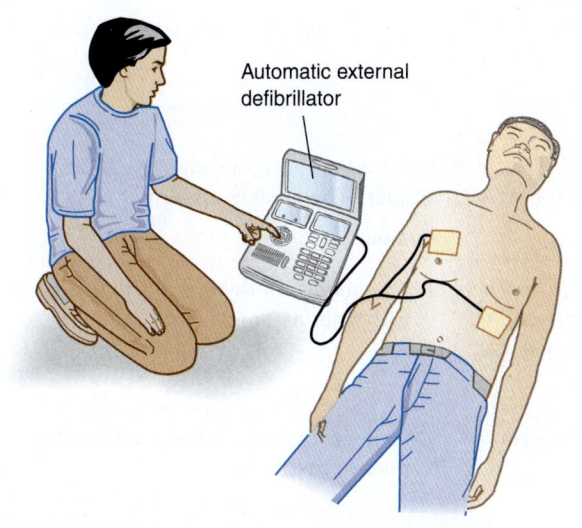

FIGURE 25.26 Automatic external defibrillator.

OTHER METHODS TO CORRECT ARRHYTHMIAS

Automatic External Defibrillators

An automatic external defibrillator (AED) is an external device that automatically analyzes rhythms. For VF or VT, it will either automatically deliver or prompt the operator to deliver an electrical shock for a shockable rhythm (Fig. 25.26). Minimally trained laypersons or hospital and rescue personnel can use these devices with little risk of injury to the patient because the AED, not the operator, analyzes the rhythm. The patient is connected to the AED with adhesive sternal-apex pads attached to cables coming from the device. This connection allows hands-free defibrillation.

AEDs are found in public places such as shopping malls, airports, stadiums, casinos, golf courses, and airplanes for immediate access. Defibrillation attempts must occur within minutes of cardiac arrest to increase chance of survival. AEDs are available for home use. They are recommended for people at high risk of sudden cardiac arrest. They are helpful for those at risk with rescue access that will take longer than 4 minutes, such as people living in rural areas, gated communities, or secured-access buildings.

> **CUE RECOGNITION 25.2**
>
> You are caring for a resident who becomes unconscious and collapses onto the bed while standing. What action do you take?
>
> *Suggested answers are at the end of the chapter.*

Cardioverter Defibrillator

A wearable cardioverter defibrillator (WCD) vest next to the skin (see https://lifevest.zoll.com) or implantable cardioverter defibrillator (ICD) or a combination pacemaker/ICD is used for patients who are at risk for sudden cardiac death or experience rapid life-threatening arrhythmias. These devices have decreased the number of deaths from these arrhythmias by analyzing and treating these heart rhythms. When a rapid life-threatening rhythm is detected that could cause death (VF), the WCD/ICD automatically delivers an electrical shock. If the arrhythmia does not convert on the initial shock, more shocks are delivered sequentially. If a device detects VT, it can cardiovert the rhythm with lower energy.

ICDs also have antitachycardia pacing ability if tachycardia rhythm is detected. ICD battery life depends on use. When battery life is low, the entire unit must be changed within a few months.

Patients with these devices can be extremely anxious about receiving shocks from them. Defibrillator or cardioversion shocks may feel like a kick in the chest. Reinforcement of patient and family education is important. To prevent problems, those with these devices should take the same precautions as discussed earlier for those with pacemakers. Provide emotional support and answer questions.

NURSING PROCESS FOR THE PATIENT WITH ARRHYTHMIAS

Data Collection

Patients at risk for arrhythmias require careful monitoring. Obtaining apical and radial pulses at frequent intervals helps detect arrhythmias. Most arrhythmias are not life threatening. A patient's report of chest pain, dizziness, or palpitations should be investigated and reported to the HCP.

Nursing Diagnoses, Planning, Implementation, and Evaluation

See "Nursing Care Plan for the Patient With Arrhythmias."

Assist the patient and family in understanding the plan of care and the reasons for the interventions. Allow them to express needs and fears. Family members are taught CPR or given information on local CPR classes, which gives them a sense of control and hope. If CPR is needed, the family can act instead of feeling helpless. The patient may feel more secure knowing that immediate help from family members is available until emergency medical help arrives.

Nursing Care Plan for the Patient With Arrhythmias

Nursing Diagnosis: Decreased Cardiac Output related to arrhythmias
Expected Outcomes: The patient's cardiac status will be stabilized. Patient will be able to perform activities of daily living (ADLs).
Evaluation of Outcomes: There is an absence of arrhythmias. The patient performs ADLs without tachycardia, chest pain, or weakness.

Intervention	Rationale	Evaluation
Monitor apical pulse, blood pressure, lung sounds, urinary output, and mental status with frequency based on stability.	*Identifies arrhythmias, heart failure, impending cardiac arrest, or shock. Dizziness, confusion, and restlessness may indicate decreased cerebral blood flow.*	Is patient free of arrhythmias with vital signs within normal limits?
Ensure that patient receives assistance with ADLs as needed and does not exceed activity tolerance.	*Reduces dyspnea and decreases oxygen demand on the myocardium.*	Does patient tolerate activity without dyspnea or chest pain?

Geriatric

Intervention	Rationale	Evaluation
Administer antiarrhythmic medications as ordered and observe for adverse reactions.	*Older patients may have decreased kidney and liver function that may lead to rapid development of toxicity.*	Does patient have signs of medication toxicity?

Nursing Diagnosis: Anxiety related to situational crisis
Expected Outcomes: The patient will be able to effectively manage anxiety. The patient will report decreased anxiety.
Evaluation of Outcomes: The patient uses effective coping mechanisms to manage anxiety. Patient expresses decreased anxiety.

Intervention	Rationale	Evaluation
Ask patient and family to identify anxiety and verbalize concerns.	*Helps correct and clarify their concerns.*	What are patient's feelings or concerns?
Explain procedures to patient and family.	*Lack of knowledge increases anxiety. This knowledge will help with compliance of therapy.*	Does patient express understanding of therapy with decreased anxiety?
Reinforce teaching of relaxation techniques such as guided imagery, muscle relaxation, and meditation.	*These measures can restore psychological and physical equilibrium and help decrease anxiety.*	Is patient successful in demonstrating relaxation techniques?

Home Health Hints

- Always have a pocket mask for cardiopulmonary resuscitation available.
- Patients prone to arrhythmias should avoid straining with bowel movements. If the patient reports straining, request a laxative or stool softener order from the HCP.
- Reinforce teaching if patient is on beta blockers and inotropic agents (e.g., digoxin) on how to take a radial pulse, because bradycardia is a major side effect. If pulse is below 60 bpm, inform the patient to call the HCP.
- Reinforce teaching for patients with a new implanted pacemaker to wear loose tops for comfort. Women can wear a small pad over the pacemaker to cushion it from a bra strap.
- Reinforce teaching for patients who are going to travel to refill medicines ahead of time.

Key Points

- The six-step process for arrhythmia interpretation includes checking regularity of the rhythm, heart rate, P waves, P-R interval, QRS interval, and QT-interval.
- An arrhythmia (or dysrhythmia) is an abnormal rhythm of the heart. They occur from disturbances in the formation of an impulse or in the conduction of the impulse.
- Treatment for bradycardia includes IV atropine; for tachycardia above 150 beats per minute includes adenosine, beta blockers, or calcium channel blockers; for atrial flutter in symptomatic patients, catheter ablation.
- Treatment for AF includes rate control with beta blockers or calcium channel blockers, pharmacological or electrical rhythm conversion, and anticoagulant therapy to reduce thrombi and stroke risk.
- CHB is a medical emergency. If the patient is symptomatic, transcutaneous pacing is needed immediately until a permanent pacemaker can be implanted.
- PVCs are treated when there are more than six per minute; they are regularly occurring, multifocal, or falling on the T wave (which can trigger life-threatening arrhythmias); or are caused by an acute MI. A beta blocker, calcium channel blocker, or antiarrhythmic medication is prescribed if needed.
- Immediate defibrillation is the best treatment for terminating VF. Each minute that passes without defibrillation reduces survival. CPR is started until the defibrillator is available.
- For VF or VT, an AED analyzes the rhythm, and either automatically delivers or prompts the operator to deliver an electrical shock.
- A WCD or ICD or a combination pacemaker/ICD is used for a patient who experiences life-threatening arrhythmias or is at risk for sudden cardiac death.

SUGGESTED ANSWERS TO CHAPTER EXERCISES

Cue Recognition

25.1: Activate your agency's resuscitation team (i.e., call a code). Obtain vital signs. Remain with the patient and provide emotional support.

25.2: Consider resident's advance directive. Then follow the ABCs, request an AED, and begin CPR as needed until AED arrives. Attach AED and follow prompts.

Critical Thinking & Clinical Judgment

Mrs. Zhang

1. You call the registered nurse (RN) or HCP while staying with the patient to provide reassurance.
2. Obtain vital signs and heart sounds, note symptoms, and obtain an ECG per agency protocol.
3. Symptoms might include lightheadedness, feeling of heart skipping, chest pain, or fatigue.
4. To alleviate symptoms, elevate the head of bed for comfort, monitor vital signs, and maintain oxygen at 2 L/min via nasal cannula per agency protocol. Remain with the patient to help alleviate anxiety. Notify the RN.
5. Possible causes include hypokalemia or ischemia leading to irritability of the heart.
6. RN, HCP, respiratory therapist.
7. Documentation should include the following:
   - 1400: Ambulated 20 feet with one assist. Vital signs stable. Stated: "Feel good. Pain zero."
   - Tolerated well. Assisted to bed. Oxygen at 2 L/min via nasal cannula.
   - 1405: See ECG strip with intermittent PVCs. Vital signs: BP 132/84 mm Hg; apical 92 bpm, irregular; R 22 breaths per minute.
   - "Pain zero. I can feel my heart skipping, it takes my breath away." RN notified.
8. Arrhythmias, hypotension, decreased oxygen saturation, chest pain

Mrs. Parker

1. A heart in VT has an ectopic focus that is initiating impulses. The heart is unable to maintain adequate cardiac output with such a rapid heart rate. The rapid and irregular heart rhythm does not allow the heart chambers time to adequately fill and empty, thereby reducing the blood volume with each beat. This in turn affects the peripheral circulation, causing the absence of palpable pulses.
2. In VT, one or more sites in the ventricle may be initiating impulses. The rapid rate of VT overrides the normal pacemaker of the heart. The rhythm can be regular or irregular. The inability of the heart to conduct impulses along normal pathways prevents the chambers from emptying and filling properly. This leads to a decreased cardiac output and can lead to cardiac arrest if the rhythm is not converted.
3. Understand advance directive status. Begin cardiopulmonary resuscitation (CPR), if applicable. Call for assistance and have 911 called.
4. Documentation should include the following: 1600: Patient found in bed unresponsive to verbal and tactile stimuli. Respirations shallow. No palpable pulses. BP 60/20 mm Hg, P 160 bpm, R 6 breaths per minute. CPR initiated. RN arrived at 1602 and 911 called.

Mr. Treacher
1. Mr. Treacher could be experiencing pacemaker malfunction.
2. Your first actions should be to obtain an ECG per agency protocol and to notify the RN or HCP. The emergency number 911 may need to be called.
3. Next, keep the head of the bed elevated and administer oxygen at 2 L/min via nasal cannula per protocol. Turn the patient onto his left side, as this may help float the pacemaker wire to the chamber wall for better contact. Monitor the patient's vital signs and symptoms and remain with patient to provide emotional support.
4. Interventions may include transfer to a hospital emergency department for assessment and reprogramming of the pacemaker or a return to surgery for manipulation or replacement of the pacemaker wires.

Additional Resources

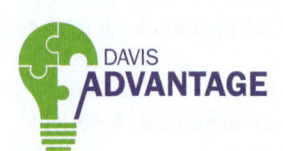

Go to Davis Advantage to complete your learning: strengthen understanding, apply your knowledge, and prepare for the Next Gen NCLEX®.

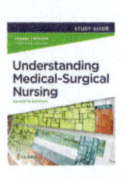

A Study Guide is also available.

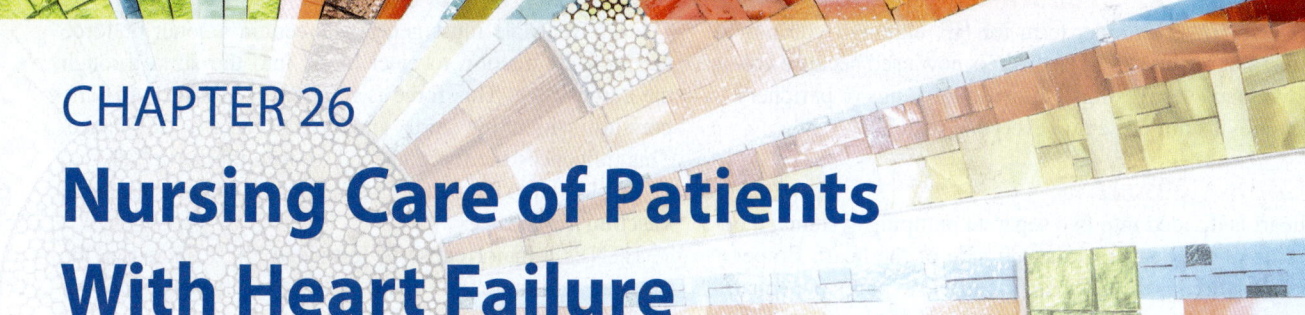

CHAPTER 26
Nursing Care of Patients With Heart Failure

Kathy Berchem

KEY TERMS

afterload (AF-ter-lohd)
cor pulmonale (KOR PUL-mah-NAH-lee)
cyanosis (SIGH-an-NOH-siss)
exertional dyspnea (ig-zur-shun-ul DISP-nee-ah)
hepatomegaly (HEP-ah-toh-MEH-gah-lee)
orthopnea (or-THOP-nee-ah)
paroxysmal nocturnal dyspnea (PEAR-ox-IS-mul knock-TURN-al DISP-nee-ah)
perfusion (pur-FEW-shun)
peripheral vascular resistance (puh-RIFF-uh-ruhl VAS-kyoo-lar ree-ZIS-tense)
preload (PREE-lohd)
pulmonary edema (PULL-muh-NARE-ee eh-DEE-muh)
splenomegaly (SPLEE-noh-MEG-ah-lee)

CHAPTER CONCEPTS

Caring
Collaboration
Comfort
Fluid and electrolytes
Oxygenation
Perfusion
Teaching and learning

LEARNING OUTCOMES

1. Describe the pathophysiology of left- and right-sided heart failure.
2. Define acute heart failure.
3. List causes of acute and chronic heart failure.
4. Identify the signs and symptoms of acute and chronic heart failure.
5. Plan nursing care for patients undergoing diagnostic tests for heart failure.
6. Explain the medical treatments used for acute and chronic heart failure.
7. Plan nursing care for acute and chronic heart failure.
8. Plan teaching for patients with heart failure and their families.

OVERVIEW OF HEART FAILURE

Heart failure (HF) is a clinical syndrome that affects **perfusion**. It occurs from the inability of the ventricle(s) to fill or pump enough blood to meet the body's oxygen and nutrient needs. It may cause dyspnea (shortness of breath), fatigue, and fluid volume overload. It can reduce the quality and length of life. The causes of HF are varied. They can include coronary artery disease (most often), myocardial infarction, cardiomyopathy, heart valve problems, and hypertension (HTN). Any heart problem can potentially lead to HF. In the older adult, the most common cause of HF is cardiac ischemia. HF may develop rapidly (acute), as with cardiogenic shock and pulmonary edema. It can also occur over time (chronic) as a result of another disorder. This could include HTN or pulmonary disease.

Incidences of HF are on the rise due to a growing aging population and treatment advances with better survival rates. According to the American Heart Association (AHA), an estimated 6.2 million people have HF with a million new cases each year. A total of 3.2 million women have HF; notably, black females have the highest incidence, prevalence, and mortality. In 2017, HF was the most common reason for hospital admission in older adults. Readmission rates for HF treatment are highest for those previously hospitalized for HF (Virani et al, 2020).

• WORD • BUILDING •
perfusion: per—throughout + fundere—pour

Congestive Heart Failure

Congestive HF is an older term for HF, although you may still hear it being used. The term *HF* is now used because volume overload ("congestion") either in the lungs or periphery (extremities) is not present in everyone with HF.

Pathophysiology

The heart is divided into two separate pumping systems: the right side of the heart and the left side of the heart. Proper cardiac functioning requires each ventricle to pump out equal amounts of blood over time. If the amount of blood returned to the heart becomes more than either ventricle can handle, the heart can no longer function effectively as a pump.

HF can be the result of systolic (contractile) dysfunction, diastolic (relaxation) dysfunction, or mixed systolic and diastolic dysfunction. Systolic dysfunction is a contractile problem in which the ventricle is unable to generate enough force to pump blood from the ventricle. Diastolic dysfunction is a problem with the ventricle's ability to relax and fill. Mixed systolic and diastolic dysfunction is a combination of the two defects.

> **LEARNING TIP**
> To understand HF, compare the failing heart to a dam in a river:
> - In a river without a dam, water flows freely; in the normal circulatory system, blood flows freely.
> - In a river with a dam, the water is blocked by the dam and builds up behind it; in HF, the failing ventricle acts like a dam in the river, causing blood to back up behind it.
> - If too much water builds up behind the dam, the riverbanks are flooded; in HF, when too much blood builds up behind a failing ventricle, either the lungs (pulmonary edema from left ventricular failure) or peripheral tissues (peripheral edema from right ventricular failure) are flooded.

Conditions causing HF can affect one or both of the heart's pumping systems. Therefore, HF can be classified as right-sided HF, left-sided HF, or biventricular HF. The left ventricle typically weakens first because it has the greatest workload in ejecting blood against the resistance in the aorta. The right and left sides of the heart's pumping system work together in a closed system. Failure of one side will usually lead to failure of the other side.

> **LEARNING TIP**
> To understand and see the effects of HF, trace the flow of blood backward from each ventricle. Along the backward path from the failing ventricle, congestion develops. This produces the signs and symptoms seen in HF. Understanding the backward path of congestion can help you identify the signs and symptoms of either right- or left-sided HF.

Left-Sided Heart Failure

The left ventricle must generate a certain amount of force during a contraction to eject blood into the aorta through the aortic valve. This force is referred to as **afterload**. The pressure within the aorta and arteries acts as resistance. This influences the force needed to open the aortic valve to pump blood into the aorta. This pressure is called **peripheral vascular resistance**.

HTN is a major cause of left-sided HF. It increases the pressure within arteries. This makes the left ventricle work harder to pump blood into the aorta. Over time, the strain caused by the increased workload causes the left ventricle to weaken and fail as an effective pump. See Table 26.1 for other causes of left-sided HF.

With left-sided HF, blood first backs up from the left ventricle into the left atrium. Then it backs up into the four pulmonary veins and lungs (Fig. 26.1). This increases pulmonary pressure. The pressure causes fluid to move into the interstitium and then into the alveoli. Alveolar edema is serious. It reduces gas exchange across the alveolar-capillary membrane, resulting in shortness of breath and cyanosis from decreased oxygenation of the blood. If the fluid buildup is severe, acute pulmonary edema occurs. This requires immediate medical treatment.

Right-Sided Heart Failure

Conditions causing right-sided HF increase the work of the right ventricle. They either increase the amount of contractile force needed or require pumping of excess blood

Table 26.1 Causes of Left-Sided Heart Failure

Cause	Primary Effect on Left Ventricular Workload
Aortic stenosis	Increased volume to pump from restricted blood outflow
Cardiomyopathy	Increased workload from impaired contractility
Coarctation of the aorta	Restricted outflow and increased resistance from narrowing of aorta
Hypertension	Resistance increased from elevated pressure
Heart muscle infection	Increased workload from damaged myocardium
Myocardial infarction	Increased workload from impaired contractility
Mitral regurgitation	Increased volume to pump from backward blood flow

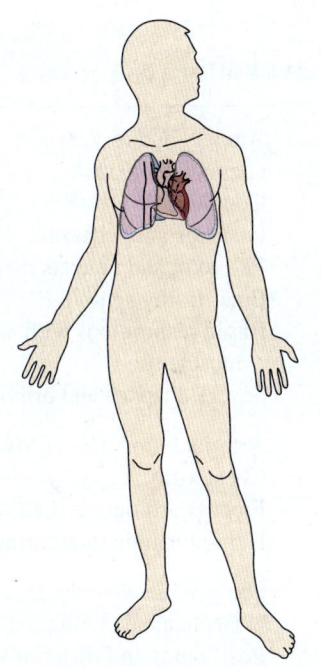

FIGURE 26.1 Left-sided heart failure. Shaded areas indicate areas of congestion from blood backup caused by the failing left side of the heart.

volume (**preload**). Causes of right-sided HF are described in Table 26.2. The major cause of right-sided HF is left-sided HF. When the left side fails, fluid backs up into the lungs. Pulmonary pressure is increased. The right ventricle must continually pump blood against this increased fluid and pressure. Over time, this strain causes it to weaken and fail as a pump. When the right ventricle hypertrophies (increases muscle mass) or fails from disorders of the lung, it is called **cor pulmonale**.

Table 26.2
Causes of Right-Sided Heart Failure

Cause	Primary Effect on Right Ventricular Workload
Atrial septal defect	Left atrial blood flow into right atrium increases right ventricular volume to pump
Cor pulmonale	Resistance increased from elevated pressure
Left-sided heart failure	Resistance increased from backup of fluid and elevated pressures
Pulmonary hypertension	Resistance increased from elevated pressure
Pulmonary valve stenosis	Increased volume to pump from restricted right ventricular blood outflow

When the right ventricle fails, it does not empty normally. A backward buildup of blood occurs in the systemic blood vessels. With the blood backed up from the right ventricle, right atrial and systemic venous blood volume increases, causing the jugular veins to become distended. Normally, they are not visible, but with the patient in a 45-degree upright position, the jugular vein distention can be seen. Edema may occur in the peripheral tissues. The abdominal organs can become distended (Fig. 26.2). Fluid congestion causes upset in the gastrointestinal (GI) tract. Anorexia, abdominal pain, and nausea can occur. As the right-sided failure progresses, blood pools in the hepatic veins. The liver becomes congested (**hepatomegaly**). Liver function is impaired. Pain occurs in the right upper quadrant of the abdomen. Systemic venous congestion also leads to distension of the spleen (**splenomegaly**).

> **LEARNING TIP**
> To understand the signs and symptoms of left-sided versus right-sided heart failure, remember that left-sided signs and symptoms are found in the lungs (Left = Lungs = L). Any signs and symptoms not related to the lungs are caused by right-sided failure.

COMPENSATORY MECHANISMS TO MAINTAIN CARDIAC OUTPUT

Compensatory mechanisms help ensure that enough blood is being pumped out of the heart. Although these mechanisms are designed to maintain cardiac output, they contribute to a cycle that, instead of being helpful, leads to further HF. Let's look at how that occurs.

When the sympathetic nervous system detects low cardiac output, it releases epinephrine and norepinephrine. This speeds up the heart rate (cardiac output = heart rate × stroke volume). Normally, this is helpful to maintain an adequate cardiac output. However, whenever the heart beats faster, the heart itself also requires more oxygen. The failing heart finds it difficult to supply this additional oxygen that it needs, thus worsening HF.

With a low cardiac output, blood flow to the kidneys is reduced. The kidneys activate the renin-angiotensin-aldosterone system to save water. Antidiuretic hormone is released from the pituitary gland to conserve water. Urine output decreases, which adds further fluid to the fluid retention problem already occurring in HF.

Over time, the heart responds to its increased workload by enlarging its chambers (dilation) and increasing its muscle mass (hypertrophy). This is known as *remodeling*. In dilation,

• WORD • BUILDING •
cor pulmonale: cor—heart + pulm—lung
hepatomegaly: hep—liver + mega—large
splenomegaly: splen—spleen + mega—large

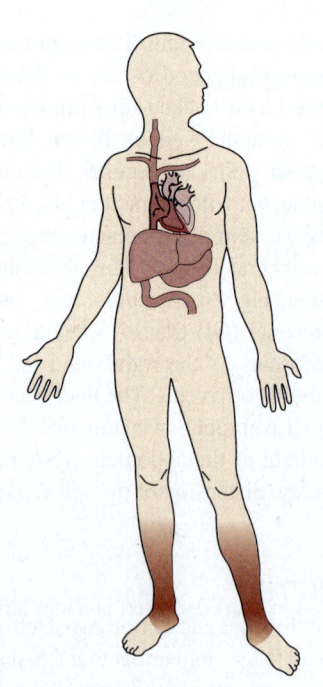

FIGURE 26.2 Right-sided heart failure. Shaded areas indicate areas of congestion from blood backup due to the failing right side of the heart.

Table 26.3
Acute Heart Failure Summary

Signs and Symptoms	Anxiety and restlessness Clammy, cold skin Coughing Crackles and wheezes Pale skin and mucous membranes Pink, frothy sputum Rapid respirations with accessory muscle use Severe dyspnea and orthopnea
Diagnostic Tests	Arterial blood gases (ABGs) Chest x-ray Electrocardiogram (ECG) Hemodynamic monitoring
Therapeutic Measures	Oxygen via cannula, mask, or mechanical ventilation Positioning in Fowler or semi-Fowler position Bedrest Frequent vital signs and urinary output Intravenous medication s (e.g., diuretics, inotropic agents, vasodilators) Treatment of underlying cause Daily weights
Priority Nursing Diagnoses	*Impaired Gas Exchange* *Decreased Cardiac Output* *Excess Fluid Volume*

the heart muscle fibers stretch, which increases the force of myocardial contractions. This stretch is known as the *Frank-Starling phenomenon*. In hypertrophy, the muscle mass of the heart increases, also creating more contractile force. Both compensatory mechanisms temporarily improve patient symptoms but also increase the heart's oxygen needs. As you now know, this further contributes to HF. In addition, the heart walls stiffen, reducing the heart's ability to effectively pump.

PULMONARY EDEMA (ACUTE HEART FAILURE)

Pulmonary edema (acute HF) is sudden, severe fluid congestion within the lung alveoli. It is life threatening. Pulmonary edema can occur with an acute event such as a myocardial infarction. It can also happen when the heart is severely stressed, causing the left ventricle to fail. Complications of pulmonary edema include arrhythmias and cardiac arrest.

Pathophysiology
Initially, pressure rises in the lung's venous blood vessels as blood builds up, causing fluid to move into the interstitial spaces. Then, with continued pressure increasing, fluid containing red blood cells leaks into the alveoli. Finally, the alveoli and airways become filled with fluid. This reduces gas exchange and oxygen levels.

Signs and Symptoms
Signs and symptoms of pulmonary edema are listed in Table 26.3. Pink, frothy sputum is the classic symptom. It is caused by lung congestion and increased pressure that cause the leaking of fluid and red blood cells into the alveoli. Compensatory mechanisms increase the heart rate and blood pressure. Then, as pulmonary edema worsens, the blood pressure can fall.

Diagnostic Tests
Diagnostic studies are listed in Table 26.3. X-rays show the congestion in the pulmonary system. Arterial blood gases (ABGs) show a decrease in partial pressure of oxygen (PaO_2). This continues to drop as the edema worsens. Partial pressure of carbon dioxide ($PaCO_2$) is increased. This causes respiratory acidosis. Hemodynamic monitoring shows elevated pulmonary pressures and a decreased cardiac output.

Therapeutic Measures
Immediate treatment is needed to prevent acute respiratory distress (see Table 26.3). The goal of therapy is to reduce the workload of the left ventricle. This will improve cardiac output and reduce the patient's anxiety. Place the patient in a semi-Fowler or Fowler position based on comfort. This reduces venous return. It also allows the lungs to expand more easily. Give oxygen as ordered. A mask is used when

higher oxygen concentrations are needed. Endotracheal intubation and mechanical ventilation may be necessary for severe cases. Medications are given intravenously to reduce fluid overload, strengthen heart contractions, reduce arterial pressure (afterload), and reduce sodium and water retention to relieve dyspnea.

Nursing Care
The patient is typically critically ill and is treated in an intensive care unit. Psychosocial care is important because the patient, if alert, will be anxious.

CHRONIC HEART FAILURE

Signs and Symptoms
Chronic HF is a progressive disorder. Signs and symptoms worsen over time (Table 26.4).

Fatigue and Weakness
Fatigue and weakness are the earliest symptoms of chronic HF. They occur from reduced oxygen reaching the tissues. The fatigue worsens during the day, especially with activity (see "Evidence-Based Practice").

Evidence-Based Practice

Clinical Question
What are the effects of nurse-led interventions on the instrumental activities of daily living (IADLs), heart failure knowledge, self-care, quality of life, and depression for HF patients with mild cognitive impairment or dementia?

Evidence
A systematic review of literature of six randomized controlled trials included 595 HF patients with a mean age of 68 years to examine the effects of nurse-led interventions for HF patient with mild cognitive impairment or dementia (Hickman et al, 2020). The nurse-led interventions included brain exercises, customized education, personalized self-care schedule, interactive problem-solving training, and association techniques to prompt self-care activities. There were no notable improvements in cognitive function and depression with these interventions. However, working memory and IADLs as well as the patient's HF knowledge, self-care, and quality of life were improved substantially.

Implications for Nursing Practice
Patients with HF who suffer from mild cognitive impairment or dementia can benefit from nurse-led interventions to improve heart failure knowledge, quality of life, and self-care activities.

Reference: Hickman, L., Ferguson, C., Davidson, P. M., Allida, S., Inglis, S., Parker, D., & Agar, M. (2020). Key elements of interventions for heart failure patients with mild cognitive impairment or dementia: A systematic review. *European Journal of Cardiovascular Nursing, 19*(1), 8–19. https://doi.org/10.1177/1474515119865755

Dyspnea
Dyspnea (shortness of breath) is a common symptom of left-sided chronic HF. It occurs from pulmonary congestion that impairs gas exchange. Dyspnea triggers compensatory mechanisms. Short, rapid respirations result. Dyspnea is classified in several ways:

- **Exertional dyspnea** is shortness of breath that increases with activity.
- **Orthopnea** is dyspnea that increases when lying flat. In an upright position, gravity holds fluid in the lower extremities. In a supine position, gravitational forces are removed, allowing fluid to move from the legs to the heart. This overwhelms the already congested pulmonary system. When orthopnea is present, two or more pillows are often used for sleeping. Data collection documentation should state the number of pillows used (e.g., "three-pillow orthopnea").
- **Paroxysmal nocturnal dyspnea** is a sudden shortness of breath that occurs after lying flat for a time. It results from excess fluid in the lungs. The sleeping person awakens with feelings of suffocation and anxiety. Relief is obtained by sitting upright for a short time, reducing the amount of fluid returning to the heart.

Cough
A chronic, dry cough is common in chronic HF. Coughing increases when lying down from increased irritation of the lung mucosa. This irritation is due to increased pulmonary congestion that occurs when gravity releases fluid in the legs that returns to the heart and lungs.

Crackles and Wheezes
Pulmonary congestion causes abnormal breath sounds. These include crackles and wheezes. Crackles are the sound of the fluid buildup in the alveoli. Wheezes occur from bronchiolar constriction from increased fluid.

Tachycardia
As discussed, low cardiac output triggers the sympathetic nervous system to increase the heart rate.

LEARNING TIP
To simulate the sound of crackles heard with a stethoscope, open a piece of Velcro or rub hair together next to your ear.

Chest Pain
Chest pain may occur from ischemia. Several factors cause ischemia. A low cardiac output does not deliver adequate oxygen to the heart muscle. Tachycardia raises the heart's

• WORD • BUILDING •
orthopnea: orth—straight + pnea—to breathe

Table 26.4
Chronic Heart Failure Summary

	Right-Sided Heart Failure	Left-Sided Heart Failure
Signs and Symptoms	Ascites Dependent peripheral edema Fatigue, weakness Gastrointestinal (e.g., anorexia, nausea, pain) Hepatomegaly Jugular vein distention Nocturia Splenomegaly Tachycardia Weight gain	Cheyne–Stokes respiration Crackles, wheezing Cyanosis Dry hacking cough, especially when supine Dyspnea on exertion Nocturia Orthopnea Paroxysmal nocturnal dyspnea Tachypnea, tachycardia
Diagnostic Tests	Arterial blood gases (ABGs) Cardiac catheterization Cardiac magnetic resonance imaging (MRI) Chest x-ray Coronary angiography Echocardiography, two-dimensional with doppler Electrocardiogram (ECG) Hemodynamic monitoring Laboratory tests: complete blood count (CBC), serum B-type natriuretic peptide (BNP), electrolytes, blood urea nitrogen (BUN), creatinine, liver function tests, thyroid-stimulating hormone, fasting blood glucose, lipid profile, ferritin, urinalysis Nuclear imaging studies Sleep study Stress testing	
Complications	Cardiogenic shock Hepatomegaly Left ventricular thrombus and emboli Pleural effusion Splenomegaly	
	Noninvasive	*Invasive*
Therapeutic Measures	Treatment of underlying cause Medication therapy (see Table 26.5) Oxygen by cannula or mask Dietary sodium restriction Fluid restriction Daily weights Cardiac rehabilitation	Pacemaker Resynchronization therapy Implantable cardioverter defibrillator (ICD) Intra-aortic balloon pump (IABP) Left ventricular assist device Total artificial heart Surgery: Coronary artery bypass graft (CABG), valvuloplasty, heart valve replacement, cardiac transplant
Priority Nursing Diagnoses	*Impaired Gas Exchange* *Decreased Cardiac Output* *Excess Fluid Volume*	

oxygen needs. Increased preload also increases the heart's workload and oxygen needs. Ischemic pain results. Pain also increases oxygen requirements. These factors all contribute to the vicious cycle of HF.

Cheyne–Stokes Respiration
Cheyne–Stokes breathing is a pattern of shallow respirations building to deep breaths followed by a period of apnea. The period of apnea occurs because deep breathing causes carbon dioxide (CO_2) levels to drop. Low CO_2 levels do not stimulate the respiratory center. The apnea may last up to 30 seconds. Then, the Cheyne–Stokes breathing pattern begins again.

Edema
Edema occurs in chronic HF. It results from systemic blood vessel congestion and, as discussed, compensatory mechanisms that save water. Systemic edema or pulmonary edema (discussed earlier) can occur. Systemic edema is seen with jugular vein distension, swelling of the legs and feet, sacral edema in the supine patient, and increased abdominal cavity fluid (ascites).

Anemia
Many patients with HF are anemic due to hemodilution from fluid overload and decreased angiotensin-converting enzyme (ACE) action. The reduced ACE action decreases erythropoietin release. This results in decreased production of red blood cells.

Nocturia
Nocturia is an increase in urine output at night during sleep. After lying down, fluid in the lower legs returns to the circulatory system. Renal blood flow and filtration are increased, resulting in greater urine production and the need to urinate frequently during the night. Nocturia may occur up to six times per night, contributing to the patient's fatigue from interrupted sleep.

Cyanosis
The skin, nailbeds, or mucous membranes may appear blue, or cyanotic, from decreased oxygenation of the blood. **Cyanosis** is a late sign of chronic HF and occurs primarily with left-sided HF.

Altered Mental Status
Reduced cardiac output decreases the amount of oxygen delivered to the brain. Restlessness, insomnia, confusion, decreased level of consciousness, and impaired memory may occur.

Malnutrition
Several factors contribute to malnutrition for those with chronic HF. Altered mental status, dyspnea, and fatigue affect eating. GI upset, anorexia, and malabsorption occur from excess fluid pressing on the GI structures (ascites).

> **CRITICAL THINKING**
>
> **Part 1: Mr. Bjorklund,** age 66, has a family history of cardiac disease. He has been hypertensive for 10 years and takes lisinopril (Zestril) daily. His baseline vital signs are blood pressure 122/78 mm Hg, pulse 80 beats per minute (bpm), respirations 18 breaths per minute, height 66 inches, and weight 170 lb. During a visit to his HCP, Mr. Bjorklund states that he has been short of breath during his daily 2-mile walk and has been using two pillows at night for sleep. His physical examination shows blood pressure 140/86 mm Hg, pulse 106 bpm, respiration 24 breaths per minute, weight 80.7 kg (178 lb), and bilateral crackles in the lung bases.
>
> 1. What signs and symptoms of heart failure (HF) does Mr. Bjorklund display?
> 2. Do the signs and symptoms reflect right- or left-sided HF?
> 3. Why are each of the signs and symptoms occurring?
> 4. Why is Mr. Bjorklund using two pillows for sleeping? What is the medical term for this?
> 5. What health-care team members might collaborate on Mr. Bjorklund's care for his HF?
>
> *Suggested answers are at the end of the chapter.*

Complications of Heart Failure
Complications of chronic HF are listed in Table 26.4. The liver and spleen enlarge from the fluid congestion. This causes impaired function, cellular death, and scarring. The elevated pressures in the capillaries of the lung can cause pleural effusion, a leakage of fluid from the capillaries of the lung into the pleural space. Thrombosis and emboli can occur as a result of poor emptying of the ventricles. This leads to stasis of blood. Aspirin or anticoagulants are often prescribed. They prevent thrombus formation in patients with HF. Cardiogenic shock is often caused by a myocardial infarction that damages the left ventricle. It occurs when the left ventricle is unable to supply the tissues with enough oxygen and nutrients to meet their needs. Cardiogenic shock is a life-threatening condition that requires immediate treatment (see Chapter 9).

Diagnostic Tests
Diagnostic tests provide evidence to support a diagnosis of chronic HF in combination with other data such as physical symptoms (see Table 26.4):

- An elevated serum B-type natriuretic peptide (BNP) or N-terminal proBNP (NT-proBNP) level along with other data can indicate HF, although this level can also be normal in some people with heart failure. BNP is made by the heart to regulate blood volume levels in order to reduce cardiac workload. When the heart works harder over time, it releases more BNP.
- Serum laboratory tests can evaluate contributing factors for HF. These include elevated serum blood urea nitrogen (BUN) and serum creatinine from renal failure, elevated

- liver enzymes from liver damage, elevated ferritin with hemochromatosis (iron overload), and thyroid function tests.
- A chest x-ray examination shows the size, shape, and any enlargement of the heart as well as congestion in the pulmonary vessels.
- Cardiac arrhythmias that precipitate and contribute to HF are diagnosed with an electrocardiogram (see Chapters 21 and 25).
- Echocardiography may measure ventricular size, wall thickness, motion, and ejection fraction and assess valvular function.
- Stress testing, cardiopulmonary exercise testing, and nuclear imaging studies show activity tolerance and severity of functional impairment, which is usually limited in HF.
- Cardiac magnetic resonance imaging (MRI) shows both moving and still pictures of the heart and major blood vessels. Cardiac structure and function are analyzed to determine treatment for cardiac disease.
- Cardiac catheterization and angiography are used to detect underlying heart disease that may be the cause of HF.
- A sleep study may be done because sleep apnea or breathing disorders can contribute to HF.
- Measurement of the pressure in the heart and lungs can be done with hemodynamic monitoring to guide medical therapy.

> ### CRITICAL THINKING
>
> **Part 2:** Mr. Bjorklund's chest x-ray examination shows an enlarged heart (cardiomegaly).
>
> 1. Why is Mr. Bjorklund's heart enlarged?
> 2. What is the significance of an enlarged heart?
>
> *Suggested answers are at the end of the chapter.*

Therapeutic Measures

The goals of treatment for chronic HF are to improve the heart's pumping ability to reduce symptoms and to reduce mortality. Treatment of HF focuses on (1) identifying and correcting the underlying cause, (2) increasing the strength of the heart's contraction, (3) maintaining optimal water and sodium balance, and (4) decreasing the heart's workload. HF management requires a team approach that may involve HCPs, case managers, nurses, dietitians, physical therapists, occupational therapists, pharmacists, social workers, and clergy. HF pathways guide treatment. HF clinics ensure quality-based outcomes while reducing treatment costs.

The severity of HF determines the patient-centered therapy selected. Noninvasive approaches are often tried first. Combination medications and multiple therapies are used for better patient outcomes. Then, as needed, invasive treatments are used.

Oxygen Therapy

One of the major problems caused by HF is a reduction in oxygen delivered to the tissues. The signs and symptoms of this are fatigue, dyspnea, altered mental status, and cyanosis. Oxygen therapy may assist in supplying tissue oxygen needs. In mild HF, oxygen may be delivered by nasal cannula. For severe heart failure, ABG values guide oxygen delivery. Masks that provide high concentrations of oxygen or mechanical ventilation can be used.

Activity

Activity tolerance is dependent on the severity of HF signs and symptoms. Severe symptoms may require bedrest until treatment reduces the symptoms. For stable HF, a regular exercise program such as walking can improve cardiac function. Patients are encouraged to stay as active as possible. A referral to a cardiac rehabilitation program is beneficial. Patients are educated on how to exercise safely and identify symptoms to prevent overexertion.

Sodium Restriction and Weight Control

Dietary sodium is restricted to decrease fluid retention. Salt substitutes often use potassium in place of sodium. The patient and HCP should discuss their use. A healthy weight range should be maintained. A dietitian can develop a plan for a low-sodium diet and weight reduction, if needed.

> ### BE SAFE!
>
> **AVOID FAILURE TO RECOGNIZE!** In severe HF, when abdominal discomfort is present, malnutrition is a concern. The patient can be anorexic. But the weight gain that occurs with fluid retention can mask the weight loss occurring from the anorexia. Monitor food intake. Ensure that weight gain from fluid retention does not allow malnutrition to go undetected.

Medication Therapy

There is no cure for chronic HF. Medications, however, can help improve symptoms and quality of life (Table 26.5). The American College of Cardiology Foundation/American Heart Association/Heart Failure Society of America 2017 guidelines recommend medication classes with various considerations for the type of HF, cardiac ejection fraction status (preserved or reduced), symptoms, and comorbidities (Yancy et al, 2017). Medication classes that may be used for a patient's individualized treatment plan are discussed.

ANGIOTENSIN-CONVERTING ENZYME INHIBITORS. ACE inhibitors vasodilate, which lowers blood pressure and reduces workload on the heart. They also prevent cardiac remodeling, which leads to progressive cardiac deterioration. ACE inhibitors can cause a dry cough that may require changing to another medication class, not another medication in the same class, to avoid this side effect.

Table 26.5
Medications Used for Heart Failure

Medication Class/Action

Angiotensin-Converting Enzyme (ACE) Inhibitors
Decreases afterload to prevent hypertension (HTN).

Examples	*Nursing Implications*
captopril (Capoten) benazepril (Lotensin) enalapril (Vasotec) fosinopril (Monopril) lisinopril (Prinivil, Zestril) moexipril (Univasc) quinapril (Accupril) perindopril (Aceon) ramipril (Altace) trandolapril (Mavik)	Check apical pulse and blood pressure (BP). If pulse is less than 60 bpm or systolic BP less than 100 mm Hg, notify health-care provider (HCP). Give 1 hour before meals. *Teaching:* Take first doses at night to adjust to lower BP. Rise slowly. Check BP weekly. Report if persistent cough or other side effects develop.

Angiotensin II Receptor Blockers (ARBs)
Block angiotensin II receptor to reduce extracellular fluid and cause vasodilation. May be used if ACE inhibitor not tolerated.

Examples	*Nursing Implications*
candesartan (Atacand) irbesartan (Avapro) losartan (Cozaar) valsartan (Diovan)	Check apical pulse and BP. If pulse is below 60 bpm or systolic BP below 100 mm Hg, notify HCP. *Teaching:* Rise slowly. Report rash, sore throat/mouth, fever, swelling, difficulty breathing, chest pain, or irregular heartbeat.

Angiotensin Receptor Neprilysin Inhibitors (ARNis)
Reduce blood volume and vasodilate to reduce cardiac workload.

Example	*Nursing Implications*
valsartan/sacubitril (Entresto)	Contraindicated with ACE inhibitors or history of angioedema. Check apical pulse and BP. If pulse is below 60 bpm or systolic BP below 100 mm Hg, notify HCP. Monitor for hyperkalemia, kidney problems, and angioedema (swelling of lips/face). *Teaching:* Rise slowly. Report cough. Seek emergency care for swelling of lips/face.

Beta-Adrenergic Blockers (Beta Blockers)
Reduce sympathetic nervous system input and cardiac remodeling; improve cardiac output to reduce symptoms; reduce disease progression and sudden death.

Examples	*Nursing Implications*
bisoprolol (Zebeta) carvedilol (Coreg) metoprolol succinate (Toprol XL)	Check apical pulse and BP. If pulse is below 60 bpm or systolic BP below 100 mm Hg, notify HCP. *Teaching:* Take pulse daily and notify HCP if below 60. Take BP biweekly. Rise slowly.

Continued

Table 26.5
Medications Used for Heart Failure—cont'd

Medication Class/Action

Loop Diuretics
Decrease fluid overload.

Potassium-Wasting

Examples	Nursing Implications
bumetanide (Bumex) furosemide (Lasix) torsemide (Demadex)	Check BP and pulse before giving. Monitor electrolyte levels (especially potassium and in those on digitalis) and fluid status (daily weight, intake and output, thirst, dry mouth, weakness, oliguria) throughout therapy. Administer per patient lifestyle (usually in the morning) to avoid nocturia.

Potassium-Sparing

Example	Nursing Implications
spironolactone (Aldactone)	Do not give a potassium-sparing diuretic if patient is hyperkalemic. *Teaching:* Report signs of hyperkalemia (e.g., weakness, fatigue, confusion, dyspnea, arrhythmias, confusion)

Thiazide Diuretics
Decrease fluid overload; potassium-wasting.

Examples	Nursing Implications
chlorothiazide (Diuril) hydrochlorothiazide (HydroDIURIL, HCTZ, Microzide) metolazone (Zaroxolyn)	Monitor potassium. *Teaching:* Do not give a potassium-wasting diuretic if patient is hypokalemic. Administer potassium supplements as ordered; if on digitalis, increased risk of toxicity with hypokalemia. Monitor weight daily, and report 2- to 3-pound change over 1 to 2 days.

Hyperpolarization-Activated Cyclic Nucleotide-Gated (HCN) Channel Blockers
Slows heart rate so heart can pump more blood with each heartbeat.

Examples	Nursing Implications
ivabradine (Corlanor)	*Teaching:* Avoid grapefruit or grapefruit juice. Take with food. Report chest pressure, heart rate below 60 or above 100, palpitations, and shortness of breath immediately. Temporary visual brightness (halos around lights, kaleidoscope colors, flashes) may occur; enter bright light slowly to allow time to adapt.

Inotropes: Cardiac Glycoside (Positive Inotrope and Negative Chronotrope)
Use recommended only for slowing rate for atrial fibrillation, if present.

Examples	Nursing Implications
digoxin (Lanoxin)	Take apical pulse for 1 minute; if below 60 bpm, notify HCP. Older patients are more susceptible to toxicity. Periodically monitor medication level and electrolytes (hypokalemia, hypomagnesemia, and hypercalcemia make patient more susceptible to toxicity). *Teaching:* Take medication exactly as directed, at the same time each day. Take pulse before taking medication; if below 60 bpm, hold and contact HCP. Report signs of digitalis toxicity: abdominal pain, anorexia, nausea, vomiting, visual changes (blurred, yellow-green halos, photophobia, diplopia), bradycardia, arrhythmias.

Table 26.5
Medications Used for Heart Failure—cont'd

Medication Class/Action

Vasodilators
Decrease afterload to prevent HTN; used for patients who cannot take ACE inhibitors.

Examples	*Nursing Implications*
isosbide dinitrate (Isorbid, Isordil) hydralazine (Apresoline) nitroglycerin	Take blood pressure and pulse before giving. Notify HCP if not within normal limits. *Teaching:* Rise slowly. Headache common initially, treated with aspirin.

> **LEARNING TIP**
> To help you identify angiotensin-converting enzyme, or ACE, inhibitors, remember that their generic names end with -*pril*.

ANGIOTENSIN II RECEPTOR BLOCKERS. ARBs are an alternative to ACE inhibitors. They inhibit the renin-angiotensin-aldosterone system. This lowers blood pressure and workload on the heart. ARBs do not produce a cough as a side effect as much as ACE inhibitors do.

ANGIOTENSIN RECEPTOR NEPRILYSIN INHIBITORS (ARNis). ARNis reduce hospitalizations and deaths from chronic HF and reduced ejection fraction. Entresto, a combination medication of valsartan/sacubitril, is often used with beta blockers and diuretics. Angioedema (swelling of lips/face) is a serious side effect of this medication that can be life-threatening. ACE inhibitors increase the risk of angioedema. They must be stopped with a 36-hour wash-out period before Entresto is started.

BETA ADRENERGIC BLOCKERS. The sympathetic nervous system acts to compensate for HF. Long-term sympathetic nervous system effects, however, are not helpful. Beta-adrenergic blockers, or beta blockers, help avoid these adverse effects. They improve cardiac output, reduce symptoms, reduce disease progression, and reduce sudden death.

ALDOSTERONE ANTAGONISTS. Spironolactone (Aldactone) blocks the effects of aldosterone, which causes retention of sodium and fluid. Potassium must be monitored carefully because spironolactone is a potassium-sparing agent. The risk of hyperkalemia increases if an ACE inhibitor or ARB is also being used.

DIURETICS. Diuretics act on various areas of the kidneys. They reduce fluid volume and increase urine output. This reduces pulmonary venous pressure. In turn, cardiac workload decreases. Diuretics are given to help prevent edema. However, edema does not need to be present for their use. A combination of diuretics may be ordered. Potassium supplements may be given with potassium-wasting diuretics. Electrolytes (especially potassium levels to prevent hypokalemia) and fluid balance (to prevent dehydration) should be carefully monitored.

> **BE SAFE!**
> ***AVOID FAILURE TO RECOGNIZE!*** Always check serum potassium levels before giving a potassium-wasting diuretic (e.g., loop diuretics furosemide [Lasix], bumetanide [Bumex], and torsemide [Demadex]) or before giving a potassium supplement. Do not give a diuretic if the potassium level is low or a potassium supplement if the potassium level is high. Notify the HCP of the laboratory value.

HYPERPOLARIZATION-ACTIVATED CYCLIC NUCLEOTIDE-GATED CHANNEL BLOCKERS. Ivabradine (Corlanor) blocks the channel controlling the heart's pacemaker current to slow the heart rate. This increases diastole and filling time, which increases cardiac output. It is used in stable heart failure to reduce the risk of hospitalization.

INOTROPIC AGENTS. Inotropic medications strengthen ventricular contraction, which increases cardiac output. Inotropic agents include digitalis (e.g., digoxin), sympathomimetics (e.g., dobutamine), and phosphodiesterase inhibitors (e.g., milrinone). Digitalis is only recommended for rate control of atrial fibrillation, if present. The sympathomimetics and phosphodiesterase inhibitors are infusions that are usually used short term for severe heart failure.

SODIUM-GLUCOSE COTRANSPORTER 2 (SGLT2) INHIBITORS. A newer class of medication for reducing hospitalizations in both diabetics and non-diabetics who have HF with reduced cardiac ejection fraction is showing great promise in the treatment of heart failure. Dapagliflozin (Farxiga) was approved for this purpose by the U.S. Food and Drug Administration in May 2020. Researchers theorize that the osmotic diuresis action of the drug relieves congestion better than other diuretics by removing more interstitial fluid.

> ### CRITICAL THINKING & CLINICAL JUDGMENT
>
> **Part 3: Mr. Bjorklund** visits his HCP. He is told to continue the ACE inhibitor and begin a diuretic as well as a 2 g sodium diet.
>
> **Critical Thinking (The Why)**
> 1. Why is the ACE inhibitor continued?
> 2. Will the ACE inhibitor affect preload or afterload?
> 3. Why is the diuretic ordered?
> 4. Why is a 2 g sodium diet ordered?
> 5. What is the goal of this prescribed treatment plan?
>
> **Clinical Judgment (The Do)**
> 6. What laboratory test result do you check before administering the diuretic?
>
> *Suggested answers are at the end of the chapter.*

PACEMAKERS AND IMPLANTABLE CARDIOVERTER DEFIBRILLATOR. Pacemakers and ICDs are used along with medication therapy for patients at risk of sudden death. Pacemakers provide an electrical impulse to pace the heart to maintain a set rate. ICDs deliver an electric countershock if a shockable life-threatening rhythm occurs.

CARDIAC RESYNCHRONIZATION THERAPY. With HF, the ventricles do not always beat in normal synchrony with each other. This results in less-effective pumping by the ventricles and reduces stroke volume. Cardiac resynchronization therapy restores normal timing of ventricular contraction. It reduces symptoms and improves quality of life. A biventricular cardiac pacing system is used. It synchronizes ventricle contraction to atrial pacing when three-chamber pacing is used. Left ventricular filling and, thus, contraction is improved. Cardiac resynchronization therapy is also available with an ICD. For more information about cardiac resynchronization devices, visit www.medtronic.com.

MECHANICAL ASSISTIVE DEVICES. Mechanical cardiopulmonary support provides temporary function to patients with impaired cardiac function or who are experiencing cardiogenic shock. Assistive devices can act as a bridge to recovery or transplantation, to destination therapy (a long-term solution when other options are not available for the failing heart), or as heart replacement. These devices include extracorporeal membrane oxygenation (ECMO), the intra-aortic balloon pump (IABP), ventricular assist devices, total artificial heart, and implantable replacement heart. Technology in this area is continually evolving. ECMO is a portable bedside device that uses extrathoracic cannulation to perform respiratory (oxygenation and carbon dioxide removal) and circulatory support (somewhat similar to cardiopulmonary bypass used during cardiac surgery).

INTRA-AORTIC BALLOON PUMP. For acute care, an IABP increases circulation to the coronary arteries and reduces the work of the heart. The pump catheter is inserted into the femoral artery and positioned in the descending aortic arch (Fig. 26.3). It is attached to a computer that senses ventricular contraction and controls the balloon. While the heart is relaxed (diastole), the balloon is inflated. This sends more blood into the coronary arteries. Just before the heart contracts (systole), the balloon deflates to allow blood to flow past. The deflation creates a suction effect. The blood flows past it with less resistance (decreased afterload) into the aorta. The IABP is inserted in a cardiac catheterization laboratory, critical care unit, or surgical suite. It is used short term for several days.

VENTRICULAR ASSIST DEVICES. Ventricular assist devices can be transcutaneous (pump located outside the body), which may be used short term after cardiac surgery or implanted mechanical devices. They assist cardiac pumping to maintain cardiac output (Fig. 26.4). They allow the failing ventricle to rest. Ventricular assist devices are used temporarily. They can be a bridge to transplantation (while patient awaits a donor heart), a bridge to recovery (for patients whose hearts may recover), or as a destination therapy (a long-term therapy) for those who are not candidates for heart transplant. These devices are referred to as *left* ventricular assist devices if only used in the left ventricle, *right*

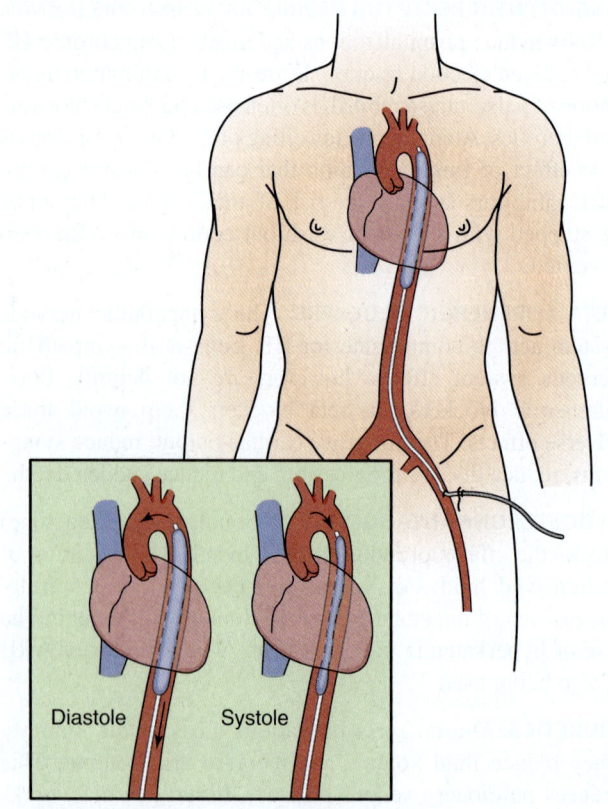

FIGURE 26.3 Intra-aortic balloon pump.

Chapter 26 Nursing Care of Patients With Heart Failure 437

ventricular assist devices if only used in the right ventricle, or *biventricular* assist devices if used in both ventricles. Two devices are used for biventricular failure.

Surgical Management
The causes of HF may be treated surgically (see Chapters 23 and 24). HF symptoms may resolve after these conditions are corrected. Surgical ventricular reconstruction reduces left ventricular volume. It might be done along with coronary artery bypass surgery. Reconstruction can reduce left ventricle end-systolic volume more than coronary artery bypass grafting (CABG) alone. Routine surgical ventricular reconstruction during CABG is not yet standard protocol, though new research demonstrates increased benefits (Rajakumar et al, 2019).

Nursing Process for the Patient With Chronic Heart Failure
Data Collection
While obtaining data for the patient with chronic HF, look at areas that can indicate the presence of HF (Table 26.6).

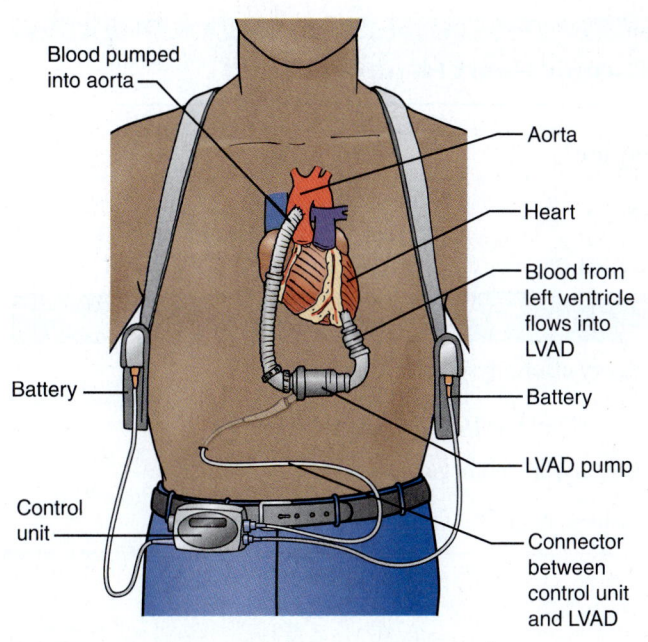

FIGURE 26.4 Schematic of a left ventricular assist device.

Table 26.6
Nursing Data Collection for the Patient With Chronic Heart Failure

	Subjective Data
Health History	
Respiratory	Lung disease? How many flights of stairs can be climbed without dyspnea? How many pillows used for sleeping? Dyspnea at rest or that awakens from sleeping?
Cardiovascular	Any cardiac disease history: hypertension, myocardial infarction, valvular problem, anemia, arrhythmias, palpitations? Chest pain: precipitating factors, severity, relieving factors? Can activities of daily living be performed? Can activities performed 6 months, 4 months, 2 months, 2 weeks ago still be done? Any dizziness (vertigo) or fainting (syncope)?
Fluid Retention	Daily sodium intake? Weight gain? Are shoes tight? Do ankles swell?
Gastrointestinal	Is appetite good? Any nausea, vomiting, or abdominal pain?
Urinary	Decrease in daytime urine output? Urinates how many times at night (nocturia)?
Neurologic	Any change in behavior?
Knowledge of Condition	What are you being treated for? What questions do you have?

Continued

Table 26.6
Nursing Data Collection for the Patient With Chronic Heart Failure—cont'd

Coping Skills	What coping techniques do you usually use? Are they effective? Who is a part of your support system?
Medications	What are all of the medications that you take?
Objective Data	
Respiratory	Tachypnea, crackles, wheezing, respiratory effort, dyspnea with exertion
Cardiovascular	Tachycardia, arrhythmias, jugular vein distention, peripheral edema (degree of pitting)
Gastrointestinal	Abdominal distention, ascites, hepatomegaly, splenomegaly
Neurologic	Confusion, decreased level of consciousness, restlessness, impaired memory
Integumentary	Cold, clammy skin; pallor; cyanosis
General	Weight
Diagnostic Tests	Review findings

Nursing Diagnoses, Planning, Implementation, and Evaluation

See "Nursing Care Plan for the Patient With Chronic Heart Failure" for common nursing diagnoses. The major focus of nursing care for chronic HF patients is to improve oxygenation and activity tolerance. This can be done by decreasing the body's need for oxygen with rest, positioning, medications, and normal fluid balance maintenance.

REST AND ACTIVITY. Reduction of the body's oxygen demands decreases the workload of the heart. A balance of rest and activity to manage signs or symptoms of oxygen deprivation is essential. The activity level of the patient is determined by the severity of the HF. During times of exertion, monitor the patient's vital signs and respiratory effort. Look for signs of oxygen deprivation. If activity intolerance develops, stop the activity.

Patients may have difficulty sleeping due to anxiety, diuretics, nocturia, orthopnea, or paroxysmal nocturnal dyspnea. Assist patients to take diuretics opposite their normal sleeping hours (Sleep nighttime hours = Diuretic early morning; Sleep daytime hours = Diuretic upon arising).

> **NURSING CARE TIP**
> To reduce nocturia, reclining 30 minutes with legs at or above heart level before bedtime helps redistribute fluid to the kidneys so that the patient can void before going to sleep instead of soon afterward for undisturbed rest.

POSITIONING. Semi-Fowler or high-Fowler position makes breathing easier. In upright positions, the lungs can expand more fully. Gravity also decreases the amount of fluid returning to the heart. This reduces the heart's workload.

FLUID RETENTION. Daily weights show fluid weight gain. It is important to detect fluid retention in this way. Edema is usually not observed until 5 to 10 pounds of extra fluid are present. A baseline weight is obtained when HF is diagnosed. Daily weights should be measured on the same scale, at the same time of day, and with the same type of clothing worn for accuracy. A good time to obtain a daily weight is in the morning after the bladder is emptied. Document daily weights. Include the date and time of the weight, the scale used, the clothing worn, and the weight measurement. At home, the patient can keep a weight journal. Tell the patient to report weight gains of 2 to 3 pounds over 1 to 2 days.

> **BE SAFE!**
> **AVOID FAILURE TO COMMUNICATE!** A patient's weight gain of 2 to 3 pounds over 1 to 2 days could be a sign of worsening HF. Recognize the importance of notifying the patient's HCP of these types of changes to prevent deterioration of their heart function.

OXYGEN CONSUMPTION. Activities that increase oxygen consumption by the heart should be avoided. Sustained tachycardia increases the oxygen needs of the heart. It should be reported promptly to the HCP for treatment. Older patients are especially vulnerable to the effects of tachycardia due to their decreased cardiac reserves. Constipation should be prevented as straining during defecation (Valsalva maneuver) increases the heart's workload by increasing venous return to the heart. Stool softeners can prevent straining.

Nursing Care Plan for the Patient With Chronic Heart Failure

Nursing Diagnosis: *Decreased Cardiac Output* related to the heart's inability to effectively pump adequate blood
Expected Outcome: The patient will demonstrate vital signs within normal limits (WNL).
Evaluation of Outcome: Are vital signs WNL without dyspnea or chest pain?

Intervention	Rationale	Evaluation
Monitor for primary signs of heart failure (HF): dyspnea, orthopnea, paroxysmal nocturnal dyspnea, fatigue, edema, and secondary signs of weight gain, jugular vein distension, lung crackles, oliguria, coughing, and clammy skin with color changes.	These signs were identified as being either primary or secondary in HF.	Does patient exhibit any of these signs of HF?
Maintain bedrest with head of bed elevated for breathing ease during an acute episode.	Bedrest with the head of the bed elevated reduces workload of the heart and eases breathing.	Does bedrest with head of the bed elevated relieve HF signs and symptoms?

Geriatric

Intervention	Rationale	Evaluation
Monitor for fatigue and depression.	Fatigue and depression can be signs of HF in the older adult.	Are fatigue or depression present?

Nursing Diagnosis: *Decreased Activity Tolerance* related to oxygen imbalance
Expected Outcome: The patient will demonstrate increased activity tolerance with vital signs WNL in response to activity.
Evaluation of Outcome: Does the patient participate in activities and maintain vital signs WNL?

Intervention	Rationale	Evaluation
Provide assistance with ADLs, rest periods, spaced activities, and conservation of energy.	Myocardial oxygen need is decreased with rest and energy conservation.	Does patient participate in activity with minimal pulse rate or electrocardiogram changes?

Geriatric

Intervention	Rationale	Evaluation
Increase time allowed to complete activities.	Independence and participation are increased if extra time is allowed for tasks.	Does patient report greater ability to complete activities with fewer symptoms?

Nursing Diagnosis: *Excess Fluid Volume* related to HF and the secondary reduction in renal blood flow for filtration.
Expected Outcomes: The patient will remain free from edema and dyspnea, have clear lung sounds, and maintain baseline weight at all times.
Evaluation of Outcomes: Does the patient have clear lung sounds with baseline weight maintained?

Intervention	Rationale	Evaluation
Monitor intake and output (I&O), edema, weight gain, jugular vein distension, and lung crackles.	Excess fluid is indicated by imbalanced I&O, edema, daily weight gain, jugular vein distension, and crackles in the lungs.	Are I&O balanced for 24 hours? Are edema, weight gain, jugular vein distension, and/or crackles present? Are they worsening or improving?
Maintain fluid and sodium restrictions as prescribed.	Sodium retains fluid and excess fluid contributes to edema.	Does patient restrict fluid and sodium intake?

To reduce fatigue, patients should be taught to alternate activity with periods of rest. This will save energy while performing activities of daily living. The occupational therapist and physical therapist can develop ways to help the patient save energy during self-care. Suggestions for conserving energy include putting frequently used objects at waist level to avoid reaching overhead, having rest periods during bathing and grooming activities, and using Velcro fasteners to make dressing easier.

LOW-SODIUM DIET AND WEIGHT CONTROL. A consult with a dietitian helps the patient and family understand how to read food labels for sodium content and plan low-sodium food menus that are appealing and easy to use. Table salt should be eliminated. Food preparers should be informed not to salt food during cooking. Spices, herbs, and lemon juice may be used to flavor unsalted foods. The patient should be aware that salt substitutes may contain potassium if that is a concern. Eating should remain pleasurable for the patient to avoid malnutrition. Do not talk *only* about foods they cannot have; discuss foods the patient likes and can still have.

For patients who are overweight, weight reduction may help eliminate the underlying cause of HF. Collaboration with a dietitian for diet counseling and support will assist patients with weight loss strategies. The body mass index and waist-to-hip ratio can guide weight loss.

If anorexia occurs in later stages of HF, patient intake should be evaluated by a dietitian. Several small meals rather than three large meals a day can decrease exertion and the heart's workload.

MEDICATIONS. HF is a progressive, chronic condition, and patients may require lifetime medication, including combination medication therapy. Taking multiple pills daily can be challenging. Financial resources, adherence to therapy regimen, and ongoing monitoring must be considered.

Diuretics. Diuretics require monitoring of patients' potassium levels and blood pressure. To prevent hypokalemia, high-potassium foods or a potassium supplements may be prescribed. If too much fluid is removed the patient may become hypotensive, and orthostatic hypotension can develop. This causes dizziness and a risk of falling. Caution patients to change positions slowly. They should dangle their legs at the bedside before standing. This will help prevent falls.

Digitalis. Before giving digitalis, the patient's apical pulse should be counted for 1 minute. This medication slows the heart rate. If the pulse is below 60 bpm, notify the HCP. Some patients are given digitalis with heart rates between 50 and 60 bpm, such as if the heart's conduction system is normal or if the rate is due to other medications such as a beta blocker. Be aware that hypokalemia can lead to toxicity even with a normal dose of digitalis. It is important to know this, as those taking digitalis often also take diuretics. Some diuretics lower potassium levels. Early signs and symptoms of digitalis toxicity include anorexia, nausea, and vomiting; bradycardia or other arrhythmias; visual problems; and mental changes. Older adults are especially prone to the toxic effects of this medication. They may exhibit confusion when levels are elevated.

Vasodilators. Medications with vasodilating effects reduce the heart's workload by decreasing vascular pressure and resistance. Blood pressure is monitored when giving vasodilators.

CUE RECOGNITION 26.1

You are caring for a patient with HF who was started on a new vasodilator medication 3 days ago. As she gets up to use the bathroom, she begins to sway and states that she is lightheaded and dizzy. What action do you take?

Suggested answers are at the end of the chapter.

Medication Education. Patients and their families are taught the purpose, side effects, and precautions for prescribed medications. Patients should understand the importance of taking their medication as prescribed, even if they do not have symptoms. A schedule should be developed so patients remember to take their medications. Explain to report side effects to the HCP. If dizziness occurs from medications that reduce blood pressure, the medications can be staggered so that they are not all taken at the same time.

OXYGEN. Oxygen therapy is prescribed by the HCP. It is guided by blood gas analysis and patient medical history and symptoms. It requires careful monitoring. For chronic HF, oxygen may be administered at 2 to 6 L/min via nasal cannula.

EDUCATION. Chronic management of HF requires patient and family understanding of the disease process, management of home oxygen therapy and medications, diet and weight control, and the continued need for immunizations, such as the annual flu shot (see "Home Health Hints"). The patient and family must recognize the importance of all of these factors to foster quality of life for the patient with chronic HF. A discussion of HF and signs and symptoms to report to the HCP using simple terms should be included in the teaching plan (Box 26.1).

COPING. Living with a chronic illness can be frustrating for both patients and their families. Identifying coping skills used by patients and their families can be used to develop a plan for coping with this current illness. Referrals to social workers, sex counselors, and nurse-managed clinics can be

Box 26.1
Patient and Family Education

Heart Failure Signs and Symptoms to Report to the Health-Care Provider
- Ankle/foot/leg edema
- Anorexia
- Dry cough
- Fatigue
- Nocturia
- Orthopnea
- Paroxysmal nocturnal dyspnea
- Shortness of breath
- Weight gain of 2 to 3 pounds over 1 to 2 days

helpful in collaborating to provide resources to maintain or improve quality of life for the patient with HF. Nurse-managed HF clinics decrease hospitalization rates and increase effective management of the therapeutic regimen.

Home Health Hints

- A telehealth unit in the home can alert the agency to signs of exacerbation such as a weight gain of 2 pounds in 24 hours. Interventions such as medication changes can then be ordered to prevent hospital admissions.
- Blood drawn for potassium level needs to be transported to the laboratory within 1 hour. Ice should not be put directly on the blood-draw tube because it can cause destruction of the cells and a false elevation in the potassium level.
- Observe for signs of oxygen deprivation and hypoxia, such as confusion, combativeness, or unusual expressions of anger.
- Measure for edema using a tape measure in centimeters on the abdominal girth, thigh, calf, and ankle. Measure at the same place each time (e.g., girth of calf at specified distance above medial malleolus). Edema can be present if the patient reports jewelry, waistband, or shoes and socks feel tighter.
- The sacrum, back, and sides of a bedridden patient should be observed for edema. These are dependent areas in the bedridden patient where fluid accumulates instead of the ankles.
- Observe the contents of medicine bottles. If pills have been cut in half, question the patient because this is often an attempt by the patient to "stretch" the medicine to decrease expenses. Refer to the social worker for financial assistance.
- Adjust medication times to fit the patient's lifestyle. A dose of diuretic too late in the day may cause frequent awakenings during the night to void. This may lead to a lack of adherence and then rehospitalization.
- For the patient on a low-sodium diet, an effective diet-teaching technique is to have the patient name the foods highest in sodium. Asking the patient to rename the list on each visit helps knowledge retention and adherence to the diet.
- Reinforce education for patients on sodium-restricted diets to use no-salt-added canned vegetables or to drain and rinse the vegetables. Herbs and spices can make them flavorful.
- Reinforce education for patients that long oxygen tubing allows movement around the home. For safety, caution about keeping the tubing out of the way and avoiding kinks in the tube.
- Reinforce education for patients and caregivers about the explosive nature of oxygen and the danger of an open flame or smoking in its presence.
- Reinforce education for patients with orthopnea that a foam wedge can be obtained from a medical equipment company to use under the head instead of pillows when sleeping.
- Reinforce education for self-management skills to reduce the odds of hospital readmission (e.g., sodium restrictions, daily weights, and warning signs of exacerbation to report).
- If an ambulance is called, teach caregivers to turn on an outside light and clear a pathway to enable the emergency technicians to get to the patient more easily.

NURSING CARE TIP

Provide written discharge instructions to all patients with HF and their caregivers. Instructions should focus on medications (stressing adherence to following the medication regimen), diet, activity level, daily weights, and follow-up appointments. They should also tell patients and caregivers to report or seek medical care for symptoms that worsen.

CLINICAL JUDGMENT

Part 4: Mr. Bjorklund talks with the nurse after his HCP prescribes that he should continue an ACE inhibitor, a diuretic, and a 2 g sodium diet.

1. What patient-centered education do you reinforce for Mr. Bjorklund based on his prescribed treatment?
2. What directions do you give him for taking his diuretic?
3. Considering that Mr. Bjorklund is on a governmental subsidy food program and receives mostly packaged food and canned vegetables, what action do you take?
4. With whom do you collaborate to assist Mr. Bjorklund with planning and understanding his new 2 g sodium diet?
5. Mr. Bjorklund tells you he weighs himself each day at the local pharmacy, so how do you address this information?

Suggested answers are at the end of the chapter.

CARDIAC TRANSPLANTATION

Cardiac transplantation is used for patients with end-stage cardiac disease (visit www.nhlbi.nih.gov). Transplant centers use selection guidelines for donors and recipients to improve survival. A multi-organ (heart, lungs, liver) transport device (e.g., Organ Care System, often called Heart in a Box) is a warm portable monitoring system that keeps the heart beating and nourished with the donor's blood in a human-like state which increases accessibility and the number of organs viable for transplant (https://www.transmedics.com).

The use of drones to deliver organs is also being explored around the world and has been shown to safely reduce waiting list times by increasing accessibility (Al-Ayyad et al, 2019).

Surgical Procedure

Once a donor heart is found, the recipient is notified, admitted to the hospital, and prepared for surgery. The general procedures for this surgery are similar to those described in Chapter 21. One of two types of cardiac transplant procedures will be performed: orthotopic or heterotopic. In the orthotopic procedure, once the patient is on cardiopulmonary bypass, the recipient's diseased heart is removed, leaving the posterior wall of the atria, superior and inferior vena cava, and pulmonary vein (Fig. 26.5). The donor's atria, aorta, and pulmonary artery are then anastomosed to the recipient's atria, aorta, and pulmonary artery. The heterotopic procedure joins the donor heart and vessels to the recipient's heart and vessels without removing the recipient's heart, so the donor heart rests in the right side of the chest.

Immunosuppressive therapy is required to prevent rejection of the transplanted heart. Medications such as cyclosporine (Neoral, Sandimmune), mycophenolate mofetil (CellCept), tacrolimus (Prograf), sirolimus (Rapamune), and prednisone are used. A high-loading dose of one of these medications begins preoperatively. The risk for rejection is highest immediately after surgery. Over time, it decreases but never goes away. Dosages of immunosuppressive medication are also highest initially after surgery and decrease with time. Lifelong antirejection therapy is required and involves the combination of medications to allow lower doses. This helps to reduce side effects. These medications may interact with foods such as grapefruit, Seville oranges, or tangelos and with herbs such as St. John's wort. Ensure patients understand what foods and herbs are contraindicated while they are taking these medications.

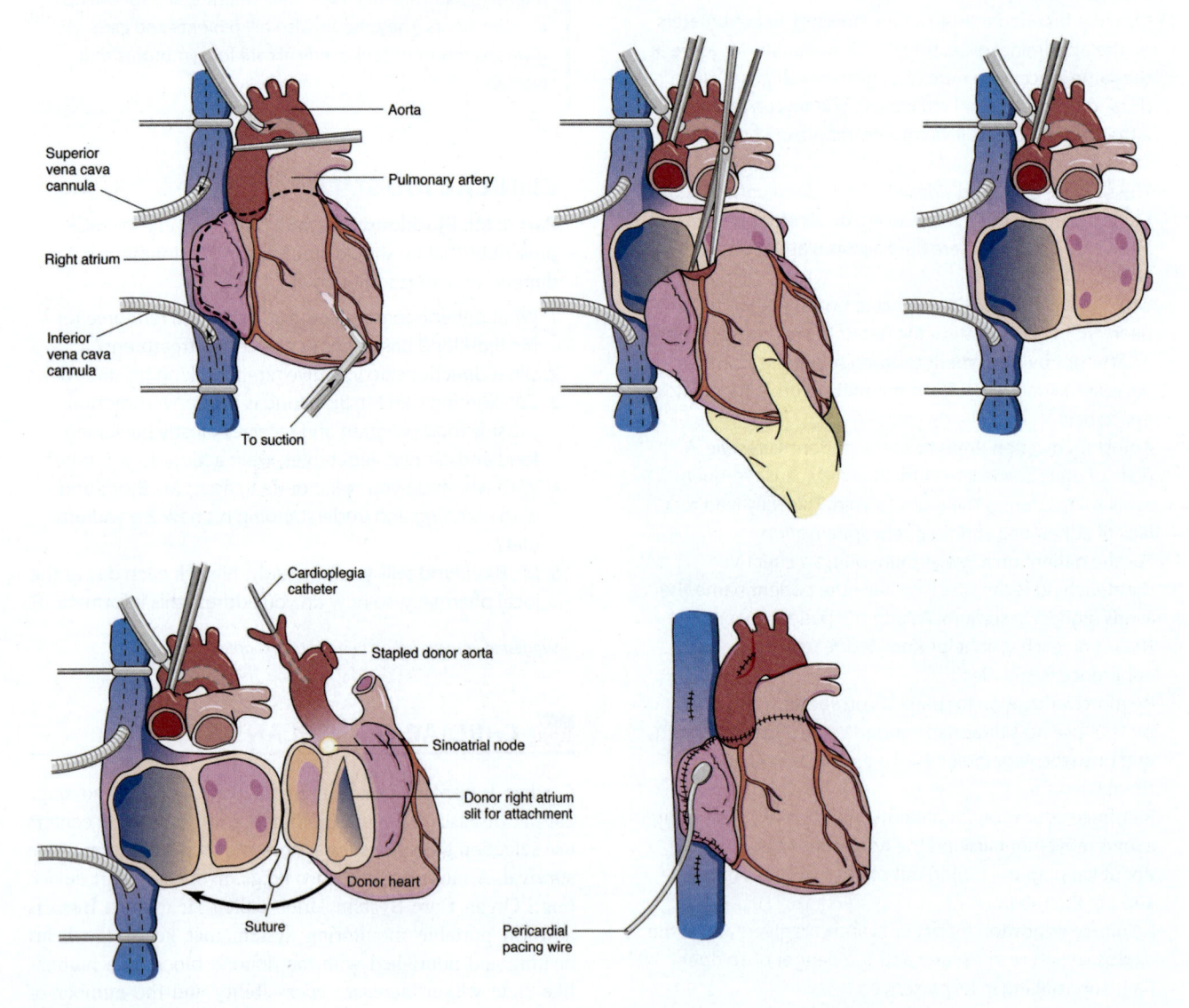

FIGURE 26.5 Heart transplantation.

Complications

Heart transplantation complications may include those associated with cardiac surgery. Heart rejection, which is the major cause of death within the first year, is another complication. To detect rejection, frequent biopsies of cardiac muscle or a newer blood test to detect activation of rejection genesis is done during the first year. If a biopsy shows damaged cells, indicating rejection, antirejection medication therapy may be modified.

Due to immunosuppressive therapy, infection and cancer may occur. The medications used for immunosuppressive therapy also may cause adverse reactions such as increased susceptibility to infections, cataracts, high cholesterol, diabetes, kidney disease, and osteoporosis.

Therapeutic Measures

After cardiopulmonary bypass ends, the patient is observed for fluid overload and receives a diuretic to aid in excretion of excessive circulating fluid. Other assessments include hourly monitoring of intake, output, and lung sounds for crackles. Weight and electrolyte levels are checked daily.

Postcardiotomy syndrome may occur from days 2 to 5 after surgery and last a few weeks. Patients may awaken normally and be oriented but exhibit mild confusion or psychosis. Pupillary reaction and motor response are assessed. The safety of the patient is maintained with side rails up, bed in low position, and nursing call light within reach. The patient is given as much rest and as little sensory stimulation as possible.

Due to postoperative pain and the continuous level of activity in the intensive care unit, sleeping is difficult. Sleep is promoted in 90-minute intervals. Dim lights and decreasing all sensory stimulation near the patient are important. In addition, listening to a favorite soothing type of music with earphones or the use of ordered narcotics for pain may also help sedate and relax the patient to allow for healing.

Temperature is monitored every 4 hours. Because immunosuppression can increase the risk of infection, any increase in temperature is immediately reported. Complete blood cell count and white blood cell results are monitored for indications of infection. If oral thrush (white patches) develops, an antifungal agent is ordered. A urine culture to diagnose a urinary tract infection is ordered if cloudy urine or urinary tract burning occurs.

Nursing Process for the Preoperative Cardiac Transplant Patient

General preoperative care is discussed in Chapter 12.

Nursing Process for the Postoperative Cardiac Transplant Patient

Data Collection

The patient is accompanied to the intensive care unit by the anesthesiologist. The intensive care nurse is given a hand-off report on the patient's surgical procedure. In addition, complications as well as hemodynamic and ventilatory management of the patient are reported. Bedside cardiac monitoring is used to detect arrythmias. A mechanical ventilator is needed for 4 to 24 hours. A temporary artificial cardiac pacemaker is connected to the epicardial pacing wires if they were placed during surgery as a precaution to treat sinus bradycardia or other arrhythmias. The patient is placed under a forced-air warming device such as a blanket for rewarming, which requires body temperature monitoring to prevent excess warming. The chest tubes fluid levels are monitored for a large increase or a sudden decrease. The nasogastric tube is attached to suction. The urinary catheter is positioned for gravity drainage. Intake and output are monitored hourly, as fluid imbalance can alter cardiac output. Cardiac transplant patients may be in isolation for their own protection, depending on the agency's policy.

A head-to-toe assessment of the patient is performed by the registered nurse, perhaps with data collection assistance by the licensed practical or licensed vocational nurse, that includes incisional dressings, tubes, and IV lines. Of importance are signs of pain, awakening, shivering, lung and heart sounds, and palpation of the entire chest and neck to detect crepitus (air in the subcutaneous tissue from opening the chest). Complete blood count, electrolytes, coagulation studies, and ABGs are monitored. Low calcium and magnesium and low or high potassium decrease cardiac contractility and cardiac output. Acidosis decreases cardiac contractility. A low cardiac output may lead to further acidosis.

After the initial transfer data collection, vital signs, oxygen saturation, and cardiac pressures are monitored and recorded every 15 to 30 minutes. Lung sounds are monitored as crackles may indicate heart failure or pulmonary edema. Sputum character is monitored. Peripheral circulation is monitored as mottling or weak pulses may indicate poor cardiac output. An electrocardiogram is obtained to detect perioperative myocardial infarction. A chest x-ray is done to check central line and endotracheal tube placement. An x-ray can also detect a pneumothorax or hemothorax, diaphragm elevation, or mediastinal widening from bleeding. At this point, the family may see the patient and receive explanations on the patient's care.

> **CUE RECOGNITION 26.2**
>
> As you are caring for your patient who is 3 days post-op cardiac transplantation, you notice that the patient's respiratory rate is 28 with shallow breaths and pale skin. What action do you take?
>
> *Suggested answers are at the end of the chapter.*

Nursing Diagnoses, Planning, Implementation, and Evaluation

Nursing diagnoses for postoperative care are discussed in "Nursing Care Plan for the Patient Undergoing Surgery" in Chapter 12. Chest pain after surgery can be frightening. Explain that chest pain can occur from the surgical incision and not be due to angina or a myocardial infarction. Assist the patient to splint the chest incision for all movement and coughing and deep breathing. This helps stabilize the incision and reduces pain.

Cardiac transplant patients may have memory deficits, cognitive dysfunction, and short attention spans resulting from long-term decreased cerebral perfusion. Reinforce education in small increments using written and video materials. Include families in educational sessions and encourage them to promote self-care by the patient. Patients usually have questions regarding sexual functioning. Referrals can be made to sex counselors. Patients need comprehensive information to comply with posttransplant care. Discharge teaching includes treatment, complications such as incisional infection, activity, medications, and enhancing quality of life. Organ rejection is possible. Instructions for anti-rejection medications and testing must be followed to prevent or detect rejection. Education on signs and symptoms to report is essential.

Coping With Cardiac Transplant

Cardiac transplant patients may have feelings of sadness and grief for the donor and the donor's family while also experiencing great elation, relief, and hope after a long wait for the transplant. Patients should be told that these feelings are normal. Emotional support may be needed.

After a cardiac transplant, patients work out in an exercise rehabilitation program. Their activity is closely monitored for signs of activity intolerance. Many patients are able to reach an activity level to play recreational sports, if desired.

Patient Perspective

Jim

I have always known that I am incredibly lucky, or more accurately, someone up there is looking out for me in spite of myself. I had always considered myself healthy, although a little overweight. I had an active job, first as a police officer and then as a probation officer doing a lot of field work. I also stayed active playing golf, kayaking, hiking, and building things around the house.

When I was on vacation with my family at age 50, cycling in Ireland, things changed, but someone was still watching over me. I had a heart attack on one of the remote trails in the Killarney National Park. My daughter was carrying aspirin as part of her preparedness. There was a doctor on the trail behind us who stayed with me and started the IV. In Ireland, the EMTs were able to give me an emergency medication that had not yet been approved in this country. After being stabilized, I was transferred to a state-of-the-art cardiac hospital in Cork with the best cardiologists and professional staff in the country.

The doctors in Ireland contacted doctors in NYC who, along with outstanding nurses and phlebotomists, ensured that my treatment continued uninterrupted when I went home. Although I was feeling stronger all the time, the New York cardiologist decided to have me wear a Holter device that detected an arrhythmia and resulted in my having an implanted defibrillator. For almost 10 years, I maintained an active lifestyle and had a real sense of invulnerability. I would joke with coworkers that in the event of a cardiac event, they would have to find the defibrillator on the wall, while had my own!

Then one day my defibrillator went off. After four more defibrillator events, an ever-increasing regimen of medications, and a short hospital stay, the doctor informed me that I had become a candidate for a heart transplant. That was an awakening.

Although I remained in denial for a couple of years despite close medical outpatient treatment, during a routine doctor visit, a nurse had to call an ambulance to take me to the emergency department. I then spent 3 months in the cardiac transplant ward attached to several bags of medicine until a heart was found. While there I had two false starts when I was prepped for an available transplant only to be told at the last minute that the doctors determined that it would not be a good fit. These events were strangely comforting because they showed that doctors were looking for perfection and not just good enough. When the heart for my transplant finally arrived, things happened extremely fast, which was good because there was little time to think about it before being sedated.

When I woke up in a different ward with different staff, I was very disoriented and unprepared for the strange feelings I was experiencing. But I was sustained by all the positive people who knew all about what I was feeling. After two days in intensive care, I was moved to post-op care where, on the next day, two physical therapists insisted that it was time to get up and walk. Although I did not believe it was possible because of all the tubes and wires coming out of my body, they persisted and got me to walk then and three times a day thereafter. After three days, my luck continued and I was released to home without the need to go to a rehabilitation program.

Right after my transplant, I was taking more than 20 medications that were closely monitored with frequent heart biopsies and other tests, but over time the number of medications has gone down to eight with less frequent testing. After less than a year, I was cleared for all activities that did not involve sudden exertion, such as sprinting or tennis, because of the heart's inability to efficiently return to a normal rhythm. During the 2020 COVID-19 pandemic, I have been in extreme isolation and have had no social contacts due to my immunosuppression from antirejection medications. The care and concern from all the medical professionals I have met during my postoperative procedures and support groups continues to sustain me. Having met them and experienced their goodness, along with having support and prayers of family and friends, confirms that there is someone up there who is looking out for me.

CRITICAL THINKING

Mrs. Lavigne, age 45 and a single mother of two, is transferred to a surgical unit 5 days after a cardiac transplant. She is withdrawn and has a poor appetite. Her vital signs are stable. When ambulating to the bathroom, she is very weak, requiring two nurses to help her. Her respiratory rate increases from 20 to 32 breaths per minute and is slightly labored. Her apical pulse increases from 88 to 103 mm Hg.

1. Is Mrs. Lavigne tolerating this activity? Why or why not?
2. List four reasons why Mrs. Lavigne has a poor appetite.
3. Explain four patient-centered nursing interventions for Mrs. Lavigne's poor appetite.
4. Give three reasons why Mrs. Lavigne is withdrawn.
5. What health-care team members might collaborate in Mrs. Lavigne's care?

Suggested answers are at the end of the chapter.

Key Points

- HF is a clinical syndrome that affects perfusion. It occurs from the inability of the ventricles to either fill or pump enough blood to meet the body's oxygen and nutrient needs. It may cause dyspnea, fatigue, and fluid volume overload.
- With left-sided HF, blood backs up from the left ventricle into the left atrium and then into the four pulmonary veins and lungs. This increases pulmonary pressure, causing fluid to move into the interstitium and then into the alveoli. Consequently, gas exchange is reduced across the alveolar capillary membrane, causing dyspnea.
- When the right ventricle fails, it does not empty normally. There is a backward buildup of blood in the systemic blood vessels. With the blood backed up from the right ventricle, right atrial and systemic venous blood volume increases.
- The major cause of right-sided HF is left-sided HF. When the left side fails, fluid backs up into the lungs. Pulmonary pressure is increased. The right ventricle must continually pump blood against this increased fluid and pressure. Over time, this strain causes the right ventricle to weaken and fail as a pump.
- Pulmonary edema (also called acute HF) is sudden, severe fluid congestion within the lung alveoli and is life threatening.
- Pink, frothy sputum is the classic symptom of pulmonary edema. It is caused by the lung congestion and increased pressure that causes leaking of fluid and red blood cells into the alveoli. Other signs and symptoms include anxiety and restlessness, clammy skin, coughing, crackles and wheezes, and rapid respirations with accessory muscle use.
- Symptoms of chronic HF include fatigue and weakness, dyspnea, cough, crackles and wheezing, tachycardia, chest pain, and edema.
- Diagnostic tests for HF include blood testing, chest x-ray, electrocardiogram, echocardiogram, stress testing and nuclear imaging studies, cardiac magnetic resonance imaging, cardiac angiography, and sleep studies.
- Treatment of HF focuses on (1) identifying and correcting the underlying cause, (2) increasing the strength of the heart's contraction, (3) maintaining optimal water and sodium balance, and (4) decreasing the heart's workload.
- Medications often in combination are used for HF (Table 26.5)
- Artificial cardiac pacemakers and wearable or implantable cardioverter defibrillators (WCDs/ICDs) are used along with medications for patients at risk of sudden death. Artificial pacemakers produce an electrical impulse to regulate the heart's conduction system. WCDs/ICDs deliver an electric countershock if a life-threatening rhythm occurs.
- Chronic management of HF requires patient and family understanding of the disease process, management of home oxygen therapy, diet and weight control, medications, and the need for immunizations such as the annual flu shot.

The author acknowledges the contributions to this chapter by Leila Cherara.

SUGGESTED ANSWERS TO CHAPTER EXERCISES

Cue Recognition

26.1: Assist patient to safely return to bed and take her BP (consider orthostatic BP if able to safely tolerate it). Report findings to HCP. Do you recognize the connection between new vasodilator and dizziness/lightheadedness from a possible low BP?

26.2: Monitor lung sounds to gather data to identify heart failure or pulmonary edema. Report findings to HCP.

Critical Thinking & Clinical Judgment
Part 1: Mr. Bjorklund

1. Signs and symptoms of heart failure (HF) include shortness of breath, two-pillow orthopnea, dry cough, tachycardia (pulse 106 bpm), tachypnea (respiration 24 breaths per minute), and bilateral crackles.
2. Left-sided HF is indicated by the findings.
3. *Shortness of breath:* fluid in the lungs impairs gas exchange; *orthopnea:* lying flat increases fluid accumulation in the

SUGGESTED ANSWERS TO CHAPTER EXERCISES—cont'd

lungs, causing dyspnea; *dry cough:* fluid in the lungs irritates the mucosal lining of the lungs; *tachycardia:* sympathetic compensation to increase cardiac output; *tachypnea:* sympathetic compensation to increase blood oxygenation; *bilateral crackles:* fluid trapped in the lungs.
4. The two pillows help reduce orthopnea by using a more upright position, which allows gravity to decrease fluid accumulation in the lungs.
5. The HCP, case manager, nurses, dietitian, physical therapist, occupational therapist, pharmacist, social worker, and clergy.

Part 2: Mr. Bjorklund
1. Mr. Bjorklund's heart is enlarged to compensate for the strain caused by increased peripheral vascular resistance from hypertension to maintain an adequate cardiac output.
2. An enlarged heart requires more oxygen, which often cannot be supplied in HF.

Part 3: Mr. Bjorklund
1. The ACE inhibitor is needed for vasodilation to reduce peripheral vascular resistance and decrease the heart's workload. This in turn prevents cardiac remodeling and improves cardiac output.
2. The ACE inhibitor will affect afterload.
3. The diuretic is ordered to decrease fluid volume, which reduces preload and decreases the heart's workload.
4. The low-sodium diet is ordered to reduce water retention, which reduces preload and decreases the heart's workload.
5. The goal is to (1) decrease the heart's workload and increase its efficiency by reducing preload and peripheral vascular resistance, and (2) decrease progression of chronic HF and improve survival.
6. Potassium needs to be monitored because diuretics can be either potassium-wasting or potassium-sparing.

Part 4: Mr. Bjorklund
1. After determining Mr. Bjorklund's knowledge base, medication education should be given on the ACE inhibitor and diuretic, including their purpose, side effects, and precautions. A schedule for taking the medications can be planned. The diuretic should be taken in the morning to avoid sleep disruption at night. Explain the purpose of a low-sodium diet and plan menus based on Mr. Bjorklund's likes and dislikes.
2. Low-sodium foods should be selected to prevent fluid retention. High-potassium foods can be included to prevent hypokalemia from the diuretic, if appropriate. Encourage Mr. Bjorklund to read food labels. He needs education on low-sodium foods. Examples include puffed rice, wheat cereals, fruits, chicken, beef, eggs, and potatoes. High-sodium foods include tomato juice, sauerkraut, softened water, buttermilk, cheese, smoked meats, canned tuna, canned soup, pickles, instant rice, and instant potatoes. High-potassium foods include salt substitutes, bran products, avocado, bananas, prunes, oranges, baked potato, sweet potato, spinach (cooked), chocolate, nuts, and molasses. Encourage patient to request low sodium or no-added-sodium foods. He can rinse canned vegetables to lower sodium.
3. Collaborate with a dietitian to help education Mr. Bjorklund on his new 2 g sodium diet.
4. Reinforce education for Mr. Bjorklund that daily weights at the same time, with similar clothing (ideally in the morning), are ideal to detect rapid weight gain from fluid. The use of diuretics may also cause weight loss. These instructions ensure accuracy of the weight so that comparison to the baseline weight detects a weight gain or loss. The guideline for reporting a weight increase is an increase of 2 to 3 pounds in 1 to 2 days.

Mrs. Lavigne
1. No, Mrs. Lavigne is not tolerating this activity, as evidenced by her increased respiratory rate and apical rate.
2. Steroids, immunosuppressive therapy, depression, and fatigue could be causing her poor appetite.
3. Nursing interventions related to Mrs. Lavigne's poor appetite could include the following: Offer small, frequent meals; have her family bring favorite foods from home; allow the patient to rest before meals; provide oral hygiene before meals; administer antiemetics before meals; and give a high-calorie meal at peak appetite.
4. Mrs. Lavigne could be withdrawn because of changes in her lifestyle as a result of her transplant, extreme fatigue, concerns regarding how she will raise her children, grieving for the donor, and fear that she will reject her new heart.
5. HCP (e.g., surgeon, physician's assistant, nurse practitioner), case manager, nurses, dietitian, physical therapist, occupational therapist, pharmacist, social worker, and clergy.

Additional Resources

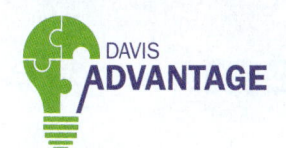

Go to Davis Advantage to complete your learning: strengthen understanding, apply your knowledge, and prepare for the Next Gen NCLEX®.

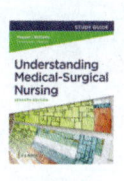

A Study Guide is also available.

UNIT SIX Understanding the Hematologic and Lymphatic Systems

CHAPTER 27
Hematologic and Lymphatic System Function, Data Collection, and Therapeutic Measures

Margaret McCormick, Lucy L. Colo, Janice L. Bradford

KEY TERMS

ecchymoses (EK-ih-MOH-sis)
hemolysis (hee-MAHL-ih-sis)
lymphedema (LIMPF-uh-DEE-mah)
petechiae (puh-TEE-kee-eye)
purpura (PURR-purr-uh)

CHAPTER CONCEPTS

Cellular regulation
Infection

LEARNING OUTCOMES

1. List the components of blood.
2. List the components of the lymphatic system.
3. Describe how changes in the blood or lymphatic systems can manifest as disease processes.
4. Describe the sequence of events in the process of blood clotting.
5. Identify data to collect when caring for a patient with a disorder of the hematologic or lymphatic system.
6. Explain laboratory and diagnostic studies that are used when evaluating the hematologic and lymphatic systems.
7. Plan nursing care for patients undergoing diagnostic tests of the hematologic or lymphatic systems.
8. List common therapeutic measures for patients with hematologic and lymphatic disorders.
9. Discuss the role of the licensed practical nurse/licensed vocational nurse in administering blood products.

NORMAL HEMATOLOGIC AND LYMPHATIC SYSTEM ANATOMY AND PHYSIOLOGY

The hematologic system includes the bone marrow, blood, and blood components. The lymphatic system includes lymph nodes; nodules, which filter pathogens for destruction; and lymph vessels, which return lymph to the blood.

Blood

The general functions of blood are transport of substances; regulation of body temperature, pH, and fluid balance; and transport of cells that offer the body protection.

The human body contains 4 to 6 L of blood. Approximately 45% is formed elements. The remainder is plasma (Fig. 27.1). All formed elements are produced from stem cells in the red bone marrow (hematopoietic tissue) found in flat bones, irregular bones, and the epiphyses of long bones (Fig. 27.2). T-lymphocyte maturation and differentiation occur in the thymus. Table 27.1 shows normal blood cell counts.

Plasma

Plasma, the transporting medium, is about 91% water. Plasma proteins are synthesized by the liver. They include clotting factors, albumin, and globulins. Clotting factors such as prothrombin and fibrinogen circulate

Chapter 27 Hematologic and Lymphatic System Function, Data Collection, and Therapeutic Measures   449

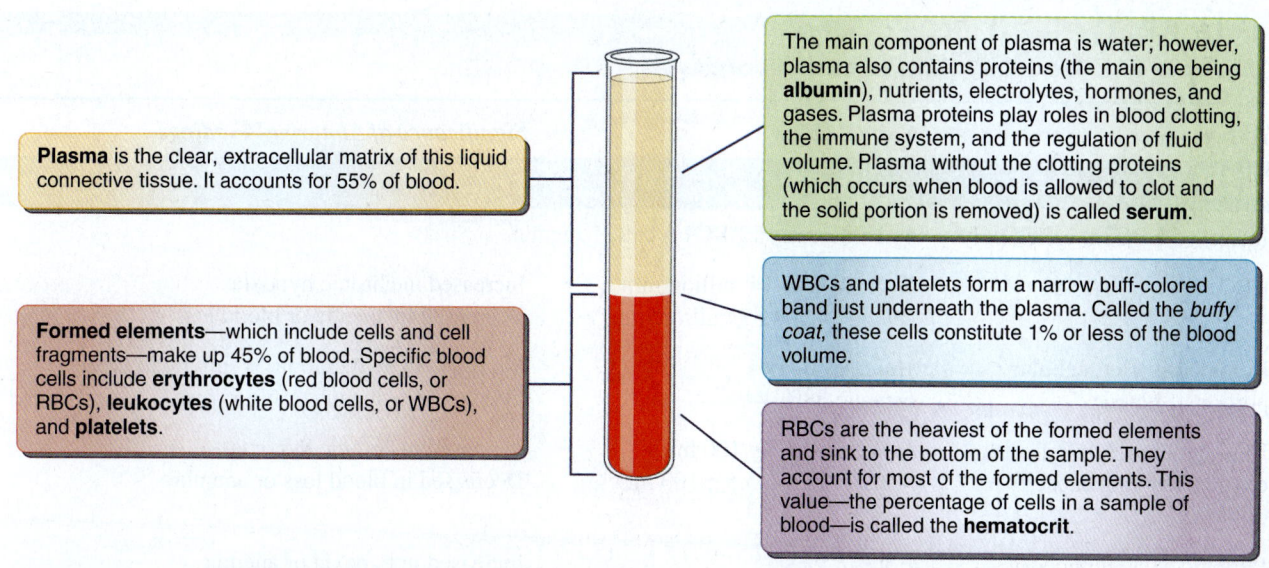

Plasma is the clear, extracellular matrix of this liquid connective tissue. It accounts for 55% of blood.

The main component of plasma is water; however, plasma also contains proteins (the main one being **albumin**), nutrients, electrolytes, hormones, and gases. Plasma proteins play roles in blood clotting, the immune system, and the regulation of fluid volume. Plasma without the clotting proteins (which occurs when blood is allowed to clot and the solid portion is removed) is called **serum**.

WBCs and platelets form a narrow buff-colored band just underneath the plasma. Called the *buffy coat*, these cells constitute 1% or less of the blood volume.

Formed elements—which include cells and cell fragments—make up 45% of blood. Specific blood cells include **erythrocytes** (red blood cells, or RBCs), **leukocytes** (white blood cells, or WBCs), and **platelets**.

RBCs are the heaviest of the formed elements and sink to the bottom of the sample. They account for most of the formed elements. This value—the percentage of cells in a sample of blood—is called the **hematocrit**.

FIGURE 27.1 Components of blood.

All blood cells can trace their beginnings to a specific type of bone marrow cell called a stem cell (also called a pluripotent stem cell). Stem cells are unspecialized cells that give rise to immature red blood cells, white blood cells, and platelet-producing cells.

Stem cell

Proerythroblast   Myeloblast   Lymphoblast   Monoblast   Megakaryoblast

The "offspring" of the stem cell divide further, ultimately becoming a mature red blood cell, white blood cell, or platelet.

Reticulocyte   Progranulocyte   Megakaryocyte

Erythrocytes   Basophil   Eosinophil   Neutrophil   Lymphocyte   Monocyte   Thrombocytes

                        Granulocytes   Agranulocytes

Red blood cells   **White blood cells**   **Platelets**

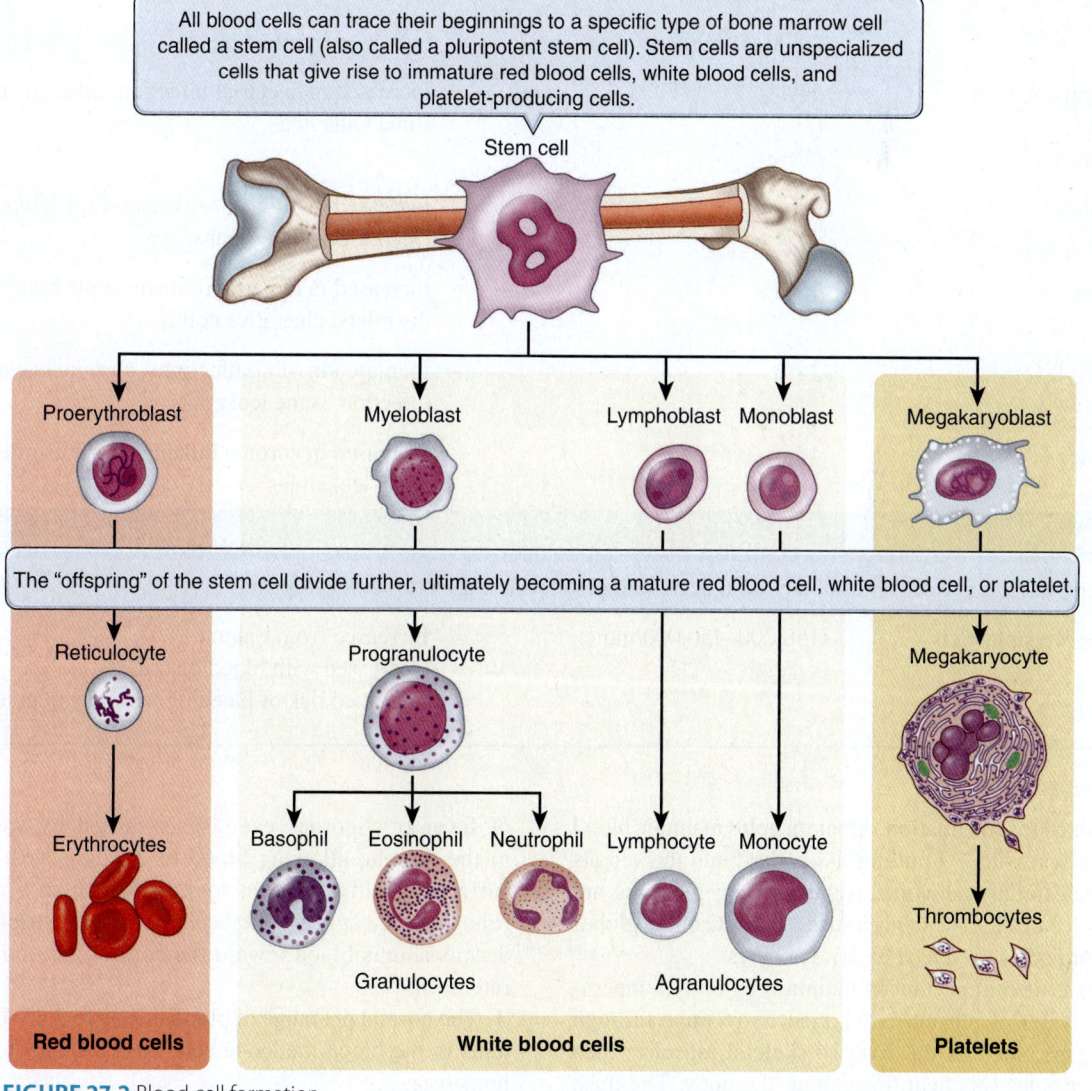

FIGURE 27.2 Blood cell formation.

Table 27.1
Review of Blood Cell Values and Disorders

Test	Normal Value	Significance of Abnormal Findings
Red Blood Cells (RBCs)		
Increased RBCs is called polycythemia; decreased RBCs is called anemia.		
RBCs	Male: 4.71–5.14 million/mm^3 Female: 4.2–4.87 million/mm^3	Increased in chronic hypoxia Decreased in anemia or blood loss
Hematocrit (Hct; cellular portion of blood)	Male: 43%–49% Female: 38%–44%	Increased in dehydration or chronic hypoxia Decreased in anemia or blood loss
Hemoglobin (Hgb; reflects oxygen-carrying capacity of blood)	Male: 14–17.3 g/100 mL Female: 11.7–15.5 g/100 mL	Increased in chronic hypoxia Decreased in blood loss or anemia
Reticulocytes (number of circulating immature RBCs)	1.5%–2.5%	Increased in hypoxia or anemia Decreased in RBC maturation defect
White Blood Cells (WBCs)		
Increased WBCs is called leukocytosis; decreased WBCs is called leukopenia.		
WBCs	4,500–11,000/mm^3	Increased in infection
Neutrophils (Bands) (Segments)	59% (3%) (56%)	Increased in bacterial infection, inflammation, some leukemias
Eosinophils	2.7%	Increased in allergic response, some leukemias Decreased in infections
Basophils	0.5%	Increased in hyperthyroidism, some bone marrow disorders, ulcerative colitis
Lymphocytes	34%	Increased in viral infections, chronic bacterial infection, some leukemias
Monocytes	4%	Increased in chronic inflammatory disorders, some leukemias
Platelets		
Increased platelets is called thrombocytosis; decreased platelets is called thrombocytopenia.		
Thrombocytes/platelets	150,000–450,000/mm^3	Increased from trauma Decreased with blood disorders Increased risk of bleeding with low platelet count

until activated for coagulation. Albumin helps maintain blood volume and pressure by pulling tissue fluid into the venous ends of the capillary networks. Alpha and beta globulins are carrier molecules for substances such as fats. Gamma globulins are antibodies produced by lymphocytes.

Plasma is also important in maintaining body temperature. The water of plasma is warmed by passage through active organs, such as the liver or skeletal muscles, then blood distributes this heat throughout the body. The flush of fever or vigorous exercise is caused by vasodilation in the dermis, allowing blood to circulate near the body surface, resulting in heat loss. A person in a cold environment may appear pale because vasoconstriction in the dermis shunts blood toward the core of the body for heat retention.

The normal pH range of blood is 7.35 to 7.45. Buffer systems in the blood moderate acid–base changes to maintain homeostasis.

Red Blood Cells

Mature red blood cells (RBCs) are biconcave disks without nuclei; they carry oxygen bonded to the iron in hemoglobin. *Oxyhemoglobin* is formed in the pulmonary capillaries when oxygen bonds to the iron in hemoglobin. Once hemoglobin gives up its oxygen to the cells of the body, it becomes *reduced hemoglobin*. The amount of hemoglobin in RBCs, the amount of iron in that hemoglobin, and the number of RBCs determine the amount of oxygen the blood can carry. Reduced oxygen-carrying capacity causes anemia. This results in symptoms such as shortness of breath and fatigue.

Hypoxia stimulates the kidneys to secrete erythropoietin. This increases the rate of RBC production and, thus, the oxygen-carrying capacity of the blood. A *reticulocyte* (immature RBC) becomes a mature RBC when it ejects its nucleus. This causes the characteristic biconcave disk shape. The presence of large numbers of reticulocytes in peripheral blood indicates an insufficient number of mature RBCs to meet the oxygen demands of the body.

Sufficient dietary intake of protein and iron to synthesize hemoglobin is required for normal production of RBCs. The vitamins folic acid and vitamin B_{12} are needed for DNA synthesis in the stem cells of the red bone marrow; mitosis is dependent on the ability to produce new sets of chromosomes. Vitamin B_{12} is called *extrinsic factor* because it comes from an extrinsic source: food. The parietal cells of the stomach lining produce *intrinsic factor*. This is a chemical that combines with vitamin B_{12} to promote its absorption in the small intestine.

RBCs live for about 120 days. After that, they become fragile and are phagocytized by fixed macrophages in the liver, spleen, and red bone marrow (Fig. 27.3). Diseases such as malaria and sickle cell anemia cause an accelerated destruction of RBCs (**hemolysis**). The resulting release of excess hemoglobin can cause the blood level of bilirubin to rise. Elevated bilirubin levels discolor the sclerae, skin, and mucous membranes to a yellowish orange hue; this condition is known as *jaundice*.

Each person has an inherited blood type. Blood type is determined by the antigens present on the RBCs. The two most important type categories are the ABO group and the Rh factor. The ABO type (A, B, O, or AB) indicates the antigens present (or not present, as in type O) on the RBCs. The plasma contains antibodies for antigens that are not present in the blood. These antibodies can interact with antigens in transfused blood if the donor's blood does not match the recipient's blood (Table 27.2). To be Rh-positive means that the D antigen is present on the RBCs; Rh-negative means that the antigen is not present. Rh-negative people do not have natural antibodies to the D antigen but will produce them if given Rh-positive blood.

White Blood Cells

White blood cells (WBCs) are larger than RBCs. They have nuclei when mature. The granular WBCs (neutrophils, eosinophils, and basophils) and the agranular WBCs (lymphocytes and monocytes) are produced in the red bone marrow; the T lymphocytes complete their development in the thymus. The T lymphocytes and B lymphocytes become activated, proliferate, and differentiate in the lymph nodes, spleen, and lymphatic nodules. Table 27.1 shows normal values and percentages for each type of WBC in a differential count. WBCs function within tissue fluid and blood. All are involved in the immune or inflammatory response to injury. Each white cell type has a different life span, but in general, they circulate only a few days before migrating into tissues where some cell types can live for years to be called back to active duty when needed.

Monocytes become macrophages in tissues, which phagocytize pathogens and viral-infected cells. Neutrophils are more numerous and phagocytize foreign materials. Eosinophils combat the effects of histamine, detoxify foreign proteins during allergic reactions, and respond to parasitic infections. Basophils release heparin and histamine as part of inflammatory reactions. There are two groups of lymphocytes: T cells and B cells. T cells may be helper, suppressor, killer, or memory T cells. B cells become memory cells and plasma cells; plasma cells produce antibodies to foreign antigens.

Platelets

Platelets are formed in the red bone marrow. They are fragments of large cells called megakaryocytes. Platelets are involved in all mechanisms of hemostasis: vascular spasm, platelet plugs, and chemical clotting. The lifespan of platelets is about 10 days.

After a platelet plug is formed, one of two pathways initiates a cascade of events to bring about coagulation. When a blood vessel or surrounding tissues *outside* the blood are damaged, the extrinsic pathway begins. When platelets adhere to damaged endothelium and release clotting factors, this initiates the *intrinsic* pathway. Either way, the result is a fibrin clot (Fig. 27.4).

Excessive clotting in the vascular system is prevented in several ways. The smooth endothelial lining of blood vessels repels platelets so that they do not stick to intact vessel walls. Heparin produced by mast cells inhibits the clotting mechanism. Antithrombin inactivates excess thrombin to prevent the clotting mechanism from becoming a vicious cycle.

Lymphatic System

The lymphatic system consists of lymph, lymph vessels, lymph nodes and nodules, the spleen, red bone marrow, and the thymus (Fig. 27.5). Functions of the lymph system include the return of tissue fluid to maintain blood volume and protecting the body against pathogens and other foreign material. (Immunity is covered in Unit 4.)

• WORD • BUILDING •

hemolysis: heme—blood + lysis—dissolution

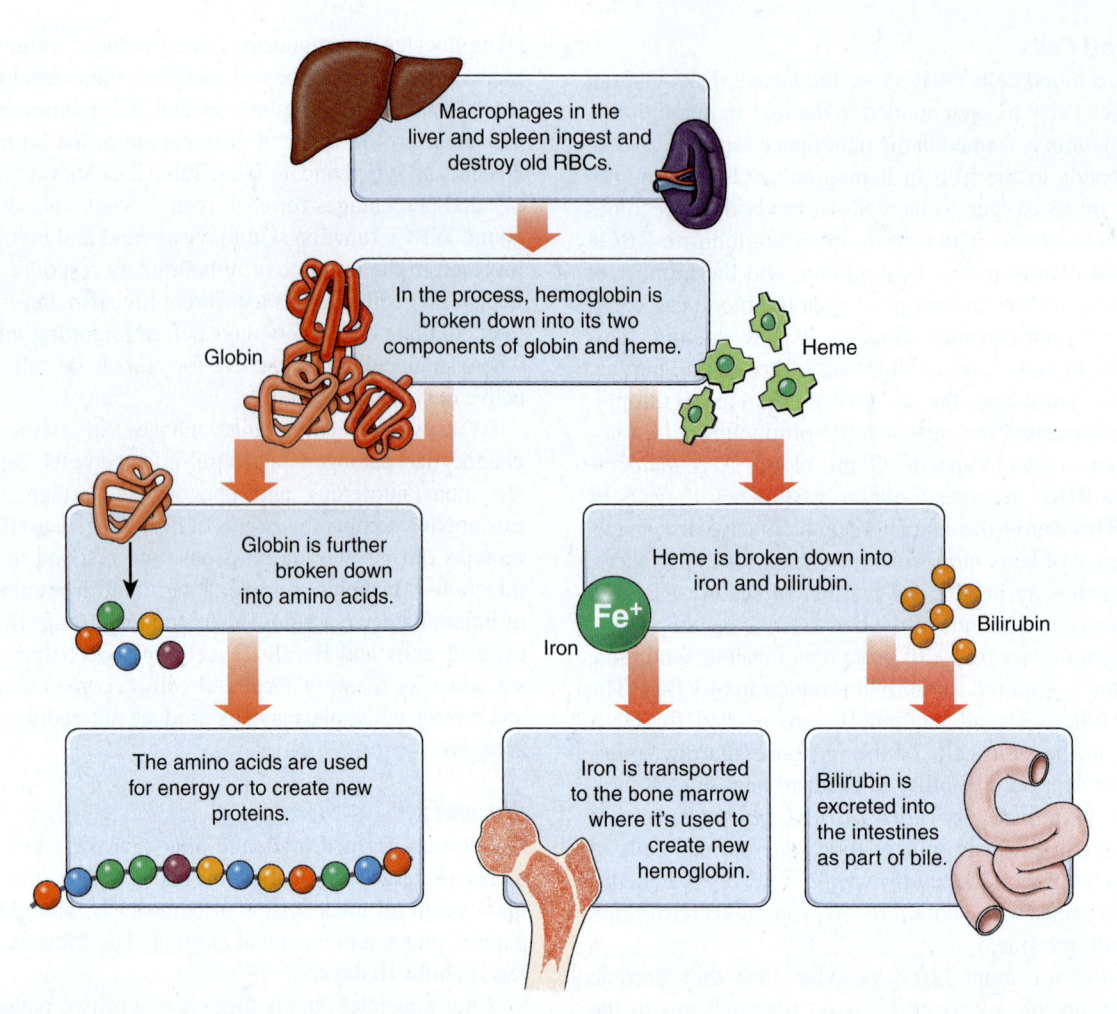

FIGURE 27.3 Breakdown of red blood cells.

Table 27.2
ABO Blood Types

Type	Antigens Present on Red Blood Cells	Antibodies Present in Plasma
A	A	Anti-B
B	B	Anti-A
AB	Both A and B	Neither anti-A nor anti-B
O	Neither A nor B	Both anti-A and anti-B

Lymphatic Vessels

Lymph is tissue fluid that has entered lymph capillaries. Lymph must be returned to the blood to maintain blood volume and blood pressure. Lymph capillaries are found in most tissue spaces. They anastomose, forming larger and larger lymph vessels, which have valves to prevent backflow. Lymph from areas below the diaphragm and the upper left half of the body enters the thoracic duct. It is returned to the blood in the left subclavian vein. Lymph from the upper right body enters the right lymphatic duct. It is returned to the blood in the right subclavian vein.

Lymph Nodes and Nodules

Lymph *nodes* are masses of lymphatic tissue along the pathways of the lymph vessels. They house activated lymphocytes and macrophages. Nodes are scattered throughout the body. They are concentrated in the cervical, axillary, and inguinal regions, where they are well situated to remove pathogens before the lymph is returned to the blood. Foreign materials are phagocytized by fixed macrophages; lymphocytes form immune responses.

Lymph *nodules* (or mucosa-associated lymphatic tissue) are small masses of lymphatic tissue found just beneath the epithelium of all mucous membranes. Mucosal-lined tracts (respiratory, digestive, urinary, and reproductive) have openings to the external environment. Any natural body opening is a potential portal of entry for pathogens. Microbes that penetrate the epithelium are usually destroyed by the macrophages in the lymph nodules. The tonsils, which protect the

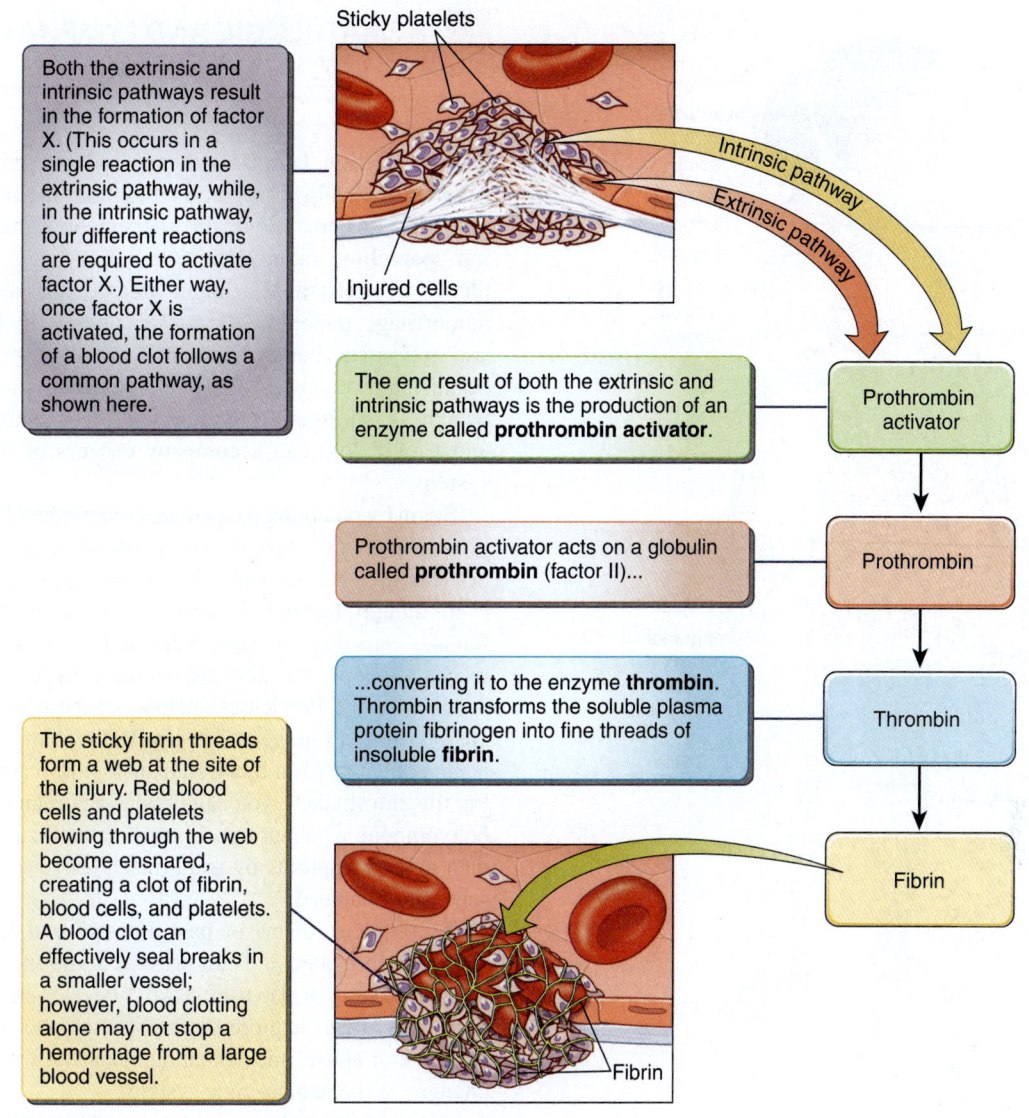

FIGURE 27.4 Formation of a blood clot.

oral and nasal portions of the pharynx, are familiar examples of lymph nodules.

Spleen

The spleen is in the upper left quadrant of the abdominal cavity, just below the diaphragm and behind the stomach. The lower rib cage protects the spleen from mechanical injury. In the fetus, the spleen produces RBCs, a function assumed by the bone marrow after birth.

The spleen has several functions after birth. It contains B cells and T cells, which conduct immune responses. It also contains fixed macrophages that phagocytize pathogens and worn or defective blood cells and platelets. The heme unit from RBC destruction forms bilirubin. Bilirubin is sent to the liver by way of portal circulation for excretion in the bile. The spleen stores up to one-third of the body's platelets.

The spleen is not considered a vital organ because other organs compensate for its functions if it must be removed. The liver and red bone marrow also remove worn RBCs from circulation. The many lymph nodes and nodules produce lymphocytes and macrophages for protection. However, a person without a spleen is somewhat more susceptible to certain bacterial infections, such as pneumonia and meningitis.

Thymus

The thymus is located in the mediastinum, anterior to the trachea. As we age, the thymus atrophies, so relatively little thymic tissue is found in adults. The thymus contains T lymphocytes (T cells) that mature and proliferate. Thymic hormones contribute to the maturation of the T cells. (Immunity is covered in Unit 4.)

Aging and the Hematologic and Lymphatic Systems

Older adults undergo a number of changes in the hematologic and lymphatic systems (Fig. 27.6).

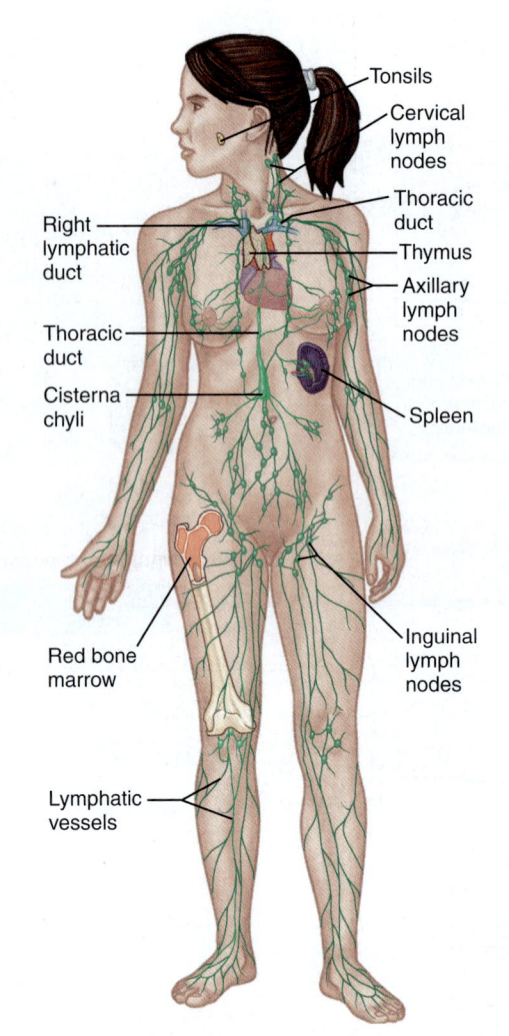

FIGURE 27.5 The lymphatic system.

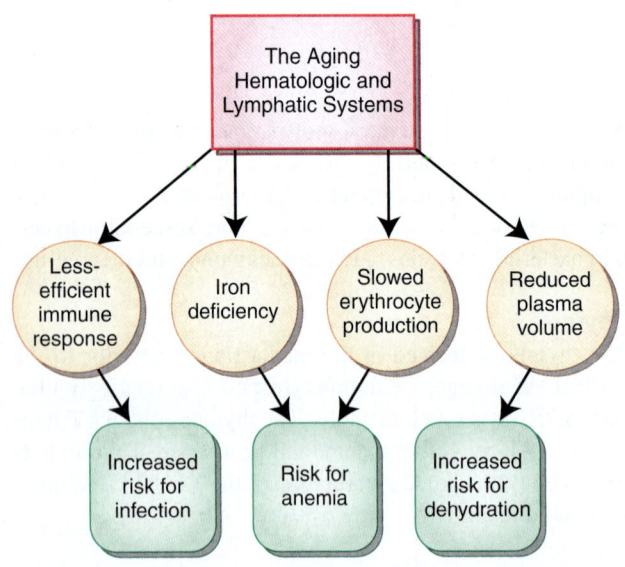

FIGURE 27.6 Effects of aging on the hematologic and lymphatic systems.

HEMATOLOGIC AND LYMPHATIC SYSTEMS DATA COLLECTION

Health History

Data collection begins with an in-depth patient history (Table 27.3). Specific problems that might be seen in patients with hematologic disorders include abnormal bleeding, **petechiae** (small purplish hemorrhagic spots under the skin), **ecchymoses** (larger areas of discoloration from hemorrhage under the skin—see images in Chapter 28), and **purpura** (hemorrhage into the skin, mucous membranes, and organs). Additional symptoms include fatigue, weakness, shortness of breath, and fever. Fatigue, malaise, and weight loss can accompany cancers of the lymphatic system.

Begin by obtaining the patient's biographical data, occupation, religion, age, sex, and ethnic background. This information can give you valuable clues to risk factors. For example, even though hemophilia almost always occurs in males, females can carry the gene. Sickle cell anemia occurs mostly in Black people but also affects those of Mediterranean or Asian ancestry. Pernicious anemia occurs most often in people of northern European ancestry. Religion may be important if the patient needs a blood transfusion. By carefully collecting this information, you can obtain important clues that will help pinpoint a patient's problem. Finally, focus on collecting data about symptoms by using the **WHAT'S UP?** format presented in Chapter 1.

A complete review of past illnesses and family history is always indicated and can provide additional information. A social history is also useful. After developing good rapport with the patient, explore dietary and alcohol intake habits, drug use or abuse, and sexual habits, all of which can cause changes in the hematologic system.

An occupational review can reveal exposure to hazardous substances that can cause bone marrow dysfunction. Certain occupations, such as working in a paint factory, tool and dye processing, and even dry cleaning, can be related to the formation of some hematologic cancers. Military history can also reveal sources of exposure that can help during the diagnostic phase for hematologic and lymphatic disorders.

Physical Examination

Hematologic and lymphatic disorders can involve almost every body system, so each system must be considered. Signs and symptoms of hematologic and lymphatic disorders can be vague, such as dyspnea or fatigue. Careful data collection will guide nursing care but may also uncover important data that should be reported to the health care provider (HCP). Table 27.4 reviews objective data that should be collected and possible interpretations of findings.

Table 27.3
Subjective Data Collection for the Hematologic and Lymphatic Systems

Questions to Ask During the Health History	Rationale/Significance
Reason for Seeking Health Care	
Why are you seeking health care?	Signs and symptoms of hematologic/lymphatic disorders may be nonspecific. Any body system can be involved.
Family History	
How is the health of your blood relatives? Does anyone in your family have any blood-related diseases?	Some blood and immune disorders are hereditary.
Diet History	
Describe your usual diet.	Dietary deficiencies can lead to anemia or altered immune responses.
Medications/Supplements	
What medications do you take? What herbs or alternative therapies do you use?	Herbs and drugs can cause adverse reactions in the blood and immune systems.
How much alcohol do you drink each day?	Excess alcohol intake can lead to folic acid–deficiency anemia.
Occupational/Exposure History	
What is your occupational history? What is your military history?	Exposure to certain hazardous substances can lead to anemias, leukemias, or other cancers.
Fatigue	
Have you noticed any change in your energy level?	Anemia and many cancers are associated with fatigue.
Bleeding Tendency	
Have you experienced nosebleeds or any other unusual bleeding? Have you had bloody or black bowel movements?	Bleeding may indicate low platelet levels or a clotting factor deficiency.
Respiratory	
Do you experience shortness of breath or faintness?	Red blood cells (RBCs) carry oxygen, so a reduced RBC count can cause dyspnea.
Integumentary	
Have you noticed any changes in your skin?	Bleeding into the skin or mucous membranes can indicate a bleeding disorder.
Lymphadenopathy	
Have you noticed swelling in your neck, armpits, or groin?	Swollen lymph nodes may indicate inflammation, infection, or some cancers.

Table 27.4
Objective Data Collection for the Hematologic and Lymphatic Systems

Abnormal Findings	Possible Hematologic/Lymphatic Causes
Vital Signs	
Fever	Poor immune function, infection
Subnormal temperature	Possible overwhelming gram-negative infection
Elevated heart rate	Blood loss
Elevated respiratory rate	Anemia, decreased oxygen supply
Level of Consciousness	
Decreased level	Hypoxia, fever, intracranial bleeding
Skin, Mucous Membranes	
Pallor	Anemia
Cyanosis	Poor oxygenation of red blood cells
Jaundice (yellow color)	Hemolysis, liver involvement
Inflammation, redness, swelling, drainage	Poor immune function, infection
Purpura, ecchymoses, petechiae	Bleeding disorder
Dry or coarse skin	Some anemias
Itching	Blood or lymph disorders, jaundice, liver involvement
Fingernails	
Striations	Anemia
Spoon-shaped nails	Anemia
Clubbed fingers	Long-term hypoxia, anemia
Abdomen	
High-pitched, tinkling bowel sounds	Intestinal obstruction
Increasing abdominal girth	Ascites, bleeding
Neck, Axillae	
Lymph nodes greater than 1 cm in size or tender nodes	**Lymphedema**, inflammation, some cancers
Sternum	
Tenderness	Bone marrow packed with abnormal cells

DIAGNOSTIC TESTS FOR THE HEMATOLOGIC AND LYMPHATIC SYSTEMS

Blood Tests
Examples of laboratory studies routinely done for patients with hematologic disorders include complete blood count (CBC), total hemoglobin (Hgb) concentration, hematocrit (Hct) level, and platelet level. See normal values in Table 27.1.

Coagulation Tests
Coagulation tests are shown in Table 27.5. Agglutination tests include ABO blood typing, Rh typing, crossmatching of blood samples, and direct antiglobulin tests (also known as the *Coombs' test*).

• WORD • BUILDING •
lymphedema: lymph—fluid found in lymphatic vessels + edema—swelling

CRITICAL THINKING & CLINICAL JUDGMENT

Mrs. Brown is on warfarin (Coumadin) therapy because of a blood clot in her leg. She has an international normalized ratio (INR) done at her HCP's office. The result is 4.

Critical Thinking (The Why)
1. How do you expect the HCP to adjust her warfarin dosage based on this result? Explain your rationale. (Use Table 27.5 and Chapter 23 to figure out the answer.)
2. What foods might be interacting with her warfarin? (Check Chapter 23 for diet information.)
3. What antidote would be used if her INR was dangerously high?

Clinical Judgment (The Do)
4. What care would you initiate if her INR was 8.2?

Suggested answers are at the end of the chapter.

LEARNING TIP

When a patient has a bacterial infection, the neutrophils, which are the most numerous of the white blood cells (WBCs), rise in number to help fight it. There are two forms of neutrophils: segmented (mature) and bands (immature). Initially, the number of segmented neutrophils rises. Then, as the infection becomes more severe, the number of immature bands will rise.

An easy way to remember this is that the WBCs are part of the body's defenses, just like the military is part of a country's defenses. When needed, sergeants who are fully trained or mature are called to assess the battle first. If they are unable to fight off the invading enemy, new recruits being trained in boot camp are called in to help.

Segmented neutrophils (called **s**egs) are like the **s**ergeants, fully mature and ready to fight. The **b**ands are like **b**oot camp recruits, immature and not fully trained. However, in an acute infection, bands keep the body from being overwhelmed by the infection and losing the battle.

As you look at the differential WBC count, if the segs are elevated but the bands are normal, the infection is probably new. If the bands are also elevated, the infection is worsening. The more elevated they are, the more severe the infection.

Lymphocytes fight viral infections and are elevated during a virus. A common pattern in the WBCs is produced for either a bacterial or viral infection. If the infection is acute bacterial:

Segs ↑ Bands ↑ Lymphocytes ↓
If the infection is viral:
Segs ↓ Bands ↓ Lymphocytes ↑

The bone marrow produces the cells most needed during the time of viral infection and reduces production of those cells least needed. When the infection is resolved, all of the cells should return to their normal production levels.

Bone Marrow Biopsy

Biopsy information can be obtained through removal of a small amount of bone marrow with a needle. Aspiration of marrow is done to obtain a specimen that can be viewed under the microscope. Purposes of this test include the diagnosis of hematologic disorders; monitoring the course of treatment; discovery of other disorders, such as primary and metastatic tumors, infectious diseases, and certain granulomas; and isolation of bacteria and other pathogens by culture.

An accurate bone marrow specimen in an adult can be obtained from the sternum, the spinous processes of the vertebrae, or the anterior or posterior iliac crest. Bone marrow biopsy is considered a minor surgical procedure. It is carried out under aseptic conditions. For iliac crest aspiration, the patient is placed comfortably on the side with the back slightly flexed. The posterior iliac crest is cleansed and covered with antiseptic solution. The skin, subcutaneous tissue, and periosteum are anesthetized with lidocaine (Xylocaine). A small incision is made to facilitate penetration with a 2- to 4-cm-long bone marrow needle. The incision is made to avoid introducing a skin plug into the marrow cavity, which can cause infection.

The nurse's role in bone marrow biopsy is multifaceted. You may need to help coordinate between the laboratory and the HCP, establish a time to do the procedure, and determine who obtains the supplies, such as the disposable bone marrow aspiration tray and specialized needles. Be sure to obtain an order for an analgesic and to administer it before the procedure. Assist with positioning the patient before and during the procedure. Afterward, observe the aspiration site for bleeding and infection. Provide emotional support to the patient before, during, and after the procedure.

Lymphangiography

Problems in the lymph system, such as lymphoma or metastatic cancers, can be evaluated using lymphangiography. This procedure involves injection of a dye into the lymphatic vessels of the hand or foot. X-ray views are then taken to determine lymph flow or blockages. X-ray examinations are repeated in 24 hours to assess lymph node involvement.

Following the procedure, the HCP may order a pressure dressing and immobilization of the injected limb to prevent bleeding at the site. Monitor the limb for swelling, circulatory changes, and changes in sensation. Warn the patient that the skin, urine, or feces may be tinged blue from the dye for about 2 days.

Lymph Node Biopsy

If a lymph node is enlarged, it may be biopsied to determine whether the cause is infection or malignancy. A biopsy is done with a needle aspiration or surgical incision. A small dressing or bandage is applied to the site. Following the procedure, review signs of bleeding and infection with the patient that should be reported to the HCP.

Table 27.5
Coagulation Studies

Test	Normal Value	Significance of Abnormal Findings
Prothrombin time (PT; affected by activity of clotting factors V, VII, and X; prothrombin; and fibrinogen)	*Male:* 9.6–11.8 seconds *Female:* 9.5–11.3 seconds *Therapeutic range:* 1.5–2.0 times normal for patient on warfarin (Coumadin) therapy	Abnormalities in these values when the patient is not receiving anticoagulant therapy can indicate liver malfunction and bleeding tendency.
International normalized ratio (INR; standardized test adopted by World Health Organization)	Less than 1.1 *Therapeutic range:* 2.0–3.0 for patient on warfarin; 3.0–4.5 for recurrent problems	When receiving anticoagulant therapy, indicates if dosage needs to be increased or decreased. See Chapter 23 for dietary (vitamin K) implications.
Activated partial thromboplastin time (aPTT; evaluates factors I, II, V, VIII, IX, X, XI, and XII)	25–39 seconds *Therapeutic range:* 1.5–2.0 times normal for patient on heparin therapy	When receiving anticoagulant therapy, indicates if dosage needs to be increased or decreased.
Bleeding time (measures time for small puncture wound to stop bleeding)	2.5–9.5 minutes	Prolonged bleeding time indicates a platelet disorder.
Capillary fragility test (tests ability of capillaries to resist rupture under pressure)	Fewer than 10 petechiae appearing in a 2-inch circle after application of a blood pressure cuff at 100 mm Hg for 5 minutes	More than 10 petechiae could be related to fragile capillaries or thrombocytopenia.

THERAPEUTIC MEASURES FOR THE HEMATOLOGIC AND LYMPHATIC SYSTEMS

Blood Administration

Blood may be administered by a registered nurse (RN) or licensed practical nurse/licensed vocational nurse (LPN/LVN), depending on the state where you practice. As an LPN/LVN, you may assist with proper identification procedures and monitoring of vital signs during the transfusion.

Blood may be obtained from donors, or individuals can donate their own blood prior to a procedure in which blood may be needed. This is called an autologous transfusion, and can reduce the risk of complications. It can be stored for up to 42 days or frozen for future use.

Table 27.6 lists blood components that may be ordered. The main goals are to administer them safely and to avoid mistakes. Make sure to use proper identifying information to ensure that the right patient is receiving the right blood products. In addition, most institutions require a special transfusion consent form to be completed and present in the patient's chart.

Special Precautions

FLUID COMPATIBILITY. Use only normal saline solution to help dilute the blood and to flush the IV lines before and

Table 27.6
Blood Products

Product	Rationale for Use
Whole blood (all blood components)	Significant blood loss due to trauma or surgery
Packed red blood cells (RBCs)	Severe anemia or blood loss
Platelets	Bleeding caused by thrombocytopenia
Albumin	Hypovolemia caused by hypoalbuminemia
Fresh frozen plasma	Provides clotting factors for bleeding disorders; occasionally used for volume replacement
Cryoprecipitates	Bleeding caused by specific missing clotting factors

after transfusions. Solutions that contain dextrose can cause RBCs to lyse (i.e., destroy their cell membranes). Solutions with calcium can cause the blood product to clump, clot, or not infuse at all.

TIMING. A transfusion must be started within 30 minutes of picking up the blood from the blood bank. Transfuse each unit of packed cells over 2 hours. If it must transfuse more slowly because of the patient's condition, make sure the unit does not hang longer than 4 hours, to prevent deterioration and bacterial growth.

FILTERING. Filters are used with blood administration tubing to prevent potentially harmful particles from entering the patient. Most often, the filter that comes with the transfusion tubing is sufficient for each unit of packed RBCs. In some situations, special filters may be needed to remove leukocytes or micro-aggregates. The blood bank can advise in these situations.

WASHED OR LEUKOCYTE-DEPLETED BLOOD. In some instances, packed RBCs are ordered as "washed." They arrive from the blood bank in a special bag. The washing process removes almost all the plasma to decrease the risk or severity of a febrile reaction. In addition, leukocyte filters may be used to completely remove all WBCs. This removal process is used when many transfusions are anticipated to decrease the risk of antigen sensitization. It can also reduce transmission of certain viruses, such as cytomegalovirus.

WARMED BLOOD. If the patient has had severe bleeding and is receiving multiple rapid transfusions, the HCP may consider a blood warmer. It works just as the name implies, warming the cold blood from the blood bank to the standard body temperature of 98.6°F (37°C). This warming helps prevent hypothermia, which can cause heart arrhythmias. It also prevents shivering, which can destroy blood cells and platelets.

Monitoring

Whether or not you actually administer the blood, you will likely participate in monitoring to prevent complications or to detect and treat them quickly if they occur. Stay with the patient for the first 15 minutes of the blood transfusion to monitor for any immediate reactions. The 15 minutes begins when the blood enters the vein. If saline solution is in the tubing, it may take several minutes before the blood reaches the patient. Check and document vital signs before starting the transfusion, after the blood has begun to infuse, and after the infusion is complete. Always follow institution guidelines for vital sign monitoring. During the transfusion, continue to monitor the patient for signs and symptoms of complications.

> **PRACTICE ANALYSIS TIP**
> Linking NCLEX-PN® to Practice
> The LPN/VN will monitor transfusion of blood products.

Complications

Quick detection of complications can be lifesaving. It is easy to think of transfusing blood components as a routine procedure because it is a common activity. Do not be fooled. *It is a serious procedure that can be life threatening if errors occur.* Regular monitoring according to institution policy can help detect complications early when treatment is most effective.

FEBRILE REACTION. By far, the most common reaction is fever (febrile reaction). It occurs up to 2% of the time. Make sure that blood never transfuses for more than 4 hours. The risk of a febrile reaction goes up with each unit of blood product given to the patient. Many times, febrile reactions occur after the transfusion is completed, but they can occur at any time. This is the reason for obtaining a set of baseline vital signs, including the patient's temperature. Once a febrile reaction begins, the most common signs are an increase in temperature and shaking chills, which can be severe. Other symptoms include headache and back pain. If febrile symptoms occur, or the temperature rises greater than 1 degree Fahrenheit, stop the transfusion and notify the HCP. Acetaminophen may be ordered. If a hemolytic reaction is not suspected, the HCP may order the transfusion to continue once the patient is more comfortable. Administering leukocyte-depleted blood can usually prevent future febrile reactions.

URTICARIAL (HIVE) REACTION. Urticarial (hive) reactions are considered minor allergic reactions, usually associated with antigens in the plasma accompanying the transfusion. There may be a fever, but the cardinal sign is the appearance of urticaria, a hive-like rash. On discovery of this reaction, stop the transfusion and notify the HCP immediately. Expect that the patient will be given a dose of an antihistamine, such as diphenhydramine (Benadryl). If the transfusion is restarted, continue to monitor the patient closely. Make sure the 4-hour administration rule is not violated.

HEMOLYTIC REACTION. The deadliest and, fortunately, rarest of the reactions is an acute hemolytic reaction. The cause of this reaction is transfusion of incompatible blood. The result is hemolysis (destruction) of RBCs. This serious reaction is usually noticed within minutes of starting the transfusion. The patient may report back pain, chest pain, chills, fever, shortness of breath, nausea, vomiting, or a feeling of impending doom. As the reaction progresses, the patient begins to show signs of shock, hypotension, oliguria, and decreased consciousness. Late signs and symptoms include those associated with disseminated intravascular coagulation (e.g., uncontrollable bleeding from many different sites at the same time, usually causing death).

At the first sign of this type of reaction, immediately stop the transfusion and stay with the patient. Institute emergency procedures to notify the supervisor, the HCP, and the blood bank. Keep the vein open with normal saline using a new tubing set (ensuring that no more incompatible blood is administered) so that emergency drugs can be administered. High volumes of fluids are administered to decrease shock and hypotension. High doses of diuretics are given to promote urine flow because the kidneys are the most likely organs to be damaged.

ANAPHYLACTIC REACTION. Anaphylactic reactions are not common but may be seen more often in patients who have received many transfusions or have had many pregnancies. Usually, the source of the anaphylaxis is sensitization to immunoglobulins passed from the donor blood product. In this type of reaction, the first milliliters of blood containing the allergens to pass into the patient's system may be enough to cause the patient to develop respiratory or cardiovascular collapse. Other more common symptoms include severe gastrointestinal cramping, vomiting, and uncontrollable diarrhea.

If the patient exhibits these signs and symptoms, stop the transfusion at once and stay with them. Have someone else notify the RN and the HCP, using institutional emergency procedures. Emergency resuscitation measures, including cardiopulmonary resuscitation (CPR) if necessary, must be instituted until the rapid response or code team arrives. Expect the patient to be intubated and receive oxygen, steroids, and other drugs as needed for life support. After the emergency has passed, this patient may need transfusions from frozen, deglycerolized blood cells.

TRANSFUSION-RELATED ACUTE LUNG INJURY. Transfusion-related acute lung injury (TRALI) is a potentially fatal syndrome caused by a blood transfusion. It is responsible for 30% of transfusion-related deaths in the United States (Cho, Modi, & Sharma, 2020). Therefore, it is critical that you recognize and report this syndrome quickly to the HCP. TRALI can be either acute or delayed—during or up to 72 hours following a blood transfusion. Prevention is key; donor plasma used in blood transfusion should be screened for anti-leukocyte antibodies and anti-neutrophil-specific antibodies.

Critically ill patients with sepsis (such as patients with COVID-19) who require massive transfusions or are on mechanical ventilation are at greater risk for TRALI. Symptoms include acute respiratory distress, SpO2 less than 90% requiring oxygen support, crackles, decreased breath sounds, and use of accessory muscles. A fever greater than 100.4°F (37°C) with hypotension and tachycardia occur. Transient leukopenia and thrombocytopenia are noted in the laboratory results. Diagnosis is based on chest x-ray showing bilateral pulmonary infiltrates without evidence of pulmonary vascular overload.

During a transfusion, if the patient develops shortness of breath, stop the transfusion immediately and notify both the HCP and blood bank. Send the unused unit of blood and tubing back to the blood bank so it can be tested for antibodies. The patient should be monitored in the ICU for 48 to 96 hours. Supplemental oxygen or mechanical ventilation may be necessary. Gradual recovery usually occurs in 2 to 4 days. The nurse should make sure that deep vein thrombosis (DVT) prophylaxis and pressure injury precautions are implemented.

TRANSFUSION-ASSOCIATED CIRCULATORY OVERLOAD. Transfusion-associated circulatory overload (TACO) is caused by rapid transfusion in a short period, particularly in older and debilitated patients. Usual signs and symptoms include chest pain, cough, frothy sputum, distended neck veins, crackles and wheezes in the lung fields, and increased heart rate. If symptoms occur, stop the transfusion and notify the HCP. Anticipate administration of diuretics, which help get rid of the excess fluid. The transfusion may be restarted later at a slower rate (see "Gerontological Issues").

> **CUE RECOGNITION 27.1**
>
> You are caring for a patient receiving an autologous blood transfusion after surgery. When entering the room, you notice that the patient is scratching their arm, leaning forward, and speaking in short sentences. What do you do?
>
> *Suggested answers are at the end of the chapter.*

> **Gerontological Issues**
>
> **Monitoring for Fluid Excess.**
> Older patients have less cardiac and renal ability to adapt to changes in blood volume and thus have a much higher risk of fluid overload with IV infusions or blood transfusions. Carefully monitor lung sounds and vital signs before, during, and after a blood transfusion. New onset of dyspnea, crackles, hypertension, or bounding pulse during any infusion should be reported to the registered nurse or HCP immediately. If an older adult requires more than one unit of blood, a diuretic may be ordered between units.

Key Points

- The human body contains 4 to 6 L of blood. Approximately 45% is formed elements; the remainder is plasma. Formed elements include RBCs, WBCs, and platelets.
- Lymph is tissue fluid that has entered lymph capillaries. Lymph must be returned to the blood to maintain blood volume and blood pressure. Lymph capillaries are found in most tissue spaces. They anastomose, forming larger and larger lymph vessels, which have valves to prevent backflow.
- Lymph nodes are masses of lymphatic tissue along the pathways of the lymph vessels. They house activated lymphocytes and macrophages. Lymph nodules are small masses of lymphatic tissue found just beneath the epithelium of all mucous membranes.
- The spleen has several functions. It contains B cells and T cells, which conduct immune responses. It also contains fixed macrophages that phagocytize pathogens and worn or defective blood cells and platelets. The spleen stores up to one-third of the body's platelets.

- The thymus is located in the mediastinum, anterior to the trachea. The thymus contains T lymphocytes (T cells) that mature and proliferate. Thymic hormones contribute to the maturation of the T cells.
- All WBCs function within tissue fluid and blood and are involved in the immune or inflammatory response.
- Platelets are involved in all mechanisms of hemostasis: vascular spasm, platelet plugs, and chemical clotting.
- After a platelet plug is formed, one of two pathways initiates a cascade of events to bring about coagulation. When a blood vessel or surrounding tissues *outside* the blood are damaged, the extrinsic pathway begins. Conversely, when platelets adhere to damaged endothelium and release clotting factors, this initiates the *intrinsic* pathway.
- Specific problems that might be seen in patients with hematologic disorders include abnormal bleeding, petechiae, ecchymoses, and purpura. Additional symptoms include fatigue, weakness, shortness of breath, and fever. Fatigue, malaise, and weight loss can accompany cancers of the lymphatic system.
- Diagnostic and laboratory tests for hematologic and lymphatic disorders include blood tests, coagulation studies, bone marrow biopsy, lymphangiography, and lymph node biopsy.
- Blood may be administered by an RN or an LPN/LVN, depending on the state in which you practice. As an LPN/LVN, you may be called on to assist with proper identification procedures and monitoring of vital signs during the transfusion.
- Whether or not you actually administer the blood, you will likely participate in monitoring to prevent complications or to detect and treat them quickly if they occur. Stay with the patient for the first 15 minutes of the blood transfusion to monitor for any immediate reactions. Check and document vital signs before starting the transfusion, after the blood has begun to infuse, and after the infusion is complete. Always follow institution guidelines for vital sign monitoring. During the transfusion, monitor the patient for signs and symptoms of complications.

SUGGESTED ANSWERS TO CHAPTER EXERCISES

Cue Recognition
27.1: Even though this blood was donated by the patient prior to surgery, they could be having an allergic reaction. There is a risk that they could develop anaphylaxis. You need to stop the blood immediately, and then notify the RN and HCP.

Critical Thinking & Clinical Judgment
Mrs. Brown
1. The HCP may decrease Mrs. Brown's warfarin dose. Note in Table 27.5 that the INR for a patient on warfarin should be 2 to 3 or, for those with chronic problems, 3 to 4.5. A value of 4 (if her blood clot is not a chronic issue) means her blood is taking too long to clot, and she needs a lower dose to avoid bleeding. Dosing is adjusted based on INR. The normal INR is <1.1. In order for the patient to be therapeutically anticoagulated, the HCP wants the dose to be two to two and a half times the control.
2. Warfarin has many food–drug interactions, especially green leafy vegetables such as kale or spinach. Teach Mrs. Brown to eat about the same amount of vitamin K–rich foods daily, to avoid wide fluctuations in her INR. It is possible that she eats a lot of vitamin K–rich foods, but a decreased intake for a day or two might have elevated her INR.
3. Warfarin decreases the synthesis of vitamin K–dependent clotting factors. The antidote for overdose is vitamin K.
4. An INR of 8.2 significantly increases bleeding risk. Notify the RN or HCP, and institute bleeding precautions. See Box 28.1, "Interventions to Prevent Bleeding," in Chapter 28.

Additional Resources

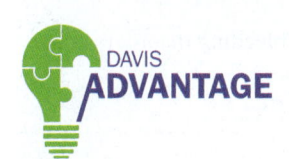

Go to Davis Advantage to complete your learning: strengthen understanding, apply your knowledge, and prepare for the Next Gen NCLEX®.

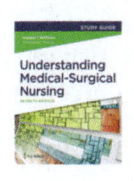

A Study Guide is also available.

CHAPTER 28
Nursing Care of Patients With Hematologic and Lymphatic Disorders

Margaret McCormick, Lucy L. Colo

KEY TERMS

anemia (ah-NEE-mee-ah)
aplastic (ay-PLAS-tik)
disseminated intravascular coagulation (dis-SEM-ih-NAY-ted IN-trah-VAS-kyoo-lar koh-AG-yoo-LAY-shun)
glossitis (gloss-SY-tis)
hemarthrosis (HEE-mar-THROH-sis)
hemolytic (HEE-moh-LIT-ik)
hemophilia (HEE-moh-FIL-ee-ah)
*idiopathic thrombocytopenic purpura (ID-ee-uh-PATH-ik THROM-boh-SY-toh-PEE-nik PURR-purr-uh)
immune thrombocytopenic purpura (ih-MEWN THROM-boh-SY-toh-PEE-nik PURR-purr-uh)
leukemia (loo-KEE-mee-ah)
lymphoma (lim-FOH-mah)
pancytopenia (PAN-sy-toh-PEE-nee-ah)
panmyelosis (PAN-my-eh-LOH-sis)
pathological fracture (PATH-uh-LAW-jik-uhl FRAK-chur)
phlebotomy (fleh-BAH-tuh-mee)
polycythemia (PAH-lee-sy-THEE-mee-ah)
splenectomy (spleh-NEK-tuh-mee)
splenomegaly (SPLEH-no-MEG-ah-lee)
thrombocytopenia (THROM-boh-SY-toh-PEE-nee-ah)

CHAPTER CONCEPTS

Cellular regulation
Comfort
Infection
Safety

LEARNING OUTCOMES

1. Explain the pathophysiology of each of the hematologic and lymphatic disorders discussed in this chapter.
2. Describe the etiologies, signs, and symptoms of each disorder.
3. Identify tests and procedures used to diagnose each of the disorders.
4. Describe current therapeutic measures for each disorder.
5. List data you should collect when caring for patients with disorders of the hematologic and lymphatic systems.
6. Plan nursing care for patients with hematologic and lymphatic disorders.
7. Explain how you will know whether your nursing interventions have been effective.
8. Describe precautions to prevent bleeding in patients with clotting disorders.
9. Identify precautions to take to prevent infection in patients at risk.
10. Identify nursing care and teaching you will provide for patients undergoing a splenectomy.

HEMATOLOGIC DISORDERS

Patients with hematologic disorders have problems related to their blood. They may have too many, too few, or defective blood cells.

- When red blood cells (RBCs) are affected, oxygen transport is also affected, causing symptoms related to poor oxygenation.
- When white blood cells (WBCs) are affected, patient is unable to effectively fight infections.
- If platelets or clotting factors are affected, bleeding disorders occur.

DISORDERS OF RED BLOOD CELLS

Anemia

The term **anemia** describes a condition in which circulating blood is deficient of RBCs, hemoglobin (Hgb), or both. Because Hgb carries oxygen, this results in a reduced capacity to deliver oxygen to

• WORD • BUILDING •
anemia: a—not + emia—blood

---

*Although *idiopathic* thrombocytopenic purpura is still in use, the newer term is *immune* thrombocytopenic purpura.

the tissues. Symptoms such as lightheadedness, dizziness, weakness, shortness of breath, or palpitations can lead the patient to seek medical help.

Pathophysiology
A decrease in the number of RBCs can be traced to three conditions: (1) impaired production of RBCs, as in aplastic anemia and nutritional deficiencies; (2) increased destruction of RBCs, as in **hemolytic** or sickle cell anemia; or (3) massive or chronic blood loss. Some anemias are related to genetic problems in certain cultures (see "Cultural Considerations"). It is important to remember that the general term *anemia* refers to a symptom or condition secondary to another problem and is not a diagnosis.

Cultural Considerations
Deficiency of the enzyme Mediterranean-type glucose-6-phosphate dehydrogenase (G6PD) causes a gender-linked genetic disease found primarily in the Middle East. G6PD deficiency affects the person's RBCs and results in anemia. It causes a hemolytic crisis when the person eats fava beans, takes aspirin or certain other drugs, or enters an acidotic or hypoxemic state. Only males have symptoms of Mediterranean-type G6PD deficiency, but some females are carriers.

Etiology
NUTRITIONAL DEFICIENCIES. Iron, folic acid, and vitamin B_{12} are all essential to the production of healthy RBCs. (See "Nutrition Notes" for more information.) A deficiency of any of these nutrients can cause anemia. *Pernicious anemia* is associated with a lack of intrinsic factor in stomach secretions, which is necessary for absorption of vitamin B_{12}.

Nutrition Notes
Understanding Common Nutritional Anemias
Nutrients required for synthesis of RBCs include iron, vitamin B_{12}, and folate. Inadequate intake of these nutrients can produce some forms of anemia. Nutrition therapy is useful; however, additional therapies may be required.

Microcytic Anemia
RBCs smaller than normal size are called *microcytic*. Inadequate intake of iron rich food, blood loss, renal disease, lead toxicity, gastrointestinal surgeries, and digestive conditions can lead to iron-deficiency anemia, the most common cause of microcytic anemia. Populations at risk include children, individuals with a family history or a genetic predisposition, and women of childbearing age.

Food sources of iron include animal meats, legumes, iron-fortified grains, dried fruits, and dark leafy greens. Vitamin C helps iron absorb into the body. Citrus, strawberry, kiwi, mango, tomato, broccoli, peppers, and cabbage are rich in vitamin C.

Iron supplements are given to treat iron deficiency. It may take 3 to 6 months to replenish iron stores. Provide iron supplements in between meals with water or vitamin C–rich food to encourage absorption. If side effects occur, provide with meals and speak with the provider to lower the dose. (National Heart, Lung, and Blood Institute, 2020).

Macrocytic Anemia
RBCs larger than normal size are called **macrocytic**. The most common cause of macrocytic anemia is deficiency of vitamin B_{12} and folate.

Vitamin B_{12} is required for DNA, RBC synthesis, and neurological function. B_{12} requires a highly specific protein-binding factor called *intrinsic factor*, secreted by the stomach. The intrinsic factor protects vitamin B_{12} from digestive enzymes and intestinal bacteria until it reaches the ileum, where the vitamin is absorbed.

Vitamin B_{12} is found in animal meats and eggs; dairy products (milk, cheese, yogurt); and vitamin B_{12}–fortified foods such as soy milk, tofu, and breakfast cereals. Strict vegetarians may be at risk and can pass this risk on to their breastfed infants. Pregnant and lactating women following a vegan diet should be evaluated for vitamin B_{12} adequacy. Vitamin B_{12} deficiency can cause irreparable nerve damage and should be considered in a person being evaluated for dementia. Patients who have had weight-loss surgery, had part of the small intestine removed, drink excessive alcohol, or have malabsorptive disorders such as inflammatory bowel disease are at risk for B_{12} deficiency. Metformin, a common oral diabetes medication, interferes with B_{12} absorption (Office of Dietary Supplements, 2020b).

Folate is required for the formation of DNA and heme, the iron-containing portion of Hgb. It is necessary for rapidly growing cells in the gastrointestinal tract, blood, and fetal tissue. Alcohol, anticonvulsants, and aspirin can interfere with folate absorption and cause anemia.

Food sources of folate include vegetables (spinach, asparagus, and Brussels sprouts), fruits (oranges and bananas), nuts, legumes, animal meats, eggs, dairy products, and fortified grains. Inadequate folate intake increases the risk for fetal neural tube defects such as spina bifida and anencephaly. Women of childbearing age should consume 400 mcg of folate daily from fortified foods or supplements in addition to a balanced diet (Office of Dietary Supplements, 2020a).

• WORD • BUILDING •

hemolysis: heme—blood + lysis—break down
hemolytic: heme—blood + lytic—break down

Signs and Symptoms

Symptoms of anemia include pallor, tachycardia, tachypnea, fatigue, and shortness of breath (Table 28.1). These symptoms occur because there are fewer functioning RBCs to carry oxygen to tissues. In addition to these symptoms, the patient with pernicious (vitamin B_{12} deficiency) anemia may experience numbness of the hands or feet, weakness, and memory problems. This is because vitamin B_{12} is needed for normal neurologic function. Pernicious anemia is also associated with an inflamed, beefy red tongue (**glossitis**). Patients with iron deficiency may have fissures at the corners of the mouth, glossitis, and spoon-shaped fingernails.

Diagnostic Tests

A complete blood count (CBC) is done to determine the number of RBCs and WBCs per cubic millimeter. Microscopic examination determines the size, color, and shape of the blood cells. Hgb and hematocrit (Hct) levels are below normal in anemia. Serum iron, ferritin, and total iron-binding capacity (TIBC) measurements are done to determine whether the anemia is due to iron deficiency. Serum folate and B_{12} levels may be measured. A bone marrow biopsy and analysis may also be done.

Patients with pernicious anemia may have antibodies to intrinsic factor, associated with poor absorption of vitamin B_{12}. Homocysteine levels may also be high in pernicious anemia. If blood loss is suspected, additional tests are done to determine the source of bleeding.

Therapeutic Measures

Treatment begins with elimination of underlying causes. Intake of the deficient nutrient can be increased in the diet or administered as a supplement (see "Nutrition Notes"). Changing cooking habits, decreasing alcohol intake, and controlling chronic diarrhea can also help correct B_{12} and folic acid deficiencies. If symptoms of anemia are acute, a blood transfusion may be needed.

Nursing Process for the Patient With Anemia

DATA COLLECTION. Monitor Hgb and Hct levels and other laboratory studies ordered. Report any downward trend. Monitor responses to therapy, the patient's fatigue level, and the patient's ability to ambulate safely and perform activities of daily living (ADLs). Monitor dyspnea and oxygen saturation, but be aware that, at lower Hgb levels, oxygen saturation values may not be accurate. Observe for pallor in the skin and conjunctivae.

NURSING DIAGNOSES, PLANNING, AND IMPLEMENTATION. Possible nursing diagnoses are listed next along with outcomes and interventions.

> **Decreased Activity Tolerance related to tissue hypoxia and dyspnea**
>
> **EXPECTED OUTCOME:** The patient will be able to tolerate activity as evidenced by ability to complete ADLs and other important activities with minimal assistance. The patient will have knowledge about conserving energy as evidenced by a verbal statement.

- Monitor vital signs before and after activity. *The patient experiencing activity intolerance may have tachycardia or an increased respiratory rate during activity. A drop in blood pressure may be caused by moving from a lying to a sitting or standing position, and may be accompanied by lightheadedness or dizziness.*
- If the pulse or respiratory rate increases more than 20% from baseline during activity, reduce the activity level. *This is caused by activation of the sympathetic nervous system compensating for the anemia and is evidence that the activity is too strenuous.*
- Plan care to conserve energy after periods of activity. *Balancing activities and rest periods helps the patient conserve energy.*
- Assist the patient with self-care activities as needed. *Assisting with ADLs helps to decrease the amount of energy expended by the patient.*
- Encourage the patient to limit visitors, telephone calls, and unnecessary interruptions *to conserve energy.*
- Administer oxygen as ordered to relieve dyspnea. *The patient with anemia does not have enough Hgb to carry oxygen to vital organs.*

> **Imbalanced Nutrition: Less Than Body Requirements related to disease, treatment, or lack of knowledge about adequate nutrition**
>
> **EXPECTED OUTCOME:** The patient will (1) have improved nutrition as evidenced by stable weight, Hgb level, and Hct level; and (2) will be able to appropriately select foods to meet nutritional requirements for anemia treatment.

- Consult a dietitian *to provide diet instruction if the anemia is caused by a dietary deficiency.*
- Teach the patient with folic acid deficiency to include foods from each food group at every meal. *A balanced diet includes adequate amounts of folic acid.*
- Instruct the patient to take supplements as ordered by the health-care provider (HCP). *Supplements replace the deficient nutrient.*
- Instruct the patient with pernicious anemia that vitamin B_{12} injections are given for life. *Oral B12 is not absorbed in pernicious anemia.*
- Instruct the patient with iron deficiency about high-iron foods and correct use of an iron supplement *to replace deficiency.* An iron supplement should be taken with vitamin C–rich foods or fluids *to enhance absorption of iron.*

- **WORD • BUILDING •**
glossitis: glos—tongue + itis—inflammation

Table 28.1
Clinical Manifestations of Anemia

Body System	Mild (Hgb 10–14 g/dL)	Moderate (Hgb 6–10 g/dL)	Severe (Hgb <6 g/dL)
Skin	None	None	Pallor, jaundice, pruritus
Eyes	None	None	Jaundiced conjunctivae and sclerae, retinal hemorrhages, blurred vision
Mouth	None	None	Glossitis, smooth tongue
Cardiovascular	Palpitations	Increased palpitations	Tachycardia, increased pulse pressure, systolic murmurs, angina, congestive heart failure, myocardial infarction
Lungs	Exertional dyspnea	Significant dyspnea	Tachypnea, orthopnea, dyspnea at rest
Neurologic	None	None	Headache, vertigo, irritability, depression, impaired thought processes
Gastrointestinal	None	None	Anorexia, hepatomegaly, splenomegaly
Musculoskeletal	None	None	Bone pain
General	None	Fatigue	Sensitivity to cold, weight loss, lethargy

- Administer oral iron 1 hour before or 2 hours after meals *to enhance absorption.*
- Instruct the patient to notify the HCP of side effects related to iron supplements such as nausea, diarrhea, constipation, and dark stools. *Some side effects require HCP attention.*
- Administer intramuscular iron injections by the Z-track method *to avoid staining of the injection site.*
- Administer liquid iron supplements with a drinking straw *to avoid staining the teeth.*

Impaired Oral Mucous Membrane Integrity related to altered dietary status

EXPECTED OUTCOME: The patient will have intact oral mucous membranes.

- Monitor condition of oral mucous membranes *to detect changes.*
- Provide oral hygiene *to keep the oral cavity clean and prevent infection.*
- Encourage soft, bland foods, *which are more tolerable until healing can occur.*
- Instruct the patient to use a soft toothbrush for oral care *because it is gentler until healing can occur.*

EVALUATION. When successfully treated, patients should be able to tolerate their usual level of activity without shortness of breath or excess fatigue. The patient should be able to explain the treatment plan and therapeutic measures for long-term prevention of problems, including dietary choices, supplements, and self-care measures. The oral mucosa will be intact.

Aplastic Anemia
Pathophysiology
Aplastic anemia differs from other types of anemia in that the bone marrow becomes fatty and cannot produce enough blood cells. It is also called *hypoplastic* anemia. The cells that are produced are normal in size and shape, but there are not enough of them to sustain life. The result is **pancytopenia**, or reduced numbers of all cells from the bone marrow, including RBCs, platelets, and WBCs. Sometimes just one type of cell is affected. Left untreated, aplastic anemia is almost always fatal.

Etiology
Aplastic anemia may be congenital—that is, the person is born with bone marrow incapable of producing the correct number of cells. It also may be due to exposure to toxic substances, such as industrial chemicals (e.g., benzenes and insecticides), chemotherapy, or radiation. Other causes include bacterial and viral infections, such as tuberculosis and hepatitis, or autoimmune disease.

• WORD • BUILDING •
aplastic: a—not + plastic—develop
pancytopenia: pan—all + cyto—cell + penia—poverty

Signs and Symptoms

The clinical features of aplastic anemia vary with the severity of bone marrow failure. As with other anemias, early symptoms include fatigue, pallor, and shortness of breath. As the disease progresses and the pancytopenia worsens, other symptoms, such as tachycardia and heart failure, may appear. Reduced platelets cause ecchymoses (Fig. 28.1) and petechiae (Fig. 28.2) on the skin surface. Blood may ooze from mucous membranes. Injection sites may progress from oozing to frank bleeding. There may be bleeding into vital organs. Reduced WBCs leads to infection. Without treatment, most patients die of infection or bleeding.

Diagnostic Tests

The diagnosis of aplastic anemia begins with a CBC. Usually, all values are very low, with the occasional exception of the RBC count, in part because of the longer life span of RBCs. Eventually, the RBCs are also depleted. If the patient has bleeding internally or externally, the RBC level can drop rapidly and dramatically. The most definitive test is a bone marrow biopsy. Because the bone marrow is essentially dead, the result may be described as a "dry tap," in which pale, fatty, yellow, fibrous bone marrow is extracted instead of the red, gelatinous bone marrow normally seen. Other diagnostic tests include TIBC and serum iron level. It is common to find both these levels elevated because the RBCs are not being produced and are not using up the stores of iron in the production of Hgb.

Therapeutic Measures

Early identification of the cause of aplastic anemia and correction of the underlying problem are important to survival. Unfortunately, it is often difficult to determine the cause. There is no way to reverse the damage. Aggressive supportive measures may be the only treatment. Most of these measures are aimed at prevention of infection and bleeding. Transfusions may be administered to replace deficient cells.

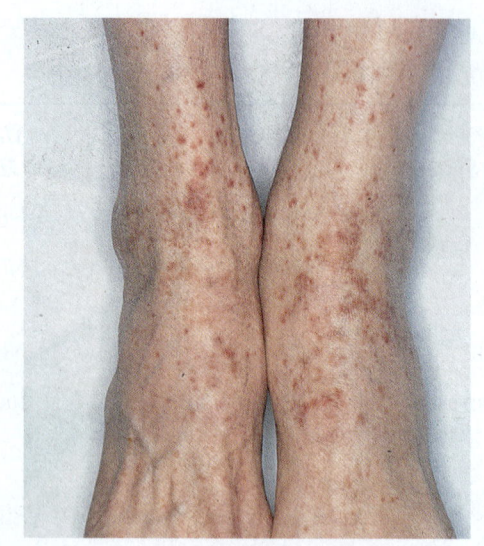

FIGURE 28.2 Petechiae on the skin (from thrombocytopenia).

Steroids may be administered to stimulate production of cells in the weakened bone marrow. Immunosuppressant agents may be given if an autoimmune disorder is the underlying cause. Occasionally, the administration of hormones may work to increase the viability of the marrow. The most effective treatment for aplastic anemia is stem cell (bone marrow) transplantation (see "Patient Perspective").

In many treatment institutions, limited success is being obtained with the use of colony-stimulating factors, natural elements that can now be produced synthetically. (You can read more about these medications in Chapter 11.) For example, epoetin alfa, a form of erythropoietin (Epogen), stimulates production of RBCs, and filgrastim (a granulocyte colony stimulator; Neupogen) stimulates production of WBCs. The major drawback is cost. Many pharmaceutical manufacturers have patient access programs that help reduce the costs of these medications.

Nursing Management

Nursing care of patients with symptoms related to reduced RBCs was presented earlier in the "Nursing Process for the Patient With Anemia" section. If the patient's platelet count is low (usually less than 20,000), place the patient on bleeding precautions (Box 28.1). If the WBC count is low, the patient must be protected from infection (Box 28.2).

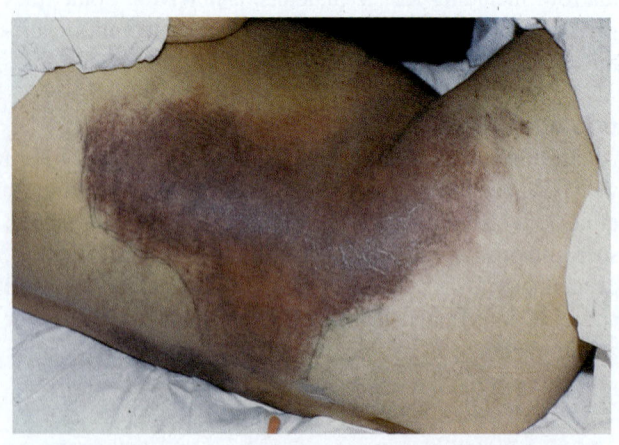

FIGURE 28.1 Ecchymoses. Extensive hemorrhage into the skin. Note how the area is outlined in pen so the nurse can determine if the area is spreading.

> **BE SAFE!**
>
> **BE VIGILANT!** Watch patients with aplastic anemia carefully for even subtle signs of bleeding, such as early skin changes or pink-tinged urine. Monitor for bleeding from IV and phlebotomy sites. Inspect skin for petechiae or ecchymoses. Monitor for subtle signs of infection; even behavior changes can signal infection in older adults. Monitor CBC. Report findings before condition worsens.

Patient Perspective

Janet

I took my daughter to the doctor for a sports physical. Later that day, I received a call telling me to take her to the university hospital immediately because she had a serious life-threatening illness. I kept telling myself and my husband that our small-town hospital must have made some sort of error. As it turned out, they had not. My daughter was diagnosed with aplastic anemia and needed a bone marrow transplant. I became obsessed with the illness, poring over every tidbit of medical information I could find. Sometimes I found myself out in the car unable to remember where I was going; sometimes I had to pull over because my eyes were filled with tears and I could no longer see.

My daughter was 16 at the time of her illness, yet it is the parents who sign consent forms and make the choices in care. When the chemotherapy was started and was running through the IV tubing, I felt like grabbing the tubing and pinching it off, yelling, "I need more time to think about this decision," but time was running out. Without a bone marrow transplant, she had about 8 months to live.

After transplantation, my daughter was in an isolation room for a month. I stayed with her every day, and at night I stayed at the inn that was attached to the hospital. If I was needed, I wanted to be no more than a minute away. I was one of the luckier parents because I had the financial means to manage this process. I thought about how horrible it would be if I had other children at home. Sometimes I would have an urge to run away and escape from it all. I attended support groups that were held on the hospital unit. I got to know a lot of other parents with sick kids, and it became very upsetting to me at times. One day parents told me how well their child was doing; the next day I saw the child's room empty and thought he must have gone home, only to find out later that he had died during the night. I wondered if my daughter would be next.

I look at my daughter now, 4 years later, alive and perfectly healthy, and I tell myself that I made the right choices for her. But she tells me that if it happens again, she will not go through chemotherapy. I wonder, is chemo worse than death?

Box 28.1
Interventions to Prevent Bleeding

- Use an electric razor instead of a safety razor for shaving.
- Use a soft toothbrush or gauze to clean the teeth. Avoid flossing.
- Avoid invasive procedures as much as possible, including enemas, douches, suppositories, and rectal temperatures.
- Avoid intramuscular injections.
- To avoid injury when checking blood pressure, pump cuff up only until pulse is obliterated.
- Avoid blood draws whenever possible. Use established access sites or group specimen collections into once-daily draws.
- Maintain pressure on IV, blood draw, and other puncture sites for 5 minutes.
- Encourage use of shoes or slippers when out of bed.
- Keep area clutter-free to prevent bumps and bruises.
- Avoid use of drugs that interfere with platelet function, such as aspirin products and NSAIDs (e.g., aspirin, ibuprofen, naproxen).
- Administer stool softeners as ordered to prevent straining to have a bowel movement.
- Move and turn patient gently to avoid bruising.
- Instruct patient to blow nose very gently and only when necessary.
- Advise patient to consult health-care provider about whether sexual intercourse is safe.

Box 28.2
Interventions for the Patient at Risk for Infection

- Place the patient in a private room.
- Ensure that all staff and visitors wash hands before entering the room.
- Teach the patient to wash hands before and after using the toilet and before and after eating.
- Teach the patient and family to wash hands before touching each other.
- Prevent staff or visitors with known infections from entering the patient's room.
- Teach the patient to not handle flowers or plants brought into the room.
- Teach the patient to avoid unwashed fruits and vegetables.
- Avoid use of indwelling urinary catheters and other invasive devices.
- Use strict aseptic technique if invasive procedures are needed.
- Use acetaminophen if an antipyretic is needed; aspirin can induce bleeding.
- Report any rise in temperature immediately.

Sickle Cell Anemia

Pathophysiology

Sickle cell anemia is an inherited anemia in which the RBCs have a mutation that makes the Hgb very sensitive to oxygen changes. When the cells sense a change in oxygen, they begin an observable physical change from their usual spherical shape to a sickle or crescent shape (Fig. 28.3). Sickled cells are very sticky, rigid, and easily cracked and broken. The abnormal shape causes the cells to become tangled in the blood vessels and organs. The result is congestion, clumping, and clotting.

As RBCs are broken, the cellular contents spill out into the general circulation. The resulting increase in the bilirubin level causes jaundice. Gallstones (cholelithiasis) may develop because of the increased amounts of bile pigments. The spleen and liver may enlarge because of the increase in retained cells and cellular materials.

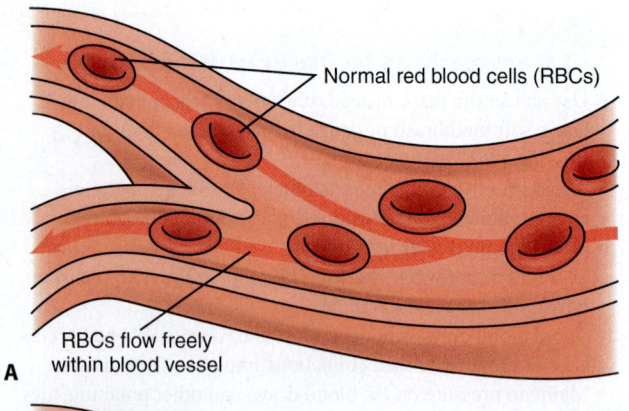

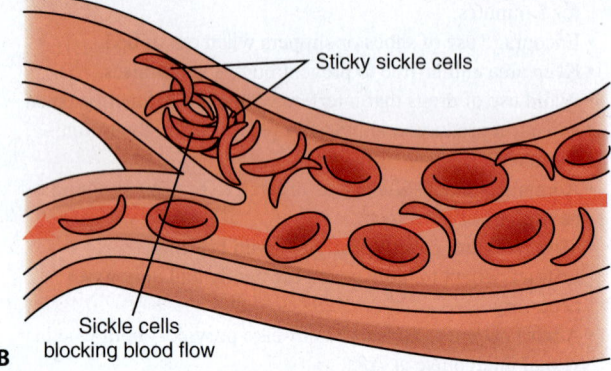

FIGURE 28.3 (A) Normal red blood cells (RBCs) flowing freely in a blood vessel. The inset image shows a cross-section of a normal RBC with normal hemoglobin (Hgb). (B) Abnormal, sickled RBCs blocking blood flow in a blood vessel. The inset image shows a cross-section of a sickle cell with abnormal (sickle) Hgb forming abnormal strands.

Cultural Considerations

Sickle cell anemia is the most common genetic disorder among Black Americans. Sickle cell anemia is also found in individuals who live in areas where malaria is endemic, such as the Caribbean, the Middle East, the Mediterranean region, Africa, and Asia. Sickle cell trait protects these populations from dying of malaria. About 1 in 13 Black babies is born with sickle cell trait in the United States, and 1 in 365 has sickle cell disease (Centers for Disease Control and Prevention, 2019).

Because the cells are fragile, their life span is significantly decreased. Normal RBCs live about 120 days. Sickled cells survive only about 10 to 20 days, an 80% to 90% decrease.

Etiology

Sickle cell disease (SCD) is an autosomal recessive hereditary disorder. This means that if both parents pass on the abnormal Hgb (sickle hemoglobin [HbS]), the child will have the disease. If only one parent passes on the abnormal Hgb, the child will have the sickle cell trait and will be able to pass on the trait (or the disease if the other parent is also affected) to their child. Symptoms do not appear in infants until after age 4 or 5 months. Up to that age, the infant is using Hgb manufactured during fetal life, which is not affected by the sickling process.

Signs and Symptoms

The sickling changes happen daily. The rapid return of the oxygen level to normal usually returns the cells to their normal shape.

Sometimes, the sickling process cannot be reversed. This sudden and severe sickling is called a *sickle cell crisis* or *vaso-occlusive crisis*. As more sickling occurs, blood flow becomes sluggish. Collection in the capillaries and veins of the joints, chest, and abdominal organs can cause infarction with resulting tissue necrosis (death) from lack of blood supply. Tissue necrosis causes pain, fever, and swelling. Spleen involvement increases infection risk. Clotting in the cerebral blood vessels can lead to stroke. Refer to Chapter 49 for detailed information on stroke.

Any condition that leads to decreased oxygenation can contribute to the development of a sickle cell crisis. Some examples include pneumonia, exposure to cold, diabetic acidosis, exercise, dehydration, and severe infection. Sickle cell anemia presents problems for the patient who needs surgery. Anesthesia and blood loss during surgery and postoperative dehydration can trigger a crisis.

Common symptoms during sickle cell crises include severe pain and swelling in the joints, especially of the elbows and knees, as the sickled cells interfere with circulation. Hands and feet may be swollen. Abdominal pain is common with swelling of the spleen and engorgement of the vital organs. Hypoxia occurs as fever and pain increase, causing the patient to breathe rapidly. A male patient may have a continuous, painful erection (priapism) from impaired blood flow through the penis. Symptoms of kidney failure occur when circulation is slowed and the kidneys become clogged with cellular debris.

Repeated crises and infarctions lead to chronic manifestations such as hand-foot syndrome, an unequal growth of fingers and toes from infarction of the small bones in the hands and feet (Fig. 28.4). Additional manifestations of SCD are shown in Figure 28.5.

The patient with sickle cell anemia has impaired quality of life. Sports and strenuous exercise may be impossible because of the risk of crisis. Crises may occur without any apparent cause. In general, crises last from 4 to 6 days. They may occur in cycles close together for a time and then become dormant for months to years. The cause of death in patients with sickle cell anemia is usually infection, stroke, or organ failure.

Diagnostic Tests

The Sickledex test shows sickling of RBCs when oxygen tension is low. Hgb electrophoresis is a test used to determine the presence of Hgb S, the abnormal form of Hgb. There is also a decreased amount of Hgb, a lowered RBC count, an elevated WBC count, and a decreased erythrocyte sedimentation rate (ESR).

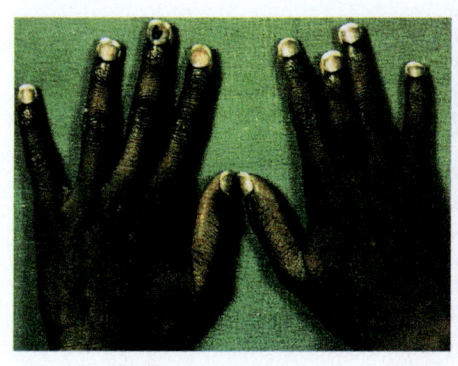

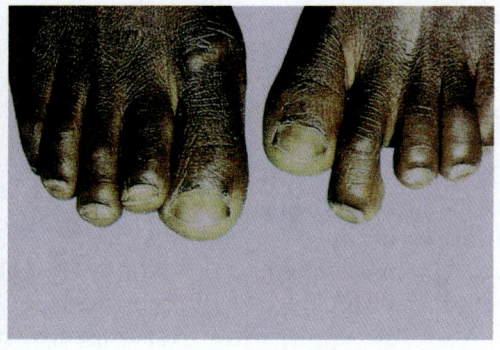

FIGURE 28.4 Hand-foot syndrome. Note different lengths of fingers and toes.

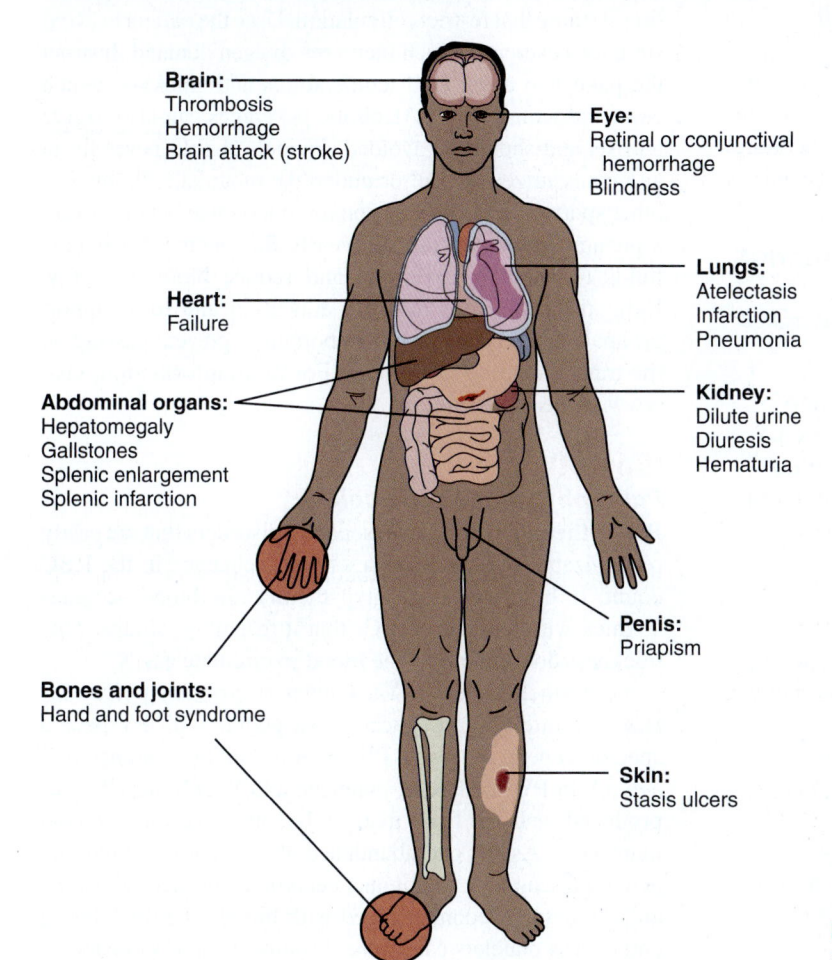

FIGURE 28.5 Clinical manifestations of sickle cell anemia.

- **Brain:** Thrombosis, Hemorrhage, Brain attack (stroke)
- **Eye:** Retinal or conjunctival hemorrhage, Blindness
- **Heart:** Failure
- **Lungs:** Atelectasis, Infarction, Pneumonia
- **Abdominal organs:** Hepatomegaly, Gallstones, Splenic enlargement, Splenic infarction
- **Kidney:** Dilute urine, Diuresis, Hematuria
- **Penis:** Priapism
- **Bones and joints:** Hand and foot syndrome
- **Skin:** Stasis ulcers

Therapeutic Measures

Treatment depends on the severity of the disease. All patients should be educated on how to prevent crises and receive supportive care when crises occur. Some patients may be placed on oral antibiotics to help prevent infections at home, decreasing the risk of crises.

During acute crises, the patient is admitted to the hospital. The nurse can anticipate that the patient will require sedation and analgesia for severe pain and blood transfusions to replace the sickled RBCs. Oxygen therapy decreases dyspnea caused by the anemia. Large amounts of oral and IV fluids are given to flush the kidneys of the by-products of the broken cellular debris. Antibiotics are used to treat infection that may have triggered the crisis.

Frequent blood transfusions, often monthly, can help supply normal blood cells. However, they can cause high levels of iron to build up in the body. Deferasirox (Jadenu) may be given to decrease the excess iron levels. Corticosteroids can reduce the need for analgesics and oxygen. Hydroxyurea (Droxia) is a drug that has been shown to decrease crises but can cause life-threatening side effects; it should also be used with caution in women of childbearing years because of the risk of birth defects. Hydroxyurea has been shown to increase the amount of fetal hemoglobin in the blood. This decreases the likelihood of RBCs sickling, helping to reduce episodes of pain, hand-foot syndrome, acute chest syndrome, and hospitalizations in individuals with SCD (Reeves et al, 2019). Patients may not adhere to hydroxyurea therapy because they do not feel different; it may take months to years to make a difference in outcomes. The U.S. Food and Drug Administration has recently approved the use of L-glutamine oral powder (Endari) to reduce the frequency of crises.

Bone marrow transplantation has shown promise in the treatment of SCD, although it is not without risk. It is the only known cure for SCD.

Nursing Process for the Patient in Sickle Cell Anemia Crisis

DATA COLLECTION. In the patient in crisis, monitor circulation in the extremities every 2 hours, including pulse oximetry, capillary refill, peripheral pulses, and temperature. Monitor neurological status. Frequent pain assessment is also essential.

NURSING DIAGNOSIS, PLANNING, AND IMPLEMENTATION

> **Risk for Ineffective Cerebral/Peripheral Tissue Perfusion related to sickled cells and infarction**
>
> **EXPECTED OUTCOME:** The patient will have adequate cerebral/peripheral tissue perfusion, as evidenced by the presence of peripheral pulses, absence of neurological changes, warm extremities, urine output within normal limits, and a capillary refill time of less than 3 seconds.

- Monitor neurological status (level of consciousness, orientation, bilateral muscle strength, pupil size, speech) *to identify any changes due to cerebrovascular thrombosis from cell debris.*
- Encourage oral fluids and assist the registered nurse (RN) to monitor IV fluids *to dilute and aid in elimination of cell debris.*
- Apply warm compresses as ordered to the painful areas, cover the patient with a blanket, and keep the room temperature above 72°F (22°C) *to reduce the vasoconstrictive effects of cold.*
- Avoid cold compresses *because they decrease circulation and can increase the number of sickled cells caught in a painful area.*
- Avoid restrictive clothing and raising the bed under the knees. *These can restrict circulation.*

> **Acute Pain related to tissue infarction**
>
> **EXPECTED OUTCOME:** The patient will state pain is at an acceptable level at all times.

- Administer opioid analgesics such as morphine as ordered *for acute pain.* (Analgesics may be given via IV route or by use of patient-controlled analgesia [PCA].)
- Administer acetaminophen (Tylenol) *to control fever.*
- Avoid giving aspirin *because it may increase acidosis, which can worsen the crisis.*
- Encourage bedrest during the acute phase of the crisis *to reduce oxygen demand.*

EVALUATION. If nursing care has been effective, the patient will state that he or she is comfortable and will not have signs of poor circulation or neurological deficits.

PATIENT EDUCATION. Determine the patient's readiness to learn. Teaching is best done during remission when the patient is not distracted by pain. Teach the patient and caregiver how to prevent acute episodes. Advise the patient to avoid tight-fitting clothing that restricts circulation. Urge the patient to avoid strenuous exercise, which increases oxygen demand. Instruct the patient to avoid cold temperatures and smoking, which cause vasoconstriction. Alcoholic beverages can also trigger a crisis and should be avoided. Patients should never fly in an unpressurized aircraft or undertake mountain climbing or other sports that can cause hypoxia. Encourage patients to get a pneumococcal vaccine and yearly flu vaccine. Encourage fluids to maintain hydration and reduce blood viscosity. Refer the patient for in-depth education and to a support group. Genetic counseling is important to prevent passing on the trait or disease to children. For more information, visit www.sicklecelldisease.org.

Polycythemia

Pathophysiology and Etiology

Polycythemia includes two separate disorders that are easily recognizable by similar characteristic changes in the RBC count. In both forms of polycythemia, the blood becomes so thick with too many RBCs that it resembles sludge. This thickness does not allow the blood to circulate easily.

Polycythemia vera (PV), known as *primary polycythemia*, is a rare type of cancer. Most people with PV have a specific genetic mutation. PV onset is usually in adults over age 50. In PV, the RBCs, platelets, and WBCs are all overproduced, and the bone marrow becomes packed with too many cells. As this overabundance of cells spills out into the general circulation, the organs become congested with cells and the tissues become packed with blood. The thick blood and excess platelets can cause thrombosis and occlusion of vessels.

In contrast, secondary polycythemia is the result of long-term hypoxia. Common coexisting conditions that may predispose a patient to secondary polycythemia include pulmonary diseases such as chronic obstructive pulmonary disease (COPD), cardiovascular problems such as chronic heart failure, living in high altitudes, and smoking. The body makes more RBCs in response to the low oxygenation associated with these conditions. Secondary polycythemia is a compensatory mechanism rather than an actual disorder.

• WORD • BUILDING •

polycythemia: poly—many + cyt—cells + emia—in the blood

Signs and Symptoms

A patient with PV commonly presents with hypertension, vision changes, headache, vertigo, dizziness, and ringing in the ears (tinnitus). Laboratory results show an increased level of all bone marrow components (RBCs, WBCs, platelets), which is called **panmyelosis**. Patients may also be at risk for developing a bleeding disorder called *acquired von Willebrand syndrome*, in which the platelets do not clump together well. The patient may have nosebleeds and bleeding gums, retinal hemorrhages, exertional dyspnea, and chest pain due to pressure exerted by the excess cells. The patient usually has a dark, flushed complexion from build-up of red cells. Intense itching is related to excess mast cells (and, therefore, histamine) in the skin. Abdominal pain with an early feeling of fullness with meals occurs because of the enlarged liver and spleen. Nearly all the symptoms in PV are caused by hypervolemia, hyperviscosity, and engorgement of capillary beds. Without treatment, patients with PV die of thrombosis or hemorrhage.

Diagnostic Tests

Diagnosis of PV is made based on a CBC and bone marrow aspiration. Laboratory tests show a Hgb level greater than 18 mg/dL, an RBC mass greater than 6 million, and a Hct level of greater than 55%. A low level of erythropoietin is present, caused by negative feedback to the kidneys, where erythropoietin is made. The bone marrow or blood may show a genetic mutation of the JAK2 or TET2 gene.

Therapeutic Measures

PV can be managed, but not cured. With ongoing treatment, patients can live normal lives. Treatment takes place in two stages. The first stage is to decrease the hyperviscosity problem. The most common first-line treatment is therapeutic **phlebotomy**. Phlebotomy involves withdrawal of blood, which is then discarded. From 350 to 500 mL of blood are removed once or twice a week, with the goal being a Hct level of about 45%. This reduces the RBC level. The patient usually feels more comfortable quickly. Repeated phlebotomies eventually cause iron-deficiency anemia. This in turn stabilizes RBC production; phlebotomies can then be reduced to every 2 to 3 months. Low-dose aspirin reduces the risk of blood clots.

Antihistamines or certain antidepressants can be used to reduce itching. Chemotherapeutic agents and radiation therapy may be used to suppress production of blood cells in some patients. Leukemia is a side effect of this therapy, so it is used only if the benefits outweigh the risks. Aspirin can reduce platelet aggregation and clotting. Other drugs that can slow cell production include interferon alpha and hydroxyurea.

Nursing Management

Explain the phlebotomy procedure and reassure the patient that the treatment will relieve the most distressing symptoms. The procedure is the same as that used for donating blood. The patient should remain active and ambulatory to help prevent thrombus formation. If bedrest is needed, passive and active range-of-motion exercises should be implemented. Monitor the patient for complications such as hypovolemia and bleeding.

If the patient has more advanced manifestations, such as an enlarged liver or spleen, offer several small meals each day so the patient will be more comfortable while still receiving adequate nutrition. A dietitian can be consulted to discuss ways to maintain good nutrition. If the patient is on drug therapy, monitor CBC and platelet counts.

Patient Education

Instruct the patient to drink at least 3 L of water daily to reduce blood viscosity. Encourage smoking cessation, avoidance of tight or restrictive clothing, and elevation of feet when resting to promote good circulation. Use of support hose when active also promotes circulation. Avoidance of very hot or cold environments can reduce complications related to impaired circulation. Avoiding hot showers and baths, and using mild soap, can help control itching. If anticoagulant or antiplatelet agents are ordered, instruct the patient about side effects to watch for and the importance of routine laboratory tests. Routine bleeding precautions are implemented (see Box 28.1). Warn the patient to stop activities at the first sign of chest pain. Instruct the patient to report chest pain, increased joint pain, decreased activity tolerance, fever, and signs of iron-deficiency anemia, such as pallor, weight loss, and dyspnea. Advise the patient to report signs or symptoms of bleeding or thrombosis immediately.

HEMORRHAGIC DISORDERS

Disseminated Intravascular Coagulation

Pathophysiology

Disseminated intravascular coagulation (DIC) involves a series of events that results in severe hemorrhage. DIC is a catastrophic, overwhelming state of accelerated clotting throughout the peripheral blood vessels. In a short period, all the clotting factors and platelet supplies are exhausted, and clots can no longer be formed. This results in bleeding from nearly every bodily route possible. DIC is not a disease; it is a syndrome that develops secondary to another severe physical problem. Once this deadly syndrome develops, the progression of symptoms is rapid.

Massive clotting in blood vessels, bleeding, and impaired perfusion all lead to organ and limb necrosis. Organs affected may include the kidneys, liver, lungs, brain, skin, and adrenal glands. DIC is usually acute in onset, although in some patients it becomes a chronic condition. The prognosis depends on early diagnosis and intervention as well as the severity of hemorrhaging. DIC has a very high mortality rate.

Etiology

DIC can develop after any condition in which the body has sustained major trauma. The sources of trauma are varied and can include an overwhelming infection (including COVID-19); obstetric complications such as abruptio placentae, amniotic fluid embolism, or a retained dead fetus; or cancer-related causes such as acute leukemia or lung cancer. Massive tissue necrosis found in severe crush or burn injuries can increase the risk of DIC. Use of street drugs such as cocaine or ecstasy can also increase risk.

Signs and Symptoms
Symptoms occur from the underlying cause and the DIC response. Abnormal bleeding without history of a serious hemorrhagic disorder is a cardinal sign of DIC. Early signs of bleeding include ecchymoses (see Fig. 28.1), petechiae (see Fig. 28.2), and bleeding from venipuncture sites. Bleeding may progress to IV sites, skin tears, surgical sites, incisions, and the GI tract and oral mucosa. Joints become painful and enlarged if bleeding into the joints occurs. All these signs and symptoms may occur at the same time. Massive bleeding may also be accompanied by nausea, vomiting, dyspnea, oliguria, convulsions, coma, shock, major organ system failure, acute respiratory distress syndrome, and severe muscle, back, and abdominal pain.

Diagnostic Tests
Initial laboratory findings in DIC include a prolonged prothrombin time (PT) and partial thromboplastin time (PTT), decreased platelet count, and increased evidence of fibrin degradation products (Table 28.2). A D-dimer test helps identify the presence of blood clots. A decrease in Hgb is the result of spilled Hgb from the increased numbers of broken RBCs. Blood urea nitrogen (BUN) may be increased if there is bleeding into the digestive tract, because digested blood is a source of urea.

Therapeutic Measures
Effective treatment of DIC depends on early recognition of the condition. Treatment is first aimed at correcting the underlying cause. Additional treatment consists of supportive interventions including oxygen, hydration, administration of blood, fresh frozen plasma (which provides both clotting factors as well as natural anticoagulants), platelets, and the infusion of cryoprecipitate (which provides clotting factors) to support hemostasis. IV heparin may be used to help prevent initial clot development. It may also be used for chronic DIC cases.

Nursing Management
Care of the patient with DIC is a nursing challenge. Monitor vital signs frequently. Be vigilant in monitoring for and reporting signs of bleeding. In addition to supportive care, focus on the prevention of further bleeding episodes. Care should be taken to avoid any trauma that might cause bleeding. Be careful not to dislodge clots from any site because another clot may not form and the patient will hemorrhage. See Box 28.1 for bleeding precautions.

Patient Education
Because a patient with DIC is often cared for in the intensive care unit, there are many opportunities for patient and family teaching. Explain all diagnostic tests to the patient and family. A large part of family education is preparing the family for what the patient may look like in terms of bleeding and bruising as well as specific equipment that may be in place. It may be helpful to enlist the aid of social workers, chaplains, and other members of the health-care team to help support the family.

> **CUE RECOGNITION 28.1**
>
> You are caring for a patient admitted with sepsis and DIC. As you are bathing her, you note a large bruise on her abdomen that was not mentioned in report. She begins to bleed from her mouth. What do you do?
>
> Suggested answers are at the end of the chapter.

> **CRITICAL THINKING**
>
> **Mrs. Johns** is admitted to your unit with DIC following the difficult delivery of her new baby.
>
> 1. What data will you collect as you care for Mrs. Johns?
> 2. What treatment do you anticipate?
> 3. What concerns is Mrs. Johns likely to have?
> 4. Mrs. Johns is to receive 300 mL of IV fresh frozen plasma over 30 minutes. How many milliliters per hour should be set on the IV controller?
> 5. With which members of the health-care team should you anticipate collaborating?
>
> Suggested answers are at the end of the chapter.

Immune Thrombocytopenic Purpura
Pathophysiology and Etiology
Acute **immune** (also called *idiopathic*) **thrombocytopenic purpura** (ITP) results from increased platelet destruction by the immune system. Any time platelet numbers are reduced, the risk for bleeding increases. Acute ITP usually affects children, whereas chronic ITP mainly affects adults over age 60.

• WORD • BUILDING •

immune thrombocytopenic purpura: immune—relating to antibodies or white blood cells + thrombo—clot + cyto—cell + penic—lack + purpura—hemorrhage in the skin

Table 28.2
Common Laboratory Abnormalities in Disseminated Intravascular Coagulation

Screening Test	Finding
Prothrombin time (PT)	Prolonged
Partial thromboplastin time (PTT)	Prolonged
Fibrinogen	Reduced
Dimers (cross-linked fibrin fragments)	Elevated

Acute ITP usually occurs after an acute viral illness such as hepatitis C virus, *Helicobacter pylori*, and HIV. In children, it may follow viral infections such as mumps or measles. It may be drug-induced or associated with pregnancy. ITP is believed to be related to an immune system dysfunction. Antibodies responsible for platelet destruction are found in most diagnosed patients.

Signs and Symptoms
ITP produces clinical changes common to all forms of **thrombocytopenia**: petechiae, ecchymoses, and bleeding from the mouth, nose, or GI tract. Bleeding may occur in vital organs such as the brain, which may prove fatal. In the acute type, onset may occur suddenly, causing easy bruising, nosebleeds, and bleeding gums. Onset of chronic ITP is usually insidious.

Diagnostic Tests
A platelet count of less than 20,000/mm^3 and a prolonged bleeding time suggest ITP. Examination of platelets under the microscope shows them to be small and immature. Anemia may be present if there has been a bleeding episode. A bone marrow aspiration may be performed to rule out other causes.

Therapeutic Measures
The goal of treatment is to have an adequate platelet count and no bleeding. Most cases of acute ITP resolve spontaneously without treatment. Initial treatment, if needed, often involves the administration of steroids. The purpose of the steroids is to prolong the life of the platelets by decreasing immune activity. Drugs to promote platelet formation such as romiplostim (Nplate) may be given. In acute situations, immunoglobulin may be given to quickly increase the blood count. Some patients receive chemotherapeutic drugs. The spleen may be removed because it is the primary site of platelet destruction. Often the patient undergoing splenectomy has tried all other courses of treatment unsuccessfully and may be having bleeding episodes. Acute bleeding episodes are treated with transfusions of blood, platelets, and vitamin K. See later in this chapter for the unique needs of the patient who has had a splenectomy.

Nursing Care
Care for the patient with ITP is the same as for any patient with a bleeding disorder. See Box 28.1 for bleeding precautions. Teach the patient to watch for and report signs and symptoms of bruising and bleeding (Box 28.3). The patient should avoid trauma and restrict activity during severe episodes.

Hemophilia
Hemophilia is a group of hereditary bleeding disorders that result from a severe lack of specific clotting factors. The two most common are hemophilia A (classic hemophilia) and hemophilia B (Christmas disease). Von Willebrand disease is another related bleeding disorder, but it represents a minority of cases and is not discussed in this chapter.

Box 28.3
Patient Education
Signs and Symptoms of Bleeding
Notify your health-care provider if the following occur:
- Easy bruising of skin
- Petechiae (small red spots on skin)
- Blood in urine
- Black tarry stools
- Bleeding from nose or gums
- Increase in vaginal bleeding
- New onset of painful joints

Pathophysiology
Recall that many different clotting factors make up the clotting mechanism. Hemophilia A accounts for 80% of all types of hemophilia. It results from a deficiency of factor VIII. Hemophilia B is a factor IX deficiency; about 15% of people with hemophilia have this type. The severity and prognosis of hemophilia depend on the degree of deficiency of the clotting factors. Mild hemophilia has the best prognosis because it does not cause spontaneous bleeding and joint deformities like severe hemophilia can.

After an injury, the person with hemophilia forms a platelet plug (which differs from a clot) at the site of an injury as would normally be expected. However, the clotting factor deficiency keeps the patient from forming a stable fibrin clot. Continued bleeding washes away the platelet plug that initially formed. Contrary to popular myth, people with hemophilia do not bleed faster and are not at risk from small scratches.

Etiology
Hemophilia A and B are inherited as X-linked recessive traits. This means that the female carrier (daughter of an affected father) has a 50% chance of transmitting the gene to each son or daughter. Daughters who receive the gene are carriers, and sons who receive the gene are born with hemophilia. It is technically possible but rare for daughters to be affected with hemophilia.

Signs and Symptoms
Bleeding occurs as a result of injury or, in severe cases, spontaneously (unprovoked by injury). Bleeding into the muscles and joints (**hemarthrosis**) is common and can cause acute pain. Severe and repeated episodes of joint hemorrhage cause joint deformities, especially in the elbows, knees, and ankles. This decreases the patient's range of motion and ability to walk. A goal of Healthy People 2030 is to reduce the proportion of persons with severe hemophilia who have more than four joint bleeds per year from 16.9% (in 2016) to 13.3% by 2030 (Office of Disease Prevention and Health Promotion, 2020).

• WORD • BUILDING •
thrombocytopenia: thrombocyte—platelet + penia—lack
hemophilia: hemo—blood + philia—to love
hemarthrosis: hem—bleeding + arthr—joint + osis—condition

In mild hemophilia, excessive bleeding is usually associated only with surgery or significant trauma. However, once a person with mild hemophilia begins to bleed, the bleeding can be just as serious as that of the patient with a more severe form.

Spontaneous bleeding can occur with more severe hemophilia. It is possible to bleed into the joints or brain without any precipitating trauma. Severe episodes can produce large subcutaneous and deep intramuscular hematomas. Major trauma can cause life-threatening bleeding.

Diagnostic Tests

In some cases of mild hemophilia, a surgical procedure or trauma is the first time a bleeding problem is noticed. Laboratory data reveal a prolonged PTT. The various clotting factor levels are measured to determine which is missing. Once the missing factor is identified, the type of hemophilia is determined, and necessary treatments can be implemented.

Therapeutic Measures

Hemophilia is not curable. However, treatment advances have improved outcomes. Many patients can now live a normal life span. Treatment is aimed at preserving mobility, preventing deformities, and increasing life expectancy. Administering the missing clotting factors stops bleeding episodes. Mild hemophilia A may be treated with injection or nasal inhalation of desmopressin (antidiuretic hormone; DDAVP). Desmopressin stimulates the body to release more clotting factors. It can be administered before dental procedures or sports. More severe hemophilia A is treated with factor VIII; hemophilia B is treated with factor IX. Each is available in powder form that is reconstituted with water and administered intravenously. Factors can be made from donated blood or using recombinant DNA technology. All blood is tested for HIV and hepatitis to protect recipients.

Fibrin sealants may be applied directly to oozing wounds. Sealants are especially helpful following dental surgeries. Blood transfusions are uncommon but may be necessary after severe trauma or surgery.

Complications occur when therapy is started too late. Minor trauma typically needs to be treated with at least 72 hours of added clotting factors; major traumas and surgeries may require up to 14 days of added factors to prevent sudden bleeding. Health-care workers should pay careful attention to the patient who says that bleeding is starting even when no outward signs are evident. The patient usually knows from experience whether bleeding is starting. If treatment is delayed at this time, the results can be disastrous. Some patients with severe disease are treated prophylactically to prevent bleeding.

Nursing Process for the Patient With Hemophilia

DATA COLLECTION. Collaborate with the RN to assess the patient and family for knowledge of the disease and its treatment and understanding of how to prevent bleeding episodes. Most patients care for themselves at home, starting their own IVs and administering treatment independently. Hospitalization is needed only for surgery or major trauma.

During an acute episode of bleeding, monitor Hgb and Hct levels carefully. Monitor factor VIII or IX levels to determine whether factor replacement has reached adequate levels. Monitor vital signs for falling blood pressure and rising pulse rate, which are signs of hypovolemic shock. Monitor all body systems for signs of bleeding (see Box 28.3). Perform a pain assessment using the **WHAT'S UP?** format.

NURSING DIAGNOSES, PLANNING AND IMPLEMENTATION

Acute Pain related to bleeding into tissues

EXPECTED OUTCOME: The patient's pain will be controlled as evidenced by verbalization that pain is relieved to a satisfactory level within a specified time frame depending on medication and route of intervention.

- Provide Rest, Ice, Compression, and Elevation (RICE) for the injured or painful body part. *These actions can help pain; ice and compression also constrict vessels and reduce bleeding.*
- Administer acetaminophen for mild pain. *Acetaminophen is safer than aspirin or NSAIDS, which can increase bleeding risk.*
- Administer opioids as prescribed for severe pain. *Analgesics are the primary way to manage moderate to severe pain.*

Risk for Bleeding related to factor deficiencies

EXPECTED OUTCOME: The patient will experience no signs or symptoms of bleeding. The patient will verbalize understanding of bleeding precautions.

- Instruct the patient on bleeding precautions and signs and symptoms of bleeding (Boxes 28.1 and 28.3). *Identification of signs of bleeding will promote early intervention and prevent injury.*
- Assist with administration of factor concentrates as ordered *to treat acute episodes of bleeding.* See Chapter 27 for transfusion of blood products.
- Apply ice or pressure on bleeding sites *to help slow bleeding.*
- Avoid intramuscular, subcutaneous, or rectal medications. *These routes can cause bleeding into tissues.*
- Instruct the patient that preventive care will be needed if surgery or dental procedures are needed. *These invasive procedures can be life threatening for the patient with hemophilia.*
- Instruct the patient to obtain emergency care in the event that bleeding occurs. *Intervention is critical for survival of an acute bleeding episode.*
- Encourage patient to obtain medical alert identification *to alert emergency providers in the event of accident or injury.*
- Teach patient to avoid contact sports *to avoid injury and bleeding risk.*
- Instruct the patient and families on community services and hemophilia treatment centers. *These nationwide centers coordinate care for patients with hemophilia.*

EVALUATION. If interventions have been effective, the patient will be comfortable. Bleeding will be prevented or complications minimized. The patient and family will be able to state appropriate measures to prevent and treat bleeding episodes. The patient will be knowledgeable about the resources available to cope with the diagnosis of hemophilia.

DISORDERS OF WHITE BLOOD CELLS

Leukemia

The term **leukemia** literally means "white blood." It was first identified in 1845 when the blood of patients was examined and found to have an excess of "colorless" cells.

Pathophysiology

Leukemia is a cancer of the WBCs that affects all age groups. Immature WBCs (blast cells) are overproduced in the bone marrow, lymph tissue, and spleen. So many abnormal cells develop and are dumped into the peripheral circulation that they tend to collect in the body tissues and organs, especially where circulation is sluggish. The cells are unable to effectively fight infection; it is common for patients to be diagnosed only after experiencing an infection that does not clear up easily with treatment.

As the disease progresses, the bone marrow continues to produce large numbers of the useless cells. The peripheral circulation is filled with them. The bone marrow is packed with blast cells. Because so many of the blood stem cells are being used to make defective WBCs, production of most other normal cells is impossible. The patient becomes anemic because of the lack of RBC production. Bleeding becomes a problem, as fewer and fewer platelets are manufactured. Most important, even though the WBC count is very high, there are few normal, mature, and active WBCs with which to fight infection. Thus, the patient often develops severe infections that do not respond to antibiotics. Without treatment, leukemia leaves the patient unable to fight infection, unable to control bleeding, and with increasing fatigue and anorexia. Untreated leukemia is almost always fatal.

Classifications

Leukemias are classified as either (1) acute or chronic and either (2) lymphoid or myeloid. Symptoms of the acute leukemias begin suddenly, and the patient is very sick. Chronic leukemias develop slowly, and patients can be surprised by the diagnosis because they may feel well. Lymphoid leukemias affect the lymphocytes. Myeloid leukemias affect monocytes, granulocytes, erythrocytes, and platelets. The most common leukemias are discussed next.

ACUTE LEUKEMIA. Acute lymphocytic leukemia (ALL) is the most common cancer in children. ALL involves abnormal growth of the lymphocyte precursors (lymphoblasts). Acute myelogenous (myeloblastic) leukemia (AML) usually affects people over age 60. AML has a poor prognosis.

The patient with acute leukemia may present with sudden onset of high fever, abnormal bleeding from the mucous membranes, petechiae, ecchymoses, and easy bruising after minor trauma. Without treatment, death usually results from infection.

CHRONIC LEUKEMIAS. Chronic lymphocytic leukemia (CLL) is the most common leukemia in adults. It predominantly affects the B and T lymphocytes. Chronic myelogenous leukemia (CML) is characterized by the Philadelphia chromosome. CML occurs most often in older adults.

Chronic leukemia usually develops in a three-phase process. The first insidious phase is characterized by anemia and mild bleeding abnormalities. During this phase, the patient often feels well and is not even aware of being sick. After a time, generally years, the disease progresses to the accelerated and acute phases, in which the scenarios are similar to the events seen in acute leukemias. Chronic leukemia is rarely cured. Rather, treatment attempts to place patients into long-term remission. Eighty-five percent of patients with CLL are alive at 5 years, and 69% of patients with CML are alive at 5 years (Cleveland Clinic, 2019).

Etiology

There is no single clear-cut cause for the development of leukemia. Risk factors include smoking, family history of leukemia, genetics (e.g., persons with Down syndrome are more likely to develop leukemia), and exposures to radiation or certain chemicals. Exposure to radiation is believed to be a factor, in part because radiologists have been found to have a higher-than-average incidence of leukemia. Some patients have developed leukemia after being treated for another type of cancer using radiation or chemotherapy.

Signs and Symptoms

Symptoms are similar for all types of leukemia. They include fever or chills caused by infection; and pallor, weakness, lethargy, shortness of breath, and malaise caused by anemia. Ecchymosis or petechiae may result from thrombocytopenia. These symptoms may be present weeks or months before the appearance of other symptoms. The patient also may have tachycardia, palpitations, and abdominal pain. Sternal pain and rib tenderness may result from crowding of bone marrow. If the leukemia has invaded the central nervous system, the patient may experience confusion, headaches, and personality changes. During the acute phase, the patient may have high fevers from infection.

Diagnostic Tests

Although a simple CBC often points toward the diagnosis, only bone marrow aspiration can show the degree of proliferation of the malignant WBCs and confirm the diagnosis of leukemia. The CBC shows a decrease in the numbers of platelets, RBCs, and mature WBCs. A lumbar puncture helps determine whether the central nervous system is involved. Genetic analysis of the peripheral blood and bone marrow components may show the presence of the Philadelphia chromosome in patients with CML.

Therapeutic Measures

CHEMOTHERAPY. Systemic chemotherapy aims to eradicate the leukemic cells and induce a remission. Remission means that the bone marrow is free to produce normally occurring cells in normal proportions without production of the immature WBCs. The type of chemotherapy used varies with the type of leukemia and the level of involvement. Occasionally, partial remission is achieved when everything looks good except for an occasional leukemic cell seen in the bone marrow. Remission is not the same as cure.

There are three phases to the treatment of acute leukemia: induction, consolidation, and maintenance. Induction is the period in which an attempt is made to get the patient into remission. This first phase is difficult because chemotherapy is given in very high doses and on an aggressive timetable. Often, the patient becomes quite ill from the treatment. The patient may feel depressed because the treatment seems worse than the disease at this stage. The nurse can help the patient deal with anemia, thrombocytopenia, and leukopenia as well as other side effects (Table 28.3; also see Box 28.2 and Chapter 11).

If the first remission is accomplished, the other phases of treatment begin. In the consolidation phase, chemotherapy is used to ensure that all leukemic cells have been eradicated from the body. Finally, the patient graduates to maintenance therapy, in which the patient is kept free of leukemic cells and in remission for a period of years (and hopefully a lifetime). This requires years of continued chemotherapy treatments, often monthly.

Chronic leukemia may be treated with oral chemotherapy, which typically is well tolerated. Chemotherapy may be needed for life to maintain remission. See Chapter 11 for information on chemotherapy.

RADIATION THERAPY. Radiation therapy is sometimes used in addition to chemotherapy for initial treatment of leukemia. It may be directed at the entire body or at specific areas where leukemic cells are collecting. (See Chapter 11.)

STEM CELL TRANSPLANT. Stem cell transplant is sometimes used to treat leukemia. Stem cells can be harvested from the peripheral blood, umbilical cord, or bone marrow. When they are from the bone marrow, it may be called a bone marrow transplant.

Preparation includes high-dose chemotherapy and/or total body irradiation. The goal is to destroy all the patient's malignant bone marrow and then, at the last possible moment, replace it with a donor's clean and healthy stem cells (allogenic transplant). Another type of transplant is known as an *autologous* transplant. It uses the patient's own diseased bone marrow, which is harvested, chemically treated and cleaned, stored, and later reinfused. Transplanted stem cells are given to the patient like a blood transfusion, typically through a central line placed in the chest. Once infused into the bloodstream, the new marrow travels to the bones, where it is hoped that it will begin to grow and function normally.

OTHER THERAPIES. Biological therapies may be used to boost the patient's immune system. They may be used to help the body attack cancer cells or to control side effects by boosting RBC or WBC production. (See Chapter 11.)

Nursing Process for the Patient With Leukemia

The patient with leukemia is at risk for many problems, including fatigue, bleeding, infection, and other complications of the disease and its treatment. The patient must understand the disease process and treatment regimen to participate in self-care. See "Nursing Care Plan for the Patient With Leukemia" for interventions to deal with these problems. Additional diagnoses include *Deficient Knowledge* and *Anxiety*. The following Web sites provide resources for patients and families with leukemia:

- American Cancer Society, www.cancer.org
- Leukemia & Lymphoma Society, www.lls.org
- National Cancer Institute, www.cancer.gov

Also see Chapter 11 for general care of the patient with cancer.

Table 28.3 Leukemia Summary

Signs and Symptoms	Fever (related to infection)
	Pallor
	Weakness, malaise
	Tachycardia
	Dyspnea
	Bone pain
	Headaches, confusion
Diagnostic Tests	Complete blood count (CBC)
	Bone marrow aspiration
	Lumbar puncture
Therapeutic Measures	Chemotherapy
	Radiation therapy
	Stem cell transplant
Priority Nursing Diagnoses	*Risk for Injury* (infection, bleeding) related to pancytopenia
	Fatigue related to decreased tissue oxygenation
	Impaired Oral Mucous Membrane Integrity related to chemotherapy and pancytopenia

> **BE SAFE!**
> **BE VIGILANT!** Monitor the patient with leukemia carefully for subtle signs of infection. With inadequate or immature white blood cells, symptoms may not be obvious. Any redness, swelling, or even slight increase in temperature should be reported.

Nursing Care Plan for the Patient With Leukemia

Nursing Diagnosis: *Risk for Infection and Bleeding* related to pancytopenia
Expected Outcomes: The patient will be free from injury and infection as evidenced by temperature within normal limits and no signs or symptoms of bleeding. Signs and symptoms of infection or bleeding will be reported promptly.
Evaluation of Outcomes: Is the patient free from infection and bleeding, or are problems reported so that quick intervention can prevent further complications?

Intervention	Rationale	Evaluation
Monitor vital signs every 4 hours and as needed.	*Elevated temperature is a sign of infection. Falling blood pressure and elevated pulse rate may indicate sepsis or blood loss.*	Are vital signs stable?
Monitor patient for swelling, redness, or purulent drainage.	*These are signs of infection and should be reported promptly.*	Are signs of infection present? Have they been reported?
Protect patient from sources of infection (see Box 28.2).	*Patient is at risk for infection.*	Are precautions being observed to prevent infection?
Observe for tarry stools, petechiae, and ecchymoses (see Box 28.3).	*These are signs of bleeding and should be reported promptly.*	Are signs of bleeding present? Have they been reported?
Protect patient from injury that could cause bleeding (see Box 28.1).	*Patient is at risk for bleeding because of reduced platelet count.*	Are precautions being observed to prevent injury and bleeding?

Nursing Diagnosis: *Fatigue* related to decreased red blood cell count and oxygenation and effects of treatments
Expected Outcome: The patient's fatigue will be controlled at a level that is acceptable to the patient as evidenced by ability to participate in activities that are important to the patient.
Evaluation of Outcome: Is the patient able to identify and participate in activities as desired?

Intervention	Rationale	Evaluation
Ask about fatigue using the **WHAT'S UP?** format.	*A good assessment establishes a baseline and aids in planning.*	Is fatigue present? To what degree?
Help patient identify activities that are important (e.g., activities of daily living [ADLs], attending a child's wedding, taking a trip). Assist in setting goals to work toward the desired activity.	*If the patient cannot do everything the patient wishes, it may help to focus on the most important things.*	Can patient identify important activities? What are they? How can you assist the patient to reach activity goals?
Encourage a balanced diet. Contact dietitian as needed.	*Poor nutrition contributes to fatigue.*	Is patient eating a balanced diet? Is weight stable?
Allow periods of rest between activities.	*Any activity (e.g., ADLs, getting x-rays, even talking) can increase fatigue.*	Is patient able to rest? Does it help?
Ensure adequate sleep. Obtain order for sleeping aid if indicated.	*Lack of sleep worsens fatigue.*	Does patient state feeling rested on awakening?
Provide for ADLs when patient is unable to do so independently.	*Extreme fatigue may prevent the patient from participating in self-care.*	Are patient's needs met even when they cannot participate?

Nursing Diagnosis: *Impaired Oral Mucous Membrane Integrity* related to chemotherapy and pancytopenia
Expected Outcomes: The patient's oral mucous membranes will remain intact, as evidenced by pink, moist, smooth tissue without ulceration. The patient will be able to eat a balanced diet.
Evaluation of Outcomes: Are oral mucous membranes intact without lesions? Is patient eating a balanced diet?

(nursing care plan continues on page 478)

Nursing Care Plan for the Patient With Leukemia—cont'd

Intervention	Rationale	Evaluation
Inspect mouth daily for redness, edema, and lesions.	Routine assessment helps identify problems early so treatment can be implemented.	Are mucous membranes intact?
Encourage adequate nutrition and fluids. Consult dietitian if indicated.	Poor nutrition and dehydration increase the risk of oral lesions.	Is patient eating and drinking?
Encourage patient to brush teeth after meals with a soft toothbrush. If irritation is severe or if the patient is at risk for bleeding, use swabs or sponge Toothettes instead of a toothbrush.	Brushing the teeth controls tooth and gum disease; a toothbrush may be too harsh if the patient is at risk for bleeding.	Is mouth care being provided after meals? Is mouth care irritating? Are alternative methods effective?
Avoid use of lemon-glycerin swabs for mouth care.	Lemon-glycerin swabs are drying to oral mucosa.	Are products used appropriately?
Obtain an order for a mouthwash containing diphenhydramine (Benadryl). Obtain an order for a topical anesthetic if mouth is very inflamed and painful.	Diphenhydramine reduces inflammation; anesthetics reduce pain.	Does mouthwash soothe pain?
Encourage patient to avoid smoking, alcohol, acidic food or drinks, extremely hot or cold foods and drinks, and commercial mouthwash.	These things can be irritating to the mucosa.	Does patient state understanding of things to avoid?
Geriatric		
Advise patient to remove dentures for cleaning and at bedtime.	Dentures left in for long periods can impair circulation and increase risk of lesions.	Are oral mucous membranes intact?

CLINICAL JUDGMENT

Mr. Washington is on your unit and undergoing initial treatment for leukemia. He is receiving high-dose chemotherapy. You enter his room and find it full of visitors.

1. What concerns do you have?
2. What do you do?
3. How can you promote patient-centered care during Mr. Washington's treatment?

Suggested answers are at the end of the chapter.

MULTIPLE MYELOMA

Multiple myeloma is a deadly cancer of the plasma cells in the bone marrow. Plasma cells are part of the immune system and make antibodies when you have an infection (see Chapter 18 for more information). Five-year survival is 51% to 74%, depending on the stage at diagnosis. Early detection can decrease the amount of pain and disability due to bony destruction and **pathological fractures**. The American Cancer Society's (2020a) estimates for multiple myeloma in the United States for 2020 are about 32,270 new cases and 12,830 deaths. It is more common in Black individuals, particularly men, and in people over age 60.

Pathophysiology

In this disorder, cancerous plasma cells in the bone marrow begin reproducing uncontrollably. The cells produce abnormal, useless antibodies instead of helpful ones. These cells also make a substance that tells the osteoclasts to speed up bone destruction. X-ray examination may show holes in the bones forming a Swiss-cheese pattern (Fig. 28.6). As more and more holes form, the integrity of the bone is compromised and weakened. Multiple myeloma usually affects the bones of the skull, pelvis, ribs, and vertebrae.

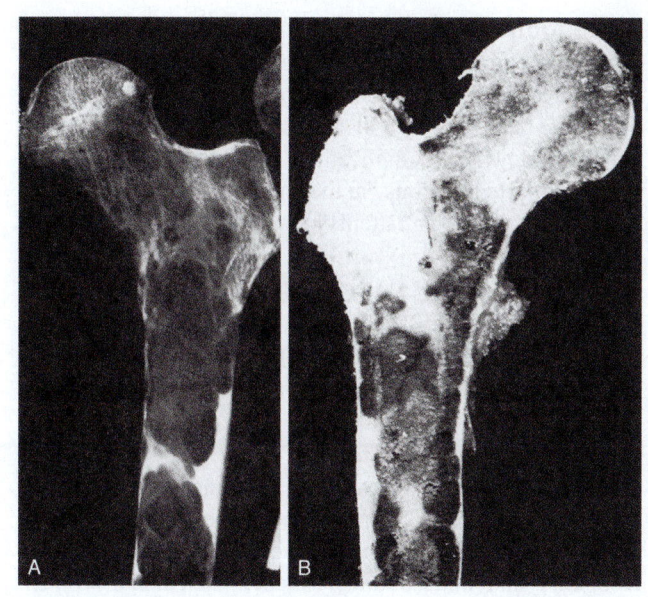

FIGURE 28.6 X-ray of bone destruction in multiple myeloma.

The plasma cells multiply uncontrollably and crowd out other cells in the bone marrow, leading to leukopenia, thrombocytopenia, and anemia. As the disease progresses, plasma cells infiltrate the major organs, including the liver, spleen, lymph nodes, lungs, adrenal glands, kidneys, skin, and GI tract. Although the overall result of the disease is the devastating destruction of the bone and widespread osteoporosis, death is often from sepsis.

Etiology
The cause of multiple myeloma is unknown. Family history of multiple myeloma may be one factor. Exposures to radiation and chemicals used in a number of industries may increase risk, though more research is needed in this area.

Signs and Symptoms
Skeletal pain is a common complaint. The patient may describe the pain as constant severe back pain that increases with exercise or movement or as pain in the ribs. Other signs and symptoms include achiness of the long bones, joint swelling and tenderness, low-grade fever, and general malaise. Sometimes evidence shows early peripheral neuropathy secondary to vertebral collapse and spinal cord compression. The patient may be unable to feel the temperature of bath water or recognize the presence of wounds and infections on the feet. In more severe cases of cord compression, the patient may lose control of bladder and bowel function. This is a true oncological emergency. Prompt emergency treatment is needed to keep the patient from becoming paralyzed.

Patients may have pathological fractures of the long bones. These are fractures that occur with no trauma (e.g., the patient breaks a leg turning over in bed or breaks a rib while sneezing). In advanced disease, the patient experiences anemia, weight loss, thoracic spinal deformities from multiple rib destruction, and a loss of height because of pathological fractures and compacting of the vertebrae.

Because calcium is mobilized from the bones and into the blood, the patient is at risk for hypercalcemia. Signs and symptoms of hypercalcemia include anorexia, nausea, vomiting, mental changes (especially confusion), seizures, weakness, and fatigue. Kidney stones may result as the excess calcium passes through the kidneys.

Patients are susceptible to infection because of compromised immune function. Pneumonia is a common finding in patients with multiple myeloma. They may develop anemia because of bone marrow dysfunction and reduced erythropoietin formation by diseased kidneys. Risk for bruising and bleeding occurs due to thrombocytopenia. Patients often develop kidney failure because the filtering capacity of the kidney becomes blocked by calcium.

Diagnostic Tests
Blood tests are done to determine levels of calcium, WBCs, RBCs, and platelets and to evaluate kidney function. Blood and urine studies are positive for M-type globulins (called *Bence–Jones proteins* when found in the urine) in 40% of patients. X-ray examinations or magnetic resonance imaging (MRI) may show changes in the lungs and diffuse osteoporosis in bones not already riddled with holes. Bone marrow biopsy is done to confirm the diagnosis and determine the stage of the disease.

Therapeutic Measures
Some people with multiple myeloma are asymptomatic and do not require treatment right away. Once treatment begins, there are two goals: (1) managing the disease and (2) managing symptoms and complications. To manage the disease, corticosteroids (prednisone or dexamethasone) and oral or IV chemotherapy agents are given. The goal of drug therapy is to suppress plasma cell proliferation. This helps decrease the amount and speed of bone destruction. Another option is high-dose chemotherapy combined with stem cell transplantation.

The second approach is control of symptoms. The patient is monitored for signs and symptoms of hypercalcemia, hyperuricemia, dehydration, respiratory infection, renal problems, and pain. The HCP may order the administration of IV bisphosphonate agents such as pamidronate (Aredia) to inhibit bone resorption. It is used to help protect bones and keep serum calcium levels controlled. Oral compounds are also available to help keep the calcium within normal limits. The goal is a serum calcium level below 10 mg/dL. If hypercalcemia occurs, the HCP will order an IV infusion of normal saline solution at a high rate, followed by regular administration of calcium-losing diuretics.

External beam irradiation may be given to especially painful areas of bone involvement. Fortunately, this treatment is quite effective, usually decreasing pain intensity in just a few days. Vigorous attention to administering pain medications during the early course of treatment greatly reduces the patient's pain levels.

The patient may need spinal surgery if vertebral collapse occurs. Because of demineralization of the bone, with resulting large amounts of calcium in the blood and urine, surgery for kidney stones and eventual dialysis for acute or chronic kidney failure may be needed.

Nursing Process for the Patient With Multiple Myeloma

The patient with multiple myeloma is at risk for many problems. See the "Nursing Care Plan for the Patient With Leukemia," which is also appropriate for patients with multiple myeloma. In addition, *Risk for Injury* is discussed shortly.

Data Collection

Monitor for fever or malaise, which can signal the onset of infection. Other conditions to be alert for include anemia, hypercalcemia, fractures, and kidney complications. Monitor intake and output, and strain urine for stones. Elevated BUN and creatinine levels will alert you to possible kidney failure. Report back pain, leg weakness, sensory loss, or loss of bowel or bladder function because these can indicate spinal cord compression. Monitor the patient for elevated CRP and low Hgb, which are associated with increased fatigue.

Nursing Diagnoses, Planning, and Implementation

> **Risk for Injury (fracture, pressure injury) related to weakened bones, complications of immobility, and complications due to hypercalcemia**
>
> **EXPECTED OUTCOME:** The patient will remain free from injury as evidenced by no fracture and no complications related to immobility or hypercalcemia.

- Keep the patient mobile. Consult physical and occupational therapy as needed. Bones in use are strongest, so the patient should remain up and moving as much as possible *to help stimulate calcium resorption and decrease demineralization.*
- Assist the patient with walking *to reduce the risk of falling or pathological fractures of the long bones.*
- If the patient is unsteady, use a walker or a support belt *to reduce the risk of falls.*
- Reposition bedridden patients every 2 hours *to prevent complications related to immobility.*
- Use a lift sheet to move the patient gently in bed *to decrease the risk of skin damage and pathological fractures.*
- Provide passive range-of-motion exercises *to maintain mobility if the patient is unable to be independently mobile.*
- Administer fluids so that daily output is never less than 1,500 mL *to flush kidneys and reduce the risk of kidney stones.*
- Teach the patient the importance of good hydration at all times *to minimize complications of hypercalcemia.* Depending on the time of year and the type and level of patient activities, the patient may need to have an intake of more than 4 L daily. Consult with HCP for amount.

Evaluation

If nursing care has been effective, the patient will be free from infection or infection will be recognized and treated promptly. The patient will avoid injury, with no fracture, skin breakdown, or complications related to hypercalcemia. See "Home Health Hints" at the end of this chapter for additional suggestions for patients being cared for at home.

LYMPHATIC DISORDERS

Lymphatic disorders include Hodgkin lymphoma and non-Hodgkin lymphomas.

Hodgkin Lymphoma

Hodgkin **lymphoma** is a cancer of the lymph system. Its distinguishing feature is the presence of Reed–Sternberg cells. This makes it different from all the other forms of lymphoma. Hodgkin lymphoma is more prevalent in men than in women. It occurs most often in young people in their 20s and 30s, and those older than age 55. Of all the lymphomas, Hodgkin lymphoma is the most curable type, even when the disease is widespread at the time of diagnosis. The 5-year survival rate is about 86% (American Cancer Society, 2020b).

Pathophysiology

Lymph nodes are made of lymphocytes and other immune tissue. Most often, Hodgkin lymphoma begins in a single lymph node, usually one of the cervical nodes of the neck. As the disease progresses, the cancer invades the lymph node chains node by node. Cancer infiltration usually follows the path of lymph fluid flow. Left untreated, other lymphoid tissues such as the spleen become infiltrated with the disease. The major organs eventually become involved.

A tentative diagnosis of Hodgkin lymphoma is based on one or more painlessly enlarged nodes in the cervical, axillary, or inguinal areas. A biopsy of several of the enlarged nodes is performed to search for the presence of Reed–Sternberg cells, which confirms the diagnosis.

Etiology

The exact cause of Hodgkin lymphoma is unknown. It is more common in people who have had mononucleosis, which is caused by the Epstein-Barr virus. Sometimes, it occurs in families, suggesting a genetic link. Patients with impaired immune function are also at higher risk, such as those with AIDS or taking immunosuppressant drugs.

Signs and Symptoms

Painless swelling in one or more of the common lymph node chains is a usual presentation. Swelling can range from barely perceptible to the size of a softball or even larger. The patient

• WORD • BUILDING •
lymphoma: lymph—fluid found in lymphatic vessels + oma—tumor

may report generalized pruritus. One other curious event, alcohol-induced pain, is occasionally present. With just a few sips of any type of alcoholic beverage, the patient may describe intense pain at the site of disease. Because the lymph nodes in the upper chest and neck are often involved, the patient may have symptoms of obstruction, such as cough, dysphagia, or stridor.

Symptoms of more advanced disease include shortness of breath, persistent low-grade fever, night sweats, fatigue, weight loss, and malaise. In older adults, enlarged lymph nodes may be less visible, so these secondary symptoms may be the only presenting symptoms. Other symptoms associated with late-stage disease include edema of the neck and face, jaundice, nerve pain, enlargement of the retroperitoneal nodes, and infiltration of the spleen; liver and bones may also be involved.

Diagnostic Tests and Staging

Diagnosis usually begins with a lymph node biopsy of the easiest lymph node to access. Lymph node biopsies are done to check for Reed–Sternberg cells, fibrosis, and necrosis. Other tests include bone marrow biopsy and aspiration, liver and spleen biopsies, chest x-ray examination, positron emission tomography (PET) scan, abdominal computed tomography (CT) scan to check for disease in the liver and spleen, lung scan, and bone scan.

Hematologic tests (e.g., CBC) may show wide variability of RBCs, indicating mild to severe anemia. The WBC count is often abnormal and extreme (either very high or very low) because of bone marrow infiltration by disease. These tests are also used for staging the disease:

- Stage I disease is limited to a single lymph node group or a single organ.
- Stage II disease occurs when two or more node regions and/or an organ are involved on the same side of the diaphragm.
- Stage III disease affects nodes and/or an organ on both sides of the diaphragm.
- Stage IV, the most serious form of the disease and the least curable, includes widely disseminated disease in both lymph nodes and other organs, such as bone marrow or liver.

Therapeutic Measures

Depending on the stage of the disease, therapy will include the use of radiation and chemotherapy. Radiation therapy is administered on an outpatient basis over a 4- to 6-week period. It can be curative for patients with stage I or stage II disease. Combinations of chemotherapy and radiation therapy are used for patients with stage III and stage IV disease. Results vary depending on the location and the stage of disease. If the disease recurs after initial treatment, stem cell transplant may be considered. Treatment-related complications such as cardiovascular disease, lung damage, increased infection risk, and secondary cancers can occur many years post-treatment (American Cancer Society, 2018). Newer targeted and immune-based therapies are being developed that have fewer side effects.

Nursing Management

Most nursing interventions are aimed at symptom management. If the patient is experiencing night sweats, interventions may include changing the gown and bed linens several times a night and helping the patient remain clean and dry. Itching can be treated with moisturizers or ointments, topical corticosteroid creams, or oral agents such as antihistamines, some antidepressants, or gabapentin. Teach the patient to avoid very hot baths, which can dry the skin and increase itching. Keeping the patient and family involved in the plan of care may help relieve anxiety.

Hodgkin lymphoma survivors can experience long-term psychosocial and health complications related to their treatment (Troy et al, 2019). The nurse should recognize that psychosocial distress can interfere with activities of daily living, quality of life, and physical health and should intervene accordingly.

If the patient experiences fatigue and activity intolerance, oxygen therapy may help. Assist with activities as needed, and teach the family how to assist as well. Teach the patient and family how to monitor for and prevent infection along with signs and symptoms to report. See Box 28.2 and Chapter 11 for nursing interventions for the patient with cancer.

Patient Education

In addition to the teaching needs above, make sure that the patient and the family know about local chapters of the American Cancer Society (www.cancer.org) and the Leukemia & Lymphoma Society (www.lls.org). Both organizations provide information, financial assistance, and counseling referral sources, which most patients find valuable.

> **CRITICAL THINKING**
>
> **Harry** is a 60-year-old nurse diagnosed with stage II Hodgkin lymphoma. He wishes to continue working at his job on a respiratory unit at the local hospital while he undergoes chemotherapy.
>
> 1. What are your priorities for Harry's care?
> 2. What concerns you about Harry working at the hospital during his treatment?
> 3. With whom can you collaborate to assist Harry?
>
> Suggested answers are at the end of the chapter.

Non-Hodgkin Lymphomas

All the other types of lymphomas are clumped into a diverse classification known as the *non-Hodgkin lymphomas* (NHLs). It is possible to sort these other types of lymphomas into different categories based on the degree of malignancy. NHLs arise in the lymphoid tissues of the body, just as Hodgkin lymphoma does, but they differ in several ways (Table 28.4). Chronic lymphocytic leukemia is a type of

Table 28.4
Hodgkin Lymphoma versus Non-Hodgkin Lymphoma

	Hodgkin Lymphoma	Non-Hodgkin Lymphomas
Age	20s–30s and over 55 years	Usually over 60 years
Incidence	Less common	More common
Prognosis	Good	Poorer
Reed–Sternberg cells	Present	Absent
Alcohol-induced pain	May be present	Absent

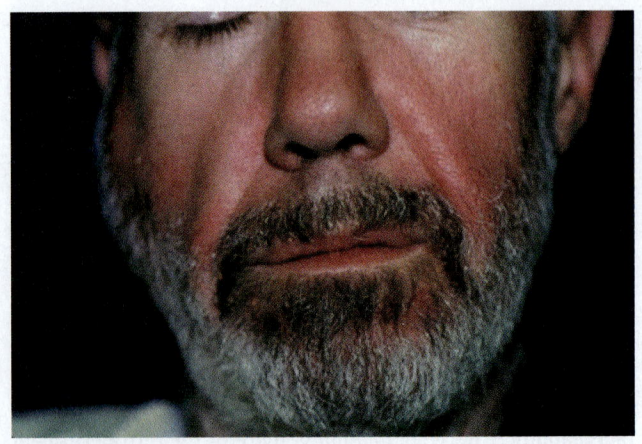

FIGURE 28.7 Non-Hodgkin lymphoma in parotid gland. Note swelling on left side of image.

lymphoma but we discussed it in the "Leukemia" section because it affects the blood instead of the lymph nodes. NHL is most common after age 60.

Pathophysiology
The most distinguishing difference is the absence of the Reed–Sternberg cells in an NHL. Instead, many of these lymphomas arise from the B cells and T cells. The B cells are involved in recognizing and destroying specific antigens. Cells specifically involved include the memory B cells and the plasma cells. The T cells also are involved in registering antigens, but there are many kinds of T cells. An abnormality in any of the T cells can result in a type of NHL. Cancerous cells are found most commonly in the lymph nodes, but they can also be found in other lymph tissues such as the tonsils, thymus, spleen, or bone marrow.

Etiology
The cause of an NHL is unclear. However, some viruses, such as the Epstein-Barr and human immunodeficiency viruses, are thought to play a role in their development. *H. pylori*, the bacterium that causes ulcers, has been associated with NHLs. Immune suppressing medications play a role, as do some herbicides and insecticides.

Signs and Symptoms
Clinical features of NHLs include enlarged, painless, rubbery lymph nodes, as well as infiltration of organs. Other symptoms are very similar to Hodgkin lymphoma. NHLs are often diagnosed later and progress more rapidly than Hodgkin lymphoma. See Figure 28.7.

Diagnostic Tests
Diagnosis is confirmed by histological evaluation of biopsied lymph nodes, tonsils, bone marrow, liver, bowel, skin, or other affected tissues. Other relevant tests include bone scans, chest x-ray, liver and spleen scans, CT, MRI, PET scan, and IV pyelogram to determine the extent of the disease. Laboratory tests include a CBC (which often indicates anemia), serum uric acid level, and liver function studies. Serum calcium level may be elevated if bone lesions are present.

Staging is very similar to staging for Hodgkin lymphoma, ranging from Stage I (one lymph node or group of nodes in the same area) to IV (widespread cancer in lymph nodes, organs, and other tissues).

Therapeutic Measures
If the patient is not experiencing symptoms, treatment may be delayed. Once initiated, treatment usually involves multimodal therapy, including the use of chemotherapy and radiation therapy in combination. Radiation therapy is given to affected areas in advanced stages of NHL. Stem cell transplant may be tried in patients with advanced disease. Newer therapies include targeted therapies and immunotherapies.

Nursing Management
You can provide emotional support by keeping the patient and family informed during the testing phase. Nursing management is similar to management of Hodgkin lymphoma. See "Nursing Management" in the earlier discussion of Hodgkin lymphoma, and Table 28.5.

SPLENIC DISORDERS

The spleen is involved in a number of disorders, including cancers of the blood, lymph, and bone marrow; hereditary conditions such as SCD; and acquired problems such as immune thrombocytopenia. Under normal circumstances, the spleen is not paid much attention; it generally performs its functions without much fanfare.

If the spleen enlarges markedly, the condition is referred to as **splenomegaly**. Other times, the spleen may or may not

• WORD • BUILDING •
splenomegaly: splen—spleen + megaly—large

Table 28.5 Lymphoma Summary

Signs and Symptoms	Swollen lymph nodes Fatigue Low-grade fever Night sweats
Diagnostic Tests	Complete blood count (CBC) Lymph node biopsy Lymphangiography Computed tomography (CT) scan
Therapeutic Measures	Chemotherapy Radiation Bone marrow or stem cell transplant
Priority Nursing Diagnoses	*Activity Intolerance, Fatigue* *Risk for Infection*

be enlarged, but the function is out of control so that too many RBCs and platelets are removed from the peripheral circulation. Sometimes, the spleen is not able to perform its job because of bleeding into the pulp of the organ, which makes it useless. Bleeding into the spleen can occur from various illnesses or from trauma. Treatment of splenomegaly is directed at the underlying disorder. Another treatment option may be splenectomy.

Splenectomy

Splenectomy is the surgical removal of the spleen. Sometimes only part of the spleen is removed; a partial splenectomy retains some splenic tissue and function. Some people have two spleens, and the second, smaller spleen can take over splenic function. Splenectomy is used to treat selected hematologic disorders, leukemias, and lymphomas, as well as after trauma or rupture. It may be done with traditional, open surgery or laparoscopically. Splenectomy is performed fairly often in the United States. However, like any surgery, it is not without risk. A new procedure being researched is splenic autotransplantation. This involves implantation of some of the removed tissue, usually in the peritoneal cavity, for return of some splenic function.

Patient Education
Explain to patients that this surgery removes the spleen, usually under general anesthesia. Inform patients that they can live a normal life after the surgery. However, tell them that they will be more prone to infection and should receive vaccines against pneumonia, meningococci, and *Haemophilus influenzae* disease, as well as a yearly influenza vaccine.

Preoperative Care
Before the surgery, ensure that the CBC and coagulation profile are completed and reported to the surgeon. Blood transfusion may be ordered to correct underlying anemia and prepare for loss of blood stored in the spleen. Vitamin K may be ordered to correct clotting factor deficiencies.

Check the patient's vital signs and collect baseline respiratory system data. Note any signs of respiratory infections such as fever, chills, crackles, wheezes, or cough. If any of these are noted, make sure that the surgeon is aware of them because surgery may need to be delayed. Teach the patient routine coughing and deep-breathing techniques to help prevent postoperative respiratory complications. See Chapter 12 for care of the patient undergoing surgery.

Postoperative Care
During the early postoperative period, watch carefully for bleeding, either external or internal. Be prepared to administer opioids for pain, usually on an around-the-clock schedule so the patient is comfortable enough to deep breathe, cough, and ambulate. After opioid administration, be sure to observe for side effects. These may include incomplete pain relief or hypoventilation. Monitor for fever every 4 hours, and expect a mild, low-grade, transient fever postoperatively. A persistent fever may indicate abscess or hematoma formation.

If the surgery was performed to decrease the numbers of cells being removed from the peripheral circulation, monitor the platelet count. Often the count begins to rise in just a few days, but it may take up to 2 weeks for the platelets to normalize.

Complications
A splenectomy can lead to complications such as bleeding, pneumonia, and atelectasis (collapsed alveoli). Respiratory problems occur because of the spleen's position close to the diaphragm and the need for a high surgical incision that is very painful. Often, the patient tries to restrict lung expansion after surgery to keep from hurting. However, this splinting behavior may leave the patient at risk for pneumonia and respiratory problems. In addition, splenectomy patients are usually more vulnerable to infection, especially influenza, because the spleen's role in the immune response is no longer filled.

Another possible complication of splenectomy includes the development of pancreatitis. Because the tail of the pancreas is close to the spleen, irritation can occur.

The most serious complication is overwhelming postsplenectomy infection (OPSI). The causative agents in OPSI include streptococci, *Neisseria* spp., and influenza bacteria (as opposed to a flu virus). OPSI can occur at any time from 1 week to 20 years after the splenectomy. Patients most at risk are those with poor immune function.

Early symptoms of OPSI include fever and malaise that seem unremarkable. However, the infection may progress within a few hours to sepsis and death. Unfortunately, OPSI can have a mortality rate as high as 70%. Be sure to include

• WORD • BUILDING •

splenectomy: splen—spleen + ectomy—excision

the signs and symptoms of OPSI in patient education. Also, stress the need to promptly obtain medical attention for the patient at the first signs and symptoms of infection. The patient should be directed to continue to receive lifetime vaccinations against these bacteria.

> ### Home Health Hints
> - Patients who are at risk for infection can place a sign on the front door of their homes to limit visitors or ask persons with colds to come back when they are well. The patient may appreciate the home health nurse giving permission to be assertive in such circumstances.
> - Teach patients with infection risk to wear gloves when gardening, avoid manicures and pedicures, avoid hot tubs, and wash hands after contact with pets, fresh flowers, or plants.
> - To prevent bruising, have the patient cut the feet off long, white sport socks and wear them on the arms. They can be hidden under long-sleeve shirts and blouses. They provide a cushion when doing activities.
> - Teach patients with thrombocytopenia to avoid contact sports and to consult with their HCP about whether sexual intercourse is safe.
> - Teach patients with thrombocytopenia to avoid over-the-counter medications unless approved by the HCP. Many such agents contain aspirin or NSAIDs.
> - Patients with sickle cell anemia usually have a lower blood pressure. It is important to report even mild hypertension in these patients.
> - Provide a high-calorie, high-protein nutritional supplement between meals. If fatigue or nausea causes poor appetite, discuss eating smaller, more frequent meals. Ask the HCP for an antiemetic order if needed.

Key Points

- Patients with hematologic disorders have problems related to the blood. When RBCs are affected, oxygen transport is also affected, causing symptoms related to poor oxygenation. When WBCs are affected, the patient cannot effectively fight infections. If platelets or clotting factors are affected, bleeding disorders occur.
- The term *anemia* describes a condition in which there is a deficiency of RBCs, Hgb, or both, in the circulating blood. Because Hgb carries oxygen, this deficiency results in a reduced capacity to deliver oxygen to the tissues. Symptoms such as weakness and shortness of breath occur.
- Aplastic anemia differs from other types of anemia in that the bone marrow becomes fatty and unable to produce enough RBCs. The cells that are produced are normal in size and shape, but there are not enough of them to sustain life. The result is reduced numbers of all cells from the bone marrow, including RBCs, platelets, and WBCs. Left untreated, aplastic anemia is almost always fatal.
- Sickle cell anemia is an inherited anemia in which the RBCs have a specific mutation. Any time a decrease in the oxygen tension is sensed, the cells begin an observable physical change from their usual spherical shape to a sickle or crescent shape. Sickled cells are very rigid and easily cracked and broken. The abnormal shape also causes the cells to become tangled in the blood vessels and organs. The result is congestion, clumping, and clotting.
- Polycythemia includes two separate disorders that are easily recognizable by similar characteristic changes in the RBC count. In both forms of polycythemia, the blood becomes so thick with too many RBCs that it resembles sludge. This thickness does not allow the blood to circulate easily.
- DIC is a catastrophic, overwhelming state of accelerated clotting throughout the peripheral blood vessels. In a short period, all the clotting factors and platelet supplies are exhausted, and clots can no longer be formed. This results in severe hemorrhage. DIC is not a disease; it is a syndrome that develops secondary to another severe physical problem. Once this deadly syndrome develops, the progression of symptoms is rapid.
- Acute immune thrombocytopenic purpura results from increased platelet destruction by the immune system. Any time platelet numbers are reduced, the risk for bleeding increases.
- Hemophilia is a group of hereditary bleeding disorders that result from a severe lack of specific clotting factors. The two most common are hemophilia A (classic hemophilia) and hemophilia B (Christmas disease).
- Leukemia is a malignant disease of the WBCs that affects all age groups. The immature WBCs (blast cells) generate rapidly in the bone marrow, lymph tissue, and spleen. The cells are abnormal and unable to effectively fight infection.
- Multiple myeloma is a deadly cancer of the plasma cells in the bone marrow. When the disease is caught in its early stages, treatment can prolong life. More important, early detection can decrease the amount of pain and disability due to bony destruction and pathological fractures.
- Hodgkin lymphoma is a cancer of the lymph system. The presence of Reed–Sternberg cells makes Hodgkin lymphoma different from all the other forms of lymphoma.
- All other types of lymphoma are grouped into a diverse classification known as the non-Hodgkin lymphomas.

SUGGESTED ANSWERS TO CHAPTER EXERCISES

Cue Recognition

28.1: Raise the head of the bed and turn her head to the side to prevent aspiration. Ensure that oxygen is running, then call for help. Do not palpate the abdomen, as this could cause further bleeding.

Critical Thinking & Clinical Judgment

Mrs. Johns

1. Monitor Mrs. Johns's vital signs and report falling blood pressure and rising pulse immediately. Inspect her skin for petechiae and ecchymoses. Outline ecchymotic areas with a marker to see whether the area is increasing in size. Monitor urine for signs of blood. Test stools for occult blood. Monitor vaginal discharge for increasing bleeding. Report any changes promptly.
2. Anticipate assisting the RN with administration of blood or blood products. Instruct Mrs. Johns in the importance of preventing injury that could cause further bleeding. Other care will be supportive.
3. Mrs. Johns will be concerned for her new baby, who is most likely on another unit or already discharged home. Allow Mrs. Johns to talk about her concerns. Arrange visits with her family and baby if permitted by her condition and her HCP.
4. $\dfrac{300 \text{ mL}}{30 \text{ min}} \bigg| \dfrac{60 \text{ min}}{1 \text{ hour}} = 600 \text{ mL per hour}$
5. Collaborate with the RN, internist, obstetrician, hematologist, neonatal nurse, husband, family, and social worker to provide holistic, patient-centered care for this new mother.

Mr. Washington

1. Because of his leukemia and treatment, Mr. Washington is at risk for infection. If he develops an infection, he will have great difficulty getting over it. With so many visitors in the room, it is likely that one or more has a cold or virus. They may not be aware of the risk this poses to Mr. Washington. Mr. Washington is probably also fatigued because of his disease, and treatment and visiting require energy.
2. You should kindly explain that although family visits are important, Mr. Washington is very susceptible to catching colds or other illnesses and that it would be best to limit visitors to one or two at a time. Point out that persons with symptoms of colds or flu should not enter the room at all. Visits should also be brief to prevent overtiring the patient.
3. Ask Mr. Washington about his preferences, and attempt to honor them if possible. He may choose one or two (healthy!) visitors to come regularly or choose a time of day when he is less fatigued to have visitors. As his nurse, you can help enforce visiting limitations so Mr. Washington does not have to feel ungracious toward his visitors.

Harry

1. Priorities for Harry include maintaining respiratory function, comfort, and infection prevention, in addition to management of chemotherapy side effects. Because Harry is a nurse, he likely has some knowledge of Hodgkin lymphoma, so be sure to determine his knowledge base before developing a teaching plan with the RN.
2. Harry will probably be fatigued from his disease, and fatigue may increase further as a side effect of treatment. Staff nursing jobs can be tiring even for healthy nurses. In addition, he will be around patients with respiratory diseases, many of whom are contagious. Because of the risk of infection secondary to the disease process and the treatment regimen, Harry might want to take a leave of absence during treatment or ask to be reassigned to an area that is less demanding and away from direct patient care until treatments have been completed.
3. In addition to routine collaborative relationships, consider collaborating with the social worker or case manager. If Harry is unable to work during his treatment, he might need assistance with applying for disability benefits.

Additional Resources

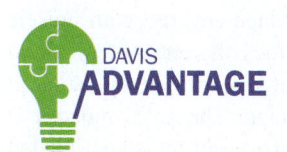

Go to Davis Advantage to complete your learning: strengthen understanding, apply your knowledge, and prepare for the Next Gen NCLEX®.

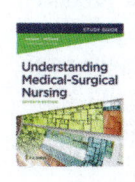

A Study Guide is also available.

UNIT SEVEN Understanding the Respiratory System

CHAPTER 29
Respiratory System Function, Data Collection, and Therapeutic Measures

Jennifer A. Otmanowski, Paula D. Hopper, Janice L. Bradford

KEY TERMS

adventitious (ad-ven-TISH-us)
apnea (AP-nee-ah)
crepitus (KREP-ih-tus)
cyanosis (SY-uh-NOH-sis)
dyspnea (DISP-nee-ah)
respiratory excursion (RES-per-uh-TOR-ee eks-KUR-shun)
retraction (rih-TRAK-shun)
thoracentesis (THOR-uh-sen-TEE-sis)
tidaling (TY-dah-ling)
tracheostomy (TRAY-key-AH-stuh-mee)
tracheotomy (TRAY-key-AH-tuh-mee)

CHAPTER CONCEPTS

Acid–base balance
Evidence-based practice
Oxygenation
Safety

LEARNING OUTCOMES

1. Describe the normal structures and functions of the respiratory system.
2. Identify how aging affects the respiratory system.
3. List data to collect when caring for a patient with a respiratory disorder.
4. Recognize expected findings when inspecting, palpating, percussing, and auscultating the chest.
5. Identify common diagnostic tests performed to diagnose disorders of the respiratory system.
6. Plan nursing care for patients undergoing each of the diagnostic tests.
7. Discuss therapeutic measures used to help patients with respiratory disorders.

NORMAL RESPIRATORY SYSTEM ANATOMY AND PHYSIOLOGY

The respiratory system is basically a tract, divided into upper and lower respiratory portions. The upper tract is above the thoracic cavity. The lower portion is within the thoracic cavity. The alveoli of the lungs are the site of gas exchange between the air and the blood of pulmonary circulation. The rest of the system moves air into and out of the lungs. Together with the cardiovascular system, the respiratory system supplies the body with oxygen and eliminates carbon dioxide.

Nose and Nasal Cavities

The nose is made mostly of bone and cartilage covered with muscle and epithelium. Hairs inside the nostrils block the entry of dust and other particles. The nasal cavities are separated at midline by the nasal septum, which is made of bone and cartilage. The nasal mucosa is highly vascular ciliated epithelium that warms and moistens inhaled air. Dust and microorganisms become trapped on mucus produced by goblet cells and are swept back into the pharynx by the cilia. Table 29.1 provides a summary of protective mechanisms in the respiratory system.

The paranasal sinuses are air cavities in the maxillary, frontal, sphenoid, and ethmoid bones that open into the nasal cavities, releasing mucus. The sinuses lessen the weight of the skull and provide resonance for the voice.

Table 29.1 Protective Mechanisms in the Respiratory System

Nasal hairs and turbinates	Trap dust and microorganisms.
Mucous membranes	Warm and moisten inhaled air; trap inhaled particles.
Cilia	Move particles toward pharynx to be swallowed or coughed out.
Irritant receptors in nose and airways	Trigger sneeze and cough to remove foreign debris.
Alveolar macrophages	Phagocytize foreign particles and bacteria.

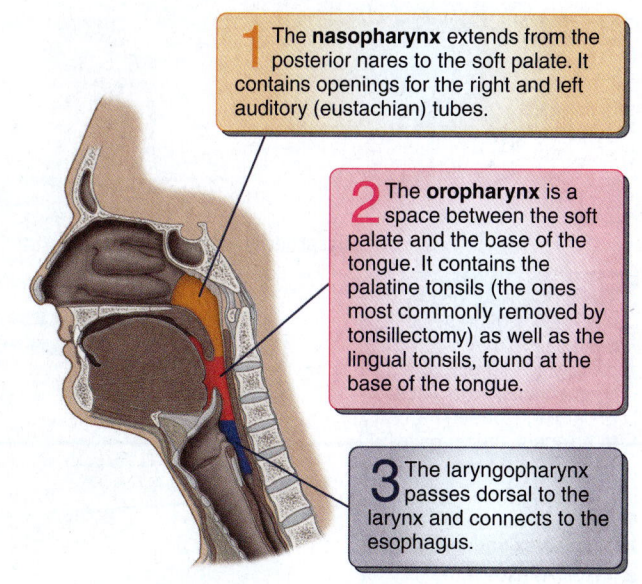

1. The **nasopharynx** extends from the posterior nares to the soft palate. It contains openings for the right and left auditory (eustachian) tubes.

2. The **oropharynx** is a space between the soft palate and the base of the tongue. It contains the palatine tonsils (the ones most commonly removed by tonsillectomy) as well as the lingual tonsils, found at the base of the tongue.

3. The **laryngopharynx** passes dorsal to the larynx and connects to the esophagus.

FIGURE 29.1 Pharynx.

Pharynx

The pharynx is posterior to the nasal and oral cavities. It has three regions (Fig. 29.1). The soft palate and uvula rise to block the nasopharynx during swallowing. The lingual tonsils, the adenoid (pharyngeal tonsil), and the palatine tonsils form a ring of lymphatic tissue around the pharynx and destroy pathogens that penetrate the mucosa.

Larynx

The larynx is the airway between the pharynx and trachea. It houses the vocal cords and produces sound that can be formed into speech. The epiglottis at the top of the larynx prevents ingested materials from entering the trachea (Fig. 29.2). The cartilaginous walls are lined with ciliated epithelium. The vagus and accessory cranial nerves innervate the larynx.

Trachea and Bronchial Tree

The trachea descends from the larynx to the primary bronchi (Fig. 29.3). The mucosa is ciliated epithelium. Mucus with trapped dust and microorganisms is swept upward toward the pharynx and swallowed.

Deeper into the bronchial tree, cartilage diminishes and smooth muscle in the walls increases. The bronchioles have no cartilage in the walls to maintain patency. Therefore, they can be closed completely by bronchoconstriction.

Lungs and Pleural Membranes

The lungs occupy the thoracic cavity on each side of the heart, extending from the clavicles to the diaphragm. They are protected by the ribs (costae). On the medial (mediastinal) surface of each lung is an indentation called the hilus. This is where the primary bronchus and the pulmonary vessels enter the lung (Fig. 29.4). A thin layer of fluid between the visceral and parietal pleural membranes provides lubrication to reduce friction during lung expansion.

The functional units of the lungs are the millions of alveoli, the air sacs where gas exchange occurs. Both the alveoli and the surrounding alveolar capillaries are made of simple squamous epithelium; their walls are only one cell in thickness to permit diffusion of gases (Fig. 29.5).

Each alveolus is lined with a thin layer of tissue fluid that is essential for the diffusion of gases. However, the surface tension of the fluid tends to make the walls of an alveolus stick together internally. Alveolar cells secrete *surfactant*, a lipoprotein that mixes with the tissue fluid and decreases surface tension to permit inflation.

Between clusters of alveoli is elastic connective tissue that can stretch during inhalation and recoil during exhalation. The recoil of this tissue allows passive exhalation without the expenditure of energy.

Mechanism of Breathing

Ventilation is the term for the movement of air into and out of the alveoli. The primary respiratory muscles are the diaphragm, inferior to the lungs, and the external intercostal muscles, between the ribs. Accessory muscles of respiration are used during exercise and times of respiratory distress. These include muscles for deep inspiration (sternocleidomastoid, scalene, pectoralis minor) and for forced expiration (internal intercostal muscles and abdominal musculature; Fig. 29.6). Respiratory centers of the brain, located in the medulla oblongata and pons, innervate muscles of respiration via the intercostal and phrenic nerves. A normal respiratory rate is 12 to 20 breaths/minute.

Ventilation is accomplished by respiratory muscle contractions, causing changes in lung volumes. Movement of air follows Boyle's law, which states that in a closed container of gases, volume and pressure are inversely related. Air moves from high-pressure to low-pressure areas.

Inhalation

Inhalation, also called *inspiration*, occurs when motor impulses from the medulla cause contraction of the respiratory

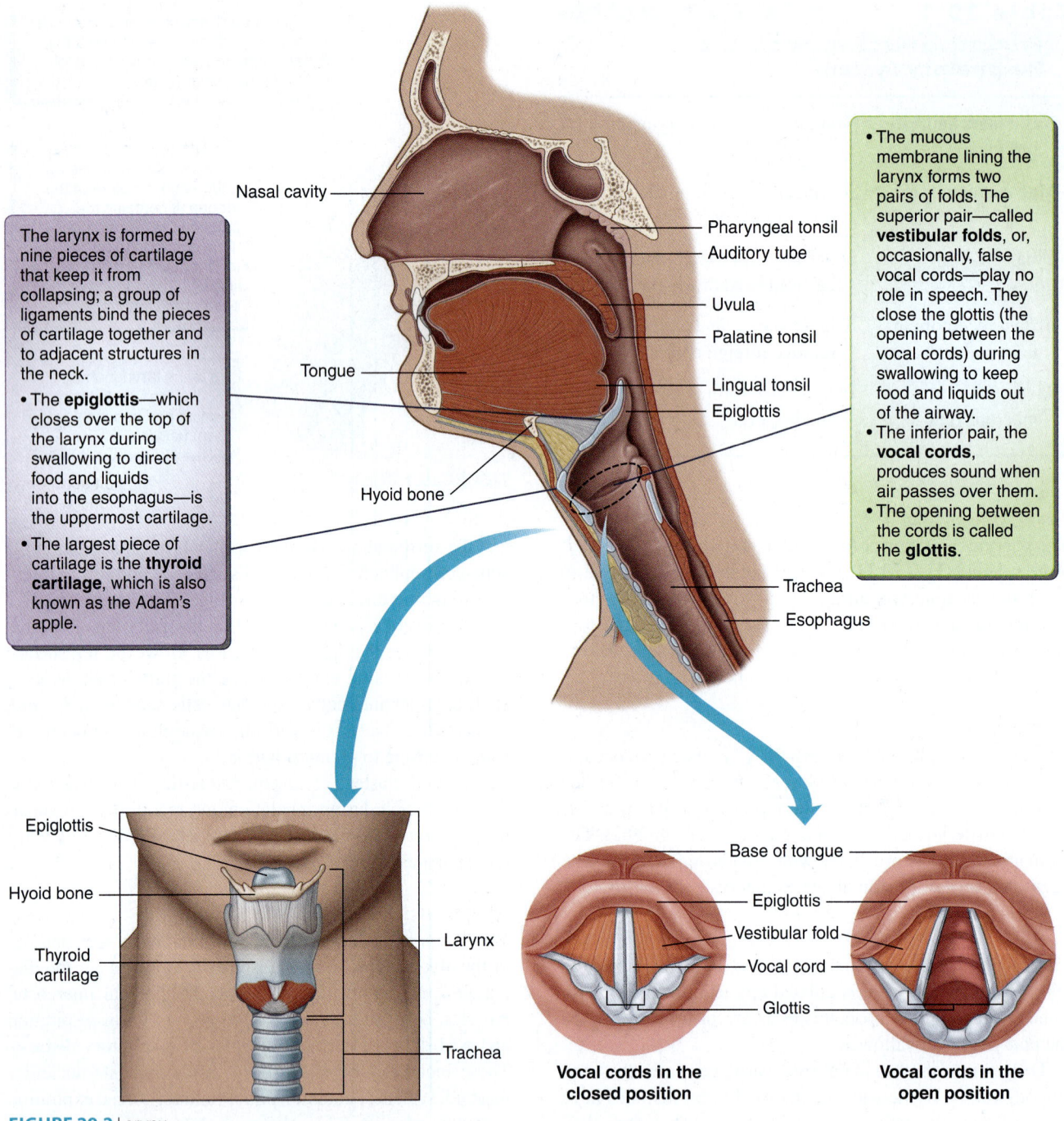

488 UNIT SEVEN Understanding the Respiratory System

The larynx is formed by nine pieces of cartilage that keep it from collapsing; a group of ligaments bind the pieces of cartilage together and to adjacent structures in the neck.
- The **epiglottis**—which closes over the top of the larynx during swallowing to direct food and liquids into the esophagus—is the uppermost cartilage.
- The largest piece of cartilage is the **thyroid cartilage**, which is also known as the Adam's apple.

- The mucous membrane lining the larynx forms two pairs of folds. The superior pair—called **vestibular folds**, or, occasionally, false vocal cords—play no role in speech. They close the glottis (the opening between the vocal cords) during swallowing to keep food and liquids out of the airway.
- The inferior pair, the **vocal cords**, produces sound when air passes over them.
- The opening between the cords is called the **glottis**.

Labels on sagittal view: Nasal cavity, Pharyngeal tonsil, Auditory tube, Uvula, Palatine tonsil, Tongue, Lingual tonsil, Epiglottis, Hyoid bone, Trachea, Esophagus

Anterior view labels: Epiglottis, Hyoid bone, Thyroid cartilage, Larynx, Trachea

Superior view labels: Base of tongue, Epiglottis, Vestibular fold, Vocal cord, Glottis

Vocal cords in the closed position

Vocal cords in the open position

FIGURE 29.2 Larynx.

muscles. Impulses travel along the phrenic nerves and cause the dome-shaped diaphragm to contract and flatten inferiorly. Intercostal nerves cause the external intercostal muscles to expand the thoracic cavity in the anteroposterior dimension. These movements then expand the pleural membranes and, therefore, the lungs as a result of adhesion from serous fluid. As the lungs expand, alveolar pressure falls below atmospheric pressure and air enters the nose and respiratory passages. A deeper inhalation requires a more forceful contraction of the respiratory muscles (including accessory inspiratory muscles) to expand the thoracic cavity and lungs even further. Ease of thoracic and lung expansion is called *compliance*.

Exhalation
Normal exhalation is a passive process. The lungs are compressed as the thoracic cavity reduces volume and the recoil of the elastic lung tissue compresses the alveoli. Alveolar pressure rises above atmospheric pressure and air is forced out of the lungs. At rest, energy is not used in exhalation because no muscle contraction is required. Forced exhalation is an active process, requiring contraction of the internal

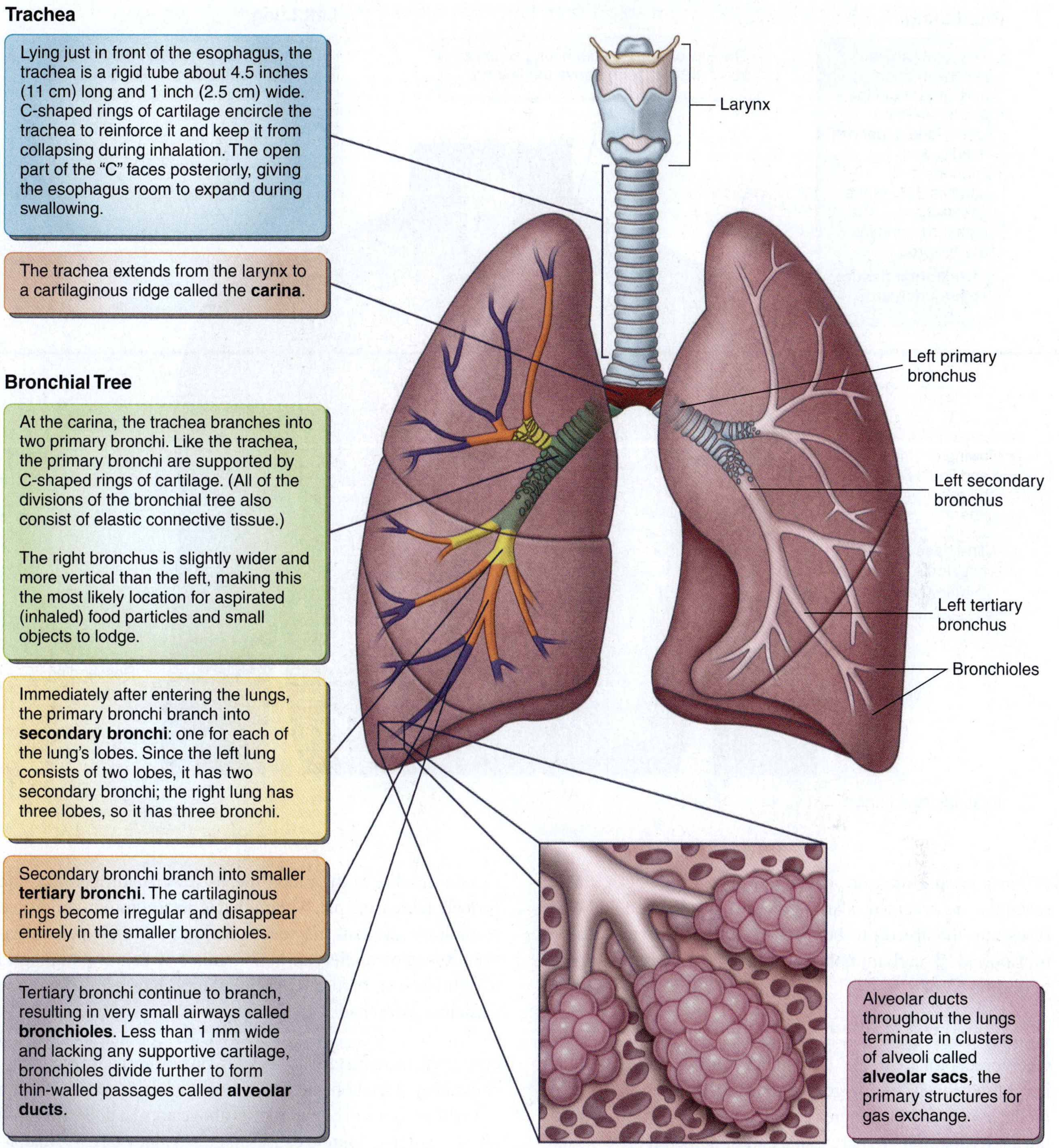

Chapter 29   Respiratory System Function, Data Collection, and Therapeutic Measures   489

Trachea

Lying just in front of the esophagus, the trachea is a rigid tube about 4.5 inches (11 cm) long and 1 inch (2.5 cm) wide. C-shaped rings of cartilage encircle the trachea to reinforce it and keep it from collapsing during inhalation. The open part of the "C" faces posteriorly, giving the esophagus room to expand during swallowing.

The trachea extends from the larynx to a cartilaginous ridge called the **carina**.

Bronchial Tree

At the carina, the trachea branches into two primary bronchi. Like the trachea, the primary bronchi are supported by C-shaped rings of cartilage. (All of the divisions of the bronchial tree also consist of elastic connective tissue.)

The right bronchus is slightly wider and more vertical than the left, making this the most likely location for aspirated (inhaled) food particles and small objects to lodge.

Immediately after entering the lungs, the primary bronchi branch into **secondary bronchi**: one for each of the lung's lobes. Since the left lung consists of two lobes, it has two secondary bronchi; the right lung has three lobes, so it has three bronchi.

Secondary bronchi branch into smaller **tertiary bronchi**. The cartilaginous rings become irregular and disappear entirely in the smaller bronchioles.

Tertiary bronchi continue to branch, resulting in very small airways called **bronchioles**. Less than 1 mm wide and lacking any supportive cartilage, bronchioles divide further to form thin-walled passages called **alveolar ducts**.

- Larynx
- Left primary bronchus
- Left secondary bronchus
- Left tertiary bronchus
- Bronchioles

Alveolar ducts throughout the lungs terminate in clusters of alveoli called **alveolar sacs**, the primary structures for gas exchange.

FIGURE 29.3 Trachea and bronchial tree.

intercostal muscles compressing the thorax and abdominal muscles that force the diaphragm superiorly, increasing compression of the lungs.

Transport of Gases in the Blood

A total of 98.5% of oxygen is carried in the blood, bound to iron of hemoglobin (Hgb) in red blood cells (RBCs). Oxyhemoglobin is formed in the lungs, where the partial pressure of oxygen (PaO_2) is high. In tissues where the PaO_2 is low, Hgb releases much of its oxygen. The remaining oxygen is dissolved in the plasma.

Most carbon dioxide (70%) is carried as bicarbonate ion in the blood plasma. These ions form when carbon dioxide enters RBCs and is converted to carbonic acid (H_2CO_3). H_2CO_3 ionizes into bicarbonate ions (HCO_3^-) and hydrogen ions (H^+). The bicarbonate ions leave the RBCs for the plasma. The remaining hydrogen ions are buffered by the Hgb in the RBCs. When the blood reaches the lungs, an area

Right Lung

The right lung is shorter, broader, and larger than the left. It has three lobes—the superior, middle, and inferior—and handles 55% of the gas exchange. The right lung contains two fissures:
- **Horizontal fissure**
- **Oblique fissure**

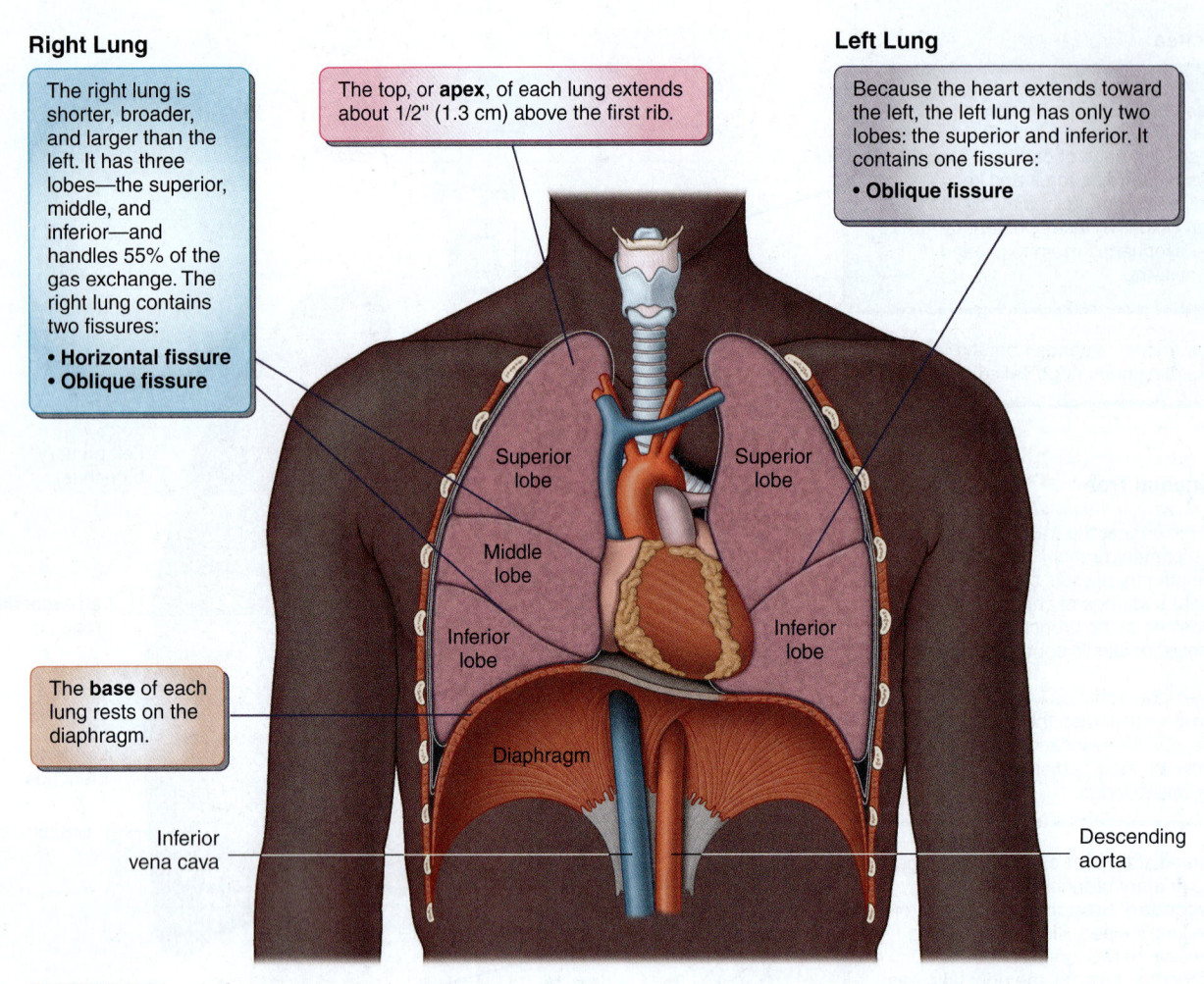

The top, or **apex**, of each lung extends about 1/2" (1.3 cm) above the first rib.

Left Lung

Because the heart extends toward the left, the left lung has only two lobes: the superior and inferior. It contains one fissure:
- **Oblique fissure**

The **base** of each lung rests on the diaphragm.

FIGURE 29.4 Lungs.

of lower partial pressure of carbon dioxide ($PaCO_2$), these reactions are reversed: Carbon dioxide is reformed and diffuses into the alveoli to be exhaled. Carbon dioxide is also transported as carbaminohemoglobin (23%) and dissolved in plasma (7%).

Chemical Regulation and Respiration
Chemoreceptors (in the carotid and aortic bodies) monitor blood levels of oxygen, carbon dioxide, and pH. The medulla responds by increasing heart and respiratory rates during hypoxemia, hypercapnia, and/or acidemia.

Respiration and Acid–Base Balance
Because of its role in regulating the amount of carbon dioxide in body fluids, the respiratory system is important in the maintenance of acid–base balance, measured by blood pH. Any decrease in the rate or efficiency of respiration permits excess carbon dioxide to accumulate in the blood. The resulting accumulation of excess hydrogen ions lowers pH. This condition is called *respiratory acidosis*. It can occur from pulmonary disease or any impairment of gas exchange in the lungs.

Respiratory alkalosis occurs when the rate of respiration increases, eliminating exhaled carbon dioxide rapidly. Less carbon dioxide in the blood means fewer hydrogen ions are formed, increasing pH. Although it is not a common condition, respiratory alkalosis may occur during states of hyperventilation caused by anxiety or hypoxemia or when acclimating to a high altitude, before RBC production increases to provide sufficient oxygenation of tissues.

The respiratory system also helps compensate for pH changes that are metabolic—that is, due to any cause other than respiratory. Metabolic acidosis occurs when the concentration of hydrogen ions in body fluids is above normal due to lowered HCO_3^- buffer. Common causes include kidney disease, uncontrolled diabetes mellitus, and severe diarrhea. Respiratory compensation involves an increase in the rate and depth of respiration to exhale more carbon dioxide. This decreases hydrogen ion formation and raises the pH toward normal. Metabolic alkalosis can be caused by overingestion of antacid medications or vomiting acidic gastric contents. Respiratory compensation involves a decrease in the breathing rate to retain carbon dioxide in the body, increasing the formation of hydrogen ions. This lowers the pH toward normal. Respiratory compensation occurs very quickly, within moments.

Respiratory compensation for an ongoing metabolic pH imbalance (such as kidney failure) cannot be complete

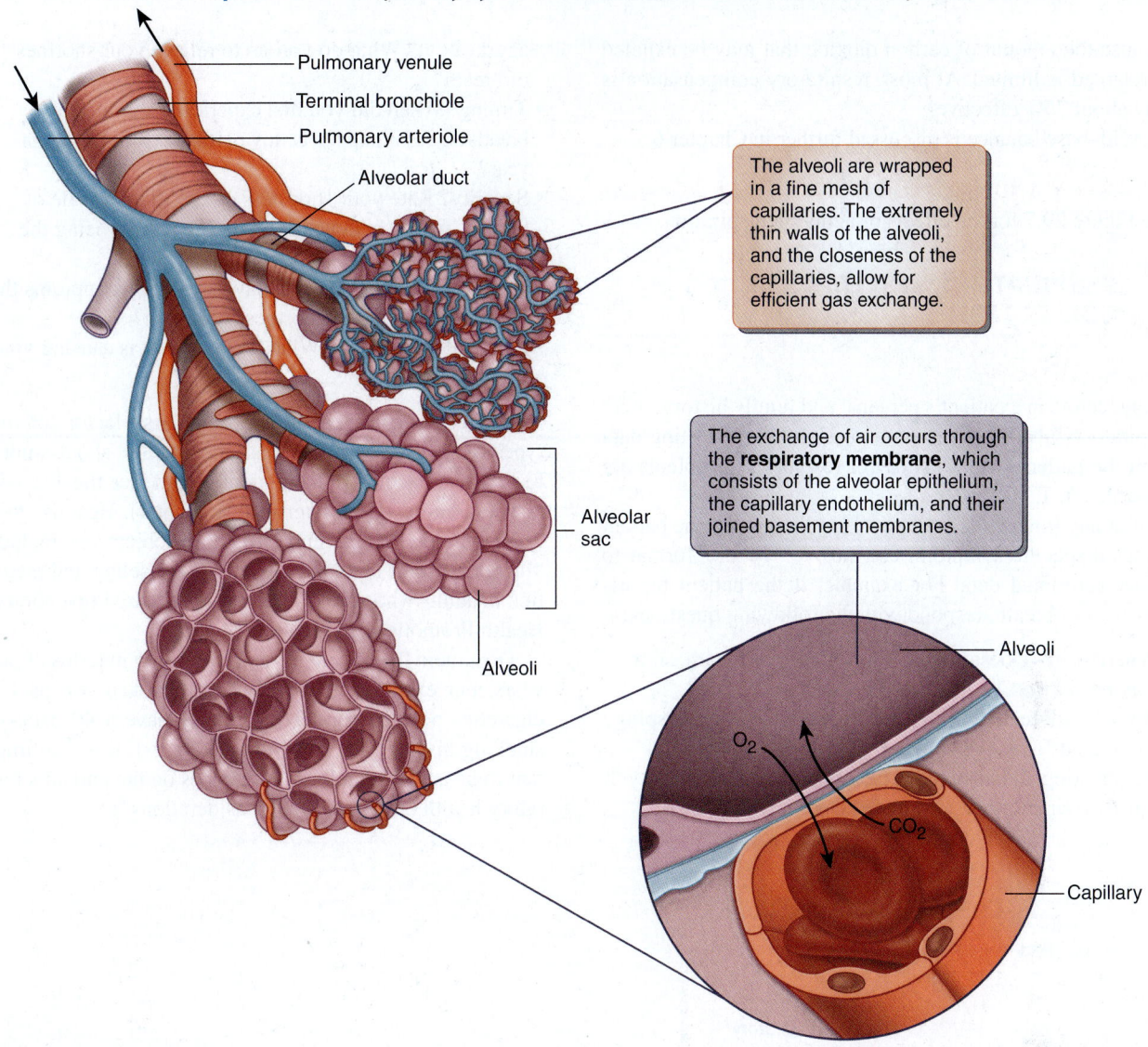

Chapter 29   Respiratory System Function, Data Collection, and Therapeutic Measures   491

- Pulmonary venule
- Terminal bronchiole
- Pulmonary arteriole
- Alveolar duct

The alveoli are wrapped in a fine mesh of capillaries. The extremely thin walls of the alveoli, and the closeness of the capillaries, allow for efficient gas exchange.

The exchange of air occurs through the **respiratory membrane**, which consists of the alveolar epithelium, the capillary endothelium, and their joined basement membranes.

- Alveolar sac
- Alveoli
- Alveoli
- O_2
- CO_2
- Capillary

FIGURE 29.5 Alveoli.

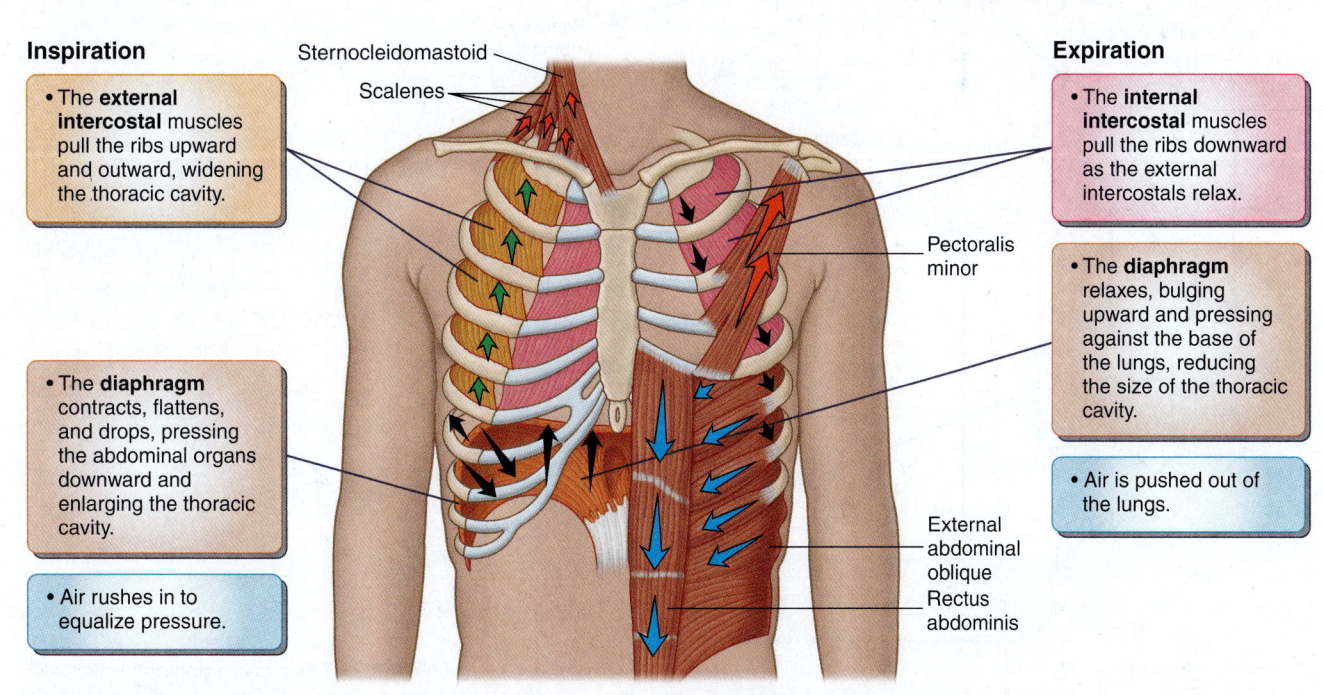

Inspiration

- The **external intercostal** muscles pull the ribs upward and outward, widening the thoracic cavity.
- The **diaphragm** contracts, flattens, and drops, pressing the abdominal organs downward and enlarging the thoracic cavity.
- Air rushes in to equalize pressure.

Sternocleidomastoid
Scalenes
Pectoralis minor
External abdominal oblique
Rectus abdominis

Expiration

- The **internal intercostal** muscles pull the ribs downward as the external intercostals relax.
- The **diaphragm** relaxes, bulging upward and pressing against the base of the lungs, reducing the size of the thoracic cavity.
- Air is pushed out of the lungs.

FIGURE 29.6 Respiratory muscles.

because the amount of carbon dioxide that may be exhaled or retained is limited. At most, respiratory compensation is only about 75% effective.

Acid–base balance is discussed further in Chapter 6.

Effects of Aging on the Respiratory System
See Figure 29.7 for the effects of aging on respiration.

RESPIRATORY SYSTEM DATA COLLECTION

Health History
Many factors in a patient's personal and family history affect respiratory function. Questions to ask while collecting data from the patient with a history of respiratory problems are presented in Table 29.2.

If at any time while you are taking the history the patient relates a specific symptom, use the **WHAT'S UP?** format to gather additional data. For example, if the patient reports shortness of breath, respond with the following questions:

- **W**here is it? (Doesn't apply to shortness of breath, so it may be skipped.)
- **H**ow does it feel? Does your breathing feel tight, gasping, painful, suffocating?
- **A**ggravating and alleviating factors? How much activity causes your shortness of breath? Does anything else aggravate it? What do you do to relieve your shortness of breath?
- **T**iming? When did you first experience shortness of breath? Does it happen at any particular time of day or year?
- **S**everity? Rate your shortness of breath on a scale of 0 to 10, with 0 being easy breathing and 10 being the worst shortness of breath you can imagine.
- **U**seful other data? Do you have any other symptoms that occur along with the shortness of breath?
- **P**atient's perception? What do you think is causing your shortness of breath?

Because smoking is such a major risk factor for many types of lung disease, it is essential to ask about smoking history and encourage the patient to quit (see the discussion of smoking cessation later in this chapter). Healthy People 2030 includes several smoking-related objectives, including "Increase use of smoking cessation counseling and medication in adults who smoke" (Office of Disease Prevention and Health Promotion, 2021).

Document the patient's smoking history in terms of pack-years. For example, if a patient has smoked two packs of cigarettes per day for 20 years, they have a 40 pack-year smoking history (2 × 20 = 40 pack-years). It is also important to be aware of cultural influences on the patient's respiratory health (see "Cultural Considerations").

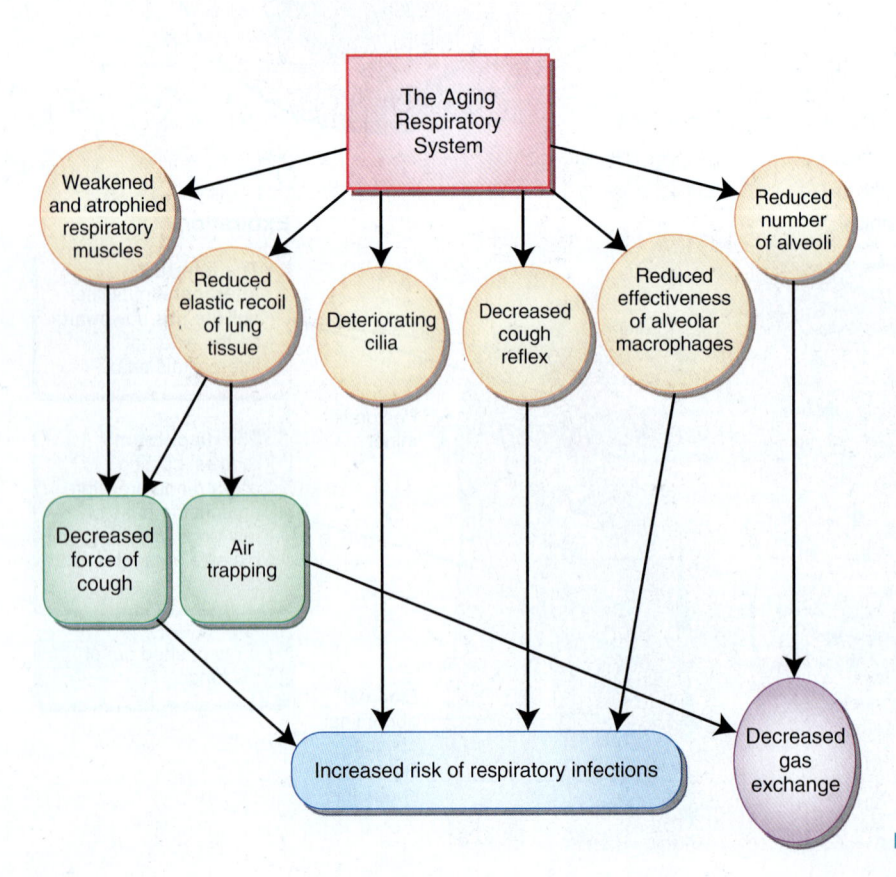

FIGURE 29.7 Effects of aging on respiration.

Table 29.2
Subjective Data Collection for the Respiratory System

Questions to Ask During the Health History	Rationale/Significance
Upper Respiratory Tract	
Do you often have headaches or sinus tenderness?	These may indicate sinusitis.
Do you often experience nosebleeds?	A history of nosebleeds may indicate an abnormality that can predispose to future nosebleeds.
Do you snore? Are you sleepy during the day?	These may be symptoms of sleep apnea.
Has your voice changed?	A voice change may indicate a variety of disorders of the nose or throat, including cancer.
Lower Respiratory Tract	
Do you have chest pain?	Chest pain can indicate a variety of respiratory or cardiac problems.
Do you ever feel short of breath, as though you can't get enough air?	Many respiratory and cardiac problems result in shortness of breath.
Do you have a cough? Is it productive?	A cough indicates respiratory irritation or excessive secretions.
What does the sputum look like?	Yellow, tan, or green sputum may accompany an infection. Blood in the sputum is usually serious; it can occur with pneumonia, tuberculosis, pulmonary embolism, or cancer.
Have you recently experienced night sweats, chills, or fever?	These are symptoms of tuberculosis.
Do you ever feel confused, light-headed, or restless?	These symptoms might indicate a low partial pressure of oxygen (PaO_2), reducing oxygen to the brain.
Have you had any chest surgeries?	This may reveal problem areas the patient has not yet mentioned.
Exposures	
Do you have any allergies that cause respiratory symptoms? How do you treat them?	The patient may take over-the-counter medications for allergies that affect respiratory function or interact with prescribed medications.
Do you smoke? How many packs per day? For how many years?	Many respiratory disorders are caused or aggravated by exposure to tobacco smoke.
Are you exposed to environmental smoke? Have you been exposed to airborne pollutants at home or work?	Pollutants such as asbestos, radon, coal dust, or chemicals can cause lung disease.
Treatments	
Do you take any medications or use inhalers (prescribed or over-the-counter) for your respiratory problems?	Information about medications gives further information about disorders, severity, and treatment. Also consider drug interactions and side effects.
Do you use home oxygen or other home respiratory treatments?	This helps determine the severity of disease and the treatment.
Family History	
Do any of your blood relatives have respiratory problems such as emphysema, asthma, or tuberculosis?	Some respiratory disorders have a hereditary tendency. Tuberculosis is contagious.

Cultural Considerations

Social determinants of health can influence the outcomes of asthma and other respiratory conditions. For example, the effects of these chronic illnesses are often worse for individuals in low-income communities. Residents may spend more time using public transportation, suffer exposures to pollutants at work, and have limited access to standard treatments and medications. Health-care providers should also be aware of variations when collecting data for cyanosis in people with darker skin pigmentation. Cyanosis and decreased blood hemoglobin levels may give the skin an ashen color instead of the bluish color seen in people with lighter skin pigmentation who have cyanosis. For a person who has darker skin pigmentation, the nurse must examine the sclerae, conjunctivae, buccal mucosa, tongue, lips, nailbeds, and palms and soles of the feet to determine if cyanosis is present.

In addition, pulse oximeters may not be accurate in darker-skinned individuals. Additional signs of respiratory status, such as difficulty breathing, increased respiratory rate, pursed-lip breathing, and cyanosis should be evaluated, documented, and treated accordingly.

Physical Examination
Inspection

Inspection begins during the nursing history and continues throughout the data collection process. Start with the nose, observing for symmetry, swelling, or other abnormalities. Note whether the patient is short of breath while speaking or moving. If the patient feels very breathless, they may speak in short sentences.

Observe the patient for use of accessory muscles of breathing (Fig. 29.8). Use of the sternocleidomastoid muscles causes shoulders to rise during labored inspiration. During forced expiration, the abdominal and intercostal muscles contract. Use of accessory muscles for breathing indicates respiratory distress. **Retraction** of the chest wall between the ribs occurs when airways are obstructed. It can indicate serious distress. When the patient inhales and air cannot easily flow into the lungs, negative pressure in the chest pulls the soft tissue between the ribs inward.

Note the color of the skin, lips, mucous membranes, and nailbeds. In light-skinned individuals, **cyanosis**, a late sign of oxygen deprivation, presents as a bluish color. In dark-skinned individuals, cyanosis may be noted as gray or whitish skin around the mouth and/or gray or bluish conjunctivae (see "Cultural Considerations"). Observe the trachea and chest for symmetry. Count the number of respirations per minute, noting depth and rhythm. Irregular respirations, or periods of **apnea** (absence of respirations), can indicate a pathological condition (Fig. 29.9). Observe the shape of the chest. Normally, the chest is about twice as wide (side to side) as it is deep (front to back). If it is more rounded, it is called a *barrel chest*, which is associated with chronic trapping of air in the lungs. See Table 29.3 for a summary of objective data.

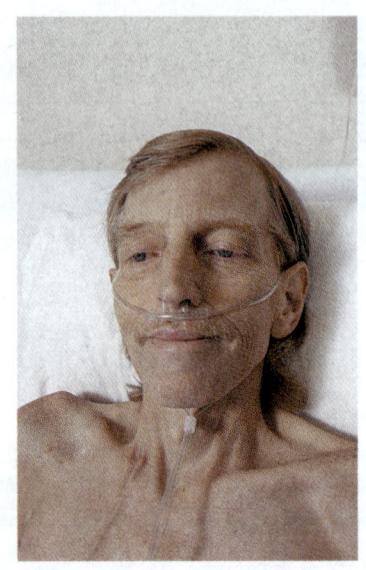

FIGURE 29.8 Accessory muscles of breathing. See the prominent sternocleidomastoid muscles. Note patient is using a nasal cannula

CUE RECOGNITION 29.1

A dark-skinned patient is reporting shortness of breath. Their pulse oximeter reading is 94%. What do you do?

Suggested answers are at the end of the chapter.

Palpation

Palpate the frontal and maxillary sinuses if sinus inflammation is suspected (Fig. 29.10). Use your thumbs to palpate gently below the eyebrows and below each cheekbone. Tenderness may indicate sinus inflammation or infection.

Respiratory excursion can also be palpated. This is a rough measurement of chest expansion on inspiration. Fig. 29.11 illustrates how to palpate for respiratory excursion. You can palpate for **crepitus** (also called *subcutaneous emphysema*) if indicated. Crepitus feels like Rice Krispies under the skin when felt with the fingers. It occurs when air leaks into subcutaneous tissues because of pneumothorax or a leaking chest tube site. Palpation is not done routinely but only when indicated by other findings.

Percussion

Percussion is typically done by the experienced nurse. It involves tapping on the anterior and posterior chest and in each intercostal space, then comparing sounds from side to side. A normal chest sounds resonant and is the same bilaterally, except over the heart. If other percussion notes are heard, they can indicate a pathological condition and should be reported.

• WORD • BUILDING •

cyanosis: cyan—dark blue + osis—condition
apnea: a—not + pnea—breath

Chapter 29 Respiratory System Function, Data Collection, and Therapeutic Measures 495

Respiratory patterns

When observing a patient's respirations, the nurse should determine their rate, rhythm, and depth. These schematic diagrams show different respiratory patterns.

Eupnea: Normal respiratory rate and rhythm

Hyperventilation: Deeper respirations; normal rate

Tachypnea: Increased respiratory rate

Bradypnea: Slow but regular respirations

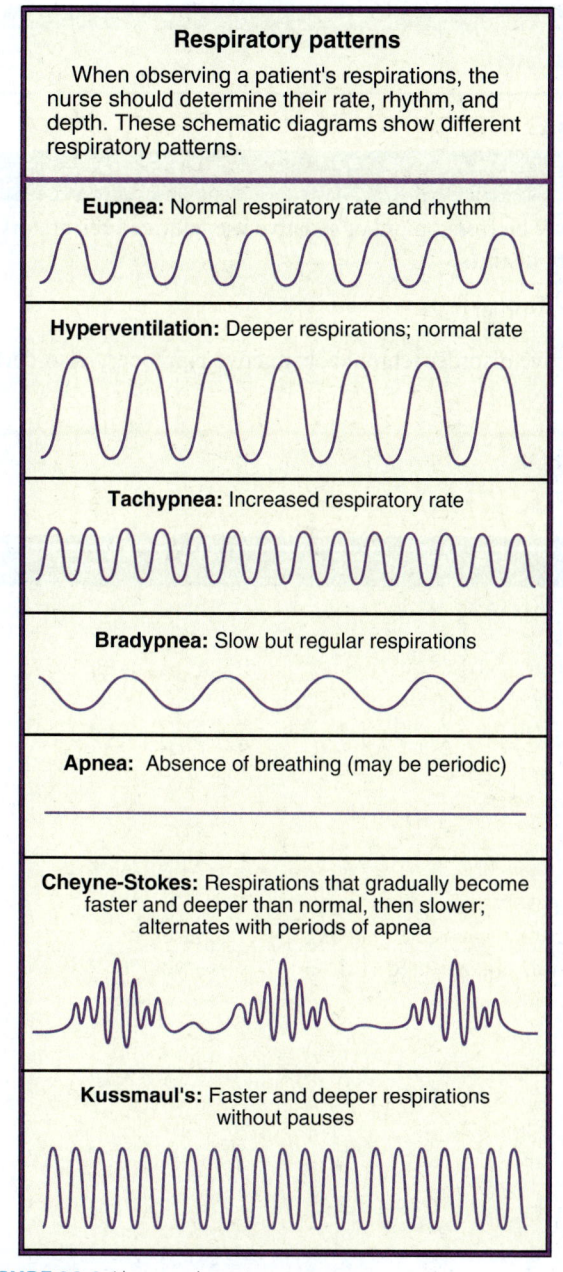

Apnea: Absence of breathing (may be periodic)

Cheyne-Stokes: Respirations that gradually become faster and deeper than normal, then slower; alternates with periods of apnea

Kussmaul's: Faster and deeper respirations without pauses

FIGURE 29.9 Abnormal respiratory patterns.

Auscultation

Auscultation provides valuable information about respiratory status. Use the diaphragm of your stethoscope to listen to the anterior, lateral, and posterior chest during an entire inspiration and expiration at each interspace (Fig. 29.12). Auscultation of the posterior chest is easiest if the patient is sitting. However, if necessary, it may be done with the patient in a side-lying position. Ask the patient to breathe deeply through the mouth to help enhance the sounds. Allow the patient to rest at intervals to prevent hyperventilation. Regular and frequent practice helps you learn to distinguish normal from abnormal breath sounds. Abnormal extra sounds (another term is **adventitious**) indicate a pathological condition. These are described in Table 29.4.

> **LEARNING TIP**
> Listen to breath sounds on all your friends and family members. Assuming they are normal, this will give you a good baseline so that when you hear an abnormal or adventitious sound on a patient, you will recognize it as "not normal."

DIAGNOSTIC TESTS FOR THE RESPIRATORY SYSTEM

Laboratory Tests
For normal values for the following laboratory tests, see Appendix B.

Blood Tests
Complete Blood Count (CBC)
Measurement of RBCs and Hgb can give information about the oxygen-carrying capacity of the blood. **Dyspnea** (shortness of breath) can be caused by a reduction in RBCs or Hgb. Elevated white blood cells (WBCs) indicate infection.

Arterial Blood Gas Analysis
Arterial blood gases (ABGs) are measured to determine the effectiveness of gas exchange. See Table 29.5 for a basic interpretation of ABGs. The blood sample is usually taken from the radial artery in the wrist by a specially trained respiratory therapist (RT) or laboratory technician. This can be painful for the patient. Place pressure on the site after the test until bleeding stops; this may take 5 minutes or more.

> **LEARNING TIP**
> If you remember that a normal blood pH is 7.35 to 7.45, then it is easy to remember that a normal partial pressure of carbon dioxide ($PaCO_2$) is 35 to 45 mm Hg.

> **LEARNING TIP**
> Remember 50! If the partial pressure of oxygen (PaO_2) falls below 50 and the partial pressure of carbon dioxide ($PaCO_2$) is above 50, the patient is in trouble, and the registered nurse or respiratory nurse should be notified. This rough analysis is helpful when a quick determination is needed.

D-Dimer
This blood test measures fibrin degradation products, present if there is a blood clot in the body. It helps diagnose the presence of a blood clot in a pulmonary artery.

• WORD • BUILDING •
dyspnea: dys—bad + pnea—breathing

Table 29.3
Objective Data Collection for the Respiratory System

Abnormal Findings	Possible Respiratory Causes
Respiratory	
Respiratory rate less than 12 or greater than 20 per minute	Respiratory depression may be from opioid or sedative use; elevated respiratory rate indicates respiratory distress
Use of accessory muscles	Restrictive or obstructive disorders
Barrel chest	Air trapping from obstructive disorder (chronic obstructive pulmonary disorder)
Adventitious sounds	See Table 29.4.
Cough	Airway irritation or secretions
Sputum	See Table 29.2.
Integumentary	
Cyanosis	Tissue hypoxia
Nail clubbing 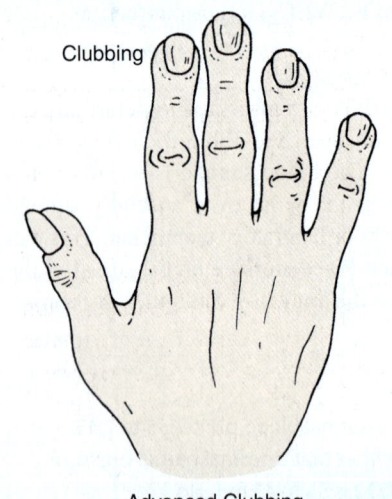	Chronic tissue hypoxia
Neurologic	
Confusion	Lack of oxygen to the brain
Gastrointestinal	
Weight loss	Dyspnea interfering with eating; use of excessive calories for breathing

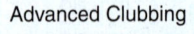

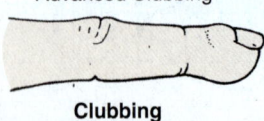

Sputum Culture and Sensitivity

A sputum culture identifies pathogens present in the sputum. The sensitivity test determines which antibiotics will be effective against those pathogens. To obtain a sputum specimen, first check the order and obtain a sterile container. Some institutions have special containers for sputum that help prevent transmission of infection to the health-care provider (HCP; Fig. 29.13). Instruct the patient to take several deep breaths and then cough sputum into the container. It is important that the patient not simply spit saliva or sinus drainage into the cup. The specimen must come from the lungs. It may be easiest to obtain a specimen first thing in

Chapter 29 Respiratory System Function, Data Collection, and Therapeutic Measures 497

the morning (after mouth care) because secretions build up during the night. Send the specimen to the laboratory immediately. If the patient is unable to cough up sputum, extra fluids or a bedside humidifier may help. An RT may be able to help obtain a specimen with a nebulized mist treatment or with a special suction catheter with a sputum trap. The HCP's order may be needed for these procedures.

> **BE SAFE!**
> **AVOID FAILURE TO RECOGNIZE!** If the HCP orders a "sputum for AFB," tuberculosis is suspected, which is caused by an acid-fast bacillus (AFB). Ask whether the patient should be placed in isolation while waiting for test results. *Always* practice standard precautions when handling laboratory specimens.

Throat Culture

A throat culture is done to determine the presence of viral or bacterial pathogens in the pharynx. Use a swab to reach into the posterior pharynx behind the uvula (without touching the patient's mouth) and swab the red area or lesions. Use a tongue blade to help hold the tongue down while obtaining the culture. Warn the patient that a gag reflex may be triggered. Once the culture has been obtained, place it in a sterile tube with culture medium, according to package instructions. Send it to the laboratory immediately for analysis.

Nasal Samples

A nasopharyngeal swab or a nasal wash can be used to identify flu or other respiratory viruses. To be accurate, it must be done in the first few days a person has symptoms. The sample may be obtained by swabbing the nasal passages or pharynx or by using a small amount of saline to wash out the nose, depending on the type of test ordered.

Oxygen Saturation

The oxygen saturation test (also called pulse oximetry, O_2 sat, or SpO_2) is a simple and noninvasive way to measure arterial

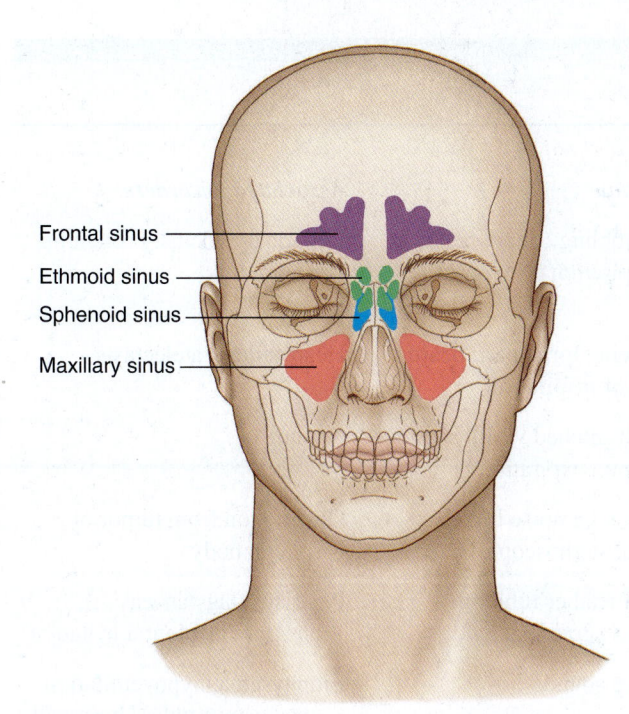

FIGURE 29.10 Paranasal sinuses.
(Labels: Frontal sinus, Ethmoid sinus, Sphenoid sinus, Maxillary sinus)

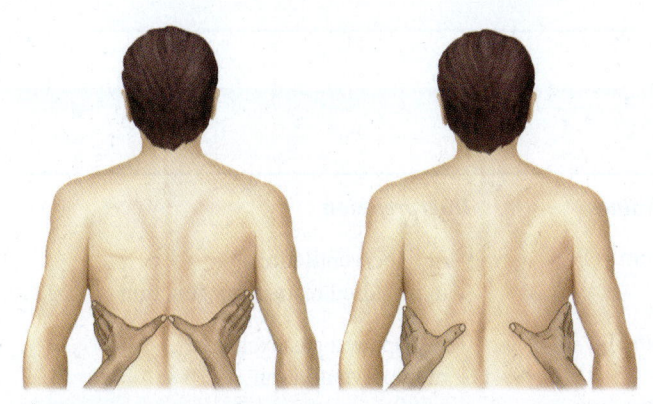

FIGURE 29.11 Palpation of respiratory excursion. Left: during exhalation. Right: after inhalation.

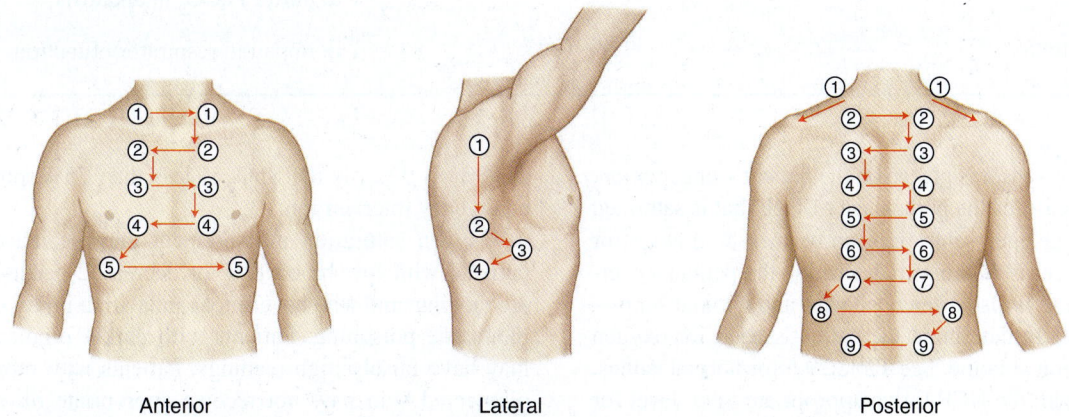

FIGURE 29.12 Auscultation of the chest. Use a systematic approach to auscultate the chest, comparing sounds from side to side.
(Anterior, Lateral, Posterior)

Table 29.4
Abnormal Lung Sounds

Abnormal (Adventitious) Sound	Cause of Sound	Description	Associated Disorders
Coarse crackles (sometimes called rales)	Fluid or secretions in airways	Moist bubbling sound, heard on inspiration or expiration	Pulmonary edema, bronchitis, pneumonia
Fine crackles (rales)	Alveoli popping open on inspiration	Velcro being torn apart, heard at end of inspiration	Heart failure, atelectasis
Wheezes	Narrowed airways	Fine high-pitched violin sound, mostly on expiration	Asthma
Stridor	Airway obstruction	Loud crowing noise heard without stethoscope	Obstruction from tumor or foreign body
Pleural friction rub	Inflamed pleura rubbing together	Sound of leather rubbing together; grating sound	Pleurisy, lung cancer, pneumonia, pleural irritation
Diminished	Decreased air movement	Faint lung sounds	Emphysema, hypoventilation, obesity, muscular chest wall
Absent	No air movement	No sounds heard	Pneumothorax, pneumonectomy, pleural effusion

Table 29.5
Arterial Blood Gas Analysis

	Normal Values	Interpretation
PaO_2 (partial pressure of oxygen)	75–100 mm Hg	↑ in hyperventilation ↓ in impaired respiratory function
$PaCO_2$ (partial pressure of carbon dioxide)	35–45 mm Hg	↑ in impaired gas exchange ↓ in hyperventilation
pH	7.35–7.45	↑ in respiratory alkalosis with low $PaCO_2$ ↓ in respiratory acidosis with high $PaCO_2$
HCO_3^- (bicarbonate ions)	22–26 mEq/L	↑ to buffer $PaCO_2$ in acidosis ↓ to buffer $PaCO_2$ in alkalosis
Oxygen saturation	95%–100%	↓ in impaired respiratory function

oxygenation. A sensor is placed on the patient's finger or ear. The sensor measures the percentage of Hgb that is saturated with oxygen. Oxygen saturation can be measured at rest or while the patient is walking to determine the patient's exercise tolerance. It is also often done with and without supplemental oxygen to determine the patient's need for oxygen supplementation at home. See Table 29.5 for normal values. Collaborate with the HCP for an appropriate SpO_2 level for your patient. Although 95% or greater is considered normal, some patients with chronic lung disease may be maintained at 90% to 92%. If the SpO_2 is less than 75%, prepare for emergency intervention.

Oxygen saturation measurement may be inaccurate in patients with low blood flow or decreased perfusion, who are moving, and who have smoke inhalation injury or carbon monoxide poisoning. Patients with darkly pigmented skin may have falsely high readings. Patients with more darkly pigmented skin may not receive appropriate oxygen therapy or medical care due to this discrepancy. These inaccuracies in oxygen saturation readings became more evident

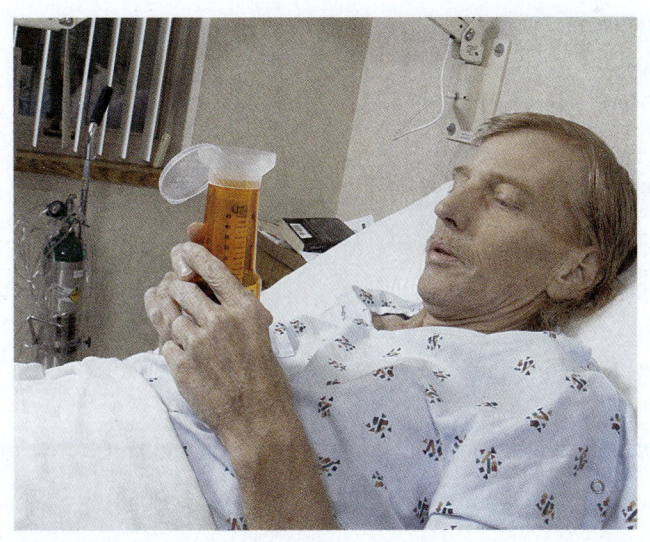

FIGURE 29.13 A special container that helps prevent transmission of infection is often used to collect sputum for culture.

during the Covid 19 epidemic. Acrylic nails may need to be removed for accurate readings. Always correlate SpO_2 results with other findings.

Capnography

The process of measuring a person's exhaled carbon dioxide level is called capnography. It provides a continuous measurement of the patient's ventilation status. It is most often used when patients are intubated. A special sensor is placed between the endotracheal (ET) tube and the ventilator to measure the exhaled carbon dioxide. Special nasal cannulas with sensors are also available. Results are displayed on a special monitor.

Other Tests

For explanations of the following diagnostic tests, see Appendix A.

Chest X-Ray Examination

A chest x-ray examination may be ordered to help diagnose a variety of pulmonary disorders. Usually, posterior-anterior (PA) and side views (lateral) are taken. If a hospitalized patient is too ill to go to the radiology department, a portable chest x-ray machine can be used at the bedside to obtain a PA view.

Computed Tomography

A computed tomography (CT) scan can show cancers, pneumonia, emphysema, and more. It may be used to obtain additional information after an abnormal chest x-ray. A spiral CT scan can be useful for evaluating trauma or blood vessel abnormalities in the chest.

Ventilation-Perfusion Scan

During a ventilation-perfusion scan (also called a lung scan or VQ scan), a radioactive substance is injected via IV route. A scan is then done to view blood flow to the lungs (perfusion). Another radioactive substance is inhaled. Scanning then shows how well gas is distributed in the lungs (ventilation). If an area of the lungs is well ventilated but has no blood supply, a pulmonary embolism is suspected. Chronic lung disease may cause poor ventilation and perfusion.

Pulmonary Function Studies

HCPs do this series of tests to determine lung volume, capacity, and flow rates. These are commonly used to help diagnose and monitor restrictive or obstructive lung disease. The patient is asked to use a special mouthpiece to blow into a cylinder that is connected to a computer. A computer printout is generated to show the results. Table 29.6 lists normal values. Some patients use handheld peak expiratory flow rate (PEFR) meters at home to monitor asthma symptoms. They might notice changes in PEFR before symptoms occur, allowing them to begin treatment before the problem becomes more serious.

Pulmonary Angiography

Pulmonary angiography involves an x-ray examination of the pulmonary vessels after IV administration of a radiopaque dye. Pulmonary angiography is used to help diagnose pulmonary embolism or other pulmonary vessel disorders. See Appendix A for pre- and postprocedure care.

Bronchoscopy

Bronchoscopy involves the use of a flexible endoscope to examine the larynx, trachea, and bronchial tree. Bronchoscopy can be used diagnostically for visualization or to obtain a biopsy specimen for examination. It can also be used therapeutically to remove an obstruction, foreign body, or thick secretions. See Appendix A for pre- and postprocedure care.

THERAPEUTIC MEASURES FOR THE RESPIRATORY SYSTEM

Smoking Cessation

Probably the *most* important intervention for preventing and treating respiratory disease is smoking cessation. Many respiratory disorders are caused or aggravated by smoking. Stopping can prevent disease from occurring or slow its progression significantly. Table 29.7 lists interventions to help patients stop smoking. Remind patients that if they have tried quitting before and failed, that does not mean that they will never be able to quit (see "Evidence-Based Practice"). Many patients try several times before quitting successfully.

Many Internet sites have information to help people stop smoking. Simply type "smoking cessation" into any search engine. Alternatively, individuals can call 800-QUIT NOW to speak with a representative who will assist with cessation strategies.

Deep Breathing and Coughing

Effective coughing can keep the airways clear of secretions. An ineffective cough is exhausting and fails to bring up secretions. Instruct the patient to take two or three deep breaths using the diaphragm. This helps get the air behind the secretions. After the third deep inhalation, have the patient hold

Table 29.6
Normal Values for Pulmonary Function Studies

Test	Definition	Normal Values*
Tidal volume (V_T)	Air inspired and expired in one breath	400–600 mL at rest
Residual volume (RV)	Air remaining in lungs after maximum exhalation	1,000–1,500 mL
Functional residual capacity (FRC)	Air remaining in lungs after normal expiration	1,800–2,300 mL
Inspiratory reserve	Amount of air beyond V_T that can be taken in with the deepest possible inhalation	2,000–3,000 mL
Expiratory reserve	Amount of air beyond V_T in the most forceful exhalation	1,000–1,500 mL
Forced vital capacity (FVC)	Maximum amount of air expired forcefully after maximum inspiration	3,000–5,000 mL
Forced expiratory volume (FEV) 1% (FEV_1/FVC)	Amount of air expired in first second of forced exhalation divided by FVC	65%–85% of the FVC
Peak expiratory flow rate (PEFR)	Maximum flow of air expired during FVC (this is a rate rather than a volume)	450 L/min

*Normal values are approximate. They are individualized based on patient's sex, height, and age.

Table 29.7
Interventions to Stop Smoking

Intervention	Rationale
Behavior modification	If the patient can identify situations associated with smoking, such as eating a meal or experiencing stress, then healthier behaviors can be substituted, such as going for a walk.
Counseling	Counseling by a health-care worker alone or in combination with other methods can greatly increase success.
Setting a quit date	The "cold turkey" (all-at-once) method is more effective than slow tapering, although the patient may choose to taper before the quit date.
Nicotine replacement therapy	Nicotine gum, patches, nasal sprays, lozenges, and inhalers can reduce withdrawal symptoms.
Drug therapy (bupropion [Zyban], varenicline [Chantix], nortriptyline [Pamelor])	Bupropion and nortriptyline interfere with smoking's effect on brain neurotransmitters. Varenicline attaches to nicotine receptors in the brain to block nicotine and reduce its pleasurable effects.
Hypnosis	Hypnosis is believed to help the person be open to the suggestion that smoking is undesirable.
Physical activity	Physical activity reduces cravings and post-cessation weight gain.
Electronic cigarettes (e-cigarettes)	Nicotine-containing e-cigarettes may help promote smoking cessation, although more research needs to be done, and e-cigarettes have not been approved by the Food and Drug Administration (FDA) for smoking cessation. Encourage patients to try the FDA-approved products first.

> **Evidence-Based Practice**
>
> **Clinical Question**
> Can nurses make a difference in helping patients stop smoking?
>
> **Evidence**
> Clinic nurses integrated the Ask, Advise, Refer strategy for smoking cessation into their routine at a Veterans Health Administration Clinic. Nurses determined the patient's smoking status, advised patients who smoked to quit, and then provided them with a list of resources. During follow-up phone calls, 19% of patients had already used at least one resource. The authors note that nurses should use every encounter as an opportunity to provide smoking cessation interventions.
>
> Reference: Boe, R., & Ridner, S. L. (2020). Connecting veterans with smoking cessation services in less than 3 minutes. *Journal of the American Association of Nurse Practitioners, 33*(8), 586–590. https://doi.org/10.1097/JXX.0000000000000433

the breath for a few seconds and then cough forcefully. This is repeated as necessary, usually every 1 to 2 hours. Good hydration can facilitate mucous removal.

Huff Coughing

Patients with chronic obstructive pulmonary disease (COPD) typically have a weak cough and airways that collapse easily. *Huff* coughing may work better for them. Instruct the patient to deep breath and cough, as just described. Instead of closing the glottis to generate a forceful cough, the patient should keep the glottis and mouth open, and use the abdominal muscles to create a series of forced expirations, moving air and mucus up the bronchial tree. This creates "huff" sounds. A short huff helps clear larger airways, and a longer huff held out for several seconds helps open and clear smaller airways. Finally, the patient should take one more controlled inhalation and produce a final huff cough to expel the mucus.

Autogenic Drainage

Autogenic drainage is a variation on deep breathing and coughing that may be more effective for patients with thick secretions that are difficult to raise, such as those with cystic fibrosis or severe COPD. It is also gentler and less likely to cause declines in oxygen saturation or uncontrolled coughing than other methods. The patient is taught to sit upright and breathe in more deeply than usual, slowly through the nose, and then hold the breath for 2 to 4 seconds. When holding the breath, the patient should keep the glottis open, to prevent airway collapse. Exhaling is done as a quiet sigh, as if trying to steam up a mirror.

Using these breathing techniques, the patient is taught three phases:

1. *Unstick*. The patient breathes out completely, then takes a slow breath, and exhales fully several times, suppressing the urge to cough. This loosens mucus in the lower airways.
2. *Collect*. The patient takes 10 to 20 slightly deeper breaths, exhaling normally, still suppressing the urge to cough. This helps move mucus up to the middle airways.
3. *Evacuate*. The patient takes 10 to 20 breaths and huff coughs to move the mucus up and out.

During the *unstick* and *collect* phases, airflow should be high enough to produce a rattle if secretions are present. This is a complex process that is typically taught by an RT.

Breathing Exercises

Breathing exercises are essential for patients with chronic lung disease. Diaphragmatic and pursed-lip breathing increase effectiveness of breathing and reduce panic when dyspnea occurs.

Diaphragmatic Breathing

The diaphragm is the major muscle of breathing. However, patients often use less-efficient accessory muscles when they are short of breath. Conscious use of the diaphragm during breathing can be relaxing and conserve energy. To reinforce diaphragmatic breathing, have the patient do the following:

1. Place one hand on the abdomen and the other on the chest.
2. Concentrate on pushing out the abdomen during inspiration and relaxing the abdomen on expiration. The chest should move very little.

Pursed-Lip Breathing

The pursed-lip breathing technique can be used any time the patient feels short of breath. It helps keep airways open during exhalation, which promotes carbon dioxide excretion. It should be done with diaphragmatic breathing. Counting during breathing also distracts the patient, reducing panic. To reinforce pursed-lip breathing have the patient do the following:

1. Inhale slowly through the nose to the count of two (using diaphragmatic breathing).
2. Exhale slowly through pursed lips to the count of four.

> **NURSING CARE TIP**
> When teaching patients to do pursed-lip breathing, try teaching them to "smell the roses" while inhaling slowly through the nose and "blow out the candle" while exhaling. If you remind them not to let the wax splatter, then they'll blow slowly and gently!

Positioning

The patient who is short of breath should be positioned to conserve energy while allowing for maximum lung expansion. Most respiratory patients do not tolerate lying flat. The patient in bed can use Fowler or semi-Fowler position to keep abdominal contents from crowding the lungs. Some patients prefer to sit in a chair while leaning forward and placing their elbows on their knees or an over-the-bed table (tripod position; Fig. 29.14).

Patients with unilateral (one-sided) lung disease can benefit from the "good lung down" lateral position. This is a side-lying position with the good lung in the dependent position. Gravity causes greater blood flow to the dependent, good lung, thereby increasing oxygen saturation. Some patients may also benefit from prone positioning.

Reducing Oxygen Consumption

Fever, anxiety, pain, and use of respiratory muscles can increase the body's demand for oxygen. Medications to treat fever, anxiety and pain should be used when appropriate along with nonpharmacological interventions such as relaxation techniques. Energy conservation techniques such as not planning activities right after a meal, doing grooming activities while sitting, and spacing out activities throughout the day can help to decrease the patient's oxygen demands.

> **NURSING CARE TIP**
> Patients at home may choose to sleep in a recliner or La-Z-Boy–type chair to keep their head elevated. Others may use a wedge under their mattress or a hospital bed.

Oxygen Therapy

Oxygen therapy is ordered by the HCP when the patient is unable to maintain oxygenation. Patients are typically placed on supplemental oxygen when their oxygen saturation is less than 90% on room air. The HCP's order should include the method of administration and the flow rate.

The role of the licensed practical nurse/licensed vocational nurse (LPN/LVN) in oxygen therapy includes monitoring the flow rate, ensuring that the cannula and tubing or other device remain properly placed, and monitoring the patient's response to treatment. If the patient becomes short of breath while on oxygen therapy, notify the RT, registered nurse (RN), or HCP. Instruct the patient to avoid smoking, using electrical equipment, and performing other activities that can cause fire in the presence of oxygen. If possible, collaborate with the RT. The RT is knowledgeable about oxygen therapy and is an excellent resource when questions arise.

> **CUE RECOGNITION 29.2**
> An older adult patient on oxygen per nasal cannula has suddenly become restless and confused. What do you do?
>
> *Suggested answers are at the end of the chapter.*

Low-Flow Devices

NASAL CANNULA. The nasal cannula is the most common method of oxygen administration. Oxygen is delivered through a flexible catheter that has two short nasal prongs (Fig. 29.15). For the nasal cannula to be most effective, the patient must

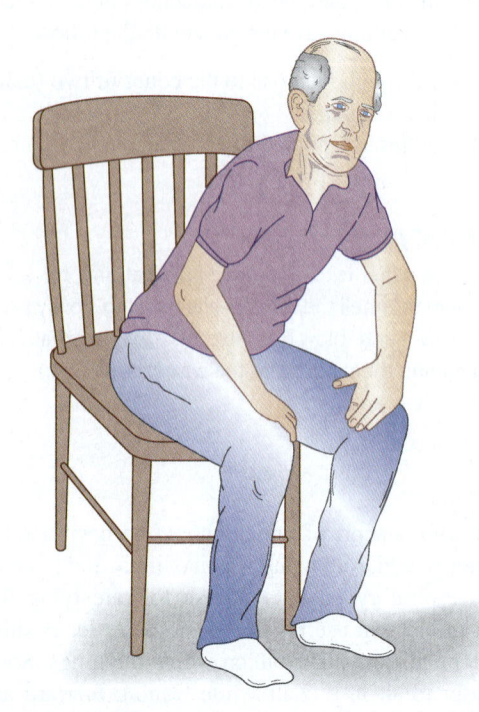

FIGURE 29.14 The tripod position may help reduce dyspnea.

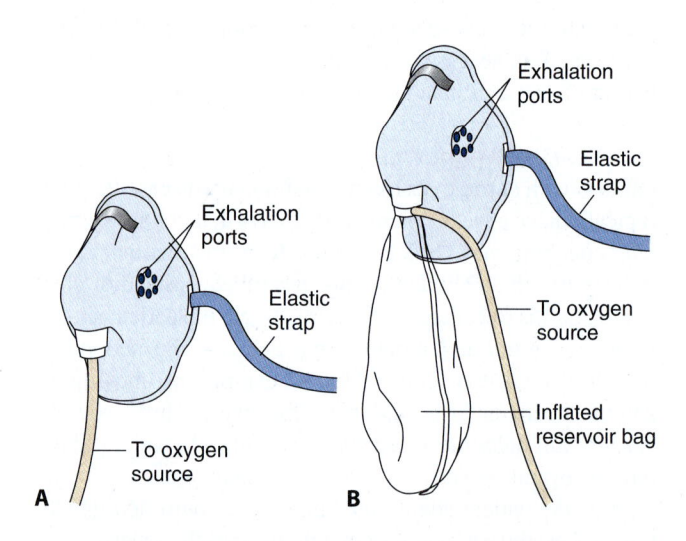

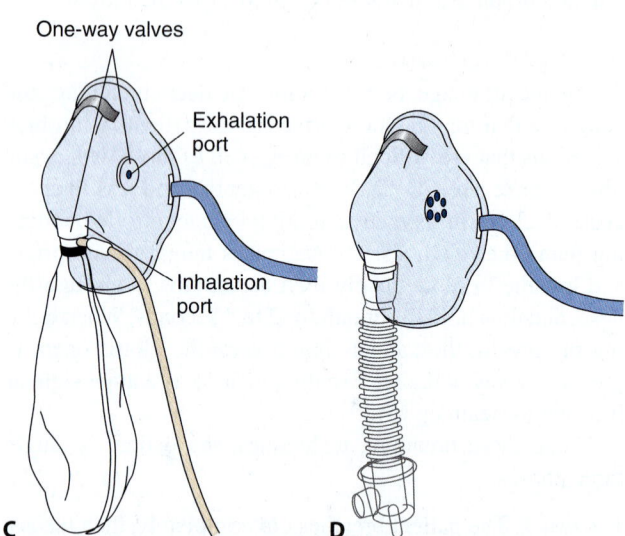

FIGURE 29.15 Oxygen masks. (A) Simple mask. (B) Partial rebreather mask. (C) Nonrebreather mask. (D) Venturi mask.

breathe through their nose. The cannula allows the patient to eat and talk. It is generally more comfortable than other methods of administration. If the nasal mucous membranes become dry, a water source can be placed on the system to humidify the oxygen. Oxygen can be delivered at 1 to 6 L per minute via a nasal cannula; special high-flow cannulas can deliver much higher rates. Patients with COPD may benefit from a special cannula with a reservoir. Oxygen is stored in the reservoir during exhalation and delivered during inhalation. Patients, therefore, receive a higher concentration of oxygen.

MASKS. Masks are used when a higher oxygen concentration is needed. However, they make some patients feel claustrophobic and must be replaced by a cannula while the patient eats.

- *Simple face mask.* A rate of 5 to 10 L/min can deliver oxygen concentrations from 40% to 60% with a simple face mask.
- *Partial rebreather mask.* A partial rebreather mask uses a reservoir bag to store oxygen. Vents on the sides of the mask allow room air to mix with oxygen. It can deliver oxygen concentrations of 50% or greater.
- *Nonrebreather mask.* A nonrebreather mask has one or both side vents closed to limit the mixing of room air with oxygen. The vents open to allow exhalation but remain closed on inhalation. The reservoir bag has a valve to store oxygen for inhalation but does not allow entry of exhaled air. It is used to deliver oxygen concentrations of 70% to 100%.

> **NURSING CARE TIP**
> When a patient is using a partial rebreather or nonrebreather mask, make sure that the reservoir bag is never allowed to collapse to less than two-thirds full.

High-Flow Devices

A Venturi mask is used for the patient who requires precise percentages of oxygen, such as the patient with chronic lung disease with CO_2 retention. A combination of entrainment ports and specified flow rates delivers exactly the right concentration of oxygen.

Transtracheal Catheter

A transtracheal catheter is a small tube surgically placed through the base of the neck directly into the trachea to deliver oxygen (Fig. 29.16). This is an attractive alternative for some patients who are on long-term oxygen therapy at home because it does not obstruct the nose or mouth. In addition, it can be easily covered with a loose scarf or collar. The patient is taught to remove and clean the catheter two or three times a day to prevent mucus obstruction. Check institution policy and procedure for specific care instructions.

Risks of Oxygen Therapy

In the past, HCPs believed that patients with COPD should never receive oxygen at rates greater than 2 L per minute because higher rates might depress breathing. With modern pulse oximetry technology, oxygen administration rates are adjusted based on the SpO_2 level. Oxygen is administered at the flow rate needed to achieve 88% to 89% saturation, depending on the HCP order.

In addition, any patient can suffer lung damage from high oxygen concentrations (greater than 50%) delivered for more than 24 hours. If a patient exhibits symptoms of dry cough, chest pain, numbness in the extremities, lethargy, or nausea, the HCP should be contacted. A PaO_2 greater than 100 mm Hg should also be reported.

Nebulized Mist Treatments

Nebulized mist treatments (NMTs) use a nebulizer to mist medication directly into the lungs (Fig. 29.17). Such topical use of medication reduces systemic side effects. Bronchodilators such as albuterol (Proventil, ProAir HFA), mixed with normal saline solution and sometimes with supplemental oxygen, are most commonly administered. Medications such as corticosteroids, mucolytics, and antibiotics may also be given. An RT or a specially trained nurse administers the NMT. The patient uses a handheld reservoir with tubing and

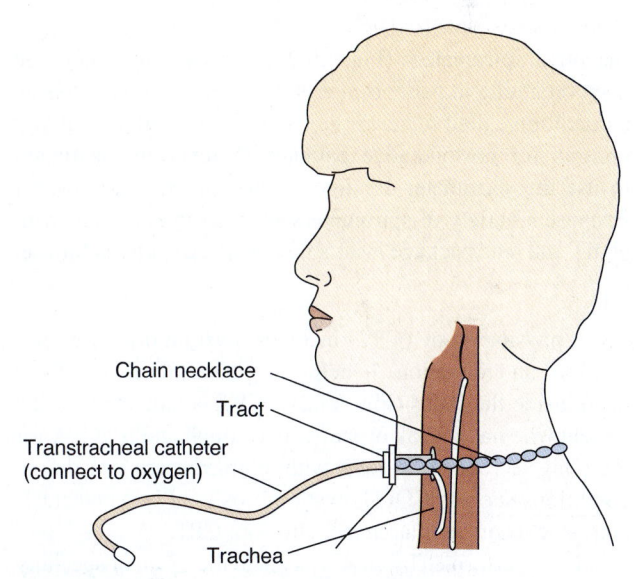

FIGURE 29.16 Transtracheal oxygen catheter.

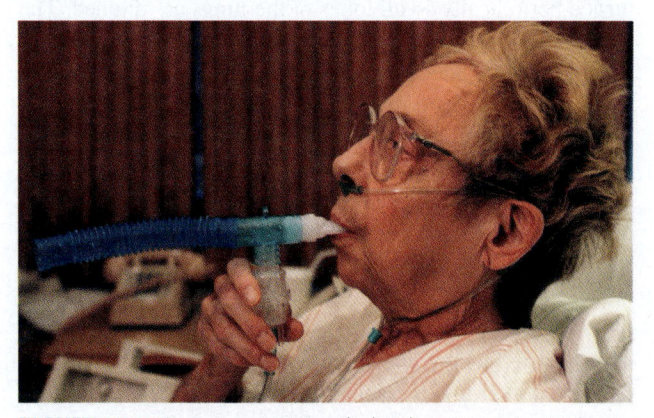

FIGURE 29.17 Patient receiving nebulized mist treatment.

a mouthpiece to breathe in the medication. Some patients are taught to administer their own NMTs at home.

Inhalers

Inhalers are another way to administer topical medication directly into the lungs, minimizing systemic side effects. Corticosteroids and bronchodilators are often administered by inhaler. Metered-dose inhalers (MDIs) use propellants to deliver medication. Fig. 29.18 shows use of a traditional MDI. Use of a spacer can increase the amount of medication that gets to the lungs (Fig. 29.19). Dry-powder inhalers (DPIs) deliver medication without the use of propellant. With so many different types of inhalers, it is important to carefully read the instructions for use before assisting a patient.

The RT or nurse must carefully instruct the patient because improper use can reduce the effectiveness of the medication. The patient should do a return demonstration so the nurse can observe the patient's technique. It is also important to teach the patient to avoid overuse of adrenergic bronchodilator inhalers. Adrenergic bronchodilators can cause severe rebound bronchoconstriction and even death when used more often than prescribed.

Incentive Spirometry

Incentive spirometers (Fig. 29.20) are used to encourage deep breathing in patients at risk for collapse of lung tissue, a condition called *atelectasis*. These devices are commonly ordered for postoperative patients. Patients are instructed to use the spirometer 10 times each hour they are awake. Because a variety of spirometers are available, consult with an RT and read package inserts for specific directions for use.

Chest Physiotherapy

Chest physiotherapy (CPT) includes postural drainage, percussion, and vibration. It helps move secretions out from deep inside the lungs (Fig. 29.21). CPT is indicated for the patient who has a weak or ineffective cough and is at risk for retaining secretions. Patients with retained secretions due to conditions such as COPD, cystic fibrosis, or bronchiectasis and patients on ventilators benefit from CPT.

CPT is performed by an RT, physical therapist, or specially trained nurse. For postural drainage, the patient is placed in various positions (head down to help drain secretions) and turned periodically so all lobes of the lungs are drained. The therapist uses cupped hands to strike the chest repeatedly (percussion), producing sound waves that are transmitted through the chest, loosening secretions. The therapist may also apply vibration to the patient's chest, using the hands or a vibrator, to loosen secretions. An NMT should be given before CPT to humidify secretions. The patient is instructed to deep breathe and cough at intervals during and after the treatment.

High-Frequency Chest Wall Oscillation Vest

The high-frequency chest wall oscillation vest (sometimes called *vest therapy*) is an alternative to CPT. Because it does not require the presence of an RT, it is less expensive over

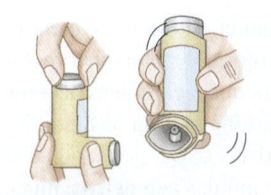

1. Gently twist the canister into the inhaler unit. Shake the inhaler and remove the cap.

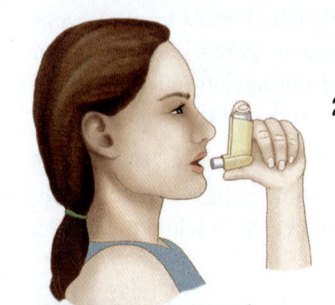

2. Exhale.

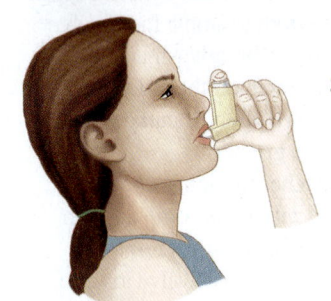

3. Place the inhaler mouthpiece in your mouth.

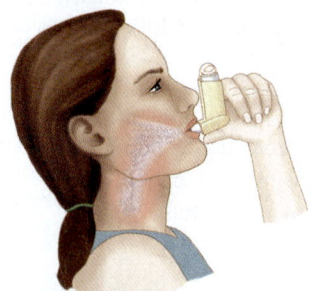

4. Press the canister down to actuate a dose of medication. As you do so, breathe in slowly and deeply. Time the dose and breath so the medication goes into the lungs and not onto the tongue.

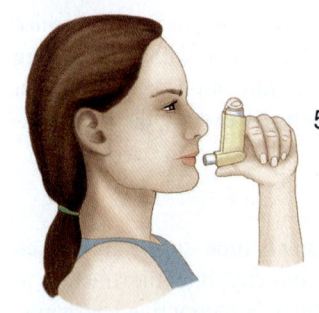

5. Hold your breath for 5–10 seconds. Repeat steps 2–4 if two puffs are ordered.

FIGURE 29.18 Instructions for use of a metered-dose inhaler. See package inserts for specific instructions because many types of inhalers are available.

time. An inflatable vest is placed on the patient. A compressor generates pulses of air into the vest to vibrate the patient's chest. Like CPT, this helps loosen secretions so they can be expectorated. The patient must cough during and after the therapy for it to be effective. It can easily be used at home.

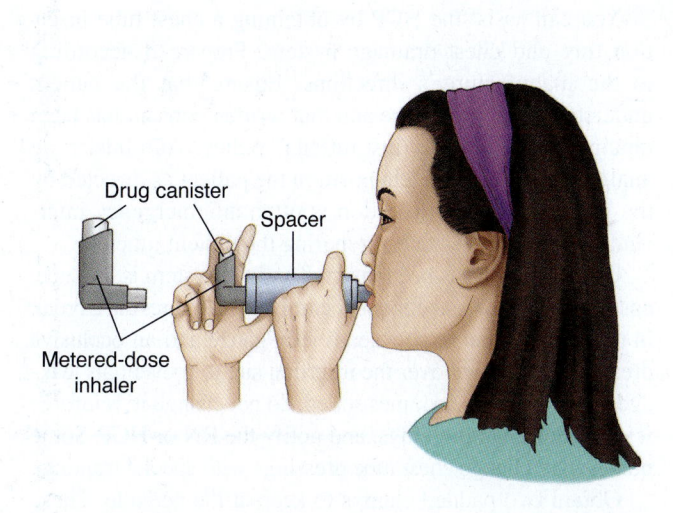

FIGURE 29.19 Use of a spacer increases the amount of medication that gets to the lungs.

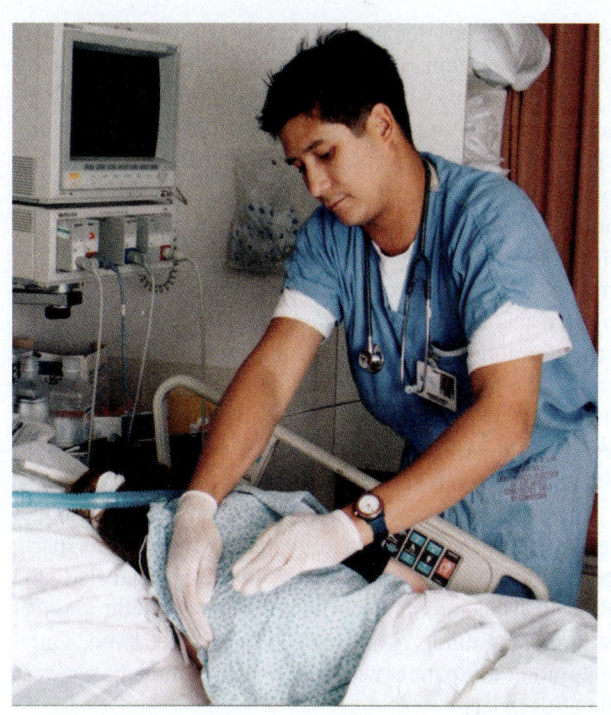

FIGURE 29.21 Patient receiving chest physiotherapy.

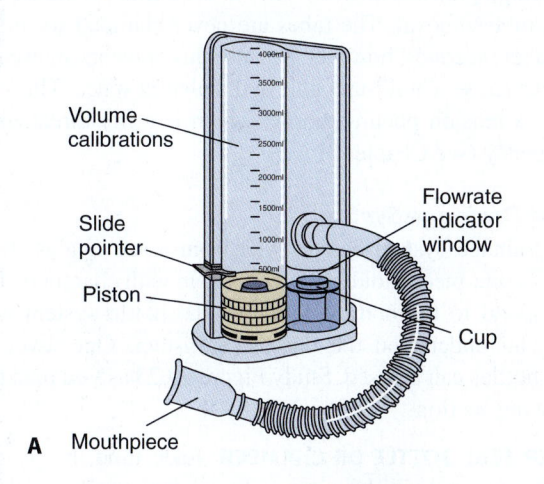

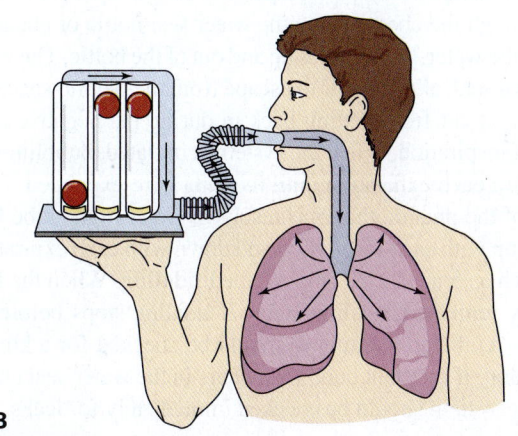

FIGURE 29.20 Incentive spirometers. (A) Voldyne volumetric deep-breathing exerciser. (B) TriFlo II incentive breathing exerciser.

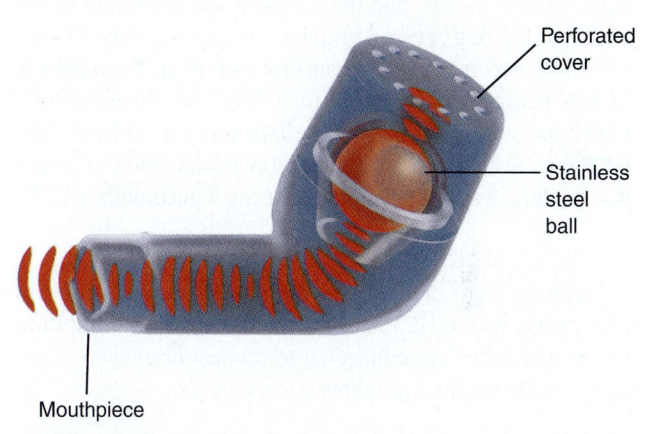

FIGURE 29.22 Flutter mucus clearance device.

When the patient blows into the mouthpiece, it makes a heavy steel ball inside bounce around in its chamber, which then sends vibrations back into the airways to help loosen mucus. Blowing into the device also creates positive pressure, which opens airways.

Thoracentesis
Thoracentesis involves the insertion of a needle into the pleural space. It is commonly done to aspirate fluid trapped in the pleural space (pleural effusion; see Chapter 31). The procedure may be diagnostic to determine the source of fluid or therapeutic to remove fluid and reduce respiratory

Vibratory Positive Expiratory Pressure Device
Another alternative to CPT is a small handheld device called a vibratory positive expiratory pressure (PEP) device. One brand is the Flutter mucus clearance device (Fig. 29.22).

• WORD • BUILDING •

thoracentesis: thoraco—chest + centesis—puncture

distress. It may also be performed to aspirate blood or air or to inject medication.

You may be asked to assist an HCP with a thoracentesis. First, verify that the patient understands the procedure and that written consent has been obtained if required by institution policy. Have the patient void before the procedure. The patient should be aware that a sensation of pressure may be felt but that severe pain is rare. Administer an analgesic, if ordered, before the procedure. Obtain a special procedure tray that has the equipment needed by the HCP. Place the patient in a sitting position, bending over a bedside table, or in a side-lying position if unable to sit. You can position yourself in front of the patient and encourage relaxation during the procedure. If you are asked to hand equipment to the HCP, be sure to keep everything sterile.

The HCP uses a local anesthetic before inserting a needle into the patient's back through the desired interspace. Specimens are withdrawn through the needle, labeled, and sent to the laboratory. A sterile container is used to collect the remaining fluid. As much as 2 L can be removed, sometimes more. The patient will usually report immediate reduction of dyspnea.

After the procedure, the HCP may apply a petroleum jelly dressing to prevent air leakage into the wound. Monitor vital signs, breath sounds, and the puncture site according to the HCP's orders (e.g., every 15 minutes times two, every 30 minutes times two, then every 4 hours for 24 hours). The patient is usually maintained on bedrest for 1 hour after the procedure. Label and send specimens to the laboratory as ordered. The HCP may order a postprocedure x-ray examination to ensure that the lung was not punctured, causing a pneumothorax.

Chest Drainage

Continuous chest drainage involves insertion of one or two chest tubes by the HCP into the pleural space to drain fluid or air. The tubes are connected to a chest drainage system that collects the fluid or allows escape of air.

Indications

Chest tubes and a chest drainage system are used when fluid or air has collected in the pleural space. This can occur with a collapsed lung (pneumothorax), pleural effusion, penetrating chest injury, or during chest surgery. These conditions are covered in Chapter 31.

Chest Tube Insertion

The HCP inserts drainage tubes through the chest wall into the pleural space either in surgery or at the bedside. If removal of air from around a collapsed lung is the goal, the tube is inserted into the upper anterior chest, in the second to fourth intercostal space. If removal of fluid or blood is the goal, such as after an injury, the tube is inserted in the lower lateral chest, in the eighth or ninth intercostal space. If a patient has both air and fluid to drain, two tubes are inserted and may be joined with a Y connector before connecting to tubing that leads to a drainage system.

You can assist the HCP by obtaining a chest tube insertion tray and chest drainage system. Prepare it according to the manufacturer's directions. Ensure that the patient understands the procedure and that written consent has been obtained according to institutional policy. Administer an analgesic as ordered. Help position the patient as directed by the HCP. Chest tube insertion is often an emergency intervention. This necessitates preparing the patient quickly.

Once the tube has been inserted and the system is in place, ensure that each connection is securely taped to prevent a break in the system. Sterile petroleum jelly gauze and an occlusive dressing are applied over the insertion site to prevent air leakage. If the dressing becomes soiled, do not change it; reinforce it with additional dressings, and notify the RN or HCP. Some nurses may change chest tube dressings with special training.

Obtain two padded clamps to keep at the bedside. These are used for clamping the chest tube if the chest drainage system becomes accidentally disconnected from the tubing, for changing the drainage system, or for a trial period before chest tube removal. The tubes are never clamped for more than a few seconds, however, because this prevents air escape and can cause a build-up of air in the pleural space. This can create a tension pneumothorax, which is a life-threatening emergency (see Chapter 31).

Chest Drainage System

The drainage system has evolved from a set of glass bottles to a one-piece molded plastic system with chambers that correspond to the bottles. Studying the bottle system will help you understand the one-piece system. One, two, or three bottles can be used. Study Figure 29.23 as you read the following sections.

WATER SEAL BOTTLE OR CHAMBER. Each time the patient exhales, trapped air also escapes the pleural space and travels through the chest tube to the water seal bottle or chamber, under the water, and bubbles up and out of the bottle. The water acts as a seal, allowing air to escape from the pleural space but preventing air from getting back in during the negative pressure of inspiration. When the system is initiated, bubbling will occur on each exhalation until the lung is re-expanded. Once most of the pneumothorax is resolved, water in the tube fluctuates up with each inspiration and down with each expiration, as much as 5 to 10 cm. This is called **tidaling**. When the lung is fully reinflated, tidaling stops. If tidaling stops before the lung is reinflated, the tubing should be checked for a kink or occlusion. If constant bubbling occurs in the water seal chamber, the system should be checked immediately for leaks.

> **LEARNING TIP**
> Do you remember blowing bubbles through a straw into a glass of water as a child? The air could escape through the water, but you could not suck the air back through the water after it escaped. A water seal chamber operates under the same principle.

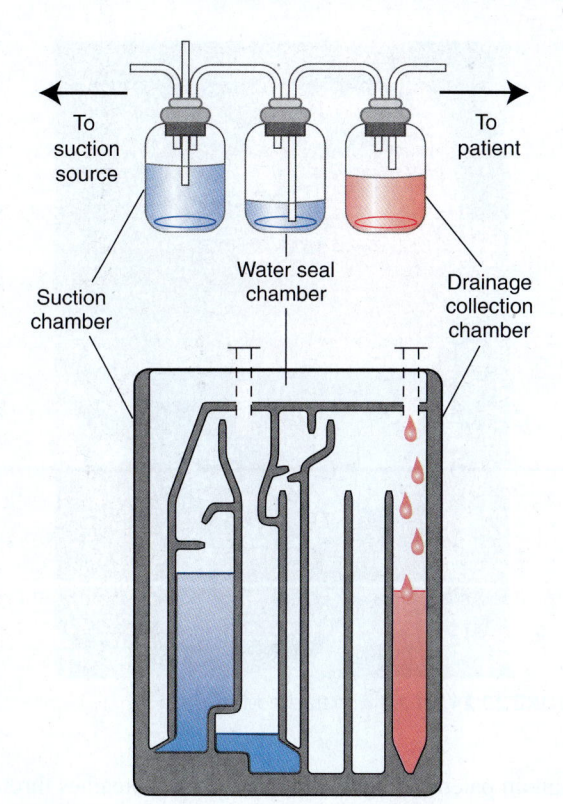

FIGURE 29.23 Pleur-evac chest drainage system.

SUCTION BOTTLE OR CHAMBER. Sometimes, a suction source is used to speed lung reinflation. A separate bottle with tubing attached to suction is used. The amount of suction depends on the level of water in the bottle, not the amount of suction set on the machine. As shown in Figure 29.23, some air is being suctioned from the atmosphere from the center straw, and some is being suctioned from the patient. The farther the straw is immersed in the water, the harder it will be for the suction to draw air from the atmosphere, creating more suction to the patient. The suction level is ordered by the HCP. It is almost always negative 20 cm of water. The suction source should be turned on far enough to cause gentle bubbling in the suction bottle or chamber. Vigorous bubbling causes water evaporation, which alters the amount of suction. If water evaporates, more must be added to maintain the correct amount of suction. Some newer one-piece systems use special suction control valves to eliminate the need for water.

DRAINAGE BOTTLE OR CHAMBER. Sometimes a third bottle is needed to catch fluid drained from the pleural space. Drainage may be from pleural effusion, chest trauma, or surgery. Sometimes, a small amount of drainage occurs because of the insertion of the chest tube. The drainage chamber is not emptied to measure drainage. Rather, the drainage level in the bottle or chamber is marked and timed each shift to monitor the amount. It is documented as output on the intake and output record. If drainage suddenly increases or becomes very bloody, notify the HCP. If the drainage chamber fills up, either the chamber or the entire unit will need to be changed, depending on the type of system.

Nursing Care for the Patient With a Chest Tube

Nursing care for a patient with a chest tube involves regular monitoring of the patient and the drainage system. See Box 29.1 for specific data collection and care. If permitted by the HCP, patients can be free to move around with the chest tube and drainage system. The drainage system must always be kept upright and below the level of the chest. If the patient must be transported, the drainage system is transported with the patient. Ask the HCP whether the patient can

Box 29.1
Care of the Patient With a Chest Drainage System

Monitor the patient according to institution policy. Start with the patient and move toward the drainage system.

Patient
1. Observe respiratory rate, effort, and symmetry.
2. Ask about shortness of breath, pain, anxiety, or other discomforts.
3. Auscultate lung sounds (lung sounds may initially be muffled or absent on the side of a collapsed lung but should gradually return to normal as the lung reinflates).
4. Confirm that dressing is intact; observe for drainage. If necessary, reinforce the dressing and notify the HCP. Do not change the dressing unless specifically ordered to and trained to do so.
5. Palpate around insertion sites for crepitus, a sign that air is leaking into the tissues.

Tubing
6. Check all tubing for kinks, breaks, or broken connections. Verify that all connections are securely taped.
7. Ensure that there are no dependent loops of tubing. Coil excess tubing on the bed.

Draining System
8. Verify that drainage system is below level of patient's chest at all times.
9. Check drainage system for cracks or leaks.
10. Check water seal chamber for correct water level and for tidaling (unless lung is reinflated). Add sterile water if evaporation has decreased level. If continuous bubbling is present, check entire system for leaks and notify registered nurse (RN) or HCP.
11. Check suction control chamber for gentle bubbling (or open to air). Confirm correct amount of water as ordered. Add water if needed.
12. Check and mark amount of drainage in collection chamber every 8 hours and as needed or as ordered. Report any marked increase in bloody drainage. Record drainage as output.
13. Document findings.
    Notify RN or HCP if any of the following occur:
    * *The patient suddenly reports increasing dyspnea.*
    * *There is a change in the patient's status.*
    * *The drainage chamber is full and needs to be changed.*

be safely transported without suction. If the answer is yes, the suction control chamber is then left open to allow air to escape. Do not clamp tubing for transport.

If a chest tube is accidentally pulled out before the pneumothorax is resolved, air can re-enter the pleural space. Contact the RN or HCP immediately if this occurs.

Stripping and Milking

You may hear about stripping or milking tubing to dislodge clots and maintain patency. Stripping is done by holding the proximal end of the tubing and using the other hand to squeeze the tubing between two fingers while sliding the fingers toward the drainage system. This is repeated on small sections of tubing until all have been stripped. However, this process can create negative pressure at the openings in the tubing that are within the pleural space. This can suck lung tissue in and cause damage. Stripping should not be done.

Milking is done by gently squeezing portions of tubing from the patient to the system without any sliding motion. This is somewhat safer for the patient but is still not done routinely. If tubing appears to be occluded, consult with the HCP for specific orders.

> **PRACTICE ANALYSIS TIP**
> **Linking NCLEX-PN® to Practice**
> The LPN/LVN will verify and process health-care provider's orders.

> **CRITICAL THINKING**
>
> **Miss Israel** has a chest tube in place for a spontaneous pneumothorax.
>
> **Critical Thinking (The Why)**
> 1. You note that the water seal chamber is bubbling vigorously. What could cause this?
>
> **Clinical Judgement (The Do)**
> 2. What should you do?
> 3. You are totaling intake and output for your 8-hour shift. There is 240 mL of serous fluid in the drainage chamber of the drainage system at 2200. At 1400, there was 190 mL. How much output should you record?
>
> *Suggested answers are at the end of the chapter.*

Removal of Chest Tube

When the reason for the chest tube is resolved, the HCP removes it and places petroleum jelly gauze and a sterile occlusive dressing over the site. Continue to watch for development of crepitus. Monitor the patient's respiratory status and dressing site.

Tracheostomy

A **tracheotomy** is a surgical opening through the base of the neck into the trachea. It is called a **tracheostomy** when it is more permanent and has a tube inserted into the opening to

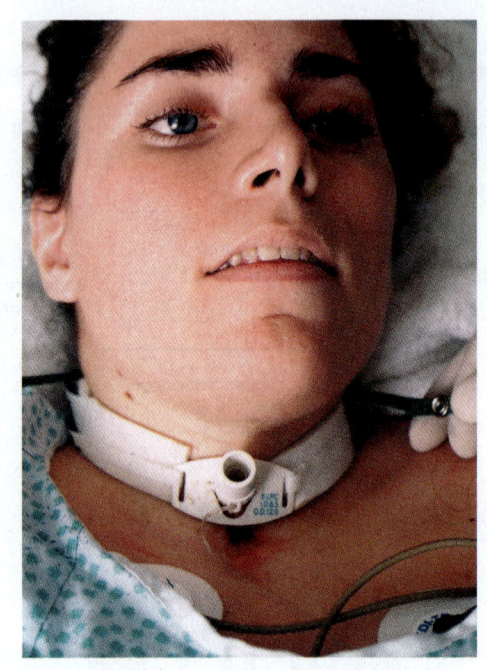

FIGURE 29.24 Patient with tracheostomy.

maintain patency (Fig. 29.24). The patient breathes through this opening, bypassing the upper airways. A tracheostomy is performed for various reasons, including in patients who have had a cancerous larynx removed, with airway obstruction caused by trauma or a tumor, who have difficulty clearing secretions from the airway, or who need prolonged mechanical ventilation.

The tracheostomy tube consists of three parts: an outer cannula, an inner cannula, and an obturator (Fig. 29.25A and B). The obturator is a guide used only during insertion of the tube. After insertion, the obturator is immediately removed and kept at the bedside (commonly in a plastic bag taped to the wall above the bed) for emergency use if the tracheostomy tube is accidentally removed. The outer cannula remains in place at all times and is secured by ties or a Velcro strap to prevent dislodging. The inner cannula is removed at intervals, usually every 8 hours and as needed for cleaning. Some newer tracheostomy tubes eliminate the need for an inner cannula.

The tube may be metal or plastic. Plastic tubes typically have disposable inner cannulas, which can be replaced rather than cleaned. Plastic tubes also may have balloon-like cuffs that are inflated to prevent air escape during mechanical ventilation. You know that the cuff is inflated if the small pilot balloon on the tubing used to inject air is inflated (see Fig. 29.25B and C). Cuffs are deflated routinely to prevent tissue damage. See "Performing Tracheostomy Care" on Davis Advantage for steps required for a routine tracheostomy cleaning.

• **WORD • BUILDING •**

tracheotomy: trach—trachea + otomy—incision
tracheostomy: trach—trachea + ostomy—opening or mouth

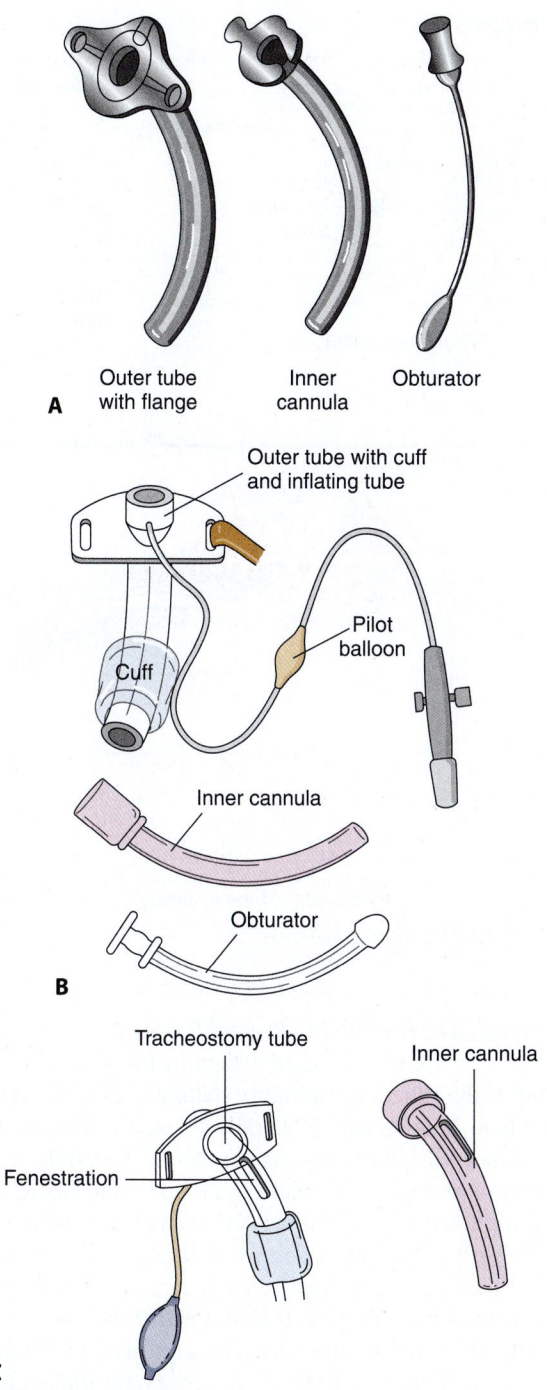

FIGURE 29.25 Tracheostomy tube. (A) Metal tube. (B) Cuffed plastic tube. (C) Fenestrated tube.

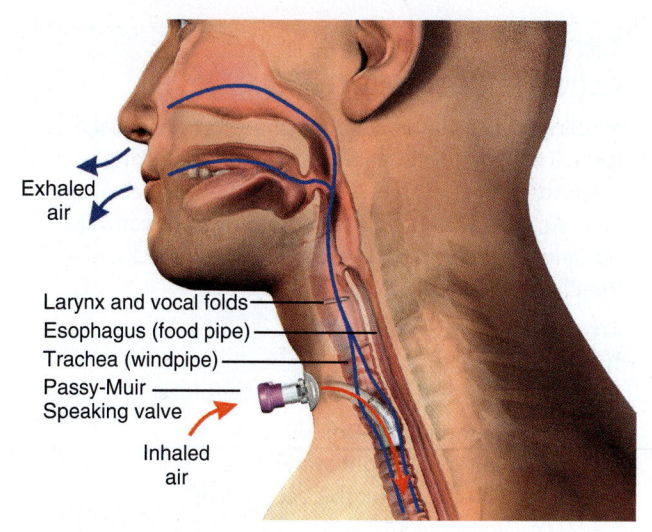

FIGURE 29.26 The Passy Muir tracheostomy speaking valve.

Communication is problematic for the patient with a tracheostomy tube because air is diverted out the tube rather than past the vocal cords and out the mouth. Fenestrated tubes are tubes with openings (fenestra) in the cannula to allow air to flow up into the larynx for speaking (see Fig. 29.25C). The patient can be taught to plug the opening of the tube while speaking to divert air through the fenestra. Another option is a valve such as the Passy Muir tracheostomy speaking valve (Fig. 29.26), which allows air to flow into the tracheostomy during inspiration. It then closes and redirects air up around the tracheostomy tube, through the vocal cords, and out the nose and mouth on expiration, allowing the patient to speak. Use of the valve eliminates the need for the patient to use a finger over the opening to speak. For the valve to be used safely and effectively, the tracheostomy tube must be small enough for air to flow around it or be fenestrated to allow air to flow up through the vocal cords. If cuffed, the cuff must be completely deflated.

> **BE SAFE!**
> **AVOID FAILURE TO RECOGNIZE!** A patient with a tracheostomy tube in place as a result of laryngectomy surgery does not have vocal cords, and the trachea no longer connects to the nose and mouth. The patient will not be able to plug the tube or use a valve to talk; plugging a laryngectomy tube would cause suffocation. Laryngectomy is covered in Chapter 30.

Some tracheostomies are permanent. However, some patients can be weaned from the tracheostomy tube when their condition has improved enough to allow breathing without it. The HCP may replace the tube with a smaller tube to prepare the patient for its removal. This allows a plug to be inserted into the tracheostomy tube at intervals to force the patient to breathe around the tube through the nose and mouth. When the tracheostomy tube has been removed, the opening may be taped shut and covered with gauze until it is healed. The gauze often becomes saturated with secretions and is changed as needed.

Nursing Process for the Patient With a Tracheostomy

See "Nursing Care Plan for the Patient With a Tracheostomy."

CRITICAL THINKING & CLINICAL JUDGMENT

Mr. Singh has a plastic, cuffed tracheostomy tube that is small enough to allow airflow around it for talking when the cuff is deflated. A friend stops by for a chat and helps Mr. Singh to plug his tracheostomy so he can talk. Mr. Singh's face turns dark red, and he gets panicky. His friend calls for help.

Critical Thinking (The Why)
1. What happened?
2. How can you help prevent this in the future?

Clinical Judgement (The Do)
3. What should you do right away?
4. How will you document this occurrence?

Suggested answers are at the end of the chapter.

Suctioning

Suctioning involves the use of a sterile flexible catheter inserted into the tracheostomy tube to remove secretions from a patient who is unable to cough effectively. This may be a patient with overwhelming secretions or a patient with a tracheostomy or ET tube who is unable to clear the tube with coughing.

The procedures for suctioning are found in your Resources on Davis Advantage. Consult a procedure manual for more detailed instruction. Remember that suctioning is both frightening and uncomfortable for a patient. Patients sometimes feel as though oxygen is being "vacuumed" from their lungs. Suctioning can cause hypoxia, vagal stimulation with resulting bradycardia, and even cardiac arrest. Suction only when necessary rather than on a routine basis. Coughing is the most effective way to clear secretions and should be encouraged if the patient is capable. Signs that suctioning is needed include crackles or wheezes heard with or without a stethoscope or a dropping oxygen saturation value. Explain each step to the patient during suctioning even if they are unresponsive.

Intubation

Some patients are intubated with a special ET tube through the nose or mouth and into the trachea (Fig. 29.27). Cardiopulmonary arrest, general anesthesia during surgery, and respiratory failure are examples of situations that may require intubation. Most intubated patients are also mechanically ventilated. Some patients have advance directives that indicate they do not wish to be intubated. You should be familiar with the patient's wishes and bring them to the attention of the HCP if necessary.

Because intubation can damage vocal cords and surrounding tissues, it is usually a short-term intervention. Patients who need long-term ventilatory support have a tracheostomy tube placed.

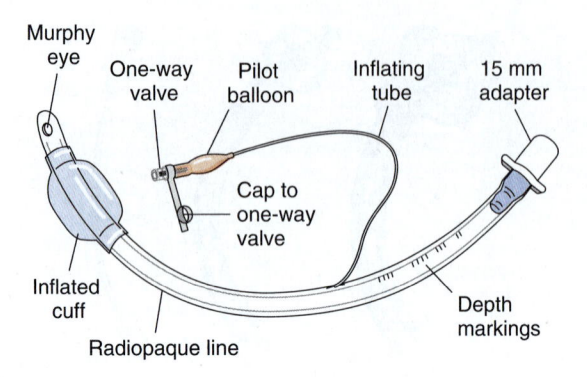

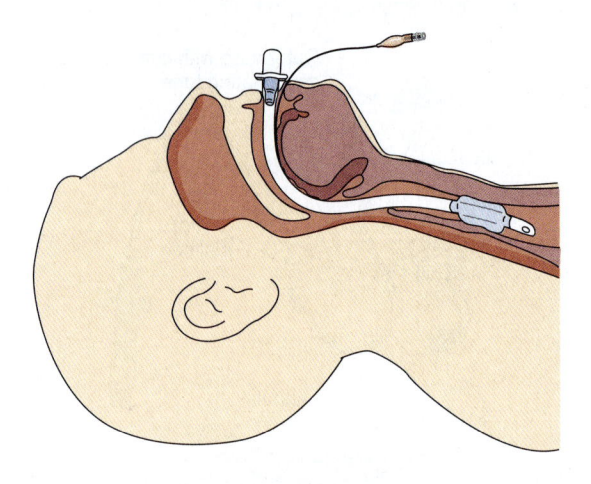

FIGURE 29.27 Endotracheal tube.

Nursing Care for the Intubated Patient

Nursing care for the intubated patient includes regular monitoring of the patient's respiratory status and tube placement. Auscultate lung sounds bilaterally to ensure that the tube has not been displaced into one bronchus. Carefully secure the tube with tape or a Velcro holder to avoid dislodging. Reposition and secure oral tubes to the opposite side of the mouth every 24 hours or according to institution policy to prevent tissue damage. Apply an adhesive skin barrier under the tape to protect the skin. If alert, instruct the patient to be careful not to pull on the tube. You may need to obtain an order for soft wrist restraints if necessary for the confused patient. Restraints can be avoided if a family member is available to sit with the patient. Many nursing interventions for the patient with a tracheostomy are also appropriate for the intubated patient. (See "Nursing Care Plan for the Patient With a Tracheostomy.")

Like tracheostomy tubes, ET tubes have a cuff (balloon-like area around the tube) to help maintain proper placement and to prevent leakage of air around the tube. Consult the RT to help monitor the cuff pressure.

Patients will need suctioning because they are unable to cough effectively with an ET tube. Visible secretions in the tube, crackles or wheezes heard with or without the

Nursing Care Plan for the Patient With a Tracheostomy

Nursing Diagnosis: *Ineffective Airway Clearance* related to excessive secretions
Expected Outcome: The patient's airway will be free of secretions as evidenced by no audible crackles or wheezes in airway and a clear cannula.
Evaluation of Outcome: Is airway free of secretions?

Intervention	Rationale	Evaluation
Auscultate lung sounds every 4 hours and as needed (prn).	*Coarse crackles or wheezes may indicate secretions in airways.*	Are coarse crackles or wheezes present?
Monitor oxygen saturation every 4 hours and prn.	*Secretions may reduce gas exchange.*	Is oxygen saturation less than 90% to 95%, indicating a problem?
Monitor and document amount, color, and character of secretions. Report change in secretions accompanied by fever.	*Purulent sputum accompanied by fever can indicate pneumonia.*	Is sputum clear or white and scant in amount? Is purulent sputum reported?
Clean tracheostomy according to agency policy.	*Cleaning helps remove excess mucus and keeps airway clear.*	Does cleaning help maintain an open airway?
Suction patient using sterile technique, only when needed.	*Suctioning clears secretions from airways. Unnecessary suctioning irritates airways.*	Is suction necessary? Is airway free of secretions after suctioning?
Provide humidified oxygen or a room humidifier.	*Humidification helps prevent drying of mucosa and secretions.*	Are mucosa moist and secretions easily removed?
Encourage patient to deep breathe and cough as able.	*Patient may be able to clear own secretions without suctioning.*	Is patient able to cough up secretions effectively?
Encourage fluids if not contraindicated.	*Fluids help hydrate secretions, making them easier to cough up.*	Is patient taking adequate fluids? Are secretions thin?
Encourage ambulation as able or turn every 2 hours.	*Movement helps mobilize secretions.*	Is patient mobilized as much as possible?

Nursing Diagnosis: *Risk for Infection* related to bypass of normal respiratory defense mechanisms and increased aspiration risk
Expected Outcome: The patient will be free of infection, as evidenced by vital signs within normal limits and clear secretions.
Evaluation of Outcome: Is patient free from symptoms of infection?

Intervention	Rationale	Evaluation
Monitor and report signs and symptoms of infection (e.g., fever, increased respiratory rate, purulent sputum, elevated white blood cell count).	*Early recognition and treatment of infection improves outcome.*	Are signs of infection present?
Use good hand hygiene practice.	*Hand hygiene is important in preventing infection.*	Do all caregivers use good hand hygiene technique?
Keep head of bed elevated 30 to 45 degrees.	*Elevation helps reduce aspiration of gastric contents, which can lead to pneumonia.*	Is the head of bed elevated?
Protect tracheostomy opening from foreign material, such as food, sprays, and powders.	*Foreign materials in the tracheostomy can cause pneumonia.*	Is the tracheostomy adequately protected?

(nursing care plan continues on page 512)

Nursing Care Plan for the Patient With a Tracheostomy

Intervention	Rationale	Evaluation
Use meticulous sterile technique for all tracheostomy care and suctioning.	Use of nonsterile technique may introduce microorganisms into the respiratory tract.	Is sterile technique used by all caregivers?
Consult with speech therapist and health-care provider (HCP) about whether to have cuff inflated or deflated on cuffed tube.	An inflated cuff can impair swallowing in some patients.	Is the cuff properly inflated or deflated according to specific orders?
Encourage a well-balanced diet. Consult dietitian prn.	A well-balanced diet enhances immune function.	Is patient eating a balanced diet or receiving adequate supplementation?

Nursing Diagnosis: *Impaired Verbal Communication* related to tracheostomy tube
Expected Outcomes: The patient will use alternate methods of communication effectively. The patient will express satisfaction with ability to communicate needs.
Evaluation of Outcomes: Is the patient able to use alternative methods to express needs?

Intervention	Rationale	Evaluation
Take time to allow patient to communicate needs.	Patient may become frustrated if hurried.	Does patient feel adequate time is given for communication of needs?
Watch for patient's nonverbal cues.	Gestures and facial expression can provide valuable cues.	Are nonverbal cues recognized?
Offer pen and paper or whiteboard (if patient is literate).	Patient may be able to write out his or her needs/concerns.	Is patient able to communicate in writing?
Use a picture board (available from speech therapy department).	The patient can point to a picture (water, toileting) that indicates need.	Is patient able to point appropriately to needs?
Collaborate with speech therapist.	Speech therapist may have additional methods for communicating with patient.	Are alternative methods effective?
Teach patient with fenestrated or small tracheostomy tube how to cover opening with a plug or clean finger to talk, or to use Passy Muir valve, according to HCP or speech therapy recommendations.	Covering the opening or using a valve diverts air into larynx and allows speech.	Is patient able to communicate in this manner?

Nursing Diagnosis: *Deficient Knowledge* related to care of new tracheostomy
Expected Outcomes: The patient and significant other will verbalize understanding of self-care, demonstrate tracheostomy self-care procedures, and state resources for help after discharge.
Evaluation of Outcomes: Are the patient and significant other able to verbalize self-care and correctly demonstrate care procedures? Can the patient state how to obtain help after discharge?

Intervention	Rationale	Evaluation
Determine patient's and significant other's baseline knowledge of self-care.	Teaching should only be initiated if a knowledge deficit exists.	Does patient exhibit knowledge of self-care?
Allow patient opportunity to share concerns about tracheostomy.	Sharing concerns helps patient to sort out feelings and problem solve.	Does patient exhibit readiness to learn self-care?

Nursing Care Plan for the Patient With a Tracheostomy

Intervention	Rationale	Evaluation
Provide follow-up with the home health nurse after discharge. Provide information on support groups.	*Patient will need to access community resources.*	Is patient receptive to having a home health nurse assist? Is patient interested in a support group?
Instruct patient and significant other in tracheostomy cleaning, deep breathing and coughing, suctioning, prevention of infection and symptoms to report to the HCP, and protection of tracheostomy from pollutants and water (no swimming, careful showering).	*Patient will need to care for self after discharge.*	Does patient verbalize understanding of self-care and demonstrate all procedures correctly?

stethoscope, or a drop in SpO_2 without another obvious cause are signs that suctioning is necessary. The ET tube suctioning procedure is sterile. It is the same as suctioning a tracheostomy tube. Most institutions have in-line suctioning devices, which are connected to the ET tube within a sterile sleeve. This maintains sterility, protects the nurse, and simplifies the suctioning procedure. Oral suction may also be necessary to keep the mouth free of secretions.

The intubated patient is often extremely anxious, especially if they are alert. Explain the purpose of all care activities. Suctioning is a particularly anxiety-producing activity. It should be explained carefully even if the patient is unresponsive.

Intubated patients are at risk of developing ventilator-associated pneumonia (VAP) because normal respiratory defense mechanisms are bypassed. Good hand hygiene and frequent mouth care to reduce risk of aspirating oral microorganisms can help prevent VAP. The head of the bed should also be kept elevated 30 to 45 degrees at all times.

Because the ET tube passes between the vocal cords, the patient is unable to speak. Provide paper and pencil or a picture board for communication. Yes/no questions can be answered by a nod or shake of the head.

Monitor ABG and oxygen saturation values and notify the HCP of changes. If oxygen values drop or the patient becomes confused or agitated, immediately check the patient for a disconnected oxygen source or excessive secretions.

If the HCP determines that the patient can breathe effectively without the tube, the tube will be removed. The patient will be slowly weaned from the ventilator first. Before tube removal, the patient's mouth and tube are suctioned, and the cuff is deflated. After removal, the patient is observed closely for laryngeal edema or respiratory distress. The patient is maintained in high-Fowler position to maximize chest expansion.

Mechanical Ventilation

Ventilators are devices that provide ventilation (respirations) for patients who are unable to breathe effectively on their own (Fig. 29.28). Ventilators use positive pressure to push oxygenated air via a cuffed ET or tracheostomy tube into the lungs at preset intervals. Patients may need mechanical ventilation after some surgeries, after cardiac or respiratory arrest, for declining ABGs related to worsening respiratory disease, or for neuromuscular disease or injury that affects the muscles of respiration.

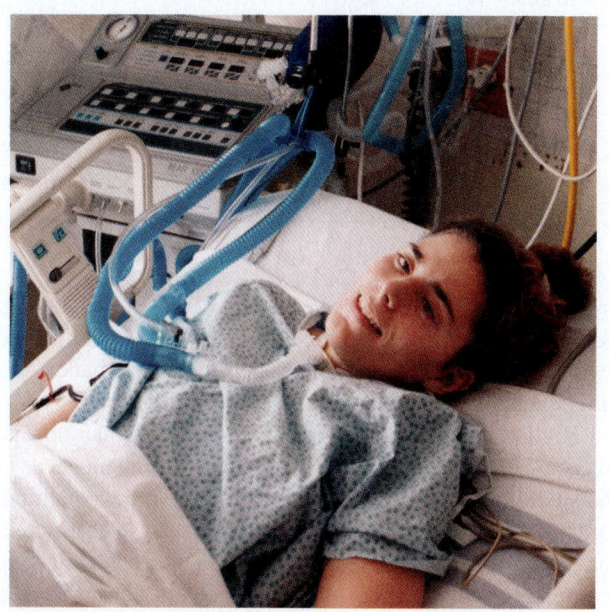

FIGURE 29.28 Patient on ventilator.

Ventilator Modes

Ventilators can control ventilation or assist the patient's own respirations. See Table 29.8 for terms related to ventilator function. There are many types and models of ventilators. Consult the respiratory care department for explanation of a patient's ventilator and to troubleshoot alarms.

Ventilator Alarms

Several types of alarms are found on ventilators. Low-pressure alarms sound if the ventilator senses reduced pressure in the

Table 29.8
Ventilator Terminology

Fraction of inspired oxygen (FIO_2)	Range: 21%–100%.
Tidal volume (V_T)	Amount of air delivered with each breath. Range: 6–8 mL/kg of ideal body weight.
Rate	Frequency of breaths delivered.
Assist control (ac) mode (also called *continuous mechanical ventilation*, or CMV)	Does all the work of breathing for the patient. Ventilator delivers a breath each time patient begins to inspire. If patient does not breathe, the machine continues to deliver a preset number of breaths per minute.
Synchronized intermittent mandatory ventilation (SIMV)	Allows patient to breathe independently but delivers a minimum number of ventilations per minute as necessary. Synchronized to patient's own respiratory pattern.
Pressure support (PS)	Provides positive pressure on inspiration to decrease the work of breathing.
Continuous positive airway pressure (CPAP)	Provides positive pressure on inspiration and expiration to keep alveoli open in a spontaneously breathing patient.
Positive end-expiratory pressure (PEEP)	Provides positive pressure on expiration to help keep small airways open.

system. Low pressure can be caused by disconnected tubing, leaks in tubing or around the ET tube, or an underinflated cuff. A low-pressure alarm may also sound if the patient has attempted to remove the tube.

High-pressure alarms sound for higher-than-normal resistance to airflow. This might occur if the patient needs to be suctioned; if the patient is biting on the tube, coughing, or trying to talk; if tubing is kinked or otherwise obstructed; or if worsening respiratory disease causes decreased lung compliance. In addition, the high-pressure alarm may be triggered if the patient is anxious and unable to time his or her breaths with those of the ventilator. Water in the tubing might also cause a high-pressure alarm. Consult with the respiratory care department for guidance in draining the tubing.

A loss-of-power alarm may signal power failure or disconnected plug. Be aware of emergency power sources and prepare to ventilate the patient manually if necessary. Volume and frequency alarms sound when tidal volume or number of breaths per minute fall outside preset parameters.

When an alarm sounds, always check the patient first. If the patient is stable, check the machine. Determine why the alarm is sounding and correct the problem quickly. If no cause can be found, call for help. If the ventilator is not functioning, disconnect the patient from the ventilator and call for help. Use a manual resuscitation bag until help arrives.

> **PRACTICE ANALYSIS TIP**
> **Linking NCLEX-PN® to Practice**
> The LPN/LVN will recognize self-limitations of task/assignments and seek assistance when needed.

Nursing Care

Before initiating mechanical ventilation, it is important for the health-care team to be aware of advance directives and consult with the patient and family. Some patients do not wish to be intubated or mechanically ventilated. Some patients accept mechanical ventilation if it is a temporary measure but not if it might be a permanent intervention.

In the past, ventilators were used only in intensive care units. Now, ventilators are seen on medical-surgical units, in nursing homes, and even in patients' homes. It is important to use a team approach when caring for a patient who is mechanically ventilated. The social worker; RT; physical, occupational, and speech therapist(s); dietitian; nurse; and HCP collaborate to provide the comprehensive care needed by the patient. RTs usually take responsibility for routine monitoring and equipment maintenance.

The nurse is responsible for monitoring the patient, ensuring that ventilator settings are maintained as prescribed, providing initial response to alarms, keeping tubing free from water accumulation, and keeping the patient's airway free from secretions. In addition, keep a manual resuscitation bag at the bedside for emergencies. Good nursing care is essential for preventing ventilator-associated complications, especially pneumonia. Keep the head of the bed at a 30- to 45-degree angle to reduce the risk of aspiration and pneumonia. Oral care with chlorhexidine mouthwash can reduce the incidence of VAP. Keep the airway clear with suctioning as needed. Good nutrition is also essential and can increase the success of eventual weaning.

Patients who are mechanically ventilated are unable to talk and can become very uncomfortable and anxious if there is no easy way to communicate. Box 29.2 provides tips for making ventilated patients feel more secure.

Box 29.2
Tips for Caring for Patients Who Are Mechanically Ventilated

- Mechanically ventilated patients report feeling panicky but less so if relatives or nursing staff are present:
  - Speak to the patient each time you enter the room and explain everything you do.
  - Encourage family to visit.
  - Answer the patient's call light and attend to ventilator alarms promptly.
  - Use restraints only as a last resort.
- Patients may have difficulty relaxing and sleeping while on a ventilator:
  - Administer sedatives or antianxiety medications as ordered. Request order if necessary.
  - Allow uninterrupted blocks of time for sleep.
- Patients with endotracheal tubes report pain and discomfort:
  - Monitor for comfort and reposition at regular intervals.
  - Be careful not to pull on the ventilator tubing.
  - Administer analgesics as ordered.
  - Provide good oral care, moistening lips with a cool washcloth and water-based lubricant.
- Suctioning is painful and frightening for patients:
  - Suction quickly and smoothly and avoid inserting the catheter too deeply.
  - Oxygenate the patient with 100% oxygen prior to suctioning.
  - Avoid the use of saline with suctioning, which can reduce oxygen saturation.
  - Allow patients to suction themselves if possible (with HCP order and appropriate instruction).
- Communication is very difficult for patients:
  - Be patient when trying to understand communication efforts.
  - Provide a pencil and paper but be aware that even writing can be exhausting.
  - Ask yes/no questions when possible. Establish a response system with the patient such as blinking (once for no, twice for yes), hand squeezes, or nodding.
  - Validate patient expressions and body language; don't assume that a patient is sad or wants to be left alone based on facial expression.
  - Make sure the call light is within reach at all times.

Source: Modified from Jablonski, R. A. S. (1995). If ventilator patients could talk. *RN, 58*(2), 32.

Noninvasive Positive-Pressure Ventilation

Noninvasive positive-pressure ventilation (NIPPV) is an alternative to intubation and mechanical ventilation for patients who are able to breathe on their own but are unable to maintain normal ABGs. Patients with severe respiratory disease, sleep apnea, or neuromuscular diseases such as amyotrophic lateral sclerosis (ALS) that weaken respiratory muscles can benefit from this treatment. Instead of the invasive ET or tracheostomy tube, NIPPV uses an external masklike device that fits over the nose or mouth and nose (Fig. 29.29). It can be successful in patients who are alert, able to cooperate, do not have excessive secretions, and are able to breathe on their own for periods of time. It can be used with or without supplemental oxygen. In an acutely ill patient, oxygen saturation is monitored.

Two basic types of NIPPV are available: continuous positive airway pressure (CPAP) and bilevel positive airway pressure (BiPAP). With CPAP, the same amount of positive pressure is maintained throughout inspiration and expiration to prevent airway collapse. In BiPAP, a higher level of positive pressure is used on inspiration, and a lower level on expiration.

Nursing Care

Monitor patients receiving NIPPV for skin irritation from the mask and gastric distention from swallowing air. Apply an adhesive skin barrier to the areas that come in contact with the mask to prevent irritation. To prevent gastric distention, place the patient in semi-Fowler position. Consult with the RT to adjust air delivery pressure if necessary. A special humidifier on the machine can reduce nose and mouth dryness. An air leak around the mask can cause air to blow in the patient's eyes, which can be irritating. If this happens, remove the mask and reposition it. Many patients do not like the tight mask covering their nose or mouth. Be patient in explaining the reason for this treatment. Check the patient frequently to help control anxiety. Be sure to ask about the patient's goals for therapy. Some patients may choose not to use NIPPV, but they must be fully aware of possible consequences.

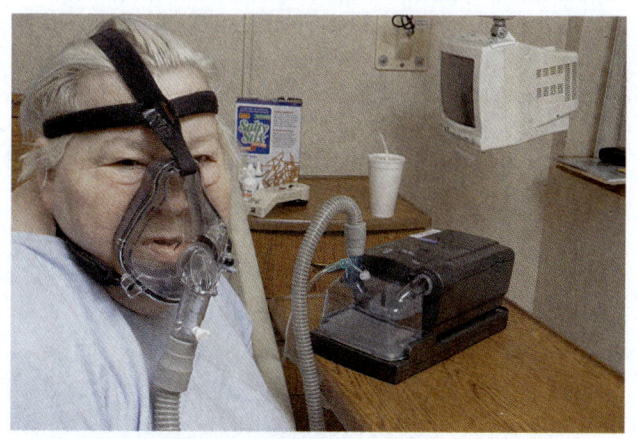

FIGURE 29.29 Noninvasive positive-pressure ventilation. Note round face from steroid use.

Patients can use NIPPV nearly continuously, removing it to eat or use the bathroom. Other patients who are able to breathe effectively on their own during the day use it only when they are sleeping. Some use it for a few days until an acute exacerbation of disease is resolved. Others continue its use indefinitely at home.

Key Points

- The respiratory system is basically a tract, divided into upper and lower respiratory portions. The upper tract is above the thoracic cavity. The lower portion is within the thoracic cavity.
- The alveoli of the lungs are the site of gas exchange between the air and the blood of pulmonary circulation; the rest of the system moves air into and out of the lungs.
- Together with the cardiovascular system, the respiratory system supplies the body with oxygen and eliminates carbon dioxide.
- Because of its role in regulating the amount of carbon dioxide in body fluids, the respiratory system is important in the maintenance of acid–base balance, measured by blood pH.
- Because smoking is such a major risk factor for many types of lung disease, it is essential to ask about smoking history and encourage the patient to quit. Document the patient's smoking history in terms of pack-years.
- Note the color of the skin, lips, mucous membranes, and nailbeds. In light-skinned individuals, cyanosis, a late sign of oxygen deprivation, presents as a bluish color. In dark-skinned individuals, cyanosis may be noted as gray or whitish skin around the mouth and/or gray or bluish conjunctivae.
- Count the number of respirations per minute, noting depth and rhythm.
- Auscultation provides valuable information about respiratory status. Use the diaphragm of your stethoscope to listen to the anterior, lateral, and posterior chest during an entire inspiration and expiration at each interspace. Auscultation of the posterior chest is easiest if the patient is sitting.
- Measurement of RBCs and Hgb can give information about the oxygen-carrying capacity of the blood. Dyspnea can be caused by a reduction in RBCs or Hgb. Elevated WBCs indicate infection.
- ABGs are measured to determine the effectiveness of gas exchange. The blood sample is usually taken from the radial artery in the wrist by a specially trained respiratory therapist or laboratory technician.
- A sputum culture identifies pathogens present in the sputum. The sensitivity test determines which antibiotics will be effective against those pathogens.
- Pulmonary function studies are a series of tests done to determine lung volume, capacity, and flow rates. These are commonly used to help diagnose and monitor restrictive or obstructive lung disease.
- Bronchoscopy involves the use of a flexible endoscope to examine the larynx, trachea, and bronchial tree. Bronchoscopy can be used diagnostically for visualization or to obtain a biopsy specimen for examination. It can also be used therapeutically to remove an obstruction, foreign body, or thick secretions.
- The pursed-lip breathing technique can be used any time the patient feels short of breath. It helps keep airways open during exhalation, which promotes carbon dioxide excretion.
- The patient who is short of breath should be positioned to conserve energy while allowing for maximum lung expansion. Most respiratory patients do not tolerate lying flat. The patient in bed can use Fowler or semi-Fowler position to keep abdominal contents from crowding the lungs.
- Oxygen therapy is ordered by the HCP when the patient is unable to maintain oxygenation. Patients are typically placed on supplemental oxygen when their oxygen saturation is less than 90% on room air.
- Continuous chest drainage involves insertion of one or two chest tubes by the HCP into the pleural space to drain fluid or air. The tubes are connected to a chest drainage system that collects the fluid or allows escape of air.
- A tracheotomy is a surgical opening through the base of the neck into the trachea. It is called a tracheostomy when it is more permanent and has a tube inserted into the opening to maintain patency.

SUGGESTED ANSWERS TO CHAPTER EXERCISES

Cue Recognition

29.1: Observe for other signs and symptoms of respiratory distress because oxygen saturation readings may not be accurate in dark-skinned individuals.

29.2: Make sure the cannula is in the patient's nose and that the tubing is not kinked or disconnected. Check pulse oximeter reading and observe for other signs and symptoms of hypoxia.

Critical Thinking & Clinical Judgment

Miss Israel

1. Bubbling in the water seal chamber indicates a leak in the system. Vigorous bubbling may indicate a large leak.
2. The HCP should be contacted immediately. After checking the patient, check the entire system for cracks or leaks and correct any problems discovered.
3. 50 mL.

Mr. Singh

1. Mr. Singh plugged his tracheostomy while the cuff was still inflated, so no air could get to his lungs. If the plug is not removed immediately, he will be totally unable to breathe.
2. To prevent this from happening in the future, teach Mr. Singh how his tracheostomy tube works and how to care for it. Show him how to check the pilot balloon if he is unsure.
3. ***Immediately*** remove the plug!
4. "Answered call for help at 12:30, found patient dark red in color, unable to breathe, trach plugged. Trach unplugged, respirations restored, vital signs stable. Patient stated he plugged trach so he could talk to his friend. Function of trach cuff explained to patient and friend. Both verbalize understanding to only plug trach when cuff is deflated or call nurse if unsure."

Additional Resources

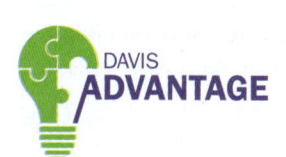

Go to Davis Advantage to complete your learning: strengthen understanding, apply your knowledge, and prepare for the Next Gen NCLEX®.

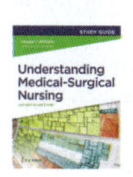

A Study Guide is also available.

CHAPTER 30
Nursing Care of Patients With Upper Respiratory Tract Disorders

Jennifer A. Otmanowski, Paula D. Hopper

KEY TERMS

dysphagia (dis-FAY-jee-ah)
epistaxis (EP-uh-STAX-is)
exudate (EKS-yoo-date)
laryngectomee (lare-in-JEK-tuh-mee)
laryngitis (lare-in-JY-tis)
myalgia (my-AL-jyah)
septoplasty (SEP-toh-plas-tee)
pharyngitis (fair-in-JY-tis)
rhinitis (ry-NY-tis)
rhinoplasty (RY-noh-plas-tee)
sinusitis (SY-nuh-SY-tis)

CHAPTER CONCEPTS

Comfort
Grief and loss
Infection
Oxygenation

LEARNING OUTCOMES

1. Explain the pathophysiology of disorders of the upper respiratory tract.
2. Describe etiologies, signs, and symptoms of disorders of the upper respiratory tract.
3. Describe current therapeutic measures for disorders of the upper respiratory tract.
4. Plan nursing care for the patient with an upper respiratory disorder.
5. Discuss how you will know whether your care has been effective.
6. Identify the special needs of the patient who has undergone a laryngectomy.

Disorders of the upper respiratory tract include problems occurring in the nose, sinuses, pharynx, larynx, and trachea. Many of these problems are minor illnesses that can be cared for at home. Others can become serious if they are not recognized and treated in a timely manner.

DISORDERS OF THE NOSE AND SINUSES

Epistaxis
Pathophysiology
Epistaxis is commonly known as a nosebleed. The nose can bleed from the anterior or posterior region. Anterior bleeds are much more common and originate from a group of vessels called the Kiesselbach plexus. Anterior bleeds are easier to locate and treat than posterior bleeds. The blood vessels of the posterior nose are larger, and bleeding can be severe and difficult to control.

Etiology
The most common cause of epistaxis is dry, cracked mucous membranes. Trauma, forceful nose blowing, nose picking, and tumors are also factors. Anything that reduces the blood's ability to clot, such as hemophilia or leukemia, regular aspirin use, anticoagulant therapy, or chemotherapy, can predispose a patient to nosebleeds. Cocaine use can also cause epistaxis, as can inhaled steroids used for respiratory conditions. High blood pressure can prolong a nosebleed but is not usually the cause.

Therapeutic Measures

Instruct a patient with a nosebleed to sit in a chair and lean forward slightly to avoid aspirating or swallowing blood. If the patient swallows blood, it will be difficult to determine the extent of bleeding. Also, it might cause nausea and vomiting. Be sure to wear gloves and follow standard precautions. Pinch the nares at the soft part of the nose together for 15 minutes (5 minutes in children) to stop bleeding. Do not release pressure during this time. Ice packs to the nose and eye area may be used to constrict the bleeding vessels.

If first aid measures cannot stop bleeding, the health-care provider (HCP) may attempt more invasive treatment. Local application of a vasoconstrictive agent such as oxymetazoline (Afrin) might be used to constrict the bleeding vessels. If the bleeding vessels can be located, the HCP may cauterize them by use of an electrical cauterizing device or by application of silver nitrate.

Gauze may be used to pack the anterior nasal cavity firmly but gently, usually with half-inch petroleum or iodoform gauze. Placement and removal of packing can be uncomfortable for the patient. If there is time, administer an analgesic before the procedure. Petroleum jelly on the packing helps prevent gauze from adhering to the nasal mucosa. If the packing is to remain in place for several days, it is coated with an antibiotic ointment to reduce the risk of infection.

Commercial products such as compressed sponges and nasal tampons are available to pack the nose. For anterior and posterior bleeds, balloon catheters such as the Rapid Rhino device can be inserted and inflated near the bleeding vessels in the nasal cavity (Fig. 30.1). The inflated balloon places pressure on the vessels to stop the bleeding. A small Foley catheter can also be used for this procedure. If these measures are not effective, materials such as a gelatin sponge or a tiny coil can be inserted into the bleeding artery. Patients who are treated for posterior bleeding are typically hospitalized until they are stable.

If the patient has lost a significant amount of blood, IV fluid replacement or a transfusion may be needed. Nosebleeds rarely cause death because blood loss lowers blood pressure, which in turn slows the bleeding. Ultimately, the cause of the epistaxis is determined and corrected if possible. Rarely, surgical correction may be necessary for repeat episodes of epistaxis.

Nursing Care for the Patient With Epistaxis

Monitor bleeding, noting the amount and color of drainage. Monitor vital signs and hemoglobin level for signs of excessive blood loss. If the patient swallows repeatedly, inspect the back of the throat for bleeding. If bleeding does not stop within 10 to 15 minutes or worsens, notify a registered nurse (RN) or HCP immediately.

If posterior packing has been used, monitor the patient for airway obstruction from a slipped device. Know how to remove the device in case of emergency. Institute comfort measures and maintain the placement of the external portion of the device. The HCP will remove the packing or catheter. Once bleeding is controlled, caution the patient not to blow the nose for up to 48 hours and to avoid nose picking. The patient should also avoid bending over, which can increase pressure in the nose. If the cause of the bleeding is dryness, the patient could use nasal saline spray or a room humidifier.

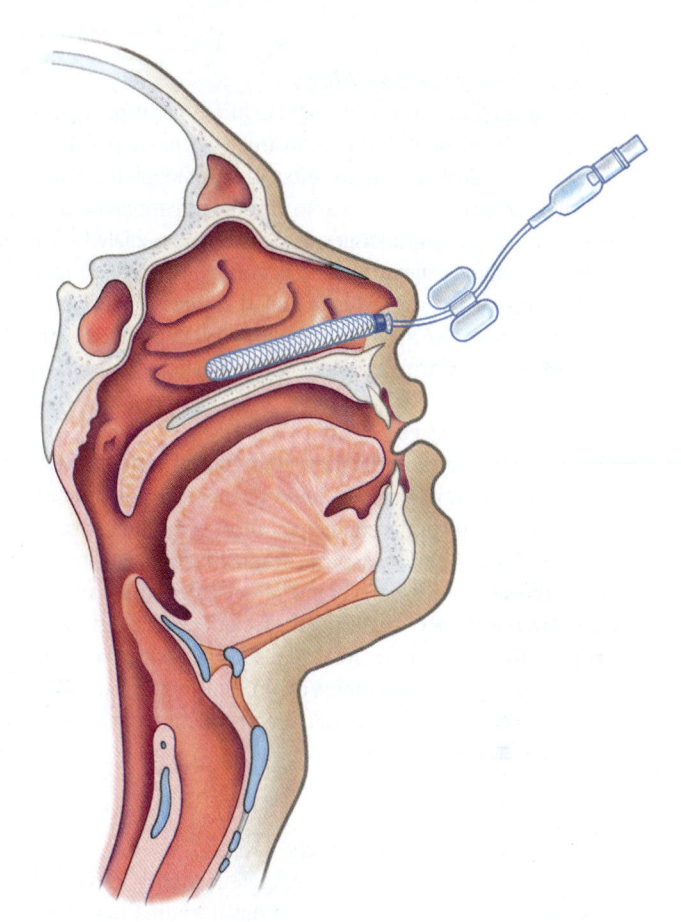

FIGURE 30.1 Rapid Rhino. Courtesy of ArthroCare, Inc., Austin, TX.

CRITICAL THINKING & CLINICAL JUDGMENT

Mr. Jondahl is brought to the emergency department with a nosebleed. His vital signs are blood pressure 140/90 mm Hg, pulse 92 beats per minute, and respirations 20 breaths per minute. He states that he has never had a nosebleed before. He denies any history of coagulation disorders. His current medications include captopril (Capoten), furosemide (Lasix), and ibuprofen (Motrin).

Critical Thinking (The Why)
1. Which of Mr. Jondahl's medications may be contributing to his nosebleed?

Clinical Judgement (The Do)
2. What should you do for Mr. Jondahl?

Suggested answers are at the end of the chapter.

Nasal Polyps
Pathophysiology and Etiology
Polyps are grapelike clusters of mucosa in the nasal passages. They are usually benign, but can obstruct the nasal passages and may be complicated by sinus infections. Although the exact cause is unknown, they are related to chronic inflammation and often occur in people with allergies. They are also associated with cystic fibrosis. Some patients with nasal polyps also have asthma and are allergic to aspirin. This is called *aspirin-exacerbated respiratory disease (AERD)*. People with AERD produce high levels of leukotrienes, which promote inflammation.

Therapeutic Measures
Control of allergy symptoms may help control polyp development. Oral antihistamines, leukotriene antagonists, or nasal corticosteroid sprays can help control symptoms. Some patients may benefit from aspirin desensitization and treatment. Antibiotics are used if there is a related sinus infection. If polyps obstruct breathing, they can be removed in an outpatient procedure under local anesthesia, using laser or endoscopic surgery. Patients must avoid aspirin products after surgery, as they increase the risk of postoperative bleeding and recurrence of the polyps.

Deviated Septum
Pathophysiology and Etiology
The septum dividing the nasal passages is slightly deviated in most adults. This may result from nasal trauma but often has no cause. Some septa may be so deviated that they block sinus drainage or interfere with breathing.

Signs and Symptoms
The patient may report a chronically stuffy nose or discomfort from blocked sinus drainage. Some patients have headaches, sinus infections, or nosebleeds.

Therapeutic Measures
Symptoms may be treated with decongestants, antihistamines, or intranasal cortisone sprays to reduce inflammation. However, if the deviated septum is causing chronic problems, a **septoplasty** can be done. This surgery involves revising or removing the deviated portion of the septum. Nasal packing is then placed to reduce bleeding. This is typically done as an outpatient surgical procedure under local anesthesia.

Nursing Care for the Patient After Septoplasty
After surgery, monitor vital signs and bleeding until the patient is stable. Excessive swallowing should alert you to check for blood running down the back of the throat. The patient will have nasal packing and a "mustache dressing" of folded gauze under the nose to catch drainage.

Most patients are discharged home once they are stable, and so the nurse will need to prepare the patient for caring for themselves at home. Box 30.1 details additional care and instructions following nasal surgery.

Box 30.1 Patient Education
Nasal Surgery

1. Your nose will feel stuffy and may drain. Change the moustache dressing as often as needed. Do *not* blow your nose. If you must sneeze, do so with your mouth open.
2. Avoid strenuous exercise, including swimming, for several weeks.
3. Drink plenty of fluids unless your health-care provider (HCP) advises otherwise.
4. Use a cool mist vaporizer to humidify air and prevent nasal drying.
5. Keep your head elevated on two pillows or sleep in a recliner chair.
6. Expect some bruising around your eyes.
7. Use an ice pack on your face to help reduce swelling and bruising.
8. Take pain medication as prescribed. Antibiotics may be prescribed if packing is in place.
9. Avoid aspirin because it can increase bleeding.
10. Request a stool softener if needed to avoid straining to have a bowel movement.
11. Call your HCP if you experience uncontrolled bleeding, excessive swelling, or a fever.
12. Avoid alcohol and smoking. Alcohol can increase congestion; smoking can delay healing.
13. Return to see your HCP for removal of packing as directed. Check hospital or surgeon policy for specific instructions.

Rhinoplasty
Rhinoplasty is surgical reconstruction of the nose, usually for cosmetic purposes or to correct deformity caused by trauma. Nursing care is similar to care for the patient after septoplasty.

Sinusitis
Pathophysiology and Etiology
Sinusitis is inflammation of the mucosa of one or more sinuses. It can be either acute or chronic. Chronic sinusitis is diagnosed if symptoms have existed for more than 3 months and are unresponsive to treatment. The maxillary and ethmoid sinuses are the most commonly affected. The inflammation is often the result of a bacterial infection. It may follow a cold or other viral upper respiratory illness. Because the mucous lining of the nose and sinuses is continuous, nasal organisms easily travel to the sinuses. When the infected mucous lining of the sinuses swells, drainage is

• WORD • BUILDING •

nasoseptoplasty: naso—nose + septo—septum + plasty—to mold, as in plastic surgery
rhinoplasty: rhin—nose + plasty—to mold, as in plastic surgery
sinusitis: sinu—sinus + itis—inflammation

blocked. Bacteria that normally reside in the sinuses multiply in the retained secretions. The most common infecting organisms are *Streptococcus pneumoniae* and *Haemophilus influenzae*. Allergies, nasal polyps, fungal infection, or intubation with a nasotracheal or nasogastric tube can increase the risk of sinusitis.

Signs and Symptoms
The patient usually has pain over the region of the affected sinuses and purulent nasal discharge. If a maxillary sinus is affected, the patient will have pain over the cheek and upper teeth. In ethmoid sinusitis, pain occurs between and behind the eyes. Pain in the forehead typically indicates frontal sinusitis. Fever may be present in acute infection, with or without generalized fatigue and foul breath.

Diagnostic Tests
Uncomplicated sinusitis may be diagnosed on the basis of symptoms alone. If repeated episodes occur, x-ray examination, nasal endoscopy, computed tomography (CT) scan, or magnetic resonance imaging (MRI) may be done to confirm the diagnosis and determine the cause. Nasal discharge may be cultured to determine appropriate antibiotic therapy.

Therapeutic Measures
Treatment is aimed at relieving pain and promoting sinus drainage. Nasal irrigation with sterile normal saline solution, or solution made at home with water that has been boiled and cooled, helps some sufferers of chronic sinusitis. Corticosteroids, usually via a nasal spray (e.g., fluticasone [Flonase]), reduce inflammation. Warm, moist packs over the affected sinus for 1 to 2 hours twice a day may help decrease inflammation. Acetaminophen or ibuprofen is given for pain and fever. Oral fluids and a room humidifier can help loosen secretions. Antihistamines dry and thicken secretions and usually are avoided. Antibiotics are not recommended for most sinus infections unless the symptoms continue after 7 days. Surgery may be necessary in cases where anatomic abnormalities are present.

Nursing Care for the Patient With Sinusitis
Instruct the patient to increase water intake to 8 to 10 glasses per day unless contraindicated. Excess water might be contraindicated in patients with fluid overload, such as those with cardiovascular or kidney disease. Pressure may be relieved if the patient maintains a semi-Fowler position, as in a reclining chair. Explain the use of warm and moist packs, analgesics, and prescribed medications. If antibiotics are ordered, instruct the patient to finish the antibiotic prescription even if they are feeling better before it is completed. Advise the patient or caregiver to call the HCP if pain becomes severe or if signs of complications, such as a change in level of consciousness, occur.

Sleep Apnea
Pathophysiology and Etiology
The patient with obstructive sleep apnea (OSA) has periods of apnea during sleep. This most often occurs when sleeping supine. The muscles of the throat relax, and the tongue and soft tissues fall back to obstruct the airway (Fig. 30.2). The resulting hypoxemia sends a signal to take a breath, causing a sudden, loud inhalation. This can occur up to 100 times an hour throughout the night. Men are affected more often

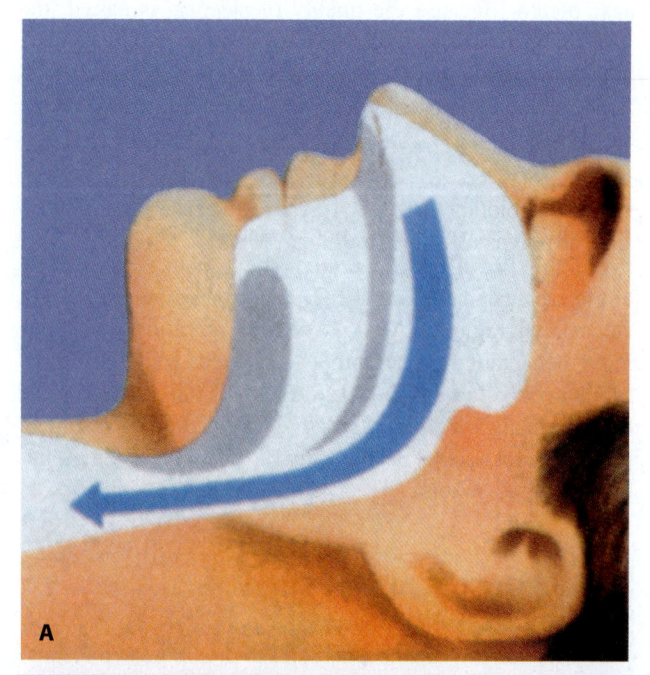

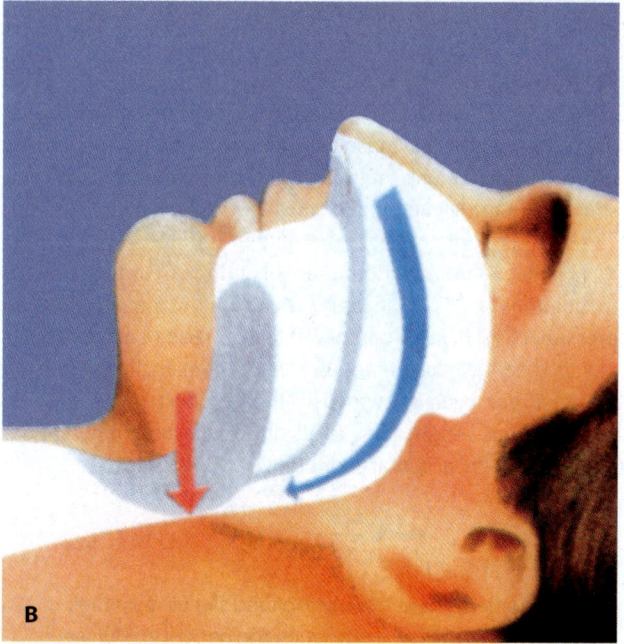

FIGURE 30.2 Obstructive sleep apnea (OSA). (A) Normal open airway. (B) Obstructed airway in OSA. Courtesy of Philips Respironics, Murrysville, PA.

than women, as are those who are overweight, are smokers, or have high arched palates or receding jawlines. OSA is associated with increased risk for heart disease, high blood pressure, stroke, and diabetes.

Signs and Symptoms
Ask the sleeping partner of someone with sleep apnea, and they will tell you that sleep apnea is noisy. When the tongue falls back and obstructs the airway, the result is total silence. When breathing resumes, it is like a very loud snore. Spouses often find themselves lying awake waiting for the next breath. Because the quality of sleep is impaired, the sufferer may awaken feeling unrested and with a headache, be sleepy throughout the day, and may have difficulty with memory and attention. Sudden sleepiness can make driving dangerous.

Diagnostic Tests
A sleep study (nocturnal polysomnography) involves an overnight stay at a sleep center. The patient is hooked up to electroencephalogram (EEG), electrocardiogram (ECG), electromyography (EMG), oxygen saturation, and eye movement monitors and then observed while sleeping. Many people find it somewhat difficult to fall asleep hooked up to so many wires, but a sedative would alter the results of the test. A less-sophisticated form of the test can sometimes be performed at home.

> **PRACTICE ANALYSIS TIP**
> Linking NCLEX-PN® to Practice
> The LPN/LVN will provide measures to promote sleep/rest.

Therapeutic Measures
Alcohol or sedatives at bedtime can worsen apnea by increasing relaxation of the muscles in the pharynx and should be avoided. The patient should avoid sleeping on the back and stop smoking. A patient can call 1-800-QUIT-NOW (1-800-784-8669) to connect with the state quit line.

Evidence-based guidelines involve three treatment recommendations: (1) weight loss, (2) continuous positive airway pressure (CPAP; see Chapter 29), and (3) use of a mandibular advancement device (a mouthpiece to advance the mandible). Exercise has been shown to lead to modest improvements even without weight loss. If all other measures have failed, surgery may be necessary to remove excess tissue.

> **NURSING CARE TIP**
> If your patients have trouble avoiding sleeping on their back, have them sew a pocket on the back of an old tee shirt and put a tennis ball in it. As soon as patients roll over onto the ball, they will quickly be back on their side!

INFECTIOUS DISORDERS

Viral Rhinitis/Common Cold
Pathophysiology and Etiology
Rhinitis (also called coryza) is inflammation of the nasal mucous membranes. The release of histamine and other substances causes vasodilation and edema. It may occur as a reaction to allergens (sometimes called *hay fever*) such as pollen, dust, molds, or some foods. It may also be caused by viral or bacterial infection. Viral rhinitis is another name for the common cold. The most common cold virus is the rhinovirus, which is contagious.

Signs and Symptoms
Common symptoms include nasal congestion, localized itching, sneezing, sore throat, and nasal discharge. Viral or bacterial rhinitis may also be accompanied by fever and malaise. Sometimes it is difficult to differentiate between a cold and influenza (flu); see Table 30.1.

Diagnostic Tests
A throat culture or rapid flu test can help identify whether symptoms are caused by the flu virus.

Prevention
Staying away from others who are ill and good hand hygiene are the best preventive measures.

Therapeutic Measures
Treatment of viral rhinitis is symptomatic. Because colds are caused by viruses, antibiotics are not effective. Inappropriate use of antibiotics can lead to antibiotic-resistant infections. Explain that taking antibiotics for a viral infection is not only ineffective but also potentially dangerous.

Acetaminophen can be used for generalized discomfort. Decongestants cause vasoconstriction, which reduces swelling and congestion. Any medications that cause vasoconstriction should be used cautiously in patients with heart disease or hypertension. Cough syrups and cold medicines should be used with caution. They do not treat the underlying cause of the cold and often contain several medications, many of which are not really needed. Teach the patient that rest and fluids are the most effective treatment (see "Nursing Care Plan for the Patient With an Upper Respiratory Infection"). Echinacea, vitamin C, and zinc are alternative remedies that might help reduce the severity or length of symptoms by supporting the immune system. However, there is not enough evidence to be sure at this time. Patients should take precautions to avoid spreading their illness to others, including handwashing and covering their nose when coughing or sneezing. (See cough etiquette guidelines in Chapter 8.)

• WORD • BUILDING •
rhinitis: rhin—nose + itis—inflammation

Table 30.1
Differentiating Respiratory Tract Infections

Signs and Symptoms	Cold	Influenza	Bacterial Infection
Onset	Slow	Sudden	Usually slow
Fever	None or low grade	Common, may exceed 101°F (38.3°C)	Common, may exceed 101°F (38.3°C)
Headache	Rare	Common	Less common
Muscle Aches	Less common	Common, may be severe	Less common
Cough	Present	Present, usually dry	Present, may be dry or productive
Chest Pain	Absent	Common	Common
Fatigue	Slight	Common, prolonged, may be severe	Common
Runny Nose	Common	Less common	Less common
Sore Throat	Common	Less common	Less common
Complications	Rare	Pneumonia	Pneumonia
Treatment	Rest and fluids	Rest and fluids, antiviral agents in some cases	Antibiotics

Evidence-Based Practice

Clinical Question
Can the common cold be prevented?

Evidence
Researchers compared one group who participated in mindfulness-based stress reduction and one group who participated in moderate exercise, to a control group. Both the mindfulness group and the exercise group experienced fewer incidences of acute respiratory infection and the common cold and missed fewer days of work than the control group.

Implications for Nursing Practice
Patients can take an active role in preventing acute respiratory infections.

Reference: Barrett, B., Hayney, M. S., Muller, D., Rake, D., Brown, R., Zgierska, A. E., Barlow, S., Hayer, S., Barnet, J. H., Torres, E. R., & Coe, C. L. (2018). Meditation or exercise for preventing acute respiratory infection (Mepari-2): A randomized controlled trial. *PLoS ONE 13*(6): e0197778. https://doi.org/10.1371/journal.pone.0197778

Pharyngitis

Pathophysiology and Etiology

Pharyngitis, or inflammation of the pharynx, is usually related to bacterial or viral infection. It may also occur from trauma to the tissues. From 5% to 15% of pharyngitis cases are caused by beta-hemolytic streptococci, commonly known as *strep throat*. If strep throat is not treated with antibiotics, it can lead to rheumatic fever, glomerulonephritis, or other serious complications.

Signs and Symptoms

The most common symptom of pharyngitis is a sore throat. Some patients may also experience **dysphagia** (difficulty swallowing). The throat appears red and swollen, and **exudate** (drainage or pus) may be present. Exudate usually signifies bacterial infection and may be accompanied by fever, chills, headache, and generalized malaise.

Diagnostic Tests

The HCP may order a rapid streptococcal antigen test or a throat culture and sensitivity test (see Chapter 29) to identify the causative organism and determine which antibiotic will be effective.

Therapeutic Measures

If the pharyngitis is bacterial, antibiotics are ordered. Penicillin is commonly used for streptococcal infection. Acetaminophen or throat lozenges may be used to relieve discomfort. Saltwater gargles (one-quarter teaspoon of salt in a glass of warm water)

• WORD • BUILDING •

pharyngitis: pharyng—pharynx + itis—inflammation
dysphagia: dys—bad + phagia—to swallow
exudate: to sweat out

Nursing Care Plan for the Patient With an Upper Respiratory Infection

Nursing Diagnosis: *Impaired Comfort* related to infectious process
Expected Outcomes: The patient will be comfortable as evidenced by statement of increased comfort and ability to swallow and sleep at night.
Evaluation of Outcomes: Does the patient express comfort? Is the patient able to sleep?

Intervention	Rationale	Evaluation
Collect data on the cause of discomfort (e.g., malaise, muscle aches, fever, sore throat).	Knowing the cause of discomfort helps guide intervention.	Can interventions be directed toward specific symptoms?
Offer acetaminophen or NSAIDs as ordered.	Analgesics relieve pain. Antipyretics relieve fever, which may contribute to discomfort.	Do analgesics/antipyretics relieve symptoms?
Offer throat lozenges, saltwater, or honey gargles as ordered for irritated throat.	Lozenges or gargles soothe irritated mucous membranes.	Do measures relieve throat irritation?
Encourage rest.	Physical stress increases need for sleep. Rest boosts immune function.	Is patient resting comfortably?
Humidified air.	A humidifier may be used but needs to be cleaned regularly. The patient can sit in the bathroom with a warm shower running for a few minutes.	Is patient's congestion lessened? Is the throat less irritated?

Nursing Diagnosis: *Hyperthermia* related to infectious process
Expected Outcomes: The patient will have a temperature lower than 103°F (39.4°C) and show no signs/symptoms of dehydration.
Evaluation of Outcomes: Is the patient's fever controlled at a safe level? Is the patient well hydrated?

Intervention	Rationale	Evaluation
Monitor temperature daily; every 4 hours if fever present.	Screening helps detect temperature changes early.	Is patient febrile?
If patient begins chilling, recheck temperature when chilling subsides.	Chilling indicates rising temperature.	Is chilling present? Should temperature be checked more often?
Monitor for signs of dehydration (e.g., dry skin and mucous membranes, thirst, weakness, hypotension).	Fever causes loss of body fluids.	Are signs of dehydration present?
Encourage oral fluids if not contraindicated.	Fluids prevent or treat dehydration.	Is patient taking fluids well?
Administer antipyretic such as acetaminophen if fever is higher than 102°F (39°C) or for discomfort.	Antipyretics reduce fever. Fever enhances immune function and so should be treated only if high, if patient has a history of febrile seizures, or if patient is uncomfortable.	Is fever higher than 102°F (39°C)? Are antipyretics indicated? Are they effective?
If fever rises above 103°F (39.4°C) in an adult, contact health-care provider (HCP).	A fever above 103°F (39.4°C) can indicate more serious infection and may require treatment.	Is fever above 103°F? Has HCP been contacted? (*Note:* Ask pediatrician about fever in a child.)

or honey mixed with warm water help soothe inflamed tissues. Encourage fluids (if not contraindicated) and rest. (See "Nursing Care Plan for the Patient With an Upper Respiratory Infection.")

Laryngitis

Pathophysiology and Etiology
Laryngitis is an inflammation of the mucous membrane lining the larynx (voice box). It can be caused by irritation from smoking, alcohol, chemical exposure, gastroesophageal reflux disease (GERD), voice strain, or a viral, fungal, or bacterial infection. It is most often associated with upper respiratory infection or voice strain. Laryngeal cancer can also cause laryngitis symptoms.

Signs and Symptoms
The most common symptom is hoarseness. Cough, dysphagia, or fever may also be present.

Diagnostic Tests
The HCP may use a tiny mirror to view the larynx. If hoarseness persists for more than 2 weeks, a laryngoscopy and biopsy may be done to rule out cancer of the larynx.

Therapeutic Measures
Treatment includes rest, fluids, humidified air, and aspirin (adults only) or acetaminophen. Antibiotics are used if bacterial infection is present. Medication to control acid reflux is used if GERD is the cause. Encourage the patient to rest the voice. Rather than having the patient whisper, encourage the use of paper and pen, texting, or dry erase board to help the patient communicate. Throat lozenges may help increase comfort. Help the patient to identify and avoid causative factors. (See "Nursing Care Plan for the Patient With an Upper Respiratory Infection.")

Tonsillitis/Adenoiditis

Pathophysiology and Etiology
The tonsils are masses of lymphoid tissue that lie on each side of the oropharynx. They filter microorganisms to protect the lungs from infection. Tonsillitis occurs when the filtering function becomes overwhelmed with a virus or bacteria and infection results. The adenoids, a mass of lymphoid tissue located at the back of the nasopharynx, can also become involved. Tonsillitis is more common in children but is more serious when it occurs in adults. Tonsillitis is usually viral, but bacteria that are commonly associated with tonsillitis include *Streptococcus* species, *Staphylococcus aureus*, *H. influenzae*, and *Pneumococcus* species.

Signs and Symptoms
Tonsillitis usually begins suddenly with a sore throat, fever, chills, and pain on swallowing. Generalized symptoms include headache, malaise, and **myalgia**. On examination, the tonsils appear red and swollen and may have yellow or white exudate on them. If the adenoids are involved, the patient may experience snoring, a nasal obstruction, and a nasal tone to the voice.

Diagnostic Tests
A throat culture is done to discover the causative organism and determine effective treatment. A white blood cell count and differential can also help identify whether the infection is viral or bacterial. A chest x-ray may be done if respiratory symptoms are present.

Therapeutic Measures
Antibiotics are prescribed for bacterial infection. Acetaminophen, lozenges, and saline gargles help promote comfort. For care of the patient who is not having a tonsillectomy, see "Nursing Care Plan for the Patient With an Upper Respiratory Infection."

If tonsillitis becomes chronic or if breathing or swallowing is affected, a tonsillectomy may be considered, although this is not a common procedure in an adult. Enlarged tonsils may contribute to obstructive sleep apnea. An adenoidectomy may be performed at the same time. After the tonsillectomy, the patient is maintained in a semi-Fowler position to reduce swelling and promote drainage. Monitor the patient for signs of bleeding (e.g., frequent swallowing, observable bleeding, coughing up aspirated blood, or vomiting blood clots) and airway patency. Encourage fluids for hydration; cold fluids may help reduce pain, and gargling with cold water may reduce minor bleeding. Red-colored drinks are avoided because they interfere with observation for bleeding. Some surgeons recommend a soft diet for up to one week. A room humidifier helps prevent drying. Keep suction equipment available for emergencies.

> **CRITICAL THINKING & CLINICAL JUDGMENT**
>
> **Mrs. Hiler** is recovering after a tonsillectomy. She is sleeping, but you notice that she swallows every few seconds. She has an IV line of normal saline solution running at 100 mL per hour.
>
> **Critical Thinking (The Why)**
> 1. What could be causing the increased swallowing?
>
> **Clinical Judgment (The Do)**
> 2. What should you do?
> 3. At how many drops per minute should her IV run if the tubing has a drop factor of 15?
>
> *Suggested answers are at the end of the chapter.*

Respiratory Viruses

Pathophysiology and Etiology
Respiratory viruses such as influenza and the coronavirus (COVID-19) are easily transmitted via droplets from

• WORD • BUILDING •

laryngitis: laryng—larynx + itis—inflammation
myalgia: myo—muscle + algia—pain

coughs and sneezes of infected people. The incubation period for influenza is 1 to 3 days, and the incubation period for COVID-19 is 2 to 14 days. Older adults and those with comorbidities such as obesity, hypertension, cardiovascular disease, and diabetes are at increased risk for complications and even death from COVID-19. Individuals at risk for complications from influenza include those with neurological conditions, cardiovascular disease, and asthma or other respiratory disease.

Prevention

According to the Centers for Disease Control and Prevention (CDC), influenza led to more than 400,000 hospitalizations and 22,000 deaths during the 2019–2020 flu seasons (CDC, 2020). COVID-19 reached pandemic levels in 2020 with 375,000 deaths occurring in the United States (CDC, 2021). Black individuals have a disproportionately high rate of COVID-19 fatality. Social determinants of health, such as poverty and race/ethnicity, can have considerable negative effect on outcomes from COVID-19.

One of the Healthy People 2030 goals is to increase the proportion of people who get the flu vaccine every year (Office of Disease Prevention and Health Promotion, 2020). The CDC (Grohskopf et al, 2020) recommends a yearly flu vaccine for anyone older than 6 months of age. Current recommendations for the COVID-19 vaccine include anyone older than 5. Medicare covers the cost of a flu shot, yet many older adults do not get one. Emphasize to older people that they will not get the flu or COVID-19 from the shot because it does not contain a live virus. Once the vaccines have been administered, it takes about 2 weeks for antibodies to develop. Because new strains develop, the flu vaccine must be given every year. Whether the COVID-19 vaccine will be recommended yearly has not yet been determined. Other important preventive measures include hand hygiene; mask wearing; keeping hands away from the mouth, nose, and eyes; avoiding people with influenza or COVID-19; and avoiding crowds when cases are prevalent. Visit www.cdc.gov/flu for more information.

> **BE SAFE!**
> **AVOID FAILURE TO RESCUE!** Patients who have had severe reactions to eggs should receive the flu vaccine in a setting where reactions can be treated. Flu vaccines contain small amounts of egg protein. While rare, reactions can be deadly.

Signs and Symptoms

Symptoms of flu include abrupt onset of fever, chills, myalgia, sore throat, cough, general malaise, and headache. Flu can last for 2 to 5 days, with malaise lasting up to several weeks. The most common symptoms of COVID-19 include cough, myalgia, and headache, with some patients reporting changes in the sense of smell or taste. Recovery from COVID-19 varies from 2 weeks to 3 to 4 months for those with more severe disease.

Complications

The most common complication of influenza is pneumonia, which may be caused by the same virus as the flu or by a secondary bacterial infection. This should be suspected if the patient has persistent fever and shortness of breath or if the lungs develop crackles or wheezes. Most deaths from COVID-19 occur as the result of respiratory failure, and patients should seek medical attention for difficulty breathing.

> **PRACTICE ANALYSIS TIP**
> **Linking NCLEX-PN® to Practice**
> The LPN/LVN will identify clients in need of immunizations (required and voluntary).

> **CUE RECOGNITION 30.1**
> You are caring for a patient in long-term care recovering from COVID-19. This morning he is short of breath with an oxygen saturation of 87% on room air. What do you do?
>
> *Suggested answers are at the end of the chapter.*

Diagnostic Tests

Viral cultures of throat or nasal swabbing can be done to identify influenza, but results may take 3 to 10 days. Rapid tests can identify the presence of flu virus in less than 15 minutes in an office setting but are less reliable than cultures. Cultures may also be done to rule out bacterial infection. Nasal swabbing is also used for COVID-19 testing. Once influenza has been identified in a geographical area, HCPs will test less often and treat on the basis of symptoms.

Therapeutic Measures

Treatment is primarily symptomatic. Acetaminophen is given for fever, headache, and myalgia. Aspirin is avoided in children because it increases the risk of Reye syndrome. Rest and fluids are essential. Antibiotics are used only if a secondary bacterial infection is present.

Antiviral medications, such as zanamivir (Relenza, an inhaled agent) and oseltamivir (Tamiflu, an oral medication), may be used for influenza to reduce the severity and duration of symptoms and should be given within 48 hours of becoming ill to be effective. Antiviral agents may also be given prophylactically to high-risk people who have not been immunized for influenza or to all residents of an institution, regardless of their vaccination status, when an influenza outbreak occurs. Patients who are at a higher risk of complications from influenza include those ages 65 and older, pregnant or postpartum women, residents of long-term care, American Indians and Alaskan Natives, obese individuals, immunocompromised individuals, and those receiving glucocorticoids or other immunosuppressive medications.

Nursing Care for the Patient With a Respiratory Virus

Older adults or other high-risk patients may be hospitalized for treatment of influenza or COVID-19. These patients are closely monitored for complications. Listen to lung sounds and vital signs every 4 hours and monitor for dehydration. Report changes to an RN or HCP. Encourage rest and fluids (if not contraindicated) and provide comfort measures. Remind families not to give aspirin to children younger than 18 because of the risk of Reye syndrome. (See "Nursing Care Plan for the Patient With an Upper Respiratory Infection.")

BE SAFE!
AVOID FAILURE TO RECOGNIZE! Between 70% and 85% of deaths from influenza occur in adults 65 and older. Recognize symptoms of decline in the older adult with influenza, such as difficulty breathing or shortness of breath, a cough that improves then worsens, confusion, weakness, or unsteadiness.

PRACTICE ANALYSIS TIP
Linking NCLEX-PN® to Practice
The LPN/LVN will identify client risk and implement interventions.

CRITICAL THINKING & CLINICAL JUDGMENT
Mrs. Murdock is a 97-year-old resident of a long-term care facility who develops flu symptoms. She is lethargic, confused, and feverish. Because of her mental status changes, you want to send her to the hospital, but her son asks you to please keep her where she is. She has a history of chronic obstructive pulmonary disease (COPD) and diabetes.

Critical Thinking (The Why)
1. What are some interventions that could help prevent influenza?
2. What is a possible cause of her confusion?

Clinical Judgment (The Do)
3. What can be done now to prevent Mrs. Murdock from developing complications?
4. What other team members should you collaborate with to provide her care?

Suggested answers are at the end of the chapter.

Other Respiratory Viruses

West Nile virus is less deadly than some flu viruses but can still cause serious complications. West Nile virus is transmitted from birds to humans by mosquitoes. It causes either no symptoms or flu-like symptoms. However, in a few people, especially older adults, it can progress to encephalitis (inflammation of the brain) and meningitis (inflammation of the covering of the brain and spinal cord). Reinforce the use of mosquito repellent and the removal of standing water where mosquitoes lay eggs. There is no specific treatment for West Nile virus. Patients who develop complications are hospitalized for supportive care.

Other viruses that have caused concern in recent years include avian influenza (bird flu), severe acute respiratory syndrome (SARS), and H1N1 (swine flu).

MALIGNANT DISORDERS

Cancer of the Larynx
Pathophysiology
Cancer of the larynx (the voice box) usually develops in the squamous cells of the mucosal epithelium. It is evaluated on the basis of the tumor-node-metastasis (TNM) staging system described in Chapter 11. It is most often a primary cancer and can spread to the lungs, liver, or lymph nodes. The prognosis for a patient with laryngeal cancer is good with early diagnosis but is poor when diagnosis and treatment are delayed.

Etiology
Risk factors for cancer of the larynx include a history of alcohol and tobacco use. Exposure to industrial chemicals or hardwood dust, chronic overuse of the voice, and a diet low in fruits and vegetables are also factors along with exposure to human papilloma virus (HPV). Men are more likely to be affected than women.

Prevention
Prevention begins with education. You can educate patients about the relationship between cancer of the larynx and use of alcohol and tobacco. It is important to remind patients to report any signs and symptoms of cancer of the larynx because delayed diagnosis may mean metastasis of the cancer and a poor prognosis. Any hoarseness that lasts longer than 2 weeks should be investigated by an HCP.

Signs and Symptoms
The most common symptom is persistent hoarseness because the vocal cords are in the larynx (Table 30.2). The patient may have throat or ear pain, shortness of breath, a chronic cough, and difficulty swallowing. Stridor (a harsh, crowing sound when the patient breathes) may indicate a tumor obstructing the airway. Late signs include weight loss and halitosis (foul breath).

Diagnostic Tests
Laryngoscopic examination and biopsy are used to diagnose and determine the stage of laryngeal cancer. CT scan, MRI, or other diagnostic tests may determine presence or extent of metastasis.

Table 30.2
Laryngeal Cancer Summary

Signs and Symptoms	Hoarse voice Pain Cough Shortness of breath Difficulty swallowing Weight loss Foul breath
Diagnostic Tests	Examination with laryngeal mirror Laryngoscopy with biopsy Additional blood and radiographic studies to detect metastasis
Therapeutic Measures	Radiation therapy Chemotherapy (adjunct to radiation or surgery) Endoscopic laser surgery to destroy tumor Partial laryngectomy (preserves some voice) Radical neck dissection with total laryngectomy (loss of voice)
Priority Nursing Diagnoses	Ineffective Airway Clearance Acute Pain Impaired Verbal Communication Risk for Imbalanced Nutrition: Less Than Body Requirements Impaired Swallowing Grieving Disturbed Body Image

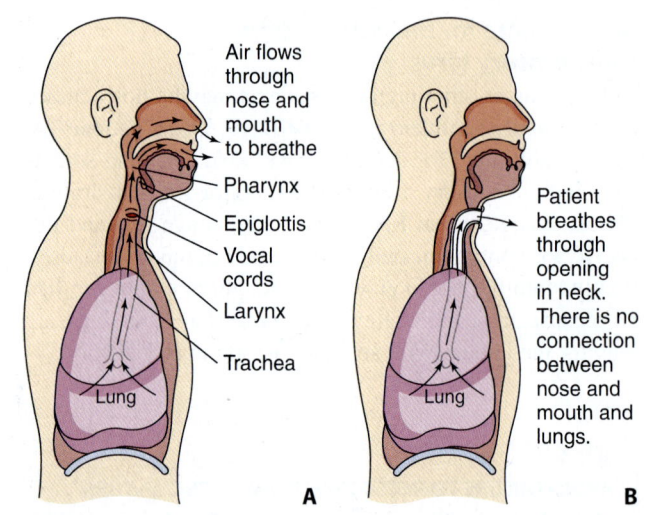

FIGURE 30.3 (A) Before laryngectomy. (B) After laryngectomy.

Therapeutic Measures

If laryngeal cancer is diagnosed early in the disease, it may be treatable with radiation therapy; this can preserve the patient's voice. Chemotherapy may be used with radiation or surgery but is not usually used alone. Surgery may be done at any stage of the disease. The larynx will be either partially or completely removed (Fig. 30.3). Laryngeal preservation surgery can be used in select patients to allow for possible swallowing and speech function. If cancer has spread beyond the larynx, a radical neck dissection, which removes adjacent muscle, lymph nodes, and tissue, may be done. Surgery can be done using laser technology, endoscopy, or traditional methods.

After a partial laryngectomy, the patient may have a permanently hoarse voice. With a total laryngectomy, the patient will have a permanent tracheostomy (called a laryngectomy) tube in place and no voice. The patient will need to learn alternative methods of communication.

Several alternatives for speech exist:

- Esophageal speech involves swallowing air and forming words as the air is regurgitated back up the esophagus.
- The electrolarynx is a battery-operated device placed against the neck that uses sound vibrations to help the patient form words. UltraVoice is an electronic device placed inside an upper denture or retainer. The patient speaks into a small microphone (Fig. 30.4A).
- Another alternative is a tracheoesophageal puncture (TEP), such as the Blom-Singer voice prosthesis, which uses a surgically implanted voice prosthesis that creates a valve between the trachea and esophagus. If the patient holds a finger over the laryngectomy, air is diverted into the esophagus and the patient forms words as the air exits the mouth (Fig. 30.4B).

All these devices require adjustment time. The patient will need support after discharge to continue to develop communication skills.

Nursing Process for the Patient Undergoing Total Laryngectomy

PREOPERATIVE CARE. In addition to routine preoperative teaching, the patient undergoing a total laryngectomy surgery must be prepared for breathing through a stoma in the neck and loss of ability to speak. Initial instruction in communication techniques should take place before surgery to prevent the patient from feeling panicky after surgery when he or she cannot speak. A variety of techniques and devices are available. Consult a speech therapist before surgery to provide a picture board, dry erase board, or paper and pencil (see Chapter 49). Instruct the patient to point to the picture that corresponds with the need or to write out his or her concern. A dietary consult is also important before surgery if the patient has been undernourished.

POSTOPERATIVE CARE
Data Collection. Collecting data about the patient's physical and psychosocial status, comfort, nutritional status, and ability to swallow is important both before and after

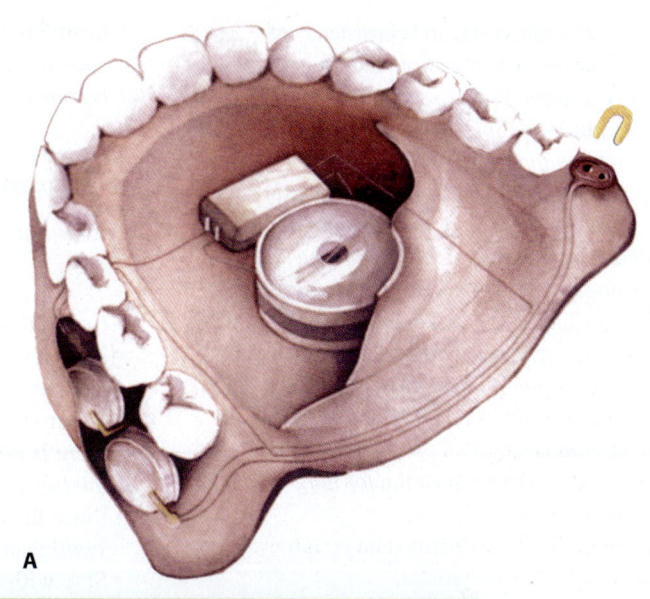

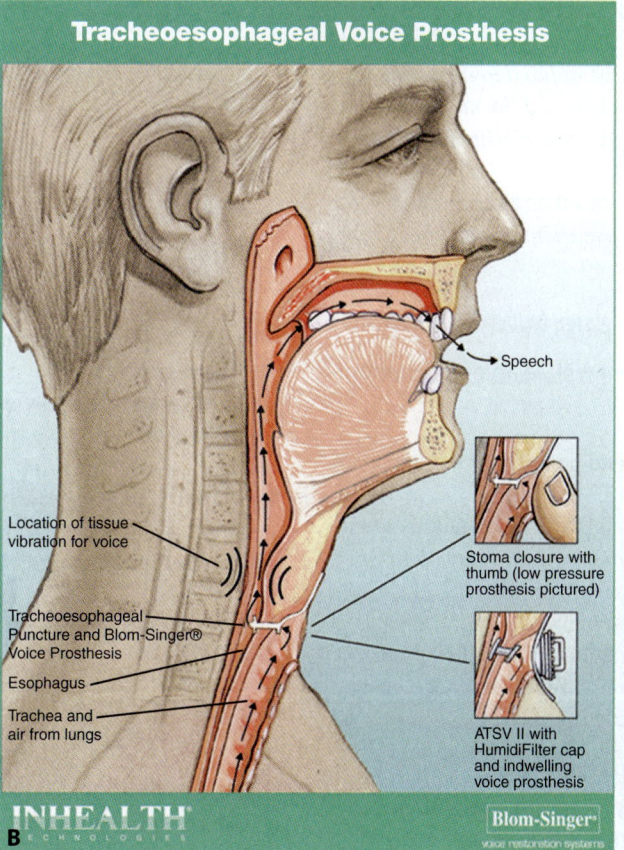

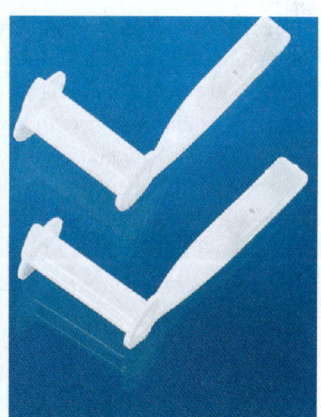

Chapter 30 Nursing Care of Patients With Upper Respiratory Tract Disorders 529

FIGURE 30.4 Devices to aid speech in the laryngectomy patient. (A) UltraVoice is an electronic device placed inside a denture or retainer; the patient speaks into a small microphone. Courtesy of UltraVoice Ltd., Newtown Square, PA. (B) The Blom-Singer voice prosthesis diverts air into the esophagus and out the mouth to form tracheoesophageal speech. Courtesy of InHealth Technologies, Carpinteria, CA.

surgery. After surgery, monitoring of airway patency and respiratory function takes priority. Monitor lung sounds, oxygen saturation, and arterial blood gases. In addition, be sure to collect data on the patient's understanding of the disease process and self-care needs after surgery. It is important to evaluate the patient's support systems and ability to cope with the partial or total loss of voice after surgery.

Nursing Diagnoses, Planning, and Implementation

Ineffective Airway Clearance related to excessive secretions and new tracheostomy/laryngectomy

EXPECTED OUTCOME: The patient will maintain a clear airway, as evidenced by clear lung sounds and ability to cough up secretions.

- Monitor and record amount, color, and consistency of secretions; vital signs; oxygen saturation; lung sounds; and signs of respiratory distress. *Visible secretions from the stoma, a drop in oxygen saturation (SpO_2), or an increase in crackles may indicate airway compromise and a need for suctioning. A change in amount or color of secretions, increased temperature, or presence of adventitious sounds can indicate infection and should be reported to the HCP immediately.*
- Provide tracheostomy care and suctioning according to agency policy (see Chapter 29) *to keep the airway clear.*
- Maintain strict sterile technique with tracheostomy care and suctioning. *Prevention of infection is essential, because the airway no longer has the protection of normal upper airway defense mechanisms.*
- Place the patient in semi-Fowler position *for lung expansion and more effective coughing.*
- Encourage the patient to deep breathe and cough every hour *to keep airway free of secretions.*
- Administer oxygen as ordered. A special tracheostomy collar should be used. *Supplemental oxygen helps maintain oxygenation. The oxygen must be applied to the stoma because there is no connection between the nose and lungs.*
- Provide room or oxygen humidification. *Humidification can help keep secretions mobile.*
- Avoid use of powders, sprays, or other airborne materials near the patient. *These can cause irritation or infection if they enter the laryngectomy.*

Impaired Verbal Communication related to loss of vocal cords

EXPECTED OUTCOME: The patient will be able to communicate their needs.

- Use a picture board or paper and pencil *so the patient can communicate without speaking.*
- Make sure the patient has a call light or bell nearby at all times. *Patients can become panicky if they have a need and no way to summon a nurse.*
- Work with the speech therapist and HCP to provide the patient with a method of communication that best fits their needs (see Fig. 30.4). *Different patients prefer different long-term communication methods.*

Risk for Imbalanced Nutrition: Less Than Body Requirements related to absence of oral feeding immediately following surgery and possible previous alcohol use or abuse

EXPECTED OUTCOME: The patient's weight will be within normal limits for height and age.

- Monitor weight. *Underweight or weight loss reflects inadequate nutrition.*
- Monitor parenteral nutrition or tube feedings after surgery until the neck has begun to heal and swallowing can be evaluated. *Nutrition must be maintained to support healing.*
- Consult a dietitian for nutrition guidance. If the patient has a history of alcohol abuse, they may have been undernourished before surgery. *You may need to advocate for the patient and ensure that they are receiving adequate calories for healing. A dietitian can assist with specific recommendations.*

Impaired Swallowing related to edema or presence of laryngectomy tube

EXPECTED OUTCOME: The patient will be able to swallow safely.

- Consult a speech therapist to assist with a swallowing assessment and recommendations. *Speech therapists are trained to assess and treat swallowing disorders.*
- Assure the patient that aspiration will not occur *because there is no longer a connection between the mouth and the lungs.*
- Place the patient in high-Fowler position *to make swallowing easier.*
- Stay with the patient during the first attempts *to eat to help alleviate anxiety.*

Situational low self-esteem related to loss of voice

EXPECTED OUTCOME: The patient will express feelings of loss and begin to plan for the future.

- Demonstrate compassion recognizing that the *inability to speak is a loss that cannot be underestimated. The patient may also be facing a career change if job-related exposure contributed to the disease or if loss of voice prevents return to a previously held job.*
- Actively listen to the patient's communication of feelings *to show your support and validate feelings.*
- Identify and involve the patient's support system. *Support of family and friends is important to the patient's long-term adjustment to a laryngectomy.*
- Contact the patient's clergy if patient wishes. *A religious counselor can help with grief and spiritual distress.*

Disturbed Body Image related to change in body structure and function

EXPECTED OUTCOME: The patient will verbalize acceptance of new laryngectomy and participate in self-care.

- Demonstrate an accepting attitude. *Patients are very aware of nurses' nonverbal behavior, and looks of distaste can be disturbing.*
- Allow the patient to share feelings if they indicate a need to do so. *This may help the patient to work through feelings about the changes to their body image.*
- With the patient's permission, contact a local support group that may have names of people who have had similar experiences who are willing to visit with the patient. *Such visitors can provide firsthand information and support.*
- Assist the patient to find ways to camouflage the change, such as scarves or necklines that conceal but do not obstruct the airway. *Camouflage can help the patient feel less conspicuous while protecting the airway.*

Evaluation. When evaluating the patient's progress toward goals, ask the following questions:

- Is the airway clear, without signs of infection or obstruction?
- Does the patient verbalize an acceptable level of comfort?
- Do the patient and significant others demonstrate understanding of self-care at home or have referrals to continue learning self-care at home?
- Does the patient indicate satisfaction with the level and quality of communication?
- Is the patient's weight stable?
- Is the patient able to swallow if taking oral nutrition?
- Is the patient able to grieve appropriately?
- Does the patient have someone to talk to if they wish to do so?
- Does the patient show acceptance of the laryngectomy by learning to care for it?

Note that many of these evaluative criteria are long term and may not be seen while the patient is hospitalized, so follow-up by a home health nurse is essential.

Patient Education. After determining the patient's readiness to learn, instruct the patient on self-care measures for the laryngectomy, including how to perform cleaning and suctioning (see Chapter 29). Instruct the patient to protect the laryngectomy from water and debris. Lightweight scarves or purchased products can protect the stoma. Involve the significant other or family whenever possible.

The patient must also be instructed to perform gentle range-of-motion exercises of the neck. Some patients may avoid extending the neck because of the location of the incision, causing muscle contracture.

Referral to a home health-care agency after discharge will provide assessment of the home environment as well as follow-up instruction. A social service referral may be made for financial or psychosocial concerns if needed. Consult with the HCP or check the local phone directory for **laryngectomee** support groups and refer the patient if appropriate. The local branch of the American Cancer Society may also be able to provide information. Assist the patient in finding resources to support alcohol and smoking cessation. Continued alcohol and tobacco use will increase the patient's risk of cancer recurrence.

To find additional information for laryngectomees, visit the National Cancer Institute Web site at www.cancer.gov.

Key Points

- Disorders of the upper respiratory tract include problems occurring in the nose, sinuses, pharynx, larynx, and trachea. Many of these problems are minor illnesses that can be cared for at home. Others can become serious if not recognized and treated in a timely manner.
- These disorders include epistaxis, nasal polyps, deviated septum, sinusitis, sleep apnea, common cold, pharyngitis, laryngitis, and tonsillitis. Influenza is in this category, and so is West Nile virus.
- If a deviated septum is causing chronic problems, a nasoseptoplasty can be done. This surgery involves revising or removing the deviated portion of the septum.
- Rhinoplasty is the surgical reconstruction of the nose, usually for cosmetic purposes. It may also be done to correct deformity caused by trauma.
- Sinusitis is inflammation of the mucosa of one or more sinuses. It can be either acute or chronic. Chronic sinusitis is diagnosed if symptoms have existed for more than 3 months and are unresponsive to treatment.
- The patient with obstructive sleep apnea has periods of apnea during sleep. It most often occurs when sleeping supine. The muscles of the throat relax, and the tongue and soft tissues fall back to obstruct the airway. The resulting hypoxemia sends a signal to take a breath, causing a sudden, loud inhalation up to 100 times an hour throughout the night.
- Respiratory viruses such as influenza and COVID-19 can cause serious complications and even death in vulnerable individuals. Patients should be encouraged to become immunized.
- Antiviral medications, such as zanamivir (Relenza, an inhaled agent) and oseltamivir (Tamiflu, an oral medication), may reduce the severity and duration of symptoms of the flu if given within 48 hours of becoming ill. Antiviral agents may also be given prophylactically to high-risk people who have not been immunized or to control outbreaks in high-risk situations, such as in long-term care facilities.
- Cancer of the larynx usually develops in the squamous cells of the mucosal epithelium. It is most often a primary cancer and can spread to the lungs, liver, or lymph nodes.
- The most common symptom is persistent hoarseness because the vocal cords are in the larynx. The patient may also have throat or ear pain, shortness of breath, a chronic cough, and difficulty swallowing. Stridor may indicate a tumor is obstructing the airway.
- If laryngeal cancer is diagnosed early in the disease, it may be treatable with radiation therapy. This treatment can preserve the patient's voice. Chemotherapy may be used with radiation or surgery, but it is not usually used alone. Surgery may be done at any stage of the disease. The larynx will be either partially or completely removed.

• WORD • BUILDING •

laryngectomee: laryng—larynx + ectome—excision (person who has undergone laryngectomy)

- After a partial laryngectomy, the patient may have a permanently hoarse voice. If a total laryngectomy is done, the patient will have a permanent tracheostomy (in this case, called a laryngectomy) tube in place and no voice. The patient will need to learn alternative methods of communication.

SUGGESTED ANSWERS TO CHAPTER EXERCISES

Cue Recognition
30.1: Roll up the head of the bed, start oxygen per your facility policy, and prepare for transfer to the hospital. Provide encouragement and emotional support to decrease anxiety.

Critical Thinking & Clinical Judgment
Mr. Jondahl
1. Explore the amount of ibuprofen being taken daily because NSDAIDs can interfere with platelet aggregation. In addition, high blood pressure can aggravate the bleeding.
2. Instruct a patient with a nosebleed to sit in a chair and lean forward slightly to avoid aspirating or swallowing blood. If the patient swallows blood, it will be difficult to assess the extent of bleeding. Wear gloves and follow standard precautions. Pinch the nares at the soft part of the nose together for 15 minutes to stop bleeding. Do not release pressure during this time. Ice packs to the nose and eye area may be used to constrict the bleeding vessels. Collaborate with the RN or HCP if these measures do not control bleeding.

Mrs. Hiler
1. Mrs. Hiler may be swallowing blood. Examine the back of her throat with a flashlight. Check vital signs for evidence of impending shock. Notify an HCP if bleeding is confirmed.
2. Continue to be vigilant for signs of bleeding (e.g., frequent swallowing or bright red blood from the mouth). Monitor for changes in vital signs and report even small changes to the RN or HCP. Contact the nurse (RN) for persistent bleeding, coughing up of aspirated blood, or vomiting of blood clots. Minor bleeding can be treated by having the patient gargle with cold water.
3. Use this formula to determine drops per minute:

$$\frac{100 \text{ mL}}{1 \text{ hour}} \times \frac{1 \text{ hour}}{60 \text{ minutes}} \times \frac{15 \text{ gtt}}{1 \text{ mL}} = 25 \text{ gtt per minute}$$

Mrs. Murdock
1. Mrs. Murdock's flu could probably have been prevented with a flu vaccination, but her son refused it because he believed it could cause her to get the flu. Good hand hygiene by staff and urging visitors not to visit when ill may have also helped.
2. Mrs. Murdock may be dehydrated.
3. If it is within 48 hours of symptom onset, an HCP may prescribe an antiviral agent to help reduce her symptoms and shorten the course of her illness. You should also monitor her closely for evidence of dehydration, bacterial infection, or pneumonia and report signs or symptoms immediately to the HCP. Monitor lung sounds and vital signs and indications of dehydration such as decreased skin turgor or dry mucous membranes and low blood pressure. In addition, you can provide fluids, acetaminophen, and deep breathing and coughing.
4. Collaborate with the HCP for medical interventions and to determine when hospitalization is necessary. Collaborate with the assistive personnel to assist the patient to take in adequate fluids and to monitor the vital signs. Collaborate with the infection control nurse and facility director on how to prevent the transmission of influenza to the other residents.

Additional Resources

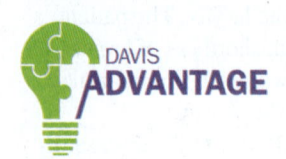

Go to Davis Advantage to complete your learning: strengthen understanding, apply your knowledge, and prepare for the Next Gen NCLEX®.

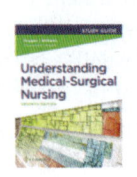

A Study Guide is also available.

CHAPTER 31
Nursing Care of Patients With Lower Respiratory Tract Disorders

Jennifer A. Otmanowski, Paula D. Hopper

KEY TERMS

anergic (AN-ur-jik)
antitussive (AN-tee-TUS-iv)
atelectasis (AT-eh-LEK-tah-sis)
atypical (ay-TIP-ih-kuhl)
blebs (BLEBS)
bronchiectasis (BRONG-key-EK-tah-sis)
bronchitis (brong-KY-tis)
bronchodilator (BRONG-koh-DY-lay-ter)
bronchospasm (BRONG-koh-spazm)
bullae (BUL-ah)
ectopic (ek-TOP-ik)
emphysema (EM-fih-SEE-mah)
empyema (EM-pye-EE-mah)
exacerbation (eg-ZAS-ur-BAY-shun)
expectorant (eks-PEK-tah-rant)
exudate (EKS-yoo-dayt)
hemoptysis (hee-MOP-tih-sis)
hemothorax (HEE-moh-THOR-aks)
induration (IN-doo-RAY-shun)
lobectomy (loh-BEK-tuh-mee)
mucolytic (MYOO-koh-LIT-ik)
paradoxical respiration (PEAR-uh-DOK-sih-kuhl RES-per-AY-shun)
pleurodesis (PLOO-roh-DEE-sis)
pneumonectomy (NOO-moh-NEK-tuh-mee)
pneumothorax (NOO-moh-THOR-aks)
polycythemia (PAW-lee-sy-THEE-mee-ah)
status asthmaticus (STAT-us az-MAT-ih-kus)
tachypnea (TAK-ip-NEE-uh)
thoracotomy (THOR-ah-KOT-ah-mee)

CHAPTER CONCEPTS

Acid–base balance
Infection
Oxygenation
Perfusion

LEARNING OUTCOMES

1. Explain the pathophysiology of each of the disorders of the lower respiratory tract.
2. Describe the etiologies, signs, and symptoms of each of the disorders.
3. Identify tests that are used to diagnose lower respiratory disorders.
4. Describe therapeutic measures used for disorders of the lower respiratory tract.
5. List data to collect when caring for patients with disorders of the lower respiratory tract.
6. Plan nursing care for patients with disorders of the lower respiratory tract.
7. Identify interventions for patients experiencing impaired gas exchange, ineffective airway clearance, or ineffective breathing pattern.
8. Explain how you will know whether your nursing interventions have been effective.

Disorders of the lower respiratory tract include problems of the lower portion of the trachea, bronchi, bronchioles, and alveoli. These disorders may be related to infection, noninfectious alterations in function, neoplasm (cancer), or trauma. Any pathological condition of the lower respiratory tract can seriously impair carbon dioxide and oxygen exchange.

INFECTIOUS DISORDERS

Acute Bronchitis

Bronchitis is an inflammation of the bronchial tree. The bronchial tree includes the right and left bronchi, secondary bronchi, and bronchioles. When the mucous membranes lining the bronchial tree become irritated and inflamed, excessive mucus is produced. The result is congested airways. Acute bronchitis is usually an isolated episode, caused by a virus. If bronchitis occurs more than 3 months out of the year for

• WORD • BUILDING •
bronchitis: bronch—airway + itis—inflammation

two consecutive years, chronic bronchitis is diagnosed. See the discussion of chronic bronchitis later in this chapter for more information that applies to both the acute and chronic forms.

Bronchiectasis

Pathophysiology

Bronchiectasis is a dilation of the bronchial airways (Fig. 31.1). The dilated areas become flabby and scarred. Bronchiectasis can remain localized or spread throughout the lungs. Secretions pool in these areas and are difficult to cough up. This creates an environment where bacteria can flourish, and infection is common.

Etiology

Bronchiectasis usually occurs secondary to another chronic respiratory disorder, such as cystic fibrosis, asthma, tuberculosis, bronchitis, or exposure to a toxin. Airway obstruction from a tumor or foreign body can also be a predisposing factor. Infection and inflammation of the airways in these underlying disorders weaken the bronchial walls and reduce ciliary function. Airway obstruction from excessive secretions then predisposes the patient to development of bronchiectasis. Vitamin D deficiency may play a role in bronchiectasis (Ferri et al, 2019).

Signs and Symptoms

The patient with bronchiectasis experiences recurrent lower respiratory infections. Sputum is copious and purulent. The accompanying cough can produce as much as 200 mL of thick, foul-smelling sputum in a single episode of coughing. Extreme airway inflammation may cause sputum to be bloody. If bronchiectasis is widespread throughout the lungs, the patient may experience dyspnea even with minimal exertion. Wheezes and crackles may be auscultated. Fever is present during active infection. Cor pulmonale (right-sided heart failure; covered in Chapter 26) and clubbing of the fingers may develop with chronic disease.

Diagnostic Tests

A chest x-ray examination is done, but it may not show early disease. A computed tomography (CT) scan provides a better view of the dilated airways. Bronchoscopy may be done, if needed. Sputum cultures determine infecting organisms and guide antibiotic therapy. Additional testing may be done to determine the cause of bronchiectasis.

Therapeutic Measures

Treatment is aimed at keeping the airways clear of secretions, controlling infection, and correcting the underlying problem, if possible. Antibiotics may be used intermittently or for prolonged periods. Azithromycin (Zithromax) may reduce **exacerbations** (acute worsening of symptoms). Measures to prevent infection, including vaccinations for flu and pneumonia, should be implemented. **Bronchodilators** relax smooth muscle in the airways to reduce obstruction. **Mucolytic** agents and **expectorants** help loosen and mobilize secretions so they can be coughed up. Bronchitol, a form of mannitol, is an inhaled mucolytic that promotes mucus clearance. It is a sugar that draws fluid into the airways to help liquefy mucus. Anti-inflammatory agents such as corticosteroids or leukotriene inhibitors reduce airway inflammation.

Chest physiotherapy (CPT) or a high-frequency chest wall oscillation vest can help mobilize secretions. Noninvasive positive-pressure ventilation (NIPPV; see Chapter 29) can help maintain oxygenation. Oxygen is used if hypoxemia is present. Oral fluids are encouraged. If the affected area of the lung is localized and symptoms are severe, surgery may be considered to remove the diseased area. Lung transplant may be considered in severe cases. Nursing care is found in "Nursing Care Plan for the Patient With a Lower Respiratory Tract Disorder."

> **NURSING CARE TIP**
> If your patient is coughing up a lot of sputum, line an emesis basin with a white tissue. This makes it easier to assess the color of the sputum and simplifies cleaning out the basin.

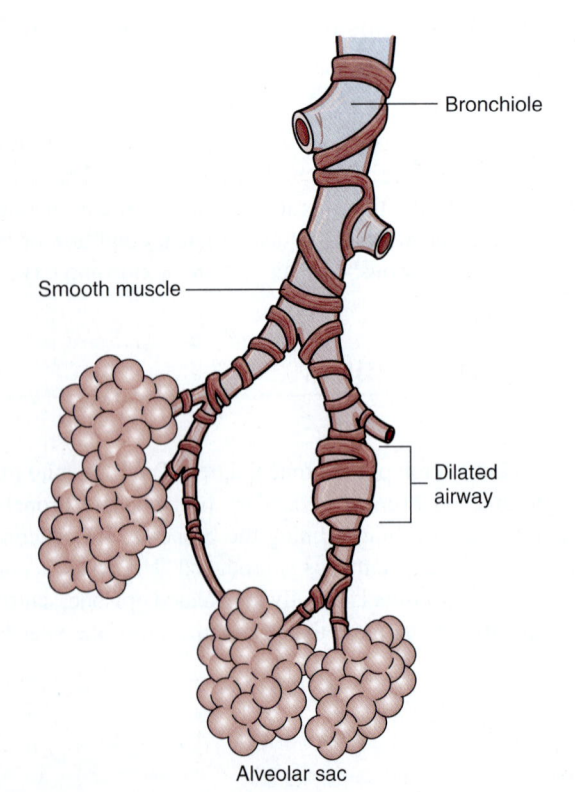

FIGURE 31.1 Bronchiectasis. Note dilated airway.

• WORD • BUILDING •
bronchiectasis: bronch—airway + ectasis—dilation or expansion
bronchodilator: broncho—airway + dilator—to expand
mucolytic: muco—mucus + lytic—break up
expectorant: ex—out of + pec—chest

Chapter 31 Nursing Care of Patients With Lower Respiratory Tract Disorders

Nursing Care Plan for the Patient With a Lower Respiratory Tract Disorder

Note: The most commonly used nursing diagnoses related to respiratory disorders are presented in the following care plan. This is not a care plan for any one respiratory disorder. Rather, use it as a reference when one of the nursing diagnoses applies to the patient, based on a thorough respiratory assessment.

Nursing Diagnosis: *Impaired Gas Exchange* related to decreased ventilation or perfusion as evidenced by partial pressure of oxygen (PaO_2) less than 80 mm Hg, partial pressure of carbon dioxide ($PaCO_2$) greater than 45 mm Hg, or peripheral capillary oxygen saturation (SpO_2) less than 90%, statement of dyspnea.
Expected Outcomes: The patient will experience improved gas exchange, as evidenced by improving arterial blood gases (ABGs) or pulse oximetry and acceptable level of dyspnea.
Evaluation of Outcomes: Are the patient's ABGs or SpO_2 improving? Does the patient state that dyspnea is resolved or controlled at an acceptable level?

Intervention	Rationale	Evaluation
Monitor ABG values and pulse oximetry as ordered.	PaO_2 less than 80 mm Hg, $PaCO_2$ greater than 45 mm Hg, or SpO_2 less than 90% indicate impaired gas exchange.	Are values within patient's baseline values?
Have the patient rate degree of dyspnea on a scale of 0 to 10, with 0 being dyspnea and 10 being worst dyspnea.	The patient's subjective report is the best measure of dyspnea; dyspnea indicates impaired gas exchange.	Is patient's degree of dyspnea within parameters that are acceptable to patient?
Assess lung sounds, respiratory rate and effort, use of accessory muscles.	Respiratory rate less than 12 per minute or more than 20 per minute or use of accessory muscles indicates distress. Diminished or adventitious lung sounds can indicate risk factors for impaired gas exchange.	Are lung sounds clear and audible? Is respiratory rate 12 to 20 per minute and unlabored?
Observe skin and mucous membranes for cyanosis.	Cyanosis indicates poor oxygenation. Oral mucous membrane cyanosis indicates serious hypoxia.	Are skin and mucous membranes cyanotic?
Monitor for confusion or changes in mental status.	Changes in mental status can signal impaired gas exchange.	Is patient alert and oriented? If not, could poor gas exchange be the reason?
Elevate head of bed or help patient to lean on over-bed table.	Upright positioning promotes lung expansion.	Did change of position relieve some distress?
Position with good lung dependent ("good lung down").	This position allows the healthier lung to be better perfused and increases gas exchange.	Is SpO_2 improved in this position?
Administer supplemental oxygen as ordered.	Supplemental oxygen decreases hypoxemia.	Is oxygen placed properly on patient? Does it provide relief from dyspnea?
Place a fan in patient's room or provide a handheld fan.	The handheld fan directed toward the face reduces feelings of breathlessness.	Is a fan available to patient, and does it help?
For severe dyspnea, ask health-care provider (HCP) about an order for IV morphine sulfate.	Low doses of IV morphine reduce anxiety and cause peripheral vasodilation, which helps relieve pulmonary edema.	Does morphine provide relief from dyspnea?
Teach patient relaxation exercises.	Relaxation exercises decrease perceived dyspnea.	Does patient use relaxation effectively?
For chronic disease, teach patient diaphragmatic and pursed-lip breathing. (See Chapter 29.)	Breathing exercises promote relaxation and increase CO_2 excretion.	Does patient use breathing exercises correctly? Do they help?

(nursing care plan continues on page 536)

Nursing Care Plan for the Patient With a Lower Respiratory Tract Disorder—cont'd

Intervention	Rationale	Evaluation
Encourage patient to stop smoking if patient is a current smoker.	Smoking is damaging to lungs and respiratory function.	Is patient receptive to smoking cessation? Are resources available?

Nursing Diagnosis: *Ineffective Airway Clearance* related to excessive secretions as evidenced by crackles or wheezes, and ineffective cough
Expected Outcome: The patient will have improved airway clearance as evidenced by clear breath sounds and ability to cough up secretions.
Evaluation of Outcome: Are the patient's breath sounds clear? Is the patient able to effectively cough up and expectorate secretions?

Intervention	Rationale	Evaluation
Assess lung sounds every 4 hours and as needed (prn).	Crackles and wheezes may indicate excess secretions in airways.	Do lung sounds indicate retained secretions?
Monitor amount, color, and consistency of sputum.	Thick, purulent sputum indicates infection and should be reported to the HCP.	Does sputum indicate infection?
Turn patient every 2 hours or encourage ambulating if able.	Movement mobilizes secretions.	Is patient mobile?
Encourage oral fluids; use cool steam room humidifier.	Hydration decreases viscosity of secretions and aids expectoration.	Is patient able to take oral fluids? Are secretions thin and easily expectorated?
Encourage patient to cough and deep breathe every hour and prn.	Controlled coughing following deep breaths is more effective in clearing the airway.	Does patient cough and deep breathe effectively?
Administer expectorants or mucolytics as ordered.	Expectorants help liquefy secretions and trigger the cough reflex.	Are expectorants effective?
If patient is unable to cough up secretions, suction per institution policy.	Suctioning is necessary to remove secretions when patient is unable to cough effectively.	Is suctioning necessary? Does it help remove secretions?
Obtain order for chest physiotherapy (CPT) or vibratory positive expiratory pressure (PEP) device, if indicated.	CPT and PEP help mobilize secretions.	Is CPT (or PEP) effective and well tolerated by patient?

Nursing Diagnosis: *Ineffective Breathing Pattern* related to anxiety or pain as evidenced by respiratory rate less than 12 per minute or greater than 24 per minute, labored or shallow respirations, and abnormal ABGs and SpO_2 values.
Expected Outcomes: The patient will maintain an effective breathing pattern as evidenced by a respiratory rate between 12 and 20 per minute that is even and unlabored, and ABG and oxygen saturation results within the patient's normal range.
Evaluation of Outcomes: Is the patient's respiratory rate within normal limits and unlabored? Does the patient's breathing pattern support normal ABG and SpO_2 values?

Intervention	Rationale	Evaluation
Assess respiratory rate, depth, and effort every 4 hours and prn.	Respirations less than 12 per minute or more than 20 per minute may indicate an ineffective pattern.	Is respiratory pattern ineffective?
Monitor ABG and oxygen saturation values.	An ineffective breathing pattern will not maintain oxygenation.	Is breathing pattern adversely affecting oxygenation?

Nursing Care Plan for the Patient With a Lower Respiratory Tract Disorder—cont'd

Intervention	Rationale	Evaluation
Determine and treat the cause of ineffective breathing pattern.	*Pain or anxiety can cause a patient to change the breathing pattern.*	Is a contributing factor identifiable and correctable?
Place patient in Fowler or semi-Fowler position.	*This allows for maximum chest expansion.*	Is patient in a comfortable position that enables adequate expansion?
Teach patient to use diaphragmatic breathing, with a regular 2-second in, 4-second out pattern.	*Breathing exercises promote relaxation and increase CO_2 excretion.*	Is patient able to demonstrate an effective breathing pattern?

Nursing Diagnosis: *Activity Intolerance* related to imbalance between oxygen supply and demand as evidenced by dyspnea or drop in SpO_2 with routine activity
Expected Outcomes: The patient will tolerate increasing activity level as appropriate based on prognosis, evidenced by stable respiratory rate and SpO_2 with activity. The patient will receive assistance with self-care until they can carry out own activities of daily living (ADLs).
Evaluation of Outcomes: Are the patient's care needs met by self or caregiver?

Intervention	Rationale	Evaluation
Assess amount of activity patient can tolerate without becoming short of breath (SOB).	*Patients should be encouraged to do as much as they can for themselves to avoid becoming deconditioned.*	What is patient able to do?
Monitor vital signs and oxygen saturation with activities.	*Respiratory and heart rates will rise and SpO_2 will drop if activity is not tolerated.*	Are vital signs and SpO_2 stable?
Allow patient to rest between activities. Bedrest may be needed during acute dyspnea.	*Even talking or eating can be exhausting to a patient who is dyspneic.*	Is patient able to catch his or her breath between activities?
Obtain bedside commode, shower chair, and handheld showerhead, if needed.	*Assistive devices can help patient conserve energy.*	Do assistive devices allow patient more independence?
Obtain portable oxygen if patient can ambulate.	*Portable oxygen may enable patient to ambulate and prevent deconditioning.*	Is patient able to ambulate and maintain SpO_2 within normal limits with portable oxygen?
Allow uninterrupted rest at night as much as possible.	*Lack of sleep can contribute to activity intolerance.*	Is patient able to sleep uninterrupted? Can interferences be delayed until morning?
Slowly increase activity as able.	*Increasing activity helps maintain muscle tone and endurance.*	Is patient able to increase a little each day? Is this a realistic goal for patient?
Refer patient with chronic lung disease to a pulmonary rehabilitation program.	*Pulmonary rehabilitation programs can help patient increase exercise tolerance.*	Is patient willing to participate in a rehabilitation program?

Pneumonia

Pneumonia is the cause of many hospital admissions each year and is a common cause of death from infection. Persons at risk for pneumonia are the very young, adults over age 65, smokers, those with chronic disease, and people with compromised immune systems, such as those with AIDS, alcoholism, or who take medications that reduce immune function. Pneumonia is categorized according to where it is acquired. For example, hospital-acquired pneumonia (HAP) is defined as pneumonia that develops at least 48 hours after a hospital admission. One type of HAP is ventilator-associated pneumonia (VAP). Health-care-associated pneumonia (HCAP) is pneumonia that develops in a person who has had recent health-care encounters such as a recent hospitalization, residency in a skilled care facility, home infusion or wound care, or chronic dialysis as well as a family member with multiple-drug-resistant organism. Risk factors for HAP include older age, intubation, chronic lung conditions, depressed consciousness, and aspiration. Community-acquired pneumonia (CAP) develops in the community and is usually less serious than other forms. Each type of pneumonia may be caused by different organisms.

Pathophysiology

Pneumonia is an acute inflammation and/or infection of the lungs that occurs when an infectious agent enters and multiplies in the lungs of a susceptible person. Infectious particles can be transmitted by the cough of an infected individual, from contaminated respiratory therapy equipment, from infections in other parts of the body, or from aspiration of bacteria from the mouth, pharynx, or stomach. Organisms from the mouth and pharynx may be related to poor oral hygiene or may be present because of a cold or influenza virus. When pathogens enter the body of a healthy person, normal respiratory defense mechanisms and the immune system prevent the development of infection. In a person who is immunocompromised, however, even microorganisms that are normally present in the oropharynx can cause an infection.

When the microorganisms multiply, they release toxins that induce inflammation in the lung tissue, causing damage to mucous and alveolar membranes. This leads to the development of edema and **exudate**, which fills the alveoli and reduces the surface area available for exchange of carbon dioxide and oxygen. Some bacteria also cause necrosis of lung tissue.

Pneumonia may be confined to one lobe (lobar pneumonia) or be scattered throughout the lungs (bronchopneumonia). Bronchopneumonia occurs more often as HAP or in the very young or old and can be quite serious. Patients may use terms such as *walking pneumonia* or *double pneumonia*. These are not medical terms, but it is helpful to understand them. *Walking pneumonia* refers to a mild infection that may not even keep the patient from working (or walking); *double* is a lay term for "bilateral."

Etiology

BACTERIAL PNEUMONIA. The most common cause of community-acquired bacterial pneumonias is *Streptococcus pneumoniae*, also called pneumococcal pneumonia. Other community-acquired infections are caused by *Staphylococcus aureus*, *Chlamydia trachomatis*, and *Mycoplasma pneumoniae*. HAPs are often antibiotic resistant and tend to be much more serious than CAPs. HAPs can be caused by *Escherichia coli*, *Haemophilus influenzae*, and *Klebsiella pneumoniae*, among others. Methicillin-resistant *Staphylococcus aureus* (MRSA), *Pseudomonas aeruginosa*, and other antibiotic-resistant pneumonias are especially difficult to treat.

VIRAL PNEUMONIA. Influenza viruses are the most common cause of viral pneumonia. The presence of viral pneumonia increases the patient's susceptibility to a secondary bacterial pneumonia. Generally, patients are less ill with viral pneumonia than with bacterial pneumonia, but they may be ill for a longer period because antibiotics are ineffective against viruses.

FUNGAL PNEUMONIA. *Candida* and *Aspergillus* are two types of fungi that can cause pneumonia. *Pneumocystis jiroveci* pneumonia (PJP) is caused by a fungus and typically causes pneumonia in patients with AIDS.

ASPIRATION PNEUMONIA. Some pneumonias are caused by aspiration of foreign substances, most often in patients with decreased levels of consciousness or impaired cough or gag reflex. These conditions can occur with alcohol ingestion, stroke, general anesthesia, seizures, gastrointestinal reflux disease (GERD), or other serious illness. Aspiration pneumonia increases risk for subsequent bacterial pneumonia.

VENTILATOR-ASSOCIATED PNEUMONIA. VAP is a type of aspiration pneumonia that develops in patients who are intubated and mechanically ventilated. The endotracheal (ET) tube keeps the glottis open so secretions can be easily aspirated into the lungs.

CHEMICAL PNEUMONIA. Inhalation of toxic chemicals can cause inflammation and tissue damage, which can lead to chemical pneumonia. This increases the risk for subsequent bacterial infection.

Prevention

Flu, COVID-19, and pneumonia vaccination are essential to preventing pneumonia. All individuals ages 6 months and older should receive the yearly flu vaccine. Check the Centers for Disease Control and Prevention (CDC; www.cdc.gov) Web site for flu, COVID-19, and pneumonia vaccine recommendations, which change frequently (see "Gerontological Issues: Respiratory Infections in Advanced Age").

Nursing care plays an important role in the prevention of HAP. Regular coughing, deep breathing, and position changes for patients on bedrest or after surgery; prevention of aspiration for patients at risk; and mouth care and good hand hygiene practices by both patients and health-care personnel can help prevent many cases.

• WORD • BUILDING •
exudate: to sweat out

Gerontological Issues

Respiratory Infections in Advanced Age

Advanced age is a significant risk factor for serious complications from respiratory infections such as influenza, pneumococcal pneumonia, and aspiration pneumonia. Therefore, it is recommended that people over age 65 and people with chronic disease have yearly influenza vaccines and two pneumococcal vaccines (a dose of pneumococcal conjugate vaccine [PCV13] first, followed by a dose of pneumococcal polysaccharide vaccine [PPSV23] a year later). Consistent oral care and twice-yearly dental cleanings are important to help prevent morbidity and mortality from aspiration pneumonia.

Several health organizations have developed "ventilator bundles" to prevent VAP in the intensive care unit (ICU). A bundle is a group of interventions that when used together can promote quality care. VAP prevention bundles usually include these measures: (1) elevation of patient's head of bed to 30 to 45 degrees, (2) daily sedation vacation and daily assessment of readiness for extubation, and (3) deep vein thrombosis (DVT) prophylaxis. Previous VAP bundles have included peptic ulcer prophylaxis, but recent studies have demonstrated that this can actually increase incidence of VAP (Kallet, 2019).

CRITICAL THINKING & CLINICAL JUDGMENT

Mr. Smith is an 86-year-old man who was watching television when he couldn't sleep one night. After seeing a commercial for toilet cleaner, he decided his own toilet could use some attention. He used bleach and ammonia "to get it really clean." The combination created toxic fumes, which caused a severe chemical pneumonia. He was brought to the emergency department in acute respiratory distress.

Critical Thinking (The Why)

1. As his nurse, what questions might you ask as you assess the cause of his pneumonia?

Clinical Judgment (The Do)

2. What can you teach Mr. Smith related to prevention of similar episodes in the future?
3. How can you be vigilant in preventing complications in Mr. Smith?

Suggested answers are at the end of the chapter.

Signs and Symptoms

Patients with pneumonia present with fever, shaking, chills, chest pain, dyspnea, fatigue, and a productive cough. Sputum is purulent or may be rust-colored or blood-tinged. Crackles and wheezes may be heard on lung auscultation because of the exudate in the alveoli and airways.

Some bacterial and many viral pneumonias cause **atypical** symptoms. The patient may experience fatigue, sore throat, dry cough, or nausea and vomiting.

Older adult patients may not exhibit expected symptoms of pneumonia. New-onset confusion or lethargy in an older patient can indicate reduced oxygenation. This should alert you to look for other symptoms or request evaluation by the health-care provider (HCP). New onset of fever or dyspnea should also cause suspicion of pneumonia in older adults.

BE SAFE!

AVOID FAILURE TO RECOGNIZE! Older adults may not experience the typical symptoms of pneumonia. Investigate any changes in cognition or activity levels.

Complications

Complications from pneumonia most commonly occur in patients with other underlying chronic diseases. Pleurisy and pleural effusion (excess fluid in the pleural space) are two of the most common complications and generally resolve within 1 to 2 weeks. **Atelectasis** (collapsed alveoli) can occur as a result of trapped secretions. It may be resolved by efforts to keep the airways clear, such as use of an incentive spirometer. Other complications result from spread of infection to other parts of the body, causing septicemia, meningitis, septic arthritis, pericarditis, or endocarditis. Treatment for each of these is antibiotics. Although antibiotics can greatly reduce the incidence of death related to pneumonia, it is still a common cause of death in older people.

Diagnostic Tests

A chest x-ray examination is done to identify the presence of pulmonary infiltrate, which is fluid leakage into the alveoli from inflammation (Fig. 31.2). In addition, sputum and blood cultures are obtained to identify the organism causing the pneumonia and determine appropriate treatment. If the patient is unable to produce a sputum specimen, a nebulized mist treatment (NMT) may be ordered to promote sputum expectoration. Nasotracheal suctioning or a bronchoscopy can be done to obtain a specimen from a very ill patient.

NURSING CARE TIP

Obtain sputum culture specimens before antibiotics are started to avoid altering culture results. The best time to obtain a specimen is first thing in the morning, before breakfast. If the patient has eaten, be sure they rinse the mouth to keep food particles out of the specimen.

• WORD • BUILDING •

atypical: a—not + typical—usual
atelectasis: atel—imperfect + ectasis—expansion

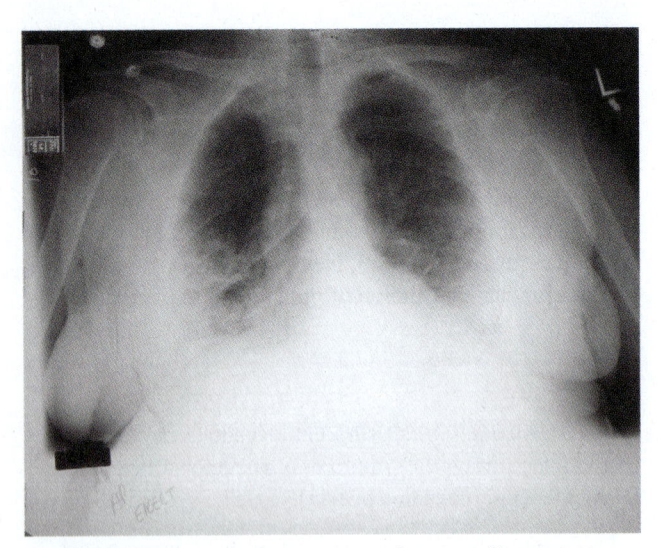

FIGURE 31.2 Chest x-ray examination showing infiltrates in pneumonia.

Therapeutic Measures

Broad-spectrum antibiotics are initiated as soon as cultures are sent to the laboratory even if results are not completed. Once the culture and sensitivity (C&S) report is available, antibiotic orders may change to more narrow-spectrum agents. Many patients can be treated with oral antibiotics as outpatients. However, hospitalization and IV therapy may be necessary in older adults or in individuals who are chronically or acutely ill. If the pneumonia is caused by a virus, rest and fluids are recommended. Occasionally, antiviral medications are used.

Expectorants, bronchodilators, and analgesics may be given for comfort and symptom relief. NMTs or metered-dose inhalers (MDIs) may be used to deliver bronchodilators. Supplemental oxygen via nasal cannula or mask is used as needed. Nursing care is found in "Nursing Care Plan for the Patient With a Lower Respiratory Tract Disorder." See Table 31.1 for a pneumonia summary.

Nursing Process for the Patient With Pneumonia

Nursing diagnoses for pneumonia include *Impaired Gas Exchange*, *Ineffective Airway Clearance*, and *Activity Intolerance*. These are found in "Nursing Care Plan for the Patient With a Lower Respiratory Tract Disorder."

Tuberculosis

Pathophysiology and Etiology

Tuberculosis (TB) is an infectious disease caused by the bacterium *Mycobacterium tuberculosis*. TB primarily affects the lungs, but the kidneys, liver, brain, and bone may be affected as well. *M. tuberculosis* is an acid-fast bacillus (AFB): When it is stained in the laboratory and then washed with an acid, the stain remains, or stays, "fast." *M. tuberculosis* can live in dark places in dried sputum for months but is killed in a few hours of direct sunlight. It is spread by inhalation of the TB bacilli from respiratory droplets (droplet nuclei) of an infected person.

Once the bacilli enter the lungs, they multiply and begin to disseminate to the lymph nodes and then to other parts of the body. The patient is then infected but may or may not go on to develop clinical (active) disease. TB infection without disease is called *latent TB infection* (LTBI). The body develops immunity, which keeps the infection under control. If the lungs are involved, the immune system surrounds the

---

Evidence-Based Practice

Clinical Question
What is the effect of yoga on quality of life, respiratory function, and symptom control in patients with asthma?

Evidence
A total of 112 patients with asthma participated, 56 in the experimental group and 56 in the control group. The experimental group attended 12 yoga sessions over 6 weeks. Post-test scores for quality of life, respiratory function, and the Asthma Control Test increased significantly in the experimental group.

Implications for Nursing Practice
Teach patients that yoga can be an effective tool in managing asthma by strengthening respiratory muscles, increasing lung capacity, and relieving shortness of breath.

Reference: Turan, G. B., & Tan, M. (2020). The effect of yoga on respiratory functions, symptom control and life quality of asthma patients: A randomized controlled study. *Complementary Therapies in Clinical Practice, 38*. https://doi.org/10.1016/j.ctcp.2019.101070

Table 31.1
Pneumonia Summary

Signs and Symptoms	Fever, chills Chest pain Dyspnea Productive cough Crackles and wheezes
Diagnostic Tests	Chest x-ray Sputum cultures
Therapeutic Measures	Antibiotics Supplemental oxygen Bronchodilators Expectorants Rest, fluids
Complications	Pleurisy Pleural effusion Atelectasis
Priority Nursing Diagnoses	Impaired Gas Exchange Ineffective Airway Clearance Decreased Activity Tolerance

infected area in the lung with neutrophils and alveolar macrophages. This creates a lesion called a *tubercle* that seals off the bacteria and prevents spread. Similar processes take place in other affected areas of the body. The bacteria within the tubercle die or become dormant, and the patient is no longer infectious. If the patient's immune system becomes compromised, however, some of the dormant bacteria can become active, causing disease. Only 5% to 10% of infected people in the United States actually develop the disease. Even then, it may not occur for many years (see "Gerontological Issues: Aging and Tuberculosis").

Gerontological Issues

Aging and Tuberculosis
The age-related decline in immune system function can decrease the effectiveness of the tuberculosis (TB) antibodies in someone who previously had latent infection. The TB bacilli can be activated, causing active disease. Because of the risk of false-negative tuberculin test results, a two-step test is recommended, with the second test done 1 to 3 weeks after the first. Decline in immune system function can also have an impact on clinical manifestations of TB. Patients may exhibit fewer symptoms, making recognition difficult.

Risk Factors

Residents and employees of prisons, nursing homes, homeless shelters, drug treatment facilities, health-care facilities, and so on have a higher risk for TB exposure and infection. Aging, AIDS, chronic drug or alcohol abuse, and certain medications (e.g., chemotherapy and some medications for rheumatoid arthritis, Crohn disease, or psoriasis) can compromise immune function and increase risk of activation. The incidence of TB has been decreasing for the past two decades, but progress is now slowing down. The effects of health disparities are apparent with 88% of TB cases occurring in racial and ethnic minority groups.

Prevention

If a hospitalized patient is known or suspected to have TB, they are placed in respiratory isolation to prevent spread to staff or other patients. Special negative-pressure isolation rooms are ventilated to the outside. Staff should wear a particulate filter respirator certified by the Centers for Disease Control and Prevention (CDC) and the National Institute for Occupational Safety and Health (NIOSH) when in the room of a patient with TB; a regular surgical mask is not effective against TB. Masks should be fitted to size of the employee's face. If the patient must travel through the hallway for tests or other activities, they must wear a mask. Additional personal protective equipment, such as gowns, gloves, or goggles, are used when contact with sputum is likely.

A vaccine against TB, the Bacillus Calmette-Guérin (BCG) vaccine, is available. It is used in areas where TB is prevalent. It is not used routinely in the United States because of the low risk for infection. Individuals who have had the vaccine will have a positive skin test for TB, so alternative methods for screening must be used.

Ultimately, prevention will come from adequate treatment of patients with TB. A current concern is the development of antibiotic-resistant strains of the TB bacillus, which can develop when patients are noncompliant with medication therapy. When antibiotics are taken intermittently or discontinued early, the more virulent (stronger) bacteria survive and multiply and become resistant to the medications being used. This multidrug-resistant TB (MDR-TB) can then be passed on to someone else. Some strains are resistant to nearly all antibiotics. These strains are called *extensively drug resistant TB* (XDR-TB). It is, therefore, vital to reinforce the importance of strict adherence to medications therapy. Patients who are at risk for nonadherence to medications therapy must have a visiting nurse or other health professional observe each dose of antibiotic taken. This is called *directly observed therapy*, or DOT. DOT transfers responsibility for making sure the medications are taken from the patient to the health-care worker. The World Health Organization reports the highest treatment success rates with DOT.

Because progress in decreasing TB cases in the United States is slowing down, Healthy People 2030 has developed a goal to reduce the rate of TB by curing people with active TB and expanding testing and treatment for latent TB (Office of Disease Prevention and Health Promotion, 2020).

Signs and Symptoms

A diagnosis of TB should be suspected when the patient presents with a cough longer than 2 or 3 weeks in duration, pain in the chest, coughing up blood or sputum, night sweats, fevers, weight loss, and/or swollen lymph nodes. As the disease progresses, progressive weight loss and dyspnea may occur. Older adults may present with less specific symptoms such as dyspnea and fatigue.

Complications

Spread of the TB bacilli throughout the body can result in pleuritis, pericarditis, peritonitis, meningitis, bone and joint infections, genitourinary or gastrointestinal (GI) infection, and infection of many other organs.

Diagnostic Tests

Routine screening for TB infection is usually done with a purified protein derivative (PPD) skin test. The PPD is injected intradermally. The test is considered positive if a raised area of **induration** occurs within 48 to 72 hours. If a

• WORD • BUILDING •

induration: in—in + durus—hard

red area appears around the induration, this is not measured. The size of induration that indicates a positive test varies based on the individual's history (Table 31.2). If a person is **anergic** (has limited ability to react to the test due to immune dysfunction), a smaller area of induration would be considered a positive result. A red area without induration is considered a negative result. A positive result indicates that a person has been exposed to TB; it does not mean that active TB disease is present.

Some health-care institutions use a two-step process for baseline testing of employees and residents. If an individual has a negative PPD test, he or she is retested in 1 to 3 weeks. Someone who was exposed many years ago may not react to the first test, which acts as a reminder to the immune system to react. In this case, the second test will be positive.

> **NURSING CARE TIP**
> You have probably had a purified protein derivative (PPD) skin test so you can do your clinical practice for school. When you have it checked, the clinician should touch your arm. Just looking at it is not adequate to judge whether there is a raised area of induration.

The QuantiFERON-TB (QFT-TB) and T-SPOT tests are blood tests that detect the cell-mediated immune response to TB bacteria in blood. Unlike the PPD skin test, these are simple blood tests and are valid in individuals who have been vaccinated against TB.

A chest x-ray is used as a screening tool in someone with a positive test. Final diagnosis is made based on sputum culture results.

Table 31.2 Classifying a Tuberculin Skin Test Reaction

Size of Induration	Considered Positive for:
5 mm or more	People infected with HIV Chest x-ray suggestive of previous TB Recent contacts of infectious TB cases Organ transplant recipients Those who are immunosuppressed for other reasons (e.g., taking immune suppressing medications)
10 mm or more	Recent immigrants (within last 5 years) from high-prevalence countries Injection drug users Residents or employees of high-risk congregate settings Mycobacteriology laboratory personnel Persons with clinical conditions that place them at high risk Children younger than age 4 Infants, children, or adolescents exposed to adults in high-risk categories People with low body weight
15 mm or more	People with no risk factors for TB

Source: Centers for Disease Control and Prevention. (2020). *Tuberculosis skin testing.* www.cdc.gov/tb/publications/factsheets/testing/skintesting.htm

> **BE SAFE!**
> **AVOID FAILURE TO COMMUNICATE!** While awaiting culture results on a patient in a facility, ask the HCP or infection control nurse whether the patient should be isolated to protect staff and other patients.

Therapeutic Measures

Treatment consists of antibiotic therapy. First-line medications have the fewest adverse effects:

- Isoniazid
- Rifampin
- Ethambutol
- Pyrazinamide

However, they can still be toxic to the liver and nervous system and have other side effects. More toxic antibiotics are reserved for cases that do not respond to first-line medication therapy. Generally, two or three antibiotics are given simultaneously to allow lower doses of each individual medications, reducing the incidence of serious side effects as well as the risk of developing resistant bacteria. Medications must be taken for 6 to 9 months or up to 2 years for MDR-TB. Because of the length of therapy and the incidence of side effects, adherence is often a problem.

Additional treatment is supportive. Rest and good nutrition are important for helping the patient's own immune system to work. Patients must be isolated until their sputum no longer contains TB bacteria. Typically, after about 2 weeks on antibiotic therapy, the patient is no longer contagious, but a sputum culture must be done to confirm this. Reinforce to the patient that they avoid being around others and use proper hand hygiene during this time period.

Approximately 80% of the TB cases in the United States progress from LTBI. Hence, the CDC now recommends treating patients with LTBI with 3 months of isoniazid plus rifapentine (Sterling et al, 2020). The CDC provides information about TB at www.cdc.gov; simply type "tuberculosis" into the search window.

Nursing Process for the Patient With Tuberculosis

DATA COLLECTION. Perform a thorough history and head-to-toe physical examination, because TB can affect many systems. Focus on collecting respiratory and psychosocial data. The severity of the disease determines the impact on the patient's lifestyle. It is also important to determine the patient's knowledge of the disease and treatment and adherence to medications.

NURSING DIAGNOSES, PLANNING, AND IMPLEMENTATION. Nursing interventions for *Impaired Gas Exchange, Ineffective Airway Clearance*, and *Activity Intolerance* are found in "Nursing Care Plan for the Patient With a Lower Respiratory Tract Disorder." Additional nursing diagnoses for the patient with TB follow.

> **Ineffective Health Management related to deficient knowledge and length of treatment**
>
> **EXPECTED OUTCOME:** The patient will follow treatment regimen and infection will be resolved, as evidenced by negative cultures.

- Assess the patient's and family's ability and intent to follow treatment regimen. *It is essential for patients to be diligent about taking their medications to eradicate the infection and to prevent spread to others.*
- Reinforce to the patient and family the need to take medications for the entire course (6 months or longer) or a drug-resistant form of disease may develop. *Patients may be more willing to adhere to treatment if they understand the rationale for taking their medications.*
- Forewarn the patient that rifampin turns urine and other body fluids red. *This might frighten the patient and prevent adherence to treatment.*
- Remind patient to report side effects of medications. *If side effects can be managed, the patient is more likely to adhere to therapy.*
- Request an order for a home health nurse. *A nurse can monitor adherence to therapy. DOT has been found to increase adherence to medication therapy.*
- Reinforce with the patient and family prevention of spreading the disease. *TB is contagious.*
- The patient should stay home and away from others for a few weeks until sputum cultures are negative.
- Have patient wear a mask when around others.
- Use a tissue to cover the mouth and nose when coughing or sneezing, and flush tissue down toilet or discard in a sealed bag.
- Use good hand-washing technique.
- Keep home and room well ventilated.

EVALUATION. If nursing care has been effective, the patient will understand the disease and the importance of taking care of self. The patient will take medications and receive follow-up care as ordered and will take measures to protect others from catching TB.

> **CRITICAL THINKING & CLINICAL JUDGMENT**
>
> **Mr. Woo,** a new resident at your long-term care facility, is being tested for tuberculosis. You check his skin test and find that the purified protein derivative (PPD) test in his forearm has a 13 mm area of induration.
>
> **Critical Thinking (The Why)**
> 1. How do you document these results?
> 2. How do you interpret them? (See Table 31.2.)
>
> **Clinical Judgment (The Do)**
> 3. What should you do?
>
> *Suggested answers are at the end of the chapter.*

RESTRICTIVE DISORDERS

Restrictive disorders are those problems that limit the ability of the patient to expand the lungs and inhale air. Restrictive disorders can be intrinsic, involving lung tissue (e.g., pulmonary fibrosis), or extrinsic, involving structures outside the lungs (e.g., pleural effusion).

Pleurisy (Pleuritis)
Pathophysiology
Recall that the visceral and parietal pleurae are the membranes that surround the lungs. Between these membranes is a small amount of serous fluid that prevents friction as the pleurae slide over each other during inhalation and exhalation. If the membranes become inflamed, they do not slide as easily. Instead of sliding, one membrane may "catch" on the other, causing it to stretch as the patient attempts to take a breath. This causes a characteristic sharp pain on inspiration. The irritation causes an increase in the formation of pleural fluid to reduce friction and decrease pain.

Etiology
Pleurisy is usually related to another underlying respiratory disorder, such as pneumonia, TB, a tumor, or trauma. Nonrespiratory disorders such as pancreatitis or certain autoimmune disorders can also result in pleurisy.

Signs and Symptoms
Pleurisy causes a sharp pain in the chest on inspiration. Pain also occurs during coughing or sneezing. Breathing may be shallow and rapid because deep breathing increases pain. The patient may also exhibit fever, chills, and an elevated white blood cell (WBC) count if the cause is infectious. A pleural friction rub is heard on auscultation.

Complications

As pleural membranes become more inflamed, serous fluid production increases, which may result in pleural effusion (see next section). If pleuritic pain is not controlled, patients have difficulty breathing deeply and coughing, which may lead to atelectasis. If the cause is an untreated bacterial infection, empyema (collection of pus in the pleural cavity) can result.

Diagnostic Tests

Diagnosis is based on signs and symptoms, including auscultation of a pleural friction rub. A chest x-ray examination, CT scan, or ultrasound and complete blood count (CBC) may be done. FVC (forced vital capacity) is reduced more than FEV_1 (forced expiratory volume in 1 second) because expansion is limited by the restrictive disorder; airways and FEV_1 may be normal. Additional testing is done to determine the underlying cause.

Therapeutic Measures

Treatment is aimed at correcting the cause. NSAIDs or opioids are given to control pain and facilitate deep breathing and coughing. The physician may perform a nerve block by injecting anesthetic near the intercostal nerves to block pain transmission. Patients may experience some pain relief when lying on the affected side.

Pleural Effusion

Pathophysiology

When excess fluid collects in the pleural space, it is called a *pleural effusion*. Fluid normally enters the pleural space from surrounding capillaries and is reabsorbed by the lymphatic system. When a pathological condition causes an increase in fluid production or inadequate reabsorption of fluid, excess fluid collects. A normal amount of pleural fluid around each lung is 1 to 15 mL. More than 25 mL of fluid is considered abnormal; in pleural effusion, as much as several liters of fluid can collect. The effusion can be either *transudative*, a watery fluid from the capillaries, or *exudative*, with fluid containing WBCs and protein from an inflammatory or infectious process.

Etiology

Like pleurisy, pleural effusion is generally caused by another lung disorder as a symptom, not a disease. Transudative effusion may result from heart failure, liver disorders, or kidney disorders. Exudative effusion more commonly occurs with lung cancer, infection, or inflammation.

Signs and Symptoms

Symptoms depend on the amount of fluid in the pleural space. The patient may or may not experience pleuritic pain. Increasing shortness of breath occurs because of the decreasing space for lung expansion. Cough and **tachypnea** may be present. A dull sound is heard when the affected area is percussed. Lung sounds are decreased or absent over the effusion, and a friction rub may be auscultated.

Diagnostic Tests

A chest x-ray or CT scan is done to determine whether pleural effusion is present. If a thoracentesis is done, fluid samples are sent to the laboratory for C&S and cytological examination. Further tests are done to determine the cause of the effusion.

Therapeutic Measures

The underlying cause should be treated, for example, diuretics for heart failure patients or antibiotics for bacterial pneumonia. If symptoms are severe, a therapeutic thoracentesis is done to remove the excess fluid from the pleural space and relieve the patient of dyspnea. (Chapter 29 discusses how to assist with a thoracentesis.) Patients usually experience immediate improvement in dyspnea following thoracentesis.

The HCP uses x-ray examinations and percussion or sometimes ultrasound to determine where to insert the needle to obtain the fluid. If the fluid accumulation is large or recurring, a chest tube may be placed to continuously drain the pleural space. Occasionally, talc or another irritating agent will be instilled via the chest tube to cause pleural membranes to adhere to each other (this is called **pleurodesis**), eliminating the pleural space and preventing future episodes of pleural effusion. Treatment of the cause of the effusion is necessary to prevent recurrence.

Empyema

Empyema is the collection of pus in the pleural space. It is a pleural effusion that is infected. Empyema is usually a complication of pneumonia, TB, or lung abscess. Symptoms, diagnosis, therapeutic measures, and nursing care are the same as the care of the patient with a pleural effusion, with an added emphasis on identifying and resolving the infection. A chest tube or surgery may be necessary to drain the area.

Pulmonary Fibrosis

Pathophysiology

Pulmonary fibrosis (PF), sometimes called interstitial lung disease, is a group of disorders that cause scarring and fibrosis of lung tissue. PF may evolve from injury to the alveoli, causing chronic inflammation; inflamed tissues are gradually replaced by fibrous connective tissue. Alveoli become thick and scarred, and gas exchange becomes difficult.

Etiology

Various factors are linked with PF, including heredity, exposure to certain viral illnesses, wood and metal dust exposure, medications, radiation therapy, and smoking. It may also be associated with some autoimmune disorders such as lupus erythematosus or rheumatoid arthritis. Chronic GERD may play a role. Often, PF is called *idiopathic PF* because no specific cause can be found.

• WORD • BUILDING •

tachypnea: tachy—rapid + pnea—breathing
pleurodesis: pleur—pleural membrane + desis—binding

Signs and Symptoms

Patients with PF experience progressive shortness of breath. Inspiratory crackles and chronic cough are present. Some experience flu-like symptoms. Fatigue is common and clubbing of fingers may be present. The average patient has a gradual decline in lung function with eventual respiratory failure and death in approximately four years.

Diagnostic Tests

A chest x-ray may show lung infiltrates. A CT scan may be done. Spirometry is done to verify that the condition is restrictive. Arterial blood gases (ABGs) may show reduced partial pressure of oxygen (PaO_2). A bronchoscopy and lung biopsy can help rule out other causes of the patient's symptoms. They can also show inflammation and fibrosis. A blood test (antinuclear antibodies [ANA] titer) shows whether an autoimmune process is involved.

Therapeutic Measures

Two new antifibrotic medications, pirfenidone (Esbriet) and nintedanib (Ofev), can reduce disease progression and preserve lung function. Patients should be encouraged to stop smoking and to avoid secondhand smoke. Oxygen is used if needed to maintain oxygenation. Patients should receive flu and pneumococcal vaccines. Aerobic and breathing exercise can help decrease dyspnea. Lung transplant may be considered for patients with few comorbidities. Pulmonary rehabilitation helps patients maintain optimum activity tolerance.

Atelectasis

Atelectasis is the collapse of alveoli. It most commonly occurs in postsurgical patients who do not cough and deep breathe effectively but can result from anything that causes hypoventilation. Areas of the lungs that are not well aerated become plugged with mucus, preventing inflation of alveoli. As a result, alveoli collapse. Compression of lung tissue from effusion or a tumor can also cause atelectasis. The focus of nursing care is on prevention. Patients should be taught the importance of coughing and deep breathing or the use of an incentive spirometer whenever the risk for hypoventilation is present. Frequent position changes and ambulation are also helpful.

Nursing Process for the Patient With a Restrictive Disorder

Data Collection

Perform a routine respiratory assessment. Monitor lung sounds for friction rub or decreasing breath sounds in the lobes. Assess pain level and vital signs. Be vigilant for increase in dyspnea or tachypnea, changes in vital signs or pulse oximetry, or increased WBC count or temperature.

Nursing Diagnoses, Planning, and Implementation

Priority nursing diagnoses are similar to those for other respiratory disorders and are addressed in "Nursing Care Plan for the Patient With a Lower Respiratory Tract Disorder."

In addition, it is essential to address pain as it can prevent the patient from breathing effectively.

> **Ineffective Breathing Pattern related to acute pain**
>
> **EXPECTED OUTCOME:** The patient will be comfortable enough to breathe deeply and cough effectively and will have a respiratory rate of 12 to 20 per minute.

- Monitor respiratory rate and depth as well as pain location and level. *Some types of pain can cause shallow respirations, especially pleuritic pain.*
- Position the patient for comfort. *Sometimes, lying on the affected side for short periods will help reduce chest wall movement and pain.*
- Administer pain medication as ordered, preferably around the clock, to prevent pain from becoming severe. *Pain must be controlled so the patient can breathe deeply and prevent further complications. Acetaminophen or NSAIDs are usually tried first because they will not suppress cough and respirations.*
- If opioids are required to control pain, carefully monitor respirations and cough. *Opioids can suppress respirations and cough, which can further complicate the underlying disorder.*
- Reinforce with the patient the importance of effective deep breathing and coughing (see Chapter 29). *This can help prevent further complications. If opioids have suppressed cough reflex, the patient will need to purposefully deep breath and cough.*
- Request an order for an incentive spirometer. *Incentive spirometry can help encourage the patient to breathe deeply.*

Evaluation

If interventions have been effective, the patient should report a decrease in dyspnea and anxiety. Pain will be controlled so that the patient is able to take deep breaths and cough effectively. Breath sounds will be clear and equal bilaterally, and the patient will be free of signs and symptoms of infection.

OBSTRUCTIVE DISORDERS

Obstructive disorders are characterized by air trapping and difficulty getting air out of the lungs. Obstructive disorders covered in this chapter include chronic obstructive pulmonary disease, emphysema, chronic bronchitis, asthma, and cystic fibrosis.

Chronic Obstructive Pulmonary Disease/Chronic Airflow Limitation

According to the American Lung Association (2021), 16.4 million adults in the United States have been diagnosed with chronic obstructive pulmonary disease (COPD). Many more likely have it but have not yet been diagnosed. Death rates in men have fallen slightly in recent years, but death rates in women are steady, due to more women smoking.

Pathophysiology

COPD is a group of pulmonary disorders characterized by difficulty exhaling. In COPD, airways are narrowed or blocked by inflammation and mucus, and there is loss of elasticity in the alveoli. Both conditions make it difficult for air to be removed from the alveoli, leading to trapping of air. More effort is required for weakened alveoli to push air out through obstructed airways (Fig. 31.3). Emphysema, chronic bronchitis, and asthma are disorders that limit airflow. A patient with COPD may have some degree of both emphysema and chronic bronchitis. Asthma may also be present, but it differs somewhat because the airway limitation in asthma is usually reversible. A patient with unremitting asthma is treated as having COPD. Airflow limitation in emphysema and bronchitis is progressive and minimally reversible (Fig. 31.4).

COPD may also be referred to as chronic airflow limitation (CAL) or chronic obstructive lung disease. COPD develops slowly and may be present for many years before symptoms become evident. It may be advanced by the time the patient seeks treatment. It is characterized by periods of relative stability and exacerbations, which may be triggered by respiratory infection or other stressors. See Table 31.3 for a COPD summary.

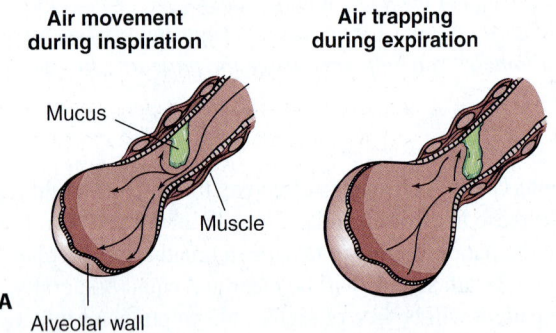

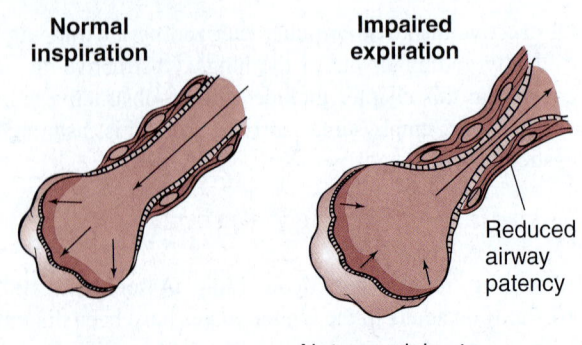

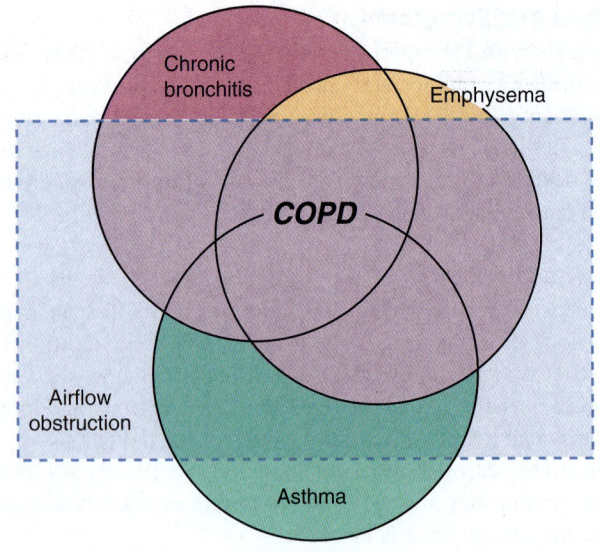

FIGURE 31.4 Chronic bronchitis and emphysema are the primary underlying disorders in COPD. Asthma also may play a role.

LEARNING TIP
Restrictive disorders cause difficulty with **i**nhalation or air entering the lungs. **O**bstructive disorders are associated with difficulty exhaling or getting air **O**ut.

CHRONIC BRONCHITIS PATHOPHYSIOLOGY. Chronic bronchitis is similar to acute bronchitis, with symptoms occurring for at least 3 months of the year for 2 consecutive years. Patients may have multiple exacerbations, each lasting 2 weeks or more. The bronchial tree becomes inflamed from inhaled irritants. Impaired ciliary function reduces the ability to remove the irritants. The mucus-producing glands in the airways become hypertrophied, producing excessive thick, tenacious mucus, which obstructs airways and traps air (Fig. 31.5). These changes lead to chronic low-grade infection.

EMPHYSEMA PATHOPHYSIOLOGY. Emphysema affects the respiratory bronchioles and alveoli distal to the terminal bronchioles, causing destruction of the alveolar walls and loss of elastic recoil (see Fig. 31.5). This also causes damage to adjacent pulmonary capillaries. Because of the loss of elastic recoil, passive exhalation is impaired and air is trapped in the alveoli. The combination of damaged alveoli and capillaries causes reduced surface area for gas exchange.

Etiology

Smoking is the single-most important risk factor for COPD. Other types of tobacco use in pipes, cigars, or water pipes as well as marijuana are also risk factors. Vaping (e-cigarettes) has also been linked to COPD. Other factors include passive (secondhand) indoor and outdoor air pollution and exposure

FIGURE 31.3 Air trapping in COPD.

• WORD • BUILDING •
emphysema: to inflate

Table 31.3 COPD Summary

Signs and Symptoms	Cough Chronic sputum production Dyspnea that occurs every day, worsens with exercise Activity intolerance Crackles, wheezes, diminished breath sounds Barrel chest Use of accessory muscles
Diagnostic Tests	Chest x-ray examination, computed tomography (CT) scan Arterial blood gas (ABG) analysis Complete blood count (CBC) Sputum analysis Spirometry Alpha-1 antitrypsin (AAT) level if hereditary deficiency suspected
Therapeutic Measures	Smoking cessation Promote healthy diet and physical activity Bronchodilators: per os, or by mouth (PO), nebulized mist treatment (NMT), metered-dose inhaler (MDI) Corticosteroids, expectorants Flu and pneumonia vaccinations Supplemental oxygen Breathing exercises Chest physiotherapy (CPT) Pulmonary rehabilitation
Priority Nursing Diagnoses	*Impaired Gas Exchange* *Ineffective Airway Clearance* *Decreased Activity Tolerance*

> **NURSING CARE TIP**
> Cyanosis may be difficult to detect in dark-skinned individuals. Check the oral mucosa, conjunctiva, and nailbeds.

Signs and Symptoms
Classic symptoms of COPD are chronic cough, with or without sputum production, and progressive dyspnea on exertion. Patients exhibit prolonged exhalation because of obstructed air passages and reduced elastic recoil. Air trapping causes the lungs to become hyperinflated, which leads to the classic barrel chest, a round, bulging chest that has the shape of a barrel.

The patient with chronic bronchitis has a chronic productive cough, shortness of breath, and activity intolerance. Symptoms may initially be worse in the winter months. Crackles and wheezing are often noted on auscultation and may improve after coughing.

The most characteristic symptom of emphysema is progressive shortness of breath, accompanied by activity intolerance. Use of accessory muscles to breathe is evident. Auscultation reveals diminished breath sounds. Remember that many patients have symptoms of both chronic bronchitis and emphysema.

ABGs may be checked during an acute exacerbation of COPD and show an increase in partial pressure of carbon dioxide ($PaCO_2$) and a low PaO_2. The patient develops **polycythemia** in response to chronic hypoxemia, which results in a ruddy skin color. Cyanosis may also be present.

In late stages of COPD, patients may lose weight and become malnourished. They have difficulty eating because of severe dyspnea, and the increased work of breathing expends more calories. Chronic hypoxemia causes release of chemicals that may also lead to weight loss. Patients use accessory muscles to breathe and tend to assume the classic tripod position to aid breathing.

Complications
Some patients with emphysema develop large air spaces within the lung tissue (**bullae**) or adjacent to the pleurae (**blebs**). Similar to blisters, they can rupture and cause the lung to collapse. Right-sided heart failure may develop because the heart has to work harder to pump blood to the diseased lungs. (See the section on cor pulmonale in Chapter 26.) Death usually results from respiratory infection or respiratory failure.

Diagnostic Tests
Information from spirometry is correlated with the history and physical examination to diagnose COPD. Spirometry is essential for diagnosis. Normally, the FEV_1 is about 70% to 80% of the FVC. In COPD, the FEV_1 following bronchodilator use is less than 70%. The patient with airflow limitation cannot forcefully exhale as much air in the first second as normally expected.

• WORD • BUILDING •
polycythemia: poly—many + cyt—cells + emia—in the blood

---

to industrial chemicals, dust, and fumes in the workplace. Studies are ongoing regarding the effects of thirdhand smoking (nicotine residue left on indoor surfaces and clothing). Some familial predisposition to chronic bronchitis has been demonstrated. A small number of individuals have an inherited deficiency of the enzyme alpha-1 antitrypsin (AAT), which causes a predisposition to the development of emphysema. Patients with this inherited tendency who also smoke have a very high risk of developing the disease. Children of smoking parents are at higher risk because of smoke exposure.

Prevention
Prevention is important because no cure for COPD is currently available. Avoidance of smoking and other inhaled irritants is vital, especially in individuals with parents or siblings with COPD. Remind your patients that e-cigarettes contain nicotine and are as addictive as other cigarettes.

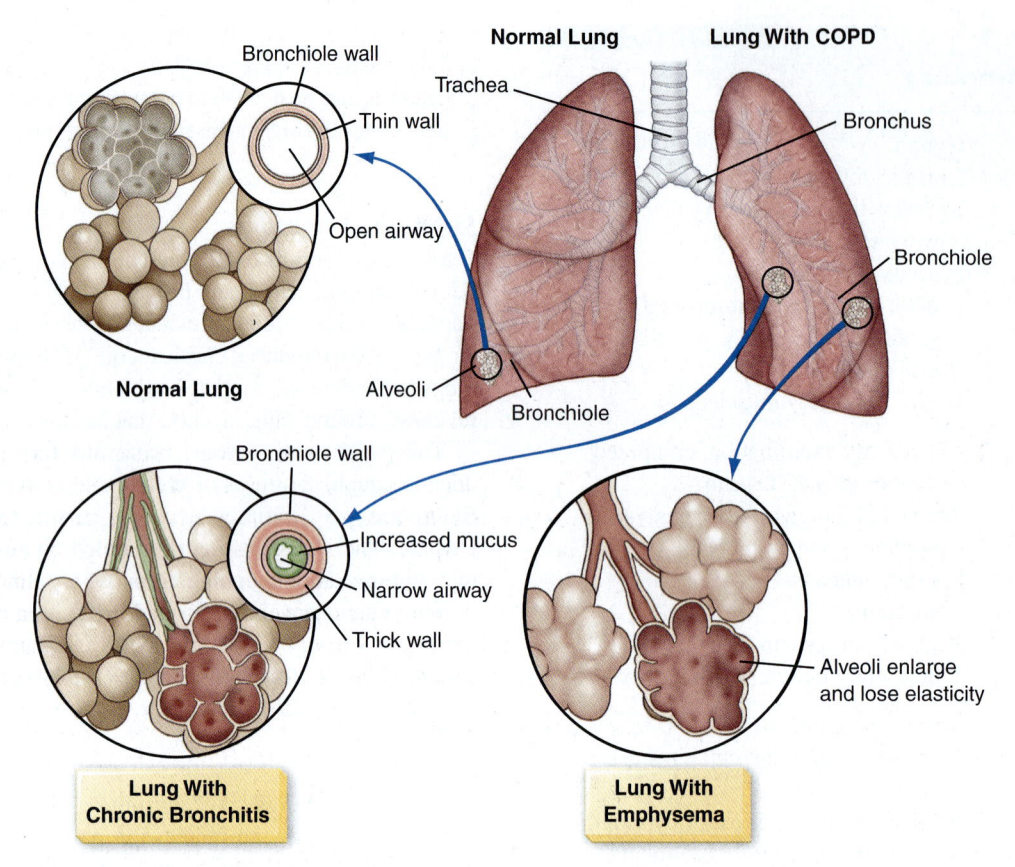

FIGURE 31.5 Normal lung versus lung with COPD.

If lung function improves after a bronchodilator, asthma is suspected rather than COPD. An AAT level is checked if deficiency is suspected, especially in patients with a family history of COPD. CBC, electrolytes, and sputum culture may be assessed during exacerbations.

COPD is classified according to spirometry results into four grades, from GOLD 1 (mild airflow limitation) to GOLD 4 (very severe airflow limitation), and into four categories (A, B, C, D) based on symptoms (Global Initiative for Chronic Obstructive Lung Disease [GOLD], 2017). So 1A would be very mild, and 4D would indicate severe disease.

Therapeutic Measures

The goals of COPD treatment, according to the GOLD guidelines, are to reduce symptoms and reduce risk of exacerbations (GOLD, 2021). In addition, the reduction of exposure to tobacco and occupational exposures should be included as a goal throughout any management program.

SMOKING CESSATION. Even late in the disease process, stopping smoking can slow disease progression and prolong life. Exposure to other respiratory contaminants should also be minimized. Hair spray, other household aerosols, and body powder should be avoided. Fig. 31.6 shows the benefits of smoking cessation. "Patient Perspective" provides a personal account from one woman who understood too late the importance of smoking cessation. See Chapter 29 for more information.

> ### Patient Perspective
> **Sarah**
> At age 17, I started the habit that would change my life. I started to smoke.
>
> At first it was just a few cigarettes, but as time passed, I smoked more and more until I reached two packs a day. This habit continued for 42 years. I disregarded all the warnings about what could happen. I was sure this would never happen to me.
>
> Now at age 75, I must do three breathing treatments a day and carry an inhaler with me at all times. I have a cough that cannot be controlled. I can no longer ride a bike with my grandchildren, play badminton, or even bowl. My lungs won't let me. Going shopping is no longer fun—it's a chore. I have to walk slowly or I can't breathe.
>
> All the things I enjoyed most I've given up because for 42 years I was a slave to cigarettes. If any of you smoke, stop now. Smell the coffee and roses without coughing.

OXYGEN. Oxygen therapy is used in patients with chronic oxygen saturation levels of 88% or less. Oxygen flow rate is titrated (adjusted) to achieve oxygen saturation between 88% and 92%. If the patient tends to retain CO_2, having a much higher saturation could reduce the respiratory drive.

Chapter 31 Nursing Care of Patients With Lower Respiratory Tract Disorders 549

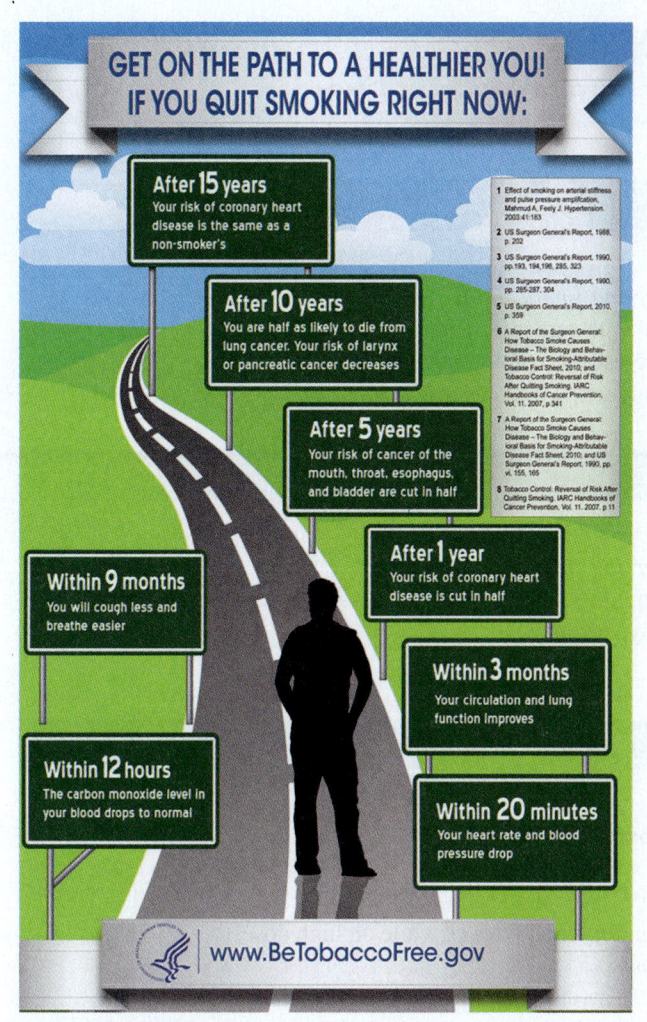

FIGURE 31.6 Benefits of smoking cessation.

But remember that our brains need oxygen! Always aim for 88% to 92% in patients with COPD and watch your patients closely. If they become drowsy or their respiratory rate falls too low, call the registered nurse (RN) or HCP.

MEDICATIONS. Medications commonly used include adrenergic and anticholinergic MDIs or NMTs to open airways, corticosteroid inhalers to control inflammation, and antibiotics when needed. **Antitussive** agents should be avoided with COPD because patients must be able to cough up secretions.

Oral theophylline bronchodilators are sometimes used but have significant side effects so are avoided if possible. Oral or IV corticosteroids are used for acute exacerbations. Replacement of AAT may be used in emphysema patients who are deficient. See Table 31.4 for a more detailed list of medications used in the treatment of COPD.

Patients with COPD should also be assessed for depression. Depression is common with chronic illness and often goes undiagnosed. Patients may not report feeling depressed but experience more physical symptoms. Antidepressant medications, if indicated, can increase quality of life for COPD patients.

Morphine or other opioids may be effective in reducing acute dyspnea and anxiety. They are reserved for end-stage disease.

SUPPORTIVE CARE. Pneumococcal and yearly influenza vaccinations are recommended to reduce the risk of respiratory infection. Advise avoidance of crowds and exposure to people with respiratory infections.

Good hydration and a cool mist humidifier help keep secretions loose. A dietitian consultation is helpful for the patient who is unable to maintain a desirable weight. Breathing exercises help improve oxygenation and reduce anxiety (see Chapter 29).

REHABILITATION. Pulmonary rehabilitation programs can help patients increase exercise tolerance and maintain a sense of well-being (Fig. 31.7). Patients exercise in a monitored environment and benefit from the support of other patients with similar problems. Some groups of pulmonary rehabilitation patients have even formed harmonica clubs! Playing their harmonicas mimics pursed-lip breathing and may strengthen the diaphragm, the major muscle of breathing.

SURGERY. Surgical removal of emphysematous lung tissue (called *lung volume reduction surgery*, or LVRS) increases the space available for good lung tissue to expand, reducing dyspnea and increasing exercise tolerance. This is a high-risk procedure but has allowed some patients to return to a more normal activity level and improved quality of life. Surgery may also be performed to remove blebs to prevent pneumothorax. Lung transplant may be an option in select patients.

ENDOBRONCHIAL VALVE. A newer treatment is similar to lung reduction surgery, but without the surgery. It is placement of a tiny one-way valve called an endobronchial valve via bronchoscopy into an area of emphysematous lung, which causes the diseased area to collapse. This allows the healthy lung tissue more space to expand, which can increase FEV_1 and exercise tolerance.

MECHANICAL VENTILATION. If ABGs worsen despite treatment, intubation and mechanical ventilation may be considered, depending on the patient's advance directive. Unfortunately, mechanical ventilation will not make a patient's disease better, and weaning may be difficult or impossible once it is initiated. Use of NIPPV (see Chapter 29) may be a good alternative for many patients.

END-OF-LIFE PLANNING. It is important to assess whether the patient has a living will or durable power of attorney for health care (see Chapter 17). COPD is a progressive disease, and patients can increase the quality of their life and death by making decisions in advance. Patients should make decisions about whether they would want to be intubated and mechanically ventilated or have cardiopulmonary

• WORD • BUILDING •

antitussive: anti—against + tussive—cough

Table 31.4 Selected Medications Used for Lower Respiratory Tract Disorders

Medication Class/Action

Adrenergic Bronchodilators

Stimulate beta receptors to dilate bronchioles.

Examples	Nursing Implications
albuterol (Ventolin, Proventil, ProAir) levalbuterol (Xopenex) metaproterenol (Alupent) pirbuterol (Maxair)	Use with care in patients with cardiac disease. Overuse can cause rebound bronchospasm. Short acting; used as rescue inhalers.

Anticholinergic Agents

Block parasympathetic response, causing bronchodilation.

Examples	Nursing Implications
ipratropium (Atrovent) tiotropium (Spiriva) umeclidinium (Incruse Ellipta) aclidinium (Tudorza Pressair)	Should be avoided with narrow-angle glaucoma and prostatic hypertrophy.

Corticosteroids

Reduce inflammation in airways.

Examples	Nursing Implications
methylprednisolone (Medrol, Solu-Medrol) prednisone triamcinolone acetonide (Azmacort) beclomethasone (Beclovent, QVAR) fluticasone (Flovent) budesonide (Pulmicort) Mometasone (Asmanex)	Must be used regularly to prevent symptoms. Never discontinue abruptly; must be tapered. Monitor blood glucose while on high doses. Teach: Rinse mouth after inhaler use to prevent local infection (candidiasis). If using glucocorticoid and adrenergic metered-dose inhalers together, use adrenergic inhaler first to open airways.
Combination agents: albuterol and ipratropium (Combivent) fluticasone and salmeterol (Advair) Fluticasone/vilanterol/umeclidinium (Trelegy Ellipta) budesonide and formoterol (Symbicort) fluticasone and vilanterol (Breo Ellipta) tiotropium/olodaterol (Stiolto Respimat) umeclidinium/vilanterol (Anoro Ellipta)	See individual agents. Salmeterol and formoterol are long-acting beta agonists that are unsafe for use alone but appear to be safer when used with inhaled corticosteroids. Use only as directed. Not for use as rescue inhalers.

Phosphodiesterase-4 Inhibitor

Reduces COPD exacerbations.

---

resuscitation (CPR) in event of a cardiac arrest. CPR is rarely successful in a patient with end-stage disease. Patients should be made aware of palliative care and hospice options and assured that they will be kept as comfortable as possible.

Nursing Process for the Patient With COPD

See "Nursing Process for the Patient With an Obstructive Disorder" and "Nursing Care Plan for the Patient With a Lower Respiratory Tract Disorder." Priority nursing diagnoses include *Impaired Gas Exchange, Ineffective Airway Clearance*, and *Activity Intolerance*.

Asthma

Asthma affects more than 260 million people worldwide (Global Initiative for Asthma [GINA], 2021) and 25 million in the United States (Asthma and Allergy Foundation

Chapter 31 Nursing Care of Patients With Lower Respiratory Tract Disorders 551

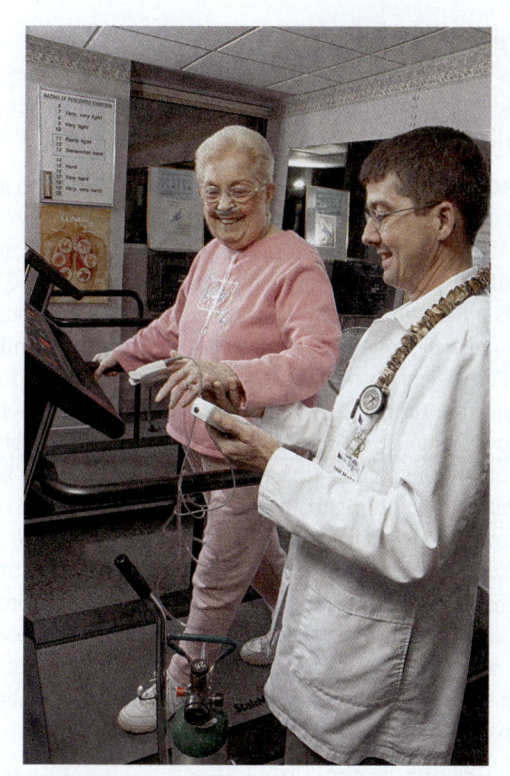

FIGURE 31.7 Patients build exercise tolerance in pulmonary rehabilitation programs. Note therapist monitoring oxygen saturation.

of America [AAFA], 2021). Rates of asthma are highest among Black individuals, who are three times more likely to die from asthma than White people. These disparities are related to social determinants of health such as poverty, city air quality, indoor allergens, health literacy, and poor health care (AAFA, 2021). With careful monitoring, education, and treatment, however, patients with asthma can manage their symptoms and lead normal lives.

Pathophysiology

Asthma is characterized by chronic inflammation of the airways and hyperresponsiveness of the bronchial smooth muscles (**bronchospasm**). This causes narrowed airways and air trapping, which is why it is considered an obstructive disorder. Inflammation occurs in part because things that trigger asthma (asthma triggers) cause the release of inflammatory substances such as histamine and leukotrienes. Symptoms are intermittent and generally reversible, with periods of normal airway function. Some people develop permanent changes in their airways, called *remodeling;* this leads to a progressive loss of lung function.

Many patients develop the disorder in childhood, and some outgrow it. However, a significant number develop symptoms again later in life. Children with asthma should be counseled that smoking can increase the risk of recurrence in adulthood. Asthma may also complicate chronic bronchitis or emphysema. Asthma is classified as mild, moderate, or severe based on the amount and type of medication required to control it (GINA, 2021).

Etiology

The tendency to develop asthma is inherited. The most common predisposing factor is the genetic tendency to be allergic to airborne allergens such as pollen or mold. Viral respiratory infections are also a contributing factor to asthma diagnosis and exacerbation. Tobacco smoke, air pollution, early use of antibiotics, and sensitization to house-dust mites and cockroaches have also been linked to asthma development.

Asthma Triggers

Once asthma develops, exposure to allergens such as dust mites, cockroaches, cat and dog dander, or pollen can trigger an acute attack. Other possible triggers include viral infection, emotional upset, exercise, stress, and certain medications (e.g., aspirin, beta blockers).

Prevention

Although asthma cannot be prevented at this time, research is ongoing to determine factors associated with its development. Current research recommendations include (1) avoidance of environmental tobacco smoke during pregnancy and a child's first year of life, (2) vaginal delivery (exposing baby to mother's vaginal flora may be beneficial), and (3) avoidance of acetaminophen and broad-spectrum antibiotics during the first year of life (GINA, 2021). There is increasing evidence for the support of a healthy diet during pregnancy to provide some protection against asthma in children. Appropriate control of childhood asthma may prevent more serious asthma in later years. Avoidance of smoking may reduce the risk of recurrence of asthma that started in childhood. To prevent acute attacks, it is important that the patient identify triggers of asthma symptoms and avoid them whenever possible. Monitoring of symptoms and compliance with prophylactic and maintenance therapy is also important. An asthma plan should be provided to the patient showing the steps required to keep asthma from getting worse, as well as guidance for when to call the HCP or go into the emergency room.

Signs and Symptoms

Asthma symptoms are intermittent and are often referred to as attacks. Attacks may last from minutes to days. Patients report wheezing, chest tightness, dyspnea, coughing, and difficulty moving air in and out of the lungs. Symptoms are often worse at night. Some patients experience coughing but no wheezing. Once initial symptoms are controlled, airways may remain hypersensitive and prone to asthma symptoms for many weeks.

On examination, you will note an increased respiratory rate as the patient attempts to compensate for narrowed airways. Inspiratory and expiratory wheezing is heard because of turbulent airflow through swollen airways with thick

• WORD • BUILDING •

bronchospasm: broncho—airway + spasm—convulsion, involuntary narrowing

secretions; wheezing may sometimes be audible even without a stethoscope. Air is trapped in the lungs, and expiration is prolonged. A cough is common and may produce thick, clear sputum. Use of accessory muscles to breathe is a sign that the attack is severe and warrants immediate attention.

Be aware that an absence of audible wheezing may not signal open airways but rather may be an ominous sign that the patient is not moving enough air to make any sound. If wheezing is not heard, use of accessory muscles and peak expiratory flow rate (PEFR) values must be carefully evaluated. Once treatment begins to open the airways, wheezing may become audible.

Complications

Status asthmaticus occurs if bronchospasm is not controlled and symptoms are prolonged. As the patient increases the respiratory rate to compensate for narrowed airways, carbon dioxide is exhaled and respiratory alkalosis occurs. If the attack is not resolved and the patient begins to tire, the patient will no longer be able to compensate. $PaCO_2$ will rise, resulting in respiratory acidosis. This can lead to respiratory failure and death if untreated.

Diagnostic Tests

Diagnosis is based on the patient's report of symptoms, physical examination, and spirometry results. PEFR and FEV_1 are reduced, especially during symptomatic periods. Asthma can be differentiated from COPD during spirometry testing by administering an adrenergic agonist (such as an albuterol inhaler) and then retesting. Asthma symptoms can generally be reversed with the medication, but COPD cannot. Allergy skin testing and increased serum immunoglobulin E and eosinophil levels indicate allergic involvement and may help determine appropriate treatment. ABGs may be evaluated during an acute severe attack.

On a long-term basis, asthma control can be evaluated using FEV_1 or PEFR measurements, frequency and severity of exacerbations and night-time awakenings, and frequency of short-acting beta-agonist use.

CRITICAL THINKING & CLINICAL JUDGMENT

Timothy is a 16-year-old whose mother brought him to the emergency department because of an asthma attack. He says he feels short of breath, but you do not hear wheezing in his lungs.

Critical Thinking (The Why)
1. What do you think could be happening?

Clinical Judgment (The Do)
2. Does Timothy really need to be in the emergency department?
3. What should you do?
4. What other team members can you collaborate with as you care for Timothy?

Suggested answers are at the end of the chapter.

Therapeutic Measures

Patients must learn to manage asthma at home. If they can monitor and manage their symptoms, acute episodes and hospitalizations can be avoided.

SELF-MONITORING. All patients benefit from learning to monitor asthma and make treatment decisions accordingly. This can be done by carefully monitoring symptoms or by monitoring of the peak expiratory flow rate, or PEFR (Fig. 31.8). PEFR is a measurement in liters per minute of the amount of air a patient can blow into a peak flowmeter from fully inflated lungs. The patient determines his or her baseline PEFR during symptom-free times. Readings can be charted to keep track of progress (Fig. 31.9). If symptoms worsen or PEFR begins to fall below the patient's baseline, the patient should begin self-treatment according to an asthma action plan (Fig. 31.10). If treatment does not improve PEFR to the expected degree, the patient is advised to go to the emergency department. PEFR results may indicate the onset of asthma before the patient experiences any obvious symptoms. Physical activity as well as breathing exercises have been shown to be beneficial for symptom management and improving the quality of life in patients with asthma.

AVOIDANCE OF TRIGGERS. The patient is instructed to identify and avoid asthma triggers. If triggers cannot be avoided, the patient can use a bronchodilator as prescribed before exposure. Inhalers can be especially useful before exercise. Animal dander and foods that cause symptoms are best avoided when possible. Eliminating carpets and curtains in bedrooms, using vinyl mattress and pillow covers, and installing a portable or central air filter can reduce dust mite exposure. Maintenance of indoor humidity between 40% and 50% can reduce mold growth. If cold air triggers symptoms, the patient should keep the nose and mouth covered when outside in cold weather. Smoking and exposure to secondhand smoke are strongly discouraged.

Aspirin and NSAIDs can cause asthma symptoms in some individuals. Beta-blocking medications (e.g., propranolol, metoprolol), used commonly for hypertension, block beta receptors in the lungs, preventing the sympathetic nervous system from promoting bronchodilation. These medications should be avoided if they make symptoms worse.

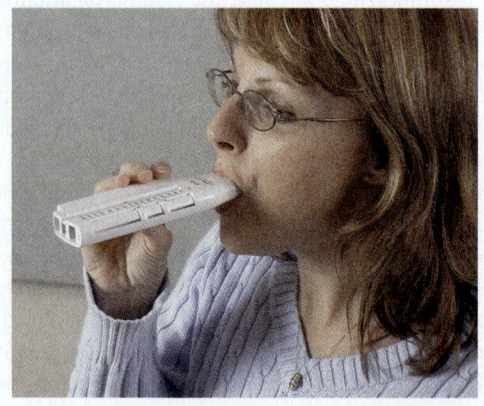

FIGURE 31.8 Patient with asthma using a peak flowmeter to monitor peak expiratory flow rate.

Chapter 31 Nursing Care of Patients With Lower Respiratory Tract Disorders

FIGURE 31.9 Peak flow chart. The green zone is 80% to 100% of the patient's normal peak flow rate. The yellow zone is 50% to 80% of normal. The red zone is less than 50% of normal. The patient works with the health-care provider to determine which actions to take when readings fall in the yellow or red zones.

FIGURE 31.10 Asthma action plan.

> **PRACTICE ANALYSIS TIP**
> Linking NCLEX-PN® to Practice
> The LPN/LVN will reinforce education to client regarding care and condition.

MEDICATIONS. Using short-acting bronchodilators alone is no longer recommended for adults and adolescents. Inhaled corticosteroids such as fluticasone (Flovent) or budesonide (Pulmicort) are generally given to control inflammation. Instruct the patient that corticosteroids must be used regularly to prevent symptoms and that they do not provide immediate symptom relief during an acute attack.

Long-acting beta agonist (LABA) bronchodilators such as salmeterol (Serevent) or formoterol (Foradil) can also help prevent symptoms by keeping airways dilated for up to 12 hours or more. They should be used in combination with inhaled corticosteroids (fluticasone and salmeterol [Advair], budesonide and formoterol [Symbicort]).

If inhaled medications do not control symptoms or if the patient has nocturnal symptoms, oral antileukotrienes may be added. Immunotherapy (allergy shots) may be used for some patients with allergic asthma.

An acute asthma attack may be treated with an inhaler (MDI or NMT) or short-acting beta agonists (SABA) IV. Oral corticosteroids (e.g., methylprednisolone, prednisone) are potent anti-inflammatory agents that are useful in an acute episode, but because of side effects, they should be avoided for long-term use. Long-term corticosteroids must be tapered before discontinuing to prevent withdrawal symptoms. (See discussion of adrenal crisis in Chapter 39.)

It is important for patients to understand the difference between long-acting maintenance medications and rescue medications and use them appropriately. Oxygen is generally not necessary because many patients hyperventilate during an acute attack. If the attack is prolonged and the patient becomes cyanotic or PaO_2 levels begin to fall, oxygen therapy will be used.

> **NURSING CARE TIP**
> Instruct the patient to contact the HCP if using more than one adrenergic MDI canister per month. This has been associated with an increased risk of death.

Nursing Process for the Patient With Asthma
See "Nursing Process for the Patient With an Obstructive Disorder" section, following the section on cystic fibrosis in this chapter. Primary nursing diagnoses include *Impaired Gas Exchange, Ineffective Airway Clearance,* and *Anxiety.* See Table 31.5 for an asthma summary.

Cystic Fibrosis
In the past, cystic fibrosis (CF) was considered a childhood disease because most affected children did not survive past puberty. However, with new treatments, patients with CF are living longer and more productive lives. Some CF patients now live into their 60s.

Pathophysiology
CF is a disorder of the exocrine glands that affects the lungs, GI tract, and sweat glands. Abnormal sodium and chloride transport across cell membranes, causing thick, tenacious secretions that cause many of the characteristic symptoms. These sticky respiratory secretions are difficult to remove and cause airway obstruction, trapping air and causing frequent infections.

Similar abnormalities in the pancreas cause blocked ducts and retained digestive enzymes. These retained enzymes digest and destroy the exocrine pancreas. The absence of digestive enzymes in the intestines causes malabsorption of essential nutrients; frequent foul-smelling, fatty stools; and excess flatus.

Patients with CF secrete sweat that is high in sodium and chloride because these electrolytes are not reabsorbed as they pass through the sweat ducts.

Etiology
CF is a genetic disorder. Both parents must be carriers of the defective gene for CF to present in a child. Patients with CF who marry are counseled on the risk of offspring having the disease.

Signs and Symptoms
Symptoms usually first appear in infancy or childhood, although a few individuals are not diagnosed until adulthood.

Table 31.5 Asthma Summary

Signs and Symptoms	Chest tightness, dyspnea, cough Wheezing
Diagnostic Tests	Spirometry, before and after bronchodilator Arterial blood gas (ABG) analysis in acute attack
Therapeutic Measures	Identification and avoidance of triggers Inhaled corticosteroids Inhaled bronchodilators Oral bronchodilators and steroids if inhaled ineffective Written asthma action plan
Complications	Status asthmaticus
Priority Nursing Diagnoses	*Impaired Gas Exchange* *Ineffective Airway Clearance* *Anxiety*

Respiratory symptoms are often the first visible manifestation of the disease and range from chronic sinusitis to production of thick, tenacious sputum. Finger clubbing is common. Over time, bouts of infection become more frequent, with eventual loss of lung function and respiratory failure.

Frequent foul-smelling stools, poor appetite, bowel obstruction, cirrhosis, cholecystitis, and cholelithiasis are associated findings. Chronic disease causes delayed sexual maturation in both males and females, and infertility is common. Death is usually the result of pulmonary complications, especially antibiotic-resistant infection.

> **PRACTICE ANALYSIS TIP**
> Linking NCLEX-PN® to Practice
> The LPN/LVN will identify signs and symptoms related to acute or chronic illness.

Diagnostic Tests

Diagnostic tests begin with genetic testing. A blood test for immunoreactive trypsinogen may show high levels in CF. A sweat chloride test determines whether sweat is high in sodium and chloride. You may recall public health campaigns that advise parents to kiss their babies and report any salty taste to their HCPs. Chest x-ray, spirometry, and GI tests also may be done.

Therapeutic Measures

Because there is no cure for CF, treatment is aimed at controlling infection and relieving symptoms. Removal of thick sputum is promoted with hydration, use of a vibratory positive expiratory pressure (PEP) device, CPT, or a high-frequency chest wall oscillation vest (see Chapter 29). All forms of smoke should be avoided. NMTs using normal or hypertonic saline or mucolytic medications may be used before CPT. An inhaled medication called *dornase alfa* (Pulmozyme) is an enzyme that breaks up and loosens mucus; it has been shown to reduce lung infections and improve lung function. Bronchitol, mentioned earlier in the section on bronchiectasis, has been approved for use in adults with CF. Inhaled beta-agonist bronchodilators help keep airways open. Ivacaftor (Kalydeco) was approved in 2020 for use in patients as young as 4 months. It is the first medication that targets the underlying cause of CF by improving the function of a protein that is defective in patients with CF. Lung transplant is a potentially promising treatment. Pulmonary rehabilitation programs help patients maintain activity tolerance.

Patients should receive a yearly flu vaccination. Antibiotics must be administered as soon as signs of infection occur. Antibiotic-resistant infections are a deadly threat to the patient with CF. Patients must be vigilant in avoiding others with infections.

Pancreatic enzyme replacement (pancrelipase [Pancrease, Viokase]) helps reduce symptoms related to malabsorption and improve nutritional status. An increase in calorie requirements necessitates a high-calorie, nutrient-dense diet. For more information, visit the Cystic Fibrosis Foundation at www.cff.org.

Nursing Process for the Patient With Cystic Fibrosis

See "Nursing Process for the Patient With an Obstructive Disorder." *Ineffective Airway Clearance* is the priority nursing diagnosis. Also, be sure to remember the special needs of the adolescent patient with this chronic, debilitating disease. Not only are normal physical growth and development delayed, but psychosocial development is also affected by repeated hospitalizations and the necessity of routine daily medication and treatments.

> **CRITICAL THINKING & CLINICAL JUDGMENT**
>
> **Mr. Jenkins** is a 36-year-old accountant with bronchiectasis secondary to cystic fibrosis. You enter his room during an episode of uncontrollable coughing and offer him support. You observe his sputum as you dispose of it—a whole coffee cup full of thick, bright yellow sputum; the smell makes you nauseated. Even after coughing, his lungs sound congested from retained secretions. You offer him mouth care before you leave his room.
>
> **Critical Thinking (The Why)**
> 1. What questions can you ask Mr. Jenkins to find out more about his cough?
> 2. What nursing diagnosis is most appropriate for Mr. Jenkins?
>
> **Clinical Judgment (The Do)**
> 3. What nursing care can you provide to enhance secretion removal?
> 4. How would you document this episode of coughing?
> 5. What other team members can you collaborate with to provide the best care for Mr. Jenkins?
> 6. To whom can you delegate the mouth care?
>
> Suggested answers are at the end of the chapter.

Nursing Process for the Patient With an Obstructive Disorder

Data Collection

Perform thorough collection of data, as presented in Chapter 29. Frequency of data collection is dictated by the severity of the patient's condition. Note orientation and level of consciousness; poor gas exchange can cause confusion and lethargy. Observe respiratory rate and effort. Observe skin and mucous membranes for cyanosis. Auscultate lungs for adventitious sounds. Monitor cough and color, viscosity, odor, and amount of sputum. Note exercise tolerance and have the patient report degree of dyspnea on a scale of 0 to 10. Monitor vital signs, oxygen saturation, and ABGs if ordered. Careful documentation allows you to be vigilant for trends in patient progress.

Nursing Diagnoses, Planning, and Implementation

A number of nursing diagnoses are appropriate for the patient with an obstructive disorder. As always, choose diagnoses based on defining characteristics and the patient's individual assessment findings.

Priority nursing diagnoses for most chronic respiratory patients include *Impaired Gas Exchange, Ineffective Airway Clearance, Ineffective Breathing Pattern*, and *Activity Intolerance*. Interventions for these diagnoses are presented in "Nursing Care Plan for the Patient With a Lower Respiratory Tract Disorder." Related diagnoses are discussed next.

Imbalanced Nutrition: Less Than Body Requirements related to poor appetite and increased calorie expenditure as evidenced by weight loss or low weight for height

EXPECTED OUTCOME: The patient's weight will be stable at desired weight for height.

- Monitor food intake and weekly weight. *Regular monitoring can help identify nutrition problems before they are severe.*
- If the patient is too dyspneic to eat, schedule rest periods and bronchodilator treatments before meals. *Eating takes a lot of energy and resting can help conserve energy before a meal. Bronchodilators can reduce dyspnea while eating.*
- Create a pleasant eating environment. *Unpleasant views or odors can spoil an appetite.*
- Provide smaller, more frequent meals of the patient's favorite foods. *Eating a lot at one time can fill up the stomach and reduce room for lung expansion.*
- Encourage family members to bring favorite foods from home for the hospitalized patient. *A large tray of unappetizing food may spoil the patient's appetite. Be sure to note sodium or other restrictions; although the patient with end-stage disease may be allowed a more lenient diet, excess sodium can cause fluid retention and increase dyspnea.*
- Consult a dietitian for liquid supplement recommendations.
- See also "Nutrition Notes."

Anxiety related to acute dyspnea as evidenced by statement of anxiety, tense appearance, and tremors

EXPECTED OUTCOME: The patient will state that anxiety is controlled; appearance of tension and tremors will be absent. The patient will use techniques to control dyspnea and anxiety when they occur.

- Stay with a patient who is acutely dyspneic and anxious. *Feeling alone during episodes of dyspnea can increase anxiety.*
- Calmly remind the patient to breathe slowly in through the nose and out through pursed lips. *During acute episodes of dyspnea, the patient may forget that breathing exercises can help.*

Nutrition Notes

Optimizing Nutrition in Patients With Respiratory Disease

Caloric requirements commonly are increased in patients with respiratory disease. When caloric intake is inadequate, the body begins to break down muscle stores, including the respiratory and GI muscles, which only worsens the problem.

Causes of inadequate food intake can include the following:

- Anorexia
- Shortness of breath
- Fatigue (too tired to eat)
- Pressure from the GI tract impinging on the chest
- Medication side effects

Many patients with COPD have carbon dioxide retention and oxygen depletion. Because fat calories produce less carbon dioxide when metabolized than do carbohydrate calories, increasing fat and decreasing carbohydrate may help. Special supplements for pulmonary patients are available. Energy and protein needs may be increased for normal maintenance of nutritional status. Nevertheless, it is important not to overfeed the patient. Excess intake can raise the demand for oxygen and the production of carbon dioxide beyond the patient's capacity to manage them.

The American Lung Association recommends the following dietary strategies:

- Eat when hunger strikes. Offer nutritionally dense, small meals five to six times a day. Eat more food earlier in the morning if more fatigued later in the day. Rest prior to eating.
- Consume a diet composed of complex carbohydrates (20 to 30 g of fiber per day), limiting simple carbohydrates; adequate, high-quality protein; and monounsaturated and polyunsaturated fats.
- Limit sodium in diet.
- Drink adequate fluids.
- Consult a registered dietitian regarding a multivitamin.
- Avoid foods that cause gas or bloating (these may include carbonated beverages, legumes, and cruciferous vegetables).
- Drink liquids between meals if drinking with meals causes early fullness.
- Add a nutrition supplement, especially a low-carbohydrate supplement such as Pulmocare, at night to help improve nutrition.

References: American Lung Association. (2020, April 1). *Nutrition and COPD.* http://www.lung.org/lung-health-and-diseases/lung-disease-lookup/copd/living-with-copd/nutrition.html; Hâncu, A. M. (2019). Nutritional status as a risk factor in COPD. *Maedica, 14*(2), 140–143. https://doi.org/10.26574/maedica.2019.14.2.140

- Reinforce relaxation exercises during times when anxiety is minimal, and remind the patient to use them during acute anxiety. *Relaxation exercises can help reduce muscle tension and distract the patient.*
- Administer antianxiety medications as ordered. *Medications can reduce anxiety but can also depress respirations, so should be used with caution.*
- Administer IV morphine as ordered (or contact RN to do so). *Morphine helps acute dyspnea and anxiety in patients with end-stage disease.*

Evaluation

If interventions have been effective, the patient will learn techniques to make breathing as comfortable as possible and will be able to cough up secretions and maintain a clear airway. The patient will be able to manage anxiety symptoms and complete activities of daily living or other desired activity without dyspnea. The patient's intake should be adequate to maintain a stable weight. If any of the patient's goals have not been met, the plan of care should be revised.

Patient Education

The patient must be aware of the contributing factors to the disease and eliminate them if possible. The patient who is a smoker should not simply be told to quit smoking but should be referred to a smoking cessation program and provided with medication, nicotine patches, or other resources and support as necessary to quit (see Chapter 29). Techniques for effective breathing and anxiety control should also be taught. A formal pulmonary rehabilitation program is an excellent resource for patient education. Always have the patient demonstrate how they use their inhaler so you can make sure they are using it correctly.

> **CRITICAL THINKING & CLINICAL JUDGMENT**
>
> **Mr. Franklin** is admitted to the respiratory unit with exacerbated COPD. He has a history of emphysema and now has an acute infection complicating his disease. His lung sounds are very diminished, and he is short of breath at rest, even on 2 L of oxygen per nasal cannula. You walk into his room to respond to his call light and find him sitting on the bedside commode with a look of panic in his eyes. He is gasping for breath, his color is gray, and his respiratory rate is 36 per minute.
>
> **Critical Thinking (The Why)**
> 1. What is happening with Mr. Franklin?
>
> **Clinical Judgment (The Do)**
> 2. What should you do first?
> 3. With whom should you collaborate in your care of Mr. Franklin?
> 4. How will you document this episode?
> 5. What can you teach Mr. Franklin to prevent an acute dyspneic episode in the future?
>
> *Suggested answers are at the end of the chapter.*

PULMONARY VASCULAR DISORDERS

Pulmonary Embolism

Pathophysiology

An embolism is a foreign object that travels through the bloodstream. It may be a blood clot, air, or fat. A pulmonary embolism (PE), sometimes called a *pulmonary thromboembolism* (PTE), is usually a blood clot that has traveled into a pulmonary artery (Fig. 31.11). Resulting obstruction of blood flow causes a ventilation-perfusion mismatch. In this case, it means that an area of the lung is well ventilated with air but has no blood flow, or perfusion. Because reduced or no blood supply is available to pick up the oxygen in the affected portion of the lung, it becomes pulmonary "dead space," causing seriously impaired gas exchange.

Occasionally, damage occurs to a portion of the lung because of lack of oxygen. This is called *lung infarction*. It is not common because oxygen is delivered to lung tissue not only from the pulmonary arteries but also via the bronchial arteries and the airways.

Etiology

Most pulmonary emboli originate in the deep veins of the lower extremities (DVT). Therefore, every effort should be made to avoid risk factors for DVT (see Chapter 23). Less common causes of PE include fat emboli from compound fractures, amniotic fluid embolism during labor and delivery, and air embolism from air entry into the bloodstream.

Prevention

Prevention of thrombi in the deep veins of the legs is the most important factor in the prevention of a PE. Advise the patient to ambulate regularly and avoid prolonged periods of sitting if possible. If a patient is at risk for DVT or PE, such as following surgery or during times of immobility, anticoagulant medications may be ordered. Intermittent pneumatic compression (IPC) or graduated compression devices are generally used. Compression devices use cuffs around the legs that fill with air and squeeze the legs, increasing blood flow. Early ambulation and leg exercises are encouraged. If a DVT is diagnosed, prompt treatment is essential to prevent PE.

Signs and Symptoms

The most common symptom of PE is a sudden onset of dyspnea for no apparent reason. The patient may be gasping for breath and appear anxious. Tachycardia, tachypnea, cough, and pleuritic chest pain may be present. Auscultation may reveal crackles or a friction rub. If lung infarction (death of lung tissue) has occurred, **hemoptysis** may also be present. Some patients have no symptoms at all. Be vigilant for the presence of risk factors and obtain immediate assistance if the cause of dyspnea might be PE. Death can occur if treatment is not fast and effective.

• WORD • BUILDING •

hemoptysis: hem—blood + ptysis—to spit

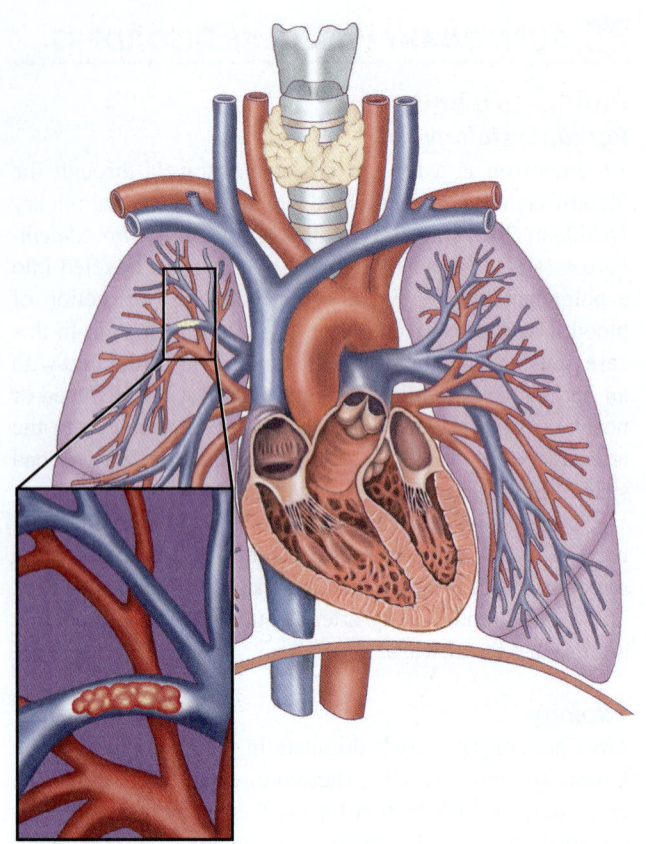

FIGURE 31.11 Pulmonary embolism.

Complications
High blood pressure within the pulmonary circulation (pulmonary hypertension) may result from arterial occlusion and lead to right ventricular failure. This occurs because the right ventricle is unable to push blood into the occluded artery. As a result, the contraction becomes weak, cardiac output falls, and the patient becomes hypotensive.

Diagnostic Tests
A D-dimer blood test can be helpful to rule out PE. Results can be obtained in less than an hour. D-dimer is a fibrin fragment that is found in the blood after any thrombus formation. It can be present in a number of disorders, but if it is negative, PE can be eliminated as a possible cause of the patient's symptoms.

A spiral CT scan with contrast dye is noninvasive and can diagnose PE quickly. If this is not available, a lung scan (ventilation-perfusion scan) is done to assess the degree of ventilation of lung tissue and the areas of blood perfusion. If an area is well ventilated but poorly perfused (i.e., a mismatch), PE is suspected.

A pulmonary angiogram is an invasive test that can outline the pulmonary vessels with a radiopaque dye injected via a cardiac catheter. It can show where blood flow is diminished or absent, suggesting an embolism.

Chest x-ray examination, electrocardiogram (ECG), ABG analysis, or magnetic resonance imaging (MRI) may also be done. However, many of these show changes only in the presence of a very large embolism or infarction.

Therapeutic Measures
Thrombolytic agents such as alteplase (Activase) or reteplase (Retavase) may be used in life-threatening emergencies to dissolve the clot; heparin or another anticoagulant is used to prevent new clots from forming. Thrombolytics must be administered within 4 to 6 hours of the clot's occurrence and are associated with risk for hemorrhage.

In patients who cannot tolerate a thrombolytic agent, the clot may be removed with a cardiac catheter, or a surgical embolectomy can be performed. The latter is a rare procedure that is reserved for emergency situations.

Oxygen is administered even if peripheral capillary oxygen saturation (SpO_2) is normal, because it may help dilate pulmonary vessels. Intubation and mechanical ventilation may be required in some cases.

Long-term use of anticoagulants follows initial treatment to prevent formation of additional clots. Medications such as heparin or rivaroxaban (Xarelto) may be used. Clotting studies must be monitored for patients receiving heparin. Sometimes heparin therapy is initiated even before a diagnosis of PE is made. It is believed that it is safer to begin therapy and then stop if PE is ruled out than to wait until all test results are available.

An oral anticoagulant is used for at least 3 to 6 months after PE to prevent recurrence. It can also be used for long-term prevention of repeated clots in patients who have risk factors that cannot be resolved. Oral therapy can begin 2 to 3 days after the heparin therapy begins. Because it has a slow onset of action, it may take several days for the full anticoagulant effect to occur. See Chapter 23 for nursing care of patients on anticoagulant therapy.

If clots are a recurring problem, a filter may be placed into the inferior vena cava via the jugular or femoral vein to trap clots traveling from the lower extremities toward the heart and lungs.

> **CUE RECOGNITION 31.1**
>
> The patient was diagnosed with a DVT and has developed shortness of breath. What do you do?
>
> *Suggested answers are at the end of the chapter.*

Nursing Process for the Patient With a Pulmonary Embolism
DATA COLLECTION. Monitor the patient for respiratory distress, including respiratory rate and effort, cyanosis, confusion, chest pain, and subjective feelings of dyspnea and anxiety. Auscultate lung sounds. Note sputum color and amount, watching especially for hemoptysis. Monitor ABGs and oxygen saturation. Monitor heart sounds and peripheral edema for signs of heart failure. Contributing factors, such as calf pain, should be noted. Remember, any sudden onset of dyspnea should be taken seriously and reported quickly. See Table 31.6 for a PE summary.

Table 31.6
Pulmonary Embolism Summary

Signs and Symptoms	Sudden-onset dyspnea, tachypnea Chest pain Tachycardia Hemoptysis Crackles History of blood clot
Diagnostic Tests	D-dimer Computed tomography (CT) scan Ventilation-perfusion lung scan Angiogram
Therapeutic Measures	Thrombolytic therapy Anticoagulants Oxygen
Complications	Pulmonary hypertension
Priority Nursing Diagnoses	*Impaired Gas Exchange* *Anxiety* *Risk for Bleeding* due to anticoagulant therapy

NURSING DIAGNOSES, PLANNING, AND IMPLEMENTATION. The priority nursing diagnosis for a patient with a PE is *Impaired Gas Exchange* (see "Nursing Care Plan for the Patient With a Lower Respiratory Tract Disorder"). Because of the impaired perfusion of the affected area of the lung, oxygen and carbon dioxide exchange are limited. *Anxiety* occurs related to dyspnea. *Risk for Bleeding* related to anticoagulant therapy is a concern once treatment is initiated (see Risk for Bleeding in Chapter 28).

CHEST TRAUMA

Pneumothorax

The term **pneumothorax** literally means "air in the chest." It is used to describe conditions in which air has entered the space between the visceral and parietal pleurae. If the pneumothorax occurs without an associated injury, it is called a *spontaneous pneumothorax*. A secondary spontaneous pneumothorax may occur due to underlying lung disease. A traumatic pneumothorax results from a penetrating chest injury. An iatrogenic (caused by medical treatment) pneumothorax results from complications of hospital procedures, such as central line insertion, pleural biopsy, or positive pressure ventilation.

Pathophysiology and Etiology

Recall that the lungs are surrounded by the visceral and parietal pleurae. These membranes are normally separated only by a thin layer of pleural fluid. Each time a breath is taken, the diaphragm descends, creating negative pressure in the thorax. This negative pressure pulls air into the lungs via the nose and mouth. If either the visceral pleura or the chest wall and parietal pleura are perforated, air will enter the pleural space, negative pressure will be lost, and the lung on the affected side will collapse (Fig. 31.12). Each time the patient takes a breath, the resulting increase in negative pressure will draw more air into the pleural space via the perforation. During exhalation, air may or may not be able to escape through the perforation.

SPONTANEOUS PRESENTATION. If no injury is present, the pneumothorax is considered spontaneous. This occurs mostly in tall, thin individuals and smokers. Patients who have had one spontaneous pneumothorax are at greater risk for a recurrence. Patients with underlying lung disease (especially emphysema) may have blister-like defects in lung tissue (called bullae or blebs) that can rupture, allowing air into the pleural space. Weakened lung tissue from lung cancer can also lead to pneumothorax.

TRAUMATIC PNEUMOTHORAX. Penetrating trauma to the chest wall and parietal pleura allows air to enter the pleural space. This can occur as a result of a knife or gunshot wound or from protruding broken ribs.

OPEN PNEUMOTHORAX. If air can enter and escape through the opening in the pleural space, it is an open pneumothorax.

CLOSED PNEUMOTHORAX. If air collects in the space and is unable to escape, a closed pneumothorax exists.

TENSION PNEUMOTHORAX. In a closed pneumothorax, air, and therefore tension, builds up in the pleural space and is unable to escape. As tension increases, pressure is placed on the heart and great vessels, pushing them away from the affected side of the chest. This is called a *mediastinal shift*. When the heart and vessels are compressed, venous return to the heart is impaired, resulting in reduced cardiac output and symptoms of shock. A tension pneumothorax is often related to the high pressures present with mechanical ventilation. It is a life-threatening emergency.

HEMOTHORAX. The term **hemothorax** refers to the presence of blood in the pleural space with or without an accompanying pneumothorax. When they occur together, it is called a *hemopneumothorax*. It is often the result of traumatic injury. Other causes include lung cancer, PE, and anticoagulant use.

Signs and Symptoms

Sudden dyspnea, chest pain, tachypnea, tachycardia, restlessness, and anxiety occur with pneumothorax. On examination, asymmetrical chest expansion on inhalation may be noted. Breath sounds may be absent or diminished on the affected side. In a "sucking" chest wound, air can be heard as it enters and leaves the wound.

• WORD • BUILDING •
pneumothorax: pneumo—air + thorax—chest
hemothorax: hem—blood + thorax—chest

x-ray examination may be done to monitor the resolution of the pneumothorax after treatment. ABGs and oxygen saturation are monitored as needed throughout the course of treatment.

Therapeutic Measures

A small pneumothorax may absorb with no treatment other than rest or high-flow oxygen, or the trapped air can be removed with a small-bore needle inserted into the pleural space. Chest tubes connected to a water seal drainage system are used to remove larger amounts of air or blood from the pleural space. See Chapter 29 for complete information about chest drainage. Smaller devices that have special one-way valves to allow air to escape but not re-enter the chest may be used for some patients who are treated at home. Some injuries require surgical repair before the pneumothorax can be resolved. Oxygen and positioning help maintain oxygenation.

If the pneumothorax is recurrent, other treatments can prevent additional episodes. Sterile talc or tetracycline injected into the pleural space via thoracentesis irritates the pleural membranes and makes them stick together. This is called *pleurodesis*, or *sclerosis*, and prevents recurrent pneumothorax. Pleurodesis is painful; prepare the patient with an analgesic before the procedure.

> **PRACTICE ANALYSIS TIP**
> **Linking NCLEX-PN® to Practice**
> The LPN/LVN will intervene to improve client respiratory status (e.g., breathing treatment, suctioning, repositioning).

Nursing Care of the Patient With a Pneumothorax

Nursing care of the hospitalized patient with a pneumothorax involves close monitoring. Frequent and thorough assessments should include level of consciousness, skin and mucous membrane color, vital signs, oxygen saturation, respiratory rate and depth, and presence of dyspnea, chest pain, restlessness, or anxiety. Regular auscultation of lung sounds provides information about reinflation of the affected lung. Be especially vigilant for signs of increasing or tension pneumothorax and report them to the HCP immediately. Nursing diagnoses to consider include *Impaired Gas Exchange, Acute Pain*, and *Anxiety*. See Chapter 29 for care of the patient with a chest tube and water seal drainage system. See Table 31.7 for a pneumothorax summary.

Rib Fractures

Etiology and Signs and Symptoms

Chest trauma is often accompanied by fractured ribs. Uncontrolled coughing, especially in the presence of osteoporosis or cancer, can also fracture ribs. Falls are a common cause of broken ribs in older people. The fourth through

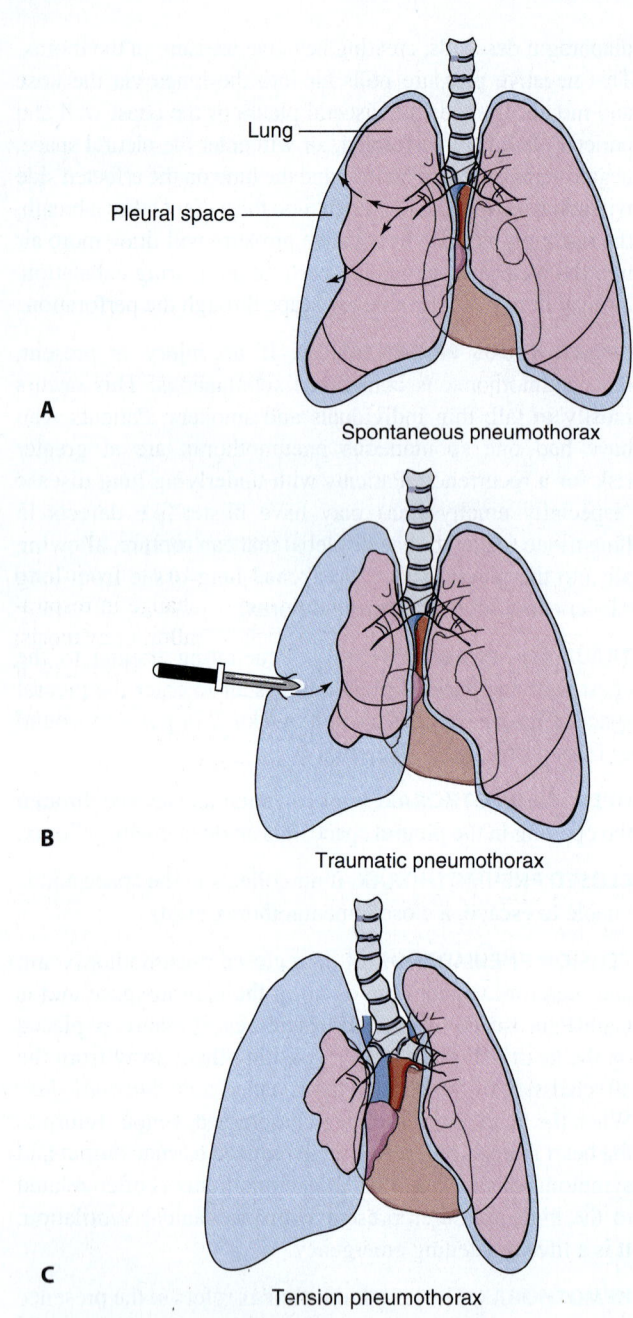

FIGURE 31.12 Types of pneumothorax. (A) Spontaneous pneumothorax. (B) Traumatic pneumothorax. (C) Tension pneumothorax with mediastinal shift.

If a tension pneumothorax develops, the patient becomes hypoxemic and hypotensive as well. The trachea may deviate to the unaffected side. Heart sounds may be muffled. Bradycardia and shock occur if emergency intervention is not provided.

Diagnostic Tests

History, physical examination, ultrasound, chest x-ray examination, and CT scan can be used to diagnose pneumothorax. In the emergency department, bedside ultrasound can shorten the time required for diagnosis and intervention and avoid the wait for a chest x-ray to be completed. Chest

Table 31.7
Pneumothorax Summary

Signs and Symptoms	Sudden-onset dyspnea, chest pain, tachypnea Asymmetrical chest expansion Diminished or absent breath sounds on affected side
Diagnostic Tests	Ultrasound Chest x-ray, computed tomography (CT) scan Arterial blood gas (ABG) analysis
Therapeutic Measures	Chest tube and water seal drainage Pleurodesis for recurrent pneumothorax
Complications	Tension pneumothorax Shock
Priority Nursing Diagnoses	*Impaired Gas Exchange* *Acute Pain* *Anxiety*

ninth ribs are the most commonly affected. Broken ribs can be painful and often prevent the patient from breathing deeply or coughing effectively, which can result in atelectasis or pneumonia. Displaced ribs can also damage abdominal organs or lung tissue, causing pneumothorax.

Therapeutic Measures
In the past, elastic rib belts were used to stabilize the ribs while healing took place. These belts are no longer used because they restrict deep breathing. Pain control is the most important treatment. Keeping the patient comfortable allows coughing and deep breathing, which prevents complications such as pneumonia and atelectasis. If traditional pain control measures such as NSAIDs or opioids are ineffective, intercostal nerve blocks may be used. Ribs heal in about 6 weeks.

Flail Chest
Pathophysiology and Etiology
When multiple ribs are fractured, the structural support of the chest is impaired. As a result, the affected part of the chest collapses with the negative pressure of inhalation and bulges with exhalation. This is called **paradoxical respiration**, which may be ineffective in ventilating the lungs and result in hypoxia.

Signs and Symptoms
The patient with a flail chest exhibits chest movement that is opposite to that usually seen with respiration. The patient is dyspneic and anxious and may also be tachypneic and tachycardic.

Therapeutic Measures
Treatment includes supplemental oxygen and analgesics. Intubation and mechanical ventilation may be necessary but are avoided, if possible, because of related risk for infection. If lung damage has occurred, treatment for a pneumothorax may be needed. Surgical stabilization of the ribs may be done in some cases.

Nursing Process for the Patient With Chest Trauma
The following nursing process is based on the stabilized patient. For emergency care of the trauma patient, see Chapter 13.

Data Collection
When caring for the patient following chest trauma, it is important to monitor respiratory status continuously. Be vigilant for any sign of worsening status, such as a change in vital signs, oxygen saturation, or lung sounds; change in respiratory rate; increase in dyspnea, chest pain, pallor, or cyanosis; development of tracheal deviation; or new onset of anxiety or restlessness. Report changes to the RN or HCP immediately. Monitor pain and condition of the chest wound, if present. Additional assessment may be necessary depending on the type of injury sustained.

Nursing Diagnoses, Planning, and Implementation
Priority nursing diagnoses for the patient with chest trauma include *Impaired Gas Exchange, Ineffective Breathing Pattern*, and *Acute Pain*. Additional diagnoses may be appropriate depending on the patient's assessment. See "Nursing Care Plan for the Patient With a Lower Respiratory Tract Disorder" for interventions for *Impaired Gas Exchange* and *Ineffective Breathing Pattern*.

Acute Pain related to chest trauma as evidenced by pain rating

EXPECTED OUTCOME: The patient will state pain is controlled and will be able to cough and deep breathe effectively.

- Administer NSAIDs or opioids as ordered. *Pain must be controlled so that the patient is able to breathe deeply and prevent atelectasis and pneumonia.*
- If opioids are used, monitor for depressed respirations and reduced cough reflex. *Depressed respirations and cough increase the risk of atelectasis and pneumonia.*
- Teach the patient to splint the chest with a pillow for coughing. *This may help reduce chest movement and pain during coughing.*

Evaluation
Are pain, anxiety, and dyspnea controlled? Are respiratory rate and SpO_2 within normal limits? Are vital signs stable? Frequent evaluation is essential so failure to progress can be quickly reported.

> **CUE RECOGNITION 31.2**
>
> An older adult female was admitted following a motor vehicle accident and is being treated for a femur fracture. She has bruising on her chest related to her seat belt. Her SpO_2 has dropped from 94% to 89%. What do you do?
>
> *Suggested answers are at the end of the chapter.*

RESPIRATORY FAILURE

Acute Respiratory Failure

Pathophysiology

Acute respiratory failure is diagnosed when the patient is unable to maintain adequate blood gas values. Hypoxemia may result from inadequate ventilation (air movement in and out of lungs) or poor oxygenation (adequate ventilation but inability to get the oxygen into the blood and, therefore, the cells), or both. Hypercapnia and respiratory acidosis occur when the diseased lungs are unable to effectively eliminate carbon dioxide.

Etiology

An acute respiratory infection in a patient with chronic obstructive disease is often the precipitating factor in acute respiratory failure. Other causes include central nervous system (CNS) disorders that affect the muscles of breathing, such as a stroke, spinal cord injury, or myasthenia gravis; inhalation of toxic substances; opioid overdose; and aspiration.

Prevention

Avoiding respiratory infections in patients with chronic respiratory disease is important. Instruct patients to notify their HCP immediately if sputum becomes purulent so treatment can be initiated.

Sedatives and narcotics should be used carefully or avoided in patients with chronic respiratory disease because these are respiratory depressants and can precipitate failure. Careful monitoring and early intervention are essential in patients at risk for respiratory failure.

Signs and Symptoms

The patient with impending respiratory failure may become restless, confused, agitated, or sleepy. ABGs show decreasing PaO_2 and pH and increasing $PaCO_2$, which lead to respiratory acidosis. The patient is cyanotic and dyspneic. Respirations become rapid and deep in an effort to blow off excess CO_2.

Diagnostic Tests

Respiratory failure is diagnosed when PaO_2 falls below 60 mm Hg or $PaCO_2$ is elevated above 50 mm Hg. Some patients with chronic respiratory disease have adapted to impaired gas exchange. In these patients, a drop in PaO_2 of 10 to 15 mm Hg is considered acute failure. Sputum cultures or chest x-ray examinations may be used to identify underlying respiratory problems. Additional tests may be done to determine nonpulmonary causes and guide treatment. Pulse oximetry is used to continuously monitor oxygen saturation. Patients cared for in ICUs may have additional monitoring, including capnography (Chapter 29).

Therapeutic Measures

Carefully observe the patient, and report significant findings to the HCP immediately. It is easy to mistakenly treat symptoms of agitation or confusion caused by hypoxia with sedatives. However, this will speed the onset of respiratory failure. Oxygen therapy via nasal cannula or mask is provided. Oxygen saturation should be maintained at 88% to 92%. Higher levels could depress the stimulus to breathe, worsening the situation.

Antidotes such as naloxone should be administered for opioid overdose or flumazenil for benzodiazepine overdose. Antibiotics are ordered if the underlying cause is a bacterial infection. Bronchodilators promote ventilation and secretion removal. Interventions for ineffective airway clearance and impaired gas exchange are initiated. Suctioning is indicated if the patient is unable to cough effectively.

> **BE SAFE!**
>
> **ACT FAST!** If PaO_2 falls below **50** and the $PaCO_2$ is above **50**, get help fast!

Acute Respiratory Distress Syndrome/Acute Lung Injury

Acute respiratory distress syndrome (ARDS) is a group of disorders that has diverse causes but similar pathophysiology, symptoms, and treatment.

Pathophysiology and Etiology

ARDS occurs because of acute lung injury (ALI), most commonly from widespread sepsis. Other causes include pneumonia, trauma, shock, narcotic overdose, inhalation of irritants, burns, pancreatitis, and aspiration. Each of these causes begins a chain of events leading to alveolocapillary damage and noncardiogenic pulmonary edema (pulmonary edema that is not caused by heart failure). ARDS usually affects patients without a previous history of lung disease.

Tired respiratory muscles in combination with edema and atelectasis reduce gas exchange and result in hypoxia. As the condition progresses, atelectasis and edema worsen, and the lungs may hemorrhage. A chest x-ray examination appears white because of the excessive fluid in the lungs.

Prevention

Early recognition and treatment of underlying disorders are important in the prevention of ARDS. Good nursing care can help reduce aspiration and some types of pneumonia.

Signs and Symptoms

The patient presents with dyspnea, tachypnea, and cyanosis. Initial respiratory alkalosis (from tachypnea) develops into acidosis as the patient tires. Fine inspiratory crackles are auscultated. The patient is often confused and lethargic. If ARDS is not reversed, eventually hypoxemia leads to decreased cardiac output, shock, and death.

Complications

Complications that can result from ARDS include heart failure, a pneumothorax related to mechanical ventilation, infection, and disseminated intravascular coagulation (DIC). The death rate for ARDS in the past was 100%. With newer treatments, it is now closer to 40%. Most patients who survive ARDS recover completely.

Diagnostic Tests

Diagnosis is made based on history of a causative injury, physical examination, chest x-ray examination, CT scan, and ABG analysis. An ECG is done to rule out a cardiac-related cause.

Therapeutic Measures

The patient with ARDS is cared for in the ICU. Treatment is supportive and aimed at the underlying cause. Oxygen therapy is adjusted based on repeated ABG results. NIPPV or intubation and mechanical ventilation are necessary in most cases, with the use of positive end-expiratory pressure (PEEP) to keep the airways open. Diuretics may be used to reduce pulmonary edema, but care must be taken to prevent fluid depletion. IV fluids are administered if blood pressure or urine output is low.

Nutritional support should be provided preferably via the enteral route. Hyperglycemia is often present during critical illnesses and should be controlled. A pulmonary artery catheter may be used to monitor hemodynamic status. If infection or sepsis is the underlying cause, antibiotics are administered. Tube feeding or parenteral nutrition maintain nutritional status while the patient is acutely ill. Positioning the patient with the less-involved lung in the dependent position ("good lung down") allows the better lung to be well perfused with blood and may increase PaO_2. Prone positioning can also increase oxygenation and reduce death rate in patients with ARDS (Aoyama et al, 2019).

Nursing Process for the Patient Experiencing Respiratory Failure

Data Collection

Assess the patient's degree of dyspnea on a scale of 0 to 10 if the patient is able to participate. Monitor respiratory rate and effort, use of accessory muscles, ABGs, and oxygen saturation values. Note the presence of cyanosis.

Monitor mental status, including restlessness, confusion, and level of consciousness, because reduced oxygenation can produce CNS symptoms. Monitor symptoms of the underlying cause of respiratory failure. If the cause is infectious, monitor temperature and WBC counts; if the infection is respiratory in origin, monitor cough and sputum.

All assessment findings should be compared with earlier data. Even subtle changes in the assessment findings can be significant and should be reported.

Nursing Diagnoses, Planning, and Implementation

Priority nursing diagnoses include *Impaired Gas Exchange, Ineffective Airway Clearance*, and *Ineffective Breathing Pattern* (see "Nursing Care Plan for the Patient With a Lower Respiratory Tract Disorder"). Related diagnoses include *Activity Intolerance, Anxiety, Risk for Acute Confusion,* and *Self-Care Deficit.*

Evaluation

If interventions have been effective, the patient will state that dyspnea is controlled. Mental status will be at baseline for the patient. Airways will be kept clear at all times, and SpO_2 and respiratory rate will be within normal limits.

> **NURSING CARE TIP**
>
> The "good lung down" position can help increase oxygenation in patients with lung disease. Gravity results in more blood in the dependent lung, where it can receive oxygen from the healthier lung tissue. The prone position may also be beneficial for patients experiencing ARDS (Meli et al, 2020).

LUNG CANCER

Lung cancer continues to be leading cause of cancer death in the United States for both men and women. However, deaths from lung cancer have declined. Lung cancer incidence has declined twice as fast in men as in women partially due to an increase in female smoking. Early detection and new treatments have also contributed to the overall decline in lung cancer.

Pathophysiology

Lung cancers originate in the respiratory tract epithelium; most originate in the lining of the bronchi (Fig. 31.13). The four major types of lung cancer are identified by the affected type of cells: small cell lung cancer (SCLC), large cell carcinoma, adenocarcinoma, and squamous cell carcinoma. The latter three types are classified as non–small cell lung cancer (NSCLC).

About 10% to 15% of lung cancers are SCLC. SCLC grows rapidly and often has metastasized by the time of diagnosis. Usually caused by smoking, it is most often found centrally near the bronchi. The patient with SCLC has a poor prognosis with average survival time of less than 1 year.

The remaining lung cancers are NSCLC. Large cell carcinoma is a rapidly growing cancer that can occur anywhere

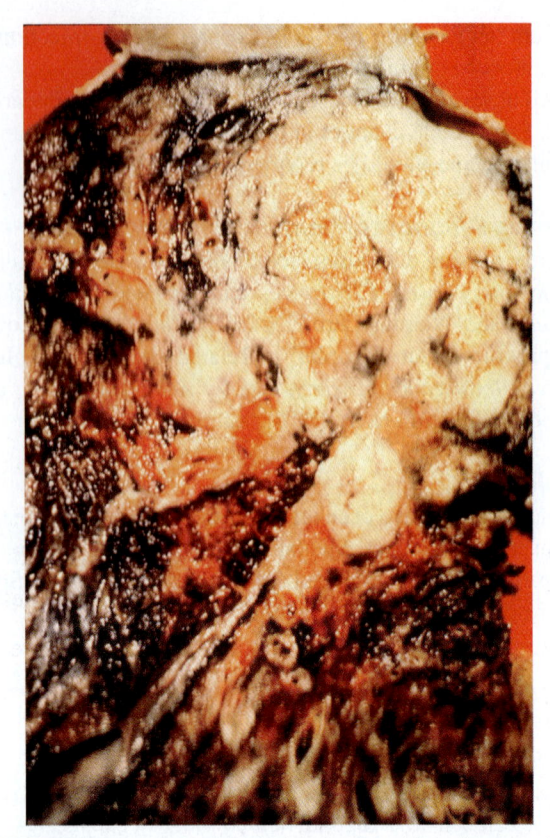

FIGURE 31.13 Cross section of a human lung. The white area in the upper lobe is cancer; the black areas indicate the patient was a smoker.

in the lungs. It metastasizes early in the disease, so these patients also have a poor prognosis.

Adenocarcinoma occurs more often in women, and most often in the peripheral lung fields. It is slow-growing but often is not diagnosed until metastasis has occurred. It is less closely linked with smoking.

Squamous cell carcinoma is the most common form of NSCLC. It usually originates in the lining of the bronchi and metastasizes late in the disease. It is associated with a history of smoking. The prognosis for individuals with squamous cell carcinoma may be better than for some other lung cancers.

Etiology

Tobacco smoke causes 80% to 90% of lung cancers. Cigarettes contain chemicals that cause DNA to mutate, creating changes in cells and development of tumors. If a patient stops smoking, the risk of lung cancer decreases significantly. Unfortunately, even with all this information, 14% of adults in the United States continue to smoke (Centers for Disease Control and Prevention, 2019).

Living with a smoker increases a nonsmoker's risk of lung cancer by 20% to 30% (National Cancer Institute, 2018). Secondhand smoke may also be related to breast cancer, nose and throat cancers, leukemia, lymphoma, and brain tumors in children. Other factors that contribute to increased lung cancer risk are exposure to asbestos, radon, arsenic, air pollution, diesel exhaust, and radiation. Genetic predisposition and a diet poor in fruits and vegetables may also be factors.

> **NURSING CARE TIP**
> Exposure to radon gas, which can be found in homes, is a significant risk factor for lung cancer. Check the Web site of the Environmental Protection Agency to find out if radon is a concern in your area. Many local health departments and hardware stores have inexpensive radon test kits available for purchase.

Prevention

The single-most important way to prevent lung cancer is to stop smoking. Many programs educate school children about the dangers of smoking. Smoking cessation programs are available for people who desire to quit. Contact your local American Cancer Society chapter for smoking cessation programs that can be recommended to patients.

Signs and Symptoms

Manifestations of lung cancer depend on the location of the tumor. Commonly, patients exhibit a persistent cough with sputum production. The patient may ignore these symptoms because they are also associated with smoking and other chronic respiratory disorders. Repeated respiratory infections may occur, producing thick, purulent sputum. Sputum may become bloody (hemoptysis). The patient may experience dyspnea. If the airway becomes obstructed by the tumor, wheezing or stridor may be heard. Late signs include chest pain, weight loss, anemia, and anorexia.

Complications

Pleural Effusion

Pleural fluid collects in the pleural space as a result of irritation or obstruction of lymphatic or venous drainage by the tumor (see earlier "Pleural Effusion" section under "Restrictive Disorders").

Superior Vena Cava Syndrome

If the tumor obstructs the superior vena cava, blood flow is interrupted, causing distention of the jugular veins and swelling of the chest, face, and neck. Diuretics may help relieve the fluid build-up. Radiation may be used to shrink the obstruction.

Ectopic Hormone Production

Some lung cancers produce **ectopic** hormones that mimic the body's own hormones. Ectopic production of antidiuretic hormone (ADH) can produce syndrome of inappropriate

• WORD • BUILDING •
ectopic: displaced

ADH (SIADH) production, with resulting fluid retention. Ectopic production of adrenocorticotropic hormone (ACTH) can cause Cushing syndrome. High calcium levels can be caused by ectopic secretion of a parathyroid-like hormone. These disorders are discussed in Chapter 39.

Atelectasis and Pneumonia

Atelectasis occurs when tumor growth prevents ventilation of areas of the lung. Patients with lung cancer also have greater risk for pneumonia. (See earlier sections on these disorders.)

Metastasis

Common sites of lung cancer metastasis include the brain, bones, opposite lung, liver, adrenal gland, and lymph nodes.

Diagnostic Tests

A complete medical history and physical examination are done to look for symptoms and risk factors for lung cancer. A chest x-ray examination is done to identify a mass. However, all tumors may not show up on x-ray. A CT or positron emission tomography (PET) scan or MRI may be done to provide more specific information about the size and location of a tumor. Sputum is analyzed for abnormal cells. Brain and bone scans are done to find metastatic lesions.

Diagnosis is confirmed with a biopsy of the lesion. A biopsy specimen may be obtained via bronchoscopy, percutaneous biopsy (a needle through the skin guided by radiograph), or mediastinoscopy (placement of an endoscope into the mediastinum to look for changes in mediastinal lymph nodes).

> **PRACTICE ANALYSIS TIP**
> Linking NCLEX-PN® to Practice
> The LPN/LVN will collect data for health history (e.g., skin integrity, height, and weight).

Therapeutic Measures

Tumors are staged based on the tumor-node-metastasis (TNM) staging system. Staging helps determine appropriate treatment (Table 31.8). If NSCLC is localized and in an early stage, it may be cured with surgical removal of the tumor. This can be accomplished with a segmental or wedge resection, which removes only the affected lung segment. A **lobectomy** (removal of a lobe) or removal of an entire lung may be done in more advanced cases (Fig. 31.14).

Chemotherapy or radiation may be done alone or in addition to surgery. Patients with Stage IV cancer may opt for using experimental medications in clinical research trials. Palliative surgery may make a patient more comfortable.

Chemotherapy is the treatment of choice in SCLC, because usually it has metastasized by the time of diagnosis. Radiation may be used in combination with chemotherapy. Surgery is not usually indicated in SCLC; the goal of treatment may be palliation of symptoms rather than cure.

Table 31.8 Stages of Lung Cancer

Stage	Characteristics
Non–Small Cell Lung Cancer	
I	Cancer in lung with no spread to lymph nodes
II	Cancer in lung and nearby lymph nodes
III	Cancer in in lung, lymph nodes, and mediastinum
IV	Cancer is in both lungs and pleurae or in distant areas
Small Cell Lung Cancer	
Limited	Cancer is limited to one side of the chest
Extensive	Cancer cells are found outside one side of the chest or in distant sites

Newer therapies for lung cancer include targeted therapies, such as monoclonal antibodies, antiangiogenesis agents, and growth factor inhibitors. Targeted therapies attack cancer cells and spare normal cells from damage. Vaccines and gene therapy are also under study to treat lung cancer. For more information about cancer treatment and nursing care, see Chapter 11.

Nursing Process for the Patient With Lung Cancer

Data Collection

Perform a complete biopsychosocial assessment of the patient with lung cancer. Assess and document respiratory rate and depth, skin and mucous membrane color, lung sounds, oxygen saturation, cough, and sputum amount and character. Ask the patient to rate the degree of pain and dyspnea on appropriate scales. Ask about appetite and weight loss as well as symptoms of other complications. Note activity tolerance and fatigue.

The patient will likely be grieving about the illness and prognosis. Assessment of the patient's coping strategies and support systems will help you plan care for psychosocial needs. The presence of a living will or durable power of attorney and the desire for assistance with end-of-life planning should be noted (see Chapter 17).

Nursing Diagnoses, Planning, and Implementation

Possible diagnoses that may be experienced by the patient with lung cancer include *Impaired Gas Exchange, Ineffective*

• WORD • BUILDING •
lobectomy: lobe—lobe (of lung) + ectomy—excision

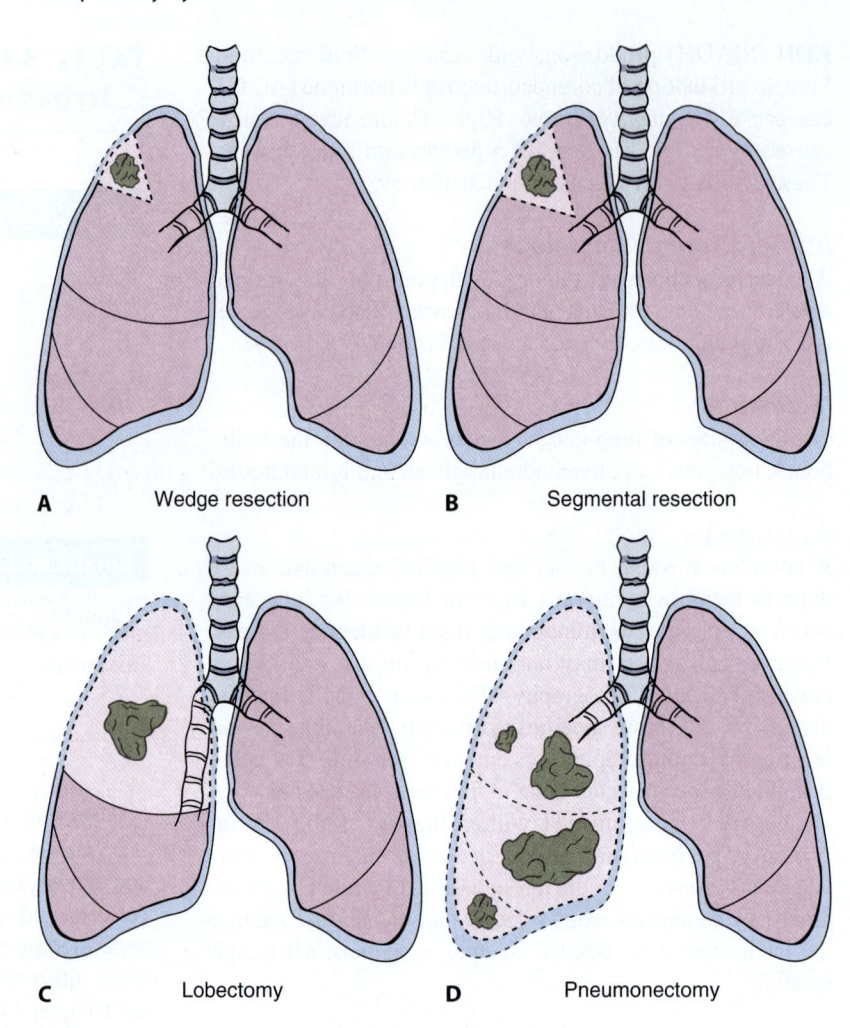

FIGURE 31.14 Types of surgeries for lung cancer. (A) Wedge resection. (B) Segmental resection. (C) Lobectomy. (D) Pneumonectomy.

Airway Clearance, Imbalanced Nutrition: Less Than Body Requirements, Pain, Constipation related to opioid use, *Grieving*, and *Activity Intolerance*. See "Nursing Care Plan for the Patient With a Lower Respiratory Tract Disorder" for care of patients with respiratory diagnoses. See Chapter 11 for interventions related to cancer diagnoses.

Evaluation

Carefully consider the patient's individual goals when evaluating care. Is the patient comfortable and free from unnecessary dyspnea? Is the airway clear and is nutrition being maintained? Are medication side effects manageable? Have patients with terminal conditions come to terms with their impending death, and have they been able to do those things most important to them before their death? See Table 31.9 for a lung cancer summary.

THORACIC SURGERY

A surgical incision made into the chest wall is called a **thoracotomy**. A thoracotomy may be performed for several reasons, including biopsy; removal of tumors, lesions, or foreign objects; repair following penetrating or crushing injury; or repair or revision of structural problems.

Pneumonectomy

A **pneumonectomy** is the surgical removal of a lung. This is usually done to treat lung cancer. It may also be used to treat severe cases of TB, bronchiectasis, or lung abscesses. Chest drainage is not usually used following a pneumonectomy because once the lung is removed, the air in the thoracic cavity is absorbed and the cavity fills with serosanguineous fluid. At about 6 months after surgery, the fluid is coagulated, and the thoracic cavity is stabilized.

Lobectomy

Lobectomy is the surgical removal of one lobe. This may be done for lung cancer, TB, or another localized problem.

Resection

Resection refers to removal of a smaller amount of lung tissue—less than one lobe. A segmental resection is the removal of one segment of a lobe; a wedge resection is removal of a small wedge of lung tissue (see Fig. 31.14).

• WORD • BUILDING •
thoracotomy: thora—chest + otomy—incision
pneumonectomy: pneum—lung + ectomy—excision

Table 31.9
Lung Cancer Summary

Signs and Symptom	Cough, hemoptysis Dyspnea, wheezing Repeat respiratory infections
Diagnostic Tests	Chest x-ray Computed tomography (CT) scan Biopsy
Therapeutic Measures	Surgery Chemotherapy Radiation Targeted therapies
Complications	Pleural effusion Superior vena cava syndrome Ectopic hormone production Atelectasis Metastasis
Priority Nursing Diagnoses	*Impaired Gas Exchange* *Ineffective Airway Clearance* *Decreased Activity Tolerance*

Video-Assisted Thoracoscopic Surgery

Video-assisted thoracoscopic surgery (VATS) is a newer technique that uses a specialized endoscope to perform surgery. It can be done with two or three small incisions, so it is much less invasive than a traditional thoracotomy, which requires opening the chest. It can be used for biopsy, staging, or treatment of tumors.

Lung Transplantation

Lung transplant can benefit patients with a variety of serious pulmonary disorders, including pulmonary hypertension, emphysema, CF, and bronchiectasis. Either a single lung, both lungs, or heart and lungs have been successfully transplanted. Better selection criteria for patients and donors along with advancements in surgical techniques have improved transplant outcomes.

Nursing Process for the Patient Undergoing Thoracic Surgery

Preoperative Nursing Care

Work with the RN to perform a thorough assessment before surgery, with a focus on the respiratory system. This gives a baseline against which to judge changes postoperatively. Routine preoperative teaching is done by the nurse in collaboration with the health-care team. The patient should understand that they will wake up in the ICU. If possible, it is helpful to have the patient and family tour the ICU before the surgery to decrease anxiety postoperatively. Prepare the patient for waking up after surgery with an ET tube connected to a ventilator, oxygen, chest tubes, IV fluids, cardiac monitor, Foley catheter, and possibly an epidural catheter for pain control. Let the patient know they will not be able to talk while the ET tube is in. Explain the use of the call light, picture board, or alternative communication techniques. Consult surgeon for specific plans.

Advise the patient that position changes and early ambulation help prevent complications following surgery. Also instruct the patient in the use of an incentive spirometer and coughing and deep-breathing techniques for after the ET tube is removed.

Postoperative Nursing Care

DATA COLLECTION. Frequent assessment of vital signs and hemodynamic stability; respiratory rate, depth, and effort; and lung sounds is performed. Remember that lung sounds are absent on the side of a pneumonectomy. An increase in pulse rate or a falling blood pressure may indicate internal bleeding and should be reported immediately. Oxygen saturation is monitored continuously. Often, patients report an immediate improvement in breathing because the pulmonary blood supply is no longer being routed to diseased lung tissue.

Assessment for tracheal deviation alerts you to the possible complication of mediastinal shift. The trachea is normally positioned straight above the sternal notch. If the trachea deviates from the midline position, the surgeon should be notified immediately. Secretions are monitored and reported to the HCP if they become thick, yellow or green, or foul smelling. ABGs are monitored closely. Chest tubes are usually present (except following pneumonectomy) and are monitored as explained in Chapter 29. Pain is assessed using a pain rating scale. Incision sites are monitored for redness, edema, or drainage. If the patient is mechanically ventilated, additional assessment of the ET tube and ventilator settings will be needed.

NURSING DIAGNOSES, PLANNING, AND IMPLEMENTATION. See "Nursing Care Plan for the Patient With a Lower Respiratory Tract Disorder" for basic interventions. Following are some additional interventions specific to the patient following thoracic surgery.

> *Ineffective Airway Clearance related to presence of ventilator, inability to cough, and sedation, as evidenced by presence of crackles and wheezes, and high-pressure ventilator alarm*
>
> **EXPECTED OUTCOME:** The patient will have a clear airway as evidenced by clear lung sounds and by absence of airway noise and high-pressure ventilator alarms.

- Suction according to agency policy. *The airway must remain free of secretions to prevent VAP and dyspnea.*
- Once extubated, remind the patient to cough and deep breathe regularly. *This helps clear the airway.*
- Administer analgesics as ordered. *Postoperative pain must be controlled for the patient to be able to cough effectively.*

Impaired Gas Exchange related to surgical intervention, opioid use, and removal of lung tissue, as evidenced by ABGs and by SpO_2 not within normal limits

EXPECTED OUTCOME: The patient's gas exchange will be within acceptable limits as evidenced by SpO_2 of 90% or above.

- Monitor SpO_2. *Interventions should maintain SpO_2 at 90% or above.*
- Reposition patient every 1 to 2 hours. Consult surgeon for specific positioning orders. *Some surgeons want patients positioned with the operative side up, and others with the operative side down. Fowler position allows room for lung expansion and helps prevent aspiration.*
- Encourage use of an incentive spirometer as ordered following extubation *to encourage the patient to deep breathe and maximize oxygenation.*
- Monitor chest tube and water seal drainage system, if used. *This helps re-expand the lung and must remain intact at all times.*
- Administer oxygen and bronchodilators as ordered *to maintain oxygenation.*

Acute Pain related to surgical procedure as evidenced by pain rating

EXPECTED OUTCOME: The patient will be comfortable as evidenced by statement or indication that pain is controlled. If the patient is unable to communicate, observe for objective signs of acute pain (e.g., increase in vital signs, restlessness).

- Administer analgesics as ordered, around the clock. *Pain control is important for the patient to be able to ambulate and deep breathe and cough effectively.*
- Monitor respiratory rate and effort if not mechanically ventilated. *Opioids depress respirations.*
- Teach the patient to splint the incision while coughing. *This can stabilize the site and reduce pain, increasing the likelihood of effective coughing.*

Risk for Infection related to intubation, Foley catheterization, surgical incision, and major surgery

EXPECTED OUTCOME: The patient will be free of signs of infection as evidenced by clean and dry incision, temperature and WBC count within normal limits, clear sputum, and clear urine.

- Monitor temperature, WBC count, incision, sputum, and urine for signs of infection *so infection can be identified and treated quickly.*
- Use standard infection control precautions, including careful hand hygiene, *because the patient is at increased risk for infection.*
- Use meticulous sterile technique for all invasive procedures (e.g., suctioning, dressing changes, catheter insertion). *This prevents introduction of pathogens.*
- Monitor nutritional intake. Consult dietitian for recommendations. *Adequate nutrients are essential for wound healing and immune function.*
- Maintain head of bed at a minimum 30-degree elevation *to help prevent aspiration of gastric contents.*
- Provide frequent oral care *to reduce risk of aspiration of oral bacteria.*
- Assist with ventilator weaning and extubation as soon as possible. *Mechanical ventilation is associated with increased risk of pneumonia.*
- Request order to remove Foley catheter as soon as possible. *Foley catheter insertion is associated with risk of urinary tract infection (UTI).*

EVALUATION. The patient's airway should remain clear, and secretions should be easily coughed up. The patient should report an acceptable comfort level and be able to cough, deep breathe, and ambulate without excessive discomfort. The patient's breathing should be unlabored, with a respiratory rate of 12 to 20 per minute. The patient's affected arm and shoulder should maintain full range of motion. Urine should be clear. Signs of infection should be absent.

Home Health Hints

- If the patient with chronic obstructive pulmonary disease (COPD) is tempted to adjust their own oxygen flow rate, equipment suppliers can put on a locking flowmeter. Increasing the flow rate can reduce hypoxic drive and cause hypoventilation if the SpO_2 is too high.
- Teach the patient with COPD to conserve energy. The patient should be encouraged to sit on a stool when cooking at the stove or doing dishes. A shower stool can be obtained from a medical supply store. Personal care activities should be spaced throughout the day.
- When a patient is using oxygen by nasal cannula, the area around the ears can become irritated or excoriated. A small sponge-type hair roller can be placed around the tubing to protect the ears. Avoid using gauze for this purpose. It can be abrasive and worsen the problem.
- Teach the patient how to use inhalers properly and have them do a return demonstration.
- When a patient requires more than one MDI, number the canisters in the order they are to be used.
- Rinse nebulizer parts with warm water after each use. Every third day, soak in 1/2 cup vinegar and 1 1/2 cup water for 20 minutes and rinse well. Air dry.
- Observe the caregiver for signs of role strain. Discuss options available and consider having a social worker consulted to assist with counseling and community resources. Contact the health-care provider to discuss your concerns and ideas.

Key Points

- Disorders of the lower respiratory tract include problems of the lower portion of the trachea, bronchi, bronchioles, and alveoli. These disorders may be related to infection, noninfectious alterations in function, neoplasm (cancer), or trauma. Any pathological condition of the lower respiratory tract can seriously impair carbon dioxide and oxygen exchange.
- Bronchitis is an inflammation of the bronchial tree. The bronchial tree includes the right and left bronchi, secondary bronchi, and bronchioles. When the mucous membranes lining the bronchial tree become irritated and inflamed, excessive mucus is produced. The result is congested airways.
- Pneumonia is an acute inflammation and/or infection of the lungs that occurs when an infectious agent enters and multiplies in the lungs of a susceptible person. Infectious particles can be transmitted by the cough of an infected individual, from contaminated respiratory therapy equipment, from infections in other parts of the body, or from aspiration of bacteria from the mouth, pharynx, or stomach.
- The most common cause of community-acquired bacterial pneumonias is *Streptococcus pneumoniae*, also called pneumococcal pneumonia.
- Hospital-acquired pneumonia can be caused by *Escherichia coli*, *Haemophilus influenzae*, and *Klebsiella pneumoniae*, among others. MRSA, *Pseudomonas aeruginosa*, and other antibiotic-resistant pneumonias are especially difficult to treat.
- Influenza viruses are the most common cause of viral pneumonia. The presence of viral pneumonia increases the patient's susceptibility to a secondary bacterial pneumonia. Generally, patients are less ill with viral pneumonia than with bacterial pneumonia, but they may be ill for a longer period because antibiotics are ineffective against viruses.
- *Candida* and *Aspergillus* are two types of fungi that can cause pneumonia. *Pneumocystis jiroveci* pneumonia is caused by a fungus and typically causes pneumonia in patients who have AIDS.
- Some pneumonias are caused by aspiration of foreign substances. This most often occurs in patients with decreased levels of consciousness or an impaired cough or gag reflex.
- Ventilator-associated pneumonia is a type of aspiration pneumonia that develops in patients who are intubated and mechanically ventilated. The endotracheal tube keeps the glottis open, so secretions can be easily aspirated into the lungs.
- Inhalation of toxic chemicals can cause inflammation and tissue damage, which can lead to chemical pneumonia. This increases the risk for subsequent bacterial infection.
- Nursing care plays an important role in the prevention of hospital-acquired pneumonia. Regular coughing, deep breathing, and position changes for patients on bedrest or after surgery, prevention of aspiration for patients at risk, and good hand hygiene practices by both patients and health-care personnel can help prevent many cases.
- The risk of ventilator-associated pneumonia can be reduced with frequent mouth care and use of a special endotracheal tube that allows continuous suctioning of secretions above the inflated cuff. All patients should be positioned with the head of the bed elevated 30 to 45 degrees to help prevent aspiration.
- Tuberculosis (TB) is an infectious disease caused by the bacterium *Mycobacterium tuberculosis*. TB primarily affects the lungs, but the kidneys, liver, brain, and bone may be affected as well. *M. tuberculosis* is an acid-fast bacillus.
- Restrictive disorders cause limited expansion of the lungs and, therefore, inspiration. Restrictive disorders can be intrinsic, involving lung tissue (such as pulmonary fibrosis), or extrinsic, involving structures outside the lungs (such as pleural effusion). Restrictive disorders include pleurisy, pleural effusion, empyema, pulmonary fibrosis, and atelectasis.

SUGGESTED ANSWERS TO CHAPTER EXERCISES

Cue Recognition
31.1: Roll up the head of the bed and quickly collect respiratory data. Apply oxygen if indicated. Notify the RN or HCP regarding possible pulmonary embolism.
31.2: Observe for other signs of respiratory distress related to chest trauma and notify HCP.

Critical Thinking & Clinical Judgment
Mr. Smith
1. A complete respiratory history is taken as described in Chapter 29. An open-ended question such as "What happened to bring you to the hospital?" elicits information about the incident. In addition, questions to determine mental status and ability to make decisions and function safely on his own are appropriate. If any concerns arise, a social service consultation will be helpful for discharge planning.
2. Mr. Smith should be instructed to always read label warnings before using any cleaning products in the future and to never mix bleach and ammonia!
3. Monitor Mr. Smith closely for signs or symptoms of bacterial pneumonia. Assist with good mouth care and maintain careful hand-washing and infection-control practices. Discourage ill visitors.

SUGGESTED ANSWERS TO CHAPTER EXERCISES—cont'd

Mr. Woo
1. Document exactly what you see: "13 mm induration at test site." Date and time your entry, and sign.
2. Mr. Woo's test is positive. He has 13 mm induration, and as a resident of a long-term care facility, he is in a high-risk group. The induration has occurred because Mr. Woo's immune system has responded to the injected antigen. Mr. Woo will need a chest x-ray and a sputum culture to confirm his diagnosis.
3. Contact Mr. Woo's HCP for orders for further testing and check with the infection control nurse about putting Mr. Woo in isolation while you await test results.

Mr. Jenkins
1. Ask questions based on the **WHAT'S UP?** format:
   - *Where* (not applicable)
   - *How* does it feel? Does the coughing cause chest pain? Are you short of breath?
   - *Aggravating and alleviating factors*. What makes the cough worse? What seems to help? Do you use any techniques at home that are helpful?
   - *Timing*. How often do you cough during a day? Is it interfering with sleep and rest?
   - *Severity*. How bad is it on a scale of 0 to 10? How much sputum are you coughing up? Is it usually this color?
   - *Useful other data*. Are you experiencing any other symptoms with your cough (such as shortness of breath, nausea, loss of appetite)?
   - *Patient's perception*. Is it better or worse than usual today? How can I help? (The patient with long-standing disease often knows what will help but is hesitant to ask.)
2. The most appropriate nursing diagnosis is *Ineffective Airway Clearance* related to excessive secretions and ineffective cough.
3. Provide hydration with oral liquids and a room humidifier to liquefy secretions. Administer expectorants as ordered. Instruct the patient in coughing and deep-breathing exercises such as autogenic drainage to increase the effectiveness of his cough. Provide good oral care following expectoration of sputum to freshen the patient's mouth. Obtain an order for CPT or a vibratory PEP device (Chapter 29) to help loosen and drain secretions.
4. "Patient expectorated 200 mL of bright yellow, foul-smelling sputum. Lungs have scattered crackles and wheezes throughout after coughing episode. Expectorant given; fluids encouraged. Mouth care provided."
5. Respiratory therapy should be involved with NMTs and assistance with airway clearance interventions. Occupational or physical therapy can help with mobilization and increasing exercise tolerance. Discharge planning may be needed to help set up home therapies or pulmonary rehabilitation. Social work or pastoral care can help with emotional distress related to having a chronic disease.
6. The assistive personnel can provide mouth care and encourage the patient to take in fluids.

Timothy
1. If Timothy is having an asthma attack, one explanation for the absence of wheezing on auscultation is that he is not moving enough air to generate the wheezing sound. If his airways are extremely tight, breath sounds may be so diminished that wheezing is not heard. This is a bad sign rather than a good one.
2. There is no way to know whether Timothy needs to be in the emergency department without further assessment. Remember that shortness of breath is very subjective and must be evaluated before discharge.
3. Collect further data. Have Timothy rate his shortness of breath. Look at his color and use of accessory muscles. Check his vital signs, peak expiratory flow rate, and oxygen saturation.
4. If Timothy's assessment findings are abnormal, call for help. The HCP may want to begin treatment quickly before further evaluation is done.
5. A respiratory therapist (RT) can be helpful with both further assessment and treatment. Collaborate with the RN to determine the cause of Timothy's problems and provide appropriate education to prevent repeat episodes.

Mr. Franklin
1. The exertion of getting onto the commode may have causes Mr. Franklin's dyspnea. When patients have trouble breathing, the brain reacts by signaling distress that can then trigger anxiety. The anxiety Mr. Franklin experienced made it even more difficult for him to breath.
2. You need to do several things at once. Begin by speaking in a calm voice and trying to help Mr. Franklin to calm himself by doing pursed-lip breathing. Assure him that you will help him and won't leave. At the same time, check his oxygen to make sure it is on the ordered number of liters and that his tubing is not kinked or disconnected. Grab the bedside table for him to lean on. Have someone bring a pulse oximeter to check his oxygen saturation. All this should take about 1 minute! Once Mr. Franklin is a bit calmer, you can find out what happened. Check his vital signs and lung sounds, and work with the RN to determine whether this represents a change in Mr. Franklin's condition that should be reported to the HCP.
3. Call for someone to page an RT to do an NMT if ordered. Also call for the RN to administer intravenous morphine if ordered.

SUGGESTED ANSWERS TO CHAPTER EXERCISES—cont'd

4. "3:00: Patient up on bedside commode (BSC), respiratory rate (RR) 36 per minute and labored, color gray, appeared very apprehensive. O_2 on at 2 L per min per nasal cannula (NC), assisted to lean on over-bed table. Encouraged pursed-lip breathing. Vital signs (VS) blood pressure 146/64 mm Hg, pulse 102 beats per minute, respirations 36 breaths per minute, SpO_2 82%. RT paged; administered as needed (prn) NMT. Breath sounds diminished, no cough. At 3:15, patient appears much calmer, RR 24 per minute and less labored, SpO_2 90%."

5. Teach Mr. Franklin that he should probably stay on bedrest until his acute exacerbation is resolved. Once he is able to start moving around, he should call for help to get up. Review his controlled breathing exercises, which he can use during movement, and encourage rest between activities.

Additional Resources

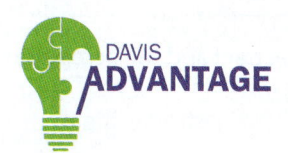

Go to Davis Advantage to complete your learning: strengthen understanding, apply your knowledge, and prepare for the Next Gen NCLEX®.

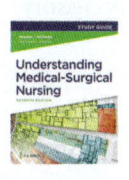

A Study Guide is also available.

UNIT EIGHT Understanding the Gastrointestinal, Hepatic, and Pancreatic Systems

CHAPTER 32
Gastrointestinal, Hepatobiliary, and Pancreatic Systems Function, Data Collection, and Therapeutic Measures

Lazette Nowicki, Janice L. Bradford

KEY TERMS

caput medusae (KAP-ut meh-DOO-sigh)
colonoscopy (KOH-lun-AW-skuh-pee)
endoscopy (EN-daw-skuh-pee)
enteral nutrition (EN-ter-uhl new-TRISH-un)
esophagogastroduodenoscopy (ee-SOFF-ah-go-GAS-troh-doo-AW-den-AW-skuh-pee)
esophagoscopy (ee-SOFF-ah-GAW-skuh-pee)
fluoroscope (FLOOR-oh-skope)
gastroscopy (gas-STRAW-skuh-pee)
gastrostomy (gas-STRAW-stoh-mee)
gavage (gah-VAZH)
icterus (ICK-ter-us)
impaction (im-PAK-shun)
jaundice (JAWN-dis)
lavage (lah-VAZH)
occult blood (oh-KULT BLUHD)
parenteral nutrition (par-EN-ter-uhl new-TRISH-un)
peristalsis (pear-ih-STALL-sis)
retrograde cholangiopancreatography (RET-roh-grade koh-LAN-jee-oh-PAN-kree-ah-TOG-rah-fee)
sigmoidoscopy (SIG-moy-DAWS-kuh-pee)
spider angioma (SPY-der AN-jee-OH-mah)
steatorrhea (STEE-ah-toh-REE-ah)
striae (STREYE-ee)

CHAPTER CONCEPTS

Elimination
Nutrition

LEARNING OUTCOMES

1. List the structures of the gastrointestinal tract and the accessory glands: liver, gallbladder, and pancreas.
2. Describe the functions of each organ of the gastrointestinal tract and the accessory glands.
3. Discuss how age affects the gastrointestinal tract and accessory glands.
4. List data to collect when caring for a patient with a disorder of the gastrointestinal system, liver, gallbladder, or pancreas.
5. Differentiate normal and abnormal data collection findings.
6. Explain techniques used to conduct a physical examination of the abdomen.
7. Assist with planning nursing care for patients having diagnostic tests of the gastrointestinal tract.
8. Explain types of nasogastric tubes and their uses.
9. Assist with planning nursing care for insertion and maintenance of nasogastric tubes.
10. Describe therapeutic measures used for patients with gastrointestinal diseases.

NORMAL GASTROINTESTINAL, HEPATOBILIARY, AND PANCREATIC SYSTEMS ANATOMY AND PHYSIOLOGY

The gastrointestinal (GI) tract (or alimentary tract) is part of the digestive system (Fig. 32.1). Digestion begins in the oral cavity and continues in the stomach and small intestine. Most nutrient absorption occurs in the small intestine. The majority of water is reabsorbed in the large intestine. Indigestible material, mainly cellulose, is eliminated from the large intestine. Accessory organs include teeth, tongue, salivary glands, liver, gallbladder, and pancreas.

Oral Cavity and Pharynx

The boundaries of the oral cavity are the hard and soft palates superiorly, the cheeks laterally, and the floor of the mouth inferiorly. Within the oral cavity are the teeth, tongue, and the openings of the ducts of the salivary glands.

The teeth begin mechanical digestion to create more surface area for the chemical digestion regulated by enzymes. The roots of the teeth are in sockets in the mandible and maxillae. The tongue is made of skeletal

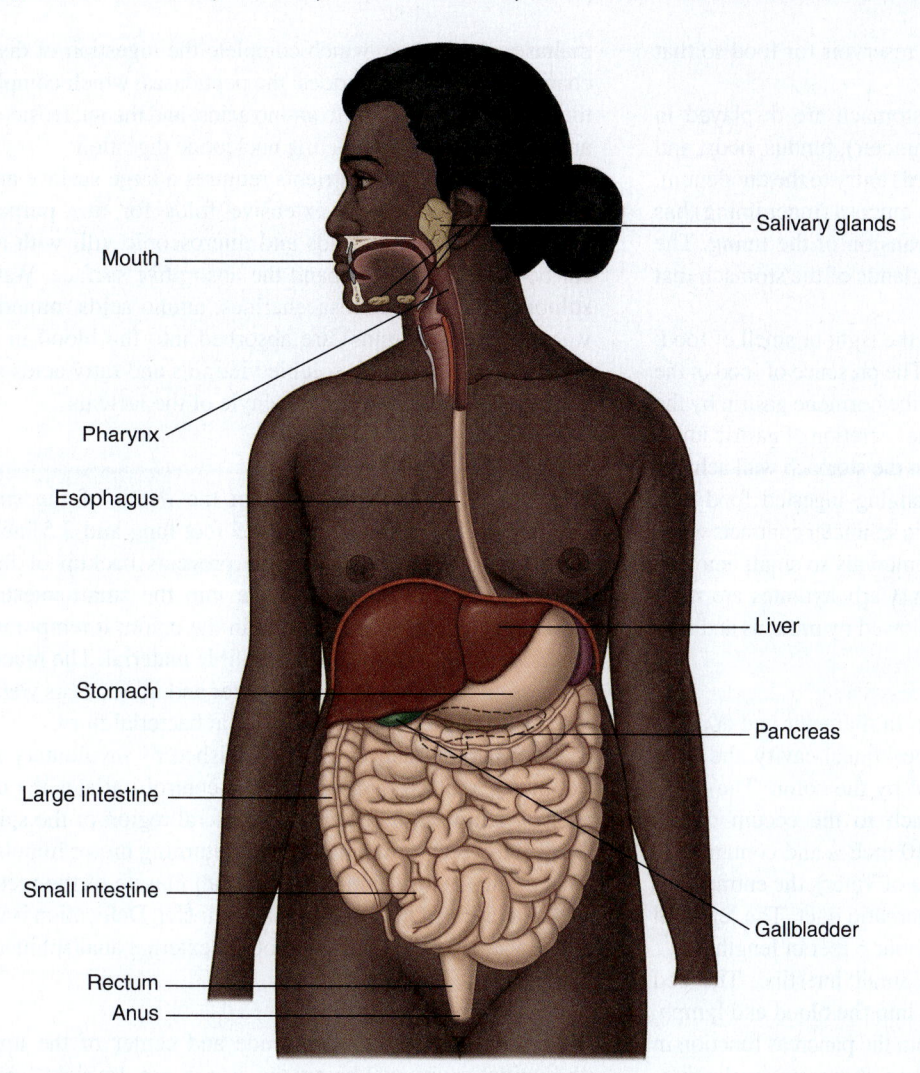

FIGURE 32.1 Digestive system.

muscle innervated by the hypoglossal nerve. Taste buds surround the base of each papilla. Innervation for tasting is by the facial, glossopharyngeal, and vagus nerves. Elevation of the tongue is the first step in swallowing.

The three pairs of salivary glands are the parotid, submandibular, and sublingual glands. Their ducts secrete saliva to the oral cavity. Salivation is a parasympathetic response mediated by the facial and glossopharyngeal nerves. Saliva is mostly water. It is used to dissolve food for gustation and moisten the food for swallowing. The only digestive enzyme in saliva that functions in the mouth is amylase, which digests starch to maltose. However, food does not remain in the mouth long enough for significant starch digestion. There is also lingual lipase. When activated by acidic pH, it begins its action in the stomach.

The pharynx is a muscular tube connecting the oral cavity to the esophagus. When a mass of food is pushed posteriorly by the tongue, the smooth muscles of the pharynx contract as part of the swallowing reflex. This reflex is regulated by the medulla and pons. The uvula closes off the nasopharynx while the epiglottis closes the opening to the larynx.

Esophagus

The esophagus is about 10 inches long. It carries ingested items from the pharynx to the stomach. No digestion takes place in the esophagus. **Peristalsis** of the muscle layer in the wall of the esophagus propels food inferiorly to the stomach. At the junction with the stomach, the lumen of the esophagus is surrounded by the lower esophageal sphincter (LES; also, cardiac sphincter, gastroesophageal sphincter, or esophageal sphincter). It is a circular, smooth muscle. The LES relaxes to permit food to enter the stomach and then contracts to prevent the backflow of stomach contents. The esophagus penetrates the diaphragm at the esophageal hiatus. The remainder of the digestive system is within the abdominopelvic cavity.

Stomach

The stomach is in the upper left abdominal quadrant, to the left of the liver and in front of the spleen. It is a J-shaped, sac-like organ that extends from the esophagus to the duodenum of the small intestine. Some digestion takes place in

• **WORD** • **BUILDING** •

peristalsis: peri—around + stellein—to place

the stomach; it serves mainly as a reservoir for food so that digestion may take place gradually.

The parts and regions of the stomach are displayed in Figure 32.2: the cardia (near its sphincter), fundus, body, and pylorus. The pylorus sphincter guards entry to the duodenum.

When the stomach is empty, the mucosa (inner lining) has folds called *rugae* that permit expansion of the lining. The mucosa contains gastric pits with glands of the stomach that produce gastric juice.

Gastric juice begins secretion at the sight or smell of food; this is a parasympathetic response. The presence of food in the stomach stimulates the secretion of the hormone gastrin by the gastric mucosa. Gastrin increases the secretion of gastric juice.

Three layers of smooth muscle in the stomach wall achieve efficient mechanical digestion, changing ingested food to a thick liquid called *chyme*. The pyloric sphincter contracts when the stomach churns and relaxes at intervals so small amounts of chyme can enter the duodenum. Carbohydrates are most readily digested by the stomach, followed by proteins and fats.

Small Intestine

The small intestine is about 1 inch in diameter and approximately 10 feet long. Within the peritoneal cavity, the coils of the small intestine are encircled by the colon. The small intestine extends from the stomach to the cecum of the colon. The duodenum is the first 10 inches and contains the hepatopancreatic ampulla (ampulla of Vater), the entrance of the common bile duct and the pancreatic duct. The jejunum is about 3 feet long; the ileum is about 6 feet in length.

Digestion is completed in the small intestine. The end products of digestion are absorbed into the blood and lymph. Bile from the liver and enzymes from the pancreas function in the small intestine (Table 32.1). When chyme enters the duodenum, the intestinal mucosa produces the enzymes sucrase, maltase, and lactase, which complete the digestion of disaccharides to monosaccharides; the peptidases, which complete the digestion of proteins to amino acids; and the nucleosidases and phosphatases, completing nucleotide digestion.

The absorption of nutrients requires a large surface area; the small intestine has extensive folds for this purpose. Macroscopic circular folds and microscopic villi with apical border microvilli expand the absorptive surface. Water-soluble nutrients (monosaccharides, amino acids, minerals, water-soluble vitamins) are absorbed into the blood in the capillary networks. Fat-soluble vitamins and fatty acids and glycerol are absorbed into the chyle of the lacteals.

Large Intestine

The large intestine extends from the ileum of the small intestine to the anus. It is about 5 feet long and 2.5 inches in diameter. The ileocecal valve prevents backup of fecal material from the large intestine into the small intestine. No further digestion takes place in the colon; it temporarily stores and then eliminates indigestible material. The mucosa absorbs significant amounts of water and minerals as well as the vitamins produced by the normal bacterial flora.

Elimination of feces is accomplished by involuntary and voluntary actions. Parasympathetic control initiates the defecation reflex from centers in the sacral region of the spinal cord. Baroreceptor input produces returning motor impulses. This causes contraction of the smooth muscle of the rectum and relaxation of the internal anal sphincter. Defecation is voluntarily controlled via actions of the external anal sphincter.

Liver

The liver occupies the right side and center of the upper abdominal cavity just below the diaphragm. Its right lobe is larger than the left lobe.

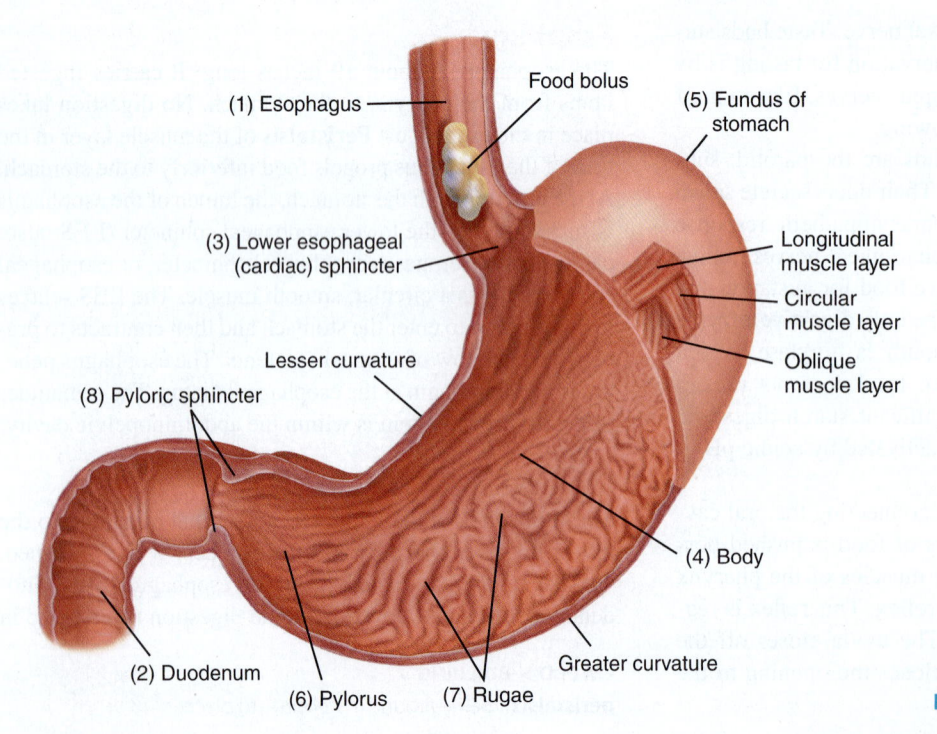

FIGURE 32.2 Parts of the stomach.

Table 32.1
Digestive Secretions

Organ	Enzyme or Other Secretion	Function	Site of Action
Salivary glands	Amylase	Converts starch to maltose	Oral cavity
Stomach	Pepsin Hydrochloric acid	Converts proteins to polypeptides Changes pepsinogen to pepsin Maintains pH of 1–2 Destroys pathogens	Stomach
Liver	Bile salts	Emulsify fats	Small intestine
Pancreas	Amylase Lipase Trypsin	Converts starch to maltose Converts emulsified fats to fatty acids and glycerol Converts polypeptides to peptides	Small intestine
Small intestine	Peptidases Sucrase, maltase, lactase	Converts peptides to amino acids Converts disaccharides to monosaccharides	Small intestine

The blood supply of the liver differs from that of other organs. The liver receives oxygenated blood by way of the hepatic artery. By way of the hepatic portal vein, blood from the abdominal digestive organs and the spleen is brought to the liver before being returned to the heart. This special pathway is called *hepatic portal circulation*. It permits the liver to regulate blood levels of nutrients or to remove potentially toxic substances such as alcohol from the blood before the blood circulates to the rest of the body. All blood leaving the liver exits via the hepatic vein.

The only digestive function of the liver is the production of bile by the hepatocytes. Bile flows to the duodenum via ducts from either the liver or gallbladder (Fig. 32.3).

Bile is mostly water and bile salts. Its excretory function is to carry bilirubin and excess cholesterol to the intestines for elimination in feces. The digestive function of bile is accomplished via bile salts, which emulsify fats in the small intestine. Emulsification is a type of mechanical digestion in which large fat globules are broken into smaller globules, producing greater surface area for chemical catabolism. Secretion of bile is stimulated by the hormone secretin. Ejection of bile from the gallbladder is stimulated by cholecystokinin.

Functions of the Liver

The liver is involved in a variety of functions, most of which involve organic molecule metabolism. These functions can be grouped into categories.

CARBOHYDRATE METABOLISM. The liver regulates the blood glucose level by storing excess glucose as glycogen and performing glycogenolysis when the blood glucose level is low. The liver also changes other monosaccharides to glucose, which is more readily used by cells for energy production.

AMINO ACID METABOLISM. The liver regulates the blood levels of amino acids based on tissue needs for protein synthesis. Of the 20 amino acids needed to produce human proteins, the liver is able to synthesize 12, called the *nonessential amino acids*, by the process of transamination. The other eight amino acids, which the liver cannot synthesize, are called the essential amino acids. Essential amino acids are required in the diet.

Excess amino acids (those not needed for protein synthesis) undergo the process of deamination in the liver; the amino group is removed, and the remaining carbon chain is converted to a simple carbohydrate used for energy production or converted to fat for energy storage. The amino groups are converted to urea, a nitrogenous waste product that is removed from the blood by the kidneys and excreted in urine.

LIPID METABOLISM. The liver forms lipoproteins for the transport of lipids in the blood to other tissues. The liver also synthesizes cholesterol and excretes excess cholesterol into bile to be eliminated in feces.

Beta oxidation is another task of the liver, in which fatty acid molecules are split into two-carbon acetyl groups. These acetyl groups may be used by the liver to produce energy, or they may be combined to form ketones to be transported to other cells for energy production.

SYNTHESIS OF PLASMA PROTEINS. The liver synthesizes albumin, clotting factors, and globulins. Albumin is the most abundant plasma protein; it maintains osmotic balance. Clotting factors produced by the liver include prothrombin and fibrinogen, which circulate in the blood until needed for coagulation. Globulin functions include becoming part of lipoproteins, acting as carriers, and acting as antibodies.

PHAGOCYTOSIS BY KUPFFER CELLS. The fixed macrophages of the liver (named *Kupffer cells* or *stellate reticuloendothelial cells*) phagocytize worn formed elements and pathogens.

FORMATION OF BILIRUBIN. Hepatocytes form bilirubin from the *heme* portion of hemoglobin removed from worn

Bile reaches the gallbladder through a series of ducts. It leaves the liver by the **right and left hepatic ducts**. These two ducts converge to form the **common hepatic duct**, which goes on to become the **common bile duct**. Bile from the liver first fills the common bile duct before backing up into the gallbladder through the **cystic duct**.

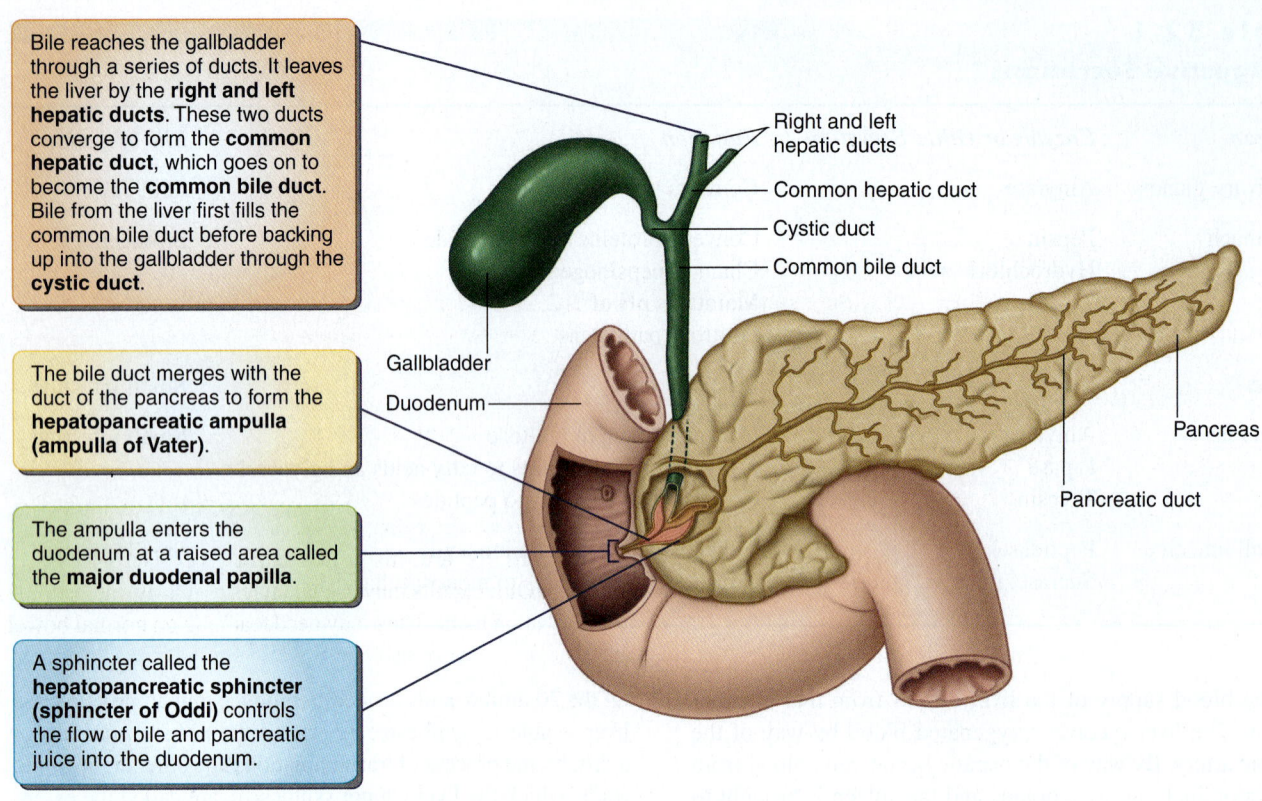

The bile duct merges with the duct of the pancreas to form the **hepatopancreatic ampulla (ampulla of Vater)**.

The ampulla enters the duodenum at a raised area called the **major duodenal papilla**.

A sphincter called the **hepatopancreatic sphincter (sphincter of Oddi)** controls the flow of bile and pancreatic juice into the duodenum.

FIGURE 32.3 Gallbladder and pancreas.

erythrocytes. They also collect bilirubin from the spleen. Bilirubin is excreted as a part of bile to be eliminated in feces.

STORAGE. The liver stores the minerals iron and copper; the fat-soluble vitamins A, D, E, and K; and the water-soluble vitamin B_{12}.

DETOXIFICATION. The liver synthesizes enzymes that convert harmful substances to less harmful ones. Alcohol and medications are examples of potentially toxic chemicals. The liver also converts ammonia from protein metabolism to urea, a less toxic substance.

ACTIVATION OF VITAMIN D. The skin, kidneys, and liver each perform a role in providing the body with activated vitamin D.

Gallbladder

The gallbladder is a muscular sac approximately 4 inches long located on the undersurface of the liver. Bile in the common hepatic duct from the liver flows through the cystic duct into the gallbladder. The gallbladder stores bile until it is needed in the small intestine (see Fig. 32.3). The gallbladder concentrates bile by absorbing water.

When fatty foods or partially digested proteins enter the duodenum, the duodenal mucosa secretes the hormone cholecystokinin. This hormone stimulates contraction of the smooth muscle of the wall of the gallbladder. Contraction of the gallbladder forces bile into the cystic duct and then into the common bile duct, which empties into the duodenum.

Pancreas

The pancreas is about 6 inches long. It is located posterior to the greater curvature of the stomach. Digestive secretions enter the duodenum either via the pancreatic duct or the alternate accessory duct (see Fig. 32.3).

The pancreatic digestive enzymes are involved in the digestion of all four of the organic molecule categories. The enzyme pancreatic amylase digests starch to maltose. Pancreatic lipase converts emulsified fats to fatty acids and monoglycerides. Trypsinogen is an inactive enzyme that is changed to active trypsin in the duodenum. Trypsin digests polypeptides to shorter chains of amino acids. Pancreatic juice also contains proteolytic enzymes: chymotrypsin, carboxypeptidase, and elastase. Ribonuclease and deoxyribonuclease, for the digestion of RNA and DNA, respectively, are contributed by the pancreas as well.

Secretion of pancreatic juice is stimulated by the hormones of the duodenal mucosa. Secretin stimulates the production of bicarbonate pancreatic juice. Cholecystokinin stimulates secretion of the pancreatic enzyme juice.

Aging and the Gastrointestinal, Hepatobiliary, and Pancreatic Systems

Many changes occur in the aging GI system (Fig. 32.4). The sense of taste is less acute. If teeth have been lost, chewing may be difficult. Periodontal disease and oral cancer increase. Secretions throughout the GI tract are reduced. Effective peristalsis diminishes because of loss of muscle elasticity and slowed motility. Indigestion episodes may

Chapter 32 GI, Hepatobiliary, and Pancreatic Systems Function, Data Collection, and Therapeutic Measures

increase, especially with loss of tone of the LES. Peptic ulcers are more common. In the colon, diverticula may form. Hemorrhoids and constipation may be problems. Colon cancer risk also increases with age.

The liver and pancreas usually continue to function well into old age. Liver damage can occur from pathogens such as hepatitis viruses or toxins such as alcohol (see "Gerontological Issues"). Gallstone formation increases. Acute pancreatitis of unknown cause is more common.

> ### Gerontological Issues
> **Medication Metabolism**
> With aging, the liver decreases in mass, volume, and blood flow. The liver metabolizes many medications, and, with impaired liver function, toxic levels of a medication can occur. Check liver function tests and review medications that are metabolized by the liver. The older adult may require a lower dosage of these medications.

GASTROINTESTINAL, HEPATOBILIARY, AND PANCREATIC SYSTEMS DATA COLLECTION

Health History

Data collection includes asking the **WHAT'S UP?** questions (see Chapter 1) (Table 32.2). Demographic data are obtained, including travel history to help diagnose the cause of GI symptoms such as diarrhea and work history for potential exposure to liver toxic chemicals.

Medications

Ask the patient about all medications, including acetaminophen, antacids, aspirin, NSAIDs, and laxatives. NSAIDs or aspirin can cause irritation and bleeding in the GI tract. Acetaminophen can be hepatotoxic. Older adults may use these medications for arthritis pain control (see "Gerontological Issues"). Older adults may use laxatives regularly and become dependent on them. They may need teaching on normal bowel patterns and laxative use.

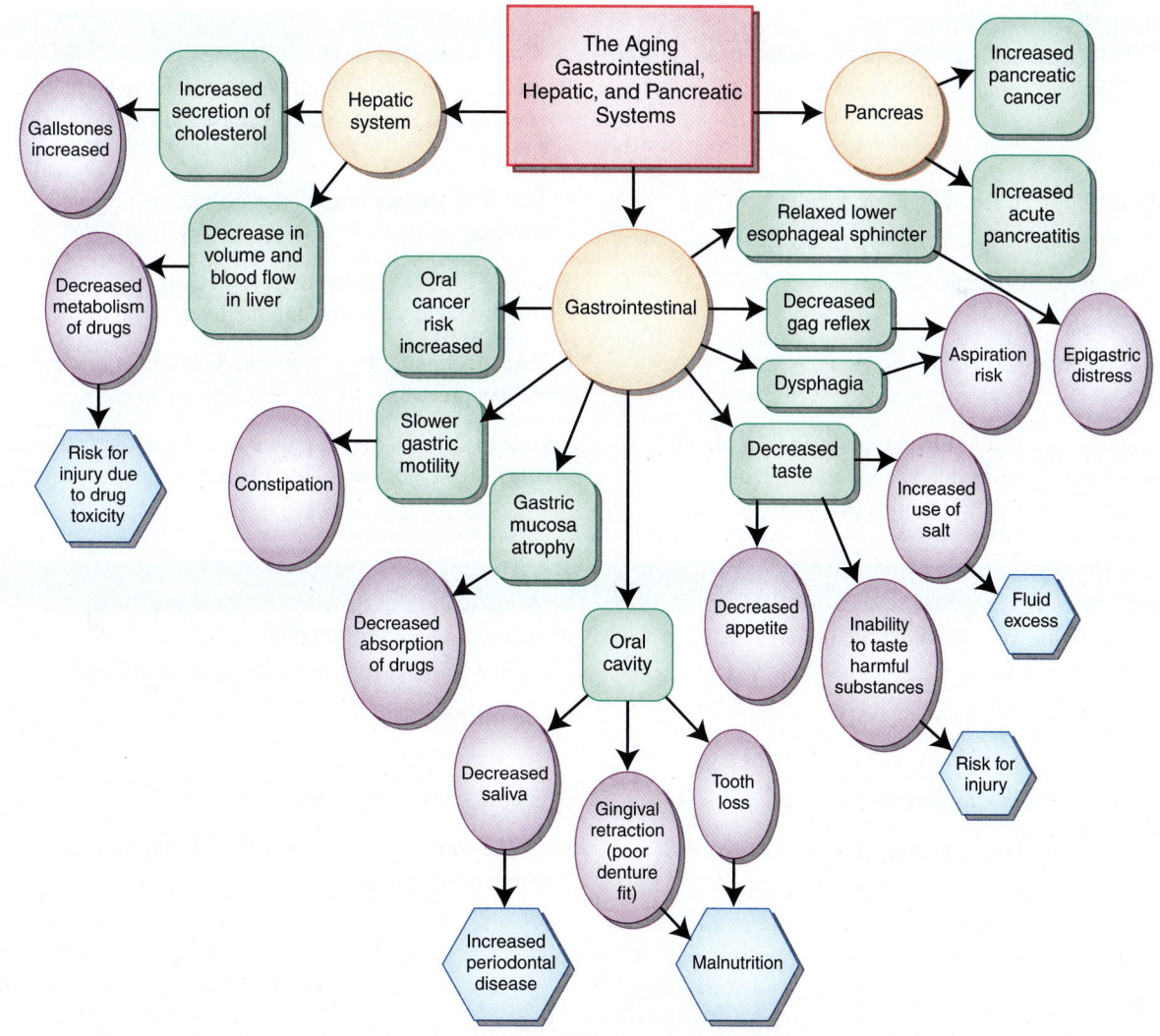

FIGURE 32.4 The effects of aging on the gastrointestinal, hepatic, and pancreatic systems are shown on this concept map.

Table 32.2
Subjective Data Collection for the Gastrointestinal, Hepatobiliary, and Pancreatic Systems

Questions to Ask During the Health History	Rationale/Significance
Gastrointestinal	
Do you have any history of gastrointestinal (GI) illnesses or surgeries?	Patient may have a recurring problem.
Nausea, vomiting, bloating, excess gas?	Can be associated with GI disorders.
Do you smoke?	Nicotine can irritate the GI mucosa. Smoking is related to esophagitis, ulcers, and GI cancers such as esophagus and mouth cancer.
What are your bowel patterns and frequency? Any changes? Stool color, consistency? Diarrhea or constipation? Bowel incontinence? Ostomy?	Changes in bowel habits could indicate new disease process. Black stools: bleeding; clay-colored stools: liver or gallbladder disease; fatty stools: pancreatic disease. Constipation may result from dehydration.
Have you had any blood in your stool or on the toilet tissue?	Blood in stool may indicate hemorrhoids, sign of cancer, or inflammatory diseases such as ulcerative colitis.
Gallbladder, Liver, and Pancreas	
Do you have abdominal pain? Do any foods cause pain?	Pain can be associated with disease of the liver, gallbladder, or pancreas. Fatty foods can cause pain in gallbladder disease.
Does your abdomen feel distended or full?	Fluid in the abdomen or ascites occurs with liver disease.
Do you bruise or bleed easily?	Bleeding is associated with liver disease, because clotting factors are made in the liver.
How much alcohol do you drink each day?	Excess alcohol intake is associated with liver disease and pancreatitis.
Have you had any recent blood transfusions or blood products, dental procedures, body piercing or tattooing, or IV injection with a potentially contaminated needle?	Breaks in skin may be the route of entry for hepatitis (type B or C) or other pathogens.
Medications	
What prescription, over-the-counter, or herbal remedies do you take?	Provides baseline information. Many medications and herbs are toxic to the liver.
Have you recently taken any NSAIDs, aspirin, anticoagulants, or steroids?	These medications can cause gastric upset and/or bleeding.
Do you routinely take laxatives or use fiber?	Patient may have dependency on laxatives.
Are you taking or have you recently taken antibiotics?	Diarrhea due to *Clostridioides difficile* can be caused by recent antibiotic use.

Table 32.2
Subjective Data Collection for the Gastrointestinal, Hepatobiliary, and Pancreatic Systems—cont'd

Questions to Ask During the Health History	Rationale/Significance
Nutrition	
Describe your usual diet. Tell me what you ate yesterday for the entire day. Do you use nutritional supplements or vitamins?	Provides information about adequacy of nutritional status. Older adults may be on a fixed income and unable to afford adequate nutrition.
Do you have any food allergies?	These may interfere with proper nutrition.
Do you have indigestion, dysphagia, heartburn, nausea, or vomiting? Have you had a change in appetite? Have you had a change in weight—gain or loss? Are there any foods that you cannot eat?	Use **WHAT'S UP?** format for further details.
Family History	
Do you have a family history of alcoholism or GI, liver, gallbladder, or pancreatic diseases?	Certain diseases are hereditary.

CLOSTRIDIOIDES DIFFICILE. Ask the patient about recent hospitalizations, antibiotic use, or uncontrolled diarrhea. Recent hospitalizations and antibiotic use are risk factors for *Clostridioides difficile* (see Chapter 8). If risk factors are present, monitor patients closely for indicators of *C. difficile* infection (e.g., diarrhea, fever, abdominal tenderness, or pain). Report these signs and symptoms to the health-care provider (HCP) promptly. *C. difficile* infection can be fatal.

CRITICAL THINKING & CLINICAL JUDGMENT

Mrs. Todd, age 74, has arthritis and takes eight aspirin daily for pain control. She is scheduled for an esophagogastroduodenoscopy (EGD) for anemia due to suspected GI bleeding.

Critical Thinking (The Why)
1. Why is Mrs. Todd having GI bleeding?

Clinical Judgment (The Do)
2. What could you do to help prevent future bleeding episodes for Mrs. Todd?
3. What nursing care will you do before and after the test?

Suggested answers are at the end of the chapter.

Nutritional History
Ask about patterns of gastric acid reflux, heartburn, indigestion, nausea, vomiting, diarrhea, constipation, flatulence, and bowel incontinence. These conditions may interfere with proper nutrition. Acid reflux can be identified by asking patients if they experience a bile taste or awaken with an unpleasant taste in their mouth.

Cultural Influences
Respecting and assisting the patient to maintain desired cultural food practices is important for nutritional maintenance (Box 32.1).

Physical Examination
Table 32.3 summarizes findings from the objective assessment of the GI, hepatobiliary, and pancreatic systems, discussed next.

Height, Weight, and Body Mass Index
The patient's height and weight are obtained for planning care. Excess waist circumferences (for women, more than 35 inches; for men, more than 40 inches) place people

Box 32.1
Cultural Nutritional Assessment

Questions to ask when performing a cultural nutritional assessment:
- What types of foods are common in your culture or community?
- What are your preferred foods?
- Which foods do you most commonly consume?
- How and where are your foods chosen and purchased?
- Who prepares the food in your household?
- Who purchases the food in your household?
- How is your food stored for future use?
- How is your food prepared before being eaten?
- What foods do you eat or avoid to maintain your health?
- What foods do you eat or avoid when you are ill?

Table 32.3
Objective Data Collection for the Gastrointestinal, Hepatobiliary, and Pancreatic Systems

Abnormal Findings	Possible Causes
Height, Weight, and Body Mass Index (BMI)	
Decreases in height, weight, and BMI	Inadequate nutrition or malabsorption problems. Recent unintentional weight loss could indicate cancer.
Oral Cavity	
Foul odor	Infection or poor oral hygiene.
A dry tongue with cracks or furrows	Dehydration, possibly due to vomiting or diarrhea.
Broken teeth or ill-fitting dentures	Trauma or poor dental care. Weight loss.
Abdominal	
Inspection	
Irregularities in contour and symmetry such as bulging or masses	Distention, tumors, hernia, abdominal aortic aneurysm, or previous surgeries.
Jaundice color, spider angiomas or caput medusae or bruising	Liver or gallbladder disease.
Scars, dressings, stoma, and ostomy appliance	Prior surgeries due to various causes.
Striae are present	The skin has been stretched with pregnancy or weight gain.
Auscultation	
Absent bowel sounds	Ileus or obstruction.
Humming sound heard over liver	Cirrhosis, indicating overloaded liver venous circulation.
Percussion	
Completed by health-care provider	Fluid, air, and masses may be in abdomen.
Palpation (Light)	
Muscle tension, rigidity, or pain	Many abdominal disorders such as appendicitis, trauma, and pancreatitis.
Ascites	Liver disease, which may increase girth as the disease worsens.
Anus	
Hemorrhoids	Increased pressure in the lower rectum such as from constipation or excess sitting.
Diarrhea	Infection, allergies or inflammatory diseases.
Skin Breakdown or rash	Diarrhea or incontinence

Table 32.4
Calculating Body Mass Index and Waist-to-Hip Ratio Measurement

To calculate body mass index (BMI) (determines percentage of body fat)	Formulas: *Pounds and inches:* weight (lb)/[height (in.)]^2 × 703 Step 1. Multiply height (in inches) by height. Step 2. Divide weight (in pounds) by Step 1 answer. Step 3. Multiply Step 2 answer by 703. *Kilograms and meters:* weight (kg)/[height (m)]^2 Step 1. Multiply height (in meters) by height. Step 2. Divide weight (in kilograms) by Step 1 answer.
BMI findings	Below 18.5: Underweight 18.5–24.9: Normal 25–29.9: Overweight 30 and over: Obese
To obtain waist-to-hip ratio measurement (determines how much fat is stored in waist, hips, and buttocks)	Step 1. Stand. Place measuring tape around bare waist at top of hip bones. Step 2. Pull snugly around the waist. Step 3. Read measurement after exhale. Step 4. Place measuring tape around hip at widest part and read measurement. Step 5. Waist measurement is divided by hip measurement.
Waist-to-hip ratio findings/risk for health complications	Female: 0.8 = low risk; 0.85 or greater = high risk Male: 0.95 = low risk; 1.0 or greater = high risk

at greater risk for diabetes and cardiovascular disease. Body mass index (BMI) is calculated to measure body fat and used along with waist-to-hip ratio measurements to determine the patient's health risk factors (Table 32.4). Healthy People 2030 goals promote healthful diets and healthy weight (Office of Disease Prevention and Health Promotion, 2021).

Oral Cavity

Oral health is very important to a person's overall health and well-being. The patient's ability to perform oral care is noted. The lips are examined for lesions, abnormal color, and symmetry. With a penlight and tongue blade, the oral cavity is inspected for inflammation, tenderness, ulcers, swelling, bleeding, discoloration, and foul breath odor. The tongue should be pink with a rough texture with no signs of dehydration, such as dryness, cracks, or furrows. The patient's gums should be pink without swelling, redness, or irregularities. Loose, broken, or absent teeth and problems with denture fit are noted. Loose teeth can become dislodged and aspirated into the airway. Broken teeth can cause pain. Ill-fitting dentures can obstruct the airway.

> **CUE RECOGNITION 32.1**
>
> Mr. Alder has just been admitted to the skilled nursing facility. During data collection, you notice he has only upper dentures and several broken teeth on the lower gums. What do you do?
>
> *Suggested answers are at the end of the chapter.*

Abdomen

Instead of following the usual inspect-palpate-percuss-auscultate (IPPA) format, abdominal examination starts with inspection, then auscultation, percussion, and palpation. This prevents palpation from altering other data collection findings.

INSPECTION. To inspect the abdomen, patients are placed in a supine position with their arms at their sides. Note type and location of any wounds, tubes, or ostomy devices.

Inspect the patient's skin for bruising, **caput medusae** (bluish purple, swollen vein pattern extending out from the navel), **jaundice** (also called **icterus**; a yellowing of the skin

• WORD • BUILDING •
caput medusae: caput—head + medusae—Medusa's snaky locks
jaundice: jaune—yellow

and the sclerae of the eyes), petechiae, scars, **striae** (commonly called *stretch marks;* light silver-colored or thin red lines on the abdomen), and **spider angiomas** (thin, reddish purple vein lines close to the skin surface). Observe for visible masses, visible movement, or peristalsis.

Jaundice is a symptom of liver or gallbladder disease and red blood cell disorders. Old red blood cells are cleared from the circulatory system by phagocytes in the spleen, liver, lymph nodes, and bone marrow. In the process, the compound heme (part of hemoglobin) is split into iron and another substance that is metabolized to bilirubin. The liver is then responsible for converting bilirubin to a water-soluble compound that can be excreted in bile. If the liver is unable to convert or conjugate bilirubin to a water-soluble compound or if bile drainage is obstructed, serum bilirubin is elevated and pigments are deposited in body tissues.

When serum bilirubin levels elevate, the patient's skin color changes to yellow. The yellow color varies from pale yellow to a striking golden orange. The color intensity is directly related to the amount of elevation of the serum bilirubin. Jaundice can be seen in body tissue and fluid where there is any amount of albumin (see "Cultural Considerations"). Pigment may occasionally be seen in cerebrospinal fluid or joint fluid. Pigment is not seen in saliva or tears. Urine becomes dark. If bile flow to the bowel is obstructed, stools will be a light clay color.

> **Cultural Considerations**
>
> To observe for jaundice in a patient with dark skin, look at the sclerae, conjunctivae, palms of hands, soles of feet, and in the buccal mucosa for patches of yellow bilirubin pigment.

The perianal and anal areas are inspected for color, rashes, scars, fissures, external hemorrhoids, and skin breakdown. Observe the patient's stool for evidence of bacteria (e.g., a foul smell), fat (e.g., stool floats on the water surface and appears greasy), pus, blood, mucus, and color. With liver or gallbladder disease, stools may be pale or clay-colored.

AUSCULTATION. Bowel sounds are soft clicks and gurgles that vary normally in frequency and rate. To listen for bowel sounds, the stethoscope is pressed lightly on the abdomen (Fig. 32.5). Bowel sounds can be categorized as normal, hyperactive, hypoactive, or absent. With a bowel obstruction, a high-pitched tinkling sound is heard proximal to the obstruction and may become muffled with abdominal distention.

Research has shown great variability in how bowel sounds are auscultated and what is heard in healthy and patient populations. These studies call into question the value of listening to bowel sounds. Further research is needed to determine if there is value in listening to bowel sounds and to standardize the auscultation method.

PERCUSSION. Percussion produces a sound that identifies the density of the organs beneath the area being percussed. It is performed by the HCP. Percussion detects fluid, air, and masses in the abdomen. It also identifies size and location of abdominal organs (especially the liver and spleen). Tympanic high-pitched sounds indicate presence of air. Dull thuds indicate fluid or solid organs.

PALPATION. Light palpation of the abdomen ends the physical assessment. If the patient is having pain, palpate that area last. Lightly depress the abdomen no more than 0.5 to 1.0 inch during the palpation using the finger pads. Note muscle tension, rigidity, masses, or expressions of pain.

Deep palpation of the abdomen is done only by the HCP. Rebound tenderness is determined by pressing down on the abdomen a few inches and quickly releasing the pressure.

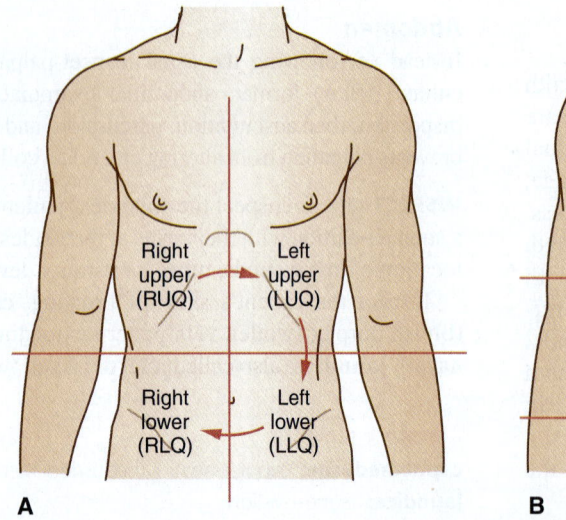

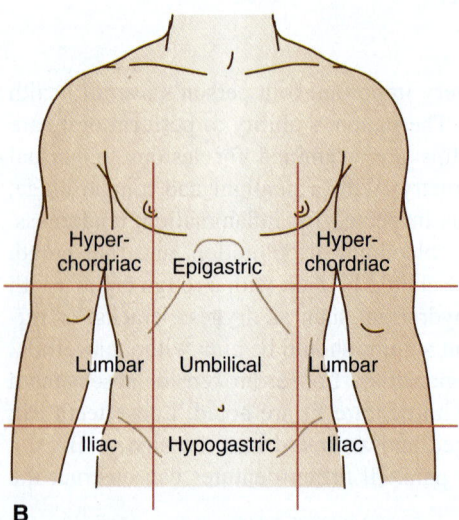

FIGURE 32.5 (A) Abdominal quadrants. Auscultation may begin from the right upper quadrant in a clockwise manner. (B) Nine abdominal regions.

If the patient feels a sharp pain during this procedure, appendicitis may be indicated.

Abdominal girth is measured by placing a tape measure around the patient's abdomen at the iliac crest. A mark is made at the measurement site so measurements are made at the same location for comparison. Abdominal girth is increased in patients with distention or conditions such as ascites (accumulation of fluid in the peritoneal cavity). When abdominal girth is abnormal, daily measurements should be monitored for changes.

DIAGNOSTIC TESTS FOR THE GASTROINTESTINAL, HEPATOBILIARY, AND PANCREATIC SYSTEMS

See Tables 32.5 and 32.6 for a summary of laboratory tests and Table 32.7 for a summary of diagnostic procedures.

Laboratory Tests

The complete blood count (CBC) reveals if anemia or infection is present. Anemia may occur with GI bleeding or cancer. Electrolyte imbalances often occur with GI illness as a result of vomiting, diarrhea, malabsorption, or use of GI suction.

Stool Tests

Stool samples can be tested for **occult blood** (blood not seen by the naked eye). A series of three tests is usually done to increase the chances of detecting blood. False-positive occult blood results can occur with bleeding gums following a dental procedure; ingestion of red meat within 3 days before testing; ingestion of fish, turnips, or horseradish; and use of medications, including anticoagulants, aspirin, colchicine, NSAIDs, steroids, and iron preparations in large doses.

Stool is collected to detect intestinal infections caused by parasites and their ova (eggs). The test usually requires a series of three stool specimens collected every second or third day. The stool specimen is collected using a tongue blade, placed in a container with a preservative, and taken immediately to the laboratory. The stool must be examined within 30 minutes of collection. False-negative results can occur if the specimen is not fresh or contains urine.

Text continued on page 588

Table 32.5
Laboratory Tests for the Gastrointestinal System

Test	Definition	Normal Range	Significance of Abnormal Findings
Carcinoembryonic Antigen (CEA)	Blood test to detect glycoproteins produced during rapid multiplication of epithelial cells.	Nonsmoker: Less than 2.5 ng/mL Smoker: Less than 5 ng/mL	Monitors response to liver and gastrointestinal (GI) cancer therapy. Serial monitoring: Elevated—recurrence or metastasis in colon and GI cancer.
Fecal Analysis			
Stool for occult blood	Stool sample tested for presence of blood.	Negative	Blood presence may indicate peptic ulcer, colorectal cancer, ulcerative colitis, hemorrhoids, or infectious diarrhea.
Stool cultures	Stool sample tested for pathogenic bacteria.	No pathogen growth	Bacterial infection, botulism.
Stool for fat (lipids)	Test measuring fat content in stool. Used to confirm diagnosis of steatorrhea.	Adult: 2–7 g per 24 hours	Increased: Malabsorptive conditions and, pancreatic disease. Decreased: Small bowel disease.
Stool for immunochemical test	Stool sample tested for presence of hidden blood.	Negative	Blood presence can be early sign of colorectal cancer, requiring further testing.
Stool for multitarget DNA	Stool sample tested for 10 biomarkers for precancerous lesions and colorectal cancer.	Negative	Precancerous lesions or colorectal cancer
Stool for ova and parasites	Stool sample tested for parasites.	No parasites, ova, or larvae	Parasitic infection

Table 32.6
Laboratory Tests for the Hepatobiliary and Pancreatic Systems

Test	Definition	Normal Range	Significance of Abnormal Findings
Blood			
Alanine aminotransferase (ALT)	ALT is an enzyme made in the liver.	*Child, adult:* Male 19–36 units/L; female 24–36 units/L *Older than 90:* Male 6–38 units/L; Female 5–24 units/L	↑ with chronic liver damage and hepatitis, or liver disease from hepatotoxic medications
Albumin	The body protein in the greatest concentration. Evaluates liver, chronic illness, and nutritional status.	*Adult:* 3.7–5.1 g/dL *Older adult:* 3.2–4.6 g/dL *Older than 90:* 2.9–4.5 g/dL	↓ in acute and chronic liver disease, kidney disease, and malnutrition
Ammonia	A by-product of protein catabolism.	*Adult:* 10–80 mcg/dL	↑ in cirrhosis and hepatitis
Amylase	Detects and evaluates treatment for pancreatitis.	*Adult, older adult:* 100–300 units/L	↑ in biliary tract disease, common bile duct obstruction or stones, pancreatitis, pancreatic ascites, cancer, cyst, or tumor ↓ in hepatic disease, pancreatectomy, and pancreatic insufficiency Some medications can increase or decrease values.
Aspartate aminotransferase (AST)	Enzyme found in large amounts in the liver and myocardial tissue, and smaller amounts in the pancreas, muscle, kidneys, red blood cells, and brain. It is released into bloodstream with tissue damage. Levels reflect degree of damage.	*Adult:* Male 20–40 units/L; female: 15–30 units/L	Greatly ↑ in acute hepatitis, especially viral, hepatocellular disease, shock, and acute pancreatitis Moderately ↑ in biliary tract obstruction, cirrhosis, chronic hepatitis, and liver tumors
Bilirubin			
• Total serum bilirubin	Evaluates liver function. Sum of conjugated, unconjugated, and delta bilirubin.	*Adult, older adult:* Less than 1.2 mg/dL	↑ in excessive red blood cell destruction, liver damage, and bile duct obstruction
• Conjugated (direct) bilirubin	Bilirubin that is conjugated in the liver (joined with glucuronic acid).	*Adult, older adult:* Less than 0.3 mg/dL	↑ with gallstones and gallbladder obstruction

Table 32.6
Laboratory Tests for the Hepatobiliary and Pancreatic Systems—cont'd

Test	Definition	Normal Range	Significance of Abnormal Findings
• Delta	Irreversibly binds to albumin. Remains elevated the longest during recovery, likely causing the persistent jaundice.	*Adult, older adult:* Less than 0.2 mg/dL	↑ with gallstones and gallbladder obstruction
• Unconjugated (indirect) bilirubin	Bilirubin in the bloodstream that has not yet passed through the liver.	*Adult, older adult:* Less than 1.1 mg/dL	↑ with excessive red blood cell destruction or liver damage, hepatitis, or cirrhosis
Calcium, total	Identifies serum calcium level, which is involved in almost all of the body's essential processes.	*Adult:* 8.2–10.2 mg/dL *Older than 90 years:* 8.2–9.6 mg/dL	↓ with acute pancreatitis, cirrhosis, malabsorption, and malnutrition
Cholesterol	Identifies 12-hour fasting serum cholesterol level.	Greater than 200 mg/dL	↑ in pancreatitis and gallbladder disease ↓ may indicate severe liver disease
Lactic dehydrogenase (LDH)	Determines level of this intracellular enzyme, which is released with injury or disease. LDH_4 and LDH_5 fraction elevates with liver damage. LDH_3 can be elevated with pancreas or spleen disorders.	*15–43 years:* 90–156 units/L *Older than 43 years:* 90–176 units/L LDH_3: 20%–26% LDH_4: 8%–16% LDH_5: 6%–16%	↑ in cirrhosis, liver cancer, pancreatitis, obstructive jaundice, and viral hepatitis
Lipase	Digestive enzymes mainly secreted by the pancreas. Released into bloodstream with pancreas damage. Serum levels diagnose pancreatic disease.	*Adult, older adult:* 0–60 units/L	↑ in pancreatic diseases, especially pancreatitis, pancreatic cancer, and acute cholecystitis
Prothrombin time (PT)	Prothrombin is a vitamin K–dependent protein produced by the liver. PT is a coagulation test measuring time for a fibrin clot to form.	*Adult:* 10–13 seconds	↑ in biliary obstruction, cirrhosis, and vitamin K deficiency
Urine			
Urine bilirubin	Detects liver disorders.	Negative	Present in cirrhosis, hepatitis, and hepatic tumor
Urobilinogen	Detects liver disorders.	Up to 1 mg/dL	↑ with hepatitis, cirrhosis, and bile duct obstruction

Table 32.7
Diagnostic Procedures for the Gastrointestinal, Hepatobiliary, and Pancreatic Systems

Procedure	Definition/Normal Findings	Significance of Abnormal Findings	Nursing Management
Noninvasive			
Barium swallow	X-ray examination of esophagus, stomach, duodenum, and jejunum using oral barium. Fluoroscope outlines organs. Normal findings: Normal organ structures.	Hiatal hernias, motility problems, polyps, foreign bodies, strictures, tumors, and ulcers	*Pretest:* Nothing by mouth (NPO) for 8 hours before test. Encourage no smoking morning of procedure. *Posttest:* Increase fluids (4 glasses). Mild laxatives may be ordered. Monitor for constipation. Stools will be white due to the barium.
Barium enema	Colon filled with barium. X-rays visualize position, movement, and filling of colon. Normal findings: Colon structures normal.	Diverticula, inflammation, obstructions, polyps, stenosis, tumors, and ulcerative colitis	*Pretest:* Low-residue diet several days before test; clear liquids 24 hours before test; NPO 8 hours before test. Laxative and enema may be given the day before the test; enema the morning of test as needed. *Posttest:* Encourage fluids (4–8 oz. glasses). Laxatives may be ordered. Stools will be white for 2–3 days. Monitor for constipation.
Computed tomography (various GI sites)	X-ray examination of GI structures using CT scanner. Normal findings: GI structures normal.	Cancer, polyps, bowel perforation or obstruction, or abscess	*Pretest:* NPO 2 to 4 hours prior to test or as ordered. Posttest: Varies depending on site.
Invasive			
Nuclear scanning: Hepatobiliary scan (biliary tract radionuclide scan, cholescintigraphy, hepatobiliary scintigraphy, hepatobiliary iminodiacetic acid [HIDA] scan, or iminodiacetic acid [IDA] scan)	Injection of small amount of IV radioactive isotope to visualize the cystic and common bile ducts of the gallbladder. Normal findings: Normal size, shape, and function of the gallbladder.	Cholecystitis, obstruction secondary to gallstones, tumor or structure, or postoperative biliary leak, fistula, or obstruction	*Pretest:* NPO 4–6 hours before test. Stop opiate-based medications 2–6 hours prior to procedure. *Posttest:* Follow organizational policies for flushing urine in first 24 hours. *Teach:* Increase fluids to flush isotope for 24–48 hours after test.

Table 32.7
Diagnostic Procedures for the Gastrointestinal, Hepatobiliary, and Pancreatic Systems—cont'd

Procedure	Definition/Normal Findings	Significance of Abnormal Findings	Nursing Management
Esophagogastroduodenoscopy (EGD)	Endoscopy allowing visualization of esophagus, stomach, and upper duodenum. Biopsy or cytology specimens can be obtained. Normal findings: Normal structures.	Inflammation, cancer, bleeding, or injury	*Pretest:* May be on a special diet 1 or 2 days prior. May have laxative and enema before the test as needed. NPO 6–8 hours before test. *Posttest:* Monitor vital signs. Keep NPO until swallow and gag reflexes are intact. Monitor for pain, bleeding, fever, and dysphagia.
Endoscopic retrograde cholangiopancreatography (ERCP)	Endoscopy allowing visualization of pancreas and common bile ducts and x-rays with contrast media. Normal findings: Normal structures without obstruction or stricture.	Gallstones, bile duct or pancreatic disease, cysts, fibrosis, pancreatitis, or tumors	*Pretest:* See EGD. *Teach:* Fast 4–8 hours before examination, and avoid anticoagulants as ordered. *Posttest:* Keep NPO until swallow and gag reflexes returns, then eat lightly for 24 hours. Monitor vital signs, contrast reaction signs, and intake and output. *Teach:* Throat will be sore with hoarseness.
Sigmoidoscopy (proctosigmoidoscopy)	Examination of distal sigmoid colon, rectum, and anal canal using a rigid or flexible endoscope (sigmoidoscope). Normal findings: Normal mucosa.	Ulcerations, punctures, lacerations, tumors, hemorrhoids, polyps, fissures, fistulas, inflammation, early malignancies, and abscesses	*Pretest:* Low-residue diet for 3 days before test; clear liquids evening before test; NPO 8 hours before test. May have laxative and/or enema the day before the test; enema morning of test. *Posttest:* Monitor vital signs and for rectal bleeding.
Colonoscopy	Visualization of lining of the lower colon through a flexible fiberoptic colonoscope. Biopsy specimen may be obtained or polyps removed. Normal findings: Normal mucosa.	Colon cancer, polyps, foreign bodies, bleeding sites, infection, vascular abnormalities, or inflammation	*Pretest:* Low-residue diet for several days before test; clear liquids evening before test; fast for 6 hours and restrict fluids 2 hours before test. Laxative and enema the evening before the test; enema morning of test as needed. *Posttest:* Monitor vital signs and for rectal bleeding.
Percutaneous liver biopsy	Needle inserted through skin into liver to obtain a small tissue sample. Normal findings: Normal liver tissue.	Liver cancer, cirrhosis, or hepatitis	*Pretest:* Consent signed. Complete blood count (CBC) and coagulation studies reviewed. *Posttest:* Monitor vital signs and biopsy site for bleeding. Give analgesics as ordered.

Stool cultures (via sterile collection technique) are done to determine the presence of pathogenic organisms in the GI tract. Stool can also be examined for lipids (fat). Excessive secretion of fecal fats (**steatorrhea**) may occur in various digestive and absorptive disorders. The stools are collected for 72 hours and stored on ice, if necessary, before transport to the laboratory.

Stool tests for colorectal screening beginning at age 45 until age 75 include an annual guaiac-based occult blood test or immunochemical test or a multitarget DNA test every 3 years.

Radiographic Tests
Barium Swallow

A barium swallow is an x-ray examination of the esophagus, stomach, duodenum, and jejunum using an oral liquid radiopaque contrast medium (barium) and a **fluoroscope** (an x-ray source and fluorescent screen between which the patient is placed) to outline the contours of the organs.

The patient usually receives nothing by mouth (NPO) for 8 hours before the procedure. Because smoking can stimulate gastric motility, the patient is discouraged from smoking the morning of the procedure. During the procedure, the patient drinks thick, chalky barium while standing in front of a fluoroscopic tube. X-ray films are taken in various positions and at specific intervals to visualize the outline of the organs. Passage of barium through the GI tract is viewed.

A laxative is usually ordered after the procedure to expel the barium and prevent constipation or a barium **impaction** (impassable mass of stone-like feces). The patient is asked to increase fluid intake to expel barium. The abdomen is checked for distention. Stool color is monitored to determine whether the barium has been completely eliminated.

Barium Enema

A barium enema is performed to visualize the position, movements, and filling of the colon. Tumors, diverticula, stenosis, obstructions, inflammation, ulcerative colitis, and polyps can be detected. If the patient has active inflammatory disease of the colon or suspected perforation or obstruction, a barium enema is contraindicated. Active GI bleeding may prohibit the use of laxatives and enemas.

The patient eats a low-residue diet for several days before the test to empty the bowel. Clear liquids only should be consumed 24 hours before the test. The patient is NPO 8 hours before the test. Laxatives, bowel-cleansing solutions, and enemas may be administered the day before the test with cleansing enemas the morning of the examination. Bowel preparation is necessary for adequate visualization during the procedure. Inadequate bowel preparation may result in poor test results or test cancellation (Fig. 32.6).

During the procedure, barium is instilled through a rectal tube with an inflated balloon or through a colostomy (with special prep and colostomy irrigation first). Fluoroscopy shows the barium's movement in the colon. The procedure takes about 15 minutes. After the test, most of the barium is removed with the rectal tube; an x-ray confirms this. The patient is allowed to use the bathroom after the procedure to expel the remaining barium. The patient is told to report any abdominal pain, bloating, or absence of stool (any of these could indicate constipation or bowel obstruction) as well as any rectal bleeding.

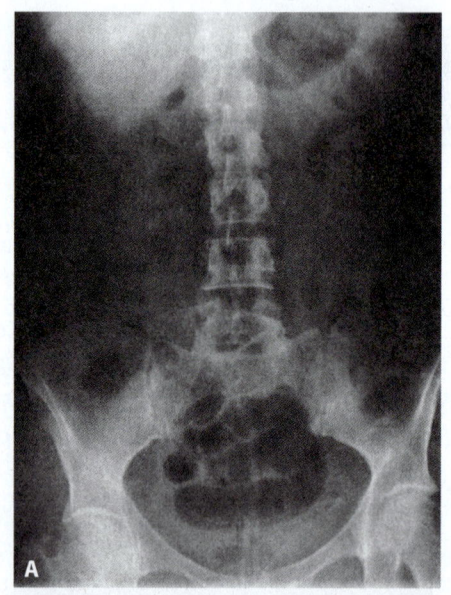

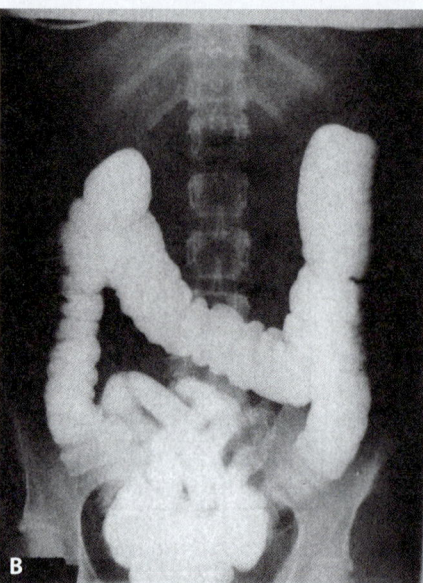

FIGURE 32.6 (A) An image of a patient who was poorly prepared for a barium enema. (B) An image of a patient who was adequately prepared for a barium enema.

• WORD • BUILDING •

steatorrhea: steato—fat + rrhea—flow
fluoroscope: fluor—a flowing + skopeìn—to look at

> **CRITICAL THINKING & CLINICAL JUDGMENT**
>
> **Mrs. Pearl** is an 85-year-old woman undergoing a barium enema for abdominal pain.
>
> **Critical Thinking (The Why)**
> 1. Why will you have concerns for Mrs. Pearl as she undergoes this test?
>
> **Clinical Judgment (The Do)**
> 2. What will you do to address your concerns for Mrs. Pearl?
> 3. What do you monitor before and after the procedure?
>
> *Suggested answers are at the end of the chapter.*

Computed Tomography Colonography

Computed tomography colonography (CTC) is a CT scan that looks at the colon. It is an option to screen for colorectal cancer every 5 years. CTC requires bowel preparation.

Nuclear Scanning

Hepatobiliary scanning primarily determines patency of the cystic and common bile ducts. It can also show hepatic and gallbladder function or gallstones. A small amount of radioactive isotope is injected. This examination can confirm cholecystitis, biliary disease, ejection problem, or obstruction.

Liver Scan

A liver scan involves injecting a slightly radioactive medium that is taken up by the liver. An instrument is passed over the liver that records the amount of material taken up by the liver and forms a composite picture of the liver. It may show tumors, masses, and abnormal size and patterns of blood vessels.

Endoscopy

Esophagogastroduodenoscopy

Esophagogastroduodenoscopy (EGD) visualizes the esophagus (**esophagoscopy**), the stomach (**gastroscopy;** Fig. 32.7), and the upper duodenum. Sedation is used to relax and ease pain during the procedure. The oropharynx is sprayed or swabbed with a local anesthetic, which may inhibit the swallow and gag reflex.

After the procedure, vital signs are monitored. If a local anesthetic in the oropharynx was used, keep the patient NPO. Check for swallow and gag reflex return before allowing fluids or food (usually within 4 hours). Patients are monitored for signs of perforation (e.g., bleeding, fever, dysphagia). Midesophageal perforation can cause referred substernal or epigastric pain. Blood loss secondary to perforation can lead to hematoma formation, which can result in cyanosis and referred back pain. Distal esophageal perforation may result in shoulder pain, dyspnea, or symptoms similar to those of a perforated ulcer. The patient may have a sore throat for a few days.

Capsule **endoscopy** makes use of a capsule with a microchip in it that is swallowed. As the capsule moves through the GI tract, pictures are taken of the stomach and small intestine to diagnose conditions such as bleeding, tumors, or Crohn disease. It is most helpful in the small intestine, which is difficult to scope because of its length and twists.

> **CUE RECOGNITION 32.2**
>
> Mrs. Flom has just returned from an EGD and reports a dry, scratchy feeling in her throat. The assistive personnel fills her water pitcher and starts to give her a drink. What action do you immediately take?
>
> *Suggested answers are at the end of the chapter.*

Endoscopic Retrograde Cholangiopancreatography

Endoscopic **retrograde cholangiopancreatography** (ERCP) shows the pancreatic and biliary ducts (Fig. 32.8). The procedure allows direct viewing, x-rays with contrast media, and intervention if needed, such as biopsy, stone or tumor removal, stricture balloon dilation, or bile duct stent placement. An endoscope is passed through the esophagus to the duodenum, where dye is injected that outlines the pancreatic and bile ducts.

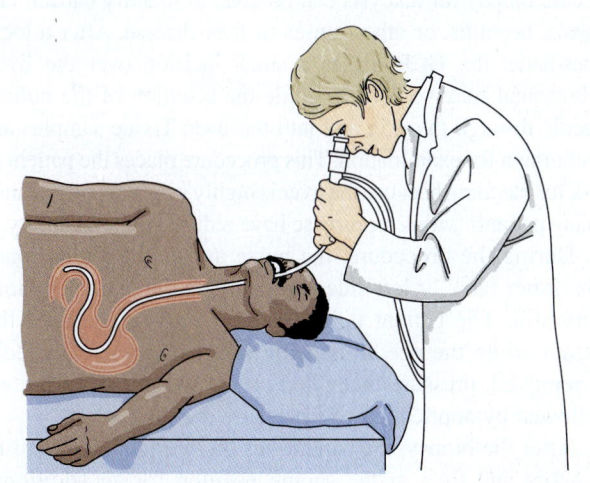

FIGURE 32.7 Gastroscopy.

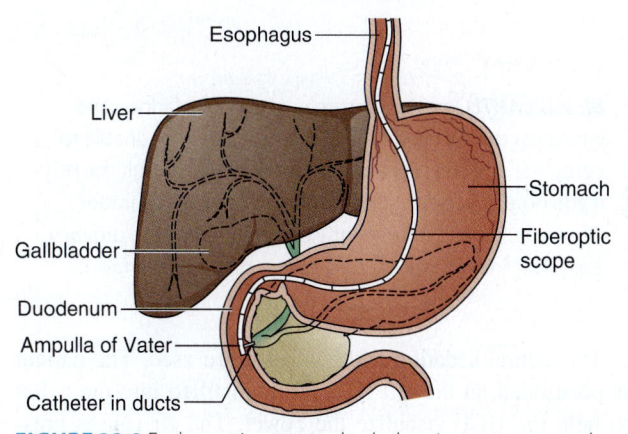

FIGURE 32.8 Endoscopic retrograde cholangiopancreatography.

Patient preparation for an ERCP is the same as for an EGD. Allergies to contrast agents are identified and reported. Ensure that ordered laboratory studies are done before the procedure and the patient has removed dentures. Postprocedure pancreatitis can develop. A pancreatic stent may be placed to prevent this issue. Follow-up care is similar to that for an EGD. Teach the patient to report increased right upper quadrant pain, fever, or chills, which may indicate infection. Reinforce teaching to report hypotension, tachycardia or rapid heart rate, increasing right upper quadrant pain, nausea, or vomiting, which may indicate perforation or the onset of pancreatitis.

Lower Gastrointestinal Endoscopy

SIGMOIDOSCOPY. **Sigmoidoscopy** is the examination of the distal sigmoid colon, the rectum, and the anal canal using a flexible endoscope (sigmoidoscope). Malignancies at an early stage can be detected, so an examination for patients ages 45 and older is recommended every 5 years until age 75.

The patient is positioned in a left lateral knee-to-chest position, allowing gravity to straighten the sigmoid colon. A rigid proctoscope is used to visualize the rectum. A flexible scope is used to permit visualization above the rectosigmoid junction. Patients are told they may feel pressure similar to with a bowel movement. During the procedure, one or more small pieces of intestinal tissue may be removed (biopsy specimens). Rectal or sigmoid polyps are removed with a snare. An electrocoagulating current is used to cauterize sites to prevent or stop bleeding. Specimens are labeled and sent to the pathology laboratory immediately for examination.

After the procedure, the patient is allowed to rest for a few minutes in the supine position to avoid orthostatic hypotension when standing. Pain and flatus may occur from instilled air. The patient is observed for signs of perforation, such as heavy bleeding, pain, and fever.

COLONOSCOPY. **Colonoscopy** provides visualization of the lining of the lower colon to identify abnormalities through a flexible endoscope, which is inserted rectally. During the colonoscopy, biopsy and fluid specimens may be obtained, polyps removed, and bleeding controlled with a laser. Examination for patients ages 45 and older is recommended every 10 years until age 75.

> **BE SAFE!**
>
> **BE VIGILANT!** Older patients may experience fatigue and weakness during bowel preparation and may be unable to complete it. Monitor the patient for distress. Consult the HCP if you note any patient distress during bowel preparation. Observe the patient frequently because defecation urgency, especially in unfamiliar surroundings, may create a fall risk.

Procedural sedation and analgesia are used. The patient is positioned on the left side. Air is instilled into the colon to help the HCP visualize the bowel. The air causes pressure and may be uncomfortable for the patient. The patient is encouraged to relax and take slow deep breaths through the nose and out the mouth. Vital signs are monitored throughout the procedure to watch for a vasovagal response, which can lead to hypotension and bradycardia.

After the procedure, the patient is monitored until stable. Hemorrhage or severe pain are immediately reported. When giving the patient discharge instructions, explain that flatus and cramping may occur for several hours after the test, that blood may be present in the stool if a biopsy specimen was taken, and to report problems to the HCP.

> ### Evidence-Based Practice
>
> **Clinical Question**
> What effect does body size have on quality of bowel preparation for colonoscopy patients?
>
> **Evidence**
> A retrospective study reviewed 9,659 patient records of patients having colonoscopies from 2012 to 2018. The results indicated that 21.3% had unacceptable colon preparations: 15% poor and 6.3% inadequate. There was no association found between increased BMI and inadequate bowel preparation. However, inadequate bowel preparation was associated with underweight females who reported constipation and with the elderly.
>
> **Implications for Nursing Practice**
> Nurses need to effectively educate patients on colonoscopy bowel preparation. The study suggests the BMI does not interfere with bowel preparation. Nurses should ensure that adequate preparation is completed for underweight females who have constipation and adults older than 70 years.
>
> *Reference:* Mohammed, R. A., & Lafi, S. Y. (2021). Effect of body size on quality of bowel preparation among patients experiencing colonoscopy. *Gastroenterology Nursing, 44*(2), 122–128. https://doi.org/10.1097/SGA.0000000000000557

Percutaneous Liver Biopsy

If less-invasive tests do not aid in diagnosis of liver disease, a needle biopsy for analysis can be done to identify cancer, cirrhosis, hepatitis, or other causes of liver disease. After a local anesthetic, the HCP makes a small incision over the liver. Ultrasound may be used to guide the insertion of the hollow needle through the skin and into the liver. Tissue samples are withdrawn for examination. This procedure places the patient at risk for bleeding because the liver is highly vascular and because many patients with liver disease have reduced clotting ability.

During the procedure, the nurse assists the patient onto his or her back or left side and instructs the patient to hold very still. The patient is instructed to exhale and hold the breath while the needle is being inserted. After the needle is removed, pressure is applied on the site up to 5 minutes, followed by application of a pressure dressing.

After the biopsy, the patient lies on the right side for 1 to 2 hours and then in the supine position for an additional 2 to 3 hours to prevent bleeding. Vital signs as well as the

Chapter 32 GI, Hepatobiliary, and Pancreatic Systems Function, Data Collection, and Therapeutic Measures

site for signs of bleeding are monitored for several hours. The patient is advised to avoid coughing or straining and to avoid exercise and heavy lifting for 1 week. Analgesics are offered for comfort as ordered.

CRITICAL THINKING & CLINICAL JUDGMENT

Mr. Wozynski is admitted with cirrhosis and jaundice. Mr. Wozynski's HCP orders a liver biopsy.

Critical Thinking (The Why)
1. What specific laboratory value can you expect to be elevated related to his jaundice?
2. Why is it important for you to check Mr. Wozynski's laboratory reports before the procedure?

Clinical Judgement (The Do)
3. What do you do immediately after the biopsy?

Suggested answers are at the end of the chapter.

THERAPEUTIC MEASURES FOR THE GASTROINTESTINAL, HEPATOBILIARY, AND PANCREATIC SYSTEMS

Gastrointestinal Intubation

GI intubation is the placement of a tube within the GI tract for therapeutic or diagnostic purposes (Fig. 32.9). When the GI tube is inserted orally into the stomach, it is an orogastric tube. When it goes from the nares into the stomach, it is a nasogastric, or NG, tube.

A variety of tubes are available with specific purposes (Table 32.8). An all-in-one NG system with multiple functions has been developed with a safety ENFit enteral connection. A reverse luer lock connection only allows tubes specifically designed for enteral feeding to be used with the tubing. Orogastric tubes reduce sinus infection risk because they do not block normal drainage of the sinuses, as can nasal tubes.

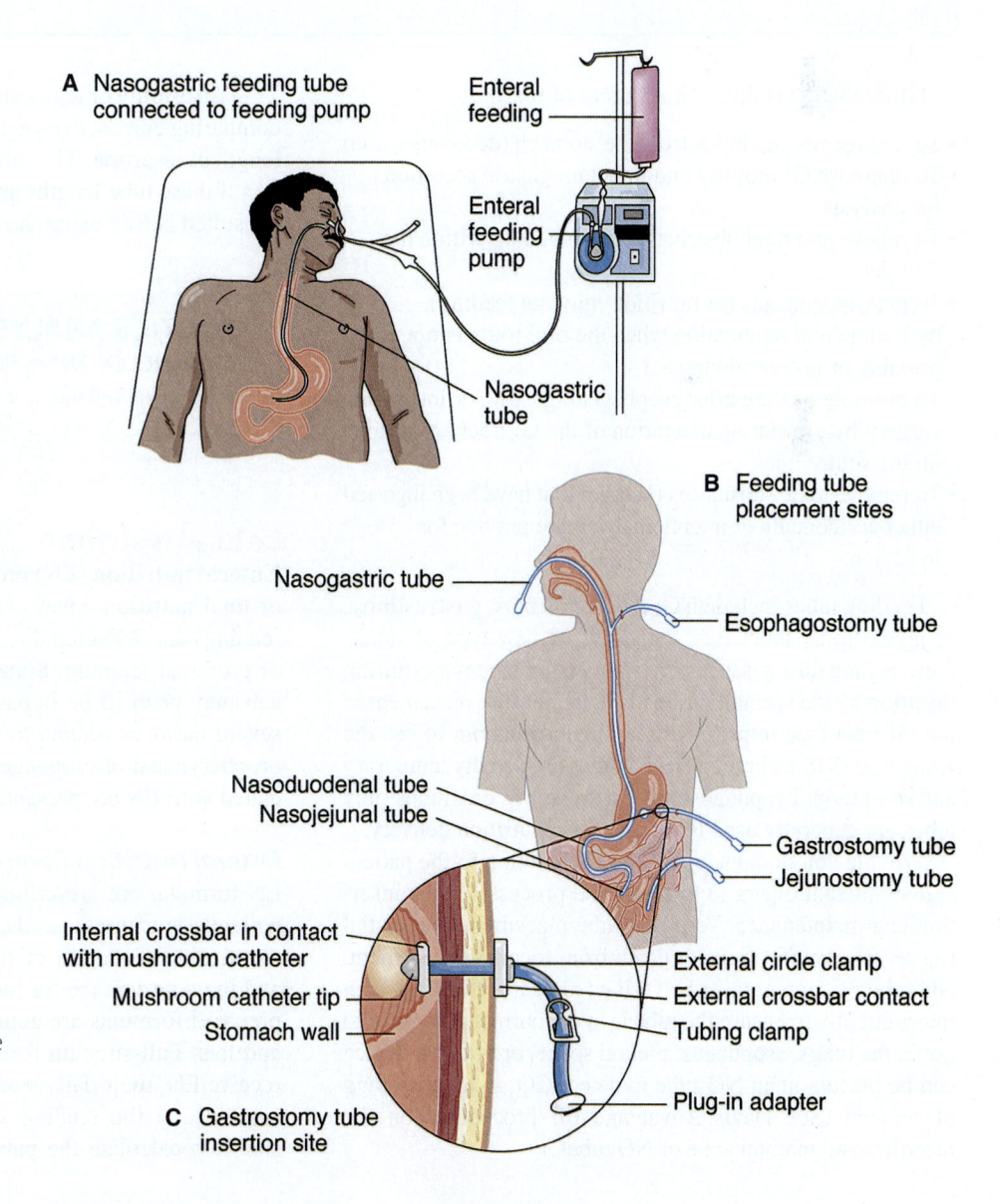

FIGURE 32.9 Feeding tubes. (A) Nasogastric tube connected to feeding tube pump. (B) Feeding tube placement sites (esophagostomy, nasointestinal, gastrostomy, and jejunostomy). (C) Gastrostomy tube insertion site.

Table 32.8
Gastric Tube Examples

Tube	Uses and Description	Nursing Considerations
Levin tube	Single lumen. May be used for gastric decompression, irrigation, lavage, and feeding.	Tube is not vented. Avoid use with continuous suction to prevent injury to stomach lining.
Sump tube	Double lumen with one lumen; an air vent prevents tube adherence to the stomach lining. Used for decompression, irrigation, lavage, feeding, and medication administration.	May be used with continuous suction because of air vent. Air vent must not be plugged off.
Weighted or nonweighted, flexible feeding tube, with or without stylets	Small-bore tube for enteral feeding only. Less injury. Can remain in place for extended periods.	Suction collapses tube. Use 10 mL syringe or greater because smaller syringe creates too much pressure, leading to possible rupture of tube. Inject 30 mL of air with a 60 mL syringe immediately before withdrawing fluid to make it easier to withdraw.

GI intubation is done for a variety of reasons:

- To remove gas and fluids from the stomach (decompression)
- To diagnose GI motility and to obtain gastric secretions for analysis
- To relieve and treat obstructions or bleeding within the GI tract
- To provide a means for nutrition (**gavage** feeding), hydration, and medication when the oral route is not possible or is contraindicated
- To promote healing after esophageal, gastric, or intestinal surgery by preventing distention of the GI tract and strain on the suture lines
- To remove toxic substances (**lavage**) that have been ingested either accidentally or intentionally and to provide for irrigation

Feeding tubes include NG, esophagostomy, **gastrostomy**, or jejunostomy tubes (see Fig. 32.9). A new type of small-bore feeding tube has a camera for viewing landmarks during insertion by the specially trained HCP to ensure placement in the GI tract (see https://www.cardinalhealth.com to see the Kangaroo IRIS technology). NG tubes are usually temporary and short term. Esophagostomy, gastrostomy, or jejunostomy tubes are generally used for longer-term nutrition delivery.

Provide emotional support and explanation to the patient and significant others to facilitate the process of tube insertion and maintenance. Verifying tube placement is essential to prevent complications or death from incorrect placement. NG tube placement must be verified after insertion and then intermittently to ensure the tube is in the correct position and not in the lungs, esophagus, pleural space, or brain. A device can be placed on an NG tube to detect CO_2 to identify lung placement. (See Davis Advantage for procedures on the insertion and maintenance of NG tubes.)

Gastrostomy or jejunostomy tube placement is verified by comparing current exposed length with documented exposed length at insertion. The tube may not be in the desired position if these tube lengths are different, so the HCP should be consulted before using the tube.

> **PRACTICE ANALYSIS TIP**
> **Linking NCLEX-PN® to Practice**
> The LPN/LVN will monitor and provide for client nutritional needs.

Enteral Nutrition

Enteral nutrition (EN) provides patients with supplemental or total nutrition when oral intake is not possible. Enteral feedings are delivered directly into the stomach, duodenum, or proximal jejunum. Sometimes, the esophagus and stomach may need to be bypassed due to inability to swallow, severe burns or trauma to the face or jaw, debilitation, and oropharyngeal or esophageal paralysis. Complications associated with EN are presented in Table 32.9.

Enteral Nutrition Formulas

EN formulas are prescribed by the HCP on the basis of the patient's nutritional needs, the consistency of the formula, the size and location of the tube, the method of delivery, and the convenience for the patient at home. Commercially prepared formulas are composed of protein, carbohydrates, and fats. Full-strength formula can be used. When patients receive EN, their daily water needs in addition to any water supplied by the feeding should be considered. Dietitians can help calculate the patient's free water needs. Water is

Table 32.9
Common Mechanical, Gastrointestinal, and Metabolic Complications of Tube-Fed Patients and Prevention Strategies

Complication	Prevention Strategies
Mechanical	
Tube irritation	Consider oral tubes and avoid nasal tubes due to sinus infection risk. Oral tubes also help prevent ventilator-associated pneumonia (VAP). Consider using a smaller or softer tube. Lubricate tube before insertion. Make sure tube is secured in place.
Tube obstruction	Flush tube with water after each use, and before and after medication administration. Do not mix medications with tube-feeding formula. Use liquid medications, if available. Crush nonliquid medications thoroughly (if crushing not contraindicated). Use infusion pump to maintain constant flow (see Fig. 32.9).
Aspiration and regurgitation	Feeding should not be started until tube placement is radiographically confirmed. Elevate head of patient's bed 30 degrees or more at all times. Discontinue feeding at least 30 to 60 minutes before treatments requiring head to be lowered (e.g., chest percussion). If patient has an endotracheal tube in place, keep cuff inflated during feeding.
Tube displacement	Place a black mark at the point where the tube, when properly placed, exits the nostril. Measure exposed length for future placement verification. If available, place CO_2 monitoring device on tube to detect displacement. For dislodgement, replace the NG tube and obtain HCP's order to confirm with x-ray imaging.
Gastrointestinal	
Cramping, distention, bloating, gas pains, nausea, vomiting, diarrhea*	Practice excellent personal hygiene when handling any feeding product. Keep formula at room temperature before feeding. Initiate and increase amount of formula gradually. Change to a lactose-free formula. Decrease fat content of formula. Administer medication therapy as ordered. Change to formula with a lower osmolality. Change to formula with a different fiber content. Evaluate medications for diarrhea side effect (e.g., antibiotics, digoxin).
Metabolic	
Dehydration	Note patient's recommended fluid requirements. Provide adequate daily water. Monitor hydration status.
Overhydration	Note patient's recommended fluid requirements. Monitor hydration status.
Hyperglycemia	Initiate feeding at a slow rate. Monitor blood glucose. Use hyperglycemic medication if needed. Select a low-carbohydrate formula.
Hypernatremia	Note patient's fluid and electrolyte status. Provide adequate fluids as ordered.

Continued

Table 32.9
Common Mechanical, Gastrointestinal, and Metabolic Complications of Tube-Fed Patients and Prevention Strategies—cont'd

Complication	Prevention Strategies
Hyponatremia	Note patient's fluid and electrolyte status. Restrict fluids as ordered. Supplement feeding with rehydration solution and saline as ordered.
Hypophosphatemia	Monitor serum level. Replenish phosphorus before refeeding as ordered.
Hypercapnia	Low-carbohydrate, high-fat formula is helpful.
Hypokalemia	Monitor potassium level. Supplement feeding with potassium as ordered.
Hyperkalemia	Reduce potassium intake as ordered. Monitor potassium level.

Source: Mazur, E. E., & Litch, N. A. (2019). *Lutz's nutrition & diet therapy* (7th ed.). Philadelphia, PA: F.A. Davis.
*The most commonly cited complication of enteral feeding is diarrhea.

the best fluid to use to flush the tube at intervals and before and after administration of medications to prevent clogging. Sterile water may be desired to prevent infection due to contaminated tap water. Use 30 mL every 4 hours to routinely flush the tube. The water used in flushing can count toward the patient's daily total water needs. Dehydration can occur if the patient's daily water needs are not met.

Method of Enteral Feeding Delivery
Feedings are administered either by gravity or by a controller pump that delivers continuous volume through the feeding tube. Gravity feedings are placed above the level of the stomach and dripped in by gravity slowly. Intermittent feedings are defined as either being delivered by a pump that runs continuously throughout the day and is discontinued each night or as a 4- to 6-hour volume of feeding given over 20 to 30 minutes. A continuous feeding administered 24 hours a day through a pump allows for small amounts to be given over a long period. Pumps are set at the specified rate to control the feeding being delivered to the patient.

When feedings are administered, patients must be positioned with the head of the bed at 30 to 45 degrees to reduce the risk of aspiration. Monitoring for the risk of aspiration is essential. Ensure proper labeling of the formula and correct feeding tube connection. Monitor the ordered beginning rate and advancement rate of the feeding to ensure nutritional needs are met.

Watch for signs that the feeding is not tolerated. Vomiting, abdominal distention, patient report of a feeling of fullness or discomfort, limited flatus or stool, diarrhea, and abnormal abdominal x-rays are indicators that the patient cannot tolerate the feeding. Research has shown that residual volumes do not reflect gastric emptying and may not be a good reflection of aspiration risk. In the study, eliminating residual volume checks did not decrease patient safety but resulted in better delivery of feeding to meet the patient's nutritional needs (Wang et al, 2019). Residual checks can result in clogged tubes, increased interruption of feeding, stoppage of a tolerated feeding in the absence of other intolerance indicators, and reduced feeding volume delivered to the patient, resulting in malnutrition. If residual checks are used, consideration can be given to raising feeding cutoff limits when other signs of intolerance are not present. Be aware of current evidence-based guidelines. Follow your agency's policy when administering enteral feedings.

If medications are administered via a feeding tube, ensure that the medication is made for the GI route. To prevent serious effects or even death, *never* interchange the routes of a medication. Obtain a new medication order if needed for the correct route form of the medication. Also understand possible medication–nutrient interactions. Some medications cannot be given with certain substances and may require feedings to be interrupted. Other medications, such as enteric-coated or sustained-release medications, *cannot* be crushed. Liquid medications should be used when possible to reduce clogging of the tube. Pharmacists and dietitians should be consulted for special considerations.

> **PRACTICE ANALYSIS TIP**
> **Linking NCLEX-PN® to Practice**
> The LPN/LVN will:
> - Insert, maintain, and remove nasogastric tube.
> - Monitor continuous or intermittent suction of nasogastric tube.
> - Provide site care for client with enteral tubes.
> - Provide feeding for client with enteral tubes.

Chapter 32 GI, Hepatobiliary, and Pancreatic Systems Function, Data Collection, and Therapeutic Measures

BE SAFE!

BE VIGILANT! Incorrect connection of enteral feeding equipment is a hazard to patient safety. An enteral feeding incorrectly connected and administered through a nonenteral system such as an IV line, peritoneal dialysis catheter, oxygen tubing, or tracheostomy tube cuff can result in patient injury or death. Worldwide equipment redesigns have been made to prevent tubing misconnections. Nurses must vigilantly ensure they understand the appropriate use of the equipment and all tubing connections they make to prevent harmful errors:

- Avoid rigging connections that may impair designed safety features.
- Package together all parts needed for enteral feeding within the agency to avoid improper equipment being selected and connected.
- Label or color-code feeding tubes and connectors within the institution.
- Verify the solution's label.
- Label enteral bags with large words such as "ALERT! For Enteral Use Only."
- Use adequate room lighting when working with equipment.
- Route tubes/catheters with different purposes in standardized directions (IV lines routed toward the patient's head; enteric lines routed toward the feet).
- If disconnection occurs, only staff familiar with equipment should make a reconnection.
- During reconnection, always trace lines back to their origins and ensure they are secure.
- During the handoff process, trace all tubes to their origin and check connections.

CRITICAL THINKING & CLINICAL JUDGEMENT

Mrs. Wood is receiving EN because of dysphagia, the cause of which is being investigated. She is not receiving any medications. You note that Mrs. Wood's tongue is bright red with deep furrows. She states her mouth is very dry. Her skin remains tented when skin turgor is checked.

Critical Thinking (The Why)
1. Why are Mrs. Wood's data collection findings present, and what do they indicate?
2. Why might Mrs. Wood be exhibiting this condition?
3. How would you document your findings?

Clinical Judgement (The Do)
4. What other data should you gather?
5. What actions do you take for this condition, and with whom do you collaborate for Mrs. Wood's condition?
6. What do you record as the total of Mrs. Wood's 8-hour intake: enteral feeding at 50 mL per hour?

Suggested answers are at the end of the chapter.

Gastrointestinal Decompression

GI decompression may be necessary when the stomach or small intestine fills with air or fluid. Swallowed air and GI secretions enter the stomach and intestines and accumulate if they are not propelled through the GI tract by peristalsis. Accumulating air or fluid causes distention, a feeling of fullness, and possibly pain in the abdomen. Gastric distention may occur after major abdominal surgery. Ambulating or turning the patient frequently can help prevent this. However, when GI decompression is necessary, an NG tube or, rarely, a nasointestinal tube may be inserted and suction applied. Nasointestinal tubes are more difficult and time consuming to place and may be uncomfortable, so they are not used often. The tube remains in place until full peristaltic activity (passage of flatus; bowel movement; no distention, bloating, or cramps) has returned. "Inserting a Nasogastric Tube" can be found in your resources on Davis Advantage.

Parenteral Nutrition

Parenteral nutrition (PN) supplies complete nutrition via a central or peripheral IV route (see Chapter 7). It is given to improve the patient's nutritional status, achieve weight gain, or enhance the healing process.

LEARNING TIP
- Patients may respond to the glucose in PN with an elevated serum glucose level. After PN is discontinued, the serum glucose levels should return to baseline levels.
- Regular insulin is ordered to control hyperglycemia during PN therapy. It can be given as an additive to the PN solution or subcutaneously per a sliding scale based on specified blood glucose monitoring results, such as every 6 hours, or both.
- The insulin type that is given for sliding scale coverage is always *regular* insulin. Can you figure out why? Because regular insulin is rapid acting, it reduces the *current* blood glucose level.

Home Health Hints
- Observe the patient's food preparation facilities to ensure the patient's nutritional needs can be met. Some older patients may have outdated or spoiled food in their refrigerators or cupboards because they are unable to see expiration dates or mold growing on foods.
- Observe and ensure that patients can use appliances to heat food safely. Patients with limited vision may not see gas flames and can ignite their clothing. If the patient can obtain and learn to use a microwave, it may be a safer cooking appliance than a stove.
- Share community nutritional support services with patients, such as Women, Infants, and Children (WIC)

- programs, nutrition sites for older adults, Meals on Wheels, school food programs, and government surplus food programs.
- Prevent a feeding tube from kinking by slipping a split straw lengthwise around the area that tends to kink and then lightly taping over the split in the straw.
- Use bent wire coat hangers over doors or closet bars for enteral feeding solution bags.
- Reinforce teaching patients to notify the home health nurse for a clogged feeding tube and not to unclog it with items such as meat tenderizer or carbonated beverages.

Key Points

- The GI tract is part of the digestive system. Digestion begins in the oral cavity and continues in the stomach and small intestine. Most absorption of nutrients takes place in the small intestine. The large intestine is where the majority of water is reabsorbed. Indigestible material, mainly cellulose, is then eliminated from the large intestine. Accessory organs include teeth, tongue, salivary glands, liver, gallbladder, and pancreas.
- The stomach serves mainly as a reservoir for food so that digestion may take place gradually.
- The only digestive function of the liver is the production of bile.
- The gallbladder stores bile until it is needed in the small intestine.
- The pancreas secretes digestive enzymes that enter the duodenum.
- Aging causes changes to the GI tract. It causes diminished sense of taste, GI secretions, and peristalsis. Older patients may have diverticula, hemorrhoids, and constipation. Liver damage can occur from hepatitis viruses or toxins such as alcohol. Gallstone formation increases. Acute pancreatitis is more common.
- During data collection, ask the patient about all medications, including acetaminophen, antacids, aspirin, NSAIDs, and laxatives.
- Abdominal examination starts with inspection, then auscultation, percussion, and palpation. This prevents palpation from altering other assessment findings.
- Abdominal girth is measured by placing a tape measure around the patient's abdomen at the iliac crest. A mark is made at the measurement site so measurements are made at the same location for comparison. Abdominal girth is increased in patients with distention or conditions such as ascites. When abdominal girth is abnormal, daily measurements should be monitored for changes.
- Diagnostic testing includes blood work, stool samples, barium swallow and enema, esophagogastroduodenoscopy, endoscopic retrograde cholangiopancreatography, colonoscopy, and gastric analysis.
- Feeding tubes include NG, esophagostomy, gastrostomy, or jejunostomy tubes. A new type of small-bore feeding tube has a camera for viewing landmarks during insertion. NG tubes are usually temporary and short term. Esophagostomy, gastrostomy, or jejunostomy tubes are generally used for longer-term nutrition delivery.
- GI decompression may be necessary when the stomach or small intestine becomes filled with air or fluid.
- Parenteral nutrition supplies complete nutrition via a central or peripheral IV route. It is given to improve the patient's nutritional status, achieve weight gain, or enhance healing.

SUGGESTED ANSWERS TO CHAPTER EXERCISES

Cue Recognition

32.1: Gather more data and determine if his upper denture fits well or is loose. Poorly fitting dentures can pose an airway risk. Gather more data to determine what type of foods Mr. Alder can chew. You may need to collaborate with the HCP and dietitian for a modified diet that he is able to eat.

32.2: Stop the assistive personnel from giving Mrs. Flom any water. Mrs. Flom had sedation, and a local anesthetic most likely was used to numb the throat. She should not have food or fluids until fully alert and the gag reflex is present to prevent aspiration.

Critical Thinking & Clinical Judgment

Mrs. Todd
1. Daily aspirin use is the most likely cause of her bleeding.
2. Medication teaching including side effects can help Mrs. Todd prevent future bleeding episodes. Mrs. Todd should be instructed to take aspirin with food to minimize GI upset and help prevent formation of ulcers. Identifying pain relief needs and consultation with the HCP will also help.
3. See Table 32.7.

Mrs. Pearl
1. Mrs. Pearl is at risk for dehydration and electrolyte loss as a result of the laxative and enema

SUGGESTED ANSWERS TO CHAPTER EXERCISES

preparation and NPO status. This risk is increased because of her age.
2. Her fluid and electrolyte status should be monitored closely. Mrs. Pearl will likely have a concern about "making it" to the bathroom during the preparation and should have a bedside commode placed within easy reach. Her call light should be answered promptly. If enemas are ordered "until clear," Mrs. Pearl will be at greater risk for fluid and electrolyte loss. If more than two or three enemas are required, the HCP should be notified. Older patients can become very fatigued during testing and test preparation. Mrs. Pearl should be allowed plenty of rest before and after the test. She may also have a concern about being able to hold the barium in her bowel during the test without having an "accident." She should be assured that the barium is held in with a balloon that is on the end of the enema catheter and that bathrooms are nearby.
3. You should monitor vital signs, fluid and electrolyte status, and passing of the barium. You should assist her to the bathroom and with ambulating until she has regained her strength. Offer fluid and foods after the procedure.

Mr. Wozynski
1. You can expect to find that Mr. Wozynski's serum bilirubin is elevated because his liver is unable to convert or conjugate bilirubin into a water-soluble compound that can be eliminated in the feces.
2. Mr. Wozynski is at risk for bleeding because the liver is highly vascular and prone to bleed when a biopsy specimen is taken. In addition, he may not be manufacturing the necessary amount of prothrombin needed for blood clotting and may bleed after the biopsy has been performed. It will be especially important to check his coagulation studies and report any elevations to the HCP before the biopsy.
3. Position Mr. Wozynski on his right side for 1 to 2 hours, then supine for 2 to 3 hours. Take vital signs frequently for several hours and observe the site for any bleeding.

Mrs. Wood
1. Dehydration.
2. Mrs. Wood's daily water needs are not being met. She is not receiving medications that would incidentally provide water during their administration.
3. Document as follows: "0800 'Mouth very dry.' Tongue bright red with deep furrows, tented turgor. Enteral feeding infusing (include solution and rate). HCP notified. K. Ohno, LVN."
4. Monitor Mrs. Wood's vital signs to look for changes such as increased heart rate, decreased blood pressure, and possibly mildly elevated temperature. Review current laboratory work, if available, for indications of dehydration such as elevated blood urea nitrogen (BUN) and elevated hematocrit (see Chapter 6).
5. Consult a dietitian and/or HCP to review Mrs. Wood's daily water needs. Divide the water needs over 24 hours, and ensure that water is administered. Ensure tubing is flushed per agency policy, and calculate water used toward daily water needs. Monitor intake and output. Continue assessing Mrs. Wood's signs and symptoms, and report abnormal findings.
6. 50 mL × 8 hours = 400 mL.

Additional Resources

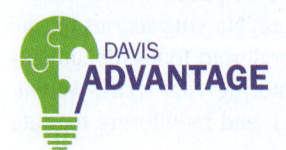

Go to Davis Advantage to complete your learning: strengthen understanding, apply your knowledge, and prepare for the Next Gen NCLEX®.

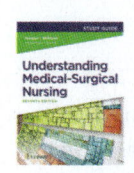

A Study Guide is also available.

CHAPTER 33
Nursing Care of Patients With Upper Gastrointestinal Disorders

Lazette V. Nowicki

KEY TERMS

anorexia (AN-uh-REK-see-ah)
aphthous stomatitis (AF-thus STOH-mah-TY-tis)
bariatric (BEAR-ee-AT-trik)
gastrectomy (gas-TREK-tuh-mee)
gastritis (gas-TRY-tis)
gastroduodenostomy (GAS-troh-DOO-oh-den-AW-stuh-mee)
gastrojejunostomy (GAS-troh-JAY-joo-NAW-stuh-mee)
Helicobacter pylori (HEH-lih-koh-back-tur PIE-lore-ee)
hiatal hernia (hy-YAY-tuhl HER-nee-ah)
obesity (oh-BEE-sih-tee)
peptic ulcer disease (PEP-tik UL-sir dih-ZEEZ)
Roux-en-Y (roo-ehn-WHY)
steatorrhea (STEE-ah-toh-REE-ah)

CHAPTER CONCEPTS

Health promotion
Nutrition
Teaching and learning

LEARNING OUTCOMES

1. Explain anorexia, nausea, and vomiting.
2. Describe therapeutic measures and nursing care for anorexia, nausea, and vomiting.
3. Describe medical, surgical, and nursing management for obesity.
4. Assist with planning nursing care for patients with acute or chronic gastritis.
5. Explain the pathophysiology, signs and symptoms, and diagnostic testing for oral and esophageal cancer, hiatal hernia, peptic ulcer disease, gastric bleeding, and gastric cancer.
6. List current pharmacological treatments used for peptic ulcer disease.
7. Assist with planning nursing care for patients with oral or esophageal cancer, hiatal hernia, peptic ulcer disease, gastric bleeding, and gastric cancer.

ANOREXIA

Anorexia is a lack of appetite. It is a symptom of many diseases. Causes include noxious food odors, certain medications (intentional or as a side effect), stress, fear, psychological problems, and infections. Prolonged anorexia can lead to serious electrolyte imbalances. These imbalances can cause cardiac arrhythmias. Ask patients what causes and improves loss of appetite to plan their care. Nursing actions for the patient with anorexia include encouraging preferred foods, documenting accurate intake and output (I&O); monitoring vital signs, weight, electrolytes, and electrocardiograms (ECGs); and monitoring the rate of an IV infusion or enteral feeding.

NAUSEA AND VOMITING

Nausea is the subjective feeling of the urge to vomit. Vomiting is the act of expelling stomach contents through the esophagus and mouth. It is a protective function to rid the body of harmful substances from the gastrointestinal (GI) tract. This reflex is controlled by the vomiting center of the brain. Stimuli and conditions that are either directly related to the GI tract or independent of it can trigger nausea and vomiting (NV). Viral GI infections, other infections, motion sickness, stress, pregnancy, medications, myocardial infarction, uremia, and other conditions may cause NV. Emesis that looks like coffee grounds occurs from bleeding in the stomach and requires further investigation. If vomiting is prolonged, dehydration and electrolyte imbalances can occur. The loss of hydrochloric acid from the stomach can result in metabolic alkalosis.

Therapeutic Measures

NV may be self-limited and require no intervention. If the cause of vomiting is known, it is treated. Antiemetics and ginger may be used to help ease nausea. For severe or prolonged vomiting, IV fluids and possibly nutrition need to be provided. Occasionally, an orogastric or nasogastric (NG) tube with suction may be ordered to decompress the stomach. After the vomiting is resolved, clear liquids are started, and the diet advanced as tolerated.

> **BE SAFE!**
> **ACT FAST!** Protection of the airway during vomiting is a priority to prevent aspiration. People at the most risk include those who are unconscious, have a gag reflex impairment, or are older and frail. Place these persons on their side when they begin to vomit. This position allows gastric contents to be expelled from the mouth rather than pooling at the back of the throat and being aspirated.

Nursing Process for the Patient With Nausea and Vomiting

Data Collection

The characteristics of the episodes of NV are noted. Medical conditions, medications, and treatments are documented to aid in diagnosing the cause. With continued vomiting, monitor and report signs of fluid deficit like weakness, thirst, dizziness, confusion, and postural hypotension.

Nursing Diagnoses, Planning, and Implementation

Nausea related to various causes

EXPECTED OUTCOME: The patient will report relief from nausea within 30 minutes of reporting nausea.

- Provide a quiet, odor-free, visually clean environment *to avoid triggering stimuli*.
- Give antiemetics as ordered *to relieve nausea*.
- Provide frequent oral care *to remove taste of emesis*.
- Reinforce teaching patient to avoid triggering fluids or foods *to prevent nausea and vomiting*.

Risk for Aspiration related to decreased gag reflex or unconsciousness with vomiting

EXPECTED OUTCOME: The patient's airway and lung sounds will remain clear at all times.

- Identify patients who are nauseated and at risk of aspiration *to plan preventive care*.
- Turn patient onto side if nauseated and vomiting *to protect airway and prevent aspiration*.

Evaluation

The patient's goals are met if nausea is not present and lung sounds remain clear.

OBESITY

Several methods can be used to diagnose a patient as overweight or obese (see Table 32.4 in Chapter 32). Factors such as gender, age, body frame size, and being an athlete with larger muscle mass can influence these measurements:

- *Ideal height-weight chart:* Weight 10% to 20% above ideal body weight is overweight; 20% or more above ideal body weight is obese.
- *Waist circumference:* Abdominal obesity for women is greater than 35 inches and for men greater than 40 inches.
- *Body mass index (BMI):* A BMI of 25 to 30 is overweight, and a BMI of >30 is obese.

Obesity is caused by a caloric intake that exceeds energy expenditure. Having a large waist results in an apple-shaped body. This is associated with greater health risks, especially for heart disease and cancer. This fat is referred to as *visceral fat*, which is metabolically more active. The metabolic activity increases substances such as triglycerides, low-density lipoprotein (LDL) cholesterol, and serum glucose that contribute to health risks.

Only a small percentage of obesity is associated with a metabolic or endocrine abnormality. Obesity can interfere with activities of daily living such as breathing or walking. Surgery can be an option for people whose BMI is above 40 or for people whose BMI is between 35 and 40 and who have obesity-related diseases such as severe sleep apnea or heart disease. A BMI greater than 30 kg/m^2 increases health risks, as it is associated with diseases called *comorbidities* (Fig. 33.1). These can include atherosclerosis, gallbladder disease, heart disease, hypertension, osteoarthritis, sleep apnea, type 2 diabetes mellitus, decreased mobility, lack of self-esteem, and depression. For more information, visit the Centers for Disease Control and Prevention (CDC) at www.cdc.gov/obesity/index.html.

Therapeutic Measures

Initial treatment for obesity is weight loss through education regarding a healthy and balanced diet, exercise, and calorie restriction. Support groups, such as Take Off Pounds Sensibly (www.tops.org) and Weight Watchers (www.weightwatchers.com), can help patients be successful. Many helpful free apps, such as MyFitnessPal, Lose It, and Fitbit, are available for mobile devices. Short-term use of medications that suppress appetite or block fat absorption may also be suggested. Healthy People 2030 has set the target of reducing adult obesity from 38.6% of adults to 36.0% (Office of Disease Prevention and Health Promotion, 2021).

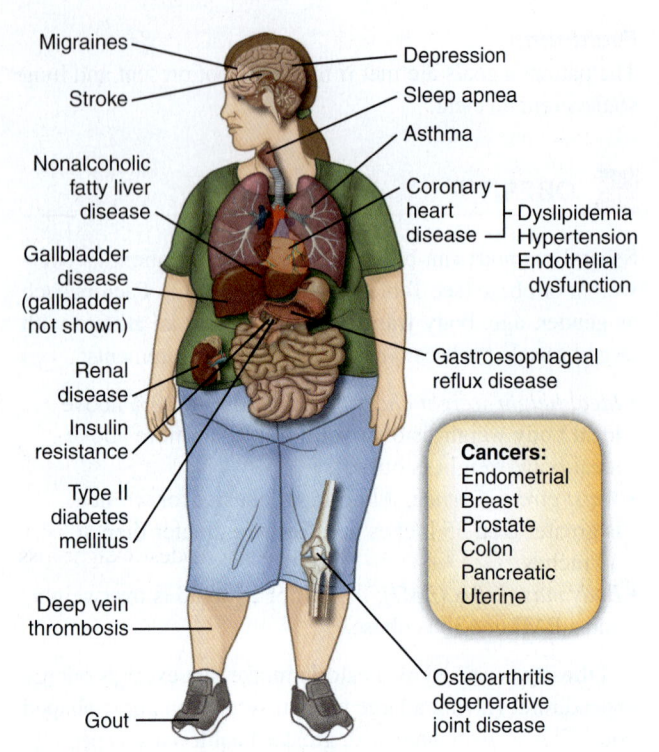

FIGURE 33.1 Comorbidities associated with obesity.

Bariatric Surgery

Patients who do not respond to medical methods of weight loss, weigh 100 or more pounds over ideal body weight, have a BMI above 40, have a BMI above 35 with comorbidities or type 2 diabetes mellitus, or have ineffectively controlled type 2 diabetes mellitus with a BMI of 30 to 35 might be candidates for surgical weight loss (see "Patient Perspective"). Screening for psychiatric and social stability is required preoperatively.

Weight loss surgery is called **bariatric** surgery (from Greek *baros* meaning "weight") or metabolic surgery by the American Diabetes Association when referring to its use to treat type 2 diabetes mellitus. Surgical techniques produce weight loss by limiting how much the stomach can hold and/or decreasing calorie and nutrient absorption (see "Nutrition Notes"). For surgical weight loss centers and procedures, visit the American Society for Metabolic and Bariatric Surgery Web site (https://asmbs.org).

Patient Perspective

Curtis
By the time I was in high school, I weighed 250 pounds, and the weight just kept building from there. I had tried many weight control programs. At age 38, I began to consider weight loss surgery. People who had had bariatric surgery pointed out the psychological aspect of how differently people treated you after weight loss. Some couples even ended up divorcing. This was a very scary aspect to me.

After much research and reaching a weight of 380 pounds, I had surgery at a bariatric surgery facility. I felt very comfortable through the presurgical testing and psychological evaluation and counseling. One of the nice features was that the facility itself was patient-friendly, with large chairs and other amenities for larger people. When I had the surgery, the first 24 hours in the critical care unit were rough. The nursing staff was very professional and understanding. The care was responsive to my needs. I think that understanding the medical field you are working in is important to promoting patient comfort. Several of my nurses had had the procedure themselves. This really helped them to know what I was experiencing.

I lost 120 pounds. My health has improved a good deal. I would do it again, even though, at about day 21, I would have said, "Never again."

As nursing professionals, it is very important to treat all patients with respect, regardless of their socioeconomic status or medical needs. I believe it is not only kind but helps in the healing and recovery processes as well. I was treated with a great deal of kindness and respect, and I greatly appreciated it. Thanks to all the professional nurses out there who do a great job!

Nutrition Notes

Supplying Nutrition in Upper Gastrointestinal Conditions

Bariatric Surgery
Candidates for bariatric surgery are counseled that the procedure is a tool to assist with weight control, along with behavioral changes, diet, and exercise. If the patient overeats, the small pouch that was created can be stretched and weight regained.

The type and amount of food intake are strictly controlled after surgery and during about 12 weeks of recovery. Long-term dietary strategies include the following:

- Choosing foods that are high protein, low fat, and low sugar
- Eating six small meals daily
- Chewing thoroughly and eating slowly
- Drinking sufficient fluids, mostly between meals
- Avoiding carbonated beverages and straws for drinking, as this introduces excess air into the gastrointestinal tract
- Taking vitamin and mineral supplements as prescribed

Common micronutrient deficiencies after gastric bypass include thiamin, vitamin B_{12}, vitamin D, iron, and copper. Intake of less than recommended amounts of calcium, magnesium, zinc, folate, and phosphorus also occurs.

Gastroesophageal Reflux Disease (GERD) and Hiatal Hernia

Guidelines to help control symptoms of GERD and hiatal hernia include the following:

- Maintaining ideal body weight
- Chewing food completely
- Avoiding high-fat, spicy, or individual trigger foods that cause symptoms, such as citrus or tomato products
- Avoiding alcohol, chocolate, coffee, peppermint, and spearmint
- Avoiding food within 3 hours of bedtime

Dumping Syndrome

Ways to decrease dumping syndrome include the following:

- Eating six small meals per day
- Eating meals that include high-protein, high-fiber complex carbohydrates, and no simple sugars
- Thickening foods with guar gum and pectin
- Avoiding fluids with meals
- Lying down for 30 to 60 minutes after meals

Gastric Cancer

If a patient has a poor prognosis after a total gastrectomy for cancer, dietary interventions should focus on symptoms the patient wishes to control. An overly restricted diet may cause the patient discomfort or distress.

See the Patient Teaching Guideline's for "Gastroesophageal Reflux and Hiatal Hernia" and "Dumping Syndrome" in your resources on Davis Advantage.

Sleeve Gastrectomy

One of the most common bariatric surgeries, laparoscopic (or open) sleeve **gastrectomy**, removes about 75% of the stomach, leaving a slim narrow tube (gastric sleeve). This reduces the stomach's volume and limits food intake at one time. It decreases the hormone ghrelin produced by the stomach that causes hunger (Fig. 33.2).

Gastric Bypass

The **Roux-en-Y** gastric bypass is a successful weight loss surgery that reduces stomach size and bypasses some of the small intestine, which reduces absorption of calories, causing weight loss (see Fig. 33.2). It is typically done laparoscopically but can be done by open surgery. First, a small stomach pouch the size of a thumb is created. This causes a quick feeling of fullness during a meal, which is the key to the success of this procedure. Next, the small intestine is divided, and the pouch is connected to the lower part of the cut small intestine to allow food to bypass the lower stomach, duodenum, and part of the jejunum. After the pouch is created, there are two entry points into the jejunum: from the pouch to the jejunum, and from the lower stomach to the duodenum and then to the jejunum. This allows for digestive juice flow to be maintained from the lower stomach into the jejunum.

Biliopancreatic Diversion With Duodenal Switch

As with sleeve gastrectomy, a small tubular pouch is created. Then, the surgeon bypasses most of the small intestine by connecting a piece of the distal small intestine to the pouch so the food goes directly to the end portion of the small intestine. The end of the bypassed small intestine is reconnected to the end portion of the small intestine so that digestive juices can mix with food (see Fig. 33.2).

Adjustable Gastric Banding

Laparoscopic adjustable gastric banding uses an inflatable silicone band around the upper portion of the stomach (see Fig. 33.2). This creates a small pouch to limit the amount of food the patient eats. The band is adjustable with a saline solution injected into the band through a port in the skin, making a larger or smaller pouch. The procedure is reversible. It is rarely used, however, owing to modest weight loss and the frequent need for surgical revision.

Intragastric Balloon

Patients who have a BMI of 30 to 40 kg/m^2 (class I obesity) and have not responded to weight loss by diet and exercise may opt for a bridge procedure of intragastric balloon placement (IGB). Three IGB devices, Orbera, Obalon, and ReShape balloons, have been approved for use in the United States. A balloon is inserted endoscopically into the stomach, filled with saline, and left in place for 6 months. The balloon restricts intake to produce weight loss. The IGB can be used alone or prior to other bariatric surgeries.

Complications of Bariatric Surgery

Complications of bariatric surgery may include NV caused by overeating or by not chewing food well, bloating, heartburn, staple disruption, obstruction, dumping syndrome, gout, gallstones, kidney stones, and osteoporosis. Protein, vitamin, and mineral deficiencies can result. Band slippage, intestinal leakage, or balloon leak or perforation can occur. (See "Complications of Gastric Surgery" later in chapter.)

Postoperative Care

Patients who have had bariatric surgery require care similar to that for most types of gastric surgeries. (See "Nursing Process for the Patient Having Gastric Surgery.") The bariatric diet, however, is very different and requires individualized dietary education. Some patients will have an NG tube placed during surgery. It is important to keep the head of the bed elevated to ensure adequate lung expansion. Patients are started on a clear liquid diet because of the small stomach pouch that has been created. Only a small amount of fluid, 30 mL, is allowed at a time and is slowly increased. The diet progresses to full liquids, pureed foods, and, finally, at about 6 weeks after surgery, regular foods, as tolerated. Patients will need to be taught to restrict the amount of food ingested

• WORD • BUILDING •

gastrectomy: gastr—stomach + ectomy—to remove

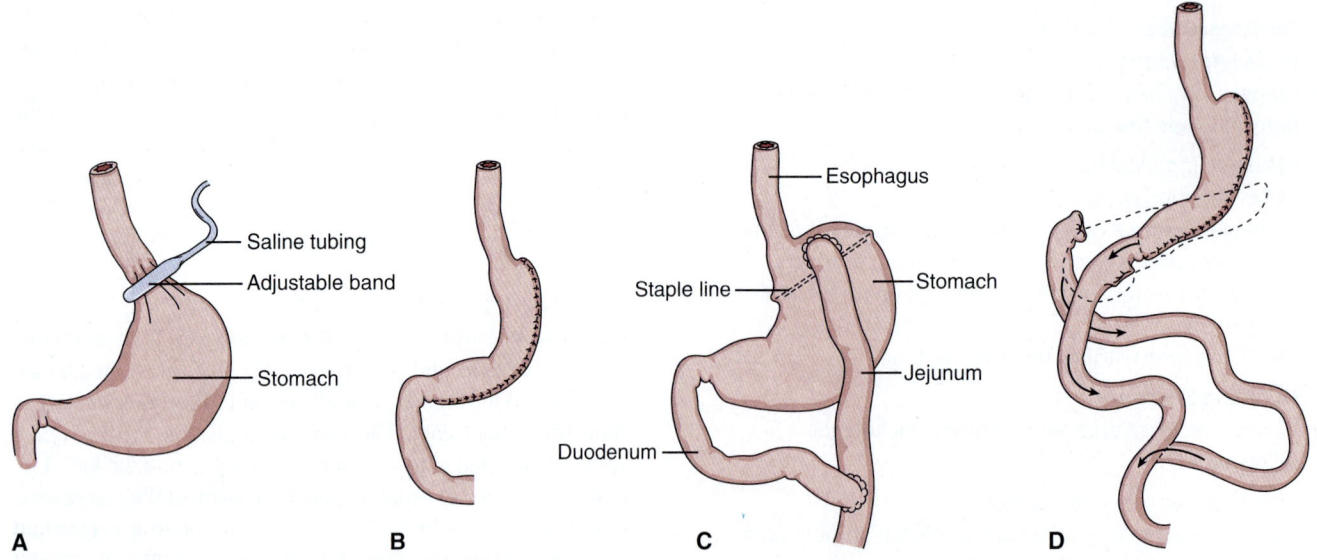

FIGURE 33.2 (A) Adjustable gastric band. (B) Sleeve gastrectomy. (C) Roux-en-Y gastric bypass. (D) Biliopancreatic diversion with duodenal switch.

at one time. Long-term follow-up is needed. Maintenance diet focuses on healthy eating and portion control. Many patients experience significant weight loss by 6 to 8 months after surgery. This can lead to a large amount of flabby skin. It is recommended that patients wait at least 1 full year before having reconstructive surgery to remove the excess skin. Psychological care may be needed for the patient and family related to weight loss and body image changes.

> **CUE RECOGNITION 33.1**
>
> A patient has had gastric bypass surgery, and a family member offers a large glass of water to the postoperative patient. What do you do?
>
> *Suggested answers are at the end of the chapter.*

Nursing Process for the Patient Who Is Obese

Data Collection
Data collection for the patient with obesity should include measurements of height, weight, and BMI and physical examination. Information about eating patterns and exercise patterns is obtained. The nurse determines if problems exist for the patient related to excess weight, such as physical limitations, social interaction issues, and personal issues (e.g., changes in sexuality or financial status). People who are overweight have an increased risk for comorbidities, which should be explored.

Nursing Diagnoses, Planning, and Implementation

> **Obesity related to caloric intake greater than metabolic needs and/or decreased activity level**
>
> **EXPECTED OUTCOME:** The patient will achieve and maintain weight loss to specified weight.

- Establish desired weight goal and monitor weight *to track progress toward goal*.
- In collaboration with a dietitian, modify eating habits and patterns *to lose weight and then maintain weight loss*.
- Establish and maintain increased activity pattern *to lose weight and maintain weight loss*.
- Discuss realistic weight loss goals of about 1 to 2 pounds (0.5 to 1 kilogram) per week *to achieve lasting weight loss effects*.
- Discuss emotions, events, and patterns of eating *to help patient identify when they are eating to satisfy an emotional need versus a physiological hunger*.
- Reinforce preoperative teaching if surgical interventions are planned *to help patient understand the procedure*.

Evaluation
The patient's goals are met if they maintain progressive weight loss to a specified weight goal and safely progress through the perioperative period if a surgical intervention is completed.

> **NURSING CARE TIP**
>
> Special bariatric equipment for providing patient-centered care includes the following:
>
> - Larger hospital bed, wheelchair, or walker
> - Patient lifting devices
> - Extra pillows to ease breathing
> - Larger hospital gowns
> - Larger blood pressure cuff

ORAL HEALTH AND DENTAL CARE

Good oral health care is important to overall health. Nutrition can be affected if oral problems interfere with eating and drinking. Respiratory illness and cardiac disease are associated with pathogens in the mouth. Regular mechanical oral hygiene is needed to remove plaque and prevent infections. Functional limitations may interfere with self-care for oral hygiene, especially for older adults (see "Gerontological Issues"). Suction toothbrushes are available for patients who cannot control secretions. The nurse should note any signs of oral inflammation or infection requiring prompt treatment. Regular dental care is important to prevent infections (Box 33.1).

Gerontological Issues
Oral Hygiene
Nurses can have a positive impact on older patients' outcomes by providing mechanical oral hygiene. Studies have shown that because mechanical oral care removes plaque, it helps prevent pneumonia and pneumonia-related death in older patients who were hospitalized or in a long-term care facility.

ORAL INFLAMMATORY DISORDERS

Aphthous Stomatitis (Canker Sores)
Aphthous stomatitis (oral inflammation) appears as small, white, painful ulcers on the inner cheeks, lips, tongue, gums, palate, or pharynx. It typically lasts for several days to 2 weeks. Triggers include injury to the mouth from biting the cheeks or dental work; a vitamin B_{12} or B_6, zinc, folate, or iron deficiency; toothpaste with sodium lauryl sulfate; stress; menstruation; or exposure to irritating foods. Application of topical corticosteroids usually shortens the healing time. A topical anesthetic such as benzocaine or lidocaine provides pain relief and makes it possible to eat with minimal pain.

Herpes Simplex Virus Type 1 Infection
Herpes simplex virus type 1 (HSV-1) infection may appear as painful cold sores or fever blisters on the face, lips, perioral area, cheeks, nose, or conjunctivae. These lesions recur over time but last only for a few days. The onset can be provoked by fever,stress, and other triggers. Viscous lidocaine can be used for pain relief. Oral or topical acyclovir help manage outbreaks. These lesions are infectious. Use standard precautions when applying ointment or giving oral care.

ORAL CANCER

Pathophysiology and Etiology
Oral cancer can occur anywhere in the mouth or throat. If detected early enough, it is curable. Oral cancer is found most commonly in patients who use alcohol or any form of tobacco.

Signs and Symptoms
Any oral sore that does not heal in 2 weeks should be assessed by the patient's health-care provider (HCP). Cancerous ulcers are often painless but may become tender as cancer progresses. In later stages, the patient may report difficulty chewing, swallowing, or speaking or have swollen cervical lymph glands.

Diagnostic Tests
Biopsy specimens are taken to identify the presence of cancer.

Therapeutic Measures
Oral cancer treatment usually involves surgery alone or in combination with radiation and/or chemotherapy. Radical or modified (preferred) neck dissection is often performed because this type of cancer frequently has metastasized to cervical lymph nodes by the time it is diagnosed (Fig. 33.3). Traditional or robotic approaches can be used to remove the tumor, lymph nodes, muscles, blood vessels, and glands. Drains are usually inserted into the incision to prevent fluid accumulation. A tracheostomy may be performed to protect the airway and prevent obstruction.

Nursing Care
See "Nursing Process for the Patient With Oral or Esophageal Cancer."

ESOPHAGEAL CANCER

Pathophysiology and Etiology
Esophageal cancer is usually detected in advanced stages because of its location near many lymph nodes that allows it to metastasize. As the cancer progresses, obstruction of the esophagus can occur, with possible perforation or fistula development that may cause aspiration. Risk factors for esophageal cancer are use of tobacco or alcohol, being overweight or obese, human papillomavirus (HPV), and Barrett's esophagus, a precancerous condition discussed later.

Signs and Symptoms
Signs and symptoms include progressive dysphagia (difficulty swallowing), weight loss, a feeling of fullness or pain in the chest after eating, or regurgitation of foods with obstruction.

Diagnostic Tests
Diagnosis of esophageal cancer is done by upper endoscopy (also known as *esophagogastroduodenoscopy* [EGD]) and a biopsy. Esophageal manometry may be done to assess esophageal motility. If metastasis is suspected, an image-guided biopsy is completed of lymph nodes and surrounding structures.

Therapeutic Measures
Treatment for esophageal cancer includes surgery (most common), radiation, chemotherapy, laser therapy, and electrocoagulation. These therapies may be used alone or

• WORD • BUILDING •

stomatitis: stoma—mouth + itis—inflammation

Box 33.1

Common Concerns in Oral Health and Dental Care

Daily and ongoing oral care is important and has been found to be linked to cardiac health.

Angular Cheilosis. A condition known as *angular cheilosis* (red, raw corners of the mouth) develops more often in older adults. It may be from infection, deficiency of riboflavin (vitamin B_2), or loss of facial profile caused by worn-down or damaged dentures or the patient not wearing their dentures. It is treated with anti-infective medications, vitamins, or new dentures.

Antibiotic Prophylaxis. Those at high risk for infective endocarditis should consult their cardiologist when having oral surgery (extractions, implants, gum surgery) to determine the need for antibiotic prophylaxis. Those with prosthetic joints do not require antibiotic prophylaxis before dental procedures unless the orthopedic surgeon prescribes them.

Dental Implants. An implant is an artificial root placed in the jawbone. The implant is usually tubular and made of titanium. Implants can be used to replace one tooth, multiple teeth, or an entire arch. They can also be used to stabilize a complete denture.

Dentures. It is helpful to have the dentist place a small identity tag in the acrylic of the denture with the person's name on it to avoid lost or mixed-up dentures, especially when the person lives in a long-term care facility.

Those with complete dentures need to be routinely screened by a dentist or dental hygienist for proper denture fit, sore areas, oral fungal infections, and oral cancer.

Gingival Recession. As people age, it is not unusual for their gingivae (gums) to recede or shrink, exposing the root surfaces of the teeth. This can lead to root sensitivity, tooth decay, or both. To protect the teeth from tooth decay because of dry mouth or gingival recession, a fluoride gel (Gel-Kam), rinse (ACT), or a prescription toothpaste with high fluoride is strongly recommended.

Gingivitis. As people get older, the gingivae have a greater tendency to bleed, a condition known as *gingivitis*. If the supporting tissues in the sockets of the teeth become inflamed, bone loss occurs, resulting in a condition known as *periodontitis* (pyorrhea). Periodontitis can lead to tooth mobility or loss.

Good oral hygiene habits cannot be overemphasized in the prevention of gum disease. Flossing every day is very important. If the patient is unable to floss because of arthritis or other conditions, an electric toothbrush or a Waterpik device is helpful.

Thrush (Candida albicans Fungus). Older adults are susceptible to oral yeast infections (*Candida albicans*) caused by certain medications, systemic conditions, or chemotherapy. Nystatin oral rinse treats this infection.

Xerostomia (Dry Mouth). As people age, they may experience a condition known as *xerostomia*. Some medications and radiation treatment of the head and neck can cause it. Xerostomia can lead to rampant tooth decay in older adults, putting their dentition at risk. Before any radiation therapy of the head or neck area, a thorough oral examination and any needed restorative dental procedures should be completed.

Although water is used as a common substitute for saliva, it does not contain the necessary compounds, such as lubricants, to protect the teeth. There are many products available for dry mouth, such as Biotene gel, ACT rinse, and sprays to help with the discomfort of dry mouth. Brushing with a high-fluoride toothpaste that is available by prescription is recommended.

Source: Dr. Ralph Kluk and Dr. Cheryl Kluk, Jackson, MI.

---

in combination. Surgical procedures include esophageal resection (esophagectomy), resection of the esophagus and anastomosis to the remaining part of the stomach (esophagogastrostomy), or use of a section of colon to replace the esophagus (esophagoenterostomy). If the tumor is inoperable, esophageal dilation, stent placement, or brachytherapy (localized high-dose radiation) can relieve dysphagia.

Nursing Process for the Patient With Oral or Esophageal Cancer

The patient with oral or esophageal cancer may undergo various forms of treatment, including chemotherapy, radiation, or surgery. Nursing care is based on the effects from these therapies (see Chapters 11 and 12). Preoperatively, the use of alcohol or tobacco is discussed and referrals to cessation programs and support groups offered as desired. Preoperative teaching includes communication methods if a tracheostomy will be placed. Postoperatively, major concerns are airway patency, pain management, swallowing ability, and fluid and nutritional needs. The airway must be monitored and secretions controlled to prevent aspiration. *Go to your resources on Davis Advantage to see the procedure for "Performing Tracheostomy Care" and review the steps required for a routine tracheostomy cleaning.* Pain is monitored, and analgesics are given as needed. A speech pathologist may perform a swallowing evaluation, and swallowing ability is monitored. IV fluids and parenteral nutrition or enteral feedings (see Chapter 32) are given to meet the patient's hydration and nutritional needs while swallowing is difficult.

HIATAL HERNIA

Pathophysiology

The esophagus passes through an opening in the diaphragm called the hiatus. A **hiatal hernia** is a condition in which the stomach slides up through the hiatus of the diaphragm into the thorax (Fig. 33.4). A sliding hiatal hernia, the most common type, occurs when the junction of the stomach and esophagus slides up into the thoracic cavity when a patient is supine and then goes back into the abdominal cavity when the patient stands upright. A paraesophageal hernia is rare but serious, as part of the stomach fundus squeezes through the hiatus and is at risk for strangulation (blood supply is cut off). Hiatal hernia occurs most commonly in smokers and in

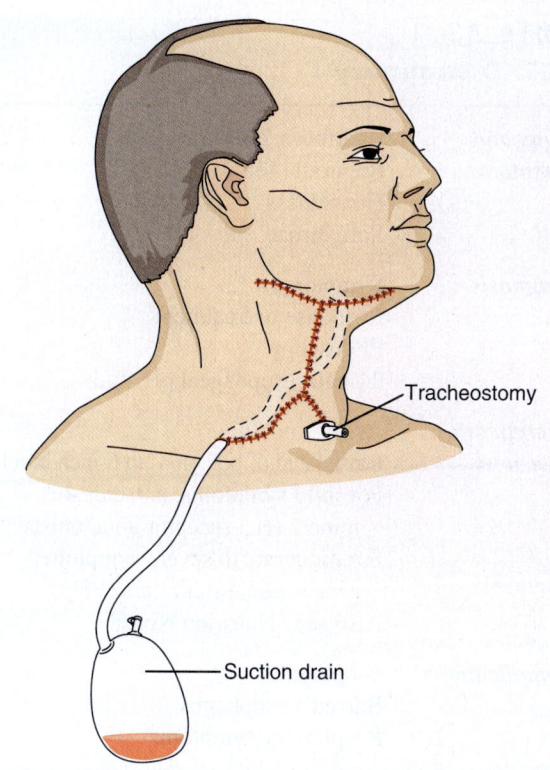

FIGURE 33.3 Radical neck dissection with tracheostomy tube and drains inserted.

those who are older than age 50, obese, or pregnant. People with hiatal hernia often have gastroesophageal reflux disease (GERD) as well (discussed later).

Signs and Symptoms
A small hernia may not produce any discomfort or require treatment. However, a large hernia can cause pain, heartburn, a feeling of fullness, or reflux, which can injure the esophagus with possible ulceration and bleeding.

Diagnostic Tests
Hiatal hernias are diagnosed by x-ray studies, endoscopy, and fluoroscopy.

Therapeutic Measures
Lifestyle changes for symptomatic hiatal hernia include not smoking and elevating the head of the bed 6 to 12 inches to prevent reflux, in addition to dietary interventions in "Nutrition Notes."

Surgical Management
Surgery is done for symptomatic hiatal hernia when gastric volvulus, strangulation, perforation, or obstruction, or respiratory complication is present. Fundoplication, in which the stomach fundus is wrapped around the lower part of the esophagus, is the most common surgical procedure performed (Fig. 33.5).

Nursing Care
The patient is taught lifestyle interventions to reduce symptoms of hiatal hernia. If the patient undergoes surgery, general postoperative nursing care is provided. Patients are monitored for dysphagia during their first postoperative meal. If dysphagia occurs, the HCP should be notified because the repair may be too tight, causing obstruction of the passage of food.

GASTROESOPHAGEAL REFLUX DISEASE

Pathophysiology
GERD is a condition in which gastric secretions reflux into the esophagus. The esophagus can be damaged by exposure to acidic secretions and digestive enzymes. GERD is caused primarily by conditions that affect ability of the lower esophageal sphincter to close tightly, such as hiatal hernia.

Signs and Symptoms
Signs and symptoms of GERD include heartburn two to three times a week, regurgitation, hoarseness, or sore throat (Table 33.1).

Diagnostic Tests
Diagnostic tests include an upper endoscopy, esophageal manometry, and pH monitoring of the lower esophagus to detect weak acid reflux.

Complications
Respiratory complications such as asthma, aspiration pneumonia, bronchospasm, laryngospasm, and chronic bronchitis can occur due to aspiration of gastric contents. GERD can

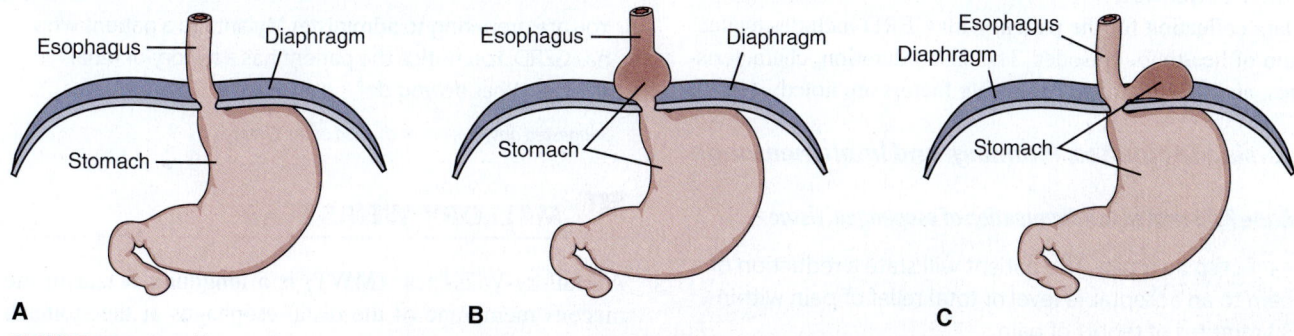

FIGURE 33.4 Hiatal hernia. (A) Normal esophagus and stomach. (B) Sliding hiatal hernia. (C) Rolling hiatal hernia.

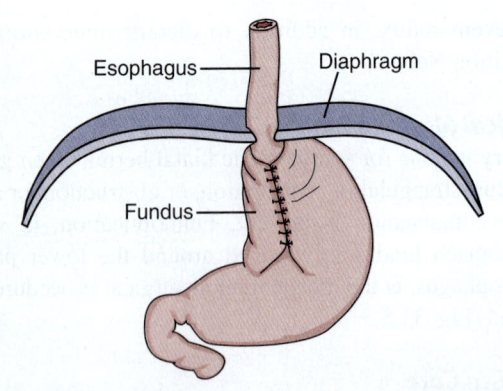

FIGURE 33.5 Hiatal hernia repair. Nissen fundoplication wraps the stomach fundus around the esophagus and then sutures it onto itself to hold it in place.

result in esophagitis (inflammation of the esophagus) due to acid reflux. Over time, this inflammation can change the epithelium of the esophagus and lead to Barrett's esophagus, a precancerous lesion that puts the patient at risk of developing esophageal cancer. Barrett's tissue can be removed during outpatient endoscopic procedures (one to three sessions) using radiofrequency ablation (the Barrx system). Normal tissue returns, and the risk of cancer is reduced.

Therapeutic Measures

Lifestyle changes are recommended first and then medications if needed (see "Nutrition Notes" and Table 33.1). If medications are not effective, a fundoplication or endoscopic procedure can be done. A minimally invasive procedure called *transoral incisionless fundoplication* (TIF) is performed through the mouth without incisions. It employs the EsophyX device to create an esophagogastric fundoplication that is up to 270 degrees and 2 to 3 cm in length. EsophyX uses an endoscope to tighten the lower esophageal sphincter, which aids in improving or eliminating GERD with good success. LINX Reflux Management System is another method to prevent reflux. A flexible band of magnets is inserted around the lower esophagus to prevent reflux of gastric contents. Stretta is an effective treatment that uses radiofrequency waves transmitted via needles into the lower esophageal sphincter muscle to form collagen contraction. This leads to a stiffer, stronger sphincter to prevent reflux.

Nursing Process for the Patient With GERD

Data Collection

Data collection for the patient with GERD includes evaluation of heartburn episodes. The onset, duration, characteristics, and precipitating or relieving factors are noted.

Nursing Diagnoses, Planning, and Implementation

Acute Pain related to inflammation of esophageal tissues

EXPECTED OUTCOME: The patient will state a reduction of pain to an acceptable level or total relief of pain within 30 minutes of report of pain.

Table 33.1 GERD Summary

Signs and Symptoms	Heartburn 2–3 times weekly Regurgitation Hoarseness Sore throat
Diagnosis	Symptoms Response to treatment Endoscopy 24-hour esophageal pH study
Therapeutic Measures	Avoid smoking Raise head of bed on 4- to 6-inch blocks For mild symptoms: antacids, histamine 2 (H_2)-receptor antagonists For moderate to severe symptoms: proton pump inhibitors (PPIs) Also see "Nutrition Notes"
Complications	Esophagitis Barrett's esophagus Respiratory symptoms
Priority Nursing Diagnoses	Acute Pain Deficient Knowledge

- Instruct the patient in lifestyle changes, including maintaining ideal weight and avoiding smoking, caffeine, peppermint, and alcohol *because they decrease functioning of the lower esophageal sphincter.*
- Instruct the patient to avoid trigger foods *to avoid pain.*
- Instruct the patient to sleep with head of bed elevated 4 to 6 inches and avoid eating 3 hours before bedtime *to prevent reflux of gastric contents into esophagus.*
- Reinforce teaching the patient about medications *to ensure appropriate use.*

Evaluation

The goal is met if the patient's pain is controlled and symptoms are relieved.

CUE RECOGNITION 33.2

You are preparing to administer Mylanta to a patient who has GERD. You notice the patient has a history of renal disease. What do you do?

Suggested answers are at the end of the chapter.

MALLORY-WEISS TEAR

A Mallory-Weiss tear (MWT) is a longitudinal tear in the mucous membrane of the distal esophagus at the stomach junction. It occurs from a sudden powerful or prolonged force due to coughing, vomiting, seizures, prolapse of the stomach into the esophagus, or cardiopulmonary resuscitation (CPR). Risk factors for developing an MWT include alcohol use and hiatal hernia. Symptoms include bright red, bloody emesis or bloody or tarry stools. The tear can be diagnosed with an EGD. Hemoglobin and hematocrit are monitored.

Treatment includes proton pump inhibitors (PPIs) and monitoring hemodynamic stability. Many tears self-heal without intervention. During endoscopy, bleeding is treated with an injection of epinephrine to constrict the blood vessel. Endoclips and thermal coagulation can be used to stop the bleeding. Excessive bleeding may occur, resulting in shock and/or the need for a fluids and blood transfusion. Persistent and reoccurring tears may be treated with angiography with transarterial embolization.

The focus of nursing care is to monitor the patient for signs of bleeding and report them. Patient teaching includes medications and the avoidance of alcohol use. See the section on gastric bleeding later in the chapter for more information.

ESOPHAGEAL VARICES

Esophageal varices are dilated blood vessels in the esophagus (see Chapter 35). Their rupture can precipitate a life-threatening event.

GASTRITIS

Gastritis is inflammation of the stomach mucosa associated with gastric mucosal injury and can be acute or chronic. Causes are listed in Box 33.2.

Acute Gastritis
Pathophysiology
Gastritis results when the protective mucosal barrier is broken down and allows autodigestion from hydrochloric acid and pepsin to occur. Inflammation results in edema of the tissue and can lead to stomach ulcers and bleeding. Untreated acute gastritis can lead to chronic gastritis.

> **Box 33.2**
> **Causes of Gastritis**
> - Alcohol use
> - Endoscopic procedures
> - Microorganisms (e.g., **Helicobacter pylori**, Salmonella)
> - Medications (e.g., aspirin, NSAIDs, corticosteroids, digitalis, chemotherapy agents)
> - Nasogastric suctioning
> - Radiation
> - Reflux of bile
> - Smoking
> - Stress (emotional, physiological)
> - Trauma
> - Crohn disease

Signs and Symptoms
The major symptom of gastritis is abdominal pain, which is often accompanied by NV. The patient may also experience abdominal tenderness, a feeling of fullness, reflux, belching, and hematemesis. If the cause of the gastritis is contaminated food, symptoms, including diarrhea, usually start within 5 to 6 hours.

Therapeutic Measures
Treatment of gastritis includes avoiding causes of gastritis such as avoiding alcohol; avoiding irritating foods; avoiding irritating medications; and treating **Helicobacter pylori** infection. Antacids, PPIs, and/or histamine 2 (H_2)-receptor antagonists are given to help control pain.

Chronic Gastritis
Chronic gastritis occurs over time and is classified as autoimmune or environmental. Identifying and treating patients with chronic gastritis is essential to prevent complications. Patients with chronic gastritis have an increased risk for developing stomach cancer.

Autoimmune Gastritis
With autoimmune gastritis, the patient can be asymptomatic or have dyspepsia or postprandial distress (after meals). It occurs in the fundus (body of stomach) and is diagnosed by endoscopy with biopsy. Autoimmune gastritis attacks the parietal cells, decreasing acid production and intrinsic factor. This causes difficulty absorbing vitamin B_{12}, leading to pernicious anemia.

Environmental Gastritis
Environmental gastritis is associated with H. pylori infection and possibly dietary factors, smoking, alcohol consumption, and chronic bile reflux. It is the most common type of chronic gastritis. The patient may be asymptomatic or have poor appetite, heartburn after eating, belching, a sour taste in the mouth, and NV. Environmental chronic gastritis can also be diagnosed by endoscopy with biopsy and gastric aspirate analysis. H. pylori infection is treated with antibiotics, PPIs, and/or H_2-receptor antagonists (Table 33.2).

Stress-Induced Gastritis
Critically ill patients may develop GI mucosal damage from ischemia. The stress response to the illness causes reduced blood flow to the stomach and small intestine, resulting in ischemia and damage to the mucosa. The damaged mucous barrier then allows acid secretions to create ulcerations. Preventive treatment is used for acutely ill patients with a high risk for GI bleeding. PPIs (oral or IV), such as pantoprazole, are used to prevent mucosal damage. H_2 blockers are used if PPIs are not tolerated. Prophylaxis treatment of stress gastritis and ulcers has decreased the occurrence of GI bleeding in critically ill patients.

• WORD • BUILDING •
gastritis: gastr—stomach + itis—inflammation

Table 33.2
Medication Regimen Examples for *H. Pylori* Infection

Type of Therapy	Included in Therapy	Examples of Therapy Options
Triple therapy	Two antibiotics + proton pump inhibitor (PPI)	Amoxicillin (Amoxil) + clarithromycin (Biaxin) + omeprazole (Prilosec) Amoxicillin (Amoxil) + clarithromycin (Biaxin) + lansoprazole (Prevacid) (available as Prevpac, combined for convenience) Amoxicillin (Amoxil) + Rifabutin (Mycobutin) + esomeprazole (Nexium)
Bismuth quadruple therapy	Two antibiotics + bismuth subsalicylate + proton pump inhibitor (PPI)	metronidazole (Flagyl) + tetracycline + bismuth subsalicylate (Pepto-Bismol) + PPI

PEPTIC ULCER DISEASE

Pathophysiology
Peptic ulcer disease (PUD) is a condition in which the lining of the stomach or duodenum is eroded, usually from infection with *H. pylori* or use of NSAIDs. The erosion may extend into the muscular layers and then occur in portions of the GI tract that are exposed to hydrochloric acid and pepsin. The erosion is due to an increase in the concentration or activity of hydrochloric acid and pepsin. The damaged mucosa is unable to secrete enough mucus to act as a barrier against the hydrochloric acid. Hypersecretion of acid creates a large amount of acid moving into the duodenum and results in more ulcers in the duodenum. Ulcers are named by their location: gastric or duodenal.

Etiology
Until 1982, the cause of peptic ulcers was poorly understood and incorrectly associated with stress, diet, and alcohol or caffeine ingestion. We now know that PUD is primarily caused by the gram-negative bacterium *H. pylori*. About half of all people worldwide are infected with *H. pylori*. North America has a low prevalence. Discovery of *H. pylori* has led to changes in treating and curing peptic ulcers. NSAID use, alcohol use, and smoking increase the risk for PUD.

Signs and Symptoms
Most patients are asymptomatic and may not experience symptoms until complications such as hemorrhage, obstruction, or perforation develop. Symptoms vary with the location of the ulcer (Table 33.3). Upper abdominal pain or discomfort is the most common symptom in patients with peptic ulcer. The pain can last for a few weeks followed by weeks or months without pain. Anorexia and NV may also occur with either ulcer location. Bleeding may occur with massive hemorrhaging or slow oozing. Patients often have low hematocrit and hemoglobin levels. Gastric or fecal occult blood may be found, depending on where the ulcers are located.

Complications
Bleeding, perforation of stomach or duodenum wall, and obstruction can occur. Bleeding can occur in varying degrees, from occult blood in stool and emesis to massive bright red bleeding. Treatment includes stopping the bleeding and replacing fluid and electrolytes. Perforation is suspected if the patient has an ulcer and develops acute, sharp, severe abdominal pain. Perforated ulcer is a medical emergency and may require surgery. Gastroduodenal contents escape through the perforation into the peritoneal cavity, causing peritonitis and hypovolemic shock. An NG tube is inserted, and IV fluids are given. Obstruction may be due to scar tissue because of repeated ulcerations and healing in a patient with chronic PUD. Obstruction frequently occurs at the pylorus, causing pain at night and vomiting. Pyloroplasty corrects the problem.

Diagnostic Tests
The presence and location of *H. pylori* can be diagnosed with several tests. With EGD, a biopsy can be taken in several places and tested for urease, which is produced by *H. pylori*. Gastric biopsy can also be done for histology to diagnosis *H. pylori* infection and associated lesions.

Table 33.3
Peptic Ulcer Disease Summary

Signs and Symptoms

Gastric ulcer	Intermittent upper abdominal burning or gnawing pain, increased 1–2 hours after meals or with food
	Variable pain pattern possibly made worse by food
	Possible malnourishment
	Bleeding (stomach secretions or stool positive for occult blood)
Duodenal ulcer	Intermittent mid-epigastric or upper abdominal burning or cramping pain, increased 2–5 hours after meals or in the middle of the night
	Relieved by food or antacids
	Patient usually well nourished
	Anorexia
	Nausea and vomiting
	Bleeding (stomach secretions or stool positive for occult blood)

Diagnostic Tests

Helicobacter pylori	Biopsy
	Urease test (during endoscopy)
	Immunoglobulin G antibody detection test for *H. pylori*
	Culture
	Urea breath test
Peptic ulcer	Esophagogastroduodenoscopy (EGD)
	Upper gastrointestinal series (barium swallow)

Therapeutic Measures

H. Pylori	Antibiotics
	Proton pump inhibitors (PPIs)
	Histamine 2 (H_2)-receptor antagonists
	Bismuth subsalicylate
Peptic ulcer	Avoid smoking, caffeine, alcohol, trigger foods
	Antacids
	PPIs
	H_2-receptor antagonists
	Sucralfate (Carafate)

Complications

Bleeding
Perforation
Obstruction

Priority Nursing Diagnoses

Acute Pain
Risk for Injury
Deficient Knowledge

Cultures of the biopsy specimen may also be done to determine antimicrobial susceptibility. Noninvasive tests include the urea breath test. It is performed by having the patient drink carbon-labeled urea. The urea is metabolized rapidly if *H. pylori* is present, allowing the carbon to be absorbed and measured in exhaled carbon dioxide. An immunoglobulin G antibody detection test for *H. pylori* identifies whether the patient is infected with *H. pylori*.

Therapeutic Measures

Several treatment options are used to cure *H. pylori* without recurrence (see Table 33.2). For better effectiveness, triple or quadruple therapy with two antibiotics to decrease resistance of the bacteria and a PPI or H_2-receptor antagonist are used. Sequential treatment lasting 14 days has better eradication rates than 10-day treatments. Bismuth subsalicylate (Pepto-Bismol) may also be used for its antibacterial effects.

PPIs are powerful agents that stop the final step of gastric acid secretion to reduce mucosa erosion and aid in healing ulcers (Table 33.4). H_2-receptor antagonists block H_2 receptors to decrease acid secretion, although they are not as powerful as PPIs. NSAIDs, alcohol, and smoking should be avoided to promote healing and prevent reoccurrence.

Nursing Process for the Patient With Peptic Ulcer Disease

Data Collection

Data are collected about the patient's PUD history and factors that trigger or relieve symptoms. The primary focus of nursing care for PUD is educating patients on the importance of diagnosis since ulcers may be caused by an infection that can be cured with antibiotics and PPIs.

Nursing Diagnoses, Planning, Implementation, and Evaluation

See "Nursing Care Plan for the Patient With Peptic Ulcer Disease."

Table 33.4 Medications Used to Promote Healing of Peptic Ulcers

Medication Class/Action	
Antisecretory Agents	
Histamine 2 (H_2)-Receptor Antagonist *Inhibit gastric acid secretion by blocking H_2-receptors on gastric parietal cells.*	
Examples cimetidine (Tagamet) famotidine (Pepcid) nizatidine (Axid)	*Nursing Indications* If giving an antacid, give it at least 1 hour before or 2 hours after an H_2-receptor antagonist because absorption may be reduced.
Proton Pump Inhibitors (PPIs) *Bind to an enzyme in the presence of acidic gastric pH, preventing final transport of hydrogen ions into the gastric lumen.*	
Examples dexlansoprazole (Dexilant) esomeprazole (Nexium) lansoprazole (Prevacid) omeprazole (Prilosec) pantoprazole (Protonix) rabeprazole (Aciphex)	*Nursing Indications* Delayed release. Capsule swallowed whole. Give before morning meal. Notify health-care provider of bleeding, diarrhea, headache, or abdominal pain.
Antacids *Increase gastric pH to reduce pepsin activity; strengthen gastric mucosal barrier and esophageal sphincter tone.*	
Examples aluminum-magnesium combinations (Riopan, Maalox, Mylanta, Gelusil) calcium carbonate (Tums, Titralac)	*Nursing Indications* Do not give aluminum and/or magnesium to patients with kidney disease. Give at least 1 hour before or 2 hours after an H_2-receptor antagonist, tetracycline, or enteric-coated tablets because absorption may be reduced. Do not give with milk. Monitor bowel movements and for signs of hypermagnesemia or hypercalcemia.
Mucosal Barrier Fortifiers *In presence of mild acid condition, form viscid and sticky gel and adhere to ulcer surface, forming a protective barrier.*	
Examples sucralfate (Carafate)	*Nursing Indications* Take on an empty stomach, 1 hour before meals and at bedtime. Monitor for constipation.

CLINICAL JUDGMENT

Mr. Smith, a patient on your medical unit, has a duodenal ulcer. His wife runs to the nursing station and says that you need to help her husband because he is in terrible pain. As you enter the room, you see Mr. Smith curled up in a knee-to-chest position on the bed. He is moaning and says he has excruciating abdominal pain.

1. What additional data do you gather?
2. What nursing actions do you complete to provide patient-centered care?
3. What emotional support do you offer to Mr. Smith?
4. What complication do you suspect Mr. Smith is experiencing?
5. What member(s) of the health-care team do you anticipate collaborating with?
6. What nursing actions do you anticipate implementing after orders from the HCP?

Suggested answers are at the end of the chapter.

GASTRIC BLEEDING

Gastric bleeding may be caused by ulcer perforation, tumors, gastric surgery, or other conditions. Bleeding peptic ulcers are the most common cause of blood loss into the stomach or intestine. Blood loss can be hidden (occult) blood in the stool, observable vomited blood (hematemesis), or black tarry stools (melena). When blood mixes with hydrochloric acid and enzymes in the stomach, a dark, granular material resembling coffee grounds is produced. This material can be vomited or passed through the GI system and mixed with stools. Melena occurs from slow bleeding in an upper GI area.

Signs and Symptoms

With mild bleeding, the patient may experience only slight weakness or diaphoresis. Severe blood loss (more than 1 L in 24 hours) may result in hypovolemic shock, with signs

Nursing Care Plan for the Patient With Peptic Ulcer Disease

Nursing Diagnosis: *Acute Pain* related to gastric mucosal erosion
Expected Outcome: The patient's pain will be relieved as evidenced by no report of pain within 30 minutes of report of pain.
Evaluation of Outcome: Is pain relieved to patient's satisfaction?

Intervention	Rationale	Evaluation
Ask about factors precipitating and relieving pain.	Peptic ulcer pain may be relieved by food, antacids, or other interventions.	Is patient able to state precipitating and relieving pain factors?
Ask patient to rate pain. Note location, onset, intensity, characteristics of pain, and nonverbal pain cues.	Prompt assessment can lead to timely intervention and relief of pain.	Does patient rate pain using scale and describe pain?
Administer medications as ordered.	Acid-suppressing medications help heal ulcer and relieve pain.	Do medications reduce patient's symptoms?
Provide small, frequent meals four to six times a day.	Small, frequent meals dilute and neutralize gastric acid.	Does patient report relief of gastric pain between meals?

Nursing Diagnosis: *Risk for Injury* related to complications of peptic ulcer activity such as hemorrhage and perforation
Expected Outcomes: The patient's vital signs will be maintained within normal limits, and bleeding or hemorrhage will be promptly detected.
Evaluation of Outcomes: Are patient's vital signs within normal limits?

Intervention	Rationale	Evaluation
Monitor for signs and symptoms of hemorrhage, such as hematemesis and melena.	Rapid assessment can lead to prompt intervention.	Does patient have any bleeding?
Monitor vital signs (e.g., blood pressure, pulse, respirations, temperature) and report abnormalities.	Severe blood loss of more than 1 L per 24 hours may cause evidence of shock, such as hypotension; weak, thready pulse; chills; palpitations; and diaphoresis.	Are vital signs normal?
Maintain intravenous infusion as ordered	Normal fluid balance prevents hypovolemia and shock due to hemorrhage.	Are intake and output balanced?

and symptoms such as hypotension; a weak, thready pulse; chills; palpitations; dizziness; confusion; and cold/clammy extremities (Table 33.5).

Therapeutic Measures

The goal of treatment for a massive GI bleed is to prevent or treat hypovolemic shock and prevent dehydration, electrolyte imbalance, and further bleeding. The following steps are taken:

- The patient is kept on nothing by mouth (NPO) status.
- Two IV lines are started to replace lost fluids and administer blood if necessary.
- A complete blood count (CBC) is obtained to determine the amount of blood lost.
- A urinary catheter may be inserted to monitor output.
- Avoid NG insertion, which does not improve patient outcomes and is not recommended.
- Oxygen therapy may be required if the patient has lost a large amount of blood.
- To prevent aspiration with vomiting, the patient is turned to the left side, and elevating the head of the bed is considered.
- The HCP may perform endoscopy (within 24 hours) to help control the bleeding and instill medications.
- Severe cases may require surgery to remove the bleeding area or ligate bleeding vessels.
- Acid suppression medications are given to decrease the secretion of gastric acid.

Table 33.5
Gastric Bleeding Summary

Signs and Symptoms	Occult blood in stool Hematemesis Melena Hypovolemic shock
Diagnostic Tests	Endoscopy Decreased hemoglobin and hematocrit
Therapeutic Measures	Hypovolemic shock: NPO (nothing by mouth), intravenous fluids, oxygen therapy Removal or ligation of bleeding area Acid suppressing medications
Complications	Hypovolemic shock
Priority Nursing Diagnoses	Deficient Fluid Volume

Nursing Process for the Patient With Gastric Bleeding

Data Collection

The nurse monitors at-risk patients for signs and symptoms of bleeding. If bleeding occurs, monitor for signs of hypovolemic shock, including hypotension, tachycardia, tachypnea, chills, palpitations, and cold/clammy extremities. Also monitor changes in level of consciousness, confusion, dry mucous membranes, fatigue, and thirst, which could indicate a decrease in circulating blood volume.

Nursing Diagnoses, Planning, and Implementation

Deficient Fluid Volume related to bleeding from GI tract via vomiting or diarrhea

EXPECTED OUTCOME: The patient's vital signs will remain within normal limits, and I&O will be balanced over 24 hours.

- Monitor color, amount, and frequency of fluid loss *to determine fluid balance changes*.
- Monitor vital signs and level of consciousness to report abnormal findings *for prompt treatment*.
- Monitor hematocrit and hemoglobin levels as ordered *to detect a decrease in circulating blood volume*.
- Obtain daily weights and monitor mucous membranes and skin turgor *to detect changes in fluid volume*.
- Avoid NG tube insertion, *as it does not improve patient outcomes*.
- Offer oral fluids or monitor IV infusions as ordered *to ensure adequate intake*.

Evaluation

If interventions have been effective, vital signs are within the normal range and the patient has a balanced I&O over 24 hours.

GASTRIC CANCER

Gastric cancer refers to malignant lesions in the stomach. It is more common in men than in women. *H. pylori* bacteria and family history can play a role in gastric cancer development. Other factors that may be associated with gastric cancer development include pernicious anemia; obesity; smoking; increased salt intake; occupational exposure to mining, metal processing, or rubber manufacturing; and alcohol. Possible protective factors include intake of fruits, vegetables, and fiber; NSAIDs; and female reproductive hormones. A poor prognosis is often associated with gastric cancer because most patients have metastasis at the time of diagnosis (see "Nutrition Notes").

Signs and Symptoms

Gastric cancer is rarely diagnosed in its early stages because symptoms do not appear until late in the disease (Table 33.6). In the early stages, there may not be any symptoms at all, and metastasis to another organ, such as the liver, may have already occurred. The symptoms of gastric cancer include weight loss, ulcer-type pain, nausea, dysphagia, melena, and early satiety. Anemia from blood loss commonly occurs.

Diagnostic Tests

Diagnosis of gastric cancer is made by upper endoscopy with biopsies.

Therapeutic Measures

Little effective medical treatment is available for gastric cancer. Eradication of *H. pylori* is done. Surgical removal, usually a total gastrectomy (Fig. 33.6), of the cancer is the most effective treatment. Typically, the cancer has already metastasized, and surgery is performed only to relieve symptoms. Chemotherapy and radiation are sometimes used in conjunction with surgery. Biological therapies with natural substances to boost the immune system might also be tried.

GASTRIC SURGERY

Two types of surgical interventions are typically used to treat upper GI diseases: subtotal gastrectomy (partial removal of the stomach) and total gastrectomy (total removal of the stomach). There are two types of subtotal gastrectomy. It is used to treat cancer or, rarely, PUD that does not respond to therapy. For a **gastroduodenostomy** (Billroth I), the distal portion of the stomach is removed, and the remainder of the stomach is anastomosed (surgically attached) to the duodenum (Fig. 33.7). A **gastrojejunostomy** (Billroth II) involves removal of a larger amount of the distal stomach and reanastomosis of the proximal remnant of the stomach to the proximal jejunum (see Fig. 33.7). Because they result in bypassing of the duodenum, either the Billroth II or Roux-en-Y (see Fig. 33.2) procedures can be used to treat duodenal ulcers. Pancreatic secretions and bile are necessary for digestion and continue to be secreted from the common bile duct even after partial gastrectomy. Total gastrectomy is the treatment for extensive gastric cancer. This surgery involves total removal of the stomach, with anastomosis of the esophagus to the jejunum (Fig. 33.6). Rarely, a vagotomy may also be performed.

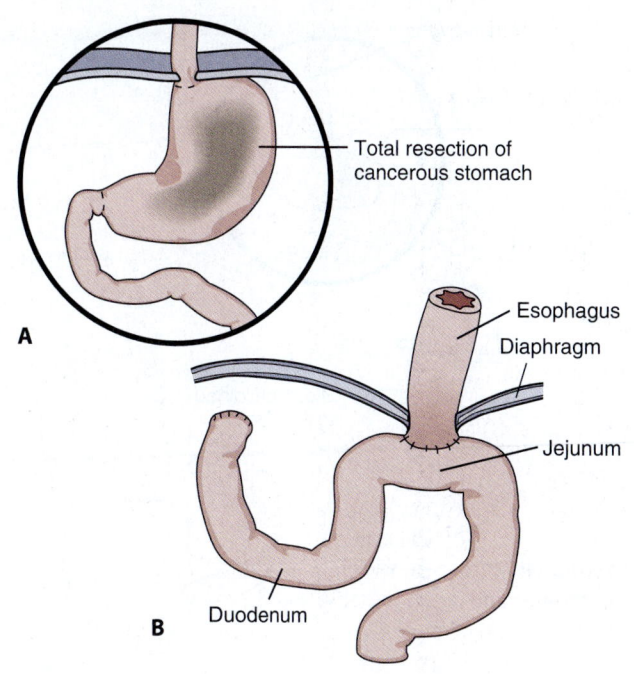

FIGURE 33.6 Total gastrectomy.

Nursing Process for the Patient Having Gastric Surgery

Data Collection

Preoperatively, identify the patient's fears or concerns to allow the provision of information on postoperative care and discharge instructions. Prophylactic antibiotics and anticoagulants are given. Postoperatively, the patient's vital signs

Table 33.6
Gastric Cancer Summary

Signs and Symptoms	Rarely detected during early stages Weight loss, ulcer-type pain, nausea, dysphagia, melena, and early satiety (symptoms can be mistaken for peptic ulcer disease) Late symptoms include involvement of other organs such as the liver
Diagnostic Tests	Upper endoscopy with biopsies
Therapeutic Measures	Surgical treatment: Subtotal or total gastrectomy Medical treatment not very effective
Complications	Related to disease and surgery (e.g., hemorrhage, acute gastric distention, nutritional problems)
Priority Nursing Diagnoses	Acute Pain Fear

• WORD • BUILDING •

gastroduodenostomy: gastro—stomach + duoden—duodenum + ostomy—mouth or opening
gastrojejunostomy: gastro—stomach + jejeun—jejunum + ostomy—mouth or opening

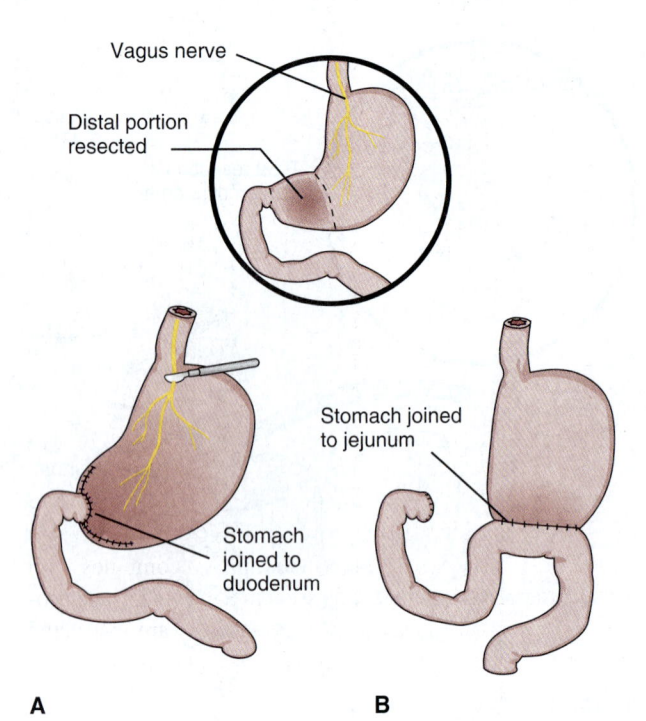

FIGURE 33.7 Subtotal gastrectomy involves removing the distal portion of the stomach. The remaining portion of the stomach is then sutured (A) to the duodenum (Billroth I procedure) or (B) to the proximal jejunum (Billroth II procedure).

are monitored as ordered. Respiratory status is carefully observed because the high location of the surgical incision may cause pain, which interferes with deep breathing and coughing. Atelectasis or pneumonia develop from guarding and shallow breathing. The patient's pain is identified and relieved, which helps the patient's ability to deep breathe or cough. The patient's IV site and infusion are monitored, and I&O are recorded. The incisional site and dressings are observed for drainage and bleeding. Early ambulation is encouraged to promote quicker recovery by improving respiratory and GI function.

Patients may have an NG tube inserted during surgery. The drainage from the NG tube is monitored for color and amount. If bleeding or excessive amounts of drainage or abdominal distention are noted, they are reported to the HCP.

BE SAFE!
BE VIGILANT! After gastric surgery, monitor the NG tube's position and drainage. Do not irrigate or reposition the NG tube to prevent damaging the suture line.

Nursing Diagnoses, Planning, and Implementation

Acute Pain related to postoperative status

EXPECTED OUTCOME: The patient will report pain is relieved or tolerable within 30 minutes of report of pain.

- Evaluate pain regularly, noting characteristics, location, and intensity on a pain rating scale *to provide information regarding patient's pain level and effectiveness of interventions.*
- Provide comfort measures such as positioning every 2 hours and back rub *to improve circulation and reduce tension associated with pain.*
- Use relaxation techniques with the patient, such as deep breathing, guided imagery, music, and distraction therapy *to enhance relaxation and improve pain relief.*
- Administer medications as ordered on a routine schedule for 24 to 48 hours *to control postoperative pain and prevent pain from becoming unbearable for patient.*
- Ensure functioning of NG tube (usually low intermittent suction) *to prevent distention and increased pain.*
- Notify HCP if pain control measures are unsuccessful *to allow revision of treatment plan.*

Fear related to body image changes, treatment, and life-threatening illness

EXPECTED OUTCOME: The patient will understand and discuss disease process and treatment options and possible outcomes of treatment before surgical procedure.

- Use open communication and convey acceptance of the patient's fears *to help patient cope with fears.*
- Reinforce teaching the disease process and treatment options *to decrease the patient's fear of the unknown.*
- Reinforce teaching about all postoperative procedures and interventions (such as medications, NG tube, drains) *to help decrease the patient's fear.*

Evaluation

If interventions have been effective, the patient will report relief or reduction of pain to a tolerable level and report that fear is reduced because of an understanding of the disease process, treatment options, and possible outcomes of treatment.

Complications of Gastric Surgery
Surgical Site Leak

Postoperative leak can occur at any suture or staple line from gastric surgeries. Signs and symptoms of a leak include fever, tachycardia and/or hypotension, and abdominal pain after gastric surgery. A CT scan or upper GI series can confirm the leak. Once confirmed, the patient is started on antibiotics, and a percutaneous drain may be used. If these are unsuccessful, surgery may be needed to correct the leak. The patient should be monitored for early signs of infection to prevent sepsis.

Gastric Distention

Symptoms of gastric distention include an enlarged abdomen, epigastric pain, tachycardia, and hypotension. The patient may report feeling full and hiccup or gag repeatedly. These symptoms must be reported to the HCP.

The HCP usually inserts the NG tube during surgery so that the suture line is not damaged. If suction is desired, an order is required. To prevent harm to the suture line, irrigating or repositioning the NG tube is not performed by the nurse. Any problems with distention or an improperly functioning NG tube are reported to the surgeon, who may need to reposition the NG tube to correct the problem. The patient's vital signs should be monitored until the patient's distention is relieved and the patient is stable.

CLINICAL JUDGMENT

Mr. Wong had gastric surgery today. He has an IV infusion of 1,000 mL dextrose 5% in 0.45 normal saline over 8 hours and an NG tube set to low intermittent suction. Mr. Wong is restless and reporting pain. His abdomen is distended. The suction canister contains no gastric output.

1. What nursing interventions, in order of priority, do you complete to help Mr. Wong?
2. What equipment do you need to provide patient-centered care for Mr. Wong?
3. As you monitor the IV, it is set for how many drops per minute with a 10-drop factor IV set?

Suggested answers are at the end of the chapter.

Dumping Syndrome

Dumping syndrome is one of the most common complications of gastric surgery. It occurs with the rapid entry of hyperosmolar food into the jejunum. The hyperosmolar food draws extracellular fluid into the small bowel from the circulating blood volume to dilute the high concentration of electrolytes and sugars. This rapid shift of fluids decreases the circulating blood volume and produces symptoms. With early dumping syndrome, the symptoms usually occur 15 to 30 minutes after eating. They include dizziness, tachycardia, fainting, sweating, nausea, vomiting, diarrhea, and abdominal cramping.

Late dumping syndrome is rare but may occur 1 to 3 hours after a meal, typically one that is high in carbohydrates. It is also known as *postprandial hyperinsulinemic hypoglycemia*. This release of insulin causes the patient to have symptoms of hypoglycemia. Symptoms include weakness, sweating, anxiety, shakiness, confusion, and tachycardia. The patient can eat some candy or drink juice containing sugar to relieve the symptoms. See "Nutrition Notes" for ways to reduce both early and late dumping syndrome. Inform the patient that these symptoms typically resolve in 7 to 12 weeks but may last for up to 6 months after gastric surgery.

Nutritional Problems

Nutritional problems that commonly occur after removal of part or all of the stomach include vitamin B_{12} and folic acid deficiency as well as reduced absorption of calcium and vitamin D. Also, rapid entry of food into the bowel often results in inadequate absorption of food.

Following gastric surgery, patients may be NPO. IV fluid provides hydration. If patients are to be NPO for any length of time, they need an alternative form of nutrition to meet their caloric and nutritional needs. After removal of the NG tube, clear fluids may be ordered with progression to full liquids and then soft foods as tolerated. Foods and fluids should be introduced into the diet gradually following gastric surgery. Eating too much or too fast can cause regurgitation.

Vitamin B_{12} deficiency may occur after some or all of the stomach is removed because intrinsic factor secretion is reduced or absent. Normally, vitamin B_{12} combines with intrinsic factor to prevent its digestion in the stomach and promote its absorption in the intestines. Patients are instructed that lifelong vitamin B_{12} replacement is required to prevent development of pernicious anemia. Vitamin B_{12} is given by the parenteral, oral, or nasal route, and dosing depends on the route. Vitamin B_{12} injections initially are given daily, then weekly, and then monthly for life. Symptoms of pernicious anemia include anemia, weakness, sore tongue, numbness and tingling, and GI upset, which should be closely monitored because they may not be reversible.

Steatorrhea

Steatorrhea is the presence of excessive fat in the stools. It is the result of rapid gastric emptying, which prevents adequate mixing of fat with pancreatic and biliary secretions. In most cases, steatorrhea can be controlled by reducing the intake of fat in the diet.

Pyloric Obstruction

Pyloric obstruction can occur after gastric surgery from scarring, edema, inflammation, or a combination of these. The signs and symptoms are vomiting, a feeling of fullness, nausea, loss of appetite, and weight loss. As the obstruction increases, it gradually becomes more difficult for the stomach to empty, and symptoms worsen. Conservative methods, such as replacing fluids and electrolytes through IV fluids and decompressing the distended stomach using an NG tube, are used first. Surgery may be necessary if conservative measures do not relieve the signs and symptoms. Pyloroplasty widens the exit of the pylorus to improve emptying of the stomach.

Key Points

- Anorexia, a lack of appetite, is a symptom of many diseases. Causes include noxious food odors, certain medications, emotional stress, fear, psychological problems, and infections.

- Nausea is the subjective feeling of the urge to vomit. Vomiting is the act of expelling stomach contents from the body through the esophagus and mouth. It is a protective function to rid the body of harmful

substances from the GI tract. If the cause of vomiting is known, it is treated.
- Initial treatment for obesity is weight loss through education regarding a healthy and balanced diet, exercise, and calorie restriction. Short-term use of medications that suppress appetite or block fat absorption may also be suggested.
- Weight loss surgery is called *bariatric surgery*. Surgical techniques produce weight loss by limiting how much the stomach can hold and/or decreasing calorie and nutrient absorption.
- Oral cancer presents as a mouth or throat sore and is often treated with radical or modified neck dissection surgery due to spread to the lymph nodes.
- Esophageal cancer is usually diagnosed in advanced stages. Surgery, chemotherapy, radiation, laser therapy, and electrocoagulation are methods used to treat esophageal cancer.
- A hiatal hernia is a condition in which the stomach slides up through the hiatus of the diaphragm into the thorax. A sliding hiatal hernia is the most common type, in which the junction of the stomach and esophagus slides up into the thoracic cavity.
- GERD is a condition in which gastric secretions reflux into the esophagus. Over time, GERD can result in esophagitis and lead to Barrett's esophagus. This is a precancerous lesion that puts the patient at risk of developing esophageal cancer.
- Acute gastritis results when the protective mucosal barrier is broken down and allows autodigestion from hydrochloric acid and pepsin to occur. Chronic gastritis can be classified as autoimmune or environmental. *H. pylori* is associated with environmental gastritis. Patients with chronic gastritis have an increased risk for developing stomach cancer.
- Peptic ulcer disease is a condition in which the lining of the stomach, pylorus, duodenum, or esophagus is eroded, usually from infection with *H. pylori*. Several treatment options are used to cure *H. pylori*. For better effectiveness, triple or quadruple therapy with antibiotics and a PPI or H_2-receptor antagonist are used.
- A perforated ulcer is a medical emergency and may require surgery. The perforation can result in peritonitis and hypovolemic shock.
- Gastric bleeding may be caused by ulcer perforation, tumors, gastric surgery, or other conditions. Bleeding peptic ulcers are the most common cause of upper GI bleeding.
- Gastric cancer refers to malignant lesions found in the stomach. It is more common in men than in women. *H. pylori* bacteria can play a role in gastric cancer development.
- Complications of gastric surgery include leaking, gastric distention, dumping syndrome, nutritional problems, pernicious anemia, steatorrhea, and pyloric obstruction.

SUGGESTED ANSWERS TO CHAPTER EXERCISES

Cue Recognition
33.1: Do not let the patient drink a large glass of water. Reinforce teaching to the patient and family of a limited (30 mL), scheduled amount of liquid allowed due to surgery.
33.2: Hold the medication because the patient has a history of renal disease, and notify HCP.

Critical Thinking & Clinical Judgment
Mr. Smith
1. Data include vital signs (looking for signs of shock); checking Mr. Smith's abdomen (looking for location of pain, tenderness, rigidity); noting vomiting and characteristics of emesis, including blood; and verifying patency of IV site access.
2. Assist Mr. Smith to a comfortable position and stay with him. Call for help. Inform the RN so the HCP can be notified immediately, and provide data regarding Mr. Smith's change in condition. Administer oxygen, monitor IV fluids, and continue to monitor vital signs. Medicate for pain as ordered.
3. Explain that you will stay with Mr. Smith as you gather data and take vital signs. Explain that you have informed the RN, who will assess Mr. Smith and report findings to the HCP. Explain that treatments ordered by the HCP will be started, including oxygen, IV fluids, and pain medication. Invite questions and have assistive personnel provide Mr. Smith with comfort needs, such as a beverage, tissues, and a chair.
4. You suspect a perforated duodenal ulcer, which is a medical-surgical emergency.
5. RN, HCP.
6. Prepare Mr. Smith for surgery by maintaining NPO (nothing by mouth) status, ensure IV access is present, verify consent is signed, obtain laboratory test results (may include complete blood count, chemistry panel, type, and cross-match for blood), and administer antibiotics as ordered.

Mr. Wong
1. Prioritize the nursing interventions:
   a. Take Mr. Wong's vital signs to determine whether he is stable. Gastric distention can cause pain, and once the distention is relieved, the pain caused by distention subsides.
   b. Check placement of Mr. Wong's NG tube by comparing the insertion length with the current length and, if ordered by the HCP, by aspirating gastric contents and verifying the pH of the contents. It is important to check for abdominal placement of Mr. Wong's NG tube to make sure it is not misplaced in the lungs. After abdominal placement is determined, if ordered, the NG tube can be connected to suction equipment. Do not reposition an NG tube in a patient who has had gastric surgery, as it could damage the surgical suture line.

SUGGESTED ANSWERS TO CHAPTER EXERCISES—cont'd

c. Next, check the suction equipment for ordered settings and to ensure that it is turned on. The suction setting normally is ordered to be on low. A whistling sound is heard when the tube is disconnected from the suction setup. The seals should be tight on the suction canister. When the tubing is hooked to suction, gastric contents should start flowing into the suction canister.

d. Check the NG tube for clogging *only if the physician orders* aspiration or irrigation to be done. If ordered, the tube is gently aspirated with a 60 mL catheter-tipped syringe. If the tube remains clogged, it is gently flushed as ordered with 10 to 20 mL of sterile normal saline.

e. After the gastric distention has been relieved, Mr. Wong's pain level is reevaluated to determine whether he needs pain medication. Considering that he is less than 1 day postoperative, he probably does.

2. Necessary equipment includes stethoscope, 60 mL catheter-tipped syringe, gloves, goggles, and normal saline for irrigation.

3. $\dfrac{1{,}000 \text{ mL}}{480 \text{ min}} \times \dfrac{10 \text{ gtt}}{\text{mL}} = \dfrac{10{,}000 \text{ drops}}{480 \text{ min}} = 21 \text{ drops/min}$

Additional Resources

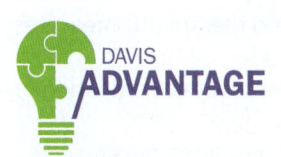

Go to Davis Advantage to complete your learning: strengthen understanding, apply your knowledge, and prepare for the Next Gen NCLEX®.

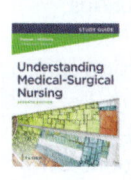

A Study Guide is also available.

CHAPTER 34
Nursing Care of Patients With Lower Gastrointestinal Disorders

Linda Rogers-Antuono

KEY TERMS

appendicitis (uh-PEN-dih-SY-tis)
colectomy (koh-LEK-tuh-me)
colitis (koh-LY-tis)
colostomy (kuh-LAW-stuh-mee)
constipation (KON-stih-PAY-shun)
diarrhea (DY-uh-REE-ah)
diverticulitis (DY-ver-tik-yoo-LY-tis)
diverticulosis (DY-ver-tik-yoo-LOH-sis)
enteritis (en-tur-EYE-tis)
fissures (FISH-ers)
fistulas (FIST-yoo-lahs)
hematochezia (HEM-uh-toh-KEE-zee-uh)
hemorrhoids (HEM-uh-royds)
hernia (HER-nee-uh)
ileostomy (IL-ee-AH-stuh-mee)
impaction (im-PAK-shun)
intussusception (IN-tuh-suh-SEP-shun)
megacolon (MEG-ah-KOH-lun)
melena (muh-LEE-nah)
obstipation (OB-stih-PAY-shun)
peristomal (PEAR-ih-STOH-muhl)
peritonitis (pear-ih-toh-NY-tis)
stoma (STOH-mah)
volvulus (VOL-view-lus)

CHAPTER CONCEPTS

Elimination
Infection
Nutrition
Teaching and learning
Tissue integrity

LEARNING OUTCOMES

1. List data to collect when caring for patients with lower gastrointestinal disorders.
2. Identify causes, signs and symptoms, and therapeutic measures of constipation and diarrhea.
3. Plan nursing care and teaching for patients with constipation or diarrhea.
4. Describe pathophysiology, therapeutic measures, nursing care, and teaching for patients with inflammatory and infectious disorders of the lower gastrointestinal tract.
5. Describe pathophysiology, therapeutic measures, nursing care, and teaching for inflammatory bowel disease.
6. Assist with planning nursing care for an abdominal hernia.
7. Assist with planning nursing care and teaching for patients with absorption disorders.
8. Describe causes, symptoms, therapeutic measures, and nursing care for intestinal obstruction.
9. Assist with planning nursing care for anorectal problems.
10. Describe causes, signs and symptoms, therapeutic measures, and nursing care for lower gastrointestinal bleeding.
11. Describe causes, signs, symptoms, therapeutic measures, and nursing care for colon cancer.
12. Assist with planning nursing care and teaching for a patient with an ostomy.
13. Discuss evaluation of nursing care for various lower gastrointestinal disorders.

The lower gastrointestinal (GI) system includes the small and large intestines, rectum, and anus.

PROBLEMS OF ELIMINATION

Constipation
Pathophysiology
Constipation occurs when the fecal mass is held in the rectal cavity for a period that is unusual for the patient or when it is eliminated fewer than three times per week. When feces are held for a prolonged time in the rectum, water continues to be absorbed from the mass. Consequently, the feces become smaller, drier, harder, and more difficult and sometimes painful to pass.

If a patient repeatedly ignores the urge to have a bowel movement (laxation), the musculature and rectal mucous membrane become insensitive to the presence of feces. Eventually, a stronger stimulus is needed to produce the peristaltic rush required for defecation. Prolonged constipation is called **obstipation**.

Etiology
There are many causes of constipation. Medications such as narcotics, tranquilizers, and antacids with aluminum decrease motility of the large intestine and may contribute to constipation. Rectal or anal conditions such as hemorrhoids or fissures may lead to a delay in defecation because of the associated pain. Metabolic or neurologic conditions such as diabetes mellitus, hyperparathyroidism, hypothyroidism, multiple sclerosis, systemic lupus erythematosus, or stroke may interfere with normal bowel innervation and function. Colon cancer may cause an obstruction that prevents normal bowel function. Low intake of dietary fiber and fluids decreases the bulk of feces and causes constipation. Decreased mobility, weakness, and fatigue, especially in older adults, reduce the strength of the muscles used for defecation, increasing the likelihood of constipation.

Signs and Symptoms
Abdominal pain and distention, indigestion, rectal pressure, a sensation of incomplete emptying, and intestinal rumbling are indications of constipation (Table 34.1). The patient may also report headache, fatigue, decreased appetite, straining at stool, and elimination of hard, dry stool.

Table 34.1
Constipation Summary

Signs and Symptoms	Abdominal pain and distention Indigestion Intestinal rumbling Rectal pressure Sensation of incomplete emptying Straining at stool Hard, dry stool
Diagnostic Tests	History Physical with rectal examination
Therapeutic Measures	High-fiber diet 2–3 L fluid daily Strengthening of abdominal muscles Exercise Bulk-forming agents Stool softeners Laxatives
Priority Nursing Diagnoses	Constipation Deficient Knowledge

Complications
A variety of problems can result from constipation. Fecal **impaction** may result when the fecal mass is so dry it cannot be passed. Pressure on the colon mucosa from a mass of stool may cause ulcers to develop. Often, small amounts of liquid stool ooze around the fecal mass, causing incontinence of liquid stools. Straining to have a bowel movement (Valsalva maneuver) can result in cardiac, neurologic, and respiratory complications. If the patient has a history of heart failure, hypertension, or recent myocardial infarction, straining can lead to cardiac rupture and death. Grossly dilated loops of the colon, known as **megacolon**, can occur proximal to the dry fecal mass and obstruct the colon. Abdominal distention occurs. In severe cases, loops of bowel can be palpated through the abdominal wall.

Diagnostic Tests
Constipation is usually self-diagnosed or diagnosed by history and physical with rectal examination. Procedures to examine causes of chronic constipation include radiographic or magnetic resonance imaging (MRI) defecography, sigmoidoscopy, colonoscopy, or anorectal manometry.

Therapeutic Measures
Treatment of constipation depends on the cause. First-line treatment for chronic constipation is bulking agents (fibers) and lifestyle modifications. These include increased physical activity, drinking more water if not contraindicated (2–3 L per day), warm water or caffeine beverage in the morning, response to the urge to defecate, and exercises to strengthen abdominal muscles. Bulk-forming agents such as psyllium (Metamucil) or stool softeners such as docusate sodium (Colace) can be tried. Laxatives for severe constipation include lubiprostone (Amitiza) and linaclotide (Linzess). Enemas and rectal suppositories are used only for severe cases and are discontinued upon resolution of an acute episode. Medications such as methylnaltrexone (Relistor) or naloxegol (Movantik) are available for opioid-induced constipation, which usually requires intervention.

Nursing Process for the Patient With Constipation
DATA COLLECTION. The patient may feel self-conscious or embarrassed when interviewed about bowel habits and history. Establish a rapport with the patient and provide privacy to gather data. Include the onset and duration of constipation, past elimination pattern, current elimination pattern, occupation, lifestyle (stress, exercise, nutrition), history of laxative or enema use, medical-surgical history, and current medications being taken. Color, consistency, and odor of the stool as well as intestinal symptoms are noted.

• WORD • BUILDING •
megacolon: mega—large + colon—colon

> ### Evidence-Based Practice
>
> **Clinical Question**
> What is the best position for defecation to promote peristalsis and prevent constipation?
>
> **Evidence**
> The preferred position for defecation in the western population is sitting. A prospective crossover study of 52 volunteers was done for 4 weeks. Bowel movement (BM) data related to straining, duration, and emptying with and without the use of a defecation posture modification device (DPMD) was collected. At baseline, 28.8% reported incomplete emptying, 44.2% experienced increased straining, and 55.8% noticed blood on their toilet paper in the past year. Utilizing the DPMD resulted in increased bowel emptiness and reduced straining patterns. Moreover, without the DPMD, participants had an increase in BM duration.
>
> **Implications for Nursing Practice**
> Use of a DPMD provides a holistic approach to preventing constipation related to posture by straightening the anal canal, decreasing straining, and increasing emptying of bowels.
>
> *Reference:* Modi, R. M., Hinton, A., Pinkhas, D., Groce, R., Meyer, M. M., Balasubramanian, G., Levine, E., & Stanich, P. P. (2019). Implementation of a defecation posture modification device: Impact on bowel movement patterns in healthy subjects. *Journal of Clinical Gastroenterology, 53*(3), 216–219. https://doi.org/10.1097/MCG.0000000000001143

After the interview, the patient's abdomen is inspected for distention and symmetry, then auscultated and palpated. Inspection of the perianal area may reveal fissures, external hemorrhoids, or irritation.

NURSING DIAGNOSES, PLANNING, AND IMPLEMENTATION.

Constipation related to irregular defecation habits

EXPECTED OUTCOME: The patient will maintain passage of soft, formed stool every 1 to 3 days without straining.

- Identify normal pattern of defecation, diet and fluid intake, medications, surgeries, and use of laxatives *to help identify factors contributing to constipation*.
- Set a specific time for defecation, such as after a meal when bowels are most active, *to facilitate the urge reflex*.
- Use a DPMD or footstool *to promote flexion of the hips, which promotes defecation*.
- Encourage a high-fiber, high-residue diet *to decrease constipation* (see "Nutrition Notes: Treating Constipation With Food Choices").
- Reinforce teaching the physiology of defecation and the importance of responding to the urge to defecate when it occurs *to help prevent constipation*.
- Reinforce teaching to increase fluid, if not contraindicated, to 2 to 3 L per day *to soften feces*.
- Reinforce teaching to increase activity through a daily walking program and abdominal exercises designed to improve the muscle tone *to improve peristalsis and promote more spontaneous defecation*.

EVALUATION. The plan has been effective if the patient has established a regular bowel function pattern (Box 34.1) and expresses satisfaction with the outcomes.

> ### PRACTICE ANALYSIS TIP
> **Linking NCLEX-PN® to Practice**
> The LPN/LVN will provide care to client with bowel or bladder management protocol.

CUE RECOGNITION 34.1
Mrs. Lopez is a 93-year-old resident in an assisted living facility. You note that she has not had a bowel movement in 5 days. What action should you take to provide patient-centered care?

Suggested answers are at the end of the chapter.

Diarrhea
Diarrhea occurs when fecal matter passes through the intestine rapidly, resulting in decreased absorption of water, electrolytes, and nutrients. Diarrhea is three or more loose or watery stools in 24 hours. Severe diarrhea can result in more than 20 bowel movements per day. Acute diarrhea usually resolves in several days. Chronic diarrhea lasts more than 14 days.

Pathophysiology and Etiology
Acute diarrhea is most often due to infections, which can lead to enteritis, and is self-limiting. The main causes of acute infectious diarrhea include viruses (norovirus, rotavirus, and adenoviruses), bacteria (*Salmonella, Campylobacter, Escherichia coli,* and *Clostridioides difficile*), and protozoa (*Cryptosporidium, Giardia,* and *Entameoba*) from contaminated food or water. Food intolerance or allergies, dairy products, wheat, sugar substitutes, excessive caffeine, and high-fat or fried foods can also cause diarrhea. Medications such as antibiotics can cause diarrhea as a side effect. Chronic diarrhea causes include inflammatory diseases such as Crohn disease or ulcerative colitis (discussed later). Radiation therapy in cancer may impair absorption, resulting in frequent, watery stools. An irritable bowel or a neurologic disorder may cause increased motility problems. Enteral feedings can result in diarrhea.

Prevention
To prevent diarrhea, proper handling, storage, and refrigeration of all fresh foods helps to minimize contact with infectious agents. Hand hygiene and cleaning of the kitchen

• WORD • BUILDING •
diarrhea: dia—through + rhea—to flow

Box 34.1
Criteria for Regular Bowel Function
- A regular time for defecation is planned.
- Fluid intake is 2 to 3 L per day.
- High-fiber and high-residue foods are added to the diet.
- A regular exercise program is followed.
- Laxative use is limited or avoided.
- Outcome is frequency of stools every 1 to 3 days and consistency of stools reported is soft and formed.

Nutrition Notes
Treating Constipation With Food Choices

Achieving the recommended fiber intake of 19 to 38 grams per day (depending on gender and age) is a matter of prudent choices at every meal. Listed here, in the first column, are examples of higher-fiber foods and, in the third column, examples of foods in the same category but with less fiber.

Higher-Fiber Foods	Grams of Fiber	Lower-Fiber Foods	Grams of Fiber
Breakfast			
All-bran buds, 1/3 cup	13	Corn flakes, 1 cup	1
Orange sections, 1 cup	4	Orange juice reconstituted from frozen concentrate, 1 cup	0
Lunch			
Chili, 1 cup	5	Chicken noodle soup, 1 cup	2
Raw apple with skin, 2¾" diameter	4	Raw apple peeled, 2¾" diameter	2
Dinner			
Whole wheat spaghetti, 1 cup cooked	6	Spaghetti, 1 cup cooked	3
Banana, 1 cup sliced	4	Watermelon, 1 cup diced	1
Totals	**36**		**9**

Other foods contribute to fiber intake. They can be evaluated via nutrition labels. Individuals who wish to correct constipation without medications should determine their present fiber intake and increase it gradually to the U.S. Department of Agriculture recommended dietary allowance while also drinking sufficient water.

as well as food preparation areas and serving items are extremely important. Enteral feedings should be given using full-strength formula rather than diluting the formula. This reduces the risk of contaminating the formula. To prevent travelers' diarrhea, routine vaccines should be up to date. In addition, specific vaccines, such as for yellow fever or typhoid, are required depending on the destination country and must be completed prior to travel. Healthy People 2030 goals include improving food-safety-related behaviors and practices (Office of Disease Prevention and Health Promotion, 2021b).

Signs and Symptoms

Diarrhea stools may be foul-smelling and contain undigested food particles and mucus (Table 34.2). The stools could contain blood or pus. Diarrhea resulting from food poisoning usually has an explosive onset and may be accompanied by nausea and vomiting. Abdominal cramping, intestinal rumbling, and thirst are common. Fever indicates an infection. Weakness and dehydration from fluid loss may occur (see "Gerontological Issues: Dehydration and Hypokalemia").

Gerontological Issues
Dehydration and Hypokalemia

Diarrhea can cause older people to quickly become dehydrated and hypokalemic because both fluid and potassium are lost in stools. The signs and symptoms of hypokalemia include muscle weakness, hypotension, anorexia, paresthesia, and drowsiness. It can also cause cardiac arrhythmias, such as atrial and ventricular tachycardia, premature ventricular contraction, and ventricular fibrillation, which can be fatal.

If the older person has decreased mobility, quick access to the bathroom is important. Because of poor muscle control, older patients may be incontinent. This might embarrass patients or cause them to hurry, which increases the risk of falls and resulting injuries such as fracture, dislocation, or hematoma. Also, because older patients' skin is more sensitive as a result of poor turgor and a reduction in subcutaneous fat layers, perirectal skin excoriation can occur secondary to the acidity and digestive enzyme content of diarrheal stools.

Table 34.2
Diarrhea Summary

Signs and Symptoms	Frequent, watery stools Abdominal cramping Distention Anorexia Intestinal rumbling
Causes	Inflammatory diseases, such as Crohn disease and ulcerative colitis Infectious organisms Recent antibiotic use Surgical procedures such as bowel resection Laxatives Enteral feedings Radiation therapy
Diagnostic Tests	History Laboratory examinations of stool
Therapeutic Measures	Replacement of fluids and electrolytes Antidiarrheal medications Antimicrobials Probiotic (Lactinex) Fecal transplant
Priority Nursing Diagnoses	Diarrhea Risk for Deficient Fluid Volume Deficient Knowledge

Diagnostic Tests

The diagnosis of diarrhea is determined by the onset and progression of the condition, presence of fever, laboratory examinations, and visual inspection of the stool for bacteria, pus, or blood.

Stool is examined for red blood cells (RBCs), white blood cells (WBCs), mucus, and appearance. Stool tests for bacterial pathogens should be completed for diarrhea lasting more than 1 week or if the patient has severe illness and/or high-risk comorbidities. Grossly bloody diarrhea should be tested for Shiga toxin to identify Shiga-toxin-producing *E. coli*. If the patient has had recent antibiotic use, testing for *C. difficile* should be done. Additional diagnostic testing for unresolved or chronic diarrhea can include cultures to identify the specific causative organism, endoscopy, colonoscopy, computed tomography (CT), and blood tests.

Therapeutic Measures

The goal of treatment is to treat the underlying condition (see "Nutrition Notes: Deciding When an Adult With Diarrhea Should Seek Medical Care"). Replacing fluids and electrolytes is important. The oral route is preferred, but IV fluid replacement may be necessary for dehydration, especially in the very young or very old. For three or more watery stools per day in the absence of fever, motility of the intestines can be decreased with the use loperamide (Imodium) or diphenoxylate (Lomotil). Bismuth subsalicylate may be used in patients with fever or dysentery. Antimicrobial agents are prescribed for some infections. If diarrhea is thought to be caused by antibiotics that change the normal flora of the bowel, a *Lactobacillus* granule probiotic supplement (Culturelle) may be used to help restore the normal flora. Fecal transplant can restore the normal intestinal flora in those who are ill or who have chronic conditions.

Nutrition Notes

Deciding When an Adult With Diarrhea Should Seek Medical Care

Most instances of diarrhea in healthy adults are self-limiting and resolve without treatment. Indications for medical care include the following:

- Lasts for more than 2 days
- Causes severe pain in the abdomen or rectum
- Fever of 102°F (38.8°C) or higher
- Produces blood in the stool or black, tarry stools
- Is accompanied by signs of dehydration
- Occurs in a person with medical conditions for which fasting, dehydration, or infectious disease is a hazard

Maintaining adequate hydration is important, and individuals should be encouraged to drink water and electrolyte-replacing beverages. Educate the person to progress to clear liquids, then to full liquids, progressing to a low-residue diet (one limited in high-fiber foods) and, finally, to a regular diet as tolerated.

Nursing Process for the Patient With Diarrhea

DATA COLLECTION. Ask the patient whether there is a known cause for the diarrhea, what the signs and symptoms are, and when they began. The patient's usual dietary habits and any changes or recent exposure to contaminated food or water are noted. Identify whether medications, such as antibiotics or laxatives, may be contributing to the diarrhea. If the patient has traveled recently, determine the geographic location and whether exposure to an infected person or someone with similar symptoms occurred. Document stool consistency, color, odor, and frequency.

Observe for symptoms of dehydration, such as tachycardia, hypotension, decreased skin turgor, weakness, thready pulse, dry mucous membranes, and oliguria. Obtain the patient's height and weight to establish a baseline. Abnormal laboratory studies that may indicate dehydration include increased serum osmolality, increased specific gravity of urine, and increased hematocrit. Decreased serum potassium may result from intestinal loss of potassium.

• WORD • BUILDING •
enteritis: entero—intestine + itis—inflammation

NURSING DIAGNOSES, PLANNING, AND IMPLEMENTATION.

Diarrhea related to infection or possible ingestion of irritating foods

EXPECTED OUTCOME: The patient will maintain formed, soft stool every 1 to 3 days.

- Obtain patient history, including medications, about diarrhea *to help identify cause.*
- Monitor and record stool characteristics, amount, and frequency *to plan care.*
- Utilize transmission precautions and consider a private patient room *to prevent infection transmission.*
- Give antidiarrheal medications as ordered *to control diarrhea.*
- Keep skin clean, dry, and protected with a moisture barrier after each bowel movement or use a fecal incontinence appliance *to protect perianal skin from contact with liquid stools and their enzymes.*
- Reinforce teaching hand hygiene by patient, family, and health-care staff *to prevent the spread of infection.*

Risk for Deficient Fluid Volume related to frequent passage of stools and insufficient fluid intake

EXPECTED OUTCOME: The patient will maintain a stable weight and vital signs, and urine output will remain within normal limits at all times.

- Weigh the patient daily and record intake and output (I&O; including diarrheal stools) *to determine fluid balance.*
- Encourage oral intake and/or maintain IV fluid replacement as ordered *to maintain fluid balance and prevent dehydration.*
- Reinforce teaching the patient signs and symptoms of dehydration to report *to allow prompt treatment.*

EVALUATION. Goals have been met if frequency of diarrheal stools is decreased and balance of fluids is achieved.

INFLAMMATORY AND INFECTIOUS DISORDERS

Many diseases of the lower GI tract are a result of inflammation in the bowel. Sometimes the inflamed areas become infected, resulting in a worsening of symptoms.

Appendicitis

Pathophysiology

Appendicitis is the inflammation of the appendix, the small, fingerlike appendage attached to the cecum of the large intestine. Because of the small size of the appendix, obstruction may occur, causing inflammation and making it susceptible to infection.

Signs and Symptoms

Abdominal pain is the most common symptom of an appendicitis. Other signs and symptoms of appendicitis include anorexia, nausea, vomiting, diarrhea, fever, and increased WBCs. Within hours of onset, the pain usually becomes localized to the right lower quadrant at the McBurney point, midway between the umbilicus and the right iliac crest (Fig. 34.1). This is one of the classic symptoms of appendicitis.

Physical examination reveals slight abdominal muscular rigidity (guarding), normal bowel sounds, and local rebound tenderness (intensification of pain when pressure is released after palpation) in the right lower quadrant of the abdomen. Sometimes there is pain in the right lower quadrant when the left lower quadrant is palpated (Rovsing sign). The patient might keep the right leg flexed for comfort and experience increased pain if the leg is straightened.

Diagnostic Tests

A complete blood count (CBC) reveals elevated leukocyte (WBC) and neutrophil counts. An ultrasound, CT scan, or MRI reveals an enlargement in the area of the cecum.

Therapeutic Measures

Surgery for nonperforated appendicitis should be performed quickly after diagnosis (within 12 hours) and can be either laparoscopic or open. Laparoscopic surgery allows for faster healing and fewer complications. The patient is NPO (nothing by mouth). The use of a heating pad, laxative, or enemas are avoided because they can cause or complicate a rupture.

If the appendix has ruptured, IV fluids and antibiotic therapy are started to treat infection and peritonitis. Surgery may be delayed for up to several weeks while the infection is resolved. If infection is present, a drain may be inserted into the abdomen by a radiologist or during surgery.

Complications

Perforation of the inflamed appendix can cause peritonitis. An abscess of the appendix can occur, which is a localized collection of pus. This is usually treated with IV antibiotics and surgical drainage. An appendectomy is done about 6 weeks later.

Peritonitis

Peritonitis is inflammation of the peritoneum that occurs from a variety of causes. It is a serious condition that can be life-threatening.

Pathophysiology and Etiology

Trauma, ischemia, or perforation in an abdominal organ causes leakage of the organ's contents into the peritoneal cavity, causing inflammation and infection. The tissues become edematous and begin leaking fluid with increasing amounts of blood, protein, cellular debris, and WBCs. The intestinal tract responds with hypermotility, soon followed by paralysis (paralytic ileus).

• WORD • BUILDING •

peritonitis: periton—pertaining to peritoneum + itis—inflammation

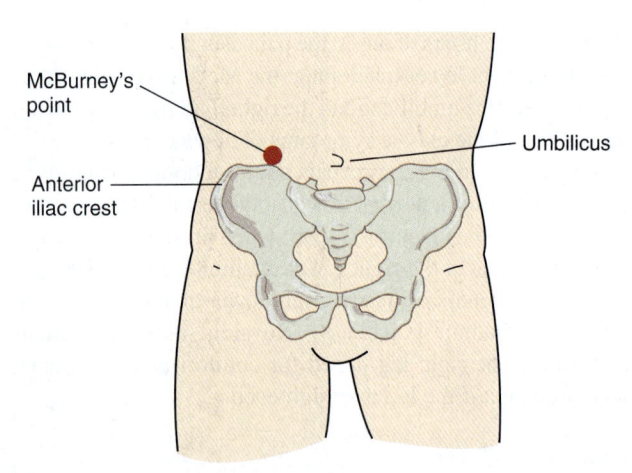

FIGURE 34.1 Pain at the McBurney point is a symptom of appendicitis.

Common causes of peritonitis that permit GI bacteria to enter the peritoneum are a ruptured appendix, peptic ulcer, gangrenous gallbladder, perforated colon, pancreatitis, peritoneal dialysis, diverticulitis, incarcerated hernia, or gangrenous small bowel. It may also be a spontaneous complication of cirrhosis due to ascites.

Signs and Symptoms
Generalized abdominal pain evolves into localized pain at the site of the perforation or leakage. The area of the abdomen that is affected is extremely tender and aggravated by movement. Rebound tenderness and abdominal rigidity (board-like) are present. Decreased peristalsis results in bloating, full feeling, anorexia, nausea and vomiting, and no bowel movement or flatus. Infection causes fever, increased WBCs, and an elevated pulse. Dehydration signs can be present. Peritonitis can cause sepsis and be life-threatening.

Diagnostic Tests
Tests include WBCs to identify elevation, an abdominal x-ray or CT scan to show distention or perforation, paracentesis and laboratory analysis to identify a causative organism, or exploratory surgery to identify the cause.

Therapeutic Measures
The patient is NPO and fluid and electrolyte replacement are crucial to correct hypovolemia and prevent or treat shock. Antibiotics are used to treat or prevent sepsis. Abdominal distention is relieved through insertion of an orogastric (or NG) tube with suction. Depending on the cause of the peritonitis, surgery may be performed to excise, drain, or repair the cause. An ostomy may be formed to divert stool, allowing resolution of the infection. After surgery, the patient usually has a wound drain, an NG tube, and a urinary catheter.

Complications
Complications of peritonitis are intestinal obstruction (discussed later), hypovolemia caused by the shift of fluid into the abdomen, and septicemia from bacteria entering the bloodstream. Shock and ultimately death may result.

Diverticulosis and Diverticulitis
Pathophysiology
A diverticulum (singular) is a small outpouching of the colon wall. **Diverticulosis** is when multiple diverticula (plural) are present without evidence of inflammation (Fig. 34.2). With increased pressure within the colon or stool trapped in a diverticulum, a tear can occur, and inflammation and infection can develop. This is called **diverticulitis**. If an abscess develops, the diverticulum may rupture, leading to peritonitis (see "Gerontological Issues: Diverticulitis").

Gerontological Issues

Diverticulitis
With aging, the incidence of diverticular disease increases as a result of chronic constipation, obesity, hiatal hernia, or atrophy of the intestinal walls. Symptoms are often not reported early because patients fear it may be cancer. Blood in the stool, which can be an indication of diverticulitis, may not be seen by the older adult because of impaired vision.

Etiology
Diverticula develop in weak places in the colon that give way under pressure. The exact cause is unknown. Low-fiber diets are thought to play a part in the development of diverticulosis, but this is not confirmed by research. Patients with chronic constipation have pressure within the bowel, which may lead to development of diverticula. Diverticulosis is most common in the sigmoid colon. A small percentage of patients with diverticulosis develop diverticulitis.

Risk Factors
People older than 60 most commonly experience diverticulitis. A diet low in fiber and high in fats and red meat, obesity, sedentary lifestyle, and smoking may increase risk for diverticulitis. Medications such as NSAIDs, opioids, and steroids can increase risk. Some health-care providers (HCPs) recommend avoiding nuts and seeds that can get caught in diverticula; however, this has not been shown to prevent diverticulitis.

Signs and Symptoms
Most people with diverticulosis never have symptoms. Steady or crampy pain in the left lower quadrant of the abdomen is the most common symptom. Nausea, vomiting, and bowel

• **WORD • BUILDING** •

diverticulosis: diverticul—blind pouch + osis—condition
diverticulitis: diverticul—blind pouch + itis—inflammation

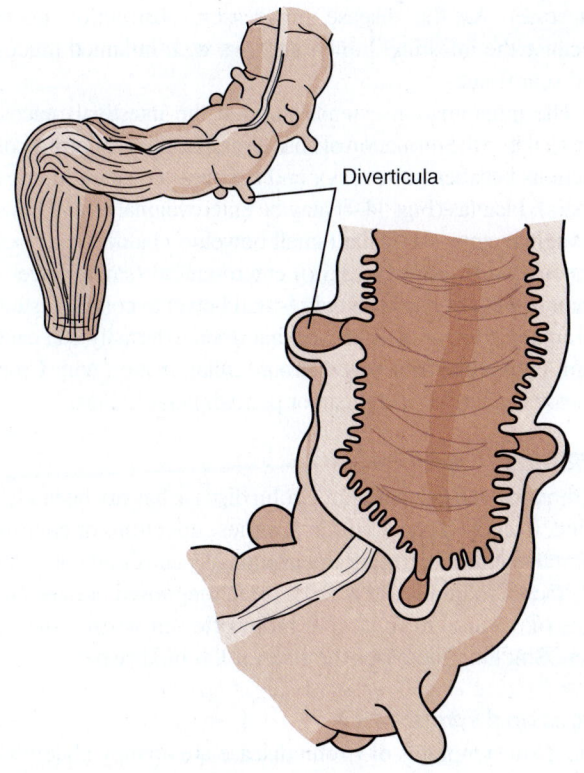

FIGURE 34.2 The presence of diverticula in diverticulosis.

habit changes with constipation can occur (Table 34.3). Other symptoms may include bleeding, fever, and fatigue.

Diagnostic Tests
Diverticulitis is confirmed with a CT scan, especially if complications such as an abscess are suspected. Diverticulosis is typically found with flexible sigmoidoscopy or colonoscopy, but these methods should not be used with diverticulitis due to the risk of perforation. WBCs are checked for infection. A stool specimen can show infection or occult blood.

Therapeutic Measures
Severity of an attack guides treatment. Home treatment is possible for mild cases. It includes over-the-counter analgesics such as acetaminophen (Tylenol), an antibiotic, and a liquid diet for 2 to 3 days. With severe diverticulitis, the patient is hospitalized for pain control, administration of IV antibiotics and fluids while being NPO, and drainage of any abscesses. When the acute period is over, a progressive diet is started.

Surgery may be considered, especially for perforation, abscess, or bowel obstruction. A bowel resection to remove the diseased area of the colon with anastomosis (reconnection) may be done. A temporary colostomy (discussed later) may be created to allow inflammation to subside and the diseased portion of the colon to rest. Later, the colostomy can be reversed and the colon reconnected.

Nursing Process for the Patient With an Inflammatory or Infectious Disorder
Data Collection
Identifying pain is essential for patients experiencing inflammation or infection. Monitor the patient closely, and notify the HCP immediately if pain increases, especially if associated with abdominal rigidity. Increased pain may indicate that the bowel has ruptured and peritonitis is developing. Abdominal distention is recorded and reported. Vital signs are monitored for fever and other signs of sepsis. Reduced urinary output, dropping blood pressure, and rising pulse rate reflect fluid volume imbalance.

Nursing Diagnoses, Planning, and Implementation

Acute Pain related to inflammatory process

EXPECTED OUTCOME: The patient will report pain is relieved or at an acceptable level within 30 minutes of report of pain.

Table 34.3
Symptoms Associated With Diverticulitis

W—Where is the pain?	Usually in the left lower quadrant
H—How does it feel? (Describe quality)	Tender, crampy, constant
A—Aggravating and alleviating factors	Constipation and low-fiber diet may aggravate; treatment of constipation may alleviate
T—Timing (onset, duration, frequency)	Gradual onset and increase in pain over several days
S—Severity (0–10)	Usually 5 to 7
U—Useful other data/associated symptoms	Intermittent rectal bleeding; straining at stool; constipation alternating with diarrhea; elevated white blood cells and sedimentation rate; elevated temperature and pulse rate; and pus, mucus, and blood in stool
P—Patient's perception	Fear of cancer diagnosis

- Have the patient rate pain using a rating scale such as 0 to 10 *to determine pain level.*
- Give analgesic or antispasmodic medications as ordered *to relieve pain.*
- Use relaxation exercises and positioning such as semi-Fowler *to reduce tension on abdomen and pain.*

Risk for Deficient Fluid Volume related to diarrhea or fluid shifting from the circulation to the peritoneal cavity

EXPECTED OUTCOME: The patient will maintain vital signs and urine output within normal limits at all times.

- Record I&O *to determine fluid balance.*
- Weigh patient daily *to determine fluid loss.*
- Monitor vital signs and urine output and report changes *to detect change from normal limits.*
- Maintain IV fluid replacement as ordered *to maintain fluid balance if output is greater than intake.*

Evaluation
The goals are met if the patient reports that pain is controlled, vital signs and urinary output remain stable, and the patient has regular, comfortable bowel elimination.

INFLAMMATORY BOWEL DISEASE

Crohn Disease
Pathophysiology
Crohn disease is an autoimmune inflammatory bowel disease (IBD) that can involve any part of the GI tract. The body has inappropriate immune response to intestinal microbes, and Crohn disease commonly affects the terminal portion of the ileum, or first part of the large intestine. The inflamed areas from Crohn disease can alternate with areas of healthy tissue (Fig. 34.3), so the inflamed areas are referred to as "skip lesions" (as they are not continuous lesions along the intestine). As the disease progresses, obstruction occurs because the intestinal lumen narrows with inflamed mucosa and scar tissue.

The inflammation extends through the intestinal mucosa. This leads to the formation of abscesses, **fistulas** (abnormal connections between structures), and **fissures** (unnatural tracts or ulcers). Fistulas (Fig. 34.4) may be enterovaginal (small bowel to vagina), enterovesicular (small bowel to bladder), enterocutaneous (small bowel to skin), entero-entero (small bowel to small bowel), or enterocolonic (small bowel to colon). Fistulas communicating with organs or that drain externally can cause pain, peritonitis, or sepsis. Chronic inflammation with Crohn disease can lead to malignant or premalignant lesions.

Etiology
Although the exact cause of Crohn disease has not been identified, it tends to occur within families. Infections or environmental agents can trigger the immune system's attack on the GI tract. Crohn disease is most often diagnosed between the ages of 15 and 30. It occurs more often in women than in men. Smoking increases the risk for Crohn disease.

Signs and Symptoms
The main symptoms of Crohn disease are crampy abdominal pain, chronic intermittent diarrhea (with or without blood), weight loss, and fatigue. Symptoms can be mild to severe and have periods of remission and exacerbations. Because crampy pains occur after eating, the patient may avoid eating to prevent pain. Lack of eating and poor absorption of nutrients result in weight loss and malnutrition. Chronic diarrhea contributes to fluid deficit and electrolyte imbalance. Inflammatory symptoms outside the GI tract can affect the eyes, liver, bile ducts, skin, and joints. Physical or psychological stress may trigger exacerbations (see "Cultural Considerations").

Cultural Considerations

In the United States, Crohn disease and ulcerative colitis are more common in White individuals, particularly people of Eastern European Jewish descent, and urban populations. The incidence of Crohn disease is increasing in Black individuals. These findings support possible hereditary and/or environmental risk factors for IBD.

Diagnostic Tests
Laboratory testing looks for anemia, infection, liver function, low albumin due to poor absorption of protein, stool infections, and occult blood. Imaging tests include multiphase CT enterography and magnetic resonance enterography (MRE), which provide detailed images of the intestines. Endoscopy (colonoscopy and sigmoidoscopy), with multiple biopsies of the diseased colon and terminal ileum, is used to confirm Crohn disease. Other tests include capsule endoscopy (swallowed camera the size of a pill), ultrasound to identify

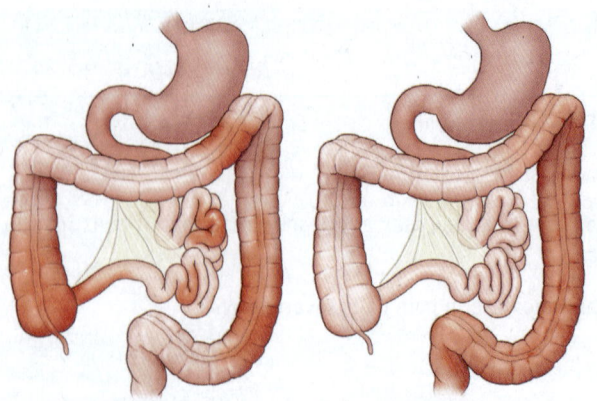

Crohn's Disease   **Ulcerative Colitis**

FIGURE 34.3 Areas affected (shaded areas) in Crohn disease and ulcerative colitis. Crohn disease can occur anywhere in the intestine with alternating healthy tissue and lesions. Ulcerative colitis occurs in the large intestine and rectum as a continuous ulceration.

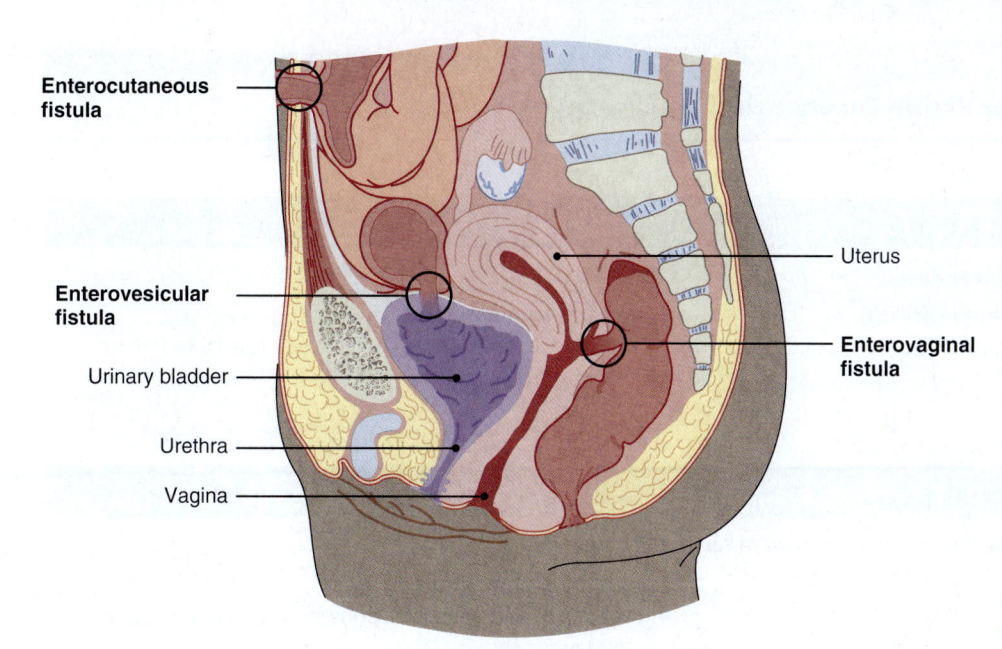

FIGURE 34.4 Fistulas are a common complication of Crohn disease.

fistulas and areas of bleeding, double balloon enteroscopy, which provides views of the inside of tissue folds, and chromoendoscopy (enhanced endoscopy that sprays blue dye into colon to illuminate any pathologic changes). Crohn disease is confirmed by granulomas in the biopsy specimen.

Therapeutic Measures

There is no cure for Crohn disease. Management is aimed at achieving and maintaining remission. Medication therapy is individualized for each patient. Medications work to decrease intestinal inflammation through different actions to promote healing of the mucosa. Classes of medications used to achieve these goals are 5-aminosalicylates, biologic response modifiers, corticosteroids, anti-inflammatory synthetic corticosteroid, and immunomodulators (Table 34.4). Medication therapy depends on the severity of the disease. For mild/low-risk Crohn disease, the first-line treatment for inducing remission is oral enteric-coated budesonide. Once remission is achieved, the steroid is tapered, then discontinued, and the patient is monitored. An ileocolonoscopy is then performed in 6 to 12 months. For patients with high-risk and moderate to severe Crohn disease, the first line of therapy includes a biologic agent (infliximab) with or without an immunomodulator (azathioprine, 6-mercaptopurine, or methotrexate). Once remission is achieved, long-term therapy with a biologic and immunomodulator are continued for 1 to 2 years. At that point, the immunomodulator may be discontinued.

Antibiotics can reduce bacterial counts in the intestine that may contribute to inflammation. Antidiarrheal medications such as diphenoxylate with atropine (Lomotil) or loperamide (Imodium) are used. Bulk-forming laxatives may reduce loose stools and skin irritation.

As complications develop, surgery may be indicated for obstruction, stricture, fistula, abscess, excessive bleeding, perforation, toxic megacolon (loss of muscle tone and dilation in colon), or symptoms that do not respond to treatment. Surgery does not cure Crohn disease because it can recur elsewhere in the GI tract. Surgical procedures may be open or laparoscopic and include strictureplasty to widen areas of stricture, resection of an affected area in the small intestine with anastomosis, **colectomy** with ileorectal anastomosis, proctectomy, or proctocolectomy (rectum and colon) with ileostomy. See details on intestinal ostomies later in this chapter. A Kock pouch is not recommended for those with Crohn disease because the disease may affect the pouch.

Healthy diet is important in overall health, but there is no special diet for Crohn disease. Dietitian referral is important for nutritional support. Adequate fluid intake is essential to prevent dehydration if diarrhea is present. Malnutrition is a concern if the small intestine is affected and nutrients are not absorbed properly. Multivitamin and mineral supplements may be needed. Foods that increase symptoms, such as dairy products, fatty food, and fresh fruits and vegetables, should be limited.

Nursing Process for the Patient With Crohn Disease

Because of the similarities between Crohn disease and ulcerative colitis, the nursing processes for both are discussed together in the "Nursing Process for the Patient With Inflammatory Bowel Disease" section that follows.

Ulcerative Colitis

Pathophysiology

Ulcerative **colitis** is similar to Crohn disease. Crohn disease, however, can occur anywhere in the GI system, whereas ulcerative colitis occurs in the large intestine and rectum

• WORD • BUILDING •

colectomy: col—pertaining to colon + ectomy—surgical excision
colitis: col—pertaining to colon + itis—inflammation

Table 34.4
Medications for Crohn Disease and/or Ulcerative Colitis

Medication/Action

5-Aminosalicylates

Decrease inflammation and suppress immune system.

Examples (may be tablets or suppositories)	**Nursing Implications**
mesalamine (Asacol HD, Canasa, Pentasa, Rowasa, Lialda)	Monitor for signs of reduced kidney function.
olsalazine (Dipentum)	Take with food.
balsalazide (Colazal)	Take with food.
sulfasalazine (Azulfidine)	Contraindicated in sulfa allergy (sulfasalazine).

Biologic Response Modifiers

Selectively target inflammatory agents to interfere with inflammatory response.

Examples	**Nursing Implications**
adalimumab (Humira)	Tuberculosis test must be done before therapy begins and annually.
certolizumab pegol (Cimzia)	
infliximab (Remicade)	Monitor for infections, bone marrow suppression, and central nervous system disorder.
ustekinumab (Stelara)	
vedolizumab (Entyvio)	

Corticosteroids

Decrease intestinal inflammation.

Examples	**Nursing Implications**
prednisone (Deltasone)	Teach patient not to stop taking medication abruptly.
methylprednisolone (Medrol, Solu-Medrol)	May increase blood sugar levels.

Anti-Inflammatory Synthetic Corticosteroid

Reduce inflammation locally for Crohn disease.

Examples	**Nursing Implications**
budesonide (Entocort EC)	*Teach:* Grapefruit and grapefruit juice should be avoided. Take in morning. Swallow whole.

Immunomodulators

Most commonly used in immunosuppression to reduce inflammation.

Examples	**Nursing Implications**
azathioprine (Imuran)	Report symptoms of infection when taking an immunomodulator.
6-mercaptopurine (6-MP, Purinethol)	Monitor for infections.
Methotrexate (Trexall)	Monitor for side effects. *Teach:* Grapefruit and grapefruit juice should be avoided. Take in morning. Swallow whole.

(see Fig. 34.3). Recurring episodes of multiple ulcerations and diffuse inflammation occur in the superficial mucosa and submucosa of the colon. The lesions spread in a continuous pattern.

Etiology

Infection, allergy, and autoimmune response are possible causes of ulcerative colitis, although an exact cause is unknown. Environmental agents such as pesticides, tobacco, radiation, and food additives may precipitate an exacerbation. Ulcerative colitis usually begins before age 30. Heredity may play a role for about a quarter of those with ulcerative colitis.

Signs and Symptoms

Diarrhea with blood or pus, abdominal and rectal pain, rectal bleeding, and fecal urgency with straining are common symptoms of ulcerative colitis (Table 34.5). Weight loss, fever, fatigue, and severe dehydration associated with passing 4 to 10 or more liquid stools a day may occur. Along with potential fluid and electrolyte imbalance, calcium is lost. Anemia often develops as a result of rectal bleeding. Symptoms are usually intermittent, with remissions lasting from weeks to years. Diet or psychological stress may trigger or worsen an attack. Other parts of the body can be affected by ulcerative colitis such as joints, skin, mouth, liver, gallbladder, and eyes.

Complications

Malnutrition occurs less often with ulcerative colitis than with Crohn disease. As with Crohn disease, other inflammatory disorders can occur. Additional complications include hemorrhage, toxic megacolon, perforation, peritonitis, osteoporosis, and increased risk for colorectal cancer.

Diagnostic Tests

A history and physical examination with laboratory tests are used to diagnose ulcerative colitis. Anemia is often present because of blood loss. Examination of stool specimens is done to rule out the presence of bacterial or amoeba organisms. The stool is positive for blood in the presence of ulcerative colitis. Electrolytes may be depleted from chronic diarrhea. Protein loss and elevated serum alkaline phosphatase are because of liver dysfunction and malabsorption. A colonoscopy to see the whole colon or a flexible sigmoidoscopy to view the lower colon is done. Biopsy specimens show inflamed cells. Barium enema, ultrasound, CT scan, and MRI are also used. Leukocyte scintigraphy, a noninvasive imaging test, uses the patient's WBCs tagged with a radioactive material to detect infection and inflammation in the colon.

Therapeutic Measures

Diet, lifestyle changes, medications, and surgery are used for treatment. Many of the medication classes used with Crohn disease are used for ulcerative colitis (see Table 34.4). Foods that cause gas or diarrhea should be avoided. Because the offending foods may be different for each patient, foods are tried in small amounts and eliminated if they cause symptoms. In general, high-fiber foods, caffeine, spicy foods, and milk products are avoided. Diarrhea may increase the need for fluids to prevent dehydration.

Surgery is considered for excessive bleeding, severe symptoms, perforation, or toxic megacolon. Because ulcerative colitis usually involves the entire large intestine, the entire colon and rectum are removed for a proctocolectomy with ileostomy (discussed later). This procedure is curative. The anal sphincter of the rectum can be preserved for an ileoanal pouch (restorative proctocolectomy). This is not curative, as the disease can return in the preserved rectum.

An ileoanal pouch does not require an ostomy pouch to be worn and is the more common surgery performed. Because the anus and sphincter are saved, stool still passes through the anus. The rectum and colon are removed. The end of the ileum, which is made into a J-shaped pouch, is attached to the anus (discussed later). A temporary ileostomy is created to allow the pouch to heal. After about 12 weeks, the ileostomy is closed. Several bowel movements per day occur. The stool is of soft consistency. Surgical complications can include a bowel obstruction or an inflammation of the pouch (pouchitis), which is treated with antibiotics. An investigational surgical technique of transanal total mesorectal excision (TaTME) has the potential to define resection margins more clearly than standard surgery through the abdomen.

Nursing Process for the Patient With Inflammatory Bowel Disease

Data Collection

A history obtained from the patient includes symptoms, including onset, duration, frequency, and severity. Ask about

Table 34.5
Inflammatory Bowel Disease Summary

Signs and Symptoms	Diarrhea Abdominal and rectal pain or cramping Rectal bleeding Fecal urgency with straining Weight loss Fluid and electrolyte imbalance Fissures, fistulas, and abscesses Arthritis and skin lesions Inflammatory eye disorders Inflammatory liver disease
Diagnostic Tests	Stool examination Endoscopy with biopsy Barium enema, ultrasound, computed tomography (CT) scan, magnetic resonance imaging (MRI) Leukocyte scintigraphy
Therapeutic Measures	Medications: see Table 34.4 Surgery if necessary Avoidance of offending foods Elemental formula or parenteral nutrition (PN) if required
Priority Nursing Diagnoses	Diarrhea Deficient Knowledge Risk for Deficient Fluid Volume Imbalanced Nutrition: Less Than Body Requirements

correlation between exacerbations of symptoms and dietary changes or stress. Note any food allergies, food intolerances, caffeine, nicotine, and alcohol intake because these stimulate the bowel and can cause cramping and diarrhea.

Identify the patient's nutritional status and signs of dehydration. Ten to 20 pounds can be lost in a 2-month period. Perianal skin should be observed for irritation and excoriation. Identification of emotional status, coping skills, and verbal and nonverbal behavior is essential. The patient may withdraw from family and friends because of frequent bowel movements. Anxiety, sleep disturbances, depression, and denial can be problems. If surgery involving an ileostomy is planned, the patient is at risk for altered body image.

Nursing Diagnoses, Planning, and Implementation

Acute Pain related to increased peristalsis and cramping

EXPECTED OUTCOME: The patient will state pain is relieved or at an acceptable level within 30 minutes of report of pain.

- Ask patient to rate pain on a scale such as 0 to 10 *to determine pain level.*
- Document the character of the pain (e.g., dull, cramping, burning) and ask whether the pain is associated with meals or other activities *to plan care.*
- Give analgesics and medications *to relieve cramping, as prescribed.*

Diarrhea related to the inflammatory process

EXPECTED OUTCOME: The patient will maintain formed, soft stool every 1 to 3 days.

- Document characteristics of stools, including color, consistency, amount, frequency, and odor *to plan care.*
- Ensure the patient has quick access to the bathroom or provide a bedside commode *to prevent incontinence.*
- Administer antidiarrheal medication as prescribed. *Controlling diarrhea controls comfort and fluid balance.*
- Keep the environment clean and odor free *to help promote comfort.*
- Reinforce teaching the patient to avoid dairy products and high-fiber foods such as whole grains and raw fruits and vegetables as well as caffeine, alcohol, and nicotine *because they stimulate intestinal motility.*

Risk for Deficient Fluid Volume related to diarrhea and insufficient fluid intake

EXPECTED OUTCOME: The patient will maintain vital signs and urine output within normal limits at all times.

- Weigh patient daily *to determine fluid loss.*
- Record I&O (including diarrhea stools) *to determine fluid balance.*
- Document and report signs of deficient fluid volume to the HCP *to allow treatment.*
- Maintain IV fluids as ordered *to maintain fluid balance.*
- Encourage fluids when acute diarrhea subsides *to maintain fluid balance.*
- Reinforce teaching the patient symptoms of dehydration to report *to allow prompt treatment.*

Anxiety related to symptoms and frequency of stools and treatment

EXPECTED OUTCOME: The patient will report that anxiety is reduced.

- Answer questions; talk in a calm, confident manner; and actively listen to the patient *to reduce anxiety, which aggravates symptoms of IBD.*

Impaired Skin Integrity related to frequent loose stools

EXPECTED OUTCOME: The patient's skin will remain intact at all times.

- Keep perianal skin clean, dry, and protected with a moisture barrier after each bowel movement *to protect perianal skin from contact with liquid stools and their enzymes.*
- Provide sitz baths, which may be comforting and helpful in keeping skin clean, *to prevent excoriation.*

Imbalanced Nutrition: Less Than Body Requirements related to malabsorption

EXPECTED OUTCOME: The patient will maintain weight within normal range for height and age.

- Weigh weekly *to detect weight loss.*
- Give special liquid (elemental) formula that is absorbed in the upper bowel as ordered *to allow the colon to rest.*
- Maintain parenteral nutrition (PN) as ordered to provide nourishment *if the patient is unable to tolerate oral intake.*

See "Nursing Care Plan for the Patient With Inflammatory Bowel Disease."

Evaluation

Goals have been met if pain is relieved, frequency of diarrhea stools is decreased, fluid and electrolyte balance is achieved, anxiety is reduced, skin is intact, and weight is within normal range for height and age.

IRRITABLE BOWEL SYNDROME

Pathophysiology

Irritable bowel syndrome (IBS) is not a disease but rather a functional problem. The colon mucosa is not damaged by the condition, and there is no increased risk of colorectal cancer. IBS is characterized by abdominal pain and altered

Nursing Care Plan for the Patient With Inflammatory Bowel Disease

Nursing Diagnosis: *Ineffective Coping* related to inflammatory bowel disease
Expected Outcome: The patient will identify strategies that promote effective coping.
Evaluation of Outcome: Is the patient able to state strategies for effective coping?

Intervention	Rationale	Evaluation
Identify patient's knowledge of the disease.	Many people have little knowledge of a disease, and accurate information is essential.	Does patient verbalize information about the disease and its effects on the body?
Encourage patient to express feelings about the disease and how it is affecting their life.	Expressing feelings about the disease and its perceived effect enables patient to talk about concerns. The health-care team can then address these concerns.	Does patient talk about feelings regarding the potential impact of the disease on their life?
Determine whether patient would like to speak with a person of similar age from the Crohn's & Colitis Foundation.	Speaking with someone close in age with the same disease lets the patient know that they are not the only person coping with this disorder. It can also help the patient learn some strategies for effectively coping with the disease.	Does patient show an interest in speaking with someone with the same disease?
Identify strategies for effective coping that are acceptable to patient.	Talking about concerns and possible solutions is a positive step. Coping strategies identified with the patient are more likely to be implemented.	Is patient able to identify strategies for effective coping that they believe will work?

bowel habits. The disorder may be classified as IBS with diarrhea, IBS with constipation, IBS mixed (diarrhea and constipation) or unclassified (meet criteria of IBS but cannot be accurately classified).

CLINICAL JUDGMENT

Judy Moore is an 18-year-old college student just diagnosed with Crohn disease.
1. What questions do you ask Judy to identify her symptoms?
2. What nursing diagnoses do you think would be relevant for Judy's condition?
3. What patient-centered care do you implement to help Judy adapt to this disease?
4. If Judy's condition were to worsen, what manifestations would be exhibited when you complete data collection?
5. With which members of the health-care team do you collaborate?

Suggested answers are at the end of the chapter.

Etiology
The cause is unknown. There is a hereditary tendency for IBS. IBS is more common in women than men and in those who are young to middle aged. Intestinal muscle contractions, nerve conduction abnormalities, immune response, intestinal inflammation, and the microbiome are influencing factors in the disorder. The nerves in the bowel are overly sensitive in people with IBS. At times of stress in daily living or with food intolerances, abnormal contractions may result. Flare-ups can be caused by infections or the menstrual cycle.

Signs and Symptoms
Patients experience chronic abdominal pain and altered bowel habits of constipation or diarrhea, which can alternate. Other symptoms include feeling of incomplete evacuation, urgency, mucus with stools, depression, and anxiety.

Diagnostic Tests
Diagnosis of IBS is based on history and physical examination along with stool examination, laboratory colonoscopy, flexible sigmoidoscopy, CT scan, or lower GI series to rule out other disorders, including lactose intolerance or celiac disease if diarrhea occurs. IBSchek is a new antibody test that identifies IBS cases that have developed two antibodies in response to exposure to a bacterial toxin found in food poisoning that results in watery diarrhea.

Therapeutic Measures
IBS is a chronic condition, but symptoms can generally be controlled with diet, lifestyle, stress management, and medication. Treatment varies on the basis of the bowel pattern. In general, adequate hydration, exercise, rest, and

avoiding food triggers, especially those that cause gas and contain gluten or FODMAPs (fermentable oligosaccharides, disaccharides, monosaccharides, and polyols), are important (see "Nutrition Notes: Low FODMAP Diet"). A high-fiber and high-bran diet and supplements (psyllium [Metamucil]) or polyethylene glycol (MiraLAX) may help to form softer, larger stools to relieve constipation. For some patients, avoiding lactose, fructan, and/or gluten can help with symptoms. Eating smaller, frequent meals can be helpful in reducing bowel contractions. Patients can keep a diary of foods eaten, stressors, and symptoms to help identify flare-up triggers. Stress management and behavioral therapy (e.g., biofeedback, hypnosis, psychotherapy) are helpful in relaxing the bowel as well as contributing to overall health. Review the Patient Teaching Guideline for "Irritable Bowel Syndrome" found in your resources on Davis Advantage.

Nutrition Notes
Low FODMAP Diet

FODMAP stands for **f**ermentable **o**ligosaccharides, **d**isaccharides, **m**onosaccharides, and **p**olyols. The Low FODMAP diet restricts certain carbohydrates that are known to cause symptoms in patients with IBS such as cramping, bloating, and diarrhea because of their poor absorption, osmotic activity, and rapid fermentation. The Low FODMAP Diet has been shown to reduce IBS symptoms.

Patients on the Low FODMAP diet should refrain from eating certain foods, such as the following:

- Fructo-oligosaccharide (fructans)—wheat, rye, onions, garlic, and artichokes
- Galacto-oligosaccharides—legumes (soybeans, chickpeas, lentils), cabbage, brussels sprouts
- Lactose—milk, dairy products, beer, and sauces
- Fructose—honey, apples, dates, mangoes, papaya, pears, watermelon, high-fructose corn syrup
- Sorbital—apples, pears, stone fruits, sugar-free mints/gum
- Mannitol—mushrooms, cauliflower, sugar free-mints/gums

Not all FODMAPs will trigger symptoms for all patients. Only those that are malabsorbed are likely to be clinically significant. Fructans and galacto-oligosaccharides (GOSs) are always malabsorbed because humans do not produce enzymes that break them down. They move unabsorbed through the GI tract and are fermented by intestinal bacteria, resulting in gas production and associated flatulence even in healthy people. There is some concern that low FODMAP disrupts the normal microbiome in the GI tract. More studies are needed to determine which diet is best for IBS.

Reference: Mazur, E. E., & Litch, N. A. (2019). *Lutz's nutrition & diet therapy* (7th ed.). Philadelphia, PA: F.A. Davis.

Medications taken depend on the type of IBS. Constipation can be treated with psyllium or polyethylene glycol. Lubiprostone (Amitiza), linaclotide (Linzess), and plecanatide (Trulance) can increase intestinal fluid secretion and improve fecal transit. Tegaserod (Zelnorm) can increase colonic motility and reduce abdominal pain. Tenapanor (Ibsrela) enhances intestinal fluid volume and movement of stool. Diarrhea is treated with loperamide (Imodium). Bile acid sequestrants, such as cholestyramine, can be used in patients with persistent diarrhea. With severe diarrhea-prominent IBS lasting 6 months, 5-hydroxytryptamine-3 (alosetron, [Lotronex]) can be used if other treatments have not been ineffective. Low-dose tricyclic antidepressants, such as desipramine (Norpramin), imipramine (Tofranil), or nortriptyline (Pamelor) are used for IBS with diarrhea because they slow movement through the intestines. Antispasmodics, such as hyoscyamine (Levbid) or dicyclomine (Bentyl), are used in IBS to relieve painful bowel spasms. Rifaximin (Xifaxan), an antibiotic, treats IBS with diarrhea if other medications have failed. Multistrain probiotics have demonstrated improvement of symptoms, although the exact strains that are most effective have yet to be determined.

Nursing Process for the Patient With Irritable Bowel Syndrome

Data Collection

Height, weight, and symptoms, including pain, are documented. Timing of the symptoms, food and fluid intake, elimination patterns, effects on self-esteem, and socialization are explored. Personal and family roles are identified as IBS is a significant cause of missed work and school, social withdrawal, and embarrassment. Patient knowledge and readiness for managing the syndrome are determined to plan care.

Nursing Diagnoses, Planning, and Implementation

Constipation related to irregular motility of GI tract

EXPECTED OUTCOME: The patient will maintain passage of soft, formed stool every 1 to 3 days without straining.

- Identify normal bowel pattern, diet and fluid intake, and medications *to help identify factors contributing to constipation for planning care.*
- Increase fluid intake, if not contraindicated, to 2 to 3 L per day *to prevent hard stools.*
- Give medication as ordered *to prevent constipation.*
- Reinforce teaching the benefits of increasing fiber in the diet *to promote soft, larger stools that are easier to pass.*

Diarrhea related to irregular motility of GI tract

EXPECTED OUTCOME: The patient will maintain formed, soft stool every 1 to 3 days.

- Obtain history and medications taken for diarrhea episodes *to help identify cause.*
- Monitor and record stool characteristics, amount, and frequency *to plan care.*

- Give antidiarrheal medications as ordered. *Controlling diarrhea controls comfort and fluid balance.*
- Keep skin clean, dry, and protected with a moisture barrier after each bowel movement *to protect perianal skin from contact with liquid stools and their enzymes.*

Readiness for Enhanced Health Self-management related to desire to manage symptoms of IBS

EXPECTED OUTCOME: The patient will state understanding of and ability to carry out preventive measures to control symptoms before discharge.

- Encourage use of food diary documenting foods eaten and timing of symptom occurrence *to identify food triggers for symptoms.*
- Consult a registered dietitian *to develop meal plan to prevent symptoms.*
- Reinforce teaching about IBS symptoms, aggravating factors, and treatments, *to promote understanding and ability to follow therapeutic regimen.*

Evaluation
The plan has been effective if the patient has regular bowel function pattern, verbalizes understanding of self-care measures, and expresses satisfaction with the outcomes.

ABDOMINAL HERNIAS

Pathophysiology and Etiology
A **hernia** is an abnormal protrusion of an organ or structure through a weakness or tear in the wall of the cavity normally containing it, such as the abdominal wall. A hernial sac is formed by the peritoneum protruding through the weakened muscle wall. Hernias occur from increased intra-abdominal pressure, such as the pressure from coughing, straining, or heavy lifting. Contents in the hernia sac can be the small or large intestine or the omentum.

Figure 34.5 illustrates the various types of hernias. Umbilical hernias are seen most often in obesity, ascites, peritoneal dialysis, or multiple pregnancies. Inguinal hernias (direct or indirect) are located in the groin where the spermatic cord in males or the round ligament in females emerges from the abdominal wall. Femoral hernias occur in the groin below the inguinal ligament and are uncommon. Ventral (incisional) hernias usually result from weakness in the abdominal wall after abdominal surgery, especially in the obese patient, if a drainage system was used or if the patient experienced poor wound healing or inadequate nutrition.

Prevention
Congenital defects cannot be prevented. Reducing strain on abdominal muscles helps prevent hernias. Those who do heavy lifting, tugging, or pushing should wear a support binder or avoid lifting. A healthy lifestyle of maintaining normal weight, not smoking, and eating high-fiber foods is recommended.

Signs and Symptoms
Unless complications occur, few symptoms are associated with hernias. An abnormal bulging can be seen in the affected area of the abdomen, especially when straining or coughing. The patient may have heaviness or dull discomfort around the hernia. The herniation may disappear when the patient lies down. If the intestinal mass easily returns to the abdominal cavity or can be manually placed back in the abdominal cavity, it is called a *reducible* hernia. When adhesions or edema occur between the sac and its contents, the hernia becomes *irreducible* or *incarcerated*.

Complications
An incarcerated hernia may become strangulated if the blood and intestinal flow are completely cut off in the trapped loop of bowel. Strangulated hernias seldom develop in adults. Incarceration leads to an intestinal obstruction and possibly gangrene and bowel perforation. Symptoms are nausea, vomiting, abdominal pain, and possibly fever.

Therapeutic Measures
Hernias are diagnosed by physical examination. Treatment options include no treatment, observation of the hernia, short-term support devices, or surgical repair. A supportive truss or brief applies pressure to keep the reduced hernia in place. Emergency surgery is needed for strangulation or the threat

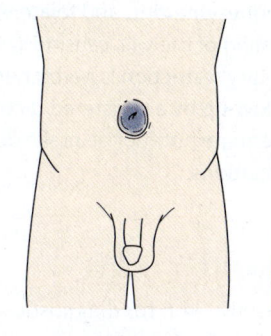

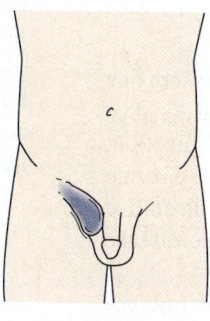

| Umbilical hernia | Direct inguinal hernia | Indirect inguinal hernia | Femoral hernia |

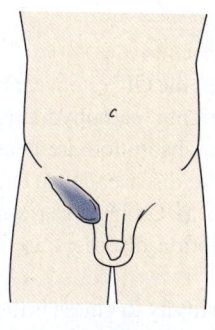

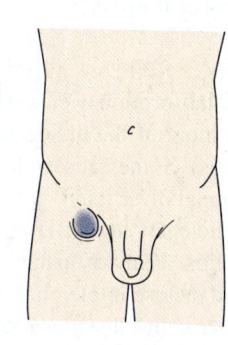

FIGURE 34.5 Types of hernias.

of bowel obstruction. Surgical repair is recommended for inguinal hernias. Surgical procedures are most often done laparoscopically and include hernioplasty (open or laparoscopically) or herniorrhaphy (open hernia repair). Herniorrhaphy involves making an incision in the abdominal wall, replacing the contents of the hernial sac, sewing the weakened tissue, and closing the opening. Hernioplasty involves replacing the hernia into the abdomen and reinforcing the weakened muscle wall with mesh. Bowel resection or a temporary colostomy may be necessary if the hernia is strangulated.

Nursing Care
The patient is instructed to avoid activities that increase intra-abdominal pressure, such as lifting heavy objects or coughing. The patient is taught to recognize signs of incarceration or strangulation and to notify the HCP immediately. If a support truss or brief has been ordered, the patient is taught to apply it before arising from bed each morning while the hernia is not protruding. Special attention should be paid to maintenance of skin integrity beneath the truss.

Postoperative Care
Care following inguinal hernia repair is similar to any abdominal postoperative care (see Chapter 12). Patients can perform deep breathing to keep lungs clear postoperatively but should avoid coughing. Coughing increases abdominal pressure and could affect the hernia repair. The male patient may experience swelling of the scrotum. Ice packs and elevation of the scrotum may be ordered to reduce the swelling. Because most patients are discharged the same day of surgery, they are taught to change the dressing and report difficulty urinating, bleeding, and signs and symptoms of infection, such as redness, incisional drainage, fever, or severe pain. The patient is also instructed to avoid lifting, driving, and sexual activities for 2 to 6 weeks, as specified by the HCP. Most patients can return to nonstrenuous work within 2 weeks.

ABSORPTION DISORDERS

The process of digestion reduces nutrients to a liquid form that can be absorbed through intestinal mucosa into the portal bloodstream. More than 8,000 mL of liquid with nutrients and electrolytes is absorbed daily, mostly proximal to the ileocecal valve.

Pathophysiology and Etiology
Malabsorption occurs when the GI system cannot absorb one or more of the major nutrients (carbohydrates, fats, or proteins). Some causes of malabsorption are ileal dysfunction, jejunal diverticula, parasitic disease, celiac disease, enzyme deficiency, and IBD such as Crohn disease and ulcerative colitis. Primary malabsorption disorders are celiac disease and lactose intolerance.

In celiac disease, a sensitivity to gluten is thought to cause malabsorption of protein. Gluten is a protein found in wheat, barley, and rye. Oats may become contaminated with gluten in the milling process of these other grains (see "Nutrition Notes: Treating Celiac Disease").

A deficiency in lactase, an enzyme that breaks down lactose (milk sugar), causes lactose intolerance. When lactose is not digested, a high concentration of it occurs in the intestines, causing an osmotic retention of water in the colon and watery stools.

Signs and Symptoms
Weight loss, fatigue, and general malaise resulting from malnutrition are associated with malabsorption disorders. Celiac disease symptoms can range from none to many in various body systems. Frequent loose, bulky, foul gray stools with an increased fat content (steatorrhea) as well as gas, bloating, and abdominal pain may occur in celiac disease. Lactose intolerance causes abdominal cramping, excessive gas, and loose stools after eating milk products.

Complications
Vitamin K deficiency and resulting hypoprothrombinemia can increase risk of bleeding. Severe calcium deficiency can cause bone pain and neuromuscular hyperirritability, including tetany. Folic acid, vitamin B_{12}, and iron deficiency can result in glossitis, stomatitis, anemia, and dry, rough skin. In celiac disease, dermatitis herpetiformis occurs, a skin rash with severe pruritus and blistering.

Nutrition Notes
Treating Celiac Disease
Celiac disease, or gluten-sensitive enteropathy, has a multifactorial etiology involving a combination of the following:
- Genetic predisposition
- Ingestion of gluten
- Autoimmune response that produces chronic inflammation of the small intestine

Treatment requires permanent elimination of wheat, rye, and barley from the diet. Gluten-free grains, such as oats, can be cross-contaminated with gluten during milling. An individual must look for a "gluten-free" claim on food packaging to ensure a food is, in fact, gluten free. People with celiac disease frequently have nutritional deficiencies of vitamins (A, D, E, and B_{12}), fiber, iron, calcium, magnesium, zinc, and folate. Absence of gluten allows the healing of the villi, causing symptoms to resolve. Because dietary restriction is permanent, instruction from and follow-up by a registered dietitian are indicated to ensure adequate nutritional intake despite the many dietary limitations.

Diagnostic Tests
See Table 34.6 for diagnostic studies used to identify malabsorption diseases. It is important to be tested before making diet changes.

Table 34.6 Diagnostic Tests for Disorders of Malabsorption

Diagnostic Test	Test Result and Associated Malabsorption Syndrome
Hematocrit	Decreased if anemia is present.
Mean corpuscular volume	Increased values found with malabsorption of vitamin B_{12}.
Upper gastrointestinal series	Thickening of the intestinal mucosa, narrowed mucosa of the terminal ileum, or a change in fecal transit time are indicative of malabsorption syndrome.
Tissue transglutaminase (tTG) antibody (IgA)	Presence indicates celiac disease.
Sudan stain for fecal fat	Malabsorption can be distinguished from maldigestion if this test shows abnormally large numbers of fat droplets.
72-hour stool collection for fat	Stool fat greater than 5 g per 24 hours after ingestion of 80 g of fat in 2 days implies a fat digestion disorder.
Biopsy	Shows flattened mucosa and loss of villi with celiac disease or IBD.

Therapeutic Measures

Celiac Disease
A consultation with a dietitian is essential to plan a gluten-free diet to relieve symptoms, promote intestinal healing, and improve nutritional status. However, because gluten is used as a filler or binder in many products, even in those labeled "wheat-free," diligence in identifying potentially offending foods is essential. The dietitian can assist with choosing safe foods.

Lactose Intolerance
Lactose intolerance is treated restricting foods that contain lactose, such as milk and milk products. Whole milk and some dairy products, such as hard cheeses (cheddar, Swiss) and yogurt, may be better tolerated. Lactase enzyme drops or tablets (e.g., Lactaid or Dairy Ease) digest about 70% of lactose in foods. They can be added to milk in liquid form or taken as a tablet before eating foods containing lactose. Vitamin D supplements may be needed.

Nursing Care
Nursing care involves monitoring fluid and electrolyte balance, nutritional status, and skin integrity. Recording daily weight and I&O helps determine whether fluid loss is occurring. Intake of electrolyte-rich fluids is encouraged to replace losses. Diet teaching is reinforced. Perianal skin is kept clean and dry, and barrier ointments are used as needed to protect the skin from excoriation.

INTESTINAL OBSTRUCTION

Intestinal obstructions occur when the flow of intestinal contents is blocked. The two types of intestinal obstruction are mechanical and nonmechanical; both can be partial or complete.

Mechanical obstruction is when a blockage occurs within the intestine from conditions causing pressure on the intestinal walls. Nonmechanical obstruction occurs when peristalsis is impaired and the intestinal contents cannot be propelled through the bowel. The severity of the obstruction depends on the area of bowel affected, the amount of occlusion within the lumen, and the amount of disturbance in the blood flow to the bowel.

Small-Bowel Obstruction
Pathophysiology
When obstruction occurs in the small bowel, intestinal contents, gas, and fluid collect proximal to the obstruction. The resulting distention stimulates gastric secretion but decreases absorption of fluids. As distention worsens, the intraluminal pressure decreases venous and arterial capillary pressure, resulting in edema, necrosis, and possible perforation of the intestinal wall.

Etiology
There are a variety of mechanical obstruction causes. Following abdominal surgery, loops of intestine may adhere to areas in the abdomen that are not healed. This may cause a kink in the bowel that occludes the intestinal flow. These adhesions, or bands of scar tissue, are the most common cause of small-bowel obstruction. They are usually acquired from previous abdominal surgery. Hernias and neoplasms are the next most common causes, followed by IBD, foreign bodies, strictures, volvulus, and intussusception. A **volvulus** occurs when the bowel twists, occluding the lumen of the intestine. **Intussusception** occurs when peristalsis causes the intestine to telescope into itself (Fig. 34.6).

Paralytic ileus is a nonmechanical obstruction that occurs when intestinal peristalsis decreases or stops because of a neuromuscular condition. Causes of nonmechanical obstructions

• WORD • BUILDING •
intussusception: intus—within + suscept—to receive

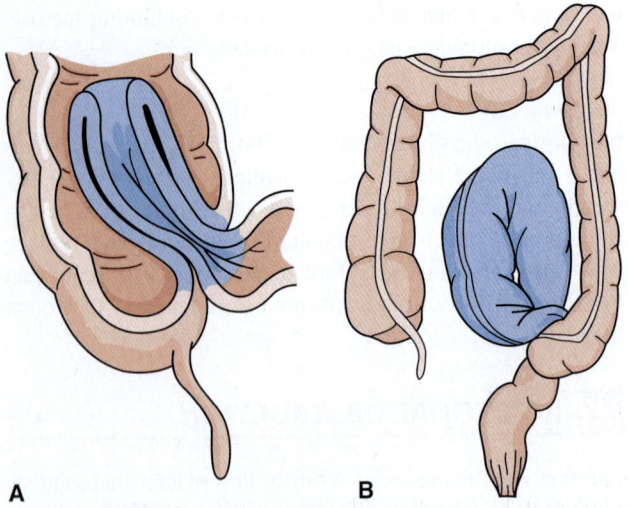

FIGURE 34.6 Mechanical bowel obstructions. (A) Intussusception. (B) Volvulus.

Table 34.7
Bowel Obstruction Summary

Signs and Symptoms	Wavelike abdominal pain Vomiting Possible fecal vomiting Blood and mucus from rectum Flatus and feces cease Bowel sounds high pitched, tinkling, or absent Abdominal distention
Diagnostic Tests	Abdominal x-ray examination Computed tomography (CT) scan Complete blood count (CBC) and electrolytes
Therapeutic Measures	Nothing by mouth (NPO) status Nasogastric tube Fluid and electrolyte replacement Parenteral nutrition (PN) as needed Medications (antiemetics, analgesics) Surgery
Priority Nursing Diagnoses	Acute Pain Risk for Deficient Fluid Volume Risk for Electrolyte Imbalance

include abdominal surgery, hypokalemia, peritonitis, spinal injuries, trauma, and vascular insufficiency.

Signs and Symptoms
The most common symptoms with acute small bowel obstruction include nausea, vomiting, cramping abdominal pain, and obstipation (inability to pass flatus or stool). As the obstruction becomes more extreme, peristaltic waves may occur to attempt to relieve the obstruction and propel the intestinal contents into the stomach. This can lead to fecal vomiting. Abdominal distention is present. Sharp, sustained pain may indicate perforation. In mechanical obstructions, high-pitched, tinkling bowel sounds are heard proximal to the obstruction and muffled or absent distal to it. In nonmechanical obstruction, bowel sounds are absent (Table 34.7).

Loss of fluid and electrolytes can lead to dehydration, with associated symptoms of extreme thirst, drowsiness, aching, and general malaise. The lower in the GI tract the obstruction is, the greater the abdominal distention. Uncorrected obstruction can lead to shock and possibly death.

Diagnostic Tests
Dilated loops of bowel are evident in radiographic studies and CT scans. If strangulation or perforation occurs, leukocytosis is evident. Hematocrit levels are elevated if the patient is dehydrated and serum electrolyte levels are decreased.

Therapeutic Measures
In most cases, the patient is NPO. Decompression of the bowel using an NG tube to suction relieves symptoms and may allow the obstruction to resolve on its own. An IV solution with electrolytes is initiated to correct fluid and electrolyte imbalance. Complete mechanical obstruction requires surgical intervention, such as removal of tumors, release of adhesions, or a bowel resection with anastomosis.

Large-Bowel Obstruction
Pathophysiology
Obstruction in the large bowel is less common and not usually as dramatic as small-bowel obstruction. Radiological examination reveals a distended colon. Dehydration occurs more slowly because of the colon's ability to absorb fluid and distend well beyond its normal full capacity. If the blood supply to the colon is cut off, the patient's life is in jeopardy because of bowel strangulation and necrosis.

Etiology
Most large-bowel obstructions occur in the sigmoid colon and are caused by carcinoma, IBD, diverticulitis, or benign tumors. Impaction of stool may also cause obstruction.

Signs and Symptoms
Symptoms of large-bowel obstruction develop slowly and depend on the location of the obstruction. If the obstruction is in the rectum or sigmoid, the only symptom may be constipation. As the loops of bowel distend, the patient may report crampy lower abdominal pain and abdominal distention. Vomiting is a late sign and may be fecal. High-pitched, tinkling bowel sounds may be heard. A localized tender area and mass may be felt on palpation. Untreated large-bowel obstructions can lead to dehydration, shock, gangrene, perforation, and peritonitis.

Therapeutic Measures

If impaction is present, enemas and manual disimpaction may be effective. Other mechanical blockages may require surgical resection of the obstructed colon. A temporary colostomy may be indicated to allow the bowel to rest and heal. Sometimes, an ileoanal anastomosis is done. A stent may be placed to expand the colon to facilitate fecal movement if surgery cannot be done immediately. A patient who is a poor surgical risk may have a cecostomy (an opening from the cecum to the abdominal wall) to allow diversion of stool. A consult with the nutrition support team to evaluate for PN should be made.

Nursing Process for the Patient With a Bowel Obstruction

Data Collection

Each quadrant of the abdomen is auscultated for bowel sounds to identify the location of the obstruction. The abdomen is palpated for distention, firmness, and tenderness. The amount and character of stool, if any, are documented. Pain is monitored using the institution's pain scale and described according to location and character, such as "crampy" or "wavelike." Vital signs are monitored for signs of infection or shock. Daily weight and I&O are monitored. Skin turgor is monitored for fluid deficit. The amount, color, and character of NG drainage are documented.

Nursing Diagnoses, Planning, and Implementation

Acute Pain related to abdominal distention

EXPECTED OUTCOME: The patient will state pain is relieved or at an acceptable level within 30 minutes of report of pain.

- Monitor pain level using rating scale *to consistently communicate pain level.*
- Give medications ordered for pain cautiously *as they may mask symptoms of perforation.*
- Maintain NPO status *to rest the bowel and promote comfort.*
- Maintain NG tube to suction *for decompression and to relieve pain.*

Risk for Deficient Fluid Volume related to vomiting

EXPECTED OUTCOME: The patient will maintain vital signs and urine output within normal limits at all times.

- Accurately monitor vital signs and I&O and report abnormal trends *to identify fluid deficit.*
- Maintain fluid replacement as ordered *to prevent dehydration.*

Risk for Electrolyte Imbalance related to suctioning

EXPECTED OUTCOME: The patient will maintain electrolytes within normal limits at all times.

- Monitor electrolyte values *to identify imbalances.*
- Monitor vital signs and watch for signs of acid–base and electrolyte imbalances such as weakness accompanied by low potassium levels *to identify imbalances for prompt treatment.*

Evaluation

Goals are met if the patient states that pain is controlled, fluid is balanced, and electrolytes are within normal limits.

CRITICAL THINKING & CLINICAL JUDGMENT

Mrs. Loos is admitted for abdominal pain. She has a history of abdominal surgery. Her abdomen is distended, firm, and tender to touch. She states that she feels nauseous.

Critical Thinking (The Why)

1. How would you know if Mrs. Loos might be developing a small-bowel obstruction?
2. Why is she at risk for developing an obstruction?
3. If she is at risk, what data should be collected?
4. What findings would be normal?
5. How would you recognize that an obstruction is developing?

Clinical Judgment (The Do)

6. What should you do if the patient's data collection findings have changed?
7. What do you document?
8. After treatment is started, what data do you collect to know the patient is improving, getting worse, or developing complications as a result of a bowel obstruction?

Suggested answers are at the end of the chapter.

ANORECTAL PROBLEMS

Hemorrhoids

Hemorrhoids are enlarged veins within the anal tissue caused by an increase in pressure in the veins, often from increased intra-abdominal pressure. Internal hemorrhoids occur above the internal sphincter, and external hemorrhoids occur below the external sphincter. Most hemorrhoids are caused by straining during bowel movements. They are common during pregnancy. Prolonged sitting or standing, obesity, and chronic constipation also contribute to hemorrhoids. Portal hypertension related to liver disease may also be a contributing factor.

Internal hemorrhoids are usually not painful unless they prolapse. They may bleed during bowel movements. External hemorrhoids cause itching and pain when inflamed and filled with blood (thrombosed). Inflammation and edema occur with thrombosis, causing severe pain and possibly infarction of the skin and mucosa over the hemorrhoid.

Treatment is aimed at preventing constipation, avoiding straining during defecation, maintaining good personal hygiene, and making lifestyle changes to relieve hemorrhoid symptoms and discomfort. Prolonged standing and sitting are avoided. Increased fluid intake and stool softeners can be used to reduce the need for straining. Daily sitz baths increase circulation to the area and aid in comfort and healing. Astringents such as witch hazel can be used for symptom relief. Anti-inflammatory medications may be tried, such as steroid creams or suppositories. Alternating ice and heat helps relieve edema and pain for thrombosed hemorrhoids. The blood clot is removed by the HCP.

If surgery is required for internal hemorrhoids, methods include rubber-band ligation using a rubber band around the hemorrhoid that cuts off the blood supply, causing the hemorrhoid to slough off into the stool; infrared coagulation that burns off the hemorrhoid; sclerotherapy that shrinks the hemorrhoid with a chemical solution; and surgical removal (hemorrhoidectomy).

If the patient has surgery, analgesics are given as needed because the many nerve endings in the anal canal can cause severe pain. Comfort measures such as a side-lying position and fresh ice packs can be used to relieve pain. After the first postoperative day, sitz baths may be ordered. Pain is managed with NSAIDs and/or acetaminophen. Opioids are avoided due to their constipating effects. Because the first bowel movement can provoke pain and anxiety, stool softeners and analgesics are administered before the first bowel movement.

Patient education includes prevention and self-care. The patient should be instructed to consume a high-fiber diet and 2 to 3 L of fluid a day for regular bowel movements. Effects and side effects, dosage, and frequency of local or topical medications should be explained.

Anal Fissures

Anal fissures are cracks or ulcers in the lining of the anal canal. They are most commonly associated with constipation and stretching of the anus with passage of hard stool, although Crohn disease or other factors may also play a role. The patient may experience bright red bleeding. Pain may be so severe that the patient delays defecation, leading to further constipation and worsening symptoms. Treatment of anal fissures involves measures to ensure soft stools to allow fissures time to heal. Sitz baths may be used to promote circulation to the area to aid in healing. Anesthetic suppositories and nonopioid analgesics may be ordered for comfort. If conservative measures are not helpful, surgical excision of the fissure may be needed.

Anorectal Abscess

An anorectal abscess is a collection of pus in the rectal area. Symptoms include pain, redness and swelling, fever, and sometimes drainage. Abscesses are treated with antibiotics and surgical incision and drainage of pus. The area may be left open to drain, with gauze packing placed to assist with drainage and healing.

Nursing care includes dressing or packing changes as ordered. Sitz baths are used to keep the area clean and promote healing, especially after bowel movements. The patient is instructed in the importance of keeping the area clean and dry. Postoperative care is similar to care following hemorrhoidectomy.

LOWER GASTROINTESTINAL BLEEDING

Etiology
Major causes of lower GI bleeding are diverticulitis, polyps (growths in the colon), anal fissures, hemorrhoids, IBD, and cancer.

Signs and Symptoms
Bleeding from the GI tract is seen in the stool. When blood has been in the GI tract for more than 8 hours and contacts hydrochloric acid, it causes **melena**, or black and tarry stools. The presence of melena indicates bleeding above or in the small bowel. Bleeding from the colon or rectum is usually bright red (**hematochezia**).

Significant blood loss causes hypotension, lightheadedness, nausea, and diaphoresis. The patient may be pale and have cool skin. The onset of tachycardia and worsening hypotension indicate hypovolemic shock and should be reported to the HCP immediately.

Diagnostic Tests
A thorough history is necessary to determine underlying disorders that may be causing the bleeding. Decreased hemoglobin and hematocrit levels result from blood loss. Stool can be tested for occult blood if it is not evident on inspection. Digital examination, CT angiography, colonoscopy, or sigmoidoscopy may be done to determine the cause of the bleeding.

Therapeutic Measures
Treatment involves correction of the cause of the bleeding. Surgery to correct diverticulosis, correct IBD, or resect cancer may be considered.

Nursing Care
Stools are checked for the presence and amount of blood. Vital signs are monitored for signs of shock. Decreasing blood pressure and rising heart rate are reported to the HCP immediately. The patient is prepared for diagnostic tests, and nursing care for the underlying disorder is provided.

> **BE SAFE!**
> **TAKE ACTION!** Many GI problems can present with bleeding. Monitor vital signs, provide fall precautions, and promptly notify the HCP for any bleeding or change in vital signs.

• WORD • BUILDING •

hematochezia: hemat—blood + chezia—in stool

COLORECTAL CANCER

Pathophysiology and Etiology

Colorectal cancer is one of the most common types of internal cancer in the United States. It originates in the epithelial lining of the colon or rectum and can occur anywhere in the large intestine. People with a personal or family history of ulcerative colitis, colon cancer, or polyps of the rectum or large intestine are at higher risk for developing cancer. Colorectal cancer has also been linked with previous gallbladder removal and dietary carcinogens. A major causative factor is lack of fiber in the diet, which prolongs fecal transit time and exposure to possible carcinogens. Also, bacterial flora is believed to be altered by excess fat, which converts steroids into compounds having carcinogenic properties. Lifestyle factors such as obesity, smoking, alcohol intake, and excessive red meat in the diet increase colon cancer risk. Healthy People 2030 has a target to reduce the incidence of colorectal cancer deaths per 100,000 population from 13.4 (as of 2018) to 8.9 in 2030 (Office of Disease Prevention and Health Promotion, 2021a).

Signs and Symptoms

Manifestations of colorectal cancer vary according to the type of tumor and the location. A change in bowel habits is the most common symptom (Table 34.8). Blood or mucus in stools may occur. All tumors cause varying degrees of obstruction. Tumors in the descending colon and rectum generally do not cause nausea or vomiting, anemia, or weight loss.

Diagnostic Tests

Screening for colorectal cancer in those older than age 45 at average risk is the best prevention. Screening guidelines can be found in Chapter 11 or at the American Cancer Society web site.

Home screening for blood in the stool can be done with a home colon cancer test kit. Immunological tests look for small amounts of blood. If blood is found, an HCP is contacted for follow-up. Most colorectal cancers are identified by biopsy done at the time of endoscopy (sigmoidoscopy or colonoscopy). New colonoscopies can use a computer-aided polyp detection system with better cancer detection rates. A colonography is a CT scan that can perform a virtual colonoscopy to view the inside of the colon. A double-barium enema is another option for screening. The carcinoembryonic antigen (CEA) blood test is used to assess response to treatment of GI cancer. CEA is present when epithelial cells rapidly divide and provides an early warning that the cancer has returned.

Therapeutic Measures

Small, localized tumors may be excised and treated during endoscopy or laparoscopy. These procedures can also be used as palliative care for patients with advanced tumors who cannot tolerate major surgery. If a tumor is causing obstruction, a stent can be placed to keep the colon open for bowel function until surgery.

Surgery is performed either to resect larger tumors and anastomose the remaining bowel or to create a fecal diversion by forming an ostomy. A variety of surgical procedures can be done depending on the location and extent of the cancer (Table 34.9 and Fig. 34.7). Medical management can include radiation therapy, chemotherapy, and monoclonal antibody therapy. When used along with surgery, increased survival rates have been demonstrated.

Monoclonal antibody therapy uses antibodies made in a laboratory that work like normal antibodies do for advanced colon cancer. They can enhance immune system function, interfere with the cancer cell's growth, or even carry treatment such as medications or radiation to cancer cells. The antibody is designed to attach to cancer cells to flag them for the immune system so they can be destroyed. Bevacizumab (Avastin) blocks the making of new blood vessels to deprive cancer cells of nourishment. Cetuximab (Erbitux) and panitumumab (Vectibix) block the cell's growth signal to stop it from growing. Additional medications used with metastatic disease are regorafenib (Stivarga), ramucirumab (Cyramza), and ziv-aflibercept (Zaltrap).

Complications

Possible complications include bleeding, complete obstruction of the colon, perforation, anastomosis leaking leading to peritonitis, and extension of the tumor to adjacent organs. Colorectal cancer can metastasize to the lymphatic system,

Table 34.8
Colon Cancer Summary

Signs and Symptoms	Change in bowel habits Blood or mucus in stools
Diagnostic Tests	Colonoscopy with biopsy and/or computer-aided polyp detection system Sigmoidoscopy with biopsy Proctosigmoidoscopy CT and MRI Barium enema Abdominal and rectal examination Fecal occult blood
Therapeutic Measures	Surgery, possibly colostomy Radiation Chemotherapy and/or radiation Medications (analgesics) Parenteral nutrition (PN) as needed Support and education
Priority Nursing Diagnoses	Acute Pain Fear Imbalanced Nutrition: Less Than Body Requirements

Table 34.9
Intestinal Surgeries

Types of Intestinal Surgery	Definition	Effect on Stool Elimination
Colectomy	Affected part of colon and nearby lymph nodes removed with laparoscope through smaller incisions.	Anastomosed ends. Stool is passed via rectum and anus.
Open colectomy	Affected part of colon and nearby lymph nodes removed through traditional incision.	Anastomosed ends. Stool is passed via rectum and anus.
Ileocolectomy	Right side of colon and diseased portion of ileum removed.	Anastomosed ends. Stool is passed via rectum and anus.
Hemicolectomy	Right or left side of colon removed.	Right: Colon attached to small intestine. Left: Anastomosed ends. Stool is passed via rectum and anus.
Total colectomy	Entire colon removed; rectum and anus remain.	Ileorectal anastomosis. Stool is passed via rectum and anus.
Total proctocolectomy	Entire colon, rectum, and sometimes anus removed.	Ileostomy. If anus left, ileal pouch-anal anastomosis and stool is passed via anus.
Rectal Cancer		
Local transanal resection: Cancer in lower area of rectum Transanal endoscopic microsurgery: Cancer higher in rectum	No incision. Rectal cancer removed through anus.	Anastomosed ends. Stool is passed via anus.
Lower anterior resection: Cancer in upper two-thirds of rectum	Affected part of colon and nearby lymph nodes removed through traditional incision.	Anastomosed ends. Stool is passed via rectum and anus.
Abdominoperineal resection: Cancer in lower one-third of rectum	Sigmoid colon, rectum, and anus removed.	Colostomy ends. Stool passed via ostomy.
Proctectomy: Cancer in lower two-thirds of rectum	All or part of rectum removed.	Coloanal anastomosis. Stool passed via anus.

lungs, peritoneum, and liver. Depending on the complication and the condition of the patient, the patient may need to wait for surgery or further treatment. See previous sections for GI bleeding and lower bowel obstruction. If perforation or anastomosis is suspected, the patient may need high-dose antibiotic therapy, ongoing laboratory monitoring, and special needs at home.

Nursing Process for the Patient With Colorectal Cancer

Data Collection

Risk factors for colorectal cancer are identified by asking questions about the patient's personal and family histories: Is there a history of IBD? What are the patient's dietary habits? What foods are usually eaten, and how much fluid is usually consumed? Prior to diagnosis, did the patient experience constipation or diarrhea? Has there been a change in bowel habits? Has mucus or blood been noted in the stools? Is there pain? Does the patient smoke, drink alcoholic beverages, exercise? Has there been a recent weight loss? If so, how much and over what period of time? Does the patient have unusual fatigue or insomnia? Stool is checked for mucus or blood.

If the patient has surgery, postoperative monitoring includes vital signs, pain, and the return of flatus and bowel movements. Lung sounds are monitored for response to coughing and deep

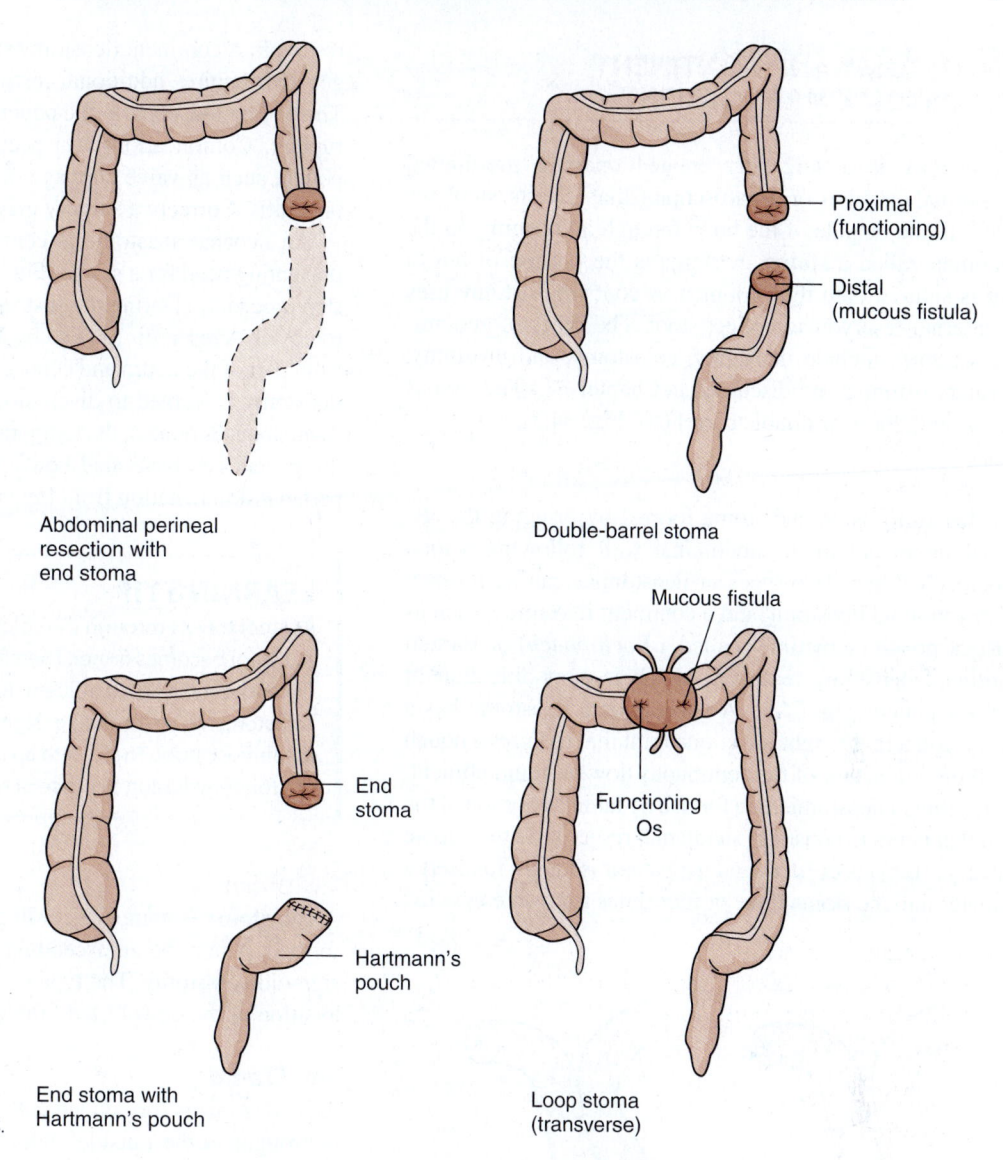

FIGURE 34.7 Types of stomas.

breathing and early ambulation. Dressings are observed for drainage. Large amounts of drainage or bleeding are reported. If a drain is inserted in the perineal wound, moderate amounts of serosanguineous (light pink) drainage are expected. If the patient has an ostomy, it is monitored (see the ostomy section later in the chapter).

Nursing Diagnoses, Planning, and Implementation

Fear related to serious threat to well-being

EXPECTED OUTCOME: The patient will state fear is reduced after information is given related to patient's condition.

- Assist patient in identifying fears *to develop plan for reducing fears.*
- Set aside time to allow the patient who so desires to talk, cry, or ask questions about the diagnosis and planned surgery *to help reduce fear.*
- Answer questions accurately *to provide a trusting relationship.*

Imbalanced Nutrition: Less Than Body Requirements related to nausea and anorexia

EXPECTED OUTCOME: The patient will maintain normal weight for height and age.

- Give antiemetics as ordered *to relieve nausea.*
- Identify foods the patient likes and provide them *to stimulate appetite.*
- Monitor PN as ordered *to provide nutrients.*
- Provide the patient with a high-protein, high-calorie diet, as ordered, that is low in residue *to decrease excessive peristalsis and minimize cramping.*

Evaluation

Expected outcomes are that the patient verbalizes less fear and attains optimum level of nutrition.

OSTOMY AND CONTINENT OSTOMY MANAGEMENT

An ostomy is a surgically created opening (traditional abdominal incision or laparoscopic) that diverts stool (or urine) to the outside of the body through an opening on the abdomen called a **stoma**. A stoma is the portion of bowel that is sutured onto the abdomen. A continent ostomy uses an internal reservoir to collect stool. The types of abdominal ostomies include ileostomy, colostomy, and urostomy. (Urinary ostomies are discussed in Chapter 37.) The stomas can be end, loop, or double barrel (see Fig. 34.7).

Ileostomy

An **ileostomy** is an end stoma formed by bringing the terminal ileum out to the abdominal wall following a total proctocolectomy. Two types of ileostomies can be formed: a conventional ileostomy and a continent ileostomy, such as a Kock pouch (sometimes called a *Koch pouch*) or Barnett continent ileostomy reservoir, which is a modification of a Kock pouch (Fig. 34.8). A conventional ileostomy has a small stoma in the right lower quadrant that requires a pouch at all times because of the continuous flow of liquid effluent.

Continent ileostomies are formed by taking a portion of the terminal ileum to construct an internal reservoir with a nipple valve. A stoma is created, and the patient is taught to insert a catheter into the stoma three or four times a day to empty the reservoir. A continent ileostomy surgical procedure takes longer and requires additional instruction for patient self-care. The patient must empty the pouch routinely to prevent pouch rupture. Complications can occur, especially for the Kock pouch, such as valve slippage or leaking, pouch rupture, or pouchitis. Corrective surgery may be required.

An ileoanal anastomosis connects the ileum to the anus, preventing need for a stoma (Fig. 34.9). This is usually a two-step procedure. During the first surgery, the diseased bowel is removed. A reservoir (named by its shape, J pouch) is formed from part of the ileum and connected to the anus. A temporary ileostomy is formed to divert stool while the reservoir heals. After about 3 months, the temporary ileostomy is reversed and the patient can have anal bowel movements. Problems with perianal skin irritation from frequent liquid stools may occur.

> **LEARNING TIP**
> As stool travels through the colon, water is absorbed and the stool becomes firmer. Therefore, an ileostomy produces the most liquid effluent, followed by an ascending colostomy. A descending or sigmoid colostomy produces the firmest stool. Those with an ileostomy are at increased risk for dehydration because of greater water loss.

Colostomy

A **colostomy** is named according to where in the bowel it is formed; it may be an ascending, transverse, descending, or sigmoid colostomy. The type of effluent is dependent on the location of the bowel used (Table 34.10).

End Stoma

An end stoma is formed when the proximal end of the bowel is brought to the outside abdominal wall. If an abdominoperineal (AP) resection is done, the rectum is removed and the proximal sigmoid or descending colon is brought out as a stoma. Another procedure involves removing the segment of diseased or injured bowel and using the proximal portion to form the stoma. The remaining limb of bowel is sutured closed and left in the peritoneal cavity so that the rectum is intact. This is called a *Hartmann pouch*, or *mucous fistula*, and may be permanent or temporary depending on the diagnosis. Because the rectum is intact, the patient may feel the urge to defecate. This is normal because the colon continues to produce mucus, fills with mucus, and alerts the patient as though stool were present.

Loop Stoma

To create a loop stoma, a loop of bowel, usually the transverse colon, is pulled to the outside abdominal wall and a

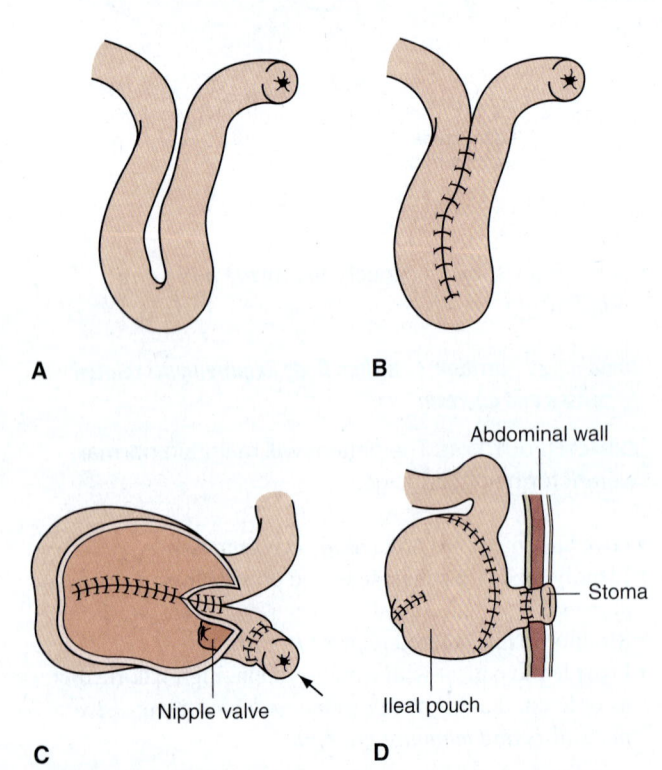

FIGURE 34.8 Surgical formation of continent ileostomy (Kock pouch). (A) Loop of terminal ileum. (B) Both limbs of ileum are brought together and sutured into a U shape. (C) Pouch created with nipple valve. (D) Pouch sutured to abdominal wall.

• WORD • BUILDING •
ileostomy: ileo—pertaining to ileum + stoma—mouth or opening
colostomy: colo—pertaining to colon + stoma—mouth or opening

bridge slipped under the loop to hold it in place. An incisional slit is made in the top of the exposed colon to allow stool to exit. The entire loop of bowel is not cut through.

Double-Barrel Stoma
With a double-barrel stoma, the bowel is completely dissected. Both ends of the colon are brought to the outside abdominal wall to form two separate stomas. The proximal stoma is the functioning stoma that expels stool. The distal stoma is called a mucous fistula because mucus produced by the bowel passes from it. A double-barrel stoma is often temporary, allowing the bowel to rest during healing after trauma or surgery.

Preoperative Care
A wound, ostomy, and continence nurse (WOCN) should be consulted before surgery. The WOCN can help prepare the patient both emotionally and physically for the surgery. The site for the stoma can then be chosen so it is visible to the patient for self-care, avoids skin or fat folds, and will not interfere with clothing. Properly planned stoma placement can prevent discomfort when sitting, inability to perform self-care, and uncomfortable, leaking, or poorly fitting appliances postoperatively. The WOCN has expertise in selecting the stoma site for the surgeon to ensure that it is easy to sit with it, care for it, and wear clothing over it. This involves observing the abdomen as the patient assumes various positions.

Routine preoperative instruction, including the importance of coughing and deep breathing, splinting, and early ambulation, is provided. Orders for cleansing of the bowel are performed to reduce the risk for infection following surgery. Unless the patient has chronic diarrhea related to IBD, an oral agent to cleanse the bowel is given.

> **LEARNING TIP**
> LPN/LVNs can obtain Wound Treatment Associate–Certified (WTA-C) through the Wound, Ostomy, and Continence Nursing Certification Board.

> **PRACTICE ANALYSIS TIP**
> **Linking NCLEX-PN® to Practice**
> The LPN/LVN will provide care to client with an ostomy (e.g., colostomy or ileostomy).

Nursing Process for the Patient With a New or Established Ostomy or Continent Ostomy
Data Collection
For a patient with a new ostomy, in addition to routine postoperative assessment, a stoma should be inspected at least every 4 hours for the first 24 hours, and then every 8 hours. The stoma should be pink to red, moist (similar to the inside of the mouth), and well-attached to the surrounding skin (Fig. 34.10). A bluish stoma indicates inadequate blood supply; a black stoma indicates necrosis. Either complication should be reported to the HCP immediately for treatment, which may require another surgery. Note edema of the stoma. The stoma size will gradually decrease over the first few weeks following surgery.

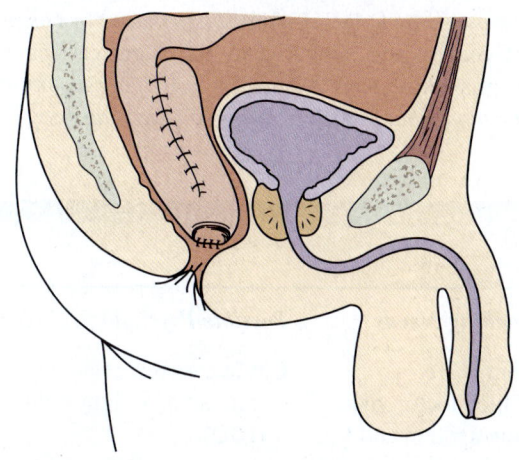

FIGURE 34.9 Ileal J pouch-anal anastomosis. The two-loop ileal pouch is simple to construct, provides adequate storage capacity, and is evacuated spontaneously and fully.

Table 34.10
Location of Stomas and Type of Effluent

Location of Stoma	Type of Effluent
Ileostomy	Liquid to mushy
Cecostomy, ascending colostomy	Liquid to mushy, foul odor
Right transverse colostomy	Mushy to semiformed
Left transverse colostomy	Semiformed, soft
Descending or sigmoid colostomy	Soft to hard formed

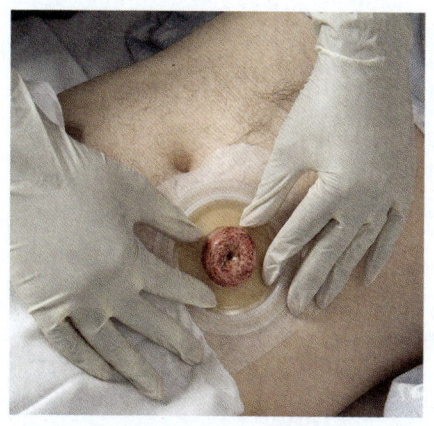

FIGURE 34.10 Normal stoma: note the moist pink to red appearance of the stoma.

For both new and established ostomies, skin is assessed for irritation around the pouch and under the pouch each time it is changed. Ostomy discharge (effluent) is monitored and documented. Unexpected changes, such as liquid stool from a descending ostomy, are reported. For the patient with a continent ostomy pouch, monitoring for regular emptying of the pouch is important to prevent rupture and leakage. The characteristics of the stool are noted for any type of continent ostomy so that problems can be reported.

Nursing Diagnoses, Planning, and Implementation
See Table 34.11.

Deficient Knowledge related to ostomy

EXPECTED OUTCOME: The patient will demonstrate how to care for ostomy.

- Determine patient readiness and ability to learn and perform self-care. *The patient experiencing pain, nausea, or vomiting is not likely to be ready to look at the ostomy or learn about ostomy care.*
- Include the caregiver in teaching if the patient is not ready or able to learn. *Short hospital stays limit teaching time and should begin soon after surgery.*
- Consult a WOCN or ostomy equipment supplier if needed *to identify appliances suited to individual patient's needs.*
- Ensure referral to a home health nurse is made *to continue teaching in the patient's home.*
- Provide special instructions or a specific type of ostomy appliance for patients with special needs, such as blindness, deafness, language barrier, severe arthritis, or other physical conditions that limit ability to perform self-care, *so they will be able to perform self-care.*
- Reinforce teaching and have patient demonstrate changing appliance *to promote self-care.*
- Reinforce teaching about diet considerations (see "Nutrition Notes: Dietary Management of Ostomies") *to help with management of ostomy.*

Disturbed Body Image related to new ostomy

EXPECTED OUTCOME: The patient will verbalize acceptance of intestinal ostomy before discharge.

- Identify knowledge of self-care of ostomies and feelings about the stoma. *Identification of misconceptions and "hearsay" knowledge is important to clarify or correct.*
- Reinforce teaching about the normal characteristics of the stoma before patient's first look. *Helping the patient understand what to expect will help relieve anxiety.*

Table 34.11
Summary of Recovery from Intestinal Surgery

Intestinal Surgery	Elimination Needs	Discharge Teaching Needs	Possible Psychological Needs
Total colectomy	Normal or continent anal passage	Continent ostomy care. Soft diet until first doctor visit. Monitor for constipation and report.	Chronic sorrow related to inflammatory bowel disease (IBD)
Hemicolectomy (right or left) or ileocolectomy	Normal, no appliance needed	Avoid stress to abdomen: heavy lifting, sit-ups. Soft diet until first doctor visit. Monitor for constipation and report.	Fear of cancer Chronic sorrow related to IBD
Partial colectomy	Normal, no appliance needed	Monitor for constipation.	Fear of cancer
Abdominoperineal resection	Pouch	Ostomy care.	Fear of cancer Body image changes
Proctosigmoidectomy	Normal, no appliance needed	Soft diet until first doctor visit. Monitor for constipation and report.	Fear of cancer
Total proctocolectomy	Continent anal passage or pouch	Continent ostomy care. Soft diet until first doctor visit. Monitor for constipation and report.	Chronic sorrow related to IBD

Readiness for Enhanced Health Self-management related to difficulty carrying out self-care measures

EXPECTED OUTCOME: The patient will demonstrate ability to perform self-care measures.

- Identify financial ability *to obtain supplies.* Most insurers, including Medicare, pay for ostomy supplies, although some limit the type of appliance and number allowed per month. Each state-funded Medicaid system is different. The type of appliance needed to eliminate leakage may not always be covered, requiring the patient either to pay the difference or wear what the insurance company will provide. If the patient has no insurance, costs can be high. Fortunately, the pouches in most two-piece systems can be washed out and reused to save money (see "Home Health Hints").
- Provide referral to case manager or social worker for financial resources *in order to obtain ostomy supplies.*

Nutrition Notes
Dietary Management of Ostomies
Ostomy patients receive a soft diet initially, progressing to a general diet as the health-care provider prescribes and is tolerated. Stringy, high-fiber foods are initially avoided. Then, they are best tried in small amounts, one at a time, until tolerance has been demonstrated. They include the following:

- Cabbage (including coleslaw and sauerkraut), corn, peas, and spinach
- Coconut, dried fruit, pineapple, and membranes on citrus fruits
- Popcorn, nuts, seeds, and skins of fruits and vegetables

Legumes, cruciferous vegetables (broccoli, brussels sprouts), eggs, fish, beer, and carbonated beverages produce excessive flatus and subsequent odor.

Low-fiber foods may be more easily tolerated:

- Applesauce and bananas
- Cheese
- Creamy peanut butter
- Pasta, white bread, and white rice

Patients with ostomies should be encouraged to:

- Drink adequate amounts of fluid.
- Eat at regular intervals.
- Chew food completely to avoid blockage of the stoma.
- Avoid foods that produce excessive gas, loose stools, offensive odors, and undesirable bulk.

Sexual Dysfunction related to body image change or erectile dysfunction

EXPECTED OUTCOME: The patient will discuss satisfying acceptable sexual practices for self and partner.

Home Health Hints
- Some ostomy supplies may be covered by insurance. Record product numbers for ease of reordering. Most companies will deliver supplies to the patient's home.
- If the patient requires a stool for occult blood test, deliver a collection device (hat) to assist with obtaining the specimen before your visit. Plan to deliver the specimen to the laboratory the day it is collected.
- Reinforce teaching patients to have supplies to change their ostomy appliance, a small plastic trash bag, and a small can of air freshener in a purse or backpack when they go out. Some patients feel more confident if they carry a change of clothes with them in their trunk.

- Ensure referral to a urologist is made if a male patient who had a low anterior resection is experiencing erectile dysfunction. *This impotence may be transient, depending on the severity of nerve damage or edema associated with the surgery.*
- Encourage the patient to discuss concerns regarding sexuality with his or her sexual partner. *Open communication may help them work through any fears or embarrassment.*
- Encourage personal hygiene, use of a pouch cover and emptying of the ostomy pouch before sexual encounters *to decrease odors, disguise pouch, and enhance experience.*

Risk for Injury related to skin and stomal complications

EXPECTED OUTCOME: The patient will remain free from injury with intact skin; red, moist stoma; and functioning ostomy.

- Identify allergies *to prevent allergic dermatitis from sensitivity to the adhesive from developing.*
- Use a protective skin paste *to prevent skin breakdown from leakage.*
- Remove tape and adhesive only when necessary, and leave pouches on for several days unless leakage occurs, *to prevent skin shearing from frequent removal.*
- Monitor for **peristomal** hernia or stomal prolapse *to detect hernias that may develop around the stoma or the stoma falling down (or out) as a result of weakened abdominal muscles and cause leakage by the change in body contours associated with the hernia.*
- Monitor stoma color and immediately report dusky or blue color, *which occurs when there is circulatory compromise.*

• WORD • BUILDING •
peristomal: peri—surrounding + stoma—mouth or opening

- Reinforce teaching the signs and symptoms of an ileostomy blockage (e.g., absent stool, abdominal cramping, edematous stoma, and stoma color that is pale or dusky) and seek medical treatment if it is not relieved *to allow it to be treated*.

Evaluation
The plan of care has been effective if the patient is able to accept the change in body image, competently care for the ostomy (or caregiver does so), carry out self-care, is satisfied with sexual practices, and describes self-care measures to prevent injury or treat complications.

> **CUE RECOGNITION 34.2**
>
> A patient with an ostomy reports itchiness around the stoma. What action do you take?
>
> Suggested answers are at the end of the chapter.

Rehabilitative Needs
Ensuring that the patient is becoming comfortable with self-care, is able to perform the ostomy appliance change, and is able to return to work or social activities as before are the goals of care. The patient can generally perform any activity they were able to do before the ostomy, including swimming.

Key Points

- Constipation occurs when the fecal mass is held in the rectal cavity for a period of time that is unusual for the patient or bowel movements occur less than three times per week. Fecal impaction may result when the fecal mass is so dry it cannot be passed. Treatment of constipation includes increased fiber intake, physical activity, exercises to strengthen abdominal muscles performed, stool softeners, laxatives, suppositories, and enemas.
- Diarrhea (three or more loose or watery stools in 24 hours) occurs when fecal matter passes through the intestine rapidly, resulting in decreased absorption of water, electrolytes, and nutrients, and causing frequent, watery stools. The most common cause of acute diarrhea is infection from contaminated food or water. Most people with diarrhea do not require treatment. Replacing fluids and electrolytes may be necessary for dehydration, especially in the very young or very old.
- Appendicitis is the inflammation of the appendix, the small, fingerlike appendage attached to the cecum of the large intestine.
- When trauma, ischemia, or perforation in an abdominal organ causes leakage of the organ's contents into the peritoneal cavity, inflammation, infection, and peritonitis result. This can be life-threatening.
- A diverticulum (singular) is a small outpouching of the bowel mucous membrane through areas of weakness in the wall of the colon. Diverticulosis is when multiple diverticula (plural) are present. If stool becomes trapped in a diverticulum, inflammation and infection can develop. This is called *diverticulitis*.
- Crohn disease is an autoimmune IBD that can involve any part of the GI tract. The inflammation extends through the intestinal mucosa. This leads to the formation of abscesses, fistulas, and fissures.
- Ulcerative colitis is similar to Crohn disease. Ulcerative colitis occurs in the large intestine and rectum.
- IBS is characterized by abdominal pain and altered bowel habits.
- A hernia is an abnormal protrusion of an organ or structure through a weakness or tear in the wall of the cavity normally containing it. Surgical repair may be needed to reduce a hernia.
- Malabsorption occurs when the GI system is unable to absorb one or more of the major nutrients. Some causes of malabsorption are celiac disease, lactose intolerance, ileal dysfunction, jejunal diverticula, parasitic disease, enzyme deficiency, and IBD such as Crohn disease and ulcerative colitis.
- Intestinal obstructions occur when the flow of intestinal contents is blocked. The two types of intestinal obstruction are mechanical and nonmechanical, both of which can be either partial or complete.
- Hemorrhoids are enlarged veins within the anal tissue. They are caused by an increase in pressure in the veins, often from increased intra-abdominal pressure.
- Anal fissures are cracks or ulcers in the lining of the anal canal. They are most commonly associated with constipation and stretching of the anus with passage of hard stool, although Crohn disease or other factors may also play a role.
- An anorectal abscess is a collection of pus in the rectal area.
- Major causes of lower GI bleeding are diverticulitis, polyps (growths in the colon), anal fissures, hemorrhoids, IBD, and cancer.
- Colorectal cancer is one of the most common types of internal cancer in the United States; a change in bowel pattern is the most common sign. People with a personal or family history of ulcerative colitis, colon cancer, or polyps of the rectum or large intestine are at higher risk for developing cancer.
- An ileostomy is an end stoma formed by bringing the terminal ileum out to the abdominal wall following a total proctocolectomy. Two types of ileostomies can be formed: a conventional ileostomy and a continent ileostomy.
- A colostomy is named according to where in the bowel it is formed; it may be an ascending, transverse, descending, or sigmoid colostomy. The type of effluent is dependent on the location of the bowel used.

SUGGESTED ANSWERS TO CHAPTER EXERCISES

Cue Recognition

34.1: You gather more data, including whether she had a bowel movement and it was inadvertently not charted; ask Mrs. Lopez if she feels constipated or has abdominal pain; and note any distention and presence or absence of bowel sounds. A digital examination may be necessary to determine if fecal impaction is present. (LVN/LPNs should check facility policies and state laws to determine if digital examination and impaction removal are allowed.) If simple constipation appears to be the problem, the medical record should be checked for as-needed laxative or enema orders. If there are no orders, contact the HCP.

34.2: Change the ostomy bag immediately to observe the skin and prevent skin breakdown from leaking stool. Itching is an indicator of leaking stool or skin irritation.

Critical Thinking & Clinical Judgment

June Moore

1. Ask about characteristics of pain (e.g., location, quality, intensity, precipitating factors, relieving factors), characteristics of bowel elimination (frequency, characteristic of stool, amount, color, consistency), nutritional status (weight loss, appetite, daily food intake, food likes/dislikes, irritating foods, fluid intake), and anxiety and coping skills (support systems, usual coping methods).
2. Appropriate nursing diagnoses include *Acute Pain* related to increased peristalsis and cramping; *Diarrhea* related to inflammatory process; *Risk for Deficient Fluid Volume* related to diarrhea and insufficient fluid intake; *Anxiety* related to symptoms and frequency of stools and treatment; *Impaired Skin Integrity* related to frequent loose stools; *Imbalanced Nutrition: Less Than Body Requirements* related to malabsorption; *Deficit Knowledge* related to new diagnosis of Crohn disease; and *Ineffective Coping* related to frequency of stools.
3. Further explore how Judy perceives that Crohn disease will affect her lifestyle. What does she know about Crohn disease? What is she concerned about? How has Crohn disease affected her ability to sleep, what she eats, her participation in sports, and her relationships with other people? Consider accommodations for classes, testing, transportation, and living arrangements. Reinforce teaching about medications. Convey a caring attitude to Judy by being accepting of her, listening actively to her concerns, and helping her to find acceptable ways to resolve them. Provide her with information that she needs about Crohn disease. Arrange to have a Crohn's & Colitis Foundation representative who has adapted well to an ostomy and who is approximately Judy's age meet with her to share coping strategies.
4. Increased frequency of stools leading to fluid volume deficit and possibly shock symptoms; bleeding leading to anemia and hypovolemia and possibly shock symptoms.
5. HCP, dietitian, psychologist, registered nurse.

Mrs. Loos

1. The first consideration is to be aware of whether the patient is at risk for a small-bowel obstruction. After abdominal surgery, loops of intestine may adhere to areas in the abdomen that are not healed, causing a kink in the bowel that occludes the intestinal flow.
2. Due to her history of abdominal surgery, she is at risk of adhesion development that can cause obstruction. If data collection findings confirm this possibility, the HCP should be contacted. Because of the nausea and the potential obstruction, withhold food and oral fluids until the HCP is consulted.
3. Begin by asking the **WHAT'S UP?** questions, including exactly where the pain is occurring, how it feels, whether there is anything that aggravates or alleviates the pain, when it started, how bad it is on a scale of 0 to 10, whether there are associated symptoms, and whether Mrs. Loos has some insight regarding the cause of her problem. Then, in this order, inspect, auscultate, and palpate; doing the examination in this order prevents palpation from changing other assessment findings. Inspect her abdomen to note distention. Listen for bowel sounds in each quadrant. Lightly palpate her abdomen, noting tenderness or rigidity. Ask when her last bowel movement was.
4. Bowel sounds normal in all quadrants, abdomen flat, soft with no tenderness, flatus present.
5. Abnormal bowel sounds, absent for a nonmechanical obstruction or a mechanical obstruction; high-pitched, tinkling bowel sounds proximal to the obstruction and absent distal to it; pain; abdominal distention.
6. Discuss findings with the registered nurse or HCP. New orders such as a nasogastric tube, NPO status, and pain management should be anticipated.
7. When documenting, answer what, why, when, where, how, and who (either explicitly or implicitly by professional knowledge, in narrative or flow sheet format) for completeness:

    What = Patient is experiencing large, firm, tender-to-touch abdomen with nausea (additional assessment data should be included).
    Why = Unknown, HCP notified
    When = Current date and time
    Where = Abdomen
    How = Unknown
    Who = S. Snyder, LPN

8. If improving, symptoms will be resolving: no nausea, abdomen soft, bowel sounds present in all quadrants, flatus present, and bowel movements normal. If condition is worsening or complications developing, symptoms will not improve. Fecal vomiting and shock may occur.

Additional Resources

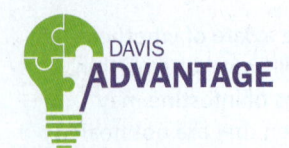

Go to Davis Advantage to complete your learning: strengthen understanding, apply your knowledge, and prepare for the Next Gen NCLEX®.

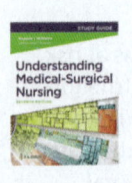

A Study Guide is also available.

CHAPTER 35
Nursing Care of Patients With Liver, Pancreatic, and Gallbladder Disorders

Lisa Price

KEY TERMS

ascites (ah-SY-teez)
asterixis (AS-tur-IK-sis)
cholecystitis (KOH-lee-sis-TY-tis)
choledocholithiasis (koh-LED-oh-koh-lih-THIGH-ah-sis)
cholelithiasis (KOH-lee-lih-THIGH-ah-sis)
cholecystolithiasis (KOH-lee-sis-to-lih-THIGH-ah-sis)
cirrhosis (sih-ROH-sis)
colic (KAW-lick)
fetor hepaticus (FEE-tur heh-PAT-tih-kus)
hepatic encephalopathy (heh-PAT-ik en-SEF-uh-LAH-pah-thee)
hepatitis (HEP-uh-TY-tis)
hepatorenal syndrome (heh-PAT-oh-REE-nuhl SIN-drohm)
laparoscopy (LAP-uh-ROS-kuh-pee)
pancreatectomy (PAN-kree-uh-TEK-tuh-mee)
pancreatitis (PAN-cree-uh-TY-tis)
portal hypertension (POR-tuhl HY-per-TEN-shun)
transjugular intrahepatic portosystemic shunt (TRANZ-jug-yoo-lur in-trah-heh-PAT-tik por-toe-sis-TEM-ik SHUNT)
varices (VAR-i-seez)

CHAPTER CONCEPTS

Cognition
Infection
Inflammation
Nutrition

LEARNING OUTCOMES

1. Explain the causes, risk factors, and pathophysiology of the various types of liver disease.
2. Describe therapeutic measures used for patients with liver disease.
3. Assist with planning nursing care for the patient experiencing a liver disorder.
4. Explain the causes, risk factors, and pathophysiology of the various pancreatic disorders.
5. Describe therapeutic measures used for patients with pancreatic disorders.
6. Assist with planning nursing care for a patient with a pancreatic disorder.
7. Explain the causes, risk factors, and pathophysiology of gallbladder disorders.
8. Describe therapeutic measures used for patients with gallbladder disorders.
9. Assist with planning nursing care for the patient with a gallbladder disorder.

DISORDERS OF THE LIVER

Hepatitis

Hepatitis is inflammation of the liver resulting from viral or bacterial infection; medications, alcohol, or chemicals toxic to the liver; and metabolic or vascular disorders. Symptoms of hepatitis range from no symptoms to life-threatening symptoms due to death of liver tissue. Viral hepatitis, which is common, is discussed here.

Pathophysiology and Etiology
Viral hepatitis is caused by one of five viruses:

- Hepatitis A virus (HAV)
- Hepatitis B virus (HBV)
- Hepatitis C virus (HCV)
- Hepatitis D virus (HDV)
- Hepatitis E virus (HEV)

The viral agents vary by mode of transmission, incubation period, symptoms, diagnostic tests, vaccines, and postexposure prophylaxis (Table 35.1). The infecting organism causes inflammation of the liver,

• WORD • BUILDING •
hepatitis: hepat—liver + itis—inflammation

Table 35.1
Viral Hepatitis Infections

	Hepatitis A (HAV)	Hepatitis B (HBV)	Hepatitis C (HCV)	Hepatitis D (HDV)	Hepatitis E (HEV)
Mode of transmission	Fecal–oral route: Fecal contact; fecal-contaminated food, water, or raw shellfish from poor hand hygiene by infected person or inadequate sanitation.	Blood or body fluids such as saliva, semen, menstrual or vaginal fluid; equipment contaminated by infected blood.	Blood or body fluids that contain blood: IV drug use is the most common. Birth from an HCV-infected mother. Rarer: Unprotected sex.	Blood or body fluids. Co-infection with HBV required for HDV replication.	Water contaminated with human feces or raw or undercooked pork, wild boar, or venison.
Incubation period	15–50 days[1]	60–150 days[2]	2 weeks to 6 months	3–7 weeks	15–60 days
Signs/symptoms, if they occur	Prodromal: Anorexia, fatigue, malaise, nausea, vomiting. Icteric: Jaundice, pale stools, pruritus, dark urine, RUQ pain.	Most asymptomatic. Prodromal: 1–2 months of fatigue, malaise, anorexia, fever, nausea, headache, RUQ pain, myalgia. Icteric: Jaundice, rashes.	Many asymptomatic. Same as HBV, but usually less severe.	Most asymptomatic. Same as HBV with coinfection but more severe.	Prodromal: anorexia, dehydration, myalgia, nausea, RUQ pain, vomiting, fever. Icteric: Jaundice, pale stools, pruritus, dark urine.
Diagnostic tests	**Anti-HAV IgM** Acute infection. **Anti-HAV IgG** Recovery and immunity to virus.	**HBsAg** Surface antigen of virus. Appears 1–10 weeks postexposure. Disappears 4–6 months after recovery. Continued presence indicates chronic infection. **Anti-HBs IgM** Antibody to surface antigen that attacks HBV. Provides immunity to HBV. **Anti-HBc IgM** Antibody to core antigen.	**Anti-HCV** Antibody to virus made after exposure/infection at unknown time. Does not provide future immunity. **HCV-RNA** Presence of replicating virus indicates current infection; done when antibody test positive. **HCV Viral Load** Monitors amount of viral RNA present at diagnosis and during treatment. **HCV genotype (1–6)** Identifies virus strain to guide treatment.	**HDV-RNA** Presence of replicating virus. **HDAg** Acute infection.	**Anti-HEV** Acute infection.

Table 35.1
Viral Hepatitis Infections—cont'd

	Hepatitis A (HAV)	Hepatitis B (HBV)	Hepatitis C (HCV)	Hepatitis D (HDV)	Hepatitis E (HEV)
		Present during acute illness and up to 6 months after recovery. **HBeAg** High HBV replication. **Anti-HBe** Slowed viral replication. Lower infectivity.			
Vaccines	Hepatitis A vaccine.	Hepatitis B vaccine.	None (due to the virus's rapid mutation rate).	Hepatitis B vaccine conveys protection if not already HBV infected.	Hepatitis E vaccine currently available in China only.
Postexposure prophylaxis (when not already immune from vaccination)	Within 2 weeks after exposure: 12 months to 40 years, hepatitis A vaccine; over 40 years or immunocompromised or with chronic liver disease, IG.[1]	Hepatitis B IG (HBIG) as soon as possible after exposure, preferably within 24 hours, and vaccination.[2]	None, due to the low risk of transmission. Follow-up with testing for HCV infection at 3–6 weeks and 4–6 months postexposure.[3]	Prevented with hepatitis B prophylaxis.	None available in United States.
High-risk groups/ activities	Travelers without vaccination to endemic areas. Persons who work with nonhuman primates; are homeless; have HIV infection or chronic liver disease; are incarcerated; men who have sex with men; and persons who use injection or noninjection drugs.[1]	Workers at risk of blood exposure, health-care workers, and correctional staff; those with multiple sexual partners; men who have sex with men; people receiving hemodialysis; those with HIV; sharing needles/ equipment; sharing toothbrushes, nail clippers, and razors.	Similar to HBV; rarely through monogamous heterosexual sex.	Same as HBV and for chronic HBV carriers.	Travelers to endemic areas.

Table 35.1
Viral Hepatitis Infections—cont'd

	Hepatitis A (HAV)	Hepatitis B (HBV)	Hepatitis C (HCV)	Hepatitis D (HDV)	Hepatitis E (HEV)
Prognosis	Acute onset with short illness. Rarely fatal.	Acute: Asymptomatic or ill for several weeks; Chronic: Can lead to potentially fatal complications of cirrhosis, liver failure, or hepatocellular carcinoma.	High cure rate with medication. Chronic: Can develop cirrhosis.	Co-infection with HBV: Mild to severe illness with recovery. Superinfection with chronic HBV: Progression to more severe disease.	Self-limiting infection. Rarely fatal but increases for pregnant women.

Anti = antibody; ALT = alanine aminotransferase; IG = immunoglobulin; IV = intravenous; RUQ = right upper quadrant.

Sources: [1]Nelson, N., Weng, M. K., Hofmeister, M. G., Moore, K. L., Doshani, M., Kamili, S., Koneru, A., Haber, P, Hagan, L., Romero, J., Schillie, S., & Harris, A. (2020). Prevention of hepatitis A virus infection in the United States: Recommendations of the Advisory Committee on Immunization Practices, 2020. Morbidity and Mortality Weekly Report, 69(5), 1–38. http://dx.doi.org/10.15585/mmwr.rr6905a1. [2]Centers for Disease Control and Prevention (2020). Viral hepatitis: Hepatitis B questions and answers for health professionals. https://www.cdc.gov/hepatitis/hbv/hbvfaq.htm. [3]Moorman, A. C., de Perio, M. A., Goldschmidt, R., Chu, C., Kuhar, D., Henderson, D. K., Naggie, S., Kamili, S., Spradling, P. R., Gordon, S. C., Russi, M. B., & Teshale, E. H. (2020). Testing and clinical management of health care personnel potentially exposed to hepatitis C virus—CDC Guidance, United States, 2020. Morbidity and Mortality Weekly Report, 69(6), 1–8. http://dx.doi.org/10.15585/mmwr.rr6906a1.

with resulting damage to liver cells and liver function. If damage involves the bile canaliculi (thin tubes that collect secreted bile), obstructive jaundice will occur. If complications do not occur, cells regenerate and normal liver function eventually resumes.

HAV, HBC, and HCV are the most common types of viral hepatitis in the United States (Centers for Disease Control and Prevention [CDC], 2020a). HCV causes the highest number of new hepatitis infections each year as well as chronic hepatitis.

HEPATITIS C VIRUS. Many people who are infected with HCV are not aware of it and can live for 20 years without symptoms. Those infected can develop chronic infection, chronic liver disease, cirrhosis, or liver cancer. Before 1992, when widespread blood supply screening began in the United States, HCV was also commonly spread through blood transfusions and organ transplants. All adults 18 years and older, pregnant women, and persons with known risk factors should be tested for HCV (CDC, 2020a). Healthy People 2030 has a goal to increase the proportion of persons who are aware they have chronic hepatitis C from 55.6% to 74.2%. Another goal is to reduce acute HCV cases from 1.0 to 0.8 per 100,000 (Office of Disease Prevention and Health Promotion, 2020).

Prevention

Hepatitis viruses are resistant to a wide range of anti-infective measures, such as drying, heat, ultraviolet light exposure, freezing, and bleach and other disinfectants. Infection control precautions should reflect the usual mode of transmission of the specific virus. The best methods for preventing transmission of hepatitis viruses are careful attention to hygiene; avoiding exposure from blood/body fluids and from high-risk groups and activities; getting available vaccinations; and using immunoglobulin (IG) and/or vaccine after an exposure (see Table 35.1).

IGs are plasma donor antibodies that circulate in the recipient's blood for up to 3 months. They do not stimulate the immune system to develop its own antibodies, so they provide only short-term passive protection. In the United States, vaccines for HAV and HBV provide permanent, active immunity by stimulating the immune system to develop a person's own antibodies. Health-care workers and those in high-risk groups should be vaccinated for HBV. Healthy People 2030 goals for HBV include increasing awareness of people infected with HBV and reducing the transmission and fatality rates (Office of Disease Prevention and Health Promotion, 2020).

Public health measures such as health education programs, licensing and supervision of public facilities, screening of blood donors and organs for transplant, and screening of food handlers are general measures to prevent the transmission of hepatitis viruses.

Signs and Symptoms

People can be asymptomatic with viral hepatitis, so many people do not know they are infected. An acute infection of hepatitis with symptom appearance often shows a typical pattern of decreased liver function, which generally occurs in three stages. During the prodromal stage, the patient may be asymptomatic or have symptoms such as fatigue, nausea,

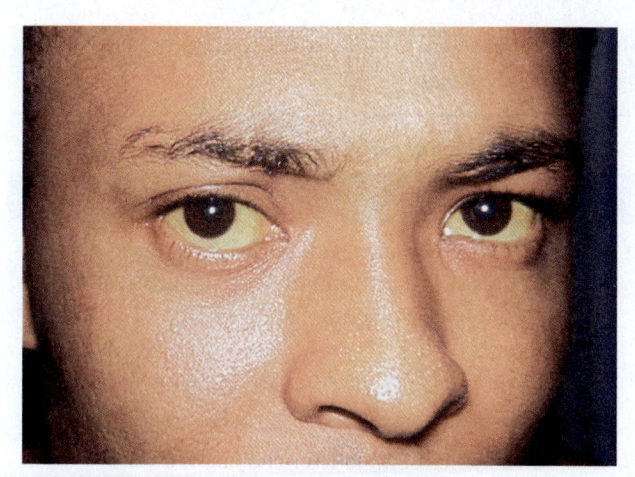

FIGURE 35.1 Jaundice of the conjunctivae and facial skin.

and vomiting (see Table 35.1). During the icteric stage, jaundice appears (Fig 35.1) and prodromal symptoms continue. The convalescent stage (posticteric) begins when the patient starts feeling better. Recovery varies and depends on the type of hepatitis. Full recovery is measured by the return to normal of liver function tests. Acute hepatitis can lead to chronic hepatitis and resulting complications.

Complications

Hepatitis may lead to fulminant (sudden and severe), acute, or chronic liver failure. Chronic infection can develop in those with HBV, HCV, and, rarely, HDV. Some people can become asymptomatic carriers of HBV or HCV and never have an active illness. However, they can infect others. They have a greater risk of developing cancer of the liver.

Diagnostic Tests

Serological tests can determine the specific virus causing the hepatitis via viral antigens. They can also identify the presence of antibodies to the virus (see Table 35.1). Serum liver enzymes, and possibly bilirubin, are elevated (Table 35.2). In patients with severe hepatitis, prothrombin time (PT) may be prolonged. An abdominal x-ray may show an enlarged liver. Liver function tests or biopsy may be done to determine liver damage and healing.

Therapeutic Measures

Treatment goals are to identify the cause of hepatitis, monitor liver status, provide symptom relief, and prevent cirrhosis development. Adequate fluid and nutrition intake are important due to nausea and vomiting. Extreme exertion should be avoided. Alcohol or medications known to be toxic to the liver should not be used (Box 35.1). Treatment for HAV and HEV infection is supportive care based on signs and symptoms. Coinfection of HBV and HDV is treated with pegylated interferon therapy plus ribavirin.

Acute HBV infection may resolve over time without treatment. See the Patient Teaching Guideline for "Hepatitis B" on Davis Advantage. If treatment is needed for chronic hepatitis B, potent antivirals that reduce viral resistance are used, such as entecavir (Baraclude) and tenofovir (Vemlidy, Viread). Pegylated interferon-alfa therapy (peginterferon alfa-2b [PEG-Intron]) may be used for a few patients. Liver transplantation may be needed.

Management of HCV infection continues to evolve as new therapies are developed. The newer direct-acting antiviral (DAA) oral medications have a high cure rate with few side effects. Various combination medication regimens are available for each HCV genotype. Examples of DAA combination medications are elbasvir plus grazoprevir (Zepatier), sofosbuvir plus ledipasvir (Harvoni), sofosbuvir plus velpatasvir (Epclusa), and glecaprevir plus pibrentasvir (Mavyret).

Nursing Process for the Patient With Hepatitis

DATA COLLECTION. Identify subjective data such as malaise, fatigue, pruritus (itching), nausea, anorexia, and right

---

Box 35.1

Common Causes of Hepatic Inflammation

Medications
- Acetaminophen (Tylenol)
- Acetylsalicylic acid (aspirin)
- Allopurinol (Zyloprim)
- Captopril (Capoten)
- Carbamazepine (Tegretol)
- Diazepam (Valium)
- Erythromycin estolate (Ilosone)
- Estrogen
- Halothane (Fluothane)
- Isoniazid (INH)
- Methotrexate (Trexall)
- Methyldopa (Aldomet)
- Oral contraceptives
- Phenobarbital (Luminal)
- Phenytoin (Dilantin)
- Sulfonamides
- Tetracycline (Sumycin)

Metabolic Disorders
- Alpha-1 antitrypsin deficiency
- Hemochromatosis (iron buildup)
- Wilson disease (copper buildup)

Toxins
- Carbon tetrachloride
- Cholecystographic dyes
- Ethyl alcohol
- Kava-containing products (herb)
- Poisonous wild mushrooms
- Toluene
- Trichloroethylene

Vascular Disorders
- Budd–Chiari syndrome (hepatic vein occlusion)
- Heart failure
- Shock

Viruses
- Cytomegalovirus
- Epstein-Barr virus
- Hepatitis A, B, C, D, E
- Herpes simplex virus
- Yellow fever

Table 35.2
Laboratory Tests for Liver Function in Hepatitis and Cirrhosis

Test	Normal Value	Significance of Abnormal Findings
Indicates Liver Damage		
Alanine aminotransferase (ALT)	**Adult** *Male:* 19–36 units/L *Female:* 24–36 units/L **Over 90 years** *Male:* 6–38 units/L *Female:* 5–24 units/L	Most specific enzyme for liver damage. Can elevate 50 times normal with death of liver cells.
Aspartate aminotransferase (AST)	**Adult, older adult** *Male:* 20–40 units/L *Female:* 15–30 units/L	Enzyme found in liver and heart. Over 500 units/L can be seen with acute hepatitis and other acute hepatocellular diseases.
Alkaline phosphatase (ALP)	**Adult** *Male:* 35–142 units/L *Female:* 25–125 units/L	Enzyme found in liver and other areas; released and elevates greatly with severe liver damage.
Measures Functioning of Liver		
Albumin	**Adult** 3.7–5.1 g/dL **Older adult** 3.2–4.6 g/dL **Over 90 years** 2.9–4.5 g/dL	Decreased because of impaired liver protein synthesis. Maintains plasma oncotic pressure, so low levels can cause edema and ascites.
Ammonia	**Adult** 10–80 mcg/dL	Increased because liver cannot metabolize this protein end product; contributes to hepatic encephalopathy.
Total bilirubin	**Adults** Less than 1.1 mg/dL	Increased because the liver is unable to use it to produce bile.
Prothrombin time (PT)	10–13 seconds Critical is greater than 27 seconds	Value prolonged. Liver can no longer make prothrombin; patient bleeds more easily.

upper quadrant (RUQ) abdominal pain. Objective data, such as baseline weight, vomiting, pale stools, dark-colored (tea-colored) urine, and jaundice, are recorded. The patient's vital signs are obtained. Fever or abnormal bruising or bleeding is reported immediately. Ask the patient about knowledge of the disease and how to prevent its spread.

NURSING DIAGNOSES, PLANNING, AND IMPLEMENTATION.

Acute Pain related to inflammation and enlargement of the liver

EXPECTED OUTCOME: The patient will state that pain level is acceptable.

- Monitor pain level using pain rating scale (e.g., 0 to 10) and ask **WHAT'S UP?** questions *to determine treatment needs.*

- Give analgesics as ordered, around the clock and as needed (prn) for intermittent breakthrough pain, recognizing that lower doses might be needed with liver dysfunction, *to control pain and prevent toxicity.*

Imbalanced Nutrition: Less Than Body Requirements related to anorexia, nausea, or vomiting

EXPECTED OUTCOME: The patient's weight will be stable and appropriate for height.

- Make dietitian referral *for development of a nutritional plan.*
- Monitor weight and nutritional intake, recording percentage of food eaten, *to determine ongoing treatment needs.*
- Administer antiemetic medications as ordered *to reduce nausea and increase appetite.*

Risk for Impaired Liver Function related to viral infection

- Monitor liver function tests and signs of liver dysfunction, including ascites, mental changes (check ammonia levels), and bleeding (check coagulation studies), *to detect liver infection*.
- Review medications for hepatotoxicity and administer carefully *to protect liver function*.
- Calculate total acetaminophen 24-hour dosage for all medications that contain it so daily limit of 2,000 mg or less is not exceeded in presence of hepatitis *to protect liver function*.
- Refer to alcohol cessation program if applicable *to preserve liver function*.

Risk for Impaired Skin Integrity related to pruritus secondary to bilirubin pigment deposits in skin

EXPECTED OUTCOME: The patient's skin will remain intact and free from secondary infection.

- Administer antihistamine such as diphenhydramine (Benadryl) as ordered *to decrease itching*.
- Encourage the patient not to scratch skin (keep fingernails trimmed) but to press firmly on the itchy area. *Scratching can damage skin and increase risk for infection*.

Ineffective Health Management related to lack of knowledge of hepatitis and its transmission and treatment

EXPECTED OUTCOME: The patient will state how to self-manage the treatment regimen for viral hepatitis and how to prevent spread of the disease.

- Determine the patient's knowledge of hepatitis *to plan teaching*.
- Reinforce teaching the patient how hepatitis affects the body and the importance of taking medications as prescribed, adequate rest, and proper nutrition *to promote recovery*.
- Reinforce teaching the importance of avoiding alcohol and other liver-toxic medications *to prevent further damage to the liver*.
- Reinforce teaching the patient and family how to prevent the spreading of the hepatitis virus, including vaccination as appropriate for family; hand washing after toileting; using soap and hot water to clean eating utensils, cookware, and food preparation surfaces; practicing safer sex (abstinence, condoms, monogamy); and not sharing needles, *because hepatitis is contagious* (see "Home Health Hints").

EVALUATION. Management of the patient with hepatitis has been successful if the patient reports pain is satisfactorily relieved; laboratory values are maintained or improved to baseline values; skin has no breaks, cuts, or tears or secondary infections; the patient can define the disease; and the patient and family understand and follow the treatment plan and transmission precautions.

Home Health Hints

- When collecting blood ammonia levels, use a chilled vacutainer. Place specimen on ice and deliver to laboratory within 10 minutes.

Abdominal Ascites
- A hospital bed at home may be needed so the patient can be positioned to aid in breathing. A health-care provider's order must be obtained for insurance coverage.
- Measure and document abdominal girth at each visit.
- Teach the patient to obtain weight on the same scale first thing in the morning and to record the weight so the nurse can document the findings.

Hepatitis
- Teach the caregiver to wear disposable gloves when cleaning the patient's bathroom. If possible, the patient should have a separate bedroom and bathroom.
- Teach the patient and caregiver to wash contaminated linens separately from household laundry and to use detergent and hot water. Presoak in cold water if soiled with blood. Rubber gloves should be worn to handle the patient's laundry.

CLINICAL JUDGMENT

Carl Young, 23, has returned from a missionary trip in Africa. He reports that during his time there, he sustained a serious laceration that required sutures. Carl also mentions his fondness for seafood and that, since his return, he has had several "feasts" that have included raw oysters. Carl states that since his return, he has lost nearly 8 pounds, is nauseated, has frequent headaches, tires easily, and is very irritable. Carl states he takes Tylenol for his headaches.

1. What information would you obtain to help you determine which type of hepatitis Carl might be experiencing?
2. What precautions will you institute for Carl until a diagnosis is made?
3. What teaching do you reinforce regarding taking Tylenol?
4. Who do you plan to collaborate with on Carl's care?
5. What teaching do you reinforce for Carl related to hepatitis?

Suggested answers are at the end of the chapter.

Acute Liver Failure

Acute liver failure is a rare but serious condition that can develop rapidly, sometimes in just 2 days. When the liver is severely damaged, its many functions are impaired. The outcome of the disease may be decided within 48 to 72 hours of diagnosis. Possible outcomes are liver recovery, need for liver transplantation, or death. See Box 35.1 for causes. Box 35.2 teaches patients ways to prevent liver damage and possible liver failure.

Box 35.2

Patient Education
Liver Failure Prevention

- Wash hands after using the bathroom and before handling food.
- Do not share personal grooming items (especially toothbrushes or razors).
- Obtain hepatitis A and B vaccines.
- Eat a balanced diet.
- Do not exceed 3,000 mg of acetaminophen in a 24-hour period or a prescribed medication with more than a 325 mg dose of acetaminophen in it.
- Review prescribed and over-the-counter medications to know which are combination medications that contain acetaminophen to prevent excessive dosage. There are more than 600 medications containing acetaminophen, such as Norco, NyQuil, Percocet, Vicodin, Tylenol with Codeine, or Tylox (see www.knowyourdose.org).
- Know how to read medicine labels and dosage found in the active ingredient list on the label. Visit www.knowyourdose.org to interactively read a medication label.
- Avoid alcohol or drink only in moderation. Do not drink alcohol if taking acetaminophen.
- Avoid exposure to blood.
- Use condoms for safer sex.
- Ensure sanitary conditions and equipment when obtaining a body piercing or tattoo.
- Do not share IV needles.

See the Patient Teaching Guideline for "Liver Failure Prevention" on Davis Advantage.

Acetaminophen Toxicity

Acetaminophen (Tylenol) overdose is the most common cause of acute liver failure. Acetaminophen intake should not exceed 3,000 mg in a 24-hour period in a person with no liver disease. The U.S. Food and Drug Administration (FDA) guidelines recommend combination of opioids and acetaminophen be limited to no more than 325 mg of acetaminophen.

For overdose of acetaminophen, activated charcoal is given to absorb acetaminophen if it is within 4 hours of ingestion and the patient is alert with an intact or protected airway. N-acetylcysteine (Acetadote) is the antidote for acetaminophen. It is effective in preventing hepatotoxicity if given within 8 hours of ingestion.

BE SAFE!

AVOID FAILURE TO RECOGNIZE! Understand how to monitor the 24-hour dosage of acetaminophen taken by a patient. Look back at the previous 24-hour time frame from the current time and add up the dosage of any acetaminophen taken alone and in combination medications. This is a floating 24-hour period, not shift times or a calendar day. The acetaminophen dose should not exceed 3,000 mg in a 24-hour period for the patient without liver disease. Teach the patient how to monitor this, too.

Signs and Symptoms

Initial symptoms of liver failure, including fatigue, gastrointestinal (GI) upset, and diarrhea, are vague and make detection difficult. As the condition worsens, symptoms become more severe; these include jaundice, hepatic **encephalopathy** (HE), bleeding, and abdominal distention. The patient may suddenly lapse into an extremely serious illness, starting with confusion and progressing to hepatic coma. Computed tomography (CT) often reveals the liver is less dense than skeletal muscles, is necrotic, and may appear nodular. Labs show a sudden elevation of liver enzymes, alanine aminotransferase (ALT), aspartate aminotransferase (AST), and bilirubin. PT is elevated; marked elevation is an ominous sign. Potassium and blood glucose levels drop.

Therapeutic Measures

Treatment is directed toward identifying the cause of the acute liver failure and stopping and reversing the damage to the liver. Most patients will require IV fluids. The patient is at risk for bleeding commonly from the GI tract and is placed on proton pump inhibitors or histamine 2 blocker. The patient needs intensive amounts of supportive care. Maintaining the airway (head elevated 30 degrees, nothing by mouth [NPO], nasogastric [NG] tube, and endotracheal intubation) is important if HE develops. An attempt is made to put the liver completely at rest. The patient is often on bedrest. Stimulation is avoided. Most medications are discontinued because they are metabolized by the liver. Nutrition may be provided via enteral or parenteral nutrition. Dialysis may be ordered if the liver damage results from an overdose of a hepatotoxic substance to filter the blood.

Nursing Process for the Patient With Acute Liver Failure

Nursing care of the patient with acute liver failure is the same as for the patient with cirrhosis, discussed next.

Chronic Liver Disease and Cirrhosis

In 2018, 4.5 million adults had chronic liver disease and cirrhosis (Villarroel et al, 2019). **Cirrhosis** is the progressive replacement of healthy liver tissue with scar tissue. It results from a chronic liver disease. There are a variety of causes of chronic liver disease (see Box 35.1). Cirrhosis is usually irreversible unless the cause is identified and treated early. Common causes of cirrhosis are chronic alcohol use, chronic hepatitis B and C, or nonalcoholic steatohepatitis (NASH). NASH is also known as fatty liver disease due to the build-up of fat in the liver. It is common in those with diabetes, obesity, heart disease, or elevated cholesterol levels.

• WORD • BUILDING •

encephalopathy: encephalo—brain + pathy—disease
cirrhosis: cirrh—orange yellow + osis—condition

> **BE SAFE!**
> **ACT FAST!** Many consequences of alcohol abuse, such as cirrhosis, can take years to develop, but that is not the case in acute alcohol toxicity. Ingesting a large quantity of ethanol (or a smaller quantity of alcohol not intended for beverages) in a short time can be fatal within a few hours. Alcohol poisoning is especially heartbreaking when, through ignorance or fear of retribution, a young person dies because they were left to "sleep it off." Education on the effects of alcohol use is an important health teaching topic for nurses.

Table 35.3 Cirrhosis Summary

Signs and Symptoms	Anorexia, nausea, weight loss Ascites Bruising and muscle cramping Weakness and fatigue Dull right upper quadrant pain Gastrointestinal bleeding Itching (from bile products deposited in skin) Jaundice Spider angiomata (central arteriole surrounded by many smaller vessels, which looks like a spider)
Diagnostic Tests	Elevated alanine aminotransferase (ALT), alkaline phosphatase (ALP), aspartate aminotransferase (AST), ammonia, bilirubin, prothrombin time (PT) Liver biopsy, CT, or MRI
Therapeutic Measures	Prevent disease progression Treat complications
Complications	Remember the pneumonic **CHEAP** (see Learning Tip)
Priority Nursing Diagnoses	*Excess Fluid Volume* *Imbalanced Nutrition: Less Than Body Requirements* *Acute Confusion*

Pathophysiology

Healthy liver cells exposed to toxins become inflamed. Then, the liver cells are infiltrated with fat and white blood cells (WBCs) and are replaced by fibrotic tissue. As the liver makes repairs, scar tissue forms. If the damage continues over years, and more and more scar tissue is created, cirrhosis can develop. Liver regeneration continues abnormally, disrupting the lobes of the liver and creating nodules. The liver becomes enlarged and hardened and lumpy instead of soft. Blood flow through the liver becomes impaired due to the nodules, resulting in portal venous hypertension and a gray color. After many years, cirrhosis can lead to liver failure.

Signs and Symptoms

Initially, symptoms may not occur with cirrhosis. As liver function becomes impaired, many signs and symptoms arise (Table 35.3). The liver may be enlarged, firm, and tender upon palpation. Laboratory values reflect progressive loss of liver function. As cirrhosis progresses, signs and symptoms of increasing loss of liver function and complications are present (Fig. 35.2).

Complications of Cirrhosis

CLOTTING DEFECTS. Blood clotting defects develop because of impaired prothrombin and fibrinogen production in the liver. Furthermore, the absence of bile salts prevents the absorption of fat-soluble vitamin K, which is essential to make certain blood-clotting factors. As a result, bruising, disseminated intravascular coagulation, or hemorrhage can occur.

PORTAL HYPERTENSION. **Portal hypertension** is persistent elevated blood pressure in the portal vein. Liver scarring obstructs blood flow in the portal vein. This causes blood to back up into surrounding blood vessels. The increased pressure causes the abdominal veins around the umbilicus to become enlarged and visible (called *caput medusae*) as well as rectal hemorrhoids, spleen enlargement (splenomegaly), and esophageal **varices** (dilated veins; Fig. 35.3).

The most serious result of portal hypertension is bleeding esophageal varices. Varices usually develop from the fundus of the stomach upward and may extend into the upper esophagus. The blood-filled, thin-walled varices may tear easily, causing severe bleeding from sudden excessive pressure, such as from coughing, vomiting, or straining.

ASCITES. **Ascites** is an accumulation of serous fluid in the peritoneal (abdominal) cavity from portal hypertension. Low production of the protein albumin by the failing liver can also allow fluid to leak from the blood vessels into the peritoneal cavity. The kidneys respond to the decreased circulating blood volume by releasing aldosterone to save sodium and thus water. Accumulated fluid in the peritoneal cavity causes a markedly enlarged abdomen. The fluid may cause severe respiratory distress as a result of elevation of the diaphragm.

HEPATIC ENCEPHALOPATHY. HE is caused by elevated ammonia, a by-product of protein metabolism, which disrupts mental status. The damaged liver is unable to convert the ammonia to urea for excretion in the urine. Signs and symptoms of HE include progressive confusion, **asterixis** (flapping tremors in the hands caused by toxins at peripheral

• WORD • BUILDING •

asterixis: a—not + sterixis—fixed position

Hepatic encephalopathy
Behavior changes
Flapping tremor
Confusion
Fetor hepaticus
Gradual progression to coma

Portal hypertension
Hemorrhoids
Ascites
Caput medusae
Enlarged spleen
Esophageal varices
Spider angiomas

Hepatorenal syndrome
Oliguria
Sodium retention

Skin
Jaundice
Itching

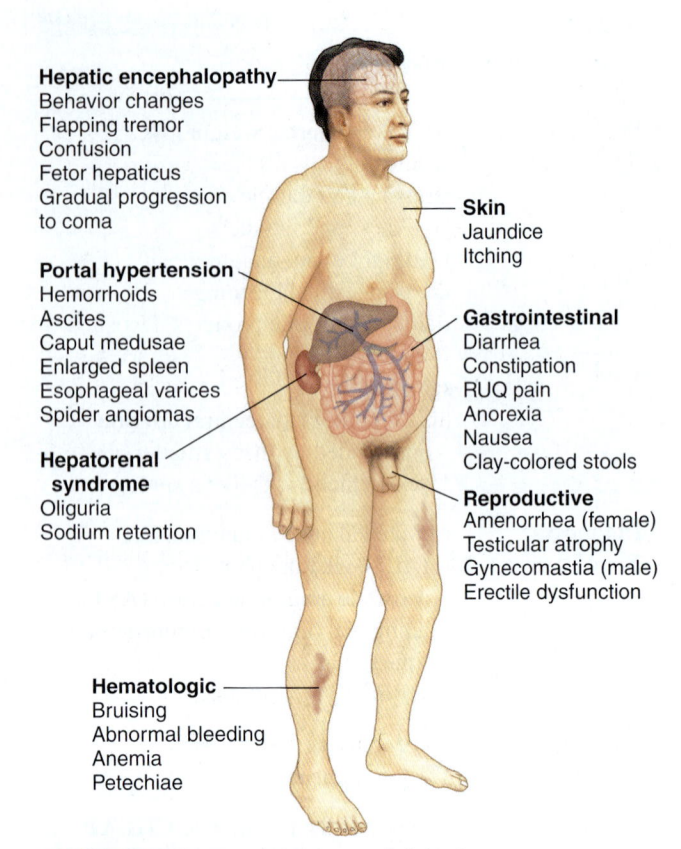

Gastrointestinal
Diarrhea
Constipation
RUQ pain
Anorexia
Nausea
Clay-colored stools

Reproductive
Amenorrhea (female)
Testicular atrophy
Gynecomastia (male)
Erectile dysfunction

Hematologic
Bruising
Abnormal bleeding
Anemia
Petechiae

FIGURE 35.2 Signs and symptoms of cirrhosis.

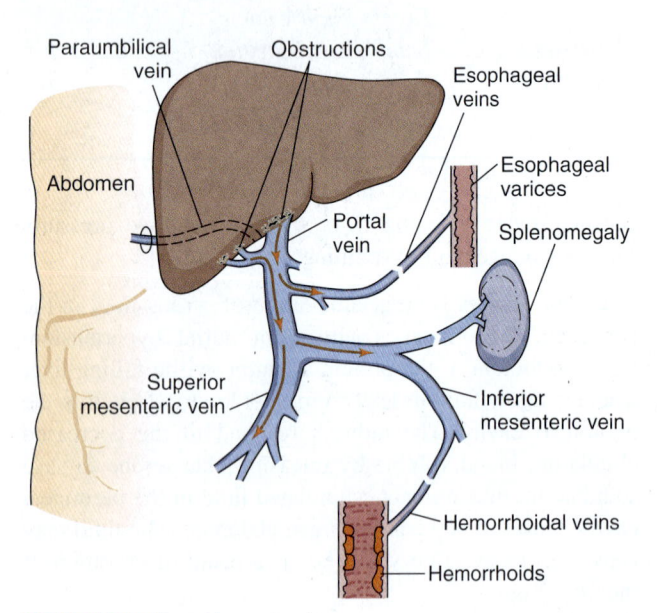

FIGURE 35.3 Portal hypertension.
(Labels: Paraumbilical vein, Obstructions, Esophageal veins, Abdomen, Esophageal varices, Portal vein, Splenomegaly, Superior mesenteric vein, Inferior mesenteric vein, Hemorrhoidal veins, Hemorrhoids)

- *Grade 1:* The patient exhibits subtle changes in personality, sleep disturbances, mood changes, and shortened attention span.
- *Grade 2:* The patient may be forgetful, seem lethargic, or behave inappropriately. Asterixis and slurred speech can occur during this stage. The patient has difficulty doing basic math or writing. The patient has moderate confusion.
- *Grade 3:* The patient is often belligerent and irritable, disoriented, somnolent, and has marked confusion. The patient is sleeping more but is arousable.
- *Grade 4:* The patient gradually loses consciousness and becomes comatose.

With treatment, as ammonia levels decrease, the patient usually gradually regains consciousness. HE represents end-stage liver failure and has a high mortality rate once coma begins.

HEPATORENAL SYNDROME. Hepatorenal syndrome is a secondary failure of the kidneys from cirrhosis. The impaired liver circulation reduces renal blood flow. Symptoms of hepatorenal syndrome include oliguria without detectable kidney damage, reduced glomerular filtration rate (GFR) with essentially no urine output or less than 200 mL per day, and nearly total sodium retention. Vasopressin and albumin can increase intravascular volume and blood flow. Liver transplant may be necessary.

> **LEARNING TIP**
> For complications of cirrhosis, remember the pneumonic **CHEAP:**
> **C:** Clotting defects
> **H:** Hepatorenal syndrome
> **E:** Encephalopathy
> **A:** Ascites
> **P:** Portal hypertension

WERNICKE–KORSAKOFF SYNDROME. Wernicke–Korsakoff syndrome is a brain disorder caused by thiamine (B_1) deficiency. Wernicke encephalopathy and Korsakoff psychosis often occur together. They are primarily diagnosed in those who abuse alcohol and occasionally in malnourished patients with no history of alcohol abuse. Wernicke encephalopathy is an acute condition resulting in confusion, delirium, visual disturbances, and ataxia. When caused by dietary deficiency, this encephalopathy can usually be successfully treated with oral or subcutaneous thiamine. Korsakoff psychosis is the result of permanent damage to the brain tissue. Administration of thiamine will not reverse this brain

• WORD • BUILDING •

fetor hepaticus: fetor—offensive odor + hepat—liver + icas—related to
hepatorenal syndrome: hepato—liver + renal—kidneys + syndrome—group of symptoms

nerves), and **fetor hepaticus** (foul breath caused by metabolic end products related to sulfur).

The five stages of HE and signs and symptoms are as follows:

- *Grade 0:* It is hard to detect this stage because there may be only minimal changes in memory, concentration, or intellectual functioning.

damage. Patients with Korsakoff psychosis display an abnormal mental state in which memory and learning are affected in an otherwise alert and responsive patient.

Diagnostic Tests

Tests that show liver damage and functioning of the liver are shown in Table 35.2. Abdominal x-ray, CT, or MRI may show ascites and enlargement of the liver. An abdominal ultrasound may show liver enlargement, or a small, nodular liver later in the disease. Esophageal varices and bleeding (discussed later in the chapter) can be detected with an esophagogastroduodenoscopy (EGD). A liver biopsy can determine the extent and nature of the liver damage (see Chapter 32).

> **NURSING CARE TIP**
>
> Patients with cirrhosis undergoing a liver biopsy need careful observation for bleeding after the procedure because of possible impaired clotting.

Therapeutic Measures

Interventions for cirrhosis are to prevent advancement of the disease and treat complications. A liver transplant may be considered if cirrhosis cannot be treated.

ASCITES. Ascites is treated with diuretics such as spironolactone (Aldactone) or furosemide (Lasix), sodium (≤2,000 mg/day) and fluid restrictions (800–1,000 mL/day), abstinence from alcohol, and albumin infusions for severe ascites. Paracentesis can be done to remove accumulated fluid from the peritoneal cavity when the fluid is compromising the patient's breathing or causing abdominal discomfort. If large amounts of fluid are removed (>5 L), albumin may be given to replace lost proteins to prevent further fluid shifting. Prophylactic antibiotics may be given to prevent GI bacteria from moving into peritoneal cavity causing infection of ascites fluid.

Ascites may be treated by the nonsurgical placement of a shunt, called a **transjugular intrahepatic portosystemic shunt** (TIPS), under fluoroscopy (Fig. 35.4). A stent is placed via the jugular vein to connect the portal vein to the hepatic vein, in the middle of the liver. This reduces portal pressure by allowing blood to bypass the liver and be carried to the heart. It reduces fluid accumulation and aids in reducing the risk of bleeding. Complications can develop with TIPS.

> **CUE RECOGNITION 35.1**
>
> Mr. Poms has cirrhosis with ascites, and you notice that he has gained 2 pounds with his daily weight this morning. As you measure his abdominal circumference, you notice it is 1 inch larger than yesterday. What do you do?
>
> *Suggested answers are at the end of the chapter.*

ESOPHAGEAL VARICES. Bleeding varices are a medical emergency, and 911 should be called. Large amounts of blood can be lost, and death can result, so screening for the

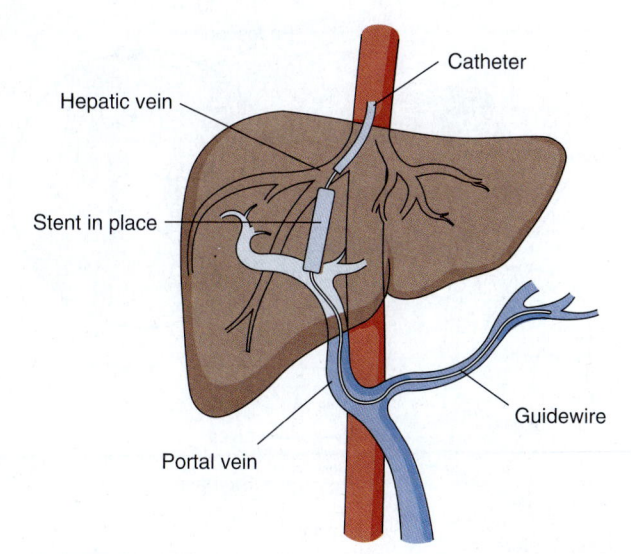

FIGURE 35.4 Transjugular intrahepatic portosystemic shunt (TIPS).

presence of varices should be done. For bleeding prevention, medications can be used such as the beta blockers propranolol (Inderal) and nadolol (Corgard). If the patient cannot tolerate the beta blockers or if they have large varices, preventative treatment can include endoscopic variceal ligation using rubber bands (Fig. 35.5).

Bleeding from esophageal varices must be stopped immediately. Bleeding varices can be treated with a vasoconstrictor such as octreotide (Sandostatin) and variceal ligation. TIPS may be recommended to reduce the pressure in the portal vein and stop the bleeding varices. A blood transfusion may be needed for lost blood volume. Antibiotics may be given to reduce the risk of infection and rebleeding from varices. A balloon tamponade can be used to temporarily stop bleeding by putting direct pressure on the bleeding varices. Rebleeding after the balloon is removed is a common problem and other treatments such as TIPS can be done.

HEPATIC ENCEPHALOPATHY. Precipitants of hepatic encephalopathy should be avoided. These include medications (narcotics, benzodiazepines, alcohol), increased ammonia production (excess protein intake or infection), dehydration, and other causes. To reduce serum ammonia levels to prevent or treat HE, the osmotic disaccharide laxative lactulose is given by mouth, NG tube, or enema (depending on how alert the patient is). It lowers the pH of the colon, inhibiting ammonia from moving into the blood so that it can be excreted in the stool and inhibiting ammonia-producing bacteria. Lactulose also causes water to be drawn into the colon, which increases ammonia's transport from the body. Antibiotics may also be given to reduce ammonia-producing

• WORD • BUILDING •

transjugular intrahepatic portosystemic shunt: trans—across + jugular—jugular vein + intra—within + hepatic—liver + porto—portal (liver circulation) + systemic—systemic (circulation) + shunt—to divert

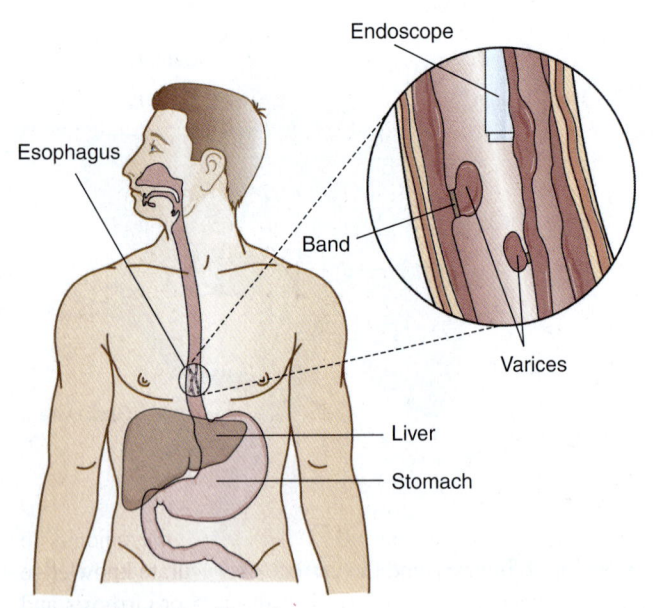

FIGURE 35.5 Variceal banding.

bacteria in the gut. Rifaximin (Xifaxan) is commonly used. Hypokalemia is often present, which increases renal ammonia production. Potassium is replaced to increase blood levels. Branched-chain amino acids can be used with some patients, although they are not standard treatment for all patients (see "Nutrition Notes: Supplying Nutrients to Patients With Liver Disease").

Nursing Process for the Patient With Acute Liver Failure, Chronic Liver Disease, or Cirrhosis

Data Collection
A complete history and physical assessment are done. Be alert to subjective symptoms of liver dysfunction, such as abdominal pain, anorexia, nausea, severe itching, and dull, aching RUQ pain. Note objective evidence of liver problems, such as jaundice, light-colored stools, ascites, ecchymosis (bruising) of the skin, GI bleeding, and any evidence of alterations in thought processes, such as confusion, disorientation, or inability to make decisions.

Nursing Diagnoses, Planning, and Implementation
Common nursing diagnoses for the patient with acute liver failure, chronic liver disease, or cirrhosis include the following:

Excess Fluid Volume related to portal hypertension and ascites

EXPECTED OUTCOME: Fluid volume will be controlled as evidenced by stable weight and abdominal girth within normal limits for the patient.

- Monitor the patient's vital signs, daily weights, and lung sounds; report changes or difficulty breathing or changes in mental status promptly *to detect fluid overload and obtain prompt treatment.*

Nutrition Notes

Supplying Nutrients to Patients With Liver Disease
A registered dietitian consultation is needed to assess nutritional status, help diagnose malnutrition, and make diet recommendations to improve nutrient intake.

Nutritional Care for Hepatitis Patients
A well-balanced diet is recommended following the principles of the 2020–2025 Dietary Guidelines for Americans. Herbal supplements and alcohol should be avoided, and vitamin/mineral supplements should be taken only under HCP supervision.

Nutritional Care for Cirrhosis Patients
Patients with cirrhosis may have a decreased appetite and be malnourished. Vitamin and mineral absorption can be impaired. The National Institute of Diabetes and Digestive and Kidney Disease recommends that patients:

- Obtain adequate calories and protein through food and nutritional supplements (either orally or by feeding tube)
- Monitor vitamin status and use appropriate supplementation
- Avoid alcohol, raw or undercooked meat, fish, and shellfish (due to bacterial infection)
- Restrict sodium

Branched-chain amino acids (isoleucine, leucine, and valine) can help improve hepatic encephalopathy. Branched-chain amino acids do not require oxidation by the liver and are available for direct use by other tissues (Varshney & Saini, 2020).

References: National Institute of Diabetes and Digestive and Kidney Disease. (2018). Eating, diet, & nutrition for cirrhosis. https://www.niddk.nih.gov/health-information/liver-disease/cirrhosis/eating-diet-nutrition; U.S. Department of Veterans Affairs. (2019). Viral hepatitis and liver disease. https://www.hepatitis.va.gov/cirrhosis/nutrition.asp; Varshney, P., & Saini, P. (2020) Role of branched chain amino acids supplementation on quality of life in liver cirrhosis patient. *Research Journal of Pharmacy and Technology, 13*(7), 3516–3519. https://doi.org/10.5958/0974-360X.2020.00622.8

- Measure intake and output, and the patient's abdominal girth (circumference) daily at the same marked location *to monitor ascites and fluid volume changes.*
- Report weight gain or increase in abdominal girth promptly *so treatment can be ordered and complications minimized.*
- Maintain a low-sodium diet and fluid restrictions *to reduce fluid retention.*
- Administer ordered diuretics as scheduled *to reduce fluid overload.*

Imbalanced Nutrition: Less Than Body Requirements related to anorexia and impaired metabolism of needed nutrients

EXPECTED OUTCOME: The patient's nutritional needs will be maintained within normal limits.

- Obtain dietitian referral *to assess for malnutrition and then develop a nutritional plan.*

- Make sure that odors and other unpleasant stimuli are eliminated *to reduce anorexia.*
- Offer the patient frequent, small, high-calorie meals *to reduce feeling of fullness that can occur with larger meals.*

Acute Confusion related to elevated ammonia levels

EXPECTED OUTCOME: The patient will remain alert and oriented to person, place, and time.

- Monitor the patient's level of consciousness and orientation often *to allow prompt treatment.*
- Monitor neuromuscular function by asking the patient to hold arms steady and straight out in front. *If asterixis, or liver flap, is present, the patient's hands will unwillingly dip and return to the horizontal position in a flapping motion due to elevated ammonia.*
- Give medications such as lactulose as scheduled *to decrease serum ammonia levels.*
- Recognize that lactulose causes loose stools but do not withhold the medication when the patient has the desired two soft or loose stools per day; report severe diarrhea. *Loose stools signify that the medication is working.*
- Question giving medications such as sedatives, opioids, and tranquilizers *because these can precipitate HE.*
- Reorient the patient to time and place if needed *to reinforce reality.*
- Provide a safe environment and implement fall precautions for the confused or unsteady patient *to prevent injury.*

Ineffective Breathing Pattern related to excess fluid in the abdomen

EXPECTED OUTCOME: The patient's respirations will be even and unlabored, 12 to 20 per minute.

- Monitor the patient's respiratory rate, rhythm, chest movement, skin color, and oxygen saturation frequently *to determine breathing pattern and its effectiveness.*
- Elevate head of the patient's bed *to give the patient's lungs maximum room for expansion.*
- Administer analgesics carefully, as ordered, if pain is causing shallow respirations. *Reducing painful breathing allows for a more effective breathing pattern.*

Risk for Deficient Fluid Volume related to bleeding esophageal varices or GI bleeding secondary to clotting disorder

EXPECTED OUTCOME: Fluid volume will remain within normal limits as evidenced by no signs of bleeding, and vital signs, weight, and fluid balance within normal limits for the patient.

- Monitor gastric secretions, stool, and urine at least every 8 hours, and report any signs of bleeding *for prompt treatment.*
- Monitor blood clotting laboratory studies such as PT and report any abnormal values *to identify risk for bleeding.*
- Avoid suctioning the patient if possible *as it can cause esophageal varices to bleed.*
- Use a small-gauge needle for injections and apply direct pressure to all puncture sites. Avoid invasive treatments *to prevent bleeding.*
- Reinforce teaching the patient to avoid forceful coughing or nose blowing, straining, vomiting, or gagging if possible. Administer medications as ordered to prevent their occurrence. *These can increase pressure and risk of bleeding varices.*

Evaluation

Nursing care has been effective if the patient is alert and oriented without signs of fluid retention, a stable weight appropriate for height has been achieved, respiratory rate is between 12 and 20 respirations per minute with no cyanosis or changes in consciousness, the patient is experiencing no bleeding or injuries, and the patient has accurate knowledge of acute liver failure, chronic liver disease, or cirrhosis and disease management requirements.

Patient Education

Reinforce teaching patients how acute liver failure, chronic liver disease, or cirrhosis affects their bodies and health. In particular, patients need to know about portal system hypertension and HE. In addition, reinforce teaching patient to do the following:

- Avoid alcohol.
- Obtain adequate rest and avoid strenuous activity.
- Use opioids, sedatives, and tranquilizers cautiously due to potential mental function impairment.
- Report bleeding; confusion, tremors, or personality changes; signs of low potassium, such as muscle cramps, nausea, or vomiting caused by diuretics; changes in weight; or other symptoms promptly.
- Maintain adequate nutrition (see "Nutrition Notes: Supplying Nutrients to Patients With Liver Disease").

CRITICAL THINKING & CLINICAL JUDGMENT

Mrs. Conner, a 76-year-old retired businesswoman, has lived alone for the past 20 years since the death of her husband. She has a history of poor nutritional habits but does not consume alcohol. She is admitted with cirrhosis. She is overweight and has type II diabetes. Her albumin level is decreased and her PT is prolonged.

Critical Thinking (The Why)
1. Why do you think that Mrs. Conner has cirrhosis?
2. Why are Mrs. Conner's albumin and PT abnormal?

Clinical Judgment (The Do)
3. What teaching do you reinforce with Mrs. Conner about two serious problems with portal hypertension?
4. What teaching do you reinforce about her care for ascites?
5. With whom do you collaborate for Mrs. Conner's care?

Suggested answers are at the end of the chapter.

Liver Transplantation

The patient with end-stage liver failure from cirrhosis, hepatitis, biliary disease, metabolic disorders, or hepatic vein obstruction may be considered for a liver transplant. The U.S. Department of Health & Human Services (2020) has processes to match organs with candidates who need transplants. Patients with urgent cases such as acute liver failure are prioritized. The patient will be evaluated for emotional and physical stability as well as acceptance of the need for daily medications for life and post-transplantation care (see "Cultural Considerations: Organ Donation").

> ### Cultural Considerations
> **Organ Donation**
> Certain considerations may need to be made for potential donor recipients who adhere to Judaism. Jewish law addresses organ transplantation from the perspectives of the recipient, the living donor, the cadaver donor, and the dying donor. If a recipient's life can be prolonged without considerable risk, transplant is ordained. For a living donor to be approved, the risk to the life of the donor must be considered. One is not obligated to donate a part of themselves unless the risk is small. The use of a cadaver for transplant is usually approved if it is saving a life. A rabbi can be helpful when making decisions regarding organ donation or transplantation.
>
> Reference: Alaluf, R. I. (2020). Organ donation in Judaism. *Experimental and Clinical Transplantation, 18*(Suppl2), 24–26. https://doi.org/10.6002/ect.rlgnsymp2020.L4

After surgical implantation of a donor liver, the patient is closely observed for evidence of donor organ rejection. The patient will be placed on medications to suppress immune system responses and prevent tissue rejection. The patient is observed for signs of impending rejection:

- Pulse greater than 100 beats per minute
- Temperature greater than 101°F (38°C)
- Reports of RUQ pain
- Increased jaundice

In addition, laboratory studies may show increased serum transaminases (ALT and AST), serum bilirubin, alkaline phosphatase (ALP), and PT. The patient who has received an organ transplant needs extended medical follow-up. Teach the patient to promptly report to the health-care provider (HCP) symptoms of infection, bleeding episodes, or RUQ pain.

Bioartificial livers with filtering membranes may be used as a short-term bridge to liver transplant. Hepatocyte transplantation via splenic artery catheter for long-term support is under study.

Cancer of the Liver

Cancer of the liver usually results from metastasis from a primary cancer at a distant location. The liver is a likely area of involvement for cancers that originated in the esophagus, lungs, breast, stomach, colon, pancreas, kidney, bladder, or skin. For some patients, the primary tumor site is the liver. Patients with history of chronic HBV or HCV, nutritional deficiencies, heavy alcohol use or smoking, and exposure to hepatotoxins have increased risk for cancer of the liver.

Symptoms of cancer of the liver include encephalopathy, abnormal bleeding, jaundice, and ascites. Laboratory tests show elevated serum ALP and alpha-fetoprotein. MRI, CT, or ultrasound are used to diagnose and monitor liver cancer. A needle biopsy can be used cautiously in some patients to determine etiology of the liver lesion.

Liver cancer is staged upon diagnosis. If found early, surgery can be curative. However, it is rarely found early. Postoperative care is similar to care for other abdominal surgeries. If surgery is not an option, the patient may receive chemotherapeutic medications by injection directly into the affected lobe of the liver or into the hepatic artery; sorafenib (Nexavar), which slows the multiplication of cancer cells; or radiation therapy. The overall survival rate for liver cancer is low. (See Chapter 11 for care of patients with cancer.)

DISORDERS OF THE PANCREAS

Pancreatitis

Pancreatitis, inflammation of the pancreas, may be either acute or chronic. The two forms of pancreatitis have different courses and are considered two different disorders.

Acute Pancreatitis
Pathophysiology

Inflammation of the pancreas appears to be caused by a process called **autodigestion**. For reasons not fully understood, pancreatic enzymes are activated while they are still in the pancreas and begin to digest the pancreas. In addition, large amounts of enzymes are released by inflamed cells. As the pancreas digests itself, chemical cascades occur. Trypsin destroys pancreatic tissue and causes vasodilation. As capillary permeability increases, fluid is lost to the retroperitoneal space, causing shock. In addition, trypsin appears to set off another chain of events that causes the conversion of prothrombin to thrombin, so that clots form.

Etiology

Acute pancreatitis (AP) is most commonly associated with heavy alcohol consumption or cholelithiasis (gallstones), although the exact mechanisms are unknown. Alcohol appears to act directly on the acinar cells of the pancreas and the pancreatic ducts to irritate and inflame the structures. Gallstones may plug the pancreatic duct and cause inflammation from excessive fluid pressure on sensitive ducts. The irritant effect of bile itself may cause inflammation. As the duct is blocked, the enzymes revert into the pancreas causing destruction of the pancreatic tissue. Elevated triglycerides, endoscopic retrograde cholangiopancreatography (ERCP) induced pancreatitis, pancreatic tumors, or, rarely, medications can cause pancreatitis. Smoking increases the risk of developing pancreatitis. Sometimes, the cause is unknown (idiopathic).

Prevention
Caution patients who drink alcohol or smoke to stop. People with biliary disease should seek medical treatment so that pancreatitis does not develop as a complication.

Signs and Symptoms
Patients with AP may present with severe pain, guarding, a rigid (board-like) abdomen, hypotension or shock, and respiratory distress from accumulation of fluid in the retroperitoneal space (Table 35.4). Pain is located in the epigastric area or left upper quadrant (LUQ), with radiation to the chest, back, and flanks. Respirations are often shallow as the patient attempts to splint the painful areas. The patient may have a low-grade fever, dry mucous membranes, and tachycardia. If primary cause is biliary, patient may report nausea and vomiting, and jaundice may be evident.

Complications
If this process continues and is severe enough, the chemical mediators leave the pancreas and cause the inflammatory process to go systemic. This can cause a decrease in fluid volume due to leakage of fluid and blood from the vessels into the tissues. This can lead to systemic inflammatory response syndrome (SIRS), cardiovascular, pulmonary (including acute respiratory distress syndrome), and acute kidney injury. SIRS is the most likely cause of death. Electrolyte imbalance, hemorrhage, peripheral vascular collapse, and infection (local or systemic) are also major concerns. The presence of Chvostek sign (twitching of facial muscles with tapping in front of ear over facial nerve) indicates neuromuscular irritability and decreased calcium levels. A purplish discoloration of the flanks (Turner sign) or a purplish discoloration around the umbilicus (Cullen sign) may occur with extensive hemorrhagic destruction of the pancreas.

Diagnostic Tests
Diagnosis of AP is made when two of these are present: abdominal pain, serum amylase (normal: 100–300 units/L), and/or serum lipase (normal: 0–60 units/L) more than three times normal. CT and MRI can also confirm the diagnosis of AP. Serum amylase rises quickly and then returns to normal in 3 to 5 days in most patients. Serum lipase is most specific for AP; it elevates and stays elevated for 8 to 14 days. Ultrasonography may show pleural effusion from local inflammatory reaction to pancreatic enzymes or a change in the size of the pancreas.

Table 35.4 Pancreatitis Summary

Signs and Symptoms	Epigastric or left upper quadrant abdominal pain Low-grade fever Nausea and vomiting
Diagnostic Tests	Elevated serum amylase and lipase CT with or without multidetector technology MRI with magnetic resonance cholangiopancreatography
Therapeutic Measures	Aggressive intravenous fluid hydration Pain control Mild acute pancreatitis: oral feeding Severe acute pancreatitis: enteral feeding
Complications	Hemorrhage, shock, sepsis, organ failure, systemic inflammatory response syndrome, infection
Priority Nursing Diagnoses	*Acute Pain* *Ineffective Breathing Pattern*

Nutrition Notes

Mild Acute Pancreatitis
Assess for and address malnutrition. Otherwise, requirements for energy and food intake remain unchanged.

Severe Acute Pancreatitis
- Enteral feedings are recommended within 24 to 48 hours to meet increased needs for energy and protein if oral feedings are not tolerated. Energy requirement is set at 25 to 30 kcal/kg body weight, glucose intake at 2 to 4 g/kg body weight, and protein at 1.2 to 1.5 g/kg body weight (Storck et al, 2019).
- Parenteral nutrition may be added to meet nutritional needs.
- Resume oral food intake as soon as possible.

Chronic Pancreatitis
Long-term pancreatic insufficiency places patients at high risk for malnutrition and requires close monitoring of nutritional status.

- Deficiencies of vitamins A, D, E, and K plus magnesium, zinc, or calcium are common and should be monitored.
- Pancreatic enzymes may be prescribed to aid digestion at mealtimes.
- Encourage abstinence from alcohol.
- If supplemental nutrition is indicated, energy requirement is set at 25 to 30 kcal/kg body weight, and protein at 1.5 g/kg body weight (Storck et al, 2019).

Reference: Storck, L. J., Imoberdof, R., & Ballmer, P. E. (2019). Nutrition in gastrointestinal disease: Liver, pancreatic, and inflammatory bowel disease. *Journal of Clinical Medicine. 8*(8), 1098. https://doi.org/10.3390/jcm8081098

Therapeutic Measures

Early aggressive IV hydration during the first 24 hours for hypovolemia treatment is recommended. In asymptomatic mild AP, oral nutrition is given (see "Nutrition Notes: Nourishing the Patient With Pancreatitis"). In moderate or severe cases, if oral feeding is not tolerated, enteral feeding is begun. If patients do not tolerate enteral feeding, parenteral nutrition can be used. Pain relief is essential especially for severe pain. Antibiotics are given for sepsis or infection. Minimally invasive debriding of necrotic tissue may be considered for symptomatic patients.

> ### CRITICAL THINKING & CLINICAL JUDGMENT
>
> **Mrs. Samuels,** an 85-year-old retired librarian, is admitted to the nursing unit from the emergency department with severe mid-epigastric pain that radiates to her back. On admission, she is noted to have guarding of the abdomen. Her medical record documents that she had an endoscopic retrograde cholangiopancreatography (ERCP) 2 days ago for recurrent episodes of RUQ abdominal pain. She has no history of excessive alcohol intake.
>
> **Critical Thinking (The Why)**
> 1. What is the most common cause of acute pancreatitis (AP)? Does Mrs. Samuels fit the description?
> 2. Why is Mrs. Samuels at risk for hemorrhage?
> 3. What laboratory test is most likely to be abnormal in early AP?
>
> **Clinical Judgment (The Do)**
> 4. What will you do to help manage Mrs. Samuels's pain?
> 5. What teaching do you reinforce about nutrition?
>
> *Suggested answers are at the end of the chapter.*

Chronic Pancreatitis
Pathophysiology

Chronic pancreatitis (CP) is a progressive fibro-inflammatory disease in which functioning pancreatic tissue is replaced with fibrotic tissue because of inflammation. Pancreatic ducts become obstructed, dilated, and, finally, atrophied. The acinar, or enzyme-producing, cells of the pancreas ulcerate in response to inflammation. The ulceration causes further tissue damage and tissue death. It also may cause cystic sacs filled with pancreatic enzymes to form on the surface of the pancreas. The pancreas becomes smaller and hardened. Progressively smaller amounts of pancreatic enzymes are produced (exocrine insufficiency). Later, islet tissue is lost, causing diabetes mellitus (endocrine insufficiency).

Etiology

Causes of CP include alcohol abuse (most common), obstructive biliary disease, and hyperlipidemia. Causes may also be idiopathic, genetic, and autoimmune related. Cigarette smoking and repeated attacks of AP are risk factors for developing CP.

Signs and Symptoms

CP may by asymptomatic. If signs and symptoms occur, they are less severe than those of AP. The patient will report epigastric or LUQ pain that worsens after eating, nausea and vomiting, weight loss, steatorrhea (greasy, foul-smelling, loose stools), and intolerance of fatty foods. The patient's history will show a pattern of exacerbations and remissions.

Complications

A variety of complications can result from CP. Abscesses and fistulas may develop when cysts filled with pancreatic enzymes burst into the abdominal cavity, causing severe inflammation and tissue necrosis. Pleural effusion may develop from inflammation under the diaphragm. Pancreatic enzymes are essential for normal nutrient absorption from the intestines. Vitamin and mineral deficiencies can develop. Fat intolerance and malabsorption syndrome with fatty stools and diarrhea may develop in response to the decreased pancreatic enzymes produced. In addition, biliary obstruction may further complicate fat absorption. As the islets of Langerhans are destroyed, diabetes mellitus results (discussed in Chapter 40). CP is a risk factor for pancreatic cancer.

Diagnostic Tests

CT scan is the preferred initial radiologic test. If inconclusive, high-quality CT using multidetector technology (CT that is fast and more detailed) or MRI with magnetic resonance cholangiopancreatography (uses magnetic fields and radio waves). Endoscopic ultrasound can be used for diagnosis, and sampling of fluid or tissue. Serum amylase and serum lipase levels will be normal or low. Fecal fat analysis shows higher than normal amounts of fat but are helpful only in late CP to identify the degree of exocrine insufficiency.

Therapeutic Measures

Treatment is aimed at promoting comfort, maintaining adequate pancreatic function and nutrition, and treating complications (see "Nutrition Notes: Nourishing the Patient With Pancreatitis"). Cessation of alcohol use is crucial to reduce pain. Other interventions to relieve pain include small low-fat meals, proton pump inhibitors, NSAIDs and analgesics, nerve block, or pancreatic enzyme supplements (Table 35.5). Patients should be advised to stop smoking. Procedures can be done to stent the pancreatic ducts or remove ductal stones (*extracorporeal shock-wave lithotripsy*). Surgery may be necessary to treat biliary disease, repair fistulas, drain cysts, or remove part of the pancreas.

• **WORD • BUILDING** •
extracorporeal shock-wave lithotripsy: extra—outside + tripsy—rub or crush

Table 35.5
Medications Used for Pancreatic and Gallbladder Disorders

Medication Class/Action

Antiemetics

Reduce nausea.

Examples	Nursing Implications
prochlorperazine (Compazine)	Contraindicated in glaucoma.
	Give antacids 2 hours before or after.
metoclopramide (Reglan)	Monitor for extrapyramidal symptoms.
	Administer 30 minutes before meals.
promethazine (Phenergan)	May be additive when used with opioids.
	Monitor intake and output, sedation, and urine retention.
ondansetron (Zofran)	Monitor for hypersensitivity.

Bile Acid Sequestrants

Bind with circulating bile acids for excretion in the stool to relieve itching.

Examples	Nursing Implications
cholestyramine (Questran, LoCholest)	Give 4–6 hours before or 1 hour after other medications.
colestipol (Colestid)	

Bile Acid Dissolution Agents

Prevent or dissolve (noncalcified) cholesterol gallstones.

Examples	Nursing Implications
ursodiol (Actigall)	Give with a full glass of water.
chenodiol (Chenix)	Aluminum antacids may reduce absorption.

Pancreatic Supplements

Replace pancreatic digestive enzymes (lipase, protease, amylase).

Examples	Nursing Implications
pancrelipase (Cotazym, Creon, Ultrase, Viokase)	Give with meals.
	Swallow whole and do not chew.

Nursing Process for the Patient With Acute or Chronic Pancreatitis

See "Nursing Care Plan for the Patient With Acute and Chronic Pancreatitis."

Data Collection

A complete history and physical assessment are done. Be alert to subjective symptoms of pancreas dysfunction, such as LUQ abdominal pain, nausea, and vomiting. Ask the patient about alcohol use, smoking, history of pancreatitis, weight loss, or steatorrhea. Note objective evidence of pancreas problems, such as fever and abnormal amylase and lipase levels.

Nursing Diagnoses, Planning, and Implementation

Common nursing diagnoses for the patient with acute pancreatitis or chronic pancreatitis include:

Imbalanced Nutrition: Less than Body Requirements related to pain, anorexia and treatment

EXPECTED OUTCOME: The patient will experience improved nutrition evidenced by stable weight.

- Monitor the patient's weight every other day *to monitor nutritional status because a loss of 1 pound of body weight occurs when the body uses 3,500 calories more than is taken in.*
- Administer pancreatic enzymes and nutritional supplements as ordered *to aid in digestion and provide adequate nutrition.*
- Reinforce teaching the patient to avoid alcohol and provide alcohol cessation resources *to prevent triggering another episode of pancreatitis.*

- Reinforce teaching the patient and family to self-monitor for symptoms of malabsorption syndrome such as fatty stools, weight loss, dry skin, or bleeding. *Absence of pancreatic enzymes causes problems with digestion of fats, carbohydrates, and proteins*

Risk for Injury related to hemorrhage or fluid and electrolyte imbalances

EXPECTED OUTCOME: The patient will experience no injury during illness.

- Monitor sodium, potassium, calcium, and magnesium levels. *Electrolyte levels can become imbalanced in pancreatitis.*
- Observe for nausea and vomiting and give antiemetics as ordered *to prevent fluid loss.*
- Observe abdomen and flanks for Cullen and Turner signs, *as these are signs of hemorrhage.*
- Measure and record intake and output *to monitor and reflect fluid balance.*
- Reinforce teaching the patient to report weakness or muscle twitching, *which may indicate electrolyte imbalance.*

Evaluation
Nursing care has been effective if the patient has improved nutrition as evidenced by a weight gain or stable body weight appropriate for height and no evidence of any injury related to hemorrhage or fluid and electrolyte imbalance.

Patient Education
Teach patients with acute or chronic pancreatitis affects their bodies and health. Teach patients to do the following:

- Avoid alcohol
- Maintain adequate nutrition (See Nutrition Notes for "Mild Acute Pancreatitis, Severe Acute Pancreatitis, and Chronic Pancreatitis")
- Avoid cigarette smoking

Nursing Care Plan for the Patient With Acute and Chronic Pancreatitis

Nursing Diagnosis: *Acute Pain* related to edema and inflammation
Expected Outcome: The patient will state pain level is tolerable within 30 minutes of pain report.
Evaluation of Outcome: Does the patient state pain level is tolerable?

Intervention	Rationale	Evaluation
Monitor patient for pain every 2 hours by asking patient to rate pain.	Intense pain is likely to occur with acute pancreatitis. A pain scale allows for consistent and individual evaluation of pain.	Does patient state that pain is tolerable?
Administer analgesics as ordered, before pain becomes severe.	Analgesics are most effective if given before pain becomes too great.	Are analgesics effective?
Assist patient to a position of comfort, usually high Fowler or leaning forward slightly.	An upright position keeps abdominal organs from pressing against the inflamed pancreas.	Does positioning promote comfort?

Nursing Diagnosis: *Ineffective Breathing Pattern* related to abdominal pressure and pain
Expected Outcome: The patient will have effective breathing pattern evidenced by unlabored respirations, 12 to 20 per minute and oxygen saturation (SaO_2) 94% or greater at all times.
Evaluation of Outcome: Are respirations unlabored and 12 to 20 per minute, and is SaO_2 94% or greater?

Intervention	Rationale	Evaluation
Observe patient's breathing pattern, including respiration depth, regularity, rate, effort, and distress, such as use of accessory muscles or intercostal muscles or SaO_2 less than 94%.	Abdominal pressure from inflammation and tissue damage under the diaphragm may cause patient to take shallow, rapid respirations, which can tire the patient.	Are patient's respirations 12 to 20 per minute, unlabored, and regular?
Administer oxygen as ordered.	Oxygen increases the SaO_2.	Is SaO_2 94% or greater?
Place patient in an upright or slightly forward-leaning position.	Relieves pressure on the diaphragm.	Is positioning effective?

Cancer of the Pancreas

Pancreatic cancer is the fourth-leading cause of cancer deaths in the United States, killing more than 46,000 people each year with an estimated 48,220 deaths in 2021 (American Cancer Society [ACS], 2021). More than 60,000 new cases of cancer of the pancreas are projected to be diagnosed in 2022 and more than 49,000 will die (ACS, 2021).

Pathophysiology

Most primary tumors of the pancreas are ductal adenocarcinomas. They occur in the exocrine (digestive secretion) parts of the pancreas. Exocrine tumors are discussed in this section because neuroendocrine pancreatic tumors are less common. The tumors in the head and body of the pancreas tend to be large. Cancer of the pancreas spreads rapidly by direct extension to the stomach, gallbladder, and duodenum. Cancer located in the body of the pancreas usually spreads farther and more rapidly than do masses in the head. Cancer of the pancreas may spread by the lymphatic and vascular systems to distant organs and lymph nodes.

Etiology

The cause of pancreatic cancer is associated most commonly with smoking followed by dietary factors (obesity, diet, coffee and alcohol intake). Other associated risk factors include work exposure to chemicals used in dry cleaning and metal industries, physical inactivity, diabetes mellitus, chronic pancreatitis, cirrhosis, *Helicobacter pylori* infection, and heredity. Prevention includes eating high-folate and lycopene fruits and vegetables and avoiding risk factors such as smoking.

Signs and Symptoms

The patient with early pancreatic cancer often does not experience signs or symptoms. When signs or symptoms appear, the cancer may have already metastasized. Epigastric or back pain, anorexia, nausea, fatigue, and malaise are early symptoms. Weight loss is the classic sign of pancreatic cancer. The patient may report abdominal pain that is worse at night. The pain is described as gnawing or boring, and it radiates to the back. The pain may be lessened by a side-lying position with the knees drawn up to the chest or by bending over when walking. The pain becomes increasingly severe and unrelenting as the cancer grows. Depression may be experienced. The patient may report a bloated feeling or fullness after eating. If the cancer obstructs the bile duct, the patient may have jaundice, pruritus, dark urine, and light-colored stools. The patient's health history may include a recent diagnosis of diabetes mellitus.

Complications

Complications may occur before or after surgical treatment. Preoperative complications include malnutrition, spread of the cancer, and gastric or duodenal obstruction. Postoperative complications include pneumonia or atelectasis, paralytic ileus, infection, breakdown of the surgical site, fistula formation, diabetes mellitus, kidney failure, and malabsorption syndrome.

Thrombophlebitis is a common complication of pancreatic cancer. As the tumor grows, by-products of the growth increase the levels of thromboplastic (clotting) factors in the blood, making clotting easier. Potential for thrombophlebitis increases if patient is on bedrest or has surgery.

Diagnostic Tests

Serum ALP, glucose, and bilirubin levels may be elevated. Amylase and lipase levels are elevated if the cancer has caused secondary pancreatitis. Blood coagulation tests, such as clotting time, are done. Carbohydrate antigen 19-9 (CA 19-9) is a tumor marker present with most pancreatic cancers. CA 19-9 can be used to monitor treatment and progression of the cancer.

CT, MRI, positron emission tomography scan (PET—radioactive material collects in cancer cells and a special camera detects the cancer cells), or ultrasonography are done to precisely locate masses in the pancreas. ERCP can be used to visualize the common ducts and to take tissue samples for microscopic analysis. Pancreatic biopsy is necessary for definitive diagnosis of pancreatic cancer. A tissue sample may be obtained by needle aspiration during ultrasonography. Staging of the cancer with **laparoscopy** and biopsy can be done to guide treatment options.

Therapeutic Measures

The prognosis for pancreatic cancer can be poor because most cases are diagnosed after the cancer has already spread. If diagnosed early enough, surgical treatment may provide a cure. If the patient's cancer has metastasized, treatment eases symptoms and provides comfort.

Curative (if all the cancer can be removed) or palliative surgery can be used. Patients generally have the best surgical outcomes when the tumor is located at the head of the pancreas. The Whipple procedure (pancreatoduodenectomy), a very complex surgery, is the most common for exocrine pancreatic cancer. This surgery removes the head of the pancreas, lymph nodes nearby, the common bile duct, the gallbladder, most of the duodenum, and parts of the stomach (Fig. 35.6). This can be done as an open or laparoscopic surgery. Postoperative problems include failure of the suture lines to hold, causing leakage of pancreatic enzymes and bile into the abdomen and other postoperative problems listed earlier in the complications section.

A distal **pancreatectomy** (removal of the tail and/or part of the pancreas body) and removal of the spleen are done for tumors in the tail of the pancreas. Also less common is a total pancreatectomy with removal of the gallbladder, a portion of the stomach, small intestine, and the spleen. However, there are more side effects with this procedure, and insulin and digestive enzymes must be used for life.

Relief of biliary obstruction can sometimes be accomplished by implanting a stent or plastic tube in the common

• **WORD • BUILDING** •

laparoscopy: laparo—pertaining to flank + scopy—to examine
pancreatectomy: pancreat—pancreas + ectomy—excision

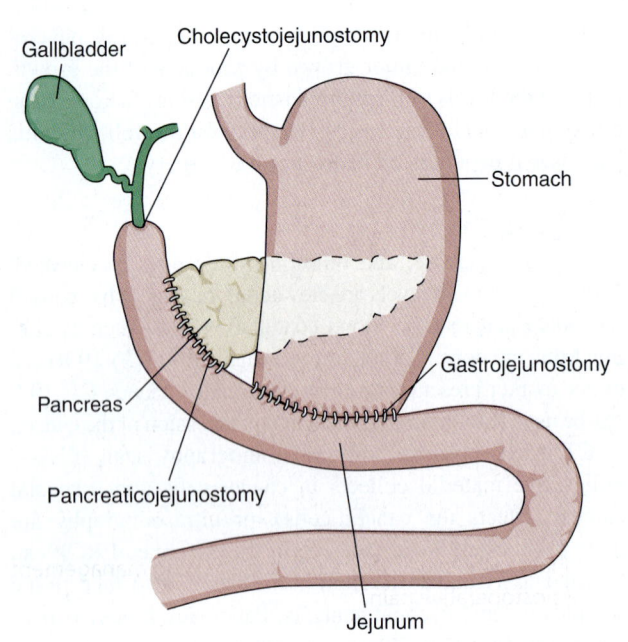

FIGURE 35.6 Pancreatoduodenectomy (Whipple procedure) for cancer of the head of the pancreas.

bile duct during an endoscopic procedure. Pain can be reduced by chemical or surgical destruction of the celiac plexus group of nerves.

Palliative surgery such as stent placement or bypass surgery for a blocked bile duct is used to promote comfort. Chemotherapy, immune therapy, and/or radiation therapy can be used to shrink or destroy the tumor, prevent metastasis, or provide symptom relief if cancer has become too widespread for surgery. (See Chapter 11 for care of patient having radiation or chemotherapy.)

Nursing Process for the Patient With Pancreatic Cancer

DATA COLLECTION. Observe the patient with cancer of the pancreas for evidence of malnutrition and fluid imbalance, including weight loss, inelastic skin turgor, nausea and vomiting, and fatty stools. Review laboratory tests, especially blood glucose, liver function studies, and clotting studies. Monitor the patient for pain. Observe the skin for bruising, scaling, and yellowing, and ask about itching. Evaluate the patient's mental status for evidence of depression.

NURSING DIAGNOSES, PLANNING, AND IMPLEMENTATION. The patient with cancer of the pancreas will have numerous problems. Interventions for the nursing diagnoses *Imbalanced Nutrition: Less Than Body Requirements* (related to inability to digest food, anorexia, nausea, and vomiting) and *Acute Pain* (related to pancreatic tumor or surgical incision) are the same as for patients with pancreatitis (see "Nursing Care Plan for the Patient With Acute and Chronic Pancreatitis" and "Nursing Process for the Patient with Acute and Chronic Pancreatitis"). Additional care is listed next. Interventions for patients with cancer, including psychosocial interventions, can be found in Chapter 11.

Risk for Deficient Fluid Volume related to nausea and vomiting

EXPECTED OUTCOME: The patient will have adequate fluid volume as evidenced by stable vital signs, elastic skin turgor, and moist mucous membranes.

- Monitor the patient's intake and output, skin turgor and mucous membranes. *Low intake increases risk of deficient fluid volume which is reflected in skin turgor and mucous membrane hydration; low output is a sign of deficient fluid.*
- Monitor vital signs and report abnormal findings. *Tachycardia, tachypnea, and low blood pressure may indicate excessive fluid loss.*
- Monitor laboratory values and report abnormal values, especially serum electrolytes. *If electrolyte values are low, the HCP may order IV replacement solutions.*

Risk for Impaired Tissue Integrity related to itching

EXPECTED OUTCOME: The patient's skin will remain intact.

- Monitor the patient for reports of itching *because scratching can cause a break in the skin.*
- Provide frequent skin care with products free of soap or alcohol *to prevent further dryness and itching.*
- Apply products such as calamine lotion as ordered *to decrease itching.*

EVALUATION. The plan of care for the patient with pancreatic cancer is successful if the patient maintains body weight within 5% of normal body weight and experiences no nausea or vomiting; states that pain remains tolerable; has urinary output greater than 30 mL/hr, elastic skin turgor, moist mucous membranes, and pulse and blood pressure within 10% of patient's baseline; and has intact skin.

PATIENT EDUCATION. Teach the patient and family self-care measures such as blood glucose monitoring, insulin administration, signs and symptoms of hyperglycemia and hypoglycemia (see Chapter 40), and the regimen for pancreatic enzyme replacement. Instruct the patient on how to manage dressing changes if they are to be discharged with tubes or drains after surgery. The patient and family should know the signs and symptoms of complications to report. A patient being cared for at home should have a referral for hospice care or home health nursing. For more information, visit the National Pancreas Foundation.

DISORDERS OF THE GALLBLADDER

Cholecystitis, Cholelithiasis, and Choledocholithiasis

Gallstones and inflammations of the gallbladder and common bile duct are the most common disorders of the biliary system.

Pathophysiology

Cholecystitis is inflammation of the gallbladder. Acute cholecystitis is a serious response to obstruction of the common bile duct by a stone, resulting in edema and inflammation. Urgent medical treatment is required generally with surgery to prevent gallbladder rupture. Chronic cholecystitis may be the result of repeated attacks of acute cholecystitis or chronic irritation from gallstones. The gallbladder then becomes fibrotic and thickened.

Cholelithiasis, also known as **cholecystolithiasis**, is the formation of gallstones in the gallbladder. The most common composition of gallstones in U.S. patients is cholesterol. **Choledocholithiasis** refers to gallstones within the common bile duct. Gallstones form when bile becomes supersaturated with a substance such as cholesterol. The substance then crystallizes, forming sludge, with continued enlargement to form stones. Another type of gallstone is a pigment stone, which is composed of calcium that forms when free bilirubin combines with calcium.

Etiology and Incidence

CHOLELITHIASIS. Causes of gallstones include aging, heredity (see "Cultural Considerations: Gallbladder Disease"), obesity, stasis of bile, frequent fasting, diabetes mellitus, cirrhosis, pregnancy, estrogen, and other medications. They occur more in women than in men. Stasis may be caused by a decreased gallbladder-emptying rate, partial obstruction in the common duct, or pregnancy. Excessive cholesterol intake combined with sedentary lifestyle is linked to an increased incidence of cholelithiasis, as are hemolytic blood disorders such as sickle cell disease and bowel disorders such as Crohn disease. Very low calorie diets (<800 kcal/day) and gastric bypass surgery are associated with gallstones.

CHOLECYSTITIS. Cholelithiasis is responsible for most cases of cholecystitis, or inflammation of the gallbladder.

Signs and Symptoms

Gallstones are asymptomatic (silent stones) and require no treatment in most people. Signs and symptoms of cholecystitis and cholelithiasis are similar. Signs include evidence of inflammation such as an elevated temperature, pulse, and respirations as well as vomiting. The patient may have a positive Murphy sign, which is the inability to take a deep breath when an examiner's fingers are pressed below the liver margin.

The epigastric pain caused by cholelithiasis may also be called biliary **colic**. The pain is a steady, aching, severe pain in the epigastrium and RUQ that may radiate back to behind the right scapula or to the right shoulder. The pain usually begins suddenly after a fatty meal and generally peaks at 1 hour and lasts less than 6 hours. The diaphoresis, nausea, and vomiting often occur with the pain. If the pain is caused by a stone in the common bile duct (choledocholithiasis), the pain may last until the stone has passed into the duodenum. Jaundice is more commonly present with acute choledocholithiasis because the common bile duct is blocked or inflamed.

> ### CRITICAL THINKING & CLINICAL JUDGMENT
>
> **Donna Stewart,** a 48-year-old woman, is suspected of having acute cholecystitis. She is 5 feet, 4 inches tall and weighs 188 pounds. After testing, the HCP recommends surgery.
>
> **Critical Thinking (The Why)**
> 1. Why was Donna at risk for developing cholecystitis?
> 2. Donna tells you that her pain started after she ate a cheeseburger with bacon on it. Why would she have pain associated with her meal?
> 3. Why would the HCP want to perform a laparoscopic cholecystectomy versus an open cholecystectomy?
>
> **Clinical Judgment (The Do)**
> 4. What teaching will you reinforce about the type of diet Donna must eat after discharge?
> 5. What teaching will you reinforce regarding management of postoperative pain?
>
> *Suggested answers are at the end of the chapter.*

The biliary colic caused by cholecystitis typically lasts 4 to 6 hours. Pain is worse with movement such as breathing. Heartburn, indigestion, and flatulence are common with chronic cholecystitis. Patients often report repeated attacks of acute cholecystitis symptoms (Table 35.6).

Complications

Complications of cholecystitis include acute cholangitis (inflammation of the bile ducts), necrosis or perforation of the gallbladder, fistulas, and adenocarcinoma of the gallbladder. A major complication of choledocholithiasis is AP if the pancreatic duct is obstructed.

Diagnostic Tests

An ultrasound of the gallbladder is the classic test done to detect stones, inflamed walls of the gallbladder, and dilated ducts. An endoscopic ultrasound can provide more detailed images of the gallbladder and bile ducts. Other tests include a CT magnetic resonance cholangiopancreatography (MRCP), or ERCP that directly visualizes the pancreatic ducts and bile ducts for the presence of stones to remove them. If ultrasonography is inconclusive, cholescintigraphy (hepatobiliary iminodiacetic acid [HIDA]) scan can be done. The patient is given IV injection of a radioactive isotope that is metabolized by the liver and excreted in the bile. The camera traces the path of the isotope through the bile ducts, gallbladder, and intestines to identify blockages.

The patient may have an elevated WBC count (normal: 5,000–10,000 cells/mm^3). If direct bilirubin is elevated

• **WORD • BUILDING** •

cholecystitis: chole—bile + cyst—bladder + itis—inflammation
cholelithiasis: chole—bile + lith—stone + iasis—condition
choledocholithiasis: chole—bile + docho—duct + lith—stone + iasis—condition
colic: colic—spasm

Table 35.6
Symptoms of Gallbladder Disorders

	Acute Cholecystitis	Chronic Cholecystitis	Cholelithiasis and Choledocholithiasis
Biliary colic	Lasts 4–6 hours Worse with movement	Only during acute attack	Sudden onset Lasts 1–3 hours Radiates to right scapula or shoulder
Jaundice	Present (if common bile duct is inflamed or blocked)	Present	
Low-grade fever	Present	Present	Present
Nausea, vomiting	Present	Only during acute attack	Present
Heartburn, indigestion, and flatulence	Not present	Present	Not present
Complications	Cholangitis Necrosis or perforation Fistulas	Empyema Fistulas Adenocarcinoma	Acute pancreatitis

> **Nutrition Notes**
>
> **Modifying the Diet for Patients With Gallbladder Disease**
>
> During an acute attack of cholecystitis, the patient may experience RUQ or epigastric pain following a large meal. For treatment of chronic cholecystitis, caused by gallstones, the patient is taught to:
>
> - Lose weight gradually, if needed, and then maintain an ideal body weight.
> - Eat a high-fiber diet with complex carbohydrates (whole grains, fruits, and vegetables), and limit simple carbohydrates (white bread, white rice, sugars).
> - Eat healthy fats, such as low-fat dairy products, lean meats, healthy monounsaturated fats (avocado and nuts), and polyunsaturated fats (vegetable oils and fish).
>
> After a cholecystectomy, a balanced low-fat, plant-based diet is often well tolerated.
>
> Reference: Barnard, N. D. (2018). Cholelithiasis. Nutrition guide for clinicians (3rd ed.). Physicians Committee for Responsible Medicine, 2018. https://nutritionguide.pcrm.org/nutritionguide/view/Nutrition_Guide_for_Clinicians/1342013/all/Cholelithiasis.

(normal: less than 0.3 mg/dL), its cause is likely obstruction in the biliary or liver areas. Liver enzymes can rise from hepatic inflammation. Serum amylase and lipase levels may be elevated if the pancreas is involved or if there is a stone in the common duct.

Therapeutic Measures

Treatment of an acute episode of cholecystitis centers on pain control with analgesics, prevention of infection, and maintenance of fluid and electrolyte balance. For some patients, bile acid dissolution agents such as ursodiol (Actigall) can be given to dissolve noncalcified cholesterol gallstones. For itching relief with jaundice from bile acid deposits in the skin, colestipol (Colestid) or cholestyramine (Questran, LoCholest) is given (see Table 35.5). If the patient has nausea and vomiting, an antiemetic may be ordered (see Table 35.5). See "Nutrition Notes: Modifying the Diet for Patients With Gallbladder Disease."

SURGERY. Treatment for cholelithiasis typically involves cholecystectomy (surgical removal of gallbladder) via laparoscopy through four small puncture wounds in the abdomen. Choledochoscopy (using endoscope) may also be used to view the common bile duct to prevent retained stones there. Patients are usually discharged within 24 hours. Laparoscopic surgery reduces recovery time.

For large stones or an infected gallbladder, a traditional open cholecystectomy may be required. A T-tube may be inserted into the common duct to ensure that bile drainage is not obstructed (Fig. 35.7). T-tube drainage is around 300 to 500 mL the first day and decreases to less than 200 mL by the third or fourth day. The patient with a traditional cholecystectomy has incisional pain that creates difficulty with coughing and deep breathing postoperatively. Patients are hospitalized for 2 to 3 days with a traditional cholecystectomy.

MEDICATION. Dissolution of small noncalcified (primarily cholesterol) stones (less than 1.5 cm) with a bile acid dissolution agent (see Table 35.5) is used for those who are not surgical candidates. Treatment with a dissolution medication may take up to 2 years, and stones often return.

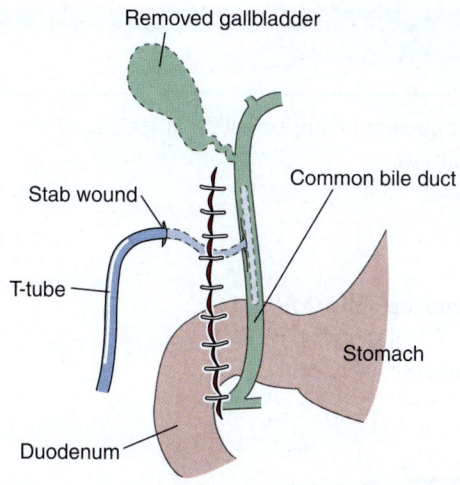

Chapter 35 Nursing Care of Patients With Liver, Pancreatic, and Gallbladder Disorders

FIGURE 35.7 T-tube to drain bile after a cholecystectomy until swelling of the duct subsides.

Evaluate laboratory studies for elevation in the WBC count or abnormalities in electrolytes or serum bilirubin levels. Weigh the patient and inspect mucous membranes, skin turgor, and urinary output for signs of dehydration. Measure intake and output, including emesis or drainage from T-tubes. Observe stools and urine for color and consistency. Obstruction of bile may result in stools that are clay-colored or have a foul, greasy appearance or in urine that is amber or tea-colored. Report these findings immediately.

NURSING DIAGNOSES, PLANNING, AND IMPLEMENTATION. Common nursing diagnoses for the patient with cholecystitis include *Acute Pain, Risk for Deficient Fluid Volume,* and *Ineffective Breathing Pattern.*

Acute Pain related to biliary colic

EXPECTED OUTCOME: The patient will rate pain as 2 or less on a 0 to 10 pain scale.

- Monitor the patient frequently for pain *to guide treatment*.
- Administer analgesics as ordered *to reduce pain*.
- Administer antispasmodics or anticholinergics as ordered *for biliary colic*.

Risk for Deficient Fluid Volume related to nausea, vomiting, or excessive tube drainage

EXPECTED OUTCOME: The patient will have adequate fluid volume as evidenced by stable vital signs, elastic skin turgor, and moist mucous membranes at all times.

- Monitor intake and output, daily weights, and skin turgor, and report changes *to monitor fluid balance*.
- Monitor T-tube drainage and record as output. Carefully observe the T-tube drainage unit to prevent kinking of the tubing. *Pressure in the biliary drainage system from poor drainage may greatly increase the patient's pain and the risk for infection.*
- Give antiemetics as ordered *to control nausea and vomiting*.
- Assist with administration of IV fluids and electrolytes as ordered if the patient is on restricted oral intake *to maintain hydration*.

Risk for Ineffective Breathing Pattern related to abdominal incision

EXPECTED OUTCOME: The patient will have effective breathing pattern with respiratory rate of 12 to 20 per minute, that is even and unlabored, and that has depth within normal limits at all times.

- Monitor respiratory rate, depth, and effort, and ability to cough effectively. *The high abdominal incision can cause pain with deep breathing and coughing.*
- Monitor pain and provide analgesics as ordered *to allow the patient to cough without pain.*

Evidence-Based Practice

Clinical Question
Do older adults (>80 years) have poorer outcomes after laparoscopic cholecystectomy compared to younger patients?

Evidence
Twelve studies encompassing 366,522 patients were reviewed. Older adults did have increased complication rates due to more complex gallbladder disease and comorbidities. Laparoscopic cholecystectomy is safe and effective with older adults and should be performed at an earlier stage to minimize poorer outcomes.

Implications for Nursing Practice
Nurses should monitor older adults closely for post-cholecystectomy complications, especially for those with underlying comorbidities.

Reference: Lord, A. C., Hicks, G., Pearce, B., Tanno, L., & Pucher, P. H. (2019). Safety and outcomes of laparoscopic cholecystectomy in the extremely elderly: A systematic review and meta-analysis. *Acta Chirurgica Belgica, 119*(6), 349–356. https://doi.org/10.1080/00015458.2019.1658356.

CUE RECOGNITION 35.2

Mrs. Garcia had an open cholecystectomy and was admitted to the surgical unit. When you gather data, you notice her respiratory rate is normal, but respirations are shallow. What do you do?

Suggested answers are at the end of the chapter.

Nursing Process for the Patient With a Gallbladder Disorder

DATA COLLECTION. Monitor the patient for pain using **WHAT'S UP?** questions. Take the patient's vital signs, particularly temperature, frequently to monitor for signs of infection.

Table 35.7
Cholecystitis Summary

Signs and Symptoms	Biliary colic: Epigastric/right upper quadrant pain, especially after a fatty meal Elevated temperature, pulse, respirations Jaundice if common bile duct blocked
Diagnostic Tests	Ultrasound, endoscopic ultrasound CT scan Magnetic resonance cholangiopancreatography (MRCP) Endoscopic retrograde cholangiopancreatography (ERCP) Cholescintigraphy (hepatobiliary iminodiacetic acid [HIDA]) White blood cell count elevated
Therapeutic Measures	Pain control Laparoscopic or open cholecystectomy Medications (see Table 35.5) Low-fat diet
Priority Nursing Diagnoses	*Acute Pain* *Risk for Ineffective Breathing Pattern* *Risk for Deficient Fluid Volume*

- Encourage the patient, as taught before surgery, to cough and deep breathe hourly while awake. *Deep breathing and coughing after any surgical procedure help prevent atelectasis and respiratory tract infections.*
- Assist the patient with splinting the abdomen when coughing *to make coughing less painful.*

EVALUATION. The plan of care for a patient with cholecystitis or cholelithiasis is successful if the patient reports tolerable pain not greater than 2 on a pain scale of 0 to 10, no weight loss, no excessive thirst, and urinary output greater than 30 mL/hour; has moist mucous membranes, elastic skin turgor, and intact skin with no warmth, redness, swelling, or purulent drainage at the wound site; no jaundice or itching; clear breath sounds; and a normal WBC count (Table 35.7).

PATIENT EDUCATION. Discharge education focuses on a high-protein, low-fat diet. Obese patients are encouraged to lose weight. After cholecystectomy, fat should be slowly reintroduced into the diet. Once the duodenum becomes accustomed to constant infusion of bile, the patient's tolerance for fat intake guides food choices.

Key Points

- Hepatitis is inflammation of the liver resulting from viral or bacterial infection; medications, alcohol, or chemicals toxic to the liver; and metabolic or vascular disorders. Symptoms of hepatitis range from no symptoms to life-threatening symptoms due to death of liver tissue.
- Hepatitis A, hepatitis B, and hepatitis C (highest number) are the most common types of viral hepatitis in the United States. Nursing interventions focus on pain management, nutrition, preventing further liver damage, and reinforcing education to the patient to manage the disease.
- Acute liver failure is a rare but serious condition that can develop rapidly, sometimes in just 2 days. When the liver is severely damaged, its many functions are impaired. The outcome of the disease may be decided within 48 to 72 hours of diagnosis. Possible outcomes are liver recovery, need for liver transplantation, or death.
- Cirrhosis is the progressive replacement of healthy liver tissue with scar tissue. It is usually irreversible unless the cause is identified and treated early. Common causes of cirrhosis are chronic alcohol use, chronic hepatitis B and C, or NASH.
- Complications of cirrhosis include blood clotting defects, portal hypertension, ascites, hepatic encephalopathy, esophageal varices, and hepatorenal syndrome. The patient with end-stage liver failure may be considered for a liver transplant.
- Cancer of the liver usually results from metastasis from a primary cancer such as the esophagus, lungs, breast, stomach, colon, pancreas, kidney, bladder, or skin.
- Acute pancreatitis (inflammation and infection of the pancreas) is most commonly associated with heavy alcohol consumption or cholelithiasis.
- Chronic pancreatitis is a progressive fibro-inflammatory disease in which functioning pancreatic tissue is replaced with fibrotic tissue because of inflammation. Pancreatic ducts become obstructed, dilated, and finally, atrophied.

Chapter 35 Nursing Care of Patients With Liver, Pancreatic, and Gallbladder Disorders

- Pancreatic cancer usually has spread before it is diagnosed. The prognosis is poor. Surgery is used as curative or palliative.
- Cholecystitis is inflammation of the gallbladder. Acute cholecystitis is a serious response to obstruction of the common bile duct by a stone, resulting in edema and inflammation. Urgent medical treatment is required with surgery to prevent gallbladder rupture.
- Chronic cholecystitis may be the result of repeated attacks of acute cholecystitis or chronic irritation from gallstones. The gallbladder then becomes fibrotic and thickened and does not empty easily or completely.
- Cholelithiasis is formation of gallstones in the gallbladder. The most common composition of gallstones in U.S. patients is cholesterol. Treatment involves laparoscopic or open cholecystectomy.

SUGGESTED ANSWERS TO CHAPTER EXERCISES

Cue Recognition

35.1: You gather more data, including vital signs and intake and output for the past 24 hours and his current medications, such as any diuretics. Then you notify the HCP of the data you have collected, which indicates excess fluid and/or worsening of Mr. Pom's ascites.

35.2: With an open cholecystectomy, the incision in high on the right side of the abdomen, and deep respirations can cause pain. You will need to adequately medicate Mrs. Garcia for postoperative pain and have her splint her incision, and then ensure that she completes turn, cough, and deep breathing exercises and uses her incentive spirometer every hour.

Critical Thinking & Clinical Judgment

Carl Young

1. During your data collection, foreign travel within the past 2 months, eating raw oysters, fatigue, nausea, and irritability suggest hepatitis A virus infection. Other data of recent possible exposure to materials contaminated with blood or body fluids and fatigue, headache, and nausea suggest hepatitis B virus infection.
2. Ensure careful hand hygiene and standard precautions when handling body fluids or feces.
3. You should reinforce teaching that any medication that is known to be hepatotoxic, such as acetaminophen, aspirin, and diazepam (Valium), should be avoided.
4. You will collaborate with infectious disease HCP, dietitian for nutritional needs, and social worker for financial information during recovery period.
5. You should teach Carl that cleanliness, especially with food preparation, is essential; that he should avoid eating raw oysters or raw or undercooked shellfish; that frequent hand washing is crucial; and that alcohol and other liver-toxic substances should be avoided. You reinforce teaching about therapeutic measures such as hydration, nutrition, rest, and any medications the HCP orders.

Mrs. Conner

1. Mrs. Conner has a history of poor nutrition, is overweight, and has diabetes. These factors put her at risk for fatty liver disease and cirrhosis.
2. The liver is damaged with cirrhosis and is unable to synthesize protein (albumin) or prothrombin. Low levels of albumin lead to edema and ascites. Patients bleed more easily with prolonged PT.
3. You will reinforce teaching Mrs. Conner that esophageal varices and ascites are the two greatest concerns for the patient with portal hypertension.
4. You will reinforce teaching Mrs. Conner that the HCP will usually order diuretics, a sodium-restricted diet, restricted fluids, and possibly IV albumin infusions. You will reinforce teaching as you complete the orders and allow for any questions about her care.
5. You will collaborate with the HCP about Mrs. Conner's health needs related to cirrhosis and comorbidities. You will collaborate with the dietitian to manage diabetes and cirrhosis.

Mrs. Samuels

1. The most common cause of AP is heavy alcohol intake. Mrs. Samuels reports no alcohol consumption, but she does have the risk factor of having had a recent ERCP, which may have dislodged a gallstone or irritated the pancreatic duct.
2. Pancreatitis may cause erosion of major blood vessels in surrounding tissue.
3. Serum amylase rises quickly and then returns to normal in 3 to 5 days. Serum lipase is thought to be more specific for AP and elevates and stays elevated for 8 to 14 days.
4. You will medicate Mrs. Samuels with opioids. Opioids are ordered because pain is intense, and pain with anxiety stimulates the autonomic nervous system, which may stimulate greater production of pancreatic enzymes. You will place Mrs. Samuels in her position of comfort, usually semi-Fowler.
5. You will reinforce teaching that oral nutrition will be used if Mrs. Samuels can tolerate it. If she cannot, enteral nutrition will be used until symptoms (pain) are resolved. Parenteral nutrition will be used only if she cannot tolerate either oral or enteral feedings.

Donna Stewart

1. Donna is at risk due to aging and obesity.
2. Gallstones can cause blockage of bile, which is needed for fat digestion. When Donna ate a high-fat meal, the gallbladder was stimulated to release bile, which was blocked by the stones. This led to pain after a high-fat meal.

SUGGESTED ANSWERS TO CHAPTER EXERCISES—cont'd

3. Laparoscopic surgery is preferred because patients are usually discharged within 24 hours after surgery, and recovery time is reduced compared to an open cholecystectomy.
4. You will reinforce teaching Donna that she must eat a low-fat diet after discharge. Eventually, she may be able to add more fats to her diet as her body adjusts to the loss of the gallbladder.
5. You will reinforce the need to take prescribed analgesics to help manage pain and aid in her postoperative recovery and ensure adequate breathing postoperatively.

Additional Resources

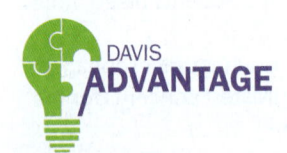

Go to Davis Advantage to complete your learning: strengthen understanding, apply your knowledge, and prepare for the Next Gen NCLEX®.

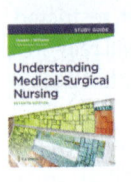

A Study Guide is also available.

UNIT NINE Understanding the Urinary System

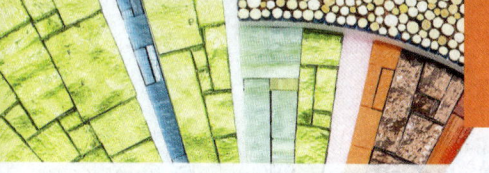

CHAPTER 36

Urinary System Function, Data Collection, and Therapeutic Measures

Maureen McDonald, Janice L. Bradford

KEY TERMS

azotemia (AY-zoh-TEE-me-ah)
cystoscopy (sis-TAH-skuh-pee)
dysuria (dis-YOO-ree-ah)
hematuria (HEE-muh-TOOR-ee-ah)
incontinence (in-CON-tin-ense)
nephrotoxic (NEF-row-TOK-sik)
nocturia (knock-TOO-ree-ah)
percutaneously (PUR-kyoo-TAY-nee-us-lee)
polyuria (pa-lee-YOO-ree-ah)
pyelogram (PIE-eh-loh-gram)

CHAPTER CONCEPTS

Caring
Elimination
Teaching and learning

LEARNING OUTCOMES

1. Identify the normal anatomy of the urinary system.
2. Describe the normal function of the urinary system.
3. Discuss the effects of aging on the urinary system.
4. Explain data to collect when caring for a patient with a disorder of the urinary system.
5. Plan preparation and postprocedure care for patients undergoing diagnostic tests of the urinary system.
6. Plan nursing care for patients with incontinence.
7. Discuss nursing actions to decrease the risk of infection in urinary catheterized patients.

NORMAL URINARY SYSTEM ANATOMY AND PHYSIOLOGY

The urinary system consists of two kidneys and two ureters, the urinary bladder, and the urethra. The kidneys form urine, and the rest of the system eliminates the urine. The purpose of urine formation is the removal of potentially toxic waste products from the blood; however, the kidneys have other equally important functions as well:

- Regulation of blood volume, pressure, and composition by excretion or conservation of water
- Regulation of the electrolyte balance of the blood by excretion or conservation of minerals
- Regulation of the acid–base balance of the blood by the excretion or conservation of ions such as hydrogen or bicarbonate
- Production of erythropoietin, which stimulates erythrocyte production in the bone marrow
- Activation of vitamin D, which maintains bone health

The process of urine formation helps maintain the normal composition, volume, and pH of blood and tissue fluid.

Kidneys

The bilateral kidneys are located against the posterior wall of the abdominal cavity. They are retroperitoneal. The superior portions of both kidneys rest on the inferior surface of the diaphragm; these portions are protected by the lower rib cage. The kidneys are cushioned by surrounding adipose tissue. This tissue is covered by a fibrous connective membrane, the renal fascia. On the medial surface of each kidney is an indentation, the hilus, where the renal artery enters and the renal vein and ureter emerge. The ureter carries urine from the kidney to the urinary bladder.

Internal Structure of the Kidney
A frontal section of the kidney shows three areas: the cortex, medulla, and pelvis (Fig. 36.1).

Blood Vessels of the Kidney
The pathway of blood flow through the kidney is an essential part of the process of urine formation. Blood enters the kidney from the renal artery and exits through the renal vein. Extensive branching within the kidney eventually leads arterial blood to each afferent arteriole. This vessel begins the microcirculation at the *nephron*, the functional unit of the kidney. The exchanges that take place in the capillaries of the nephrons form urine from blood plasma.

Nephrons
Urine is formed in the approximately 1 million nephrons per kidney. The two major parts of a nephron are the renal corpuscle with glomerulus and the renal tubule with peritubular capillaries (Fig. 36.2). These are the two sites of exchange between blood plasma and urinary filtrate within the nephron. All parts of the renal tubule are surrounded by the peritubular capillaries. The capillaries arise from the efferent arteriole and receive the materials reabsorbed by the renal tubules.

Formation of Urine
Urine formation involves three processes: glomerular filtration, tubular reabsorption, and tubular secretion.

Glomerular Filtration
In glomerular filtration, blood pressure forces water and small solutes out of the glomeruli and into Bowman capsules. This fluid is called *renal filtrate* (Fig. 36.3).

Tubular Reabsorption and Secretion
Exiting the glomerular capsule, renal filtrate enters the renal tubules. Tubular reabsorption is the recovery of useful materials from the renal filtrate and their return to the blood in the peritubular capillaries (Table 36.1). In tubular secretion, substances are actively secreted from the blood in the peritubular capillaries into the filtrate in the renal tubules.

The Kidneys and Acid–Base Balance
Other than exhalation of carbon dioxide by the respiratory system, the kidneys are the organs most responsible for maintaining the normal pH range of blood and tissue fluid. They compensate for the pH changes that are part of normal body metabolism or the result of disease. In acidosis, the kidneys secrete more hydrogen ions into the renal filtrate and return more bicarbonate ions back to the blood. When body fluids become too alkaline, the kidneys return hydrogen ions to the blood and excrete bicarbonate ions in urine.

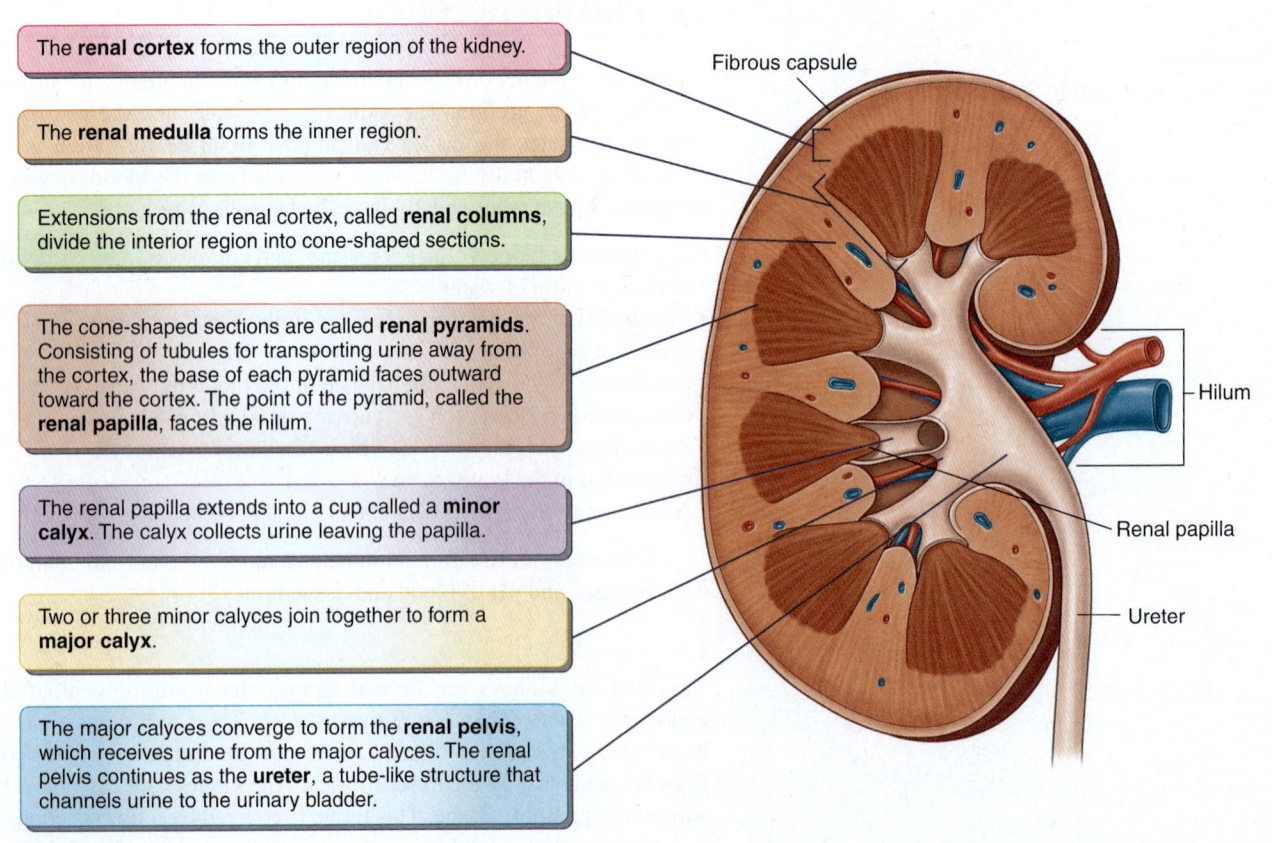

- The **renal cortex** forms the outer region of the kidney.
- The **renal medulla** forms the inner region.
- Extensions from the renal cortex, called **renal columns**, divide the interior region into cone-shaped sections.
- The cone-shaped sections are called **renal pyramids**. Consisting of tubules for transporting urine away from the cortex, the base of each pyramid faces outward toward the cortex. The point of the pyramid, called the **renal papilla**, faces the hilum.
- The renal papilla extends into a cup called a **minor calyx**. The calyx collects urine leaving the papilla.
- Two or three minor calyces join together to form a **major calyx**.
- The major calyces converge to form the **renal pelvis**, which receives urine from the major calyces. The renal pelvis continues as the **ureter**, a tube-like structure that channels urine to the urinary bladder.

Labels on figure: Fibrous capsule, Hilum, Renal papilla, Ureter

FIGURE 36.1 Interior of the kidney.

Chapter 36 Urinary System Function, Data Collection, and Therapeutic Measures

1 In the cortex, a series of **afferent arterioles** arise from the smaller arteries. Each afferent arteriole supplies blood to one nephron.

2 Each afferent arteriole branches into a cluster of capillaries called a **glomerulus**. The glomerulus is enclosed by the glomerular capsule, which will be discussed later in this chapter.

3 Blood leaves the glomerulus through an **efferent arteriole**.

4 The efferent arteriole leads to a network of capillaries around the renal tubules called **peritubular capillaries**. These capillaries pick up water and solutes reabsorbed by the renal tubules.

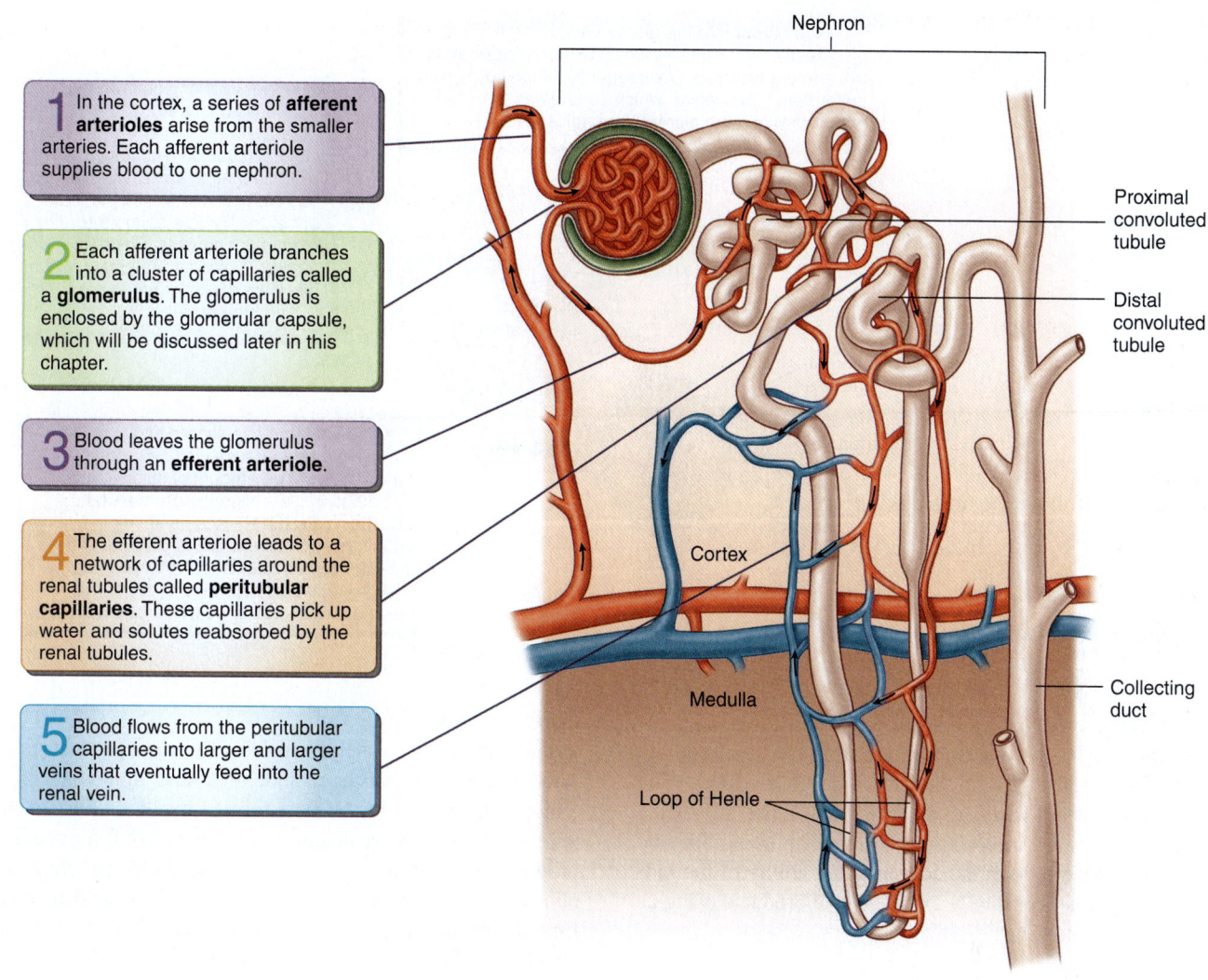

5 Blood flows from the peritubular capillaries into larger and larger veins that eventually feed into the renal vein.

FIGURE 36.2 Nephron.

Elimination of Urine

The ureters, urinary bladder, and urethra do not change the composition or volume of urine but are responsible for its elimination from the body.

Ureters

The ureters are behind the peritoneum of the dorsal abdominal cavity. Each extends from the hilus of a kidney to the lower, posterior side of the urinary bladder. The smooth muscle in the wall of the ureter contracts in peristaltic waves to propel urine toward the urinary bladder. As the bladder fills, it expands and compresses the lower ends of the ureters to prevent urine backflow.

Urinary Bladder and Urethra

The urinary bladder is a muscular sac inside the peritoneum just posterior to the pubic symphysis. In women, the bladder is anterior and inferior to the uterus; in men, the bladder is superior to the prostate gland. The functions of the bladder are the temporary storage of urine and its elimination. The female urethra is a tube about 1.5 inches (4 cm) long that carries urine from the bladder to the small urethral orifice (opening) on the perineum between the clitoris and vagina. The male urethra averages about 8.6 inches (22 cm) long and carries urine from the bladder to the opening at the end of the penis.

Urination Reflex

Urination (micturition) is a spinal cord reflex over which voluntary control may be exerted. Muscles involved include the detrusor of the bladder wall and two urethral sphincters.

Characteristics of Urine

Amount

Normal urinary output is 1,000 to 2,000 mL per 24 hours. Any changes in fluid intake or other fluid output (such as sweating) affect this volume.

Color

The color of urine is referred to as straw or amber. Dilute urine is a light color. Concentrated urine is dark amber and indicates dehydration. Freshly voided urine is normally clear. Cloudy urine may indicate an infection.

FIGURE 36.3 Glomerular filtration.

1. Blood flows into the glomerulus through the afferent arteriole, which is much larger than the efferent arteriole. Consequently, blood flows in faster than it can leave, which contributes to higher pressure within the glomerular capillaries.

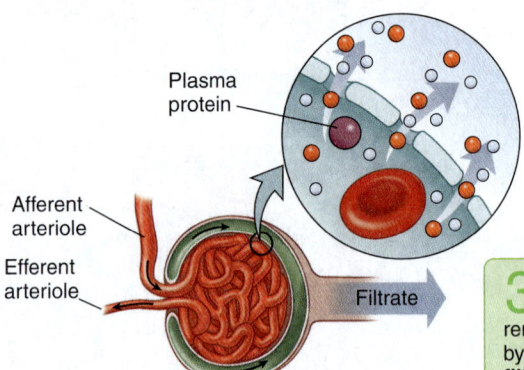

2. The walls of glomerular capillaries are dotted with pores, allowing water and small solutes (such as electrolytes, glucose, amino acids, vitamins, and nitrogenous wastes) to filter out of the blood and into the glomerular capsule. Blood cells and most plasma proteins, however, are too large to pass through the pores.

3. The fluid that has filtered into the glomerular capsule flows into the renal tubules. The amount of fluid filtered by both kidneys—called the **glomerular filtration rate (GFR)**—equals about 180 liters each day, which is 60 times more than the body's total blood volume. The body reabsorbs about 99% of this filtrate, leaving 1 to 2 liters to be excreted as urine.

Specific Gravity

Specific gravity is a measure of the dissolved materials in urine. The specific gravity of urine is 1.005 to 1.030. (The specific gravity of distilled water is 1.000.) The higher the specific gravity, the more dissolved material present. Specific gravity of urine reflects the concentrating ability of the kidneys. They must constantly excrete waste products using as little water as possible.

pH

The pH range of urine is 4.5 to 8.0, with an average of 6.0. Diet has the greatest influence on urine pH. A vegetarian diet results in alkaline urine; a high-protein diet results in acidic urine.

Constituents

Urine is about 95% water, the solvent for waste products and salts. Nitrogenous wastes include urea (and ammonia), creatinine, and uric acid. Urea is formed by liver cells when excess amino acids are deaminated (metabolized) for energy production. Creatinine is a product of metabolism of creatine phosphate, an energy source in muscles. Uric acid results from the metabolism of nucleic acids. Other solutes, such as enzymes and hormones, are present in small quantities.

Aging and the Urinary System

With age, the number of nephrons in the kidneys decreases, often by half by age 70 or 80 (Fig. 36.4). The glomerular filtration rate (GFR) also decreases (see "Gerontological Issues"),

Table 36.1
Effects of Hormones on the Kidneys

Hormone (Gland)	Function
Aldosterone (adrenal cortex)	Promotes reabsorption of sodium ions from the filtrate to the blood and excretion of potassium ions into the filtrate. Water is reabsorbed after the reabsorption of sodium.
Antidiuretic hormone (posterior pituitary)	Promotes reabsorption of water from the filtrate to the blood.
Atrial natriuretic hormone (atria of heart)	Decreases reabsorption of sodium ions, which remain in the filtrate. More sodium and water are eliminated in urine.
Parathyroid hormone (parathyroid glands)	Promotes reabsorption of calcium ions from filtrate to blood and excretion of phosphate ions into filtrate.

Source: Scanlon, V. C., & Sanders, T. (2019). *Essentials of anatomy and physiology* (8th ed.). Philadelphia, PA: F.A. Davis.

owing in part to arteriosclerosis and diminished renal blood flow. The urinary bladder decreases in size, and the tone of the detrusor muscle decreases. These changes may result in the need to urinate more often or in residual urine in the bladder after voiding. Older adults often experience more infections of the urinary tract.

> **Gerontological Issues**
>
> **Age-Related Renal Changes**
> These changes typically occur in the renal system as people age:
> - Decreased filtration efficiency of the kidneys affects the body's ability to eliminate drugs
> - Decreased renal function slows the excretion of certain medications, so they remain in the body longer
>
> Consequently, dehydration, common in older adults, and changes in renal function are a serious consideration for individuals in this age group who need medication therapy. The risk of adverse medication reactions, such as toxicity and overdose, increases. It can be important to monitor kidney function (such as serum creatinine and blood urea nitrogen [BUN] levels) in an older adult receiving medication therapy.

URINARY SYSTEM DATA COLLECTION

Health History

If the patient has impaired kidney function, head-to-toe data collection is needed because kidney disease can affect every system of the body. Table 36.2 describes sample questions to ask for a health history to use along with the **WHAT'S UP?** format (see Chapter 1) for symptoms.

Physical Examination

Table 36.3 lists objective data to collect on all body systems. Many disease states may precipitate kidney disease such as diabetes, gout, hypertension, and neoplasms. Other factors include excessive use of over-the-counter analgesics, infections, or manipulation of the urinary tract during procedures. Key signs and symptoms include costovertebral angle pain, flank pain, **dysuria**, and back and leg pain. The patient may have peripheral edema and periorbital edema in the morning. The skin may be pale, itchy, and dry. Electrolyte abnormalities may cause arrhythmias or seizures. The patient's level of consciousness may be altered, ranging from lethargy to coma. High-frequency deafness may occur with hereditary nephritis. Cardiovascular friction rubs may be heard in uremic patients. The lungs may fill with fluid and crackles heard in the lungs.

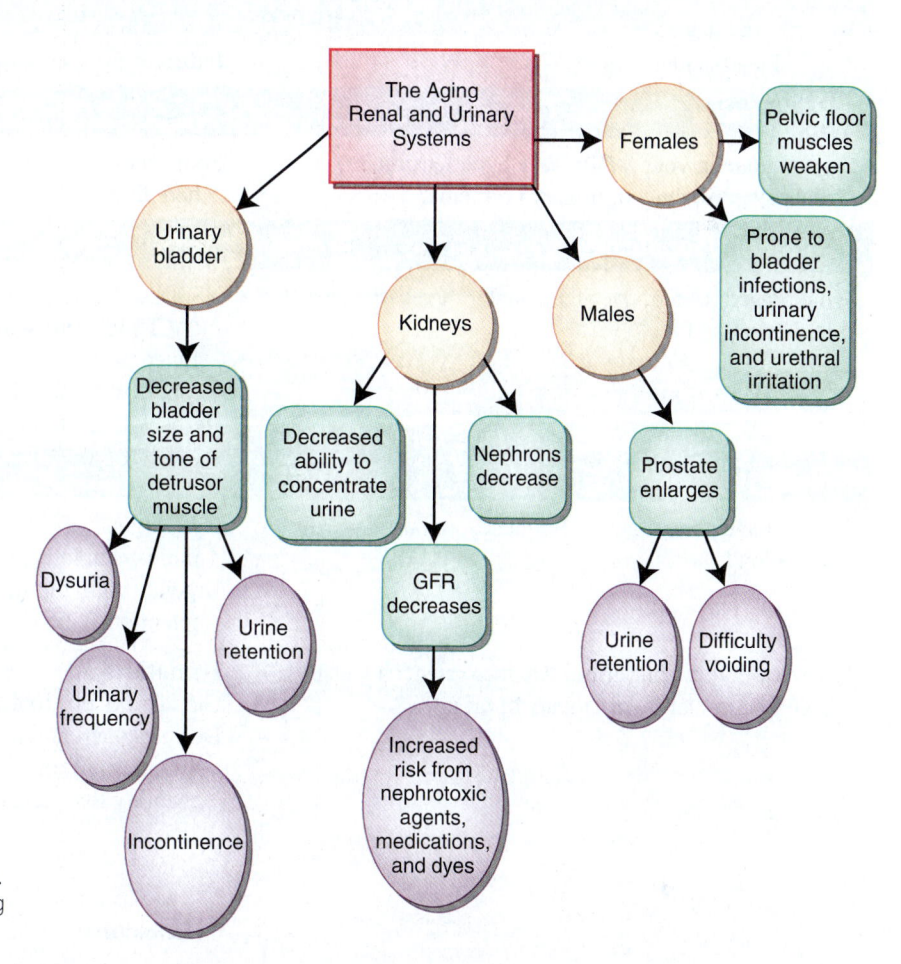

FIGURE 36.4 Aging and the urinary system. This concept map shows effects of the aging process on the urinary system.

Table 36.2
Subjective Data Collection for the Urinary System

Questions to Ask During a Health History	Rationale/Significance
Allergies	
Any allergies to antibiotics, contrast media, or dyes?	Allergies to medications such as antibiotics, contrast media, and dyes can result in impaired kidney function.
Lifestyle Habits	
Do you smoke?	Tobacco use increases risk of bladder cancer.
Occupation	
Any exposure to chemicals in jobs or hobbies?	Exposure to nephrotoxic chemicals can cause cancer (e.g., bladder: arsenic, chemicals to make dyes, leather, rubber, paint, textiles; kidney: cadmium, herbicides, trichloroethylene).
Medical History	
What medical conditions have you been diagnosed with?	Diabetes and hypertension are common causes of chronic kidney disease. Streptococcal infection (strep throat) may precede renal disease. Lupus can cause glomerulonephritis in up to 50% of those with lupus.
Surgical History	
Any kidney/bladder surgery?	Indicates prior conditions to correlate with current condition.
Family History	
Does anyone in your family have hypertension, diabetes, or kidney or urinary problems?	Some causes of renal conditions and renal disorders are hereditary.
Medications/Supplements	
What prescription or over-the-counter medications or herbs do you take?	NSAIDs, vasopressors, and angiotensin-converting enzyme (ACE) inhibitors can impair renal perfusion and kidney function. Nephrotoxic drugs can damage kidneys. Herbs with aristolochic acid may be renal toxic.
Renal/Urinary Issues	
Do you have pain, urgency, frequency, or burning with urination?	Pain, urgency, frequency, or burning with urination can indicate an infection. Urgency with diminished amounts of urine suggests urinary retention.
Is there blood in your urine? Are there any changes in color, odor, clarity, or amount of urine?	**Hematuria** may indicate infection or cancer. Cloudy urine or foul odor indicates possible infection. Decreased amount may indicate renal disease; increased amount (**polyuria**) may indicate diabetes mellitus or inability to concentrate urine.

• WORD • BUILDING •

hematuria: hemat—blood + uria—urine

Table 36.2
Subjective Data Collection for the Urinary System—cont'd

Questions to Ask During a Health History	Rationale/Significance
Do you have difficulty starting urine stream, **nocturia**, incontinence, or a urinary catheter?	Difficulty starting urination may indicate prostate obstruction. Nocturia can occur with loss of kidney's concentrating ability, nephrotic syndrome, diabetes, and heart failure.
Do you have pain in the costovertebral angle (area formed by rib cage and vertebral column)?	Renal calculus (stone) may produce a dull ache in kidney area or colicky pain radiating to genital area or leg on affected side.
Do you have swelling in the ankles or around eyes?	Edema occurs with fluid retention; periorbital edema is noted around eyes in the morning.
Nutrition/Fluid Balance	
Describe your appetite, weight loss/gain, fluid intake, and usual diet.	Anorexia occurs with renal disease. Fluid retention can result in weight gain. Large intake of protein or dairy products may lead to kidney stone formation.

Table 36.3
Objective Data Collection for the Urinary System

Possible Abnormal Findings	Possible Causes
Vital Signs	
Hypertension	Renal disease
Elevated respiratory rate	Fluid volume overload
Irregular heart rate/rhythm	Hyperkalemia; magnesium or calcium imbalance
Level of Consciousness	
Decreased level	Fluid or electrolyte imbalances, urinary tract infection (UTI)
Neurologic	
Diminished deep tendon reflexes, hyperesthesia, paresthesia, peripheral neuropathy	Altered fluid balance; increased urea, creatinine, ammonia, or parathyroid hormone
Skin	
Pallor, yellow or gray	Anemia, chronic kidney disease
Skin crystals (uremic frost)	**Azotemia**
Excoriation	Pruritus, dryness
Poor turgor	Dehydration
Eyes	
Conjunctival pallor	Anemia

Continued

• WORD • BUILDING •

nocturia: nox—night + uria—urine

Table 36.3
Objective Data Collection for the Urinary System—cont'd

Possible Abnormal Findings	Possible Causes
Cardiovascular	
Weight gain	Fluid retention
Edema, jugular vein distention, pulmonary edema	Increased fluid volume, decreased serum albumin
Friction rub	Azotemia resulting in uremic pericarditis
Respiratory	
Shortness of breath, tachypnea, crackles	Fluid volume overload
Kussmaul respirations	Metabolic acidosis seen in renal disease
Hematologic	
Anemia	Decreased erythropoietin production
Bruising, bleeding	Thrombocytopenia
Gastrointestinal	
Uremic fetor (urine breath odor)	Ammonia from urea breakdown
Constipation, diarrhea	Renal disease
Urinary	
Anuria (less than 100 mL urine/24 hours)	Acute or end-stage renal disease
Oliguria (100–400 mL/24 hours)	Severe dehydration, shock, transfusion reaction, end-stage renal disease
Incontinence	Urological or neurologic disease
Polyuria (more than 3 L/24 hours)	Diabetes mellitus, diabetes insipidus, diuretics, caffeine, ethanol, excessive intake, UTI
Musculoskeletal	
Fractures	Bone and mineral disease from low calcium, high phosphorus, decreased activated vitamin D

Daily Weights
Weight is the best indicator of fluid balance in the body. Patients with renal disease often have fluid imbalances. Weigh the patient at the same time each day, in the same or similar clothing, and with the same scale. Look for trends in weight gain or loss. If the patient's daily weight continues to increase, fluid is being retained and should be reported.

Intake and Output
The patient with kidney disease is usually on fluid restriction. Intake and output (I&O) should be carefully measured. Intake includes oral, IV, tube feeding, and other fluids. Output includes urine, emesis, nasogastric effluent, chest tube drainage, wound drainage if it is copious, and any other drainage.

I&O totals are recorded and analyzed usually every 8 to 12 hours or hourly for unstable patients. The nurse notes trends in retention or loss of fluid to report to the healthcare provider (HCP). Accurate documentation is vital. The HCP may prescribe IV fluids and medications based on I&O results.

CLINICAL JUDGMENT
Mr. Nolan is a 74-year-old resident who has a urinary drainage system in place. As you empty Mr. Nolan's urinary drainage bag after 4 hours, you find that it has 50 mL of concentrated urine in it.

1. What data do you collect?
2. What actions do you take?

Suggested answers are at the end of the chapter.

DIAGNOSTIC TESTS FOR THE URINARY SYSTEM

Laboratory Tests

Urine Tests

URINALYSIS. A urinalysis (urine analysis) is a common diagnostic test for kidney disease, the urinary system, and systemic diseases that affect the kidneys (Table 36.4).

A urine specimen for routine analysis may be collected at any time of day; however, the first-morning specimen is best. First-morning specimens are concentrated and more likely to contain abnormal constituents if they are present. The specimen should be examined within 1 hour of collection or refrigerated. Urine standing at room temperature longer than 2 hours has more bacteria present, a change in pH, and hemolysis of red blood cells (RBCs) and should not be used. A random urine specimen collected for cytology should not be a first-morning specimen due to changes in epithelial cells in urine held overnight. If a urinalysis is ordered for a patient with an indwelling urinary catheter, the nurse obtains the sterile urine specimen from the drainage system (see the procedure "Urine Specimen Collection from Urinary Drainage System" on Davis Advantage).

Composite urine specimens (e.g., a 24-hour urine test) are collected usually over 2 to 24 hours; Table 36.5 lists collection steps (also see the procedure "Collecting a 24-hour Urine Specimen" on Davis Advantage). These specimens examine urine for components such as catecholamines, creatinine, electrolytes, glucose, 17-ketosteroids, minerals, protein, and urea nitrogen. These specimens require refrigeration as they are being collected. Preservatives may be added to the collection container for some tests.

> **CUE RECOGNITION 36.1**
>
> You are to obtain a urine specimen from a female patient with hematuria who is on her menses. What action do you take?
>
> *Suggested answers are at the end of the chapter.*

Table 36.4
Urinalysis

Components	Normal Results	Significance of Abnormal Results
Color of urine	Light yellow to deep amber	Dark amber: Dehydration Brown or green: Excessive bilirubin Orange: Use of phenazopyridine (Pyridium) Red or pink: Hemoglobin present Smoky: Hematuria
Appearance	Clear	Cloudiness: Amorphous phosphates, bacteria, blood, fat, white blood cells, urates
Odor of urine	Aromatic	Infection: Foul smell Diabetic ketoacidosis: Fruity odor
pH	4.5 to 8.0	Low pH: Diarrhea, metabolic acidosis, starvation High pH: Infection, renal disease, vomiting
Specific gravity	1.005 to 1.03	Low specific gravity: Diabetes insipidus, excessive fluid intake High specific gravity: Dehydration, heart failure, shock Specific gravity fixed at 1.010: Kidney dysfunction
Protein	Negative; 24-hour urine: 30 to 150 mg	Damage to glomerulus creates persistent proteinuria creating foamy urine; significant sign of renal disease. Intermittent protein results from strenuous exercise, dehydration, or fever. Vaginal secretions can produce a positive reading.
Glucose	Negative	Diabetes mellitus, excessive glucose intake, or low renal threshold for glucose reabsorption
Ketones	Negative	Diabetes mellitus, carb-free diets, dehydration, severe diarrhea, starvation breaks body fats into ketones, vomiting

Continued

Table 36.4
Urinalysis—cont'd

Components	Normal Results	Significance of Abnormal Results
Bilirubin	Negative	Liver disorders that cause jaundice; may appear in the urine before jaundice is visible
Urobilinogen	Up to 1 mg/dL	Increased: Cirrhosis, hemolytic anemia, heart failure, hepatitis, infectious mononucleosis, malaria
Nitrite	Negative	Infection
Leukocyte esterase	Negative	Infection
Red blood cells	Less than 5/hpf (high-power field)	Cancer, infection, kidney stones, renal disease, trauma
White blood cells	Less than 5/hpf	Infection or inflammation
Casts	None to rare	Formation of tube-shaped proteins (molds or casts of the tubule). Indicate renal disease or infection. There are nine types of casts (e.g., hyaline, RBC, WBC, bacterial, fatty) that are reflective of the problem.

Table 36.5
Laboratory Tests for the Urinary System

Test	Definition/Normal Value	Significance of Abnormal Findings
Urine Studies		
Residual urine	Amount of urine left in the bladder after voiding. *Normal value:* Less than 50 mL (increases with age)	Bladder ultrasound determines amount of urine after voiding. Increased residual volume may occur in urethral strictures, sphincter impairment, or neurogenic bladder.
Urine culture and sensitivity (urine C&S)	Identifies number of bacteria or yeast in urine, causative organism of urinary tract infection, and most effective medication to use. *Normal value:* Negative: None. Positive: 100,000 or more/mL of urine.	Urine must be collected before antibiotic treatment begins to avoid altering results. Use of a tampon or catheterized specimen may be ordered to avoid risk of contamination if female patient is menstruating.
Urine volume/24 hr; urine creatinine; urine creatinine clearance	Measures amount of urine creatinine and the amount of creatinine cleared from blood in a specified time (often 24 hr) by comparing amount of creatinine in blood with creatinine in urine. *Normal urine volume*: Adults: 800–2,500 mL (average 1,200 mL) *Normal urine creatinine:* Male: 14–26 mg/kg/24 hr Female: 11–20 mg/kg/24 hr	Creatinine clearance is computed in the laboratory and is expressed in volume of blood that is cleared of creatinine in 1 minute. Minimum creatinine clearance of 10 mL per minute is needed to live without dialysis. Collection key points: To begin the test, patient is directed to urinate and discard the urine (bladder is empty). This time is recorded and becomes the test start time.

Table 36.5
Laboratory Tests for the Urinary System—cont'd

Test	Definition/Normal Value	Significance of Abnormal Findings
	Normal Creatinine Clearance: Male: 85–125 mL/min/1.73 m² Female: 75–115 mL/min/1.73 m² For each decade after 40 years: Decrease of 6–7 mL/min/1.73 m²	All urine voided is collected for 24 hours (or specified time frame) in a large container provided by the laboratory and kept refrigerated or on ice. Remind patient/staff to save all urine for accurate results. Exactly 24 hours after test began, patient is to void again (empty bladder). This urine is added to the container and the test ends.
Urine cytology	Microscopic examination of urine to detect atypical epithelial cells shed from the surface of the urinary tract. Normal value: No abnormal cells or inclusions seen	Used to screen those at high risk for cancer in the urinary system. Atypical cells indicate need for further testing.
Bladder tumor antigen (a bladder cancer marker)	Measurement of a protein produced by bladder tumor cells. Normal value: Negative	Bladder cancer
Nuclear matrix protein 22 (NMP22; a bladder cancer marker)	Measurement of a protein deposited into urine during nuclear disruption (apoptosis) of bladder cells. Normal value: Negative = Less than 6 units/mL	Bladder cancer
Blood Chemistry Studies—Kidney Function		
Blood urea nitrogen (BUN)	Urea is a waste product of protein metabolism that is excreted by the kidneys. Normal value: Adult: 8–21 mg/dL Over age 90: 10–31 mg/dL	Not as sensitive an indicator of kidney function as creatinine level because BUN is affected by increased protein intake, dehydration, and other factors in the body. Elevated level: Kidney disease, shock, severe heart failure, dehydration, high-protein diet, gastrointestinal bleeding, steroid use.
Creatinine	Creatinine is a waste product from muscle metabolism and is steadily released into the bloodstream. Normal value: Male: 0.61–1.21 mg/dL Female: 0.51–1.11 mg/dL	Very good indicator of kidney function. The higher the creatinine level, the more impaired the kidney function.
BUN-to-creatinine ratio	Evaluates hydration status. Normal value: 10:1 to 20:1	An elevated ratio occurs in hypovolemia. A normal ratio with an elevated BUN and creatinine occurs in intrinsic renal disease.
Cystatin C (Cys C)	Proteinase inhibitor produced by all nucleated cells, filtered out of blood by the glomerulus membrane. Marker for kidney damage and monitors function in kidney transplant. Normal value: Age 1 to 50 years: 0.56–0.9 mg/L 50 years and older: 0.58–1.08 mg/L	Cystatin C is a sensitive marker that reflects glomerular filtration rate independent of weight, height, diet, age, gender, and muscle mass. Cystatin C level increases with impaired renal function.

Continued

Table 36.5
Laboratory Tests for the Urinary System—cont'd

Test	Definition/Normal Value	Significance of Abnormal Findings
Uric acid	Uric acid is an end product of purine metabolism and the breakdown of body proteins. It can be used to identify the cause of renal calculi. *Normal value:* Adult male: 4–8 mg/dL Adult female: 2.5–7 mg/dL Male older than 60 years: 4.2–8.2 mg/dL Female older than 60 years: 3.5–7.3 mg/dL	Elevated uric acid levels can be caused by renal disease.
Blood Chemistry Studies		
Albumin	Plasma protein maintaining oncotic pressure in vascular system. *Normal value:* Age 20 to 40 years: 3.7–5.1 g/dL Age 41 to 60 years: 3.4–4.8 g/dL Age 61 to 90 years: 3.2–4.6 g/dL Age older than 90 years: 2.9–4.5 g/dL	Low level occurs in nephrotic syndrome and renal disease and leads to edema.
Bicarbonate (HCO_3^-)	An alkaline ion that indicates status of acid–base system. Reabsorbed and excreted by the kidneys. *Normal value:* Arterial: 22–26 mmol/L	With renal disease, metabolic acidosis and low serum HCO_3^- levels can occur.
Calcium, total (Ca^{2+})	Main mineral stored in bones and teeth. Regulated by vitamin D and parathyroid glands. Aids in muscle contraction, neurotransmission, and blood clotting. *Normal value:* Adult: 8.2–10.2 mg/dL Adult older than 90 years: 8.2–9.6 mg/dL	Decreased in renal disease, causing bone and mineral disease.
Magnesium	Found in bone and intracellularly and excreted by the kidney. *Normal value:* 1.6–2.2 mg/dL	Elevated in chronic renal disease; can result in lethargy, nausea, vomiting, and slurred speech.
Phosphorus	Mineral found in bone, teeth, bloodstream, and cells. Many functions. *Normal value:* 2.5–4.5 mg/dL	Phosphorus balance is inversely related to calcium balance. Increased in renal disease.
Potassium (K^+)	Intracellular electrolyte excreted by kidneys. *Normal value:* 3.5–5.3 mEq/L	In renal disease, K^+ is one of the first electrolytes to become abnormal. Level greater than 6 mEq/L can lead to muscle weakness and cardiac arrhythmias.
Sodium (Na^+)	Extracellular electrolyte related to hydration status. *Normal value:* 135–145 mEq/L	Remains within normal range until late stages of renal disease. Increased with azotemia and dehydration. Decreased with fluid retention (dilutional effect) and nephrotic syndrome. Monitor for seizures with values below 120 or above 160 mEq/L.

Renal Function Tests

Several blood and urine tests reflect kidney function (see Table 36.5). If the kidneys are not filtering adequately, serum values, such as for creatinine and blood urea nitrogen (BUN), will be elevated because they are not excreted. These tests are useful because they provide information about the severity of a patient's kidney disease as well as the response to treatments. Renal function test values may remain within the normal range until the GFR is less than 50% of normal.

Diagnostic Tests

Table 36.6 summarizes diagnostic tests for the urinary system.

Table 36.6
Diagnostic Tests for the Urinary System

Procedure	Uses and Possible Abnormal Findings	Nursing Management
Bladder ultrasound scan	Portable ultrasound instrument computes urine volume, bladder wall thickness, bladder calculi, tumors, diverticula.	Used at the bedside to determine urine retention or postresidual voiding to reduce need for catheterization.
Renal ultrasonography	Congenital disorders of the kidney, abscesses, hydronephrosis, kidney stones or tumors, kidney enlargement, structural changes with chronic infection.	No special preparation or aftercare. No radiation exposure.
Kidney-ureter-bladder x-ray	Renal calculi, kidney size, masses in the kidney.	If done as preliminary study, bowel prep may be done.
Computed tomographic (CT) scan (with/without contrast media)	Uses radiation for imaging: abdominal and pelvic organs, kidneys, ureters, bladder for abscesses, cysts, kidney size, lymph node enlargement, malignant masses, metastases, tumors; nonfunctioning kidneys, obstructions, infections, renal stones.	Identify allergies if contrast media to be used.
Magnetic resonance imaging (MRI) (with/without contrast media)	Staging of cancers of the kidney, bladder, prostate.	Nonradiation imaging of organs using magnetic fields and radio waves.
IV **pyelogram:** X-ray examination of renal tissue, calyces, pelvises, ureters, and bladder with contrast media.	Abnormal size or shape of kidneys, absent kidneys, polycystic kidney disease, tumors, hydronephrosis, renovascular hypertension (Fig. 36.5).	*Precare:* Instructions may include taking a laxative the evening before the test or being NPO after midnight prior to the test. *Postcare:* Monitor urine output.
Renal angiography or arteriogram with contrast media	Visualizes renal blood vessels. Hypervascular tumors, renal cysts, renal artery stenosis, renal artery aneurysms, pyelonephritis, obstructions, renal infarction, renal trauma evaluation. May be used during renal angioplasty.	*Precare:* Laxatives may be given the evening before the test. *Postcare:* Bedrest up to 12 hours to prevent bleeding at injection site. Check distal pulses in leg every 30–60 minutes and monitor vital signs and dressing frequently. *Teach:* Do not bend leg or raise head of bed more than 45 degrees.

Continued

• WORD • BUILDING •

pyelogram: pyelo—pelvis of the kidney + gram—radiograph

Table 36.6
Diagnostic Tests for the Urinary System—cont'd

Nephrotomogram: Series of x-rays with contrast media creating three-dimensional image of the kidney	Renal cysts, tumors, areas of nonperfusion, renal fractures or lacerations following renal trauma.	*Precare:* Laxatives may be given the evening before the test. *Postcare:* Maintain hydration.
Renal scan	Assesses kidneys' ability to perfuse blood and secrete urine. Renovascular hypertension diagnosis; kidney function; renal blood flow; glomerular filtration rate; tubular function; excretion of urine; kidney size and shape; abscesses, cysts, and tumors, which may appear as cold spots because of nonfunctioning kidney tissue. Determination of vascular supply to the kidneys in patients with renal trauma, dissecting aneurysm, and other disorders affecting blood flow to the kidneys.	*Precare:* Determine if patient's medications will interfere with test (NSAIDs or antihypertensives). Patient may be asked to drink two glasses of water before test. If captopril is given, monitor for hypotension.
Renal biopsy	Microscopic examination of kidney tissue for diagnosis or treatment of renal disorder, benign and malignant masses, causes of renal disease, renal transplant rejection, lupus.	*Precare:* NPO 6–8 hours. Mild sedative given. *Postcare:* Vital signs, urine output, and signs of bleeding are monitored. *Teach:* No heavy lifting for 2 weeks.
Cystoscopy and pyelogram: Minor surgical procedure with lighted fiberoptic cystoscope	Diagnostic: Inspect inside of bladder, collect urine specimen from either kidney, take x-rays or biopsy growths. Therapeutic: Remove small bladder tumors, polyps, stones from bladder/ureters; dilation of ureters; treat enlarged prostate or congenital abnormalities.	*Precare:* Surgical preparation. *Postcare:* Measure urine output to detect urine retention from swelling of urinary meatus. Encourage fluid intake. *Teach:* Expect initial voidings to be blood tinged and dysuria to be present for 24 hours.
Cystogram or voiding cystourethrogram: X-ray of bladder/lower urinary tract with contrast media or radioisotope instilled into bladder via catheter or cystoscope	Evaluates bladder filling and emptying. Incomplete bladder emptying, distention, reflux, obstruction to urine outflow identified.	*Precare:* None. *Postcare:* Bright red urine, fever, or persistent discomfort should be reported to HCP. *Teach:* After the scan, can have slight dysuria and pink urine for 1–2 days.

Contrast-Induced Acute Kidney Injury

Contrast media used in diagnostic testing and procedures can be **nephrotoxic** in the presence of risk factors and cause contrast-induced acute kidney injury (CI-AKI) within 48 hours of contrast exposure. CI-AKI is usually asymptomatic, with a decline in renal function as shown by a rise in serum creatinine. Treatment is the same as for acute kidney injury (see Chapter 37).

Risk factors for contrast-induced acute kidney injury are impaired kidney function with a low GFR that may be increased by diabetes. Creatinine levels are checked before the procedure. A risk assessment should be done before testing regarding allergies/allergic reactions, diabetes, kidney

• WORD • BUILDING •

cystoscopy: cysto—bladder + scopy—to examine

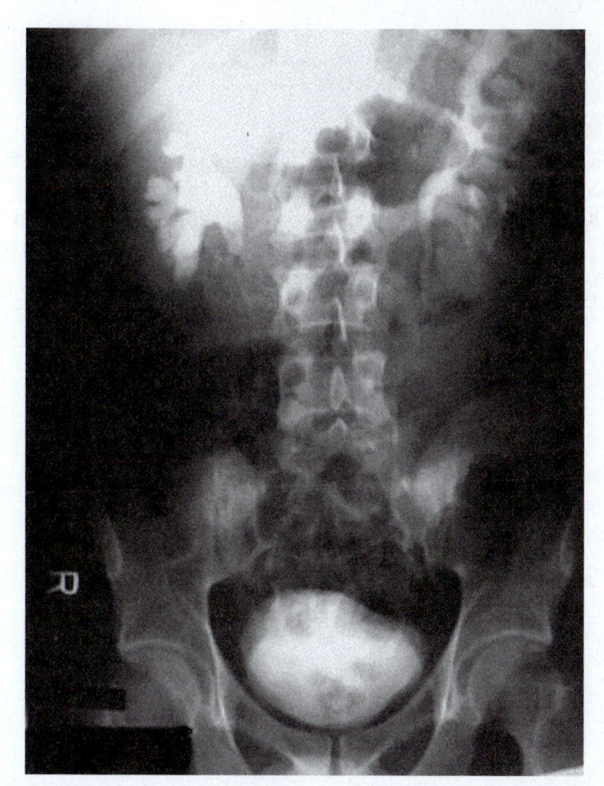

FIGURE 36.5 IV pyelogram x-ray. Contrast media injected intravenously with x-ray images taken as the contrast is excreted by the kidneys.

disease, other medical conditions, and use of oral metformin hydrochloride (Glucophage) and other medications (e.g., anti-inflammatories, antibiotics, antifungals, immunosuppressives). When contrast media are being used for high-risk patients, metformin hydrochloride should not be given before and for 48 hours after administration of the contrast media. Lactic acidosis could develop if acute kidney injury occurs. IV hydration with normal saline is one of the main preventive measures used. Research is being done on the use of statin therapy prior to the injection of contrast media for high-risk patients.

Renal Biopsy

A renal biopsy diagnoses or provides information about kidney disease. A CT scan or ultrasound is done first to locate the kidney. A small section of the renal cortex is obtained for laboratory analysis either **percutaneously** (local anesthetic, needle through skin) or with a small flank incision. Patients with bleeding tendencies, uncontrolled hypertension, or a solitary kidney generally do not undergo renal biopsy. Prior to the biopsy a complete blood count and coagulation studies are obtained. No anticoagulants can be taken. For a biopsy through the flank area, the patient is in the prone position with a sandbag under the abdomen. While the needle is inserted the patient does not breathe, to prevent the kidney from moving. Afterwards, a pressure dressing is applied.

Vital signs and urine output are monitored. Signs of bleeding are reported immediately: grossly bloody urine, falling blood pressure, and increasing pulse.

Nursing Process for Diagnostic Tests of the Urinary System

Identified contraindications to testing are reported to the HCP. The patient's baseline understanding of testing procedures is determined to plan teaching sessions.

Nursing Diagnoses, Planning, and Implementation

Anxiety related to unfamiliar environment, diagnostic test, or health status

EXPECTED OUTCOME: The patient will have reduced anxiety about a procedure or test.

- Encourage the patient to verbalize feelings, concerns, or specific stressors *to develop an individualized coping plan.*
- Maintain a calm, supportive, and confident environment and manner when interacting with the patient *to reduce anxiety.*
- Instruct the patient in relaxation techniques and facilitate their use along with family support *to reduce anxiety.*

Deficient Knowledge related to diagnostic test or procedure and health status

EXPECTED OUTCOME: The patient will report understanding of the diagnostic test or procedure prior to its occurrence.

- Collect data on the patient's understanding of the diagnostic test or procedure *to provide a baseline for teaching.*
- Explain all diagnostic test related activities and correct any misconceptions the patient has *to facilitate trust, reduce anxiety, and promote cooperation.*

Impaired Urinary Elimination related to complications from urinary system diagnostic tests

EXPECTED OUTCOME: The patient will maintain urine output greater than 30 mL per hour in the postprocedure period.

- Observe the patient for hypersensitivity reactions to contrast media (e.g., pruritus, rashes, breathing difficulties, generalized edema, urinary retention) *to detect possible reaction and protect renal function.*
- Monitor serum creatinine level, GFR, and fluid I&O postprocedure and report abnormalities to HCP *to ensure adequate renal function.*

Evaluation

If interventions have been effective, the patient will have reduced anxiety, increased understanding of the procedure, and urine output greater than 30 mL per hour.

• WORD • BUILDING •

percutaneous: per—through + cutaneous—skin

THERAPEUTIC MEASURES FOR THE URINARY SYSTEM

Management of Urinary Incontinence

Urinary **incontinence** is defined as involuntary leakage of urine. There are several types of incontinence. The incidence is rising and affects both men and women. Urinary incontinence is underreported because many people are embarrassed to talk about the problem. Most people do not seek treatment until their quality of life is affected. With incontinence, a voiding diary should be kept for several days to show when incontinence occurs and the predisposing events. A urologist specializing in incontinence, or a continence clinic can provide treatment.

Disability-Associated Incontinence

This type of incontinence can cause the inability to get to the toilet because of environmental barriers, physical limitations, loss of memory, or disorientation. People with disability-associated incontinence are often dependent on others. This dependence can be a common cause of incontinence in those who are institutionalized if they must await assistance.

Overflow Incontinence

Overflow incontinence is involuntary loss of urine associated with bladder overdistention. It occurs with acute or chronic urinary distention with dribbling of urine. The bladder cannot empty normally despite frequent urine loss. Spinal cord injuries or enlarged prostate can be a cause.

Stress Incontinence

Stress incontinence is the involuntary loss of less than 50 mL of urine associated with increasing abdominal pressure during coughing, laughing, sneezing, or other physical activities. Stress incontinence can occur in women after childbirth and menopause. In men, stress incontinence may be seen after prostatectomy and radiation. Kegel exercises can increase perineal muscle tone for both stress and urge incontinence (Box 36.1).

Urge Incontinence

Urge incontinence is the involuntary loss of urine associated with an abrupt and strong desire to void. The patient typically reports being "unable to make it to the bathroom in time." It is the most common type of urinary incontinence in older adults.

Total Incontinence

Total incontinence is a continuous and unpredictable loss of urine. It usually results from neurologic impairment, surgery, trauma, or a malformation of the ureter. Bladder training has been proven ineffective. The nurse's priority is to keep the patient clean and dry using absorptive products. For some males, an external condom catheter can be effective. External female catheter devices can be used to accurately monitor urine output in females (Mueller, 2019).

Box 36.1 Patient Education

Kegel Exercises

Kegel exercises can make the pelvic floor muscles stronger to control the bladder and bowels in men and women.

1. To establish awareness of pelvic muscle function, the patient should "pull in" the muscles in the perineum as if to control urination or passing gas. The muscles of the buttocks, inner thigh, and abdomen should remain relaxed along with normal breathing.
2. To identify the correct muscles to tighten, the patient should tighten the muscles that control urination. The patient should feel the muscles tighten and move upward. It can be helpful to use an analogy of an elevator: Start squeezing at the bottom floor and then squeeze upward to the top floor.
3. With an empty bladder, the patient is instructed to tighten the pelvic floor muscles for 8 seconds, followed by 10 seconds of relaxation.
4. Encourage the patient to perform three sets of 10 to 15 repetitions daily. The patient should avoid doing the exercises while urinating because pelvic floor muscles can be weakened or urine retained, increasing risk of urinary tract infection. Results may occur in several weeks or a few months.

Nursing Process for the Patient With Incontinence

The medical diagnoses of stress and urge incontinence are also nursing diagnoses. See "Nursing Care Plan for the Patient With Stress or Urge Incontinence" and "Nursing Care Plan for the Patient With Disability-Associated Incontinence."

Management of Urine Retention

Urinary retention is the inability to empty the bladder completely during attempts to void. It can be acute, with a sudden onset of retention and anuria, or chronic, with a slower onset of retention of urine and oliguria. Acute retention often results from surgery. It is caused by anesthesia, medications, or local trauma to the urinary structures. Acute retention can be a medical emergency causing extreme pain, an enlarged bladder, and the possibility of acute kidney injury or bladder rupture. Chronic urine retention may be related to an enlarged prostate gland, diabetes, pregnancy, a medication effect, strictures, or other obstruction of the urinary tract.

If the patient has a feeling of fullness but is unable to urinate, the nurse gently palpates the suprapubic area to identify a full bladder. An empty bladder is not palpable. When a fluid-filled bladder is percussed, a dull sound is heard over the bladder. A bedside bladder ultrasound scan can be done to determine the volume of urine in the bladder (see Table 36.6; Fig. 36.6). The scan is painless, noninvasive, and requires no patient preparation. The bladder scan may be used instead of catheterization after the patient urinates to determine the amount of urine remaining in the bladder. Normally, the bladder contains less than 50 mL after urination. A residual volume of 150 to 200 mL of urine indicates a need for treatment for urine retention.

Nursing Care Plan for the Patient With Stress, Urge or Disability-Associated Urinary Incontinence

Nursing Diagnosis: *Stress Urinary Incontinence* or *Urge Urinary Incontinence* related to decreased tone of perineal muscles; *Disability-Associated Urinary Incontinence* related to interference with voiding
Expected Outcomes: The patient will be continent.
Evaluation of Outcomes: Is the patient continent?

Urinary Incontinence

Intervention	Rationale	Evaluation
Collect incontinence data with a patient voiding journal.	*A journal helps identify the severity and timing of incontinence.*	Did patient create a voiding journal?
Identify potential acute causes of incontinence (e.g., urinary tract infection [UTI], constipation or impaction, medication effect, or decreased fluid intake).	*There are many treatable causes of incontinence.*	Does patient have any treatable causes of incontinence?

Stress or Urge Urinary Incontinence

Intervention	Rationale	Evaluation
Reinforce teaching on how to perform Kegel exercises (see Box 36.1).	*Kegel exercises increase perineal muscle tone to help prevent incontinence.*	Does patient correctly explain how to perform Kegel exercises?
For urge incontinence, reinforce teaching of urge inhibition techniques (distraction) with relaxation breathing.	*Distraction techniques can help patients reach the bathroom in time to prevent incontinence.*	Do distraction techniques help patient prevent incontinence?
Refer patient to a continence clinic, an incontinence provider, and/or support group (e.g., National Association for Continence, www.nafc.org).	*Incontinence specialists use medical or surgical interventions to treat incontinence. Support groups provide teaching and assistance with embarrassment.*	Does patient understand what resources are available to further assist with treatment and support for incontinence?

Disability-Associated Urinary Incontinence

Intervention	Rationale	Evaluation
Identify if clothing inhibits timely voiding. Velcro fasteners or sweatshirts and sweatpants can be easy to remove.	*Some clothing can be difficult to remove for older adults, resulting in incontinence before the clothing can be removed.*	Does patient have easy-to-remove clothing?
Identify obstacles to urine receptacle, such as poor lighting, an in-use bathroom, or lack of assistive devices: three-in-one commode, female, male or no-spill urinal.	*Obstacles can make it impossible for patient to reach or use a voiding receptacle in time to prevent incontinence.*	Does patient have ready access to an appropriate voiding receptacle?
Use prompted voiding techniques: checking patient regularly; providing positive reinforcement if dry; prompting patient to toilet when awakens, every 2 hours, and before sleep; and praising patient after toileting.	*Maintaining a regular toileting schedule will help patient remain continent.*	Does patient remain continent?

(nursing care plan continues on page 692)

Nursing Care Plan for the Patient With Stress, Urge or Disability-Associated Urinary Incontinence—cont'd

Geriatric

Provide prompt assistance for voiding request.	Timing of the urge for voiding signal in older adults does not allow the patient the ability to wait for assistance.	Is prompt assistance provided, allowing patient to remain continent?

Urinary Catheters

Indwelling Catheters

Indwelling urinary catheters can be used for justifiable reasons, such as burns, shock, heart failure, or urinary tract obstruction. Urinary incontinence is not a justification for insertion of an indwelling urinary catheter. Indwelling catheters result in UTIs the longer they are in place. The incidence of infection is decreased when intermittent straight urinary catheterization is used instead of an indwelling urinary catheter.

With an indwelling urinary catheter, bacteria enter the bladder mainly in one of two ways: (1) through the outlet at the end of the collection bag contaminating the urine, which is then inadvertently drained back into the bladder, or (2) around the catheter up the urethra and into the bladder (Box 36.2). Routine perineal care during the daily bath is enough to minimize infection from an indwelling urinary catheter (see also "Home Health Hints").

Intermittent Catheterization

For the patient who is unable to void, the best intervention is intermittent catheterization. Those who are postoperative, have a neurologic disorder, or experience urine retention may benefit from intermittent catheterization. The risk of infection is reduced if the bladder is not allowed to overfill. Intermittent catheterization involves the use of a straight plastic or rubber catheter that is inserted into the urethra about every 3 hours to empty the bladder. After the bladder is empty, the catheter is removed. Patients may be taught to do intermittent self-catheterization (ISC) at home. Patients doing ISC may be taught to wash and reuse the same catheter when they are in their own environment. In the health-care agency, however, sterile technique and equipment are used.

Suprapubic Catheter

After certain surgeries of the urinary tract and in some long-term situations, a suprapubic catheter may be used. This indwelling catheter is inserted through a surgical incision in the lower abdomen directly into the bladder. Nursing care of a suprapubic catheter involves keeping the area clean and dry, changing the dressing as needed when the site is new, and keeping the catheter taped to prevent tension. A skin barrier such as Stomahesive may help protect the skin from urine leakage. Other care is the same as for any indwelling urinary catheter.

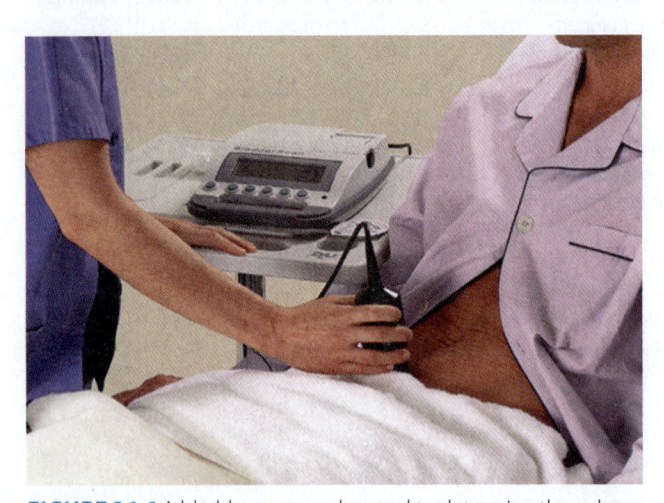

FIGURE 36.6 A bladder scan can be used to determine the volume of urine in a patient's bladder.

Box 36.2

Guidelines for Care of the Patient With an Indwelling Urinary Catheter

1. Maintain a closed system. Do not separate the catheter from the tubing of the bag. Instead, sterilely collect specimens and irrigate through the specimen port in the tubing.
2. Secure the catheter with tape or fastener as directed. This decreases traction on and movements of the catheter that can move bacteria into the bladder.
3. Encourage fluid consumption to naturally irrigate the catheter if fluids are not contraindicated.
4. Use aseptic technique when emptying the collection bag by washing hands, wearing clean gloves, and using a clean container for single-patient use to collect urine.
5. Wash the perineum with soap and water once a day and again after bowel incontinence.
6. Keep the tubing coiled on the bed and positioned to allow free urine flow. Keep the catheter bag below the level of the bladder at all times.
7. Do not clamp catheters. Clamping a catheter results in obstruction and increases risk of infection. Periodic clamping has not been found to be effective in bladder retraining.
8. Replace the urine collection system as required.
9. Remove indwelling catheters as soon as possible to reduce risk of infection.

PRACTICE ANALYSIS TIP
Linking NCLEX-PN® to Practice
The LPN/LVN will:
- Collect specimen for diagnostic testing (e.g., urine).
- Check for urinary retention (bladder scan, ultrasound, palpation).
- Insert, maintain, and remove urinary catheter.
- Provide care to client with bladder management protocol.

Home Health Hints
- Secure pets in another room when performing sterile procedures such as urinary catheter changes. When inserting a urinary catheter, use a flashlight as needed. Have an extra catheter kit and a sterile specimen container available.
- Reinforce teaching to the patient and caregiver to keep water to drink next to the patient to maintain hydration. TV commercials can be a reminder to take sips.
- Reinforce teaching for the nurse to be notified if the catheter becomes plugged as well as how to take the catheter out if it becomes plugged and the nurse is not readily available. Leave a syringe to deflate the balloon with instructions not to cut the balloon valve stem.
- When teaching females self-catheterization, have them stand with one foot on the toilet, if able, during the catheterization.
- Reinforce teaching to patient or caregiver on how to switch drainage bags from a large bag to a leg bag if desired for ambulation. When unattached to the urinary drainage system, an extra drainage bag should be cleansed with a solution of 1 part white vinegar and 3 parts water (¼ cup vinegar, ¾ cup water) or a solution of 1 part bleach to 10 parts water (1/4 cup bleach, 2½ cups water).

BE SAFE!
AVOID FAILURE TO RESCUE! After an uncircumcised male is catheterized, the foreskin must be properly repositioned over the glans penis. It cannot be left retracted, as this can cause injury. If left retracted, subsequent swelling may make it impossible to pull the foreskin over the glans penis later. This can cause ischemia of the glans penis, a medical emergency. The HCP must be notified immediately. An emergency circumcision may be needed if the foreskin cannot be properly positioned. Always ensure that the foreskin is positioned properly after catheterization or perineal care.

Key Points

- The urinary system consists of two kidneys and two ureters, the urinary bladder, and the urethra. The kidneys form urine and the rest of the system eliminates urine.
- The purpose of urine formation is the removal of potentially toxic waste products from the blood. The kidneys regulate blood pressure, electrolyte balance, acid–base balance, formation of erythropoietin, and activation of vitamin D.
- With age, the number of nephrons in the kidneys decreases, often to half the original number by age 70 or 80. The glomerular filtration rate also decreases. The urinary bladder decreases in size, and the tone of the detrusor muscle decreases. This may result in the need to urinate more often or in residual urine in the bladder after voiding. Older adults are also more subject to infections of the urinary tract.
- Hypertension and diabetes are the most common causes of renal problems.
- If the patient has impaired kidney function, head-to-toe data collection is needed because kidney disease can affect every system of the body.
- Common symptoms of kidney disease include dull ache in the back, flank pain, hematuria, and painful urination. Other signs include periorbital edema, peripheral edema, fever, chills, itchy dry skin, changes in level of consciousness, and alterations in voiding pattern.
- Weight is the best indicator of fluid balance in the body. Weigh the patient at the same time each day, in the same or similar clothing, and with the same scale. Look for trends in weight gain or loss related to fluid balance.
- Intake and output should be carefully measured. Intake includes oral, IV, irrigation, tube feeding, and other fluids. Output includes urine, emesis, nasogastric effluent, wound drainage if it is copious, and any other drainage.
- A urinalysis is a commonly performed diagnostic test for the urinary system, kidney disease, and systemic diseases that may affect the kidneys.
- Several blood and urine tests reflect kidney function. If the kidneys are not filtering adequately, the serum test values, such as the creatinine and blood urea nitrogen, will be elevated. A renal biopsy diagnoses or provides information about kidney disease.
- Contrast media used in diagnostic testing and procedures can be nephrotoxic and cause contrast-induced acute kidney injury within 48 hours.
- Urinary incontinence is defined as the involuntary leakage of urine. Types of incontinence include disability associated, overflow, stress, urge, and total.

- Urinary retention is the inability to empty the bladder completely during attempts to void. It can be acute, with a sudden onset of retention and no urine output, or chronic, with a slower onset of retention of urine and some urine being expelled. Acute retention often results from surgery. It can be a medical emergency causing extreme pain, an enlarged bladder, and the possibility of acute kidney injury or bladder rupture.
- Chronic urine retention may be related to an enlarged prostate gland, diabetes, pregnancy, a medication effect, strictures, or other causes of obstruction of the urinary tract.
- A bedside bladder ultrasound scan identifies the volume of urine in the bladder with sound waves. The result guides the need for urinary catheterization, thereby reducing unnecessary catheterizations and associated risks.
- Indwelling urinary catheters can be used for justifiable reasons, such as burns, shock, heart failure, or urinary tract obstruction. Urinary incontinence is *not* a justification for insertion of an indwelling urinary catheter.
- Indwelling catheters increase the risk of infection and result in urinary tract infection the longer they are in place.
- Patients who have had surgery, have a neurologic disorder, or experience urine retention may benefit from intermittent catheterization. The risk of infection is reduced if the bladder is not allowed to overfill.

SUGGESTED ANSWERS TO CHAPTER EXERCISES

Cue Recognition

36.1: Obtain an order for the patient to use a tampon or have a straight catheterization to obtain a urine specimen and prevent contamination.

Critical Thinking & Clinical Judgment

Mr. Nolan

A total of 50 mL of concentrated urine for 4 hours is not normal or adequate output. Further investigation is needed to identify potential causes for the low output. If a problem is identified, inform the HCP. Consider the following data to collect:

1. Mr. Nolan's diagnosis? Is he now experiencing acute kidney injury? Is he severely dehydrated? Ask if anyone emptied Mr. Nolan's urinary bag without recording the output? Look at the trends in Mr. Nolan's intake and output record. Is his intake adequate? Has his output been decreasing? Is this a change? Look at trends in daily weights. Is Mr. Nolan's weight increasing due to fluid retention? Is this an expected finding?
2. Listen to Mr. Nolan's lung sounds for crackles. Check for edema. Do findings indicate fluid retention? Palpate Mr. Nolan's bladder. Is it distended? Is the catheter blocked?

Additional Resources

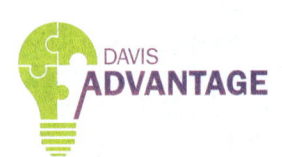

Go to Davis Advantage to complete your learning: strengthen understanding, apply your knowledge, and prepare for the Next Gen NCLEX®.

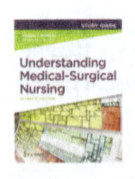

A Study Guide is also available.

CHAPTER 37
Nursing Care of Patients With Disorders of the Urinary System

Maureen McDonald

KEY TERMS

anuria (an-YOO-ree-ah)
azotemia (AH-zoh-TEE-mee-ah)
calculi (KAL-kyoo-lye)
cystitis (sis-TY-tis)
glomerulonephritis (gloh-MUR-yoo-loh-neh-FRY-tis)
hemodialysis (HEE-moh-dy-AH-lih-sis)
hydronephrosis (HY-droh-neh-FROH-sis)
nephrectomy (neh-FREK-tuh-mee)
nephrolithotomy (NEH-froh-lih-THAH-tuh-mee)
nephropathy (neh-FROP-uh-thee)
nephrosclerosis (NEH-froh-skleh-ROH-sis)
nephrostomy (neh-FRAW-stoh-mee)
nephrotoxins (NEH-froh-TOK-sins)
oliguria (AW-lih-GYOO-ree-ah)
peritoneal dialysis (PEAR-ih-toh-NEE-uhl dy-AL-ih-sis)
polyuria (PAH-lee-YOOR-ee-ah)
pyelonephritis (PY-eh-loh-neh-FRY-tis)
stent (STENT)
uremia (yoo-REE-mee-ah)
urethritis (YOO-reh-THRY-tis)
urethroplasty (yoo-REE-throw-PLAS-tee)
urosepsis (YOO-roh-SEP-sis)

CHAPTER CONCEPTS

Caring
Elimination
Fluid and electrolytes
Infection
Teaching and learning

LEARNING OUTCOMES

1. Explain the predisposing causes, symptoms, laboratory abnormalities, and treatment of urinary tract infections.
2. Explain the predisposing causes, symptoms, treatment, and teaching for kidney stones.
3. List risk factors and signs and symptoms of cancer of the bladder.
4. List risk factors and signs and symptoms of cancer of the kidneys.
5. Discuss nursing care for a patient with an ileal conduit or continent reservoir.
6. Explain the pathophysiology and nursing care for diabetic nephropathy, nephrosclerosis, hydronephrosis, and glomerulonephritis.
7. Describe the signs and symptoms for patients with acute kidney injury.
8. Describe the signs and symptoms for patients with chronic kidney disease.
9. Plan nursing care for patients with acute kidney injury.
10. Plan nursing care for patients with chronic kidney disease.
11. Discuss nursing care for a vascular access site.
12. Plan nursing care for patients on hemodialysis.
13. Plan nursing care for patients on peritoneal dialysis.

Disorders of the urinary tract involve the urethra, bladder, ureters, and kidneys. These disorders include infection, obstruction, cancer, hereditary disorders, and metabolic, traumatic, or chronic diseases. Some disorders lead to chronic kidney disease (CKD) if not treated.

URINARY TRACT INFECTIONS

The urinary tract is a sterile environment. A urinary tract infection (UTI) is the invasion of the urinary tract by bacteria. UTIs are most often caused by an ascending infection, starting at the external urinary meatus and moving up toward the bladder and kidneys. Most UTIs are caused by the bacterium *Escherichia coli*, commonly found in feces. Other less common pathogens include *Staphylococcus saprophyticus*, *Klebsiella* spp., and *Enterobacter*. Lower UTIs include urethritis, prostatitis, and cystitis. Upper UTIs include pyelonephritis and ureteritis. UTIs are the most common health-acquired infection (HAI). People who have had a UTI often develop repeat infections. It is important that education on how to prevent repeat UTIs is provided.

Risk Factors for Urinary Tract Infections

- *Aging* increases the incidence of UTIs due to diminished immune function, diabetes, estrogen decline in women, enlarged prostate that obstructs urine flow in men, or a neurogenic bladder that fails to completely empty. UTI is the most common cause of acute bacterial sepsis in patients older than 65.
- *Contamination in the perineal and urethral areas*, which can ascend the urinary tract, may occur from genital piercing; fecal soiling; sexual intercourse that massages bacteria into the urinary meatus; or infections such as vaginitis, epididymitis, or prostatitis.
- *Faulty valves causing reflux of urine* do not maintain one-way urine flow along the urinary tract. Reflux can be congenital or acquired because of previous infections.
- *Female anatomic and genetic differences* make women more susceptible to UTIs because of the short length of the female urethra and its proximity to the vagina and anus. Some women with recurrent UTIs have a shorter distance from the urethra to anus. Genetic factors may play a role in women who have a certain phenotype for developing UTIs.
- *Instrumentation infection* occurs from instruments or tubes inserted into the urinary meatus. The most common cause of instrumentation infection is insertion of a urinary catheter. Bacteria ascend around or within the catheter. Bacterial colonization begins within 48 hours of indwelling catheter insertion.
- *Previous UTIs* might provide a reservoir of bacteria that can cause reinfection.
- *Stasis of urine* in the bladder results from voiding infrequently or obstruction. Urine stasis promotes bacterial growth, which can ascend to higher structures.

> **NURSING CARE TIP**
>
> When caring for a patient at risk for an internal catheter-associated urinary tract infection (CAUTI), limit the use of a urinary catheter, always use infection control procedures, and discontinue use as soon as possible. CAUTI is a Never Event—that is, hospitals will not be paid by Medicare for the costs of care provided if this condition occurs during hospitalization.
>
> An external female catheter, the Purewick (www.pure wickathome.com), keeps females who are incontinent dry without being invasive. This reduces the risk of CAUTI. The Purewick is an external sponge/suction catheter that is placed between the labia and the gluteus muscles. It is attached to a suction device at the lowest setting to absorb and wick away the urine.

Signs and Symptoms

UTIs are characterized by shared signs and symptoms along with location-specific symptoms (Table 37.1). Decline in mental status and fever in a patient with an indwelling

Table 37.1
Urinary Tract Infection (Urethritis, Cystitis, Pyelonephritis) Summary

Signs and Symptoms	All: Voiding urgency, frequency, and burning; cloudy, foul-smelling urine; hematuria Older adult: Fatigue, confusion, and delirium Cystitis: Pelvic pain or pressure Pyelonephritis: Costovertebral tenderness, high fever, chills, nausea/vomiting
Diagnostic Tests	Urinalysis: White blood cells, red blood cells, casts, bacteria, positive for nitrites Urine culture: Positive
Therapeutic Measures	Antimicrobial for causative organism Encourage fluids Phenazopyridine (Pyridium)
Complications	Pyelonephritis Urosepsis
Priority Nursing Diagnoses	Acute Pain Impaired Urinary Elimination Ineffective Health Maintenance Behaviors

catheter meets diagnostic criteria for a UTI. In older adults, the typical presenting symptom is generalized fatigue. New-onset confusion or delirium may be present in the older adult, but a fever may not be.

Types of Urinary Tract Infections
Urethritis

Urethritis is inflammation of the urethra caused by a chemical irritant, bacterial infection, trauma, or exposure to a sexually transmitted infection (STI). Posttraumatic urethritis can occur with intermittent catheterization or instrumentation of the urethra. Bubble bath, bath salts, and spermicidal agents are urethral irritants and should be avoided by anyone with a history of UTI. Gonorrhea and chlamydia are STIs that can cause urethritis in men.

Signs and symptoms of urethritis are listed in Table 37.1. The male patient may have discharge from the penis. Urinalysis and urine culture are used to diagnose urethritis. It is treated on the basis of the cause. In cases of sexual transmission, the sexual partner(s) must also be treated. Phenazopyridine (Pyridium),

• WORD • BUILDING •

urethritis: urethr—urethra (canal that discharges urine from bladder) + itis—inflammation

a urinary analgesic, treats dysuria. Explain to the patient that urine turns orange while taking phenazopyridine.

Cystitis

Cystitis is inflammation of the bladder wall, usually caused by a bacterial infection. *E. coli* causes most UTIs. Cystitis can also result from catheter use, chemical irritants, medications, or radiation therapy. Chronic interstitial cystitis, or painful bladder syndrome, has no known cause. Signs and symptoms are listed in Table 37.1. Urinalysis or sometimes cystoscopy is used for diagnosis. Urinalysis findings for cystitis include cloudy urine, WBCs, bacteria, sometimes red blood cells (RBCs), positive nitrites, and positive leukocyte esterase (pyuria). Urine culture and sensitivity are done if indicated. Bacterial cystitis is often treated with nitrofurantoin (Macrobid, Macrodantin), sulfamethoxazole and trimethoprim (Bactrim, Septra), or fosfomycin (Monurol). Instruct patient to finish all prescribed medications to prevent bacterial resistance and have a follow-up urinalysis or culture. Encourage fluids to flush the bladder.

Pyelonephritis

Pyelonephritis is infection of one or both kidneys, which can be serious. Bacteria can travel from the ureters to the bladder and then up to the kidneys. Young women and older adults experience this infection most. Risk factors for uncomplicated pyelonephritis include a history of UTIs within the past year, sexual intercourse, or spermicide use. Complicated pyelonephritis risk factors are diabetes, weak immune system, or structural or obstruction problems. In addition to shared UTI signs and symptoms, high fever, chills, nausea/vomiting, flank pain, and costovertebral tenderness (tenderness at the angle where rib and vertebrae join with palpation) indicate pyelonephritis. Urinalysis shows cloudy urine, bacteria, WBCs, pyuria, positive nitrites, and casts. The urine culture will have 100,000 or more colony-forming units (CFU) per milliliter. In acutely ill patients, blood cultures may be obtained. Antibiotics are given orally or, if the patient is hospitalized, intravenously (Table 37.2). After treatment, there is usually no lasting kidney damage. However, frequent kidney infections can result in scarring and loss of kidney function.

Urosepsis

Urosepsis is sepsis caused by a UTI. Septic shock and death can result so prompt treatment is essential. Older adults are at greater risk for urosepsis.

Nursing Process for the Patient With a Urinary Tract Infection

Data Collection

Ask what the patient's usual pattern of voiding is and if changes have occurred. Document the presence of a catheter, recent urinary instrumentation, or surgery. Note the presence of signs or symptoms (see Table 37.1). Inspect the urine for volume, color, concentration, cloudiness, blood, or foul odor. Review urinalysis and culture results.

Nursing Diagnoses, Planning, and Implementation

Acute Pain related to inflammation and infection of urinary structures

EXPECTED OUTCOME: The patient will report relief from pain and discomfort.

- Administer phenazopyridine (Pyridium) as ordered *to relieve pain*.
- Apply heat to suprapubic area *to relieve discomfort*.

Ineffective Health Maintenance Behaviors related to lack of knowledge on preventing and resolving UTIs

EXPECTED OUTCOME: The patient will state understanding of prevention of UTIs and be free from UTIs.

- Suggest eating foods that may prevent UTIs, including polyphenols (cranberry or blueberry products, coffee, black tea, and dark chocolate) *for potential preventive action against UTIs*.
- Reinforce teaching to drink fluids, including water to produce clear light-yellow urine, *to prevent dehydration and flush bacteria from urinary tract*.
- Reinforce teaching to void as soon as the urge occurs or every 3 hours while awake *to empty the bladder and lower bacterial counts, reduce stasis, and prevent infection*.
- Reinforce teaching females to wipe from front to back *to prevent spreading bacteria from anal area to urinary meatus*.
- Reinforce teaching females to wear cotton crotch underwear and avoid constricting clothing such as tight jeans *to allow air circulation to reduce moisture*.
- Reinforce teaching to avoid perfumed feminine hygiene products, bubble bath and bath salts, scented toilet paper, and tub baths, *which can irritate the urethra or introduce bacteria into the urinary meatus*.
- Reinforce teaching to void after sexual intercourse *to flush bacteria from the urinary tract that entered the urinary meatus*.
- Reinforce teaching signs and symptoms of UTI to report *to detect UTI*.
- Reinforce teaching to finish all prescribed antibiotic medications as directed *to prevent recurrent infection or resistance to antibiotics*.

Evaluation

The outcomes have been met if the patient verbalizes relief of pain and burning, and describes ways to prevent UTI.

• **WORD • BUILDING** •

cystitis: cyst—closed sac containing fluid + itis—inflammation
pyelonephritis: pyelo—pelvis + nephr—kidney + itis—inflammation
urosepsis: uro—urine + sepsis—infection in the blood

Table 37.2
Medications Used to Treat Urinary Tract Infections

Medication Class/Action

Antibiotics

Effective against E. coli and Enterococcus faecalis

Example	Nursing Implications
fosfomycin (Monurol)	Dissolve packet in ½ cup of cool water to drink immediately. Teach: Only 1 dose is needed for UTI. Diarrhea is a common side effect that subsides when medication is stopped.

Effective against E. coli, enterococci, Staphylococcus aureus, Klebsiella spp., and Enterobacter

Example	Nursing Implications
nitrofurantoin (Macrobid, Macrodantin)	Teach: Avoid taking with antacids. Take with food or milk and full glass of water.

Beta-Lactam Antibiotics

Effective against Escherichia coli, Klebsiella spp., and Serratia

Example	Nursing Implications
ceftriaxone (Rocephin) cefepime (Maxipime) aztreonam (Azactam)	Check allergies and renal function.

Fluoroquinolones

Effective against E. coli, Klebsiella spp., Pseudomonas, and other organisms.

Example	Nursing Implications
ciprofloxacin (Cipro) levofloxacin (Levaquin)	Do not give if pregnant. Absorption may be decreased if given within 2 hr of aluminum antacids. Give with large amounts of water. Teach: Avoid sunlight or wear sunscreen of 30 HPF or more. Report tendon aches promptly as tendon may rupture.

Sulfonamides

Effective against E. coli; used for uncomplicated UTIs.

Example	Nursing Implications
trimethoprim-sulfamethoxazole (Bactrim, Septra)	Do not give if allergic to sulfa. Do not give if pregnant. Dose may need adjustment with renal disease. Teach: Avoid sunlight or wear sunscreen of 30 SPF or more. Take with large amounts of water.

Urinary Analgesic

Topical analgesic that relieves pain urgency and frequency associated with UTI.

Example	Nursing Implications
phenazopyridine (Pyridium)	Urine color changes to red-orange. Avoid in renal insufficiency. Changes urine glucose testing.

CRITICAL THINKING & CLINICAL JUDGMENT

Mrs. Milan is a 25-year-old woman who, after a weekend getaway with her husband, notices symptoms of dysuria, frequency, and urgency. She visits her health-care provider (HCP) and is diagnosed with a UTI. She is placed on an oral antibiotic.

Critical Thinking (The Why)
1. What predisposed Mrs. Milan to developing a UTI?
2. What urinalysis findings would you expect for Mrs. Milan?

Clinical Judgment (The Do)
3. What education do you provide to Mrs. Milan to prevent UTIs?
4. What do you include in Mrs. Milan's teaching plan for her therapeutic regimen?

Suggested answers are at the end of the chapter.

UROLOGICAL OBSTRUCTIONS

Urinary tract obstruction interferes with the flow of urine along the urinary tract. It can develop rapidly or slowly. Obstruction can be partial or complete or unilateral or bilateral. It is always a significant problem as urine will back up from the point of the blockage, eventually distending the kidney (**hydronephrosis**) and increasing pressure on the structures of the kidney. If not relieved, this pressure can damage the kidney, impair its function, and ultimately lead to CKD.

Urethral Strictures

A urethral stricture is a narrowing of the lumen of the urethra from scar tissue. It creates a diminished urinary stream, dysuria, frequency, and frequent UTIs. Strictures occur from injury, STIs, tissue trauma from use of catheters or surgical instruments, cancer, or an enlarged prostate (see Chapter 43). Treatment of a urethral stricture includes catheterization to drain the obstructed urine; mechanical dilation by the urologist, who inserts dilators over a wire to stretch open the urethra; endoscopic urethrotomy, which removes the stricture; surgical repair (**urethroplasty**); or implantation of a **stent** (hollow tube).

Renal Calculi (Urolithiasis)

Renal calculi (urolithiasis) are stones (**calculi;** one stone is a *calculus*) in the urinary tract. They usually form in the kidney (nephrolithiasis; Fig. 37.1) but may form in the ureter (ureterolithiasis).

Pathophysiology
Crystals start to form when (1) urine is too concentrated, resulting in high levels of calcium, oxalate (from plants), phosphorus or uric acid; and (2) substances such as citrate that inhibit stone formation are low. Crystals bind together

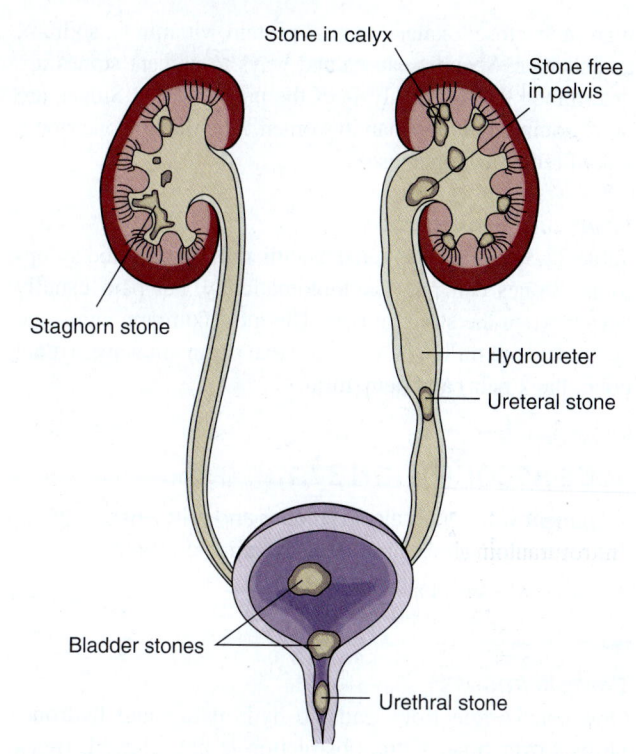

FIGURE 37.1 Location of calculi in the urinary tract.

with other substances and form a calculus that enlarges and is not flushed from the urinary tract. The four main types of stones are calcium (with oxalate or phosphate), uric acid, struvite (rare, large, fast-growing stone found in alkaline urine caused by bacteria in chronic UTIs), and cystine (rare stone; hereditary; cystine is an amino acid found in foods). Most stones are made of calcium oxalate. Renal calculi can form in the renal pelvis and calyces, or in the ureter or bladder. They range from the size of a grain of salt to staghorn (fill renal pelvis and extend into at least 2 calyces and are caused by urease-producing bacteria in chronic UTIs).

Etiology
Stone formation has numerous causes, some related specifically to the type of stone. Nonmodifiable risk factors include genetics, family history of stones, and medical conditions such as cystinuria, diabetes mellitus, gout (men), hypertension, certain intestinal disorders or bypass surgery, obesity, chronically high urine pH, or chronic UTI. Modifiable risk factors include inadequate fluid intake or excessive sweating from environment or exercise (concentrates urine); medications such as aspirin, indinavir (Crixivan), topiramate (Trokendi XR, Topamax), triamterene (Dyrenium), vitamin C supplements and vitamin D; calcium supplements between meals; dietary pattern; diet low in calcium, phytate, and potassium; or diet

• WORD • BUILDING •

hydronephrosis: hydro—pertaining to water + nephrosis—degenerative change in kidney

urethroplasty: urethro—urethra + plasty—surgical repair

high in fructose, oxalate, animal protein, vitamin C, sodium, and sucrose. Specific causes and ways to prevent stones are determined through analysis of the passed stone. Stones are more common in men than in women. After having one stone, risk of recurrence increases

Signs and Symptoms
Table 37.3 summarizes renal calculi and its signs and symptoms. Stones can pass asymptomatically, but pain usually occurs when the stone moves. The most common signs and symptoms are mild to severe pain that occurs in waves (renal colic, flank pain) and hematuria.

> **CUE RECOGNITION 37.1**
> A patient with renal calculus moans and yells when experiencing renal colic. What action do you take?
> *Suggested answers are at the end of the chapter.*

Complications
Obstructed urine flow leads to hydroureter and hydronephrosis over time. If the obstruction is not relieved, shock and sepsis can occur. Damage from the pressure can occur, causing CKD.

Prevention
Adequate hydration (2–3 quarts) daily is recommended to prevent concentrated urine. Sweetened beverages and grapefruit juice should be avoided. The Dietary Approaches to Stop Hypertension (DASH) eating plan and Mediterranean diet are recommended. For dietary guidelines, see "Nutrition Notes." Encourage the patient to walk, which promotes the excretion of stones and reduces bone calcium resorption (release). Urocit-K (potassium citrate), which restores chemicals in the urine that prevent crystals from forming to prevent calcium oxalate and uric acid stones, might be prescribed.

> **Nutrition Notes**
> **Calcium oxalate stones.** To prevent oxalate stones, limit sodium and animal protein, and consume adequate calcium to bind with oxalate. If a low-oxalate diet is prescribed, many foods may be restricted, including beets, chocolate, spinach, rhubarb, nuts, peanuts, and sweet potatoes.
> **Calcium phosphate stones.** Reducing dietary sodium and animal protein, avoiding cola beverages, and getting adequate calcium help prevent these stones.
> **Uric acid stones.** Renal calculi can be a complication of gout, which is a disorder of purine metabolism. Limit high-purine foods such as organ meats, anchovies, herring, sardines, alcoholic beverages, and gravy. Increasing fruits and vegetables may reduce uric acid stone formation.

Table 37.3 Renal Calculi Summary

Signs and Symptoms	*Nephrolithiasis:* Costovertebral angle pain Hematuria *Ureterolithiasis:* Severe, colicky (wavelike) pain from obstructed urine flow Flank, side, or lower abdomen pain radiating to genitalia Intense urge to void Frequency, dysuria, reduced output Hematuria due to irritation from stone Nausea/vomiting with severe pain *Bladder stones:* Hematuria Oliguria with obstruction of bladder outlet
Diagnostic Tests	Computed tomography (CT) Renal ultrasound Abdominal x-ray *Blood tests:* Calcium, uric acid, blood urea nitrogen (BUN), creatinine *Urinalysis:* Hematuria, crystals, urine pH Two 24-hour urine collections
Therapeutic Measures	*Small stones:* Hydration, analgesics, alpha blocker (Tamsulosin) *Large stones, symptomatic:* IV fluids Pain control Thiazide diuretic Allopurinol (Zylorprim) Lithotripsy Surgery: Percutaneous nephrolithotomy, ureteroscopy, cystoscopy, cystolitholapaxy
Complications	UTI Hydroureter Hydronephrosis Shock Sepsis Chronic kidney disease
Priority Nursing Diagnoses	*Acute Pain* *Risk for Infection* *Deficient Knowledge*

Diagnostic Tests
Blood tests (i.e. BUN, creatinine) assess renal function and urinalysis assesses for hematuria and infection. Imaging tests for renal stones and hydronephrosis include noncontrast

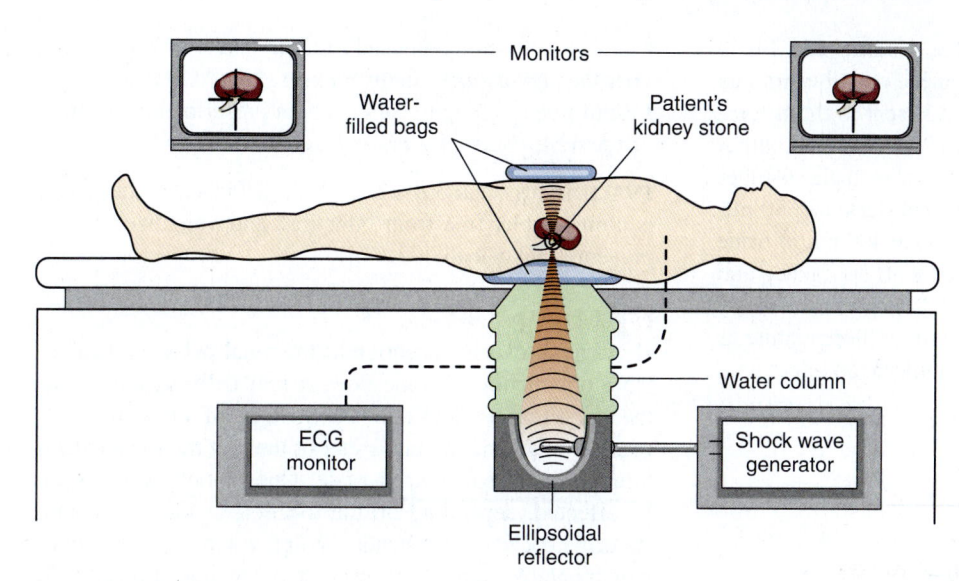

FIGURE 37.2 Extracorporeal shock-wave lithotripsy.

computed tomography (CT) or renal ultrasound (preferred for pregnant women) initially. Less commonly used tests include abdominopelvic x-ray, magnetic resonance imaging (MRI), and IV pyelography.

Therapeutic Measures

Renal calculi, usually less than 10 mm, are treated medically, if possible, with hydration and medication for pain. Most small stones can be flushed out during urination. All urine must be strained by the patient or health-care staff to detect passage of stones and for stone analysis. Treatment includes drinking 2 to 3 quarts of fluids; NSAIDs such as ibuprofen (Motrin) for the pain of renal colic, or opioids if NSAIDs are contraindicated, as in CKD or when pain is unrelieved with NSAIDs; and an alpha-blocker medication (such as tamsulosin [Flomax]) to relax ureter muscles. Patients who develop severe renal colic are usually admitted to the hospital for hydration with IV fluids and pain medication.

Surgical intervention may be needed depending on the location and size of the stone (often larger than 10 mm) or when obstruction or infection is present, urinary function is impaired, severe pain continues, or the patient is unable to pass the stone. Only rarely is open surgery required.

CYSTOSCOPY. For stones within the bladder, cystoscopy (wire basket removal) is used for small stones and cystolitholapaxy for larger stones. In cystolitholapaxy, an instrument is inserted through the urethra to the bladder to crush the stone. The stone is then washed out with an irrigating solution. See postoperative care for cystoscopy in Chapter 36.

URETEROSCOPY. The ureteroscope is inserted into the bladder and advanced along the ureter to view the stone. The stone is then removed with a wire basket or broken up with a laser or electrohydraulic energy to be flushed out in the urine. A stent may be placed for up to 2 weeks. Postoperative care is similar to cystoscopy care.

LITHOTRIPSY. Lithotripsy uses sound shock waves or laser energy to break the stone into small fragments. Examples of types of lithotripsy include shock-wave lithotripsy (SWL), laser lithotripsy, and percutaneous ultrasonic lithotripsy.

For SWL, the patient is sedated or anesthetized. Ultrasonic shock waves applied outside the body are focused on the stone to break it up into sandlike particles (Fig. 37.2). The particles are then flushed out with urination over time, with varying degrees of discomfort or pain. Occasionally, a stent is placed in the ureter to facilitate the passage of the stone fragments. SWL is most effective with calcium stones 1 centimeter or smaller that are in the kidney. After the outpatient procedure, the patient is usually discharged. Blood-tinged urine (pink) for about 1 to 3 days and back soreness for several days are common. Bruising may occur on the back or abdomen. Discharge instructions include increase fluid intake to help flush out the stone particles, strain all urine to catch stone fragments for analysis, and notify the HCP for problems.

PERCUTANEOUS NEPHROLITHOTOMY. For kidney stones that are large and cannot be removed with SWL, a percutaneous **nephrolithotomy** is performed. A small incision is made in the back through which a nephroscope is inserted into the area of the kidney where the stone is located. The stone is broken up and removed. A temporary **nephrostomy** tube or stent might be placed to help ensure unobstructed urine flow.

Nursing Process for the Patient With Renal Calculi

DATA COLLECTION. The health history may identify a family or patient history of previous stone formation. The patient is asked about a recent history of UTI, diet or activity changes, or other risk factors for renal calculi. If the cause is identified, specific education can be provided to help prevent recurrent calculi.

• WORD • BUILDING •
lithotripsy: litho-stones + tripso-breaking stones
nephrolithotomy: nephro—kidney + lith—stone + otomy—incision
nephrostomy: nephr—pertaining to the kidney + ostomy—surgically formed artificial opening to the outside

Patients with stones may experience extreme pain. Flank pain may radiate to the genitals. All urine must be strained to detect stones. If a stone is found, it is sent to the laboratory for analysis. Precise measurement of intake and output (I&O) is important. Obstruction may occur at the bladder neck or urethra. With obstruction, **anuria** (less than 50 mL of urine output daily) or **oliguria** (less than 400 mL of urine output daily) might occur. Obstruction is an emergency and must be reported and treated immediately to preserve kidney function. Urine is observed for hematuria. Temperature is monitored for elevation, which could indicate an infection.

CUE RECOGNITION 37.2

A patient with a ureterolithiasis asks you to empty the urinal. What action do you take?

Suggested answers are at the end of the chapter.

NURSING DIAGNOSIS, PLANNING, AND IMPLEMENTATION.

Acute Pain related to the presence of, obstruction by, or movement of a stone within the urinary tract

EXPECTED OUTCOME: The patient will verbalize relief of pain at tolerable level within 30 minutes of report of pain.

- Monitor location and severity of pain using a pain rating scale such as 0 to 10. *Renal colic pain typically occurs in the flank or costovertebral angle and may radiate to the abdominal, pelvic, and genital areas.*
- Administer medication for pain as ordered *to promote comfort.*
- Apply heat to painful area *to reduce pain and promote comfort.*
- Encourage ambulation *to facilitate the passage of the stone through the urinary system.*

Risk for Infection related to the introduction of bacteria from obstructed urinary flow and instrumentation

EXPECTED OUTCOME: The patient will remain infection free.

- Monitor temperature and urine amount, color, clarity, and odor and report abnormal findings *as abnormalities may indicate infection.*
- Encourage fluid intake *to flush bacteria and stones.*

Deficient Knowledge related to lack of knowledge of prevention of stone recurrence and diet

EXPECTED OUTCOME: The patient will verbalize an understanding of how to prevent renal calculi.

- Ask about patient's understanding of how to prevent renal calculi *to establish baseline knowledge.*
- Consult dietitian after stone analysis and reinforce diet teaching *to prevent formation of specific types of stones.*
- Reinforce teaching on need for fluid intake of 2 to 3 quarts per day. *Dilute urine helps prevent stone formation.*
- Reinforce teaching to patient about prescribed medication *to prevent recurrence of renal stones.*

EVALUATION. Outcomes have been achieved if the patient is comfortable, free from infection, and verbalizes how to prevent renal calculi.

Hydronephrosis

Hydronephrosis is distention of the renal pelvis and calices from obstruction of urine flow. It is usually treatable once the condition is detected. Obstruction of urine flow can result from a stricture in a ureter or the urethra, renal calculi, tumors, or an enlarged prostate. One or both kidneys can be affected, depending on the location of the obstruction. As urine backs up it distends the ureter and then the kidney, which enlarges, and pressure increases within it (Fig. 37.3). Unrelieved pressure within the kidneys causes the kidneys to become sacs filled with urine instead of functioning kidneys. In a matter of hours, the blood vessels and renal tubules can be damaged extensively if the pressure is not relieved.

If the onset of obstruction is gradual, the patient initially may be asymptomatic. If the obstruction progresses, flank and back pain may occur. A UTI may develop with symptoms of frequency, urgency, and dysuria.

Immediate treatment of hydronephrosis is to relieve the urinary retention, often by inserting a urinary catheter. The cause of the obstruction must be treated medically or surgically. A stent may be placed inside a ureter during cystoscopy to ensure passage of urine as the ureter heals (Fig. 37.4). To relive pressure within the kidney and prevent kidney damage, a nephrostomy tube can be inserted directly into the kidney pelvis to drain urine into a collecting bag (see Fig. 37.4). This tube exits through an incision in the flank area. Monitor the nephrostomy tube to ensure it drains adequately. It should not be kinked or clamped, which would result in continuation of the hydronephrosis and possible kidney damage.

I&O is carefully measured. If both a nephrostomy tube and urinary catheter are present, output from each should be measured and documented separately. Urine retention must be recognized and reported promptly.

TUMORS OF THE RENAL SYSTEM

Cancer of the Bladder

Cancer of the bladder is the most common cancer of the urinary tract. The American Cancer Society (2021a) estimates that, in 2021, new cases of bladder cancer were more than 83,730 in the United States. Bladder cancer occurs most commonly in men and in adults over 55, with the average age being 73.

- **WORD** • **BUILDING** •

anuria: an—without + uria—urine
oliguria: olig—small + uria—urine

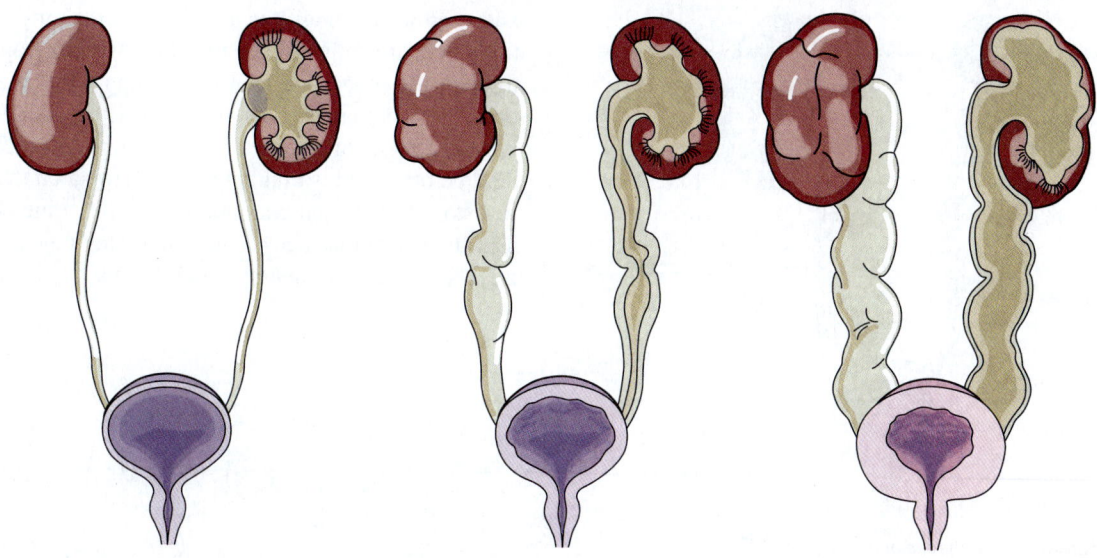

FIGURE 37.3 Hydronephrosis. Progressive thickening of bladder wall and dilation of ureters and kidneys result from obstruction of urine flow.

Pathophysiology

Cancer of the bladder often starts as a benign growth on the bladder wall that undergoes cancerous changes. Most bladder cancers begin in the inner lining of the bladder called the *urothelium*. They are called *transition cell cancers*. They come in a variety of forms and can behave in different ways. Some occur as small, wartlike growths on the inside of the bladder. Others form large tumors that grow into the muscle wall of the bladder and require surgical removal. If the cancer affects only the inner lining of the bladder, it is known as a *superficial* cancer. If it has spread to the muscle wall, it is called an *invasive* cancer. Common sites for bladder cancer metastasis include the liver, bones, and lungs.

Etiology

There is a strong correlation between cigarette smoking and bladder cancer. Those who smoke develop bladder cancer twice as often as people who do not smoke. Specific chemicals that cause bladder cancer have been found in cigarette smoke. The lung absorbs chemicals from smoking tobacco. These chemicals are passed to the kidneys through the bloodstream and collect in the urine. From there, they accumulate in the urine and damage the cells that line the bladder. Exposure to industrial pollution, such as aniline dyes, benzidine and naphthylamine, leather finishers, metal machinery, and petroleum-processing products, also increases the incidence of bladder cancer. It can take about 25 years after the exposure to these chemicals for bladder cancer to develop.

Signs and Symptoms

Cancer of the bladder usually causes painless hematuria. The urine may appear dark or reddish in color. Initially the bleeding is intermittent, which often causes the patient to delay seeking treatment. As cancer progresses, the patient develops frank hematuria, bladder irritability, urine retention from clots obstructing the urethra, and fistula formation (an opening between the bladder and an adjoining structure such as the vagina or bowel). Other symptoms include pelvic pain, pain in the lower back, painful urination, changes in bladder habits, and inability to void.

Diagnostic Tests

Cystoscopy with biopsy is the preferred diagnostic test for bladder cancer and to determine if it is in the muscle of the bladder wall. A urinalysis can show the presence of blood. A urine culture determines if an infection is causing the symptoms which are similar to those of bladder cancer. Urine for cytology looks for precancer or cancer cells with a microscope. Urine tumor marker testing looks for substances associated with bladder cancer such as bladder tumor-associated antigen (BTA), carcinoembryonic antigen (CEA), nuclear matrix protein 22 (NMP22) or chromosome changes. Imaging tests may also be done to look at the urinary tract.

Therapeutic Measures

Treatment depends on the type and staging (severity) of the bladder cancer. For early-stage cancers that affect the inside lining of the bladder, intravesical therapy with chemotherapy or immunotherapy may be used. Chemotherapeutic agents are instilled into the bladder through a urinary catheter, allowed to dwell, and then removed along with the catheter. Bacillus Calmette-Guérin (BCG) therapy is used in the bladder to trigger the immune system to attack the BCG germ as well as cancer cells. BCG may reduce the reoccurrence of bladder cancer. Photodynamic therapy, in which medications are given that make tumors sensitive to light, may be used. Light applied to the tumor area then kills the cancer cells.

Surgery is often used and can be combined with other treatments. There are several surgical treatment options. Transurethral resection of bladder tumor using a

704 UNIT NINE Understanding the Urinary System

and used as a conduit for urine. The remaining portions of the bowel are sutured back together. The surgeon is careful to keep the blood and neurologic supply intact to the section of bowel that has been removed. The isolated section of bowel is closed off on one end, the ureters are stitched into it, and the other end is brought out as a stoma on the abdomen (urostomy) that then continuously drains urine (Fig. 37.5). The urine from an ileal conduit contains mucus because it travels through the ileum, which normally secretes mucus.

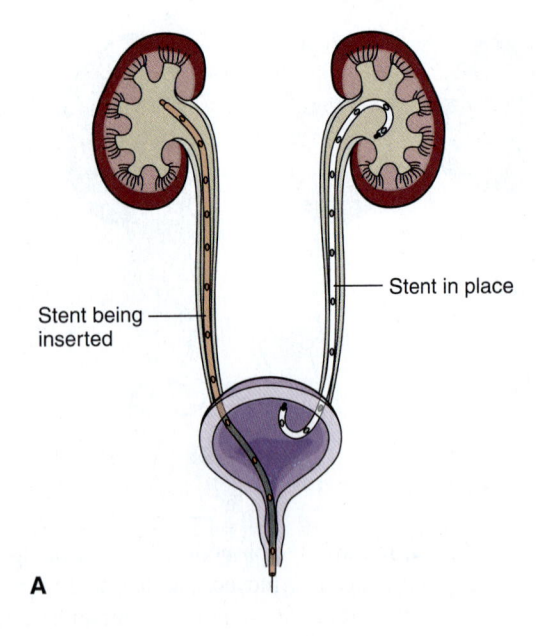

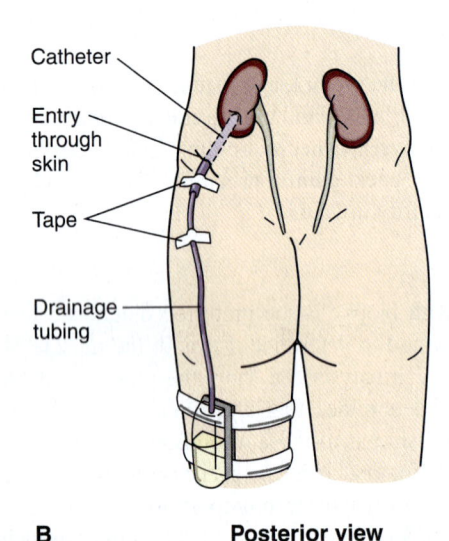

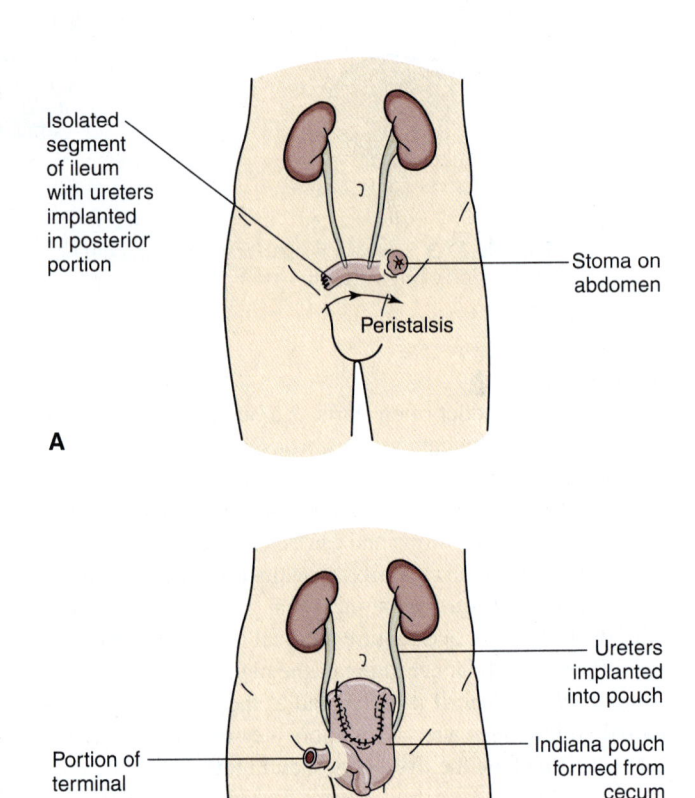

FIGURE 37.4 (A) Ureteral stents. (B) Nephrostomy tube inserted into renal pelvis; catheter exits through an incision on flank.

resectoscope with fulguration (destruction of tissue with electrical current) may be done to burn off cancerous tissue that has not invaded the muscle of the bladder wall. Alternately, a laser can be used with the resectoscope to destroy the tumor tissue. Robotic and laparoscopic surgical techniques may be used. Partial cystectomy can be done if cancer is limited to one area. If it is not, then radical cystectomy to remove the entire bladder and surrounding lymph nodes and other structures is needed. Reconstructive surgery is done after a radical cystectomy to create one of the types of urinary diversion (urine is stored and leaves the body in a different way).

INCONTINENT URINARY DIVERSION. An ileal conduit is used mainly for patients who have other health issues, the inability to care for a continent diversion, or a limited life span. A 6- to 8-inch section of the ileum or colon is removed

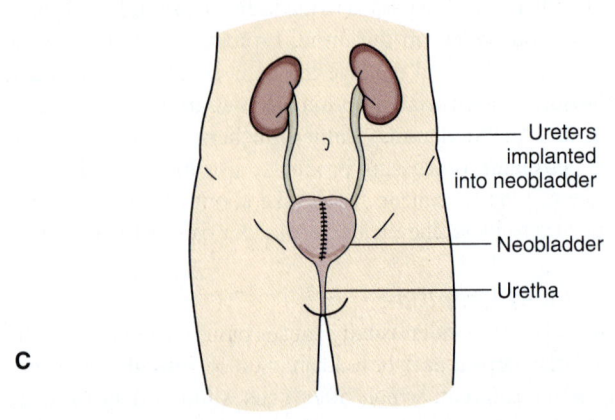

FIGURE 37.5 Urinary diversion surgery. (A) Ileal conduit. (B) Indiana pouch. (C) Orthotopic neobladder.

The patient must wear an ostomy bag to collect urine as urine continually flows from the stoma. This is why it is referred to as an incontinent urinary diversion.

CONTINENT URINARY DIVERSION. Continent urinary diversion surgeries do not require use of an ostomy bag. Instead, they require lifelong self-catheterization on a set schedule to empty the urine. They are not done as frequently today as in the past due to the development of the orthotopic neobladder. One type of a continent diversion is the Indiana pouch, which has a reservoir created using a portion of the ascending colon and terminal ileum with the ileocecal valve keeping the urine inside the reservoir (see Fig. 37.5).

ORTHOTOPIC NEOBLADDER. This continent urinary diversion surgery involves formation of an orthotopic bladder using a section of the intestine to make a neobladder (*neo* = "new") and implanting both the ureters and the urethra into the neobladder (see Fig. 37.5). It may be the preferred type of diversion because it does not require an ostomy bag or lifelong catheterization. After this surgery, the patient can void through the urethra, although incontinence may be an issue, especially at night, and intermittent catheterization may be needed.

Nursing Care

Nursing care of the postoperative urological patient is similar to care following a major surgical procedure (see Chapter 12). Urine output is monitored. Obstruction of urine output must be reported to prevent complications. A consultation with a nurse who specializes in wound, ostomy, and continence (WOC) care or an ostomy support group may be helpful before and after surgery. The patient is taught to monitor the stoma and care for the urinary diversion and surrounding skin after surgery. This may involve wearing an ostomy appliance or frequently draining the continent pouch with a catheter. Be sensitive to the patient's anxiety about caring for the urinary diversion. Body image disturbance may occur because of the change in body function. Assist the patient with coping interventions and learning signs and symptoms of infection to report.

Cancer of the Kidney

Cancer of the kidney is among the 10 most common cancers in both men and women. The American Cancer Society (2021b) estimate for 2021 is for more than 76,080 new cases of kidney cancer in the United States. Kidney cancer is diagnosed most often in those age 65 to 74. Men have twice the incidence of women. Risk factors include smoking, obesity, hypertension, long-term kidney dialysis, genetics (although rarely), and exposure to radiation, asbestos, and industrial pollution.

Signs and Symptoms

The three classic symptoms of kidney cancer are hematuria, dull pain in the flank area, and a mass in the area. Less specific symptoms include fever, weight loss, night sweats, hypertension, anemia, polycythemia, swelling in the legs, fatigue, anorexia, and constipation. Often the cancer has metastasized before it is diagnosed because the kidney has a large volume of circulating blood, which increases the risk of cancer spread. In addition, the disease has few early symptoms. Symptoms of metastasis may be the first evidence of kidney cancer and include weight loss, cough, bone fractures, liver abnormalities, and increasing weakness.

Diagnostic Tests

Diagnostic tests include a cystoscopy and pyelogram, ultrasound examination of the kidneys, CT scan of the abdomen, and MRI. A definitive diagnosis is made with a renal biopsy.

Therapeutic Measures

Surgery is the commonly used treatment for cancer of the kidney. A radical **nephrectomy** removes the entire kidney along with the adrenal gland and other surrounding structures, including fascia, fat, and lymph nodes. In nephron-sparing surgery, only the tumor is removed, and the healthy part of the kidney is saved. Radiation therapy, immunotherapy, or chemotherapy may be used after the surgery.

Nursing Care

After nephrectomy, postoperative nursing care mirrors that of any major surgery (see Chapter 12). Monitor urine output. Report changes in urine amount or color, bleeding, or signs of infection. The patient should be monitored for shortness of breath or diminished breath sounds on the affected side. Surgically induced or spontaneous pneumothorax may occur after a nephrectomy. Reinforce discharge teaching for wound care, pain management, medications, and follow-up care.

RENAL SYSTEM TRAUMA

Causes of trauma to the kidney, ureters, and bladder include motor vehicle accidents, sports injuries, falls, and gunshot and stab wounds. Bladder trauma or rupture may occur with pelvic fractures or trauma from a blow to the lower abdomen when the bladder is full. Data collection includes a history of the injury and inspection of the abdomen and flank for asymmetry, bruising, or swelling. Flank or abdominal pain, hematuria, and inability to void may be present. Diagnostic tests include urinalysis, ultrasound, CT, and MRI. Treatment depends on the injury and may include a urinary catheter or surgical intervention. Nursing care includes monitoring vital signs, pain management, measuring I&O, and monitoring IV fluids.

POLYCYSTIC KIDNEY DISEASE

Polycystic kidney disease is a hereditary disorder that can result in CKD. It is characterized by formation of multiple cysts in the kidney that can eventually replace normal kidney

• WORD • BUILDING •

nephrectomy: nephr—kidney + ectomy—excision

structures. The cysts are grapelike and contain serous fluid, blood, or urine. The patient typically first shows signs of the disease in adulthood. The initial symptoms include a dull heaviness in the flank or lumbar region and hematuria. Other symptoms include hypertension and UTIs. The renal cysts are diagnosed with ultrasound imaging. Treatment includes antihypertensive medications, dietary sodium restriction, and daily fluid intake of more than 3 liters. There is no treatment to stop the progression of polycystic kidney disease. As the disease progresses, the patient will likely develop CKD (discussed later) and require kidney replacement therapy. Because polycystic kidney disease is hereditary, patients should be offered genetic counseling.

CHRONIC RENAL DISEASES

Diabetic Nephropathy

Diabetes is the most common cause of CKD and end-stage kidney disease. Diabetic **nephropathy**, one type of diabetic kidney disease, is caused by years of damage from elevated glucose levels to the small blood vessels in the kidneys. Risk factors for diabetic nephropathy include chronic hyperglycemia, hypertension, high cholesterol, genetic predisposition, and smoking. Careful control of blood glucose levels, hypertension, and weight; not smoking; and careful use or avoidance of NSAIDs reduces the risk of nephropathy in patients with diabetes.

Pathophysiology
Multiple factors contribute to diabetic nephropathy. It begins with increased osmotic pressure from hyperglycemia, increased diuresis and compensatory cell growth and expansion, and increased glomerular filtration rate (GFR). Widespread atherosclerotic changes occur in the blood vessels of patients with diabetes, decreasing the blood supply to the kidney. Abnormal thickening of glomerular capillaries damages the glomerulus, allowing protein to leak into urine. Patients with diabetes also commonly develop pyelonephritis and renal scarring. Another complication of diabetes, neurogenic bladder, causes incomplete bladder emptying. This results in urine retention, which can cause infection, further damaging the kidneys. The patient can lose large amounts of protein (e.g., albumin) in the urine and develop nephrotic syndrome. This causes massive edema because of the resultant low levels of albumin in the blood.

Symptoms
The progression of nephropathy is marked by persistently elevated albuminuria advancing to proteinuria. Hypertension accelerates renal damage. As diabetic nephropathy progresses, GFR decreases, waste products accumulate, and eventually the patient may develop CKD.

Complications
The risk of cardiovascular disease is significant as protein spilling in the urine progresses.

Diagnostic Tests
Diabetic nephropathy is diagnosed by monitoring the patient with diabetes for onset of albuminuria or protein spillage in the urine, an early sign of the disease. A kidney biopsy may be done.

Therapeutic Measures
In the early stages of diabetic nephropathy, strict control of blood glucose levels (A1C less than 7%) and blood pressure helps slow the progress of the disease and reduce symptoms. Angiotensin-converting enzyme (ACE) inhibitors or angiotensin II receptor blockers (ARBs) are prescribed for hypertension. Statins are prescribed for cholesterol and proteinuria reduction. A healthy lifestyle should be encouraged to help manage this disease. As the disease progresses, kidney replacement therapy (dialysis or kidney transplant) may be needed.

Nephrotic Syndrome

Nephrotic syndrome is the excretion of 3.5 grams or more of protein in the urine per day. In nephrotic syndrome, large amounts of protein are lost in the urine from increased glomerular membrane permeability. As a result, serum albumin and total serum protein are decreased. Normally, albumin and other serum proteins maintain fluid within the vascular space. When levels of these proteins are low, fluid leaks from the blood vessels into tissues, resulting in edema. With very low levels of protein, ascites and massive widespread edema (anasarca) occur. In response to the low protein levels, the liver produces lipoproteins. As a result, serum cholesterol, low-density lipoproteins, and triglyceride levels are elevated. Urine may appear foamy from lipoproteinemia. Loss of immunoglobulins may lead to increased susceptibility to infection. Acute kidney injury, endocrine dysfunction, and thrombotic disease can occur.

Complications of nephrotic syndrome include impaired immune function, protein imbalances, and most important, increased blood coagulation. The latter is due to urinary loss of clotting inhibitors such as antithrombin III and plasminogen along with the loss of protein.

Treatment is focused on the cause and symptoms of nephrotic syndrome. ACE inhibitors or ARBs are prescribed to reduce pressure in the glomerulus and slow protein excretion. To reduce edema, loop diuretics and sodium intake restriction (2 grams/day) are used. Protein intake is guided by the severity of urinary protein loss. Statins to lower lipids may be tried. Anticoagulants are given for thrombosis prevention. In some cases, corticosteroids may be used to reduce inflammation.

Nursing care focuses on edema, protein intake, and preventing infection. For edema, daily weights, careful I&O measurements, and abdominal girth measurements are documented.

• WORD • BUILDING •

nephropathy: nephro—pertaining to the kidney + pathy—disease

Edematous tissue must be protected from injury. Preventing protein malnutrition is challenging but important to maintaining normal body functions. Referral to a dietitian is essential. Infection control measures are implemented.

Nephrosclerosis

Hypertension damages kidneys by causing sclerotic changes in the small arteries and arterioles, such as arteriosclerosis with thickening and hardening of the renal blood vessels (**nephrosclerosis**). Arteriosclerotic changes in the blood vessels of the kidneys decrease blood supply to the kidney (ischemia of the kidney), which can eventually destroy the organ. The remaining nephrons try to compensate with vasodilation to increase blood flow to the glomeruli. This results in increased glomerular pressure and filtration, which thickens the blood vessels. High pressure in the kidneys causes the vessels to weaken and hemorrhage. Large areas of the kidney become damaged. Symptoms of nephrosclerosis include proteinuria, hyaline casts in the urine, and, as it progresses, symptoms of CKD. Treatment for nephrosclerosis is antihypertensive medication, a low-sodium diet, and eventually dialysis. The priority nursing diagnosis for the patient with nephrosclerosis is *Ineffective Health Maintenance Behaviors* with a goal of managing hypertension. Arteriosclerosis increases risk of myocardial infarctions and cerebrovascular accidents.

> ### CLINICAL JUDGMENT
>
> **Mr. Stevens,** who is 55 years old, is admitted to the intensive care unit with uncontrolled hypertension and nephrosclerosis. His blood pressure is controlled by IV medication. His laboratory tests show protein and hyaline casts in the urine.
>
> 1. What data do you collect for your shift evaluation of Mr. Stevens's condition?
> 2. What renal function tests do you review?
> 3. What education do you reinforce for Mr. Stevens?
>
> *Suggested answers are at the end of the chapter.*

GLOMERULONEPHRITIS

Pathophysiology

Glomerulonephritis is an inflammatory disease of the filtering unit of the kidney, the glomerulus. It can be caused by a variety of factors, including immunological abnormalities, infectious agents, systemic disease, toxins, and vascular disorders. Inflammation occurs because of the deposition of antigen–antibody complexes in the basement membrane of the glomerulus or from antibodies that specifically attack the basement membrane. The resulting immune reaction in the glomerulus causes further inflammation, which in turn causes the glomerulus to be more porous, allowing proteins, WBCs, and RBCs to leak into the urine. Nephrotic syndrome can occur.

Etiology

Acute Poststreptococcal Glomerulonephritis

Glomerulonephritis is most commonly associated with a group A beta-hemolytic streptococcal infection 6 to 10 days after a streptococcal infection of the throat or skin. This is the most common cause in children and young adults. Antibodies form complexes with the streptococcal antigen and are deposited in the basement membrane of the glomerulus, inducing damage from inflammation. Edema, oliguria, and hypertension result.

Goodpasture Syndrome

Occasionally, glomerulonephritis is caused by an autoimmune response. In this case, for unknown reasons antibodies form against a person's own glomerular basement membrane. Glomerulonephritis caused by an autoimmune response usually progresses rapidly and leads to CKD.

Chronic Glomerulonephritis

Chronic glomerulonephritis occurs over years because of glomerular inflammatory disease. There may be no history of renal disease before the diagnosis. Often, proteinuria and hematuria may have been noted before the diagnosis. Systemic lupus erythematosus and type 1 diabetes mellitus may precede chronic glomerular injury. It is often discovered during an examination for another concern. Ultrasound, CT scan, or renal biopsy is used to diagnose the cause.

Symptoms

Symptoms of glomerulonephritis include hematuria, proteinuria, electrolyte imbalances, renal insufficiency, edema, hypertension, and thrombotic events (Table 37.4). Edema may begin around the eyes (periorbital edema) and face and progress to the abdomen (ascites), lungs (pleural effusion), and extremities. Flank pain may be present.

Complications

Adults who develop glomerulonephritis may recover renal function or progress to chronic glomerulonephritis. Some patients develop rapidly progressive glomerulonephritis. This can quickly lead to acute renal injury. Chronic glomerulonephritis is a slow process characterized by hypertension, gradual loss of renal function, and eventual CKD.

Diagnostic Tests

Glomerulonephritis is diagnosed with urinalysis, which shows protein, casts, or RBCs. Urine is dark or cola-colored from old RBCs and may be foamy because of proteinuria. Serum blood urea nitrogen (BUN) and serum creatinine

• WORD • BUILDING •

nephrosclerosis: nephro—pertaining to the kidney + sclerosis—hardening

glomerulonephritis: glomerulo—glomerulus + nephr—kidney + itis—inflammation

Table 37.4
Glomerulonephritis Summary

Signs and Symptoms	Fluid volume overload Hypertension Electrolyte imbalances Edema Periorbital edema Flank pain
Diagnostic Tests	Urinalysis shows red cells, white blood cells, protein, and casts Urine dark or cola-colored Foamy urine Serum creatinine elevated Serum blood urea nitrogen (BUN) elevated Renal biopsy
Therapeutic Measures	Symptomatic treatment NSAIDs Steroids Antibiotics prophylactically as needed
Complications	Chronic kidney disease
Priority Nursing Diagnoses	*Excess Fluid Volume*

levels may be elevated. Kidney ultrasound, x-ray, or biopsy may be done to determine abnormal kidney shape, size, blood flow, inflammation, or scarring of the glomeruli.

Therapeutic Measures

Most cases of acute glomerulonephritis resolve spontaneously in about a week, but some cases progress to CKD. Sodium and fluid restrictions may be ordered, along with diuretics to treat fluid retention. Medications may be given to control hypertension. If associated with a streptococcal infection, antibiotics are given. If fluid overload is severe, dialysis may be required.

Nursing Care

Nursing care for a patient with glomerulonephritis focuses on symptom relief. Vital signs are monitored because the patient may be critically ill. During the acute phase, rest is encouraged. Edema is controlled with fluid and sodium intake restrictions. Protein intake may be restricted if the kidneys are not filtering protein waste products (as shown by increased serum BUN and serum creatinine levels). Additional care is discussed in the section on CKD. Teaching the patient how to prevent glomerulonephritis is important. Antibiotics for diagnosed streptococcal throat infections should be prescribed to prevent glomerulonephritis.

ACUTE KIDNEY INJURY OR CHRONIC KIDNEY DISEASE

Kidney disease is diagnosed when the kidneys are no longer functioning adequately to maintain normal body processes and homeostasis. This results in dysfunction in almost all body systems because of imbalances in fluid, electrolytes, and calcium levels as well as impaired RBC formation and decreased elimination of waste products. Kidney disease can be acute (acute kidney injury) with sudden onset of symptoms, or it can be chronic (CKD), occurring gradually over time. For more information on the kidney, visit the American Kidney Fund (www.kidneyfund.org), the National Kidney Foundation (www.kidney.org), and the American Association of Kidney Patients (www.aakp.org).

Acute Kidney Injury

Acute kidney injury (AKI) is the sudden (hours to days) loss of the kidneys' ability to clear waste products and regulate fluid and electrolyte balance. Rapid accumulation of toxic wastes from protein metabolism in the blood (**azotemia**) occurs. Serum creatinine level and serum urea level (measured by BUN) are elevated. AKI may or may not be associated with reduced urine output. Many patients with AKI recover completely; others have a decline in kidney function.

Pathophysiology

AKI has three major mechanisms of injury: hypoperfusion, direct tissue injury, and hypersensitivity reactions causing renal inflammation. Rapid damage to the kidney causes waste products to accumulate in the bloodstream. The patient may become oliguric depending on the cause. Potassium imbalances may lead to arrhythmias and require immediate dialysis. AKI can affect other organs, leading to organ dysfunction.

AKI may progress through four stages (if urine output decreases), with an intrarenal cause taking a longer recovery time because there is actual renal damage.

> **NURSING CARE TIP**
> To protect patients' kidneys, be aware of the following:
> **Patient's Renal Function**
> • Estimated glomerular filtration rate (eGFR; best indicator)
> • Serum creatinine
> • Serum blood urea nitrogen (BUN) levels
> **Nephrotoxic Substances**
> • Diagnostic contrast agents
> • Medications, such as IV aminoglycosides (gentamicin [Garamycin], tobramycin [Tobrex]), amikacin (Amikin), cisplatin (Platinol), and vancomycin [Vancocin]).

• WORD • BUILDING •

azotemia: azo—nitrogenous waste products + temia—blood

- Chemicals, such as arsenic, carbon tetrachloride, lead, and mercuric chloride
- NSAIDs such as aspirin, ibuprofen, and naproxen, which can be harmful to the kidneys

Protective Measures Including the Following
- Before administering nephrotoxic contrast media or medications, check serum GFR and serum creatinine levels and report abnormalities to the HCP.
- With contrast media tests, ensure patients are not dehydrated. For at-risk patients (decreased GFR with or without diabetes or comorbidities), hydrate with IV fluids before and after the test. Avoid NSAIDs.
- Ensure peak/trough levels of nephrotoxic medications are monitored per institutional policy.

INITIATING PHASE. In this onset phase, an event occurs that causes AKI. It begins at the time of renal injury and lasts until the occurrence of symptoms. This phase lasts for hours to days.

OLIGURIC PHASE. In the oliguric phase, less than 400 mL of urine is produced in 24 hours. Fifty percent of those with AKI experience this phase, which occurs from 24 hours to 7 days after the initial phase and can last 2 weeks to several months. Renal function recovery decreases as the phase continues.

In the oliguric phase, fluid is retained, electrolytes become imbalanced, and waste products are not excreted as urine output decreases. Signs of fluid volume overload occur. Serum potassium rises while sodium is lost in the urine, creating normal or low serum sodium level. The longer the phase lasts, the more symptoms increase, including metabolic acidosis from reduced hydrogen ion excretion and sodium bicarbonate levels, increased phosphate and decreased calcium levels, abnormal blood cells (RBCs, WBCs, platelets), neurologic effects such as confusion, seizures, and coma, and effects on all body systems as is seen in CKD (discussed later).

DIURETIC PHASE. As the kidneys begin to excrete waste products again, 1 to 3 L/day of urine is produced. Osmotic diuresis occurs from the elevated waste products (urea), which the body is attempting to eliminate. The kidneys are not yet able to concentrate urine, so dehydration and hypotension are a concern. It is important to monitor for hypovolemia, hyponatremia, hypokalemia, and hypotension in this phase. Serum BUN and serum creatinine levels are high until the end of this phase. This phase may last 1 to 3 weeks.

RECOVERY PHASE. In this final phase, recovery begins as the GFR rises. Serum waste product levels (BUN, creatinine) decrease greatly within the first 2 weeks of this phase. This phase can last up to a year. Those who recover usually do so without complications. Older adults are more at risk for reduced recovery of renal function. In those who do not recover their renal function, CKD occurs.

Etiology

AKI is often classified as prerenal, intrarenal, or postrenal. These categories relate to the causes leading to the injury. Each category is associated with the location of the cause in the kidney. Understanding the cause can point to the direction of treatment plans helpful to the patient.

PRERENAL INJURY. Prerenal (before the kidney) injury, the most common cause of AKI, occurs when a decrease or interruption of blood supply to the kidneys impairs filtration. This may be due to decreased blood pressure from dehydration, surgery, blood loss, shock, or trauma to or blockage in the arteries that carry blood to the kidneys. Use of NSAIDs and cyclooxygenase-2 (COX) inhibitors can also lead to prerenal injury. They impair the autoregulatory responses of the kidney by blocking prostaglandin, necessary for renal perfusion.

Prerenal injury is diagnosed by evaluating possible causes. To determine if dehydration is the cause, an IV fluid challenge can be given. With increased IV fluid, more blood volume flows to the kidneys, which increases urine output and waste product filtering. An arteriogram of the renal arteries determines if the blood supply to the kidneys is decreased or blocked; angioplasty may then be used to open the blockage.

INTRARENAL INJURY. Intrarenal (inside the kidney) injury occurs with damage to the nephrons inside the kidney. The most common causes are ischemia, toxins, and reduced blood flow that lead to acute tubular necrosis (tubular cells die). Other causes are infections leading to glomerulonephritis, trauma to the kidney, exposure to **nephrotoxins**, reactions to contrast agents or medications (causing acute interstitial nephritis), and severe muscle injury, which releases substances that harm the kidneys.

A number of substances can be toxic to the kidneys (nephrotoxic) when they enter the body (Table 37.5). Kidney damage is most likely to occur when these substances enter the body in high concentrations or when pre-existing kidney damage is present for some other reason. Many commonly administered medications can be nephrotoxic. For example, aminoglycosides are nephrotoxic antibiotics; when they are administered, peaks and troughs of the drugs are carefully monitored to avoid toxic levels.

POSTRENAL INJURY. Postrenal (after the kidney) injury is associated with an obstruction that blocks the flow of urine out of the body. Only 5% of AKIs are classified as postrenal. The blood supply to the kidneys and nephron function may be normal, but urine cannot drain out of the kidney. This results in the backup of urine and impaired nephron function. Common causes are kidney stones, tumors of the ureters or bladder, and an enlarged prostate that blocks the flow of urine. Surgical intervention may be needed to correct the problem.

• **WORD** • **BUILDING** •
nephrotoxin: nephro—kidney + toxin—poison

Table 37.5
Common Nephrotoxins

Antibiotics	Aminoglycosides Amphotericin B Cephalosporins Sulfonamides Tetracyclines
Analgesics	Acetaminophen NSAIDs Salicylates
Other Medications	Angiotensin-converting enzyme (ACE) inhibitors Amphetamines Cisplatin Dextran Heroin Interleukin-2 Mannitol
Heavy Metals	Arsenic Copper Gold Lead Lithium Mercury
Contrast Media	Contrast agents used for diagnostic testing
Organic Solvents	Gasoline Glycols Kerosene Tetrachloroethylene Turpentine

Therapeutic Measures

AKI is treated by correcting the cause if possible. Prevention of permanent damage is the goal of treatment. Signs and symptoms are managed as they develop, and supportive care is given. Treatment may include restoring fluid and electrolyte balance, discontinuing nephrotoxic drugs, bypassing urinary tract obstructions with catheters to relieve urine retention, or using short-term continuous renal replacement therapy to filter blood and restore potassium and other electrolytes to normal. The care of the patient with AKI is similar to care of the patient with CKD.

CONTINUOUS RENAL REPLACEMENT THERAPY. Continuous renal replacement therapy (CRRT) is used to remove fluid and solutes in a controlled, continuous manner in unstable patients with AKI. Unstable patients may not be able to tolerate the rapid fluid shifts that occur in **hemodialysis**, so CRRT provides an alternative therapy that results in less dramatic fluid shifting. CRRT is not as complex as hemodialysis. It can be done for more than a month, if needed, via temporary vascular access. During CRRT, a permeable hemofilter is attached to the vascular access. Blood flows through the hemofilter as excess fluids and solutes move into a collection bag. The remaining blood returns to the patient via the venous access. Replacement fluid and electrolytes can be given through the vascular access. Monitoring hourly vital signs, vascular access, I&O, electrolytes, and daily weights is important.

Chronic Kidney Disease

Kidney disease is the eighth leading cause of death in the United States (CDC, 2020; see "Evidence-Based Practice"). CKD affects about 37 million people, and the incidence is on the rise (CDC, 2021). Many people are unaware they have kidney disease (Healthy People, 2030). CKD is a gradual, progressive, irreversible deterioration in renal function in which the body is unable to maintain metabolic, fluid, and electrolyte balance. The result is accumulation of nitrogenous waste products in the blood and **uremia**. CKD affects each body system (Table 37.6).

Evidence-Based Practice

Clinical Question
What is the cumulative impact of social determinants of health on mortality in U.S. adults with CKD and diabetes?

Evidence
This study analyzed data from the 2005 through 2014 National Health and Nutrition Examination Surveys for 1,376 adults who had diabetes and CKD to look at the effect that social determinants of health had on mortality. Social determinates of health relate to socioeconomic; psychosocial; neighborhood environment; and political, cultural, and economic factors that people experience during their lifetime. This analysis looked at family income to poverty ratio, food insecurity, and depression. It was found that these social determinants had a cumulative effect on mortality that increased by 41% for each additional social determinant. Depression was independently associated with mortality (Ozieh et al, 2021).

Implications for Nursing Practice
An awareness of social determinants of health, and screening for them as well as for depression in CKD patients, to plan interventions or make referrals (e.g., for Meals on Wheels or mental health services) may help reduce mortality for CKD patients.

Reference: Ozieh, M. N., Garacci, E., Walker, R. J., Palatnik, A., & Egede, L. E. (2021). The cumulative impact of social determinants of health factors on mortality in adults with diabetes and chronic kidney disease. *BMC Nephrology, 22*(1), 76. https://doi.org/10.1186/s12882-021-02277-2

• WORD • BUILDING •

hemodialysis: hemo—blood + dialysis—passage of a solute through a membrane

uremia: ur—urea + emia—in the blood

Table 37.6
Chronic Kidney Disease Summary

Signs and Symptoms	See Figure 37.6.
Diagnostic Tests/Findings	Glomerular filtration rate decreased pH—Metabolic acidosis RBCs decreased Elevated: Serum blood urea nitrogen, creatinine, magnesium, potassium Urinalysis abnormal Urine sodium level less than 10 mEq/L
Therapeutic Measures	Diet and Fluid Restriction Dialysis Transplant
Complications	Accelerated atherosclerosis Anemia Anorexia Dry itchy skin, ecchymosis Headache Heart failure Hypertension Impotence Osteomalacia Osteoporosis Platelet dysfunction Pulmonary edema Uremic encephalopathy Uremic pericarditis
Priority Nursing Diagnoses	*Excess Fluid Volume* *Decreased Activity Tolerance* *Impaired Skin Integrity*

Table 37.7
Stages of Chronic Kidney Disease

Stage	Kidney Function Description	Glomerular Filtration Rate (GFR) mL/min
1	Slight decrease	90 or greater
2	Mild decrease	60–89
3a	Moderate decrease	45–59
3b	Moderate decrease	30–44
4	Severe decrease	15–29
5	Dialysis/Transplant	Less than 15

Healthy People 2030 has 14 objectives related to CKD, including its goal of reducing the burden of chronic kidney disease and related complications (Office of Disease Prevention and Health Promotion, 2020).

Pathophysiology
When a large proportion of the body's nephrons are damaged or destroyed, AKI or CKD occurs. As the nephrons die off, the undamaged ones increase their work capacity. The patient may experience significant kidney damage without showing symptoms. CKD is a progressive disease process. In the early, or silent, stage (decreased renal reserve), the patient is usually without symptoms, even though up to 50% of nephron function may have been lost (Table 37.7).

The renal insufficiency stage occurs when the patient has lost 75% of nephron function and some signs of mild kidney disease are present. Anemia and the inability to concentrate urine may occur. Serum BUN and serum creatinine levels are slightly elevated. These patients are at risk for further damage caused by infection, dehydration, medications, heart failure, and use of contrast media. The goal of care is to prevent further damage, if possible, through control of blood glucose levels and blood pressure.

End-stage renal disease occurs when 90% of the nephrons are lost. Patients at this stage experience chronic and persistent abnormal kidney function. Serum BUN and serum creatinine levels are always elevated. These patients may make urine but not filter out the waste products, or urine production may cease. Dialysis or a kidney transplant is required for survival.

Uremia (urea in the blood) is present in CKD. Patients eventually develop problems in all body systems (Table 37.8). If left untreated, the patient with uremia will die within a short time.

Etiology
The causes of CKD are numerous. The most common include diabetes mellitus resulting in diabetic nephropathy, chronic high blood pressure causing nephrosclerosis, glomerulonephritis, and autoimmune diseases. Social determinants of health influence development and progression of CKD.

Symptoms of Kidney Disease
Patients with either AKI or CKD have multiple symptoms. Figure 37.6 illustrates symptoms; some of the more common ones are explained next.

Disturbance in Water Balance
Disturbances in the removal and regulation of water balance in the body occur with exhibition of signs of fluid accumulation. Edema, an early symptom, is seen in the extremities, abdomen, and sacral area when supine. Patients may report shortness of breath. Crackles and wheezes (signs of fluid accumulation) may be present on auscultation of the lungs. The patient may be hypertensive. These patients may produce a large amount of dilute urine (**polyuria**), small amounts of urine (oliguria), or no urine (anuria).

• WORD • BUILDING •

polyuria: poly—much + uria—urine

Table 37.8
Effects of Chronic Kidney Disease on Body Systems

Body System	Disease Process
Cardiovascular	Angina due to coronary artery disease, anemia Arrhythmias due to electrolyte imbalance, coronary artery disease Edema due to fluid overload and a decrease in osmotic pressure Heart failure due to fluid overload, left ventricular failure Hypertension due to fluid overload and accelerated arteriosclerosis Pericarditis due to presence of waste products in the pericardial sac
Gastrointestinal	Stomatitis due to fluid restriction, presence of waste products in the mouth, secondary infections Anorexia, nausea, vomiting due to uremia Gastritis/gastrointestinal bleeding due to urea decomposition in gastrointestinal tract releasing ammonia that irritates and ulcerates the stomach or bowel; patient is also under stress, increasing ulcer formation, and may have platelet dysfunction Constipation due to electrolyte imbalances, decrease in fluid intake, decrease in activity, phosphate binders Diarrhea, hypermotility due to electrolyte imbalance
Hematopoietic	Anemia due to impaired synthesis of erythropoietin, a substance needed by the bone marrow to stimulate formation of red blood cells (RBCs); also due to decreased life span of RBCs from uremia and interference in folic acid action Bleeding tendency due to abnormal platelet function from effects of uremia Prone to infection due to a decrease in immune system function from uremia; renal patients can rapidly become septic and die from septic shock
Integumentary	Dry, itchy, inflamed skin due to calcium-phosphate deposits in the skin Pale yellow skin color due to urobilins, which give urine its yellow color Skin will have an odor of urine because skin is an organ of excretion and the body attempts to remove toxins Decreased function of oil and sweat glands
Neurologic	Confusion due to uremic encephalopathy from increased urea and metabolic acids Peripheral neuropathy due to effects of waste products on neurologic system Cerebrovascular accidents due to accelerated atherosclerosis
Pulmonary	Pleurisy/pleural effusion due to waste products in the pleural space, causing inflammation with pleurisy pain and collection of fluid resulting in effusion
Reproductive	Loss of libido, impotence, amenorrhea, infertility due to a decrease in hormone production
Skeletal	Bone and mineral disease due to hyperphosphatemia and hypocalcemia

Disturbance in Electrolyte Balance

As kidney function decreases, the kidneys lose their ability to absorb and excrete electrolytes. If the kidneys are unable to maintain normal amounts of electrolytes in the blood, these substances can accumulate at high levels and become life threatening.

When the kidneys are unable to regulate sodium levels adequately, the patient may show signs of hypernatremia (excessive sodium in the blood), which causes water retention, edema, and hypertension. Hyponatremia (too little sodium) may result if too much sodium is lost. This can occur when the patient has experienced prolonged episodes of vomiting or diarrhea or is urinating large amounts of diluted urine. Patients with hyponatremia may show signs of confusion. Sodium levels may be normal, or they may be low due to dilution from excess fluid.

Hyperkalemia (adult potassium level greater than 5.3 mEq/L) can be life threatening if the level goes above 6.5 mEq/L (Earl, 2020). The patient may experience arrhythmias or cardiac arrest. Patients with hyperkalemia report muscle weakness, abdominal cramping, and diarrhea. They may be confused or disinterested in care. Patients with hyperkalemia should be placed on a cardiac monitor and observed for cardiac arrhythmias during treatment to reduce the potassium level.

Oral cavity
  Stomatitis
  Bad taste in mouth

Cardiovascular system
  Hypertension
  Heart failure
  Arrhythmias

Gastrointestinal system
  Anorexia
  Nausea
  Vomiting
  Gastrointestinal bleeding
  Ulcers

Reproductive system
  Sexual dysfunction
  Infertility

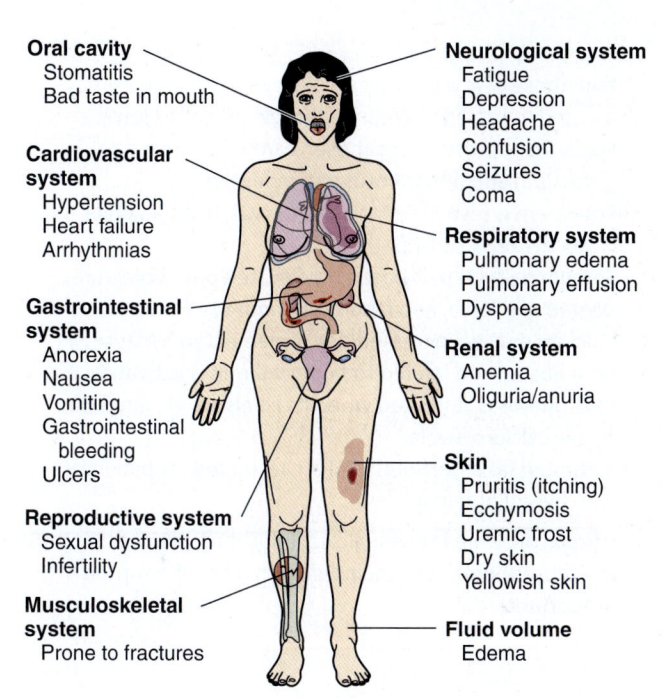

Musculoskeletal system
  Prone to fractures

Neurological system
  Fatigue
  Depression
  Headache
  Confusion
  Seizures
  Coma

Respiratory system
  Pulmonary edema
  Pulmonary effusion
  Dyspnea

Renal system
  Anemia
  Oliguria/anuria

Skin
  Pruritis (itching)
  Ecchymosis
  Uremic frost
  Dry skin
  Yellowish skin

Fluid volume
  Edema

FIGURE 37.6 Symptoms of chronic kidney disease.

A high potassium level in the patient with CKD may be caused by a diet high in potassium-rich foods, medications, injuries (releasing potassium from the cells), or blood transfusions. Monitor daily patient laboratory values and report abnormalities. Providing dietary education on foods to avoid that are high in potassium and evaluation of the patient's medications is extremely important (Box 37.1). The emergency and definitive treatment for hyperkalemia is hemodialysis. IV insulin with glucose (to prevent hypoglycemia from the insulin) may be used as a temporary measure to drive excess potassium quickly into the cells.

For maintenance therapy to reduce potassium, sodium polystyrene sulfonate (Kayexalate), patiromer (Veltassa), or sodium zirconium cyclosilicate (SZC; Lokelma) can be used. Sodium polystyrene sulfonate is given either orally or as a retention enema; it exchanges sodium for potassium in the gastrointestinal (GI) tract to then be eliminated in the stool. Since it is associated with serious risks of intestinal ischemia or thrombosis and GI ulcers and perforation it is not as commonly used as before. Patiromer (Veltassa) given orally exchanges sodium for potassium in the GI tract to then be eliminated in the stool. SZC an oral medication binds with potassium in the GI tract for elimination in the stool.

Calcium levels decrease because the kidneys are unable to produce the hormone that activates vitamin D, the vitamin needed for calcium absorption. Hypocalcemia exists when the calcium level falls below 8.5 mg/dL. Hyperphosphatemia (greater than 5 mg/dL) is associated with a low calcium level. These imbalances cause the bones to release calcium, increasing the risk of fractures. Regular ambulation is important to prevent further calcium loss from the bone. Many patients who are on dialysis develop hypercalcemia due to secondary hyperparathyroidism (excess release of parathyroid hormone). Medication may be prescribed to reduce excess levels of parathyroid hormone, which then reduces calcium levels.

Phosphates are found in many foods. Medication to bind phosphates (phosphate binders) is taken by patients with high phosphate levels. Patients must take these medications with each meal so they can bind with the phosphates in the food and be eliminated in the stool. High phosphorus levels may cause severe itching, and then produce open sores from the scratching, creating the risk of infection. Patients also may have muscle cramps and aches.

Disturbance of Removal of Waste Products

With azotemia (rapid accumulation of toxic wastes in the blood), patients may show signs of weakness and fatigue, confusion, seizures, twitching movements of extremities (asterixis), nausea, vomiting, and lack of appetite. They may report a metallic or bad taste in the mouth, and there may be the odor of urine on the patient's breath. The patient may have yellowish skin and report itching due to urea crystals on the skin. Dialysis to remove excessive waste products in the blood is the only treatment for the underlying causes of these symptoms.

Disturbance in Maintaining Acid–Base Balance

Hydrogen ion excretion is affected, causing a disturbance in the acid–base balance that results in metabolic acidosis. Patients may report headache, fatigue, weakness, nausea, vomiting, and lack of appetite. As metabolic acidosis progresses, the patient displays lethargy, stupor, and coma. Respirations become fast and deep as the lungs attempt to blow off carbon dioxide to correct the acidosis (Kussmaul respirations). See Chapter 6 for a detailed discussion of acid–base balance.

Disturbance in Hematologic Function

Anemia is seen mainly in CKD, which causes disturbances in blood cells over time. Damaged kidneys do not produce adequate erythropoietin, the hormone that stimulates RBC

Box 37.1
Foods High in Potassium

- Beans: Kidney, lentils, lima, navy, northern, pinto, refried, soy
- Chocolate
- Dairy products: Cheese, ice cream, milk, yogurt
- Dried fruit: Apricots, dates, figs, prunes, raisins
- Fruit: Avocado, banana, kiwi, mango, melons (cantaloupe, honeydew), nectarine, oranges, orange juice, papaya, pumpkin, tomato paste
- Juice: Carrot, prune, tomato, vegetable
- Nuts
- Salt substitutes
- Seeds
- Vegetables: Beet greens, potatoes (chips, sweet, white, yams), spinach, squash

production. Nutritional deficiencies and blood loss during dialysis also contribute to anemia. Injections of epoetin (Epogen, Procrit), a synthetic form of erythropoietin, can help restore RBC production and prevent anemia. Impaired WBC and immune functions contribute to an increased risk for infection. The patient should be protected from potential sources of infection. Impaired platelet function creates a risk for bleeding. The patient should be protected from injury, and signs of bleeding, such as blood in stool or emesis, must be reported.

Therapeutic Measures for Kidney Disease

Renal insufficiency and chronic kidney disease are treated based on symptoms with a restricted diet and fluid intake, medications, and careful monitoring for onset of serious problems or kidney failure (stage 5) that warrants kidney replacement therapy (dialysis or transplant). A kidney transplant can return the patient to a nearly normal state of health and functioning.

Diet

Dietary recommendations are individualized by the dietitian and HCP based on the patient's needs. Most patients are given iron, folic acid, vitamins, and minerals to supplement the restricted diet (see "Nutrition Notes: Understanding Dietary Changes in Renal Disease"). Because restrictions are complex, the diet may frustrate patients. The dietitian should be consulted for education and assistance. The nurse can help the patient identify foods they like within the diet plan.

Nutrition Notes

Understanding Dietary Changes in Chronic Kidney Disease

Patients with CKD can have complex dietary requirements and need the guidance of a dietitian who specializes in renal treatment. Dietary restrictions vary according to the patient's renal disease type and treatment. Renal diets are individualized. Educating patients to associate adherence to their diet with relief of symptoms is important. General guidelines include the following:

- Fluid restriction may vary daily according to urine output. Patients receiving hemodialysis may have 1,000 mL daily plus the previous day's urine output, if they still void.
- Adequate caloric intake is needed to maintain ideal body weight and protein stores. Simple carbohydrates and monounsaturated and polyunsaturated fats are given freely because their end products, carbon dioxide and water, are less likely to tax the kidney than protein.
- A low-protein diet is prescribed when the patient has renal function impairment to reduce damage to the nephrons. Protein is increased for dialysis to compensate for losses into the dialysate solution. Proteins of high biological value (eggs and meat) can be prescribed because they are more easily converted to body protein than those of low biological value. Vegetarian diets may be used to provide adequate protein as well as lower lipids. Plant proteins are chosen carefully to manage potassium and phosphorus serum levels.
- Potassium is restricted for patients with hyperkalemia when the cause is CKD.
- Sodium restriction is based on elevated blood pressure, degree of edema, and laboratory findings.
- Calcium may be increased or supplemented because of poor absorption related to faulty vitamin D activation.
- Phosphorus is restricted when its levels are elevated due to low calcium levels.
- Saturated fat and cholesterol are restricted for patients with hyperlipidemia.

Renal diets are individualized. Educating patients to associate adherence to their diet with relief of symptoms is important.

Medications

Early in the disease, diuretics are given to increase output. ACE inhibitors, ARBs, calcium channel blockers, or beta blockers may be used to control hypertension. Phosphate binders are given with meals (they must be given at the beginning of the meal to effectively bind with the phosphate in the food) to reduce phosphate levels. Calcium and vitamin D supplements are used to raise calcium levels. Both the active and storage forms of vitamin D should be considered to decrease fractures, cancer, and infection rates and to improve cardiac function. Medications are used to lower potassium levels if needed. All medication therapy is closely monitored because diseased kidneys are unable to effectively remove medications from the body. As renal function decreases, the patient who requires insulin may need smaller doses of some long-acting insulins.

Dialysis

Dialysis is started when the patient develops symptoms of severe fluid overload, elevated potassium levels, acidosis, pericarditis, vomiting, lethargy, fatigue, or symptoms of uremia that are life-threatening. Both peritoneal dialysis and hemodialysis involve the movement and diffusion of particles from an area of high concentration to an area of low concentration through a semipermeable membrane. Substances move from blood through the semipermeable membrane into the dialysate. Fluid and electrolyte imbalances can be corrected with dialysis. Dialysis can also be used to treat medication overdoses.

Research is ongoing in the development of a wearable artificial kidney to provide mobility and freedom from hemodialysis sessions and also for a bioartificial kidney for implantation.

HEMODIALYSIS. Hemodialysis involves the use of an artificial kidney to remove waste products and excess fluid from the patient's blood. During the dialysis procedure, the patient's blood and the dialyzing solution flow in opposite directions through the dialyzer. The dialysate contains electrolytes and fluid that resembles blood plasma. The patient's blood with metabolic waste products, excess fluid, and electrolytes is on the other side of the enclosed semipermeable membrane. The waste products from the patient's blood move into the dialysate by diffusion through the membrane because of the difference in their concentrations. The dialysate solution carries the waste products away, and the cleansed blood is returned to the patient's body intravenously (Fig. 37.7). A hemodialysis treatment is typically prescribed for 3 or 4 hours several times a week at a hemodialysis center (Fig. 37.8). Self-care hemodialysis is offered in some centers. Patients often do better when involved in treatments. Participation can range from doing some tasks to conducting the entire dialysis session after training. Hemodialysis can also be done at home with training.

Hemodialysis is not without side effects, as fluid and electrolyte levels drop rapidly. After treatment, the patient may have muscle cramps, and feel lethargic, weak, and fatigued. Sudden drops in blood pressure may cause the patient to become dizzy and nauseated. Cardiac arrhythmias and angina may occur. Patients are given large amounts of heparin, an anticoagulant, to keep the blood from clotting while it is in the dialyzer. Bleeding can occur from the puncture sites or other areas if injury occurs. Box 37.2 reviews nursing care for hemodialysis.

Vascular Access. Long-term hemodialysis requires a permanent way to access the bloodstream for blood removal and return to the body during dialysis. Typical permanent vascular access options are an arteriovenous (AV) fistula (considered to be the gold standard) or a vascular access graft. Grafts are more prone to clotting and infection. Fistulas or grafts are placed in the arm when possible.

> **NURSING CARE TIP**
> It is important to save the veins of patients with chronic kidney disease for possible future fistula creation. The nondominant patient arm should not be used for IV lines, blood draws, or blood pressure to avoid damage to the veins because it will likely be the arm used for the fistula.

Early referral to a nephrologist can allow for the establishment of vascular access so that it is matured (strong) before the need for dialysis. If this does not occur, then a temporary

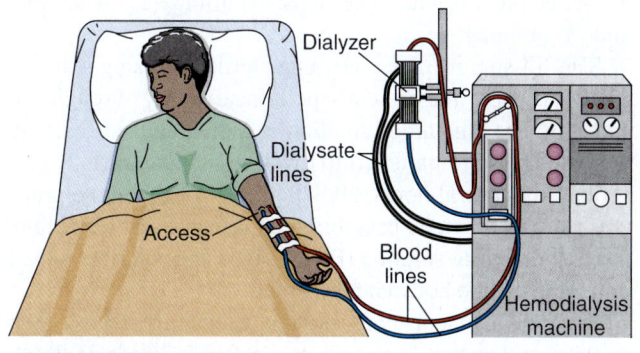

FIGURE 37.7 Hemodialysis.

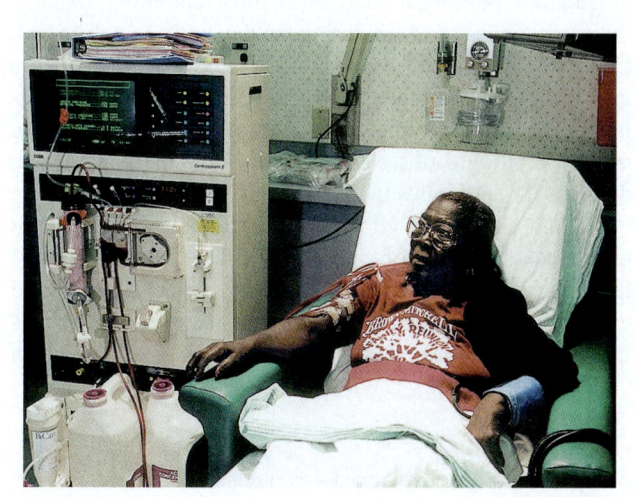

FIGURE 37.8 Patient undergoing hemodialysis at dialysis center.

Box 37.2
Nursing Care for Hemodialysis

1. Consult with the HCP about medications to hold before hemodialysis. Some medications, such as antihypertensives, can be harmful when they become effective during dialysis and can reduce blood pressure to dangerously low levels. Other medications can be dialyzed out of the body, losing their effect.
2. Ensure that the patient is weighed both before and after dialysis to document the weight loss from the fluid removal.
3. If the patient has laboratory tests ordered and blood needs to be drawn, coordinate this process with the dialysis nurse, who can obtain the blood samples and save the patient unnecessary needlesticks. To prevent painful needlesticks or other invasive procedures, a device that creates vibration to disrupt pain transmission can be held on the skin above the site of the procedure for 30 seconds. It is easy and fast to do, and patients are very appreciative. Some patients have their own devices and can teach you about it! An example of a pain-blocking vibration device can be seen at https://paincarelabs.com/buzzy.
4. Provide morning care early. Provide breakfast before dialysis if the patient tolerates eating before dialysis. For some patients, eating can cause hypotension by diverting blood flow to the GI system for digestion during dialysis.
5. When the patient returns from dialysis, weigh the patient, monitor the access site for bleeding, and monitor vital signs to ensure they are stable. Administer medications that were held if not contraindicated and vital signs are stable.
6. Protect the patient's dialysis access at all times, as outlined in Box 37.3.

access is used until a fistula or graft is placed and usable. A central venous catheter with two or three ports (the third port can be used for medications by trained staff) is placed in a central vein for temporary access. Central catheters should not be used long term because of the risk of infection.

An AV fistula is made by opening and joining a vein and artery together under the skin to create an area with greater blood volume for the dialysis machine to pull from (Fig. 37.9). AV fistulas may take several weeks to mature. The vascular surgeon determines when the fistula is mature for use.

An AV graft uses a tube made of synthetic material to attach to an artery and a vein. Two needles are inserted into the graft to access the patient's blood. Traditional graft material is not self-sealing and requires time for tissue growth to serve as a plug for the hole that the needles make before it can be used. This may take 1 to 2 weeks. Immediate-access vascular access grafts are self-sealing and do not require tissue growth, so they can be used often within 24 hours after surgical implantation. This self-sealing property decreases postdialysis bleeding, which reduces the time required for the dialysis session.

Vascular Access Care. Postoperatively, neurovascular checks are performed hourly. Neurovascular checks include extremity movement and sensation, presence of numbness or tingling, pulses, temperature, color, and capillary refill (normally less than 3 seconds). The extremity is elevated postoperatively. Range-of-motion exercises are encouraged. Vascular surgery pain is usually mild unless there is an occlusion. Dressings or incisions are checked, and any drainage, hematoma, or infection is documented and reported as needed. If a pulse is absent or weak or the extremity is cool or dusky, the HCP is notified immediately. AV fistulas or grafts can cause distal ischemia or "steal syndrome" because too much arterial blood is being "stolen" from the distal extremity. This is usually observed postoperatively and may require surgical correction to restore blood flow.

AV fistulas and grafts are checked every 4 hours for patency by the nurse by palpating to feel the thrill (a vibration) and auscultating to hear the bruit (swishing sound) at the site of the graft or fistula. Decrease or cessation of bruit or thrill indicates an occlusion. If a thrill or bruit is diminished or not present, the HCP is notified immediately. The site must be carefully monitored per institution policy to detect clotting or problems. Early detection of clotting allows the surgeon an opportunity to save the access by performing a declotting procedure rather than a total revision.

The extremity in which the access is placed should be protected. Do not use it for blood draws or IV fluids. Special care of the access is taught to the patient, as it is the patient's only way to eliminate waste (Box 37.3). The patient is taught to check patency daily.

PERITONEAL DIALYSIS. **Peritoneal dialysis** is continuous dialysis performed by the patient or family in the home. The peritoneal membrane is the semipermeable membrane across which excess wastes and fluids move from blood in peritoneal vessels into a dialysate solution that has been instilled into the peritoneal cavity. A peritoneal catheter is placed into the peritoneal space between the two layers of the peritoneum below the waistline. This catheter is used to perform an exchange process with three steps: (1) filling, (2) dwell time, and (3) draining.

The fill step involves instilling sterile dialyzing solution (dialysate) into the patient's peritoneal cavity through the catheter. The amount of solution is individualized by body weight. The solution is left to dwell in the abdomen as prescribed for several hours, allowing time for the waste products from the blood to pass through the peritoneal membrane into the dialysate solution (Fig. 37.10). The solution is then drained from the body and discarded.

Several treatment plans use this exchange process. The treatment plan that best suits the patient's needs is determined by the patient and the dialysis team. Continuous ambulatory peritoneal dialysis is most common. Usually, three exchanges are done during the day and one before bed. Other treatment plans use a computerized machine called a *cycler* to regulate exchanges during sleep. Sometimes, medications are added to dialyzing solutions, such as heparin to prevent clotting of the catheter, insulin for the patient with diabetes, or antibiotics to treat infection.

Patient and family education is extremely important for peritoneal dialysis to be successful. The patient must be taught and able to demonstrate ability to do a successful exchange. Sterile technique while performing exchanges is imperative, and the exchanges should be done in a clean

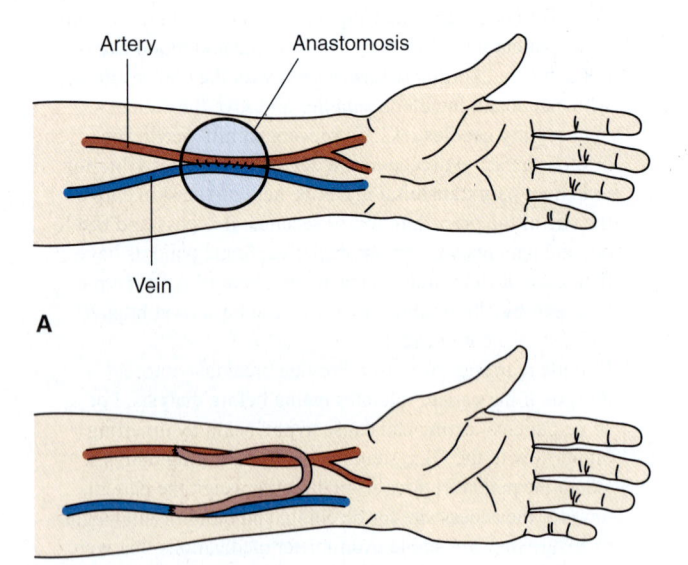

FIGURE 37.9 Hemodialysis access sites. (A) Arteriovenous fistula. (B) Arteriovenous graft.

• WORD • BUILDING •

peritoneal dialysis: peritoneal—peritoneum + dialysis— passage of a solution through a membrane

Box 37.3
Care of Blood Access Fistula or Graft

Fistulas or grafts that are created for dialysis access should not be used for any purpose other than dialysis.

1. Watch for signs of bleeding or infection at the access site.
2. Gently palpate the site for a thrill (vibration or pulsing feeling) that indicates adequate blood flow through the access site.
3. Listen for a bruit (swishing sound) at the access site by placing the diaphragm of a stethoscope gently on the site.
4. Do not take a blood pressure, use a tourniquet, draw blood, give an injection, or start any IV lines in an arm with an access site.
5. Many hospitals have indicators (such as a red arm bracelet) to signify that an arm should be protected. A sign above the bed may also be used.
6. Reinforce teaching to keep the access site clean and not to bump or cut it.
7. Reinforce teaching to follow weight restrictions for lifting with the access arm.
8. Reinforce teaching to avoid wearing constrictive clothing or jewelry over the access site.
9. Reinforce teaching to avoid prolonged bending of or sleeping on the arm with an access site.
10. Notify the HCP if signs of bleeding, reduced circulation, or infection occur in an access site extremity (e.g., coldness, numbness, weakness, redness, fever, drainage, or swelling).

environment. A major complication is peritonitis (infection of the peritoneum), which can be life threatening, most commonly related to poor technique when connecting the bag of dialyzing solution to the peritoneal catheter. The first sign of peritonitis is usually abdominal pain. (See Chapter 34 for signs and symptoms of peritonitis.) If symptoms occur, the patient must contact the HCP immediately so antibiotic treatment can begin. The patient should be taught to care for the exit site (the site where the catheter comes out of the abdomen) and inspect both the site and the dialysate solution for signs of infection.

Dietary education is also important. A dietitian can assist the patient in appropriate choices for adequate calories, protein, and potassium intake. The patient using peritoneal dialysis typically has fewer dietary and fluid restrictions than the patient on hemodialysis because peritoneal dialysis is continuous and maintains serum waste levels. Proteins are lost through the peritoneal membrane into the dialysate fluid, so increased dietary protein is needed.

LEARNING TIP

Therapy	Hemodialysis	Peritoneal dialysis	Continuous renal replacement therapy
Patient access	Vascular access	Peritoneal catheter	Temporary vascular access
Equipment	Specialized dialyzer	No dialyzer	Hemofilter
Training	Dialysis nurse	Patient	ICU nurse
Timing	Intermittent	Continuous	Continuous
Solute removal	Osmosis/Diffusion	Osmosis/Diffusion	Convection
Dialysate	Yes	Yes	No
Cardiovascular effects	Hypotension	Rare	Rare

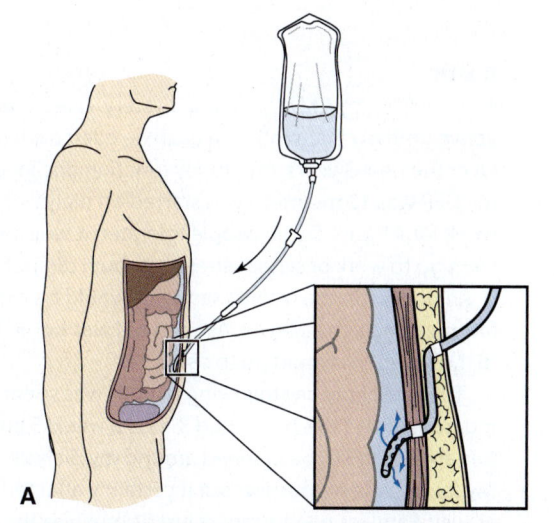

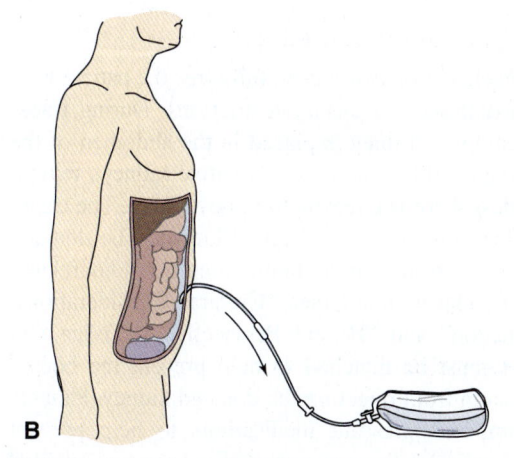

FIGURE 37.10 (A) Peritoneal dialysis works inside the body. Dialysis solution flows through a tube into the abdominal cavity, where it collects waste products from the blood. (B) Periodically, the used dialysis solution is drained from the abdominal cavity, carrying away waste products and excess water from the blood.

CLINICAL JUDGMENT

Mrs. Jackson is a single, 66-year-old woman with a 20-year history of type 2 diabetes, hypertension, hyperlipidemia, chronic anemia, and a total knee replacement. She has been diagnosed with CKD. She is being admitted to a medical unit from the emergency department for treatment of shortness of breath and CKD. Treatment will include hemodialysis. Mrs. Jackson has increasing shortness of breath, pitting edema, and a urine output of 375 mL yesterday. She is having premature ventricular contractions on the cardiac monitor. Her admitting serum laboratory values are sodium (Na) 131, potassium (K) 6, chloride (Cl) 97, calcium (Ca) 10, iron (Fe) 64, WBC 4,000, RBC 3.12, hemoglobin (Hgb) 10.1, hematocrit (Hct) 32, creatinine 2.2, and BUN 38. Her blood glucose levels yesterday were as follows: 0700, 154 mg/dL; noon, 142 mg/dL; 1700, 188 mg/dL. She has sliding-scale insulin coverage. An echocardiogram and chest x-ray will be done. She is having a two-tailed subclavian catheter placed for vascular access. Mrs. Jackson is withdrawn and quiet.

1. What is the first thing you do after getting the admitting handoff report?
2. What data do you report to the HCP?
3. What do you say to Mrs. Jackson regarding her withdrawn behavior?
4. What do you identify related to Mrs. Jackson's understanding of her self-care needs?
5. What teaching do you reinforce for the scheduled diagnostic tests?
6. What nursing care do you provide for the vascular access?
7. What type of prescribed insulin do you prepare for sliding-scale insulin coverage? Why?
8. With what members of the health-care team do you collaborate?

Suggested answers are at the end of the chapter.

Kidney Transplantation

Kidney transplantation can successfully free the patient with CKD from dialysis and dietary restrictions. During transplantation, a donor kidney is placed in the abdomen of the recipient (Fig. 37.11). The patient's native kidneys remain in place unless there is a reason to remove them. The transplanted kidney functions as a normal kidney. The donated kidney can come from a living family member, a nonrelated donor, or a cadaver donor (see "Cultural Considerations: Organ Donation" and "Patient Perspective"). Tissue and blood types must be matched to help prevent the body's immune system from rejecting the donated kidney. Patients receive immunosuppressant medications to help prevent rejection, usually for the rest of the life of the transplanted kidney. Sometimes even with medications, the body rejects the kidney and the patient requires dialysis.

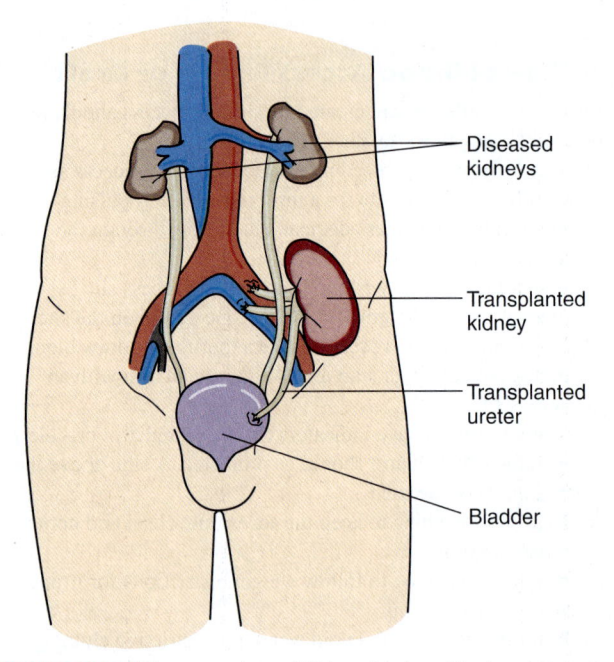

FIGURE 37.11 The transplanted kidney is placed in the abdomen.

Cultural Considerations

Organ Donation
- Some cultural groups believe that the body must be kept intact after death and may oppose the removal of body parts or organ donation. Many organizations have policies in place to discuss organ donation with all families, which can be both jarring to the family and viewed as disrespectful. Nurses can help to prepare families for these conversations by alerting them to these standard policies and reassuring them that their choices will be respected.

Patient Perspective

Garth
The cause of my CKD remains a mystery. I was healthy and active until my first symptom of ankle edema occurred. Over the next 3 years, my kidney function declined. When my GFR was 12 mL/min, I was started on dialysis 3 days a week for 4 hours. Some people tolerated it well and could even go to work or school afterward, but I did not tolerate it. An hour after the dialysis session, I would be extremely fatigued and ache all over. As soon as I was home from the dialysis center, I would go to sleep.

The rest of my day following dialysis was spent recovering from it, and this happened 3 days a week! Family activities always had to be planned around my dialysis schedule. My family was supportive, but it certainly affected them as well. Families need support just as much as the patient. I was on the kidney transplant waiting list for two and half years. I had just begun the training for home dialysis when I got the call that a kidney was available. I was overjoyed, but sad for the donor, who was on life support. My transplant surgery went smoothly. My own kidneys were left in place. The new kidney began making urine right away. In the recovery room, my urinary catheter bag was nearly full! It was liquid gold to me! The morning after surgery, I felt wonderful. I had so much energy and was walking up and down the halls, outpacing the nurses. They told me to slow down, but I felt so good for the first time in years that nothing slowed me down. The registered nurse transplant coordinator, pharmacist, and dietitian all taught me about follow-up care, my two antirejection medications that I must take for the life of the transplanted kidney, and healthy eating. I no longer had a daily 1,000 mL fluid limit (which is not much!) or dietary restrictions, which was fantastic! My recovery progressed with no complications. I had frequent follow-up laboratory work and clinic visits in the beginning. Seven years later, all is well. I take my antihypertensive, statin, and antirejection medications faithfully, and I have yearly nephrology clinic visits and monthly laboratory work. I am grateful to the donor and the donor's family for the gift I received.

Nursing Process for the Patient With Kidney Disease

Data Collection

Kidney disease progressively affects all body systems. With short-term AKI, some effects do not have time to develop. Nursing care for AKI is similar to CKD nursing care for the effects that have occurred. In CKD, more effects are seen because the disease has time to progress. Signs and symptoms vary depending on the severity of CKD and its cause (Fig. 37.6). Data should be collected for signs and symptoms in all body systems. Family history of kidney disease and patient history of health problems such as hypertension, diabetes, systemic erythematous lupus, or urinary disorders are noted in the history. Also noted are medications the patient takes because they may be nephrotoxic and require adjustments. Recent changes in weight are documented.

Nursing Diagnosis, Planning, Intervention, and Evaluation

Decreased Activity Tolerance related to anemia secondary to impaired synthesis of erythropoietin by the kidneys

EXPECTED OUTCOME: The patient will be able to perform activities important to him or her.

- Monitor hemoglobin (Hgb) and hematocrit (Hct) and for presence of pale mucous membranes, dyspnea, or chest pain *to detect anemia to report*.
- Schedule rest periods for patient between activities *to reduce fatigue and increase energy*.

Impaired Skin Integrity related to dryness, excess fluid, and crystal deposits

EXPECTED OUTCOME: The patient will maintain intact skin.

- Observe skin for open areas and signs of infection *to detect problems*.
- Bathe with tepid water, oils, or oatmeal and apply lotion afterwards *to reduce skin crystals to decrease itching and promote comfort*.

Risk for Infection related to impaired immune system function

EXPECTED OUTCOME: The patient will not develop infection, as evidenced by WBCs and temperature within normal limits as well as no signs and symptoms of infection.

- Monitor for signs and symptoms of infection *to report promptly to HCP*.
- Protect patient from sources of active infection, including caregivers, roommates, or visitors and ensure vaccinations are up to date *to reduce risk for infection*.
- Reinforce teaching of handwashing techniques to patient and caregivers *to help control spread of infection*.
- Reinforce teaching of signs and symptoms of infection to patient and family *to promptly report to HCP*.

Risk for Injury related to bleeding tendency from platelet dysfunction, use of heparin during dialysis, or gastrointestinal (GI) bleeding

EXPECTED OUTCOME: The patient will be free from bleeding, or it is detected and stopped quickly.

- Observe for blood in stool or emesis, easy bruising, or bleeding from mucous membranes or puncture sites *to report immediately*.
- Monitor Hgb, Hct, clotting studies, and platelets, and report abnormal values *to detect bleeding*.
- Reinforce teaching for patient to prevent injury *to prevent bleeding*.

Imbalanced Nutrition: Less Than Body Requirements related to restricted diet, anorexia, nausea, vomiting, and stomatitis secondary to effect of excessive urea on the GI system

EXPECTED OUTCOME: The patient will maintain ideal weight, and serum protein and albumin levels will be within normal limits.

- Monitor weekly weight and serum protein and albumin levels *to detect levels to report*.
- Renal diets may have restrictions such as low-protein *to decrease formation of waste products (urea, creatinine)*.

Nursing Care Plan for the Patient With Chronic Kidney Disease

Nursing Diagnosis: *Excess Fluid Volume* related to kidney's inability to excrete fluid
Expected Outcomes: Fluid volume will be stable as evidenced by stable weight, absence of edema, clear lung sounds, and blood pressure within the patient's normal parameters.
Evaluation of Outcomes: Is weight stable? Is edema absent? Are lungs clear? Is blood pressure within the patient's normal parameters?

Intervention	Rationale	Evaluation
Monitor weight daily at same time; report gain of more than 2 pounds.	*Those retaining fluid will have weight gain.*	Is weight stable? Should HCP be notified of change?
Monitor intake and output and for presence of edema.	*This reveals degree of fluid retention.*	Is intake more than output? Is edema present? Are these changes?
Monitor and report crackles in lungs, shortness of breath, frothy sputum, jugular vein distention, tachycardia, arrythmias.	*These are symptoms of heart failure that may accompany fluid overload.*	Are symptoms of heart failure present?
Reinforce teaching to maintain sodium and fluid restrictions as ordered.	*For those on dialysis, fluid intake is restricted so that weight gains are no more than 1 to 3 kg between dialysis sessions.*	Does patient understand and maintain sodium and fluid restriction?

- Consult dietitian for calorie count need and renal diet restrictions *to develop a dietary plan.*
- Provide frequent oral care *to reduce urine taste in mouth and enhance appetite.*
- Offer antiemetics before meals and frequent small meals *to prevent nausea.*

Evaluation

Outcomes have been achieved if the patient maintains intact skin, does not develop infection, is free from bleeding, and maintains ideal weight.
See also "Nursing Care Plan for the Patient With Chronic Kidney Disease."

Key Points

- UTIs are most often an ascending infection, starting at the external urinary meatus and moving up toward the bladder and kidneys, that are frequently caused by the bacterium *Escherichia coli*, which is commonly found in feces.
- Lower UTIs include urethritis, prostatitis, and cystitis. Upper UTIs include pyelonephritis and ureteritis. UTIs are the most common hospital-acquired infection.
- Older adults have an increased incidence of UTIs due to diminished immune function, diabetes, and a neurogenic bladder that fails to completely empty.
- Renal calculi (urolithiasis) are stones in the urinary tract that usually begin in the kidney (nephrolithiasis) but can be found in the ureter (ureterolithiasis). IV fluids, NSAIDs, and lithotripsy (sound shock waves or laser energy to break the stone into small fragments) treat renal calculi.
- Hydronephrosis (distention of the renal pelvis and calices) results from obstruction of urine flow in the urinary tract. This increases pressure on the structures of the kidney, which can damage the kidney, impair its function, and ultimately lead to acute or chronic kidney disease. Obstruction causes are stricture in a ureter or the urethra, renal calculi, tumors, or an enlarged prostate.
- Cancer of the bladder often starts as a benign growth on the bladder wall that undergoes cancerous changes. Some cancers occur as small, wartlike growths on the inside of the bladder. Others form large tumors that grow into the muscle wall of the bladder and require surgical removal.
- Those who smoke develop bladder cancer twice as often as people who do not smoke.
- Urinary diversion is used after a cystectomy: urostomy or ileal conduit (section of the ileum or colon becomes conduit for urine); continent urinary diversion (ileum made into a reservoir for urine with ureters implanted into the side), which requires self-catheterization at 4-hour intervals; orthotopic neobladder (section of intestine made into a neobladder with ureters and urethra implanted into the neobladder), which allows the patient to void through the urethra.
- Risk factors for kidney cancer include smoking, obesity, hypertension, long-term kidney dialysis, genetics (rare), and exposure to radiation, asbestos, and industrial pollution.
- Causes of trauma to the kidney, ureters, and bladder include motor vehicle accidents, sports injuries, falls, and gunshot and stab wounds.

- Polycystic kidney disease is a hereditary disorder. Multiple cysts in the kidney can eventually replace normal kidney structures resulting in CKD.
- Diabetic nephropathy is the most common cause of CKD. It is a long-term complication of diabetes mellitus in which the small blood vessels in the kidneys are damaged. Risk factors include hypertension, genetic predisposition, smoking, and chronic hyperglycemia. Careful control of blood glucose levels reduces the risk of nephropathy.
- Nephrotic syndrome is the excretion of 3.5 grams or more of protein in urine per day in which large amounts of protein are lost in the urine from increased glomerular membrane permeability. As a result, serum albumin, total serum protein, and anticlotting proteins are decreased.
- Hypertension damages the kidneys by causing sclerotic changes in the small arteries and arterioles (nephrosclerosis).
- Glomerulonephritis, an inflammatory disease of the glomerulus, can be caused by a variety of factors, including immunological abnormalities, toxins, vascular disorders, and systemic diseases.
- Kidney disease is diagnosed when waste products (BUN, creatinine) are no longer effectively being eliminated and their blood levels rise. This effects all body systems as a result of imbalances in fluid, electrolytes, and calcium levels, as well as impaired RBC formation and decreased elimination of waste products. Kidney disease can be acute, due to kidney injury (AKI), or chronic (CKD), occurring gradually over time.
- Contrast agents used during diagnostic tests can cause kidney damage, especially when the patient is dehydrated, the glomerular filtration rate is below 60 mL/min, or there is pre-existing renal damage.
- CRRT is used to remove fluid and solutes in a controlled, continuous manner in unstable patients with AKI. Unstable patients may not be able to tolerate the rapid fluid shifts that occur in hemodialysis, so CRRT provides an alternative therapy that results in less dramatic fluid shifting.
- Hemodialysis uses an artificial kidney to remove waste products and excess fluid from the patient's blood. The patient must be weighed before and after dialysis, and vital signs must be monitored to detect hypotension.
- Peritoneal dialysis provides continuous dialysis treatment and is done by the patient or caregiver in the home. The peritoneal membrane is the semipermeable membrane across which excess wastes and fluids move from blood in peritoneal vessels into a dialysate solution that has been instilled into the peritoneal cavity. The dialysate solution is drained after a prescribed time frame and the process begins again.
- A transplanted kidney functions as a normal kidney does. The donated kidney can come from a living family member, a nonrelated donor, or a cadaver donor. The donor kidney is placed in the lower abdomen of the recipient.

SUGGESTED ANSWERS TO CHAPTER EXERCISES

Cue Recognition

37.1: Ask the patient to describe and rate the pain from 0 to 10. Administer prescribed pain medication.

37.2: Strain *all* urine to identify any stones that may have been passed, as that is the patient's ticket to being discharged! Send all stones or stone fragments for analysis.

Critical Thinking & Clinical Judgment

Mrs. Milan
1. Sexual intercourse can be a predisposing factor to UTI.
2. The urinalysis will show WBCs, bacteria, RBCs, and positive nitrites.
3. Mrs. Milan should be informed to urinate after intercourse, drink adequate fluids to maintain light-yellow urine color; void regularly; wipe from front to back; wear cotton crotch underwear; avoid constricting clothing such as tight jeans; and avoid perfumed feminine hygiene products, bubble bath and bath salts, scented toilet paper, and tub baths.
4. The teaching plan includes the need to take all the antibiotics until gone, even if she feels better, to ensure that the infection is resolved so it does not return or create resistant bacteria and to return for a urine culture after the therapy.

Mr. Stevens
1. Weight, I&O, blood pressure.
2. Serum BUN, serum creatinine, and serum potassium levels.
3. Mr. Stevens should learn about his antihypertensive medications, a low-sodium diet, fluid restrictions, and importance of follow-up visits.

Mrs. Jackson
1. Collect data beginning with Mrs. Jackson's breathing and respiratory status. Address the cardiovascular system to see how she is tolerating the arrhythmia. Then obtain Mrs. Jackson's weight and I&O to monitor fluid balance.
2. Data to report: Shortness of breath and pitting edema (fluid overload); urine output 375 mL yesterday (CKD); premature ventricular contractions (elevated potassium). Decreased serum sodium (dilutional effect of excess fluid). Elevated serum potassium (retained in CKD). Decreased WBCs (low due to CKD). Decreased RBCs, Hgb, and Hct (anemia). Elevated serum creatinine and BUN (not excreted adequately in CKD). Elevated blood glucose (diabetes).
3. Therapeutic communication suggestions: "Mrs. Jackson, would you like to talk about your diagnosis?" "How do you feel about your diagnosis?" "Do you have questions or concerns?" "What are your usual coping methods?" Provide explanations for procedures and interventions to her.

SUGGESTED ANSWERS TO CHAPTER EXERCISES—cont'd

4. Determine Mrs. Jackson's understanding of what CKD is, how it is treated, how to follow the renal diet and fluid restrictions, and the action and importance of medications. Identify barriers to self-care and her support systems.
5. Teaching reinforcement includes that the chest x-ray and echocardiogram require no preparation and are not painful.
6. A two-tailed subclavian vascular access is dedicated for hemodialysis. It will not be used for any other purpose. The site will be observed for signs of infection (e.g., redness, warmth, swelling, tenderness, drainage, fever).
7. Regular insulin, which is a rapid-acting insulin. It is the only type of insulin used for sliding-scale coverage. A sliding scale is used to treat current blood glucose levels. Therefore, a rapid-acting insulin must be used to affect a current blood glucose level. Sliding-scale insulin is ordered at intervals to treat an elevated blood glucose level according to ordered parameters.
8. The registered nurse, surgeon, nephrologist, dietitian, pharmacist, and social worker.

Additional Resources

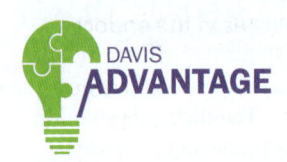

Go to Davis Advantage to complete your learning: strengthen understanding, apply your knowledge, and prepare for the Next Gen NCLEX®.

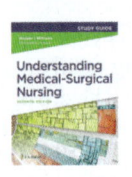

A Study Guide is also available.

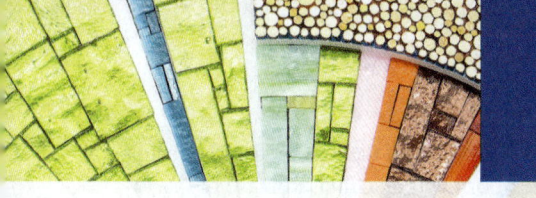

UNIT TEN Understanding the Endocrine System

CHAPTER 38
Endocrine System Function and Data Collection

Alene Homan, Paula D. Hopper, Janice L. Bradford

KEY TERMS

affect (AF-fekt)
antagonist (an-TAG-uh-nist)
exophthalmos (EKS-off-THAL-mus)
gluconeogenesis (GLOO-koh-NEE-oh-JEN-iss-iss)
negative feedback (NEG-uh-TIV FEED-bak)
positive feedback (POS-uh-TIV FEED-bak)

CHAPTER CONCEPTS

Cellular regulation
Fluid and electrolyte balance

LEARNING OUTCOMES

1. Identify the glands of the endocrine system.
2. Explain the function of each of the hormones in the endocrine system.
3. Describe the effects of aging on endocrine system function.
4. List data to collect when caring for a patient with a disorder of the endocrine system.
5. Plan nursing care for patients undergoing testing for an endocrine disorder.

NORMAL ENDOCRINE SYSTEM ANATOMY AND PHYSIOLOGY

The endocrine system consists of the endocrine (ductless) glands, which secrete hormones. Unlike other organ systems, the glands of the endocrine system are anatomically separate (Fig. 38.1). Their hormones are involved in fluid balance; metabolism, energy balance, growth, and development; contraction of smooth and cardiac muscle; glandular secretion; reproduction; and the establishment of circadian rhythms (sleep–wake cycle). Each hormone is secreted in response to a specific stimulus, is circulated by the blood, and affects target cells that have receptors for that hormone. Some hormones are secreted in response to hormones from other endocrine glands. Most hormone levels are regulated by **negative feedback** systems.

Hypothalamus and Pituitary Gland

The hypothalamus connects the nervous system to the endocrine system via the pituitary gland (hypophysis). The hypothalamus is above the midbrain, and the pituitary gland is suspended from the hypothalamus by a short stalk (Fig. 38.2). There are two primary lobes, or portions, of the pituitary gland: anterior and posterior.

Anterior Pituitary Gland
The anterior pituitary gland secretes its hormones in response to releasing hormones from the hypothalamus (Fig. 38.3).

Secretion of growth hormone (GH) is regulated by growth hormone–releasing hormone (GHRH) and by growth hormone–inhibiting hormone (GHIH, or somatostatin), both produced by the hypothalamus. See Figure 38.3 for functions of GH.

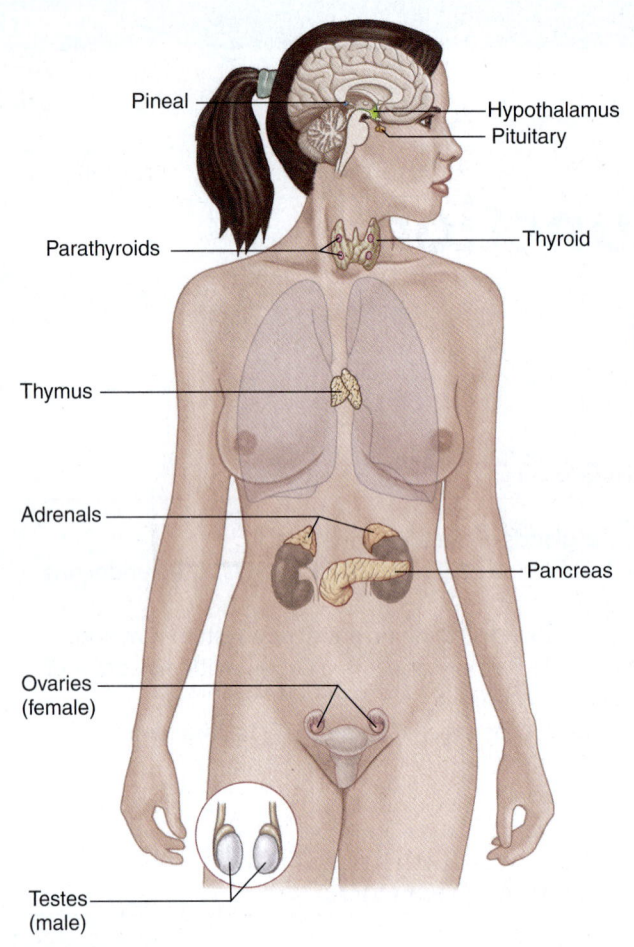

FIGURE 38.1 Endocrine organs.

Thyroid-stimulating hormone (TSH) stimulates growth and secretions of the thyroid gland. TSH secretion is stimulated by thyrotropin-releasing hormone (TRH).

Adrenocorticotropic hormone (ACTH) stimulates secretion of cortisol and related hormones from the adrenal cortex. Corticotropin-releasing hormone (CRH) from the hypothalamus stimulates the release of ACTH. CRH is produced during any type of stress such as injury, disease, exercise, or hypoglycemia.

See Figure 38.3 for other hormones of the anterior pituitary gland.

Posterior Pituitary Gland

The posterior pituitary gland stores and releases antidiuretic hormone (ADH; sometimes called *vasopressin*) and oxytocin (Fig. 38.4). Axon tracts from the hypothalamus transmit the hormones to the posterior pituitary and signal their release.

ADH increases water reabsorption by the kidney tubules, which decreases urine output. The water is reabsorbed back into the blood, thereby maintaining normal blood volume and pressure. In cases of great fluid loss, such as severe hemorrhage, the large amount of ADH secreted is especially important because it causes arteriole vasoconstriction, which increases blood pressure to homeostatic levels.

Oxytocin causes contractions of the myometrium to bring about delivery of a newborn and placenta. Release of oxytocin operates on a **positive feedback** loop. During breastfeeding, the subsequent release of oxytocin causes contraction of the smooth muscle cells around the mammary ducts. This release of milk is called *milk ejection* (or letdown).

Thyroid Gland

The thyroid gland consists of two lobes connected by a piece of tissue called the *isthmus* (Fig. 38.5). Three hormones are produced by the thyroid gland: triiodothyronine (T_3), thyroxine (T_4), and calcitonin.

T_3 and T_4 increase metabolism of glucose and fatty acids, which increases energy and heat production. They are essential for normal physical growth, mental development, and reproductive maturation. Sufficient iodine intake is required for T_3 and T_4 production.

The direct stimulus for secretion of T_3 and T_4 is TSH from the anterior pituitary. A decrease in metabolic rate causes the hypothalamus to secrete TRH. TRH stimulates the anterior pituitary to secrete TSH, which stimulates the thyroid to increase secretion of T_3 and T_4. This then increases energy production and raises the metabolic rate. Negative feedback decreases the secretion of TRH from the hypothalamus until the metabolic rate decreases again.

The third thyroid hormone, calcitonin, targets bone tissue and is especially important during childhood when bone growth is accelerated. Resorption of calcium and phosphorous into the blood is inhibited by calcitonin so than these minerals are retained in the bones, and blood levels of calcium and phosphorous are decreased. This one function of calcitonin has two important results: the maintenance of normal blood levels of calcium and phosphate, and the maintenance of a strong, stable bone matrix. The stimulus for secretion of calcitonin is hypercalcemia.

> **LEARNING TIP**
> Confused between resorption and reabsorption? *Resorption* breaks down bone tissue and releases calcium ions into circulation when parathyroid hormone is secreted. *Reabsorption* is the process of absorbing a substance into the blood again, such as when antidiuretic hormone causes water to be reabsorbed from the kidney tubules back into the blood supply.

> **LEARNING TIP**
> An easy way to remember the function of calcitonin is to remember calciTONin TONes down serum calcium.

• WORD • BUILDING •

antidiuretic hormone: anti—against + diuretic—relating to urination

Chapter 38 Endocrine System Function and Data Collection 725

The tiny, pea-sized pituitary gland sits just underneath the hypothalamus. It lies cradled in the sella turcica, a cavity within the sphenoid bone.

Pituitary gland

Neurons within the hypothalamus synthesize various hormones. Some, called **releasing hormones**, stimulate the anterior pituitary to secrete its hormones. Others, called **inhibiting hormones**, suppress hormone secretion by the anterior pituitary.

Hypothalamus
Optic chiasm
Anterior pituitary
Posterior pituitary

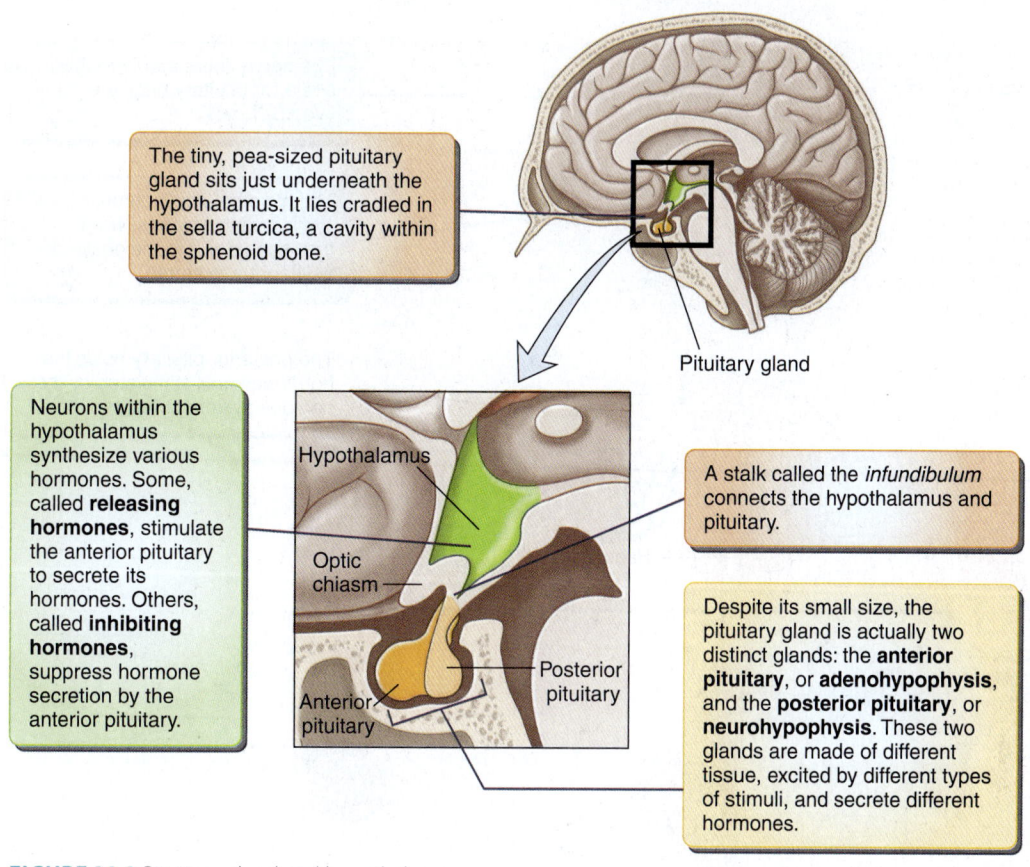

A stalk called the *infundibulum* connects the hypothalamus and pituitary.

Despite its small size, the pituitary gland is actually two distinct glands: the **anterior pituitary**, or **adenohypophysis**, and the **posterior pituitary**, or **neurohypophysis**. These two glands are made of different tissue, excited by different types of stimuli, and secrete different hormones.

FIGURE 38.2 Pituitary gland and hypothalamus.

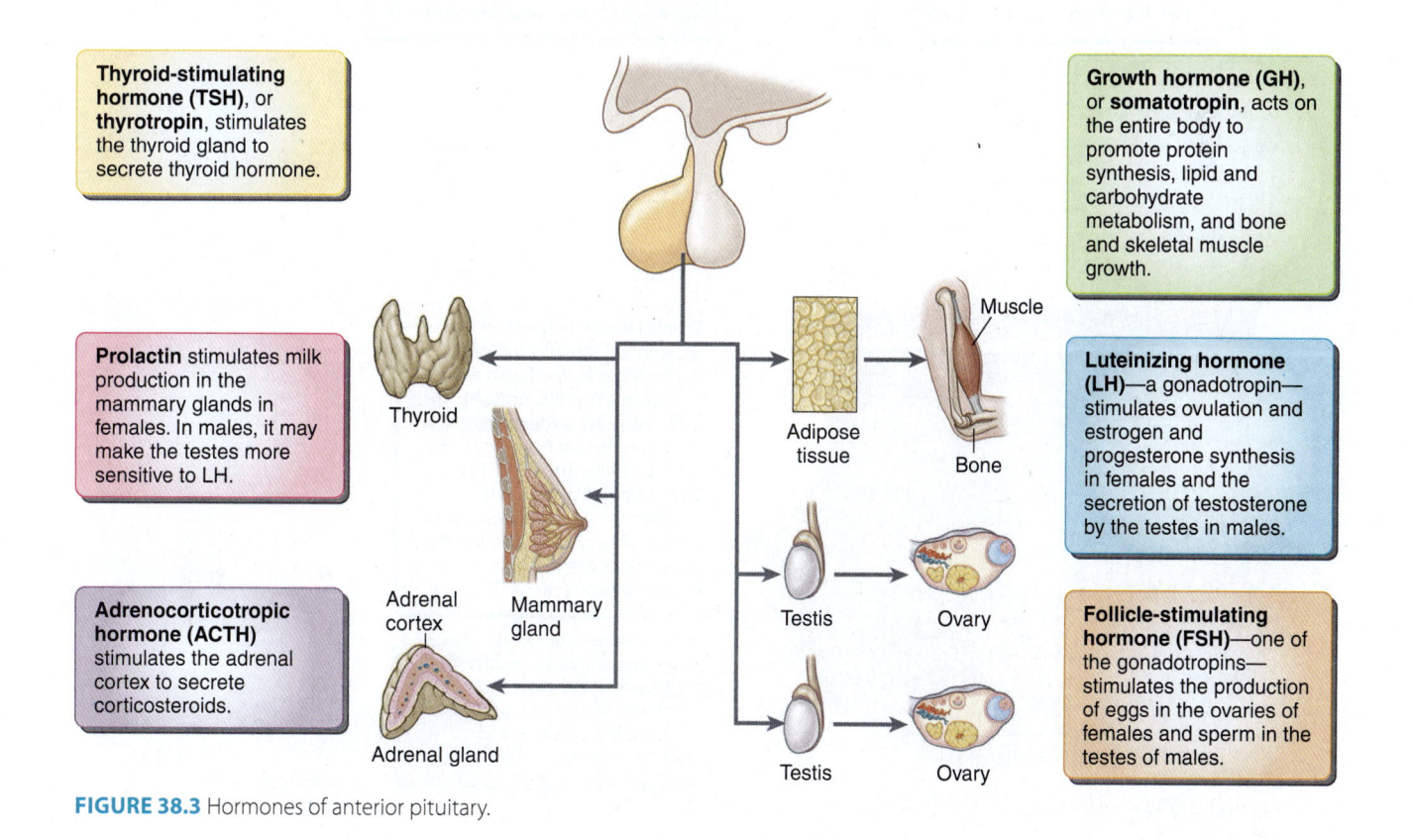

Thyroid-stimulating hormone (TSH), or **thyrotropin**, stimulates the thyroid gland to secrete thyroid hormone.

Prolactin stimulates milk production in the mammary glands in females. In males, it may make the testes more sensitive to LH.

Adrenocorticotropic hormone (ACTH) stimulates the adrenal cortex to secrete corticosteroids.

Thyroid
Adrenal cortex
Mammary gland
Adrenal gland
Adipose tissue
Muscle
Bone
Testis
Ovary
Testis
Ovary

Growth hormone (GH), or **somatotropin**, acts on the entire body to promote protein synthesis, lipid and carbohydrate metabolism, and bone and skeletal muscle growth.

Luteinizing hormone (LH)—a gonadotropin—stimulates ovulation and estrogen and progesterone synthesis in females and the secretion of testosterone by the testes in males.

Follicle-stimulating hormone (FSH)—one of the gonadotropins—stimulates the production of eggs in the ovaries of females and sperm in the testes of males.

FIGURE 38.3 Hormones of anterior pituitary.

UNIT TEN Understanding the Endocrine System

- The nerve fibers that form the posterior pituitary originate in the hypothalamus.
- The hypothalamic neurons synthesize hormones, which they send down to the posterior pituitary to be stored.
- The posterior pituitary holds the hormones until stimulated by the nervous system to release them.
- **Oxytocin** stimulates contraction of the uterus during childbirth. It also triggers the release of milk from the breasts during lactation.
- **Antidiuretic hormone (ADH)** acts on the kidneys to reduce urine volume and prevent dehydration. ADH is also called **vasopressin**.

FIGURE 38.4 Posterior pituitary and hormones.

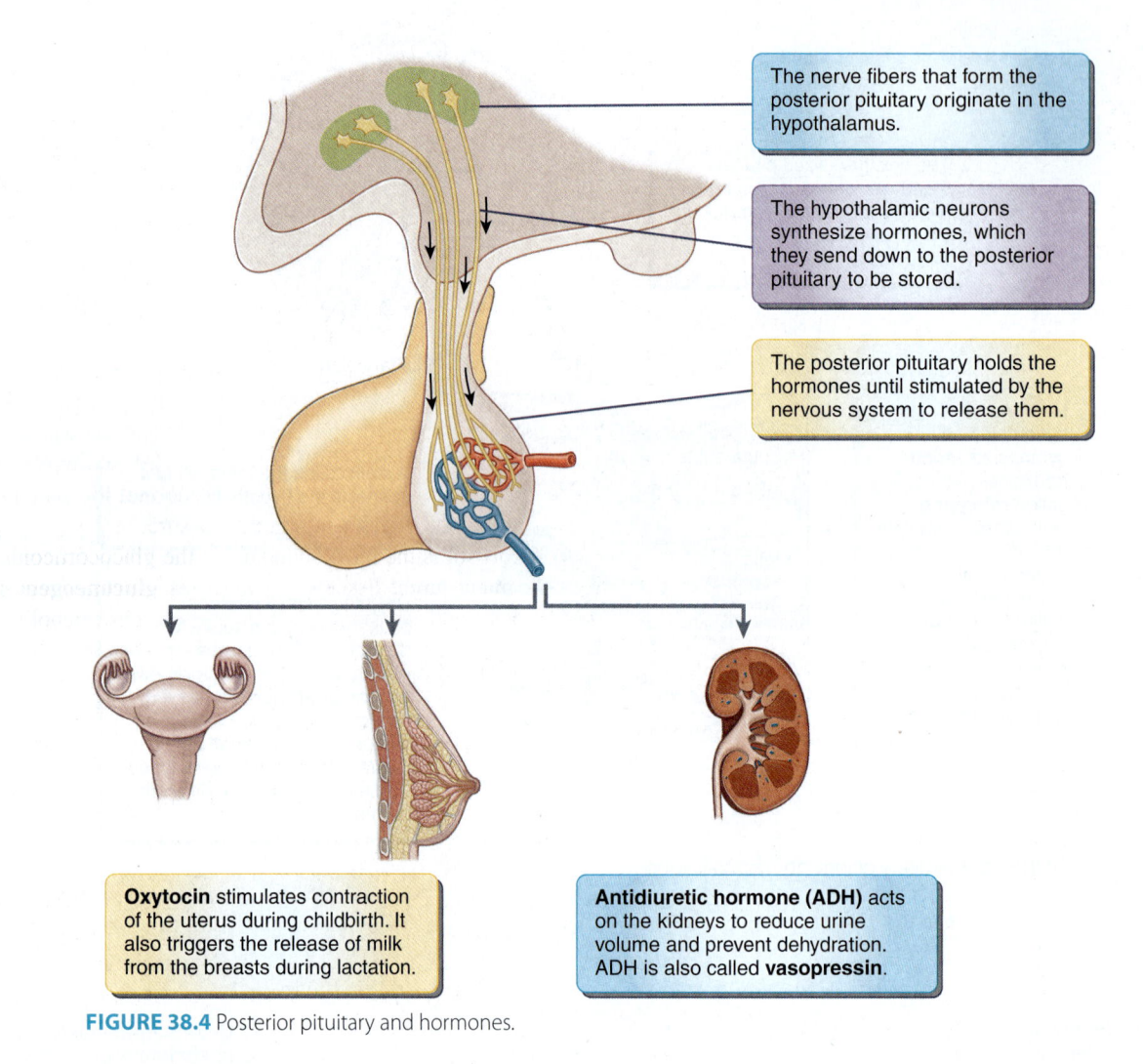

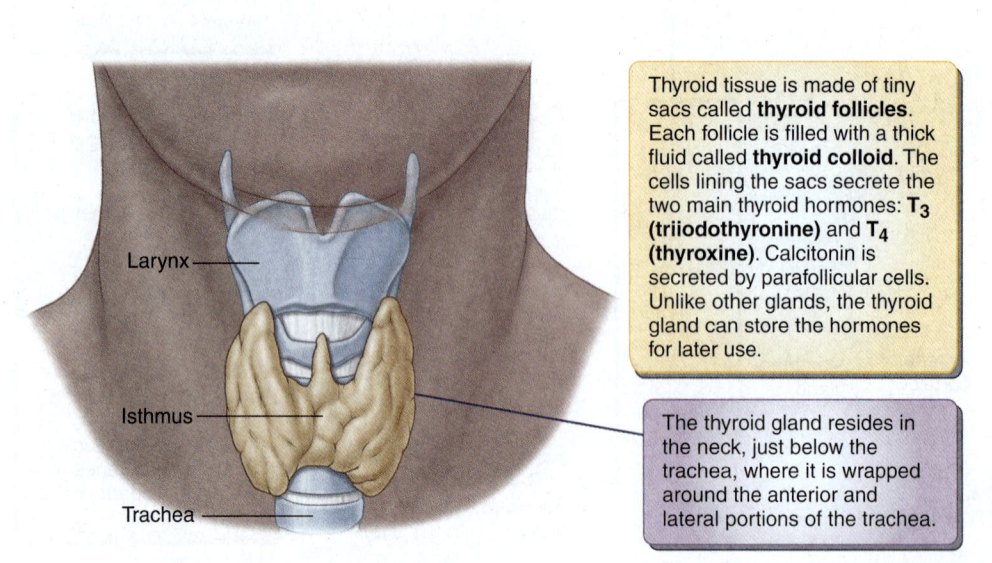

- Thyroid tissue is made of tiny sacs called **thyroid follicles**. Each follicle is filled with a thick fluid called **thyroid colloid**. The cells lining the sacs secrete the two main thyroid hormones: T_3 (triiodothyronine) and T_4 (thyroxine). Calcitonin is secreted by parafollicular cells. Unlike other glands, the thyroid gland can store the hormones for later use.
- The thyroid gland resides in the neck, just below the trachea, where it is wrapped around the anterior and lateral portions of the trachea.

Larynx
Isthmus
Trachea

FIGURE 38.5 Thyroid. ADD Calcitonin is secreted by parafollicular cells.

Parathyroid Glands

There are usually four parathyroid glands, two on the back of each lobe of the thyroid gland (Fig. 38.6). They produce parathyroid hormone (or parathormone, PTH), an **antagonist** to calcitonin. Besides bone, the target organs of PTH are the small intestine and kidneys. The overall effect of PTH is to raise the blood calcium level and lower the blood phosphate level.

Homeostasis of blood calcium level is regulated by calcitonin (from the thyroid) and PTH. Calcium ion delivery through the blood is essential for normal excitability of neurons and muscle cells and for the process of blood clotting.

Adrenal Glands

The adrenal glands are located superior to each kidney. The inner adrenal medulla is surrounded by an outer adrenal cortex (Fig. 38.7).

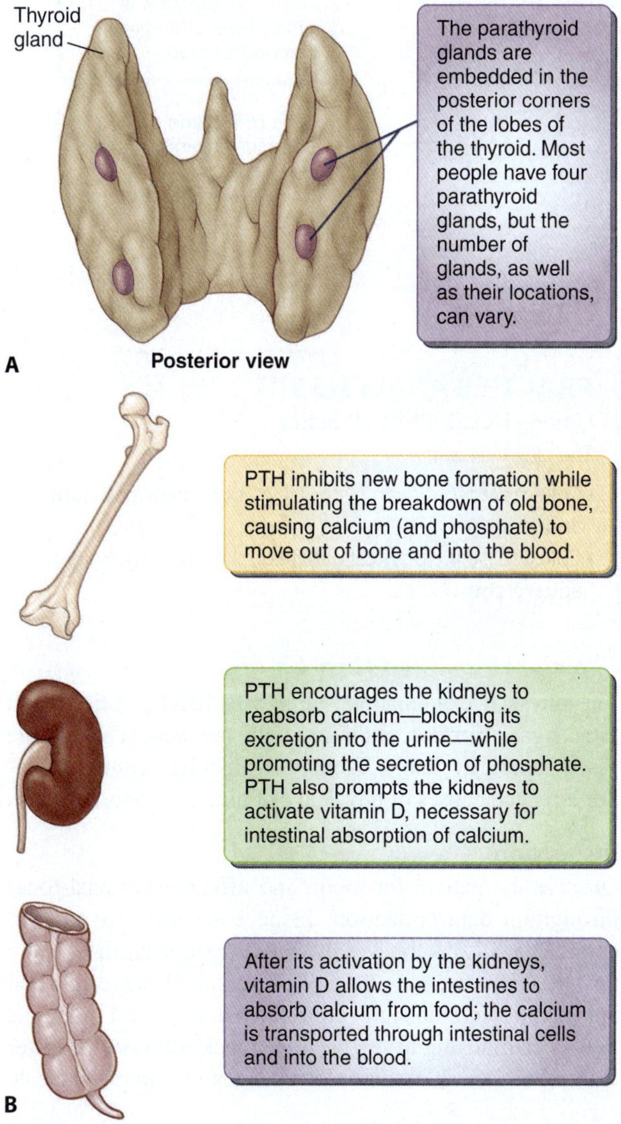

Adrenal Medulla

The catecholamines (epinephrine and norepinephrine), released by the adrenal medulla, are sympathomimetic, meaning they mimic the sympathetic nervous system. During stress, the hypothalamus stimulates their release to prolong the body's stress (fight-or-flight) response.

Adrenal Cortex

The adrenal cortex secretes three types of steroid hormones: mineralocorticoids, glucocorticoids, and gonadocorticoids ("sex steroids").

Aldosterone is the most abundant of the mineralocorticoids, and its target organs are the kidneys. Aldosterone promotes the reabsorption of sodium ions and the excretion of potassium ions by the kidney tubules. As sodium ions are reabsorbed, water follows; this is important for maintaining normal blood volume and blood pressure.

Cortisol is the most abundant of the glucocorticoids and has many target tissues. It stimulates **gluconeogenesis** in the liver and increases lipolysis and protein catabolism for energy production. By providing energy sources to body tissues, cortisol ensures that glucose will be available for the brain (glucose-sparing effect).

Cortisol release is increased during response to stress. The hypothalamus causes secretion of ACTH by the anterior pituitary, which increases cortisol secretion by the adrenal cortex. The resultant increase in energy availability is necessary for stress-induced changes. Cortisol also has an anti-inflammatory effect. However, excess cortisol decreases the immune response and can delay healing of damaged tissue.

The gonadocorticoids are small amounts of male androgens. In females, they are converted to estrogens. They are the only source of estrogen after menopause. In both genders, they contribute to libido (sexual desire).

Pancreas

The pancreas is both an exocrine and endocrine gland. As an endocrine gland, the pancreas secretes insulin and glucagon for blood glucose homeostasis. It also secretes somatostatin, which inhibits both insulin and glucagon (Fig. 38.8).

Hypoglycemia stimulates alpha cells to release glucagon. Glucagon raises blood glucose, making it available to cells.

Hyperglycemia stimulates beta cells to release insulin. Insulin increases the movement of glucose from the blood into cells. This lowers blood glucose and makes glucose available to cells for energy.

Blood glucose normally increases after meals, especially those high in carbohydrates. Insulin and glucagon function as antagonists; normal secretion of both hormones ensures a

• WORD • BUILDING •

antagonist: ant—against + agonist—promotes a function
gluconeogenesis: gluco—glucose + neo—new + genesis—formation
lipolysis: lipo—fat + lysis—breakdown

FIGURE 38.6 (A) Parathyroid. (B) Effectors/targets of parathyroid hormone.

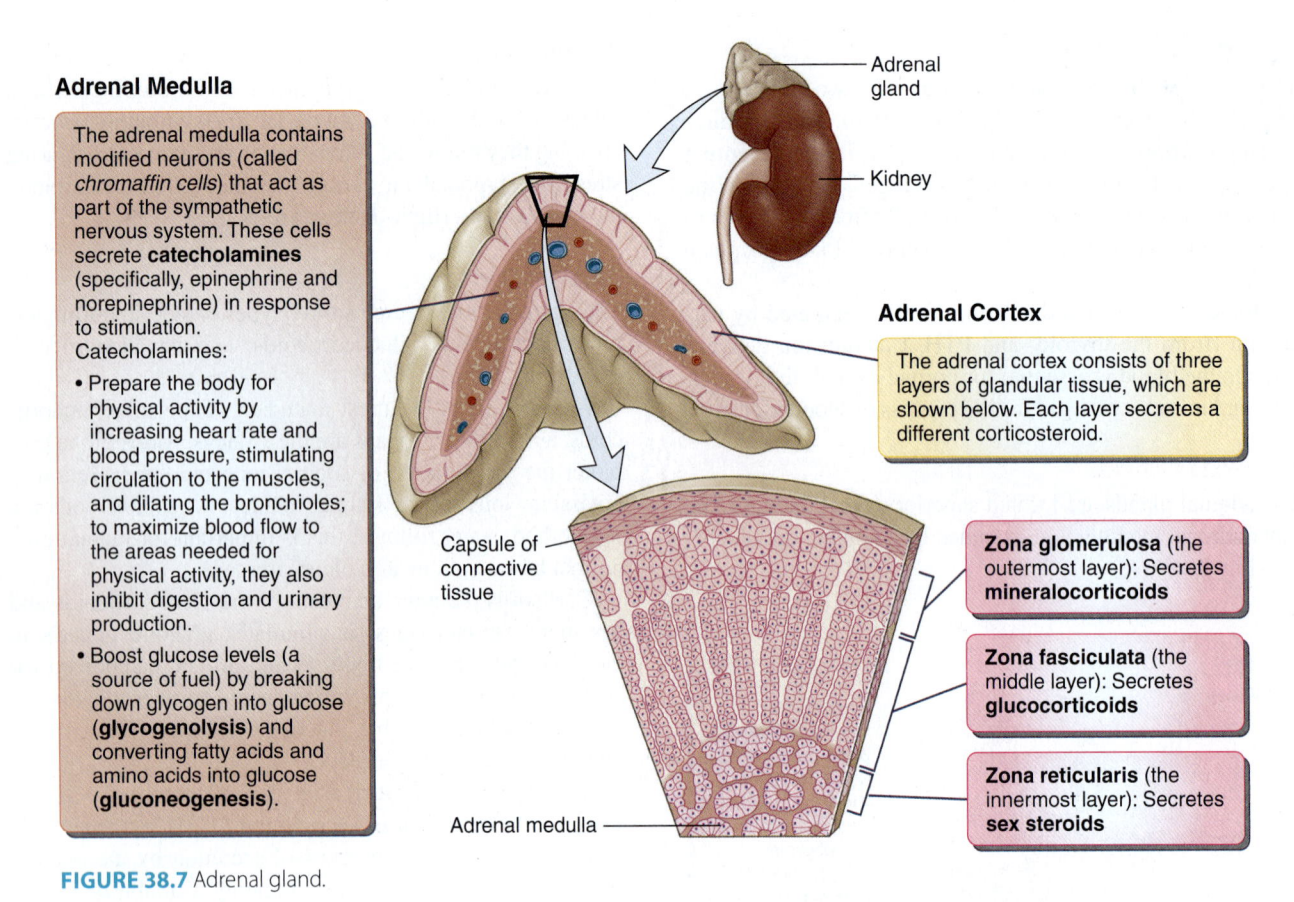

Adrenal Medulla

The adrenal medulla contains modified neurons (called *chromaffin cells*) that act as part of the sympathetic nervous system. These cells secrete **catecholamines** (specifically, epinephrine and norepinephrine) in response to stimulation.
Catecholamines:

- Prepare the body for physical activity by increasing heart rate and blood pressure, stimulating circulation to the muscles, and dilating the bronchioles; to maximize blood flow to the areas needed for physical activity, they also inhibit digestion and urinary production.
- Boost glucose levels (a source of fuel) by breaking down glycogen into glucose (**glycogenolysis**) and converting fatty acids and amino acids into glucose (**gluconeogenesis**).

Adrenal Cortex

The adrenal cortex consists of three layers of glandular tissue, which are shown below. Each layer secretes a different corticosteroid.

Zona glomerulosa (the outermost layer): Secretes **mineralocorticoids**

Zona fasciculata (the middle layer): Secretes **glucocorticoids**

Zona reticularis (the innermost layer): Secretes **sex steroids**

FIGURE 38.7 Adrenal gland.

blood glucose level that varies within normal limits (Fig. 38.9). Table 38.1 reviews endocrine hormone function.

Aging and the Endocrine System

Most of the endocrine glands decrease secretion with age, but normal aging usually does not lead to serious hormone deficiencies or illness (Fig. 38.10). In men there is usually a decrease in testosterone and in women a decrease in estrogen. Unless specific pathological conditions develop, the endocrine system continues to function adequately in old age.

ENDOCRINE SYSTEM DATA COLLECTION

Health History

When performing a health history, a number of questions can be asked to detect an endocrine problem. Often, however, you might be aware of a history of an endocrine disorder, such as diabetes or hypothyroidism. When a disorder exists or is suspected, you can do more focused data collection. Data collection related to individual disorders is provided in Chapters 39 and 40. Table 38.2 offers general questions that can help you identify new problem areas. If the data reveal abnormalities, they should be reported to the registered nurse or health-care provider (HCP).

> **PRACTICE ANALYSIS TIP**
> Linking NCLEX-PN® to Practice
> The LPN/LVN will:
> - Collect data for health history (e.g., skin integrity, height, and weight).
> - Collect baseline physical data (e.g., skin integrity, height, and weight).

Physical Examination

The physical examination starts with height, weight, and vital signs. Compare findings with the patient's baseline assessment if available. Table 38.3 includes common endocrine-related causes of physical examination abnormalities.

Inspection

Observe the patient for mood and **affect** (emotional tone) throughout data collection. Inspect the neck for thyroid enlargement. Look for eyes that bulge (**exophthalmos**). Note posture, body fat, and presence of tremor. Observe skin and hair texture and moisture. Note the presence of a moonlike face or "buffalo hump" on the upper back. Observe the lower extremities for skin and color changes that might indicate

• WORD • BUILDING •

exophthalmos: exo—outward + ophthalmos—relating to the eye

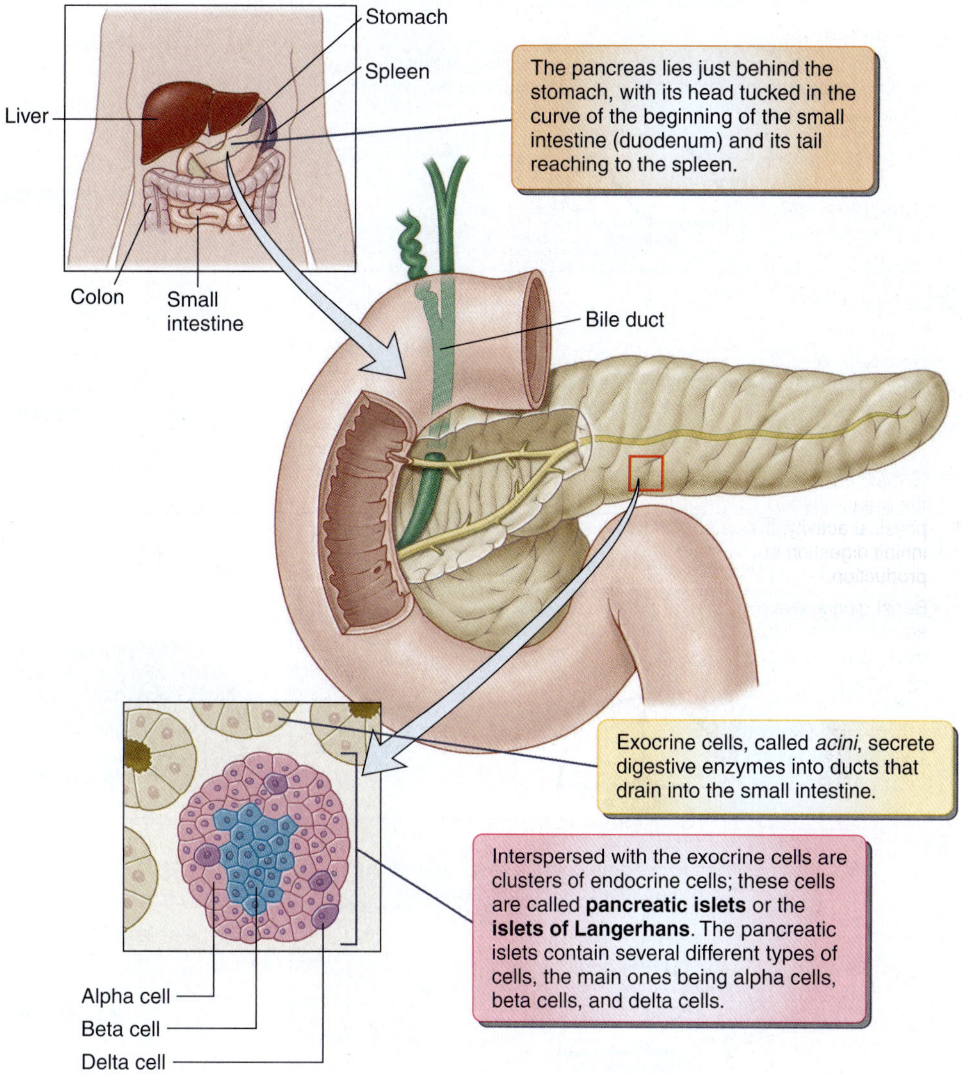

Stomach
Spleen
Liver
Colon
Small intestine
The pancreas lies just behind the stomach, with its head tucked in the curve of the beginning of the small intestine (duodenum) and its tail reaching to the spleen.
Bile duct
Exocrine cells, called *acini*, secrete digestive enzymes into ducts that drain into the small intestine.
Interspersed with the exocrine cells are clusters of endocrine cells; these cells are called **pancreatic islets** or the **islets of Langerhans**. The pancreatic islets contain several different types of cells, the main ones being alpha cells, beta cells, and delta cells.
Alpha cell
Beta cell
Delta cell

FIGURE 38.8 Pancreas.

circulatory impairment. See Table 38.3 for the rationales for these observations.

Palpation

The thyroid gland is the only palpable endocrine gland. The licensed practical nurse/licensed vocational nurse (LPN/LVN) may assist an HCP to palpate the thyroid gland. The practitioner stands behind or in front of the seated patient and palpates the gland while the patient swallows a sip of water. The LPN/LVN can assist with positioning the patient, providing water, and instructing the patient to take a sip of water and hold it in their mouth until told to swallow. The thyroid gland should never be palpated in a patient with uncontrolled hyperthyroidism because palpation can stimulate secretion of additional thyroid hormone and cause thyrotoxic crisis (see Chapter 39).

Palpate all peripheral pulses. The posterior tibial and dorsalis pedis pulses may be diminished in patients with circulatory impairment. Palpate skin turgor by gently pinching a small piece of skin. The sternum is a good place to check. If a "tent" of skin remains in place, the patient may be dehydrated as a result of water loss, as in ADH deficiency.

Auscultation and Percussion

Auscultation and percussion are not usually part of an endocrine assessment.

CUE RECOGNITION 38.1

You are caring for a patient who states they are experiencing chronic numbness and pain in their hands and feet. What history should you collect from the patient?

Suggested answers are at the end of the chapter.

DIAGNOSTIC TESTS FOR THE ENDOCRINE SYSTEM

Hormone Tests

Serum Hormone Levels

Many hormones can be measured from a simple blood specimen, useful in diagnosing hypofunctioning or hyperfunctioning gland states. See Table 38.4 for commonly measured hormones.

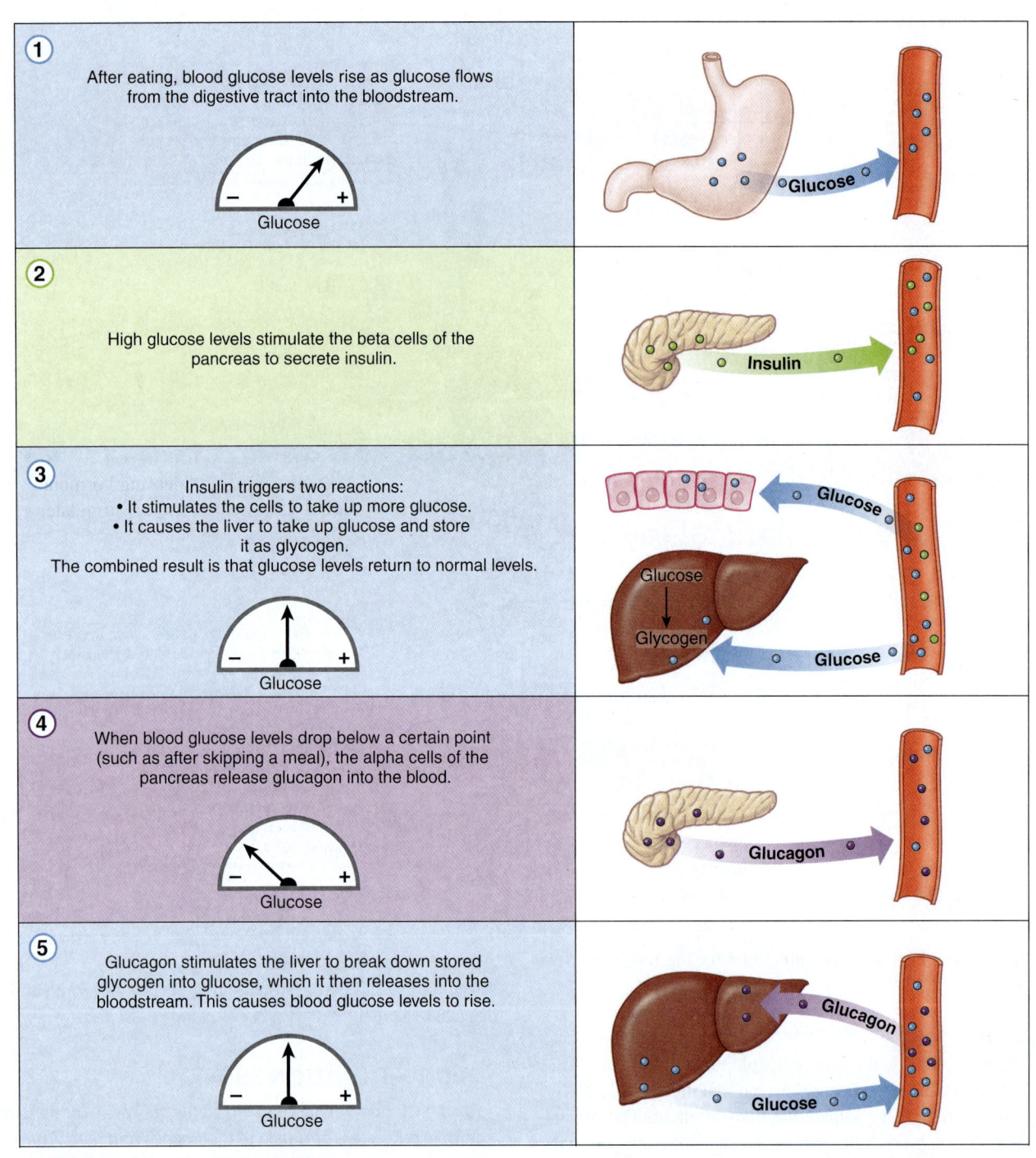

FIGURE 38.9 Regulation of blood glucose.

Stimulation Tests
Stimulation tests may also help determine endocrine gland function. For this type of test, a substance is injected to stimulate a gland. The hormone secreted by that gland is then measured in the blood to determine how well it responded to the stimulation. For example, in a TRH stimulation test, TRH is injected. If the pituitary gland responds appropriately, TSH is secreted. If the thyroid gland responds appropriately to TSH, T_3 and T_4 levels rise. Failure of TRH to stimulate TSH and thyroid hormone indicates a pituitary or thyroid condition. Further studies might be done to determine the cause.

Suppression Tests
Suppression tests are the opposite of stimulating tests. For this type of test, a substance is injected to suppress a hormone's release. For example, if dexamethasone (a steroid hormone) is injected, cortisol release from the adrenal cortex is expected to be suppressed via a negative feedback mechanism. If this does not occur, adrenal cortex dysfunction is suspected.

Table 38.1
Review of Endocrine Function

Hormone	Function(s)	Regulation of Secretion
Hormones of the Posterior Pituitary Gland		
Antidiuretic hormone (ADH, or vasopressin)	Increases water reabsorption by the kidney tubules (water returns to the blood) Causes vasoconstriction (in large amounts)	Decreased water content in the body stimulates secretion Alcohol inhibits secretion
Oxytocin	Promotes contraction of myometrium of uterus (during labor) Promotes release of milk from mammary glands	Nerve impulses from hypothalamus, the result of stretching of cervix or stimulation of nipple Secretion from placenta at the end of gestation—stimulus unknown
Hormones of the Anterior Pituitary Gland		
Growth hormone (GH)	Increases rate of mitosis Increases amino acid transport into cells Increases rate of protein synthesis Increases use of fats for energy	Growth hormone–releasing hormone (GHRH; hypothalamus) stimulates secretion Growth hormone–inhibiting hormone (GHIH, or somatostatin; hypothalamus) inhibits secretion
Thyroid-stimulating hormone (TSH)	Increases secretion of triiodothyronine (T_3) and thyroxine (T_4) by thyroid gland	Thyrotropin-releasing hormone (TRH; hypothalamus)
Adrenocorticotropic hormone (ACTH)	Increases secretion of cortisol by the adrenal cortex	Corticotropin-releasing hormone (CRH; hypothalamus)
Prolactin	Stimulates milk production by the mammary glands	Prolactin-releasing hormone (PRH; hypothalamus) stimulates secretion Prolactin-inhibiting hormone (PIH; hypothalamus) inhibits secretion
Follicle-stimulating hormone (FSH)	*In women:* Initiates growth of ova in ovarian follicles Increases secretion of estrogen by follicle cells *In men:* Initiates sperm production in the testes	Gonadotropin-releasing hormone (GnRH; hypothalamus) stimulates secretion Inhibin (ovaries) inhibits secretion GnRH (hypothalamus) stimulates secretion Inhibin (testes) inhibits secretion
Luteinizing hormone (LH)	*In women:* Causes ovulation Causes the ruptured ovarian follicle to become the corpus luteum Increases secretion of progesterone by the corpus luteum *In men:* Increases secretion of testosterone by the interstitial cells of the testes	GnRH (hypothalamus) GnRH (hypothalamus)

Continued

Table 38.1
Review of Endocrine Function—cont'd

Hormone	Function(s)	Regulation of Secretion
Hormones of the Thyroid Gland		
Thyroxine and triiodothyronine (T_4 and T_3) Calcitonin	Increase energy production from all food types Increase rate of protein synthesis Decrease the reabsorption of calcium and phosphate from bones to blood	TSH (anterior pituitary) Hypercalcemia
Hormones of the Parathyroid Glands		
Parathyroid hormone (PTH; parathormone)	Increases the resorption of calcium and phosphate from bone to blood Increases absorption of calcium and phosphate by the small intestine Increases the reabsorption of calcium and the excretion of phosphate by the kidneys; activates vitamin D	Hypocalcemia stimulates secretion Hypercalcemia inhibits secretion
Hormones of the Adrenal Medulla		
Epinephrine, norepinephrine	Increases heart rate and force of contraction Dilates bronchioles Decreases peristalsis Increases conversion of glycogen in glucose in the liver Causes vasodilation in skeletal muscles Causes vasoconstriction in skin and viscera Increases use of fats for energy Increases the rate of cell respiration	Sympathetic impulses from the hypothalamus in stress situations
Hormones of the Intestine (Incretins)		
Glucagon-like peptide (GLP-1) Gastric inhibitory polypeptide (GIP)	Regulate blood sugar by increasing insulin secretion and decreasing glucagon secretion from the pancreas	Food ingestion
Hormones of the Pancreas		
Glucagon (alpha cells)	Increases conversion of glycogen to glucose in the liver Increases the use of excess amino acids and fats for energy	Hypoglycemia
Insulin (beta cells)	Increases glucose transport into cells and the use of glucose for energy production Increases the conversion of excess glucose to glycogen in the liver and muscles Increases amino acid and fatty acid transport into cells, and their use in synthesis reactions	Hyperglycemia
Somatostatin (delta cells)	Decreases secretion of insulin and glucagon Slows absorption of nutrients	Rising levels of insulin and glucagon

Table 38.1
Review of Endocrine Function—cont'd

Hormone	Function(s)	Regulation of Secretion
Hormones of the Adrenal Cortex		
Aldosterone (mineralocorticoid)	Increases reabsorption of Na^+ (sodium) ions by the kidneys to the blood Increases excretion of K^+ (potassium) ions by the kidneys in urine	Low blood Na^+ level Low blood volume or blood pressure High blood K^+ level
Cortisol (glucocorticoid) Gonadocorticoid	Increases use of fats and excess amino acids for energy Decreases use of glucose for energy (except for the brain) Increases conversion of glucose to glycogen in the liver Anti-inflammatory effect: stabilizes lysosomes and blocks the effects of histamine *In women:* Converted to estrogens. *In both genders:* Contributes to libido (sexual desire).	ACTH (anterior pituitary) during physiological stress Gonadotropic releasing hormone (GnRH; hypothalamus)

Source: Adapted from Scanlon, V. C., & Sanders, T. (2019). *Essentials of anatomy and physiology* (8th ed.). Philadelphia, PA: F.A. Davis.

CRITICAL THINKING

Ms. Hackworth is tired all the time. The nurse practitioner orders a thyroid-stimulating hormone level drawn. The result is higher than normal.

1. You call Ms. Hackworth to come in to the clinic for further evaluation. She asks, "If my thyroid level is high, then why am I so tired?" How should you respond?
2. After further testing, the nurse practitioner places Ms. Hackworth on levothyroxine (Synthroid) 50 mcg daily. Her pharmacist supplies Synthroid 0.05 mg. Is her dose correct?

Suggested answers are at the end of the chapter.

Urine Tests

Sometimes it is helpful to measure the amount of hormone or hormone by-product excreted in the urine during a 24-hour period. One example is the urine test for cortisol. It can help diagnose Cushing syndrome and Addison disease. Go to your resources in Davis Advantage for the procedure for collecting a 24-hour urine specimen.

Other Laboratory Tests

Some laboratory tests may indirectly reflect the function of an endocrine gland. For example, a serum calcium level helps indicate PTH or calcitonin secretion, and a blood glucose level reflects insulin secretion.

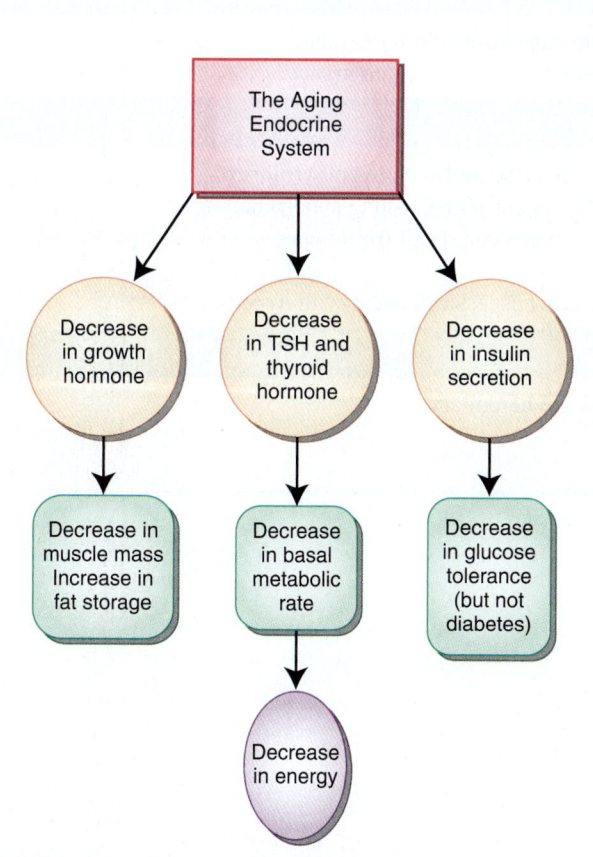

FIGURE 38.10 Effects of aging on the endocrine system.

Table 38.2
Subjective Data Collection for the Endocrine System

Questions to Ask During the Health History	Rationale/Significance
Neuromuscular	
Have you noticed muscle spasms or twitching?	These symptoms may be associated with syndrome of inappropriate antidiuretic hormone (SIADH) secretion or calcium depletion resulting from hypoparathyroidism.
Do you have numbness, tingling, or pain in your feet, legs, or hands?	These can be associated with neuropathy resulting from diabetes mellitus. Numbness and tingling can also indicate hypocalcemia related to hypoparathyroidism.
Nutrition/Fluid Balance	
Have you gained or lost weight without trying?	Actual weight gain may be associated with hypothyroidism. Weight gain due to water retention may result from Cushing syndrome or SIADH. Weight loss may result from uncontrolled diabetes or hyperthyroidism. Weight loss due to dehydration may be related to Addison disease.
Have you noticed excessive thirst or urination?	Excessive thirst and urination are classic symptoms of diabetes mellitus and diabetes insipidus.
Have you noticed a change in your energy level?	Lack of energy may be associated with uncontrolled diabetes, hypothyroidism, hyperthyroidism, Addison disease, or pituitary disorders.
Metabolic	
Do you generally tolerate changes in environmental temperature?	Hypothyroidism can cause cold intolerance. Hyperthyroidism can cause heat intolerance.
Mood/Memory	
Have you noticed a change in your mood or memory?	Mental function may be dull with hypothyroidism. Mood swings can occur with Cushing syndrome. Agitation or confusion can result from hypoglycemia in a person with diabetes. Irritability and nervousness can occur with hyperthyroidism.
Family History	
Does anyone in your family have a thyroid problem, diabetes, or another endocrine disorder?	Some disorders are hereditary.

Table 38.3
Objective Data Collection for the Endocrine System

Abnormal Finding	Possible Endocrine-Related Causes
Mood	
Depressed mood or affect	Hypothyroidism
Nervousness	Hyperthyroidism, pheochromocytoma
Agitation	Low blood glucose level
Irritability	Hyperthyroidism
Nutrition/Fluid Balance	
Weight gain	Decreased metabolic rate in hypothyroidism and Cushing syndrome; water retention in syndrome of inappropriate antidiuretic hormone (SIADH) and Cushing syndrome.
Weight loss	Increased metabolic rate in hyperthyroidism; uncontrolled diabetes
Poor skin turgor	Dehydration due to water loss in Addison disease
Integumentary	
Hyperpigmentation of skin	Addison disease
Dry, scaly skin	Hypothyroidism
Dusky lower extremities with weak peripheral pulses	Circulatory changes in diabetes mellitus
Thin, fragile skin with striae (stretch marks)	Cushing syndrome
Vital Signs	
Change in pulse rate or temperature	Elevated due to increased metabolic rate in hyperthyroidism. Decreased due to slowed metabolic rate in hypothyroidism
Elevated blood pressure	Increased catecholamine release in pheochromocytoma or fluid retention in Cushing syndrome
Decreased blood pressure	Sodium and water loss in Addison disease
Neuromuscular	
Tremor	Hyperthyroidism, hypoglycemia, or pheochromocytoma
Numbness, tingling, pain	Diabetes mellitus, hypocalcemia
Head and Neck	
Exophthalmos (bulging eyes)	Fat deposits and edema behind the eyes in Graves disease
Fat pads on neck and shoulders ("buffalo hump"), round "moon" face	Accumulation of fat in Cushing syndrome
Enlarged thyroid gland	Excessive stimulation by thyroid-stimulating hormone in hypothyroidism or hyperthyroidism

Table 38.4
Common Endocrine-Related Laboratory Tests

Test	Normal Values*	Significance of Abnormal Findings
Thyroid Tests		
Thyroid-stimulating hormone	0.4–4.2 microinternational units/mL	↑ in primary hypothyroidism ↓ in primary hyperthyroidism
Triiodothyronine (T_3), total	70–204 ng/dL	↓ in hypothyroidism ↑ in hyperthyroidism
Triiodothyronine (T_3), free	260–480 pg/dL	
Thyroxine (T_4), total	*Male:* 4.6–10.5 mcg/dL *Female:* 5.5–11 mcg/dL	↓ in hypothyroidism ↑ in hyperthyroidism
Thyroxine (T_4), free	0.8–1.5 ng/dL	
Parathyroid Tests		
Parathyroid hormone	8–24 pg/mL	↑ in primary hyperparathyroidism ↓ in primary hypoparathyroidism, parathyroid trauma during thyroid surgery
Calcium, blood	8.2–10.2 mg/100 mL *Over age 90:* 8.2–9.6 mg/dL	↑ in some cancers, hyperparathyroidism ↓ in hypoparathyroidism
Phosphorus	2.5–4.5 mg/dL	↑ in hypoparathyroidism ↓ in hyperparathyroidism
Pituitary Tests		
Growth hormone	*Male:* 0–5 ng/mL *Female:* 0–10 ng/mL	↑ in acromegaly ↓ in small stature
Antidiuretic hormone (vasopressin)	0–4.7 pg/mL	↑ in syndrome of inappropriate antidiuretic hormone (SIADH) secretion ↓ in diabetes insipidus
Urine specific gravity	1.001–1.029	↓ in diabetes insipidus
Adrenocorticotropic hormone (ACTH)	9–52 pg/mL in a.m. *Women on oral contraceptives:* 5–29 pg/mL	↑ in Addison disease ↓ in Cushing syndrome, long-term corticosteroid therapy
Adrenal Tests		
Aldosterone	*Supine:* 3–16 ng/dL *Upright:* 7–30 ng/dL	↑ in heart failure, chronic obstructive pulmonary disease (COPD), hypovolemia ↓ in Addison disease, hypoaldosteronism
Cortisol, blood	5–25 mcg/dL at 0800 3–16 mcg/dL at 1600	↑ in Cushing syndrome, stress ↓ in Addison disease, steroid withdrawal
Cortisol, urine	3.5–45 mcg/24 hr	↑ in Cushing syndrome, stress ↓ in Addison disease, steroid withdrawal

Table 38.4
Common Endocrine-Related Laboratory Tests—cont'd

Test	Normal Values*	Significance of Abnormal Findings
Pancreas Tests		
Fasting blood glucose (FBG)	70–100 mg/dL	↑ in stress, Cushing syndrome 100–125 mg/dL = prediabetes 126 mg/dL or greater = diabetes mellitus ↓ in hypoglycemia, Addison disease
Ketones, blood and urine	Negative	Positive in acidosis, fasting or starvation, diabetic ketoacidosis
Oral glucose tolerance test	Blood glucose level less than 140 mg/dL at 2 hr	140–199 mg/dL at 2 hr = prediabetes 200 mg/dL or greater at 2 hr = diabetes mellitus
Glycosylated hemoglobin	Less than 5.7%	5.7%–6.4% = prediabetes 6.5% or greater = diabetes mellitus

*All normal values are for a fasting test.

Nuclear Scanning

Thyroid Scan
A thyroid scan may be done to determine presence of tumors or nodules. For this test, radioactive material is given orally or by injection. The material is taken up by the thyroid gland. After a specified time, the thyroid gland is scanned with a scintillation camera. The scan will show hot spots (nodules), which are not malignant, or cold spots (areas that do not take up the radioactivity), which indicate malignancy. Cold spots can then be biopsied to confirm a diagnosis. Because such a small amount of radioactive material is used, risk to the patient is minimal. The test takes approximately 30 minutes to complete. See Appendix A (Nuclear Scan) for nursing care pre- and postprocedure.

Radioactive Iodine Uptake
A radioactive iodine uptake test is similar to a thyroid scan and is done to evaluate thyroid function. Several scans are taken over a 24-hour period after administration of radioactive iodine. The amount of iodine taken up by the thyroid indicates the activity of the gland. This is especially helpful in diagnosing hyperthyroidism.

PET Scan
Positron emission tomography (PET) scanning is another type of scan that can be done to differentiate between benign and malignant endocrine tumors. PET scans are helpful because they can show metabolic changes in organs or tissues.

Radiographic Tests
A computed tomography (CT) scan or magnetic resonance imaging (MRI) may be done to locate a tumor or identify hypertrophy (enlargement) of a gland.

Ultrasound
Ultrasound may be done of the thyroid or parathyroid glands to determine whether they are enlarged or to find masses.

Biopsy
Biopsy is done to obtain tissue to examine for possible cancerous cells. The thyroid gland can be biopsied either by needle aspiration under local anesthesia or using a surgical incision.

Key Points

- The endocrine system consists of the endocrine glands that secrete hormones. Their hormones are involved in fluid balance, metabolism, energy balance, growth, and development; contraction of smooth and cardiac muscle; glandular secretion; reproduction; and the establishment of circadian rhythms.
- The endocrine glands include the hypothalamus, anterior and posterior pituitary glands, thyroid, parathyroids, adrenals (medulla and cortex), and pancreas.
- The posterior pituitary gland stores and releases ADH (sometimes called vasopressin) and oxytocin.
  - ADH increases water reabsorption by the kidney tubules, reducing urine output. The water is reabsorbed back into the blood, maintaining blood volume and pressure.
  - Oxytocin causes contractions of the myometrium for delivery of a newborn and placenta.

- TSH stimulates growth and secretions of the thyroid gland: T_3, T_4, and calcitonin.
  - T_3 and T_4 increase cellular respiration of glucose and fatty acids, increasing metabolism. They are essential for normal physical growth, mental development, and reproductive maturation. Sufficient iodine intake is required for T_3 and T_4 production.
  - Calcitonin targets bone tissue and is important during childhood to support rapid bone growth. Resorption of calcium and phosphorous into the blood is inhibited by calcitonin, so minerals stay in the bone and do not accumulate in the blood.
- There are usually four parathyroid glands, two on the back of each lobe of the thyroid gland. They produce PTH, an antagonist to calcitonin. The overall effect of PTH is to raise the blood calcium level and lower the blood phosphate level.
- The adrenal medulla releases catecholamines (epinephrine and norepinephrine) that mimic the sympathetic nervous system. During stress, the hypothalamus stimulates their release to prolong the body's fight-or-flight response.
- ACTH stimulates secretion of cortisol and related hormones from the adrenal cortex: mineralocorticoids, glucocorticoids, and gonadocorticoids ("sex steroids").
  - Mineralocorticoids maintain normal blood volume and blood pressure.
  - Glucocorticoids provide energy to tissues and control the stress response.
  - Gonadocorticoids contribute to sexual desire.
- The pancreas is both an exocrine and endocrine gland. As an endocrine gland, it secretes insulin and glucagon for blood glucose homeostasis as well as somatostatin, which inhibits both insulin and glucagon.
  - Insulin decreases blood glucose and glucagon increases blood glucose.
- Most endocrine glands decrease secretion with age, but normal aging does not typically cause serious hormone deficiencies or illness. Men usually have a decrease in testosterone and women usually have a decrease in estrogen. Unless specific pathological conditions develop, the endocrine system continues to function adequately in old age.
- When performing a health history, a number of questions can be asked to determine whether an endocrine problem exists. Often, you might be aware of a history of an endocrine disorder, such as diabetes or hypothyroidism. When a disorder exists or is suspected, you can do more focused data collection.
- Many hormones can be measured from a simple blood specimen, which can help diagnose hypofunctioning or hyperfunctioning gland states.

SUGGESTED ANSWERS TO CHAPTER EXERCISES

Cue Recognition
38.1: Do you have a history of diabetes?

Critical Thinking & Clinical Judgment
Ms. Hackworth

1. "It's not your thyroid hormone that is high. It's your thyroid-stimulating hormone. That means your pituitary gland has to work extra hard to try to stimulate your thyroid gland."
2. Yes, her dose is correct.
$$\frac{50 \text{ mcg}}{} \times \frac{1 \text{ mg}}{1{,}000 \text{ mcg}} = 0.05 \text{ mg}$$

Additional Resources

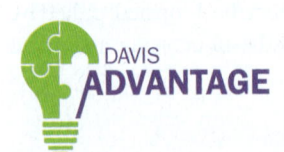

Go to Davis Advantage to complete your learning: strengthen understanding, apply your knowledge, and prepare for the Next Gen NCLEX®.

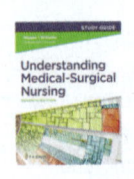

A Study Guide is also available.

CHAPTER 39
Nursing Care of Patients With Disorders of the Endocrine System

Alene Homan, Paula D. Hopper

KEY TERMS

amenorrhea (ay-MEN-uh-REE-ah)
ectopic (ek-TOP-ik)
euthyroid (yoo-THIGH-royd)
goitrogenic (GOY-troh-JEN-ik)
goitrogens (GOY-troh-jenz)
hyperplasia (HY-per-PLAY-zee-ah)
hypophysectomy (HY-pah-fi-SEK-tuh-mee)
myxedema (MIK-suh-DEE-mah)
nocturia (nok-TYOO-ree-ah)
osmolality (ahs-moh-LAL-ih-tee)
pheochromocytoma (FEE-oh-KROH-moh-sigh-TOH-mah)
polydipsia (PAH-lee-DIP-see-ah)
polyuria (PAH-lee-YOO-ree-ah)
tetany (TET-uh-nee)
tropic (TRO-pik)

CHAPTER CONCEPTS

Cellular regulation
Fluid and electrolyte balance
Growth and development
Nutrition

LEARNING OUTCOMES

1. Identify disorders caused by variations in the hormones of the pituitary, thyroid, parathyroid, and adrenal glands.
2. Explain the pathophysiology of each of the endocrine disorders presented.
3. Describe the etiologies, signs, and symptoms of each of the endocrine disorders.
4. Describe current therapeutic measures used for each of the selected endocrine disorders.
5. List data to collect when caring for patients with each of the endocrine disorders discussed.
6. Plan nursing care for patients with each of the disorders.
7. Explain how you will know if nursing interventions have been effective.

The endocrine system is subject to a variety of disorders. Although the causes vary, the pathophysiology usually involves either too little or too much hormone activity. Insufficient hormone activity may be the result of hypofunction of an endocrine gland or insensitivity of the target tissue to its hormone. Excessive hormone activity may be the result of a hyperactive gland, **ectopic** hormone production, or self-administration of too much replacement hormone (Table 39.1). If you remember the function of each hormone in the body, understanding the problems involved with an altered amount of each hormone becomes easier.

Most endocrine disorders are either primary or secondary. A primary disorder is a problem within the gland that is out of balance. Secondary disorders are caused by problems outside the gland, such as an imbalance in a **tropic** hormone, certain drugs, trauma, surgery, or a problem in the feedback mechanism. For example, if the thyroid gland is diseased and causing hypothyroidism, it is considered a primary problem. Sometimes hypothyroidism is caused by a lack of thyroid-stimulating hormone from the pituitary gland, even though the thyroid gland is healthy. This is considered a secondary problem.

> ### LEARNING TIP
> Learn the normal function of each gland and hormone (Chapter 38), then slow it down for disorders that have decreased function or secretion and speed it up for disorders that have increased function or secretion.

Table 39.1
Causes of Endocrine Problems

Insufficient hormone activity	Gland hypofunction
	Lack of tropic or stimulating hormone
	Target tissue insensitivity to hormone
Excess hormone activity	Gland hyperfunction
	Excess tropic or stimulating hormone
	Ectopic hormone production
	Self-administration of too much replacement hormone

PITUITARY DISORDERS

Pituitary disorders often involve several hormone imbalances at once. They are caused by general hypopituitarism or hyperpituitarism. Problems involving all the pituitary hormones at once, however, are rare. For simplicity, imbalances are considered separately here.

Disorders Related to Antidiuretic Hormone Imbalance

Antidiuretic hormone (ADH; also called *arginine vasopressin* [AVP]) is synthesized in the hypothalamus and stored and secreted by the posterior pituitary gland. Recall that ADH is responsible for reabsorption of water by the distal tubules and collecting ducts in the kidneys. A decrease in ADH activity results in diabetes insipidus (DI). An increase in ADH activity is called *syndrome of inappropriate antidiuretic hormone* (SIADH). Table 39.2 compares DI and SIADH. Note how symptoms of too little ADH (water loss) are the opposite of symptoms of too much ADH (water retention).

Diabetes Insipidus

PATHOPHYSIOLOGY. It is important to understand that DI is unrelated to diabetes mellitus. Diabetes *mellitus* is caused by insulin-resistant tissue or insufficient insulin production. Diabetes *insipidus* is caused by a deficiency of ADH. If ADH is lacking, adequate reabsorption of water is prevented, leading to diuresis (increased production of urine). Patients can urinate from 3 to 15 L per day, leading to dehydration and increased serum **osmolality** (concentrated blood). The increased osmolality and decreased blood pressure normally trigger ADH secretion, which causes water retention and dilutes the blood; in patients with DI, this does not happen. Increased osmolality also leads to extreme thirst, which usually causes the patient to drink enough fluids to maintain fluid balance. In an unconscious patient or a patient with a defective thirst mechanism, however, dehydration can quickly occur if the problem is not recognized and corrected.

ETIOLOGY. DI has a variety of causes. Tumors, trauma, or other problems in the hypothalamus or pituitary gland can lead to decreased production or release of ADH. Surgery in the area of the pituitary and certain drugs, such as glucocorticoids or alcohol, can also cause DI.

SIGNS AND SYMPTOMS. The patient with DI experiences frequent urination (**polyuria**) and night urination (**nocturia**). This results in high serum osmolality and low urine osmolality. Urine specific gravity is decreased, making the urine dilute and light in color.

The patient experiences extreme thirst (**polydipsia**) and consumes large volumes of water. Often patients crave ice-cold water. If urine output exceeds fluid intake, dehydration occurs, with characteristic symptoms of hypotension, poor skin turgor, and weakness. Hypovolemic shock occurs if fluid balance is not restored. Dehydration and electrolyte imbalances can result in a decrease in level of consciousness and death if the problem is not corrected.

DIAGNOSTIC TESTS. Diagnosis is based initially on a history of risk factors and reported symptoms. Urine specific gravity will be less than 1.005 (normal: 1.005 to 1.030) and can be monitored by laboratory tests or by using reagent strips at the bedside. Plasma and urine osmolality are measured and compared with each other. Serum sodium level appears high. The actual amount of sodium in the blood may be normal but seems elevated in relation to the decreased amount of water. Computed tomography (CT) scanning or magnetic resonance imaging (MRI) is used to determine whether a pituitary tumor is present.

A water-deprivation test may be done in which the patient is deprived of water for up to 6 hours. Body weight and urine osmolality are tested hourly. If the urine is still diluted when the patient is not drinking and the patient loses weight because of volume depletion, DI is suspected.

ADH levels can be measured in plasma or urine after administration of hypertonic saline or fluid restriction. The normal response would be elevated ADH; if it is not elevated, DI is suspected. The urine glucose level may also be checked to rule out diabetes mellitus.

THERAPEUTIC MEASURES. Hypotonic IV fluids, such as 0.45% saline solution, may be ordered to replace intravascular volume without adding extra sodium. IV fluids are especially important if the patient is unable to take oral fluids.

Medical treatment of DI involves replacement of ADH. In acute cases, vasopressin, a synthetic form of ADH, is given via the IV or subcutaneous route, along with IV fluid replacement. In patients who require long-term therapy, synthetic ADH (desmopressin, or DDAVP) can be administered orally, subcutaneously, or intranasally. Thiazide diuretics may decrease urine flow in the absence of ADH (even though they

• WORD • BUILDING •
polyuria: poly—much + uria—urine
nocturia: noct—night + uria—urine
polydipsia: poly—much + dipsia—thirst

Table 39.2
Antidiuretic Hormone Disorders Summary

	Insufficient Antidiuretic Hormone	Excess Antidiuretic Hormone
Disorder	Diabetes insipidus	Syndrome of inappropriate antidiuretic hormone
Signs and Symptoms	Polyuria, polydipsia, dehydration, dilute urine	Fluid retention, weight gain, concentrated urine
Diagnostic Tests	Urine specific gravity, urine and plasma osmolality, water deprivation test	Serum and urine sodium and osmolality, water load test
Therapeutic Measures	Synthetic antidiuretic hormone replacement	Treat cause
Priority Nursing Diagnoses	Deficient Fluid Volume	Excess Fluid Volume

usually are used to increase urine output). If a pituitary tumor is involved, treatment usually entails removal of the pituitary gland (**hypophysectomy**).

NURSING PROCESS FOR THE PATIENT WITH DIABETES INSIPIDUS.

Data Collection. When collecting data for a patient with DI, pay special attention to fluid balance. Daily weights are the most reliable method for monitoring the amount of fluid that is being lost. Taking accurate intake and output (I&O) measurements is also helpful. Skin turgor will be poor, and mucous membranes will be dry and sticky if the patient is becoming dehydrated. Monitor skin integrity because dehydration increases risk of breakdown. Monitor vital signs for signs of shock. Use a reagent strip (dipstick) or urinometer to measure urine specific gravities. Monitor serum electrolytes and osmolality as ordered and watch for changes in level of consciousness. Determine the patient's understanding of their disease and treatment. Once treatment is initiated, continue to monitor fluid balance, being especially alert to signs of fluid overload.

> **LEARNING TIP**
> Remember from Chapter 6 that "a pint's (about) a pound the world around." If your patient has lost 4 pounds, that is 4 pints, or a half gallon, of extra water!

Nursing Diagnoses, Planning, and Implementation

> **Deficient Fluid Volume related to failure of regulatory mechanisms**
>
> **EXPECTED OUTCOME:** The patient's fluid balance will be maintained as evidenced by urine specific gravity between 1.005 and 1.030, skin turgor within normal limits, and stable daily weight.

- Monitor daily weight, I&O, vital signs, and urine specific gravity. *Decreased weight, output greater than intake, low blood pressure, elevated pulse rate, and high urine specific gravity can all indicate fluid deficit.*
- Monitor patient for restlessness or weakness. *These can indicate significant fluid deficit with electrolyte imbalance.*
- Provide free access to oral fluids. If the patient's thirst mechanism is not intact, give the patient fluids every hour. *Oral fluids are essential to replace the excess lost in diuresis.*
- Report a significant drop in blood pressure and an increase in pulse rate to the registered nurse (RN) or health-care provider (HCP), *as these may be signs of hypovolemic shock.*
- Encourage the patient to participate in maintaining I&O records, monitoring weight, and checking urine specific gravity, if able. *This involves the patient and helps prepare them for self-monitoring at home.*
- Teach the patient to monitor daily weights at home; losses or gains of greater than 2 pounds in a day should be reported to the HCP. *Weight loss or gain can indicate fluid imbalance and the need for a change in medication regimen.*
- Advise the patient to wear identification, such as a medical alert bracelet, that identifies the disorder. *Faster treatment can be initiated if emergency personnel are aware of a DI diagnosis.*

Evaluation. If treatment has been effective, signs of dehydration will be absent, and weight and vital signs will be stable.

> **LEARNING TIP**
> An easy way to remember the pathophysiology of diabetes in**SIP**idus is that patients are thirsty and **SIP** water constantly because the lack of ADH is causing water loss.

Syndrome of Inappropriate Antidiuretic Hormone

PATHOPHYSIOLOGY. SIADH results from too much ADH in the body. This causes excess water to be reabsorbed by the kidney tubules and collecting ducts and back into the blood, leading to decreased urine output and fluid overload. As fluid builds up in the bloodstream, osmolality decreases, and the blood becomes diluted. Normally, decreased serum osmolality inhibits release of ADH. In SIADH, however, ADH continues to be released, adding to the fluid overload.

ETIOLOGY. Causes of SIADH can be categorized into four groups: nervous system disorders such as head trauma and meningitis, cancers such as lung and brain cancer (some tumors actually secrete an ADH-like substance), pulmonary diseases such as cystic fibrosis and chronic obstructive pulmonary disease (COPD), and medications such as antipsychotics and histamines. Whatever the cause of SIADH is, the result is increased secretion of ADH, which results in fluid overload.

SIGNS AND SYMPTOMS. Symptoms of SIADH include symptoms of fluid overload, such as weight gain (usually without edema) and dilutional hyponatremia (Box 39.1). The actual amount of sodium in the blood may be normal, but it appears to be low because of the diluting effect of the extra fluid. Serum osmolality is less than 275 mOsm/kg. The urine is concentrated because water is not being excreted. Electrolyte imbalance can cause muscle cramps and weakness. Because the osmolality of the blood is low, fluid can leak out of the vessels and cause brain swelling. If untreated, this results in lethargy, confusion, seizures, coma, and death.

DIAGNOSTIC TESTS. Serum sodium and osmolality are low, and urine sodium and osmolality are high. Serum ADH is high. Additional testing may be done to diagnose the cause.

THERAPEUTIC MEASURES. Treatment is aimed at the underlying cause. If a tumor is secreting ADH, surgical removal may be indicated. Symptoms can be alleviated by restricting fluids to 800 to 1000 mL per 24 hours. Hypertonic saline fluids may be administered via IV, and an oral sodium tablet may be prescribed to maintain the serum sodium level. A loop diuretic such as furosemide (Lasix) increases water excretion. A vasopressin receptor antagonist such as conivaptan (Vaprisol) may be used to block the action of ADH in the kidney.

Box 39.1
Manifestations of Dilutional Hyponatremia

- Bounding pulse
- Elevated or normal blood pressure
- Muscle weakness
- Headache
- Personality changes
- Nausea
- Diarrhea
- Convulsions
- Coma

NURSING PROCESS FOR THE PATIENT WITH SIADH

Data Collection. Excess fluid volume with hyponatremia is the primary concern for the patient with SIADH. To monitor fluid balance, check vital signs, daily weight, I&O, urine specific gravity, and skin turgor. Edema and pulmonary crackles are not typically present. Determine the patient's ability to maintain a fluid restriction. Monitor level of consciousness and neuromuscular function. Monitor laboratory tests, including serum sodium level, as ordered by the HCP. Determine the patient's understanding of the disease process and treatment.

Nursing Diagnoses, Planning, and Implementation

Excess Fluid Volume related to compromised regulatory mechanism

EXPECTED OUTCOME: The patient's fluid balance will be maintained as evidenced by weight, I&O, and serum sodium within normal limits.

- Monitor daily weight, I&O, vital signs, and laboratory values. *Increased weight, intake greater than output, elevated blood pressure, bounding pulse, and low serum sodium may all indicate fluid overload.*
- Maintain fluid restriction as ordered *to reduce serum dilution and normalize serum sodium.*
- Offer hard candy *to reduce sensation of thirst.*
- Provide ice chips (count as half the volume of fluid; that is, 100 mL of ice chips equals approximately 50 mL of water). *Ice chips take longer to consume than water and may be more satisfying to some patients.*
- Provide calibrated cups *to help the patient maintain the restriction independently if able.*
- Allow the patient to participate in planning the types and times of fluid intake. *Fluid restriction is unpleasant for patients; patients who feel control may be more likely to comply.*
- Report a change in level of consciousness immediately and monitor the patient for seizures. *These are signs of serious fluid imbalance.*
- Instruct the patient to report any weight gain greater than 2 pounds in 1 day, a decrease in urine output, or acute thirst. *These are signs of fluid overload or risk for overload.*
- Encourage use of a medical alert bracelet or other identification *so emergency personnel will be aware of SIADH.*

Evaluation. Weight should stabilize at the pre-illness level once treatment is begun. Serum sodium level should be within normal limits.

CRITICAL THINKING

Mrs. Jackson is a 78-year-old woman who has just returned to your unit after hip surgery. During the next 2 days, you notice that her weight increases from 118 to 124 pounds and that she seems lethargic. You check her ankles and sacrum for edema but find none. In the afternoon, her son rushes out of the room and tells you she is becoming confused, adding that this is not like her at all.

1. What may be the cause of Mrs. Jackson's change in mental status?
2. Based on her weight gain, about how much water is Mrs. Jackson retaining?
3. What may have caused Mrs. Jackson's 6-pound weight gain?
4. Why will Mrs. Jackson be put on fluid restriction?
5. Considering Mrs. Jackson's change in mental status, which team members should now be included in Mrs. Jackson's care?

Suggested answers are at the end of the chapter.

Disorders Related to Growth Hormone Imbalance

Growth hormone (GH), also called *somatotropin*, is responsible for normal growth of bones, cartilage, and soft tissue. GH is synthesized and secreted by the anterior pituitary gland. Excess or deficiency may be related to a more generalized problem with the pituitary gland or hypothalamus. A deficit of GH results in growth failure if not corrected in childhood, and a variety of problems in adulthood. Excess GH results in gigantism (Fig. 39.1) or acromegaly.

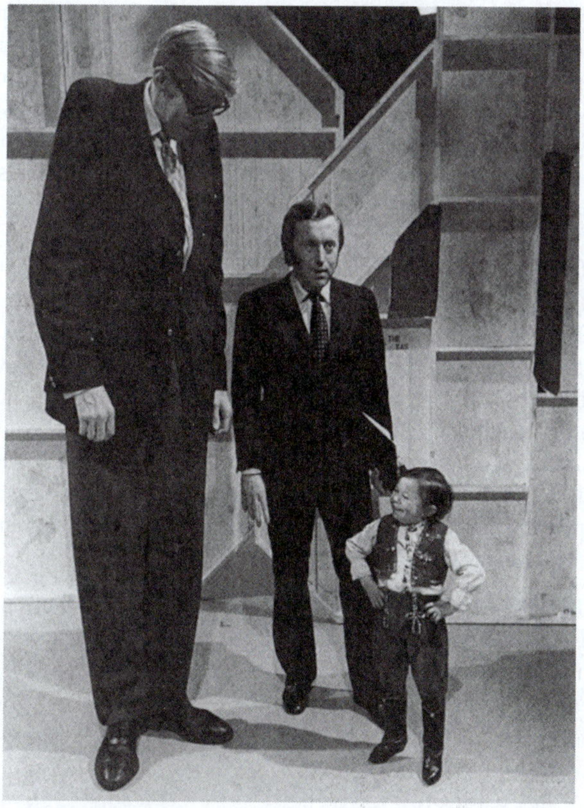

FIGURE 39.1 Gigantism and dwarfism.

Growth Hormone Deficiency

PATHOPHYSIOLOGY. When GH is deficient in childhood, a rare condition called *growth failure* or *short stature* occurs. In the past, this condition was called *dwarfism* (see Fig. 39.1). Deficiency of GH in adults does not affect growth, but we now know the hormone has important functions even during adulthood.

ETIOLOGY. GH deficiency may be due to tumors, surgery, heredity, or trauma to the pituitary gland or hypothalamus. It may also be deficient in some cases of neglect or severe emotional stress. Malnutrition is the most common cause worldwide. Sometimes the cause is not known (see "Cultural Considerations").

> ### Cultural Considerations
> **Ellis–van Creveld Syndrome** is prevalent among the Amish communities of Lancaster County, Pennsylvania. This inherited type of dwarfism is characterized by short stature and an extra digit on each hand, with some affected people having a congenital heart defect and nervous system involvement resulting in a degree of mental disability.

SIGNS AND SYMPTOMS. Children may grow to only 3 to 4 feet in height but have normal body proportions. Sexual maturation may be slowed, related to involvement of additional pituitary hormones.

In adults, symptoms of GH deficiency include fatigue, weakness, excess body fat, decreased muscle and bone mass, sexual dysfunction, high cholesterol, and increased risk for cardiovascular and cerebrovascular disease. Headaches, mental slowness, and psychological disturbances may also occur. All of these signs and symptoms can lead to decreased quality of life.

DIAGNOSTIC TESTS. GH levels in the blood can be measured by a routine laboratory test, but the results may be unreliable because GH is not evenly secreted over the course of a day. A more reliable test is a GH stimulation test that measures GH in response to induced hypoglycemia. An MRI scan can help determine the presence of a tumor; radiographic studies may be used to determine bone age. Genetic testing may also be done.

THERAPEUTIC MEASURES. Treatment of GH deficiency is administration of GH. In the past, GH was derived from human pituitary glands, so treatment was expensive and risky. Now GH, or somatropin (Humatrope, Serostim), can be made in a laboratory using recombinant DNA technology, so it is more readily available to those who need it. It is administered by subcutaneous injection. Surgery may be indicated if a tumor is the cause.

NURSING CARE OF THE PATIENT WITH GROWTH HORMONE DEFICIENCY. If GH deficiency has been present since childhood, most related problems will not be new to the patient. The priority for the nurse then is to approach the patient with respect while asking about current problems that may need attention. If the diagnosis is new, the patient may need to learn to self-administer somatropin. Collaborate with the RN to educate the patient on what to expect and how to administer the medication.

An excellent resource for people with short stature is the Little People of America organization (www.lpaonline.org).

> ## CRITICAL THINKING
>
> **Three siblings** were adopted into a loving home after having been in several foster homes. After a year in their new home, each child suddenly grew 6 to 8 inches. What do you think happened?
>
> *Suggested answers are at the end of the chapter.*

Acromegaly

Acromegaly is a rare excess of GH that affects adults, usually in their 40s. If GH excess occurs in children, the result is gigantism.

PATHOPHYSIOLOGY. Acromegaly occurs because of overproduction of GH in an adult. Bones increase in size, leading to enlargement of facial features, hands, and feet. Long bones grow in width but not length because the epiphyseal disks are closed. Subcutaneous connective tissue increases, causing a fleshy appearance. Internal organs and glands enlarge. Impaired tolerance of carbohydrates leads to elevated blood glucose.

ETIOLOGY. Excess secretion of GH can be caused by pituitary **hyperplasia**, a benign pituitary tumor, or excess of GH-releasing hormone (GH-RH) due to hypothalamic dysfunction.

SIGNS AND SYMPTOMS. Symptoms develop very slowly, and the disorder may be present for years before it is recognized. Often, the first symptom noticed is a change in ring or shoe size. The nose, jaw, brow, hands, and feet enlarge (Fig. 39.2). Teeth may be displaced, causing difficulty chewing, or dentures may no longer fit. The tongue becomes thick, causing difficulty in speaking and swallowing (dysphagia). The patient may develop sleep apnea. If a tumor is the cause, visual disturbances can occur because of tumor pressure on the optic nerve, and headaches result from pressure on the brain. Diabetes mellitus may develop because GH increases blood glucose and causes an increased workload for the pancreas (see Chapter 40). With treatment, soft tissues reduce in size, but bone growth is permanent.

DIAGNOSTIC TESTS. GH levels are measured. A CT scan or an MRI is done to locate a pituitary tumor.

THERAPEUTIC MEASURES. Treatment may include medications to block GH or hypophysectomy. Radiation may be indicated if a tumor is the cause.

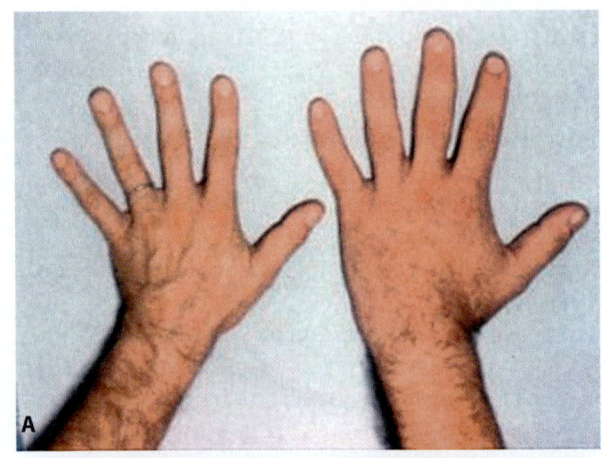

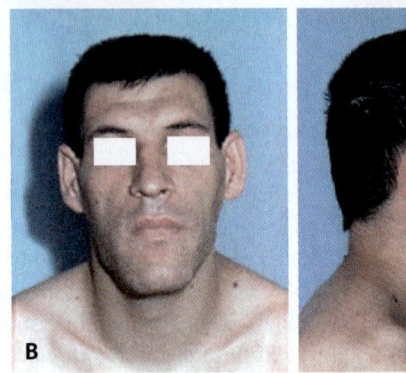

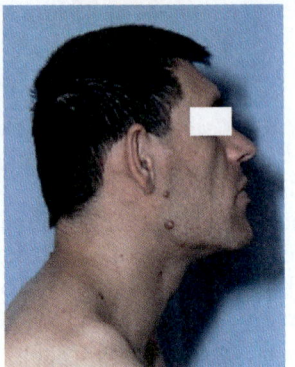

FIGURE 39.2 Patient with acromegaly. (A) Hands and (B) face.

Pituitary Tumors

Most tumors of the pituitary gland are benign adenomas. However, even benign tumors in the brain can cause many symptoms, including visual disturbances, symptoms of increased pressure in the brain, and symptoms related to hormone imbalances, as described earlier. Treatment for pituitary tumors is usually hypophysectomy. Radiation may also be used, either alone or as an adjunct to surgery.

Nursing Care of the Patient Undergoing Hypophysectomy

Removal of the pituitary gland is called *hypophysectomy*. The procedure is most often done using minimally invasive endoscopic surgery, via the nose or a small incision just under the upper lip. This allows access through the sphenoid sinus to the pituitary gland, without disturbing brain tissue. Figure 39.3 shows the transsphenoidal approach through the upper lip. Some large tumors may require transfrontal craniotomy (entry through the frontal bone of the skull).

PREOPERATIVE CARE. Make sure the patient understands the HCP's explanation of surgery. Collect and document baseline neurological data. Prepare the patient for what to expect following surgery. Explain that it will be important after

• WORD • BUILDING •

hyperplasia: hyper—excessive + plasia—formation or deviation

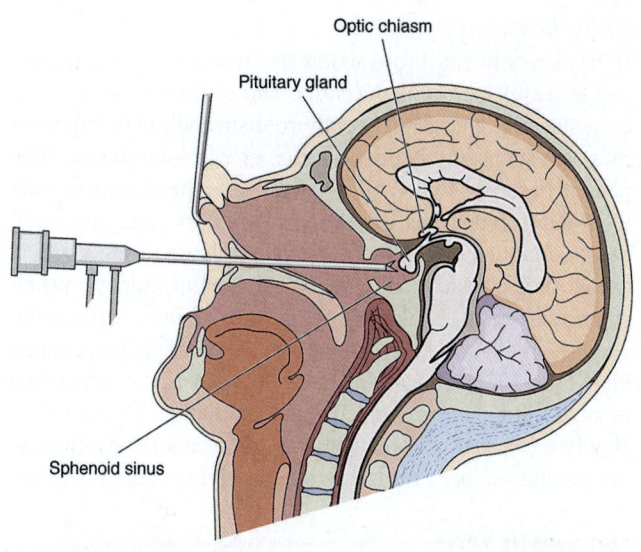

FIGURE 39.3 Transsphenoidal approach to pituitary gland for hypophysectomy.

surgery to avoid actions that increase pressure on the surgical site, such as coughing, sneezing, nose blowing, straining to move bowels, or bending from the waist. Because coughing can raise intracranial pressure and is contraindicated, instruct the patient in deep-breathing exercises or use of an incentive spirometer. Patients can usually expect to stay in the hospital about one day.

POSTOPERATIVE CARE. Monitor neurologic status to identify changes from baseline data. Check urine for specific gravity because DI can occur following pituitary surgery. If a patient has had transsphenoidal surgery, nasal packing and a "mustache dressing" will be present. These are left in place and not removed unless ordered by the HCP. Monitor the dressing for signs of cerebrospinal fluid (CSF) leakage. CSF contains glucose, so glucose testing strips can be used to determine whether drainage is CSF or nasal discharge. Remind the patient to avoid actions that increase pressure on the surgical site. The patient is placed on hormone replacement therapy after hypophysectomy. Pituitary hormones are difficult to replace, so target hormones are generally given. These may include thyroid hormones, glucocorticoids, intranasal desmopressin, and sex hormones.

PATIENT EDUCATION. Instruct the patient before discharge according to agency guidelines. These usually include instructions to prevent increased pressure on the surgical site as well as instructions on how to administer the hormones and side effects to report. Examples include the following:

- Expect a small amount of bloody or mucous drainage from your nose.
- If you must blow your nose, do so very gently. Blowing can injure the surgical site and cause bleeding or spinal fluid leakage.
- Take stool softeners as needed to prevent straining for bowel movements.
- Take cough suppressants as directed to prevent coughing.
- If an upper lip incision was used, wait until the incision line is healed to brush teeth with a toothbrush. Floss and mouth rinses can be used instead.
- Take all medications as prescribed. You will be on lifelong hormone therapy to replace the hormones made by your pituitary gland.
- Call immediately if you develop a fever, a small amount of bloody drainage from the incision site, clear drainage, unusual thirst, unusually frequent urination (a sign of diabetes insipidus), or any other symptoms that concern you.

DISORDERS OF THE THYROID GLAND

Triiodothyronine (T_3) and thyroxine (T_4) are hormones secreted by the thyroid gland. These hormones are collectively referred to as the *thyroid hormones* (THs). Deficient secretion of TH results in hypothyroidism; excess TH results in hyperthyroidism. The thyroid gland also secretes calcitonin, discussed in Chapter 38. For more information, visit the American Thyroid Association (www.thyroid.org).

Hypothyroidism

Hypothyroidism occurs primarily in women older than 50. If hypothyroidism occurs in an infant, severe problems with growth and development occur. All babies born in the United States are tested for hypothyroidism at birth.

Pathophysiology

Primary hypothyroidism occurs when the thyroid gland fails to produce enough TH even though enough thyroid-stimulating hormone (TSH) is secreted by the pituitary gland. The pituitary gland responds to the low level of TH by producing more TSH. Secondary hypothyroidism is caused by low levels of TSH, which fail to stimulate release of TH. Tertiary hypothyroidism results from inadequate release of thyrotropin-releasing hormone (TRH), secreted by the hypothalamus. Most cases of hypothyroidism are primary (Table 39.3).

Table 39.3
Thyroid Hormone Abnormalities

	Hyperthyroidism	Hypothyroidism
Primary	↑ thyroid hormone (TH) ↓ thyroid-stimulating hormone (TSH)	↓ TH ↑ TSH
Secondary (pituitary cause)	↑ TH ↑ TSH	↓ TH ↓ TSH

Because thyroid hormones are responsible for metabolism, low levels result in a slowed metabolic rate, which causes many of the characteristic symptoms of hypothyroidism.

Etiology

Primary hypothyroidism may be a result of a congenital defect, inflammation of the thyroid gland, or iodine deficiency. Hashimoto thyroiditis, also called *chronic lymphocytic thyroiditis*, is an autoimmune disorder that eventually destroys thyroid tissue, leading to hypothyroidism. Secondary or tertiary hypothyroidism can be caused by a pituitary or hypothalamic lesion. Hypothyroidism can also result from treatment of hyperthyroidism, either with medication or thyroidectomy. Lithium, a medication used to treat bipolar disorder, can cause hypothyroidism by reducing thyroid hormone release.

Signs and Symptoms

Manifestations are related to the reduced metabolic rate and include fatigue, weight gain, bradycardia, constipation, mental dullness, feeling cold, shortness of breath, decreased sweating, and dry skin and hair (see "Patient Perspective" and Table 39.4). Heart failure may occur because of decreased pumping strength of the heart. Altered fat metabolism causes hyperlipidemia, which can lead to cardiovascular disease. In advanced disease, **myxedema** develops, which is a nonpitting edema of the face, hands, and feet.

Patient Perspective

Mary

When I turned 40-something, I began to notice a few changes in my body. I seemed to be easily fatigued, but I attributed that to moving our family across country and all the adjustments that needed to be made. I also noticed weight gain, most notably around my waist. Again, I thought, "Well, I *am* 40-something," but it seemed no matter how much I exercised and watched what I ate, I couldn't lose weight. Worse, I was gaining! One day a friend of mine pointed out that I always seemed tired. Each time she called to do something, my reply was always the same, "I'd love to, but not today. I'm just so tired."

Things started to get worse. I began losing hair by the handfuls each time I shampooed. I began to notice dry skin (I thought it was just our hard water) and constipation (I thought I had irritable bowel syndrome). Finally, I went to the doctor for a physical, including laboratory tests, which included TSH and free T_4. The diagnosis came back: I had hypothyroidism and was started on levothyroxine (Synthroid). I noticed the effect on my energy almost immediately. Now I can exercise effectively. I have lost nearly all the weight I gained, and my husband no longer complains about having to clean out the drain in our shower every time I wash my hair. I am thankful for the diagnosis and treatment because I feel like myself again.

Complications

If the metabolic rate drops so low that it becomes life threatening, the result is myxedema coma. This occurs in patients with long-standing, untreated hypothyroidism and can be triggered by stress such as infection, trauma, or exposure to cold. The patient becomes hypothermic, with a temperature less than 95°F (35°C), and has decreased respiratory rate, depressed mental function, and lethargy. Blood glucose drops. Cardiac output drops, which can reduce perfusion of kidneys. Death can occur because of heart or respiratory failure. If you note changes in mental status or vital signs in your patient, contact the RN or HCP immediately. Treatment of myxedema coma involves intubation and mechanical ventilation. The patient is slowly rewarmed with blankets. IV fluids and IV levothyroxine (Synthroid) are given, and the underlying cause is treated.

Diagnostic Tests

The levels of T_3 and T_4 are low, and the level of TSH may be high or low, depending on the cause of the hypothyroidism. If the pituitary gland is functioning normally, TSH is elevated in an attempt to stimulate an increase in TH. Serum cholesterol and triglycerides are elevated. Antibodies are usually present in autoimmune disease.

Therapeutic Measures

Primary hypothyroidism is easily treated with oral thyroid replacement hormone. Most patients now take synthetic thyroid hormone (levothyroxine [Synthroid]). Doses are started low and slowly increased to prevent symptoms of hyperthyroidism or cardiac complications.

CUE RECOGNITION 39.1

While doing vital signs on a patient at the clinic where you work, you note that your patient's pulse rate is 48 and temperature is 95.6. Their affect is depressed, and they report steady weight gain. You note they are prescribed levothyroxine. What should you do?

Suggested answers are at the end of the chapter.

Nursing Process for the Patient With Hypothyroidism

DATA COLLECTION. Ask the patient about increased fatigue, weight gain, feeling cold, constipation, and shortness of breath. Check vital signs and weight, and check for dry skin and hair. Observe for mental dullness, or for memory loss in older adults. Do not palpate the thyroid gland; this is a function of the HCP. Determine whether the patient is on medication for hypothyroidism and verify that the patient is taking it as prescribed.

For nursing care of the patient with constipation, see Chapter 34. For skin care, see Chapter 54.

• WORD • BUILDING •

myxedema: myx—mucus + edema—swelling

Table 39.4
Symptoms of Thyroid Disorders

Hypothyroidism	*Hyperthyroidism*
Cardiovascular	
Bradycardia, decreased cardiac output, cool skin, cold intolerance	Tachycardia, palpitations, increased cardiac output, warm skin, heat intolerance
Neurologic	
Lethargy, slowed movements, memory loss, confusion	Fatigue, restlessness, hyperactive reflexes, tremor, insomnia, emotional instability
Pulmonary	
Dyspnea, hypoventilation	Dyspnea
Integumentary	
Cool, dry skin; brittle, dry hair	Diaphoresis; warm, moist skin; fine, soft hair
Gastrointestinal	
Decreased appetite, weight gain, constipation, increased serum lipid levels	Increased appetite, weight loss, frequent stools, decreased serum lipid levels
Skeletal	
Increased bone density but poor bone quality and increased fracture risk	Reduced bone density, increased fracture risk
Reproductive	
Decreased libido, erectile dysfunction	Decreased libido, erectile dysfunction, amenorrhea

Nursing Care Plan for the Patient With Hypothyroidism

Nursing Diagnosis: *Fatigue* related to reduced metabolic rate
Expected Outcomes: The patient will (1) report lessening fatigue after treatment is initiated and (2) be able to carry out usual activities of daily living.
Evaluation of Outcomes: (1) Does patient report lessening fatigue? (2) Is patient able to carry out activities of daily living?

Intervention	Rationale	Evaluation
Assist patient with self-care activities.	*Patients with fatigue may have difficulty carrying out activities independently.*	Are patient's self-care needs being met? Is assistance needed?
Allow for rest between activities.	*Rest periods will enable patient to conserve energy for activities.*	Does patient state rest is adequate?
Slowly increase patient's activities as medication begins to be effective.	*As thyroid replacement therapy becomes effective, patient's fatigue will lessen.*	Does patient tolerate increases in activity?
Geriatric		
When getting older patients up, watch for orthostatic hypotension.	*Orthostatic hypotension is common in older adults and may cause falls.*	Does patient's blood pressure drop when changing positions?

(nursing care plan continues on page 748)

Nursing Care Plan for the Patient With Hypothyroidism—cont'd

Nursing Diagnosis: *Imbalanced Nutrition: More Than Body Requirements* related to decreased metabolic rate
Expected Outcomes: (1) Nutrition will be balanced as evidenced by return to patient's pre-illness weight. (2) The patient will verbalize understanding of dietary recommendations.
Evaluation of Outcomes: (1) Is the patient approaching pre-illness weight? (2) Is the patient able to explain dietary recommendations and a plan for implementation?

Intervention	Rationale	Evaluation
Weigh weekly and record.	*Weekly weights record progress. Daily weights are not necessary.*	Is patient approaching ideal weight?
Consult dietitian for therapeutic diet until hypothyroidism is controlled.	*The dietitian can provide food choices for gradual weight loss if necessary.*	Does patient verbalize understanding of and ability to follow diet?
Geriatric		
Allow patient to help determine acceptable diet modifications.	*Older patients may have long-standing dietary habits that are hard to change.*	Is patient satisfied with weight loss plan?

CRITICAL THINKING

Mrs. Maino is a 59-year-old woman who is tired all the time and has gained 16 pounds during the past year. Laboratory results show low T_3 and T_4 and elevated TSH levels. Her HCP prescribes levothyroxine by mouth (PO).

1. Why is Mrs. Maino's TSH elevated?
2. What will happen to Mrs. Maino's caloric requirements as she begins treatment? Why?
3. The nurse asks you to teach Mrs. Maino to check her pulse. Why is this important?
4. Which team members are important to involve in Mrs. Maino's care?

Suggested answers are at the end of the chapter.

PATIENT EDUCATION. Collaborate with the RN to instruct the patient in the importance of consistent use of thyroid replacement medication and regular blood tests to monitor TSH. Ensure that the patient has the means to obtain the medication. The patient needs to be aware that too much TH will cause symptoms of hyperthyroidism. Such symptoms should be reported to the HCP immediately. In addition, if the patient is experiencing mental status changes, discuss the need to avoid driving or operating machinery until symptoms are resolved.

CUE RECOGNITION 39.2

You are caring for a patient being treated for hypothyroidism. The patient states she has become intolerant to heat, her heart is flip-flopping, and she feel very nervous. What do you do?

Suggested answers are at the end of the chapter.

Hyperthyroidism

Hyperthyroidism is most common in women. Graves disease, one cause of hyperthyroidism, is more common in young women. Multinodular goiter, another cause, more often occurs in older women.

Pathophysiology

Hyperthyroidism results in excessive amounts of circulating TH. The term *thyrotoxicosis* is used to describe the effects of excess thyroid hormone. Primary hyperthyroidism occurs when a problem within the thyroid gland causes excess hormone release. Secondary hyperthyroidism occurs because of excess TSH release from the pituitary gland, causing overstimulation of the thyroid gland. Tertiary hyperthyroidism is caused by excess TRH from the hypothalamus. A high level of TH increases the metabolic rate. It also increases the number of beta-adrenergic receptor sites in the body, which enhances the activity of epinephrine and norepinephrine. The resulting fight-or-flight response is the cause of many of the symptoms of hyperthyroidism.

Etiology

A variety of disorders can cause hyperthyroidism. Graves disease, the most common cause, is an autoimmune disorder in which thyroid-stimulating antibodies cause the thyroid gland to make too much TH.

Other causes include thyroid nodules that secrete excess TH (multinodular goiter and toxic adenoma), inflammation of the thyroid (thyroiditis), or a thyroid tumor. A pituitary tumor can secrete excess TSH, which overstimulates the thyroid gland. Patients taking TH for hypothyroidism may take too much. Each of these problems can cause excess circulating TH and symptoms of hyperthyroidism.

Women who smoke nearly double their risk of Graves disease. Heredity can also play a role in autoimmune hyperthyroidism.

Signs and Symptoms

Many signs and symptoms are related to the hypermetabolic state, such as heat intolerance, increased appetite with weight loss, and increased frequency of bowel movements. Nervousness, tremor, tachycardia, and palpitations are caused by the increase in sympathetic nervous system activity and may be more common in younger patients. Heart failure can occur because of tachycardia and the resulting inefficient pumping of the heart. See additional signs and symptoms in Table 39.4.

Without treatment, the patient can become manic or psychotic. Additional signs that occur only with Graves disease include thickening of the skin on the anterior legs and exophthalmos (bulging of the eyes; Fig. 39.4). Exophthalmos is caused by muscle swelling and fat expansion behind the eyes. Other eye changes include photophobia and blurred or double vision.

Older adult patients may not have the typical signs and symptoms of hyperthyroidism, so be especially alert for this. These patients may present with heart failure, atrial fibrillation, fatigue, apathy, and depression.

Complications

THYROTOXIC CRISIS. Thyrotoxic crisis (sometimes called *thyroid storm*) is a severe hyperthyroid state that can occur in hyperthyroid people who are untreated or who develop another illness or stressor. It also may occur after thyroid surgery in patients who have been inadequately prepared with antithyroid medication. Thyrotoxic crisis can result in death in as little as 2 hours if untreated. Symptoms include tachycardia, high fever, extreme hypertension (with eventual heart failure and hypotension), dehydration, restlessness, delirium, or coma.

If thyrotoxic crisis occurs, treatment is first directed toward relieving the life-threatening symptoms. Acetaminophen is given for the fever. Aspirin is avoided because it binds with the same serum protein as T_4, freeing additional T_4 into the circulation. IV fluids and a cooling blanket may be ordered to cool the patient. A beta-adrenergic blocker such as propranolol is given for tachycardia and symptom control. Oxygen is administered, and the head of the bed is elevated because the high metabolic rate requires more oxygen. Once symptoms are controlled and the patient is safe, the underlying thyroid problem is treated.

HYPOTHYROIDISM. Another complication of hyperthyroidism can be hypothyroidism. This can occur because of long-term disease or as a result of treatment. Patients with a history of hyperthyroidism should be monitored for recurrent hyperthyroidism or the onset of hypothyroidism.

Diagnostic Tests

Serum levels of T_3 and T_4 are elevated. TSH is low in primary hyperthyroidism or high if the cause is pituitary. A radioactive iodine uptake test or a thyroid scan can be done to determine hyperactivity of the gland or to locate a nodule or tumor. The thyroid gland may be enlarged; palpation of the thyroid in a patient suspected to have hyperthyroidism should only be performed by an HCP. Thyroid-stimulating immunoglobulin is present in Graves disease.

Therapeutic Measures

Methimazole (Tapazole) inhibits the synthesis of TH, but it may take several months to be effective and must be continued for 12 to 18 months. Beta blockers relieve sympathetic nervous system symptoms. Calcium and vitamin D are given to protect bones.

Radioactive iodine (^{131}I, or RAI) may be used to destroy a portion of the thyroid gland. The patient takes one oral dose of RAI. Dietary iodine normally goes to the thyroid gland, where it is used to make TH. When RAI is given, the radioactivity destroys some of the cells that make TH.

Sometimes medications or RAI alone can control hyperthyroidism. If this does not occur, surgery is planned. Prior to surgery, antithyroid medications are prescribed to calm the thyroid. They help slow the heart rate and reduce other symptoms, making surgery safer. Oral iodine reduces the vascularity of the thyroid gland, decreasing the risk of bleeding during surgery. Adequate preparation of the patient is important because a **euthyroid** state helps prevent a postoperative thyrotoxic crisis.

Thyroidectomy can be done with a traditional, open approach or with minimally invasive techniques that use a combination of a tiny incision and an endoscope. Patients can usually go home the same day and have a faster recovery time with minimally invasive surgery. The surgeon may choose to leave some of the thyroid gland intact, to continue to secrete some hormone. Following surgery, the patient will likely be hypothyroid and will require thyroid replacement hormone (levothyroxine [Synthroid]). Nursing care of the patient undergoing a thyroidectomy is discussed later in this chapter.

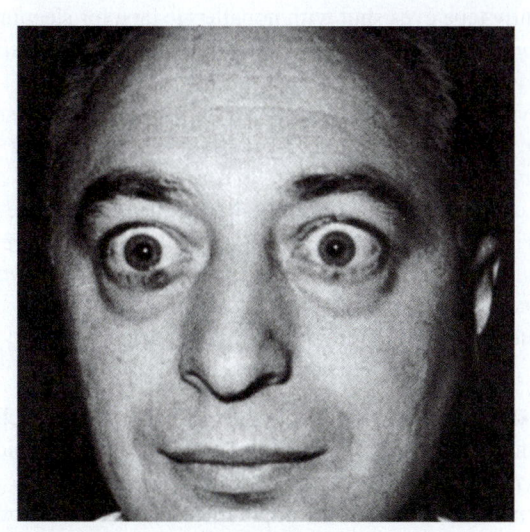

FIGURE 39.4 Exophthalmos caused by Graves disease.

• WORD • BUILDING •
euthyroid: eu—normal, healthy + thyroid

If vision is impaired from exophthalmos, surgical orbital decompression can be done. Current endoscopic techniques have made this a safer option than in the past. In 2020, the U.S. Food and Drug Administration (FDA) approved the drug teprotumumab-trbw (Tepezza) to treat thyroid eye disease. Teprotumumab blocks the receptors that cause swelling of muscle tissue and expanding fat behind the eye.

Nursing Process for the Patient With Hyperthyroidism

DATA COLLECTION. Monitor the patient with hyperthyroidism closely until normal thyroid activity is restored. Check vital signs and lung sounds, and report changes to the RN or HCP. Ask about level of anxiety and ability to cope with symptoms. Monitor weight, bowel function, and ability to sleep. Observe the eyes for risk for injury caused by exophthalmos, and note degree of muscle weakness. Never palpate the thyroid gland of a patient with hyperthyroidism because palpation can stimulate release of TH and precipitate a thyrotoxic crisis.

NURSING DIAGNOSES, PLANNING, AND IMPLEMENTATION.

Hyperthermia related to hypermetabolic state

EXPECTED OUTCOME: The patient's body temperature will be within normal limits.

- Monitor temperature. *Temperature may be elevated due to hypermetabolic state.*
- Administer acetaminophen as ordered (avoid aspirin) to reduce temperature. *Acetaminophen relieves fever by acting on heat regulation center in the hypothalamus. Aspirin can cause an increase in circulating TH.*
- Apply cooling blanket as ordered. *External cooling may be needed if acetaminophen is not effective.*
- If a cooling blanket is needed, set it to 1 to 2 degrees below current temperature, and wrap the extremities with towels to prevent shivering, *which can further increase temperature.*
- Offer fluids *to replace fluids lost through diaphoresis.*

Diarrhea related to increase in peristalsis

See Chapter 34 for nursing care of the patient with diarrhea.

Imbalanced Nutrition: Less Than Body Requirements related to increased metabolism

EXPECTED OUTCOME: The patient will have balanced nutrition as evidenced by stable weight in proportion to height.

- Determine healthy weight for height *so that the expected outcome is realistic for the patient.*
- Monitor weight weekly *to make sure interventions are working.*
- Consult dietitian for high-calorie diet and supplements *to meet caloric requirements.*

Disturbed Sleep Pattern related to sympathetic stimulation

EXPECTED OUTCOME: The patient will have improved sleep as evidenced by stating feeling rested upon awakening.

- Provide a quiet, restful environment *to help the patient to fall asleep.*
- Ask the patient if music or earplugs are desired *to mask environmental noise.*
- Administer propranolol or sedative as ordered *to reduce sympathetic stimulation and calm patient.*

Anxiety related to sympathetic stimulation

EXPECTED OUTCOME: The patient will experience reduced anxiety as evidenced by the patient's statement that anxiety is controlled.

- Provide the patient with accurate information about the disorder and treatment and explain that proper treatment will correct symptoms. *Fear of the unknown can produce anxiety.*
- Administer propranolol or antianxiety agent as ordered *to reduce sympathetic stimulation and calm patient.*
- Offer massage, music, or other relaxation techniques preferred by the patient. *These may promote relaxation.*

Risk for Injury related to hypermetabolic state and bone and eye involvement

EXPECTED OUTCOME: The patient will remain safe and without injury.

- Report changes in vital signs to RN or HCP. *Prompt treatment can reduce complications.*
- Encourage all patients with Graves disease to stop smoking if they are smokers. *Smoking is a risk factor for exophthalmos.*
- Administer lubricating saline eye drops as ordered *to protect eyes from drying.*
- Advise use of dark, tight-fitting glasses *to protect eyes from light and injury.*
- Gently tape eyes shut with nonallergic tape for sleeping. *Exophthalmos may prevent the patient from fully closing the eyes.*
- Elevate the head of the bed *to reduce edema behind the eyes.*
- Provide a low-sodium diet. *This may decrease edema behind the eyes.*
- Teach the patient to notify the HCP immediately if eye pain or vision changes occur. *These can be signs of pressure from edema on optic nerve, which can cause permanent damage if not corrected.*
- Protect from injury and falls. *Reduced bone density increases risk for fractures.*

PATIENT EDUCATION. Collaborate with the RN to teach the patient about the disease and symptoms of hyperthyroidism or hypothyroidism to report. Also teach the patient how to take medications and the importance of routine follow-up laboratory testing.

EVALUATION. If the plan of care is effective, the patient will remain free from complications and injury. Vital signs will be within normal limits. Diarrhea will be controlled, and complications of diarrhea such as skin breakdown and dehydration will be avoided. The patient's weight should remain stable. The patient should report that they are rested on awakening and that anxiety is controlled.

> **LEARNING TIP**
> To understand signs and symptoms of thyroid disorders, think of the thyroid as a furnace. Hyperthyroidism is a hot furnace and hypothyroidism is a cold furnace.

Nursing Care of the Patient Receiving Radioactive Iodine

If RAI is used, it is usually given orally in one dose. If the dose is high, such as for the patient with thyroid cancer, the patient is hospitalized. Patients receiving lower doses may be treated as outpatients. Limit time spent with the patient, and maintain a safe distance when providing direct care (see Chapter 11). Pregnant caregivers should avoid caring for patients receiving RAI. Urine, vomitus, and other body secretions are contaminated and should be disposed of according to hospital policy. Flush the toilet twice after disposal of contaminated material. The radiation safety officer and hospital policy should be consulted for specific precautions.

At home, the patient is instructed to avoid close contact with family members and to use careful hand hygiene after urinating. Oral contact with others should be avoided and eating utensils should be washed thoroughly with soap and water. Pregnancy should be avoided for a year. Hospital teaching protocols should be used for patient teaching. The amount of time patients must avoid contact with others depends on the dose of radiation received. If the treatment is administered for hyperthyroidism, symptoms should subside in about 6 to 8 weeks.

Side effects can include sore throat, dry mouth or eyes, and nausea. Sore throat is easily treated with acetaminophen, and nausea usually lasts only a day or two. Dry eyes can be relieved with moisturizing eye drops. Encourage the patient to drink plenty of fluids and void frequently to help remove RAI from the body and reduce radiation exposure to the bladder. In addition, the patient should be aware of symptoms of hypothyroidism to report because hypothyroidism can occur up to 15 years after the treatment.

Goiter
Pathophysiology and Etiology

Enlargement of the thyroid gland is called a *goiter*. The thyroid gland may enlarge in response to increased TSH levels or to the autoimmune process that occurs in Graves disease. TSH is elevated in response to low TH, iodine deficiency, pregnancy, or viral, genetic, or other conditions. When a goiter is caused by iodine deficiency or other environmental factors, it is called an *endemic* goiter.

Some medications are **goitrogens.** These substances interfere with the body's use of iodine. Some **goitrogenic** medications include propylthiouracil, sulfonamides, lithium, and salicylates (aspirin).

A goiter can be associated with a hyperthyroid, hypothyroid, or euthyroid state. A goiter that occurs with hyperthyroidism is sometimes called a toxic goiter. Once the cause of the goiter is removed, the gland usually returns to normal size.

Signs and Symptoms

The thyroid gland is enlarged, and swelling may be apparent at the base of the neck (Fig. 39.5). Alternatively, the gland may enlarge posteriorly, which can interfere with swallowing or breathing. The patient may have a full sensation in the neck. Symptoms of hypothyroidism or hyperthyroidism may be present.

Diagnostic Tests

Serum TSH, T_3, and T_4 levels are measured to determine thyroid function. An ultrasound or a thyroid scan may be done to determine the cause or evaluate the size of the gland.

Therapeutic Measures

Treatment is aimed at the cause. Consult the HCP if goitrogenic medications are used. If iodine deficiency is a problem, it is added to the diet with supplements or iodized salt.

> **Nutrition Notes**
>
> **Iodine Deficiency.** Iodine is an essential element, needed by the thyroid to produce hormones. Iodine is found in soil and seawater at various levels throughout the world. Foods differ in their iodine content depending on the concentration of iodine in the soil and water. If an individual consumes inadequate iodine, the thyroid must work harder to produce hormones and may enlarge, creating a goiter. The United States fortifies salt with iodine. Globally, approximately 30% of people are at risk for iodine deficiency (American Thyroid Association, 2019). Consuming a wide variety of foods normally prevents a deficiency in iodine. Good sources of iodine in the diet include seaweed, breads made with iodate dough conditioners, cod, Greek yogurt, oysters, milk, and iodized salt (National Institutes of Health, 2020).
>
> **Iodine Excess.** The American Thyroid Association (2019) recommends against the ingestion of supplements that contain iodine and kelp. Excessive iodine may cause thyroid dysfunction.
>
> *References:* American Thyroid Association. (2019). Iodine deficiency. www.thyroid.org/iodine-deficiency; National Institute of Health. (2020). Iodine: Fact sheet for health professionals. https://ods.od.nih.gov/factsheets/Iodine-HealthProfessional.

• WORD • BUILDING •

goitrogenic: goitro—goiter + genic—producing

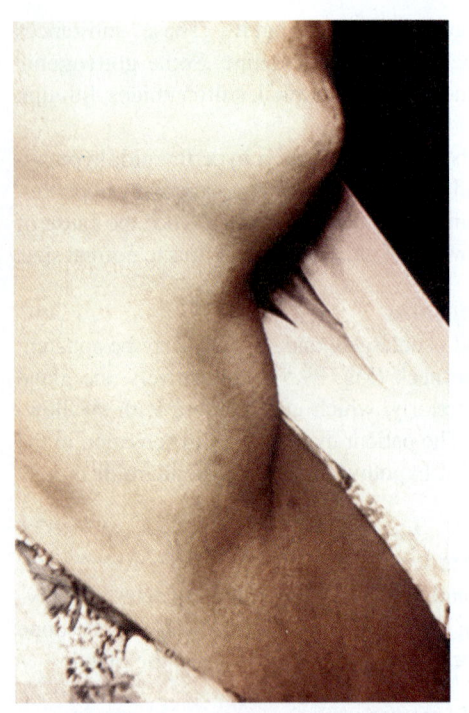

FIGURE 39.5 Goiter caused by iodine deficiency.

Hypothyroidism or hyperthyroidism is treated if indicated. Levothyroxine (Synthroid) may be given to reduce TSH levels via negative feedback. RAI therapy or thyroidectomy may be needed to treat hyperthyroid symptoms or if the enlarged gland is interfering with breathing or swallowing.

Nursing Care for the Patient With a Goiter
Be careful to monitor the effect of the goiter on breathing and swallowing. Stridor, a whistling sound, may be heard if the airway is obstructed. Stridor is an ominous sign and should be reported to the HCP immediately. If the patient experiences difficulty swallowing, notify the HCP and collaborate with the dietitian to provide soft foods that are easy to swallow. A swallowing study might be ordered. This will assist a speech pathologist or other expert in making specific recommendations for safe swallowing.

> **CUE RECOGNITION 39.3**
> You are caring for a patient with a goiter. The patient begins to have stridorous respirations. What should you do?
>
> *Suggested answers are at the end of the chapter.*

Cancer of the Thyroid Gland
Thyroid cancer is the most common cancer of the endocrine system. Women are affected more often than men. However, most tumors of the thyroid gland are not malignant. See Chapter 11 for cancer pathophysiology.

Etiology
Thyroid hyperplasia or exposure to radiation (see "Cultural Considerations: Chernobyl Nuclear Disaster") can lead to thyroid cancer. The tendency to develop some forms of thyroid cancer may be inherited.

> **Cultural Considerations**
> **Chernobyl Nuclear Disaster**
> Because of the Chernobyl nuclear disaster in Ukraine in 1986, children and adolescents who lived in the area at the time have a high risk for pituitary, thyroid, and parathyroid disorders and cancers. The proximity of Estonia, Latvia, Lithuania, Poland, and other Eastern European countries to Russia places these populations at risk as well. Be alert for endocrine disorders among immigrants and long-term visitors from these areas and assist patients to arrange genetic counseling for those who desire it.

Signs and Symptoms
A hard, painless nodule may be palpable on the thyroid gland. Difficulty breathing or swallowing, persistent cough, or changes in the voice may occur if the tumor is near the esophagus and trachea. Most patients with cancer of the thyroid have normal TH levels.

Diagnostic Tests
A thyroid scan shows a "cold" nodule. This is because malignant tumors of the thyroid do not take up RAI administered for the scan. A "hot" nodule indicates a benign tumor. A fine-needle aspiration biopsy confirms the diagnosis.

Therapeutic Measures
A partial or total thyroidectomy may be done. Chemotherapy, RAI therapy, or external beam radiation may also be used, alone or following surgery.

Nursing Care
Nursing care is determined by the symptoms the patient is experiencing. See Chapter 11 for care of the patient with cancer.

> **Evidence-Based Practice**
> **Clinical Question**
> Does weight affect thyroid function?
>
> **Evidence**
> A researcher reviewed more than 100 publications and was able to relate obesity as a contributive factor for younger adults developing thyroid cancer. In 2016, nearly one in four new obesity-related thyroid cancer patients were individuals age 20 to 44 years (Berger, 2018).

> **Implications for Nursing Practice**
> Although being overweight is known to have serious health consequences, it is now known to put persons at risk for thyroid cancer as well. It is important to encourage persons to eat healthy diets and manage weight to prevent serious negative health outcomes, including thyroid cancer.
>
> *References:* Berger, N. (2018). Young adult cancer: Influence of the obesity pandemic. *Obesity Review, 26*(4), 641–650; Obesity is shifting cancer to young adults (2018). *Oncology Times, 40*(8), 15.

Nursing Process for the Patient Undergoing Thyroidectomy

A thyroidectomy may be performed for cancer of the thyroid gland, for hyperthyroidism, or if the patient is suffering from dyspnea or dysphagia from a goiter. See Chapter 12 for general care of a patient having surgery.

A total thyroidectomy is usually performed if cancer is present. After a total thyroidectomy, lifelong replacement hormone must be taken. A subtotal (partial) thyroidectomy might be done for hyperthyroidism, leaving a portion of the thyroid gland to continue to secrete TH.

Preoperative Care

The patient should be in a euthyroid state before a thyroidectomy to avoid complications during and after surgery. This is accomplished with the use of antithyroid medication such as methimazole (Tapazole). A saturated solution of potassium iodide may also be administered to decrease the size and vascularity of the gland, reducing the risk of bleeding during surgery.

Collect baseline vital signs and document voice quality, so you can compare findings postoperatively. Explain what the patient can expect before, during, and after surgery. Preoperative teaching should include how to perform gentle range-of-motion exercises of the neck, support the neck during position changes, and use an incentive spirometer after surgery.

Postoperative Care

DATA COLLECTION. Monitor vital signs, oxygen saturation, drain (if present), and dressing every 15 minutes initially, progressing to every 4 hours, as directed, if the patient is stable. Decreased blood pressure with increased pulse can indicate shock related to blood loss. Tachycardia and fever, along with mental status changes, can indicate thyrotoxic crisis. Check the back of the neck for pooling of blood. Because of the location of the surgery, observe for signs of respiratory distress, including an increase in respiratory rate, dyspnea, or stridor. Ask the patient to speak to detect hoarseness of the voice, which can indicate trauma to the recurrent laryngeal nerve. Monitor the patient's serum calcium levels and watch for evidence of tetany (discussed later in this chapter). Report abnormal findings to the RN or HCP immediately.

NURSING DIAGNOSES, PLANNING, AND IMPLEMENTATION

Risk for Ineffective Airway Clearance related to edema at surgical site

EXPECTED OUTCOME: The patient will maintain a clear airway as evidenced by unlabored respirations without stridor.

- Notify HCP about respiratory distress immediately; keep a tracheostomy set at the bedside. *Although uncommon, a tracheostomy may be needed in an emergency if edema obstructs the airway.*
- Maintain the patient in a semi-Fowler position *to help reduce edema at the surgical site and maximize respiratory effort.*
- Monitor neck dressing. *If the dressing seems to get tighter, it may be a sign that the patient's neck is swelling, which could impair the airway.*
- Use a room humidifier or humidified oxygen *to keep airways and secretions moist.*
- Remind the patient to do coughing and deep-breathing exercises every hour. *This keeps the airway clear of secretions.*
- Have suction equipment available *in case the patient cannot cough up secretions effectively.*
- Encourage the patient to use the incentive spirometer *to assist with deep breathing.*
- Check the patient's swallowing and gag reflexes before offering clear liquids *to guard against aspiration.*

Risk for Injury (tetany, thyrotoxic crisis) related to surgical procedure

EXPECTED OUTCOME: Complications will be recognized and treated quickly.

- Monitor the patient for muscle spasms or numbness or tingling around the mouth, and report immediately if they occur. *These are symptoms of tetany, which must be treated immediately. Tetany is most likely to occur 24 to 72 hours postoperatively.*
- Monitor vital signs often, and report changes immediately. *Elevated vital signs may be signs of thyrotoxic crisis, which is most likely to occur up to 18 hours postoperatively.*

Acute Pain related to surgical procedure

EXPECTED OUTCOME: The patient's pain will be controlled as evidenced by the patient stating that his or her pain rating is acceptable.

- Administer acetaminophen or opioids as ordered. Avoid aspirin products. *Aspirin binds to the same protein as thyroid hormone and can precipitate a thyrotoxic crisis. Aspirin can also cause bleeding.*
- Use pillows or sandbags to support the patient's head. *Unexpected movement may be painful.*

Ineffective Health Self-Management related to knowledge deficit

EXPECTED OUTCOME: The patient will be able to effectively manage self-care needs as evidenced by the patient verbalizing understanding of self-care including ROM exercises, diet, and importance of follow-up care.

- Teach the patient to do gentle range-of-motion exercises, avoiding hyperextension of the neck, which can cause strain on the incision line. *Avoidance of neck movement due to pain can result in contracture.*
- Consult dietitian to assist the patient with potential dietary changes needed following surgery. *With correction of metabolic alterations, dietary needs may be significantly altered.*
- Teach the patient the importance of follow-up care *to avoid complications:*
  - How to administer replacement hormone if ordered
  - How to change the dressing and to report bleeding or signs of infection at the site
  - Immediately reporting unusual irritability, fever, palpitations, or signs of tetany
  - Follow-up laboratory work for thyroid function and medication adjustment

EVALUATION. If the plan has been effective, complications caused by surgery will not occur or will be recognized and reported early. Pain will be prevented or controlled, and the patient will demonstrate understanding of postoperative self-care.

Complications of Thyroid Surgery

THYROTOXIC CRISIS. Thyrotoxic crisis can result from manipulation of the thyroid gland during surgery, with the subsequent release of large amounts of TH. This is a rare complication since the use of antithyroid drugs before surgery has become routine. For more information on thyrotoxic crisis, see the section on hyperthyroidism earlier in this chapter.

TETANY. Tetany is caused by low serum calcium and characterized by tingling in the fingers and perioral area (around the mouth), muscle spasms, twitching, and cardiac arrhythmias. Muscle spasms in the larynx can lead to respiratory obstruction.

Tetany can occur if the parathyroid glands are accidentally removed during thyroid surgery. Because of the proximity of the parathyroid glands to the thyroid, it is sometimes difficult for the surgeon to avoid them. In the absence of the parathyroid hormone (PTH), serum calcium levels drop and tetany results. IV calcium gluconate is given to treat acute tetany.

> **BE SAFE!**
> **AVOID FAILURE TO RESCUE!** You can prevent potential life-threatening tetany in a postoperative patient following thyroidectomy by monitoring for statements of tingling in hands and face, muscle spasms, twitching, and by noting irregular heart rhythm. Any evidence of tetany must be reported immediately to ensure proper medical treatment is begun to prevent the patient from developing life-threatening respiratory obstruction.

DISORDERS OF THE PARATHYROID GLANDS

Recall that the parathyroid glands secrete PTH in response to low serum calcium levels. PTH raises serum calcium levels by promoting calcium movement from bones to blood, increasing absorption of dietary calcium, and increasing resorption of calcium by the kidneys. Decreased PTH activity is called *hypoparathyroidism.* Increased PTH activity is called *hyperparathyroidism.*

Hypoparathyroidism

Pathophysiology

A decrease in PTH causes a decrease in bone resorption of calcium, calcium absorption by the gastrointestinal tract, and resorption in the kidneys. This means that calcium stays in the bones instead of moving into the blood, and more calcium is excreted from the body, causing decreased serum calcium level, or hypocalcemia. As calcium levels fall, phosphate levels rise.

Etiology

The most common causes of hypoparathyroidism are heredity and the accidental removal of the parathyroid glands during thyroidectomy or other neck surgeries. Hypoparathyroidism also occurs following purposeful removal of the parathyroid glands for hyperparathyroidism or cancer. Another cause is hypomagnesemia, which impairs secretion of PTH. Hypomagnesemia can occur with chronic alcoholism or certain nutritional problems.

Signs and Symptoms

Calcium plays an important role in nerve cell stability. Hypocalcemia causes neuromuscular irritability. In acute cases, tetany can occur, with numbness and tingling of the fingers, tongue, and lips; muscle spasms; and twitching (Table 39.5). Positive Chvostek and Trousseau signs are early indications of tetany. See Figures 6.4 and 6.5 in Chapter 6 for illustrations of these tests.

Chronic hypocalcemia can lead to lethargy; calcifications in the brain, leading to psychosis; cataracts; and convulsions. Bone changes may be evident on x-ray examination. Electrocardiogram (ECG) changes and heart failure can develop because of the importance of calcium to cardiac function. Death can result from laryngospasm if treatment is not effective.

Diagnostic Tests

Laboratory studies show decreased serum calcium and PTH levels and increased serum phosphorus. An ECG is done to evaluate cardiac function. Radiographs show bone changes.

Therapeutic Measures

Acute cases of hypoparathyroidism are treated with IV calcium gluconate. Long-term treatment includes a high-calcium diet (see Chapter 6, Table 6.3, for foods high in calcium), with oral calcium and vitamin D supplements. Magnesium is given if hypomagnesemia is present.

Table 39.5
Parathyroid Disorders Summary

	Insufficient Parathyroid Hormone	**Excess Parathyroid Hormone**
Disorder	Hypoparathyroidism	Hyperparathyroidism
Signs and Symptoms	Hypocalcemia, neuromuscular irritability, tetany, positive Chvostek and Trousseau signs	Hypercalcemia, fatigue, pathological fractures
Diagnostic Tests	Serum parathyroid hormone, calcium, and phosphate	Serum parathyroid hormone, calcium, and phosphate
Therapeutic Measures	Calcium and vitamin D replacement; high-calcium, low-phosphorus diet	Calcitonin, parathyroidectomy
Priority Nursing Diagnoses	*Risk for Injury* related to tetany	*Risk for Injury* related to bone demineralization

Nursing Process for the Patient With Hypoparathyroidism

DATA COLLECTION. The patient at risk for hypoparathyroidism should be closely monitored for symptoms of tetany. If you suspect tetany, check for Chvostek and Trousseau signs. Monitor respirations closely for stridor, a sign of laryngospasm.

NURSING DIAGNOSES, PLANNING, AND IMPLEMENTATION.

Risk for Injury (tetany) related to calcium imbalance

EXPECTED OUTCOME: The patient will remain free from injury. Signs of tetany will be recognized and treated quickly.

- Monitor the patient for signs of tetany, and report immediately to RN or HCP *so that treatment can begin quickly.*
- Make sure a tracheostomy set, endotracheal tube, and IV calcium are available *for emergency use if laryngospasm occurs.*
- Consult a dietitian for high-calcium diet teaching. *The patient may need a lifelong high-calcium diet.*
- Teach the patient about the importance of long-term diet, medication therapy, and follow-up laboratory testing. *The patient needs to understand self-care for follow-up at home.*

EVALUATION. Injury is prevented through careful management, and early recognition and reporting of signs and symptoms of tetany. The patient should be able to describe correct treatment and self-care measures for home.

Hyperparathyroidism
Pathophysiology
Overactivity of one or more of the parathyroid glands causes an increase in PTH, with a subsequent increase in the serum calcium level (hypercalcemia). This is achieved through movement of calcium out of the bones and into the blood, absorption in the small intestine, and reabsorption by the kidneys. PTH also promotes phosphorus excretion by the kidneys.

Etiology
Hyperparathyroidism is usually the result of hyperplasia or a benign tumor of the parathyroid glands. It may also be hereditary. Parathyroid cancer is rare. Secondary hyperparathyroidism occurs when the parathyroid glands secrete excessive PTH in response to low serum calcium levels. Serum calcium may be reduced in kidney disease because of the kidneys' failure to activate vitamin D. Vitamin D is necessary for absorption of calcium in the small intestine.

Signs and Symptoms
Signs and symptoms of hyperparathyroidism are caused primarily by the increase in the serum calcium level, although many patients are asymptomatic. Symptoms include fatigue, depression, confusion, increased urination, anorexia, nausea, vomiting, kidney stones, and cardiac arrhythmias. The increased serum calcium level also causes gastrin secretion, resulting in abdominal pain and peptic ulcers. Because calcium is removed from bones, bone and joint pain and pathological fractures can occur. Severe hypercalcemia can result in coma and cardiac arrest.

Diagnostic Tests
Laboratory studies include serum calcium, phosphorus, and PTH levels. Radiographs or bone density testing may show decreased bone density. A 24-hour urine test might be used to test how much calcium is being excreted in the urine. Nuclear scanning or ultrasound may be used to help locate the parathyroid glands if surgical removal is planned.

Therapeutic Measures
Mild hyperparathyroidism with asymptomatic hypercalcemia may be treated conservatively, with extra fluids to dilute calcium, monitoring for bone changes and decline in renal

function, and weight-bearing exercise to keep calcium in the bones. Oral calcium and vitamin D supplements may be prescribed, but calcium levels must be monitored closely. Estrogen therapy might be used in women, although side effects must be considered. Cinacalcet (Sensipar) is a newer drug that acts like calcium in the blood, fooling the parathyroid glands into reducing PTH secretion.

In acute hypercalcemia, IV normal saline is given to hydrate the patient. Furosemide (Lasix) is given to increase renal excretion of calcium. Cinacalcet (Sensipar) is a drug that mimics calcium circulating in the blood, and can be administered to reduce PTH release from the parathyroids. Biphosphonates (such as alendronate/Fosamax) or calcitonin (Fortical) may be given to prevent calcium release from bones. These drugs are covered in Chapter 46.

Surgery may be done to remove diseased parathyroid glands (parathyroidectomy). If possible, some parathyroid tissue is left intact to secrete PTH. Minimally invasive radio-guided parathyroidectomy can be done under local anesthesia through a small incision.

Preoperative and postoperative care is similar to that of the patient undergoing thyroid surgery, with special attention paid to calcium and PTH levels. The patient will likely be on calcium and vitamin D supplements following surgery.

Nursing Process for the Patient With Hyperparathyroidism

DATA COLLECTION. Collect data related to symptoms of hypercalcemia, including muscle weakness, lethargy, bone pain, anorexia, nausea, vomiting, behavioral changes, and renal insufficiency. Monitor serum calcium levels as ordered.

NURSING DIAGNOSES, PLANNING, AND IMPLEMENTATION. Nursing diagnoses depend on data collected. *Risk for Injury* usually takes priority.

> **Risk for Injury (fracture, complications of hypercalcemia) related to calcium imbalance**
>
> **EXPECTED OUTCOME:** The patient will remain free from injury.

- Monitor the patient for signs or symptoms of calcium imbalance and report promptly. *Prompt treatment can prevent serious complications.*
- Encourage oral fluids *to prevent dehydration and kidney stones and promote excrete calcium.*
- Encourage strengthening and weight-bearing exercises *to help keep calcium in the bones.*
- Provide a safe environment for ambulation; assist the patient with ambulation if needed. *A fall could result in fracture if bones are demineralized.*
- Encourage smoking cessation. *Smoking causes bone loss.*
- Teach the patient symptoms to report and use of long-term medications *so that the patient can manage self-care at home.*

EVALUATION. If the plan is effective, symptoms of hypercalcemia will be recognized and reported quickly, and complications and injury will be prevented.

DISORDERS OF THE ADRENAL GLANDS

Adrenal disorders can involve the adrenal medulla or the adrenal cortex. A rare tumor of the adrenal medulla, called a **pheochromocytoma**, causes hypersecretion of epinephrine and norepinephrine. Hyposecretion of epinephrine is rare and generally causes no symptoms. Hypersecretion of cortisol from the adrenal cortex results in Cushing syndrome. Hypofunction of the adrenal cortex results in Addison disease.

Pheochromocytoma

Pathophysiology

A pheochromocytoma is a rare tumor of the adrenal medulla that secretes excess catecholamines (epinephrine and norepinephrine). Most pheochromocytomas are benign.

Etiology

Most cases of pheochromocytoma have no known cause. About one-third of cases are hereditary.

Signs and Symptoms

Because norepinephrine is the fight-or-flight hormone, patients with a pheochromocytoma have exaggerated fight-or-flight symptoms. Manifestations include hypertension, tachycardia (with heart rate greater than 100 beats per minute), palpitations, tremor, diaphoresis, feeling of apprehension, and severe pounding headache. The most prominent characteristic is intermittent unstable hypertension. Diastolic pressure may be greater than 115 mm Hg. If hypertension and tachycardia are not controlled, the patient is at risk for stroke, heart attack and heart failure, vision changes, seizures, psychosis, and organ damage.

Diagnostic Tests

Patients with a suspected pheochromocytoma will have a 24-hour urine test for metanephrines and vanillylmandelic acid (VMA). These are end products of catecholamine metabolism. A blood test for metanephrines may also be done. If results are elevated, a CT scan, MRI, or nuclear scan is done to locate the tumor.

Therapeutic Measures

Treatment for pheochromocytoma is surgical removal of one or both adrenal glands. Calcium channel blockers, alpha blockers, and beta blockers are used to control symptoms. Teach the patient to avoid caffeine and other stimulants prior to surgery. Foods high in tyramine such as aged cheeses, beer, wine, and chocolate can also exacerbate symptoms and should be avoided.

After surgery, the patient is at risk for unstable blood pressure and hypoglycemia. Monitor vital signs and blood

• WORD • BUILDING •

pheochromocytoma: pheo—dark + chromo—color + cyt—cell + oma—tumor

glucose, and report variations from normal. If both adrenal glands have been entirely removed, the patient will require lifelong replacement hormones. (See section on adrenalectomy later in this chapter.)

Adrenocortical Insufficiency/Addison Disease

Adrenocortical insufficiency (AI) is the insufficient production of the hormones of the adrenal cortex. Primary AI is called Addison disease.

Pathophysiology

AI is associated with reduced levels of cortisol, aldosterone, or both hormones. A deficiency in androgens may also exist. In primary disease, adrenocorticotropic hormone (ACTH) levels from the pituitary gland can be elevated in an attempt to stimulate the adrenal cortex to synthesize more hormone. In secondary disease, deficient ACTH fails to stimulate adrenal steroid synthesis. In most cases, the adrenal glands are atrophied, small, and misshapen and are unable to produce adequate amounts of hormone.

Etiology

Addison disease is thought to be an autoimmune disease; that is, the gland destroys itself in response to conditions such as tuberculosis, fungal infection, infection related to AIDS, or metastatic cancer. It can also be associated with other autoimmune diseases. Bilateral adrenalectomy also results in AI.

Secondary AI may be caused by dysfunction of the pituitary gland or hypothalamus. In addition, prolonged use of corticosteroid drugs can depress ACTH and corticotropin-releasing hormone production, which in turn reduces steroid hormone production. A patient receiving long-term corticosteroid therapy is particularly at risk for AI if the drugs are abruptly discontinued. Because the pituitary gland has been suppressed for a prolonged period, it may take up to a year before ACTH is produced normally again.

> **NURSING CARE TIP**
> Long-term corticosteroid therapy should always be tapered slowly to avoid adrenal crisis.

Signs and Symptoms

The most significant sign of Addison disease is hypotension, which is related to the lack of aldosterone. Remember that aldosterone causes sodium and water retention in the kidney and potassium loss. If aldosterone is deficient, sodium and water are lost and hypotension and tachycardia result. Low cortisol levels cause hypoglycemia, weakness, fatigue, weight loss, confusion, and psychosis. In primary AI, increased ACTH may produce hyperpigmentation of the skin, causing the patient to have a tanned or bronze appearance. Anorexia, nausea, and vomiting may also occur, possibly as the result of electrolyte imbalances. Women may have decreased body hair because of low androgen levels. Patients may report craving salt.

Complications

If a patient with AI is exposed to stress, such as infection, trauma, or psychological pressure, the body may be unable to respond normally with secretion of additional cortisol (our natural stress hormone), and an adrenal crisis can occur. Loss of large amounts of sodium and water and the resulting fluid volume deficit cause profound hypotension, dehydration, and tachycardia. Potassium retention can cause cardiac arrhythmias. Hypoglycemia may be severe. Coma and death result if treatment is not initiated. Treatment of adrenal crisis involves rapidly restoring fluid volume and cortisol levels. IV fluids (containing glucose) and large doses of IV glucocorticoids are administered. Electrolytes are replaced as needed. The cause of the crisis should be identified and treated.

> **PRACTICE ANALYSIS TIP**
> Linking NCLEX-PN® to Practice
> The LPN/LVN will assist client to cope with/adapt to stressful events and changes in health status.

Diagnostic Tests

Serum and urine cortisol and blood glucose levels are all low. Blood urea nitrogen (BUN) and hematocrit levels may appear elevated because of dehydration. Antibodies may be present in the blood in autoimmune disease. An ACTH stimulation test helps determine whether adrenal glands are functioning. Serum sodium and potassium levels are monitored. CT scan or an MRI may be done to evaluate the size of the adrenal glands or to locate a pituitary tumor in secondary disease.

Therapeutic Measures

Long-term treatment consists of replacement of glucocorticoids (hydrocortisone) and mineralocorticoids (fludrocortisone [Florinef]). Some patients also receive androgen therapy. Patients will need hormone replacement therapy for the rest of their lives. Hormones are given in divided doses, with two-thirds of the daily dose given in the morning and one-third in the evening to mimic the body's own daily rhythm. Remember that steroid hormones are our natural stress hormones and so are naturally elevated during times of stress. Therefore, during times of stress or illness, doses need to be increased to two to three times normal. The patient may also be placed on a high-sodium diet. If the patient is ill and cannot tolerate oral medication, hormones must be injected.

Nursing Process for the Patient With Addison Disease

DATA COLLECTION. Determine the patient's understanding of Addison disease and adherence to the treatment regimen. Monitor vital signs and daily weights or I&O to track fluid status. Monitor serum glucose levels and symptoms of hyperkalemia and hyponatremia. Report changes in mental status. If the patient is in crisis, monitor vital signs closely and report any signs of fluid volume deficit such as orthostatic hypotension or poor skin turgor to the HCP immediately.

NURSING DIAGNOSES, PLANNING, AND IMPLEMENTATION

Risk for Deficient Fluid Volume related to deficient adrenal cortical hormones

EXPECTED OUTCOME: The patient's fluid volume will be stable as evidenced by stable weights and vital signs, and skin turgor within normal limits.

- Monitor vital signs, and report change promptly. *Hypotension and tachycardia indicate hypovolemia.*
- Monitor fluid status, and report changes promptly *to prevent complications of fluid deficit.*
- Administer steroid replacements as ordered *to maintain fluid and electrolyte balance.*

Ineffective Health Self-Management related to deficient knowledge about self-care of Addison disease

EXPECTED OUTCOME: The patient will verbalize understanding of self-monitoring and self-medication at home.

- Reinforce the importance of taking hormone replacements as ordered. Ensure that the patient has access to the medication. *The patient who does not secrete endogenous adrenocortical hormones must rely on replacements for survival. If patient has access and understands reason for therapy, there is a better chance for adherence.*
- Help the patient identify the causes and symptoms of stress and explain the need to increase medication dosage during times of stress or illness according to the HCP's instructions. *Because these hormones are normally increased during times of stress, it is important that the patient understand how to increase the dose during stress to prevent adrenal crisis.*
- Advise the patient that he or she may need to increase salt intake in hot weather *because of fluid and salt losses.*
- Advise medical alert identification. *A patient in adrenal crisis may not be able to provide a medical history to emergency personnel, and identification can prevent delay of treatment.*
- If ordered by the HCP, teach the patient and family members how to use an emergency intramuscular (IM) hydrocortisone injection kit. *IM medication may be needed during stress or times when the patient is unable to take oral medications.*

EVALUATION. If nursing care is effective, the patient's fluid status will be stable, and the patient and family will be able to carry out proper self-care of Addison disease.

Cushing Syndrome

Cushing syndrome is caused by exposure to excess cortisol. This can occur because of an adrenal or pituitary gland problem, or from treatment with exogenous corticosteroids. See Table 39.6 for a comparison of adrenal insufficiency and Cushing syndrome. When it is caused by a pituitary tumor, it is called *Cushing disease*, a subset of Cushing syndrome.

Pathophysiology

Recall that cortisol, aldosterone, and androgens are the three steroid hormones secreted by the adrenal cortex. Cortisol is essential for survival and is normally secreted in a diurnal rhythm, with levels increasing in the early morning. Secretion is increased during times of stress. In Cushing syndrome, cortisol is hypersecreted without regard to stress or time of day. When levels of cortisol are very high, effects related to excess aldosterone and androgens are also seen.

Table 39.6

Adrenal Cortex Hormone Summary

	Hypofunction	Hyperfunction
Disorder	Adrenocortical insufficiency, Addison disease	Cushing syndrome
Signs and Symptoms	Sodium and water loss, hypotension, hypoglycemia, fatigue	Weight gain, sodium and water retention, hyperglycemia, buffalo hump, moon face
Diagnostic Tests	Serum and urine cortisol	Serum and urine cortisol
Therapeutic Measures	Glucocorticoid and mineralocorticoid replacement	Alter steroid therapy dose or schedule, surgery if tumor
Priority Nursing Diagnoses	Risk for Deficient Fluid Volume	Risk for Excess Fluid Volume Risk for Unstable Blood Glucose Level Risk for Infection

LEARNING TIP
An easy way to remember the hormones of the adrenal cortex is to think *salt*, *sugar*, and *sex*. Aldosterone promotes salt retention, cortisol affects sugar (carbohydrate) metabolism, and androgens are sex hormones.

Etiology
Cushing syndrome can be caused by hypersecretion of ACTH by the pituitary gland. This is most often the result of a benign pituitary adenoma. Sometimes ACTH is produced by a tumor in the lungs or other organs. The high levels of ACTH cause adrenal hyperplasia, which in turn increases production and release of cortisol. A problem within the adrenal gland, such as an adrenal adenoma or carcinoma, can also produce excess cortisol.

The most common cause of Cushing syndrome is prolonged use of glucocorticoid medication (e.g., prednisone) for chronic inflammatory disorders such as rheumatoid arthritis, COPD, and Crohn disease. The use of smaller doses of glucocorticoids (in inhalers for asthma) or topical creams does not usually cause a problem.

Signs and Symptoms
Most signs and symptoms of Cushing syndrome are related to excess cortisol levels. Weight gain, central obesity with thin arms and legs, fat pads on the upper back (buffalo hump), and a round, moon-shaped face result from deposits of adipose tissue at these sites (Fig. 39.6).

Cortisol also causes insulin resistance and stimulates gluconeogenesis, which results in glucose intolerance. Some patients develop secondary diabetes mellitus (see Chapter 40). Muscle wasting and thin skin with purple striae occur as a result of cortisol's catabolic effect on tissues. The older patient may already have muscle atrophy and thinner skin due to normal aging, and Cushing syndrome may cause further deterioration. Catabolic effects on bone lead to osteoporosis, pathological fractures, and back pain from compression fractures of the vertebrae. This is especially concerning for the female patient who may already have age-related osteoporosis. Because cortisol has anti-inflammatory and immunosuppressive actions, the patient is at risk for infection. Hyperpigmentation of the skin may occur. About half of patients develop mental status changes, from irritability to psychosis (sometimes referred to as *steroid psychosis*). Sodium and water retention are related to the mineralocorticoid effect. As sodium is retained, potassium is lost in the urine, causing hypokalemia. (See Chapter 6 to review these electrolyte imbalances.) Androgen effects include acne, growth of facial hair, and **amenorrhea** (absence of menses) in women.

Diagnostic Tests
Suspicion of Cushing syndrome may initially be based on a cushingoid appearance and history of taking steroid medication. Plasma and urine cortisol and plasma ACTH are measured. A 24-hour urine test for cortisol may be collected. Levels of cortisol in the saliva may also be measured. A dexamethasone suppression test may be done. Serum potassium is measured. Additional tests to locate the cause of excess endogenous cortisol may be done.

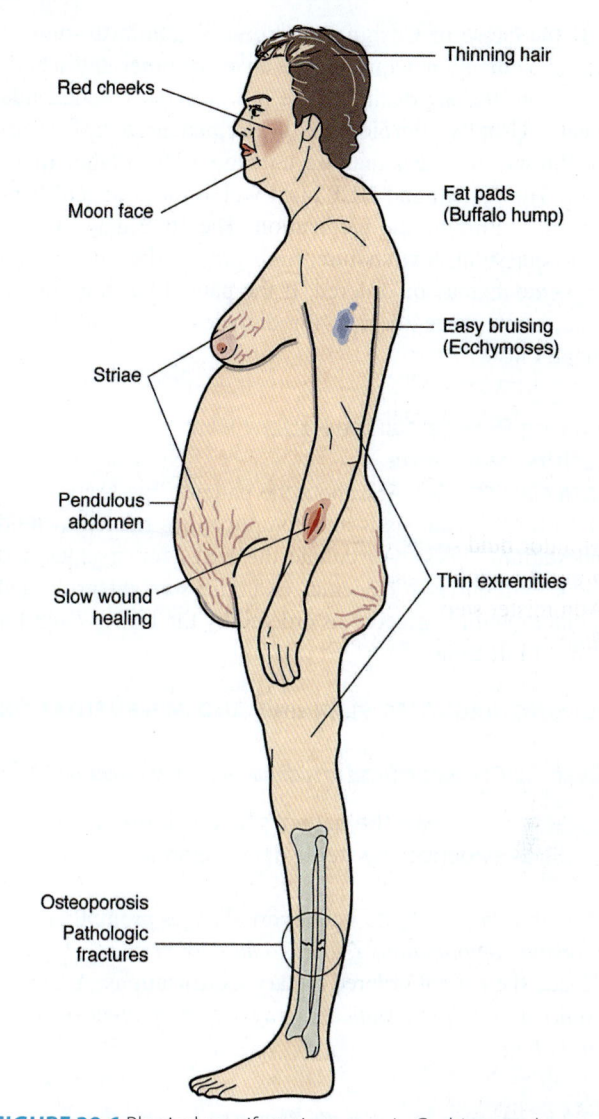

FIGURE 39.6 Physical manifestations seen in Cushing syndrome.

Therapeutic Measures
If a pituitary or ACTH-secreting tumor is present, surgical removal or radiation therapy to the pituitary gland may be employed. If the adrenal glands are the primary cause of the problem, radiation or removal of the adrenal gland or glands may be necessary. Drugs such as ketoconazole (usually used to treat fungal infection) can block production of adrenal steroids.

• WORD • BUILDING •
adenoma: aden—gland + oma—tumor
amenorrhea: a—not + men—month + orrhea—flow

If the cause of Cushing syndrome is administration of steroid medication, a lower dose, an every-other-day schedule, or once-a-day dosing in the morning may reduce side effects. Usually, steroids are prescribed as a last resort for chronic disorders that are unresponsive to other treatment. The patient and HCP must weigh the risks and benefits of continuing the medication. The HCP may order a high-potassium, low-sodium, high-protein diet. Potassium supplements may be ordered. If the patient has high blood sugar, appropriate therapy for diabetes is instituted (see Chapter 40).

Nursing Process for the Patient With Cushing Syndrome

DATA COLLECTION. Ask about the patient's medication history. Monitor vital signs and complications related to fluid and sodium excess. Auscultate the lungs for crackles and check extremities for edema. Examine skin integrity, and monitor capillary glucose as ordered by the HCP. Watch for signs of infection.

NURSING DIAGNOSES, PLANNING, AND IMPLEMENTATION

Excess Fluid Volume related to sodium and water retention

EXPECTED OUTCOME: The patient's fluid volume will be stable as evidenced by stable daily weights.

- Monitor daily weights, and report changes promptly *to prevent complications related to fluid excess.*
- Teach the patient ordered dietary modifications. *A low-sodium, high-potassium diet may help keep electrolytes in balance.*

Risk for Impaired Skin Integrity (thin, fragile skin) related to protein breakdown

EXPECTED OUTCOME: The patient's skin will remain intact.

- Observe skin and monitor for breakdown with every position change. *Early recognition and treatment of a problem can prevent further breakdown.*
- Assist the patient in changing positions at least every 2 hours *to prevent pressure injuries.*
- Use a lift sheet to move the patient in bed *to prevent friction and shear.*
- Avoid harsh soaps and hot water. *These can dry skin and increase risk for injury.*
- Use moisturizing cream *to keep skin from drying.*
- Secure IVs and dressings without tape if possible. *Tape removal can tear fragile skin.*
- Consider a specialty pressure-reducing mattress if the patient is very thin or unable to move frequently *to reduce the risk of pressure injury.*
- Consult a dietitian if nutritional status is poor. *Poor nutrition further increases risk for skin breakdown and poor healing.*

Risk for Infection related to immune suppression

EXPECTED OUTCOME: The patient will be free from infection as evidenced by a white blood cell count and temperature within normal limits.

- Monitor the patient for signs of infection and report promptly *so appropriate treatment can be ordered.*
- Use good hand hygiene before and after patient care. *Hand washing is important in reducing exposure to pathogens.*
- Instruct the patient in good hand washing and in the importance of avoiding others who are ill. *A patient with an impaired immune system is more likely to contract illness from others.*
- Consult a dietitian if nutritional status is poor. *Poor nutrition further impairs immune function.*
- Encourage flu and pneumonia vaccinations *to help prevent illness in event of exposure.*

Risk for Unstable Blood Glucose Level related to impaired glucose tolerance

EXPECTED OUTCOME: The patient's blood glucose level will remain within normal limits.

- If hyperglycemia occurs, be prepared to administer insulin *because oral hypoglycemics are not usually effective in Cushing syndrome.*
- Refer the patient and family to diabetes education classes *because diabetes is a complex disease that requires knowledge of self-care.*

See Chapter 40 for care of the patient with diabetes.

Disturbed Body Image related to cushingoid appearance

EXPECTED OUTCOME: The patient will express feelings of acceptance of self.

- Approach the patient with an attitude of acceptance and caring *to help develop a trusting nurse–patient relationship.*
- Provide an opportunity for the patient to verbalize feelings. *Expressing feelings may help reduce anxiety.*

EVALUATION. If care has been effective, complications of fluid overload will be recognized and treated early. The patient will have intact skin and be free from signs of infection. The patient will demonstrate skill in self-care of diabetes if indicated and will verbalize acceptance of self despite changes in appearance.

Nursing Care of the Patient Undergoing Adrenalectomy

Preoperative Care

Monitor the patient for electrolyte imbalance and hyperglycemia. Abnormalities must be corrected before surgery. To prevent adrenal crisis, glucocorticoids are administered because removal of the adrenals causes a sudden drop in adrenal hormones. Prepare the patient for adrenalectomy or hypophysectomy, depending on which surgery will be performed.

Postoperative Care

See "Nursing Care of the Patient Undergoing Hypophysectomy" earlier in this chapter. Following adrenalectomy, the patient receives routine postoperative care. The patient is closely monitored for changes in fluid and electrolyte balance and adrenal crisis. Patients who undergo bilateral adrenalectomy must take replacement glucocorticoid and mineralocorticoid hormones for the rest of their life. If only one adrenal gland is removed, the remaining gland should eventually produce enough hormone to enable the patient to discontinue replacement hormone.

See Table 39.7 for a summary of endocrine disorders and Table 39.8 for a summary of medications used for endocrine disorders.

Table 39.7
Summary of Endocrine Disorders

Hormone	Hypofunction	Hyperfunction
Antidiuretic hormone	Diabetes insipidus	Syndrome of inappropriate antidiuretic hormone
Growth hormone	Short stature	Acromegaly, gigantism
Thyroid hormone	Hypothyroidism	Hyperthyroidism
Epinephrine	Rare	Pheochromocytoma (hypertension)
Parathyroid hormone	Hypoparathyroidism	Hyperparathyroidism
Cortisol	Addison disease	Cushing syndrome

Table 39.8
Medications Used for Endocrine Disorders

Medication Class/Action

Medications for Antidiuretic Hormone (ADH) Disorders

Replace or block ADH.

Examples
desmopressin (DDAVP—inhaled, oral, IV, subcutaneous): Replaces ADH
demeclocycline (Declomycin—oral): Reduces ADH release

Nursing Implications
Check daily weights and urine specific gravity.
Do not give demeclocycline with dairy products or antacids.

Medications for Growth Hormone (GH) Disorders

Replace or block GH.

Examples
bromocriptine (Parlodel): Reduces GH release
octreotide (Sandostatin): Suppresses GH
pegvisomant (Somavert): Blocks the effect of GH on receptor sites
somatropin (Humatrope): Replaces GH

Nursing Implications
Monitor blood pressure, serum GH.
Teach patient self-administration.
Monitor growth.

Medications for Thyroid Disorders

Replace or block thyroid hormones.

Examples
levothyroxine (Synthroid): Replaces thyroxine (T_4)
propylthiouracil: Inhibits synthesis of thyroid hormones
methimazole (Tapazole): Inhibits synthesis of thyroid hormones

Nursing Implications
Monitor vital signs and thyroid laboratory results.
Monitor white blood cell count and differential, thyroid function, liver function.

Continued

Table 39.8 Medications Used for Endocrine Disorders—cont'd

Medication Class/Action

Medications for Adrenal Disorders

Replace adrenal hormones.

Examples
hydrocortisone: Replaces cortisol in adrenal insufficiency
fludrocortisone (Florinef): Replaces aldosterone in adrenal insufficiency

Nursing Implications
Teach patient to take with food and not to discontinue abruptly.
Monitor daily weights, vital signs, and serum potassium.

CLINICAL JUDGMENT

Judy Freberg is a 28-year-old female with Addison disease who is seen at the clinic where you work. Her symptoms are generally well controlled with medication but today she states that she has not been feeling well. She tearfully reports that her husband has filed for divorce and is demanding she move out of the marital home immediately.

1. Judy states she is feeling dizzy and her heart is skipping beats. What data should you collect?
2. With whom can you collaborate to help Judy through this stressful time in her life?
3. While you are checking Judy's vital signs, she becomes lightheaded, and her speech becomes slow and slurred. Her blood pressure is 86/40, and her heart rate is 116. How should you respond?
4. The HCP orders hydrocortisone 100 mg intramuscularly STAT and admission to the hospital. You report to the admitting nurse. Prepare an SBAR report.
5. The hydrocortisone is supplied as a vial with 250 mg powder, which you must dilute in 2 mL of saline. How much will you draw up for injection?
6. How can Judy prevent adrenal crises in the future?
7. What could have happened if Judy had not sought care at this time?

Suggested answers are at the end of the chapter.

Key Points

- The endocrine system is subject to a variety of disorders. The pathophysiology usually involves either too little or too much hormone activity. Insufficient hormone activity may be the result of hypofunction of an endocrine gland or insensitivity of the target tissue to its hormone. Excessive hormone activity may be the result of a hyperactive gland, ectopic hormone production, or self-administration of too much replacement hormone.
- ADH is synthesized in the hypothalamus and stored and secreted by the posterior pituitary gland. A decrease in ADH activity results in diabetes insipidus. An increase in ADH activity results in SIADH. Symptoms of too little ADH (water loss) are the opposite of symptoms of too much ADH (water retention).
- If ADH is lacking, adequate reabsorption of water is prevented, leading to diuresis. Patients can urinate from 3 to 15 L per day. This leads to dehydration and increased serum osmolality (concentrated blood). Increased osmolality also leads to extreme thirst, which usually causes the patient to drink enough fluids to maintain fluid balance. In an unconscious patient or a patient with a defective thirst mechanism, however, dehydration can quickly occur if the problem is not recognized and corrected.
- SIADH results from too much ADH in the body. This causes excess water to be reabsorbed by the kidney tubules and collecting ducts and back into the blood, leading to decreased urine output and fluid overload. As fluid builds up in the bloodstream, osmolality decreases, and the blood becomes diluted.
- An excess or deficiency of GH may be related to a more generalized problem with the pituitary gland or hypothalamus. A deficit of GH results in short stature, if not corrected in childhood, and a variety of problems in adulthood. Excess GH results in gigantism or acromegaly.
- Primary hypothyroidism occurs when the thyroid gland fails to produce enough TH even though enough TSH is being secreted by the pituitary gland. The pituitary gland responds to the low level of TH by producing more TSH. Because THs are responsible for metabolism, low levels of these hormones result in a slowed metabolic rate, which causes many of the characteristic symptoms of hypothyroidism.
- Hyperthyroidism results in excessive amounts of circulating TH (thyrotoxicosis). Primary hyperthyroidism occurs when a problem within the thyroid gland causes excess hormone release. A high level of TH increases the metabolic rate.

There is also an increase in the activity of epinephrine and norepinephrine. The resulting fight-or-flight response is the cause of many of the symptoms of hyperthyroidism.
- Thyrotoxic crisis (sometimes called *thyroid storm*) is a severe hyperthyroid state that can occur in hyperthyroid people who are untreated or who develop another illness or stressor. It also may occur after thyroid surgery in patients who have been inadequately prepared with antithyroid medication. Thyrotoxic crisis can result in death in as little as 2 hours if untreated.
- Enlargement of the thyroid gland is called a *goiter*. The thyroid gland may enlarge in response to increased TSH levels or sometimes in response to the autoimmune process that occurs in Graves disease.
- Decreased PTH activity is called *hypoparathyroidism*. A decrease in PTH causes a decrease in bone resorption of calcium, a decrease in calcium absorption by the gastrointestinal tract, and decreased resorption in the kidneys. The result is a decreased serum calcium level called *hypocalcemia*. As calcium levels fall, phosphate levels rise.
- Increased PTH activity is called **hyperparathyroidism.** Overactivity of one or more of the parathyroid glands causes an increase in PTH, with a subsequent increase in the serum calcium level (hypercalcemia).
- Adrenal disorders can involve the adrenal medulla or the adrenal cortex. A rare tumor of the adrenal medulla, called a *pheochromocytoma*, causes hypersecretion of epinephrine and norepinephrine. Hyposecretion of epinephrine is rare and generally causes no symptoms. Hypersecretion of cortisol from the adrenal cortex results in Cushing syndrome. Hypofunction of the adrenal cortex results in Addison disease.

SUGGESTED ANSWERS TO CHAPTER EXERCISES

Cue Recognition
39.1: These are signs of uncontrolled hypothyroidism. Verify that the patient has been taking the levothyroxine as ordered. Be careful to ask with a nonjudgmental tone, so the patient is truthful. Notify the HCP about your findings. The HCP will want to do thyroid laboratory testing and change the dose or make sure the patient is able to access the medication if they have not been taking it.
39.2: Report patient statements to HCP, as the patient may have treatment-related hyperthyroidism.
39.3: Elevate head of the bed, evaluate for respiratory distress, and notify HCP immediately.

Critical Thinking & Clinical Judgment
Mrs. Jackson
1. Possibly opioid use for postoperative pain and/or brain swelling from SIADH.
2. Remember that a pint is (about) a pound. A pint is 2 cups, or 480 mL:
3. $\dfrac{6 \text{ pounds}}{1 \text{ pound}} \times 480 \text{ mL} = 2{,}880 \text{ mL or almost 3 L}$
4. Anesthesia can cause SIADH, which leads to decreased urine output and fluid retention.
5. Fluid restriction will decrease amount of fluid in the circulating blood volume.
6. The RN and HCP should be notified of Mrs. Jackson's change of condition.

Three Siblings
The children's GH secretion was probably suppressed because of psychosocial stress. Once the children felt secure in a loving environment, GH levels returned to normal.

Mrs. Maino
1. Mrs. Maino's TSH levels are elevated because her pituitary gland is working overtime to try to stimulate the underactive thyroid gland.
2. Mrs. Maino's metabolism has been slow, so she has been burning fewer calories. When she starts on thyroid replacement hormone, her metabolic rate will return to normal, and she will need more calories. Intake of calories should be balanced with possible need for weight loss.
3. If Mrs. Maino receives too much TH, she will have symptoms of hyperthyroidism, including an increased pulse rate. She should know how to check her pulse and to call her HCP if it is elevated.
4. The nurse, HCP, and dietitian are essential. A physical therapist may be helpful if mobilization and exercise recommendations are needed. A social worker or discharge planner can help with discharge needs.

Judy Freberg
1. Vital signs: Temperature, heart rate and quality for a full minute, respirations and blood pressure.
2. Social services can arrange for a counselor to help Judy cope with her personal circumstances.
3. Make sure that she is safe—have her lie down, and call for the HCP immediately.
4. **S**—28-year-old female with history of Addison disease became dizzy with slurred speech during clinic visit. BP 85/40, heart rate 116. Being admitted immediately.
   B—She is usually well controlled on medication but has been having some personal stressors that may have precipitated this crisis.
   A—She is at risk for deficient fluid volume, hyponatremia, hyperkalemia, and hypoglycemia.
   R—The priority is monitoring her fluid and electrolyte status. Please consult with social services to help her manage her stress. She will need education on how to adjust her medication during stress or illness.
5. $100 \text{ mg} \times \dfrac{2 \text{ mL}}{250 \text{ mg}} = 0.8 \text{ mL}$

SUGGESTED ANSWERS TO CHAPTER EXERCISES—cont'd

6. Judy needs instruction on why and how to increase her doses of hydrocortisone and fludrocortisone when she is ill or stressed.

7. Fluid volume deficit, hyponatremia, hyperkalemia, and hypoglycemia, which can lead to coma and death.

Additional Resources

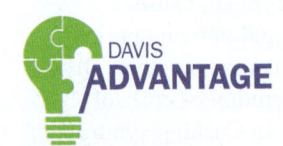

Go to Davis Advantage to complete your learning: strengthen understanding, apply your knowledge, and prepare for the Next Gen NCLEX®.

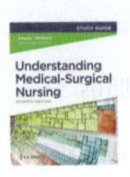

A Study Guide is also available.

CHAPTER 40
Nursing Care of Patients With Disorders of the Endocrine Pancreas

Paula D. Hopper

KEY TERMS

diabetes mellitus (DYE-ah-BEE-tis mel-EYE-tus)
endogenous (en-DAH-jen-us)
gastroparesis (GAS-troh-puh-REE-sus)
glycosuria (GLY-kos-YOO-ree-ah)
hyperglycemia (HY-per-gly-SEE-mee-ah)
hypoglycemia (HY-poh-gly-SEE-mee-ah)
ketoacidosis (KEE-toh-as-ih-DOH-sis)
Kussmaul respirations (KOOS-mahl RES-per-AY-shuns)
nephropathy (neh-FRAH-puh-thee)
neuropathy (new-RAH-puh-thee)
nocturia (nok-TYOO-ree-ah)
polydipsia (PAH-lee-DIP-see-ah)
polyphagia (PAH-lee-FAY-jee-ah)
polyuria (PAH-lee-YOO-ree-ah)
postprandial (POHST-PRAN-dee-uhl)
preprandial (PREE-PRAN-dee-uhl)
retinopathy (RET-ih-NAH-puh-thee)

CHAPTER CONCEPTS

Acid–base balance
Cellular regulation
Collaboration
Fluid and electrolyte balance
Health promotion
Nutrition
Self-care

LEARNING OUTCOMES

1. Explain the pathophysiologies of type 1 and type 2 diabetes mellitus.
2. Identify risk factors for type 1 and type 2 diabetes mellitus.
3. Describe the signs and symptoms of diabetes mellitus.
4. Describe causes, signs and symptoms, and treatment of high and low blood glucose levels.
5. Discuss how diabetes mellitus increases risk of complications such as heart disease, blindness, and kidney failure.
6. Identify diagnostic tests to diagnose and monitor diabetes mellitus and its complications.
7. Identify therapeutic measures to help control blood glucose levels with diabetes mellitus.
8. Differentiate the action of insulin and oral hypoglycemic agents in lowering blood glucose.
9. Plan nursing care and education for the patient with diabetes mellitus.
10. List measures to increase safety of the patient with diabetes mellitus undergoing surgery.
11. Explain reactive hypoglycemia and its treatment.

DIABETES MELLITUS

Diabetes mellitus is a group of metabolic diseases in which defects in insulin secretion or action result in elevated blood (or plasma) glucose (**hyperglycemia**). Be careful not to confuse diabetes mellitus with diabetes insipidus, which is a disorder of antidiuretic hormone (see Chapter 39). In this chapter, *diabetes* or *DM* refers to diabetes mellitus. According to the most recent Centers for Disease Control and Prevention (CDC) data, 34.3 million people in the United States have DM, representing 13% of U.S. adults. Another 34% of U.S. adults have prediabetes. Direct and indirect costs of diabetes for the nation total $327 billion per year (CDC, 2020).

• WORD • BUILDING •
diabetes mellitus: diabetes—passing through + mellitus—sweet
hyperglycemia: hyper—excessive + glyc—glucose + emia—in the blood

Diabetes is a serious disease that can cause complications such as blindness, kidney failure, heart attack, stroke, and cognitive decline. It is a leading cause of lower limb amputations in the United States. With education and self-care, patients with diabetes can prevent or delay complications and lead full, productive lives. Nurses play a major role in helping patients learn effective self-care.

Pathophysiology and Etiology

Body tissues, and the cells that compose them, use glucose for energy. Glucose is a simple sugar provided by the foods we eat. When carbohydrates are eaten, they are digested into sugars, including glucose, which is absorbed into the bloodstream and delivered to cells. Carbohydrates provide most of the energy used by the body. Glucose can enter the cells only with the help of insulin, a hormone produced by the beta cells in the islets of Langerhans of the pancreas (Fig. 40.1). When insulin encounters the cell membrane, it combines with a receptor that allows activation of special glucose transporters in the membrane. By helping glucose enter the body's cells, insulin (1) allows glucose to be used for energy, (2) lowers the glucose level in the blood, and (3) helps the body store excess glucose in the liver and muscles in the form of glycogen.

Another hormone, glucagon, is produced by the alpha cells in the islets of Langerhans. Glucagon raises the blood glucose (BG) when needed by releasing stored glucose from the liver and muscles. Insulin and glucagon work together to keep the BG at a constant level.

Diabetes results from deficient production of insulin by the beta cells in the pancreas, from resistance of the body's cells to insulin, or both. When glucose is unable to enter body cells, it stays in the bloodstream; hyperglycemia results, and the cells are denied their energy source. Abnormal glucagon secretion also plays a role in type 2 diabetes (see Fig. 40.1).

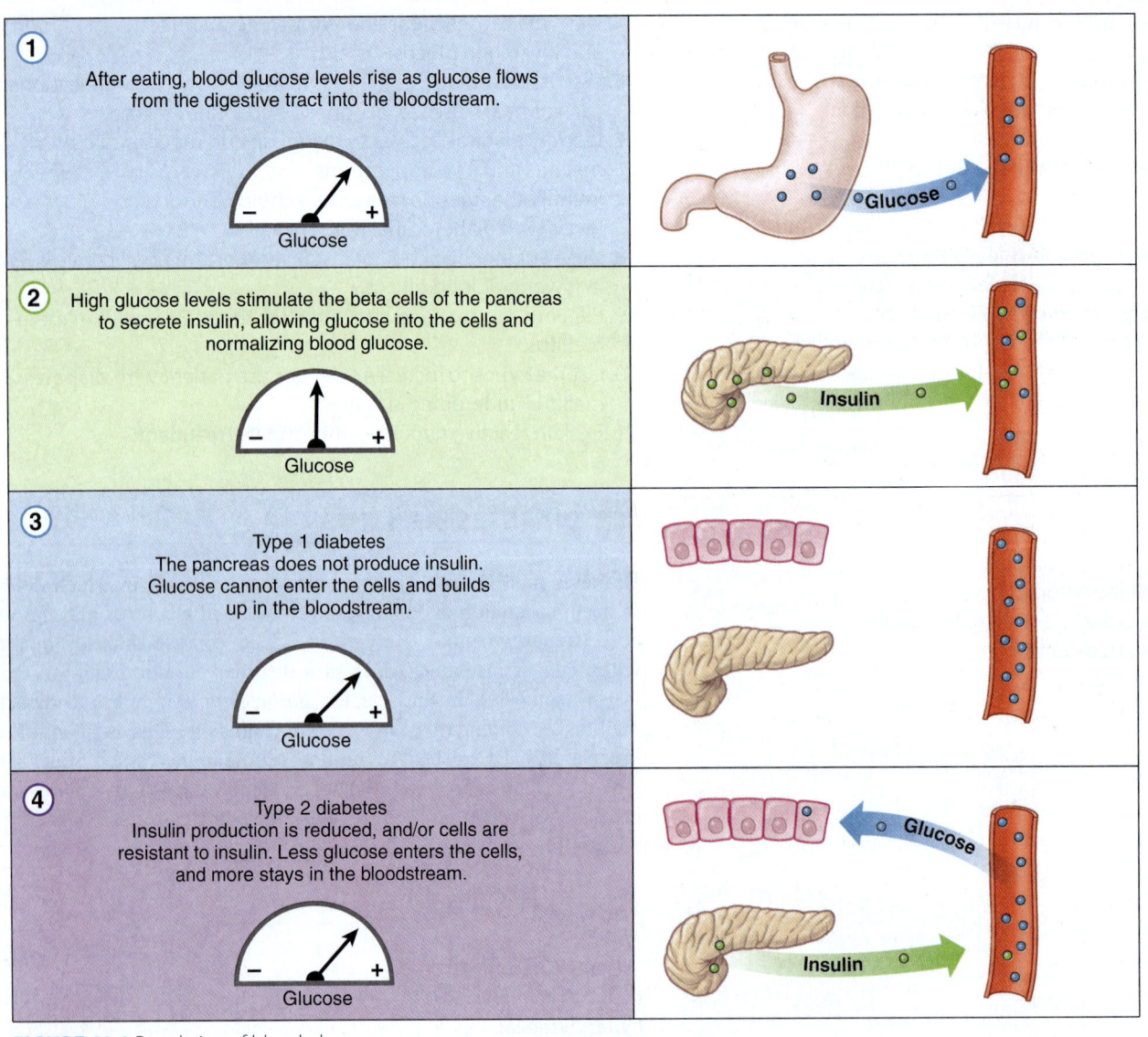

FIGURE 40.1 Regulation of blood glucose.

Types of Diabetes

Type 1 Diabetes

Type 1 diabetes (formerly called *juvenile diabetes* or *insulin-dependent diabetes mellitus* [IDDM]) is caused by destruction of the beta cells in the islets of Langerhans of the pancreas. It is usually diagnosed in childhood, but onset can also occur in adults. When the beta cells are destroyed, they are unable to produce insulin. Insulin must then be injected for the body to use food for energy. Only about 5% of people with diabetes have type 1 diabetes.

It is believed that the pancreas may attack itself following certain viral infections or administration of certain drugs. This is called an *autoimmune response*. Up to 90% of patients newly diagnosed with type 1 diabetes have islet cell antibodies in their blood. These antibodies might be present for years before actual symptoms of diabetes develop. Some people with type 1 diabetes cases have a genetic predisposition to its development. The patient diagnosed with type 1 diabetes is most often young, thin, and prone to develop ketoacidosis (discussed later) when BG is elevated. Table 40.1 provides a comparison of type 1 and type 2 diabetes.

Type 2 Diabetes

Ninety-five percent of people with diabetes in the United States have type 2 diabetes (formerly called *adult-onset diabetes* or *non-insulin-dependent diabetes mellitus* [NIDDM]). In type 2 diabetes, tissues are resistant to insulin. Early in disease development, insulin levels rise in an attempt to normalize blood glucose. As the disease progresses, insulin production diminishes. Oral medication can help boost insulin production or decrease tissue resistance. The pancreas eventually wears out, leading to little or no insulin secretion. When this occurs, the patient with type 2 diabetes will require insulin injections. The need for insulin does not mean the patient has type 1 diabetes. He or she has type 2 diabetes and needs insulin to control the BG level.

Heredity is a factor in most cases of type 2 diabetes. Obesity is a major contributing factor. Often, the patient with a new diagnosis of type 2 diabetes is obese, relates a family history of diabetes, and has had a recent life stressor, such as the death of a family member, illness, or loss of a job (see "Patient Perspective: Jim").

Patient Perspective

Jim

I am a 70-year-old White man of European descent. I was diagnosed with type 2 diabetes 5 years ago, and it was a complete shock. At the time, I considered myself moderately overweight, moderately active, and in reasonably good general health. My physician assistant took the time to explain how he reached the diagnosis (my hemoglobin A1c [HbA_{1c}] was 11.7, and my fasting blood glucose [BG] was 221) and what we could do together to address it. Having him take the time to have this discussion gave me reassurance that I would not face this new reality alone.

He gave me a booklet detailing the carb content of common foods and instructed me to limit my total carb intake to about 6 to 8 units a day. He prescribed 1,000 mg of metformin daily, with 2.5 mg of lisinopril for kidney protection and 20 mg of atorvastatin as a precaution against future heart disease.

I followed his dietary recommendations religiously. I lost 40 pounds and 6 inches off my waist over the following 6 months! At the end of 18 months, I had reduced my HbA_{1c} to 5.4 and my average fasting BG to about 85. Now, 5 years later, my weight has leveled off at about 140 pounds, my HbA_{1c} is 5.0, and I am no longer taking any diabetes medication! The physician assistant keeps me on the lisinopril and atorvastatin as a precaution against future diabetes-related complications.

Table 40.1

Comparison of Type 1 and Type 2 Diabetes

	Type 1	Type 2
Onset	Rapid	Slow
Age at onset	Usually younger than 40	Usually older than 40
Risk factors	Virus, autoimmune response, heredity	Heredity, obesity
Usual body type	Lean	Overweight or obese
High blood glucose complication	Ketoacidosis	Hyperosmolar hyperglycemic state; may develop ketoacidosis later in disease
Treatment	Diet, exercise; must have insulin to survive	Diet, exercise; may need oral hypoglycemic agents or insulin to control blood glucose level

> I would never say that this kind of control has been easy. I struggle to keep a disciplined approach to my eating and to intentionally find ways to stay active. But whenever I feel deprived or start to get lazy, I think of the consequences of uncontrolled diabetes. I don't want to face them, ever.

> **SELF-CARE TIP**
> Drink more water! Type 2 diabetes has been linked to drinking sweetened drinks. Research has also linked type 2 diabetes with consumption of diet drinks sweetened with artificial sweeteners. Water, unsweetened teas, and sparkling waters are healthier choices.

Increasing numbers of children and adolescents are developing type 2 diabetes. In the past, type 2 diabetes occurred almost exclusively in adults. This is related to increasing obesity and decreasing activity levels in children today. Earlier onset of diabetes increases the risk of early complications and death.

Gestational Diabetes

Gestational diabetes mellitus (GDM) occurs in up to 1 in 10 pregnancies, especially in women with risk factors for type 2 diabetes. The extra metabolic demands of pregnancy trigger the onset of diabetes. BG usually returns to normal after delivery, but the mother has a higher risk of developing type 2 diabetes. If the mother with GDM is overweight, she should be counseled that weight loss and exercise will decrease her risk of developing diabetes. Mothers with GDM require specialized care and should be referred to an expert in this area.

Prediabetes

Prediabetes refers to BG levels that are above normal but do not meet the criteria for diagnosing diabetes. Prediabetes occurs before the onset of type 2 diabetes. It is diagnosed by evaluating fasting BG level, oral glucose tolerance test (see "Diagnostic Tests" section), or hemoglobin A1c (HgA_{1c}). It is important to identify patients with prediabetes, because with lifestyle changes progression to type 2 diabetes can be prevented.

Other Types of Diabetes

Secondary diabetes can develop as a result of another chronic illness that damages the islet cells, such as pancreatitis or cystic fibrosis. Prolonged use of some drugs, such as steroid hormones, phenytoin (Dilantin), thiazide diuretics, and thyroid hormone, can also impair insulin action and raise BG. Less common causes include pancreatic trauma and other endocrine disorders.

Metabolic Syndrome

Prediabetes has been linked to a condition called *metabolic syndrome*. According to the American Heart Association (2021), metabolic syndrome affects about 23% of adults. It is diagnosed when at least three of the following criteria are met:

1. Abdominal obesity (measured by waist circumference): men—greater than 40 inches; women—greater than 35 inches
2. Fasting blood triglycerides 150 mg/dL or higher
3. Blood high-density lipoprotein (HDL) cholesterol: men—less than 40 mg/dL; women—less than 50 mg/dL
4. Blood pressure 130/85 mm Hg or higher
5. Fasting glucose 100 mg/dL or higher

Other risk factors include physical inactivity, aging, hormonal imbalances, and genetic predisposition. A major factor is the growing obesity epidemic in the United States.

Any patient who fits this profile should be monitored closely for the onset of type 2 diabetes and heart disease. Patients should be counseled on the importance of a heart-healthy diet, weight loss, physical activity, and control of glucose, blood pressure, and cholesterol levels.

Signs and Symptoms

Classic symptoms of diabetes (all types) include **polydipsia** (excessive thirst), **polyuria** (excessive urination), and **polyphagia** (excessive hunger). Extra glucose in the blood increases serum concentration, or osmolality. The renal tubules cannot reabsorb all the extra glucose filtered by the glomeruli, and **glycosuria** results. Large amounts of body water are required to excrete this glucose, causing polyuria, **nocturia** (nighttime urination), and dehydration. Increased osmolality and dehydration cause polydipsia. Because glucose cannot enter the cells, they starve, causing polyphagia. High BG can also cause fatigue, blurred vision, abdominal pain, and headaches. Ketones (acidic by-products of fat breakdown) can build up in the blood and urine of patients with type 1 diabetes or late in the course of type 2 diabetes (**ketoacidosis**).

> **LEARNING TIP**
> Remember the three classic symptoms of diabetes with the *Three Ps:* **p**olydipsia, **p**olyuria, and **p**olyphagia.

• WORD • BUILDING •

polydipsia: poly—many or much + dipsia—thirst
polyuria: poly—many or much + uria—urine
polyphagia: poly—many or much + phagia—to eat
glycosuria: glyc—glucose + uria—urine
nocturia: noc—by night + uria—urine
ketoacidosis: keto—ketones + acid—acidic + osis—condition

Diagnostic Tests

Fasting Blood Glucose Level
Diagnosis of diabetes is based on BG levels measured by a laboratory. Normal fasting BG level is less than 100 mg/dL. When fasting BG (drawn after at least 8 hours without eating) is 126 mg/dL or higher, diabetes is diagnosed. A second test may be required if the first test is not clearly diagnostic. If the fasting BG is between 100 and 125 mg/dL, the patient has impaired fasting glucose (IFG) and prediabetes (Fig. 40.2).

Random Blood Glucose
Sometimes, it is not feasible to check fasting BG. Random BG (RPG) is checked without regard to the last meal. Diabetes is diagnosed if the RPG is 200 mg/dL or greater, with symptoms of diabetes.

Oral Glucose Tolerance Test
Another test to diagnose diabetes is the oral glucose tolerance test (OGTT). An OGTT measures BG at intervals after the patient drinks a concentrated solution containing the equivalent to 75 grams of glucose. Diabetes is diagnosed when the BG level is 200 mg/dL or higher after 2 hours. A result between 140 and 199 mg/dL at 2 hours indicates a diagnosis of impaired glucose tolerance (IGT) and prediabetes (see Fig. 40.2).

Glycohemoglobin
The glycohemoglobin test, referred to in this chapter as the *glycosylated hemoglobin*, or HbA_{1c}, is used to diagnose diabetes and monitor diabetes control. Glucose in the blood attaches to hemoglobin in the red blood cells, which live about 3 months. When this attached glucose is measured, it reflects average BG level for the previous 2 to 3 months. This is helpful when BG levels fluctuate and a single measurement would be misleading. It also assists in monitoring the effectiveness of a patient's treatment plan. A normal HbA_{1c} is less than 5.7%. An HbA_{1c} of 6.5% or higher is diagnostic for diabetes. An HbA_{1c} between 5.7% and 6.5% indicates prediabetes. Once diagnosed, most patients are advised to keep their HbA_{1c} below 7% (see Fig. 40.2).

Newer methods allow this test to be done in a healthcare provider's (HCP's) office while the patient waits. See Table 40.2 for average fasting BG levels based on HbA_{1c} results.

Glycohemoglobin testing might be inaccurate in some people, such as those with anemia. These patients may instead be tested for fructosamine, a similar test that indicates glucose levels over a period of 1 to 2 weeks instead of 3 months.

Healthy People 2030 has a goal to "reduce the proportion of adults with diabetes who have an A1c value above 9%" (Office of Disease Prevention and Health Promotion, 2020). In the years 2013 through 2016, 18.7% of adults over age 18 had an A1c value above 9%. The Healthy People goal is to reduce this number to 11.6% by 2030.

Estimated Average Glucose
Some HCPs use a calculation to convert HbA_{1c} results to estimated average glucose (eAG) numbers, which may be more meaningful to patients. The formula is as follows:

$$28.7 \times HbA_{1c} - 46.7 = eAG$$

Here is an example for a patient whose HbA_{1c} is 8.6:

$$28.7 \times 8.6 - 46.7 = 200.12$$

This result can be rounded to 200 mg/dL.

Additional Tests
Because diabetes affects so many body systems, additional tests recommended for baseline data include a lipid profile, serum creatinine and urine microalbumin levels to monitor kidney function, urinalysis, and electrocardiogram.

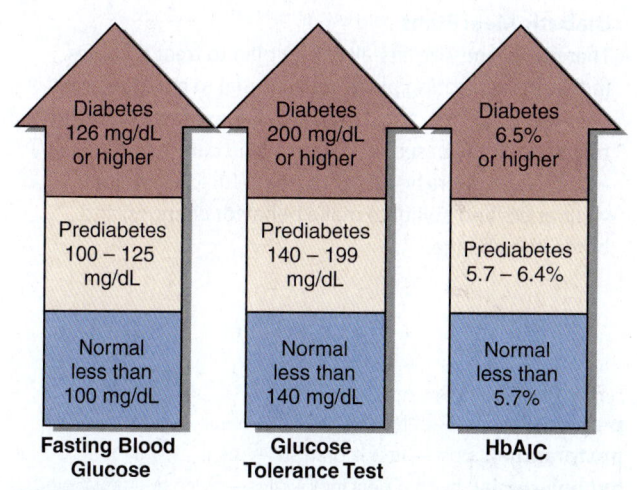

FIGURE 40.2 Tests used to determine whether a patient has normal blood glucose levels, high-risk prediabetes, or diabetes include fasting blood glucose, oral glucose tolerance, and hemoglobin A1c.

Table 40.2
Correlation Between HbA_{1c} and Mean Fasting Blood Glucose

HbA_{1c} (%)	Fasting Blood Glucose (mg/dL)
6	126
7	154
8	183
9	212
10	240
11	269
12	298

CRITICAL THINKING & CLINICAL JUDGMENT

Mr. McMillan is a 50-year-old patient brought into the emergency department with extreme fatigue and dehydration. After the HCP sees him, you ask Mr. McMillan some additional questions. Based on his answers, you request that the HCP add a random glucose level to the laboratory tests ordered. The result is 1,400 mg/dL.

Critical Thinking (The Why)
1. What questions would you ask Mr. McMillan if you suspected diabetes?
2. Why was Mr. McMillan fatigued?
3. Why was he dehydrated?

Clinical Judgment (The Do)
4. Mr. McMillan refuses to be admitted to the hospital because he has no insurance. What can you do? What concerns do you have?
5. What complications should you warn Mr. McMillan about if he does not follow his treatment plan?

Suggested answers are at the end of the chapter.

Prevention

It is possible to prevent type 2 diabetes. Research shows that patients who have prediabetes can prevent or delay the onset of diabetes with loss of 7% of body weight and moderate physical activity for at least 150 minutes per week (American Diabetes Association [ADA], 2021). Use of the diabetes medication metformin can also help prevent diabetes in patients with prediabetes. Patients at risk should have their BG level checked regularly. Research studies are ongoing to try to find ways to prevent type 1 diabetes once antibodies have been detected.

Therapeutic Measures

The only cure for diabetes is a pancreas or islet cell transplant, but these are risky procedures and are not always effective. However, diabetes can be controlled. Treatment begins with diet and exercise. Insulin is added for patients with type 1 diabetes, and for those with type 2 diabetes, insulin or oral or injectable hypoglycemic medication is added as needed. Weight loss is essential for patients who have type 2 diabetes and are overweight or obese. BG monitoring and education are also important for good diabetes control. To monitor the effectiveness of treatment, patients should have regular health-care follow-up visits.

Goals of Treatment

The ADA (2021) suggests the following goals and recommendations for most non-pregnant adults to prevent or delay complications of diabetes:

- HbA$_{1c}$ (every 3 to 6 months): Less than 7%
- HbA$_{1c}$: Less than 8% for patients with a history of severe hypoglycemia, complications, or short life expectancy
- **Preprandial** capillary glucose: 80 to 130 mg/dL
- Peak **postprandial** capillary glucose: Less than 180 mg/dL

Target levels for blood glucose are different in hospitalized patients. Because of the risk for cardiovascular disease, the ADA also recommends maintaining blood pressure of less than 130/80 mm Hg, if it can be done safely. All goals should be adjusted to individual circumstances. For example, the patient who is unable to feel symptoms of **hypoglycemia** (low BG) might have a higher preprandial glucose goal to prevent undetected hypoglycemic episodes.

> **PRACTICE ANALYSIS TIP**
> Linking NCLEX-PN® to Practice
> The LPN/LVN performs blood glucose monitoring.

Nutrition Therapy

Because the patient with diabetes has a limited amount of insulin, either **endogenous** (from within the body) or injected, it is important to eat foods that will not exceed the insulin's ability to carry it into the cells. Because carbohydrates contribute most to the BG level, the amount of carbohydrate consumed is especially important. If a patient eats a small amount of carbohydrate one day and a large amount the next, BG will fluctuate, leading to complications. It is possible to create a more flexible nutrition plan if the patient can test BG frequently at home and adjust treatment accordingly.

The ADA recommends a complete assessment by a specially trained dietitian and an individualized nutrition therapy plan and teaching (see "Nutrition Notes"). The education of the patient with diabetes is an ongoing process that may take months and cannot be accomplished in a single visit or with a paper handout or referral to a Web site.

> **Nutrition Notes**
> **Diabetic Meal Plans**
> There is no one-size-fits-all eating plan to treat diabetes. Individualized eating plans are essential to manage glucose levels, weight, and cardiovascular risk factors. Eating plans should be based on personal and cultural preferences, health literacy, access to healthful food choices, willingness and ability to make behavior changes, and barriers to change.

• WORD • BUILDING •

preprandial: pre—before + prandial—meal
postprandial: post—after + prandial—meal
hypoglycemia: hypo—deficient + glyc—glucose + emia—in the blood
endogenous: endo—within + genous—to produce

Overall goals and strategies differ by type of diabetes. In general:
- Patients with type 1 diabetes need to prevent wide swings in BG levels through careful timing of meals and snacks in relation to insulin therapy and activity.
- Patients with type 2 diabetes use diet modifications with medication as needed to maintain near-normal glucose, blood pressure, and lipid levels and to lose weight as needed.

A registered dietitian creates a meal plan based on the patient's abilities, past dietary habits, and commitment. Several meal-planning approaches are described next.

Create Your Plate
The University of Idaho's method of meal planning divides a plate into three parts: one half and two quarters. Half the plate is filled with nonstarchy vegetables. One quarter is filled with starchy foods. The last quarter is used for proteins. A serving of fruit and an 8-ounce glass of low-fat milk complete the meal (Fig. 40.3). Examples of foods suitable for each section of the plate are provided at https://www.extension.uidaho.edu/diabetesplate/planning/index.html.

Carbohydrate Counting
Carbohydrates have the greatest influence on BG levels. The total grams of carbohydrates directly affects diabetes control. Only carbohydrates are counted with this system, but patients are counseled to choose the same amount of protein each day and to choose low-fat foods. Reading labels is mandatory (e.g., fat-free products are higher in carbohydrates than the items they replace). Patients are taught to read food labels (a carbohydrate choice is 15 grams of carbohydrate) and prescribed a number of carbohydrates choices for each meal and snack.

Carbohydrate choices include starch, fruit, milk, or sweets (Table 40.3). This method offers more flexibility in food choices than do other approaches.

Carbohydrate counting may entail the following:
- Weighing and measuring food
- Keeping food records
- Monitoring BG before and after eating
- Controlling body weight

Patients should maintain their carbohydrate intake at the same level each day to keep BG as close to normal as possible.

Glycemic Index/Glycemic Load
All carbohydrates are not metabolized equally. Foods containing equal amounts of carbohydrate affect BG levels differently. The glycemic *index* (GI) is a value assigned to foods according to the speed and degree of change they produce in BG levels. The standard is set with glucose having a value of 100; other foods are then compared with glucose. For example, corn flakes have a GI of 81, and cooked carrots have a GI of 39. A GI less than 55 is low, 56 to 69 is moderate, and 70 to 100 is high. When determining how portion size affects the GI of a food, a glycemic *load* (GL) is calculated by multiplying GI times the carbohydrate per serving divided by 100. A 1-cup serving of corn flakes has 24 g of carbohydrate, and a 1-cup serving of boiled cooked carrots has 5 g of carbohydrates; therefore, the GL of corn flakes is 19.44 and of cooked carrots is 1.9. A GL of less than 10 is considered low, 11 to 19 is medium, and 20 or greater is high. Carrots are appropriate for individuals following a low GI/GL diet. Motivated patients can incorporate low GI/GL foods into the successful management of their disease.

References: Evert, A. B., Dennison, M., Gardner, C. D., Garvey, W. T., Lau, K. K., MacLeod, J., Mitri, J., Pereira, R. F., Rawlings, K., Robinson, S., Saslow, L., Uelmen, S., Urbanski, P. B., & Yancy Jr., W. S. (2019). Nutrition therapy for adults with diabetes or prediabetes: A consensus report. *Diabetes Care, 42*(5), 731–754.
Gray, A., & Threlkeld, R. J. (2019). Nutritional recommendations for individuals with diabetes. In Feingold, K. R., et al., eds., *Endotext [Internet]*. South Dartmouth, MA: MDText.com. https://www.ncbi.nlm.nih.gov/books/NBK279012.
Harvard Health Publishing. (2020, January 6). *Glycemic index for 60+ foods*. https://www.health.harvard.edu/diseases-and-conditions/glycemic-index-and-glycemic-load-for-100-foods.
University of California–San Francisco. (2020). *Counting carbohydrates*. https://dtc.ucsf.edu/living-with-diabetes/diet-and-nutrition/understanding-carbohydrates/counting-carbohydrates.
University of Idaho. (2019). *What's on your plate?* Retrieved from https://www.extension.uidaho.edu/diabetesplate/index.html.

Weight Loss
Weight loss can help the patient with type 2 diabetes control BG, blood pressure, and blood lipid levels. Weight loss can even help prevent the need for medication in some patients. In obese patients who have difficulty losing weight with usual measures, metabolic (weight loss or bariatric) surgery may be considered. There are several metabolic surgeries that may be effective; see Chapter 33 for more information.

Exercise
Exercise lowers BG by reducing insulin resistance and improving insulin action in the muscles and liver. The effects

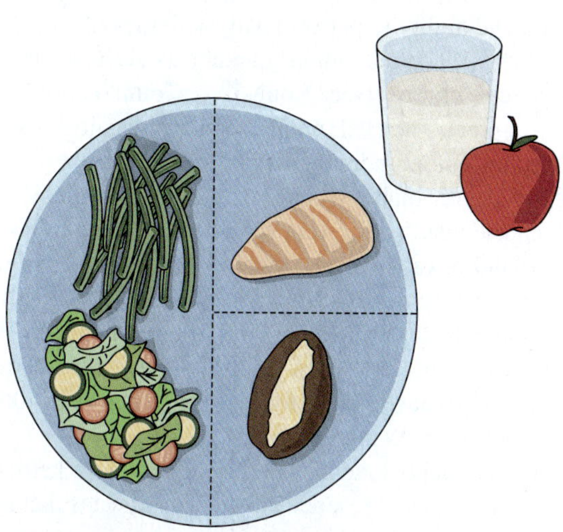

FIGURE 40.3 An example of the diabetes plate method.

Table 40.3 Example of Carbohydrate Counting

Prescribed Carbohydrate Choices (1,200 to 1,500 kilocalories/day)	Carbohydrate Selected*
Breakfast	
3	¾ cup dry cereal 8 oz skim milk ½ cup unsweetened orange juice
Lunch	
3	8 oz regular cola 1 cup melon 1 slice whole-wheat bread
Dinner	
3	½ cup cooked potato ½ cup corn ½ cup regular ice cream
Snack	
1	8 oz skim milk

*Additional proteins and fats are added in moderate amounts but need not be counted. Each item selected is approximately 15 grams carbohydrate or 1 carb exchange.

can last up to 48 hours. Exercise also improves blood lipid levels and circulation, important because diabetes increases risk of cardiovascular disease. Patients are instructed to engage in moderate aerobic exercise at least 150 minutes per week, at least 3 days in a week. In addition, it is important to avoid a sedentary lifestyle and to interrupt prolonged sitting with light activity at least every 30 minutes. Resistance exercise two to three times weekly also improves glycemic control, strength, and ability to perform daily activities (ADA, 2021).

Patients with complications of diabetes must be careful in their exercise choices (see "Long-Term Complications" later in this chapter). The HCP or an exercise physiologist should be consulted for an individualized exercise plan.

Persons with diabetes who take insulin or medications that increase insulin secretion should check their BG before exercise and always carry a quick source of glucose when exercising in case the BG drops too low. They should also be cautious about exercising at the time of day when their BG is at its lowest point (i.e., when insulin or medication action is peaking) and to have a carbohydrate snack before exercising if BG is less than 90 mg/dL.

Caution patients to avoid exercise if they have ketones in their blood or urine. Presence of ketones indicates that insufficient insulin is available and glycogen may be released during exercise, further increasing the serum glucose.

Medication

INSULIN. The person with type 1 diabetes has no endogenous insulin and thus must inject insulin daily. At this time, insulin cannot be taken by mouth because it is a protein and gets digested. A form of oral insulin is being tested. Inhaled insulin is available but is not widely used. Insulin is typically given subcutaneously; fast-acting insulin may be ordered via the intramuscular or IV route in urgent situations. Several types of insulin are available with various onsets and durations of action. The type and administration schedule are determined by the HCP in collaboration with the patient based on the patient's lifestyle and willingness to spend time on monitoring and injections. In general, more frequent injections lead to better glucose control.

Site Rotation. Insulin injections should be given in a different subcutaneous site with each dose to avoid tissue injury. A sample rotation chart is shown in Figure 40.4. Because each area absorbs insulin at a slightly different rate, it is advisable to use one area for a week, then move on to the next area. Within that area, each injection should be spaced at least 2 inches from the previous injection. Some experts recommend using primarily the abdomen for more uniform absorption. Aspirating for blood before injection and rubbing the site after injection are not recommended with insulin.

Insulin Pumps. Patients who desire tighter control of BG levels and a more flexible lifestyle may use an electronic insulin pump (Fig. 40.5). A pump delivers short- or rapid-acting insulin via a tiny catheter continuously in small (basal) amounts. The catheter is placed in subcutaneous tissue and remains for 2 to 3 days. The patient can program a bolus of insulin for before meals or snacks. This provides insulin

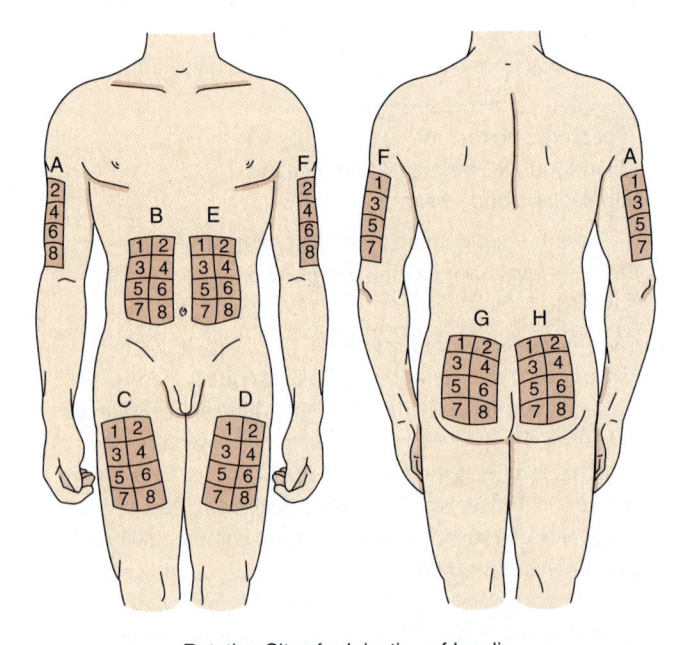

Rotation Sites for Injection of Insulin

FIGURE 40.4 Sample insulin rotation chart.

> **Cultural Considerations**
>
> Blacks, Latinx and Hispanic individuals, American Indians, Pacific Islanders, and some Asian Americans have a higher risk for type 2 diabetes than White individuals (CDC, 2020). The "standard" diabetic diet may need significant adjustment to include foods from various cultures. A typical food exchange list may prove unhelpful because it may not include foods common in a patient's culture. In such cases, the patient may be considered nonadherent to therapy when, in reality, the HCP has not considered cultural food preferences. Helping the patient choose a meal plan that considers their culture is important. Resources include www.diabetes.org and www.eatright.org.

levels that are more like those of a person without diabetes. A pump is worn on the abdomen or buttocks. Some models receive input from continuous glucose monitors or can even connect with a smartphone.

Insulin Sources. Insulin is synthetically produced in a laboratory. It is either identical to human insulin or different by one or two amino acids (called *insulin analogs*). In the past, insulin was derived from cows and pigs; this type of insulin is no longer available in the United States but may be available from other countries. Be careful to check the source when preparing insulin for injection, especially if you work in home health-care situations in which patients could purchase their insulin online from another country. Insulins from different sources may act slightly differently. Some people may be allergic to beef or pork preparations or refuse them based on cultural beliefs.

Onset, Peak, and Duration. Once insulin is injected, a period elapses before it begins to lower BG. This time is called the *onset of action*. The *peak action* occurs when the insulin is working its hardest and BG is at its lowest point. During this peak time, the patient is most at risk for an episode of low BG. *Duration of action* is the length of time the insulin works before it is used up. Onset, peak, and duration are determined by whether insulin is short, intermediate, or long acting (Table 40.4). It is important for the individual with diabetes and the nurse to be aware of the onset, peak, and duration of any insulin given. This informs decisions about certain situations, such as when to give insulin in relation to meals, when to exercise, and when to be alert to low BG symptoms.

Insulin Regimens. Patients work with their HCPs to determine the best regimen to meet their needs and fit their lifestyles. Some patients are only willing to take one or two injections a day. More patients are now choosing to take more frequent injections to achieve better, tighter control of BG. These patients are often taught to adjust their insulin dose based on BG level and the amount of carbohydrate eaten. Although patients who choose tight control must be more cautious about risk for hypoglycemia, it can significantly reduce the risk of long-term complications.

A common regimen called *basal-bolus therapy* mimics normal insulin secretion. It consists of an injection of a basal insulin (such as insulin glargine [Lantus]) once a day, often at bedtime, to provide a constant small amount of insulin in the bloodstream. Then an injection of very short-acting insulin (such as insulin lispro [Humalog]) is given before meals to mimic the extra insulin that is secreted normally with meals.

Sliding-Scale Insulin. Some patients receive varying doses of short-acting insulin before meals based on BG reading. An example of a sliding scale might read as follows: "BG less than 140, 0 units; BG 141–170, 2 units; BG 171–200, 4 units; greater than 200, call HCP." A scale is useful when the patient is ill and glucose levels are unstable or when adjustments need to be made. However, routine use of sliding-scale insulin is not recommended because, although it corrects an already-high BG, it is preferable to prevent hyperglycemia before it happens with routine insulin doses. A better approach is to take short-acting insulin before each meal based on its carbohydrate content.

Mixing Insulins. When two insulins need to be given at the same time, they can often be mixed to prevent multiple injections. Preset mixtures of intermediate- and short-acting insulins are also available. Some insulins cannot be mixed, so always know your insulins!

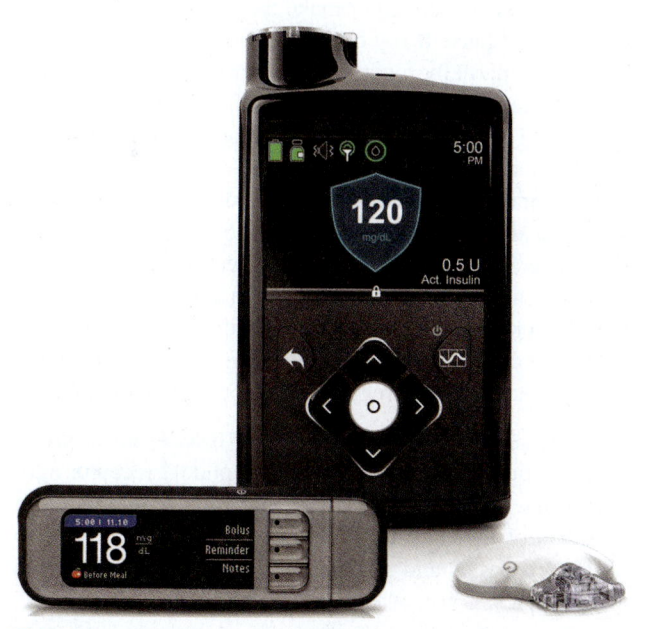

FIGURE 40.5 Insulin pump. (Courtesy of Medtronic MiniMed, Inc.)

> **NURSING CARE TIP**
>
> Inform your patients that unopened insulin vials should be stored between 36°F and 46°F (2°C and 8°C). Insulin should not be placed in a freezer. The vial currently in use can be stored at room temperature, avoiding sunny windows and steamy bathrooms.

Table 40.4
Onset, Peak, and Duration of Insulins

Insulin Type	Example	Onset	Peak	Duration	When to Give
Very short acting	Insulin lispro (Humalog) Insulin aspart (NovoLog) Insulin glulisine (Apidra)	15 min	1–2 hr	2–4 hr	Not more than 15 minutes before meal
	Inhaled insulin (Afrezza)	12–15 min	30 min	3 hr	
Short acting	Insulin regular (Humulin R, Novolin R)	30 min	2–3 hr	3–6 hr	Not more than 30 minutes before meal
Intermediate acting	Insulin neutral protamine Hagedorn (NPH) (Humulin N, Novolin N)	2–4 hr	4–12 hr	12–18 hr	Not more than 30 minutes before meal
Long acting basal	Insulin glargine (Lantus AE) Insulin detemir (Levemir)	1–2 hr	No peak	Up to 24 hr	The same time each day

Adapted from American Diabetes Association. *Insulin Basics*. https://www.diabetes.org/healthy-living/medication-treatments/insulin-other-injectables/insulin-basics. Accessed January 11, 2022.
Note: All times are approximate. Different brands may vary slightly.
A variety of premixed formulas are also available.

CLINICAL JUDGMENT

Mrs. Evans is a 78-year-old woman with type 2 diabetes who resides in the long-term care facility at which you work. She is on 42 units of insulin glargine (Lantus) every evening and 10 units of insulin lispro (Humalog) before each meal.

1. What time should you administer her Lantus insulin? If she eats her meals at 0800, 1200, and 1700, when should her Humalog insulin be administered? (*Hint:* See Table 40.4.)
2. At what times of day should you remind her to be alert for symptoms of low blood glucose?
3. What should you do if Mrs. Evans feels ill and misses her lunch?
4. Mrs. Evans receives an apple with her meal but cannot eat it because her dentures do not fit well. She is on a carbohydrate-counting meal plan. What should you do?

Suggested answers are at the end of the chapter.

ORAL HYPOGLYCEMIC MEDICATION. The patient with type 2 diabetes may be able to control BG with nutrition therapy and exercise alone. If needed, oral hypoglycemic medication or insulin will be prescribed. Oral hypoglycemic agents are not insulin pills but work to produce more insulin (e.g., by stimulating the pancreas) or make the tissues more sensitive to insulin. Because many oral hypoglycemic agents depend on at least a partially functioning pancreas, they are not useful for patients with type 1 diabetes. Table 40.5 lists commonly used oral hypoglycemic agents and their mechanisms of action.

Most oral hypoglycemic agents should be administered before meals. Care should be taken to prevent passage of more than 30 minutes between medication administration and the meal because this may result in a hypoglycemic episode. Check individual drugs for specific timing. If the BG level is not controlled with an oral hypoglycemic agent, insulin may be added to the regimen, with or without oral agents.

INJECTABLE HYPOGLYCEMIC MEDICATION. A newer group of medications is the glucagon-like peptide-1 receptor agonists. These are injectable drugs that were first isolated in the saliva of the Gila monster, a poisonous lizard native to the United States and Mexico. See Table 40.5 for actions and examples.

Table 40.5
Medications for Type 2 Diabetes Mellitus

Medication Class/Action

Alpha-Glucosidase Inhibitors (AGIs)—Oral

Lower postprandial glucose by reducing rate of carbohydrate digestion and absorption.

Examples	Nursing Implications
acarbose (Precose) miglitol (Glyset)	Give at start of each meal. No weight gain or hypoglycemia risk. Multiple dosing is less convenient. If used in combination with another drug and hypoglycemia occurs, treat with milk or glucose tablets, not table sugar.

DPP-4 Inhibitor—Oral

Inhibits DPP-4, an enzyme that breaks incretins. Incretins are hormones secreted by the gastrointestinal system in response to food; they reduce glucagon secretion and increase insulin synthesis and release.

Examples	Nursing Implications
sitagliptin (Januvia) saxagliptin (Onglyza) linagliptin (Tradjenta)	Administer once a day. Only works when blood glucose is high, so does not cause hypoglycemia when used alone. Watch for allergic reactions.

Biguanide—Oral

Decreases glucose production by liver; increases glucose uptake by muscle.

Examples	Nursing Implications
metformin (Glucophage, Glucophage XR, Fortamet, Riomet, Glumetza)	Give with meals. May enhance weight loss. Withhold if patient is having tests involving contrast dye. Contraindicated in renal and hepatic disease and heart failure. Monitor serum creatinine level. Notify health-care provider of early symptoms of lactic acidosis (e.g., hyperventilation, myalgia, malaise).

Sulfonylureas—Oral

Stimulate insulin secretion by pancreas and increase insulin receptor sensitivity.

Examples	Nursing Implications
glipizide (Glucotrol) glimepiride (Amaryl) glyburide (Micronase, Diabeta, Glynase Prestab)	Monitor patient for hypoglycemia. Teach patient to avoid alcohol.

Glucagon-like peptide-1 receptor agonists—Injected

Mimic natural incretins in the body to (1) stimulate insulin release and (2) reduce glucagon release in response to nutrients in the intestine.

Examples	Nursing Implications
exenatide (Byetta, Bydureon) liraglutide (Victoza) dulaglutide (Trulicity) semaglutide (Ozempic)	Administered as a subcutaneous injection. Check individual agent information or Web sites for instructions on use of pens and auto-injectors. May promote weight loss. Slows gastric emptying, so may alter absorption of oral medications.

Continued

Table 40.5
Medications for Type 2 Diabetes Mellitus—cont'd

Medication Class/Action

Sodium-Glucose Cotransporter-2 (SGLT2) Inhibitors—Oral

Reduce reabsorption of glucose by kidneys, increasing glucose excretion in urine.

Examples	Nursing Implications
canagliflozin (Invokana) empagliflozin (Jardiance) dapagliflozin (Farxiga)	Monitor for hypotension, hyperkalemia, urinary tract infection, and vaginal yeast infection. Monitor renal function.

Multiple combination agents are available. See individual medications.

Another injectable drug, pramlintide (Symlin), may be used with insulin. It is a synthetic analog of amylin, a naturally occurring hormone that reduces glucose levels following meals. It may also promote weight loss in individuals who are overweight. Patients using Symlin have an increased risk of hypoglycemia.

NATURAL REMEDIES. Many herbs and other natural remedies have been promoted for diabetes treatment. Some patients have tried cinnamon for blood sugar control, but no scientific evidence exists of efficacy. If your patient wishes to try a natural remedy, it is essential to encourage a conversation with their HCP first.

Self-Monitoring of Blood Glucose

Home blood glucose testing is an important part of diabetes management for all patients with type 1 diabetes and for many with type 2. A variety of BG monitors are on the market at reasonable prices (Fig. 40.6). Most of the cost involved in monitoring is in the test strips that must be used. Health insurance programs may cover this cost.

Self-monitoring of blood glucose (SMBG) schedules are based on specific patient needs and abilities. A patient taking multiple daily injections of insulin will usually test before meals and snacks, occasionally postprandially, at bedtime, before exercise, when experiencing low BG and following treatment for low BG, and before critical activities such as driving (ADA, 2021). Less-frequent schedules may be prescribed for patients who are unable or unwilling to test so often or for patients with type 2 diabetes who take oral hypoglycemic agents.

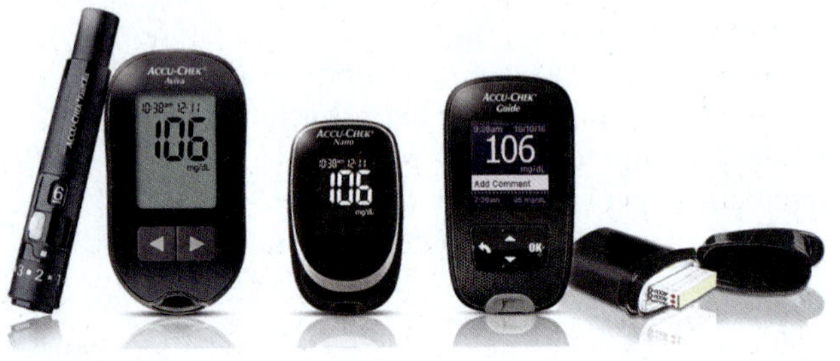

Another option is continuously monitoring glucose in interstitial fluid via a small catheter inserted under the skin. The device records the glucose level at frequent intervals on a monitor or smartphone. It can be set to alarm if the BG is out of range.

The diabetes provider should be consulted for desirable BG ranges because these may differ for each patient. The ADA (2021) recommends a preprandial goal of 80 to 130 mg/dL for most patients. Patients who are prone to hypoglycemia or small children or older adults may have higher goal ranges, such as 100 to 150 mg/dL. Lower BG levels for these populations could increase the risk of hypoglycemia.

An important aspect of SMBG is interpretation of results. Monitoring is useless if the results are not used to improve BG control. The patient should be instructed to keep a diary of BG levels (Fig. 40.7). Some patients have computer software that graphs results. The patient may be taught by a diabetes educator to interpret the trends in the results, or the diary may be taken on a regular basis to the HCP for interpretation and adjustment of the treatment plan.

Urine Glucose and Ketone Monitoring

Urine also may be tested for glucose and for ketones. Urine glucose testing was done routinely before the development of SMBG. A variety of dipsticks and tape products are available for urine testing. Glucose in the urine makes the patient aware that the BG is elevated, but the actual level is unknown. Most people have glucose in their urine when their BG is more than about 180 mg/dL, although this is highly variable. It is difficult to base treatment on urine glucose levels, so routine urine testing for glucose is no longer recommended.

Urine should be tested for ketones (ketonuria) during acute illness or stress, when BG levels are elevated in ketosis-prone patients, or when symptoms of ketoacidosis are present (see later in this chapter). If ketones are present, the patient knows an insulin deficiency is present and should notify HCP. Patients with type 1 diabetes are most at risk for developing ketoacidosis; however, it is wise for the patient

FIGURE 40.6 Glucose meters.

Day		Breakfast	Lunch	Supper	Bedtime	Urine Ketones	Notes
Sunday	Time	7:00	11:30	6:00	11:00		
	Glucose	186	108	116	142		
	Insulin	10 units Humalog	10 units Humalog	10 units Humalog	32 units Lantus		
Monday	Time	7:30	12:00	6:00	10:30	6:00-neg	Ate cake at Betty's party at 3 pm-oops!
	Glucose	171	97	302	180		
	Insulin	10 units Humalog	10 units Humalog	10 units Humalog	32 units Lantus		
Tuesday	Time						
	Glucose						
	Insulin						

FIGURE 40.7 Sample diary of blood glucose results and insulin use.

with type 2 diabetes to test for ketones if risk factors are present. Table 40.6 provides a review of diabetes symptoms, diagnosis, and treatment.

Transplant

If the patient is evaluated to be an appropriate candidate, a pancreas transplant may be considered. This is especially beneficial in the patient with kidney disease, who can receive both a kidney and pancreas transplant at the same time. Another promising treatment is the implantation of pancreatic islet cells.

Table 40.6
Diabetes Summary

Signs and Symptoms	Polyuria Polydipsia Polyphagia Fatigue Blurred vision Headache
Diagnostic Tests	Fasting blood glucose (BG) HbA_{1c} (glycosylated hemoglobin) Oral glucose tolerance test (OGTT) Additional testing for complications
Therapeutic Measures	Nutrition therapy Exercise Insulin Oral hypoglycemic medication Self-monitoring of BG levels Education
Complications	Hypoglycemia, hyperglycemia Diabetic ketoacidosis, hyperosmolar hyperglycemia Long-term complications
Priority Nursing Diagnosis	*Risk for Unstable Blood Glucose Level*

Acute Complications of Diabetes

A person with diabetes is at risk for a variety of complications. Acute complications related to high and low BG levels are treatable and can be prevented with appropriate care.

Hyperglycemia

When calories eaten exceed insulin available or glucose used, high BG (hyperglycemia) occurs. A common cause of hyperglycemia is eating more than the meal plan prescribes. Another major cause is stress. Stress causes the release of counterregulatory hormones, including epinephrine, cortisol, growth hormone, and glucagon. These hormones all increase the BG level. In a person without diabetes, this is an adaptive function. However, the patient with diabetes is unable to compensate for the increased BG with increased insulin secretion, and hyperglycemia results.

Patients must be able to recognize signs and symptoms of high BG levels and know what to do if they occur (Table 40.7). For many patients, these may be similar to the symptoms they experienced when they were first diagnosed with diabetes. Chronic high BG levels can lead to long-term complications (discussed later in this chapter).

MORNING HYPERGLYCEMIA. Sometimes, patients experience elevated morning BG levels even though they have not eaten all night. *Dawn phenomenon* is caused by normal hormone fluctuation during the night as well as release of stored glucose, leading to morning hyperglycemia. The *Somogyi effect* occurs when BG drops too low during the night due to a missed snack or too much insulin. The body responds by releasing counterregulatory hormones (epinephrine, glucagon, corticosteroids, growth hormone), which then cause rebound hyperglycemia in the morning.

The patient might be asked to monitor BG between 0200 and 0400 for a few days in addition to bedtime and morning testing to assess for the Somogyi effect or the dawn phenomenon. The patient and HCP will work together to adjust meal and insulin timing and stabilize BG.

Hypoglycemia

Low BG, or hypoglycemia, occurs when there is not enough glucose available in relation to circulating insulin. This is sometimes referred to as an *insulin reaction*. Common causes

Table 40.7
Comparison of High and Low Blood Glucose Levels

	Hyperglycemia	*Hypoglycemia*
Causes	Overeating Stress Illness Too little insulin or medication	Undereating, skipping a meal Too much insulin or medication Exercise Alcohol
Symptoms	Polyuria Polydipsia Polyphagia Blurred vision Headache Lethargy Abdominal pain Ketonuria Coma	Hunger Sweating Tremor Blurred vision Headache Irritability Confusion Seizures Coma
Treatment	Confirm hyperglycemia with glucose meter; if patient is at risk, check urine for ketones and increase fluid intake. Determine cause of hyperglycemia and teach prevention. Return to prescribed treatment plan if applicable. Call health-care provider (HCP) for medication adjustment if indicated or if blood glucose exceeds 180 mg/dL for 2 days. Call HCP if patient is ill or vomiting.	Confirm hypoglycemia with glucose meter (if able). Administer 15 g fast-acting carbohydrate. Recheck glucose in 15 minutes. If still low, readminister carbohydrate. Continue cycle of checking glucose and administering fast sugar until hypoglycemia subsides. If symptoms worsen, call HCP or emergency help. Administer glucagon or dextrose 50% via intravenous route if ordered. Determine cause of hypoglycemia and teach prevention.

of hypoglycemia are skipping a meal, exercising more than usual, or accidentally administering too much insulin. An occasional hypoglycemic episode, treated promptly, should not lead to chronic complications. Repeated or extremely low BG levels can cause neurologic damage because there is not enough glucose for brain function. It is, therefore, important to teach patients and families how to recognize, prevent, and treat low BG (see Table 40.7).

Occasionally, symptoms occur because of a rapid drop in BG, although actual glucose is normal or high. Initial symptoms of hypoglycemia are caused by activation of the sympathetic nervous system and may include hunger, sweating, pallor, tremor, palpitations, and headache. As hypoglycemia progresses, the brain is deprived of glucose (called *neuroglycopenia*). Neurologic symptoms, such as irritability, confusion, seizures, and coma, may occur.

The ADA (2021) recognizes three levels of hypoglycemia:

- Level 1 hypoglycemia is defined as a BG level less than 70 mg/dL, although patients may feel symptoms at higher or lower levels. It should be treated immediately.
- Level 2 hypoglycemia is defined as BG less than 54 mg/dL, which may be accompanied by neurologic symptoms such as agitation or confusion.
- Level 3 hypoglycemia is defined as "a severe event characterized by altered mental and/or physical status requiring assistance for treatment of hypoglycemia" (ADA, 2021, S80) (see "Patient Perspective: Dave").

Patient Perspective

Dave

Right after eating lunch, I headed for the woods on a cloudy mid-March afternoon. I began sawing firewood, splitting it, and loading up the trailer. I did not take insulin with lunch like I normally would because the extra activity increases the risk of hypoglycemia. I've had type 1 diabetes for nearly 60 years, so I have a lot of experience with hypoglycemia. After a short time of working, I began to sense that feeling. For me, it is an interruption of clear thinking. I immediately stopped work, went to my stash of hard candies and shoved 10 pieces into my mouth, and began to head home. My house is only a very short distance from the woods. I started up the tractor and headed home. As I pulled down the trail to the main road, the tractor quit. I spent maybe 2 minutes attempting to start it, then, with a sense of apprehension, I decided to walk the short distance to the house. Six hours later, I awakened in the emergency department. I had decided after walking only 40 yards to lie down in my neighbor's yard and take a nap. I obviously do not remember any of this. The neighbor had arrived home and saw a body in her yard and called for help. My body temperature was so low that the emergency department staff was not sure if I would make it. I still feel blessed and thankful to God that I survived this experience and have learned valuable lessons. I never cut wood alone anymore. I began using a continuous glucose monitor and an insulin pump that has a threshold suspend feature that stops the flow of insulin in the event of hypoglycemia.

BE SAFE!
AVOID FAILURE TO RECOGNIZE! You can prevent hypoglycemia in patients with awareness of who is at risk and when they are most at risk, as well as monitoring for early symptoms. If you recognize symptoms such as shaking or hunger and respond quickly, you can prevent more serious complications for your patient.

CRITICAL THINKING
Jeff is a 16-year-old with type 1 diabetes who is having trouble with repeated episodes of hypoglycemia. He says he has not had this problem before, and it is interfering with his new job. What questions might you ask as you collect data to help him figure out how to prevent future episodes?

Suggested answers are at the end of the chapter.

To treat hypoglycemia, administer a "fast sugar" (15 to 20 grams of carbohydrate that will enter the bloodstream quickly). Examples of fast sugars include the following:

- 4 oz orange juice
- 4 oz regular (not diet) soda
- 8 oz low-fat milk
- Miniature box of raisins
- Commercial glucose tablets or gel
- Six to eight hard candies

If the patient is not alert or is unable to safely swallow (level 2 or 3 hypoglycemia), subcutaneous glucagon can be given. A newer form is glucagon nasal powder (Baqsimi). If the patient is hospitalized, IV 50% dextrose can be administered by the registered nurse (RN). Recheck the BG in 15 minutes. If it does not return to at least 70 mg/dL, repeat the procedure every 15 minutes until 70 mg/dL is reached, even if the patient is feeling better. Do not overtreat with too much sugar because doing so can cause hyperglycemia and rebound hypoglycemia.

If you find someone with symptoms of altered BG but are unable to identify whether it is high or low, do a BG test. However, if the patient has neurologic symptoms, treat for low BG immediately. The BG may then be checked and further treatment provided as indicated.

NURSING CARE TIP
Avoid temptation to add sugar to orange juice to treat hypoglycemia. Adding sugar can raise the blood glucose (BG) too much. Also avoid giving sugar that has fat or protein in it (such as chocolate or peanut butter) because fat or protein will slow down digestion of the sugar and delay recovery of the BG level.

Once the hypoglycemic episode is resolved, the patient should eat a complex carbohydrate to prevent recurrence, unless they will have a meal within 30 minutes. If symptoms worsen, call 911 or contact the RN or HCP. Always be aware of agency protocol for treating hypoglycemia.

Some older adult patients with poor autonomic nervous system function or patients taking beta-adrenergic blocking medication such as propranolol or atenolol (which block the sympathetic response) may not feel the symptoms of hypoglycemia. These patients should check glucose levels more often and maintain a safe range to prevent hypoglycemic episodes. Other patients at higher risk of hypoglycemia include those being treated with insulin, patients with longstanding diabetes, older age, and those with cognitive impairment who might have difficulty recognizing or responding to symptoms.

All people with diabetes should be instructed to keep a fast sugar in their purse or pocket at all times. Fast sugars may also be stored in bedside tables, cars, and desks at work.

CUE RECOGNITION 40.1
You are caring for a patient with diabetes. You enter her room and find her agitated. She has not been agitated previously. What do you do?

Suggested answers are at the end of the chapter.

Diabetic Ketoacidosis
PATHOPHYSIOLOGY. Diabetic ketoacidosis (DKA) occurs when BG levels are very high and insulin is deficient. This most commonly occurs in people with type 1 diabetes but may occur in type 2 diabetes when insulin deficiency exists, usually late in the disease process. DKA symptoms are often the reason a person with undiagnosed type 1 diabetes first seeks help. It may also be the result of stress or illness in a person with previously diagnosed diabetes. With insufficient insulin to allow glucose into cells, the cells starve. The body then breaks down fat to be used for energy, which releases an acid substance called *ketones*. As ketones build up in the blood, ketoacidosis occurs.

The body attempts to compensate for acidosis by deepening respirations to blow off excess carbon dioxide. Because carbon dioxide combines with water in the body to form carbonic acid, blowing off carbon dioxide is like blowing off acid. (See the section on metabolic acidosis in Chapter 6.) This deep, sighing respiratory pattern is called **Kussmaul respirations.** The expired air has a fruity odor caused by the ketones and may be mistaken for alcohol. Some nurses have likened the odor to Juicy Fruit chewing gum.

With such high BG and accompanying polyuria, the body becomes dehydrated very quickly. Tachycardia, hypotension, and shock result. Acidosis also causes potassium to leave the cells and accumulate in the blood (hyperkalemia). Potassium is lost in large amounts in urine, which can lead to hypokalemia. The combination of dehydration, potassium imbalance, and acidosis causes flu-like symptoms, including abdominal pain and vomiting. The patient loses consciousness and death occurs if DKA is not treated. The mortality rate for DKA is about 2%.

THERAPEUTIC MEASURES. Treatment includes IV fluids, IV or subcutaneous insulin, and BG monitoring, often initially in an intensive care unit setting. Glucose is added to the IV when the BG drops to about 180 mg/dL to avoid hypoglycemia. Potassium should also be monitored closely, as normal levels are essential to cardiac function. Arterial blood gases help monitor acidosis. The cause of the DKA should be identified and treated.

Prevention of ketoacidosis involves careful monitoring of BG levels at home. Teach at-risk patients to use a urine dipstick (Ketostix) to check for ketones if BG is elevated or if they are ill or under stress. If ketones are present, the HCP should be notified. Instruct patients never to stop their insulin without an HCP's supervision.

Hyperosmolar Hyperglycemic State

PATHOPHYSIOLOGY. Hyperosmolar hyperglycemic state (HHS; also called *hyperosmolar hyperglycemic nonketotic syndrome* [HHNKS]) occurs mainly in type 2 diabetes, when BG levels are high and the patient has reduced fluid intake as a result of stress or illness. Because the person with type 2 diabetes has some insulin production, cells do not starve, and DKA usually does not occur. HHS occurs more often in older adults.

As BG level rises (hyperglycemia), polyuria causes profound dehydration, producing the hyperosmolar (concentrated) state. BG may rise as high as 1,500 mg/dL, and electrolyte imbalances occur. Because ketoacidosis is not present, the patient may not feel as physically ill as the patient with DKA and may delay seeking treatment. Symptoms of HHS develop slowly and include extreme thirst, lethargy, and mental confusion. Shock, coma, and death occur if it is left untreated. The mortality rate for HHS is much higher than for DKA, in part because of the underlying problems and age of the patient.

THERAPEUTIC MEASURES. Treatment includes IV fluids and insulin as well as glucose monitoring. Electrolytes are closely monitored. The cause of HHS should be identified and treated. HHS can be prevented with careful monitoring of glucose levels at home. Instruct patients to drink plenty of sugar-free fluids if BG levels are beginning to rise, especially in times of stress and illness. They should also know when to call their HCP with high BG results.

> **CUE RECOGNITION 40.2**
>
> You are caring for a patient with hyperglycemia. His blood pressure this morning was 146/88 mm Hg. Eight hours later, it is 122/70 mm Hg. What should you do?
>
> *Suggested answers are at the end of the chapter.*

Long-Term Complications

Over time, chronic hyperglycemia causes serious complications in persons with diabetes, affecting the circulatory system, eyes, kidneys, skin, and nerves. Most of the complications involve either the large blood vessels in the body (*macrovascular* complications) or the tiny blood vessels, such as those in the eyes or kidneys (*microvascular* complications). In addition to the effects of diabetes and elevated glucose on complications, smoking significantly increases risk of complications.

The Diabetes Control and Complications Trial (DCCT), a large classic research study completed in 1993, showed that individuals with type 1 diabetes who maintain tight control of BG experience fewer long-term microvascular complications than individuals who take traditional care of their diabetes (Diabetes Control and Complications Trial Research Group, 1993). Follow-up studies show continued benefits from tight control. Similarly, the United Kingdom Prospective Diabetes Study (UKPDS), completed in 1998, showed that individuals with type 2 diabetes who maintain an HbA_{1c} below 7% can significantly reduce complications. In fact, for every percentage of decrease in HbA_{1c}, there were 25% fewer deaths from diabetes-related complications (United Kingdom Prospective Diabetes Study Group, 1998). Unfortunately, tight control can be accompanied by an increased risk of hypoglycemia, and even tight control does not guarantee the prevention of all long-term complications.

Macrovascular Complications

CIRCULATORY SYSTEM. People with diabetes develop atherosclerosis and arteriosclerosis faster than the general population. They are more likely to have hypertension and elevated low-density lipoprotein (LDL) cholesterol and triglyceride levels. High BG can also affect platelet function, leading to increased clotting. These problems lead to a higher incidence of stroke, heart attack, and poor circulation in the feet and legs. The risk of cardiovascular disease and stroke is two to four times more common in persons with diabetes than in the general population.

Control of BG, blood pressure, and cholesterol levels are vital to help prevent these deadly complications. Patients should also avoid smoking, maintain normal weight, and exercise regularly. All patients should be evaluated by their HCP for treatment with aspirin or other antiplatelet medication, angiotensin-converting enzyme (ACE) inhibitor or angiotensin-receptor blocker (ARB) therapy for blood pressure control, and statin therapy for control of blood lipids.

Microvascular Complications

EYES. Small blood vessels can become diseased, eventually leading to some degree of retinopathy in most patients with diabetes. **Retinopathy** involves damage to the tiny blood vessels that supply the eye. Small hemorrhages occur, which can cause blindness if not corrected. Diabetes is a leading cause of new cases of blindness in U.S. adults ages 18 to 64 (CDC, 2020). Good control of BG and blood pressure can reduce the risk of retinopathy. Laser surgery may help improve vision after hemorrhages. Diabetes is also associated with a higher incidence of cataracts and glaucoma. Patients with diabetes should have a yearly dilated eye examination.

KIDNEYS. Nephropathy is caused by damage to the tiny blood vessels in the kidneys. Diabetes is the leading cause of end-stage renal (kidney) disease (ESRD) in the United States. Latino, Black, and American Indian individuals have the highest risk. A primary risk factor for diabetic nephropathy is poor control of BG. If nephropathy occurs, the kidneys are unable to remove waste products and excess fluid from the blood. When the kidneys have lost most of their function, patients may have their blood cleansed artificially by either hemodialysis or peritoneal dialysis (see Chapter 37). The only cure for ESRD is a kidney transplant.

Patients should be taught the importance of BG and blood pressure control to prevent or delay kidney disease. ACE inhibitor and ARB medications slow the development of kidney problems in patients with diabetes. Routine urine tests check for albumin in the urine. A renal dietitian should work with the patient and HCP to determine the best diet for protecting the kidneys.

Nerve Complications

Another complication of diabetes is **neuropathy**, which is damage to nerves as a result of chronic hyperglycemia. Neuropathy can cause numbness and pain in the extremities, erectile dysfunction (impotence) in men, sexual dysfunction in women, **gastroparesis** (delayed stomach emptying), and other problems. Unfortunately, neuropathic pain is difficult to treat with traditional analgesics. Anticonvulsant agents gabapentin (Neurontin) and pregabalin (Lyrica) help reduce painful nerve impulses. Certain antidepressant agents may also help control nerve pain. Tight control of BG levels can delay onset and help manage neuropathy.

Infection

People with diabetes are prone to infection for several reasons. If injuries occur, healing may be slow because of impaired circulation. They may have limited blood supply to heal the wound or fight an infection. For the same reason, it may be difficult for IV antibiotics to reach an infected site, and topical antibiotics may be preferable. In the presence of hyperglycemia, white blood cells become sluggish and ineffective, further reducing the body's ability to fight infection.

The incidence of periodontal (gum) disease, caused by bacteria in plaque, is also increased in individuals with diabetes. Patients must be taught to maintain good oral hygiene and make regular visits to the dentist. The ADA and CDC recommend all patients with diabetes follow guidelines for routine vaccinations against flu, pneumonia, human papillomavirus, herpes zoster, tetanus/diphtheria/pertussis, and hepatitis B (ADA, 2021).

Foot Complications

The combination of macrovascular disease, neuropathy, and risk for infection makes patients with diabetes prone to foot problems. Consider the patient who has no feeling in the feet because of neuropathy. If the patient has a foot injury, they may not notice right away. Vascular disease prevents good blood supply from warding off infection and promoting healing. If infection sets in, it is slow to resolve and may progress to necrosis and gangrene. Pressure points on the feet also increase the risk for pressure injuries (Fig. 40.8). Neuropathy can also lead to deformities of the feet, further increasing the risk of injuries.

For these reasons, diabetes is the leading cause of nontraumatic amputation of the lower extremities in the United States. Teaching patients how to care for their feet and prevent complications is an important role for the licensed practical nurse/licensed vocational nurse (LPN/LVN); see Box 40.1. If sores are noted, the patient should not delay in seeking treatment. During routine visits to the HCP, teach the patient to be sure to remove shoes and socks so the feet can be thoroughly examined. The HCP or diabetes specialist can test sensation in the feet with tiny filaments. Loss of protective sensation is an early risk factor for amputation, so any reduction in sensation is a warning sign that extra care must be taken. Patients should be referred to a podiatrist (foot doctor) or specialized wound treatment center if problems occur.

• WORD • BUILDING •

retinopathy: retino—nervous tissue of the eye + pathy—illness
nephropathy: nephro—of the kidney + pathy—illness
neuropathy: neuro—nervous system + pathy—illness
gastroparesis: gastro—stomach + paresis—partial paralysis

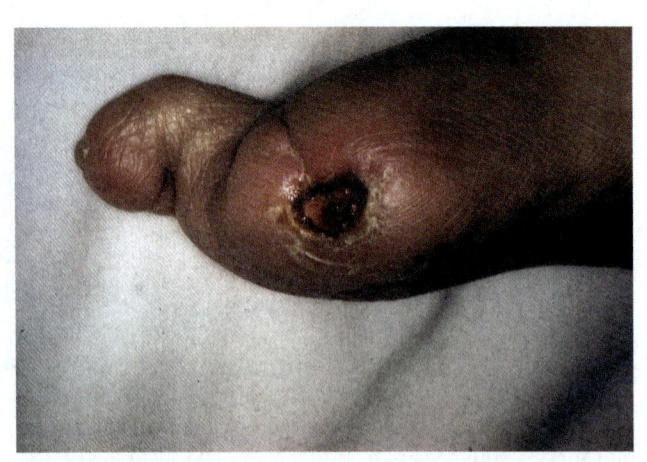

FIGURE 40.8 Diabetic foot ulcer at site of amputated toe.

Box 40.1
Foot Care Tips

- Wash and dry feet every day. Use warm (not hot) water to avoid burns.
- Apply lotion that does not contain alcohol, avoiding areas between toes.
- Inspect feet for sores or red areas daily (have a family member help if necessary).
- Report any abnormalities immediately.
- Wear leather shoes and white or light-colored cotton socks.
- Never go barefoot.
- Avoid garters and tight socks.
- Avoid crossing legs.
- Cut toenails to natural shape of nail (not into corners).
- See a podiatrist for calluses or problem toenails (avoid "bathroom surgery").
- Have feet checked at least yearly (preferably three to four times a year) for sensation loss.

NURSING CARE TIP
When collecting routine patient data, **always** look carefully at your patients' feet. Remove shoes and socks, examine all skin surfaces, and look between toes. Report any redness, lesions, or other suspicious areas. **You** could make the difference between a small, treatable wound and amputation!

NURSING CARE TIP
Encourage patients to wear white or light-colored socks. One woman did not know she had a wound on her foot until she saw blood coming through her white cotton socks.

CRITICAL THINKING & CLINICAL JUDGMENT

Mr. Jones is a 54-year-old banker with type 2 diabetes admitted to your unit with a tiny red area on his right heel. His admitting blood glucose is 360 mg/dL. The lesion is so small you wonder what the fuss is about. While asking about the lesion, you find that he wore a new pair of shoes to work all day about a month ago and has been avoiding seeing his HCP about the resulting red area. He is placed on IV antibiotics, and, within 3 days, the red area has broken open and has yellow drainage. He is sent home with topical antibiotics and crutches, to be followed by a visiting nurse. The wound takes 6 months to fully heal.

Critical Thinking (The Why)
1. List three risk factors for foot problems.
2. Why did the sore take so long to heal?
3. Why do you think crutches are necessary?
4. Why might topical antibiotics work better than IV antibiotics?
5. What could have happened if Mr. Jones had not sought care?
6. What team members can you collaborate with on Mr. Jones's care?

Clinical Judgment (The Do)
7. The nurse documents the following description of Mr. Jones's wound: "Small red open area on heel, with yellow drainage on dressing." What is wrong with this charting? How can you improve it?
8. What information is essential to give to Mr. Jones for his care at home?

Suggested answers are at the end of the chapter.

Special Considerations for the Patient Undergoing Surgery

Surgery is a stressor. The counterregulatory hormones released during stress cause the BG to rise, even if the patient has been fasting. High BG levels interfere with immune function and healing and can increase the patient's risk for infection. Critically ill patients do not tolerate low BG. Glucose levels in critically ill hospitalized patients should typically be maintained between 140 and 180 mg/dL, preferably with use of IV insulin (ADA, 2021). All patients are different, however, and the HCP should be consulted for specific target glucose levels. Patients who are fasting prior to surgery or other procedures will need specific insulin or oral hypoglycemic orders. Basal insulins or some oral agents may still be needed even if the patient is not eating.

Often, patients are placed on IV infusions of glucose and insulin, during and immediately after surgery, in place of longer-acting insulins. Monitor BG levels every 2 to 4 hours or as ordered and monitor carefully for signs and symptoms of hypoglycemia or hyperglycemia. If a patient uses a pump at home, check with a diabetes resource nurse to determine whether they can continue use during hospitalization.

Patients not previously on insulin may be placed on insulin during and after surgery. They can generally return to their presurgical treatment plan after the stress of surgery is past.

Nursing Process for the Patient With Diabetes Mellitus

Data Collection

A complete nursing history and physical examination should be carried out because diabetes affects every body system. Some focus areas are listed in Table 40.8. Social determinants of health, such as the patient's income; educational level; availability of health insurance; and ability to access health care, medications, testing supplies, and appropriate foods, impact the patient's management of their diabetes. These parameters should be determined and included in the plan of care. In addition, determine each patient's knowledge of diabetes and its care so that appropriate teaching can be carried out.

> **PRACTICE ANALYSIS TIP**
> Linking NCLEX-PN® to Practice
> The LPN/VN will explore reasons for client noncompliance with treatment plan.

Nursing Diagnoses, Planning, and Implementation

Because diabetes affects so many different areas, nearly any nursing diagnosis may be appropriate. See "Nursing Care Plan for the Patient With Diabetes Mellitus" for an example of the diagnosis *Risk for Unstable Blood Glucose Level*. The actual presence of the defining characteristics should be confirmed with the patient before choosing any nursing diagnosis.

Diabetes affects not only the person with the disease but the entire family. Once diagnoses have been identified, planning should include both the patient and family members. The desired outcomes for the plan of care are for the patient to know about and become able to care for their disease and prevent complications. Consult the dietitian, social worker, certified diabetes educator, home health nurse, outpatient education programs, and other resources as needed (see "Home Health Hints").

Evaluation

The best indicator of the success of a care plan for diabetes is controlled BG and HbA_{1c} within target levels. The patient should be without symptoms of hypoglycemia or hyperglycemia and able to state what to do if they occur. Long-term complications should be minimized. Another important indicator is the patient's statement of satisfaction and comfort with the plan and their ability to carry it out each day.

> **PRACTICE ANALYSIS TIP**
> Linking NCLEX-PN® to Practice
> The LPN/VN reinforces education to client regarding medications.

Diabetes Self-Management Education

The individual with diabetes must receive diabetes self-management education. No amount of care from an HCP or nurse can replace the self-care required of the person with

Table 40.8
Data Collection for the Patient With Diabetes Mellitus

Subjective Data	• Age and symptoms at onset • Understanding of diabetes (type 1 or type 2) and self-care • Current treatment plan (medication, nutrition therapy, exercise) and adherence to plan • Frequency of blood glucose (BG) self-monitoring and pattern of BG levels (check diary if patient has kept one) • History of diabetes-related complications • History of depression or anxiety • Involvement of family or other support systems • Presence of food or housing insecurity • Ability to access medications and supplies
Objective Data	• Vital signs • Height, weight, body mass index • Skin: Integrity, turgor, condition of injection sites • Feet: Pulses, color, temperature, skin integrity, pressure points, sensation • Laboratory results: BG, HbA_{1c}, creatinine, lipid profile, albuminuria, urine and serum ketones

Nursing Care Plan for the Patient With Diabetes Mellitus

Nursing Diagnosis: *Risk for Unstable Blood Glucose Level*
Expected Outcomes: The patient will maintain at all times an HbA$_{1c}$ less than 7%, a preprandial glucose of 80 to 130 mg/dL, and a postprandial glucose less than 180 mg/dL. The critically ill hospitalized patient treated with insulin will maintain BG measurements between 140 and 180 mg/dL. Verify specific individualized goals with HCP.
Evaluation of Outcomes: Are BG levels within predetermined parameters? Does the patient show an understanding of diabetes self-care?

Intervention	Rationale	Evaluation
Determine knowledge of diabetes self-care.	*Teaching should be initiated only if a knowledge deficit exists.*	Does patient exhibit knowledge of diabetes self-care?
Assist patient to collaborate with HCP to determine appropriate BG targets and action to be taken if BG level is too high or too low.	*Appropriate BG levels may be different for each patient. The patient should know what BG levels require notification of the HCP.*	Does patient state appropriate BG levels and action to take if glucose is high or low?
Teach patient to assess glucose levels before meals and at bedtime or as ordered by HCP. Ensure that patient obtains glucose monitor and instruction for home use.	*Good BG control depends on knowledge of glucose levels and trends.*	Does patient demonstrate correct use of glucose monitor or state how monitor and instruction will be obtained?
In a hospitalized patient who is taking nothing by mouth (NPO), check glucose level every 4 to 6 hours around the clock. Check patient receiving intravenous insulin every 30 minutes to 2 hours.	*Regular BG monitoring is needed for insulin administration and maintaining glucose levels within target parameters.*	Is BG monitoring carried out on an appropriate schedule? Are glucose readings within target range?
Collaborate with RN to teach patient how to administer insulin or oral hypoglycemic in relation to BG results and meals. Replace any uneaten carbohydrate foods to prevent hypoglycemia.	*If most medications are taken without appropriate food to supply calories, hypoglycemia can occur. Check individual medication for specific instructions.*	Does patient state appropriate meal and medication schedule?
Assist with teaching technique for administering insulin if indicated.	*Patient and family will be administering insulin independently at home.*	Does patient demonstrate correct injection technique?
Observe for symptoms of hypoglycemia and hyperglycemia, and treat as needed. Teach causes, prevention, cue recognition, and treatment of hypoglycemia and hyperglycemia.	*If patient has a good understanding of hypoglycemia and hyperglycemia, most episodes can be prevented. If hypoglycemia or hyperglycemia does occur, prompt treatment is essential to prevent complications.*	Does patient state causes, prevention, symptoms, and treatment of hypo- and hyperglycemia? Does patient carry fast sugar at all times?
Administer 15 to 20 g of glucose or carbohydrate if BG level falls below 70 mg/dL or according to institution hypoglycemia guidelines. Contact registered nurse or HCP if BG is above 180 mg/dL.	*A fast sugar provides prompt treatment of hypoglycemia to prevent complications. Glucose levels over 180 mg/dL are associated with poor outcomes.*	Does fast sugar resolve hypoglycemic episode within 15 minutes? If not, repeat. Are glucose levels within safe range?
Collaborate with dietitian for nutrition therapy instruction.	*The dietitian is trained to assess patient preferences and provide in-depth meal plan instruction.*	Is patient able to state plan for obtaining appropriate meals?

Nursing Care Plan for the Patient With Diabetes Mellitus—cont'd

Intervention	Rationale	Evaluation
Teach patient on insulin to eat additional complex (not fast-acting) carbohydrate before exercise if glucose is less than 90 mg/dL, and to have access to carbohydrates before, during, and after exercise.	*Exercise can further lower BG.*	Does patient state appropriate plan for maintaining glucose levels during exercise?
Collaborate with social worker or case manager as needed.	*Some patients may not have the resources or support to carry out effective self-care.*	Does patient state availability of adequate resources for self-care at home?
Provide patient with information for obtaining comprehensive diabetes education.	*Instruction provided in the hospital usually is not comprehensive. Outpatient diabetes classes can provide additional self-care and health promotion information.*	Does patient state plan for obtaining further diabetes education after discharge?
Assist patient to obtain medical alert card or tag that identifies diabetes.	*If the patient is ever unresponsive for any reason, the HCP would need to be aware of diabetes condition.*	Does patient state plan to carry or wear identification at all times?
Geriatric		
Determine ability to see and manipulate syringe, glucose monitor, and other equipment. Obtain assistive devices as needed.	*The older adult patient may have poor eyesight or other sensory deficits.*	Is patient able to manipulate equipment to safely care for self?

diabetes. The involvement of family or significant others is also important for the successful treatment and well-being of the person with diabetes.

If the patient is hospitalized at diagnosis, initial instruction is done in the hospital. However, hospital stays are so short, you cannot waste any time. Begin determining baseline knowledge and teaching as soon as the patient is feeling physically well enough to learn. Depending on your state nurse practice act, this may be the responsibility of the primary or registered nurse, although aspects may be delegated to the LPN/LVN. Some hospitals have a certified diabetes educator who provides classroom or bedside instruction. The dietitian should be contacted to provide nutrition instruction.

Most hospitals have policies or management plans describing instruction to be provided by the nurse. Generally, this encompasses *survival skills*, including the basic information the patient needs initially to survive at home: medication administration; glucose monitoring; meal plan basics; and causes, symptoms, and treatment of high or low BG levels. A variety of helpful aids, such as pamphlets and videos, are available. Diabetes equipment suppliers provide kits that are full of samples and information. These are a significant help when you are teaching a patient. Also advise the patient to purchase a medical alert bracelet or necklace.

Home Health Hints

- Call the patient the day before performing a venipuncture for a fasting BG and remind them not to eat after midnight.
- Record a blood sugar at every visit. If patient has not yet checked their BG, have them take it while you are there. This will allow you to see whether the patient can use the glucometer independently, that the glucometer is working, and that the patient has adequate strips and lancets. If supplies are needed, assist the patient in ordering.
- Some home glucose monitoring devices have a memory that you can access during the visit. It gives the date, time, and BG result. This is a good indication of adherence with self-monitoring performed by patient or caregiver.
- Even if the patient has had diabetes for many years, observe them preparing and injecting their insulin. This provides an opportunity to praise good technique, correct bad habits, and ensure that the patient's vision is still adequate to perform this task.

- Patients with newly diagnosed diabetes may be anxious and overwhelmed. Have the patient repeat instructions to you and perform return demonstrations.
- Store prefilled syringes in the refrigerator flat or with needles pointing up. This prevents crystals from settling and clogging the needles. Allow syringes to reach room temperature before injecting.
- If the patient has a visual or dexterity problem, suggest a syringe magnifier or a prefilled insulin pen. A referral to occupational therapy may also be appropriate.
- Patients with vision problems can become isolated and depressed. Assist your patient with obtaining vision aids that can help improve social outlets.
- Encourage the patient not to skip meals. Assist the patient to identify easy but nutritious meals, such as frozen dinners that are low in sodium. Another option is home-delivered meals such as Meals on Wheels.
- Assist patients to discard used syringes and needles in a hard plastic container (e.g., a laundry detergent bottle with a screw top) if red needle boxes are not available.
- Advise patients to use a mirror to look at the bottom of the feet or have a family member examine the patient's feet regularly.
- Teach patients to wear comfortable shoes and avoid sandals, high heels, and flip flops. If necessary, the HCP can request a podiatry consult. A podiatrist can arrange for the patient to be measured and fitted with special shoes that reduce pressure on problem areas. Special shoes may be covered by Medicare.
- Teach patients to keep a pair of nonskid slippers at the bedside. If the patient needs to get up in the night to use the restroom, putting on secure slippers can help prevent the possibility of stepping on something and causing a foot injury.
- Advise the caregiver that hot water heaters should be set below 120°F (48.8°C) to avoid a possible burn, because many patients with diabetes have decreased skin sensation.

It is difficult to teach glucose monitoring with the variety of monitors available. Many drugstores and medical supply stores not only sell the monitors but also provide training for the patient and family. You can obtain this information by calling local medical suppliers or by contacting the certified diabetes educator or discharge planner at your institution.

After discharge, the patient should be referred to outpatient diabetes classes for further instruction. If classes are unavailable or if the patient is unable to leave home, a referral to a visiting nurse should be made. It is usually advisable to have a nurse present for the patient's first insulin injection at home. The Association of Diabetes Care and Education Specialists (ADCES, 2020) recommends that diabetes self-management education include information about the following:

- Healthy eating
- Being active
- Monitoring
- Taking medication
- Problem solving
- Reducing risks
- Healthy coping

The ADA has helpful resources for both you and your patients at www.diabetes.org. You can find the ADCES at www.diabeteseducator.org.

Because many people with diabetes are older, it is important to be aware of the special needs of the older population (see "Gerontological Issues").

REACTIVE HYPOGLYCEMIA

Reactive hypoglycemia, also called postprandial hypoglycemia, occurs when BG drops below a normal level following meals, usually below 50 mg/dL. Hypoglycemia is most often a complication of diabetes treatment, but at times it may occur without the presence of diabetes. It may be a warning sign of impending diabetes.

Pathophysiology and Etiology
Low BG can occur as an overreaction of the pancreas to eating. The pancreas senses the BG level rising and produces more insulin than is necessary for the use of that glucose. As a result, the BG drops below normal due to abnormally low levels of glucagon or, alternatively, to high levels of insulin. True reactive hypoglycemia is a rare condition and many "hypoglycemic" episodes are instead related to activation of the sympathetic nervous system for other reasons, without true hypoglycemia.

Signs and Symptoms
Low BG causes release of epinephrine, which in turn causes the BG to rise. Epinephrine release causes a fight-or-flight reaction, which may produce shaking, sweating, and palpitations. Headache, chills, and confusion may also occur. Symptoms are the same as those described earlier related to hypoglycemia in diabetes.

Diagnosis
Patients can test for hypoglycemia with a home glucose monitor when they have symptoms. These results may then be taken to the HCP for interpretation.

Therapeutic Measures
Treatment includes frequent small meals and avoidance of fasting. Simple sugars can aggravate symptoms. High-fiber foods, complex carbohydrates, and proteins are recommended.

Evidence-Based Practice

Clinical Question
Are meditative movement exercises effective for glucose control in patients with diabetes?

Evidence
A systematic review in India of 21 studies found that meditative exercise (yoga, tai chi, and qigong) "significantly improved FBG, HbA$_{1c}$, postprandial BG, total cholesterol, LDL-C, and HDL-C (in patients with type 2 diabetes). No improvement was found in BMI."

Implications for Nursing Practice
This systematic review shows promising results for the use of meditative movements in diabetes treatment. Such exercises reduce sedentary time and may also help manage stress levels. There is no evidence, however, that meditative movement can replace aerobic and resistance exercises. Collaborate with the HCP to encourage appropriate patients to incorporate meditative movement into their treatment regimens.

Reference: Xia, T., Yang, Y., Li, W., Tang, Z., Huang, Q., Li, Z., & Guo, Y. (2020). Meditative movements for patients with type 2 diabetes: A systematic review and meta-analysis. *Hindawi Evidence-Based Complementary and Alternative Medicine*. https://doi.org/10.1155/2020/5745013

Gerontological Issues

Diabetes and Older Adults.
Diabetes care can be a challenge for many older adults:

- Blood glucose goals can be relaxed in some older adults, as long as acute hyperglycemic complications are avoided.
- Older adults with diabetes should be assessed for cognitive impairment and depression; both conditions can make self-management difficult.
- Syringe magnifiers and talking glucose meters are available for those with impaired vision.
- Family members can be taught to draw up a week's supply of insulin for the patient to store in the refrigerator. Family members should also be able to recognize signs and symptoms of hypo- and hyperglycemia.
- Home meal programs can help ensure an adequate diet.
- Older adults should have an emergency call system in the home and regular contact with family members or other support people.

Key Points

- Diabetes mellitus is a group of diseases with defects in insulin secretion or action that cause elevated BG (hyperglycemia).
- Type 1 diabetes destroyed beta cells in the pancreas that are unable to produce insulin. Insulin must be injected so the body can use food for energy.
- In type 2 diabetes, tissues resist insulin, made by the pancreas but in inadequate amounts. As the disease advances, the pancreas eventually wears out and stops producing insulin. This leads to the need for injections.
- Many children and adolescents are developing type 2 diabetes, which once only affected adults. Increasing obesity and decreasing activity levels in children today have contributed to this epidemic.
- In GDM, the metabolic demands of pregnancy trigger diabetes. BG typically normalizes after delivery, but the mother remains at elevated type 2 diabetes risk.
- With prediabetes, BG levels are above normal but do not meet the criteria for diabetes. Prediabetes occurs before the onset of type 2 diabetes.
- Classic symptoms of diabetes include polydipsia (excessive thirst), polyuria (excessive urination), and polyphagia (excessive hunger).
- Diagnostic tests for diabetes mellitus include fasting BG, random BG, oral glucose tolerance test, and glycohemoglobin.
- Research studies have shown that patients who have prediabetes can prevent or delay the onset of diabetes with weight loss and a regimen of moderate physical activity.
- Treatment begins with diet and exercise. Insulin is added for patients with type 1 diabetes. Those with type 2 diabetes may need insulin or oral hypoglycemic medication.
- Weight loss is essential for overweight or obese patients who have type 2. BG monitoring and education are also important for good diabetes control.
- The patient with diabetes must not exceed the insulin's ability to carry food energy into the cells. They must be especially important to limit carbohydrate intake.
- Personalized eating plans help patients manage glucose levels, weight, and cardiovascular risk factors. These diets should be based on personal and cultural preferences, health literacy, access to healthful food choices, willingness and ability to make behavioral changes, and existing and possible barriers to change.
- Exercise lowers BG by reducing insulin resistance and improving insulin action in the muscles and liver. Physical activity also boosts blood lipid levels and circulation, important because diabetes increases risk of cardiovascular disease.

- With type 1 diabetes, insulin is typically given subcutaneously. Fast-acting insulin may be ordered via the intramuscular or IV route in urgent situations.
- A common regimen called *basal-bolus therapy* mimics normal insulin secretion.
- Home blood glucose testing facilitates diabetes management for all patients with type 1 diabetes and for many with type 2.
- Urine should be tested for ketones (ketonuria) during acute illness or stress, when BG levels are elevated in ketosis-prone patients, or when symptoms of ketoacidosis are present.
- When calories eaten exceed insulin available or glucose used, high BG (hyperglycemia) occurs.
- Stress causes the release of counter-regulatory hormones, including epinephrine, cortisol, growth hormone, and glucagon. These hormones all increase the BG level.
- Low BG, or hypoglycemia, occurs when there is not enough glucose available in relation to circulating insulin. Common causes are skipping a meal, exercising more than usual, or accidentally administering too much insulin.
- To treat hypoglycemia, administer a fast sugar (15 to 20 grams of carbohydrate that will enter the bloodstream quickly), such as 4 oz orange juice, 4 oz regular (not diet) soda, or 8 oz low-fat milk.
- Diabetic ketoacidosis occurs when BG levels are very high and insulin is deficient. This most commonly occurs in people with type 1 diabetes, but it may occur in type 2 diabetes when insulin deficiency exists, usually late in the disease process.
- Hyperosmolar hyperglycemic state (also called *hyperosmolar hyperglycemic nonketotic syndrome*) occurs mainly in type 2 diabetes, when BG levels are high and the patient has reduced fluid intake as a result of stress or illness.
- Over time, chronic hyperglycemia causes a variety of serious complications in persons with diabetes involving the circulatory system, eyes, kidneys, skin, and nerves.
- Effective diabetes education includes instruction on healthy eating, being active, monitoring blood glucose, taking medication, problem solving, reducing risks, and healthy coping.
- The best indicator of the success of a care plan for diabetes is controlled BG and HbA_{1c} within target levels. The patient should be without symptoms of hypoglycemia or hyperglycemia and able to state what to do if they do occur. The patient should be satisfied with the care plan and have minimal long-term complications of the disease.

SUGGESTED ANSWERS TO CHAPTER EXERCISES

Cue Recognition
40.1: Check blood glucose.
40.2: Consider hyperosmolar hyperglycemia as a possible cause and look for other signs of dehydration. Notify the RN or HCP.

Critical Thinking & Clinical Judgment
Mr. McMillan
1. "Have you been eating or drinking more than usual? Have you been urinating more than usual? Do you get up at night to urinate? How is your appetite? Does anyone in your family have diabetes?"
2. Fatigue occurs because the glucose cannot enter the cells without insulin, so they are starving.
3. Mr. McMillan is dehydrated because he is losing excessive amounts of urine as his kidneys lose excess glucose.
4. Mr. McMillan needs acute care. Some options are to call the case manager to determine if there are resources to help pay for his care. Many hospitals offer free care to patients in need or provide assistance in signing up for Medicaid. Find out what resources Mr. McMillan has at home. Can someone assist him? Can he return to the hospital for diabetes classes? Is home care an option? Does he have resources to purchase medications?
5. Depending on the type of diabetes, Mr. McMillan is at very high risk for hyperosmolar hyperglycemia or diabetic ketoacidosis. Either can lead to death if he is not treated. He is also at risk for long-term complications.

Mrs. Evans
1. Insulin glargine (Lantus) should be given the same time each day. The order says each evening; any time in the evening is okay as long as it is consistent. Insulin lispro (Humalog) is very fast acting, so it should be given no more than 15 minutes before eating, ideally when her food is ready to eat so no delay can occur.
2. She should be alert for low blood glucose (BG) 30 to 90 minutes after she receives each Humalog dose, the peak action time for Humalog. Eating her meal after her insulin dose should prevent hypoglycemia.
3. If Mrs. Evans receives insulin and misses her meal, she will likely develop hypoglycemia. If you know she is not feeling well, it would be best to hold her insulin for that meal until you speak with the HCP.
4. She can eat another fruit that has the same amount of carbohydrate. Applesauce, canned sugar-free peaches or pears, or other soft fruits would be appropriate.

Jeff
What kind of new job is it? What schedule is he working? Is it more physically strenuous than his previous job? Does it interfere with his usual meal schedule? What other changes has he experienced in his life that may have affected his BG?

Mr. Jones
1. Poor circulation, neuropathy, and slow wound healing place Mr. Jones at risk for problems.

2. Circulation to the foot may be poor, and white blood cells are sluggish if the BG is high.
3. Any pressure on the foot while walking may further impair circulation. He should not bear weight on the affected foot.
4. If circulation to the area is poor, IV antibiotics may not reach the sore.
5. An unrecognized foot wound can lead to infection, necrosis, and even amputation.
6. Mr. Jones might benefit from involvement with a wound care nurse, dietitian, certified diabetes educator, and home health nurse. Collaborate with the HCP for the need for a referral to a comprehensive diabetes education center.
7. "Small red open area on right posterior heel, 1 cm × 1.5 cm, 2 mm deep, 2 cm area of yellow drainage on dressing." In addition, many agencies are now taking instant photos of wounds to include in the chart. If no camera is available, a drawing of the size and shape is helpful.
8. Mr. Jones must know how to care for his feet (see Box 40.1), how to change his dressing, how to monitor the wound, and when to contact the HCP. He also should understand the importance of tight control in preventing additional problems, and work with the HCP to determine BG goals and treatment.

Additional Resources

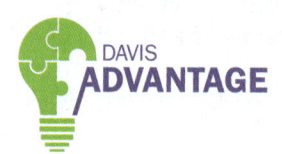

Go to Davis Advantage to complete your learning: strengthen understanding, apply your knowledge, and prepare for the Next Gen NCLEX®.

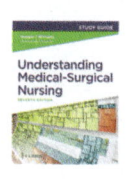

A Study Guide is also available.

UNIT ELEVEN Understanding the Genitourinary and Reproductive Systems

CHAPTER 41
Genitourinary and Reproductive Systems Function and Data Collection

Rebecca Ericson, Jan Bradford

KEY TERMS

adnexa (ad-NEK-sah)
bimanual (by-MAN-yoo-uhl)
circumcised (SIR-kum-sized)
colposcopy (kul-PAHS-koh-pee)
conization (KOH-ni-ZAY-shun)
culdoscopy (kul-DOS-koh-pee)
curet (kyoo-RET)
cystic (SIS-tik)
ejaculation (ee-JAK-yoo-LAY-shun)
epispadias (EP-ih-SPAY-dee-ahz)
erection (ee-REK-shun)
gravida (GRA-vid-ah)
gynecomastia (GY-neh-koh-MAS-tee-ah)
hydrocele (HY-droh-seel)
hypospadias (HY-poh-SPAY-dee-ahz)
hysterosalpingogram (HISS-tur-oh-SAL-ping-oh-gram)
hysteroscopy (HISS-tur-AH-skoh-pee)
insufflation (in-suf-LAY-shun)
libido (lih-BEE-doh)
mammography (mah-MAH-grah-fee)
menarche (meh-NAR-kee)
menopause (MEN-oh-pawz)
orgasm (OR-gazm)
para (PAR-ah)
salpingoscopy (SAL-pin-GOS-koh-pee)
transillumination (TRANS-ih-loo-mih-NAY-shun)
varicocele (VAR-ih-koh-seel)

CHAPTER CONCEPTS

Health promotion
Sexuality

LEARNING OUTCOMES

1. Explain the normal structures and functions of the reproductive system.
2. Identify the effects of aging on the reproductive system.
3. List data to collect when caring for a patient with a disorder of the reproductive system.
4. Identify commonly performed tests used to diagnose disorders of the reproductive system.
5. Plan nursing care for patients undergoing each of the diagnostic tests.

NORMAL GENITOURINARY AND REPRODUCTIVE SYSTEMS ANATOMY AND PHYSIOLOGY

The male and female reproductive systems produce gametes (sperm and egg cells [ova]) and facilitate the union of gametes in fertilization following sexual intercourse. The uterus provides for the developing embryo/fetus until birth.

Female Reproductive System

The female reproductive system consists of paired ovaries and fallopian tubes, a single uterus and vagina, and external genitalia (Fig. 41.1). The mammary glands are considered accessory organs to the system.

Ovaries

The ovaries are a pair of oval structures, about 5 cm long and 2.5 cm wide, located on either side of the uterus in the pelvic cavity. The ovarian ligaments and the broad ligament help keep the ovaries and uterus in position.

The ovaries produce egg cells by oogenesis (meiosis), which begins and then pauses in the fetus, resumes at puberty, and ends at menopause. This process is cyclical. Typically, one mature ovum with its 23 chromosomes is produced and released approximately every 28 days, under hormonal control. Ovarian follicles produce estrogen and later, as the corpus luteum, secrete progesterone as well.

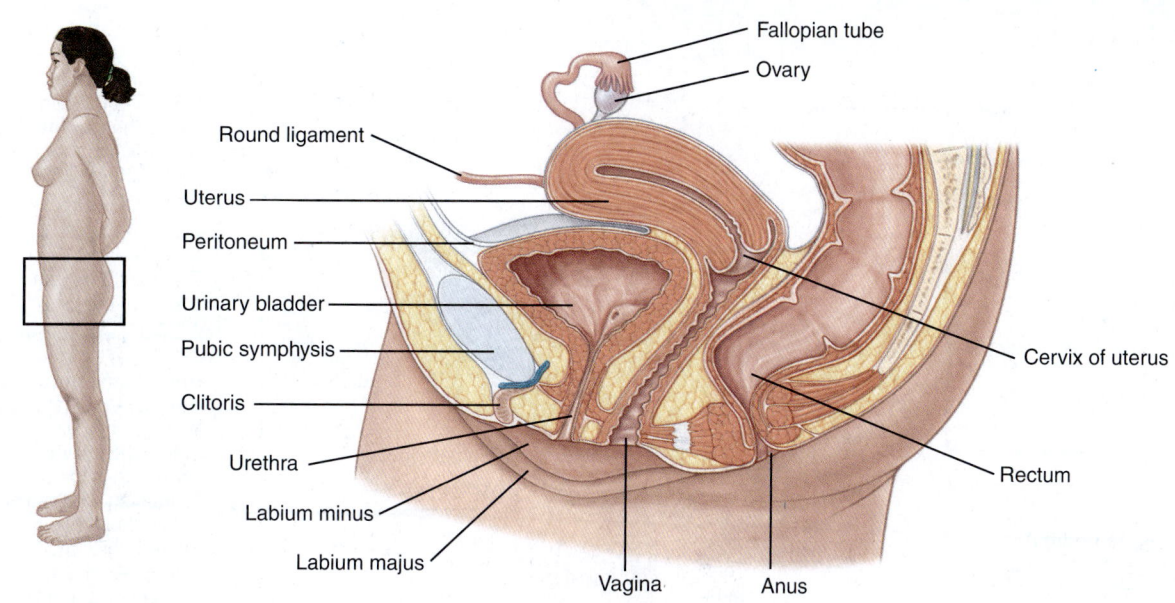

FIGURE 41.1 Female reproductive system in a midsagittal section.

Fallopian Tubes
Each fallopian (uterine) tube is about 10 cm in length and extends from near the ovary to the uterus (Fig. 41.2). Its fimbriae draw an ovum into the tube, and ciliated epithelium transport the ovum (or zygote, if fertilized) toward the uterus.

Uterus
The uterus is a muscular organ about 8 cm long and 5 cm wide. Ligaments help keep the uterus in position, tilted anteriorly over the top of the bladder. During pregnancy, the uterus increases greatly in size and contains the placenta, which nourishes the fetus until birth. Rising oxytocin levels increases uterine contractions to bring about birth.

The uterus is divided into three layers: the external perimetrium, the myometrium, and the internal endometrium. The endometrium is a highly vascular mucous membrane, part of which is lost and regenerated with each menstrual cycle. During pregnancy, the endometrium helps form the maternal side of the placenta.

Vagina
The vagina extends from the uterine cervix to the vaginal orifice in the perineum. It lies between the urethra and the rectum.

After puberty, the vaginal mucosa is relatively resistant to infection. The normal bacterial flora of the vagina creates an acidic pH, which prevents microbial growth. While present, the hymen provides mechanical protection.

External Genitalia
Also called the *vulva*, the female external genitalia include the clitoris, mons pubis, and labia majora and minora (Fig. 41.3).

Mammary Glands
Enclosed within the breasts and surrounded by adipose tissue, the mammary glands produce milk after pregnancy (Fig. 41.4). During pregnancy, high levels of estrogen and progesterone prepare the glands for milk production. Prolactin causes the production of milk after pregnancy. Breastfeeding stimulates the release of oxytocin, which in turn stimulates the release of milk and contraction of the uterine muscle.

The Ovarian and Menstrual Cycles
The female reproductive cycles depend on follicle-stimulating hormone (FSH), luteinizing hormone (LH), estrogen, and progesterone (Table 41.1). These hormones bring about changes in the ovaries and uterus.

The menstrual cycle begins with the loss of the endometrium during menstruation, which lasts an average of 5 days. After the endometrium begins to proliferate again due to estrogen, FSH increases and several ovarian follicles begin to develop, although typically only one will dominate. The secretion of LH also increases, peaking to cause ovulation.

After ovulation, the ruptured follicle becomes the corpus luteum, which begins to secrete progesterone in addition to estrogen. Progesterone stimulates further development of the endometrium. If the ovum is not fertilized, the secretion of progesterone decreases. Without progesterone, the endometrium cannot be maintained and begins to slough off in menstruation. FSH secretion begins to increase as estrogen and progesterone decrease, and the cycle begins again. An average cycle is 28 days, but it is normal to have a cycle that is shorter or longer.

Male Reproductive System
The male reproductive system consists of bilateral testes and a series of tubules, ducts, and glands. The glands contribute secretions to the sperm, producing semen.

Fallopian Tubes

A narrow isthmus is the portion of the fallopian tube closest to the uterus.

The middle portion of the tube, called the **ampulla**, is the usual site of egg fertilization. Cilia line the inside of the tube. Their beating movements, combined with peristaltic contractions of the tube, propel an egg toward the uterus.

The distal funnel-shaped end of the fallopian tube is called the **infundibulum**. The fallopian tube does not attach directly to the ovary. Instead, finger-like projections called **fimbriae** fan over the ovary.

Uterus

The curved upper portion of the uterus is called the **fundus**. The upper two corners of the uterus connect with the fallopian tubes.

The central region of the uterus is the **body**.

The inferior end is the **cervix**. A passageway through the cervix, called the **cervical canal**, links the uterus to the vagina. Glands within the cervical canal secrete thick mucus; during ovulation, the mucus thins to allow sperm to pass.

Labels on figure: Ovary, Fimbriae, Broad ligament, Cervical canal, Endometrium, Myometrium

Vagina

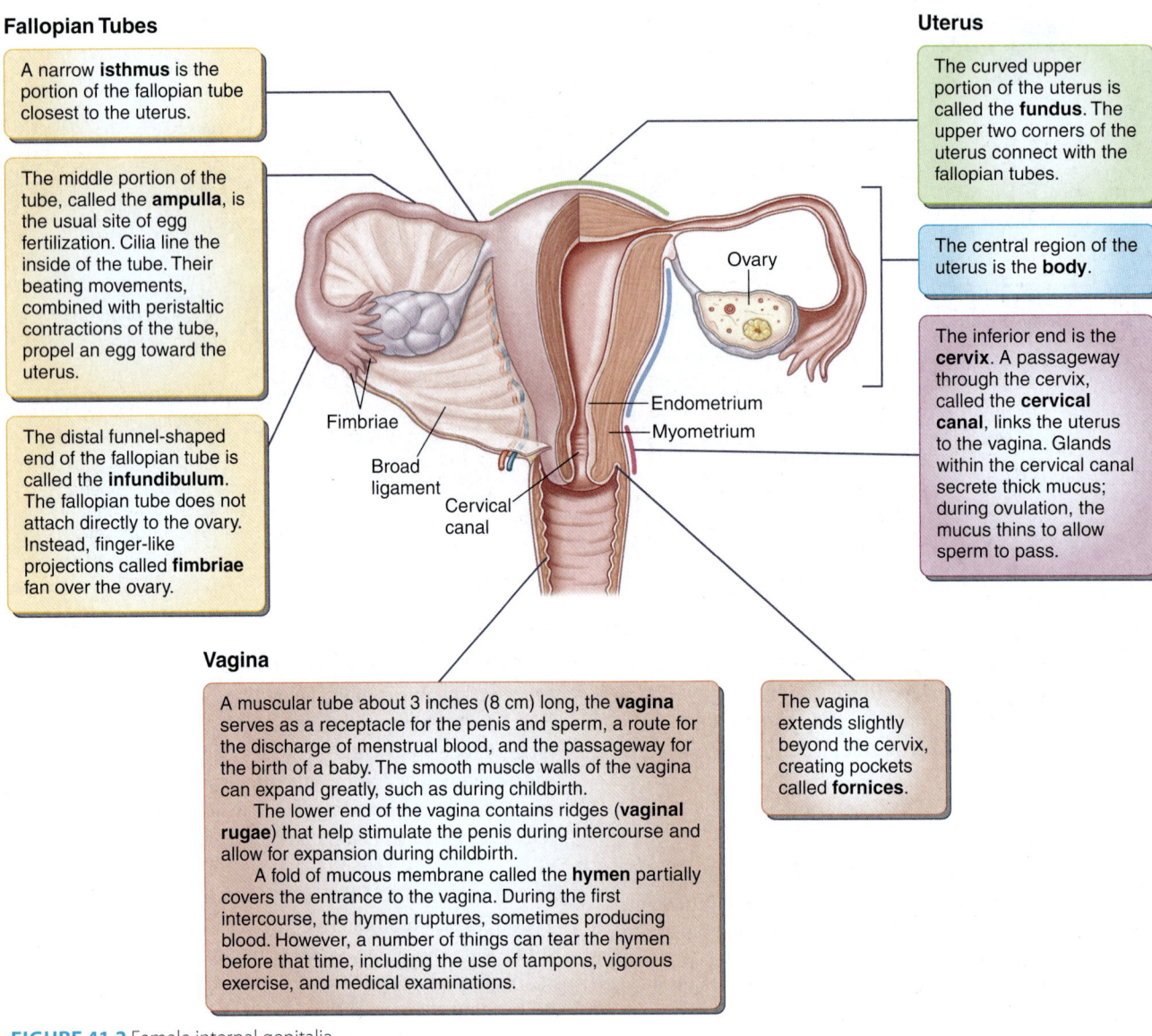

A muscular tube about 3 inches (8 cm) long, the **vagina** serves as a receptacle for the penis and sperm, a route for the discharge of menstrual blood, and the passageway for the birth of a baby. The smooth muscle walls of the vagina can expand greatly, such as during childbirth.

The lower end of the vagina contains ridges (**vaginal rugae**) that help stimulate the penis during intercourse and allow for expansion during childbirth.

A fold of mucous membrane called the **hymen** partially covers the entrance to the vagina. During the first intercourse, the hymen ruptures, sometimes producing blood. However, a number of things can tear the hymen before that time, including the use of tampons, vigorous exercise, and medical examinations.

The vagina extends slightly beyond the cervix, creating pockets called **fornices**.

FIGURE 41.2 Female internal genitalia.

Testes

The testes are located in the scrotum between the upper thighs, where the temperature is slightly lower than body temperature. This is necessary for production of viable sperm. Each testis is about 5 cm long and 3 cm wide and contains the seminiferous tubules in which spermatogenesis (meiosis) takes place. In contrast to oogenesis, once started at puberty, spermatogenesis is a constant rather than cyclical process and usually continues throughout life. FSH initiates spermatogenesis. LH stimulates the secretion of testosterone, which contributes to the maturation of sperm. The secretion of inhibin is stimulated by testosterone; inhibin decreases the secretion of FSH, which helps keep the rate of spermatogenesis fairly constant. The functions of these hormones are summarized in Table 41.2.

Epididymis, Ductus Deferens, and Ejaculatory Ducts

A series of ducts lead sperm into and through the pelvic cavity where secretions are added; semen then exits the body via the urethra. The comma-shaped epididymis is a tube about 6 meters long coiled on the posterior side of a testis. Smooth muscle within its wall propels sperm from the testes into the ductus deferens. Also called the *vas deferens*, the ductus deferens extends from the epididymis in the scrotum to the ejaculatory duct within the pelvic cavity. Each of the two ejaculatory ducts receives sperm from the ductus deferens and the secretion of the seminal vesicle bilaterally. Both ejaculatory ducts propel semen through the urethra.

Seminal Vesicles, Prostate Gland, and Bulbourethral Glands

The male reproductive system includes bilateral seminal vesicles and bulbourethral glands and a singular prostate (Fig. 41.5).

The mostly alkaline secretions of the male reproductive glands ensure that many sperm remain viable in the acidic environment of the vagina. The normal bacterial flora of the

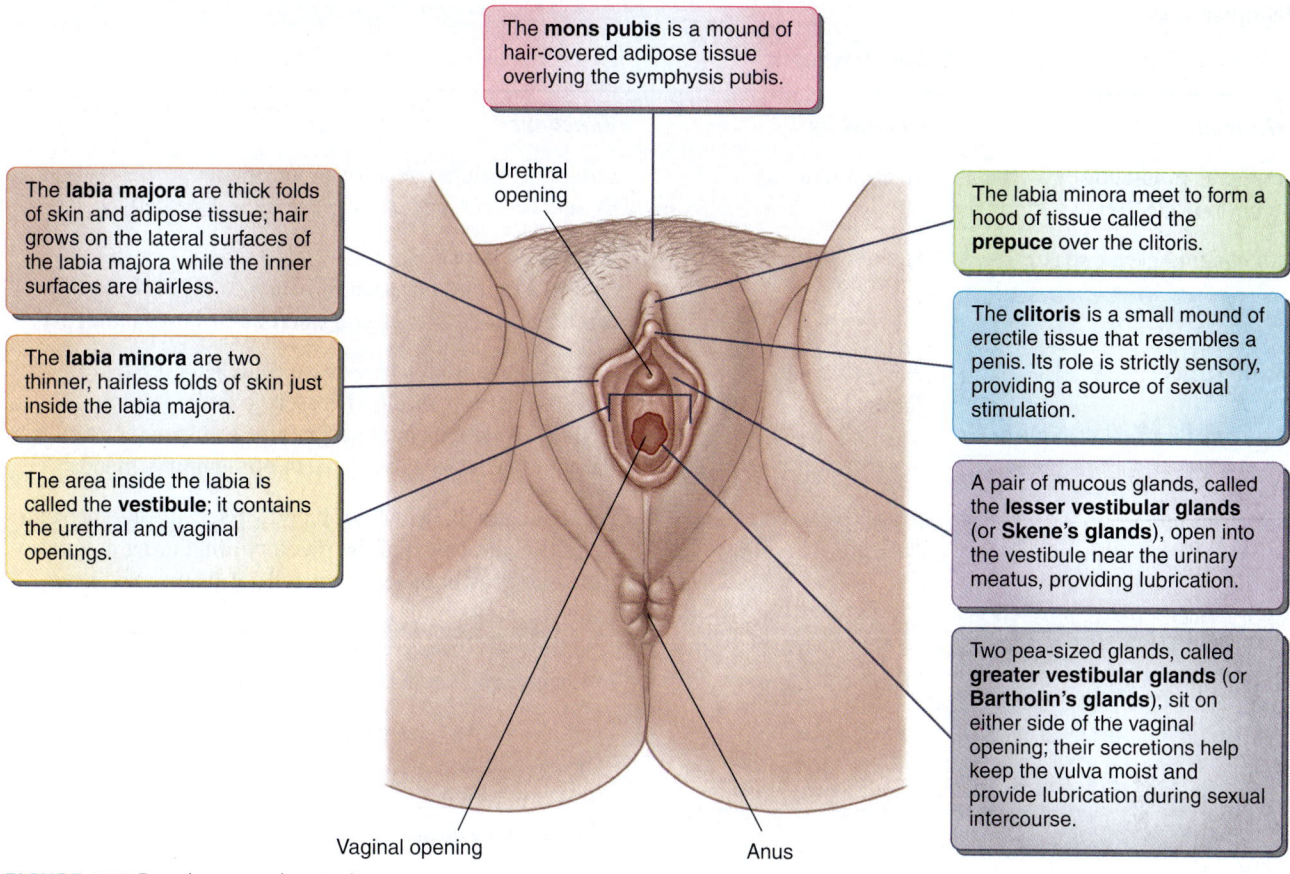

Chapter 41 Genitourinary and Reproductive Systems Function and Data Collection 793

The **mons pubis** is a mound of hair-covered adipose tissue overlying the symphysis pubis.

The **labia majora** are thick folds of skin and adipose tissue; hair grows on the lateral surfaces of the labia majora while the inner surfaces are hairless.

The **labia minora** are two thinner, hairless folds of skin just inside the labia majora.

The area inside the labia is called the **vestibule**; it contains the urethral and vaginal openings.

The labia minora meet to form a hood of tissue called the **prepuce** over the clitoris.

The **clitoris** is a small mound of erectile tissue that resembles a penis. Its role is strictly sensory, providing a source of sexual stimulation.

A pair of mucous glands, called the **lesser vestibular glands** (or **Skene's glands**), open into the vestibule near the urinary meatus, providing lubrication.

Two pea-sized glands, called **greater vestibular glands** (or **Bartholin's glands**), sit on either side of the vaginal opening; their secretions help keep the vulva moist and provide lubrication during sexual intercourse.

Urethral opening
Vaginal opening
Anus

FIGURE 41.3 Female external genitalia.

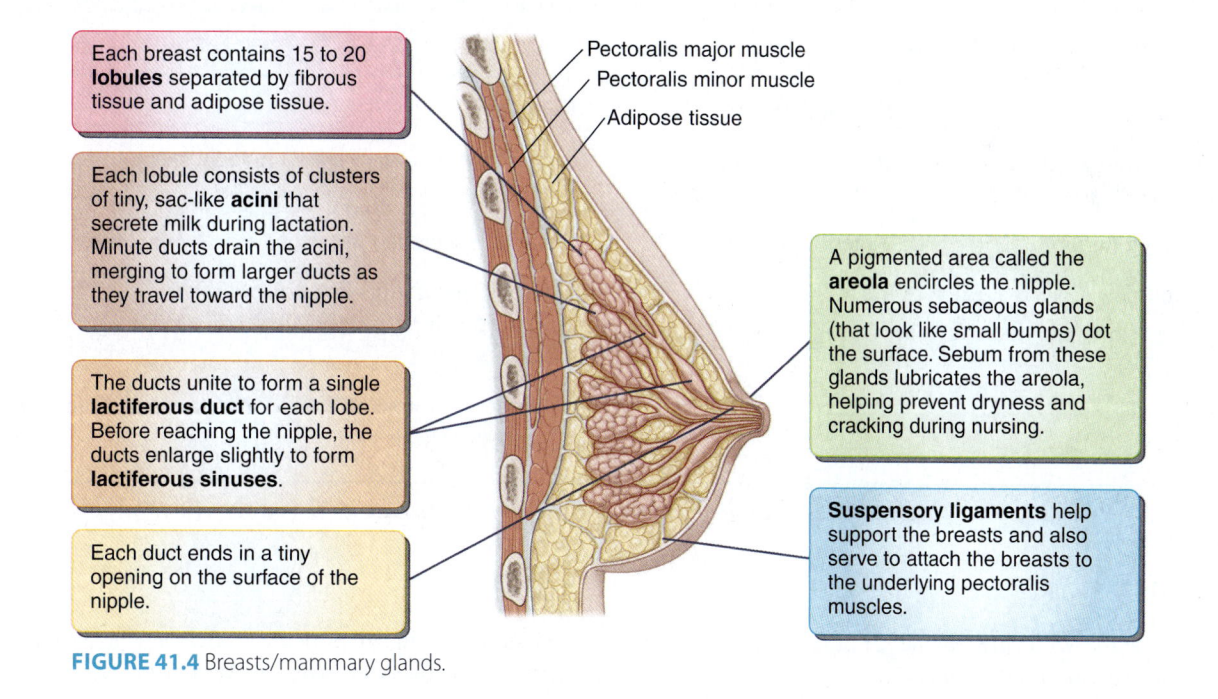

Each breast contains 15 to 20 **lobules** separated by fibrous tissue and adipose tissue.

Each lobule consists of clusters of tiny, sac-like **acini** that secrete milk during lactation. Minute ducts drain the acini, merging to form larger ducts as they travel toward the nipple.

The ducts unite to form a single **lactiferous duct** for each lobe. Before reaching the nipple, the ducts enlarge slightly to form **lactiferous sinuses**.

Each duct ends in a tiny opening on the surface of the nipple.

Pectoralis major muscle
Pectoralis minor muscle
Adipose tissue

A pigmented area called the **areola** encircles the nipple. Numerous sebaceous glands (that look like small bumps) dot the surface. Sebum from these glands lubricates the areola, helping prevent dryness and cracking during nursing.

Suspensory ligaments help support the breasts and also serve to attach the breasts to the underlying pectoralis muscles.

FIGURE 41.4 Breasts/mammary glands.

Table 41.1
Hormones of Female Reproduction

Hormone	Secreted By	Functions
Follicle-stimulating hormone (FSH)	Anterior pituitary	Initiates development of ovarian follicles Stimulates secretion of estrogen by follicle cells
Luteinizing hormone (LH)	Anterior pituitary	Causes ovulation Converts ruptured ovarian follicle into corpus luteum Stimulates secretion of progesterone by corpus luteum
Estrogen	Ovary (follicle) Placenta	Promotes maturation of ovarian follicles Promotes growth of blood vessels in endometrium Initiates development of secondary sex characteristics Promotes growth of duct system of mammary glands
Progesterone	Ovary (corpus luteum) Placenta	Promotes further growth of blood vessels in endometrium Inhibits contractions of the myometrium during pregnancy Promotes growth of secretory cells of mammary glands
Inhibin	Ovary (corpus luteum)	Decreases secretion of FSH toward end of cycle
Prolactin	Anterior pituitary	Promotes production of milk after birth
Oxytocin	Posterior pituitary	Promotes uterine contractions during labor; release of breast milk

Source: Scanlon, V. C., & Sanders, T. (2019). *Essentials of anatomy and physiology* (8th ed.). Philadelphia, PA: F.A. Davis.

Table 41.2
Hormones of Male Reproduction

Hormone	Secreted By	Functions
Follicle-stimulating hormone (FSH)	Anterior pituitary	Initiates production of sperm in the testes
Luteinizing hormone (LH)	Anterior pituitary	Stimulates secretion of testosterone by the testes
Testosterone	Testes	Promotes maturation of sperm Initiates development of male secondary sex characteristics
Inhibin	Testes	Decreases secretion of FSH to maintain a constant rate of spermatogenesis

Source: Scanlon, V. C., & Sanders, T. (2019). *Essentials of anatomy and physiology* (8th ed.). Philadelphia, PA: F.A. Davis.

vagina create the acidic pH, but the pH of semen is about 7.4 and permits sperm to remain motile.

Urethra and Penis

The urethra is the last of the male reproductive ducts; its longest portion is within the penis. The penis is an external genital organ; its distal end is called the glans penis. When uncircumcised, the glans penis is covered with a fold of skin called the prepuce, or foreskin. Within the penis are three areas of erectile or cavernous tissue (Fig. 41.6).

When blood flow through these sinuses is minimal, the penis is flaccid (soft). Sexual stimulation causes the arterioles of the penis to dilate; the sinuses fill with blood, and the penis becomes erect and firm. This is brought about by

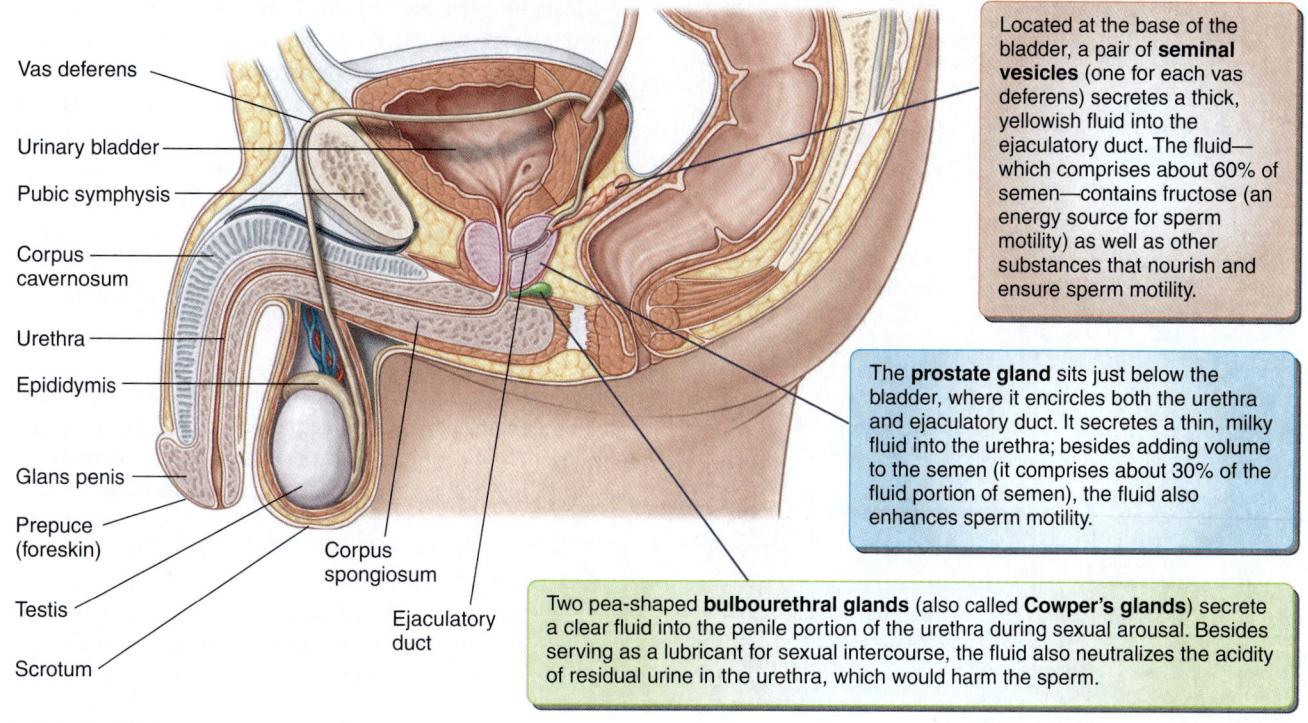

Chapter 41　Genitourinary and Reproductive Systems Function and Data Collection　795

Labels (Figure 41.5):
- Vas deferens
- Urinary bladder
- Pubic symphysis
- Corpus cavernosum
- Urethra
- Epididymis
- Glans penis
- Prepuce (foreskin)
- Testis
- Scrotum
- Corpus spongiosum
- Ejaculatory duct

Callouts (Figure 41.5):

Located at the base of the bladder, a pair of **seminal vesicles** (one for each vas deferens) secretes a thick, yellowish fluid into the ejaculatory duct. The fluid—which comprises about 60% of semen—contains fructose (an energy source for sperm motility) as well as other substances that nourish and ensure sperm motility.

The **prostate gland** sits just below the bladder, where it encircles both the urethra and ejaculatory duct. It secretes a thin, milky fluid into the urethra; besides adding volume to the semen (it comprises about 30% of the fluid portion of semen), the fluid also enhances sperm motility.

Two pea-shaped **bulbourethral glands** (also called **Cowper's glands**) secrete a clear fluid into the penile portion of the urethra during sexual arousal. Besides serving as a lubricant for sexual intercourse, the fluid also neutralizes the acidity of residual urine in the urethra, which would harm the sperm.

FIGURE 41.5 Male accessory glands.

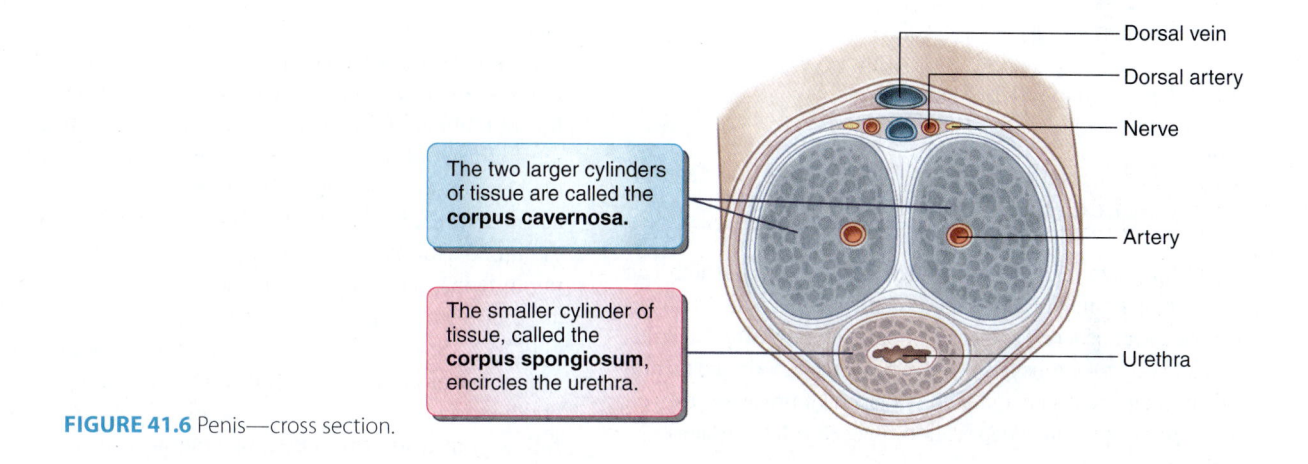

Labels (Figure 41.6):
- Dorsal vein
- Dorsal artery
- Nerve
- Artery
- Urethra

The two larger cylinders of tissue are called the **corpus cavernosa**.

The smaller cylinder of tissue, called the **corpus spongiosum**, encircles the urethra.

FIGURE 41.6 Penis—cross section.

parasympathetic impulses. The culmination of sexual stimulation is **ejaculation** (the expelling of semen from the urethra with force). This is brought about by peristalsis of the reproductive ducts and contraction of the prostate gland.

Spermatozoa
The head of the sperm cell contains 23 chromosomes. The midpiece connects the head to the flagellum. Sperm form in the seminiferous tubules of a testis and are stored in the epididymis.

Aging and the Reproductive System
Women have a definite end to reproductive capability called **menopause,** which occurs when menses has ceased for 12 months. Menopause usually occurs between the ages of 45 and 55. Estrogen secretion decreases, and ovulation and menstrual cycles become irregular and finally cease. The decrease in estrogen has other effects as well. Figure 41.7 presents a concept map on the effects the aging process has on the reproductive system for both men and women.

For most men, testosterone secretion continues throughout life, as does sperm production, although both diminish with advancing age. Perhaps the most common reproductive problem for older men is enlargement of the prostate gland, called *benign prostatic hyperplasia*.

• WORD • BUILDING •

menopause: men—month + pause—stop

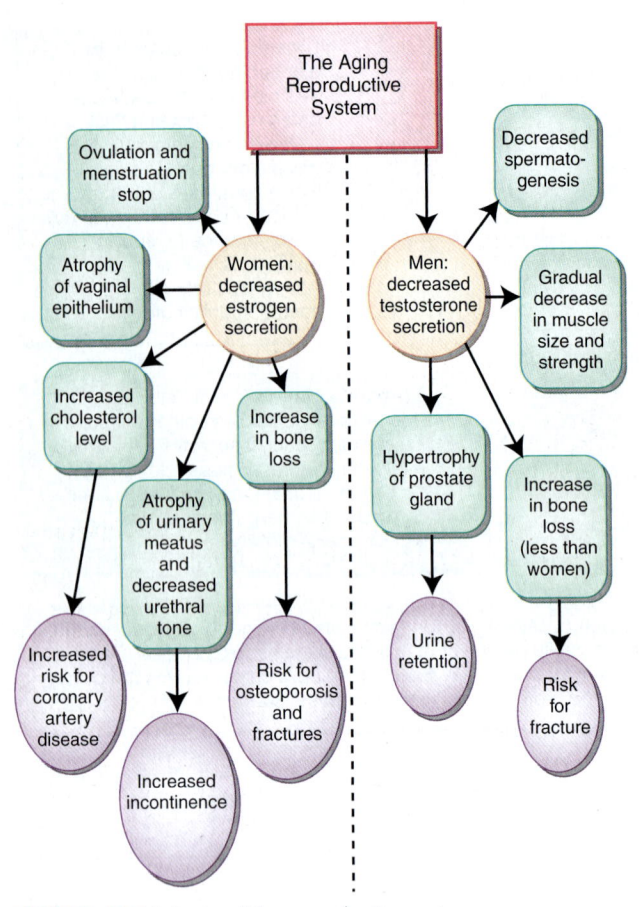

FIGURE 41.7 Aging and the reproductive system.

FEMALE REPRODUCTIVE SYSTEM DATA COLLECTION

Collecting data related to a women's reproductive health can seem challenging because of the complex relationship of physical and psychosocial factors. Hormones not only affect a multitude of body functions but also can influence moods and mental functioning. Reproduction involves physical processes as well as relationships, role identification, and self-esteem issues.

Normal Function Baselines

Knowing about expected functioning of the reproductive system is your best preparation for data collection. Regular, relatively pain-free shedding of the endometrial lining of the uterus (menstruation) is expected from puberty through midlife. Intercourse is normally expected to be free of pain and infection, to occur when desired by both partners, to be satisfying, and generally to result in pregnancy within a few months unless precautions are taken. A pregnancy is expected to last approximately 40 weeks and to produce a healthy child. Physical and psychological sexual characteristics and function, including **libido** (sexual desire), are expected to be adequately maintained by hormones. Sexual functioning, desire, and fertility are expected to change throughout the process of aging. Individuals may vary somewhat from these expected descriptions. Chapter 42 further defines specific female reproductive system disorders.

Much of what happens in female reproductive system disorders occurs inside the body and may not show external signs. Skill in asking appropriate questions, documenting patient statements, and describing observations is essential. Descriptions of symptoms should be thorough. Follow the *WHAT'S UP?* format described in Chapter 1. Because many signs and symptoms of reproductive system disorders occur in a cyclic fashion, you or the health-care provider (HCP) may ask the patient to keep an accurate written record of occurrences, noting times and dates to identify patterns.

Health History

Subjective data related to the female reproductive system include general personal information as well as menstrual, obstetrical, gynecological, sexual, family, and psychosocial histories. See Table 41.3 for specific data to collect.

> **NURSING CARE TIP**
> It is helpful to have women maintain a monthly calendar of their menstrual cycles and bring it to any appointment during which discussion of the cycle may take place.

An obstetrical history includes number of pregnancies, pregnancy outcomes, and complications. These are generally documented using abbreviations of Latin words: G (for the Latin word *gravida*) = number of pregnancies; P (for the Latin word *para*) = births, whether alive or stillborn (regardless of number of fetuses) after 20 weeks' gestation; A (from the Latin word *abortus*) = abortions, whether spontaneous or therapeutic; a spontaneous abortion is sometimes called a *miscarriage*. Roman numerals follow the letters to specify the number of each. For example, three pregnancies resulting in twins, one single birth, and one spontaneous abortion are recorded as GIII, PII, AI. This may also be written as G3P2A1. Some hospitals use additional notations, such as number of premature or full-term births, number of living children, and number of therapeutic abortions. Be sure to follow your institution's documentation policy.

> **LEARNING TIP**
> Remember the word *gravida* by thinking of gravity and knowing that a woman typically is heavier when pregnant.

Many nurses feel awkward asking reproductive history questions, and patients may also feel uneasy with this line of questioning. A matter-of-fact attitude, an assurance of confidentiality, and an adequate explanation about why the information is needed tend to encourage patient comfort and cooperation.

Breast Examination
Palpation

Palpation is the most important technique for breast examination because it can be used to identify alterations from

Table 41.3
Subjective Data Collection for the Female Reproductive System

Questions to Ask During the Health History	Rationale/Significance
Personal History	
Have you ever been diagnosed or treated for any health problems?	Data may reveal general state of health, knowledge/practice of health promotion behaviors, meaning of health, and expectations related to care.
Have you had any recent weight changes?	Weight changes may reflect physical or psychological pathology.
Are you experiencing pain? (Use **WHAT'S UP?** questions if patient reports pain.)	Subjective indication of pain may signal a variety of disorders.
Do you have any allergies? (If so, what is the agent/type of reaction?)	Allergy status should always be assessed to guide possible intervention should treatment be needed.
Are you using any medications (prescription, over-the-counter, herbal remedies)?	A medication list may lead to health issues not yet revealed and may guide possible interventions should treatment be needed.
Do you smoke, consume caffeine, drink alcohol, or use recreational drugs? How much/how often?	Recreational behaviors can indicate risk of health disorders. Smoking increases risk of coagulation disorders with use of contraceptives containing estrogen in women over age 35.
Do you exercise? What type of exercise do you do? How often?	Exercise is recognized as an activity that improves health status, in general, and for many disorders.
How many hours of sleep do you get in a 24-hour period? Do you feel you get enough rest?	May indicate state of health or lead to discussion of social issues that lead to stress and, ultimately, physical disorders.
Do you feel under stress? How do you deal with stress?	Can indicate social issues that may lead to physical disorders.
Have you been hit, kicked, slapped, or made to do anything sexually against your will since your last visit?	Abuse screening should be considered during all primary care visits; may indicate need for intervention or guide care.
Menstrual History	
At what age did you begin menstruating (**menarche**)? How often do you menstruate, and how long do your periods last? How heavy is your flow?	May reveal abnormalities of cycle and lead to a diagnosis of benign/malignant tumors, endometriosis, pregnancy, anemia, and endocrine disorders.
At what age did you enter menopause [if applicable]? If menopausal, has bone density screening been done? What is your calcium/vitamin D intake?	May determine need for bone density screening and teaching related to calcium and vitamin D intake.
Obstetric/Gynecological History	
How many pregnancies and deliveries have you had? Were they full term or preterm? Were your deliveries vaginal or by cesarean section? How much did your largest baby weigh? Did you have any complications following your deliveries?	May indicate health of reproductive system, knowledge/meaning of health maintenance practice, and risk for disease.
Have you had previous treatment/surgery on your reproductive organs?	May indicate past health issues related to the reproductive organs and need for current evaluation related to issues.

Continued

Table 41.3
Subjective Data Collection for the Female Reproductive System—cont'd

Questions to Ask During the Health History	Rationale/Significance
Have you had any itching of your perineum, or have you noted any unusual vaginal discharge (describe)?	Subjective report of itching or discharge may indicate disorder of inflammation or lead to diagnosis of a sexually transmitted infection (STI).
When was your last Pap/pelvic examination? What were the results?	May reflect meaning of health and guide current care.
Do you do breast self-examination? How often? Have you noticed any breast changes? When was your last mammogram [if applicable]?	If changes have been noted by the patient, they should be evaluated by the primary care provider for possible pathology.
Did you breastfeed? How long?	Breastfeeding may offer some protection against breast cancer. If patient is currently breastfeeding, may help guide care and diagnosis.
Sexual History	
Are you sexually active? How many partners do you have? Of what gender? What is your lifetime number of partners? Is your sexual activity satisfying?	May indicate risk of STIs and/or unintended pregnancy as well as state of sexual satisfaction/intimacy.
At what age did you become sexually active? What contraceptive method(s) do you use (if sexually active with a male)? How do you use them? How long have you used this method?	Early onset of sexual activity increases risk of STIs and cervical cancer. May reflect meaning of health, high-risk health behaviors, and risk for unintended pregnancy or STI. Asking length of use of a particular method allows determination of need for replacement, as in an intrauterine device, or need for a bone density examination.
Have you ever been diagnosed with an STI? If so, when, what type, and how was it treated? Are you aware if the treatment was successful?	May indicate high-risk sexual behavior patterns or potential for active disease and, therefore, indicate need for diagnostic testing and treatment.
Family History	
Do you have a family history of cardiovascular problems, cancer, osteoporosis, diabetes, or thyroid abnormalities?	May indicate underlying cause of or risk for sexual/physical abnormalities of the reproductive system.
Psychosocial History	
Are you married or in a significant relationship? Is the relationship satisfying?	Relevant to determine financial, social, and emotional support.

normal consistency, confirm the presence of lumps, and locate areas of tenderness. Even mammograms are not sensitive enough to detect a small percentage of masses that can be felt by the patient or HCP.

Breast Self-Examination

Self-palpation during breast self-examination (BSE), if done regularly and thoroughly, may be even more sensitive than HCP or nurse palpation. Often, the patient becomes so familiar with her own breasts that she is more likely to notice subtle changes that an HCP might overlook. Because recent studies of BSE have failed to show a reduction in cancer deaths, some HCPs are now simply urging women to be familiar with their breasts and report changes rather than teaching them to do monthly examinations. Other providers, however, continue to teach and recommend monthly BSE because they have seen it make a significant difference for many women. Table 41.4 lists additional objective data to collect.

Table 41.4
Objective Data Collection for the Female Reproductive System

Physical Examination Findings	Possible Abnormal Findings/Causes
Clinical Breast Examination (CBE) Observe and palpate for swelling, lumps, skin changes, and nipple exudate.	Changes may indicate breast cancer or fibrocystic breast disease.
External Genitalia Observe for color, symmetry, hair distribution, lesions, swelling, and exudate.	Changes may indicate vulvar cancer, developmental abnormalities, infection, or injury.
Vagina Observe for shape, bulges, color changes, lesions, and exudate.	Changes may indicate infection, structural abnormalities, or injury.
Internal Genitalia (performed by trained personnel) Palpate for tenderness, size, shape, and mobility. Observe for color, lesions, exudate, and bleeding.	Changes may indicate infection, structural abnormalities, cervical cancer, polyps, endometriosis, fibroid/malignant tumors, pregnancy, or injury.
Perineum Observe for lesions and shape.	Abnormalities may indicate infection, structural abnormalities, or injury.
Anus Observe for shape, color changes, and lesions.	Abnormalities can indicate hemorrhoids or injury.
Inguinal Nodes Palpate for swelling and tenderness.	May indicate infectious process or regional malignancy.

Note: A female physical examination is typically done by an HCP or other trained provider.

Patient Education

If BSE is done monthly, a good time to perform it is 1 week after menses when swelling of normal breast tissue is at a minimum. For women who no longer have a regular menstrual period, any regular monthly schedule is fine. Although most women's breasts are not exactly the same size, marked differences between breasts or a change in the size of one breast should be checked with an HCP. Puckering or dimpling of skin, asymmetrical movement, and different pointing position of the nipples should also be reported. Whether breasts are examined in parallel lines, a spiral formation, or a wedge pattern is not important. It is important, however, for the examination to be methodical and cover all areas of the breast, including the tail of Spence, which extends into the axilla (Fig. 41.8).

> **NURSING CARE TIP**
> Some women do breast self-examination the day their electric bill (or other bill) arrives each month because it is a dependable monthly reminder.

> **CRITICAL THINKING & CLINICAL JUDGMENT**
>
> **Jill,** age 24, states, "Why should I do breast exams at my age? I probably won't get breast cancer until I'm older, if I get it at all."
>
> **Critical Thinking (The Why)**
> 1. Why is it important for Jill to become familiar with her own breasts?
>
> **Clinical Judgment (The Do)**
> 2. What should your response to Jill include?
> 3. Why would this be a good time to provide education about health maintenance?
>
> *Suggested answers are at the end of the chapter.*

Diagnostic Tests of the Breasts
Ultrasound and Mammography

Ultrasound can determine the density of the tissues and map the breast structures. This is mainly useful for distinguishing

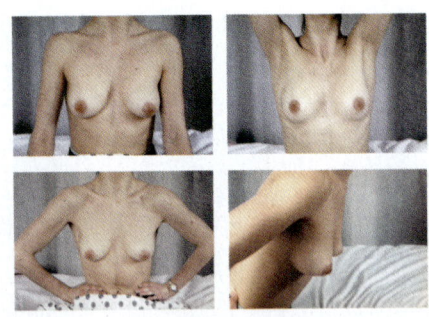

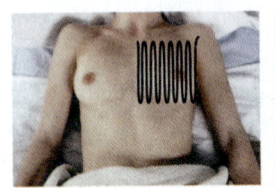

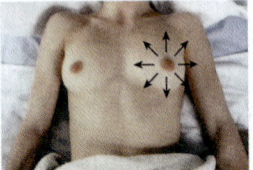

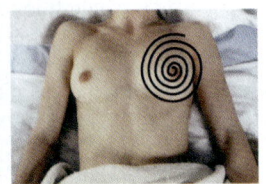

FIGURE 41.8 Breast self-examination.

fluid-filled (**cystic**) lumps from solid tumors. It can also be used to guide a needle for fine-needle aspiration of cystic fluid or core needle biopsies.

Mammography is a radiographic (x-ray) examination of the breasts. A special machine spreads and flattens the breast tissue to a thin layer to more effectively show benign and malignant growths that might be hidden by breast structures on typical chest examination (Fig. 41.9). Digital technology is available and may be more effective in detecting cancers in younger women and those with dense breasts. The procedure is the same for a digital mammogram, but the image is computerized, allowing the radiologist to look more closely at problem areas.

The American Cancer Society (2021) recommends the following for average risk women:

- Women aged 40 to 44 have the option to start screening mammogram yearly.
- Women aged 45 to 54 should get mammograms yearly.
- Women aged 55 and older can switch to every other year or continue yearly.
- All women should be familiar with how their breasts normally look and feel and should report any changes to an HCP right away. A regular clinical breast examination (CBE) and BSE are not recommended.
- All women should understand what to expect when getting a mammogram for breast cancer screening.

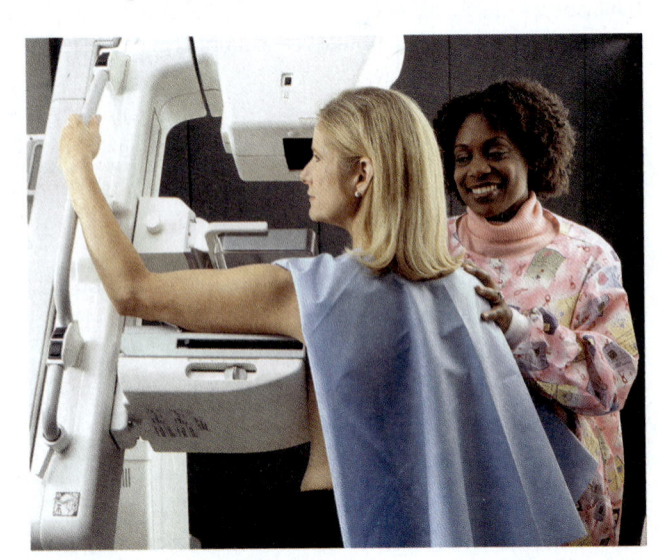

Magnetic resonance imaging (MRI) and a mammogram every year are recommended for women with a high risk for breast cancer, such as those with *BRCA1* or *BRCA2* genetic mutations or a strong family history. See Chapter 11 for more information.

Advise patients preparing for mammography to bathe and not to apply deodorant, powder, or any other substance to the upper body because these can cause false shadows on the test.

Thermography, Computed Tomography Scan, and MRI

Several other methods for diagnosis of breast disorders are available but not commonly used. Thermography maps the breast using photographic paper that records temperature variations throughout the tissue in different colors. A computed tomography (CT) scan or MRI offers precise location of tumors without displacement caused by flattening the breast for a mammogram.

Biopsy

If suspicious lesions are found, they will be further assessed with a biopsy. This may be done by surgically removing a

FIGURE 41.9 Mammogram machine.

• **WORD** • **BUILDING** •
cystic: baglike
mammography: mammo—breast + graphy—recording

portion of tissue or by aspirating fluid or cells through a needle that is placed into the lesion.

Monitoring of the patient's psychological condition during breast diagnosis procedures is essential. Most women know someone who has had breast cancer. Although breast cancer screening procedures can seem routine to health-care workers, they can be the cause of much anxiety for patients and their families. An understanding and calm nurse who can explain the procedures can help the assessment phase to be less traumatic.

> **BE SAFE!**
> **BE VIGILANT!** Be sure to label specimen containers right away while still with the patient!

Laboratory Tests
A blood test can be done to identify mutations in *BRCA1* and *BRCA2*, genes that are associated with breast and ovarian cancer. By reviewing a woman's family history, risk factors can be determined, and testing can be offered. Women who test positive for either gene can discuss preventive treatments with their HCPs and also make their sisters and daughters aware of potential risk.

Bone Health Data Collection
Bone health assessment is important for women of all ages. Teaching women early about the importance of dietary intake of foods rich in calcium and vitamin D, physical activity, not smoking, and limiting alcohol intake will benefit them later in life. Vitamin D needs may depend on the degree of sun exposure. Women of childbearing age produce estrogen, which helps prevent bone loss and works with calcium and other minerals to build bone. As women age and approach menopause, estrogen production slowly decreases, which slows building and remodeling of bone. Menopausal women produce very little estrogen and thus have little bone protection. In fact, the body tends to break down more bone than it rebuilds. At this point of life, dietary calcium and vitamin D requirements increase unless the woman is on hormone replacement therapy.

The U.S. Preventive Services Task Force (USPSTF) issued a research-based statement in 2018 recommending against supplementation with vitamin D of 400 IU or less and calcium of 1,000 mg or less, noting that it does not prevent fractures and may increase incidence of kidney stones. Results from studies using higher doses are inconclusive. More research is needed in this area, but for now, women should aim to get recommended calcium and vitamin D amounts through diet. The USPSTF also notes that exercise is effective to prevent falls that lead to fractures in older adults. If a woman is diagnosed with osteoporosis, she should speak to her HCP about a treatment plan. Table 41.5 provides recommendations for calcium and vitamin D intake from the National Institutes of Health's Office of Dietary Supplements. See Chapter 6 for the calcium content of selected foods.

Diagnostic Tests of the Bones
In addition to being encouraged to increase the dietary intake of calcium and vitamin D, menopausal women older than age 50 who are not on hormone replacement therapy should be assessed for bone loss. The National Osteoporosis Foundation recommends bone density testing for all women older than 65 and for younger postmenopausal women at high risk (see Chapter 46).

The best test for bone density is a dual-energy x-ray absorptiometry (DEXA) scan, which measures bone density at the hip or spine. This specialized x-ray takes only 5 to 10 minutes to complete. A quantitative computed tomography (QCT) scan can also determine bone density. Pharmacies or other outpatient facilities may offer tests of peripheral locations such as the heel. These are less sensitive but still provide useful information that can be followed with more extensive testing if indicated.

Additional Diagnostic Tests of the Female Reproductive System
Hormone Tests
Hormone tests are commonly used to assess endocrine system function as it relates to reproduction. Tests can measure potential fertility, find reasons for abnormal menses, assess hormone-producing tumors, and determine efficacy of treatments to adjust hormone levels. Some hormone tests are time-specific, so samples can be rendered useless if not gathered within that range.

Consult institution policy for specific instructions for each test. Explain the procedure to the patient and provide support. Women who are undergoing hormone tests may feel embarrassed, worried about their femininity and potential fertility, and depressed because of repeated tests. Some may fear loss of their significant other's love (and perhaps the relationship) if they are diagnosed with alterations in hormone levels or function that lead to infertility.

Pelvic Examination
The pelvic examination allows visual inspection of the vagina and cervix as well as sampling of mucus, discharge, cells, and exudates. Palpation of portions of the reproductive system and some treatments may also be done as part of the procedure (Fig. 41.10).

Be prepared to assist the HCP with the examination. Explain the procedure as you set out supplies according to policy or HCP preference. Have the patient empty her bladder, remove her clothing, and change into a gown (socks can remain on and often give a woman a bit of comfort!). When the HCP is ready, assist the patient into the lithotomy position, with feet in stirrups. If the HCP is using a metal speculum, run it under warm water to make it a little more comfortable for the patient. Have the patient take a deep breath and blow out to help her relax as the speculum is inserted. Being in

Table 41.5
Adult Calcium and Vitamin D Recommendations

Age (years)	Male	Female	Pregnant	Lactating
Recommended Dietary Allowances for Calcium				
14–18 years	1,300 mg	1,300 mg	1,300 mg	1,300 mg
19–50 years	1,000 mg	1,000 mg	1,000 mg	1,000 mg
51–70 years	1,000 mg	1,200 mg	—	—
71 years or older	1,200 mg	1,200 mg	—	—
Recommended Dietary Allowances for Vitamin D				
14–18 years	600 IU (15 mcg)	600 IU (15 mcg)	600 IU (15 mcg)	600 IU (15 mcg)
19–50 years	600 IU (15 mcg)	600 IU (15 mcg)	600 IU (15 mcg)	600 IU (15 mcg)
51–70 years	600 IU (15 mcg)	600 IU (15 mcg)	—	—
71 years or older	800 IU (20 mcg)	800 IU (20 mcg)	—	—

Source: Office of Dietary Supplements, National Institutes of Health. (Updated 2021). Vitamin D fact sheet for professionals. https://ods.od.nih.gov/factsheets/VitaminD-HealthProfessional; and Office of Dietary Supplements, National Institutes of Health. (Updated 2021). Calcium fact sheet for professionals. https://ods.od.nih.gov/factsheets/Calcium-HealthProfessional

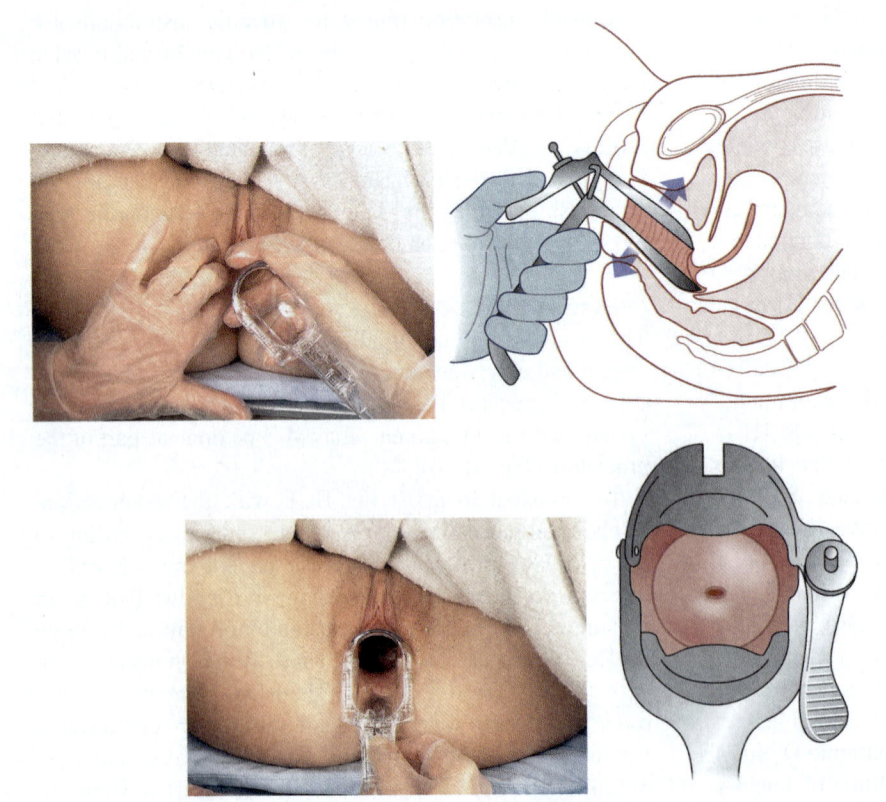

FIGURE 41.10 Pelvic examination with Pap smear.

lithotomy position may make some women feel embarrassed and exposed. Be sure to provide privacy. Ideally, the examination table faces away from the door.

Bimanual Palpation

Because much of the reproductive system is not visible even with a speculum, **bimanual** palpation is often done during a pelvic examination. One hand is placed on the abdomen and the other gloved hand is inserted deeply into the vagina. The uterus and **adnexa** are moved about between the two hands to feel the size, shape, and consistency of the uterus and adnexa and to check for any abnormal growths.

Explain the procedure and support the patient. Some women may be fearful, embarrassed, or tense and may find the procedure uncomfortable (see "Patient Perspective"). Active relaxation strategies may decrease discomfort.

Patient Perspective

Jacqueline

I am a sexual assault nurse examiner. When patients come to see me, they are in crisis, unsure how or what to feel and whom to trust. They are very apprehensive. As patients give me the history of their assaults, they begin to trust me. They see someone who is interested in them and who believes them. By the time I start the head-to-toe physical examination, they know they are safe. Often, when I am performing the physical examination, I start small talk and take an interest in their lives that has nothing to do with the assault. When they are discharged from my care, they are more animated, talkative, and sometimes smiling.

The patient I remember the most is a child whose father was molesting her when her mother went to work. She was about 6 years old. When she came to the hospital, she wasn't talking to anybody, let alone a nurse in a scary hospital at midnight. I spent 4 hours with this child. We colored, played, and talked about her brothers. By the end of the night, she allowed me to examine her, and she trusted me enough to let the physician come in and look at her. Unfortunately, in her young life, she had a reason to be scared. Her life became much worse before it got better. Her father tried to kill her mother and himself because the abuse had been discovered as a result of this.

So many of us have grown up with pop culture television, and we think of forensic examiners as professionals working with dead people. In fact, forensic nursing is caring for patients as it applies to the law. As a sexual assault nurse examiner, I care for people who have experienced interpersonal violence. I care for this special population of patients through the nursing process. I care not only for their physical trauma but also for their spiritual needs, and I collect evidence for the prosecution of a crime. I advocate for patients' safety needs, and I help provide for their physical needs. I provide a bridge to the legal and mental health systems.

I began forensic nursing years ago when the concept was still new. We were navigating uncharted waters and were unsure what the result would bring. What we quickly learned is that when you deliver good nursing care to patients, the result can be a positive change in their lives. That is the reward of the job: making a positive difference in patients' lives and giving them some tools to help in their recovery process. Having the patient and family look at you and say, "Thank you for helping me," is what we all went into nursing for.

Being a sexual assault nurse examiner has made me become a more empathetic person, a more compassionate nurse, and a better citizen of my community.

PRACTICE ANALYSIS TIP

Linking NCLEX-PN® to Practice

The LPN/LVN assists with the performance of a diagnostic or invasive procedure.

Cytology

Cytology is the study of cells taken as tissue samples. Cells required for microscopic examination can be removed from the reproductive system in several ways. During a Papanicolaou (Pap) smear, one or more small samples are gently scraped away from the surface of the cervical canal. These cells are smeared or rolled onto microscope slides and sprayed with a fixative to preserve them for viewing or placed into a fixative solution for later preparation and viewing in a lab. Cells may also be collected by **conization**, removing a small cone-shaped sample from the cervical canal, or punch biopsy, which removes a small core of cells. Endometrial biopsy specimens are samples of cells taken from the lining of the uterus by scraping with a small spoon-shaped tool called a **curet** inserted through the cervix. Small biopsy specimens may be taken by cutting or removing a suspicious lesion. Cells can be observed for changes indicative of hormonal secretion, cellular maturation, or abnormalities seen with viral growths and cancerous or precancerous conditions. Results are reported simply as "normal," "unclear," or "abnormal."

NURSING CARE. Consult the procedure manual or HCP concerning specific types of instruments to set up for biopsies and Pap smears. Cells die and degrade rapidly once removed from the patient, so they must be packaged securely for transport to laboratory facilities. Always label specimens carefully.

• **WORD** • **BUILDING** •

bimanual: bi—two + manual—hands
adnexa: ad—together + nexa—to tie (usually refers to ovaries and tubes)
conization: coniz—cone-forming + ation—process

Prepare the patient by explaining the procedure and providing support. The woman may be fearful of cancer or other abnormality. Removal of the sample may cause pain, bleeding, swelling, or, later, inflammation, so the patient is monitored after the procedure and alerted to report these complications if they occur. After the procedure, document the woman's status on the chart and record that the sample was sent to the laboratory. Advise the woman that if results are unclear or abnormal, additional testing will be done. Assure her that abnormal results have many causes and typically do not mean a cancer diagnosis.

> **PRACTICE ANALYSIS TIP**
> Linking NCLEX-PN® to Practice
> The LPN/LVN will provide emotional support to the client.

> **CRITICAL THINKING & CLINICAL JUDGMENT**
>
> **Reproductive Data Collection**
>
> **Critical Thinking (The Why)**
> How might the age of the patient change your approach and plans for the patients in the following scenarios?
>
> **Clinical Judgment (The Do)**
> What teaching would you reinforce for each of these patients?
>
> 1. A 2-year-old child is brought into the clinic by her mother because she has a foul-smelling discharge coming from her perineal area and a slight yellowish discharge from her vagina.
> 2. A 21-year-old woman comes to the HCP office where you work to renew her birth control pill prescription. Your employer enforces regular checks for cervical changes by renewing the prescription only after a Pap smear is done. As you start setting out the Pap smear materials, your patient expresses reluctance to have it done today because she is so sore already.
> 3. Your 56-year-old patient comes in to "get things checked out" because she has pain every time that she and her husband have intercourse.
>
> *Suggested answers are at the end of the chapter.*

Swabs and Smears

Swabs and smears are done to determine which microorganisms are causing infection and, consequently, which antibiotics should be used. If infection is suspected, add sample collection materials, including swabs, slides, and sterile saline in site-specific receptacles, and a gonorrhea/*Chlamydia* collection kit, to the pelvic examination equipment. *Chlamydia* samples are especially difficult to transport to laboratories, and special kits are available for this pathogen. Some microorganisms, such as yeasts and *Trichomonas*, can be identified well from smears on slides. Wet mounts are smears of discharge spread onto a slide. These must be taken to the microscope immediately after they are obtained. Sodium chloride and potassium hydroxide are dropped onto individual wet-mount slides before they dry to aid identification of some microorganisms. Support the patient, who may be anxious about possible sexually transmitted infections (STIs) and effects on relationships.

Sonography

Ultrasound assessment (also called *sonography*) may be done to determine size, shape, development, and density of structures associated with the female reproductive system as well as fetal measurements and some types of prenatal diagnoses. This procedure is especially useful for differentiating cysts from solid tumors and locating ectopic pregnancies and intrauterine devices. Ultrasound may be used to guide needles for obtaining samples of fluid or cells. External or vaginal transducers may be used to send and receive the signals. Vaginal transducers are placed in a plastic sheath before insertion. A full bladder may be required for some ultrasound tests.

Explain the procedure and support the patient. The pressure of the transducer on the skin or in the vagina may be painful if adjacent structures are inflamed or swollen or the bladder is full.

Radiographic Procedures

Several radiographic procedures may be used to diagnose reproductive system problems. CT scan and MRI are used to locate tumors of the reproductive system. Structures of the female reproductive system may also be outlined by taking x-ray pictures of cavities that have been filled with a radiopaque substance. During a **hysterosalpingogram**, dye is injected into the uterus until it comes out the ends of the fallopian tubes. This test is useful for identifying congenital abnormalities in the shape or structure of the uterus and blockages of the fallopian tubes.

NURSING CARE. Prepare the patient for a radiographic test according to agency policy, which may include a laxative, suppository, or enema. Ensure the patient understands the procedure and appropriate consents are signed as required. Ask about allergies to dye or iodine. Notify the supervisor immediately if the patient reports an allergy. After the procedure, collect data on signs and symptoms such as nausea, light-headedness, and signs of allergic reaction and promote comfort, because some cramping can occur. Discharge teaching should include signs of infection and advice that

• WORD • BUILDING •

hysterosalpingogram: hystero—womb + salpingo—tube + gram—record

the x-ray dye can stain clothing. Provide a perineal pad following the procedure and advise the patient to wear a perineal pad until vaginal drainage stops.

> **NURSING CARE TIP**
> If you are assisting a patient prepare for a breast examination, place the patient in an upright sitting position for the first part of the examination so the shape and symmetry of the breasts can be assessed, and then later assist the patient into a supine position.

Endoscopic Examinations

Several types of endoscopic examinations visually inspect internal areas to diagnose (and sometimes treat) reproductive system disorders. The names of the tests vary according to the area inspected, but all generally make use of a fiber-optic light and lens system inserted through a tube called a *cannula* into a small incision. A laparoscopy is done to view the abdominal cavity and is useful for identifying problems such as endometriosis (Fig. 41.11). A **salpingoscopy** is performed to see the inside of the fallopian tubes. A **hysteroscopy** is done to see the inside of the uterus. A binocular microscope is used with an endoscope that is introduced into the vagina to closely study lesions of the cervix during a **colposcopy**. During **culdoscopy**, an endoscope is introduced into the vagina and through a small incision in the vagina into the cul-de-sac of Douglas, a cavity behind the uterus, to observe for abnormalities in this region (Fig. 41.12).

NURSING CARE. Preoperatively, the patient is prepared for an endoscopic examination according to agency protocol. This involves asking the patient whether she has fasted as instructed, assessing vital signs, recording the time of last voiding, helping the patient into a gown, and ensuring the consent form has been signed. General anesthesia may be given for some endoscopic procedures. Explain what to expect and provide support for the woman. She may be anxious about possible disorders.

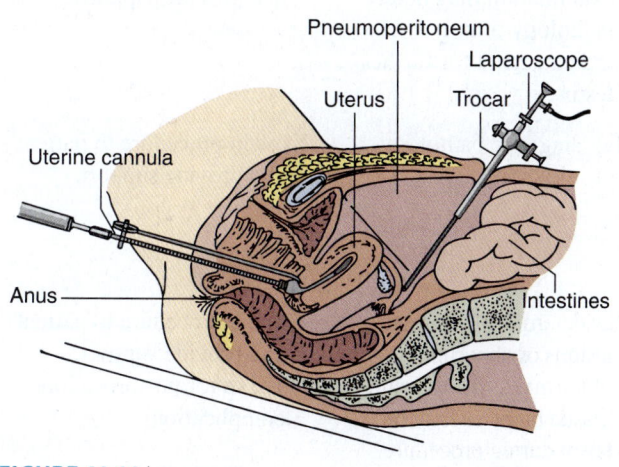

FIGURE 41.11 Laparoscopy.

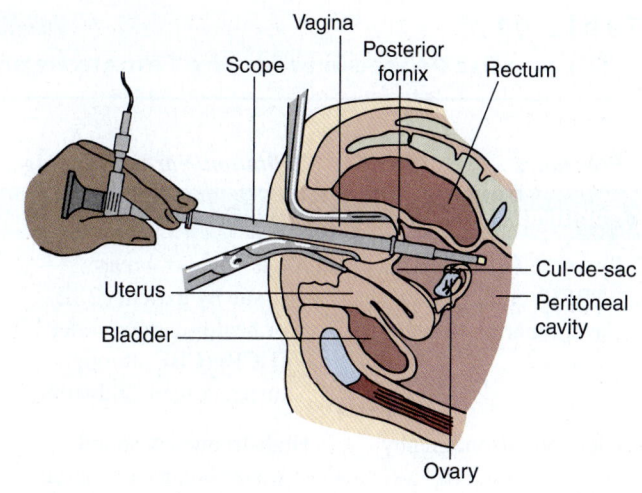

FIGURE 41.12 Culdoscopy.

Postoperatively, provide comfort measures. The woman may experience pain in the neck, shoulders, and upper back if carbon dioxide (CO_2) gas was pumped into the body compartment being examined. This is called **insufflation** and increases the distance between structures, so that it is easier for the HCP to visualize them. If small incisions were made through the abdominal wall for insertion of the endoscope and for insufflation, a Band-Aid or small dressing is applied.

PATIENT EDUCATION. Advise the patient to observe the incision sites for redness, bleeding, or drainage, notifying the HCP promptly if these occur. The patient will need to visit the HCP as directed for suture removal. If the endoscopic procedure was done transvaginally, provide a perineal pad following the procedure and advise the patient to wear a pad until the drainage stops. Also, instruct the patient to report any bright bleeding after the operative day and to report any fever or foul-smelling discharge. Table 41.6 provides a summary of diagnostic tests.

MALE REPRODUCTIVE SYSTEM DATA COLLECTION

As with the female reproductive system, the male reproductive system is a complex interaction of physical and psychosocial factors. Men sometimes find it much more difficult to talk about or admit to having problems related to reproductive health than women do. From toilet training through adulthood, men are expected to exhibit behaviors associated with maleness. Unfortunately, by the time some boys reach manhood, their male identity is often defined by the successful functioning of their sex organs.

• WORD • BUILDING •
salpingoscopy: salpingo—tube + scopy—looking
hysteroscopy: hystero—womb + scopy—looking
colposcopy: colpo—vagina + scopy—looking
culdoscopy: culdo—cul de sac + scopy—looking
insufflation: in + suffl—to blow + ation—process

Table 41.6
Diagnostic Procedures for the Female Reproductive System

Procedure	Definition/Normal Finding	Significance of Abnormal Findings	Nursing Management
Noninvasive			
Breast self-examination (BSE) or clinical breast examination (CBE)	Assessment of breast tissue by patient (BSE) or health-care provider (HCP) (CBE) through inspection and palpation	Abnormal findings during physical examination may indicate pathology and indicate need for further assessment.	Educate about appropriate technique and observe a return demonstration of BSE.
Ultrasound/sonography	High-frequency sound waves bounce off tissue to map tissue structure and determine tissue density. Also may be used to guide biopsy procedure.	May help determine abnormal lesions, abnormalities of tissue structure, or presence of abnormal fluid volume.	Follow institutional guidelines for patient preparation and support, which may be determined by testing goals.
Mammography	Radiographic examination of tissue. X-ray may be used with dye contrast injected before procedure.	May help to determine abnormal lesions or abnormalities of normal tissue structure.	Educate patient not to apply lotions, powders, or deodorant before test.
Thermography, computed tomography (CT) scan, magnetic resonance imaging (MRI)	Precise pictures of tissue using temperature (thermography), x-ray (CT scan), or radiofrequency (MRI)	May help to determine abnormal lesions or abnormalities of normal tissue structure.	Ask patients about metal or wire inside their body before MRI because the procedure may be contraindicated.
Hormonal tests	Assessment of endocrine function related to reproduction	Abnormal hormone levels may identify fertility potential, reasons for abnormal menses, hormone-producing tumors, or need for hormone replacement.	Explain procedure to patient and provide support.
Invasive			
Pelvic examination or bimanual examination	Inspection and palpation of external/internal reproductive organs by HCP	Abnormal physical examination may detect pathology or may indicate need for further testing.	Explain procedure to patient and provide support.
Biopsy, cytology, swabs, or smears	Obtainment of body cells/tissue through aspiration or excision or by swabbing/scrapping of tissue/exudate	May diagnose pathology or infection.	Explain procedure to patient and provide support.
Endoscopy or laparoscopy	Use of fiber-optic light and lens system to inspect internal structures	May determine abnormal lesions or abnormalities of normal tissue structure. Tissue biopsies may be taken during procedure.	Explain procedure to patient and provide support. Observe for postprocedure complications.

One of the important first steps in collecting data on the male reproductive system is to provide a comfortable, nonjudgmental, confidential atmosphere for discussion. This means you must first be knowledgeable and comfortable with sexual issues. Although it may be challenging to ask questions about **erection** or ejaculation history, such questions may allow men to talk about difficulties they are experiencing. Be open and straightforward with all questions and answers. It may be necessary at times to use more commonly expressed sexual words instead of medical terminology. You will discover that many men do not know the function of their prostate gland or the difference between ejaculation and **orgasm.** Use the encounter as an opportunity to teach men the facts about their own sexual functioning.

> **PRACTICE ANALYSIS TIP**
> Linking NCLEX-PN® to Practice
> The LPN/LVN will identify barriers to communication.

Health History

Some basic questions to ask a male patient during reproductive data collection are found in Table 41.7. As mentioned earlier, a professional, matter-of-fact attitude, along with an explanation as to why the questions are necessary, can put both you and the patient at ease while collecting data.

> **PRACTICE ANALYSIS TIP**
> Linking NCLEX-PN® to Practice
> The LPN/LVN will collect data for health history (e.g., skin integrity, height, and weight).

> **CUE RECOGNITION 41.1**
> You are answering the triage line when a patient calls her HCP's office 3 days after a transvaginal endoscopic procedure to report that she woke up this morning with a moderate amount of bright red bleeding on her pad. What do you do?
> *Suggested answers are at the end of the chapter.*

Physical Examination

The physical examination is generally performed by an HCP trained in physical assessments. The examination begins with the patient's general appearance. He is observed for male patterns of hair growth on the head, face, chest, arms, and legs. Normal male pubic hair pattern is in a triangular shape, with hair growth up toward the umbilicus. The patient's height and muscle mass are noted. Men are commonly taller than 5 feet, 6 inches; weigh more than 135 pounds; and have shoulders that are broader than their hips. The presence of excess breast tissue may indicate **gynecomastia**, from an excess of female hormones. Abnormal findings in either hair patterns or muscle mass often indicate a hormone imbalance.

The penis, scrotum, and testes (testicles) are examined by observation and palpation with the examiner sitting in front of a standing patient. On observation, the penis is normally flaccid (soft) and hanging straight down. The size can vary greatly and should not be a concern unless it is unusually small (microphallus) or edematous. The left testis typically hangs slightly lower in the scrotum than the right.

The penis is examined for warts, sores (evidence of STIs), swelling, curves, or lumps along the shaft. The examiner also makes sure the urethral opening is at the tip of the penis and not on the underside of the shaft (**hypospadias**) or on the dorsum of the shaft (**epispadias**). If the man is not **circumcised** (surgical removal of the foreskin), the foreskin should be pulled back carefully, and the glans inspected for signs of inflammation or foul-smelling discharge. The HCP should be sure to replace the foreskin in the forward position after the examination is completed.

The scrotum and testes are carefully examined and palpated. Both testes should be present and a normal size (approximately 2 to 4 cm). The testes are egg shaped and should feel smooth and rubbery when lightly palpated between the thumb and fingers. The epididymis can be felt along the top edge and posterior section of each testis. The testes and scrotum are palpated for lumps, cysts, or tumors. If a fluid-filled mass (**hydrocele**) is found, further evaluation should be done.

A simple noninvasive test called **transillumination** determines whether a mass is fluid-filled or solid. With the room lights out, a flashlight is held behind the scrotum. If the mass is fluid, a red glow appears; if it is solid, it appears opaque. Each spermatic cord (made up of veins, arteries, lymphatics, nerves, and the vas deferens) is palpated and should feel firm and threadlike. If a condition called a **varicocele** is present, the area feels like a bag of worms. A varicocele, or swelling of the veins of the spermatic cord, is one of the most common causes of male infertility.

> **NURSING CARE TIP**
> Wrap the flashlight with clear plastic wrap to decrease the risk of contamination. Change the wrap between patients.

• WORD • BUILDING •

gynecomastia: gyneco—female + mastia—breast
hypospadias: hypo—under + spadias—span, to draw
epispadias: epi—upon + spadias—span, to draw
circumcised: circum—around + cised—cut
hydrocele: hydro—water + cele—hernia
transillumination: trans—across + illumin—light + ation—process
varicocele: varico—twisted vein + cele—swelling

Table 41.7
Subjective Data Collection for the Male Reproductive System and Sexual Health

Questions to Ask During the Health History	Rationale/Significance
Medication	
Are you using any medications (prescription, over-the-counter, and herbal remedies)? How much/how often? (For medications that affect sexual desire, erection, or ejaculation, see Chapter 43.)	Loss of sexual desire, erection, ejaculation, orgasm, or fertility can occur as a result of some medication use.
Family History	
Do you have a family history of genetically transmitted diseases (e.g., heart problems, hypertension, diabetes, cancer)? Did your mother use diethylstilbestrol (DES) during pregnancy?	These conditions put men at high risk for circulation problems that interfere with erections or congenital anomalies of reproductive organs.
Personal Habits and Health Promotion Behaviors	
Do you smoke, consume caffeine, drink alcohol, use recreational drugs, or use steroids? How much/how often? Do you use hot tubs, engage in long-distance drives, or ride a bike? How much/how often? Do you use contraceptives? What type of contraceptives do you use? How do you use them? Do you do testicular self-examinations (TSEs)? Have you noticed any changes in your testicles or other reproductive organs?	These habits may lead to decreased blood flow to penis, loss of erection; decreased testosterone (male hormone) interferes with erection and fertility; excessive heat decreases sperm production. Data will reveal knowledge/practice of health promotion behaviors, meaning of health, and history of changes or abnormalities.
Personal Health History	
Did you have mumps during adolescence, or have you recently had an infection or fever?	Some infectious processes may lead to decreased sperm production.
Mental Health	
Are you experiencing stress? How do you deal with stress? Are you having problems with a sexual partner? Have you ever or are you experiencing performance anxiety or depression?	Decreased sexual desire and ability to have an erection may result from mental and/or emotional stress.
Circulatory/Respiratory	
Have you ever been diagnosed with or treated for heart problems/surgery, high blood pressure, sickle cell disease, lung disease, or sleep apnea?	Decreased circulation can lead to inability to have a usable erection; decreased respiratory function can result in activity intolerance or loss of erection.
Gastrointestinal	
Have you ever been diagnosed with or treated for liver infection/disease or bowel problems?	Liver infections/disease can lead to decreased testosterone and increased estrogen production, and loss of erection; gastrointestinal/bowel problems can lead to pain or loss of desire; surgery may result in loss of blood flow or innervation.

Table 41.7
Subjective Data Collection for the Male Reproductive System and Sexual Health—cont'd

Questions to Ask During the Health History	Rationale/Significance
Musculoskeletal	
Do you have painful joints, pelvic/lower back pain, or nerve damage?	Pain; loss of desire; limited movement/positions; and loss of erection, ejaculation, and orgasm may result from musculoskeletal problems.
Neurologic	
Have you ever experienced a stroke or suffered from multiple sclerosis, Parkinson disease, or other neurologic disorders?	Limited movement/positions, loss of sensations, and loss of control can result from neurologic problems.
Metabolic/Endocrine	
Have you ever suffered from diabetes, obesity, or thyroid problems?	Diabetes mellitus can result in circulation problems, retrograde ejaculation, and nerve damage; obesity can result in decreased male hormones and excess female hormones.
Genitourinary	
Have you ever been diagnosed with a congenital deformity of the penis/testicles, suffered from prostate problems, or experienced erection/ejaculation problems? Have you ever been diagnosed with a sexually transmitted infection? When, what type, and how was it treated? Are you aware if treatment was successful? Do you have any lesions, pain, discharge, or swelling of the reproductive organs? Have you noticed any abnormalities/changes in size, shape, or color of your external reproductive organs? If so, describe.	Difficulty with erection, penetration problems, retrograde ejaculation, or infertility may be associated with genitourinary abnormalities, stress, or medication use. Lesions, pain, discharge, swelling, or other abnormalities of the external reproductive organs may indicate infection, structural abnormalities such as varicocele, or other disease processes such as cancer.
Do you practice monthly TSEs?	Adolescent and adult men should be encouraged to perform monthly TSEs as a cancer prevention measure.
For patients older than age 50: When was the last time you had a prostate examination?	A digital rectal examination (DRE) should be a regular part of a man's routine physical after age 50. Prostate cancer is treatable when detected early.
Sexual Practices	
Are you sexually active? How many partners do you have? Of what gender? Is the amount/type of sexual activity satisfying?	Some sexual practices can lead to a decrease in quality and quantity of sperm that reach the female egg.

The male patient is examined for inguinal hernias by pressing up through the scrotum into each of the inguinal rings while asking him to cough or bear down. Each side is examined separately while he is in the standing position. A hernia feels like a pulsation against the examiner's fingertips.

A digital rectal examination (DRE) may be done by an experienced practitioner. During DRE, the prostate gland is palpated by inserting a gloved, lubricated finger into the rectum while the man is in the Sims position or standing and bending at a right angle over the examination table. The entire posterior lobe of the gland can be felt this way. The gland should feel slightly firm and without any lumps. If the prostate gland is very hard or soft, feels enlarged, or contains any lumps, a rectal ultrasound with needle biopsy may be ordered. A swollen, painful prostate generally indicates that an infection is present.

Table 41.8
Objective Data Collection for the Male Reproductive System

Physical Examination Findings	Possible Abnormal Findings/Causes
Clinical Breast Examination (CBE) Observe and palpate for presence of swelling, lumps, skin changes, and nipple exudates.	Changes may indicate breast cancer, although it is rare in males.
Glans of Penis Observe for lesions, exudate, and tenderness. Observe for placement of the urethra. If foreskin is present, attempt to reduce to observe for lesions, exudate, and inflammation. (Be sure to replace when finished to prevent paraphimosis.)	Lesions, exudate, and tenderness can indicate presence of infective or disease process and injury. Epispadias/hypospadias may be noted when observing for placement of the urethra.
Shaft of Penis Observe for lesions, tenderness, and shape.	Lesions, exudate, and tenderness can indicate presence of infectious or disease process or injury. Irregularity of shape may indicate structural abnormalities/disease.
Scrotum Visualize and palpate for swelling, pain, and lesions.	Inguinal herniation may be noted. Swelling may occur with heart or renal failure, local inflammation, or injury.
Testes Palpate for descent, pain, lesions, size, and shape, consistency. Palpate for lesions/swelling of epididymitis.	Absence of palpated testes may indicate nondescent. Testicular lesion can indicate testicular cancer. Swelling and pain can indicate infectious process.
Spermatic Cord Palpate for swelling, size, consistency, and pain.	Presence of swelling or pain can indicate infection or varicocele.
Inguinal Ring (examination performed by trained personnel) Palpate for bulge and pain.	Bulge or pain may indicate inguinal hernia.
Inguinal Lymph Nodes Palpate for swelling and pain.	Swelling or pain may indicate infectious process or regional malignancy.
Digital Rectal Examination (DRE; performed by trained personnel) Observe external rectum for lesions and exudate. Palpate for pain, swelling, and penile exudate.	Pain, swelling, or exudate may indicate benign changes, infectious process, cancer, or injury.

Note: A male physical examination is typically done by an HCP or other trained provider.

Many men are under the impression that if they have had prostate surgery, the gland has been completely removed. When simple surgery is performed, prostate tissue is left in the body and will begin to regrow over time. This prostatic tissue can become cancerous and needs to be monitored with a yearly DRE.

Remind all men aged 50 and older to talk to their HCPs about prostate cancer screening. There are many pros and cons to screening, and each man should make a decision that is best for him. Table 41.8 provides a summary of objective data to collect for the male reproductive system.

Testicular Self-Examination

All men after puberty should do a monthly testicular self-examination (TSE) to detect any tumors or other changes in the scrotum (Fig. 41.13). See Box 41.1 for instructions that can be used to teach a man how to examine his testicles.

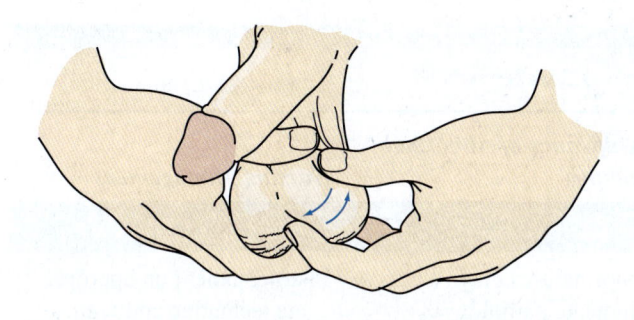

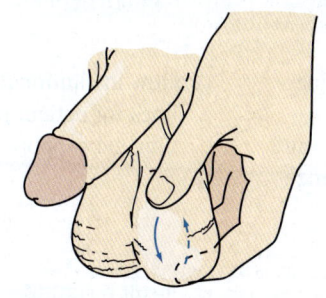

FIGURE 41.13 Testicular self-examination.

Box 41.1

Guidelines for Monthly Testicular Self-Examination

A testicular self-examination is easiest during or right after a warm shower or bath, when the scrotum is relaxed and the testicles are hanging low. Choose the same day each month to do the examination.

1. Raise the penis up out of the way and look for any difference in size or shape of each side of the scrotum (sac). The left side usually hangs a little lower than the right.
2. Using both hands, hold the scrotum in the palms. Begin, one at a time, to gently roll each testicle between the thumb and first three fingers, feeling for any lumps or hard spots.
3. Identify the parts. The testicles should feel round, smooth, and egg-shaped. The epididymis along the top and back side should feel soft and a little bit tender. The spermatic cord runs from the epididymis and usually feels firm, smooth, and movable.
4. See an HCP immediately if you feel any lumps or unusual changes.

CRITICAL THINKING & CLINICAL JUDGMENT

Tony is a 20-year-old who reports a "bump" on his right testicle. He comes into the health clinic and asks whether he can take any medication for his "disease."

Critical Thinking (The Why)
1. What might be going on with Tony?

Clinical Judgment (The Do)
2. What would be the best action?
3. What should you include in your data collection?

Suggested answers are at the end of the chapter.

Breast Self-Examination
Although breast cancer in men is rare, it can occur. Men, like women, should be familiar with their breasts and report changes.

Diagnostic Tests of the Male Reproductive System

Ultrasound
An ultrasound may be done to diagnose or evaluate various male reproductive or genitourinary problems. Transrectal ultrasound can help diagnose prostate cancer. For this procedure, a rectal probe transducer is inserted into the rectum; sound waves are used to evaluate the prostate gland.

Pelvic or scrotal ultrasound helps evaluate and locate masses. Ultrasound may also be done to guide a needle during a fine-needle biopsy. Explain the procedure to the patient. An enema may be ordered before the procedure. No special aftercare is needed.

Cystourethrography
A cystourethrogram may be done to evaluate the degree of obstruction by an enlarged prostate gland. For this procedure, a Foley catheter is inserted, and a dye is injected into the bladder. Radiographs are taken with the dye in the bladder and while voiding after the catheter has been removed. Explain the procedure to the patient and ask about allergies to dyes. Instruct the patient to void before the procedure. A sedative or analgesic may be ordered to help the patient relax during the procedure. If an analgesic is used, the patient must have someone drive him home.

After the procedure, intake and output are measured for 24 hours. Alteration from the patient's normal pattern, such as blood in urine or absence of urination, is reported to the HCP. Fluids are encouraged to promote excretion of dye. A warm, moist cloth held over the urethra can assist with mild pain.

Laboratory Tests
PROSTATE-SPECIFIC ANTIGEN. Prostate-specific antigen (PSA) is a glycoprotein produced by prostate cells. The normal value of PSA is less than 4 ng/mL. An elevated level indicates prostatic hypertrophy or cancer.

PROSTATIC ACID PHOSPHATASE. Prostatic acid phosphatase (PAP) is an enzyme that affects metabolism of prostate cancer cells. The normal value of PAP is less than 3 ng/mL. An elevated level may indicate prostate cancer.

OTHER TESTS. If prostate cancer is suspected or diagnosed, additional tests may be done. Acid phosphatase may be elevated in metastatic prostate cancer. Alkaline phosphatase and serum calcium levels may be elevated if metastasis to the bone has occurred. Table 41.9 summarizes diagnostic procedures.

Tests for Infertility
Various hormone levels may be measured, including FSH, LH, testosterone, and adrenocorticotropic hormone (ACTH),

Table 41.9
Diagnostic Procedures for the Male Reproductive System

Procedure	Definition/Normal Finding	Significance of Abnormal Findings	Nursing Management
Noninvasive			
Testicular self-examination (TSE)	Palpation of testes by patient.	Abnormalities may indicate pathology and require further evaluation.	Instruct patient on appropriate technique and witness a return demonstration.
Ultrasound	High-frequency sound waves bounce off tissue to map tissue structure and determine tissue density. Also may be used to guide biopsy procedure.	May help to determine abnormal lesions, abnormalities of tissue structure, or presence of abnormal fluid volume.	Follow institutional guidelines for patient preparation and support.
Hormonal tests and antigen level testing	Blood test to measure hormone or antigen levels.	Abnormal hormone levels may reflect fertility potential. Abnormal antigen levels may indicate pathology.	Consult institutional policies for specific instructions for each test. Explain procedure to patient and provide support.
Invasive			
Digital rectal examination (DRE)	Palpation of internal reproductive organs, especially prostate gland, through rectum.	Abnormal physical examination may indicate pathology and indicates need for further testing.	Educate patient about procedure and provide support.
Cystourethrography	Insertion of a Foley catheter and dye into the bladder to evaluate for obstruction (usually an enlarged prostate) by radiography.	Obstruction may cause difficulty with urination.	Educate patient about the procedure and postprocedure care. Instruct patient to void before procedure. Measure intake and output for 24 hours following procedure. Observe for allergic reaction.

to help determine causes of infertility in male patients. Semen analysis may provide information about causes of infertility or evaluate whether a vasectomy has been effective. Semen may be analyzed for sperm count, motility, and shape. Other tests determine whether the semen contains adequate nutrients to support sperm, whether antibodies to the sperm are present, and whether sperm can penetrate an ovum.

NURSING CARE. The patient is instructed to refrain from ejaculation for 3 days before collecting the semen sample to avoid altering findings. Generally, specimens are collected on three separate occasions over a period of 4 to 6 days. Masturbation and ejaculation directly into a sterile container are recommended to avoid loss of semen. Condoms and lubricants should be avoided. The sample should be taken to the laboratory within 1 hour of collection. Additional tests of the male reproductive system are discussed in Chapter 43.

TRANSGENDER POPULATION DATA COLLECTION

Transgender is a term used to describe individuals who identify with a gender that does not match their gender at birth. When assessing patients who identify as transgender, use a nonjudgmental approach and begin by asking the name they like to be called, which may differ from the name on their medical record. Transgender patients may be in different stages of gender-confirming surgery or may have decided to opt out of surgery. Patients transitioning from male to female may be prescribed a combination of estrogen and medications that decrease androgen levels. Patients transitioning from female to male may be taking testosterone. The transgender patient should receive the appropriate tests related to the gender assigned at birth. For example, a male converting to female will still need a prostate examination. Transgender individuals face many health disparities related to discrimination, lack of cultural competence of providers, and socioeconomic barriers. The transgender population has a high rate of unemployment and suicide; they are often victims of violence. Transgender youth may experience bullying in school. A psychosocial assessment and depression screening should be completed (Hashemi et al, 2018).

Key Points

- The female reproductive system consists of paired ovaries and fallopian tubes, a single uterus and vagina, and external genitalia. Mammary glands may be considered accessory organs.
- The ovaries produce egg cells by oogenesis (meiosis), which begins and then pauses in the fetus, resumes at puberty, and ends at menopause in a cyclical process.
- Each fallopian tube extends from near the ovary to the uterus.
- During pregnancy, the uterus increases greatly in size and contains the placenta, which nourishes the fetus until birth.
- The female external genitalia include the clitoris, mons pubis, and labia majora and minora.
- The mammary glands produce milk after pregnancy.
- The male reproductive system consists of bilateral testes and a series of tubules, ducts, and glands that contribute secretions to the sperm, producing semen.
- The testes are located in the scrotum between the upper thighs, where the temperature is slightly lower than body temperature. This is necessary to produce viable sperm.
- A series of ducts lead sperm into and through the pelvic cavity where secretions are added. Semen exits the body via the urethra.
- The urethra is the last of the male reproductive ducts. Its longest portion is within the penis. The penis is an external genital organ. Its distal end is called the glans penis. When uncircumcised, the glans penis is covered with a fold of skin called the prepuce, or foreskin.
- The reproductive capability of women ends with menopause.
- For most men, testosterone secretion and sperm production continue throughout life. Prostate enlargement is the most common age-related reproductive concern.
- Subjective data related to the female reproductive system include general personal information and menstrual, obstetrical, gynecological, sexual, family, and psychosocial histories.
- Many nurses feel awkward asking reproductive history questions, and patients may also feel uneasy with these questions. An open, honest approach can encourage the patient to feel comfortable.
- Diagnostic tests for the female reproductive system include ultrasound of the breasts and uterus, mammography (a radiographic [x-ray] examination of the breasts), blood tests for *BRCA1* and *BRCA2* and ovarian cancer, bone density testing, and hormone testing.
- The pelvic examination allows visual inspection of the vagina and cervix, as well as sampling of mucus, discharge, cells, and exudates. Palpation of portions of the reproductive system and some treatments may also be done as part of the procedure.
- Male reproductive diagnostic tests include digital rectal examination of the prostate, testicular examination, ultrasound of the prostate, cystourethrogram, blood tests for PSA, and other tests.
- Transgender individuals may be taking medications such as estrogen, testosterone, or medications that decrease androgen levels. Transgender individuals will need screenings based on their gender assigned at birth.

SUGGESTED ANSWERS TO CHAPTER EXERCISES

Cue Recognition
41.1: Have the patient come in for an evaluation.

Critical Thinking & Clinical Judgment
Jill
1. Knowing her breasts and reporting changes are essential so that she can report any changes or abnormalities to her HCP.
2. The answer should include basic breast health statistics and risks as well as proper assessment practice and techniques, as discussed in this chapter. She should be informed that, although monthly BSE is not absolutely necessary, technique should be demonstrated and a return demonstration done during the visit.
3. Questions about breast health and self-assessment practices provide an opportunity for the nurse to educate a patient about health facts and technique. Patient questions can also be a cue to patient readiness and willingness to learn

Reproductive Data Collection

1. Calm fears. Explain simply. Allow the parent to stay with the child during the examination if appropriate. Consider whether it is possible that the child has been abused. If so, evidence needs to be collected and a report filed with the appropriate child protection authorities. Check with your supervisor if you believe this is a possibility. Let the child know that this is a normal part of the body that is to be protected and taken care of.
2. Assess knowledge and maturity. Prepare the patient for a Pap smear and for swabs and smears. Explain the procedure while getting supplies ready. Explain that vaginal soreness usually needs to be treated and that the HCP must know more about the problem to do so effectively. Explain that inflammation can interfere with Pap smear results, so testing may have to be repeated after treatment. Explain culture and sensitivity testing. Remind patient about risk reduction and that oral contraceptives do not prevent STIs.
3. Try to put the woman at ease through general conversation. Set out supplies for a Pap smear (if needed) and for swabs and smears. Explain the procedure while getting supplies ready. Discuss aging and the effects of decreased estrogen in general and specifically on vaginal tissues. Inform her that there are several ways to deal with problems resulting from decreased estrogen, such as oral hormonal replacements, water-soluble vaginal lubricants, vaginal creams, estrogen patches, and selective estrogen receptor modulators.

Tony

1. Palpable scrotal changes can result from a variety of reproductive and/or genitourinary abnormalities. Before Tony's question can be answered, a complete history needs to be obtained and a clinical examination of the genitalia performed.
2. Collect a history from Tony.
3. The history should explore the following:
   - Whether testicular self-examinations are regularly performed and whether any other changes are noted
   - Whether Tony is sexually active and has recently or in the past been knowingly exposed to an STI
   - When Tony first felt the bump
   - Whether there has been pain associated with the bump or exudate noted from the penis

The assessment, done by an HCP, should include the following:

- Visual inspection of the size, shape, symmetry, and color of the scrotum and its contents
- Palpation to assess for abnormalities and pain
- Cultures to rule out STIs
- An inguinal examination to rule out herniation

Ultimately, based on the patient's report, a testicular tumor should be ruled out.

Additional Resources

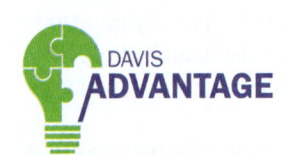

Go to Davis Advantage to complete your learning: strengthen understanding, apply your knowledge, and prepare for the Next Gen NCLEX®.

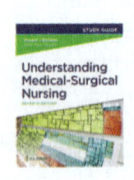

A Study Guide is also available.

CHAPTER 42
Nursing Care of Women With Reproductive System Disorders

Sarah Holda, Laura L. McCully

KEY TERMS

agenesis (ay-JEN-uh-sis)
amenorrhea (AY-men-oh-REE-ah)
anteflexion (AN-tee-FLEK-shun)
anteversion (AN-tee-VER-zhun)
augmentation (AWG-men-TAY-shun)
colporrhaphy (kohl-POOR-ah-fee)
contraceptive (KON-truh-SEP-tiv)
cryotherapy (KRY-oh-THER-uh-pee)
culdocentesis (KUL-doh-sen-TEE-sis)
culdotomy (kul-DOT-uh-mee)
cystocele (SIS-toh-seel)
dermoid (DER-moyd)
dilation and curettage (DIL-AY-shun and kyoor-e-TAHZH)
dysmenorrhea (DIS-men-oh-REE-ah)
dyspareunia (DIS-puh-ROO-nee-ah)
dysplasia (dis-PLAY-zee-ah)
fibrocystic (FY-broh-SIS-tik)
hypertrophy (hy-PER-truh-fee)
hypoplasia (HY-poh-PLAY-zee-ah)
hysterectomy (HISS-tuh-REK-tuh-mee)
hysterotomy (HISS-tuh-RAH-tuh-mee)
imperforate (im-PER-foh-rate)
in vitro fertilization (in VEE-troh FER-ti-li-ZAY-shun)
laparotomy (LAP-uh-RAH-tuh-mee)
leiomyoma (LYE-oh-my-OH-mah)
lumpectomy (lump-EK-tuh-mee)
mammoplasty (MAM-oh-PLAS-tee)
marsupialization (mar-SOO-pee-al-ih-ZAY-shun)
mastalgia (mass-TAL-jee-ah)
mastectomy (mass-TEK-tuh-mee)
mastitis (mass-TY-tis)
mastopexy (MAS-toh-PEKS-ee)
myomectomy (MY-oh-MEK-tuh-mee)
oophorectomy (oo-fur-EK-tuh-mee)
perimenopause (PER-ee-MEN-oh-PAWS)
phytoestrogens (FY-toh-ES-troh-jenz)
postcoital (post-KOH-ih-tal)
rectocele (REK-toh-seel)

retroflexion (REH-troh-FLEK-shun)
retrograde (REH-troh-grade)
retroversion (REH-troh-VER-zhun)
salpingectomy (sal-pin-JEK-tuh-mee)
teratoma (ter-uh-TOH-muh)
vaginitis (VAJ-in-EYE-tis)
vaginosis (VAJ-in-OH-sis)

LEARNING OUTCOMES

1. Explain the pathophysiology of each of the disorders of the female reproductive system.
2. Describe the etiologies, signs, and symptoms of each disorder.
3. Identify tests used to diagnose female disorders.
4. Describe current therapeutic management for each disorder.
5. List data to collect when caring for patients with disorders of the female reproductive system.
6. Plan nursing care for female patients with reproductive disorders.
7. Explain how you will know whether nursing interventions have been effective.
8. Compare different forms of contraceptives and their effectiveness.

CHAPTER CONCEPTS

Family
Health promotion
Reproduction and sexuality
Self

Reproductive system disorders can be frightening, irritating, frustrating, embarrassing, and, in some cases, fatal. They involve not just body parts but also roles, relationships, and sense of identity and purpose in life. Nurses can play an important role in helping women with these disorders. Many ongoing research studies focus on aspects of women's health. The Nurses' Health Study, conducted at Harvard Medical School, is a large ongoing study on many topics related to women's health. You can learn about it at www.nurseshealthstudy.org.

BREAST DISORDERS

Benign Breast Disorders

Cyclic Breast Discomfort

PATHOPHYSIOLOGY, ETIOLOGIES, AND SIGNS AND SYMPTOMS. The most common breast symptoms result from cyclic variations in hormone levels. Swelling, tenderness, and sometimes pain (**mastalgia**) can be related to hormone-mediated changes within the breast tissues that prepare them for their potential role of breastfeeding.

THERAPEUTIC MEASURES. If persistent or severe, these symptoms can be treated with oral contraceptives that modify hormone levels or NSAIDs to control pain. Explaining that cyclic discomfort is temporary and not from a disease process helps to reduce anxiety.

Fibrocystic Breast Disease

PATHOPHYSIOLOGY, ETIOLOGIES, AND SIGNS AND SYMPTOMS. Fibrocystic breast disease is common in women between the ages of 30 and 50. An excess response of the cells in the breasts to hormonal stimulation (especially estrogen) can cause long-term changes, resulting in replacement of normal tissue with fibrous tissue. This makes the breasts feel hard, lumpy, and sometimes painful. Overdevelopment of cells and blockage of ducts can form cysts around fluid, resulting in green or brownish drainage. These changes often occur during the reproductive years and can be responses to hormonal variations during the menstrual cycle. Fibrocystic changes usually subside with menopause.

DIAGNOSIS. Fibrocystic breast changes can be identified on palpation. A mammogram or ultrasound may be done to aid in diagnosis. A biopsy may be done to rule out cancer.

THERAPEUTIC MEASURES. Treatment for fibrocystic breast changes is based on patient symptoms. Often, no treatment is necessary. Analgesics (primarily NSAIDs) and use of a supportive bra can help reduce discomfort. Herbal remedies, such as evening primrose oil, or supplemental vitamin E therapy may offer symptomatic relief, but these therapies remain controversial. Limitation of dietary fat and caffeine and addition of oral contraceptive use may help control hormonal changes.

Although fibrocystic changes are not cancerous, more frequent mammography or ultrasound may be advised because these changes can make it more difficult to feel early cancerous lumps during breast examination. Some types of breast cysts are associated with a higher cancer risk. Needle aspiration may be used to treat cystic lesions.

Mastitis

PATHOPHYSIOLOGY, ETIOLOGIES, AND SIGNS AND SYMPTOMS. Mastitis is breast inflammation that may also involve infection. It occurs as a result of injury and possible introduction of bacteria into the breast. This condition most commonly occurs while breastfeeding. The breast becomes swollen, hot, red, and painful; an abscess can form.

THERAPEUTIC MEASURES. Mastitis can be treated either with antibiotics or rarely by incision and drainage of the abscessed area. NSAIDs, warm packs, and breast supports are often used to control pain and swelling.

NURSING CARE AND PATIENT EDUCATION. Advise the patient to wash hands carefully to prevent the spread of infection. If the patient is breastfeeding, it is often continued to promote drainage of the breast, mother–infant bonding, and infant nutrition. For more information about mastitis during breastfeeding, refer to your maternity text.

Malignant Breast Disorders

Pathophysiology and Etiology

Breast cancer is an abnormal growth of breast cells. It can arise from the milk-producing glands, the ductal system, or the fatty and connective tissues of the breast. It is the second most diagnosed cancer in women (Centers for Disease Control and Prevention, 2020).

Research has identified many factors that increase the risk of breast cancer in women. These include increasing age; being Black, Asian, or Latina; personal or family history of breast cancer; being overweight or obese; alcohol use; smoking; hormone replacement therapy; early menarche; late menopause; and first pregnancy after age 30. There are also many emerging risk factors being identified, such as low vitamin D levels, eating grilled meats with low intake of fruits and vegetables, and exposure to certain chemicals used in gardening. See more at www.breastcancer.org/risk/factors.

Signs and Symptoms

A lump or thickening of breast tissue or change in the shape or contour of a breast can indicate breast cancer. A tumor can cause dimpling of the overlying skin (called *peau d'orange*, or orange skin) or retraction of the nipple. Clear or bloody nipple discharge can occur. Swelling, tenderness, or discoloration of the breast can indicate inflammatory breast cancer, a rare but deadly form. Breast symptoms have many causes and should be investigated by a health-care provider (HCP).

Prevention

Breast cancer risk can be reduced by exercising, moderating fat and alcohol consumption, and using nonhormonal methods for birth control and menopausal symptoms. Breastfeeding may also reduce risk, even in women who have late first pregnancies. However, many factors cannot be controlled, so the importance of early detection cannot be overemphasized. Certain genes (*BRCA1* and *BRCA2*) are linked with susceptibility to breast cancer.

• WORD • BUILDING •

mastalgia: mast—breast + algia—pain
fibrocystic: fibro—fibrous + cystic—sac-like
mastitis: mast—breast + itis—inflammation

Genetic testing offers the possibility of very early identification of women at the highest risk of developing breast cancer (as well as ovarian cancer for those with *BRCA1*). These women can then be monitored closely for breast changes and receive early treatment if cancer develops. Some women choose to have bilateral prophylactic (risk-reducing) mastectomy.

Before genetic testing, patients should be counseled by a professional who is qualified to explain and interpret the results. It is also important to review risks and benefits of testing. Some insurance plans do not cover the cost of such testing. More information regarding *BRCA* testing can be found at www.cancer.gov.

Diagnostic Tests

Breast self-examination (BSE) and clinical breast examination (CBE) may play an important role in cancer identification. Cancerous growths tend to be harder, less mobile, less painful, and more irregularly shaped. They also have less clearly defined borders than benign growths. The most common location for a malignant tumor is in the upper outer quadrant of the breast, but they can occur anywhere in the breast tissue. The prognosis is good for women who have breast cancer removed in early stages but gets worse when treatment begins during later stages of the disease process. Teaching and encouraging regular use of BSE and appropriate use of mammography can save lives. See Chapter 41 for more about BSE and for explanations about diagnostic tests used to assist in determining whether tumors of the breast are malignant.

Staging

The spread (metastasis) of cancerous cells from the primary site to other areas of the body by way of the blood or lymph is denoted by staging classifications 0 to IV (see Chapter 11). Lower numbers indicate less cancer spread.

Therapeutic Measures

Treatment options for breast cancer are surgery, radiation therapy, chemotherapy, hormone therapy, targeted therapies, and immunotherapy. These may be used separately or in combination depending on the condition of the patient and the stage of the disease. Patients may also choose complementary and holistic therapies, to be used in tandem with traditional treatments.

SURGERY. A **lumpectomy** removes just the tumor and a margin around it. A **mastectomy** may be partial (removing only part of the breast), simple (removing the breast tissue of one or both breasts), or radical (removing breast tissue, underlying muscle, and surrounding lymph nodes). The amount of tissue removed varies depending on the size, nature, and invasiveness of the cancer. Surgical practice has shifted from radical mastectomies to more breast-conserving surgeries with the addition of radiation therapy, resulting in survival rates similar to those for radical mastectomy. Surgeries to remove cancerous breast tissue can be disfiguring and have profound effects on a patient's body image and self-esteem.

RADIATION THERAPY. Radiation can be administered externally or internally to attack the rapidly dividing cells of a tumor. Although radiation affects all rapidly dividing cells in its path, including healthy cells, radiation to an area of the breast just surrounding the tumor bed reduces the incidence of side effects. It is often used after surgery to reduce the risk of cancer recurrence or spread.

CHEMOTHERAPY. Chemotherapy kills all rapidly dividing cells, not just breast cancer cells, which leads to many side effects. It may be used alone or in combination with other therapies. Newer chemotherapy options use higher doses over a shorter treatment period to reduce side effects (see Chapter 11).

HORMONE THERAPY. Hormone therapy may be used to deprive cancer cells of hormones that stimulate their growth. Because breast cancer cells are often estrogen-sensitive, this may be accomplished by decreasing circulating estrogen levels with drugs or by blocking the use of estrogen by cancer cells. Interference with estrogen levels, however, may produce menopausal symptoms and increase the risk of osteoporosis and heart disease. Table 42.1 lists estrogen antagonists.

TARGETED THERAPIES. Targeted therapies attack specific molecular agents or pathways involved in the development of cancer. Some targeted therapies are given to intensify positive body responses (e.g., stimulate the immune system) or to decrease negative body responses. Because they target cancer cells, they are less toxic to normal cells. Examples include biological response modifiers such as interferons, tumor necrosis factor, interleukins, and various experimental immunotherapy formulations. Some drugs, such as trastuzumab (Herceptin), pertuzumab (Perjeta), and lapatinib (Tykerb), target the protein HER2, found on the surface of breast cancer cells,

IMMUNOTHERAPIES. Immunotherapy is a newer field of breast cancer treatment that uses the body's immune system to fight cancer. Immunotherapy may be combined with chemotherapy.

ALTERNATIVE THERAPIES. Alternative therapies are also available for many cancers. See Chapter 5 for information about helping patients evaluate alternative and complementary therapies. The American Cancer Society and cancer treatment centers also have staff who can answer questions about experimental and alternative therapies and discuss research findings. For more information about breast cancer, visit the American Cancer Society at www.cancer.org.

• WORD • BUILDING •

lumpectomy: lump + ec—away + tomy—cutting
mastectomy: mast—breast + ec—away + tomy—cutting

Table 42.1
Medications for Disorders Related to Hormonal Alterations (Breast Disorders, Menstrual Disorders, Menopause)

Medication Class/Action

Contraceptives

Interfere with the release of gonadotropin-releasing hormone (GnRH), luteinizing hormone (LH), and follicle-stimulating hormone (FSH); also maintain stable hormonal levels, relax uterus, and limit endometrial proliferation.

Examples	Nursing Implications
Progesterone and estrogen *Oral:* norethindrone acetate and ethinyl estradiol (Loestrin) drospirenone and ethinyl estradiol (Yasmin, Yaz) levonorgestrel and ethinyl estradiol (Aviane) ethinyl estradiol/norgestimate (Ortho Tri-Cyclen) *Patch:* norelgestromin and ethinyl estradiol (Ortho Evra) *Vaginal ring:* etonogestrel and ethinyl estradiol (NuvaRing) **Progesterone only** norethindrone (Micronor) medroxyprogesterone Acetate (Depo-Provera) levonorgestrel-releasing intrauterine system (Mirena, Skyla, Kyleena) etonogestrel implant (Nexplanon)	*Teach:* About use and side effects (see ACHES Learning Tip). Smoking increases risk of blood clots; advise to stop smoking while on these medications.

Hormone Replacement Therapy (HRT)

Interferes with GnRH, LH, and FSH release; maintains stable hormonal levels, relaxes uterus, limits endometrial proliferation, promotes vasomotor stability, prevents bone loss.

Examples	Nursing Implications
Progesterone and estrogen: conjugated estrogens and medroxyprogesterone (Prempro) estradiol and norethindrone acetate (Activella) **Estrogen only** conjugated estrogens (Premarin, Cenestin) estradiol (Estrace, Climara) **Vaginal preparations** conjugated estrogens (Premarin cream) estradiol (Estrace cream, Vagifem, Estring) **Progesterone only** norethindrone (Micronor) medroxyprogesterone acetate (Provera) **Estrogen and testosterone** esterified estrogens and methyltestosterone (Estratest)	*Teach:* About use and side effects (see ACHES Learning Tip). Smoking increases risk of blood clots; advise to stop smoking while on these medications.

Estrogen Antagonists

Inhibit growth of estrogen-dependent tumors.

Examples	Nursing Implications
tamoxifen (Nolvadex) anastrozole (Arimidex) toremifene (Fareston) exemestane (Aromasin) letrozole (Femara) fulvestrant (Faslodex)	Promote use of nonhormonal contraceptives during use. *Teach:* Report vaginal bleeding, leg cramps, shortness of breath, and weakness. Smoking increases risk of blood clots; advise to stop smoking during use.

Nursing Care

See "Nursing Care Plan for the Patient Undergoing a Mastectomy." In addition to the diagnoses covered, the patient will need preoperative teaching and support, and care for postoperative pain. See Chapters 10 and 12, respectively, for additional interventions for pain and patients undergoing surgery, including drain care. Table 42.2 provides a breast cancer summary.

Nursing Care Plan for the Patient Undergoing a Mastectomy

Nursing Diagnosis: *Risk for Ineffective Peripheral Tissue Perfusion* related to damage to blood and lymph vessels and tension at surgical incision site
Expected Outcome: The patient's incision will heal by primary intention without excessive bleeding or swelling.
Evaluation of Outcome: Are edges of the incision well approximated, with scant bleeding/serous drainage and mild edema/erythema?

Intervention	Rationale	Evaluation
Monitor vital signs and SpO$_2$ according to agency policy and as necessary.	Vital signs and SpO$_2$ affect tissue perfusion and oxygenation.	Are vital signs and SpO$_2$ stable and within normal range? Are extremities pink and warm?
Avoid use of the affected arm for blood pressures, venipunctures, and injections. Place a wrist band or signage to alert staff to avoid using affected arm.	Restrictive and invasive procedures might further compromise tissue integrity of the arm.	Is arm protected?
Monitor incision for bleeding, amount and color of drainage, and swelling. Empty drain device every two hours or as needed. Document drainage amount and characteristics according to agency policy.	Excessive bleeding or swelling can compromise tissue perfusion.	Does incisional area look swollen, smooth, or shiny? Are drainage amount and color appropriate?
Measure circumference of both arms daily and compare. Report changes.	Swelling causes an increase in circumference and impairs circulation.	Is affected arm larger than unaffected arm?
Elevate affected arm higher than heart whenever possible if swelling occurs.	Gravity aids fluid return to the heart.	Does elevation reduce swelling?
Place items where patient can easily reach them.	Excessive movement of the affected arm may exert tension on incision and increase bleeding.	Can patient reach items without abducting the arm more than 90 degrees?
Reinforce postmastectomy exercises of affected arm according to agency protocol. Ensure that patient has written instructions for home use.	Appropriate exercise promotes circulation, preserves muscle and joint function, and increases self-care ability.	Is patient moving arm appropriately and gradually increasing range of motion and self-care ability?
Reinforce postoperative teaching about self-care and signs and symptoms of ineffective healing to report.	Early recognition and intervention help prevent the development of serious complications.	Does patient demonstrate and verbalize understanding of appropriate postoperative self-care?

(nursing care plan continues on page 820)

Nursing Care Plan for the Patient Undergoing a Mastectomy—cont'd

Nursing Diagnosis: *Risk for Ineffective Coping* related to cancer threat and body image disturbance
Expected Outcomes: The patient will verbalize ability to cope and will seek help and support appropriately.
Evaluation of Outcomes: Does the patient take an interest in care of condition? Does the patient ask appropriate questions related to care and verbalize appropriate concerns?

Intervention	Rationale	Evaluation
Observe patient's interest in self-care, ability to problem solve, and level of family or other support.	*Poor self-care, poor problem-solving skills, and lack of support may indicate a risk for ineffective coping.*	Does patient solve problems appropriately? Are family members or other support persons present? Is patient taking an active interest in her personal appearance?
Use therapeutic communication and listening skills to allow patient to share concerns.	*Loss of a breast disturbs many aspects of body image, and cancer threatens one's sense of security and stability in life.*	Is patient able to share concerns with nurse or other appropriate person?
Help patient remember previous successes in coping and strategies used.	*Memory of prior success can encourage hope for future success.*	Does patient possess appropriate coping strategies?
Provide accurate information about surgery and postoperative care, according to agency policy. Make sure patient's questions and concerns have been addressed by registered nurse or surgeon.	*Fear of the unknown can increase anxiety and reduce coping.*	Does patient relate understanding of follow-up treatment?
Refer to appropriate agencies for further support as needed (e.g., American Cancer Society, Reach to Recovery, local support groups).	*Social support can assist individuals to meet their needs while developing effective coping skills and strategies.*	Does patient have resources to call on as needed?

Table 42.2
Breast Cancer Summary

Signs and Symptoms	Swelling, tenderness, pain, redness Palpable lumps Leakage of fluid/blood from nipple Changes in contour of skin of breast/nipple
Diagnostic Tests and Findings	Breast self-examination (BSE) and clinical breast examination (CBE) Mammography Excisional/fine-needle biopsy
Therapeutic Measures	Lumpectomy, mastectomy, breast reconstruction Radiation Chemotherapy Hormone therapy Targeted therapy Immunotherapy
Complications	Metastasis Significant treatment side effects Profound negative effect on patient's self-image.
Priority Nursing Diagnoses	*Risk for Ineffective Peripheral Tissue Perfusion* *Ineffective Coping*

CLINICAL JUDGMENT

Julie, age 32, reports pain and grapelike "lumps" in her breasts, and her nurse practitioner diagnoses fibrocystic changes.

1. What questions would you ask to collect additional data related to Julie's symptoms?
2. What information can you provide for Julie to help her control her symptoms?
3. What can Julie do to remain vigilant for more concerning changes in her breasts?

Suggested answers are at the end of the chapter.

Breast Modification Surgeries

Mammoplasty is surgical modification of the breast and may be done to restore a normal shape after removal of cancerous tissues. Many women also have elective mammoplasty to change the size or appearance of breasts. Body image is an important component of quality of life.

Breast Reduction and Mastopexy

Generally, in breast reduction operations, the nipple is separated from the surrounding tissue except for a small section with the blood vessels and nerves that supply it (Fig. 42.1). A large wedge of tissue is removed from the bottom of the breast, the edges are sewn together, and the nipple is reimplanted in a higher position. This not only decreases the overall size of the breast, which may help with back, neck, and head pain, but also corrects excessive sagging—a common problem for women with large breasts.

A **mastopexy** involves the removal of some skin and fat with subsequent repair and suturing so that the breast tissues are held higher on the chest to correct sagging breasts. This procedure usually does not remove as much tissue as a breast reduction.

Augmentation and Reconstruction Mammoplasty

Augmentation is a surgery to increase the size of the breasts. An implant—a bag containing either saline solution

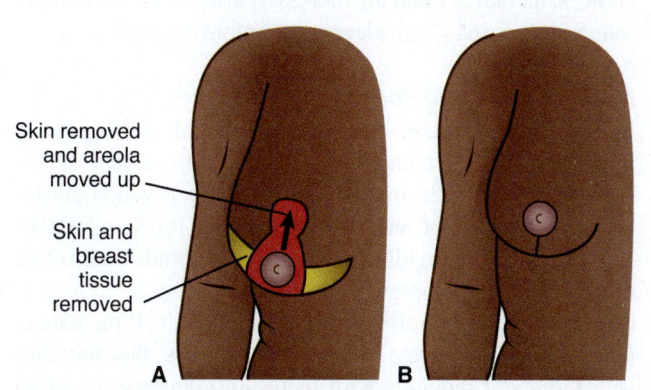

FIGURE 42.1 Breast reduction. (A) Skin and tissue removed; areola moved up. (B) Postoperative scars fade over time.

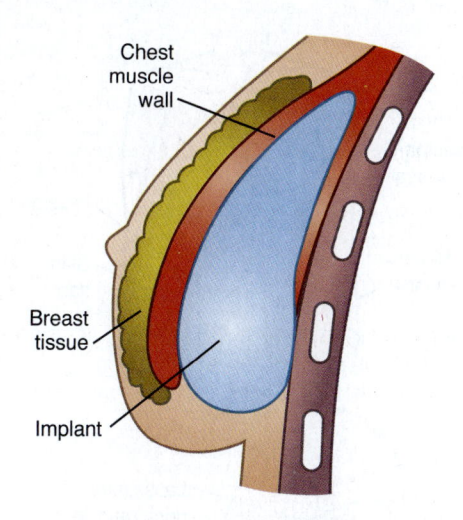

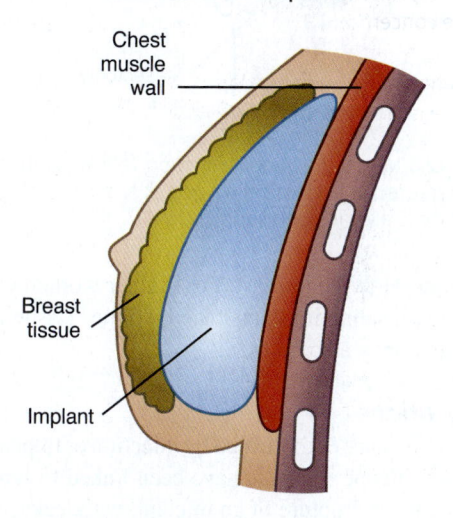

FIGURE 42.2 Breast implants. (A) Implant above pectoralis major and minor muscles. (B) Implant between pectoralis major and minor muscles.

or silicone gel or a transplanted portion of the patient's own body tissues from another area—is inserted through an incision and positioned either under or over the pectoral muscles (Fig. 42.2).

For reconstructive mammoplasty, use of the patient's own tissues is generally safer than use of artificial implants because no foreign material is introduced into the body. For situations in which significant amounts of tissue are needed for reconstruction, a portion of tissue may be moved from one area of the body to another as a pedicle graft. *Pedicle* literally means "little foot" because the graft remains attached to a stalk (containing the blood vessels and nerves) somewhat resembling a little leg with a foot (the graft) attached.

Figure 42.3 shows two options for mastectomy reconstruction surgery. Using the patient's own tissue can create

• WORD • BUILDING •

mammoplasty: mamm(o)—breast + plasty—to mold
mastopexy: masto—breast + pexy—fixation

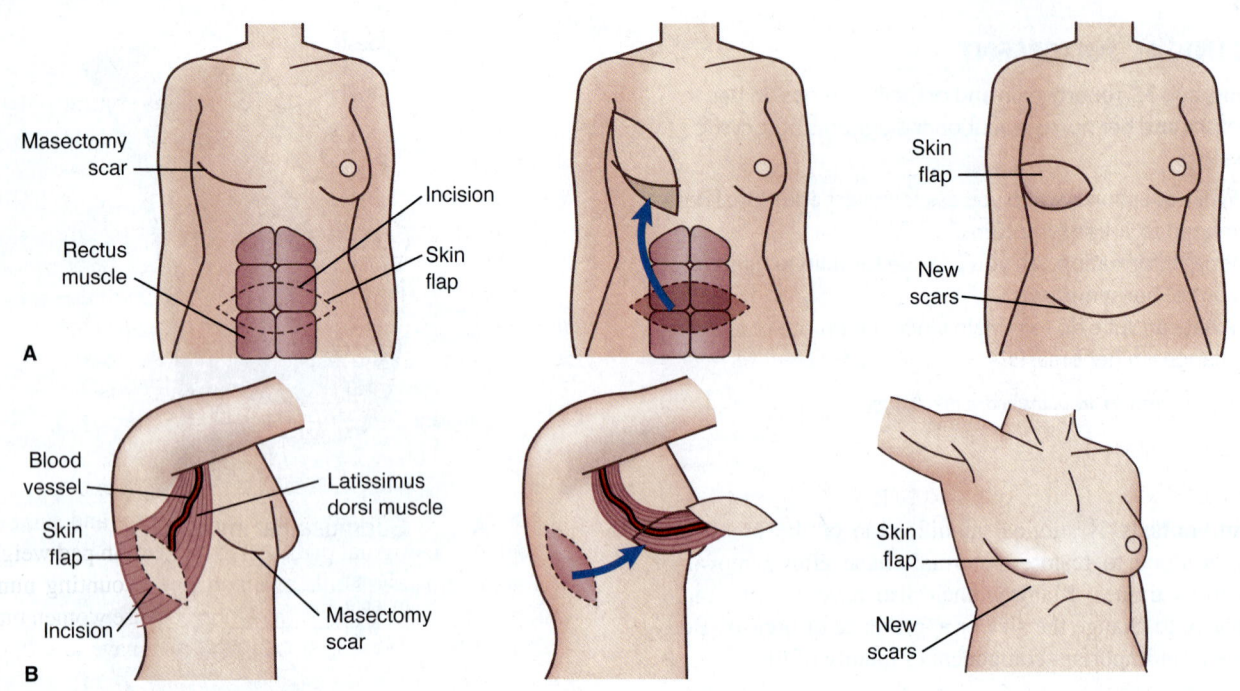

FIGURE 42.3 Mastectomy reconstruction. (A) Latissimus dorsi flap uses skin, blood vessels, and muscle to create new breast-like tissue. (B) Transverse rectus abdominal muscle, skin, and vessels can be pulled through abdomen to breast area or separated and moved to breast area (attaching a local blood supply).

a more natural feeling breast. For thinner women with little excess tissue, saline implants may be done. Tissue from the buttock area may also be used.

Complications
Any surgery can be complicated by infection or impaired healing. Some silicone implants have been linked to lymphoma, a type of cancer. Rupture of an implant, with leakage of contents, may require removal and replacement of the implant.

Nursing Care and Patient Education
Carefully monitor the healing process when changing dressings and explain to the patient how to monitor healing, because not all tissues successfully attach at the new site. Failure of attachment can require surgical revision. Signs of poor attachment include unnatural color of the incision, graft, or surrounding tissues; swelling; drainage; gaping incision lines; and sloughing of the graft or edges of the site.

MENSTRUAL DISORDERS

Premenstrual Syndrome and Premenstrual Dysphoric Disorder
Pathophysiology, Etiologies, and Signs and Symptoms
Premenstrual syndrome (PMS) is a recurrent problem for many women. Although the exact cause is not understood, ovarian hormones, aldosterone, and neurotransmitters such as monoamine oxidase and serotonin are believed to play a role. Symptoms include water retention; headaches; discomfort in joints, muscles, and breasts; changes in affect, concentration, and coordination; and sensory changes. Few women have serious PMS that affects work or relationships.

Premenstrual dysphoric disorder (PMDD) is a condition like PMS but much more severe. Women experience symptoms of depression, irritability, and tension before menstruation. They may have mood swings, feelings of hopelessness, and suicidal ideation. As is the case for PMS, the exact cause is unknown.

Therapeutic Measures
A variety of drugs have been given to combat PMS and PMDD with varying degrees of success. Some commonly used medications include NSAIDs, hormonal contraceptives, antidepressants, and diuretics as well as supplements of calcium, magnesium, vitamin E, and vitamin B_6. Patients should be warned that dosages of vitamins should not be increased without professional advice because vitamins are medications as well as nutrients. High doses of some vitamins can lead to physiological damage. Regular exercise and healthy choices, including reducing intake of caffeine, alcohol, sugar, salt, and smoking, help alleviate symptoms as well.

Nursing Care and Patient Education
Being understanding and nonjudgmental is especially important. Some women who suffer with severe symptoms may have been treated as if they are psychologically impaired because of outdated ideas about PMS or PMDD. You can help by providing educational materials on lifestyle measures and encouraging the patient to engage in regular exercise and develop stress management skills. If the patient is experiencing severe depression, discuss the possibility of suicidal thoughts with increasing depression during the second half of the menstrual cycle. Counsel the patient who has suicidal thoughts to call 911 or seek medical care immediately.

Flow and Cycle Disorders

Pathophysiology, Etiologies, and Signs and Symptoms

There are many types of menstrual abnormalities (Table 42.3). Causes can include stress, pregnancy, hormonal imbalances, metabolic imbalances (such as obesity, anorexia nervosa, and excessive exercise), tumors (both benign and malignant), infections, organ diseases (such as liver, kidney, or thyroid disease), blood or bone marrow abnormalities, and the presence of foreign bodies in the uterus (such as intrauterine devices [IUDs]). Menstrual abnormalities can be distressing, often resulting in anemia, persistent fatigue, and sexual dysfunction. Establishment of a comfortable and open professional relationship between a woman and her nurse or HCP is essential for communication about such concerns.

Diagnostic Tests

Appropriate testing to determine the cause of menstrual abnormalities involves a thorough history and physical examination. Papanicolaou (Pap) smear, cervical and vaginal cultures, laparoscopy, ultrasound, imaging studies, endometrial biopsy, pregnancy testing, urine testing, and blood testing may be done to screen for disorders that influence menstrual cycle and flow.

Table 42.3
Menstrual Flow Disorders

Disorder	Description
Amenorrhea	Menses absent for more than 6 months or three cycles in a row Called *primary amenorrhea* when menarche has not occurred by age 17 Called *secondary amenorrhea* when menses are absent after menarche
Hypermenorrhea	Menses lasting longer than 7 days
Hypomenorrhea	Less than the expected amount of menstrual bleeding
Menometrorrhagia (also called metromenorrhagia)	Overly long, heavy, and irregular menses
Menorrhagia	Passing more than 80 mL of blood per menses
Oligomenorrhea	Menstrual cycles of more than 35 days
Polymenorrhea	Menses more frequently than 21-day intervals

Therapeutic Measures

Medical treatment of menstrual disorders often involves manipulation of hormone levels with birth control pills or use of NSAIDs. Surgical treatment can involve **dilation and curettage** (D&C), laser ablation of endometrial tissue, and **hysterectomy** (removal of the uterus). During D&C, the cervix is first dilated (opened wider); a curette (a sharp, spoonlike instrument) is then inserted through the cervix and used to scoop out the inner lining of the uterus. Laser ablation involves targeted burning of endometrial tissue so that scar tissue forms that does not bleed. Hysterectomy is a last-resort treatment and is described later in this chapter.

Nursing Care

The only accurate way to estimate menstrual flow is to weigh used sanitary pads (sealed in a biohazard bag) and subtract the weight of the original pads. A 1-g increase in pad weight equals approximately 1 mL of blood loss. Counting numbers of pads used is much less accurate, because women may change pads at different intervals. You may have to rely on a woman's report of blood loss. Be sure to include "patient estimate" when you document.

D&C is typically done as an outpatient procedure. Women can expect some cramping and spotting or light bleeding for a few days afterward.

Dysmenorrhea

Pathophysiology, Etiologies, and Signs and Symptoms

Painful menstruation, or **dysmenorrhea**, is a common problem in women. Primary dysmenorrhea (menstrual cramps) is not pathological and is thought to be caused mainly by the action of endogenous prostaglandins that stimulate uterine contractions, producing cramping pain. Secondary dysmenorrhea is caused by a reproductive tract disorder such as endometriosis, pelvic infection, retroversion of the uterus, or fibroid tumors.

Diagnostic Tests

Hormonal tests of estrogen and progesterone levels may be evaluated for primary dysmenorrhea. Additional tests such as laparoscopic examination, imaging studies, biopsies, or cultures may be required for investigation of secondary dysmenorrhea.

Therapeutic Measures

Primary dysmenorrhea can be treated with drugs that inhibit prostaglandin synthesis, such as aspirin and NSAIDs. Correction of secondary causes of dysmenorrhea may include such measures as hormonal adjustment with oral contraceptives or hormone replacement therapy, D&C, or other surgical or medical intervention based on the cause.

• WORD • BUILDING •

dilation and curettage: dilat(e)—to widen + ation—the process of + curet—scoop + tage—doing
hysterectomy: hyster—womb + ec—away + tomy—cutting
dysmenorrhea: dys—painful + men(o)—month + rrhea—flow

Nursing Care and Patient Education

Regular exercise and stress management may help reduce symptoms. A warm heating pad to the abdomen or a warm bath can reduce discomfort. If dysmenorrhea is related to uterine retroversion, assuming a knee-to-chest position may relieve the discomfort. Sudden development of dysmenorrhea in a woman with no previous menstrual discomfort should always be investigated.

Endometriosis
Pathophysiology, Etiologies, and Signs and Symptoms

Endometriosis is a condition in which functioning endometrial tissue is located outside the uterus (Fig. 42.4). One cause is **retrograde** menstruation, backward leakage of blood and tissue into the fallopian tubes and pelvic cavity. Wayward endometriotic cells then grow into tissues such as the intestinal walls, ovaries, and other abdominal structures. On a cyclic basis, mediated by ovarian hormones, these cells build up and slough as they would in the uterus. However, sloughing and bleeding occur in the enclosed abdominal cavity or into the tissues they have invaded. Accumulation of blood and cells can result in pain, swelling, damage to abdominal organs and structures, scar tissue development, and infertility. During diagnostic testing, the HCP may note blue-black "powder burns" or brownish "chocolate cysts," cysts filled with old blood.

Therapeutic Measures

Surgical intervention may be required, especially if scar tissue develops into tight bands that impede sections of bowel or ureters. Reduction of estrogen and prevention of ovulation either with medications or by surgical removal of the ovaries can be effective but result in infertility and menopausal symptoms. Analgesics may be required for pain.

Nursing Care and Patient Education

The severity and persistence of the pain of endometriosis can lead to reliance on pain medication, so it is important to teach patients alternative and complementary pain relief strategies such as relaxation exercises and application of heat to the abdomen or back.

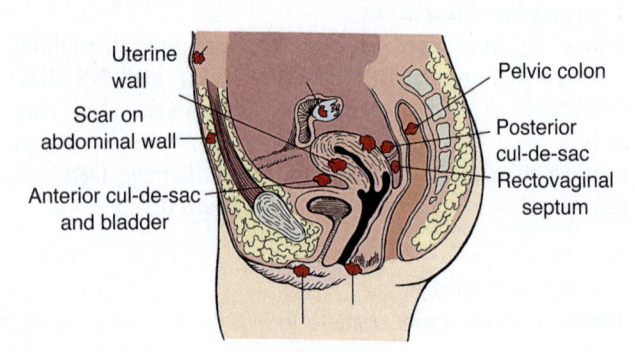

FIGURE 42.4 Possible sites of endometriosis.

Menopause
Pathophysiology and Signs and Symptoms

Menopause is the permanent cessation of menstrual cycles resulting from decreased hormone production. Related uncomfortable symptoms and conditions can occur with this natural phase of aging. The climacteric (**perimenopause**) is the period of gradual decline in hormone production before the permanent end of menses. It may last from months to years. Perimenopausal physical symptoms vary widely. They can include erratic menses, atrophy of urogenital tissues with a marked decrease in the amount of natural lubrication, a pH shift toward alkalinity (encouraging yeast overgrowth), and vasomotor instability resulting in hot flashes and night sweats.

Estrogen protects women against several disease processes. The risk of heart disease and osteoporosis increases with declining estrogen production. Mental changes can occur because of the complex interplay of reproductive hormones and neurotransmitters. It is important to acknowledge symptoms such as irritability, anxiety, insomnia, memory problems, and mild depression as a normal, temporary result of hormonal changes so that perimenopausal women do not doubt their sanity.

Therapeutic Measures

Hormone replacement therapy (HRT), also known as menopausal hormone therapy (MHT), is a decision that should be made based on an individual's personal history, family history, and risk factors. HRT has many potential benefits, including decreased vasomotor symptoms and improved sleep, bone health, and mood. However, increased breast cancer risk, blood clot risk, and cardiac risk must also be considered. Each woman should discuss with her HCP whether HRT is appropriate for her if symptoms of menopause are not tolerable. If hormonal therapy is not appropriate, treatment with lifestyle changes, herbal supplements, or certain antidepressants may be alternatives. Estrogen alone is indicated only for women who have had a hysterectomy. All other women should receive progesterone along with estrogen. HRT can be administered orally, vaginally, or transdermally. See Table 42.1 for examples.

Dietary changes that include **phytoestrogens** (present in foods and herbs such as soy, tofu, flax seeds, black cohosh, and dong quai) may provide some of the benefits of estrogen replacement without HRT. However, even phytoestrogens have some risk. Women should discuss food and herb supplements with their HCP before using them.

Prevention of osteoporosis begins in early adulthood, long before perimenopause. Fair-skinned, thin women are at greatest risk for bone loss. Throughout life, adequate intake

• WORD • BUILDING •

retrograde: retro—backward + grade—step
perimenopause: peri—around + men(o)—month + pause—stopping
phytoestrogens: phyto—plant + estrogens—hormones

of calcium and vitamin D (preferably from foods) and regular weight-bearing exercise help to maximize bone mass. At menopause, some women may receive treatment with bone-building medications such as alendronate (Fosamax) to slow bone loss.

Complications

It is important to note that resumed vaginal bleeding after menstruation has ceased can signify an endometrial cell disorder caused by benign changes, such as polyps, or malignant changes of internal reproductive organs. Any bleeding that occurs following previous cessation should always be investigated.

Nursing Care and Patient Education

Teach perimenopausal women that they can plan for hot flashes by dressing in layers of clothing that may be removed. Vaginal symptoms can be treated with a water-soluble moisture restorer or lubricant or with an estrogen cream (following prescription directions). Eating a healthy diet that is light in caffeine, sugar, and alcohol can help women better control their bodies and minds. Looking forward to new challenges rather than backward to the past may help to counteract hormone-related depressive tendencies. It is important to remind perimenopausal women that they may still be fertile even after several months of **amenorrhea**. To prevent conception, women need to continue to practice birth control until they receive confirmation from their HCP that menopause is complete. Table 42.4 provides a summary of menstrual disorders.

> **CLINICAL JUDGMENT**
>
> **Lola**, age 53, has been experiencing menopausal hot flashes during the afternoons as she works in her office.
>
> 1. What self-care measures can you suggest to help with her symptoms?
> 2. If she considers hormone replacement therapy, what information should you share with her?
> 3. With whom should you collaborate to help Lola decide what to do?
>
> *Suggested answers are at the end of the chapter.*

IRRITATIONS AND INFLAMMATIONS OF THE VAGINA AND VULVA

Pathophysiology

The normal vaginal environment is a balanced ecosystem with a pH of less than 4.2 as a result of lactic acid and hydrogen peroxide production by vaginal cells. This acidic pH protects against growth of many pathogenic microorganisms. A variety of microorganisms normally coexist unless the ecological balance is destroyed. Candidiasis, bacterial vaginosis, and cytolytic vaginitis are all instances of overgrowth of normally present, nonpathogenic microorganisms. Trichomoniasis also is included because it can be transmitted nonsexually (on fomites, such as toilet seats) as well as sexually, and it grows well when the vaginal environment is disturbed. See Chapter 44 for information on sexually transmitted infections (STIs).

Table 42.4 Menstrual Disorders Summary

Signs and Symptoms	Increase or decrease in menstrual flow Increased pain with menses or generalized abdominal pain Fluid retention Headaches Breast pain, lesions, swelling Mood changes
Diagnostic Tests	Hormone levels Pregnancy test Pap smear Cervical/vaginal cultures Urine testing Ultrasound Laparoscopy Biopsy
Therapeutic Measures	Medication to stabilize hormone levels NSAIDs Dilation and curettage (D&C), laser ablation, hysterectomy Treatment of underlying causes Vitamin/mineral supplements Diuretics, serotonin reuptake inhibitors (SSRIs), dietary changes
Priority Nursing Diagnoses	*Deficient Fluid Volume* related to increased bleeding *Acute Pain* related to uterine cramping *Deficient Knowledge* related to self-care measures

Etiology

Several conditions can predispose women to an overgrowth of normal microbes. These include poor nutrition (especially diets high in simple sugars), inconsistent control of blood glucose levels in patients with diabetes, stress, pregnancy, marked hormonal fluctuations, pH changes, prolonged overheating of the genital area with little aeration (as happens with sitting still for long periods in restrictive clothing), and changes in the balance of vaginal flora types because of antibiotic treatment or douching. Patients who have a

• WORD • BUILDING •

amenorrhea: a—without + men(o)—month + rrhea—flow

compromised immune system can experience overgrowth of resident microbes; conversely, vaginal infections can make women more susceptible to STIs, such as gonorrhea and HIV. Frequent and persistent yeast infections can be one sign of HIV infection. **Vaginosis** (overgrowth) and **vaginitis** (inflammation) can sometimes produce irritation and inflammation in the male sexual partner as well, leading to urethritis, excoriation, and penile inflammation or lesions.

Signs and Symptoms
Common signs and symptoms include itching, burning, redness, foul odor, and vaginal discharge. Table 42.5 lists signs and symptoms of common vaginal irritations and inflammations that are not generally sexually transmitted.

Diagnosis
Typically, a pelvic examination is done with samples obtained for examination, pH, and culture.

Therapeutic Measures
A variety of anti-infective medications are used for these disorders (Table 42.6). If the male partner is not also treated, he may reactivate the problem for the woman. Therefore, several types of medication come in "partner packs" for both partners to use.

Nursing Care
The patient may feel embarrassed to talk about what is bothering her. A safe way to begin with most patients is to say, "Hello. What can I write on your chart as the reason for your visit today?" If embarrassment is evident, commenting that you need to know what materials to put out for examination purposes often defuses an uncomfortable situation. As you set up supplies for a pelvic examination, you can explain that some information is needed to determine how to treat the problem (see Chapter 41). Ask about vaginal discharge or other signs and symptoms using the **WHAT'S UP?** format (Chapter 1). Allow for privacy while she changes into a gown. Return to the room if requested as a chaperone, assistant, and support for the woman.

> **NURSING CARE TIP**
> If wet-mount slides are made, they must be taken to the laboratory immediately while still wet. Use standard precautions to transport samples. Although samples may be taken for culture, the HCP may prescribe medication before the results are returned because such irritations are so uncomfortable.

> **NURSING CARE TIP**
> Assure patients that all information is confidential. However, some communicable infections require mandatory reporting. See www.cdc.gov and your local state regulations.

Vaginal inflammations and infections may require oral medication or local application of medication in cream, suppository, or douche form. You may apply this for some women who cannot do so themselves (such as in an extended care facility), but typically you will teach patients to self-administer. Anatomically, the vagina slopes back toward the sacrum for about the length of an adult finger (although it can stretch longer). Application is best when the patient is lying down ready to sleep because vaginal medications tend to run out when the patient stands or sits. Medicated douches may be administered to a hospitalized patient sitting on a bedpan in bed in the semi-Fowler position. Patients may self-administer while sitting on a toilet. Most vaginal medications come with an applicator that either injects a dose of medication or pushes a firm shaped dose of medication off the end of the tube when the plunger is depressed. Consult the instructions supplied with the medication. Instruct patients to use all the medication as prescribed and wear an absorbent pad to prevent staining of clothing.

TOXIC SHOCK SYNDROME

Pathophysiology and Etiology
Toxic shock syndrome (TSS) is often associated with super-absorbent tampon use during menstruation but can also occur with use of diaphragms, cervical caps, or nasal packings. Less commonly, TSS can occur in individuals following recent surgery or cuts or burns on the skin. It is a severe systemic infection with strains of *Staphylococcus aureus* that produce toxins. The effect of the toxin on the liver, kidneys, lungs, and circulatory system makes TSS a life-threatening condition. A *streptococcal* infection can cause a similar syndrome.

Signs and Symptoms
Individuals with TSS may experience a sudden high fever with sore throat, headache, dizziness, confusion, low blood pressure, redness of the palms and soles of the feet, rash, blisters, and petechiae. Muscle pain and weakness as well as gastrointestinal upset have been reported. Signs and symptoms of TSS should be reported to an HCP immediately.

Prevention
Tampon makers have removed the highly absorbent fibers that were most often associated with the syndrome from their product lines, and TSS is now rare. Women can also reduce their risk of developing TSS by substituting sanitary pads for tampons at least part of the time, such as at night; changing tampons every 4 hours; washing hands carefully before inserting anything into the vagina; not leaving female barrier contraceptives in place for longer than needed; and

• WORD • BUILDING •
vaginosis: vagin—vagina + osis—condition
vaginitis: vagin—vagina + itis—inflammation

Table 42.5
Common Vaginal Irritations and Inflammations

Disorder and Etiology	Signs and Symptoms	Discharge/Examination	Diagnostic Tests	Usual Treatment
Candidiasis: *Candida albicans, C. glabrata,* or *C. tropicalis* overgrowth	Burning, itching, redness of vulva; burning on urination	White, cottage cheese appearance	Wet-mount slides (yeasts look like tiny, budding tree branches); may be cultured	Antifungal agents (drugs mostly ending in *-azole*)
Bacterial vaginosis: *Gardnerella vaginalis, Mycoplasma,* or anaerobe overgrowth	None or vulvar or vaginal irritation	White or gray, homogeneous, foul-smelling discharge; pH higher than 4.5	Wet-mount slides show "clue cells" or release fishy odor when potassium hydroxide is applied	Metronidazole, tinidazole, or clindamycin
Trichomoniasis: *Trichomonas vaginalis* (may be transmitted by inanimate objects or sexually)	Itching, irritation, foul odor, redness, dysuria	Discharge may be frothy; pH higher than 4.5; "strawberry cervix" resulting from petechiae	Wet-mount slides treated with normal saline show motile cells with flagella (like tiny whips); may also be cultured	Metronidazole or tinidazole
Cytolytic vaginosis: *Lactobacilli* overgrowth, stress, some medications	Burning, irritation, pain with intercourse	Nonodorous, thick, white, pasty, or dry and flaking	Lower than normal pH as tested with pH indicator tape (or litmus strip); may be cultured	Depends on cause; alkaline douches may be prescribed
Contact vulvovaginitis: Contact with allergens or irritating chemicals such as contraceptive creams or bubble baths	Itching, burning, redness	Generally, no change from normal discharge, though may be increased	History and physical information, recent contact with chemicals	Avoidance of the offending substance; warm sitz baths or application of hydrocortisone cream
Atrophic vaginitis: Estrogen levels too low to support estrogen-sensitive vaginal tissues	Vulvovaginal irritation, dryness, dyspareunia, increased tendency for resident microbe overgrowth	May have little or increased discharge; discharge may be watery, yellow, or green; may be blood tinged	Maturation index may be determined during Pap test to identify atrophic cellular changes, but diagnosis is usually by history and physical information	Hormone replacement therapy (oral, patch, or vulvovaginal cream) or water-soluble lubricant replacing vaginal lubricants

avoiding tampons or female barrier contraceptives in the first 12 weeks after giving birth. If skin wounds are present, they should be kept clean and covered, and not be exposed to hot tubs, swimming pools, or other bodies of water.

Diagnostic Tests
Blood and urine will be collected for cultures as well as to look for signs of shock. The vagina or throat may be cultured. X-rays or a CT scan may be ordered to determine organ involvement.

Therapeutic Measures
Patients with TSS are hospitalized. Antibiotics are administered for infection. Intravenous fluids and medication can be used to manage blood pressure and treat shock and organ failure.

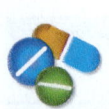

Table 42.6
Medications for Irritations and Inflammations of the Vagina and Vulva

Medication Class/Action

Antibiotics

Inhibit bacterial protein synthesis.

Examples	Nursing Implications
clindamycin (Cleocin)	Teach: Correct use. Use as directed, even if symptoms cease. Report change in symptoms.

Antifungals

Believed to bind to sterol in fungal cell membrane, thereby altering cell permeability.

Examples	Nursing Implications
fluconazole (Diflucan) miconazole (Monistat) terconazole (Terazol) clotrimazole (Gyne-Lotrimin)	Teach: Correct use. Use as directed, even if symptoms cease. Report change in symptoms.

Antiprotozoal

Enters cells of microorganisms that contain nitroreductase; interferes with DNA synthesis and causes cell death.

Examples	Nursing Implications
metronidazole (Flagyl)	Teach: Avoid alcohol use while on medication and for 48 hours after completion. Concurrent use of alcohol and metronidazole will induce severe nausea and vomiting. Use as directed, even if symptoms cease. Take with meals. Treat partner.

Nursing Care and Patient Education

All menstruating women should be taught measures to prevent TSS. They should also be taught to recognize symptoms of TSS because early identification and treatment can save lives. See care of the patient with septic shock in Chapter 9.

DISORDERS RELATED TO THE DEVELOPMENT OF THE GENITAL ORGANS

Pathophysiology, Etiologies, and Signs and Symptoms

Several types of congenital malformations of the reproductive organs can affect the health of female patients, caused by environmental factors during pregnancy or genetic factors. They may require medical or surgical treatment at some point in life. **Agenesis** of structures (such as the vagina) means that they never developed. **Hypoplasia** of reproductive tract portions means that they are underdeveloped, such as a very small uterus. **Imperforate** means that expected openings do not exist. This can occur when the hymen over the vagina does not have an opening. Blind pouches may exist where cavities should meet but do not.

Many malformations are discovered during childhood or early adolescence, but some are identified when patients seek medical help because of dysmenorrhea, **dyspareunia** (pain with intercourse), infertility, repeated spontaneous abortions (miscarriages), or preterm labor.

Diagnostic Tests

Procedures such as ultrasonography (USN), hysterosalpingography (HSG), computed tomography (CT) scan, magnetic resonance imaging (MRI), and endoscopy may be used to determine the type and extent of developmental defects.

• WORD • BUILDING •

agenesis: a—without + genesis—production
hypoplasia: hypo—little + plasia—shape (or form)
imperforate: im—not + perforate—pierced
dyspareunia: dys—painful or abnormal + pareunia—mating

Therapeutic Measures
Some defects, such as an imperforate hymen, can be repaired surgically, while others cannot. Depending on the type and location of the defect, surgeries may be endoscopic or by incision.

Nursing Care
Patients who have these problems may struggle with self-esteem issues, such as feeling that they are incomplete or have been cheated of something they desire. Show that you are willing to listen if and when the patient wishes to talk, while allowing her as much privacy as she desires.

DISPLACEMENT DISORDERS

Pathophysiology and Etiologies
The pelvic organs are suspended in the pelvis by ligaments and supported by muscles and fascia. The pubococcygeus muscle runs from the pubis to the coccyx and supplies support from below. Pregnancies (especially those producing large babies) and rapid or traumatic deliveries may result in stretching and injury of the supporting structures. This can cause displacement of the uterus, vagina, bladder, or bowel from a normal position.

Some children have defective muscular support of the pelvic organs, and prolapse is more prevalent in some families. Such observations seem to suggest that congenital defects and genetic inheritance influence displacement disorders, even without pregnancy. Scarring from STIs may also be a factor. Aging generally increases the problem because effects of gravity over time contribute to stretching, and lower estrogen levels weaken estrogen-dependent supportive tissues. Chronic constipation, obesity, and lack of exercise also worsen these problems.

Diagnostic Tests
Ultrasonography, hysterosalpingography, CT scan, MRI, and endoscopy may be used to determine the type and extent of displacement disorders.

Therapeutic Measures
A *pessary* is a supportive (usually ring-shaped) device placed in the vagina to help support the pelvic organs. A pessary is usually removed daily at bedtime for cleaning, but some are designed to remain in the vagina for months. The woman returns to the HCP for a recheck after an initial period of pessary use to determine whether it is causing pressure damage to tissues. Because the pessary is a foreign object in the vagina, increased vaginal discharge can be expected. Discharge should not be pink, bloody, or purulent. Another noninvasive intervention is use of Kegel exercises (see "Nursing Process for the Woman With a Displacement Disorder"). If noninvasive interventions are not effective, surgery may be required.

Cystocele
Pathophysiology and Signs and Symptoms
Cystocele occurs when the bladder sags into the vaginal space because of inadequate support (Fig. 42.5A). Pelvic pressure and stress incontinence are common with this condition.

Therapeutic Measures
Kegel exercises or the use of a pessary may help. If these measures are ineffective, anterior **colporrhaphy**, which is a surgical repair of the anterior portion of the vagina, may be needed. Another possible surgical treatment involves resuspending the bladder.

Rectocele
Pathophysiology and Signs and Symptoms
Rectocele occurs when a portion of the rectum sags into the vagina because of inadequate support (see Fig. 42.5B). A feeling of pelvic pressure as well as fecal incontinence, constipation, and hemorrhoids can result.

Therapeutic Measures
Kegel exercises can help strengthen the supporting muscles. The patient should maintain bowel regularity with a high-fiber diet to avoid further discomfort and sagging from bowel overdistention. Posterior colporrhaphy may be necessary to correct this problem.

Uterine Position Disorders
Pathophysiology and Signs and Symptoms
The most common variations in position of the uterus are **anteversion, anteflexion, retroversion**, and **retroflexion** (Fig. 42.6). In anteversion, the uterus lies too far forward, and in retroversion, it lies too far back. In anteflexion, the upper portion of the uterus bends forward, and in retroflexion, it bends backward.

Symptoms that can result from these uterine displacements include painful menstruation and intercourse, infertility, and repeated spontaneous abortion.

Therapeutic Measures
A pessary may correct some positional problems. If infertility or recurrent spontaneous abortion is involved or the condition is very painful, surgery to correct the condition may be necessary.

• WORD • BUILDING •

cystocele: cysto—bag (bladder) + cele—hernia
colporrhaphy: colpo—vagina + rrhaphy—suture
rectocele: recto—rectum + cele—hernia
anteversion: ante—front + version—turning
anteflexion: ante—front + flexion—bending
retroversion: retro—back + version—turning
retroflexion: retro—back + flexion—bending

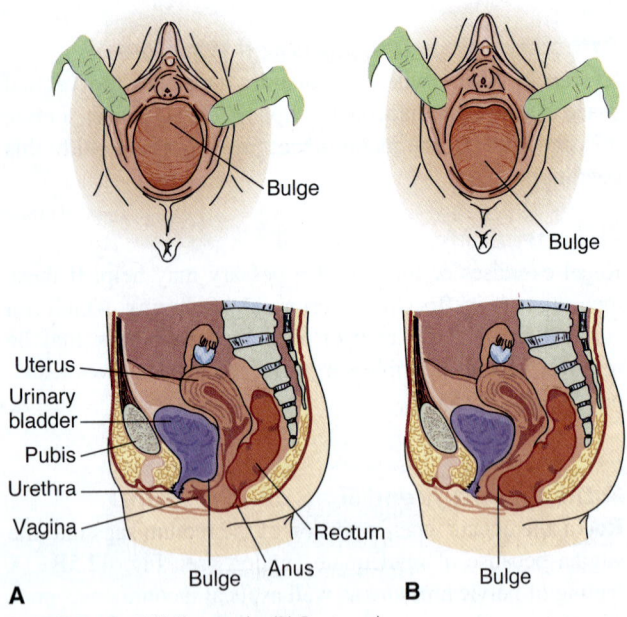

FIGURE 42.5 (A) Cystocele. (B) Rectocele.

Uterine Prolapse
Pathophysiology
Uterine prolapse occurs when the uterus sags into the vagina. The amount of prolapse can vary and increase over time because of the effects of gravity, poor pelvic support, and excessive lifting or straining. See Figure 42.7 for degrees of prolapse.

Signs and Symptoms
Uterine prolapse can be very uncomfortable, resulting in back pain, pelvic pain, pain with intercourse (or inability to have intercourse), urinary incontinence, constipation, and development of hemorrhoids. Pressure on the uterus can compromise circulation, resulting in tissue necrosis. Vaginal vault prolapse can also occur in women who have had a hysterectomy, so that the vagina turns inside out and sags downward, causing similar signs and symptoms. This condition typically requires surgical resuspension.

Therapeutic Measures
Some minor uterine displacements may be treated with use of a pessary. Kegel exercises may be more effective in prevention than in treatment of uterine prolapse because, once the tissues become stretched sufficiently for the uterus to sag into the vagina, the continued weight of the uterus prevents adequate contraction of the muscles. Surgery may be done to correct the prolapse. Although the uterus can be resuspended by shortening the muscles and fascia, hysterectomy is the more common treatment unless further childbearing is desired.

Nursing Process for the Woman With a Displacement Disorder
Data Collection
Women may present with statements of feeling a lump or bulge, or in severe cases may state, "something is falling out." Ask about urinary incontinence or difficulty urinating.

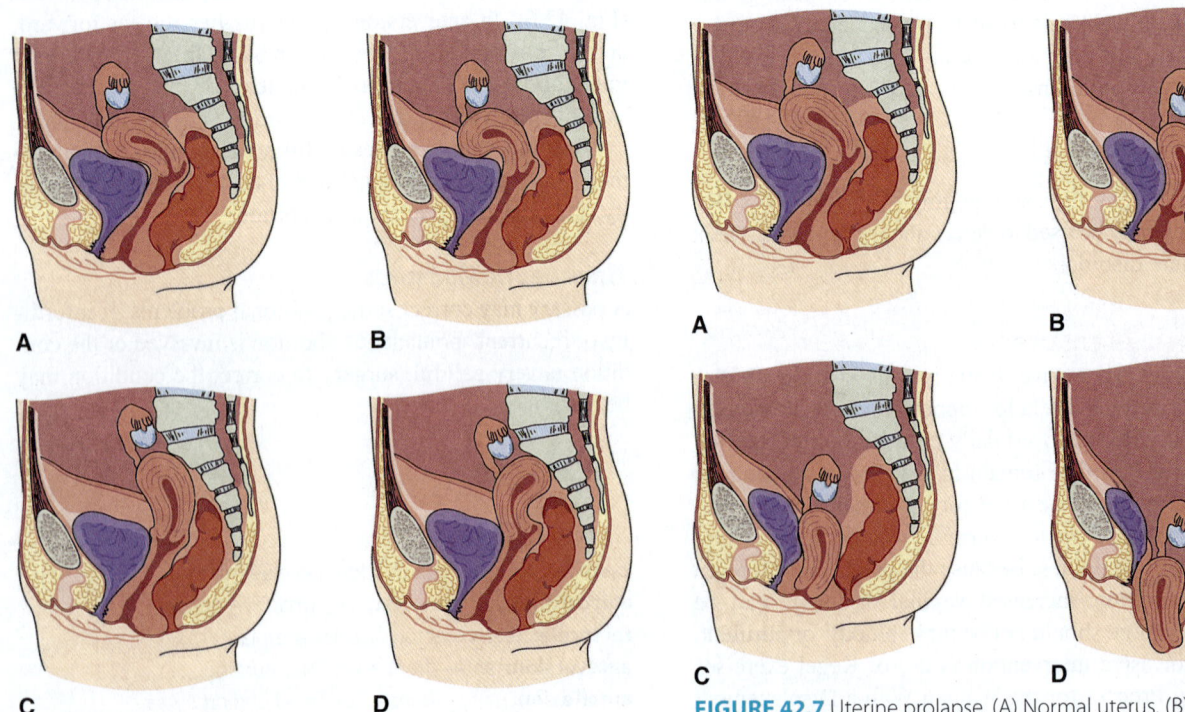

FIGURE 42.6 Uterine positions. (A) Anteversion. (B) Anteflexion. (C) Retroversion. (D) Retroflexion.

FIGURE 42.7 Uterine prolapse. (A) Normal uterus. (B) First-degree prolapse: descent within the vagina. (C) Second-degree prolapse. (D) Third-degree prolapse: vagina is completely everted.

Determine if she is experiencing back pain or pain with menstruation or intercourse. Do symptoms worsen as the day progresses? Ask the **WHAT'S UP?** questions. Physical examination will be carried out by the HCP.

Nursing Diagnosis
A variety of nursing diagnoses may be applicable, such as *Pain, Urinary Incontinence, Constipation, Sexual Dysfunction*, or *Grieving* related to alteration in reproductive status.

Implementation and Patient Education
Advise women to eat a healthy diet to avoid obesity and constipation. Also collaborate to teach Kegel exercises to keep the pubococcygeus muscle strong and able to support the organs in the pelvic cavity. One way to do Kegel exercises follows:

1. To find the pubococcygeus muscle, tighten while urinating so that the flow of urine stops.
2. Squeeze the muscle that stopped urinary flow tightly, holding for 10 seconds and totally relaxing the muscle afterward. Repeat 15 times per day.
3. Practice controlling the muscle by contracting and relaxing it to move the pelvic floor upward and downward very slowly. Thinking of an elevator helps some women. Repeat this 15 times per day.

> **NURSING CARE TIP**
> Teach women to do Kegel exercises during the day, such as while waiting in lines, to use otherwise wasted time to promote their health. Another suggestion is to plan specific times of day or activities that would include Kegel exercises, such as while in a car or working at a computer. Kegel exercises can be done anywhere and are not apparent to anyone watching.

See Table 42.7 for a summary of displacement disorders.

Evaluation
Evaluation depends on the woman's specific concerns. Is she satisfied with her care? Is she able to manage her discomfort?

FERTILITY DISORDERS

Infertility is a complicated problem with many causes. Some couples with infertility may have multiple reproductive problems. Both male and female partners should be examined. (See Chapter 43 for greater detail on male reproductive system disorders.) Table 42.8 provides a summary of fertility disorders and diagnostic tests.

Therapeutic Measures
Treatment of infertility is designed to ensure that an adequate amount of sperm and an ovum can be in proximity in the

Table 42.7
Displacement Disorders Summary

Signs and Symptoms	Pain with menses or sexual intercourse Infertility Spontaneous abortion or preterm labor Prolapse of uterus, bladder, or rectum into vagina or outside of body
Diagnostic Tests	Physical examination Ultrasound Hysterosalpingography Computed tomography (CT) scan or magnetic resonance imaging (MRI) Endoscopy
Therapeutic Measures	Kegel exercises Surgery Hormone supplements
Priority Nursing Diagnoses	*Acute* or *Chronic Pain* related to structural abnormality or surgery *Urge Urinary Incontinence* or *Constipation* related to structural abnormalities *Sexual Dysfunction* related to disturbance in self-concept *Grieving* related to absence or loss of reproductive status

most conducive environment for fertilization. Removal of barriers such as scar tissue may require surgery. Depending on the results of blood tests and a **postcoital** test (described in Table 42.8), adjustments of environmental factors may involve such actions as sperm washing to avoid destructive antigen–antibody responses, changing the pH of the seminal fluid to encourage sperm motility, treating the female partner to prevent substances in her genital tract fluids from disabling the sperm, or adjusting her hormone levels. The number of sperm or ova available can be increased with fertility drugs or hormone preparations. Infertility treatments are quite complicated and expensive and change periodically as a result of ongoing research.

In vitro fertilization (IVF) involves bringing ova and sperm together outside the bodies of the participants. Ova may be harvested using a long needle or an endoscope after hormonal preparation of the woman. Sperm can be obtained through masturbation; intercourse with a nonlubricated, nonspermicidal condom; or electrical stimulation of ejaculation

• **WORD • BUILDING** •
postcoital: post—after + coital—pertaining to intercourse
in vitro fertilization: in—inside + vitro—glass + fertiliz—fruitful + ation—process

Table 42.8
Female Fertility Disorders

Pathophysiology/Etiology	Diagnostic Tests
Ovulation	
Possible anatomic and physiological abnormalities of ovaries Hormonal imbalances related to hypothalamus, thyroid, or adrenal glands Polycystic ovary syndrome (PCOS)	Basal body temperature charting Midluteal serum progesterone blood levels Luteinizing hormone (LH) levels Blood or urine testing Ultrasound monitoring of a follicle for evidence of release of ovum Endometrial biopsy Observation of male hair distribution Other hormone testing as indicated
Tubal	
Possible obstruction of the fallopian tubes resulting from anatomic variations, scarring, or adhesions; prior surgeries; or inflammatory processes involving other abdominal tissues	Hysterosalpingography (see Chapter 41) Laparoscopy
Uterine	
Possible abnormalities in shape or blockages within the uterus (rare cause of infertility but a potential cause of pregnancy loss before maturity) Menstrual disorders involving the endometrium	Hysteroscopy (see Chapter 41) Removal of tissue samples using curet or endoscope
Other Sources	
Possible reproductive environmental factors such as destructive antigen–antibody responses Inappropriate pH of seminal fluid for maximal sperm motility Substances in genital tract fluids that disable sperm	Postcoital test: Couple is advised to have intercourse when LH and estrogen levels are high; then a specimen of cervical mucus is taken from the woman 2 to 12 hours later for analysis of reproductive environment

for patients with spinal cord injuries. Once fertilized, the ova are implanted in the woman's uterus.

There are many variations on IVF. The HCP may use intrauterine insemination (IUI) to place a semen sample from the male partner closer to the ovum via a small catheter. Gamete intrafallopian transfer (GIFT) involves mixing sperm and eggs together and transferring to the fallopian tube. In zygote intrafallopian transfer (ZIFT), fertilization of gametes occurs outside of the body; the fertilized egg is placed into a woman's fallopian tube to travel to the uterus.

When measures to improve the chances of conception using the partners' own gametes are unsuccessful, gametes from donors may be used. Artificial insemination by injecting another man's sperm into the woman's genital tract is the simplest of the donor procedures. Ova also may be harvested from a donor woman and used for IVF using the male partner's sperm if possible. Both procedures allow for genetic inheritance from one member of the couple. If genetic inheritance is not possible or desirable (as with familial disease carriers), both donor sperm and ova may be used for IVF to be transferred into the female patient. Surrogacy is a situation in which an embryo from one couple is placed into a "host" mother for growth of a baby for the couple.

Nursing Care and Education of the Patient Undergoing Fertility Testing and Treatment

An understanding attitude by the nurse is very important because infertility can be a cause of low self-esteem as well as strain on a relationship. Patients who have been undergoing diagnostic testing or treatment for infertility can become discouraged with the process and the expense, especially if it has been ineffective. Having to plan one's sexual activity around an HCP's directions can compromise feelings of spontaneity, enjoyment, and privacy.

On the first infertility investigation visit, the nurse may provide information to the woman about keeping a precise record of her oral temperatures with a basal thermometer each morning on awakening, before any other activity. The first day of her menses is day 1 on the temperature chart. Changing levels of hormones result in slight temperature changes, which can be used to identify when ovulation is occurring and when hormone levels should be tested. Because many factors can influence temperature and cycles, explain that it may take a few months of recording to clearly identify her pattern.

You may assist with office procedures such as endometrial biopsy, which can be done during a pelvic examination 2 or 3 days before menses is expected. A pregnancy test should be done before this procedure to avoid interfering with a pregnancy. The woman may receive pain medication and regional anesthesia for the procedure. Some women experience a vasovagal response to the biopsy, causing dizziness and faintness. This goes away after the biopsy.

If infertility was caused by something the patient perceives as avoidable, such as an STI, she may feel guilt in addition to psychological discomfort. Patients may experience repeated disappointments. The beginning of menses can signal a time of mourning for these couples. Depression may result after failed IVF attempts. Strained relationships may develop between marriage partners, especially if they disagree about the value of testing or the importance of having biological children.

In IVF, usually couples decide to implant more than the desired number of embryos because it is expected that not all will survive; this approach is more cost effective with less physical risk for the mother. However, it may require the heart-wrenching decision of whether to "reduce" (abort) extra pregnancies or risk having more than the desired number of children at once as a result of fertility treatments. As the nurse, you can provide emotional support and refer women to resources such as an IVF support group.

REPRODUCTIVE LIFE PLANNING

Reproductive life planning is a more comprehensive term than *contraception* and implies reasoned decisions related to pregnancy timing and whether to have children. Healthy People 2030 has a goal to reduce unintended pregnancies to 36.5% by 2030; in 2013, 43% of pregnancies in women ages 15 to 44 years were unintended. Both women who have unintended pregnancies and their children have more mental health problems than do their counterparts who have intended pregnancies, and children are more likely to have physical health problems and to struggle in school (Office of Disease Prevention and Health Promotion, 2020). Nurses can contribute to the overall health and quality of life for women and families by helping them to find the resources they need to make informed choices.

Many types of birth control are available, and several additional types are in developmental and testing stages. General categories of agents are discussed in this section. Understanding of the different types of contraceptives can assist the nurse in answering patient questions and helping them find additional information.

Methods are introduced in the order of usual effectiveness, from most to least effective (with the exception that experimental methods are discussed at the end regardless of efficacy). Consult your clinic or HCP for an approved, current comparison list of methods for distribution.

For some women, the distinction of whether a birth control method prevents conception or only interferes with implantation or maintenance of a pregnancy is an important factor in their decision. If a patient believes life begins at conception, any action other than prevention of conception would be considered equivalent to abortion.

Intrauterine Devices

The presence of a foreign object in the uterus prevents sperm from reaching an egg. Those that contain progestin also alter cervical mucous causing sperm to have difficulty moving through the environment. IUDs are generally made from a form of plastic. They may contain copper wire (such as ParaGard) or a supply of a progestin (e.g., Mirena) that is slowly released into the system to further alter the uterine environment to hinder fertilization or implantation.

Advantages, Disadvantages, Side Effects, and Risks

The main advantage of an IUD is continuous contraception without the necessity of remembering to take medication and without the side effects associated with medications. The following IUD brands contain the hormone levonorgestrel. ParaGard is effective for 10 years, and Mirena and Kyleena are effective for 5 years. Skyla is effective for 3 years. The IUDs with progestins may help lighten and potentially eliminate menstrual bleeding in women who have a history of anemia or heavy menstrual flow.

Disadvantages are changes in menstrual bleeding, cramping, and increased risk of pelvic inflammatory disease (PID). Rarely, an IUD has caused a uterine perforation. IUDs should be avoided in women with uterine abnormalities, those with PID, and those who currently have STIs. Expulsion or displacement of the IUD can occur, so women should be taught to feel for the presence of the external string before intercourse.

Insertion Procedure

Insertion of an IUD typically is done in an HCP's office, usually during the first 7 days of the menstrual cycle because the cervix is slightly dilated at this time. The IUD is inserted into the cervix through a tube that comes packaged with the IUD, which temporarily holds the IUD flat or folded for insertion. When the IUD is pushed out the end of the tube, it springs into a shape that helps to keep it inside the uterus. One potential danger of IUD insertion is vasovagal reflex stimulation (described in association with endometrial biopsy).

Oral Contraceptives

Oral **contraceptive** medications are among the most widely used forms of birth control in North America. Most contain an estrogen and a progestin in combination, although some (mini-pills) contain only progestin. Some prevent conception by inhibiting ovulation or changing the environment of the reproductive tract to inhibit sperm activity. Others do not prevent conception but make implantation less likely and hasten the breakdown of the corpus luteum so that pregnancy-sustaining hormones are not produced. Many adverse effects that occurred in the past have been overcome by adjustment of dosage levels.

Oral contraceptives can also be used in some instances to regulate irregular menses, decrease menorrhagia or dysmenorrhea, or decrease symptoms associated with endometriosis or cyclic breast changes. Oral contraceptives do not prevent STIs; advise women about the risks of contracting STIs and using condoms for prevention while taking an oral contraceptive.

Advantages, Disadvantages, Side Effects, and Risks

Oral contraceptives are very effective. Improvement of dysmenorrhea, endometriosis, increased regularity of menses, and decrease in menstrual flow may occur; however, some women experience menstrual changes such as amenorrhea, irregular or prolonged menses, and intermenstrual spotting.

Oral contraceptives require commitment because irregular use decreases effectiveness. To encourage regular use, oral contraceptives are generally dispensed in containers labeled with the days of the week. Some companies include unmedicated pills in the package to be taken during the time of hormone cessation for menses so that the woman only must remember to take a daily pill, instead of timing the taking of the pills with her cycle. Women should speak to their HCPs to determine which method is best for them.

Some women experience side effects such as acne, fluid retention, headaches, breast swelling and discomfort, midcycle bleeding, and sometimes depression. Use of an oral contraceptive also has some risks. Higher rates of blood clot formation, stroke, high blood pressure, heart attack, and worsening of diabetes are rare occurrences with some hormonal contraceptives. These are generally related to preexisting risk factors. Women who smoke or have diabetes, high blood pressure, heart disease, or a history of thrombophlebitis should receive information about the risks of oral contraceptives and alternative methods of contraception.

Oral contraceptives decrease the risk of endometrial and ovarian cancer. However, there is a slight increase in risk of breast cancer and cervical **dysplasia** (cell changes that may become cancerous) and cancer. Women should be advised to have regular Pap smears while taking oral contraceptives.

Many medications alter the effectiveness of oral contraceptives. Women should be warned to alert HCPs and pharmacists that they are using oral contraceptives when a new medication is started or a regular medication is discontinued. Use of hormonal contraceptives increases the risk of vitamin B deficiencies, so a healthy diet with good sources of B vitamins is advisable.

> **LEARNING TIP**
> Side effects of oral contraceptives can be serious. Teach your patient to watch for "ACHES" and to contact her HCP immediately if they occur. ACHES stands for:
>
> **A**bdominal pain
> **C**hest pain
> **H**eadache
> **E**ye pain
> **S**evere leg pain

Contraceptive Implant and Injectable Medications

Contraceptive implants are small permeable tubes surgically implanted through a small incision under the skin; they slowly release hormones for long-term contraception. Implants have been used with varying success; an example is etonogestrel implant (Nexplanon).

Medroxyprogesterone acetate (Depo-Provera) is a contraceptive agent available in a slow-release *depot* form that can be injected intramuscularly. Medication is continuously released for 3 months. Both forms contain progesterone only.

Advantages, Disadvantages, Side Effects, and Risks

The main advantage of injections and implants is that the woman does not have to remember to take daily medication. Disadvantages are that the medications may not be immediately effective, so another method may be necessary for 1 to 2 weeks after the initial injection. Another disadvantage is that fertility may not return for several months to 1 year after discontinuation.

Alterations in menstrual flow, especially amenorrhea, are the most common side effects with both depot medications and implants. Weight gain of 5 to 10 pounds is also common, which can lead to discontinuation of use. Other side effects and risks are similar to other oral contraceptives that contain progesterone only.

Estrogen-Progestin Contraceptive Ring

An estrogen-progestin contraceptive ring (NuvaRing) works in much the same manner as other hormonal contraceptives by slowly releasing hormones. The user inserts the ring into the vagina. The ring is left in place for 3 weeks; it is then removed for 1 week for menses to occur, after which a new ring is placed.

• **WORD** • **BUILDING** •

contraceptive: contra—against + ceptive—taking in (conceiving)

dysplasia: dys—painful or abnormal + plasia—shape or form

Advantages, Disadvantages, Side Effects, and Risks

Not having to remember daily medication can be an advantage of the contraceptive ring. However, failing to remove it at the right time may disrupt the regularity of the menstrual cycles. With consistent use, it is very effective in preventing pregnancy. Because it does not provide a barrier over the cervix, there is less risk of infection than with a diaphragm or cervical cap. A common side effect is an increase in normal vaginal discharge. Other side effects and risks are similar to other low-dose hormonal contraceptives.

Transdermal Contraceptive Patch

Transdermal patches contain estrogen and progestin (Xulane). The patch is placed on the abdomen, upper arm, or buttock after a menstrual period and left in place for 1 week. A new patch is placed on the body each week for 3 weeks. After 3 weeks, the patch is removed and not replaced for 1 week for menses to occur.

Advantages, Disadvantages, Side Effects, and Risks

The contraceptive patch has been found to be similar to oral contraceptives in effectiveness, side effects, and risks, but with the advantage of not having to remember to take a pill each day. The patch remains in place during bathing, swimming, and other activities.

> **CLINICAL JUDGMENT**
>
> **Jessica,** who appears about 13 years old, announces loudly at the clinic reception desk that she is "ready to be a responsible adult" and would like some birth control.
>
> 1. What information should be gathered from her?
> 2. What do you think she needs to know before making a decision?
> 3. How can you base your teaching on her desire to be a responsible adult?
>
> *Suggested answers are at the end of the chapter.*

Barrier Methods

Barrier methods of birth control are less effective in preventing pregnancy than most of the previously mentioned methods when used alone. Barriers are intended to prevent sperm from reaching the ovum. Used in combination, barrier methods with spermicidal preparations have effectiveness close to that of oral contraceptives. Barrier methods and spermicidal preparations may be purchased without a prescription.

Condoms

Condoms are barriers that are used once and then discarded into an appropriate waste receptacle. Condoms used with contraceptive jelly or spermicide are most effective at decreasing risk of pregnancy. They should be stored in a cool, dry place before use, as heat or pressure can weaken them. Storage in a wallet or glove compartment is not advised. Petroleum-based substances, such as Vaseline, can also weaken condoms, so use of water-soluble lubricants (preferably spermicides) should be advised.

ADVANTAGES, DISADVANTAGES, SIDE EFFECTS, AND RISKS OF MALE CONDOMS. Male condoms have long been used for contraception because they are a relatively inexpensive, reversible method that men can control at the time of intercourse. Most condoms also provide barrier protection against transmission of STIs.

The main disadvantages of condom use are interruption of foreplay for application, decreased sensation, and the possibility of slippage or breakage during intercourse. These disadvantages may be overcome with application of the condom by the female partner as a part of foreplay; use of lubricated or textured condoms to increase sensation; use of the correct size condom with a reservoir or application that leaves about a half-inch at the tip of the condom loose enough to serve as a reservoir for semen (Fig. 42.8); and removal from the vagina before relaxation of the erection.

ADVANTAGES, DISADVANTAGES, SIDE EFFECTS, AND RISKS OF FEMALE CONDOMS. Female condoms allow female initiation of contraception and provide some barrier protection against STIs. Coverage of the labia by the condom may provide more of a barrier than male condoms (Fig. 42.9). Disadvantages are similar to those of male condoms; they are also more expensive than male condoms.

Diaphragms and Cervical Caps

Diaphragms and cervical caps work in the same manner as condoms, by blocking the entry of sperm through the cervix (Fig. 42.10). The barrier effect is enhanced by simultaneous

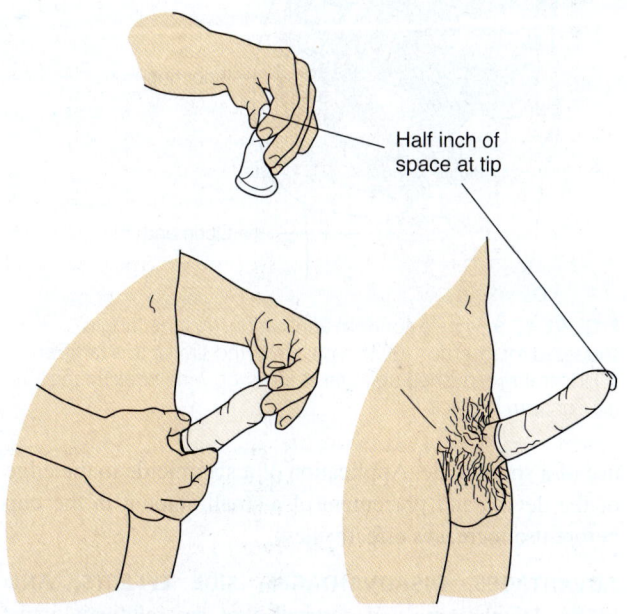

FIGURE 42.8 Correct application of a male condom.

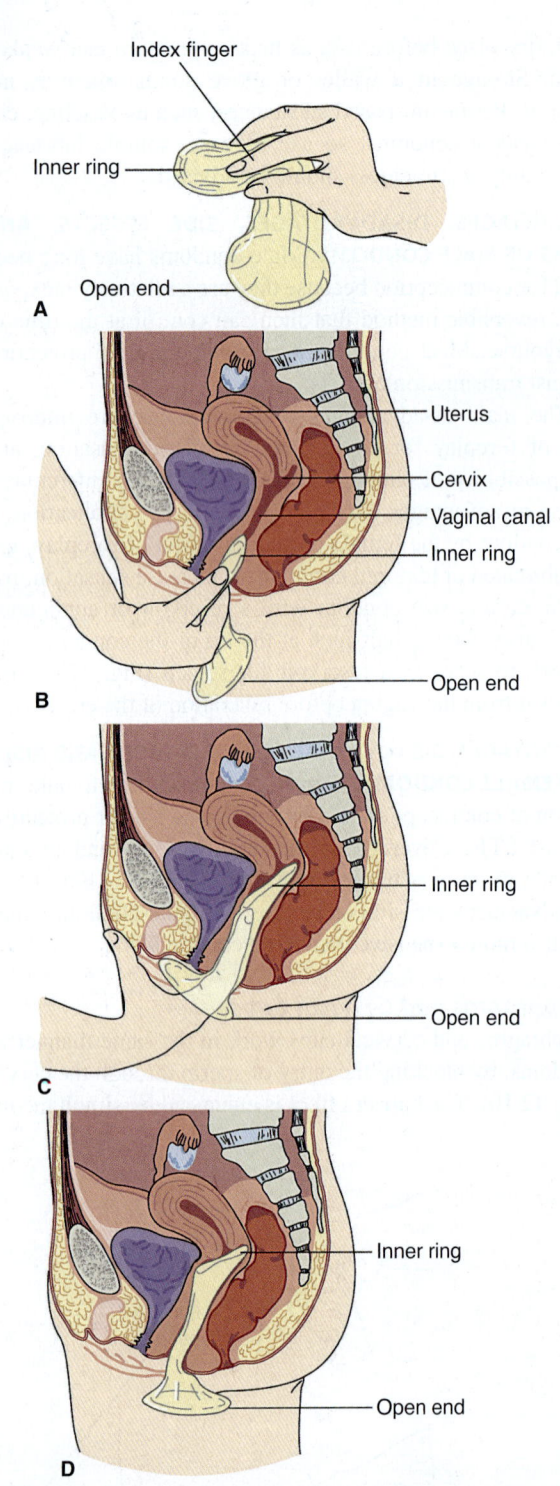

FIGURE 42.9 Female condom application. (A) Inner ring is squeezed for insertion. (B) Sheath is inserted similar to a tampon. (C) Inner ring is pushed up as far as it can go with index finger. (D) Condom in place.

use of a spermicide. Application of a spermicide to the edge of the device and placement of a small amount in the cup before use increases effectiveness.

ADVANTAGES, DISADVANTAGES, SIDE EFFECTS, AND RISKS. Diaphragms and cervical caps are relatively inexpensive, are female-initiated, and work without systemic

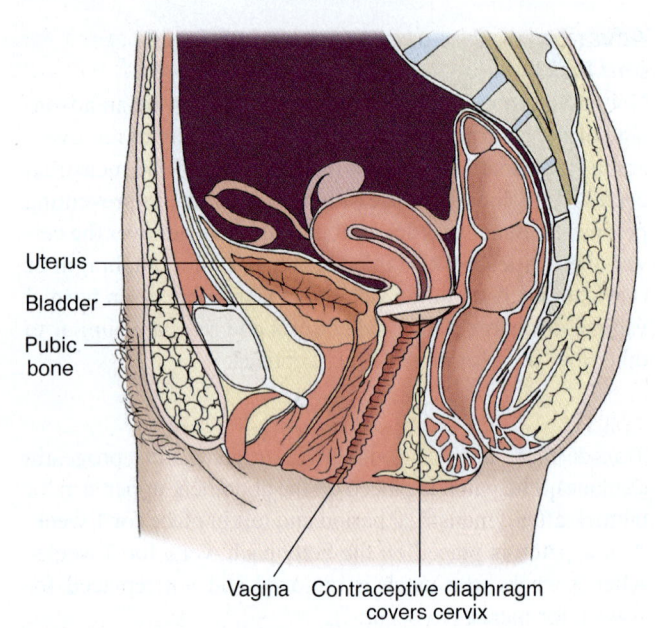

FIGURE 42.10 Contraceptive diaphragm.

medication. Diaphragms and cervical caps require initial fitting and a prescription, may need refitting after childbirth and weight loss or gain, and can last for years. They should be replaced periodically based on manufacturer recommendations or with evidence of hardening, cracking, or thin spots. They need to be washed with soap and water, dried, and stored in a case away from heat and sunlight between uses.

Women and their partners can experience irritation or allergic reaction to the spermicide or the contraceptive device material, which would require changing birth control methods. These methods require that the device be inserted before intercourse and left in place for several hours afterward. (See package inserts for specific recommendations.) An increase in incidence of urinary tract infection has been reported with use of the diaphragm, and risk of TSS increases with prolonged uninterrupted use of cervical barriers. Adequate fluid intake, voiding shortly after intercourse, and removal of the device as directed after intercourse help to prevent potential problems. If urinary tract infections recur with the diaphragm, changing to a cervical cap may decrease the occurrence by reducing pressure against the bladder through the anterior vagina.

Spermicides

Spermicidal agents may be used alone, although use in combination with a barrier method is much more effective. They come in a variety of forms, such as creams, gels, foams, and suppositories, that kill or disable sperm so that fertilization does not occur.

Advantages, Disadvantages, Side Effects, and Risks

Spermicidal preparations are relatively inexpensive and can be male- or female-initiated. They do not produce systemic effects, and no hormones are involved. Spermicides require application before each act of intercourse, and some patients consider them somewhat messy. Many contain the same ingredient: nonoxynol 9. If genital irritation or a rash occurs with a spermicide, the patient should read labels carefully to avoid future contact with the same ingredient.

Natural Family Planning

Periodic abstinence (natural family planning) is less effective than the previously described methods. Couples control their fertility by restricting intercourse to "safe periods" during which risk of conception is low. Many signs can be assessed to determine "safe" days, including temperature changes, cervical consistency and mucus changes, calendar timing, and awareness of symptoms of fertility.

Slight body temperature changes can indicate ovulation. During the first half of the menstrual cycle, the temperature remains low, with a marked drop just before ovulation occurs. With ovulation, the temperature rises and stays higher for the last half of the cycle. Women who use this assessment method should use a basal body temperature thermometer when they awaken, before doing anything else, and record it on a chart.

Cervical consistency and mucus changes also help pinpoint ovulation. As hormone levels change, the consistency of cervical mucus changes. As ovulation approaches, the amount of mucus increases and becomes more clear, thin, slippery, and stretchable than at other times of the month. Around the time of ovulation, the cervix becomes softer to touch and more open than at other times of the cycle.

Following the calendar can work fairly well if a woman's menstrual periods are regular, but becoming aware of her pattern may take time. Symptoms such as breast tenderness and midcycle discomfort (*mittelschmerz*) can also help identify ovulation. Users of this method should be advised to abstain from intercourse for approximately 3 days before ovulation and 3 to 4 days after because the sperm and ovum can survive for a long period in the female genital tract.

Advantages and Disadvantages

The advantage of this method is that it requires no expense or medication. For those who adhere to Catholicism, it is the only birth control method currently approved by the Catholic Church. The disadvantages are that it requires the cooperation of both partners and may interfere with spontaneity of sexual expression. It is generally not very effective as a means of birth control. It may be difficult to accurately identify ovulation times because infectious and inflammatory processes can affect temperature readings, infections and feminine hygiene products can affect cervical mucus, and irregularity of flow and symptoms may make prediction difficult.

Least Effective Methods
Coitus Interruptus
Coitus interruptus involves removal of the penis from the vagina before ejaculation occurs. Although this method requires no expense or preparation, it is not very effective. Excellent control of ejaculation is required, and even the small amount of sperm present in pre-ejaculatory fluid can result in pregnancy.

Postcoital Douching
The intended purpose of postcoital douching is to wash sperm out of the reproductive tract or to kill or immobilize sperm that the douche solution contacts. This is relatively inexpensive and female-initiated, but it is not very effective. Sperm move very rapidly once deposited, and douching may push the sperm upward.

Lactational Amenorrhea Method (Breastfeeding)
Breastfeeding is sometimes used as a method of birth control because the high blood levels of prolactin that occur with breastfeeding may suppress ovulation. This may be effective in the first 6 months after delivery. It requires "full or nearly full" breastfeeding and that the woman has not experienced her first postpartum menses (any bleeding 56 days postpartum). This method costs nothing but is not very effective. Prolactin levels can vary widely, and ovulation may resume at any time without any noticeable signs, resulting in pregnancy before a menstrual period occurs.

Sterilization

Permanent sterilization can be accomplished by interrupting the fallopian tubes, interrupting the vas deferens (by vasectomy, as discussed in Chapter 43), or removing the uterus (hysterectomy). Tubal interruption (tubal ligation or "getting the tubes tied") may be done by tying a suture or placing a ring or clip around each fallopian tube, coagulating a section of the tubes, or surgically removing a portion of the tube and suturing the ends. These procedures are usually done by laparoscope in an outpatient setting, as an additional procedure performed during a caesarean delivery, or within a few days after a vaginal delivery.

Advantages, Disadvantages, Side Effects, and Risks
Although sterilization is not absolutely certain to be permanent, the failure rate is low and has decreased with newer surgical methods.

Patient Education
Patients should be advised by their surgeon about the complications of the surgery and reversal options before they sign a consent form for sterilization. If any uncertainty about the surgery is evident, the HCP should be notified promptly.

PREGNANCY TERMINATION

Termination of pregnancy (abortion) is a difficult topic. Discussions are often charged with emotion. Both prolife and prochoice advocates argue based on human rights—the former on rights of the fetus and the latter on rights of the mother—because of the humanity of each party. In the United States, abortions are legal in the first and second trimesters of pregnancy.

Reasons for Therapeutic Abortion
Ectopic Pregnancy
An ectopic pregnancy is the implantation of a fertilized ovum in an area other than the uterus. This can occur because of an abnormally shaped uterus or fallopian tubes that are obstructed as a result of abnormal development, scarring from STIs or other inflammatory processes, or for unknown reasons. It is a life-threatening situation for the mother; currently, a therapeutic abortion is the only treatment.

Prenatal Abnormalities
Development of a variety of prenatal testing methods has introduced the possibility of knowing many things about a baby before birth. Prenatal testing may be done using ultrasound, samples of fluid taken from the amniotic sac or the placental villi, or blood samples from the mother. From these tests, some genetic diseases and congenital deformities can be identified. After anomalies are diagnosed, some patients choose to abort the baby. This is a very difficult decision, even in instances in which the baby has a fatal defect that will not allow it to live outside the uterus. It is important to provide information about abortion, as well as alternatives to abortion and possible treatments for the child, when a patient has a serious prenatal diagnosis. No one should feel pressured to make the decision quickly to abort, but legal requirements and increasing risk for the mother may limit the time to decide. Abortion because of fetal abnormality may result in grieving and guilt for the patient and her family.

Methods of Abortion
Several methods are available, determined primarily by the length of the gestation and the goal of inflicting as little trauma to the mother's reproductive system as possible while still inducing pregnancy loss. Time periods for the different abortion methods and the allowable reasons for legal abortion vary according to the laws of the state, province, or country.

Chemical Agents
For emergency contraception, treatment consists of postcoital administration of sufficient estrogen and progestin, or levonorgestrel (Plan B, also sometimes called the "morning-after pill"), to prevent ovulation and possibly to prevent fertilization if ovulation has already occurred. The drug also prevents a fertilized ovum from implanting in the uterine lining. If a fertilized ovum has already implanted when the patient takes the drug, the pregnancy will not be terminated. For this reason, there is disagreement about whether Plan B is a form of contraception or a form of abortion.

Plan B is available at pharmacies without a prescription. Typically, it is used after unexpected, unprotected sexual intercourse (as with sexual assault) or with unexpected risk of conception (as with condom failure). For the medication to be effective, the initial dose must be taken within 5 days of intercourse; but sooner is better. Because no advance planning is required before intercourse, Plan B can be misused as a casual form of birth control. Patients who use it in this way need education about more appropriate birth control methods. Side effects of Plan B can include nausea, vomiting, headaches, and breast tenderness.

Another type of postcoital medication prevents binding of progestins at their receptors, causing a chemically induced abortion up to the 10th week of pregnancy, and is known as a *medical abortion*. Medication can be given orally and/or vaginally. You may recall the controversial RU-486, or mifepristone (Mifeprex). Mifepristone causes the blockage of progesterone from the uterine lining, causing the lining to break down. The patient is also given a dose of misoprostol, which causes the uterus to empty. It must be used within 70 days after the first day of the woman's last period. Pregnancy must be confirmed along with how far pregnant a woman is before medical abortion. Nausea and cramping can accompany expulsion of the uterine contents.

Abortion Methods for Early Pregnancy
Early in a pregnancy (during approximately the first 13 weeks), pregnancy termination will likely take place using menstrual extraction or vacuum aspiration. Menstrual extraction is removal of the endometrial lining by manual suction and can be done during the first 7 weeks following the last menstrual period. This can be done without anesthesia or cervical dilation by inserting a small cannula into the cervix and aspirating with a large syringe. Vacuum aspiration is a similar process used from confirmation of pregnancy through the first 13 weeks. It requires cervical dilation and usually is done with local anesthesia. The patient returns home 1 to 4 hours after the procedure.

Abortion Methods for Later Pregnancy
During the second trimester, dilation and evacuation (D&E) may be performed. The fetus is much larger, so more dilation is required. In this procedure, the cervix is first softened with oral or local mifepristone or misoprostol. Dilation can be accomplished by inserting an absorbent rod (usually Dilopan). This absorbs fluid and swells, gradually dilating the cervix and stimulating labor contractions. The uterine contents are aspirated and removed with forceps. This is done as an outpatient procedure, usually under regional or local anesthesia. Prostaglandin is another option administered either by suppository into the vagina or by injection into the amniotic sac; this induces uterine contractions and results in delivery a few hours later. Unfortunately, a live fetus too premature to survive may be born by this method and continue to breathe for a time.

Hysterotomy involves removal of the uterine contents through an abdominal incision in the same manner as a

• WORD • BUILDING •

hysterotomy: hystero—womb + tomy—cutting

cesarean delivery. This procedure is rarely done for pregnancy termination.

Risks and Complications

Abortion involves risks. Some are the same risks inherent in childbirth, such as possible hemorrhage or introduction of infection. However, additional risks are related to the interruption of natural processes and the aggressiveness with which the products of conception are removed during abortion. During an uncomplicated childbirth, the uterine lining is not scraped or forcefully emptied by suction. Natural hormonal preparation for term childbirth contributes to uterine contraction after the birth, which decreases blood loss. With abortion, this process is interrupted. Artificial dilation of the cervix or introduction of instruments may cause injury. Injured tissues can become sites for growth of microorganisms. Finally, infertility as a result of complications related to abortion, although relatively uncommon, is a risk.

Some possible physical complications following abortion are injuries to the uterus or cervix, excessive bleeding, infection, retention of some products of conception, and possible failure of abortion. Rarely, second-trimester abortions can be complicated by amniotic fluid embolism, in which amniotic fluid is absorbed into the uterine circulation because of disruption of placental attachments with instruments. Amniotic fluid in the mother's circulatory system can result in circulatory collapse and disseminated intravascular coagulation (DIC). DIC is a serious derangement of the body's blood clotting controls and, although rare, can be fatal.

Nursing Care and Patient Education

Care after abortion is very important. Patients rarely stay overnight, and complications can occur after discharge. Patients should be carefully monitored after the procedure for signs of bleeding. Instruct the patient that bleeding should not exceed a heavy period, that passage of clots larger than a quarter may signify complications, and that discharge should not become foul-smelling. Patients should be given a phone number to call 24 hours per day, 7 days per week, in case fever, chills, excessive bleeding, or foul-smelling discharge occur. The patient should be advised to abstain from sexual intercourse for the time specified by the HCP (usually about 3 weeks).

Some women feel relief after abortion. However, a grief response is also common, even if the baby was unwanted and the patient does not have strong beliefs against abortion. There is debate about frequency of postabortion syndrome or whether such a condition exists. However, loss and trauma have occurred in any case and can result in higher rates of anxiety, depression, substance use disorders, and suicidal behavior (Reardon, 2018). Availability of psychological counseling for women after abortion is very important. Women should be given a number to call for support if they wish to do so. The need for birth control should be determined.

Ethical Issues

Ethically, an individual nurse should not be required to assist in treatment that demands they act in a way that contradicts personal moral beliefs. This would violate the nurse's rights. However, the nurse also has an ethical duty to care to patients for whom they are responsible. It is wise for nurses who have moral objections to abortion to carefully choose their work setting. For example, choosing to work in day surgery in a hospital that performs abortions and refusing to care for abortion patients is not a legitimate option. Nurses can positively influence the abortion situation by teaching about family planning, which may lower the number of requests for abortions or becoming involved with agencies that help women find viable alternatives.

TUMORS OF THE REPRODUCTIVE SYSTEM

Benign Growths

Fibroid Tumors

PATHOPHYSIOLOGY AND ETIOLOGY. A fibroid tumor, or **leiomyoma** (plural: leiomyomas or leiomyomata), is a benign tumor made up of endometrial cells that have implanted on or within the walls of the uterus. Although the exact cause is unknown, heredity and hormones play a role.

SIGNS AND SYMPTOMS. Small fibroid tumors may cause no symptoms at all; other tumors can grow very large and may cause pain or menstrual disorders, and interfere with fertility. If they exert pressure on the bladder or bowel, urinary frequency or constipation may occur. Pressure on the blood supply to tissues can result in tissue necrosis.

DIAGNOSTIC TESTS. If a woman has symptoms of a fibroid tumor, an abdominal or transvaginal ultrasound will be performed. Blood tests may be done to identify hormone imbalances or anemia due to bleeding. If necessary, magnetic resonance imaging may be done, or other imaging studies such as hysteroscopy or hysterosalpingography (see Chapter 41).

THERAPEUTIC MEASURES. Because fibroid tumors are estrogen-sensitive, medical treatment may involve hormone suppression. Uterine artery embolization (also called fibroid embolization) introduces tiny spongelike particles into the artery that supplies the fibroid. This cuts off the blood supply to the tumor and causes it to shrink. Surgical options include myomectomy or hysterectomy. **Myomectomy** is removal of only the fibroid tumor, chosen to preserve fertility. Myomectomy may be done surgically through an abdominal or vaginal incision or with a laser introduced through a laparoscope. Hysterectomy may be necessary for large fibroids or those that cause severe bleeding or discomfort.

• WORD • BUILDING •
leiomyoma: leio—smooth + myom(a)—fibroid
myomectomy: myom(a)—fibroid + ec—away + tomy—cutting

Polyps

PATHOPHYSIOLOGY, ETIOLOGY, AND SYMPTOMS. Polyps are benign growths that grow inside the uterus or on the cervix. They may bleed after intercourse or between menstrual cycles. They are generally teardrop-shaped and attached by a stalk. The cause is unknown, but estrogen plays a role in their development.

THERAPEUTIC MEASURES. Polyps are generally removed vaginally or transcervically by separating the stalk from the uterus and stopping the bleeding with chemical, electrical, or laser cautery. Removal of polyps in the vagina can be done without anesthetic in an HCP's office. Removal of polyps transcervically requires cervical dilation and is more likely to be done in a hospital with anesthesia.

Reproductive System Cysts

PATHOPHYSIOLOGY, ETIOLOGIES, AND SIGNS AND SYMPTOMS. Several types of cysts affect women's health. Ovarian cysts are associated with incomplete ovulation, **hypertrophy** of the corpus luteum after ovulation, and inflammation of the ovary. Most ovarian cysts eventually shrink spontaneously and merely cause discomfort for a time. "Chocolate" cysts are formed when endometrial cells bleed into an enclosed space, such as with endometriosis. They are filled with old blood that has become the color of chocolate. Cystadenomas are benign growths that sometimes undergo cellular transformation and become cancerous. Any pelvic mass in a postmenopausal woman should be investigated for malignancy.

THERAPEUTIC MEASURES. Most cysts are not surgically removed, but excessive size, interference with fertility, and high cancer potential may make needle drainage, biopsy, laparoscopic surgery, or **laparotomy** necessary. If cysts are painful, heat application to the abdomen or back can promote comfort.

Polycystic Ovary Syndrome

PATHOPHYSIOLOGY AND ETIOLOGY. Polycystic ovary syndrome (PCOS) is a complex endocrine disorder of unknown etiology. Many symptoms of PCOS result from insulin resistance with excessive insulin levels in the blood that stimulates secretion of androgens by the ovaries. Heredity and inflammation also contribute.

SIGNS AND SYMPTOMS. Women with PCOS often have infertility, obesity, and menstrual disturbances. They also may have masculinization (including excess hair growth). They have increased risk of diabetes mellitus, elevated blood pressure, coronary artery disease, depression, and endometrial cancer, among other problems. Obesity increases risk for complications.

DIAGNOSTIC TESTS. Diagnostic tests can include blood tests to rule out other causes of endocrine abnormality and determine lipid levels and glucose tolerance. A pelvic examination can help identify abnormal growths. Transvaginal ultrasound helps identify abnormalities in the uterus and ovaries.

THERAPEUTIC MEASURES. Medical treatments can involve blood pressure medications, lipid control medications, and oral hypoglycemic agents such as metformin (Glucophage). Diet and exercise may be recommended for weight reduction, control of lipid levels, and cardiac health. Oral contraceptives may be used to normalize hormone levels and protect the endometrium for those who do not plan to conceive. Ovulation-inducing medication may be used for women who desire to conceive; treatment with metformin may also prompt ovulation. If masculinization is a problem, antiandrogen medication such as spironolactone (Aldactone) may be prescribed. See "Evidence-Based Practice."

If medications and lifestyle changes are ineffective, laparoscopic surgery or laser treatments may be used to trigger ovulation or destroy some of the cysts.

Evidence-Based Practice

Clinical Question
Does cinnamon help control blood sugar in women with polycystic ovary syndrome?

Evidence
A systematic review of studies looking at the use of cinnamon supplementation for blood sugar control in polycystic ovary syndrome (PCOS) found that "cinnamon supplementation significantly reduced" insulin resistance in women with PCOS (Heshmati et al, 2020). Other studies have also found cinnamon can reduce insulin resistance in type 2 diabetes.

Implications for Nursing Practice
You can encourage your patients with PCOS to talk to their HCPs about adding cinnamon to their treatment. This should not be done without HCP involvement, because even natural substances can interact with medications, and dosage recommendations may vary.

References: Hendre, A., Sontakke, A., Patil, S., & Phatak, R. (2019). Effect of cinnamon supplementation on fasting blood glucose and insulin resistance in patients with type 2 diabetes. *Pravara Medical Review, 11*(2), 4–8; Heshmati, J., Sepidarkish, M., Morvaridzadeh, M., Farsi, F., Tripathi, N., Razavi, M., & Rezaeinejad, M. (2020). The effect of cinnamon supplementation on glycemic control in women with polycystic ovary syndrome: A systematic review and meta-analysis. *Journal of Food Biochemistry, 45*(1), e13543. https://doi.org/10.1111/jfbc.13543.

Bartholin Cysts

PATHOPHYSIOLOGY, ETIOLOGY, AND SIGNS AND SYMPTOMS. Bartholin glands are located on each side of the vaginal opening and secrete lubricating fluid. If a gland becomes obstructed, a cyst results. If the cyst becomes infected

• **WORD • BUILDING** •

hypertrophy: hyper—too much + trophy—nourishment (growth)
laparotomy: laparo(o)—abdominal wall + tomy—cutting

(abscessed), it can be very painful. A small Bartholin cyst may be asymptomatic. Infection of the cyst can cause pain with sitting and with intercourse.

THERAPEUTIC MEASURES. Sitz baths can help a small cyst to rupture on its own or promote healing after incision and drainage (I&D). I&D can alleviate the discomfort of a larger infected cyst. Antibiotics may be prescribed. If Bartholin cyst formation occurs repeatedly, **marsupialization** (the surgical formation of a permanent opening in a gland to facilitate drainage) may be recommended.

Dermoid Cysts

PATHOPHYSIOLOGY, ETIOLOGY, AND SIGNS AND SYMPTOMS. Rarely and for unknown reasons, a **dermoid** cyst (also called a cystic **teratoma**) may develop from a germinal cell of an ovary. This cell divides and differentiates into various tissue types such as skin, teeth, bones, hair, and even extremities in a disordered arrangement. This type of cyst may grow quite large and may occur on both ovaries at the same time.

THERAPEUTIC MEASURES. Dermoid cysts are removed by laparoscopy or laparotomy. If the cyst contains glandular tissue that is secreting hormones, adjustment of hormone levels to normal may take some time. Although most dermoid cysts are benign, some are malignant, especially in postmenopausal women, so a biopsy is generally done on the tissue.

NURSING CARE. Growth of a dermoid cyst can be a frightening experience. Reassurance that this is a disordered group of cells identical to the other cells in her body, rather than a deformed baby, is important.

Malignant Disorders

Malignancies can occur in all parts of the reproductive system and at all ages. Although reproductive system cancers are more common in older women, ovarian tumors can occur even in young girls. Both male and female children of women who were given diethylstilbesterol (DES) between 1940 and 1971 to prevent pregnancy complications have experienced a high incidence of developmental defects and cancers of the reproductive organs.

This section presents a general overview of the most common cancers. If investigated and treated early enough, cure is often possible.

Vulvar Cancer

PATHOPHYSIOLOGY, ETIOLOGY, AND SIGNS AND SYMPTOMS. Although vulvar cancer is not common, alertness to changes in visible parts of the reproductive system such as the vulva can result in early diagnosis, require less drastic treatment, and end with more positive results. Persistent itching of the vulva or appearance of white or red patches, rough areas, skin ulcers, or wartlike growths should not be ignored; these can be signs of precancerous or cancerous changes. Risk factors for vulvar cancer include exposure to human papillomavirus, precancerous or cancerous changes of the genitalia, immune system depression, and smoking.

DIAGNOSTIC TESTS. Regular pelvic and physical examinations can identify lesions. Biopsy of suspicious lesions is necessary to diagnose vulvar cancer.

THERAPEUTIC MEASURES. If discovered early, vulvar cancer may be treated with removal or destruction of cancerous cells. If diagnosed late, it may require surgical removal of the entire vulva and associated lymph nodes (a radical vulvectomy) with subsequent skin grafting from other areas of the body for repair. Radiation, chemotherapy, immunotherapy, and targeted therapy may also be used.

> **LEARNING TIP**
> "Three C" changes that may indicate cancer are changes in **c**olor, **c**ontour, and **c**onsistency of a tissue.

Cervical Cancer

PATHOPHYSIOLOGY. Changes in cervical cells discovered with a Pap smear are called *cervical dysplasia*. Without treatment, severe dysplasia can become cancerous.

ETIOLOGIES. Abnormal cells are almost always caused by human papillomavirus (HPV). Other factors include multiple sex partners, three or more pregnancies, smoking, being overweight, a compromised immune system, and infection with chlamydia, gonorrhea, syphilis, or HIV/AIDS.

SIGNS AND SYMPTOMS. Although some women experience slight spotting or serosanguineous discharge with cervical cancer, many are asymptomatic until the cancer is widespread. Stages of cervical cancer range from stage I (confined to the cervix) to stage IV (spread to other areas of the body).

DIAGNOSTIC TESTS. Pap smears (Chapters 11 and 41) are the best method of screening for cervical cancer currently available. A Pap smear determines the degree of cellular change, or dysplasia. Women can also do self-checks for HPV with a home kit. Colposcopy is done to obtain more information following an abnormal Pap smear (Chapter 41). Imaging studies may be done to assist with staging of the cancer. Women can usually stop having routine Pap smears at age 65 if they have had normal tests for three years in a row.

THERAPEUTIC MEASURES. Treatments for preinvasive neoplasias include **cryotherapy** (freezing), laser therapy (burning), and surgical removal of the involved area with a loop

• **WORD • BUILDING •**

marsupialization: marsupial—pouch + ization—process of making
dermoid: derm—skin + oid—form
teratoma: terat—monster + oma—growth
cryotherapy: cryo—cold + therapy—treatment

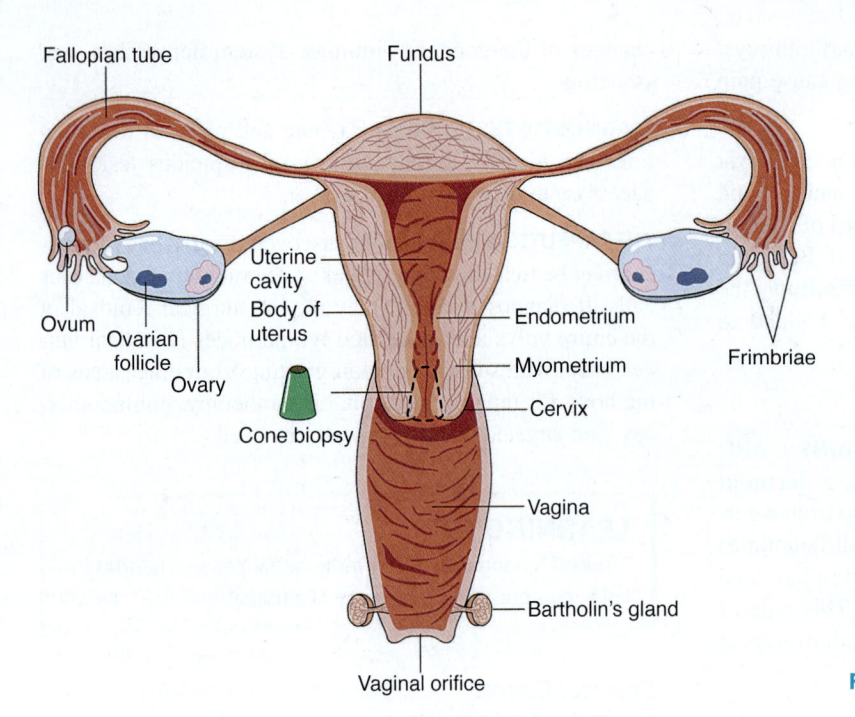

FIGURE 42.11 Conization.

excision instrument or by conization (Fig. 42.11). All these procedures are done through the vagina, with no external incisions. After these treatments, the patient is advised not to douche, use tampons, or have intercourse for approximately 2 weeks to allow healing to take place. Advise her to report immediately if fever, bloody vaginal discharge, or foul-smelling vaginal discharge occurs. For invasive cancers, hysterectomy, radiation implant, or chemotherapy may be done.

PREVENTION. An HPV vaccination (Gardasil) can protect against many types of HPV. It is recommended for both males and females aged 9 to 26, regardless of sexual activity status or exposure to HPV.

Endometrial Cancer

PATHOPHYSIOLOGY, ETIOLOGIES, AND SIGNS AND SYMPTOMS. Endometrial cancer is the most common type of uterine cancer and typically develops in response to relative estrogen excess. Abrupt changes in bleeding patterns, especially bleeding in a menopausal woman, can indicate endometrial cancer. Estrogen excess can develop for many reasons. Estrogen levels fluctuate widely in the perimenopausal period. Obesity results in increased estrogen production that is not balanced by progestins. Estrogen replacement therapy for menopausal symptoms without addition of progestins has been associated with an increase in endometrial cancer. Addition of a progestin may decrease the risk of endometrial cancer to less than that of untreated women. Additional risk factors include never being pregnant and older age.

DIAGNOSTIC TESTS. Diagnosis is generally done by endometrial biopsy. Transvaginal ultrasound or hysteroscopy may also be performed.

THERAPEUTIC MEASURES. Depending on the stage of endometrial cancer and metastasis, treatment with hysterectomy, radiation, or chemotherapy may be used.

Ovarian Cancer

PATHOPHYSIOLOGY AND ETIOLOGY. Ovarian cancer is an insidious killer because cellular changes in the ovaries are often asymptomatic until cancer advances. We know little about what prompts malignant changes in these cells. Risk factors include early menarche and late menopause, long-term estrogen replacement therapy, family history of ovarian cancer, and older age. Birth control pills may reduce risk.

SIGNS AND SYMPTOMS. Symptoms may be vague, and include weight loss, urinary frequency, pelvic pain, and gastrointestinal problem such as a bloated feeling, constipation, and early satiety.

DIAGNOSTIC TESTS. Identification of abnormal growths on the ovaries may begin with bimanual examination, so it is important for women, especially older women, to continue regular pelvic exams even if they are not sexually active or have had a hysterectomy. Various blood tests measuring tumor marker substances, ultrasonography, CT scan, and MRI may be used to assist in diagnosis. Removal of an ovary to test for cancer may be done.

THERAPEUTIC MEASURES. Treatment may involve surgical removal of the ovaries (and sometimes the uterus) by laparoscopy or laparotomy. Sometimes ovaries are removed to prevent the disease in women who have a high familial risk. Estrogen-blocking therapy can reduce stimulation of cancer cells. Radiation and combination chemotherapy may also be used.

Nursing Care of Patients With Malignant Disorders

Women with gynecological cancers have unique needs because of the nature of the disease. Body image disturbance, anxiety, depression, and concerns about sexuality may occur. You can collaborate with a social worker, case manager, clergy, or psychologist to help women cope. You can assist with locating a support group if the patient is interested. See Chapter 11 for care of patients receiving radiation or chemotherapy. See the next section for patients undergoing surgery. See Table 42.9 for a summary of tumors of the reproductive system.

GYNECOLOGICAL SURGERY

Endoscopic Surgeries

Many surgeries performed on the reproductive system can be done using an endoscope. These instruments contain magnifying lenses and a light source and often also include tiny tools for performing surgery, removing small areas of diseased tissue and samples, suction, and cauterizing bleeding vessels. Because endoscopic surgeries require tiny incisions (usually less than 1 inch long), these procedures carry less tissue disruption, less risk of infection, and less bleeding than traditional surgical techniques. Recuperation is usually faster and with fewer complications. However, not all surgeries can be managed in this way.

Laparoscopies are the most common endoscopic surgical procedure for women's reproductive system surgeries. This method provides access to the abdominal cavity and anterior portions of the reproductive organs for tubal ligations and repairs, removal of ectopic pregnancy, removal of small tumors or endometriotic tissue, and aspiration of fluid-filled cysts.

Minimally invasive robotic surgery uses computers and robots (see Chapter 12). This method allows the surgeon to make several of 1 cm to 2 cm incisions to gain access and three-dimensional visualization into the pelvic cavity. Gynecologically, this method can be used for hysterectomy and myomectomy. The benefits of this method compared to other surgical methods include a shorter hospital stay and less pain and scarring for the patient. There is also less risk of infection, less blood loss, fewer transfusions, faster recoveries, and quicker return to normal activities.

Culdoscopies provide access to the area at the back of the uterus. A **culdotomy**, an incision into the upper posterior portion of the vagina, is necessary to insert the cannula. A **culdocentesis**, the removal of fluid from the cul-de-sac of Douglas, may be done during a culdoscopy. Aftercare is similar to that for a laparoscopy. The patient should be informed that a small amount of vaginal spotting may be expected from the incision but that heavy, purulent, or foul-smelling discharge should be reported because it could indicate infection.

Colposcopies typically are used to screen, diagnose, or treat problems of the cervix. A binocular microscope attached to the scope cannula is introduced into the vagina so the HCP can examine dysplastic cells while in their normal place and treat cervical dysplasia.

Hysteroscopy may be used to treat problems within the uterus. Removal of polyps and other growths, modification of congenital malformations such as septa (walls of tissue where there should be none), and laser ablation of endometrial tissue may all be done during hysteroscopy. The endoscope may be inserted farther into the fallopian tubes to perform a salpingoscopy, allowing surgical or laser opening of blocked tubes.

Nursing Care and Patient Education

Postoperative care involves careful monitoring for possible excessive internal bleeding, including vital signs, skin color and temperature, and pain. Discharge teaching includes instruction about signs of complications, medications, and when and where to go for suture removal.

Table 42.9 Tumors of the Reproductive System Summary

Signs and Symptoms	Menstrual pain/dysfunction Infertility Constipation Vaginal bleeding Abdominal/perineal pain or swelling Androgen characteristics Obesity Diabetes Coronary artery disease
Diagnostic Tests	Physical examination Laparoscopy Ultrasound Computed tomography (CT) scan or magnetic resonance imaging (MRI) Biopsy Hormone levels
Therapeutic Measures	Surgery Chemical, electrical, or laser cautery Oral contraceptives and medications Incision, drainage, marsupialization Chemotherapy Radiation therapy
Priority Nursing Diagnoses	*Acute* or *Chronic Pain* related to lesion/surgery *Urge Urinary Incontinence* or *Constipation* related to lesion or surgery *Disturbed Body Image* related to body structure abnormality *Sexual Dysfunction* related to disturbance in self-concept

Hysterectomy

Removal of the uterus (hysterectomy) may be done for a variety of reasons, including abnormally heavy or painful menstruation, large fibroid or other benign tumors, severe uterine prolapse, and cancer of the uterus. It should not be done as a sterilization procedure because the risks involved in hysterectomy are much greater than the risks associated with tubal ligation. The surgery can be done through an abdominal incision (total abdominal hysterectomy [TAH]), vaginally, laparoscopically, or robotically. The vagina is left intact, and the proximal end (which had been attached to the uterus) is sutured, forming a blind pouch. Although less vaginal lubrication is present after hysterectomy, nerve routes are maintained, and satisfactory sexual intercourse is expected to continue.

There are three types of hysterectomy: *Total hysterectomy* is the removal of the uterus and cervix. *Supracervical hysterectomy* (also known as partial or subtotal) removes just the upper part of the uterus, while the cervix is left in place. A *radical hysterectomy* involves the removal of the whole uterus, the tissue on both sides of the cervix, and the upper part of the vagina.

Sometimes, the choice is made to remove the fallopian tubes (**salpingectomy**) and ovaries (**oophorectomy**), known as a *bilateral salpingo-oophorectomy* (BSO). If the ovaries are removed, the woman undergoes immediate menopause. She may suffer from symptoms associated with menopause, including increased risks of cardiovascular disease and osteoporosis. Estrogen replacement therapy is typically given until the age of natural menopause. If removal of the ovaries is done because of the presence of estrogen-dependent cancer, then estrogen replacement is not usually feasible. You can assist with education about management of menopausal symptoms as well as by providing emotional support.

See "Nursing Care Plan for the Patient Undergoing Hysterectomy" for nursing care specific to hysterectomy. In addition to the nursing diagnoses covered, monitor for *Acute Pain, Delayed Surgical Recovery, Anxiety, and Constipation*. See Chapters 10 and 12, respectively, for additional interventions for pain and postoperative patients, and Chapter 34 for interventions for constipation.

CUE RECOGNITION 42.1

Your patient is 12 hours post–total abdominal hysterectomy. You administer her pain medication as ordered, but an hour later she is still in pain. What do you do?

Suggested answer are at the end of the chapter.

• **WORD • BUILDING** •
salpingectomy: salpingo—tubal + ec—from + tomy—cutting
oophorectomy: oophor—ovary + ec—from + tomy—cutting

Nursing Care Plan for the Patient Undergoing Hysterectomy

Nursing Diagnosis: *Grieving* related to change in body image and loss of reproductive ability
Expected Outcome: The patient will adjust to life change; accept assistance from others
Evaluation of Outcome: Does the patient talk about her feelings? Does she talk about plans to seek out assistance from a support group or friends and family?

Intervention	Rationale	Evaluation
Develop a trusting relationship with the patient.	A trusting relationship is essential to communication.	Does patient show trust? Is she willing to talk with nurse or others?
Listen to the woman's story; she may want to talk about her children or her desire for children.	Reproductive status is very important to some women. Hysterectomy may be especially difficult for premenopausal women.	Does she wish to share her experiences?
Help the woman identify coping strategies that have worked in the past.	Strategies that have worked in the past are more likely to be useful in the future.	Can she identify two or three helpful strategies?
Provide information about local support groups.	If the information is readily available, it may be easier for her to follow up.	Does she follow up or state plans to do so?
Help the patient set goals for the future.	Setting goals for the future can help her look forward instead of backward.	Does she identify goals?
If indicated, request a referral for counseling.	Some patients may need more personalized assistance.	Is counseling indicated? Is referral obtained?

Nursing Care Plan for the Patient Undergoing Hysterectomy—cont'd

Nursing Diagnosis: *Risk for Urinary Retention* related to manipulation of the bladder and ureters during surgery, anticholinergic drugs, fluid intake changes, and fear of pain
Expected Outcome: The patient will void 30 mL/hr or more without difficulty.
Evaluation of Outcome: Is the patient able to void and effectively empty bladder when voiding? Is the patient voiding at least 30 mL/hr?

Intervention	Rationale	Evaluation
Monitor urinary output after surgery. Report to registered nurse or HCP if less than 30 mL/hr or unable to void.	Inadequate urinary output can be an evidence of dehydration, low glomerular perfusion, kidney dysfunction, damage to ureter, or urinary retention.	Is output greater than 30 mL/hour? Is patient able to void without discomfort?
Determine bladder fullness using Doppler monitoring or scratch test (listening with a stethoscope, lightly scratch abdomen as you move downward from xiphoid until you hear change in sound indicating top of the bladder).	Urine retention can cause infection and damage to kidneys, ureters, and bladder. The scratch test and Doppler monitoring cause less discomfort and pressure than palpation of the abdominal incision area.	Does patient feel she is emptying fully when voiding? Does Doppler or scratch test indicate residual urine after voiding?
Medicate for pain on a fixed schedule for operative day and first postoperative day (unless patient declines).	Maintenance of a consistent blood level of medication in the immediate postoperative period provides relief of pain and promotes voiding without fear of discomfort.	Does patient state that she is comfortable?

Key Points

- Most breast symptoms, such as pain, swelling, and tenderness result from cyclic variations in hormone levels.
- Fibrocystic breast disease occurs when breast cells have an exaggerated response to hormones such as estrogen, causing pain and hard lumps.
- Mastitis is breast infection with inflammation from injury and introduction of bacteria into the breast, most commonly with breastfeeding.
- Breast cancer, the most common cancer in women, is an abnormal growth of breast cells.
- Breast cancer may be treated with surgery, radiation therapy, chemotherapy, hormone therapy, targeted therapy, or a combination of these.
- Mammoplasty is surgical modification of the breast to restore a normal shape after removal of cancerous tissues or to change breast size or appearance.
- The many types of menstrual abnormalities can be caused by stress, pregnancy, hormonal imbalances, metabolic imbalances, benign or malignant tumors, infections, liver, kidney or thyroid diseases, blood or bone marrow abnormalities, and foreign bodies in the uterus.
- Medical treatment of menstrual disorders often starts with hormone level adjustments or use of NSAIDs. Surgical treatment can involve D&C, laser ablation of endometrial tissue, and hysterectomy.
- Painful menstruation, or dysmenorrhea, may be primary or secondary. Primary dysmenorrhea likely results from endogenous prostaglandins that stimulate uterine contractions, producing cramping pain. Secondary dysmenorrhea is caused by endometriosis, pelvic infection, retroversion of the uterus, fibroid tumors, or another reproductive tract disorder.
- PMS is a recurrent problem for many women. Symptoms include water retention; headaches; discomfort in joints, muscles, and breasts; changes in affect, concentration, and coordination; and sensory changes.
- PDD is like PMS but much more severe, with symptoms of depression, irritability, tension before menstruation, mood swings, feelings of hopelessness, and suicidal ideation.
- Endometriosis causes pain, infertility, development of scar tissue, swelling, and organ damage because of functioning endometrial tissue located outside the uterus.
- Menopause is the permanent cessation of menstrual cycles from decreased hormone production, a natural part of aging that may cause uncomfortable symptoms.
- TSS is most often associated with superabsorbent tampon use during menstruation. TSS is a life-threatening systemic infection with strains of *Staphylococcus aureus* or *Streptococcus* that produce toxins.

- Cystocele occurs when the bladder prolapses into the vaginal space because of inadequate support. A feeling of pelvic pressure and stress incontinence are common with this condition.
- Rectocele occurs when a portion of the rectum prolapses into the vagina because of inadequate support. This causes pelvic pressure, fecal incontinence, constipation, and hemorrhoids.
- Uterine prolapse occurs when the uterus prolapses into the vagina. Hysterectomy is the most common treatment.
- Infertility is a complicated problem with many causes that may result from either male or female partners.
- *Reproductive life planning* is a more comprehensive term than *contraception* that implies reasoned decisions about pregnancy.
- Types of effective contraception include oral contraceptives (birth control pills), implants and injectable medicines, estrogen-progestin ring, transdermal contraceptive patch, barrier methods, condoms, diaphragms and cervical caps, spermicides, intrauterine devices, and natural family planning. Tubal ligation also prevents pregnancy.
- Therapeutic abortions may be performed for several reasons, including ectopic pregnancy or prenatal abnormalities.
- A fibroid tumor, or leiomyoma, is a benign tumor made up of endometrial cells that have implanted on or within the walls of the uterus. These tumors can grow very large and may cause pain or menstrual disorders, exert pressure on the bladder or bowel, cause necrosis because of pressure on the blood supply to tissues, and interfere with fertility. Although the exact cause is unknown, heredity and hormones play a role.
- Cysts of the ovaries can result from incomplete ovulation, hypertrophy of the corpus luteum after ovulation, or inflammation of the ovary. Most ovarian cysts eventually shrink.
- Polycystic ovary syndrome is a complex abnormality of endocrine balance of unknown etiology. Multiple cysts on the ovaries are the characteristic symptom along with too much or too little hair, insulin resistance, diabetes, irregular menses, hypertension, coronary artery disease, depression, endometrial cancer, and infertility.
- Changes in cervical cells are called *cervical dysplasia*. Abnormal cells are most often caused by human papillomavirus. Without treatment, severe dysplasia can turn into invasive cancer.
- Endometrial cancer is the most common type of uterine cancer. Abrupt changes in bleeding patterns, especially bleeding in a menopausal woman, can indicate endometrial cancer.

SUGGESTED ANSWERS TO CHAPTER EXERCISES

Cue Recognition
42.1: Use the **WHAT'S UP** format to collect data related to the pain. Examine her abdomen and incision or dressing. Report findings to the RN. Keep in mind that the pain may be more than just postsurgical pain and may even represent a serious complication of surgery.

Critical Thinking & Clinical Judgment
Julie
1. Use the **WHAT'S UP?** format to gather data about Julie's symptoms: How long have you been noticing the lumps? Do you do breast self-examination? Has there been a change in the characteristics of the lumps? Are the lumps mobile or fixed? Have you noticed any breast skin or nipple changes? Have you noticed any leakage of fluid or blood from your breasts? Are you breastfeeding, or have you recently delivered an infant? Have you had a fever? Are the pain and lumps related to your menstrual cycle? Is there anything that makes the symptoms better or worse? Document your findings.
2. Collaborate with the registered nurse or nurse practitioner to teach Julie to continue to do BSE because she is the best person to detect changes. Provide information about limiting fat and caffeine in her diet to help reduce symptoms. Reinforce any information or treatments provided by the nurse practitioner.
3. If Julie is doing BSE every month, then she knows her breasts better than anyone. She should be vigilant for changes that do not feel like her usual tissue.

Lola
1. Interventions that can help control Lola's discomfort related to hot flashes include possible HRT, including phytoestrogens in her diet under her HCP's direction; limiting caffeinated beverages, sugar, and alcohol; dressing in layers so that some may be removed as needed; and lowering the thermostat if possible.
2. Information that should be shared with Lola concerning HRT includes the risks as well as benefits according to most recent data. Check your workplace for prepared pamphlets and other information.
3. Collaborate with the HCP, because even herbal remedies can interact with medications and should be recommended by an HCP.

Jessica
1. Some important information from Jessica would include her true age (state and province laws vary concerning birth control for minors), her intentions, her family situation, whether she is already sexually active, and what information she wants.
2. She needs to know that being sexually active involves more risks than just pregnancy. Discussion of STIs is vital.

Early sexual activity may also be associated with abuse and psychological suffering. The choices of birth control should be explained, including the risks, effectiveness, disadvantages, and advantages of each method. Follow clinic protocol to determine your role in teaching the patient.

3. Potential scenarios can be presented for her "responsible" consideration, such as the following: What would she do if contraceptive failure resulted in a pregnancy? How would she feel if she contracted an incurable or permanently damaging STI that she might pass on to someone else? How would she react to a breakup with her partner after she has engaged in sexual intercourse? Ask about her goals and plans in life. Counseling that evidences concern for the individual at this stage may do a lot to postpone sexual activity until the patient is more mature. It is important for her to realize that choosing to delay sexual activity at this time may be the most responsible and health-promoting life decision she can make. If the HCP does order contraception, ensure that Jessica has the resources to obtain contraception.

Additional Resources

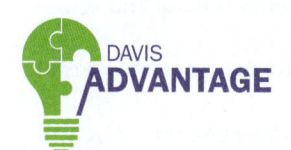

Go to Davis Advantage to complete your learning: strengthen understanding, apply your knowledge, and prepare for the Next Gen NCLEX®.

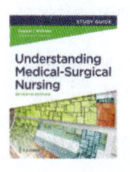

A Study Guide is also available.

CHAPTER 43
Nursing Care of Male Patients With Genitourinary Disorders

Debra K. Hadfield, Jaime Crabb

KEY TERMS

cryptorchidism (kript-OR-ki-dizm)
epididymitis (EP-i-DID-i-MY-tis)
erectile dysfunction (ee-REK-tile dis-FUNK-shun)
hydrocele (HY-droh-seel)
orchiectomy (or-ki-EK-toh-mee)
orchitis (or-KY-tis)
paraphimosis (PAR-uh-fih-MOH-sis)
phimosis (fih-MOH-sis)
priapism (PRY-uh-pizm)
prostatectomy (PRAHS-tah-TEK-tuh-mee)
prostatitis (PRAHS-tuh-TY-tis)
retrograde (REH-troh-GRADE)
suprapubic (SOO-pruh-PEW-bik)
urodynamic (YOO-roh-dy-NAM-ik)
urosepsis (YOO-roh-SEP-sis)
vasectomy (va-SEK-tuh-mee)

CHAPTER CONCEPTS

Elimination
Health promotion
Sexuality

LEARNING OUTCOMES

1. Explain pathophysiology of each male genitourinary and reproductive disorder discussed.
2. Describe the etiologies, signs and symptoms, and treatments of prostate disorders.
3. Plan nursing care for men with genitourinary and reproductive disorders.
4. Describe disorders of the testicles and penis and how they affect sexual function.
5. List selected physical and emotional causes of erectile dysfunction.
6. Discuss the nurse's role in helping men cope with loss of sexual function.
7. Identify disorders of the male reproductive system that interfere with fertility.
8. List treatment options available for male infertility.

Problems affecting the male genitourinary system may be sensitive in nature for both the patient and the nurse because of the sexual nature of the male anatomy. To provide holistic care, the nurse must acknowledge patient sexuality and become skilled in collecting data and caring for problems related to sexual and genitourinary health. The nurse has a unique opportunity to provide important sexual health-care teaching. Discussions about sexual health can be positive learning experiences for both the patient and the nurse if approached in an appropriate manner.

PROSTATE DISORDERS

The prostate gland sits at the base of the bladder and wraps around the upper part of the male urethra like a ring. The primary purpose of the prostate is to provide alkaline secretions to semen and aid in ejaculation. The prostate often increases in size with age. The prostate does not contain any hormones; however, many men fear that prostate problems and treatment will cause problems with their erections or sexual activities.

Prostatitis

Pathophysiology

Prostatitis, or inflammation of the prostate gland, can occur any time after puberty. It can be chronic or a single, acute episode. The inflammation causes the prostate gland to swell, which causes pain, especially when standing. It can eventually lead to difficulty in passing urine because of an inward pressure on the urethra and restricted urine flow.

Etiology

There are four basic types of prostatitis: (1) acute bacterial prostatitis, (2) chronic bacterial prostatitis, (3) chronic prostatitis/chronic pelvic pain syndrome, and (4) asymptomatic inflammatory prostatitis. Bacterial prostatitis is most common in older men. It results in edema and inflammation of all or part of the prostate gland.

Any bacteria that can cause a urinary tract infection (UTI) can also cause acute or chronic bacterial prostatitis. Common bacteria are organisms such as *Escherichia coli* and *Staphylococcus aureus*. Sexually transmitted infections (STIs) can also cause prostatitis. The prostate gland may become infected by the following means:

- Bacteria ascending the urethra
- Infected urine refluxing from the bladder into the prostatic ducts
- Bacteria in the blood or lymph supply infecting the gland
- Surgical instrumentation or other forms of urethral trauma introducing pathogens

Prevention

Ways to prevent prostatitis are regularly and completely emptying the bladder to prevent UTIs, avoiding excess alcohol (a bladder irritant), and avoiding high-risk sexual practices, such as multiple partners.

Signs and Symptoms

The most common symptoms occur with any UTI: urgency, frequency, hesitancy, dribbling, and dysuria. Because of the location and function of the prostate gland, the patient may report low-back, perineal, and postejaculation pain. Other symptoms include nocturia, fever, and chills.

Complications

One complication of acute bacterial prostatitis is urinary retention. If the prostate is extremely swollen, the bladder cannot be completely emptied. Another complication may be a temporary problem with erections. Ascending infections, prostatic abscess, epididymitis, and prostatic calculi (stones) are some of the more serious and rare complications of prostatitis.

Diagnostic Tests

Initial diagnosis is based on symptoms. The first test is a digital rectal examination of the prostate. The health-care provider (HCP) examines the prostate gland by inserting a lubricated, gloved finger into the rectum. Findings may include a warm, irregular, swollen, or painful prostate gland. A urine culture tests for bacteria. The examiner may massage the prostate gland to express prostate secretions, which can be tested for bacteria and white blood cells. Cystoscopy, visualization of the urethra and bladder, may be done to rule out other urological conditions.

Therapeutic Measures

Acute bacterial prostatitis is treated with antibiotics. Additional treatments may include anti-inflammatory agents, stool softeners to reduce straining with bowel movements, warm sitz baths, prostatic massage, and dietary changes such as decreasing spicy foods and alcohol. Alpha-adrenergic blockers such as alfuzosin (Uroxatral) can help relax the bladder neck and reduce pain with urination (Table 43.1). Some patients need prostate surgery to remove the obstruction.

> **BE SAFE!**
> **BE VIGILANT!** Patients with prostate disorders should avoid alpha-adrenergic agonist and anticholinergic medications, which can cause urine retention.

Nursing Process for the Patient With Prostatitis

DATA COLLECTION. Begin collecting data by asking the patient to describe signs and symptoms that indicate evidence of a UTI, such as sudden fever, chills, and reports of urgency, frequency, hesitancy, dysuria, and nocturia. The patient may also have pain in the lower back, in the perineum, or after ejaculating. Ask the patient whether he has ever had a UTI or prostate infection. Ask about sexual history to determine the risk of STIs. Be sure to check for urinary retention from obstruction. Obtain a urine culture and assist with collection of the prostate secretion specimen as needed.

> **PRACTICE ANALYSIS TIP**
> Linking NCLEX-PN® to Practice
> The LPN/LVN will monitor diagnostic or laboratory test results.

NURSING DIAGNOSES, PLANNING, AND IMPLEMENTATION.

> *Urinary Retention related to obstruction evidenced by residual urine in bladder after voiding*
>
> **EXPECTED OUTCOME:** The patient will be able to void effectively as evidenced by residual urine of less than 25% of bladder capacity.

- Evaluate the patient's medications for urinary retention as a side effect. *Many medications, especially those with anticholinergic effects, can cause urinary retention.*

• WORD • BUILDING •

prostatitis: prostat—prostate gland + itis—inflammation

Table 43.1
Medication Used to Treat Disorders of the Male Reproductive Organs

Medication Class/Action

Testosterone Suppressing/Blocking Agents

Examples	Nursing Implications
Initially stimulates and then inhibits follicle-stimulating hormone (FSH) and luteinizing hormone (LH) to suppress testosterone: leuprolide (Lupron) *Analog to luteinizing-releasing hormone; works on pituitary to decrease FSH to decrease sex hormones:* goserelin (Zoladex) *Inhibits androgen uptake and/or binding in tissues:* flutamide (Eulexin)	Store drug at room temperature and protect from light. Monitor for side effects. Inject into upper abdominal wall. Do not aspirate syringe. Monitor hepatic function tests. *Teach:* Signs and symptoms may increase initially. Medication may increase testosterone initially and thus increase symptoms. Urine color changes to amber/yellow green. Avoid excess exposure to sun. Promptly report side effects.

Alpha-Adrenergic Antagonists and Alpha-Reductase Inhibitors

Alpha-Adrenergic Antagonists
Relax smooth muscle and produce vasodilatation.

Examples	Nursing Implications
tamsulosin (Flomax) terazosin (Hytrin) alfuzosin (Uroxatral) doxazosin (Cardura)	Monitor blood pressure/pulse. *Teach:* Dizziness may occur with onset of use. Report side effects. Do not to crush or chew tablets. Do not drive or use heavy machinery.

Alpha-Reductase Inhibitors
Inhibit enzyme responsible for formation of potent androgen from testosterone.

Examples	Nursing Implications
finasteride (Proscar) dutasteride (Avodart)	Obtain baseline prostate-specific antigen (PSA) and perform DRE before use. Caution with liver dysfunction. *Teach:* Side effects. Do not to chew or crush tablets.

Vasodilators, Smooth Muscle Relaxers, and Hormone Replacement

Examples	Nursing Implications
Relax smooth muscle and produce vasodilation: sildenafil (Viagra) tadalafil (Cialis) vardenafil (Levitra)	Some are taken daily and help with symptoms of BPH Check cardiovascular status before use; may be contraindicated. *Teach:* Avoid use when taking nitroglycerin preparations. Take about 1 hour before sexual activity (may be taken 30 minutes to 4 hours before). If erection lasts more than 4 hours, seek emergency care.

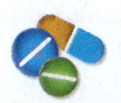

Table 43.1
Medication Used to Treat Disorders of the Male Reproductive Organs—cont'd

Medication Class/Action	
Relax smooth muscle and produce vasodilation: alprostadil (Caverject injection or MUSE suppository) prostaglandin E1 *Herbal vasodilator:* yohimbine	Monitor vital signs. Check for medical conditions before use. Monitor blood pressure as well as renal and hepatic function. *Teach:* Erection should occur in 2 to 5 minutes and should not last more than 4 hours. Report side effects immediately.
Testosterone replacement; produce androgen effects: testosterone transdermal (Testoderm, Androderm) testosterone cypionate (DEPO-testosterone injection)	Rule out cancer before use. Monitor hepatic function and red blood cell count. *Teach:* Report side effects, prolonged erection, or difficulty urinating. Women should avoid contact with medication.

- With suspicion of urine retention, determine residual urine volume by catheterizing patient (according to HCP order) or obtaining a bladder ultrasound immediately after voiding. *Incomplete emptying of the bladder may lead to increased discomfort or ascending infection.*
- Have patient complete a bladder log including patterns of elimination and related symptoms as well as volume/type of fluid consumed for 3 to 7 days. *This will provide an objective verification of intake and output volumes and aid in determination of urinary retention.*
- Educate the patient about avoidance of risk factors for urine retention (e.g., alpha-adrenergic agonists, anticholinergic agents, overfilling of the bladder). *These are modifiable variables that may limit retention of urine.*
- Report urine retention to the registered nurse (RN) or HCP. *Catheterization may be needed to empty the bladder and prevent complications.*
- Educate the patient about avoidance of sexual activities that increase the risk of STIs and the importance of fully treating an STI. *STIs can cause multiple complications, including prostatitis and infertility.*
- Encourage timed voiding to reduce UTI (voiding every 2 to 3 hours during the day).
- Double voiding may help some men empty the bladder. Have the patient try to void again a few minutes after each void.

Deficient Knowledge about cause, treatment, and prevention of prostatitis

EXPECTED OUTCOME: The patient will verbalize understanding of the disorder and demonstrate appropriate self-care.

- Determine the patient's current knowledge and understanding about cause and treatment of prostatitis. *This will allow for additional and/or correct information to be provided about the disorder for appropriate understanding.*
- Provide the patient with additional and/or correct information about the cause and treatment of prostatitis. *This will allow the patient to have a full understanding of the etiology and care related to the disorder and increase likelihood of patient adherence to treatment.*
- Teach avoidance of risk factors such as urinary catheterization, poor hygiene, risky sexual practices, and excessive intake of bladder irritants such as alcohol, caffeine, or citrus juices. *Avoiding risk factors is important to resolving or preventing prostatitis.*
- Encourage the patient to wash his hands and sitz bath equipment before and after each treatment *to prevent infection.*
- Encourage the patient to empty his bladder every 2 to 3 hours even if he does not feel the urge to urinate. *An overstretched bladder increases risk of infection.*
- Encourage fluids up to 2,500 to 3,000 mL/day unless contraindicated by heart failure or other chronic illness. *Fluids help flush the bladder and prevent infection.*
- Include patient's partner in care. *Some treatment options may also include treatment of the partner (e.g., for STIs such as gonorrhea, chlamydiosis, or trichomoniasis; see Chapter 44).*
- Explain use of antibiotics as directed and advise the patient to take the complete course of medication even if he is feeling better. *The entire course of antibiotics is essential to fully treat bacterial infection and prevent development of antibiotic-resistant bacteria.*

Acute Pain related to swelling and irritation of the prostate gland as evidenced by pain rating

EXPECTED OUTCOME: The patient's pain will be controlled as evidenced by the patient's statement that comfort is at an acceptable level.

- Use a culturally appropriate pain scale to help the patient identify his comfort level. *This will aid in understanding the comfort level as defined by the patient and aid in guiding appropriate interventions.*
- Encourage appropriate use of anti-inflammatory medication as ordered. *This will decrease inflammation and promote comfort.*
- Encourage use of comfort measures such as warm sitz baths, sitting on a pillow, or prostatic massage, as needed. *These measures help to decrease swelling and promote patient comfort.*
- Teach the patient to avoid irritants, such as spicy and acidic foods, alcohol, or caffeine. *These irritants can exacerbate symptoms.*
- Consult the HCP about the need for stool softeners. *Firm stool will further irritate the prostate during defecation and increase discomfort.*

EVALUATION. A clean urine culture with the absence of all symptoms of prostatitis is the desired outcome. If interventions have been effective, the patient will have an acceptable comfort level and understand the cause and treatment plan. Prevention of chronic prostatitis can generally be achieved with patient education.

Benign Prostatic Hyperplasia

Enlargement of the prostate gland is a normal process in older men. Benign prostatic hyperplasia (BPH) is a common nonmalignant growth of the prostate that gradually causes urinary obstruction. According to current data, BPH does not increase risk of cancer of the prostate.

Pathophysiology

A slow increase in the number of cells in the prostate gland is generally the result of aging and the male hormone dihydrotestosterone. As the size of the prostate gland increases, it begins to compress or put pressure on the urethra. This narrowing of the urethra makes it difficult to empty the bladder. Eventually the narrowing causes an obstruction, which leads to urine retention or distention of the kidney with urine (hydronephrosis).

The location of the enlargement, rather than the size, determines symptoms. A small growth in the prostate gland closest to the urethra can cause more problems with urination than a larger growth in the outer portion of the gland. BPH typically begins in the center of the gland, causing urinary symptoms early in the disease process.

Etiology

There is no known cause of BPH other than normal aging. Some men think they may have caused the problem by certain sexual practices; however, there is no scientific proof of that at this time. Obesity may play a role in increasing risk. Exercise can reduce risk.

Signs and Symptoms

Symptoms of BPH are identified in two ways: problems related to obstruction or problems related to irritation. Symptoms related to obstruction include a decrease in the size or force of the urinary stream, difficulty in starting a stream, dribbling after urination is complete, urinary retention, and a feeling that the bladder is not empty. The patient may also experience overflow incontinence or an interrupted stream, in which the urine stops midstream and then starts again.

Symptoms related to irritation include nocturia, dysuria, and urgency. HCPs may use a standardized symptom score index tool with patients to monitor symptoms and determine treatment options.

Complications

When BPH is untreated and obstruction is prolonged, serious complications can occur. Urine that sits in the bladder for too long can back up into the kidneys, causing hydronephrosis, renal insufficiency, or **urosepsis** (UTI with septicemia). It can also damage the bladder walls, leading to bladder dysfunction, recurrent UTIs, or calculi (stones). Acute urine retention with total inability to urinate can occur. This is a medical emergency that requires catheterization.

> **NURSING CARE TIP**
> It can be difficult to catheterize a man with an enlarged prostate gland. If you try once and are unable to advance the catheter, contact the RN or HCP.

> **PRACTICE ANALYSIS TIP**
> **Linking NCLEX-PN® to Practice**
> The LPN/LVN will recognize and report change in client condition.

> **BE SAFE!**
> **AVOID FAILURE TO RECOGNIZE!** Check for urine output per facility protocol. Lack of urine output in a patient with BPH could indicate obstruction. This is a medical emergency and must be reported immediately.

Diagnostic Tests

The first test is usually digital rectal examination of the prostate to check for enlargement and whether the gland is hard, lumpy, or "boggy" (soft and spongy). A normal prostate should be fairly firm and smooth. Additional tests include urinalysis, blood urea nitrogen (BUN), serum creatinine, and prostate-specific antigen (PSA). Secondary tests include **urodynamic** flow studies, which may show a decreased urine flow rate. Transrectal ultrasound of the prostate and cystoscopy can reflect structural abnormalities.

• WORD • BUILDING •

urosepsis: uro—urine + sepsis—systemic infection
urodynamic: uro—urine + dynamic—force

Therapeutic Measures

If the patient has no symptoms or mild symptoms, the current medical approach is "watchful waiting." The HCP watches for any increase in symptoms that suggest the urethra is becoming obstructed. Treatment of symptoms may include use of a catheter (indwelling or intermittent), encouraging oral fluids, and antibiotics for UTI.

Conservative medical treatment includes the use of medication to either relax the smooth muscles of the prostate and bladder neck or block the male hormone to prevent or shrink tissue growth. Alpha-adrenergic antagonists, such as tamsulosin (Flomax) and alfuzosin (Uroxatral), are medications that relax the smooth muscles. They are also used to treat high blood pressure, so patients must work closely with their HCPs to avoid overdose or the negative side effects of postural hypotension (see Table 43.1).

The most used medications to block the action of the male hormone in the prostate gland are finasteride (Proscar) and dutasteride (Avodart). These medications must be taken on a long-term, continuous basis to achieve results (see Table 43.1). Conservative measures are used initially unless the patient is experiencing recurring infections, repeated gross hematuria, bladder or kidney damage, evidence of cancer, or unsatisfactory lifestyle changes.

Nonsurgical invasive treatments are available; however, some are experimental and may have limited accessibility. Nonsurgical treatments include transurethral microwave therapy (heat is applied directly to the gland to inhibit growth), transurethral needle ablation (radiofrequency waves are used to destroy excess prostate tissue), and high-intensity focused ultrasound (radio or sound waves are used to destroy parts of the prostate). Urethral stents can be used to open the passageway for urine obstructions.

Complementary and Alternative Therapies

Some herbal supplements, such as *Hypoxis rooperi*, saw palmetto, and pygeum africanum, have been used for management of BPH. However, research has been unable to show any benefit with these or other herbs, and the American Urological Association recommends against their use (McVary, 2021). Acupuncture is currently under clinical investigation as a treatment for BPH.

Surgical Treatment

Because so many other treatments are available now, surgery is not needed as often as in the past. When symptoms are severe enough to require surgery, several types are available.

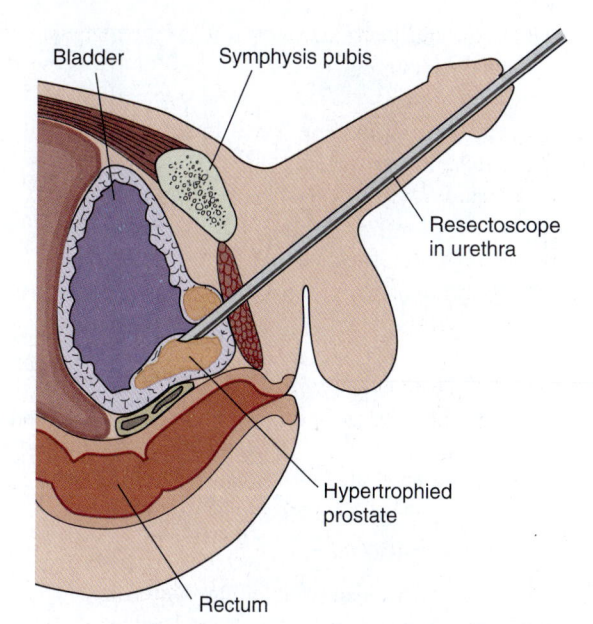

TRANSURETHRAL RESECTION OF THE PROSTATE. Transurethral resection of the prostate (TURP) is used most often to relieve obstruction caused by an enlarged prostate (Fig. 43.1). Several other transurethral options also exist. Transurethral incision of the prostate (TUIP) uses surgical incisions into the gland to relieve obstruction. Transurethral ultrasound-guided laser-induced prostatectomy (TULIP) uses a laser.

FIGURE 43.1 Transurethral resection of the prostate.

For TURP, the patient is anesthetized. The surgery is performed using an instrument called a resectoscope. The resectoscope is inserted into the urethra, and the prostate gland is shaved away a small piece at a time. Special surgical instruments are used to "vaporize" or "microwave" the pieces and cut down on the amount of bleeding during surgery. During routine TURP, the shaved tissue is flushed out with an irrigating solution. They are sent to the laboratory to be analyzed for possible evidence of cancer. The prostate gland is not completely removed but sliced away from the urethra. The prostatic tissue that remains eventually grows back. It can cause obstruction again later. Patients need to be reminded to continue with yearly prostate examinations.

Bleeding occurs during a TURP. A Foley catheter will be inserted and left in place with 30 to 60 mL of sterile water inflating the balloon. The catheter is secured tightly to the leg or abdomen, and the overinflated balloon in the bladder helps to tamponade (compress) the prostate area and stop bleeding. Irrigation solution generally flows continuously (Fig. 43.2); manual irrigation may be done for the first 24 hours to help remove clots and shaved prostate tissue and to maintain catheter patency. The Foley catheter is removed after the danger of hemorrhage has passed.

You may need to save "serial urines" (multiple consecutive urine samples) to monitor for bleeding. To do this, each time the patient urinates or the catheter bag is emptied, save a sample of urine in a transparent cup. Place it in a safe place, such as on a shelf in the bathroom. With each subsequent urination, place the new cup to the right of the previous cup.

• WORD • BUILDING •

su: retro—backward + grade—step

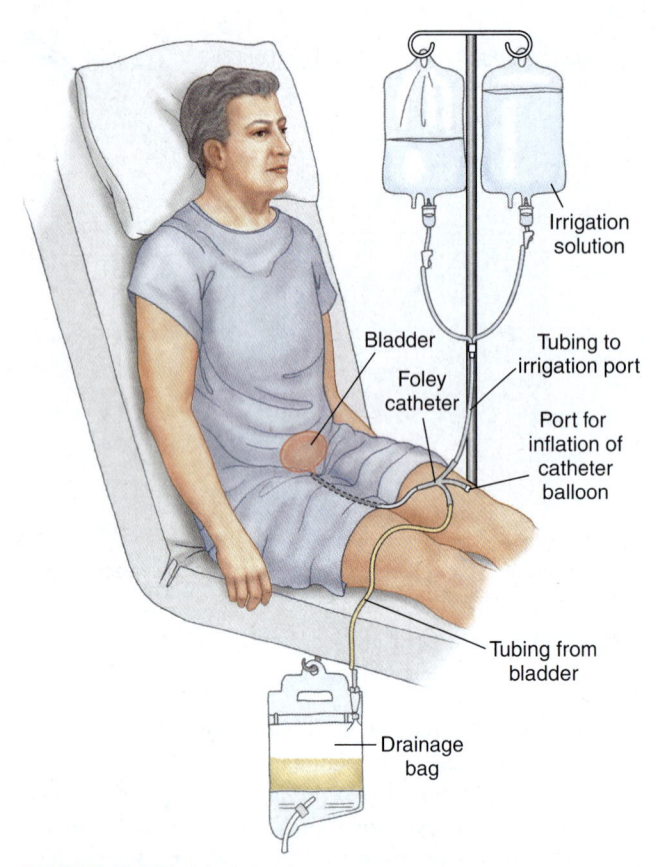

FIGURE 43.2 Bladder irrigation.

When five or six cups are lined up, you can start over at the left side, replacing the oldest cup with the newest one. This allows the nurse or HCP to examine the urine for progressively less blood with each void.

Complications associated with prostate surgery depend on the type and extent of the procedure performed. The main medical complications include clot formation, bladder spasms, and infection. Analgesics or antispasmodics (such as belladonna and opium [B&O] suppository) can be given for pain. Less common complications are urinary incontinence, hemorrhage, and erectile dysfunction (see "Nursing Care Plan for the Postsurgical Patient Having Transurethral Resection of the Prostate for Benign Prostatic Hyperplasia").

> **PRACTICE ANALYSIS TIP**
> **Linking NCLEX-PN® to Practice**
> The LPN/LVN will monitor client response to procedures and treatments.

> **PRACTICE ANALYSIS TIP**
> **Linking NCLEX-PN® to Practice**
> The LPN/LVN will assist with care for client before and after surgical procedure.

> **CUE RECOGNITION 43.1**
> You are caring for a patient who is 18 hours post-TURP. You enter the room. He is standing at the window, and you see an increase in blood and clots in the catheter collection bag. What do you do?
>
> *Suggested answers are at the end of the chapter.*

Retrograde ejaculation is a common result of prostate surgery. When any of the prostate gland is removed, the amount of semen produced decreases. Also, part of the ejaculatory ducts may be removed, resulting in less semen pushed outside the body. Instead, it "falls back" into the bladder. This causes no harm. The semen is simply passed during the next urination.

It is important to understand that erection, ejaculation, and orgasm are all separate actions. Erection means the penis becomes hard, ejaculation is the release of semen, and orgasm is felt as pulsations along the urethra. Unless additional problems are present, the patient continues to have erections and orgasmic sensations but decreased or no ejaculation.

RADICAL PROSTATECTOMY. When the prostate gland is very large, causes obstruction, or is cancerous, a radical **prostatectomy** may be performed to remove the entire prostate gland.

Open Prostatectomy. Several approaches may be taken during traditional radical surgery (Fig. 43.3). In the **suprapubic** approach, an incision is made through the lower abdomen into the bladder. The gland is removed and the urethra is reattached to the bladder. The retropubic approach is similar, except with no incision into the bladder. A perineal prostatectomy involves an incision between the scrotum and anus to remove the gland. This procedure is rarely done because of the increased risk of contamination of the incision (close to the rectum). There is also risk of urinary incontinence, erectile dysfunction, or injury to the rectum.

An open prostatectomy means a longer hospital stay compared with other BPH surgeries. The presence of a suprapubic catheter (placed in the lower abdomen to drain the bladder) and care for an abdominal incision increase the length of stay and risk for complications. Follow-up home health care for wound and catheter care is important for these patients.

Minimally Invasive Prostatectomy. Newer techniques use laparoscopy and tiny robot arms to perform radical prostatectomy through five small "porthole" incisions in the abdomen. The surgeon makes all the decisions about the surgery while guiding the robotic arms from a computer. The robotic

• WORD • BUILDING •

prostatectomy: prostat—prostate gland + ectomy—excision
suprapubic: supra—above + pubic—pubic bone

Nursing Care Plan for the Postsurgical Patient Having Transurethral Resection of the Prostate for Benign Prostatic Hyperplasia

Nursing Diagnosis: *Risk for Bleeding* related to surgical intervention
Expected Outcome: The patient's bleeding will be minimal as evidenced by urine becoming progressively clearer.
Evaluation of Outcome: Is urine clearing? Is bleeding reported promptly?

Intervention	Rationale	Evaluation
Closely monitor urinary output in terms of amount, color, and presence of clots at least every hour for the first 24 to 48 hours postoperatively. Monitor serial urines. If clots increase or urine becomes bright red, report to RN or HCP.	*Careful monitoring and reporting of changes can help prevent major complications.*	Is urine showing progressively less blood and clots, and is it clearer with each void?
Explain to the patient that some bloody urine is normal after a TURP, as long as it does not suddenly get much worse. Also explain that a little blood mixed with irrigating fluid in a Foley bag may look worse than it actually is.	*Seeing the catheter bag filled with bloody drainage may be upsetting to the patient or his family.*	Is the patient aware of what to expect in a Foley bag?
Encourage the patient to drink up to 2,500 mL/day (unless contraindicated by other medical conditions) of water, noncitrus juices, and other noncaffeinated, nonalcoholic beverages.	*Increasing urine flow can help flush blood from the bladder.*	Is the patient drinking adequate amounts?
Teach the patient to avoid constipation (e.g., suggest stool softener, fluids, prune juice) and heavy lifting.	*These can increase pressure in the abdomen and increase risk of bleeding.*	Does the patient verbalize understanding of instructions?
Advise patient to lie down if urine becomes bright red or has large clots.	*Activity can increase bleeding.*	Does the patient reduce activity if bleeding increases?
Teach the patient to avoid aspirin and NSAIDs until risk of bleeding is over.	*Aspirin and NSAIDs inhibit platelet function and increase risk of bleeding.*	Does the patient verbalize understanding?

Nursing Diagnosis: *Urge Urinary Incontinence* related to poor sphincter control as evidenced by inability to control urination
Expected Outcome: The patient will be able to prevent incontinence.
Evaluation of Outcome: Is the patient experiencing incontinence?

Intervention	Rationale	Evaluation
Teach Kegel (pelvic floor) exercises (see Chapter 42), to be practiced every time the patient urinates and throughout the day.	*Kegel exercises strengthen muscle tone to hold urine after the catheter is removed.*	Is the patient able to start and stop urine stream?
Discuss use of a condom catheter or penile pads.	*These can keep the patient dry until incontinence can be controlled.*	Does the patient indicate an informed choice of incontinence products?
Instruct patient to continue drinking 2,000 to 4,000 mL of noncaffeinated, nonalcoholic beverages each day.	*Adequate nonirritating fluid intake is important for healing and preventing UTI.*	Does the patient drink adequate fluids even though his bladder dribbles?
Encourage the patient to discuss long-term (longer than 6 months) incontinence problems with the HCP.	*The patient may need to learn self-catheterization or try medication.*	Does the patient verbalize understanding of what to do if incontinence continues?

(nursing care plan continues on page 856)

Nursing Care Plan for the Postsurgical Patient Having Transurethral Resection of the Prostate for Benign Prostatic Hyperplasia—cont'd

Intervention	Rationale	Evaluation
Refer the patient to national incontinence support group if indicated.	*Support groups can provide information and emotional support.*	Does the patient show interest in a support group?

Nursing Diagnosis: *Deficient Knowledge* related to lack of experience with postoperative restrictions and care
Expected Outcomes: The patient will avoid activities that increase intra-abdominal pressure resulting in excessive bleeding. The patient will verbalize understanding of how to prevent postoperative infection.
Evaluation of Outcomes: Does the patient verbalize understanding of how to prevent bleeding? Is infection prevented?

Intervention	Rationale	Evaluation
Teach the patient to avoid lifting heavy objects (more than 10 pounds), stair climbing, driving, strenuous exercise, constipation, straining during bowel movements, and sexual activities until approved by the HCP (about 6 weeks).	*Heavy lifting or straining can disrupt the healing process and result in tissue damage or excess bleeding.*	Does the patient verbalize understanding of reasons for limitation of heavy lifting and straining?
Instruct the patient on proper catheter care if the patient will be discharged with a catheter. Include the following information: Keep catheter tubing secured to abdomen or thigh and keep bag below bladder; wash catheter/meatus junction with soap and water once daily; use clean technique with good hand hygiene to change from leg bag to night drainage bag; report signs and symptoms of UTI to HCP immediately; and encourage oral fluids.	*UTIs are extremely dangerous and can cause death following genitourinary surgery in an older patient.*	Can the patient give a return demonstration of proper catheter care? Is the patient free from signs and symptoms of infection?
Teach the patient to report bleeding that is not stopping with rest, fever, swelling, or difficulty urinating to HCP promptly.	*These are signs of complications that may require prompt medical intervention.*	Does the patient verbalize understanding of signs and symptoms to report?

Nursing Diagnosis: *Anxiety* related to concerns over loss of sexual functioning following prostate surgery as evidenced by patient statement
Expected Outcomes: The patient will verbalize normal sexual changes that happen after prostate surgery. The patient will identify available support systems if needed.
Evaluation of Outcomes: Is the patient able to verbalize understanding of expected body function after prostate surgery? Does the patient access support systems?

Intervention	Rationale	Evaluation
Explain to the patient that he will probably have retrograde ejaculation into the bladder after surgery. It is not harmful, and semen will come out when he urinates.	*Removal of the prostate gland often results in retrograde ejaculation.*	Does the patient understand what will happen when he ejaculates?
Instruct the patient to talk with the urologist if erection problems occur.	*Urologists who specialize in treatment of erectile dysfunction can provide information and treatment.*	Is the patient aware of local support services?

arms allow for precision and an ability to maneuver in small areas. The robotic surgery is much less invasive than open prostatectomy. Patients experience better results with less postoperative bleeding, incontinence, and nerve damage as well as shorter hospital stays.

Nursing Process for the Patient With BPH Who Undergoes a TURP Procedure

DATA COLLECTION. Ask the patient whether he has ever had treatment or surgery for prostate trouble. Determine amount and type of fluid intake per day. Ask whether the patient has noticed symptoms of BPH. Monitor output. If the patient is not catheterized, ensure urine retention is managed appropriately.

NURSING DIAGNOSES, PLANNING, AND INTERVENTIONS. For nursing care of the patient following TURP, see "Nursing Care Plan for the Postsurgical Patient Having Transurethral Resection of the Prostate for Benign Prostatic Hyperplasia." Each patient experience is different. Care plans must be individualized. Keep in mind that most of these patients are older and have secondary medical problems such as cardiovascular disease.

EVALUATION. A patient should be discharged home with minimal bladder discomfort, light pink to clear urine, no evidence of UTI, and knowledge related to self-care at home. Home health-care nursing may be required if the patient lives alone or does not have the capacity to provide for meals, toileting, or transportation for the follow-up visit. Table 43.2 provides a summary of BPH.

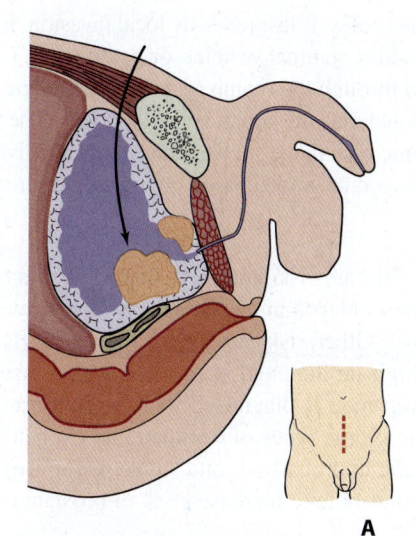

FIGURE 43.3 (A) Suprapubic prostatectomy. (B) Retropubic prostatectomy. (C) Perineal prostatectomy.

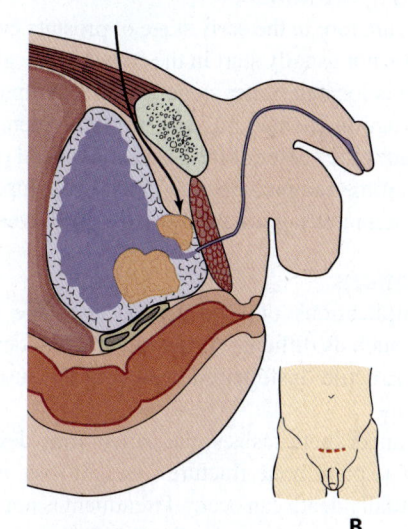

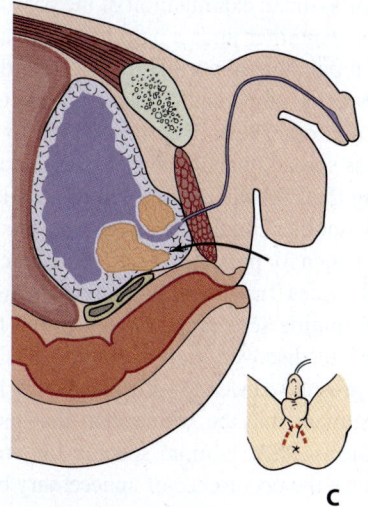

CRITICAL THINKING & CLINICAL JUDGMENT

Mr. Atkinson is a 68-year-old Black farmer with an enlarged prostate gland. He lives on a 75-acre farm with his wife and one son. He is scheduled for a transurethral resection of the prostate in 6 weeks. Mr. Atkinson is currently taking terazosin (Hytrin). His HCP wants him to increase his dose from 2 to 5 mg daily until surgery.

Critical Thinking (The Why)
1. Why is Mr. Atkinson taking tetrazosin?

Clinical Judgment (The Do)
2. Mr. Atkinson has a bottle of tetrazosin at home of 2 mg tablets. How should you instruct him to take his medication? What side effect should he be advised to watch for?
3. What special postoperative instructions should he be given because of his occupation?
4. What should you tell him if he asks about how the surgery will affect his sexual activities?
5. What other health-care team members can you collaborate with and anticipate Mr. Atkinson might need while in the hospital or when he goes home?

Suggested answers are at the end of the chapter.

Table 43.2
Benign Prostatic Hyperplasia Summary

Signs and Symptoms	*Related to obstruction:* Decrease in size/force of stream, difficulty in starting stream, dribbling, interrupted stream, urinary retention, overflow incontinence *Related to irritation:* Nocturia, dysuria, urgency
Diagnostic Tests	*Primary:* Digital rectal examination, urinalysis, blood urea nitrogen (BUN), serum creatinine, prostate-specific antigen (PSA) *Secondary:* Urodynamic flow studies, transrectal ultrasound, cystoscopy
Therapeutic Measures	*Conservative:* Alpha-adrenergic blockers, testosterone blockers *Nonsurgical:* Transurethral microwave therapy, prostatic balloon, prostatic stents *Transurethral:* Transurethral incision of the prostate (TUIP), transurethral ultrasound-guided laser-induced prostatectomy (TULIP), transurethral resection of the prostate (TURP) *Radical prostatectomy:* Suprapubic, retropubic, perineal, laparoscopic, or robotic resection
Complications	Ascending or localized infection Injury to surrounding tissues during surgery Impaired sexual function related to tissue injury
Priority Postoperative Nursing Diagnoses	Risk for Bleeding Acute Pain (see Chapter 10) Urge Urinary Incontinence Deficient Knowledge Anxiety

Cancer of the Prostate

Cancer of the prostate is the most common cancer in American men. Most prostate cancers grow very slowly and often do not cause a major threat to health or life. Many treatment options are available, and the prognosis is often very good.

Pathophysiology

Prostate cancer depends on testosterone to grow. The cancer cells are usually slow growing. They begin in the posterior (back) or lateral (side) part of the gland. The cancer spreads by one of three routes. If it spreads by local invasion, it will move into the bladder, seminal vesicles, or peritoneum. Cancer may also spread through the lymph system to the pelvic nodes and may travel as far as the supraclavicular nodes. The third route is through the vascular system to bone, lung, and liver. Prostate cancer is staged or graded based on the growth or spread.

Etiology

Age is the primary risk factor. Prostate cancer is found most often in men older than age 65 and is rare in men younger than age 40. Other risk factors are higher levels of testosterone, a high-fat diet, and immediate family history. About one in seven men is diagnosed with prostate cancer during his lifetime. Some types of occupational exposures (e.g., to polyaromatic hydrocarbons and smoke from fire) have been found to contribute to increased risk of prostate cancer.

Signs and Symptoms

Symptoms are rare in the early stage of prostate cancer as the growth does not usually start in the center of the gland where the urethra is located. Later stages include symptoms of urinary obstruction, hematuria, and urinary retention as the tumor invades the center of the gland. Advanced (metastatic) stage symptoms can include pain in the back, hip, abdomen, or bone; anemia; weakness; weight loss; and overall fatigue.

Complications

Early complications of prostate cancer relate to bladder problems, such as difficulty urinating and bladder or kidney infection. Erectile dysfunction can occur because of cancer or treatment.

If the cancer metastasizes, the patient may develop problems such as pain, bone fractures, weight loss, and depression; eventually death can occur if treatment is not successful.

Diagnostic Tests

A routine digital rectal examination of the prostate is the first test; often the examiner finds a hard lump or hardened prostate lobe. If a palpable abnormality is found, the HCP may order a transrectal ultrasound and biopsy for confirmation. Bone scans and other tests may be ordered to determine if the cancer has spread outside the prostate gland.

Measuring the PSA via a blood sample can indicate prostate cancer or another conditions. In the past, the PSA test was used to screen men for prostate cancer. More recently, the U.S. Preventive Services Task Force withdrew this recommendation because routine screening was not found to save lives. Screening led to discovery and treatment of slow-growing, noninvasive prostate cancers. If prostate cancer is not aggressive, the treatment may be worse than the disease. A new blood test, the IsoPSA, is more specific for prostate cancer and may reduce the occurrence of unnecessary biopsies.

Therapeutic Measures

Prostate cancer in the early stages may be treated with testosterone-suppressing medications, such as leuprolide (Lupron) or goserelin (Zoladex), or with drugs that block testosterone's action on the prostate gland, such as bicalutamide (Casodex). Surgery, such as TURP or radical prostatectomy, or a combination of medication and radiation therapy may be done. In later stages, the treatment is usually a radical prostatectomy, radiation therapy, or implantation of radioactive "seeds" into the prostate (brachytherapy). The immune stimulant sipuleucel-T (Provenge) slows the growth and aggressiveness of some prostate cancers.

Metastatic prostate cancer treatment involves relief of symptoms through blocking testosterone by bilateral **orchiectomy**, administration of antiandrogen (flutamide [Eulexin]), or use of agents such as leuprolide and goserelin. Sometimes chemotherapy is used to help relieve symptoms resulting from spread of the cancer.

Unfortunately, any therapy that reduces androgen activity in a man can cause side effects, such as hot flashes, breast tenderness and growth, impaired sexual function, osteoporosis, and loss of muscle mass. These, in turn, can cause significant concerns with body image.

RADICAL PROSTATECTOMY. A radical prostatectomy (described earlier in this chapter) is done for patients with cancer of the prostate or when the gland is too large to resect using a less invasive method.

The patient returns from surgery with a large indwelling catheter in the urethra and potentially a suprapubic catheter. A wound drain may be placed to remove fluids and promote wound healing from the inside outward. Keep dressings, drains, and incisions clean and dry according to institution policy using sterile technique.

Radical prostatectomy has more potential complications than any other treatment option, including hemorrhage, infection, loss of urinary control, and erectile dysfunction.

Patient Education
All men older than 40 should be educated regarding prostate screening, including the risks and benefits of screening.

> **LEARNING TIP**
> *BPH:* Starts in the center of the prostate gland where the urethra is located; urinary symptoms start early in the disease process; prostate feels large, soft, and "boggy" (spongy).
> *Prostate Cancer:* Starts in the posterior and lateral parts of the prostate gland; urinary symptoms start late in the disease process as the tumor invades the center of the gland where the urethra is located; prostate feels normal size, hard, or has a hard lump or hard lobe.

> **PRACTICE ANALYSIS TIP**
> **Linking NCLEX-PN® to Practice**
> The LPN/LVN will reinforce client education about procedures and treatments.

PENILE DISORDERS

Problems of the penis, aside from those caused by STIs, are fairly rare but may cause great concern and worry for the patient. Many men have difficulty seeking help for such a private topic. It is important to be sensitive when collecting data or providing care for these patients.

Peyronie Disease
Peyronie disease gives the penis a curved or crooked look when it is erect. Fibrous bands or plaques form mainly on the dorsal (top) part of the layer of tissue that surrounds one of the corpora cavernosa of the penis. The plaque may be caused by injury or inflammation of the penile tissue and may come and go spontaneously. Thick plaques can cause curvature, pain with erection, difficulty in vaginal penetration, and erectile dysfunction. When conservative treatments such as oral vitamin E, colchicine, or potassium aminobenzoate do not work, surgery may be needed to remove the plaque. Another option is injections to break down the scar tissue. Patients need to be reassured that the problem is not life threatening and can be treated.

Priapism
Priapism is a painful erection that lasts longer than 4 hours. If not relieved, it can become a medical emergency. The small veins in the corpora cavernosa spasm, so blood cannot drain back out of the penis as it should. When the blood cannot drain, penile tissue does not get oxygen. Permanent tissue damage can result. There may be a complete loss of erection ability after the priapism episode. Prolonged priapism can also prevent the patient from passing urine, which can lead to painful bladder and kidney problems. Some causes of priapism are sickle cell anemia, leukemia, widespread cancer, spinal cord injury or tumors, and use of medications to manage erectile dysfunction (such as sildenafil [Viagra]) or recreational drugs (such as crack cocaine). Treatment in the emergency department may include ice packs, sedatives, analgesics, injection of medications directly into the penis to relax the vein spasms, needle aspiration, and irrigation of the corpora. Surgery to implant a shunt that reroutes blood flow can also be done.

Phimosis and Paraphimosis
Phimosis is a condition in which the foreskin of an uncircumcised male becomes so tight that it is difficult or impossible to pull back away from the glans (head) of the penis for cleaning. Smegma, a cottage cheese–like secretion made by the glands of the foreskin, becomes trapped under the foreskin, a prime place for the growth of bacterial and yeast infections. Antibiotics and warm soaks may be ordered for infection. Topical steroid ointment and stretching exercises

• WORD • BUILDING •
orchiectomy: orchi—testicles + ectomy—excision
priapism: priap—phallus + ism—condition of
phimosis: phimo—muzzling + osis—condition

for the foreskin may be prescribed. A circumcision may be recommended if the problem continues. Phimosis is generally prevented by teaching uncircumcised males to pull the foreskin back carefully, wash with mild soap and water daily, and replace the foreskin to its normal position.

Paraphimosis occurs when the uncircumcised foreskin is pulled back, during intercourse or bathing, and not replaced in a forward position. This can lead to compression of vessels of the penis and potentially gangrene. Prevention requires good hygiene and returning the foreskin back over the glans of the penis when it has been retracted.

Cancer of the Penis

Cancer of the penis has been found in men who were not circumcised as infants or adolescents and who have acquired the human papillomavirus (HPV). The tumor is typically a squamous cell carcinoma that may look like a small, round raised wart, induration, or red area. This form of cancer can be spread to a sexual partner. Several research studies have found a link between cancer of the penis and cancer of the uterine cervix. Cancer of the penis may be treated with minor surgery, such as a circumcision or laser removal of the growth. If the cancer has spread, sections of the penis may be surgically removed. Penile reconstruction can be done, if necessary, after surgery. Radiation or chemotherapy may also be done. Teach male patients the importance of early reporting of any lesions, HPV vaccination, and good hygiene if not circumcised.

> **CUE RECOGNITION 43.2**
>
> The assistive personnel just finished **Mr. Cooper's** bed bath and he is now complaining of discomfort at the tip of his penis. You notice that the foreskin was not replaced after his bath. What do you do?
>
> *Suggested answers are at the end of the chapter.*

TESTICULAR DISORDERS

Cryptorchidism

Cryptorchidism (undescended testicles) is a congenital condition in which an infant is born with one or both of his testicles not in the scrotum. The testicles normally descend into the scrotum in the last 1 to 2 months before a male is born. Often, undescended testicles descend into the scrotum on their own in the first few months of life. If they do not descend during that time, surgery should be done to correct the problem, typically before age 1. Testicles that are not brought down into the scrotum may lead to infertility. Also, the risk of testicular cancer is higher if the condition is not corrected before the child reaches his teen years.

Hydrocele

A **hydrocele** is a painless collection of fluid in the scrotal sac. The cause is not known. It can happen at any point during a man's lifetime. No treatment is necessary unless the hydrocele is so large that it causes discomfort or embarrassment or threatens the blood supply to the testicles. In cases requiring treatment, the patient may have surgery to remove the hydrocele or a needle aspiration of the fluid.

Varicocele

A varicocele is a condition sometimes called *varicose veins of the scrotum*. The main blood supply to the testicles travels along the spermatic cord. The veins become dilated, and when the man is standing, the area in the scrotum begins to feel like a "bag of worms." The patient may report a pulling sensation, a dull ache, or scrotal pain. The sensations are most often felt when standing up. Most varicoceles occur on the left side because of the way the scrotal vein enters at a sharp angle from the left renal vein.

A varicocele is often not discovered until a couple is unable to conceive. It is believed that the varicose veins may increase the temperature of the testicles and cause damage to the sperm. The most successful treatment is surgical repair of the varicose veins.

Epididymitis

The epididymis is a small tube along the back of the testicles where sperm is matured for its last 10 to 12 days before it is ready to be ejaculated. **Epididymitis** is inflammation or infection of the epididymis that can be caused by bacteria, viruses, parasites, chemicals, or trauma. Risk factors include sexual or nonsexual contact, STIs, a complication of some urological procedures, or reflux (backflow) of urine. The problem can also be associated with prostate infections. It is usually painful, with the scrotal skin being tender, red, and warm to the touch.

Epididymitis is treated with antibiotics; the partner is also treated if it was sexually transmitted. Depending on the severity of the pain, the patient may be placed on bedrest with the scrotum elevated, possibly on ice packs, and given analgesics. The pain and tenderness usually go away in about a week, although the swelling may last for several weeks. Complications include chronic epididymitis, abscess formation, and sterility.

Orchitis

Orchitis is a rare inflammation or infection of the testicles. The problem may be caused by trauma or infection from epididymitis, UTIs, STIs, or systemic diseases such as influenza, infectious mononucleosis, tuberculosis, gout, pneumonia, or mumps (after puberty). The patient has swollen,

> • WORD • BUILDING •
>
> **paraphimosis:** para—abnormal + phimo—muzzling + osis—condition
> **cryptorchidism:** crypt—hidden + orchid—testicle + ism—condition
> **hydrocele:** hydro—water + cele—swelling
> **epididymitis:** epididymis + itis—inflammation
> **orchitis:** orch—testicle + itis—inflammation

extremely tender testicles; red scrotal skin; and a fever. Interventions are essentially the same as for epididymitis. Sterility is a complication of orchitis caused by mumps. This complication can be prevented by giving boys the mumps vaccine at an early age.

Cancer of the Testicles

Pathophysiology and Etiology

Cancer of the testicles is the most common cancer in men between ages 15 and 35 in the United States. The etiology of testicular cancer is unknown. Some known risk factors are cryptorchidism, family history, White race, and high socioeconomic status. Some older studies showed a link between testicular cancer and a mother's use of diethylstilbesterol (DES; an estrogen preparation once used to prevent spontaneous abortion) while pregnant. However, current research has not shown this risk to be significant. The tumors are mostly a germ cell type of cancer.

Prevention

The best prevention is early detection with a monthly testicular self-examination (TSE). The American Cancer Society does not necessarily recommend monthly TSE for all men. This is because not enough studies have been done to show that it reduces death. However, men should be aware of what is normal for them so that they can recognize changes if they occur. The TSE procedure is simple and easy to learn. It makes sense to teach it to all men until more data are available. See Chapter 41 for instructions on TSE.

Signs and Symptoms

Early warning signs of cancer can include a small, usually painless lump on the testicle. The patient may also notice that the scrotum is swollen and feels heavy. Some tumors produce hormones that cause breast enlargement and tenderness.

Complications

Emotional complications can range from fear of cancer and death to feelings of loss of masculine body image and sexual function. Physical complications may involve dealing with pain and the effects of metastasis to areas such as the lungs, abdomen, or lymph nodes. Other less common areas of cancer spread are the liver, brain, and bone.

Diagnostic Tests

When a lump is found, several laboratory and radiographic tests are done. An ultrasound of the testicles is done first to differentiate a possible tumor from a hydrocele or other noncancerous condition. Blood is drawn to look for tumor markers. An example of a tumor marker for testicular cancer is human chorionic gonadotropin (hCG). A surgical biopsy or removal of the testicle is done to determine the stage of the tumor. If cancer is confirmed, a chest x-ray examination is done to look for spread to the lungs. A scan of the lymph nodes, liver, brain, and bones also may be ordered. Testicular tumors are staged according to the TNM (tumor-node-metastasis) classification of malignant tumors system introduced in Chapter 11.

Therapeutic Measures

Intervention depends on the stage of the cancer. All treatment begins with complete removal of the cancerous testicles, spermatic cord, and local lymph nodes. Based on the stage of the cancer, radiation or chemotherapy may be done in addition to surgery. If the cancer is found in the beginning stages, the chances for complete recovery are very good. All patients should have regular follow-up testing.

Nursing Care

Nursing care is directed first at prevention, by teaching young men to practice TSE and to see their HCP if they notice changes. If a diagnosis of cancer has been made, provide emotional support for the patient. Patients who want to have children should be encouraged to make deposits in a sperm bank before surgery or treatment. The patient and his partner may have many questions about sexual activities as they go through treatment. Encourage them to talk with their HCP or a sex therapist about ways to express love and tenderness toward one another. Helping patients deal with pain and the side effects of chemotherapy or radiation therapy are also important nursing interventions. See Chapter 11 for care of the patient with cancer.

> **CRITICAL THINKING & CLINICAL JUDGMENT**
>
> **Mr. Cunningham** is a 23-year-old college student engaged to be married next spring. While taking a shower one day, he discovers a lump on his left testicle.
>
> **Critical Thinking (The Why)**
> 1. What advice is appropriate for Mr. Cunningham?
> 2. What are the treatment options if Mr. Cunningham has testicular cancer?
>
> **Clinical Judgment (The Do)**
> 3. How can you help Mr. Cunningham cope with the diagnosis?
>
> *Suggested answers are at the end of the chapter.*

SEXUAL FUNCTIONING

Vasectomy

A **vasectomy** uses tiny clamps or cauterization to seal off the vas deferens and prevent sperm from reaching the outside of the body (Fig. 43.4). This 15- to 30-minute surgery is done through a small puncture in the upper part of the scrotum. It is performed as an outpatient procedure and is intended for men who do not want to reproduce. The patient should

• WORD • BUILDING •

vasectomy: vas—vas deferens + ectomy—excision

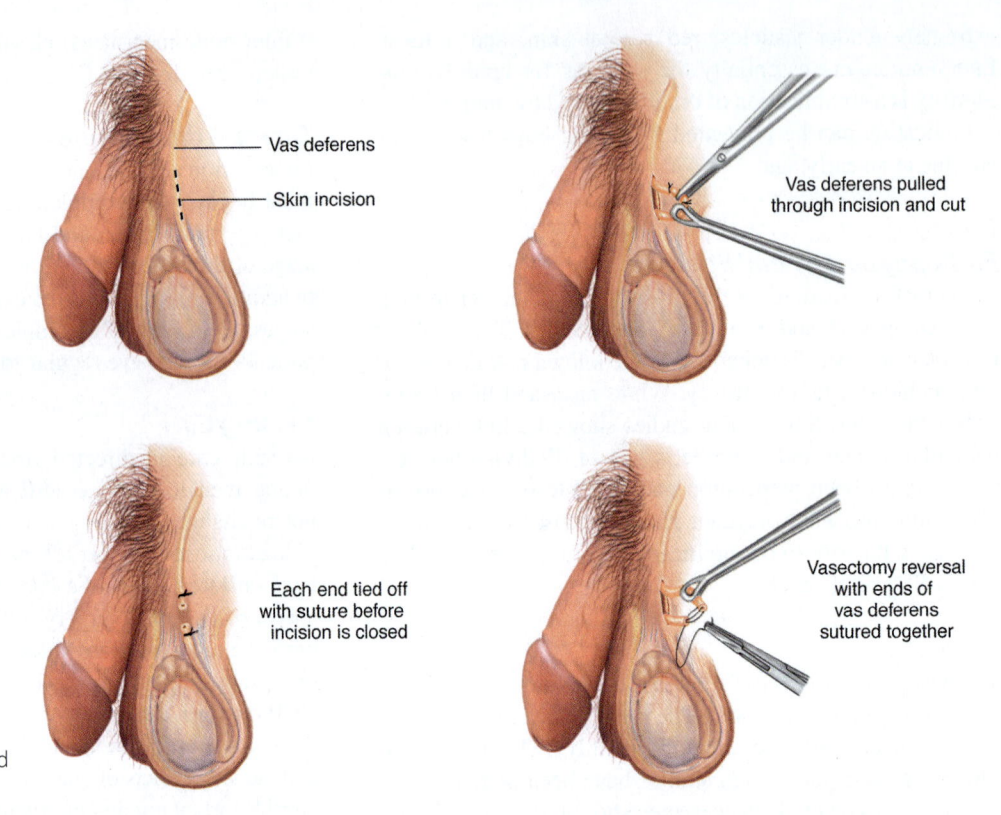

FIGURE 43.4 Vasectomy and reversal.

carefully discuss the surgery with his physician so that he has a clear understanding of the results of the procedure.

After the procedure, the testicles continue to produce sperm and the male hormone testosterone. The prostate gland, along with the seminal vesicles, still ejaculates semen, but it does not contain sperm. There should be no major change in the way the ejaculate looks or feels after the procedure. The patient should be encouraged to use another birth control method for about 3 months after surgery to be sure there are no sperm left in the tract above the surgical site. A semen sample should be evaluated for the absence of sperm before the procedure is considered successful. Sperm continue to be produced in the testicles but are absorbed by the body.

Vasectomy Reversal

Sometimes a man may decide he wants to have more children and asks to have a vasectomy reversed. The surgical procedure to reverse a vasectomy is called a *vasovasostomy*. Using microscopic instruments, the surgeon reconnects the vas deferens. If this is not possible, the surgeon may reconnect the vas deferens to the epididymis. During the surgery, the physician typically tries to determine whether the testicles are still producing good sperm. Vasectomy reversal is more successful if it is done soon after the vasectomy. Success rates drop as the period between vasectomy and reversal grows longer.

Erectile Dysfunction

A problem getting or keeping an erection can happen at any age. It has been a concern of men and their partners for centuries. It is a unique problem because it affects not only the man but his partner as well. Most men experience temporary erectile dysfunction at some point, caused by stress, illness, fatigue, or excessive use of alcohol or drugs. When the problem becomes persistent, it is time to seek medical help.

Before the 1980s, 90% of men who went to their HCPs for help were told the problem was emotional, not physical. Because of improved testing methods, however, researchers now believe that 80% to 90% of erection problems have a physical cause.

Pathophysiology

The term *impotence* means "powerlessness." This term is being replaced with the more accurate term **erectile dysfunction**, or ED, which describes a physical condition. Erectile dysfunction means that a man cannot obtain or keep a functional erection that is firm enough and lasts long enough for satisfactory sexual intercourse. A functional erection requires several conditions:

1. *Circulatory system.* The blood supply coming into the penis from the arteries must be sufficient to fill the corpus cavernosa (spongy erectile tissue inside the penis), causing the penis to become rigid. The veins in the penis must then be able to constrict to trap the blood in the corporal bodies to keep the penis erect. The most common cause of erectile dysfunction is failure in the circulatory system.
2. *Nervous system.* Both the sympathetic and parasympathetic nerves are involved in the erection, ejaculation, orgasm, and resting phases of the penile

response cycle. Many nerve receptors and transmitters in the spinal cord and the penis must be intact for a usable erection. Spinal cord injury is the most common neurologic cause of erectile dysfunction.

3. *Hormonal system.* There are three basic male hormones involved with an erection. The most important hormone, testosterone, affects a man's sex drive and desire. Luteinizing hormone (LH) stimulates testosterone production. Prolactin in large amounts may block testosterone.
4. *Limbic system.* This is the center in the brain that affects how we feel emotionally. It works with our five senses to stimulate the desire for sex.

All these systems can be influenced by physical, emotional, and chemical factors. A thorough data collection is important to determine the cause of erectile dysfunction.

Etiology

Erectile dysfunction has many psychological and physical causes. It can also be caused by many medications and chemicals that interfere with desire, blood supply, or nerve transmission (Table 43.3). The most common types of medications that cause problems are those prescribed for high blood pressure and cardiovascular disease. Obstructive sleep apnea has been found to be related to erectile dysfunction, but it is unclear which condition might come first.

Diagnostic Tests

In the first step of the assessment process, the HCP obtains a history, including medical-surgical history; use of medications, including any substance abuse; lifestyle patterns; and sexual history. During physical examination, the HCP looks for evidence of genital disorders, hormonal imbalance (such as hair patterns or enlarged breasts), surgical interventions, decreased circulation, and lack of nerve sensation. Blood tests evaluate glucose levels; testosterone; evidence of liver, heart, or kidney disorders; signs of infection; or blood disorders. Some HCPs may use intracorporeal injection of vasoactive medications that can create an erection to test the blood flow in the penis. A psychosocial evaluation may be recommended to rule out relational or emotional problems that may contribute to erectile dysfunction or affect the treatment outcome.

A second level of testing may involve the use of vascular flow studies to locate areas where either the blood vessels are narrowed or the veins allow the blood to drain out of the penis too rapidly. Other testing can monitor erections during sleep. A healthy man typically has erections every 60 to 70 minutes while he sleeps. Absence of erections during sleep indicates a physical cause for erectile dysfunction. Because of the expense of vascular flow studies and sleep studies, they are used on a limited basis.

Therapeutic Measures

One of the most important treatment options begins with a couple being able to share intimate communication. No matter what is causing the problem, if the patient and his partner

Table 43.3
Causes of Erectile Dysfunction

Psychological	Stress
	Anxiety
	Depression
	Fatigue
Urological	Peyronie disease
	Kidney failure
	Treatment for prostate disease
Endocrine	Low testosterone levels
	Diabetes mellitus
Respiratory	Obstructive sleep apnea
Cardiovascular	Heart disease
	Atherosclerosis
	Metabolic syndrome
	Stroke
Neurologic	Spinal cord injury
	Parkinson disease
	Multiple sclerosis
Lifestyle	Tobacco use
	Alcohol use
	Drug use (e.g., cannabis, cocaine, others)
	Excessive caffeine use
	Obesity
Medications*	Angiotensin-converting enzyme (ACE) inhibitors
	Antianxiety agents
	Antidepressants
	Antihistamines
	Antineoplastic agents
	Beta blockers
	Diuretics
	Estrogen
	Histamine (H_2) antagonists
	Muscle relaxants
	NSAIDs
	Opioids
	Drugs for Parkinson disease

Note: Not all drugs in a category cause erectile dysfunction.

are not touching, talking, and sharing feelings, treatment options will have limited success.

When the problem has clearly been identified as psychological, counseling or therapy is the treatment of choice. If long-term therapy has been tried with only limited success, the addition of oral medication or even intracorporeal injection therapy may be added to provide a boost in confidence and self-esteem. Medical treatment for physical erection problems begins with conservative, nonsurgical treatment. It then progresses to surgical options if needed. See Table 43.1 for additional information on medications.

MEDICATION CHANGES. Sometimes all that is needed to correct the problem is a change in medication. It is important for the patient to talk with his HCP before stopping any medication. Some men have stopped taking their blood pressure medication because it interfered with their sexual activity and have risked causing a stroke or heart attack.

ORAL MEDICATIONS. Oral medications (sildenafil [Viagra], tadalafil [Cialis], and vardenafil [Levitra]) are now the first line of therapy to treat erectile dysfunction. These medications relax the arterioles and cavernous tissue, allowing more blood to flow into the penis in response to sexual stimulation. The pill is usually taken 30 to 60 minutes before anticipated sexual intercourse. Priapism is a potential side effect of these mediations; men should be educated and informed to seek medical care immediately if this occurs. Men using nitrate medication (antianginal agents) should avoid using the pills because of risk for severe low blood pressure.

> **BE SAFE!**
> **AVOID FAILURE TO COMMUNICATE!** Be sure to educate the patient on the symptoms of priapism. This is a **medical emergency** and should be reported immediately.

HORMONE TREATMENT. If the patient's testosterone level is low, replacement hormone may be needed. The HCP should first examine the patient carefully for evidence of prostate cancer; testosterone replacement can cause the cancer to grow and spread. Testosterone replacement can be given by intramuscular injection, topical gel, or transdermal patch. Testosterone levels must be monitored closely for both positive and negative effects.

HERBAL REMEDIES. Several herbal remedies may be effective, including yohimbine, dehydroepiandrosterone (DHEA; a steroid hormone), ginseng, ginkgo, and others. Herbal remedies have side effects, just like prescription medications. They should not be taken without an HCP's recommendation.

INJECTED MEDICATIONS. After careful evaluation, a patient or his partner may be taught how to inject a medication into the penis using a 26- or 27-gauge needle on a tuberculin syringe or a prefilled autoinjector. The injections are nearly painless and produce a natural erection in 10 to 15 minutes. The most serious side effect is priapism, which requires immediate reversal in a physician's office or emergency room. See Be Safe! regarding priapism.

TRANSURETHRAL SUPPOSITORY. To facilitate medication dispersion and absorption, a patient may choose to use a suppository. The patient is instructed to urinate before use of the suppository. A tiny pellet (microsuppository) is inserted into the urethra using a specialized single-dose applicator. The medication usually begins to work in 5 to 10 minutes. The effects last for about 30 to 60 minutes.

OTHER NONSURGICAL TREATMENTS. Patients who do not want or cannot afford expensive medical treatment can consider a variety of mechanical sexual aids. Men should be encouraged to talk with an HCP or qualified sex therapist before trying these alternatives.

Suction devices are one nonsurgical treatment option. An external cylinder vacuum device fits over the penis and draws blood up into the corporeal bodies, causing an erection. A penile ring is slipped onto the base of the penis. Once the cylinder is removed, sexual intercourse can begin. Special care must be taken to remove the ring within 15 to 20 minutes to prevent tissue damage.

SURGICAL TREATMENTS

Penile Implants (Prostheses). Penile implants are a pair of solid or fluid-filled chambers surgically placed into the corporeal bodies in the penis to produce erection. Implants may be noninflatable or inflatable (Fig. 43.5).

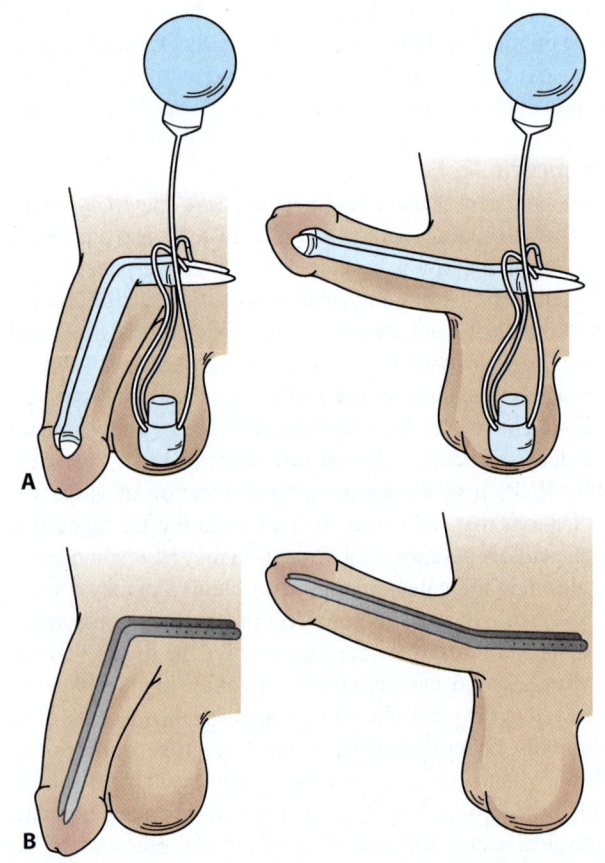

FIGURE 43.5 Penile implants. (A) Inflatable penile implant. Inflatable cylinders are implanted in the penis, the small hydraulic pump in the scrotum, and the fluid-filled reservoir in the lower abdomen. Sterile radiopaque saline from the reservoir fills the cylinders to provide an erection. (B) Malleable penile implant. Malleable rods are implanted into the penis. The penis is always firm, but the rods can be bent close to the body when erection is not desired.

Vascular Surgery. If a younger man has an erection problem caused by poor blood flow into the penis or from blood leaking out of the penis, rapidly causing the loss of the erection, corrective surgery may be performed. A bypass graft may be done to increase blood flow into the penis or to go around a blockage (e.g., as occurs with Peyronie disease).

Nursing Process for the Patient With Erectile Dysfunction

DATA COLLECTION. Your role as a nurse may vary based on work setting. It is always appropriate to ask a man if he has concerns related to sexual health using a matter-of-fact communication style. It may encourage him to talk further. It is important to provide privacy and confidentiality. Ask questions about possible psychosocial causes, such as use of medications, street drugs, alcohol, or nicotine. If a problem is identified, alert the HCP, who will give a more thorough assessment.

NURSING DIAGNOSES, PLANNING, AND IMPLEMENTATION

Sexual Dysfunction related to physical or psychosocial alterations

EXPECTED OUTCOME: The patient will verbalize understanding of the cause and treatment options for erectile dysfunction.

- Determine the patient and partner's current knowledge and understanding about cause and treatment of the disorder. *This will allow for additional and/or correct information to be provided about sexual dysfunction for appropriate understanding.*
- Provide patient and partner with additional and/or correct information about cause and treatment of disorder. *This allows patient to fully understand the etiology and care related to the disorder and increase likelihood of patient adherence to and success of treatment.*
- Refer the patient and partner (as appropriate) for medical treatment, psychological treatment, or counseling. *An individualized treatment plan (determined by the etiology) is needed to move toward restoration of sexual functioning.*

EVALUATION. The best indicator of a positive outcome is restoration of erectile function with a verbal account of understanding the disorder and satisfaction with the treatment process. Sometimes the physical problem is easier to correct than the emotional scars that the problem has created. It is important to evaluate both the physiological and emotional outcomes of treatment.

PATIENT EDUCATION. The nurse plays an important role in public education related to erectile dysfunction. Men need to know that they are not alone with their problem. More than 30 million men in the United States experience ongoing problems with erections. Usually, the cause is physical. Help is available through HCPs who specialize in treating erectile dysfunction. See Table 43.4 for a summary of male sexual dysfunction.

Table 43.4 Male Sexual Dysfunction Summary

Signs and Symptoms	Report of problems with obtaining and keeping an erection Reported dissatisfaction with sexual performance
Diagnostic Tests	*Primary:* History, physical, review of current medications *Secondary:* Vascular flow evaluation, sleep studies
Therapeutic Measures	Counseling Medication to increase blood flow to the penis or hormone treatment Sexual device techniques Surgical implants or repair of structural disorders
Priority Nursing Diagnosis	Sexual Dysfunction

CRITICAL THINKING & CLINICAL JUDGMENT

Mr. Kittle presents to the clinic saying that he is not able to sustain an erection long enough for sexual intercourse that is satisfactory for himself and his partner.

Critical Thinking (The Why)
1. What are some possible reasons for Mr. Kittle's problem?

Clinical Judgment (The Do)
2. You have never had a patient tell you his sexual problems, and you feel a little uncomfortable. How should you respond?
3. What will your data collection include?
4. What is an appropriate role for the licensed practical nurse/licensed vocational nurse in helping Mr. Kittle?

Suggested answers are at the end of the chapter.

Infertility

A growing number of couples in the United States are having difficulty conceiving children. Several factors can interfere with a man's ability to father a child.

Physiology

Many conditions must be present in the man for conception. Endocrine function, autonomic nervous system function, and male reproductive structures must all be functioning properly. Normal healthy sperm in a concentration of at least 20 million per milliliter of semen are needed.

Etiology
The factors related to infertility are divided into three general categories: pretesticular, testicular, and post-testicular.

PRETESTICULAR (ENDOCRINE) FACTORS. The first factor involves proper functioning of the hypothalamus, pituitary gland, and testicles. These endocrine functions are complex and represent a rare cause of infertility. Examples of endocrine causes include pituitary or adrenal tumors, thyroid problems, or uncontrolled diabetes.

TESTICULAR FACTORS. The two most common causes of male infertility are varicoceles (40% to 50%) and idiopathic causes (40%). It is believed that a varicocele lowers the sperm count by raising the blood flow and temperature in the testicles. Sperm cannot live if the temperature is too high or too low.

Congenital anomalies such as Klinefelter syndrome (a chromosomal defect) or cryptorchidism result in absent or damaged testicles. Certain disease or inflammatory processes may damage the storage area (e.g., epididymitis) or the testicles themselves (e.g., mumps orchitis). Any high fever or viral infection can interfere with the production of sperm for up to 3 months.

Medications, radiation, substance abuse, environmental hazards, and lifestyle practices have all been identified as factors that can interfere with spermatogenesis (sperm production). Excessive use of hot tubs and saunas, tight jeans, and long-haul truck driving can all raise the temperature level in the scrotum to an extent that decreases sperm production.

POST-TESTICULAR FACTORS. The most common factor in post-testicular infertility is surgery or injury along the pathway from the testicles to the outside of the man's body. Examples of surgical causes are vasectomy, bladder neck reconstruction, pelvic lymph node removal, or surgery that causes retrograde ejaculation. Congenital anomalies and infections may also cause infertility problems.

Prevention
Prevention involves possible lifestyle changes to avoid excessive heat to the scrotum, substance abuse, exposure to toxins, and environmental hazards. Problems related to medication or infections should also be discussed with the HCP.

Signs and Symptoms
A couple is considered infertile if they have been unsuccessful at becoming pregnant after at least 1 year of unprotected intercourse. If pregnancy has occurred during the year but there was no delivery, the problem usually is considered a female rather than a male factor.

Diagnosis
Diagnosis begins with a detailed history and physical examination that looks for known male causes of infertility.

HISTORY. Initial data collection includes frequency of intercourse, timing (according to ovulation cycle), use of contraceptives, problems with premature ejaculation, and erection problems. Use of hot tubs or saunas; tight jeans; use of nicotine, caffeine, alcohol, or cannabis; and the desire for children on the part of the man are all determined. High stress, long periods of sitting, and exposure to environmental toxins are determined. The patient also may be questioned about STIs, endocrine problems, congenital urinary problems, serious illnesses or groin injuries, cancer, and treatment with chemotherapy or radiation.

PHYSICAL EXAMINATION. The HCP will observe for normal hair pattern and growth, muscle development, size of testicles, and any evidence of a varicocele or hydrocele.

DIAGNOSTIC TESTS. Analysis is done on several semen specimens to see if they contain the amount and type of healthy sperm needed for a pregnancy. Infection should be ruled out. Several other tests may be done, including hormone tests, genetic testing, and ultrasound, depending on the level of desire and the financial resources of the couple. Many insurance companies do not pay for testing or treatment for infertility.

Therapeutic Measures
Treatment may be as simple as making a change in sexual or lifestyle practices. Surgery to correct a varicocele or obstruction may be done. If the couple can handle the emotional and financial strain, they may try a variety of in vitro fertilization (IVF) procedures. IVF is very costly, and success rates vary. Another option that may be presented to the couple is adoption.

You can play an important role in the emotional support a couple needs during infertility studies. It is important that the couple feel comfortable in communicating their feelings and frustrations with one another and their HCP. It also may help them to attend a support group designed for couples experiencing infertility.

Key Points

- Prostatitis, or inflammation of the prostate gland, can occur any time after puberty as a chronic issue acute episode. The inflammation causes the prostate gland to swell, resulting in pain, especially when standing, and difficulty passing urine with progression.
- BPH occurs due to slow increase in the number of cells in the prostate gland starting in the center of the gland. It generally results from aging and the male hormone dihydrotestosterone. As the gland size increases, it puts pressure on the urethra. This narrowing makes it difficult to empty the bladder and eventually causes obstruction.
- When BPH is untreated, prolonged obstruction can cause serious complications. Urine trapped in the bladder can

- back up into kidneys, causing hydronephrosis, renal insufficiency, or urosepsis.
- TURP is used to relieve obstruction caused by an enlarged prostate. Several other transurethral options also exist. Transurethral incision of the prostate uses surgical incisions into the gland to relieve obstruction. Transurethral ultrasound-guided laser-induced prostatectomy uses a laser to relieve obstruction.
- When the prostate gland is very large, causes obstruction, or is cancerous, a radical prostatectomy may be performed to remove the entire prostate gland.
- Prostate cancer depends on testosterone to grow. The cancer cells are usually slow growing. They begin in the posterior or lateral part of the gland. The cancer spreads by local invasion, the lymph system, or the vascular system to the bone, lung, and liver.
- Prostate cancer in the early stages may be treated with testosterone-suppressing medications, such as leuprolide (Lupron) or goserelin (Zoladex), or with drugs that block testosterone's action on the prostate gland, such as bicalutamide (Casodex). Surgery, such as TURP or radical prostatectomy, or a combination of medication and radiation therapy may be done.
- Priapism is a painful erection that lasts longer than 4 hours. If not relieved, it can become a medical emergency. Small veins in the corpora cavernosa spasm, so blood cannot drain back out of the penis as it should. This can cause permanent tissue damage from lack of oxygen.
- Phimosis is a condition in which the foreskin of an uncircumcised male becomes so tight that it is difficult or impossible to pull back away from the glans (head) of the penis. It may make it impossible to clean the area under the foreskin.
- Paraphimosis occurs when the uncircumcised foreskin is pulled back, during intercourse or bathing, and is not replaced in a forward position over the glans of the penis. This can compress the penis vessels and lead to gangrene.
- Penile cancer has occurred in men who were not circumcised as infants or adolescents or who have acquired HPV. The tumor is typically a squamous cell carcinoma. It may look like a small, round raised wart, induration, or red area. This form of cancer can be spread to a sexual partner.
- Cryptorchidism (undescended testicles) is a congenital condition in which an infant boy is born with one or both of his testicles not in the scrotum. Testicles that are not brought down into the scrotum may lead to infertility. Also, the risk of testicular cancer is higher if the condition is not corrected before the child reaches his teen years.
- A hydrocele is a painless collection of fluid in the scrotal sac with unknown cause. It can happen at any point during a man's lifetime. No treatment is necessary unless the hydrocele causes discomfort or embarrassment or threatens the blood supply to the testicles.
- A varicocele is a condition sometimes called *varicose veins of the scrotum*. The main blood supply to the testicles travels along the spermatic cord. The veins become dilated and may cause a pulling sensation, a dull ache, or scrotal pain.
- Epididymitis is inflammation or infection of the epididymis that can be caused by bacteria, viruses, parasites, chemicals, or trauma. Risk factors include sexual or nonsexual contact, STIs, a complication of some urological procedures, or reflux of urine. The problem can also be associated with prostate infections. It is usually painful, with the scrotal skin being tender, red, and warm to the touch.
- Orchitis is a rare inflammation or infection of the testicles from trauma or infection from epididymitis, urinary tract infections, STIs, or systemic diseases such as influenza, infectious mononucleosis, tuberculosis, gout, pneumonia, or mumps (after puberty).
- Cancer of the testicles is the most common cancer in men between ages 15 and 35 in the United States. The etiology of testicular cancer is unknown. Some of the known risk factors are cryptorchidism, family history, white race, and high socioeconomic status.
- A vasectomy uses tiny clamps or cauterization to seal off the vas deferens to prevent sperm from reaching the outside of the body. This 15- to 30-minute surgery is done through a small puncture in the upper part of the scrotum. It is performed as an outpatient procedure and is intended for men not to reproduce.
- After the vasectomy, the testicles continue to produce sperm and the male hormone testosterone. The prostate gland, along with the seminal vesicles, still ejaculates semen. However, the semen does not contain sperm.
- Sometimes a man may decide he wants to have more children and asks to have a vasectomy reversed. The surgical procedure to reverse a vasectomy is called a vasovasostomy. Using microscopic instruments, the surgeon reconnects the vas deferens.
- Erectile dysfunction means that a man cannot obtain or keep a functional erection that is appropriately firm and lasts long enough for satisfactory sexual intercourse. Erectile dysfunction has many psychological and physical causes. It can also be caused by many medications and chemicals that interfere with desire, blood supply, or nerve transmission.
- Infertility is a concern for many couples. Many conditions must be present in the man for conception to occur. Endocrine function, autonomic nervous system function, and male reproductive structures must all be functioning properly. Normal healthy sperm in a concentration of at least 20 million per milliliter of semen are needed.
- The factors related to infertility are divided into three general categories: pretesticular, testicular, and post-testicular.

SUGGESTED ANSWERS TO CHAPTER EXERCISES

Cue Recognition
43.1: Assist the patient back to bed and report changes immediately to RN or HCP.
43.2: Gently replace the foreskin and speak with the assistive personnel about the importance of replacing the foreskin after cleansing.

Critical Thinking & Clinical Judgment
Mr. Atkinson
1. Because Mr. Atkinson's prostate is enlarged, he may be having trouble emptying his bladder. Terazosin acts by relaxing the muscles in the prostate as well as the opening of the bladder to increase urine flow.
2. $\frac{1.5 \text{ mg}}{2 \text{ mg}} \times 1 \text{ tablet} = 2.5$ tablets

   Mr. Atkinson should be alert for signs of hypotension, such as dizziness or lightheadedness upon arising. He should not drive until effects and side effects of the medication are known.
3. Mr. Atkinson should be instructed not to lift anything heavier than 10 pounds for the first 6 weeks. He will not be able to plow or drive for the first 6 weeks. It is important that his son understand his father's limitations and how important it is for him or someone else to assist with the farm chores.
4. Mr. Atkinson will notice a change in his ejaculation (either very little ejaculate or none at all). If he was able to have an erection before surgery, the chances are very good that he will continue to be able to have intercourse; however, he may have little to no ejaculation.
5. A home health-care nurse can assist Mr. Atkinson with care at home, such as catheter care and removal, possible dribbling postsurgery, and reinforcement of activity level. A dietitian can help with dietary instructions related to foods high in dietary fiber and fluids to avoid such as caffeine, citrus juices, and alcohol beverages.

Mr. Cunningham
1. Mr. Cunningham should be encouraged to see his HCP immediately for an evaluation to rule out testicular cancer.
2. Depending on the stage of the cancer, he will have the cancerous testicle, cord, and lymph nodes removed. He may need chemotherapy or radiation treatments as well.
3. Mr. Cunningham should be encouraged to make deposits at a certified sperm bank before any treatments. It is also important to include his partner and his family in the decision-making process. They should be encouraged to share their feelings and concerns with one another. Cancer support groups may also be helpful to Mr. Cunningham.

Mr. Kittle
There are many possible causes for Mr. Kittle's problem, including anxiety/depression, cardiovascular issues, or alcohol use (see Table 43.3).

1. It is okay to "pretend" here! Act like you are perfectly comfortable and that you hear this sort of thing every day. (Of course, you would never pretend to know something you don't—it is always okay to say you don't know.) Have a matter-of-fact communication style. If you get nervous and forget what questions you should ask, start with something general such as, "Can you tell me more about your symptoms?"
2. Begin collecting psychosocial data to identify presence of stress, fear, depression, fatigue, or problems with interpersonal relationships; also ask about medication, alcohol, and nicotine use. Assure him you will alert the HCP to follow up with further assessment.
3. After alerting the HCP, encourage Mr. Kittle to share openly so that an accurate diagnosis can be made. Reassure Mr. Kittle that many men have the same problem and that he is not alone. Let him know there are many treatments available and that his HCP will work with him to find what is best for him.

Additional Resources

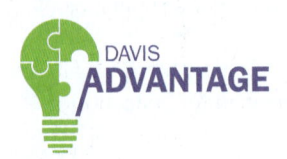

Go to Davis Advantage to complete your learning: strengthen understanding, apply your knowledge, and prepare for the Next Gen NCLEX®.

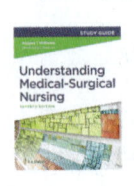

A Study Guide is also available.

CHAPTER 44
Nursing Care of Patients With Sexually Transmitted Infections

Michelle Corona, Laura L. McCully

KEY TERMS

cervicitis (SIR-vih-SY-tis)
chancre (SHANK-er)
condylomata acuminata (KON-dih-LOH-mah-tah ah-KYOO-min-AH-tah)
condylomatous (KON-dih-LOH-mah-tus)
conjunctivitis (kon-JUNK-tih-VY-tis)
cytotoxic (SY-toh-TOK-sik)
electrocautery (ee-LEK-troh-CAW-tur-ee)
endometritis (EN-doh-meh-TRY-tis)
exudate (EKS-yoo-dayt)
gummas (GUH-mahs)
hepatosplenomegaly (heh-PAT-oh-SPLEH-noh-MEG-ah-lee)
herpetic (her-PET-ik)
lymphadenopathy (lim-FAH-deh-NAH-puh-thee)
mucopurulent cervicitis (MYOO-koh-PURE-u-lent SIR-vih-SY-tis)
ophthalmia neonatorum (awf-THAL-mee-ah NEE-oh-nuh-TOR-uhm)
proctitis (prok-TY-tis)
puerperal (pyoo-UR-pur-uhl)
sacral radiculopathy (SAY-krul ra-DIK-yoo-LAH-puh-thee)
salpingitis (SAL-pin-JY-tis)
serological (SEAR-uh-LAH-jik-uhl)
stigma (stig-mah)
urethritis (YOO-reh-THRY-tis)
verrucous (veh-ROO-kus)
vesicular (veh-SIK-yoo-lur)
vulvovaginitis (VUL-voh-VAJ-ih-NY-tis)

CHAPTER CONCEPTS

Health promotion
Infection
Sexuality

LEARNING OUTCOMES

1. Identify pathogens involved with each of the common sexually transmitted infections (STIs).
2. Describe the signs and symptoms of each of the common STIs.
3. Plan teaching to promote STI prevention and facilitate necessary treatments.
4. Describe treatment options for common STIs and potential treatment problems.
5. Plan tailored patient-centered nursing care for patients with STIs.
6. Explain how to evaluate if nursing interventions are effective.

Sexually transmitted infections (STIs) can be passed from one individual to another through intimate contact with the genitals, mouth, or rectum. Some STIs are also spread by other routes, such as blood or body fluids. A nurse's best protection against diseases from blood and body fluids of infected patients is the strict practice of standard precautions and good hand hygiene.

The Office of Disease Prevention and Health Promotion creates 10-year health objectives for the United States, a public health initiative called Healthy People. In 2018, the nation witnessed some of the highest rates of chlamydia, gonorrhea, and syphilis ever recorded (Centers for Disease Control and Prevention [CDC], 2019). Healthy People 2030 continues to focus on reducing rates of STIs and improving well-being of patients with STIs. Physically, STIs can cause tremendous suffering because of pain, scarring of genitourinary structures, damage to other body organs, infertility, nervous system damage, development of cancer, and adverse pregnancy outcomes including birth defects and even death of infected patients and sometimes their children. Coexistence of more than one STI in an individual is also common. Many infections and syndromes are associated with STIs. Common STIs are discussed in this chapter; HIV and AIDS are discussed in Chapter 20.

Psychologically and socially, STIs have profound effects on individuals, families, and relationships. **Stigma** is a mark of shame, and patients with STIs may feel stigmatized from their peers, families, and even their health-care providers (HCPs). Patients may experience feelings of guilt about passing on an incurable infection to a loved one. The sexual partners of patients with an STI may feel betrayed because they could be infected by an intimate encounter. These feelings are just some of the emotional consequences of STIs.

Risk factors for STIs include the following:

- Inconsistent/inappropriate use of a condom for each anal, oral, or vaginal sex act
- Sexual activity with multiple and/or anonymous partners
- Use of mind-altering substances prior to and during sexual activity, such as drugs or alcohol
- Social determinants of health, such as poverty and unstable housing

One of the most important ways to help those who experience STIs is by being kind, nonjudgmental, and sensitive to the patient's communication. Maintaining an open posture and eye contact (if appropriate for the patient's culture) relays a sense of openness and willingness to talk. These open and active communication techniques preserve the possibility of continuing health promotion with these individuals in the future, particularly for vulnerable populations. For more information on STIs, visit www.cdc.gov/std/healthcomm/fact_sheets.htm.

> **BE SAFE!**
> **AVOID FAILURE TO COMMUNICATE!** You can prevent further spread of STIs by informing your patients about safer sex methods and supplies, as well as possible signs and symptoms. Instruct patients to refrain from sexual contact until they have a confirmed diagnosis of an STI and are receiving treatment.

DISORDERS AND SYNDROMES RELATED TO SEXUALLY TRANSMITTED INFECTIONS

Vulvovaginitis

Vulvovaginitis is an inflammation of the vulva and vagina. It can be asymptomatic or involve redness, itching, burning, excoriation, pain, swelling of the vagina and labia, and/or discharge. A variety of sexually and nonsexually transmitted infectious agents can cause vulvovaginitis. The odor, consistency, and color of the discharge vary with the different microbes involved. Nonsexually transmitted vaginitis, vulvovaginitis, and vaginosis are described in Chapter 42. Bartholin glands, which produce vaginal lubrication, can develop abscesses as a result of infection with STIs, such as gonorrhea and chlamydia, or nonsexually transmitted microbes.

Urethritis

Both STIs and nonsexually transmitted microorganisms can cause **urethritis** in men and women. In men, inflammation of the urethra, prostate, and epididymis can result in difficult, painful, and frequent urination and a urethral discharge. Discharge may be clear, cloudy, or yellow. Women may suffer from urethritis and have similar symptoms or lack of symptoms. In addition to urethritis, women may also develop mucopurulent cervicitis. Some causative agents for urethritis include *Neisseria gonorrhoeae, Chlamydia trachomatis, Mycoplasma genitalium, Ureaplasma urealyticum, Trichomonas vaginalis, Candida albicans*, and herpes simplex virus. *M. genitalium* is the most common cause of persistent or recurrent nongonococcal urethritis.

Mucopurulent Cervicitis

Mucopurulent cervicitis (MPC) is an inflammation of the cervix. It may produce mucopurulent yellow discharge or **exudate** on the cervix or have no noticeable symptoms. Some women experience intermenstrual bleeding, typically after sexual activity. MPC can be caused by the same organisms that cause urethritis. MPC during pregnancy can result in **conjunctivitis** and pneumonia in newborns. It can also cause **puerperal** infection in the mother. If not treated promptly, MPC may spread up the genital tract to become pelvic inflammatory disease (PID).

Pelvic Inflammatory Disease

Pathophysiology and Etiology

PID is an infection of the upper genital tract that can cause chronic pelvic pain due to inflammation. The primary sources of infection include *C. trachomatis* and *N. gonorrhoeae*. It may also result from any organism associated with an STI or normal vaginal flora. These organisms can invade the endocervical canal, resulting in inflammation of the cervix (**cervicitis**), and move upward, resulting in infection of the endometrium (**endometritis**), fallopian tubes (**salpingitis**), and pelvic cavity. The chronic inflammation results in extensive scarring and adhesions, which can cause infertility and increase the risk of ectopic pregnancy. Increased risk for PID occurs with a history of multiple sexual partners, STIs, substance abuse, frequent vaginal douching, and insertion of an intrauterine device (IUD).

Signs and Symptoms

Women may present with lower abdominal pain and tenderness, purulent vaginal discharge or vaginal bleeding, pain with sexual intercourse, fever, nausea and vomiting, and pain with urination. They may also present with no symptoms. Findings during physical examination include adnexal tenderness upon palpation and pain in the uterus and cervix when moved during a bimanual examination.

• WORD • BUILDING •

vulvovaginitis: vulvo—vulva + vagin—vagina + itis—inflammation
urethritis: ureth—urethra + itis—inflammation
mucopurulent cervicitis: muco—involving mucus + purulent—involving pus + cervic—cervix + itis—inflammation
conjunctivitis: conjunctiv(a)—lining of the eyelids and sclera of the eye + itis—inflammation
puerperal: puer—child + parere—to give birth
cervicitis: cervic—cervix + itis—inflammation
endometritis: endo—inside + metr—womb + itis—inflammation
salpingitis: salping—tube + itis—inflammation

Diagnostic Tests
To diagnose PID, HCPs obtain a medical history and perform a pelvic exam. Additionally, providers may obtain urinalysis, ultrasonography, endometrial biopsy, laparoscopy and/or vaginal fluid for microscopy. STIs can be identified through positive culture. Urinary tract infection may need to be ruled out.

Therapeutic Measures
With serious infection, hospitalization and IV antibiotics may be needed. IV therapy can be changed to oral therapy after 48 hours if status improves. Outpatient therapy with oral antibiotics is used with minor infections. Laparoscopic surgery may be done to release adhesions and reduce complications. Testing and treatment for other STIs should be considered for both the patient and partner. Education on the cause of the infection and prevention of future episodes is critical for the patient's and their partner(s)'s sexual health.

Proctitis and Enteritis
Proctitis is inflammation of the rectum and anus that may result in pain, discharge, and/or tenesmus. It may result from nonsexually transmitted microbes or STIs and is prevalent among those who practice anal intercourse, particularly the receptive partner. The most common causative organisms are *C. trachomatis*, *N. gonorrhoeae*, *T. pallidum*, and herpes. Enteritis is inflammation of the lining of the intestine that may occur from contamination during anal intercourse. *Giardia lamblia* is the most common infecting organism. Care of patients who have gastrointestinal disorders is discussed in Unit 8.

Genital Ulcers
Genital ulcers are formed when papules or macules erode and leave painful, raw, pitted, or excoriated areas on or around the genitals. Not all genital ulcers are caused by STIs. STIs that can produce genital ulcers include syphilis, herpes, and HIV. Although the ulcerations can look similar in these STIs, a distinctive difference is that a syphilitic ulcer is painless. Genital ulcers from one type of STI may increase the risk of infection with other STIs during sexual activity. Open ulcers present easy access for the infecting organism.

Cellular Changes
Cellular changes can also be caused by STIs, including **condylomatous** (wartlike) growths and dysplasia (presence of abnormal cells) or neoplasia (abnormal growth of tissue). These may result in precancerous or cancerous conditions. Herpes viruses, HIV, and human papillomavirus have all been linked to the development of cancer.

SEXUALLY TRANSMITTED INFECTIONS

Chlamydia
Etiology and Signs and Symptoms
Chlamydia, the most common STI in the United States, is caused by the bacteria *C. trachomatis*. (Table 44.1 provides a summary of this and other common STIs.) Contact with secretions during anal, vaginal, and/or oral sex can transmit *C. trachomatis*, which has several strains. Chlamydia is often asymptomatic ("silent") in women but can cause urethritis, MPC, conjunctivitis, PID, and Fitz-Hugh-Curtis syndrome, a surface inflammation of the liver related to chronic PID. This inflammation can cause nausea, vomiting, and sharp pain at the base of the ribs that sometimes radiates to the right shoulder and arm. As a frequent cause of PID and infertility, chlamydia also increases the risk of ectopic pregnancy. The infection can be passed from mother to baby during birth, resulting in neonatal pneumonia and conjunctivitis. Chlamydial infections also increase the risk of HIV acquisition.

Lymphogranuloma venereum (LGV) is caused by some strains of *C. trachomatis*. LGV is more common in tropical climates or among people who emigrated from tropical areas. This disease can cause urethritis and proctitis. It inflames lymph nodes that drain the pelvic area, resulting in draining sores and fistula development. Scarring can complicate vaginal deliveries.

Diagnostic Tests
Several tests for chlamydia are available. Samples are gathered in a special collection tube to send to a laboratory for processing, which may include culturing or nucleic acid amplification testing (NAAT). NAAT identifies the presence of chlamydial DNA or RNA in urine, cervical, or urethral specimens. If the HCP is performing a Papanicolaou (Pap) test, the chlamydia NAAT screening can be done with the ThinPrep specimen. The CDC recommends that all sexually active females younger than 25, older women with risk factors such as new or multiple sex partners, and women with sex partners who have had an STI be tested annually.

Therapeutic Measures
Antibiotics are given to treat chlamydia in adults and their sexual partners (Table 44.2). Many U.S. jurisdictions allow for partners of patients with confirmed chlamydial or gonococcal infections to receive treatment without examination by an HCP. This type of treatment is known as *expedited partner therapy* (EPT) and was established as an additional strategy to prevent further spread of certain STIs.

Erythromycin or azithromycin is used during pregnancy because other antibiotics may pose a risk to the fetus. Use of an erythromycin ophthalmic ointment is recommended to treat the neonate shortly after birth to prevent conjunctivitis, though efficacy for prevention of chlamydial ophthalmia is unclear. Institutional policies and state regulations determine whether administration of the medications requires specific consent of the parents.

• WORD • BUILDING •
proctitis: proc—anus + itis—inflammation
condylomatous: condyl—rounded projection + oma(t)— growth + ous—like

Table 44.1
Common Sexually Transmitted Infections Summary

	Chlamydia	*Gonorrhea*	*Syphilis*	*Trichomoniasis*	*Herpes Simplex*	*Condylomata (HPV)*
Signs and Symptoms	Conjunctivitis; in men, urethritis, epididymitis, prostatitis; in women, MPC, urethritis	In men, urethritis, penile discharge, epididymitis, prostatitis; in women, MPC, urethritis, abnormal menses	*Primary syphilis:* chancre; *secondary syphilis:* flu-like symptoms, rashes, condylomatous growths	Genital redness, swelling, itching, burning, foul discharge; in men, urethritis, prostatitis; in women, "strawberry cervix"	Vesicles/ulcerations in mouth, genitals, flu-like symptoms, lymphadenopathy, urethritis, cystitis, MPC	Fleshy tumors, primarily on genitalia
Diagnostic Tests	NAAT culture, urine	NAAT culture, urine	VDRL test, ELISA, RPR test, FTA-ABS	Microscopic examination	Culture, Western blot, ELISA	Visualization of lesions, biopsy
Therapeutic Measures	Antibiotics (see Table 44.2)	Antibiotics (see Table 44.2)	Penicillin	Metronidazole (Flagyl) or tinidazole (Tindamax)	Antiviral medication (see Table 44.2)	Wart removal, topical therapies, interferon therapy
Complications	Fitz-Hugh-Curtis syndrome, increased susceptibility to HIV infection, PID, infertility, transmission to baby at birth, co-infection with gonorrhea	PID, disseminated gonococcal infection, Fitz-Hugh-Curtis syndrome, transmission to baby at birth, co-infection with chlamydia	Tertiary syphilis; gumma damage to heart, circulatory system, nervous system; transmission to fetus during pregnancy	Preterm delivery, infertility, increased risk of HIV transmission	Lifelong infection, disseminated infection, nervous system invasion, increased risk of cervical cancer, transmission to baby at birth	Long-term complications are rare

Note: ELISA = enzyme-linked immunosorbent assay; FTA-ABS = fluorescent treponemal antibody absorption; HPV = human papillomavirus; MPC = mucopurulent cervicitis; NAAT = nucleic acid amplification testing; PID = pelvic inflammatory disease; RPR = rapid plasma reagin; VDRL = Venereal Disease Research Laboratory.

Gonorrhea

Etiology and Signs and Symptoms

N. gonorrhoeae, the organism that causes gonococcal infections, is the second-most reported STI. Transmission can occur through anal, vaginal, or oral sex, or through childbirth from mother to infant. It can produce a variety of signs and symptoms or remain asymptomatic. Men may experience dysuria; white, yellow, or green urethral discharge; and/or scrotal pain. Women often have either no noticeable symptoms or mild clinical presentation, so the gonococcal infection may be mistaken for another urogenital condition. Women who do have signs and symptoms may experience dysuria, abnormal discharge, MPC, or abnormal menstrual symptoms such as bleeding between periods. Many cases

Table 44.2
Medications Used to Treat Sexually Transmitted Infections

Medication Class/Action	
Chlamydia Antibiotics	
Macrolides *Inhibit bacterial protein synthesis.*	
Examples erythromycin azithromycin	**Nursing Implications** Administer on empty stomach. Do not administer with antacids. Use caution with hepatic disorders.
Tetracyclines *Inhibits protein synthesis by binding to ribosomes.*	
Example doxycycline	**Nursing Implications** Do not administer during pregnancy due to bone/teeth effects. Do not give with antacids or dairy products. Administer on empty stomach. Teach: Avoid unnecessary exposure to sunlight.
Penicillin *Binds to bacterial cell wall, causing cell death.*	
Example amoxicillin	**Nursing Implications** May make birth control pills less effective.
Fluoroquinolones *Inhibit cell wall synthesis.*	
Examples ofloxacin levofloxacin	**Nursing Implications** Safety under age 18 is not established. Do not administer with antacids. Use caution with other medications and with renal, hepatic, or central nervous system (CNS) disorders. All quinolones have a black box warning for potential tendinitis, tendon rupture, peripheral neuropathy, and CNS effects. Teach patients to stop taking the medication and call their physician for any signs or symptoms. Contraindicated in pregnancy. Avoid use in patients with a history of myasthenia gravis.
Gonorrhea Antibiotics	
Cephalosporins *Inhibit cell wall synthesis.*	
Examples ceftriaxone cefixime	**Nursing Implications** Use caution with penicillin allergies or renal or hepatic dysfunction. Teach: Avoid excess sun exposure.
Syphilis Antibiotics	
Penicillin *Inhibits cell wall synthesis.*	
Examples penicillin G	**Nursing Implications** Administer deep intramuscularly or slow intravenously. Apply ice packs to injection site as needed.

Continued

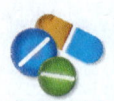

Table 44.2
Medications Used to Treat Sexually Transmitted Infections —cont'd

Medication Class/Action	
	Administer orally on empty stomach.
	Avoid tetracycline in children and pregnant women.
	Teach:
	Report fever/rash.
Tetracyclines	
Examples	**Nursing Implications**
tetracycline	See above under *Tetracyclines*.
doxycycline	
Trichomoniasis Amebicides/Antiprotozoals	
Bind to DNA to inhibit synthesis and cause cell death.	
Examples	**Nursing Implications**
metronidazole (Flagyl)	Administer with food.
tinidazole (Tindamax)	Treat partner as well as patient.
	Teach:
	Avoid alcohol; abstain for a minimum of 48 hours following treatment to prevent severe flu-like reaction.
Herpes Antivirals	
Inhibit DNA synthesis.	
Examples	**Nursing Implications**
acyclovir	Use systemic preparations cautiously with CNS, hepatic, or renal disorders.
valacyclovir	Infuse IV slowly.
famciclovir	Maintain hydration.
	Caution patient that viral transmission can still occur during treatment.
	Some patients take daily as suppressive therapy.
Genital Warts—Acidic Agents	
Acids burn and erode affected area.	
Examples	**Nursing Implications**
trichloroacetic acid (TCA)	*Teach:*
bichloracetic acid (BCA)	Return for repeated applications as needed.
	Avoid medication contact with eyes or tissue surrounding lesion.
Genital Warts—Antimitotic Agent	
Exact mechanism of action unknown. Causes necrosis of wart tissue.	
Examples	**Nursing Implications**
podofilox solution	Can be applied by patient at home with cotton-tipped applicator.
	Teach:
	Apply to warts only and allow to dry completely, or as ordered by health-care provider.
Genital Warts—Antiviral/Immune Response Modifier	
Stimulates patient's immune system to destroy warts.	
Example	**Nursing Implications**
imiquimod	Can be applied by patient at home.
	May take up to 16 weeks to completely clear warts.
	Teach:
	Apply thin film to clean dry skin at bedtime, as ordered by provider.

of PID are caused by gonorrhea. Gonorrhea can also cause Fitz-Hugh-Curtis syndrome. Fever, nausea, vomiting, and lower abdominal pain may be present. Gonorrhea may infect the throat and the rectum. The associated symptoms include sore throat, rectal discharge, itching, bleeding, or pain during bowel elimination. In addition, it may cause disseminated gonococcal infection, resulting in inflammation of the joints, skin, meninges, and lining of the heart.

Infants born to mothers who have gonorrhea can develop **ophthalmia neonatorum.** This involves inflammation of the conjunctivae and deeper parts of the eye and can result in blindness. All newborns are treated with erythromycin ophthalmic ointment to prevent this complication. The newborn may also experience a gonococcal infection at other sites following birth. Infections may develop where fetal scalp monitors were attached during labor, and infections of the nose, lungs, and rectum may also occur.

Diagnostic Tests

Diagnosis is made by microscopic examination of smears and cultures of the discharge or identification of bacterial DNA (NAAT) from urine, the vagina, or the endocervix. Testing can also be obtained with ThinPrep if a Pap specimen is collected.

Therapeutic Measures

Development of antibiotic resistance in *N. gonorrhoeae* and co-infection with other microorganisms, such as *C. trachomatis*, has complicated treatment. Dual therapies from different antibiotic classes are recommended for gonorrhea (see Table 44.2). It is important that the patient's partner is treated as well. If permissible within the local jurisdiction, partners of patients with confirmed gonococcal infections may be able to be treated using EPT.

Ophthalmia neonatorum can be prevented by use of erythromycin eye ointment. It is recommended that all infants be treated shortly after birth regardless of the diagnostic status of the mother. The treatment is simple and may prevent a devastating outcome for the newborn. Institutional policies and state regulations determine whether administration of the ointment requires consent of the parents.

> **BE SAFE!**
> **AVOID FAILURE TO COMMUNICATE!** If available in your area, collaborate with the patient and the HCP to provide EPT for the patient's partner.

Syphilis

Pathophysiology, Etiology, and Signs and Symptoms

Syphilis is an ancient infection that has not disappeared, although it is overshadowed by more common STIs. Its progression and clinical manifestations occur in stages. The primary stage begins with the entry of the *Treponema pallidum* spirochete through the skin or mucous membranes. Between 10 and 90 days later, a papule develops at the site of entry and then sloughs off, leaving a painless, red, ulcerated area called a **chancre** (Fig. 44.1). Chancres can also develop in other areas of the body at this time. Chancre formation typically is the only symptom of this stage of syphilis. The chancre eventually heals, but the spirochete remains active in the infected individual and can be passed on to others.

Secondary syphilis begins when a rough red or reddish-brown rash appears on the body, primarily on the palms and soles of the feet. This stage causes general physical problems such as flu-like symptoms, joint pain, hair loss, mouth sores, **lymphadenopathy**, and condylomatous growths in moist areas of the body.

Serious damage can occur if syphilis is untreated in the early stages. Untreated patients will enter the latent stage, where they no longer experience any signs or symptoms. This stage is divided into two substages, early and late latent. Those within the early latent period were infected with *T. pallidum* within the prior 12 months. Individuals infected for more than 12 months have entered the late latent stage, which can last for years.

About 15% of infected individuals progress to the tertiary (or late) stage, up to 10 to 30 years later. At this stage, it can involve any organ system of the body (CDC, 2017). The spirochete can form **gummas**, or rubbery tumors that can break down and ulcerate, leaving holes in body tissues. Gummas can damage the heart, bones, liver, circulatory system, and nervous system (called *neurosyphilis*). Ulceration of gummas can destroy areas of vital tissue and lead to mental and physical disability or early death.

Congenital Syphilis

Syphilis can be passed to unborn children of women who carry the spirochete. Congenital syphilis can result in **hepatosplenomegaly**, increase in bilirubin, destruction of red blood cells, birth defects (especially of the face), lymphadenopathy, and a baby who can transmit the spirochete through nasal drainage. If left untreated, syphilis during pregnancy can cause lesions in fetal organs, resulting in higher rates of spontaneous abortion, stillbirth, and premature birth.

Diagnostic Tests

Several tests for syphilis exist, and a combination is necessary for accurate diagnosis. **Serological** (blood) tests include nontreponemal and treponemal tests. The Venereal Disease

• WORD • BUILDING •

ophthalmia neonatorum: ophthalmia—eye disease + neonatorum—of the newborn
lymphadenopathy: lymph—lymph nodes + adeno—node + pathy—disorder
gummas: from the word meaning "rubber"—rubbery tumors
hepatosplenomegaly: hepato—liver + spleno—spleen + megaly—enlargement
serological: sero—blood + logical—science

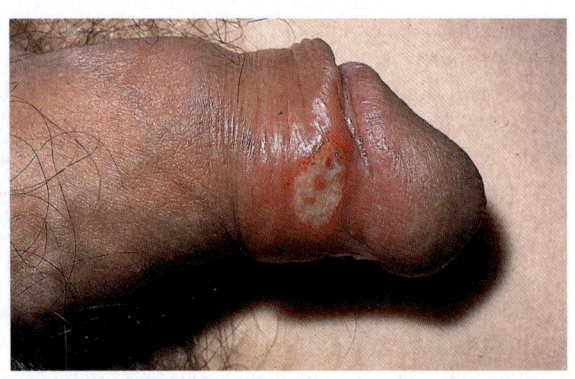

FIGURE 44.1 Syphilis chancre.

Research Laboratory (VDRL) test and the rapid plasma reagin (RPR) test are nontreponemal tests that indirectly check for syphilis by detecting the presence of antibodies to *Treponema*. Diagnosis of neurosyphilis is even more difficult because some testing of cerebrospinal fluid may result in false-negative results. Fluorescent treponemal antibody absorbed (FTA-ABS), *T. pallidum* passive particle agglutination assay (TP-PA), and other various enzyme immunoassays are treponemal tests that directly detect for the bacterium responsible for syphilis (CDC, 2017). These newer methods reduce the risk of false results. Latent syphilis infections can be detected by serologic testing even when patients have no symptoms.

Therapeutic Measures
Penicillin G is the treatment of choice for patients diagnosed with syphilis (see Table 44.2). The preparation, dosage, and duration of treatment is determined by the symptoms and stage of syphilis. For those allergic to penicillin, doxycycline and tetracycline are treatment options.

> **BE SAFE!**
> **AVOID FAILURE TO RESCUE!** You can prevent medication errors by asking patients about their allergy history. If a patient is prescribed antibiotics for an STI, be sure to confirm they do not have an allergy or sensitivity to that class of medications or related class.

Trichomoniasis
Pathophysiology and Etiology
Trichomoniasis is an STI caused by a protozoan parasite, *Trichomonas vaginalis*. It is more common in women than in men, particularly those ages 40 and older. Likewise, it is more common in Black women than in White non-Latina women. Individuals seeking care at an STI clinic and those who are incarcerated have a higher prevalence than the general population. Patients infected with *T. vaginalis* are often asymptomatic and can remain infected for long periods of time, and those patients are also at an increased risk of HIV acquisition and transmission. Trichomoniasis is most often transmitted through vaginal intercourse.

Signs and Symptoms
Symptoms include redness, swelling, itching, and burning of the genital area; pain with intercourse and voiding; and a frothy, foul-smelling discharge that can be clear, white, yellowish, or greenish. Men with trichomonal infection can develop prostatitis and infertility. Women who are pregnant risk preterm delivery and babies with low birth weights.

Diagnostic Tests
A Pap smear, NAAT, or antigen testing can be done on secretions or on urine in men. Visualization of the cervix during female pelvic examination shows a characteristic "strawberry cervix." When wet-mount slides of discharge are viewed under a microscope, organisms can be identified by motility and whiplike flagella. Because trichomoniasis can produce abnormal Pap readings, more frequent tests will provide adequate surveillance of cellular changes.

Therapeutic Measures
Metronidazole (Flagyl) or tinidazole (Tindamax) are used to treat trichomoniasis (see Table 44.2). Because some people carry the organism without symptoms, sexual partners should also be treated regardless of symptoms.

> **CRITICAL THINKING & CLINICAL JUDGMENT**
>
> **Kerri** presents to the health clinic with a report of generalized redness, swelling, itching, and burning of her external genitalia. Following history and physical and microscopic examinations, trichomoniasis is diagnosed. Kerri is upset, stating she has been in a monogamous relationship for 2 years.
>
> **Critical Thinking (The Why)**
> 1. What should your response to Kerri include?
> 2. What patient education is important for Kerri?
>
> **Clinical Judgment (The Do)**
> 3. Kerri is placed on metronidazole (Flagyl), but you are uncomfortable with the dose prescribed, so you look it up. How do you approach the HCP with an apparent error?
>
> Suggested answers are at the end of the chapter.

Herpes
Pathophysiology, Etiology, and Signs and Symptoms
Herpes infection is caused by the herpes simplex virus types 1 and 2 (HSV-1 and HSV-2). Herpes viruses affect the skin and nervous system. HSV can lie dormant in nervous system tissues and reactivate when the body undergoes stress, fever, or immune system compromise. Both HSV-1 and HSV-2 can cause fever blisters of the mouth (Fig. 44.2) and genital lesions. However, HSV-1 is more frequently associated with oral lesions and HSV-2 with genital lesions.

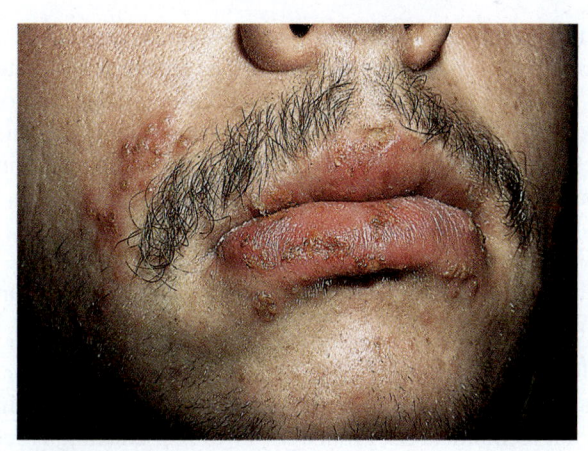

FIGURE 44.2 Herpes simplex.

Genital HSV-2 outbreaks are more severe than genital HSV-1 outbreaks. After infection, vesicles develop, spontaneously rupture, and produce painful ulceration of underlying skin tissues. Asymptomatic latent periods are generally interspersed between **vesicular** outbreaks. Although less common, the virus may be transmitted during latent periods through shedding.

An initial outbreak following infection with HSV typically occurs 2 days to 2 weeks after exposure and can produce a flu-like condition. Urethritis, cystitis, or MPC with vaginal discharge can also occur. Infection of the spinal nerve roots by HSV can result in **sacral radiculopathy** (damage of the sacral spinal nerves), causing retention of urine and feces. Although rare, disseminated herpes infection can result in inflammation of the spinal cord, meninges, nerve pathways, and lymph nodes as well as urethral strictures and increased risk for development of cervical cancer in women.

Despite roughly 12% of individuals ages 14 to 49 years having HSV-2 worldwide, most babies born to women with HSV do not develop **herpetic** disease (World Health Organization, 2020). If infected, the baby's skin, eyes, mucous membranes, and nervous system can be involved, and death from disseminated herpes infection is possible. The greatest risk of herpes transmission from mother to child during pregnancy occurs if the mother acquires HSV in her third trimester and/or has an active genital lesion at the time of delivery.

Diagnostic Tests

Clinical diagnosis of herpes can be difficult due to the lack of clinical manifestations in many HSV infected persons. Testing requires special viral collection kits for swabbed or scraped specimens from lesions. Cell cultures and PCR are the preferred HSV tests. Follow the directions on the viral collection kit as well as institutional policies. Blood tests are used to test specifically for HSV-1 or HSV-2 antibodies.

Therapeutic Measures

There is currently no known cure for herpes infection, although antiviral medications may be given to decrease the severity and frequency of symptoms (see Table 44.2).

The same discussion and treatment options should be had with patients who only test positive with blood testing. Pregnant women with a history of HSV are treated prophylactically with antiviral medication starting at 36 weeks' gestation (CDC, 2021b). If an active genital lesion is present when a woman is close to the time of delivery, a cesarean delivery will likely be performed. However, an active lesion at any time during pregnancy poses a risk for transmission. See "Nursing Care Plan for the Patient With a Sexually Transmitted Infection" later in the chapter.

Human Papillomavirus

Human papillomavirus (HPV) can be either high risk or low risk. More than 100 types of HPV have been identified. Many HPV types can be spontaneously cleared from the body by the immune system and do not cause tissue damage. However, several strains have been closely linked to the development of cancers. High-risk HPV can cause cervical, vaginal, and vulvar cancers in women, penile cancers in men, and anal and oropharyngeal cancers in both men and women. Low-risk HPV does not cause cancer but can cause genital warts (condyloma).

The Gardasil vaccine was introduced in 2006 for the prevention of four types of HPV. The current 9-valent Gardasil formulation protects against the low-risk types 6 and 11, which cause 90% of genital warts, and high-risk types 16, 18, 31, 33, 45, 52, and 58, known to cause 70% of cervical cancers. Women and men can receive the vaccine between the ages of 9 and 26, with age 11 or 12 being the recommend age for routine vaccination. If the vaccine is initiated between 9 and 14, only two doses are needed. The second dose is administered 6 to 12 months after the first dose. If initiated on or after a child turns 15, then the three-dose schedule is recommended. The first dose is given, followed by the second dose 2 months after initiation, and the third dose 6 months after initiation (Meites et al, 2016). After submission of a supplemental application, the Federal Drug Administration (FDA) approved the use of Gardasil 9 in a larger age group. This includes both men and women 27 to 45 years old (FDA, 2018).

Genital Warts (Low-Risk HPV)

SIGNS AND SYMPTOMS. **Condylomata acuminata** (genital warts) is a common sexually transmitted viral infection. Infection with HPV produces condylomata, soft, raised, **verrucous** fleshy tumors that may have fingerlike projections and resemble cauliflower (Fig. 44.3). Lesions most commonly develop on the external genitalia and perineum as well as on the internal vaginal wall and cervix in women

- WORD • BUILDING •

herpetic: herpet—herpes + ic—pertaining to
condylomata acuminata: condyl—rounded projection + oma—growth + ta—pluralizes the word (singular form is condyloma) + acuminata—genital growths
verrucous: verruc—wart + ous—like

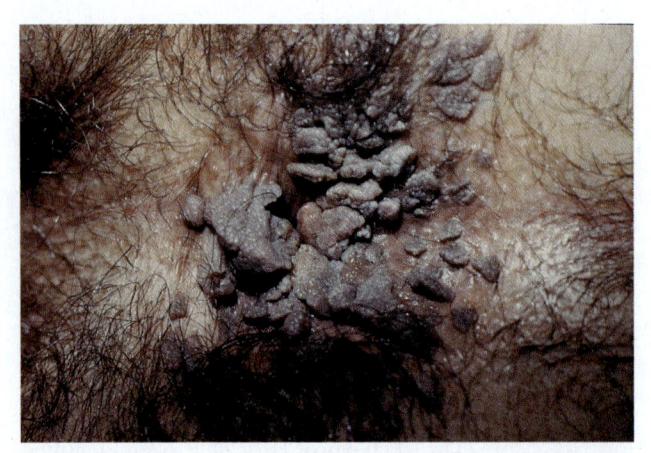

FIGURE 44.3 Condylomata, commonly known as genital warts.

but can also develop on other areas of the body after contact with the virus. Some people remain asymptomatic but can still transmit the infection.

The time from exposure to the development of the warts, known as the latent period, can last from a few weeks to a few years. HPV can be passed from a pregnant woman to her fetus, resulting in HPV infection of the baby's respiratory tract. In pregnant women, genital warts tend to grow more rapidly and bleed more easily with injury than in nonpregnant women. Vaginal delivery is an option unless warts block the pelvic outlet or would cause excessive bleeding.

DIAGNOSTIC TESTS. Diagnosis of condyloma is usually by visual inspection. Biopsy can be used to confirm diagnosis but is only done if lesions are atypical. HPV testing is not recommended for condyloma since the results are not reliable.

THERAPEUTIC MEASURES. There is currently no known cure for HPV. Genital warts can be treated by freezing, burning, or chemically destroying them or by manipulating the patient's immune system to attack the virus. Cryotherapy (freezing) of the warts can be done by touching each wart with a cryoprobe or a liquid nitrogen–soaked swab. Warts may also be burned or electrocoagulated with an **electrocautery** or a laser. Heat causes the proteins to coagulate, resulting in death of the wart tissue. Several topical agents are also available (see Table 44.2).

Some treatment options are not appropriate for use during pregnancy because of their **cytotoxic** effects, which might damage the fetus. However, cryosurgery and laser destruction of wart tissue are available for pregnant women. All treatments may require multiple applications and generally result in discomfort as the warts degenerate, ulcerate, and slough over a long period. Wart removal does not cure the infection, and new wart growth can occur after treatment.

HOME CARE. Patients who have genital warts burned off need to recuperate at home. Multiple areas may be treated. If the burns are near the urethra or rectum, the patient may need a Foley catheter inserted to avoid contamination and irritation of the lesions after treatment. The patient is instructed to increase dietary fiber and fluids to prevent constipation. Consult HCP for care of burns. Teach the patient to premedicate for pain as needed and use sterile technique for dressing changes.

High-Risk HPV

High-risk HPV is known to cause cervical, anal, penile, and oropharyngeal cancers.

DIAGNOSIS. Testing can be performed using conventional Pap or liquid-based Pap cytologic tests. Annual screening is not recommended. From ages 21 to 29, screening is recommended every 3 years. From 30 to 65, screening may continue every 3 years or Pap tests with high-risk HPV co-testing every 5 years.

TREATMENT. If the results of the Pap test are abnormal, follow-up care should be provided by the HCP. Depending on the severity of the findings, repeating the Pap, a colposcopy, a diagnostic excision of the lesion, or hysterectomy may be done.

Hepatitis B and C

Hepatitis B and C infections are caused by the hepatitis virus and result in liver inflammation. These hepatitis strains can be transmitted through sexual contact with blood and body fluids. During pregnancy, hepatitis B virus may be transmitted to the unborn baby. This can result in acute hepatitis and the possibility of becoming a chronic carrier of hepatitis B. See Chapter 35 for a full discussion on hepatitis.

Genital Parasites
Etiology and Signs and Symptoms

Genital parasites are not a true STI but may be transmitted during close body contact. The two most common parasites are pubic lice (*Phthirus pubis*, commonly called "crabs" because of the shape of the lice) and scabies (*Sarcoptes scabiei*). These parasites cause itching, redness, and, for scabies, tracks under the skin where the females burrow to lay their eggs.

Diagnostic Tests

History, physical examination, and visualization or magnification of parasites aid diagnosis.

Therapeutic Measures

Parasites are treated with topical insecticides such as permethrin (Elimite or Acticin) for scabies or malathion (Ovide) for pubic lice. Advise the patient to refer to package inserts for application instructions and precautions to avoid reinfection.

• WORD • BUILDING •

electrocautery: electro—electrical + cautery—branding iron
cytotoxic: cyto—cell + toxic—poison

> **BE SAFE!**
> **AVOID FAILURE TO COMMUNICATE!** The nurse may be required to facilitate the reporting and public health follow-up of STIs by filling in patient information on an STI reporting form and placing the form in the patient's chart for completion by the HCP. The requirements for reporting STIs vary in different states, provinces, and countries. In some areas, laboratories are also required to submit a report form for positive reportable STI results. The report form has spaces for listing of sexual contacts that should be notified of possible STI exposure. Depending on state law, contacts may be notified by the HCP, patient, or a public health authority.

NURSING PROCESS FOR SEXUALLY TRANSMITTED INFECTIONS

Data Collection

STIs are usually assessed, diagnosed, and treated in HCP offices and in clinics. It is important to evaluate the patient's reason for seeking care with every outpatient visit. Sometimes patients visit clinics or HCP offices for stated reasons other than STIs, yet their real concern is an STI.

If a patient presents with signs and symptoms that could lead to an STI diagnosis, inquire about irritation, pain, lesions, or discharge in the genital region. Explain to the patient that you need to know what examination supplies to prepare for an appropriate assessment, as this may allow them to share concerns and true reasons for the visit. Establishing rapport and conveying acceptance may also facilitate communication. You may be asked to be present during the examination to assist the HCP and to serve as a chaperone or patient support person.

STIs may also be discovered in hospitalized patients. Nurses are often the ones who bathe and provide perineal care to patients. It is important to be aware of signs and symptoms in older adults as well as younger people (see "Gerontological Issues"). Unusual discharge, redness, blisters, swollen areas, ulcers, and evidence of parasites in the genital area may be observed during patient care. STI awareness can also sensitize you to the possible significance of patient reports of persistent pelvic pain, dysuria, discharges, and rectal soreness. Such problems should be accurately documented and reported so that further investigation and treatment can take place.

> **CUE RECOGNITION 44.1**
> You are performing perineal care for your older adult client and note that the perineum is swollen, red, and blistered. What do you do?
>
> *Suggested answers are at the end of the chapter.*

Nursing Diagnoses, Planning, and Implementation

See "Nursing Care Plan for the Patient With a Sexually Transmitted Infection."

Special Population Considerations

Individuals who belong to the lesbian, gay, bisexual, transgender, queer (LGBTQ) community or other sexual minorities face challenges with access to health care. They face discrimination, whether intentional or by lack of knowledge regarding their specific health concerns. Nurses can practice some inclusive strategies that include creating an environment that demonstrates inclusivity, using gender-neutral language, and engaging in cultural sensitivity and competency training for LGBTQ health care. Nurses can display LGBTQ-specific patient education readily in the clinical areas and speak in an empathetic, nonjudgmental way to build a rapport of trust and compassion between themselves and their patients (Gay and Lesbian Medical Association, 2006; Landry 2017).

Black men make up 48% of new HIV cases in the United States. Death from HIV is higher in this ethnic/racial group than in any other ethnic/racial group. Black men are less likely to have access to care and to receive prescriptions for antiretroviral drugs for HIV. Compared to other ethnic/racial groups, Black men and Black women have higher rates of other STIs including chlamydia, gonorrhea, and syphilis. Factors such as lack of employment, poverty, lack of education, distrust of the health-care system, and lack of access to health care make it difficult for some racial/ethnic minorities to maintain sexual health (CDC, 2018).

Antimicrobial Resistance (AMR)

Pathogens develop resistance to the medications and therapies prescribed to eliminate them from a patient's body. Many STIs have developed resistance, such as chlamydia, gonorrhea, trichomoniasis, syphilis, and *M. genitalium*. AMR makes treatment difficult and can lead to complications in patients. Nurses can help prevent STIs from occurring through education of safer sex practices and ways to access screening and treatment for infections. They can also educate patients on the importance of taking all their medication to treat an STI to prevent organisms from becoming resistant to that specific antibiotic (CDC, 2021a; Ladenheim, 2018).

> **PRACTICE ANALYSIS TIP**
> **Linking NCLEX-PN® to Practice**
> The LPN/LVN will reinforce education to client regarding medications.

> **Gerontological Issues**
> **Older Adults and Sexual Activity**
> Older adults retain interest in and engage in sex. Do not assume that an older adult is not sexually active even if they are single or widowed. Those who enjoyed active and fulfilling sex lives with a previous spouse or partner may seek that in new relationships. Older adults who engage in high-risk sexual behaviors (e.g., multiple partners, genital-anal sex, no use of barriers during sexual intercourse) are at risk for STIs.

NURSING CARE TIP

Neighbors, friends, or family members may seek information from you because they know nurses are educated about health issues. Such questions may be stated in indirect terms, such as "I have a friend who is having a problem." You can provide accurate information and stress the importance of diagnosis and treatment to prevent the serious consequences of untreated STIs without asking probing or embarrassing questions.

CRITICAL THINKING & CLINICAL JUDGMENT

Stephanie is sitting in the examination room of the clinic where you work. She comments, "I am new to this area, and I've heard that there are three guys in this town who have syphilis and are spreading it around. Is that true?"

Critical Thinking (The Why)
1. What are some patient concerns this question might reflect?
2. You find out that Stephanie knows very little about syphilis. List in outline form a teaching plan that includes the information that is important for Stephanie to know about syphilis.

Clinical Judgment (The Do)
3. What type of environment is best to discuss potentially sensitive information?
4. If after talking to Stephanie you believe she might be experiencing symptoms of an STI, what actions would you take, and with whom would you collaborate to provide care?

Suggested answers are at the end of the chapter.

Nursing Care Plan for the Patient With a Sexually Transmitted Infection

Nursing Diagnosis: *Risk for Infection* (transmission to others) related to lack of knowledge about transmission, symptoms, and treatment
Expected Outcome: The patient will verbalize understanding of measures to prevent transmission to others.
Evaluation of Outcome: Does the patient verbalize understanding of transmission prevention? Does the patient practice preventive behaviors?

Intervention	Rationale	Evaluation
Collect data regarding patient's understanding of transmission, symptoms, complications, and treatment of STIs.	New instruction should be based on patient's previous knowledge.	Is patient's current understanding accurate? What teaching is needed?
Collect data about whether patient is engaging in high-risk behaviors.	If patient continues to engage in high-risk behaviors, risk is high for infection of others.	Is patient protecting self and others appropriately?
Use standard precautions and strict aseptic technique for procedures involving blood and body fluids.	The health-care team, in addition to other patient contacts, must be protected.	Are standard precautions observed?
Instruct patient in appropriate strategies to reduce risk of infecting others, including abstinence, monogamy (if no active infection), use of barrier methods and spermicides, and adherence to treatment regimen (Table 44.3).	These measures may help prevent transmission of infection to others.	Does patient verbalize understanding of methods to prevent transmission and intent to practice them?
Teach patient signs and symptoms of STIs to report immediately.	Prompt treatment of patient and their partners further reduces risk of transmission of infection.	Does patient verbalize understanding of signs and symptoms to report?
Explain importance of a follow-up evaluation.	Follow-up is essential to affirm that treatment was successful.	Does patient make a follow-up appointment?

Table 44.3
Barrier Methods for Safer Sex

Barrier	Related Information
Male condoms	Latex condoms are less likely than other types to break during intercourse. Lubrication decreases the chance of breakage during use. Only water-soluble lubricants should be used because substances such as petroleum jelly (Vaseline) may weaken the condom. Condoms should never be inflated to test them; doing so can weaken them. Condoms should be applied only when the penis is erect. Condoms should have a reservoir tip or should be applied while holding about a half inch of tip flat between the fingertips to allow room for ejaculate; otherwise, the condom might break. The penis should be withdrawn after ejaculation and before the erection begins to subside while holding the condom securely around the penis to avoid spillage. Condoms should never be reused and should be discarded properly after use so that others will not come in contact with contents.
Female condoms	Female condoms should be applied before any penetration occurs; even pre-ejaculation fluid can contain microorganisms. Lubrication decreases the chance of breakage during use, but only water-soluble lubricants should be used because substances such as petroleum jelly (Vaseline) may weaken the condom. Female condoms should never be reused and should be discarded properly after use so that others will not come in contact with contents.
Cervical caps or diaphragms	These may provide some protection for the cervix only. They are not effective barriers against sexually transmitted infections (STIs).
Rubber gloves, rubber dental dams, split (opened) male condoms	Dental dams are latex or polyurethane sheets. These may provide some barrier protection for manual and oral sex. Although some groups suggest that male condoms may be split down one side and opened or that rubber dental dam material may be taped over areas that have lesions to avoid direct contact with blood and body fluid, this very high-risk behavior is not recommended.

Key Points

- Patients with an STI are at greater risk for acquiring other STIs.
- Vulvovaginitis is an inflammation of the vulva and vagina caused by a variety of sexually and nonsexually transmitted infectious agents.
- Both STIs and nonsexually transmitted microorganisms cause urethritis in men and women.
- MPC is an inflammation of the cervix. It may produce a mucopurulent yellow exudate on the cervix or may have no noticeable symptoms.
- Proctitis is inflammation of the rectum and anus. It may be due to either nonsexually transmitted microbes or STIs. It is especially prevalent among those who practice anal intercourse. Enteritis may occur.
- Genital ulcers are formed when papules or macules erode and leave painful, raw, pitted, or excoriated areas on or around the genitals. Not all genital ulcers are caused by STIs. STIs that can produce genital ulcers include syphilis, herpes, and HIV. Syphilitic ulcers are painless.
- PID is an infection of the upper genital tract that can cause chronic pelvic pain due to inflammation.
- Chlamydia is a commonly diagnosed STI in the United States. It is often asymptomatic in women, but it can cause urethritis, MPC, PID, and conjunctivitis.
- Gonorrhea is caused by the bacterium *N. gonorrhoeae*. Transmission can occur vaginally, rectally, orally, via contact with other mucous membranes. Men may be asymptomatic or may have urethritis with a yellow urethral discharge. Women may have either no noticeable symptoms or have urethritis, MPC, or abnormal menstrual symptoms such as bleeding between periods or during sex.
- Newborns born to mothers who have gonorrhea can develop ophthalmia neonatorum. This involves inflammation of the conjunctivae and deeper parts of the eye and can result

- in blindness. All newborns are treated with erythromycin ophthalmic ointment for prevention.
- Syphilis occurs in three stages that develop over weeks to years and can be fatal if untreated. If left untreated, syphilis during pregnancy can cause lesions in various organs of the unborn baby and result in higher rates of spontaneous abortion, stillbirth, and premature birth.
- Trichomoniasis is an STI caused by a protozoan parasite *T. vaginalis*. Symptoms include redness, swelling, itching, and burning of the genital area; pain with intercourse and voiding; and a frothy, foul-smelling discharge that can be clear, white, yellowish, or greenish.
- Herpes infection is caused by the herpes simplex virus types 1 and 2 (HSV-1 and HSV-2). HSV-1 is more frequently associated with oral lesions and HSV-2 with genital lesions.
- HPV can be either high risk or low risk. High-risk HPV can cause cervical, vaginal, and vulvar cancers in women; penile cancers in men; and anal and oropharyngeal cancers in both men and women. Low-risk HPV does not cause cancer but can cause genital warts (condyloma).
- Genital parasites are not a true STI, but they may be transmitted during close body contact.
- One of the most important ways you can help those who experience STIs is by being kind, nonjudgmental, and using therapeutic communication.
- Patients who suspect or have confirmed cases of STIs should be instructed to avoid any sexual contact until they are treated and encourage their partners to be screened. For those participating jurisdictions, partners of patients who have chlamydia or gonorrhea may be eligible for expedited partner therapy.

SUGGESTED ANSWERS TO CHAPTER EXERCISES

Cue Recognition
44.1: Notify the RN or HCP. Do not assume because the patient is an older adult that they do not have an STI.

Critical Thinking & Clinical Judgment
Kerri
1. Explain to Kerri that trichomoniasis is often an STI but that the organism that causes the infection can be transmitted through infected articles during nonsexual contact and can survive a long time outside the body. Also explain that a person can be asymptomatic for many years following exposure to the organism before an outbreak occurs. Her partner could also have an undiagnosed infection.
2. Teach Kerri that treatment should be provided to her partner regardless of symptoms. Also, reinfection may occur if both partners are not treated. Teach her how the infection is spread and how to avoid it in the future. She and her partner should use condoms or remain abstinent until treatment is effectively completed. Be sure to tell her that she should abstain from alcohol while on metronidazole and for at least 48 hours following its completion. Patients who drink alcohol while taking it are very likely to vomit.
3. You don't want to assume the HCP is wrong. An approach might sound something like, "I wanted to confirm your order for this patient because I noticed in the drug guide that the usual dose is 2 grams, but I see you have written it for 4 grams."

Stephanie
1. Concerns might include (a) the wish to speak with a health-care worker, (b) uncertainty about whether patient information will be kept confidential (give assurance that if you knew about anyone with syphilis, it would be your professional responsibility to keep it confidential), (c) fear that she might have become infected through heterosexual contact, (d) a desire to protect herself by avoiding those who have syphilis, and (e) a desire for information about syphilis and its transmission routes.
2. The teaching plan might include information about the spirochete that causes syphilis, signs and symptoms, diagnostic tests, means of transmission, strategies for risk reduction, treatment, research, and rights and responsibilities of those who have the disease.
3. Discussing private matters such as sexual preferences and practices of patients should be done in a private room. Despite her questions regarding other people within the community, Stephanie might really be asking questions for herself. Providing a quiet, private space to have an open conversation is the best environment.
4. If you believe that Stephanie might be experiencing symptoms of an STI, you would discuss the diagnostic testing available and recommend screening based on her clinical presentation. You would need to collaborate with the health-care provider to have a full assessment and examination completed.

Additional Resources

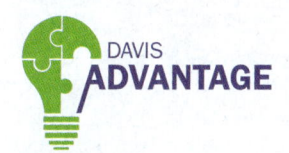

Go to Davis Advantage to complete your learning: strengthen understanding, apply your knowledge, and prepare for the Next Gen NCLEX®.

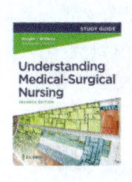

A Study Guide is also available.

UNIT TWELVE Understanding the Musculoskeletal System

CHAPTER 45
Musculoskeletal Function and Data Collection

Suzanne Sutton, Janice L. Bradford

KEY TERMS

arthrocentesis (AR-throw-sen-TEE-sis)
arthrogram (AR-throw-gram)
arthroscopy (ar-THRAH-skuh-pee)
articular (ar-TIK-yoo-lar)
bursae (BUR-sah)
crepitation (crep-ih-TAY-shun)
diaphysis (dye-AFF-uh-sis)
epiphyses (e-PIFF-uh-sees)
gout (GOWT)
hemarthrosis (heem-ar-THROW-sis)
osteoblast (ahs-TEE-oh-blast)
osteoclast (ahs-TEE-oh-clast)
periosteum (PEAR-ih-ahs-TEE-um)
resorption (ree-SORP-shun)
synarthrosis (sin-AR-throw-sis)
synovitis (sin-oh-VY-tis)

CHAPTER CONCEPTS

Caring
Mobility
Teaching and learning

LEARNING OUTCOMES

1. Explain the anatomy and function of the musculoskeletal system.
2. Describe the effects of aging on the musculoskeletal system.
3. List subjective data that are collected when caring for a patient with a disorder of the musculoskeletal system.
4. List objective data to collect for a patient with a disorder of the musculoskeletal system.
5. List areas included for neurovascular data collection for the musculoskeletal system.
6. Identify diagnostic tests for musculoskeletal problems.
7. Describe the nursing care provided for patients undergoing diagnostic tests of the musculoskeletal system.

MUSCULOSKELETAL SYSTEM ANATOMY AND PHYSIOLOGY

The skeletal and muscular systems can be considered as one system because together they move the body. The skeleton is the framework of the body to which the voluntary muscles are attached. The framework includes the joints, or articulations, between bones. Contraction of a muscle stabilizes or changes the angle of a joint. Movement would not be possible without the proper functioning of the nervous, cardiovascular, and respiratory systems. Voluntary muscles require nerve impulses to contract, a continuous supply of blood provided by the circulatory system, and oxygen provided by the respiratory system.

MUSCULOSKELETAL SYSTEM TISSUES AND THEIR FUNCTIONS

The tissues that make up the skeletal system are primarily bone tissue, **articular** (joint) cartilage (cushions joint and reduces friction), and fibrous connective tissue that forms the ligaments (that connect bone to bone) and other structures within joints. Tissues of the muscular system include skeletal muscle tissue and fibrous connective tissue. Fibrous connective tissue forms tendons that connect muscle to bone and *fasciae* (the strong membranes enclosing individual muscles).

Besides its role in movement, the skeleton has other functions. It protects organs and tissues from mechanical injury. The brain is protected by the skull, and the heart and lungs are protected by the thoracic cage. Flat and irregular bones as well as the ends of long bones contain red bone marrow, the hematopoietic (blood-forming) tissue. These bones also store excess calcium, which may undergo **resorption** (bone broken down with minerals including calcium released into blood) for blood calcium homeostasis. Calcium in the blood is needed for blood clotting and for the proper functioning of nerves and muscles.

Although the primary function of the muscular system is to move or stabilize the skeleton, the voluntary muscles collectively contribute significantly to heat production, which maintains normal body temperature. Another important function of the muscular system is to aid in the return of blood from the legs through muscular compression on the leg veins.

Bone Tissue and Bone Growth

Bone tissue is composed of bone cells, called *osteocytes*, within a strong, nonliving matrix made of calcium salts and the protein collagen. In compact bone, the osteocytes and matrix are in precise, densely structured arrangements called *osteons*. In spongy bone, the arrangement of cells and matrix is irregular and sparse, resembling a sponge. Compact bone forms the diaphyses (shafts) of the long bones, covers the spongy bone of the epiphyses of long bones, and covers the spongy bone that forms the bulk of short, flat, and irregular bones. The **periosteum** (connective tissue) covers all outer bone surfaces except at the joints, where cartilage covers the end of the bone. The periosteum provides protection, is involved in bone growth and repair (producing osteoblasts) and participates in the blood supply of bone.

Osteoblasts produce bone matrix during growth and replace matrix during normal remodeling or in repair of fractures. Other cells called **osteoclasts** resorb bone matrix when more calcium is needed in the blood or during repair when excess bone must be removed as bone changes shape.

The growth of bone from fetal life until final adult height depends on many factors. Proper nutrition (particularly vitamins and minerals) provides the raw material to produce bone matrix, comprising calcium, phosphorus, and protein. Vitamin D is essential for the efficient absorption of calcium and phosphorus in the small intestine. Vitamins A and C are required for the production process of bone matrix. Hormones directly needed for growth include growth hormone (GH) from the anterior pituitary gland, thyroxine from the thyroid gland, and insulin from the pancreas. GH increases mitosis and protein synthesis. Thyroxine stimulates osteoblasts and increases energy production. Insulin is essential for the efficient use of glucose to provide energy. If a child is lacking any of these hormones, growth is slower, and the child may not reach his or her genetic potential for height.

Bone is not a fixed tissue, even when growth in height has ceased. Calcium and phosphate are constantly being removed and replaced (remodeled) to maintain normal blood levels of these minerals. Parathyroid hormone, secreted by the parathyroid glands, increases the removal of calcium and phosphate from bones. The hormone calcitonin from the thyroid gland promotes the retention of calcium in bones.

Structure of the Skeleton

The 206 bones of the adult human skeleton are in two divisions: the axial and appendicular skeletons (Fig. 45.1; axial in white, appendicular in turquoise). The axial bones are flat or irregular bones and contain red bone marrow (hematopoietic tissue). Within the appendicular skeleton, the limbs consist of long bones (except the carpals, tarsals, and patella). All long bones have the same general structure: a central **diaphysis**, or shaft, with two ends called **epiphyses.**

Skull

The skull consists of eight cranial bones and 14 facial bones. It also contains the three auditory bones found in each middle ear cavity. All the joints between the cranial bones and between most of the facial bones are immovable joints called sutures (**synarthrosis**).

Vertebral Column

The vertebral column (or spinal column) is made of 33 individual bones called *vertebrae* (Fig. 45.2). *Atlas*, the first of seven cervical vertebra, articulates with the occipital bone of the skull and forms a pivot joint with the *axis*, the second cervical vertebra. The 12 thoracic vertebrae articulate with the posterior ends of the ribs. The five lumbar vertebrae are the largest and strongest. The *sacrum*, consisting of five fused sacral vertebrae, articulates with the *os coxae* at the sacroiliac joints. The coccyx, composed of four fused coccygeal vertebrae, serves as an attachment point for some muscles of the perineum.

The vertebrae as a unit form a flexible backbone that supports the trunk and head and that contains and protects the spinal cord. Spinal nerves and vessels exit via intervertebral foramina. Intervertebral discs cushion and permit movement of the column.

Thoracic Cage

The thoracic cage consists of 12 pairs of ribs and the sternum that protect the heart and lungs as well as upper abdominal organs, such as the liver and spleen, from mechanical injury. During breathing, the flexible thoracic cage is pulled upward and outward by the external intercostal muscles to expand the chest cavity and bring about inhalation.

Synovial Joints

The primary joints of the appendicular skeleton are summarized in Table 45.1. All freely movable joints (diarthroses) are synovial joints (Fig. 45.3). Many synovial joints also have **bursae** (small sacs of synovial fluid between the joint and structures that cross over the joint). Bursae lessen wear in areas of friction.

• WORD • BUILDING •

periosteum: peri—surrounding + osteo—bone
osteoblast: osteo—bone + blastanō—germinate
osteoclast: osteo—bone + klastēs—breaker
epiphyses: epi—upon + phyein—to grow
synarthrosis: sun—together + arthrosis—jointing

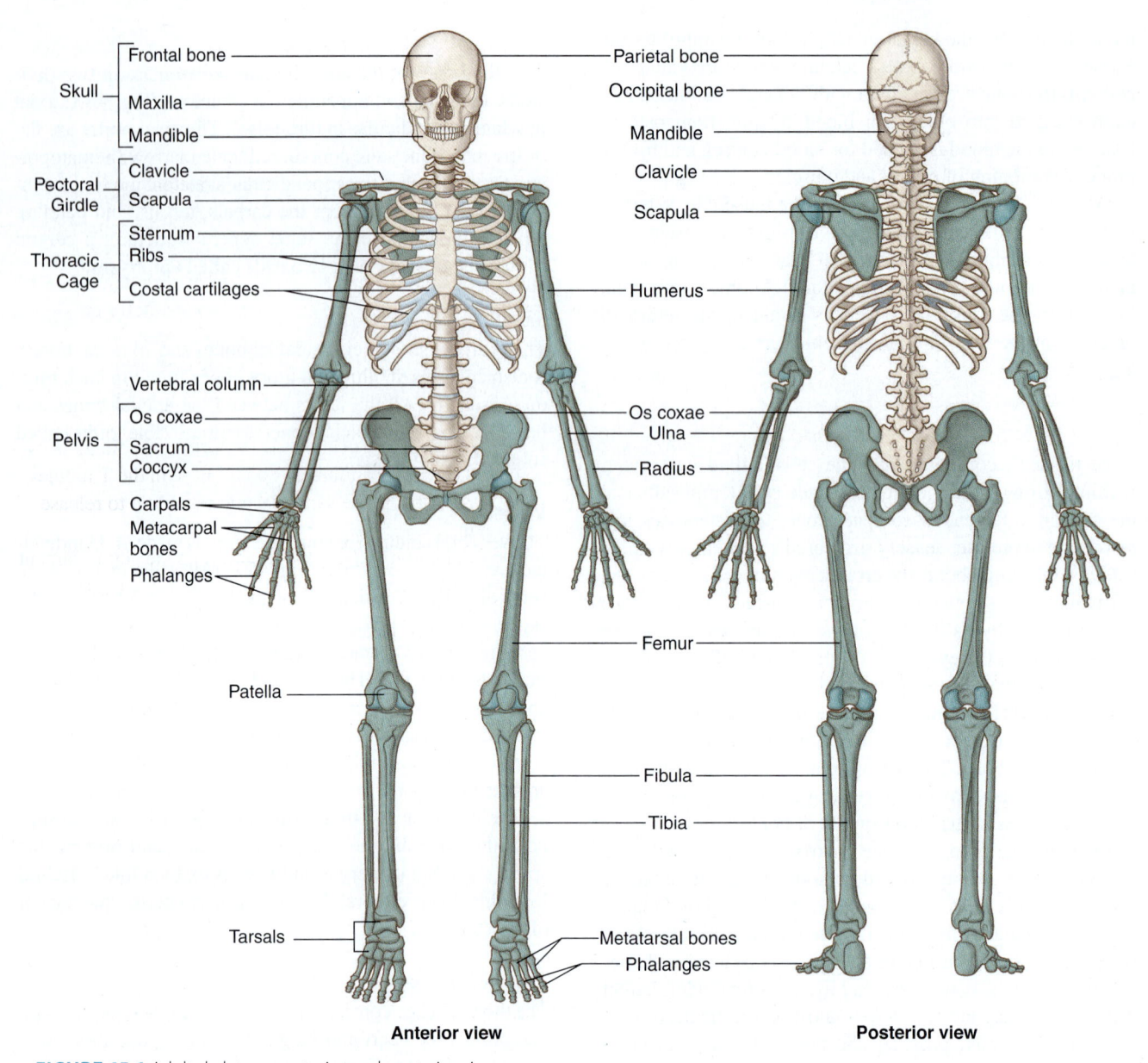

FIGURE 45.1 Adult skeleton—anterior and posterior views.

Muscle Structure and Arrangements

One muscle can consist of thousands of skeletal muscle cells (fibers), which are specialized for contraction. When a muscle contracts, it shortens and exerts force on a bone. Each muscle fiber receives its own motor nerve ending. The number of fibers that contract depends on workload. Muscles are anchored to bones by tendons made of fibrous connective tissue. A muscle usually has at least two tendons, each attached to a different bone. The more stationary muscle attachment is called its *origin;* the more movable attachment is the *insertion.* The muscle itself crosses the joint formed by the two bones to which it is attached. When the muscle contracts, it pulls on the insertion, moving the bone in the intended direction. The muscle causing the action is termed the *agonist.*

The body has approximately 700 skeletal muscles (Fig. 45.4). Their general arrangement is the agonist with opposing antagonists and the cooperative synergists. Without synergism, balance and fine motor control for writing or talking would be difficult, if not impossible.

ROLE OF THE NERVOUS SYSTEM

Skeletal muscles are voluntary: conscious control initiates nerve impulses to cause contraction. Nerve impulses originate in the motor areas of the frontal lobes of the cerebral cortex. The coordination of voluntary movement is a function of the cerebellum. Neurons in the central nervous system (CNS) act involuntarily to regulate muscle tone, the state of slight contraction usually present in muscles. Healthy muscle tone is important for posture and coordination.

Chapter 45 Musculoskeletal Function and Data Collection 887

Five Sections of the Vertebral Column

- Cervical vertebrae (7 vertebrae)
- Thoracic vertebrae (12 vertebrae)
- Lumbar vertebrae (5 vertebrae)
- Sacrum (5 fused vertebrae)
- Coccyx (4 fused vertebrae)

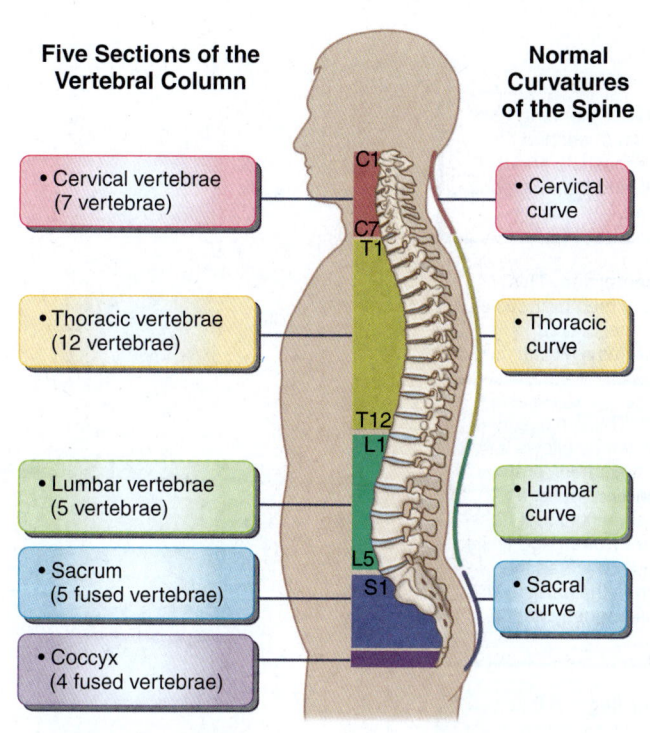

Normal Curvatures of the Spine

- Cervical curve
- Thoracic curve
- Lumbar curve
- Sacral curve

FIGURE 45.2 Vertebral column.

Table 45.1 Joints of the Appendicular Skeleton

Type of Joint and Description	Examples
Symphysis—disk of fibrous cartilage between bones	Between vertebrae Between pubic bones
Ball and socket—movement in all planes	Scapula and humerus (shoulder) Pelvic bone and femur (hip)
Hinge—movement in one plane	Humerus and ulna (elbow) Femur and tibia (knee) Between phalanges (fingers and toes)
Combined hinge and planar	Temporal bone and mandible (lower jaw)
Pivot—rotation	Atlas and axis (neck) Radius and ulna (distal to elbow)
Gliding—side-to-side movement	Between carpals (wrist)
Saddle—movement in several planes	Carpometacarpal of thumb

Source: Modified from Scanlon, V. C., & Sanders, T. (2019). *Essentials of anatomy and physiology* (8th ed.). Philadelphia, PA: F.A. Davis.

Neuromuscular Junction

Each muscle fiber has its own motor neuron ending. The neuromuscular junction is the termination of the motor neuron at the muscle fiber (synapse). The neuron releases the neurotransmitter acetylcholine (ACh), signaling the muscle to contract. Figure 45.5 illustrates the following steps:

1. When an impulse reaches the end of a motor neuron, it causes small vesicles in the axon terminal to release the neurotransmitter (chemical messenger) ACh into the synaptic cleft (narrow space between the motor neuron and muscle fiber).
2. The ACh diffuses across the synaptic cleft, where it stimulates receptors in the sarcolemma (muscle fiber membrane).
3. This sends an electrical impulse over the sarcolemma and inward along the T tubules. The impulse in the T tubules causes the sacs in the sarcoplasmic reticulum to release calcium.
4. The calcium binds with the troponin on the actin filament to expose attachment points. In response, the myosin heads of the thick filaments grab onto the thin filaments and muscle contraction occurs.

If a muscle has little work to do, few of its many muscle fibers contract; but if the muscle has more work, more muscle fibers contract.

AGING AND THE MUSCULOSKELETAL SYSTEM

The amount of calcium in bones depends on several factors. Good nutrition is certainly one, but age is another, especially for women. One function of estrogen (and testosterone in men) is the maintenance of a strong bone matrix. For women, after menopause, bone matrix loses more calcium than is replaced. The loss can be offset by weight-bearing physical exercise, which stimulates bone matrix deposition, increasing bone density.

Weight-bearing joints are also subject to damage after many years. Often the articular cartilage wears down and becomes rough, leading to pain and stiffness.

Muscle strength declines with age as protein synthesis decreases. Such loss of strength need not be exaggerated because aging muscles also benefit from regular exercise. Furthermore, maintenance of muscle strength reduces falls and accidents. Figure 45.6 presents a concept map that shows the effects the aging process has on the musculoskeletal system.

MUSCULOSKELETAL SYSTEM DATA COLLECTION

Health History

Subjective data collection on the patient begins with a history that includes the condition's impact on the patient's life (Table 45.2). The **WHAT'S UP?** model can be used to collect data about pain (see Chapter 1).

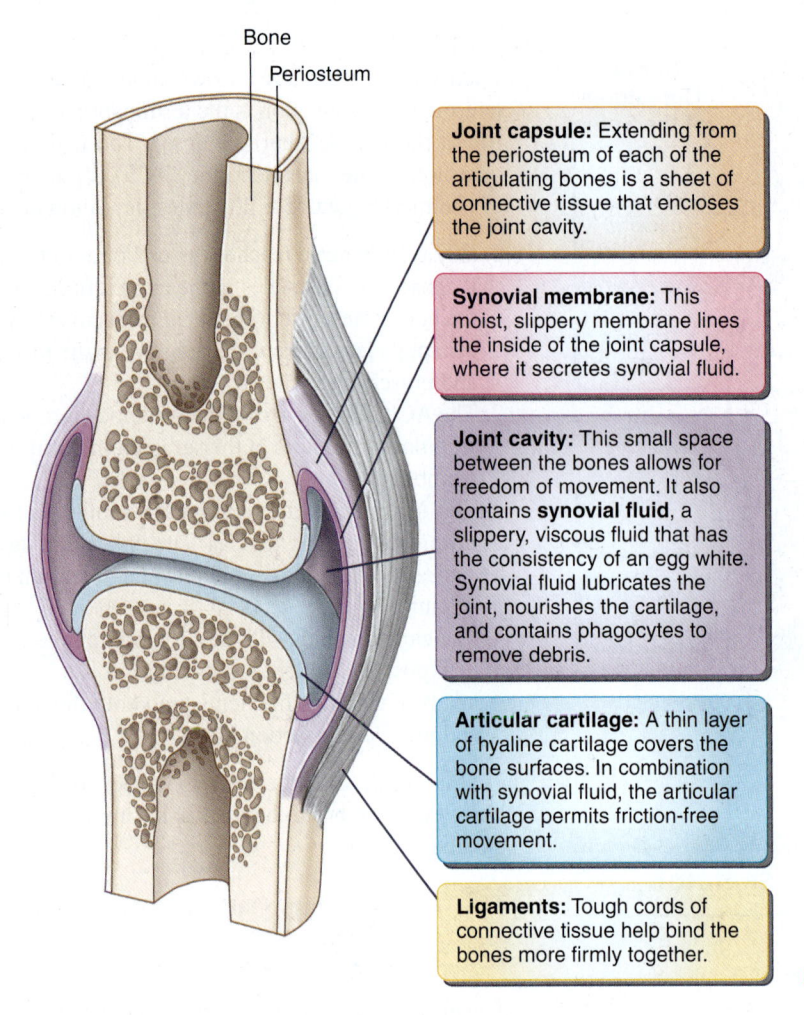

FIGURE 45.3 Synovial joints.

Joint capsule: Extending from the periosteum of each of the articulating bones is a sheet of connective tissue that encloses the joint cavity.

Synovial membrane: This moist, slippery membrane lines the inside of the joint capsule, where it secretes synovial fluid.

Joint cavity: This small space between the bones allows for freedom of movement. It also contains **synovial fluid**, a slippery, viscous fluid that has the consistency of an egg white. Synovial fluid lubricates the joint, nourishes the cartilage, and contains phagocytes to remove debris.

Articular cartilage: A thin layer of hyaline cartilage covers the bone surfaces. In combination with synovial fluid, the articular cartilage permits friction-free movement.

Ligaments: Tough cords of connective tissue help bind the bones more firmly together.

Deformities resulting from arthritis or other musculoskeletal disorders can affect a patient's body image and self-concept and may result in social withdrawal (see Chapter 46). Chronic pain may keep the patient from working or socializing. Data collection should include questions related to the psychological effects of the musculoskeletal disorder. Ask about the patient's support systems. Determine ability to cope by asking what previous coping strategies were used for other life stressors. As needed, consult social work, clergy, or support groups to meet the psychosocial needs of the patient.

Physical Examination

Objective musculoskeletal data collection includes three important areas: inspection, range of motion (ROM), and muscle tone and palpation (Table 45.3). If the patient can walk, inspect posture and gait, noting poor posture or alterations in movement, such as limping. Note the use of mobility aids, such as a cane or walker. Document other gross deformities, such as unequal limbs, malalignment, or contractures. Spinal deformities are especially significant as they can compromise breathing and balance. Inspect the joints and muscles of the arms, hands, legs, and feet for deformity, redness, and swelling. Listen for **crepitation** (grating sound as joint or bone moves). Also note the patient's general nutritional status (e.g., normal, obese, emaciated).

Observe ROM and muscle tone as the patient performs activities of daily living. To check ROM in the hands, ask the patient to touch each finger, one by one, to the thumb (known as *opposition*) and then make a fist. Note the size, shape, strength, and tone of muscles. Evaluate bilateral muscle strength by asking the patient to grip your hands. This enables you to feel the strength and equality. The push of an extremity against your hand generally indicates muscle strength. A physical therapist or an occupational therapist performs a more detailed assessment.

Next, gently palpate the skin for warmth and tenderness in the areas of swelling and in areas where the patient reported pain. Reddened joints are palpated for **synovitis** (swollen synovial tissue within the joint) or the presence of bony nodes. Joints and muscles may seem healthy but can be tender when palpated. Frequent neurovascular checks are

• WORD • BUILDING •
synovitis: synovia—joint + itis—inflammation

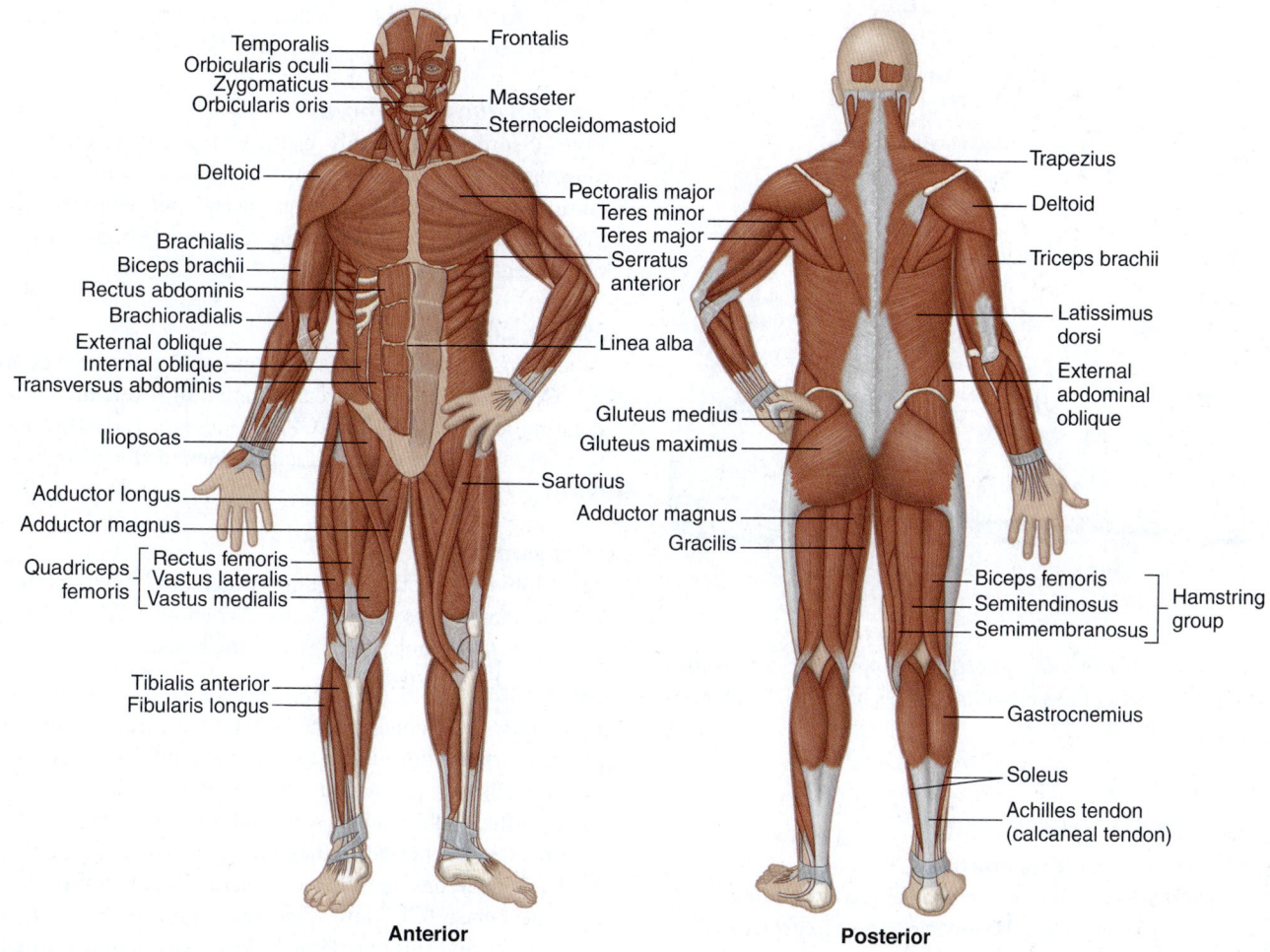

FIGURE 45.4 Superficial muscles.

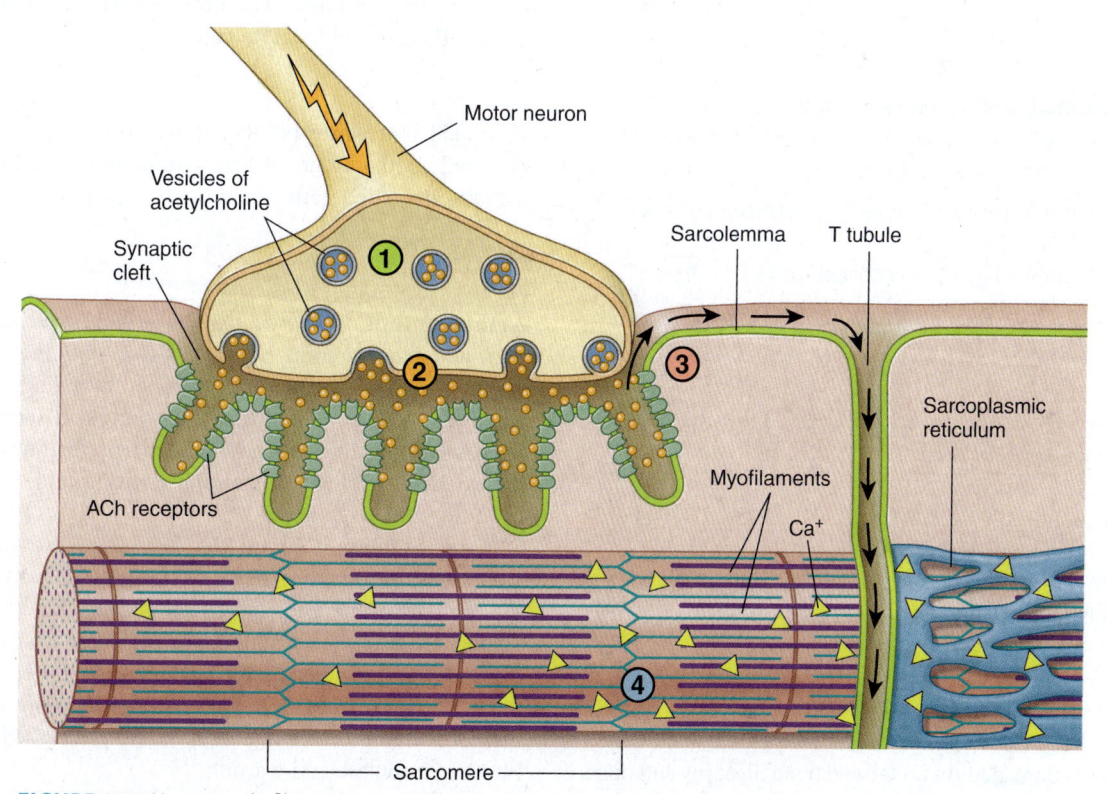

FIGURE 45.5 How muscle fibers contract. (See *Neuromuscular Junction* on page 887 for explanation of numbered steps.)

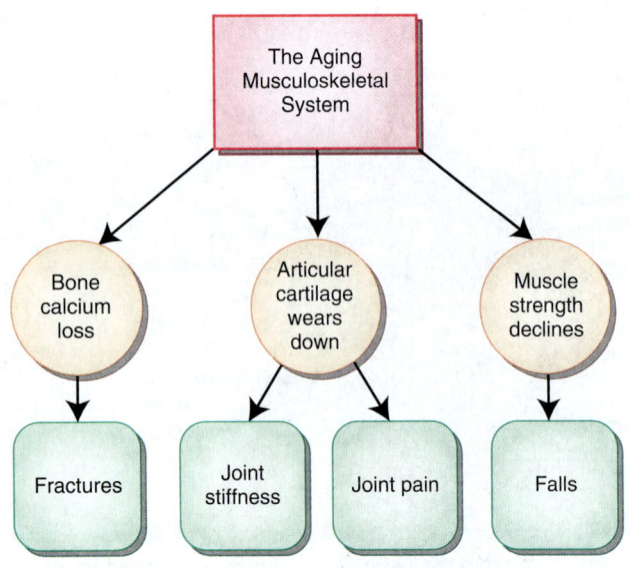

FIGURE 45.6 Aging and the musculoskeletal system.

needed with the risk of circulation impairment, which may occur if the patient has a fracture or has had musculoskeletal surgery (Table 45.4).

> **PRACTICE ANALYSIS TIP**
> **Linking NCLEX-PN® to Practice**
> The LPN/LVN will perform focused data collection based on client condition (e.g., neurological checks, circulatory checks).

CLINICAL JUDGMENT
Mrs. O'Donnell, age 80, is brought to the emergency department with a fractured left hip. She is positioned for comfort while you collect data.
1. What health history and subjective data do you collect for Mrs. O'Donnell?
2. What objective data do you collect for Mrs. O'Donnell?

Suggested answers are at the end of the chapter.

DIAGNOSTIC TESTS FOR THE MUSCULOSKELETAL SYSTEM

Diagnosis of musculoskeletal problems is assisted by laboratory tests and diagnostic imaging and procedures (Table 45.5, Table 45.6). Specific tests for connective tissue diseases are described in Chapter 46.

Laboratory Tests
Alkaline Phosphatase
Alkaline phosphatase (ALP) is an enzyme that increases when bone is damaged. In metabolic bone diseases and bone cancer, ALP increases to reflect osteoblast (bone-forming cell) activity.

Calcium and Phosphorus
Bone disorders commonly cause changes in calcium and phosphorus (or phosphate) levels. In a healthy person, calcium and phosphorus have an inverse relationship. This means that when serum calcium increases, serum phosphorus decreases, and vice versa.

Muscle Enzymes
When muscle tissue is damaged, many serum enzymes are released into the bloodstream, including skeletal muscle creatine kinase (CK-MM [CK3]), aldolase (ALD), aspartate aminotransferase (AST), and lactate dehydrogenase (LDH).

Myoglobin
Myoglobin is a protein found in striated (skeletal or cardiac) muscle that causes its red color. When skeletal muscle is damaged, myoglobin levels rise in the blood.

RHABDOMYOLYSIS. Rhabdomyolysis is a very serious, potentially fatal condition associated with muscle destruction due to an injury (such as crush syndrome), high fever, convulsions, or prolonged muscle compression. It commonly affects older adults who fall and lie in one position for an extended period as they are alone and cannot get up. If the patient has muscle destruction, watch for elevated creatine kinase (CK) up to five times greater than normal, myoglobin, and serum potassium levels to monitor for rhabdomyolysis. Observe for dark urine, muscle weakness, and myalgia (muscle pain). The goal of treatment is to restore normal fluid and electrolyte balance.

Uric Acid
Uric acid is a waste product found in the blood normally excreted in the urine. When serum uric acid levels rise, a condition called **gout** can occur (Chapter 46).

Diagnostic Procedures
Arthrocentesis
Arthrocentesis is a procedure in which synovial fluid is aspirated from a joint for analysis or to relieve pressure (improves pain and mobility). The fluid build-up often occurs secondary to an inflammatory process such as bursitis. Analysis of the synovial fluid can help diagnose crystals, **hemarthrosis** (blood in the joint cavity), noninflammatory conditions, and septic arthritis.

Using aseptic technique, the health-care provider (HCP) administers a local anesthetic. A needle is used to aspirate the contents of the joint space. For analysis, the fluid is sent to the laboratory. If required, the HCP can instill medications such as corticosteroids, anti-inflammatories, or antibiotics. The site is covered with a sterile dressing to prevent infection. Monitor the injection site for increased bruising, bleeding, redness, and warmth.

Table 45.2
Subjective Data Collection for the Musculoskeletal System

Questions to Ask During the Health History	Rationale/Significance
Demographic	
What is your age, gender, socioeconomic status?	Increased age, being female, and lower socioeconomic status can increase risk of musculoskeletal injury/problems.
What is your occupation?	Enables discharge planning if occupation may be affected by condition.
Where do you live geographically?	Regions where sunlight is limited increases the risk of vitamin D deficiency, leading to increased risk for skeletal injuries.
Prior Health History	
Do you have allergies?	Prevents exposure to medication or compounds used in diagnostic tests, treatments, and therapies.
What prior medical conditions, surgeries, or problems with anesthesia (e.g., malignant hyperthermia) have you had?	Identifies any pre-existing conditions that may influence the musculoskeletal system.
What activities do you participate in, and how often?	Provides baseline information about the patient's activity level before the problem.
What risk factors for musculoskeletal problems are present (e.g., smoking, sedentary lifestyle, weight gains/losses)?	Smoking and a sedentary lifestyle are risk factors for musculoskeletal problems.
What is your nutritional intake?	Nutritional intake of calcium and vitamin D influences some musculoskeletal disorders.
What is your family's medical history?	Some musculoskeletal conditions or anesthesia problems have genetic and familial tendencies.
Injury or Present Concern	
What is the history of the injury or current concern?	Provides information that helps in the diagnosis of the problem as well as possible complications of the injury.
What is your pain level (use pain assessment scale)? What medications, treatments, and procedures are used to alleviate pain?	Pain or related stiffness and tenderness may be acute or chronic and may limit the patient in everyday life.
Psychosocial	
Are deformities, changes in body image, or self-concept present?	The patient may need assistance with strategies to cope with the stress of a possible chronic musculoskeletal condition.
What coping skills do you use? Whom do you consider your support system?	Some musculoskeletal conditions require lifestyle alterations that can cause increased stress and difficulties in coping.

CUE RECOGNITION 45.1

You are visiting a home health patient who had an arthrocentesis of his right shoulder 3 days ago. You note red streaks that are warm to the touch down the patient's affected arm. What action do you take?

Suggested answers are at the end of the chapter.

Arthroscopy

An arthroscope allows the surgeon to directly visualize a joint using a small tube. The knee and shoulder are the joints most often evaluated. Because **arthroscopy** is an invasive

• WORD • BUILDING •

arthroscopy: arthro—joint + scopy—to examine

Table 45.3
Objective Data Collection for the Musculoskeletal System

Abnormal Findings	Possible Causes
Circulation	
Decreased capillary refill	Impaired circulation
Diminished or absent pulses	Compartment syndrome, fractures, trauma
Ecchymosis	Fractures, trauma
Swelling	Arthritis, infection, fractures, trauma
Skin color: Lighter pigmentation – Pale; reddened Darker pigmentation – Pale palms or soles; Purplish/Blue, Eggplant color	Impaired circulation: inflammation, infection
Skin temperature: Cool; warm	Impaired circulation: inflammation, infection
Neuromuscular	
Impaired movement	Compartment syndrome, trauma
Weakness	Compartment syndrome, trauma
Musculoskeletal	
Extremities: Asymmetry, contractures, crepitation, deformity, malalignment, unequal limbs	Arthritis, fractures, trauma
Impaired range of motion	Arthritis, dislocation, fractures, trauma
Altered gait	Arthritis, fractures, osteoporosis, trauma
Deformed posture	Osteoporosis, spinal deformity

procedure performed under local or light general anesthesia, the patient is treated in a same-day surgery setting.

The surgeon makes a small incision to insert the scope and visualize the joints. Other incisions may be needed for other tools. The joint is moved through ROM so tears, defects, or other soft tissue damage can be observed and/or repaired through the scope using special instrumentation. Depending on procedure, a bulky or small dressing with an elastic bandage may be applied.

The perianesthesia care nurse monitors the neurovascular status of the surgical limb frequently (see Table 45.4). A mild analgesic usually relieves pain. The patient resumes activities as ordered, usually within 24 to 48 hours. If a surgical repair was performed, the patient may have activity restrictions and require a stronger analgesic. In this case, the surgeon sees the patient in 1 week to check for complications and progress. Although complications are uncommon, explain to the patient to report these signs to the HCP: thrombophlebitis (extremity warmth, redness, swelling, tenderness, pain), infection (fever or warmth, pain, redness, swelling at surgical site), and increased joint pain. Physical or occupational therapy may be ordered (see "Home Health Hints").

CUE RECOGNITION 45.2
You are caring for a resident who had a left knee arthroscopy. You note his left lower leg is warm to the touch. What action do you take?

Suggested answers are at the end of the chapter.

BE SAFE!
AVOID FAILURE TO RECOGNIZE! You can prevent your patient from having a serious postoperative complication by recognizing signs and symptoms of infection early. If you respond when you notice warmth, redness, pain, or swelling, you can prevent further complications. Be vigilant during frequent observations of your patients.

Bone or Muscle Biopsy
Bone or muscle tissue can be extracted for microscopic examination to confirm cancer, damage (muscle biopsy), infection (bone biopsy), or inflammation. Afterwards, a sterile pressure dressing is applied because bone is highly

Table 45.4
Neurovascular Data Collection

Monitor	Report
Neuro	
Movement	Alterations in movement
Pain	Disproportionate to the injury; unrelieved with narcotics
Sensation	Alterations in feeling; tingling or paresthesia
Vascular	
Capillary refill	Nailbed that does not blanch in 3–5 seconds
Pulses	Diminished or absent distal pulses
Skin color	Pallor, cyanosis, redness, or discoloration
Swelling	Tight, shiny skin
Temperature	Unusual coolness or warmth

vascular. The nurse monitors the biopsy site for bleeding, swelling, and hematoma formation. Increased pain that is unresponsive to analgesic medication may indicate bleeding into the soft tissue. Vital signs and neurovascular checks are monitored (see Table 45.4).

Bone Density Scan
A bone density test measures bone strength. There are several types of scans. One that uses a special x-ray process is the dual-energy x-ray absorptiometry (DEXA), which measures the spine, hip, and total body bone density. DEXA is used to diagnose osteoporosis (see Chapter 46). Other types of scans examine the heel, fingers, or wrist.

Computed Tomography
Computed tomography (CT) scan can help diagnose problems of the joints or vertebral column (Fig. 45.7).

Magnetic Resonance Imaging
Magnetic resonance imaging (MRI) diagnoses musculoskeletal problems, especially involving soft tissue. An MRI is more accurate than a CT scan for diagnosing issues affecting the vertebral column (Fig. 45.8). If the patient has had previous spinal surgery, a contrast medium is used. Before the test, determine whether the patient has any cardiac or orthopedic implants and whether they are designated MR safe

Table 45.5
Laboratory Tests for the Musculoskeletal System

Test (Serum)	Normal Value	Significance of Abnormal Findings
Alkaline phosphatase (ALP), total	*Male:* 35–142 units/L *Female:* 25–125 units/L	↑ in Paget disease, metastatic bone cancer, new bone formation
Calcium, total	8.4–10.2 mg/dL	↑ in bone cancer, extended immobilization, hypophosphatemia, Paget disease ↓ in hyperphosphatemia, nutritional deficiency, osteomalacia
Creatine kinase (CK)	*Male:* 50–204 units/L *Female:* 36–160 units/L	↑ in cellular destruction of cells that store CK, intramuscular injections
CK3 (CK-MM) isoenzyme	96%–100%	↑ in conditions that cause cellular damage
Phosphorus	2.5–4.5 mg/dL	↑ in hypocalcemia, bone cancer ↓ in hypercalcemia, gout, vitamin D deficiency
Myoglobin	*Male:* 28–72 ng/mL *Female:* 25–58 ng/mL	↑ in skeletal muscle destruction
Uric acid	*Male:* 4–8 mg/dL *Female:* 2.5–7 mg/dL Over 60 years: *Male:* 4.2–8.2 mg/dL *Female:* 3.5–7.3 mg/dL	↑ in gout

Table 45.6
Diagnostic Procedures for the Musculoskeletal System

Procedure	Definition	Significance of Abnormal Findings	Nursing Management (if applicable)
Noninvasive			
X-rays	Visualization of skeletal abnormality or deformity, dense or inflamed tissues, and joints.	Guides treatment plan and information for care. *Example:* Broken ribs demand increased attention to respiratory system.	Inform patient of what to expect during ordered procedures.
Computed tomography	Radiographic "slices" of bone or soft tissue images.	Shows bone cancer, damage, fractures, and infections.	Before test, nothing by mouth (NPO) for 4 hours. If contrast used: Ask if history of reaction to contrast medium (reaction to iodine-based contrast dye is not the same as a shellfish allergy, as iodine is not an allergen [Long et al, 2019]).
Magnetic resonance imaging (MRI)	Electromagnets provide a three-dimensional visualization of the area.	Shows bone, joint, and soft tissue abnormalities.	Screen for contraindications to MRI such as certain metals or implants, claustrophobia, and allergy to contrast medium, if used. Inform patient of the need to lie still and the noise of the machine during the procedure.
Ultrasonography	Visualizes bone or soft tissue using sound waves.		Inform the patient that the jelly-like conducting substance will feel cold when applied.
Nerve conduction studies	Electromyography (EMG) is the electrical testing of nerves and muscles.	Alterations usually indicate a problem with the nerves or the muscles.	Explain that there may be some discomfort during nerve and muscle stimulation as well as when needles are inserted (if needed).
Invasive arthrography	Air or a contrast medium is injected into a synovial joint which is then x-rayed.	Aids in the diagnosis of joint abnormalities.	Inform patient that the test is uncomfortable during injection. Joint swelling is common after the procedure. Apply ice and elevate limb. Rest extremity for 12–24 hours after procedure.
Myelogram	Visualizes the spine and spinal cord. May use injection of a contrast medium.	Identifies spinal problems.	Postprocedure: Monitor for headache and nausea. Maximum head raise is 45 degrees for 3 hours or as ordered.
Nuclear medicine scans	Radioisotope is injected to help visualize bone and other soft tissue abnormalities.	Finding a "hot spot" usually indicates metastases or bone infection.	Explain test is not dangerous and may take up to 90 minutes.

Chapter 45 Musculoskeletal Function and Data Collection 895

Table 45.6
Diagnostic Procedures for the Musculoskeletal System—cont'd

Procedure	Definition	Significance of Abnormal Findings	Nursing Management (if applicable)
Gallium/thallium scans	A radioactive element is injected that migrates to bone, and inflammatory tissue.	Gallium concentrates in areas of tumors, inflammation, and infections. Thallium detects osteosarcoma.	Verify if agency recommends that children and pregnant women stay a few feet away from the patient for the first 48 hours.
Arthroscopy	Provides direct visualization of a joint and its capsule using an instrument inserted into the joint space.	Identifies joint abnormalities.	Perform neurovascular checks. Apply ice, and keep limb elevated to minimize swelling (if ordered).
Arthrocentesis	Withdrawal of synovial fluid from a joint space. Used for analysis of synovial fluid or reduction of excess fluid pressure.	Arthritis, bleeding, gout, infection, and inflammation.	Monitor patient for infection, inflammation, or hemarthrosis.
Bone or muscle biopsy	Needle aspiration (closed) or surgical extraction (open) of bone or muscle tissue.	Bone tumors, infection, lymphoma, and leukemia.	Monitor site of biopsy for bleeding. Provide wound care for open biopsy. Perform neurovascular checks as needed.

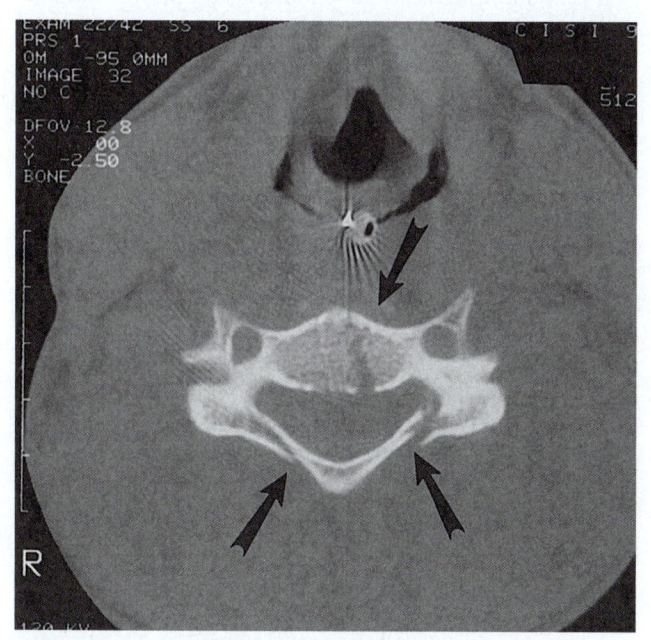

FIGURE 45.7 Computed tomography (CT) scan of fifth cervical vertebra showing a burst fracture of the vertebral body (*top arrow*) and both laminae (*bottom arrows*).

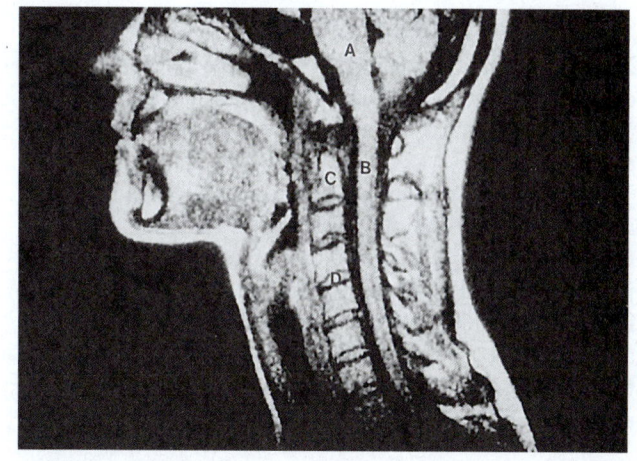

FIGURE 45.8 Magnetic resonance image (MRI) of a normal cervical spine. (A) Cerebellum. (B) Spinal cord. (C) Marrow of C2 vertebral body. (D) C4–C5 intervertebral disk.

(no hazard), MR conditional (able to carefully use MRI), or MR unsafe (unacceptable risk). It cannot be assumed that a cardiac implant prevents an MRI from being performed. Studies show that people with non-MRI conditional cardiac devices can safely have MRIs (Gupta et al, 2020).

Inform HCP if the patient has a cardiac device or orthopedic implant. See patient teaching guidelines for screening and preparation information for MRI on Davis Advantage.

Myelography
Myelography is usually reserved for patients unable to have a CT scan or MRI or for complicated spinal surgery revisions. Inform patients that they may be positioned head down briefly to allow injected contrast medium to flow up to the level of the neck.

Nerve Conduction Studies

Electromyography (EMG) measures a muscle's electrical impulses. This study helps diagnosis muscle diseases or nerve damage, which may follow a traumatic injury. Instruct the patient not to apply lotions before the test and to remove all jewelry. Occasionally, slight discomfort and bruising may occur at the site. Warm compresses or mild analgesics can be offered for pain relief.

Nuclear Medicine Scans

A bone scan allows visualization of the entire skeleton. The patient is injected with a radioisotope that is attracted to bone and travels to bone tissue. Images are taken at intervals to see how the radioisotope has collected in the bone. Gallium and thallium are radioisotope examples. Gallium concentrates in areas of tumors, inflammation, and infections. Thallium identifies bone cancer, especially osteosarcoma.

Patients are instructed to remove all jewelry before the test. For an accurate test, the patient must be able to lie still for up to 90 minutes during scanning. Patients who are older, restless, agitated, or in pain may find this test uncomfortable. Sedatives or analgesics may have to be administered before or during the procedure.

The HCP looks for "hot spots" on the test results created by increased circulation in abnormal bone areas that concentrates the radioactive substance there. Hot spots indicate bone disease.

Radiographs (X-Rays)

X-ray examination is used to determine bone alignment, density, erosion, swelling, and soft tissue damage (e.g., ligaments and tendons) because of alterations in bone position and spacing.

Arthrogram (or arthrography) is an x-ray examination of a synovial joint, most often the knee or shoulder, after joint trauma. Air or a contrast medium is injected into a synovial joint, which is then x-rayed. Inform the patient that the test is uncomfortable during injection. Joint swelling is common after the procedure. Apply ice, elevate the limb, and inform the patient to rest the joint for 12 to 24 hours after procedure as ordered.

Ultrasonography

Sound waves are used to detect osteomyelitis (bone infection), soft tissue disorders, traumatic joint injuries, and surgical hardware placement.

CRITICAL THINKING & CLINICAL JUDGMENT

Mrs. Gardenio, 84 years old, fell when using a step stool in her home as she was getting ready to attend her church's worship service. She was taken to the hospital, where it was determined that she had a femoral neck fracture of her left hip.

Critical Thinking (The Why)

1. What tests may be performed to identify the condition creating her problem?

Clinical Judgment (The Do)

2. What data do you obtain from Mrs. Gardenio?
3. Mrs. Gardenio is to receive morphine 4 mg by intramuscular injection now. You have available morphine 5 mg/mL. How many milliliters do you give?

    You collect data on Mrs. Gardenio's left leg 2 hours later. You are not able to palpate a pedal pulse. Her left foot is cool to the touch.
4. What action do you take now?

    You determine that there is only a very faint weak pulse present.
5. What action do you take based on your data collection?

    After a successful hip repair, Mrs. Gardenio's recovery progresses well with the assistance of the health-care team.
6. With what health-care team members do you collaborate during Mrs. Gardenio's postoperative care?
7. What discharge teaching should you reinforce for home safety for Mrs. Gardenio?

Suggested answers are at the end of the chapter.

Home Health Hints

According to the Social Security Act, to be considered homebound, a Medicare patient must meet the following criteria:

1. Because of illness or injury, the patient needs supportive devices such as crutches, canes, wheelchairs, and walkers; the use of special transportation; or the assistance of another person to leave their place of residence. Leaving the home may be contraindicated because of a patient's medical condition.
2. There must also exist a normal inability to leave home, and leaving home must require a considerable and taxing effort.

- If the patient is not homebound, services such as physical and occupational therapy can be performed in an outpatient setting.
- Observe patients performing their activities of daily living to determine functional abilities. Observe the patient's dress and hygiene. Do not rely on self-report of functional abilities. Older patients may hide their deficits out of fear that they will not be allowed to stay in their homes.
- If the home health nurse identifies that the patient is at risk for falls or if the patient has had recent falls, request a physical therapy referral. Inform the patient of the benefit in removing loose rugs that could be a trip hazard.
- Reinforce teaching to caregivers to use sand or cat box litter on icy steps to increase traction, preventing slips and falls.

• WORD • BUILDING •
arthrogram: arthro—joint + gram—diagram

Key Points

- The skeletal and muscular systems move the body together. Voluntary muscles are attached to the skeleton, which includes the spaces between bones (joints).
- Bone tissue, articular cartilage, and fibrous connective tissue that forms the ligaments and other structures within joints make up the skeleton.
- Muscle comprises skeletal muscle tissue and fibrous connective tissue.
- The skeleton helps us move and protects organs and tissues from injury.
- The muscles move the skeleton and keep it stable, help maintain normal body temperature, and allow venous return from the legs through compression.
- Skeletal muscles are voluntary, or consciously controlled. Nerve impulses originate in the motor areas of the frontal lobes of the cerebral cortex. Coordination of voluntary movement is a function of the cerebellum.
- For postmenopausal women, the bone matrix loses more calcium than is replaced.
- Weight-bearing joints are subject to damage after many years. Often the articular cartilage wears down and becomes rough, leading to pain and stiffness. Muscle strength declines with age as protein synthesis decreases.
- Subjective data collection on the patient begins with a history that includes the condition's impact on the patient's life. Three areas of musculoskeletal data collection are important: inspection, range of motion, and muscle tone and palpation.
- Laboratory tests to diagnose musculoskeletal system problems include alkaline phosphatase, calcium, phosphorus, muscle enzymes, myoglobin, and uric acid.
- Arthrocentesis is a procedure in which synovial fluid is aspirated from a joint for analysis or pressure relief. The fluid buildup may be caused by an inflammation such as bursitis.
- An arthroscope allows the surgeon to directly visualize a joint.
- Bone or muscle tissue can be extracted for microscopic examination to confirm cancer, damage, inflammation, or infection.
- A bone density scan measures bone strength in the total body or areas such as the spine, hip, heel, fingers, or wrist.
- CT scan diagnoses joint or vertebral column disorders.
- MRI diagnoses musculoskeletal disorder, especially those involving soft tissue.
- Myelography is reserved for patients who need spine surgery revisions or who cannot have an MRI or CT scan.
- Electromyography measures a muscle's electrical impulses to diagnose nerve or muscle damage after trauma.
- A nuclear bone scan allows visualization of the entire skeleton through injection of a radioisotope that accumulates in the bone.
- X-ray examination determines bone alignment, density, erosion, swelling, and soft tissue damage (e.g., ligaments and tendons) from alterations in bone position and spacing.
- Arthrogram (or arthrography) is an x-ray examination of a synovial joint. Air or a contrast medium is injected into a synovial joint, which is then x-rayed.
- Ultrasounds detect osteomyelitis (bone infection), soft tissue disorders, traumatic joint injuries, and surgical hardware placement.

SUGGESTED ANSWERS TO CHAPTER EXERCISES

Cue Recognition
45.1: Collect data including vital signs and temperature, pain level, neurovascular checks of the extremity, and the aspiration site. Report findings to the registered nurse or HCP.

45.2: Collect data including pain level, neurovascular checks of the extremity, and measure of the circumference of the lower leg. Notify HCP immediately.

Critical Thinking & Clinical Judgment
Mrs. O'Donnell
1. Determine whether Mrs. O'Donnell has any allergies to medications, how and when the injury occurred, whether she has had any previous surgeries, what medications she takes, her medical history, and any past problems she or her family may have had with anesthesia.
2. Inspect and compare her left leg with her right leg, including limb length, deformity, pain, loss of range of motion, edema, and ecchymosis. Perform neurovascular checks, including movement, sensation (numbness/tingling), presence of pulses, skin temperature, color, and capillary refill.

Mrs. Gardenio
1. X-ray examinations, bone scans, bone density tests, and laboratory tests, including serum alkaline phosphatase, calcium, phosphorus, thyroid, and vitamin D levels, are tests that might be performed.
2. Identify Mrs. Gardenio's age, allergies, nutritional intake, what she was doing at the time of the injury, whether anything like this has happened before, whether anything similar has happened to any of her relatives, her pain level, when she ate last, her medications, her medical history, and whether she uses tobacco products.
3. Unit analysis method:

$$\frac{4 \text{ mg}}{1} \cdot \frac{1 \text{ mL}}{5 \text{ mg}} = \frac{4 \text{ mL}}{5} = 0.8 \text{ mL}$$

SUGGESTED ANSWERS TO CHAPTER EXERCISES—cont'd

4. You obtain a doppler probe in order to listen for the pulse.
5. Notify the registered nurse or the HCP immediately as intervention is needed to save the limb and ensure circulation is normal.
6. HCP, clergy, dietitian occupational therapist, pharmacist, physical therapist, social worker or case manager.
7. Discuss home safety and ways to avoid the use of a step stool to keep the patient free from injury.

Additional Resources

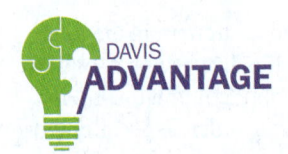

Go to Davis Advantage to complete your learning: strengthen understanding, apply your knowledge, and prepare for the Next Gen NCLEX®.

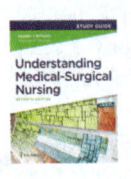

A Study Guide is also available.

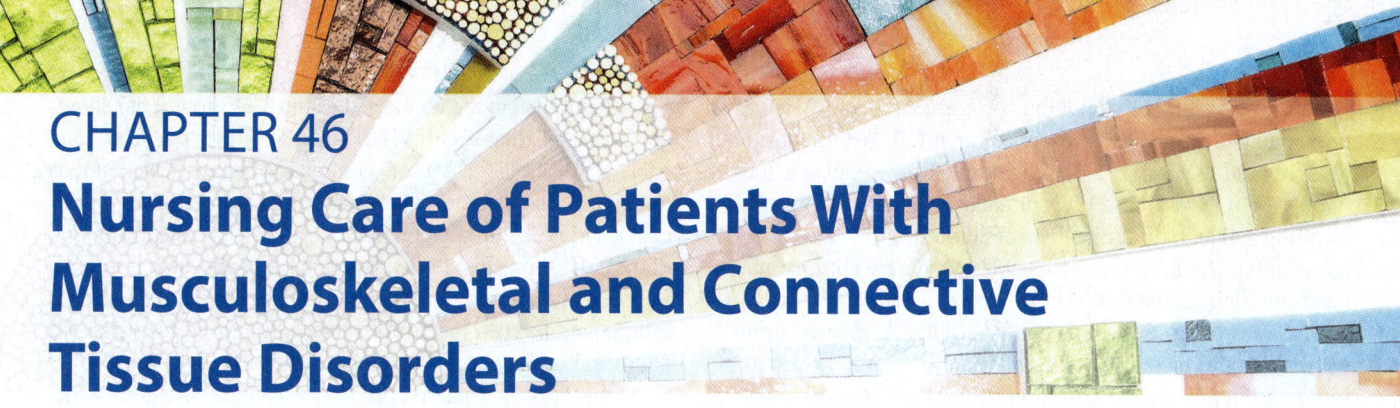

CHAPTER 46
Nursing Care of Patients With Musculoskeletal and Connective Tissue Disorders

Suzanne Sutton

KEY TERMS

arthritis (ar-THRY-tis)
arthroplasty (AR-throw-PLAS-tee)
avascular necrosis (ah-VAS-cue-lar neh-KROW-sis)
fasciotomy (fash-ee-OTT-oh-mee)
hemipelvectomy (heh-mee-pel-VEC-tuh-mee)
hyperuricemia (HY-purr-yoor-eh-SEE-mee-ah)
osteomyelitis (OSS-tee-oh-my-eh-LY-tis)
osteosarcoma (OSS-tee-oh-sar-KOH-mah)
replantation (ree-plan-TAY-shun)
rhabdomyolysis (RAB-doe-my-OLL-e-sis)
synovitis (sin-oh-VY-tis)

CHAPTER CONCEPTS

Comfort
Mobility
Teaching and learning

LEARNING OUTCOMES

1. Explain the pathophysiology, signs and symptoms, and complications of fractures.
2. Plan nursing care for a patient in a splint, cast, traction, or external fixation.
3. Describe the causes and prevention of osteomyelitis.
4. Plan nursing care for osteomyelitis.
5. Describe risk factors, pathophysiology, treatment, and nursing care for osteoporosis.
6. Describe the pathophysiology, treatment, and nursing care for gout.
7. Compare the care for osteoarthritis and rheumatoid arthritis.
8. Plan nursing care for the patient with a fractured hip.
9. Plan nursing care for a patient having a total joint replacement.
10. Explain patient teaching for a patient with a lower extremity amputation and prosthesis.

BONE AND SOFT TISSUE DISORDERS

Strains

A strain is a soft tissue injury that occurs when a muscle or tendon is excessively stretched. Causes of strains include falls, excessive exercise, and lifting heavy items. A mild strain causes minimal inflammation with swelling and tenderness. A moderate strain involves partial tearing of muscle or tendon fibers, causing pain and inability to move the affected body part. The most severe strain occurs when a muscle or tendon is ruptured, with separation of muscle from muscle, tendon from muscle, or tendon from bone. This can cause severe pain and disability.

RICE is an acronym for *R*est, *I*ce, *C*ompression, and *E*levation, which is the therapy for strain injuries. Immediately after a strain, the injured area should be *R*ested to protect it. *I*ce should be applied for 15 to 20 minutes, four times a day to decrease swelling and pain. Applying an elastic bandage for *C*ompression and *E*levating the affected area (if appropriate) supports the strained area and reduces swelling. After swelling stops, heat application (15 to 30 minutes four times a day) increases blood flow to the injured area for healing. Activity is limited until the soft tissue heals. NSAIDs and muscle relaxants may be prescribed. Severe strains may need surgical repair.

Sprains

A sprain is excessive stretching of ligaments from twisting movements during sports, exercise, or a fall. A mild sprain involves the tearing of a few ligament fibers, causing tenderness. RICE and NSAIDs are used for several days until swelling and pain diminish. In a moderate sprain, more fibers are torn but the joint remains stable. Moderate sprains may need immobilization with a brace or cast. A moderate sprain is uncomfortable, especially with activity. A severe sprain causes instability of the joint and usually requires surgical intervention for tissue repair or grafting. Pain and inflammation restrict mobility.

Dislocations

A dislocation is a common injury in which the ends of the bones (joints) are moved out of their normal position, usually caused by trauma or a disease such as rheumatoid arthritis. Severe pain, loss of range of motion of the joint, and joint deformity occur. Keep the joint immobile and apply ice. Immediate medical treatment is required to preserve function. Do not move the joint, as blood vessels, muscles, and nerves could be damaged.

> ### BE SAFE!
> **BE VIGILANT!** For patients with disease processes that could result in a dislocation or fracture, careful moving is essential. Use lifting devices such as draw sheets and mechanical devices when moving a patient rather than pulling on the patient's extremities to avoid patient injury. Follow institutional policy for moving patients to avoid patient injury and liability for a patient's injury.

Bursitis

Bursae (fluid-filled sacs) cushion tendons during movement to prevent friction between bone and tendon. Several joints have bursae (e.g., shoulder, elbow, hip, knee, ankle, heel). Inflammation of a bursa is called *bursitis*. It occurs from **arthritis**, gout, repetitive movement, infection, or sleeping on one's side that compresses the shoulder bursa. Prevention is key because bursitis may become harder to cure over time. Educate patients to stretch and strengthen muscles, move frequently, avoid repetitive movements for long periods, use cushioned seats, and avoid leaning on the elbows.

Symptoms of bursitis include achy pain, stiffness, swelling, redness, or burning pain over the joint area that worsens with activity. Usually, pain decreases in about a week. The condition can become chronic if it lasts more than 6 months. Treatment includes resting the joint and applying ice several times per day until joint warmth is gone, then switching to heat. Elevating the joint, ultrasound, massage, NSAIDs, antibiotics for infection, and physical therapy may also be used.

Rotator Cuff Injury

Short tendons that are connected to muscles around the shoulder form the rotator cuff. The cuff covers the top, front, and back of the shoulder. Muscle contraction causes these tendons to tighten and move or rotate the shoulder. Various cuff injuries can occur. With chronic impingement syndrome, the top tendon of the cuff (supraspinatus tendon) and bursae become impinged in the narrow space under the acromion bone. This causes inflammation when the arm is repeatedly moved forward, and pain results. Over time, the tendon can tear from the bone.

Symptoms of rotator cuff injury include shoulder ache, increased pain with lifting arm, pain that worsens at night, weakness, and limited range of motion. Magnetic resonance imaging (MRI) diagnoses the injury. For minor injury, resting the shoulder, ice, NSAIDs, and physical therapy are recommended. For severe injury, arthroscopic surgery relieves impingement or repairs the tear. A sling or special brace is worn after surgery. Physical therapy is prescribed for rehabilitation.

Carpal Tunnel Syndrome

Carpal tunnel syndrome results in compression of the median nerve within the carpal tunnel caused by swelling, which can result from edema, trauma, rheumatoid arthritis, or repetitive hand movements (repetitive motion injury) used in some occupations such as typing. Preventive measures include alternating nonrepetitive tasks with repetitive movements and using ergonomically appropriate devices to minimize the pressure placed in the area of the wrist. Slow-onset finger, hand, and arm pain and numbness may occur. Painful tingling and paresthesia may also be present. Eventually, fine motor deficits and then muscle weakness may develop. Diagnosis is based on signs and symptoms, patient history, and a positive Phalen test (numbness with wrist flexion). Electromyography detects nerve abnormalities.

Treatment initially aims to relieve the inflammation and rest the wrist using a splint. NSAIDs or cortisone injection into the tunnel reduce inflammation and pain. Endoscopic or open incision surgery may be needed to release the median nerve from compression. After surgery, elevate the patient's hand. Explain the use of a splint as ordered. Teach the patient to restrict lifting for several weeks and report symptoms of neurovascular compromise such as numbness and tingling, coolness, lack of pulse, pale skin or nailbeds, or limited movement. Physical therapy helps recover extremity function.

Fractures

A fracture is a break in a bone that can be minor and treated on an ambulatory basis or complex and treated with surgical intervention and rehabilitation.

Pathophysiology

Bone is a dynamic, changing tissue. When it is broken, the body immediately begins to repair the injury (Fig. 46.1). For an adult, within 48 to 72 hours after the injury,

• **WORD** • **BUILDING** •
arthritis: arthr(on)—joint + itis—inflammation

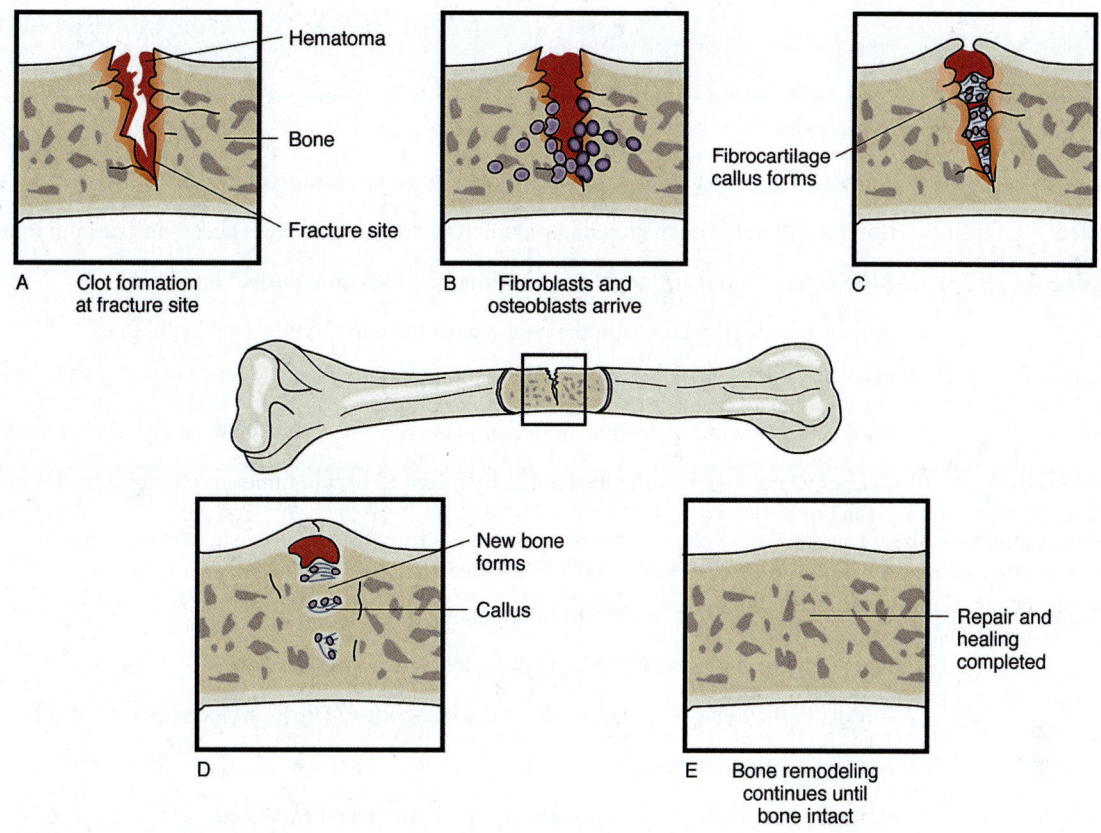

FIGURE 46.1 Fracture healing phases.

a hematoma (blood clot) forms at the fracture site because bone has a rich blood supply. Various cells that begin the healing process are attracted to the damaged bone. In about a week, a nonbony union called a *callus* develops and is seen on x-ray examination. As healing continues, osteoclasts (bone-destroying cells) resorb necrotic bone, and osteoblasts (bone-building cells) make new bone as a replacement. This process is referred to as bone remodeling. Young, healthy adult bone completely heals in about 6 weeks; however, it can take up to a year before the whole process of remodeling is complete. An older person's bones take longer to heal. Adequate nutrition that includes vitamins, minerals, and protein is essential to heal fractures (see Chapter 45).

Etiology and Types
Fractures are caused by a fall, an accident, or a crushing injury. Bone disease, such as osteoporosis; metastatic bone cancer; malnutrition; and regular intake of carbonated beverages containing phosphoric acid (which may interfere with calcium absorption) can lead to fractures. Side effects from some medications can cause a decrease in bone density, resulting in fracture. When fractures result from disease, they are referred to as pathological fractures.

There are many types of fractures (Table 46.1). Fractures can be described by the way the bone breaks (spiral or oblique; Fig. 46.2). In a complete fracture, the bone is broken into two pieces. Complete fractures have the potential to be life threatening, as sharp bone fragments can sever blood vessels and nerves. In an incomplete fracture, the bone does not divide in two. With a displaced fracture, bone sections are out of alignment. In a closed fracture, the bone does not disrupt the skin. In an open fracture, the bone breaks through the skin, creating infection risk.

Signs and Symptoms
This section focuses on fractures of upper and lower extremities. If the patient sustains a hairline (microscopic) fracture, signs and symptoms are not readily observable. The patient may report tenderness over the site of the injury or more severe pain when moving the affected part of the body. The patient with a hip fracture usually experiences pain either in the groin area (the hip is a deep joint) or at the back of the knee (referred pain). If the fracture is complete, the limb is often shortened because of contraction of the muscles pulling on the bone sections.

In addition to pain, patients with complex fractures experience limb rotation or deformity and shortening of the limb (if a limb bone is broken). Range of motion is decreased. With movement, a continuous grating sound (crepitation) caused by bone fragments rubbing on each other may be heard. Do not move the extremity, as damage could occur to nerves and blood vessels.

Inspect the skin for intactness. An open fracture creates a wound. A patient with a closed fracture may have

Table 46.1
Types of Fractures

Fracture Type	Description
Avulsion	A piece of bone is torn away from the main bone while still attached to a ligament or tendon.
Comminuted	Bone is splintered or shattered into numerous fragments. Often occurs in crushing injuries.
Impacted	Bone is forcibly pushed together, resulting in bone being pushed into bone.
Greenstick	Bone is bent and fractures on the outer arc of the bend. Often seen in children.
Interarticular	Fracture involves bones within a joint.
Displaced	Bone pieces are out of normal alignment. One or more pieces may be out of alignment.
Pathological (also called *neoplastic*)	Caused when bone is weakened either by pressure from a tumor or an actual tumor within the bone.
Spiral	Fracture curves around the shaft of the bone.
Longitudinal	Fracture occurs along the length of the bone.
Oblique	Fracture occurs diagonally or at an oblique angle across the bone.
Stress	Results in the bone being fractured across one cortex. This is an incomplete fracture.
Transverse	Bone is fractured horizontally.
Depressed	Bone is pushed inward. Often seen with skull and facial fractures.

ecchymosis (bruising) over the fractured bone from bleeding into the soft underlying tissue. Swelling may also be present and can impair blood flow, causing marked neurovascular compromise.

CUE RECOGNITION 46.1

You are caring for a patient with an open fracture to the left foot that required surgery. What priority care do you provide to prevent a complication?

Suggested answers are at the end of the chapter.

Diagnostic Tests

An x-ray can visualize bone fractures, malalignment, or disruption. A computed tomography (CT) scan detects fractures of complex areas such as the hip and pelvis. MRI shows the extent of associated soft tissue damage. Serum calcium level may be ordered to determine baseline values for bone repairs. With moderate to severe bleeding, hemoglobin and hematocrit levels are checked.

Emergency Treatment

Box 46.1 describes urgent care for the patient with an extremity fracture. A patient with a fracture often has other injuries. Observe the patient for respiratory distress, bleeding, and head or spine injury. Emergency care for these problems is provided prior to fracture care.

LEARNING TIP
For emergency care of a suspected fracture, do not try to reposition the limb. Remember: *Splint it as it lies*. Ensure that the limb is secured above and below the fracture to minimize movement.

Fracture Management

The goals of fracture management are reduction (alignment) of bone ends; immobilization of the fractured bone; preservation or restoration of surrounding soft tissue structures, such as vessels, tendons, ligaments, and muscles; prevention of deformity or further injury; preservation or restoration of function; promotion of early healing; and pain relief.

CLOSED REDUCTION. Closed reduction is the most common treatment for simple fractures. Analgesia and/or procedural sedation is given before the procedure. While manually pulling on the bone (limb), the health-care provider (HCP) manipulates the bone ends into alignment. An x-ray confirms that the bone ends are aligned before the area is immobilized by a splint or cast.

SPLINTS. An elastic wrap and splint may be used to immobilize the bone during the healing phase. Splints are used when there is a wound to care for or a need to allow for swelling. Perform neurovascular checks hourly to monitor adequate

FIGURE 46.2 Types of fractures.

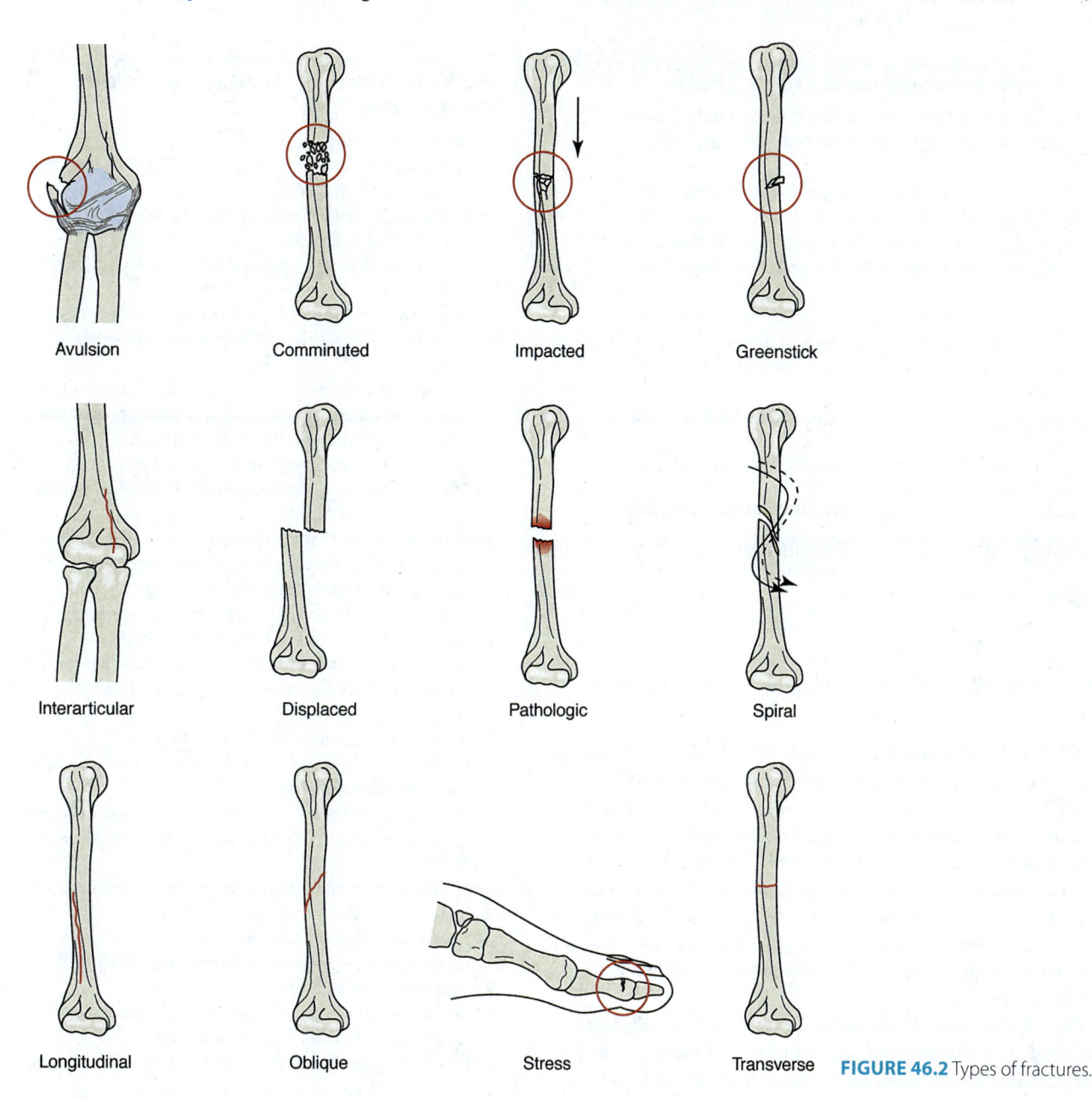

Avulsion, Comminuted, Impacted, Greenstick, Interarticular, Displaced, Pathologic, Spiral, Longitudinal, Oblique, Stress, Transverse

blood flow to the area until the concern for swelling is over (see Chapter 45).

CASTS. Casts provide stronger support than splints for fractured bones. Plaster or fiberglass casts are typically used. As casts dry, heat is produced. Plaster cast drying can take 24 to 72 hours. The plaster cast is dry when it is hard, firm, odorless, and shiny white. Synthetic material casts such as fiberglass harden quickly and dry in less than 2 hours. Box 46.2 and Figure 46.3 present care for a patient with a cast.

A serious complication of a too-tight cast is compartment syndrome (discussed later). If the cast becomes too tight, it must be cut (bivalved) with a cast saw, per HCP orders, to relieve pressure and prevent necrosis of the underlying skin. If a wound is present or an odor is detected, a window opening into the cast is created to allow treatment of the skin. When wound care is not being provided, the cast window should always be taped in place to prevent the skin from "popping up" through the window and developing pressure points and ischemia.

TRACTION. Traction is the application of a pulling force with prescribed weights to part of the body to position and hold bone fragments in correct alignment. Advances in orthopedic surgery have made traction primarily a temporary measure. Buck traction is *skin traction*, with 5- to 10-pound (2.2 to 4.5 kg) weights; it is used for patients with hip fractures to relieve muscle spasms and stabilize the fracture until surgery can be performed. *Skeletal traction* uses pins, wires, or tongs inserted into the bone for bone alignment as the fracture heals. Extremity skeletal traction is maintained with

Box 46.1

Urgent Management of Fractures

1. Immediately immobilize the affected limb. If movement is required for splinting, support the limb above and below the fracture.
2. Unless there is bleeding, apply splints and padding above and below the fracture site, directly over the clothing. For bleeding, the site may need to be seen before pressure can be applied to the origin of the bleeding. Keep the patient covered to preserve body heat.
3. If the fracture is in the leg, the other leg can be used as a splint by bandaging both legs together if needed. An arm can be bandaged to the chest or put into a sling to minimize further tissue damage.
4. Monitor color, warmth, circulation, and movement of the limb distal to the fracture.
5. For an open fracture, cover protruding bone with a clean (sterile preferred) dressing.
6. Do not attempt to straighten or realign a fractured extremity. Move the affected limb as little as necessary.
7. If not in a hospital, transport for emergency medical care as soon as possible.

Box 46.2

Nursing Interventions for a Patient With a Cast

1. Monitor the following:
   a. Neurovascular checks 1 to 2 hours for 24 hours, then four times a day and as needed
   b. Cast for tightness (ask patient), and ask patient to move all digits distal to the cast
   c. Patient comments about the cast to take action to prevent complications
2. Fiberglass casts dry within 15 to 30 minutes. Plaster casts may take 24 to 36 hours to dry. With newly applied casts, when drying:
   a. Do not grasp a wet cast to hold or move it. Use only the palms of the hands, as finger pressure on a wet cast can cause pressure points on the inside cast surface.
   b. Position cast on absorbent surface; do not place it on a surface that can cause an indentation. Placing on a pillow while drying traps heat and increases thermal injury risk.
   c. Inform the patient that the cast creates heat when drying. Thermal injuries can occur. Ensure a cast air dries (may require 24 to 72 hours for complete drying). Do not cover a cast, but keep it open to the air. Do not use drying aids such as hot blow dryers, which add more heat.
   d. If the patient is lying, assist the patient to turn every 1 to 2 hours to prevent flattening of a plaster cast surface during drying.
3. Reduce swelling (essential for the first 48 hours):
   a. Elevate extremity above the patient's heart level. Elevate casted arm while walking.
   b. Ice cast (first 48 hours). Can use ice packs, bags of frozen vegetables or leakproof plastic bags of ice wrapped with a towel.
   c. For casted arm, pump fingers 10 times per hour while awake.
4. Maintain tissue integrity within the cast:
   a. Check visible skin for signs of impaired integrity.
   b. Ensure cast edges are smooth; cover with stockinet or gauze to prevent skin rubbing.
   c. Educate patient to keep cast dry; during bathing, cover with plastic and rubber band or tape ends.
   d. Monitor for signs of infection, such as foul odor, warmth, redness, and pain.
   e. Do not use skin products on affected limb.
   f. Monitor visible blood on the surface of the cast. Outline area with a pen to observe for increasing size. Shadowing of blood not quite reaching the surface of the cast is common but also should be circled and monitored.
   g. Never place an object inside the cast, and instruct patient not to do so. Explain the risk of tissue damage and infection.
   h. For itching, teach patient to try a blow dryer to blow cool air into the cast or tapping on the cast. Diphenhydramine may be helpful.

20- to 40-pound (9 to 18 kg) weights that must hang freely at all times.

OPEN REDUCTION WITH INTERNAL FIXATION. The fractured bone ends are reduced (aligned) by direct visualization through a surgical incision (open reduction). Bone ends are held in place by internal fixation devices such as metal plates and screws or by a prosthesis with a femoral component similar to that used for total joint replacement (Fig. 46.4). For hip surgery, the internal fixation device remains after the fracture heals. For ankle or long-bone surgery, hardware may need to be removed after healing due to loosening or pain.

One of the most common indications for this surgical procedure is a fractured hip involving the proximal femur. Hip fractures affect older adults more than any other age group. Healthy People 2030 has an objective to reduce hip fractures among older adults (Office of Disease Prevention and Health Promotion, 2020). Open reduction with internal fixation of the hip allows early ambulation while the bone is healing. Monitor pain level and give analgesics for postoperative pain especially prior to activity such as physical therapy. Use a fracture bedpan as needed for ease and comfort. Apply thigh-high compression stockings or sequential compression device to unaffected limb as ordered. Remind the patient to practice leg exercises, and promote early ambulation as ordered. Administer anticoagulants as ordered to prevent blood clots.

EXTERNAL FIXATION. External fixation is used when bone damage is severe, as in crushed or splintered fractures, or if the bone has numerous breaks. After the fracture is reduced, the surgeon inserts pins into the bone. The pins are held in place by an external metal frame to prevent bone movement (Fig. 46.5). External fixation allows visualization of soft tissue damage that also requires treatment. See "Nursing Care Plan for the Patient With External Fixation of the Lower Extremity."

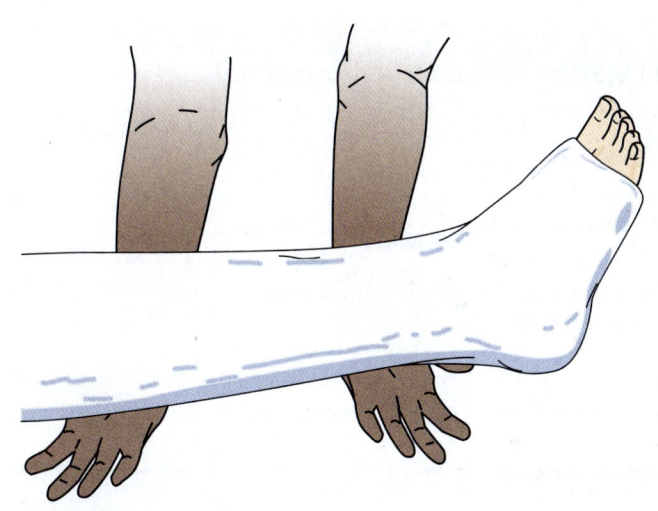

Chapter 46   Nursing Care of Patients With Musculoskeletal and Connective Tissue Disorders

FIGURE 46.3 A wet plaster cast is moved with the palms of the hand to prevent making indentations in the plaster that could become pressure points.

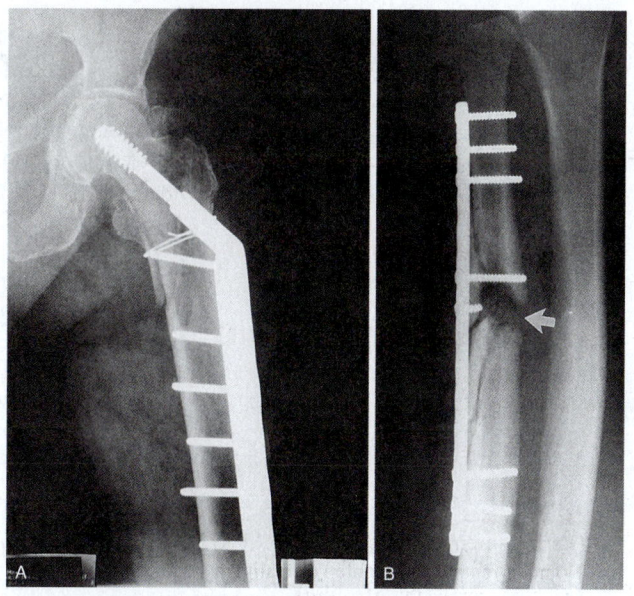

FIGURE 46.4 Internal fixation. (A) Intertrochanteric fracture of the hip with fracture fixation via a side plate and screw combination device. (B) Side plate and screw fixation of radial fracture.

CLINICAL JUDGMENT

Mrs. Martinez, a rehabilitation center resident, was found at 1900 lying on her left side, moaning and holding her left leg. She cried out with any movement and said she fell and her leg hurts. Vital signs are blood pressure 150/84 mm Hg, pulse 100 beats per minute, and respirations 20 breaths per minute. Her left leg is noticeably shorter than her right leg. The supervisor notified paramedics and the HCP. The licensed practical nurse (LPN) remained with Mrs. Martinez and instructed her not to move until help arrived. The LPN got blankets and a pillow for her head. At 1925, the paramedics took Mrs. Martinez to the hospital, where she was diagnosed as having an incomplete femoral neck (hip) fracture. Five pounds of Buck traction until surgery the next morning was applied.

1. How does the LPN at the rehabilitation center document Mrs. Martinez's fall?
2. What data does the nurse at the hospital monitor for the Buck traction on Mrs. Martinez?

Suggested answers are at the end of the chapter.

CRITICAL THINKING

Mr. Schnell, age 18, was in a motor vehicle accident that resulted in a fractured pelvis and an open right femoral fracture.

1. Identify four priority nursing diagnoses related to Mr. Schnell's care.
2. What are nursing interventions and rationales for these diagnoses?

Suggested answers are at the end of the chapter.

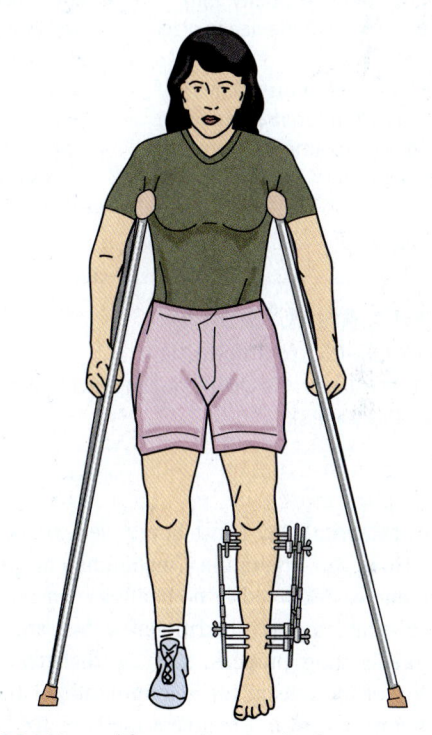

FIGURE 46.5 External fixation for complex fractures and wound care.

NURSING CARE TIP

When moving a limb that has an external fixation device, grasp the device and lift, raise, or move the limb as needed. Grasping the device reduces movement of the healing bone, lessening both trauma to the healing site and pain with movement. Care must be taken not to loosen any fasteners holding the pins in place.

Nursing Care Plan for the Patient With External Fixation of the Lower Extremity

Nursing Diagnosis: *Risk for Infection* related to open skin at pin site
Expected Outcome: The patient does not develop an infection.
Evaluation of Outcome: Does the patient remain free from infection?

Intervention	Rationale	Evaluation
Inspect pin sites and dressings for signs of infection (e.g., warmth, redness, heat, edema, drainage, pain).	Early and frequent inspection allows for timely intervention to prevent infection.	Are pin sites infected?
Provide pin-site care per agency policy using strict aseptic technique.	The pin is a pathway for microorganisms to directly enter bone tissue and cause osteomyelitis. Aseptic technique reduces risk of infection.	Are pin sites clean with no crusting?

Nursing Diagnosis: *Impaired Physical Mobility* related to the limb injury
Expected Outcome: The patient will maintain desired level of mobility and activity.
Evaluation of Outcome: Has the patient maintained desired level of mobility and activity?

Intervention	Rationale	Evaluation
Monitor the patient's mobility with external fixation (EF) device in place.	Data concerning the patient's abilities allow intervention planning.	Does the patient transfer and ambulate with or without assistance?
Collaborate with other disciplines in educating patient on moving limb with EF device to ambulate and transfer safely.	Physiotherapy can provide initial teaching or reinforce education needed to promote ambulation (e.g., with crutch walking).	Has the patient used information learned from other disciplines to move the extremity with EF device?

> **PRACTICE ANALYSIS TIP**
> **Linking NCLEX-PN® to Practice**
> The LPN/LVN will use safe client handling techniques (e.g., body mechanics).

NONUNION MODALITIES. Most bones heal properly with treatment. However, malunion (malalignment of healed bone) or nonunion (delayed or no healing) can occur. Bone healing is affected by age, nutritional status, and diseases that alter the healing process, such as diabetes mellitus. Identification of the reason for nonunion allows the appropriate treatment selection. Treatment methods for nonunion can include electrical bone stimulation, bone grafting, or external fixation.

Complications of Fractures

Monitor the patient for possible complications. Although rare, acute compartment syndrome or fat embolism syndrome (more common with fractures of long bones) can be life-threatening complications of fractures.

NEUROVASCULAR STATUS. Neurovascular checks are done to detect abnormalities. Decreased or absent pulses, cool skin temperature, and dusky color indicate circulation problems. Numbness and tingling and decreased sensation and mobility indicate neurologic changes. These findings should be reported to the HCP right away.

HEMORRHAGE. Bone is highly vascular. Damage to or surgery on bone (particularly the femur) can cause bleeding. Monitor for bleeding and monitor vital signs.

INFECTION. Trauma can lead to infection, especially when the skin, the body's first line of defense, is not intact. Wound infections, pin-site infections, drainage tube infections, and **osteomyelitis** (bone infection) can occur.

THROMBOEMBOLIC COMPLICATIONS. Deep vein thrombosis (DVT) or pulmonary embolus (see Chapter 31) can develop in patients having orthopedic surgery. Leg exercises, early ambulation, and prophylactic anticoagulant therapy (such as with rivaroxaban [Xarelto], dalteparin [Fragmin], apixaban [Eliquis], or enoxaparin [Lovenox]) help to prevent them.

ACUTE COMPARTMENT SYNDROME. Compartments are sheaths of fibrous tissue that support and partition nerves, muscles, and blood vessels, primarily in the extremities (Fig. 46.6). Each extremity has several compartments. Acute

• WORD • BUILDING •
osteomyelitis: osteo—bone + myel—bone marrow + itis—inflammation

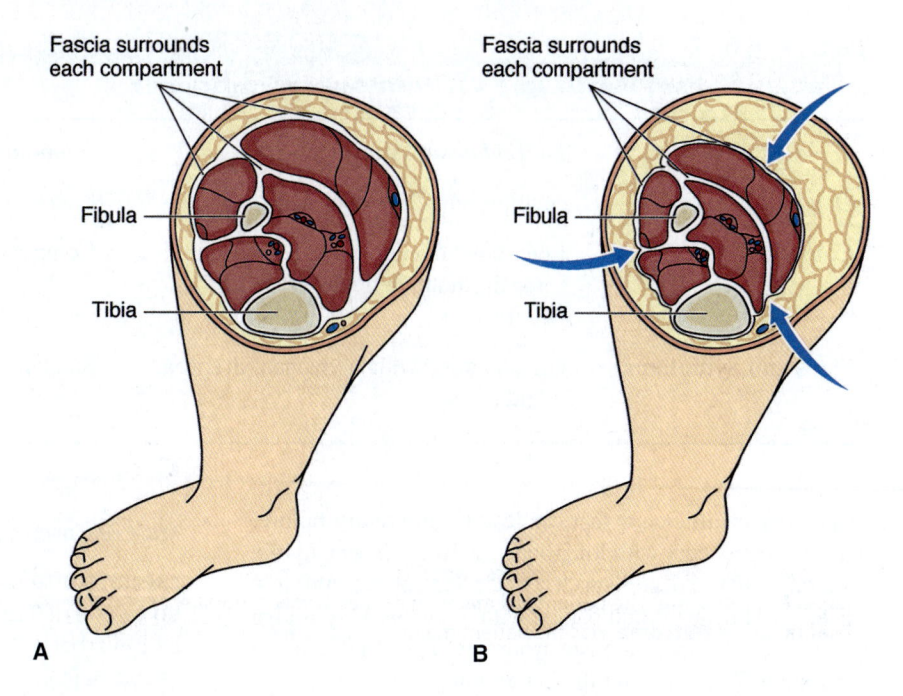

FIGURE 46.6 (A) Lower leg compartments. Each compartment contains muscles, an artery, a vein, and a nerve. (B) Compartment syndrome. Increased pressure in a compartment compresses structures within the compartment.

compartment syndrome is a limb-threatening condition in which pressure in limb compartments increases. This causes reduced circulation to the compartment's muscles and nerves. Trauma, tight splints, casts, or dressings are common causes.

The early symptom of acute compartment syndrome is the patient's report of severe, increasing pain that is not relieved with opioids and occurs more in active movements than passive movements. Decreased sensation follows before ischemia becomes severe. To save the limb, report early symptoms immediately! In severe acute compartment syndrome, the patient may have the six *P*s if treatment did not prevent late symptoms:

1. Pain (severe, unrelenting, and increased with passive stretching)
2. Paresthesia (painful tingling or burning)
3. Pallor (but there may be warmth or redness over the area)
4. Paralysis (late symptom)
5. Pulselessness (late and ominous sign)
6. Poikilothermia (temperature matches environment, i.e., the extremity is cool to touch).

CUE RECOGNITION 46.2

You are caring for a patient with a femur fracture who reports pain that has increased to a 10/10 in the extremity. You note a decreased pulse in the patient's lower extremity. What action do you take?

Suggested answers are at the end of the chapter.

Immediate pressure relief is the goal, achieved by removing the source of pressure. The HCP may bivalve the cast or perform a **fasciotomy**, which is an incision into the fascia enclosing the compartment. Fasciotomy allows compartment tissue the ability to expand, which relieves the pressure. These surgical incisions are left open until the pressure decreases, then are closed. If this condition continues without pressure relief, tissue necrosis, infection, Volkmann contracture (permanent flexion of hand at the wrist), **rhabdomyolysis** (muscle breakdown releases myoglobin, which is harmful to the kidneys), or acute kidney injury may result.

CLINICAL JUDGMENT

Mr. Kardos has a fracture of his right tibia, which required application of a cast 3 hours ago. His toes are edematous. He received 1 mg of hydromorphone (Dilaudid) intravenously for pain of 6. Now, 30 minutes later, he is reporting unrelieved pain of 8.

1. What data do you collect now?
2. What recommendation do you make during your ISBARR communication with the HCP?

Suggested answers are at the end of the chapter.

FAT EMBOLISM SYNDROME. Fat embolism syndrome is a serious complication of fractures. Small fat droplets are released from yellow bone marrow into the bloodstream (Table 46.2). These droplets travel to the lung fields, causing

• WORD • BUILDING •
fasciotomy: fascia—fibrous tissue + otomy—opening into
rhabdomyolysis: rhabdo—striped + myo—muscle + lysis—break down

Table 46.2
Fat Embolism Syndrome vs. Pulmonary Embolism

	Fat Embolism Syndrome	*Pulmonary Embolism*
Origin	Multiple small fat droplets	Large blood clot or fat globule
Cause	Long-bone fractures; surgical fracture repair; multiple fractures Hip fracture	Complication of deep vein thrombosis
Signs and Symptoms	Gradual onset with tachypnea, dyspnea, and cyanosis	Sudden onset, shortness of breath, and chest pain

respiratory insufficiency that can lead to respiratory failure. This process occurs with long-bone fractures (especially the femoral shaft) and perhaps when the patient has multiple fractures. The older adult patient with a fractured hip is also at a high risk for fat embolism syndrome. This condition can occur up to 72 hours after the initial injury.

The three primary manifestations of fat embolism syndrome are respiratory failure, cerebral involvement, and skin petechiae. Pulmonary dysfunction is the earliest sign and includes tachypnea, dyspnea, and cyanosis. Cerebral changes are often seen and include confusion or drowsiness. A petechial (red, measles-like) rash may occur on the chest, neck, and axilla. Conjunctiva appears in some patients. Other signs include tachycardia, fever, and retinal changes. If a fat embolism is suspected, notify the HCP immediately. Treatment interventions may include the following:

1. Promote oxygenation by administering oxygen at 2 L/min via nasal cannula and apply a pulse oximeter.
2. Place the patient in high-Fowler position or raise the head of the bed as tolerated.
3. Maintain bedrest and minimize movement of the extremity.
4. Obtain arterial blood gas.
5. Initiate venous access for medications.
6. Administer corticosteroids.
7. Prepare patient for a chest x-ray and an MRI of the brain.
8. Provide emotional support and a calm environment.

Nursing Process for the Patient With a Fracture
Caring for the patient with a fracture requires collaborative care with other health-care team members.

DATA COLLECTION. Frequent checking of neurovascular status (e.g., circulation, sensation, mobility) distal to a fracture is vital to detect problems (see Chapter 45). Pain is monitored using appropriate pain rating scales.

NURSING DIAGNOSES, PLANNING, AND IMPLEMENTATION. Determination of the appropriate nursing diagnosis depends on the location and type of fracture. See the "Open Reduction With Internal Fixation" section for nursing interventions.

Acute Pain related to bone fracture or movement

EXPECTED OUTCOME: The patient will report pain relief on a scale of 0 to 10 or be rated as pain-free using a nonverbal pain rating scale for those who cannot report pain.

- Identify pain level using appropriate pain rating scale *to establish baseline for further interventions.* (See "Nursing Care Tip.")
- Provide regularly scheduled pain rating to determine need for analgesics for those who cannot report pain *to ensure pain is being relieved.*
- Administer analgesics and NSAIDs as ordered *to relieve pain and swelling.*
- Ensure proper positioning and alignment *to promote pain relief and promote future functioning of body part.*
- Explain use of appropriate complementary methods for pain relief, such as heat or cold therapy, guided imagery, distraction, massage therapy, *to maximize relief of pain.*

Impaired Physical Mobility related to bone fracture or pain

EXPECTED OUTCOME: The patient will demonstrate increased mobility.

- Observe the patient's mobility level *to provide baseline data.*
- Utilize other disciplines, such as occupational and physiotherapy, and equipment, such as crutches, as needed, *to encourage and promote patient mobility.*
- Provide pain management prior to mobility *to improve ability to move.*
- Encourage independence *to prevent contributing to immobility.*
- Encourage active range-of-motion exercises *to prevent or minimize alteration in joint function while immobile.*
- Provide chair seat 3 inches above height of knee and raised toilet seat or commode with arms *to improve the ability of the older adult to stand up from seated position.*

Risk for Peripheral Neurovascular Dysfunction related to increased tissue volume or restrictive envelope

EXPECTED OUTCOME: The patient will maintain peripheral pulses, warm skin, sensation, and ability to move extremity.

- Monitor for swelling of affected extremity (especially if the patient has a cast, splint, or tight dressing) *to detect complications.*
- Monitor for compartment syndrome signs and symptoms (swelling, increasing pain even after analgesics) *to allow prompt reporting of abnormalities to HCP.*
- Report abnormalities immediately *to allow prompt treatment and prevent complications.*
- Administer anti-inflammatory as ordered *to reduce pain and swelling.*
- Apply cold therapy to fracture site as ordered *to decrease swelling and pain.*

EVALUATION. The outcome is met if the patient reports or demonstrates that pain is within tolerable levels on a pain rating scale, peripheral pulses, warm skin, sensation, and the ability to move extremity are maintained, and the patient demonstrates increased physical mobility.

PATIENT EDUCATION. For the patient with a cast, teach cast care (see Box 46.2), wound care if needed, and care of the extremity after cast removal (Box 46.3). Teach patient signs and symptoms of infection to report. Explain the importance of adequate intake of protein, calories, vitamins, and minerals in healing.

> **PRACTICE ANALYSIS TIP**
> **Linking NCLEX-PN® to Practice**
> The LPN/LVN will:
> - Provide care to an immobilized client based on need.
> - Reinforce education to client regarding care and condition.

Osteomyelitis

Osteomyelitis is an infection of bone that can be either acute (lasts less than 4 weeks) or chronic (lasts more than 4 weeks).

> **Box 46.3**
> **Extremity Care After Cast Removal**
> - Cleanse skin by soaking rather than rubbing skin to remove dry scales.
> - The extremity may be weak, with decreased range of motion. Move it gently and use analgesics as needed.
> - Support extremity when resting with pillows until strength and range of motion return.
> - Ensure active and passive range of motion are performed as recommended by physical therapist.

> **NURSING CARE TIP**
> - A patient who is confused or comatose may not be able to report pain. This can be problematic, as the most reliable indicator of pain is the patient's report. Nonverbal indicators (e.g., grimacing, restlessness, elevated blood pressure, and heart rate) are not reliable for pain identification and should not be used to assume the absence of pain.
> - Use pain assessment tools designed for those who are cognitively impaired to ensure their pain is adequately relieved. The Pain Assessment in Advanced Dementia (PAINAD) scale, for example, was developed for this purpose. Share pain research findings with institution administrators to establish policies that support proactive pain management for all patients.
> - Prevent pain by anticipating it and treating it in advance. This can be done by recognizing causes of pain and understanding that the effects of mild but repetitive pain (as in turning several times a day) can adversely affect the patient (e.g., by leading to exhaustion).
> - Causes of pain include conditions or diseases (such as fractures, trauma, or cancer), procedures (such as surgery, turning, or wound care), and biomedical devices (such as fixation devices, wound drains, urinary catheters, nasogastric tubes, and chest tubes).
> - With few patients routinely being medicated before painful procedures (some of which, like turning, may be done several times a day), patients who are confused or comatose are at greater risk for lack of pain relief. To keep patients comfortable, administer analgesics as ordered before painful procedures and on a regular basis when pain is assumed to be present. For anticipated pain, use the acronym APP (assume pain present).

Pathophysiology
Bone infection results from invasion of bacteria into the bone and surrounding soft tissues. Inflammation occurs, followed by ischemia (decreased blood flow; Fig. 46.7). Bone tissue becomes necrotic (dies), which impairs healing and furthers infection, often as a bone abscess.

Etiology
Injury to the body, such as an open fracture, allows pathogens direct access to bone tissue. Infection in another part of the body can travel to a bone. For instance, a patient with a total hip replacement may acquire osteomyelitis from a urinary tract infection. The most common pathogen causing osteomyelitis is *Staphylococcus aureus*.

Signs and Symptoms
The patient with acute osteomyelitis has site pain, redness, warmth, and swelling as well as fever. Ulceration, drainage, and localized pain are signs and symptoms of chronic osteomyelitis.

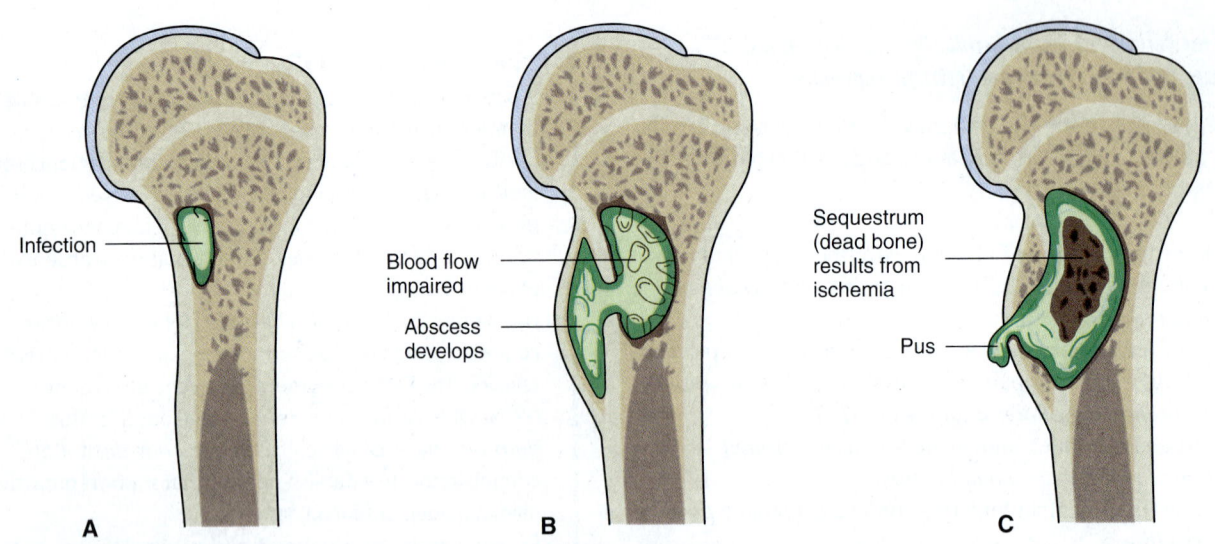

FIGURE 46.7 Sequence of osteomyelitis development. (A) Infection begins. (B) Blood flow is blocked in the area of infection. An abscess with pus forms. (C) Bone dies within the infection site, and pus formation continues.

Diagnostic Tests

The patient with osteomyelitis may have an elevated white blood cell count, an elevated erythrocyte sedimentation rate (ESR), positive bone biopsy for infection, and positive blood cultures. MRIs, x-rays, and CT scans show infected areas.

Therapeutic Measures

Infection in bone tissue is difficult to resolve. Treatment is individualized. Curative therapy can include surgical debridement, reconstruction, and antibiotics. Palliative therapy is provided with chronic suppressive antibiotic therapy. Amputation is used for patients who have severe infections that have not responded to one or more of the conventional treatments.

Nursing Care

Patients on long-term IV antibiotics can receive them at home. The home health nurse provides education on action, side effects, toxicity, interactions, and precautions for antibiotic therapy. If a soft tissue wound is present, sterile technique is used for dressing changes. The home health nurse educates the patient and family on how to perform dressing changes, the importance of hand hygiene before dressing changes, and how to avoid the spread of pathogens.

Osteoporosis

Osteoporosis (porous bone) is a metabolic disorder characterized by low bone mass and deterioration of bone structure, resulting in fragile bones that are prone to fracture. The spine, wrist, and hip are most commonly involved, although all bones can be affected.

Prevalence

More than 54 million Americans have osteoporosis or low bone density (National Osteoporosis Foundation, 2021). Women are at greatest risk because their bones are smaller than men's bones. As the U.S. population ages, incidence and cost of osteoporosis will rise. Healthy People 2030 osteoporosis objectives strive to increase the proportion of older adults who get screened for osteoporosis, reduce the proportion of adults with osteoporosis, and increase the proportion of older adults who get treated for osteoporosis after a fracture (Office of Disease Prevention and Health Promotion, 2020). This is important because hip or vertebral fractures are associated with reduced quality of life, increased disability, and increased risk of death, especially within the year after a hip fracture.

Pathophysiology

Bone is living tissue that is constantly resorbing (breaking down) old bone tissue (osteoclast cells) and building new bone tissue (osteoblast cells). Normally, the bone remodeling process is balanced. In osteoporosis, there is an imbalance. Bone density (mass) peaks between ages 30 and 35. After these peak years, the rate of bone breakdown exceeds the rate of bone buildup. For postmenopausal women, decreased estrogen appears to slow the absorption of calcium, leading to increased bone loss.

Types and Risk Factors

Osteoporosis is categorized as either primary or secondary. Primary osteoporosis, the most common, is not associated with another disease. Some risk factors for primary osteoporosis cannot be modified, such as age, White or Asian ethnicity, family history of osteoporosis or fractures, female gender, history of fractures, low testosterone and estrogen in men, postmenopausal status, and small-boned, petite body build.

Modifiable risk factors for osteoporosis can be reduced with lifestyle changes. These include anorexia nervosa, cigarette smoking, excessive alcohol use, nutrition (e.g., low calcium or vitamin D intake; excessive caffeine, protein, or sodium intake), and sedentary lifestyle.

Secondary osteoporosis results from an associated medical condition or procedure, such as hyperparathyroidism; renal dialysis; medication therapy with steroids, certain antiseizure medications, sleeping medications, aluminum-containing antacids, hormones for endometriosis, or cancer medications; and prolonged immobility, such as from a spinal cord injury.

Prevention

To protect against osteoporosis, healthy lifestyle and nutritional habits that build bone are especially important through age 30, before bone mass begins to decrease. These habits include consuming recommended amounts of calcium (1,000 mg/day for ages 19 to 50 and 1,200 mg/day for ages 50 and over) and vitamin D (600 IU [15 mcg]/day for ages 1 to 70 and 800 IU [20 mcg] for ages 71 and over) (National Institutes of Health, 2021). Additional healthy habits include performing weight-bearing exercises, avoiding alcohol, and not smoking.

Signs and Symptoms

Most people do not realize they have osteoporosis until they fracture a bone, have vertebral compression fractures, lose height (up to 6 inches), or develop a forward curvature of the spine (kyphosis). Pain may not be present. The patient may be embarrassed by the change in body image and curtail social activities. Some patients cannot find clothes that fit comfortably.

General effects of the disease go beyond the obvious bone deformities, often affecting quality of life and causing acute or chronic pain. Physiological effects can include decreased respiratory capacity due to spinal deformities. It can be difficult to expand the lungs because of curvature of the spine or painful vertebral fractures. This can increase fatigue and the risk of pneumonia. Osteoporosis can be associated with chronic obstructive pulmonary disease (COPD) because of limited activity related to dyspnea and corticosteroid therapy (which breaks down bone).

Functional abilities (activities of daily living [ADLs] and instrumental ADLs [activities individuals do to function independently and care for self, e.g., finances, shopping, meals, housekeeping, laundry, transportation, telephone communication]) may be limited, increasing the patient's dependence. Emotional effects relate to body image changes, depression, or fear of breaking a bone such as during intimacy. Socialization may be reduced because of activity limitations or fear of injury. Because these effects are interrelated, data should be collected on the whole person, not just the disease, for treatment that will improve quality of life.

Diagnostic Tests

Dual-energy x-ray absorptiometry (DEXA) is the standard screening tool to measure bone density (see "Gerontological Issues: Osteoporosis"). This noninvasive scan is a low-dose x-ray and takes about 5 minutes to perform while the patient lies on a table. The DEXA scan identifies low bone density at the hip and spine. It also can show response to treatment.

Serum calcium and vitamin D values can decrease, and serum phosphorus may be increased. With severe bone loss, alkaline phosphatase levels may be elevated, confirming bone damage.

> **Gerontological Issues**
>
> **Osteoporosis**
> Bone mineral density testing can help determine the risk of fractures for residents in long-term care. Providing treatment for osteoporosis can reduce the risk of hip fractures.

Therapeutic Measures

There is no cure for osteoporosis, but it can be treated. The cornerstone of treatment for osteoporosis is medication and controlling risk factors to prevent bone loss.

MEDICATION. Supplements and medication are used for prevention or treatment. These include calcium supplements, vitamin D, antiresorptive medications, and bone-forming medications.

If serum calcium falls below normal levels, the parathyroid glands stimulate bone to release calcium into the bloodstream. The result is demineralized bone. Therefore, calcium supplements to maintain normal levels and prevent bone loss are important. The patient is taught to drink plenty of fluids to prevent calcium-based urinary stones. Vitamin D supplementation, to aid calcium absorption, also may be needed. This is especially important for patients who have reduced exposure to sunlight (e.g., residents of long-term care facilities or northern geographical areas) or who cannot metabolize vitamin D.

Antiresorptive Medications. Bisphosphonates bind to bone and suppress osteoclast activity to prevent or reduce bone breakdown in osteoporosis. They include alendronate (Fosamax, Fosamax Plus D), ibandronate (Boniva), risedronate (Actonel, Actonel with calcium), and zoledronic acid (Reclast).

Side effects of bisphosphonates include bone, muscle, or joint pain; gastrointestinal upset; gastric ulcers; and, rarely, osteonecrosis (bone death) of the jaw. Reinforce teaching on exactly how to take the medication to reduce side effects. The tablet or solution form is taken after arising in the morning on an empty stomach with 6 to 8 ounces of water only. The patient should wait 30 minutes before taking other medications. To prevent esophageal reactions, the patient should remain upright for at least 30 minutes after taking the medication. Older adults should be monitored for increased risk of gastrointestinal reactions.

The synthetic thyroid hormone calcitonin (Fortical, Miacalcin) treats osteoporosis by decreasing bone loss. It is used for women who have been menopausal for 5 years.

The monoclonal antibody denosumab (Prolia) inhibits the protein that signals bone removal. Raloxifene (Evista) is a selective estrogen receptor modulator (SERM) that increases bone mass by 2% to 3% each year. SERM medications are designed to mimic estrogen in some parts of the body while blocking its effects elsewhere.

Estrogen therapy may be used to prevent the bone loss that occurs with menopause as estrogen levels fall. However, other treatments are usually considered first due to risk factors associated with estrogen therapy.

Anabolic (Bone-Forming) Medications. Teriparatide (Forteo) is used for men and women who are at great risk for fracture. Teriparatide increases bone mass by increasing the action and number of osteoblasts that form bone. It should not be taken for more than 2 years.

DIET. Increasing calcium and vitamin D intake are the main dietary considerations. Inform patients of foods that are high in calcium, such as dairy products, sardines, salmon, fortified breakfast cereals, and dark green, leafy vegetables.

EXERCISE. Weight-bearing exercise, especially walking, stimulates bone building. The patient should wear well-supporting, nonskid shoes and avoid uneven surfaces that could cause falls. Exercise such as weight training is also beneficial (see "Gerontological Issues: Falls").

> ### Gerontological Issues
> **Falls**
> Falls become more common as people age. Exercise that focuses on strength, balance, agility, and coordination is one way of reducing falls in older adults.

Fall Prevention
Osteoporotic bone may cause a pathological fracture, in which the hip breaks and causes a fall. On the other hand, a fall can cause a hip or other fracture. Therefore, fall prevention programs in health-care facilities are important. A walker or cane can provide support during ambulation.

For the patient's home, the patient and caregivers are taught to create a hazard-free environment, without slippery floors, rugs, clutter, and other obstacles.

> **PRACTICE ANALYSIS TIP**
> **Linking NCLEX-PN® to Practice**
> The LPN/LVN will:
> - Provide for mobility needs (e.g., ambulation, range of motion, transfer, repositioning, use of adaptive equipment).
> - Ensure availability and safe functioning of client care equipment.

Nursing Care
Nursing care for osteoporosis focuses on education for prevention, providing pain relief and support for symptoms, and medication teaching. For more information, visit the National Osteoporosis Foundation at www.nof.org.

Paget Disease
Paget disease is a rare metabolic bone disease. Increased breakdown and formation of bone results in weak, abnormal bones. This causes severe bone pain, deformities and fractures, and osteoarthritis. There is no cure for Paget disease. Older adults and men are mainly affected. X-rays show bones with punched-out areas. Increased serum alkaline phosphatase levels occur due to osteoblast activity. NSAIDs are given for pain control, and bisphosphonates reduce bone resorption. Calcitonin (Fortical, Miacalcin) decreases bone loss. Exercise helps maintain bone health and joint mobility. Nursing care promotes pain relief, teaching, and quality of life.

Bone Cancer
Bone tumors may be benign or malignant. Malignant tumors are primary (begin in the bone) or metastatic (migrate to bone from another site). Metastatic lesions often affect older adults.

Osteosarcoma, or osteogenic sarcoma, is the most common malignant bone tumor. It occurs mainly in the ends of long bones, usually near the knees. It typically affects young people between ages 10 and 25 and males more than females. Swelling, bone pain, and/or pathological bone injury are common symptoms. It is treated with chemotherapy and radiation.

Ewing sarcoma is a rare bone tumor or tumor of the soft tissue around bone. In addition to bone pain and swelling, low-grade fever, fatigue, and weight loss are common. The legs, pelvis, ribs, arms, and spine are affected, most often in those ages 10 to 20. Chemotherapy and radiation are used; then, if necessary, surgery is performed.

Primary malignant tumors that occur in the prostate, breast, lung, and thyroid gland are called *bone-seeking cancers* because they migrate to bone more than any other primary cancers do. With metastasis, multiple sites in the bone are typically seen. Pathological fractures and severe pain are major concerns in managing metastatic disease (see Chapter 11).

Signs and Symptoms
Primary tumors cause pain and swelling at the site. A tender, palpable mass is often present. Metastatic disease is not as visible, but the patient reports diffuse severe pain, eventually leading to marked disability.

Diagnostic Tests
Diagnosis of bone cancer is made with x-ray, CT scan, bone scan, bone biopsy, positron emission tomography (PET) or PET-CT scan, or MRI (see Chapter 45). Patients with metastatic disease have elevated alkaline phosphatase

• WORD • BUILDING •
osteosarcoma: osteo—bone + sarc—flesh + oma—tumor

levels and possibly an elevated ESR, indicating secondary tissue inflammation.

Therapeutic Measures
Treatment of primary bone tumors is usually surgery with chemotherapy or radiation. Chemotherapy and surgical excision of the affected bone with bone grafting or amputation of the affected limb are common treatments for osteosarcoma. For patients with Ewing sarcoma or early osteosarcoma, external radiation may be the treatment of choice to reduce tumor size and pain. For metastatic bone disease, surgery is not appropriate. External radiation is given, primarily for palliation to shrink the tumor and reduce pain.

Nursing Care
Nursing care for the patient with bone cancer is similar to care for other types of cancer (see Chapter 11). Care of the postoperative patient is similar to that for any patient undergoing musculoskeletal surgery. Monitoring the neurovascular status of the operative limb is a vital nursing intervention (see Chapters 12 and 45).

CONNECTIVE TISSUE DISORDERS

Connective tissue disorders comprise more than 100 diseases in which the major signs and symptoms result from joint involvement. Some affect only one part of the body; others affect many body organs and systems. Gout, osteoarthritis, and rheumatoid arthritis are discussed.

Gout
Gout is an easily treated systemic connective tissue disorder occurring from the build-up of uric acid. Men, especially those middle aged and older, are most affected.

Pathophysiology
Uric acid is a waste product resulting from the breakdown of proteins (purines) in the body. Urate crystals are formed because of excessive uric acid build-up (**hyperuricemia**). They are deposited in joints and other connective tissues, causing severe inflammation (Fig. 46.8). The inflammation may resolve in several days, with or without treatment. Urate deposits (tophi) occasionally appear under the skin (outer ear, commonly) or in the kidneys or urinary system, causing stone (calculi) formation (see Chapter 37).

Etiology and Types
Primary gout, the most common type, is caused by an inherited problem with purine metabolism. Uric acid production is greater than the kidneys' ability to excrete it. Therefore, the amount of uric acid in the blood increases. Acute attacks of gout may be triggered by stress, alcohol consumption, illness, trauma, dieting, or certain medications such as aspirin and diuretics.

Uric acid is also increased in secondary gout. However, the increase is related to a health issue. Examples include renal insufficiency or medications, such as diuretic therapy and certain chemotherapeutic agents.

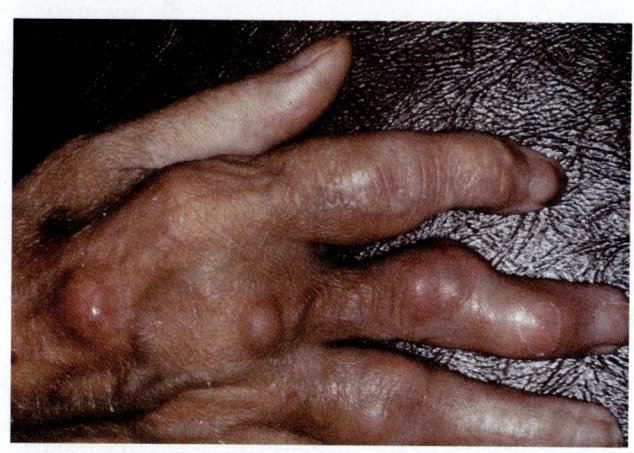

FIGURE 46.8 Gout: subcutaneous nontender lesions near joints.

Signs and Symptoms
When an "attack" of acute gout occurs, the patient has severe pain and inflammation due to the uric acid crystals in one or more small joints, usually the great toe. The joint is swollen, red, hot, and usually too painful to be touched.

Patients with chronic gout may not have obvious signs and symptoms. Renal stones can develop from elevated uric acid.

Diagnostic Tests
Diagnosis of gout is based on an elevated serum uric acid level. Joint fluid aspiration analysis can also identify uric acid crystals in the synovial fluid.

Therapeutic Measures
Medication therapy is the first-line treatment for primary gout. Treatment for secondary gout involves management of the underlying cause. For an acute gout episode, NSAIDs, colchicine (Colcrys), or steroids are prescribed until the joint inflammatory response subsides. Chronic gout patients for whom other medications are not effective may be helped by pegloticase (Krystexxa) by IV infusion every 2 weeks for about 6 months.

Uricosuric medications are used to prevent increased serum uric acid levels. Febuxostat (Uloric) and allopurinol (Zyloprim) decrease uric acid production. Probenecid (Benemid) increases renal excretion of uric acid. Serum uric acid level is monitored during medication use.

Prevention and Nursing Care
Interventions for patient education to help prevent gout include the following:

- Drink plenty of fluids, especially water.
- Consider eating cherries or drinking cherry juice.
- Avoid high-purine (protein) foods, like organ meats, shellfish, and oily fish (e.g., sardines).

• WORD • BUILDING •

hyperuricemia: hyper—excessive + uric—uric acid + emia—in blood

- Avoid alcohol.
- Avoid all forms of acetylsalicylic acid (aspirin) and medications containing it.
- Avoid diuretics.
- Avoid excessive physical or emotional stress.

Osteoarthritis

Osteoarthritis (OA) is the most common type of arthritis, affecting more than 32.5 million people in the United States (Centers for Disease Control and Prevention, 2020). It is more common with age and in women especially over age 50. OA is also known as *degenerative joint disease*.

Pathophysiology

OA is a disease of the joint that affects all the joint's structures (Table 46.3). The cartilage and bone ends slowly break down. The joint space narrows, bone spurs develop, and

Table 46.3
Osteoarthritis and Rheumatoid Arthritis Summary

	Osteoarthritis	Rheumatoid Arthritis
Pathophysiology	Articular cartilage and bone ends deteriorate. Joint is inflamed.	Inflammatory cells cause synovitis. Synovium becomes thick and fluid accumulates, causing swelling and pain. Joint becomes deformed.
Etiology	*Primary (idiopathic):* • Cause unknown. • Risk factors include age, obesity, activities causing joint stress. *Secondary:* • Causes include trauma, sepsis, congenital abnormalities, metabolic disorders, rheumatoid arthritis.	Periodontal disease may be a cause. Is an autoimmune disease. Can occur at any age (including juvenile rheumatoid arthritis). Familial history possible.
Signs and Symptoms	Joint pain and stiffness occur. Pain increases with activity and decreases with rest. Nodes on joints of fingers appear (Heberden nodes, Bouchard nodes).	Symptoms vary according to disease process. *Early symptoms:* • Bilateral and symmetrical joint inflammation • Redness, warmth, swelling, stiffness, pain • Stiffness after resting (morning stiffness) • Activity decreases pain and stiffness • Low-grade fever, weakness, fatigue, anorexia (mild weight loss) • Organ system involvement *Late symptoms:* • Joint deformity • Secondary osteoporosis
Therapeutic Measures	Medication • NSAIDs • Acetaminophen • Muscle relaxants. Balanced rest and exercise Splinting of joint to promote rest Heat and cold Weight loss Complementary therapies Surgery for total joint replacement	Medication • Antibiotics • NSAIDs • Biological response modifier • Prednisone • Disease-modifying antirheumatic drug (DMARD) • T-cell modulators Heat and cold Balanced rest and activity Surgery for total joint replacement
Priority Nursing Diagnoses	*Acute Pain* *Impaired Physical Mobility* *Disturbed Body Image*	*Acute Pain* *Self-Care Deficit(s)* *Fatigue*

the joint lining becomes inflamed. Ligaments and tendons may also be affected. The body's repair process is not able to overcome this loss of cartilage and bone. Weight-bearing joints (e.g., hips and knees), hands, and the vertebral column are most often affected (Fig. 46.9).

Etiology
Risk factors for OA include heredity, obesity, and physical activities that create mechanical stress on synovial joints, such as long periods of standing or repetitive motions. OA may also develop because of trauma, sepsis, congenital anomalies, certain metabolic diseases, or rheumatoid arthritis.

Signs and Symptoms
Pain and stiffness, especially upon arising, commonly occur. Joint pain and swelling increase after activity. Stiffness is reduced with movement. The patient usually seeks medical attention when symptoms are severe or range of motion is limited while performing everyday activities. Painful bony nodes on the finger joint, called Heberden and Bouchard nodes, may occur. Women tend to have these more often than men. If the vertebral column is involved, the patient reports radiating pain and muscle spasms in the extremity innervated by the area affected.

Diagnostic Tests
X-ray examinations can outline the joint structure and detect bone changes. MRI is helpful in showing joint structure abnormalities. Analysis of synovial fluid aids in the diagnosis of OA.

Evidence-Based Practice

Clinical Question
Can exercise effectively relieve chronic low back pain?

Evidence
In this systematic review, 89 studies were examined for the effectiveness of exercise for relieving nonspecific chronic low back pain (Owen et al, 2020). The results showed that resistance training and aerobic exercise training were most effective in relieving this type of pain.

Implications for Nursing Practice
Nurses can encourage patient participation in exercise programs to improve strength/resistance and coordination/stabilization.

Reference: Owen, P. J., Miller, C. T., Verswijveren, S. J., Tagliaferri, S. D., Brisby, H., Bowe, S. J., & Belavy, D. L. (2020). Which specific modes of exercise training are most effective for treating low back pain? Network meta-analysis. *British Journal of Sports Medicine, 54*(21), 1279–1287.

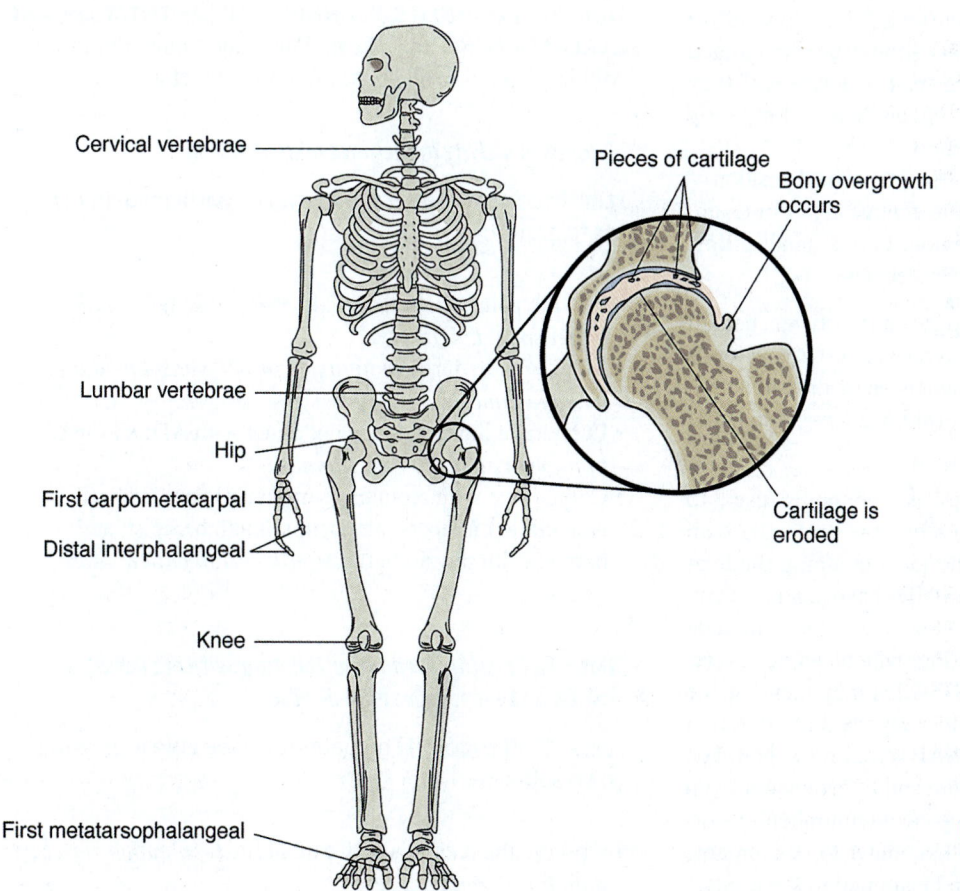

FIGURE 46.9 Common joints affected by osteoarthritis and the changes that result in the joint.

CLINICAL JUDGMENT

Mr. Finn, a 59-year-old hardware store manager, is 5′ 11″ and weighs 250 pounds. He visits his HCP because of knee pain. He has noticed that it is becoming increasingly difficult to bend to pick up heavy boxes, and reports knee stiffness, especially in the morning. The HCP suspects osteoarthritis.

1. What data collection questions do you ask Mr. Finn?
2. What risk factors do you identify that Mr. Finn has?
3. What patient-centered care interventions do you provide for Mr. Finn?
4. What health-care team members do you collaborate with?

Suggested answers are at the end of the chapter.

Therapeutic Measures

There is no cure for OA. Symptom control is the focus of treatment. An interdisciplinary approach is needed to prevent decreased mobility and preserve joint function.

EXERCISE. Joint pain from OA tends to decrease with rest, so pain is less severe in the morning. Activities should be scheduled at this time. A severely inflamed joint may be splinted by the occupational therapist or physical therapist to promote rest to a selected joint. However, rest must be balanced with exercise to prevent muscle atrophy from disuse. Exercise has been identified to maintain general health and weight, range of motion, and muscle strength, while decreasing anxiety and depression. To minimize muscle atrophy and to stabilize and protect arthritic joints, patients should be encouraged to perform exercises to strengthen their quadriceps if they have OA of the knee. Yoga and tai chi are helpful for gently stretching the joints to reduce stiffness.

Joints should always be placed in their functional position—that is, a position that does not lead to contractures. For example, to prevent excessive neck flexion, only a small pillow should be placed under the head when sleeping.

WEIGHT CONTROL. Obese or overweight patients benefit from losing weight to decrease stress on weight-bearing joints and thereby reduce pain. If the patient is on medications that can alter fluid volumes (corticosteroids), a low-sodium diet may be appropriate.

MEDICATION. Medication therapy is commonly used to reduce pain in patients with OA. Often, it is combined with other pain-reducing therapies. The most common medications are NSAIDs (Table 46.4). NSAIDs have analgesic and anti-inflammatory effects. Common side effects include gastrointestinal distress and bleeding, which can be severe, and sodium and fluid retention. NSAIDs may increase the risk of cardiovascular events, such as myocardial infarction or stroke. Older patients taking NSAIDs routinely should be carefully monitored for heart failure and hypertension from fluid retention. Analgesics such as acetaminophen or corticosteroids may be used. Over-the-counter topical creams such as capsaicin (Arthricare) can be applied to the joints.

Synvisc-One (one injection) or SYNVISC (three injections) is injected directly into osteoarthritic knees to replace the cushioning synovial fluid. Pain can be relieved and flexibility restored for up to 6 months.

HEAT AND COLD. The patient with OA usually prefers heat therapy unless the joint is acutely inflamed. Hot packs, warm compresses, warm showers, moist heating pads, and paraffin dips provide sources of heat. Cold therapy may alter cutaneous pain receptors, thereby decreasing pain. Cold packs should be applied for no longer than 20 minutes at a time, as they narrow blood vessels.

COMPLEMENTARY AND ALTERNATIVE THERAPIES. Complementary and alternative therapies can reduce pain. Acupressure, acupuncture, hydrotherapy, imagery, music therapy, massage, and other holistic modalities that foster the mind–body–spirit connection work well for many people.

SURGERY. If the patient's pain cannot be managed successfully, a total joint replacement may be indicated. Total joint replacement is the most common type of arthroplasty (see later section on musculoskeletal surgery).

Nursing Process for the Patient With Osteoarthritis

DATA COLLECTION. The patient's report of pain is documented. Affected joints are observed for signs of inflammation or deformity. Also examined are joint function, ADL performance, and mobility.

NURSING DIAGNOSES, PLANNING, IMPLEMENTATION, AND EVALUATION. See the "Acute Pain" and "Impaired Physical Mobility" nursing diagnoses for Bone Fracture.

Decreased Activity Intolerance related to pain

EXPECTED OUTCOME: The patient will participate in ADLs as tolerated.

- Provide pain relief measures before activity *to enable an increase in activity level.*
- Monitor pain during activity *to provide baseline data to manage pain.*
- Encourage independence but assist with ADLs as needed *to prevent patient exhaustion.*
- Collaborate with an interdisciplinary team, such as pain clinic members, an occupational therapist, and home health physiotherapist, *to develop patient plan of care.*

Bathing, Dressing, Feeding, or Toileting Self-Care Deficit related to degenerative joint disease

EXPECTED OUTCOME: The patient will be able to provide own self-care.

- Observe the patient's self-care abilities *to gather baseline data for planning care.*

Table 46.4
Common Medications Used to Treat Connective Tissue Diseases: Osteoarthritis, Rheumatoid Arthritis, and Others

Medication Class/Action

Biological Response Modifiers

Interleukin-1 inhibitors that reduce inflammation and cartilage degradation.

Examples
anakinra (Kineret)

Nursing Implications
Monitor neutrophils.

Corticosteroids

Reduce inflammation and swelling.

Examples
prednisone (Deltasone, Orasone)

Nursing Implications
Take daily weight.
Monitor intake and output.
Monitor for infection.
Give with food/milk.
Recommend patient obtain medic alert ID.
Not used for osteoarthritis.

Disease-Modifying Antirheumatic Drugs (DMARDs)

For use in rheumatoid arthritis and ankylosing spondylitis; reduce symptoms, prevent joint damage, and preserve joint function by suppressing immune or inflammatory systems. Slow-acting and may take months for effect; other medications used to control symptoms until effective. Effect ends when medication stopped.

Pyrimidine Synthesis Inhibitors

Examples
leflunomide (Arava)

Nursing Implications
Screen for tuberculosis before starting.
Monitor blood pressure, complete blood count, liver function.
Teach patient to report rash promptly.

Gold Preparations

Examples
auranofin (Ridaura)
aurothioglucose (Solganal)

Nursing Implications
Give test dose and monitor for allergic reaction for about 1 hour.
Laboratory testing for gold toxicity recommended.

Immunosuppressives

Examples
azathioprine (Imuran)
cyclophosphamide (Cytoxan)
cyclosporine (Sandimmune, Neoral)
leflunomide (Arava; *for rheumatoid arthritis only*)
methotrexate (Otrexyom, Rasuvo, Xatmep)
d-penicillamine (Cuprimine, Depen)

Nursing Implications
Protect from infection.
Monitor for infections.

Tumor Necrosis Factor Inhibitors

Examples
adalimumab (Humira)
adalimumab-adaz (Hyrimoz)
adalimumab-adbm (Cyltezo)
adalimumab-afzb (Abrilada)

Nursing Implications
Screen for tuberculosis.

Continued

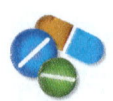

Table 46.4
Common Medications Used to Treat Connective Tissue Diseases: Osteoarthritis, Rheumatoid Arthritis, and Others—cont'd

Medication Class/Action	
adalimumab-atto (Amjevita) adalimumab-bwwd (Hadlima) etanercept (Enbrel) etanercept-szzs (Erelzi) etanercept-ykro (Eticovo) golimumab (Simponi) inflizimab (Remicade) infliximab-dyyb (Inflectra)	

Antimalarials

Examples	Nursing Implications
chloroquine (Aralen) hydroxychloroquine (Plaquenil)	Report vision problems. Promote safety due to dizziness.

NSAIDs

Block activity of enzyme cyclooxygenase (COX-1, COX-2), which makes prostaglandins that produce inflammation, fever, and pain; support platelets; and protect stomach lining (COX-1 only).

Examples	Nursing Implications
acetylsalicylic acid (aspirin) diclofenac sodium (Voltaren) etodolac (Lodine; *for osteoarthritis only*) ibuprofen (Motrin) indomethacin (Indocin) meloxicam (Mobic) naproxen (Aleve, Naprosyn) oxaprozin (Daypro) nabumetone (Relafen) sulindac (Clinoril)	Those with asthma at higher risk for allergic reaction. Explain risk of gastrointestinal bleeding.

T-Cell Modulators

Reduce activation of T cells in the inflammatory process.

Examples	Nursing Implications
abatacept (Orencia)	Screen for tuberculosis. Use silicone-free syringe only. Infuse over 30 minutes. Monitor for serious infections.

- Encourage independence *to decrease feelings of despair about being unable to care for self.*
- Assist when necessary *to minimize frustration when the patient cannot perform self-care.*
- Reinforce teaching about assistive devices to help with ADL living *to promote self-care.*
- Collaborate with an interdisciplinary team, such as a home health nurse, occupational therapist, or physiotherapist, *to acquire assistive devices and use alternate resources.*

Disturbed Body Image related to changes in joint function and structure

EXPECTED OUTCOME: The patient will demonstrate acceptance of changes in body image.

- Encourage the patient to discuss feelings and concerns *to allow the nurse to understand what the patient is experiencing.*

- Provide information and clarify misconceptions *to ensure that the patient is aware of expected problems and concerns.*
- Encourage socialization *to improve patient's perceptions of how they appear to others.*

Chronic Sorrow related to body image changes, altered role, pain, and ongoing losses

EXPECTED OUTCOME: The patient will verbalize improvement in feelings of sorrow.

- Observe patient's affect and mood connected to pain and loss *to provide baseline data.*
- Allow time to discuss feelings and anticipate trigger events *to ensure the patient is aware of what may increase feelings of sorrow.*
- Encourage use of interdisciplinary team, such as a social worker, psychologist, clergy, or spiritual adviser, *to provide alternative methods of dealing with sorrow.*
- Encourage use of support groups *to enable the patient to discuss concerns with others experiencing the same problems.*

EVALUATION. Outcomes are met if the patient rates pain at a tolerable level on an appropriate pain scale, demonstrates improved physical mobility, participates in ADLs, provides self-care, demonstrates acceptance of changes in body image, and verbalizes improvement in feelings of sorrow.

PATIENT EDUCATION. A vital function of each member of the health-care team is health teaching. The patient with OA is seldom admitted to the hospital for treatment of OA unless surgery is scheduled. However, many patients with OA are admitted for other reasons. Their OA needs must also be considered in the plan of care. Most patients residing in long-term care facilities have OA, which can affect their participation in ADLs and recreational activities.

Patients should be taught ways to protect their joints and conserve energy. For educational materials and self-help courses, visit the Arthritis Foundation at www.arthritis.org.

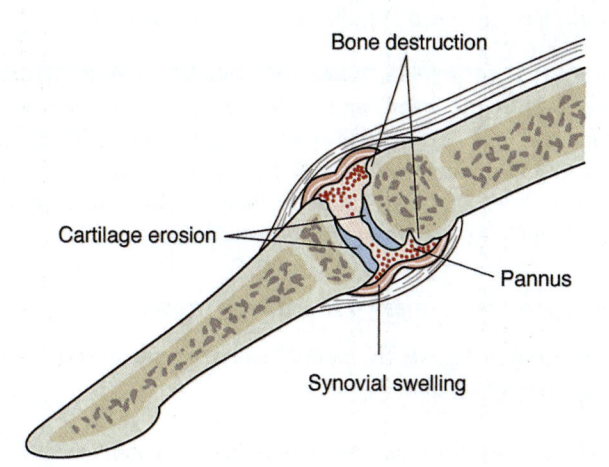

FIGURE 46.10 Rheumatoid arthritis.

Rheumatoid Arthritis

Rheumatoid arthritis (RA) is a chronic, progressive, systemic inflammatory disease that destroys synovial joints and other connective tissues, including major organs.

Pathophysiology

Inflammatory cells and chemicals cause **synovitis**, an inflammation of the synovium (the lining of the joint capsule). As the inflammation progresses, the synovium becomes thick. Fluid accumulation causes joint swelling and pain. A destructive pannus (new synovial tissue growth infiltrated with inflammatory cells) erodes the joint cartilage and eventually destroys the bone within the joint (Fig. 46.10). Ultimately, the pannus is converted to bony tissue, resulting in loss of mobility. Joint deformity and bone loss are common in late RA (see Table 46.3).

Any connective tissue may be affected in RA, including blood vessels, nerves, kidneys, pericardium, lungs, and subcutaneous tissue. Dysfunction or failure of the organ or system can occur. Death can result if the disease does not respond to treatment.

Many patients experience spontaneous remissions and exacerbations (flare-ups) of RA. Symptoms may disappear without treatment for months or years. Then the disease flares up just as unpredictably, often due to physical or emotional stress.

Etiology

RA affects people with a family history of the disease two to three times more often than it affects others. Antibiotic prescriptions have been associated with a 60% increased risk of RA, although it is unknown if that effect results from the antibiotic itself or the infection being treated (Sultan et al, 2019). Oral pathogens may cause RA. Studies show that symptoms of RA improve with antibiotic treatment. In RA, an autoimmune response occurs that affects the synovial membrane of the joints. Antibodies (called *rheumatoid factor*; RF) are often found in patients with RA. It is suggested that these antibodies join with other antibodies and form antibody complexes. These complexes lodge in synovium and other connective tissues, causing local and systemic inflammation. They may be responsible for the destructive changes of RA in body tissues.

Signs and Symptoms

Signs and symptoms vary because the disease presents differently in each patient. In general, the signs and symptoms can be divided into early and late manifestations.

The typical pattern of joint inflammation is bilateral and symmetrical. The disease usually begins in the upper extremities and progresses to other joints over many years (Fig. 46.11). Affected joints are slightly reddened, warm, swollen, stiff, and painful. The patient with RA often has morning stiffness lasting for up to an hour. Those with severe disease may report having stiffness all day. Generally, activity decreases pain and stiffness.

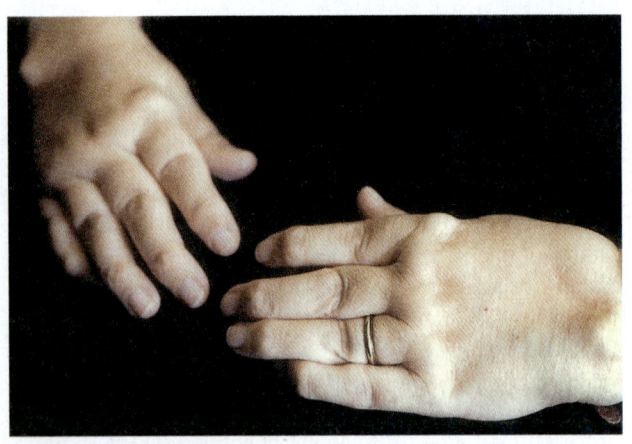

FIGURE 46.11 Joint abnormalities in hands of patient with rheumatoid arthritis.

Because of the systemic nature of RA, the patient may have a low-grade fever, malaise, depression, lymphadenopathy, weakness, fatigue, anorexia, and weight loss. As the disease worsens, major organs or body systems are affected. Joint deformities occur as a late symptom. Secondary osteoporosis (bone loss) can lead to fractures.

Diagnostic Tests

No specific diagnostic test confirms RA. An increase in white blood cells and platelets is typical. Immunological test findings for patients with RA usually include the following:

- Presence of RF in serum
- Decreased red blood cell count
- Decreased C4 complement
- Increased ESR
- Positive antinuclear antibody test
- Positive C-reactive protein test

RF can indicate the aggressiveness of the disease. However, it is not specific to RA. The ESR test screens for inflammation. It measures the amount of time it takes for red blood cells to settle to the bottom of a test tube. In the presence of inflammation, red blood cells settle faster in the tube. Therefore, the ESR increases with the presence of inflammation. It also evaluates the effectiveness of treatment. If the disease responds to treatment, the ESR decreases.

> **LEARNING TIP**
> For those with rheumatoid arthritis, a verbal "Nice to meet you" greeting instead of a handshake avoids the pain caused by a handshake, even a weak one.

X-ray examination and MRI detect joint damage and bone loss, especially in the vertebral column. A bone or joint scan assesses the extent of joint involvement throughout the body. With arthrocentesis, synovial fluid is cloudy, milky, or dark yellow with inflammatory cells present.

Therapeutic Measures

Antibiotics may improve the symptoms of RA. Chronic joint pain can interfere with mobility or the ability to perform ADLs. Medication therapy can relieve or reduce pain as well as slow the progression of the disease. Disease-modifying antirheumatic drugs (DMARDs) can prevent joint destruction, deformity, and disability with early single or combination medication use. NSAIDs and corticosteroids are also used (see Table 46.4). Many of these medications have potentially serious side effects, such as severe infection, and must be monitored carefully.

Complementary therapies that may help decrease inflammation or pain include capsaicin cream, fish oil, and antioxidants such as vitamin C, vitamin E, and beta carotene (see Chapter 5).

HEAT AND COLD. Heat applications or hot showers help decrease joint stiffness and make exercise easier for the patient. For acutely inflamed, or "hot," joints, cold applications may be best. A program that balances rest and exercise is most beneficial for the patient.

SURGERY. If nonsurgical approaches are not effective in relieving arthritic pain, the patient may have a total joint replacement (discussed later).

Nursing Process for the Patient With Rheumatoid Arthritis

DATA COLLECTION. A complete history and physical examination are needed for the patient with RA, as the disease can involve every system of the body. In addition to identifying physical signs and symptoms, explore the patient's psychosocial, functional, and vocational needs.

After having the disease for approximately 15 years, fewer than half of RA patients are totally independent in their ADLs. These limitations may place a burden on family members, who must be included in the care of the patient with RA. Many patients with the disease are young or middle-aged. RA can impair their ability to work, depending on the type of job they have. Occupational therapy assesses the patient's work skills to determine the need for changes in the workplace or a need to train for a new type of work.

NURSING DIAGNOSES, PLANNING, AND IMPLEMENTATION. See the "Acute Pain" and "Impaired Physical Mobility" nursing diagnoses for Bone Fracture and "Bathing, Dressing, Feeding, Toileting Self-Care Deficit" and "Disturbed Body Image" in the "Nursing Diagnoses, Planning, Implementation, and Evaluation" section under Osteoarthritis.

Fatigue related to chronic pain and limited mobility

EXPECTED OUTCOME: The patient will have decreased episodes of fatigue.

- Monitor levels of fatigue through the day *to determine patient's reaction to various activities.*

- Provide assistance as required *to conserve the patient's energy.*
- Ensure regular rest periods throughout the day *to avoid overexerting the patient.*
- Reinforce teaching energy conservation techniques *to reduce workload.*
- Reinforce teaching the patient the need to delegate *to avoid overexertion.*

EVALUATION. The outcomes are met if the patient has pain relief within acceptable levels on a pain rating scale, improved physical mobility, ability to provide self-care, acceptance of changes in body image, and decreased episodes of fatigue.

PATIENT EDUCATION. The patient with RA needs extensive patient education regarding the disease process, medication management, and the comprehensive plan of care. In collaboration with health-care team members, help the patient plan a daily schedule that balances rest and exercise. A vocational counselor may be necessary for job training if the patient needs to pursue a different occupation. Patients who are unable to work may be able to qualify for disability benefits through the federal Social Security program. Inform the patient about community resources such as support groups (visit www.arthritis.org).

CLINICAL JUDGMENT

Mrs. Harris is a 48-year-old nurse who has had upper extremity joint pain and swelling for about 4 years. She was recently diagnosed with rheumatoid arthritis but has no systemic involvement. She has extreme fatigue at this time and is concerned that she will have to give up providing direct patient care on a busy medical unit in the local hospital.

1. What questions do you ask Mrs. Harris about her illness?
2. What do you discuss with Mrs. Harris about pain management?
3. What complications do you look for in Mrs. Harris?

Suggested answers are at the end of the chapter.

MUSCULOSKELETAL SURGERY

Some health problems cannot be managed conservatively and require surgery. The most common orthopedic surgeries are discussed here.

Total Joint Replacement

Total joint replacement (TJR) is most often performed for patients who have some type of connective tissue disease in which their joints become severely deteriorated. TJR may also be needed for cancer, trauma, or after long-term steroid therapy. Long-term use of steroids, trauma, and complications of joint replacement can cause **avascular necrosis**, a condition in which bone tissue dies (usually the femoral head) because of impaired blood supply. Advanced avascular necrosis is very painful and usually does not respond to conservative pain relief measures. The primary goal of TJR is to relieve severe chronic pain and improve ability to carry out ADLs when no other treatment is successful.

Total hip replacement and total knee replacement are the most common replacement surgeries. Any synovial joint can be replaced. Another term used for joint replacement is **arthroplasty**. The prosthetic components are made of ceramic, polyethylene, or metal. Most implants are cementless and are secured by the patient's bone as it grafts and connects to the porous prosthesis. Cemented prostheses are used when bone health is poor, such as in osteoporosis. The incision is closed with internal dissolvable sutures, skin glue, and skin sealer. Skin staples may be used.

Total Hip Replacement

Total hip replacement (THR) uses an acetabular cup inserted into the pelvic acetabulum and a femoral stem and head inserted into the femur to replace the femoral neck and head (Fig. 46.12). Various surgical approaches for THR can be done by surgeons, which then require differences in postoperative hip care and precautions. These approaches include posterior, anterior-lateral, and anterior. Tranexamic acid, an antifibrinolytic agent, may be given to reduce blood loss during surgery. A prophylactic antibiotic, usually given 1 hour prior to incision time, reduces the chance of an infection. The patient's length of stay may be 1 to 3 days, although outpatient procedures are growing. In a study, THRs were found to last 25 years in 58% of patients (Evans et al, 2019).

PREOPERATIVE CARE. THR is an elective procedure. It is scheduled to allow time for preoperative teaching and screening. A case manager (e.g., registered nurse or social worker) may assess the patient's needs and support systems available postoperatively. The patient is taught about the procedure and what to expect postoperatively. Preoperative exercises to perform to help strengthen the operative leg may be explained by a physical therapist.

A preoperative autologous (self) blood donation by a patient may be ordered in the event a postoperative blood transfusion is needed due to blood loss in surgery. This can reassure patients who are concerned about receiving donor blood.

Preoperative preparation at home the night before surgery includes a shower and hair wash with no shaving of the skin to prevent microabrasions that could harbor bacteria. The patient is given prepackaged antibacterial skin cleansing cloths to use the night before and the day of surgery in the area illustrated on a diagram of the body.

Preoperatively, the nurse obtains a patient history, including allergies and medications, and checks the neurovascular status of the operative extremity, level of pain, and mobility.

• WORD • BUILDING •
arthroplasty: arthro—joint + plasty—creation of

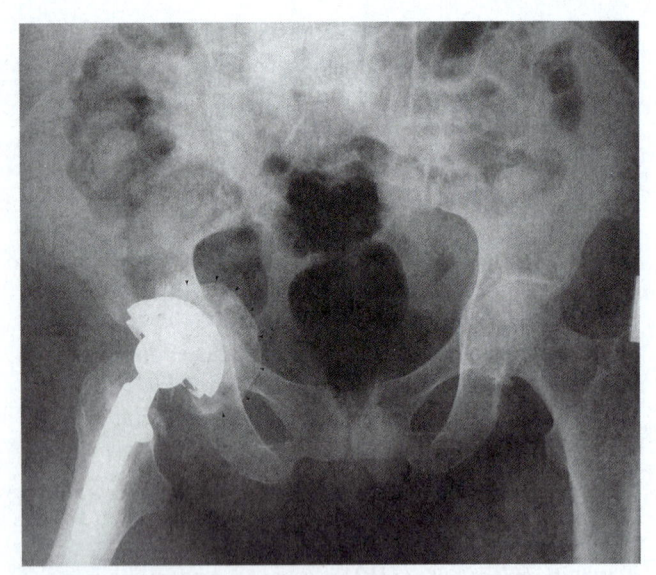

FIGURE 46.12 Total hip arthroplasty of arthritic right hip.

POSTOPERATIVE. Care for the patient having a THR is interdisciplinary. Pain is managed with IV, IM, or oral analgesics, including paracetamol (Tylenol) and NSAIDs. Cold and heat therapy are used in 15- to 20-minute intervals. Within 2 hours after return to the patient's hospital room, the physical therapist and occupational therapist will assist the patient with ambulation sessions that may include getting in and out of bed, standing, sitting, and walking every 2 hours and with managing assistive devices such as a walker, a cane, an elevated toilet seat, a long-handled shoehorn, and a sponge. In addition to providing general postoperative care that all patients undergoing general or epidural anesthesia require, plan and implement interventions to help prevent the common complications of THR (see Chapter 12).

Hip Dislocation. The most common postoperative complication for the patient having a posterior or anterior-lateral THR is subluxation (partial dislocation) or total dislocation. Dislocation occurs when the femoral component becomes dislodged from the acetabular cup. Often, if a dislocation occurs, there is an audible "pop" followed by immediate pain in the affected hip. In addition to pain, the patient experiences shortening and possibly internal rotation of the surgical leg. If these signs and symptoms occur, notify the surgeon immediately and keep the patient in bed. Under anesthesia, the surgeon manually manipulates the hip back into alignment.

Preventing dislocation is a major nursing responsibility. Correct positioning of the surgical leg is critical. The primary goals are to prevent hip adduction (across the body's midline) and hyperflexion (bending forward more than 90 degrees). The patient is informed to use two regular pillows (one proximal and one distal) between the legs when sleeping and turn to the side of the body per HCP preference. When turning, it is important that the hip and legs turn together to minimize the chance of dislocation. Supporting the leg with a pillow during turning is required to decrease the chance of dislocation. Ensure that the patient does not adduct or hyperflex the surgical hip during transfer to a chair.

To prevent hyperflexion, when sitting, ensure the patient is using a straight-back chair with arm rests and educate the patient to avoid chairs lower than knee height (Fig. 46.13). The toilet seat is also raised. Patients are instructed not to bend forward more than 90 degrees.

Skin Breakdown. Because most patients having THR are older, skin breakdown prevention is a major part of postoperative care. Early ambulation is helpful. Protect the heels, elbows, and the sacrum, which can break down within 24 hours (see Chapter 54). Assisting the patient to use the toilet every 2 hours and using a protective barrier cream help prevent skin problems related to incontinence. Adequate diet and hydration are also important to prevent skin breakdown.

Infection. Orthopedic surgery patients are at an increased risk for infection because of the nature of the surgery. Increased age also is a risk factor. When performing dressing changes, observe the incision for signs and symptoms of infection (e.g., redness, swelling, warmth, odor, pain, or yellow, green, or brown-tinged drainage). Monitor the patient's temperature. An older patient with an infection might not experience a fever but may exhibit confusion due to the infection.

CLINICAL JUDGMENT

Mrs. Adam is 78 years old and had a left total hip replacement. When changing the surgical dressing, the home health nurse notices a purulent discharge. Cefaclor (Ceclor) 500 mg by mouth every 8 hours is ordered. Cefaclor is available as a 375 mg/5 mL suspension. How many milliliters should Mrs. Adam be given?

Suggested answers are at the end of the chapter.

Bleeding. The patient might need salvaged operative, autologous, or postoperative blood. By using orthopedic patient autotransfusion (such as OrthoPAT) during surgery, about 50% of lost blood can be recovered and saved for reinfusion into the same patient. Postoperatively, blood can be replaced

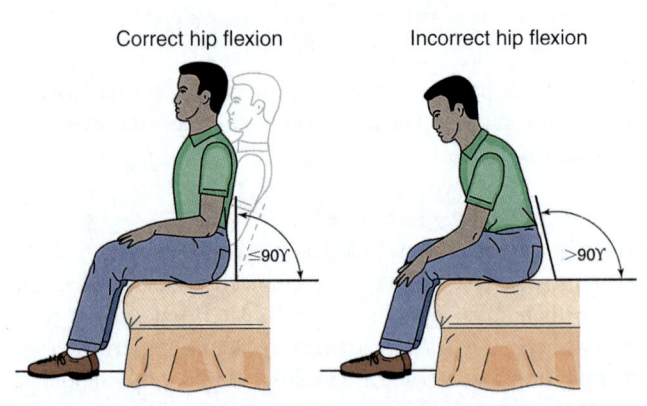

FIGURE 46.13 Hip flexion after total hip replacement should be 90 degrees or less to prevent dislocation.

by collecting shed blood via suction into a reservoir and then filtering and reinfusing it within 6 hours of collection. Surgical drains (e.g., Hemovac or Jackson-Pratt) are not recommended for routine use. Monitor for blood loss and signs of shock. Monitor dressings for drainage and report large or unexpected amounts.

Neurovascular Compromise. For any musculoskeletal surgery or injury, frequent neurovascular checks for circulation (e.g., color, warmth, pulses), sensation, and movement are performed distal to the surgical procedure or injury (and compared with the unaffected side) when vital signs are checked. The procedure and significance of these checks are described in Chapter 45.

Venous Thromboembolitic Complications. Patients having hip surgery are at greatest risk for DVT or pulmonary embolus. An anticoagulant medication is given to help prevent blood clot formation. In addition, thigh-high compression stockings and intermittent pneumatic compression devices may be used (see Chapter 12).

> **BE SAFE!**
> **BE VIGILANT!** When giving low molecular weight heparin medications such as enoxaparin (Lovenox) or dalteparin (Fragmin), to avoid possible tissue necrosis, medication should be administered in the abdomen subcutaneously. The air bubble should not be removed from the prefilled syringe before administration to ensure the entire dose is given. To minimize bruising, do not rub injection site after administration.

Because DVT occurs mostly in the lower extremities, leg exercises taught preoperatively are started in the immediate postoperative period and continued until the patient is fully ambulatory.

DISCHARGE. When the patient is medically stable, they are discharged home for about 2 weeks of in-home physical therapy and then receive outpatient physical therapy for 4 to 6 weeks for strengthening and fall prevention or else are discharged to a facility for short-term rehabilitation. Before hospital discharge, the interdisciplinary team provides patient education for home safety, including no use of throw rugs, no extension cords near walkways, safety measures to prevent falls in the shower, and any hip precautions that need to be used until the surgeon reevaluates the patient at the 6- to 8-week follow-up visit (Box 46.4). Posterior or anterior-lateral hip replacements require the use of safety precautions to prevent hip dislocation since muscles are cut that reduce hip stability. The surgeon may not specify any hip precautions for anterior hip replacements as there is little risk of hip dislocation since no muscles are cut during this surgical approach. Other surgeons may prescribe some hip precautions for this approach. The patient should follow their surgeons' directions.

Box 46.4

Patient Education After Posterior Total Hip Replacement

Reinforce education for patients to prevent hip dislocation as specified by the HCP after a posterior or anterior-lateral THR:
- Keep legs abducted (away from center of body) with pillows.
- Sleep with pillows between legs to prevent abduction and on side specified by HCP.
- Do not bend at the waist (hip) more than 90 degrees per HCP's instructions.
- Rise from a sitting position by pushing straight up off the chair or bed without leaning forward.
- Use a walker, if desired, to assist walking.
- Physiotherapy and occupational therapy can provide equipment that aids in putting on socks and shoes.
- Sexual activity can occur per HCP instructions when tolerated, provided hip safety measures are followed.

Patient Perspective

Bruce

I found my total joint replacement (TJR) surgery for hip osteoarthritis at age 71 to be easy and uneventful. Two years earlier, I had a total shoulder replacement, which also went smoothly and immediately relieved my shoulder pain from the arthritis. The shoulder rehabilitation was a month longer and more intense than for the total hip replacement. I found the shoulder replacement initially limited the performance of my ADLs more than did the hip replacement.

To prep for the hip surgery, I was instructed to shower the night before surgery and use antibacterial wipes over the surgical area and repeat the morning of surgery. My surgery took 2 hours, then I was back in my room and offered the option of being discharged that day (imagine that, the same day!) or the next day after 4 hours of "joint camp"—intense physical therapy (PT)/occupational therapy (OT) instruction and therapy. I went home after the joint camp and started 2 weeks of home PT (2 times a week) and 6 weeks of regular PT (3 times weekly). I had to be careful to prevent hip dislocation while doing my assigned exercises. I transferred from bed and ambulated into a chair with assistance about 4 hours after surgery. Later that night, I used a walker to ambulate up and down the hospital corridors. I used a cane for a month until I felt secure enough to walk without falling.

The most important thing my nurses did for me was to pay attention to my pain level to make sure I could get up and walk to start the healing process. The nurses were also attentive to getting me up and moving, a vital process in healing, and in establishing a rapport with me. The nurses also took time to make sure I understood the discharge procedures and what I was and was not to do when arriving home. My pain level after surgery was 8 out of 10. I was prescribed acetaminophen/hydrocodone (Norco) for pain relief at home.

I was able to walk, ride in the car, and climb stairs immediately with minimal pain, although I was told to limit the use of stairs. I had to have the transport person lift my leg into the car for my ride home from the hospital. Six months later, I am pain-free, and the numbness in my left quad is starting to resolve. The surgeon said it would take a year to fully heal. I did not start driving until about 4 weeks after surgery because it took time to rebuild the strength in my legs.

My recovery has gone smoothly, but it will require perseverance and 6 more months of exercise for a full recovery. It likely helped that I am married to a former ortho nurse. Nurses rock! I am happy I had the surgeries done so I can live pain-free while I exercise and play golf.

Total Knee Replacement

The knee is the second-most commonly replaced joint. It requires three components for total replacement: a femoral component, a tibial component, and a patellar button (Fig. 46.14). For patients who do not yet need a total replacement, partial knee resurfacing is available.

Nursing care for the patient with a total knee replacement (TKR) is similar to that required for a patient with a THR, except that dislocation and preventive positioning are not concerns. After surgery, a bulky dressing and possibly a surgical drain are in place. Again, it is important to monitor for bleeding along with usual postoperative interventions. Medical complications described for THR, such as DVT and infection, may occur with knee replacement.

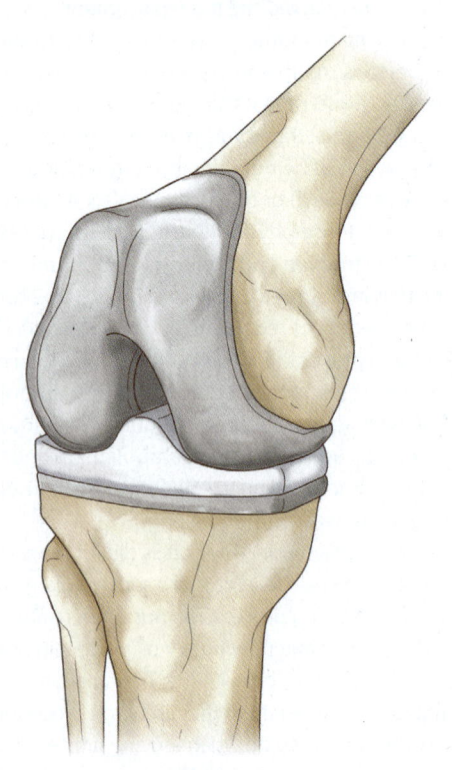

Amputation

An amputation is the removal of a body part. It can be as limited as removing part of a finger or as devastating as removing nearly half the body. Amputations may be *surgical* as a result of disease or *traumatic* as a result of an accident.

Surgical Amputation

The main reason for surgical amputations is ischemia from peripheral vascular disease in the older adult. The rate of lower extremity amputation is much higher in diabetic than nondiabetic patients (see Chapter 40). Surgical amputations may also be done for bone tumors, thermal injuries (e.g., frostbite, electric shock), crushing injuries, congenital problems, or infections.

Traumatic Amputation

Traumatic amputations occur from accidents. Industrial machinery, motor vehicles, lawn mowers, chain saws, and snow blowers are common causes of accidental amputation. In these patients the amputated part is usually healthy, so attempts at **replantation** can occur. Fingers are the most common replantations. Pre-hospital care of the severed body part is discussed in Chapter 13. The surgical procedure is performed by specialists who operate using a microscope. Nerves, vessels, and muscle must be reattached.

Levels of Amputation

The most common surgical amputation site is the lower extremity. The more proximal the amputation, the more disability is present. Loss of the great toe affects balance and gait. If the lower leg is amputated, a below-the-knee amputation is preferred over an above-the-knee amputation to preserve joint function. The higher the level of amputation, the more energy required for ambulation. Hip disarticulation (removal through the hip joint) and **hemipelvectomy** (removal through part of the pelvis) are reserved for young patients with cancer or severe trauma.

Upper extremity amputations are usually more significant than lower extremity amputations and more often result from trauma. The arms and hands are necessary for performing ADLs. Early replacement with a prosthesis is crucial to regain function in the patient with an upper extremity amputation.

Preoperative Care

Patients scheduled for elective amputations have the advantage of time for preoperative teaching, prosthesis fitting, grieving, and adjustment to the loss of part of their body.

Total knee replacement

FIGURE 46.14 Total knee replacement.

• WORD • BUILDING •

replantation: re—again + plant—to plant + ation—process
hemipelvectomy: hemi—half + pelv—pelvis + ectomy—removal of

Preoperatively, the patient should be referred to a certified prosthetist-orthotist to begin plans for replacing the removed body part with a prosthesis. Preoperative teaching is started in the surgeon's office. Postoperative and rehabilitative care is reviewed with the patient and family or significant other.

Patients experiencing a traumatic amputation cannot prepare for the significant changes that result from the accident. Preoperative care involves addressing both physical needs and significant psychological and emotional concerns, which continue postoperatively.

Disturbed Body Image is a common nursing diagnosis for the patient having an amputation. If possible, it is helpful for the preoperative patient to meet with a rehabilitated amputee. Note the patient's reaction to having an amputation. Expect that the patient will experience many of the stages of loss and grieving. Support systems and coping mechanisms are identified to help the patient through the surgery and postoperative period. Ensure that appropriate support is provided by other disciplines, such as social work and clergy.

Postoperative Care

In addition to the general postoperative care described here, plan and implement interventions to help prevent postoperative complications, including hemorrhage and infection (see Chapter 12).

PREVENTION OF INFECTION AND HEMORRHAGE. When a patient loses part of the body, because of either trauma or surgery, blood vessels are severed or damaged. The patient returns from surgery with a large pressure dressing secured with an elastic wrap. Monitor the closest proximal pulse between the heart and the amputated body part for strength. Compare findings with the nonsurgical extremity. Check the bulky dressing for bloody drainage. If blood is on the dressing when the patient is admitted to the postanesthesia care or surgical unit, circle, date, and time the area of drainage and closely monitor for enlargement. If bleeding continues, notify the surgeon immediately. A tourniquet should be readily available in case severe hemorrhage occurs.

After the dressing is removed, observe for adequate perfusion to the skin flap at the end of the residual limb, referred to as the *stump*. The skin should not be lighter or darker than the skin pigmentation in a patient who has dark skin. It should be pink in a patient who has light skin. The residual limb temperature should be warm but not hot to touch.

Infection of the wound can be problematic, especially if the infection enters the bone (osteomyelitis). Inspect the wound for intense redness or drainage. Localized infections usually do not cause an increase in body temperature. If temperature is elevated, it could indicate a serious wound infection or systemic infection. Traumatic amputations are at risk for infection due to the nature of the injury and the likelihood of exposure to environmental pathogens from the source of the amputation.

PAIN CONTROL. Phantom pain arises from the spinal cord and brain. The patient reports severe pain, usually distal to the removed body part, described as intense burning, cramping, shooting, stabbing, or throbbing. Never doubt that a patient is experiencing phantom pain. Phantom sensation is different from phantom pain in that with phantom sensation the patient feels as if the limb is still present rather than feeling pain. Phantom pain can be triggered by touching the residual limb, fatigue, emotional stress, or weather changes. It can improve over time.

Treat phantom pain with prescribed medication and complementary and alternative therapies. Medications used include anticonvulsants, such as gabapentin (Gralise, Neurontin) or pregabalin (Lyrica); beta-blocking agents, such as propranolol (Inderal); and antidepressants, such as amitriptyline (Elavil). To complement traditional therapy, alternative therapies may be useful, including biofeedback, nerve stimulation, myo-electric prosthesis, massage, mirror box (watching unaffected limb while moving), imagery, acupuncture, and spinal cord or brain stimulation (during which a small electric current is used). Future therapy may involve virtual reality goggles (during which it appears as if no amputation occurred).

MOBILITY AND AMBULATION. To reduce surgical swelling, cold application may be ordered. Alternatively, the residual limb may be elevated on a pillow for less than 24 hours. Continued elevation can lead to flexion contractures, especially with a below-the-knee or above-the-knee amputation. If the hip becomes contracted (abnormal shortening of muscle or scar tissue), the patient will not be able to use a prosthesis to walk. Check the limb periodically to ensure that it lies completely flat on the bed. The patient should avoid positions of flexion, such as sitting for long periods. If the patient is able, lying prone (on the stomach) for 30 minutes four times daily helps prevent hip contracture.

Postoperative care after amputation is interdisciplinary. It often requires an extensive rehabilitation program. The physical therapist teaches the patient muscle-strengthening exercises that help with ambulation and transfers and prevent flexion contractures. A trapeze bar on an overhead bed frame aids in strengthening the arms and helps the patient move around in bed.

PROSTHESIS CARE. The residual limb must be prepared for wearing the prosthesis. A temporary prosthesis may be worn until the swelling subsides. A shrinker sock is commonly used to decrease swelling and prepare the residual limb for the prosthesis. It is also worn with the prosthesis. It is important to perform neurovascular checks and check the residual limb for infection and alterations in tissue integrity each time the shrinker sock is removed.

The prosthesis requires special care. The patient should be taught to do the following:

- Clean the prosthesis socket with mild soap and water and then dry it.
- Clean inserts and liners regularly.
- Use garters to keep socks in place.
- Grease prosthesis parts as instructed by prosthetist.
- Replace shoes when worn out with shoes of the same height and type.

LIFESTYLE ADAPTATION. The patient may feel that life will be markedly changed as a result of amputation. The case manager may recommend job counseling with a vocational analyst or specialized case manager. With technological advances in prostheses, most patients who worked before surgery can return to their jobs after surgery. Many patients with amputations can continue many of the recreational hobbies they were able to do before surgery.

A supportive family or significant other is vital to help the patient adjust to body image change. Consider the need for a sexual counselor or psychologist if indicated. For any patient with an amputation, help the patient set realistic expectations.

For the patient who is not a candidate for a prosthesis, home adaptations for a wheelchair may be needed. The patient must have access to toileting facilities and areas necessary for self-care (see "Home Health Hints"). Structural changes in the living environment may be needed before the patient can be discharged from rehabilitation.

Home Health Hints

- If equipment or modifications to the home are needed following hospitalization for an orthopedic adaptation, it is best if they can be obtained or arranged before discharge.
- The home health nurse frequently removes staples and sutures. Always have several of each type of removal device on hand. Remember that staples, scissors, and other sharp items must be disposed of in a biohazard container or sturdy plastic container such as a detergent bottle.

- Physical and occupational therapy are often ordered for the orthopedic patient discharged from the hospital to help with strengthening, ambulation, ADLs, and access to and use of assistive devices (e.g., raised toilet seats, handheld reachers, walkers, canes, wheelchairs, and handrails).
- For safety have the patient remove all throw rugs, unnecessary furniture, and other possible fall hazards in the home.
- Reinforce teaching for the patient to wear flat, sturdy, rubber-soled shoes to prevent slipping, tripping, or turning an ankle.
- Reinforce to the patient to wear padded cycling gloves if the walker makes hands sore.
- Reinforce teaching for the patient that the risk of deep vein thrombosis (DVT) after hip or knee surgery is highest by the postoperative day five and that the risk persists for up to 12 weeks. Teach the patient to be alert for such signs as warmth, redness, edema, and increased pain of the affected leg.
- Reinforce instruction for the patient on how to put on their open-toed compression stockings more easily. Using a plastic bag, instruct the patient to tie a knot on the closed end. Slip the bag over the foot, and then put the stocking on over the bag. Once the stocking is on over the heel, the patient or caregiver can grab the knot in the plastic bag and pull the bag out through the toe opening.
- Reinforce teaching for the patient or a family member on how to give their injections to prevent DVT formation. If the patient cannot do this, the home health nurse can make visits to administer the injections.

Key Points

- Soft tissue injuries include sprains, strains, dislocations, bursitis, rotator cuff injury, and carpal tunnel syndrome.
- Fractures (a bone break) are caused by a fall, an accident, or a crushing injury. Bone disease, such as osteoporosis, metastatic bone cancer, malnutrition, and regular intake of carbonated beverages containing phosphoric acid (may interfere with calcium absorption) and some medications can cause fractures.
- A patient with a fracture often has other injuries. Observe for respiratory distress, bleeding, and head or spine injury.
- Treatment for fractures includes closed reduction, splints, casts, or traction and surgery called an *open reduction internal fixation*.
- External fixation is used for severe bone damage or numerous breaks.
- Although rare, acute compartment syndrome and fat embolism syndrome (more common with fractures of long bones) can be life threatening. Other complications include infection, hemorrhage, neurovascular impairment, thrombosis, and embolus.
- Osteomyelitis is an infection of bone that can be either acute (lasts less than 4 weeks) or chronic (lasts more than 4 weeks). Curative therapy can include surgical debridement, reconstruction, and antibiotics. Amputation may be necessary.
- Osteoporosis (porous bone) is a metabolic disorder with low bone mass and deterioration of bone structure, resulting in fragile bones that are prone to fracture.
- There is no cure for osteoporosis, but it can be treated. The cornerstone of treatment for osteoporosis is medication, nutrition, and controlling risk factors to prevent bone loss.
- Osteosarcoma, or osteogenic sarcoma, and Ewing sarcoma are common primary malignant bone tumors and usually affect young people between ages 10 and 25. Primary malignant tumors occurring in the prostate, breast, lung, and thyroid gland are called *bone-seeking cancers* because they migrate to bone more than any other primary cancer does.
- Gout is a systemic connective tissue disorder occurring from build-up of uric acid. Men, especially those middle-aged and older, are most affected.

- OA is a disease of the joint that affects all the joint's structures. Weight-bearing joints, hands, and the vertebral column are most often affected.
- Most patients residing in long-term care facilities also have OA, which can affect their participation in activities of daily living and recreational activities.
- RA is a chronic, progressive, systemic inflammatory disease that destroys synovial joints and connective tissues, including major organs. Dysfunction or failure of any organ or system can occur.
- Many patients experience spontaneous remissions and exacerbations (flare-ups) of RA.
- TJR is most often performed for patients who have some type of connective tissue disease in which their joints become severely deteriorated.
- Preventing hip dislocation after a THR is a primary nursing responsibility. Correct positioning of the surgical leg is critical: prevent hip adduction (across the body's midline) and hyperflexion (bending forward more than 90 degrees).
- The knee is the second-most commonly replaced joint with a femoral component, a tibial component, and a patellar button.
- The main reason for surgical amputations is ischemia from peripheral vascular disease in the older adult. Lower extremity amputation is higher in the diabetic patient than in the nondiabetic patient.
- *Disturbed body image* is a common nursing diagnosis for the patient having an amputation. Support systems and coping mechanisms are identified that can help the patient through the surgery and postoperative period.
- After amputation, the residual limb (stump) must be prepared for wearing the prosthesis. A temporary prosthesis may be worn until the swelling subsides.

SUGGESTED ANSWERS TO CHAPTER EXERCISES

Cue Recognition

46.1: Implementation of infection control interventions such as handwashing and sterile dressing changes to prevent infection.

46.2: Consider the patient may have compartment syndrome and contact HCP immediately.

Critical Thinking & Clinical Judgment

Mrs. Martinez

1. When documenting, answer the questions what, why, where, who, and how to make the charting complete.
   What = Patient found on the floor on her left side, moaning and holding her left leg, crying out with any movement.
   Why = Fall
   When = Date/time: 7/2, 1000
   Where = Day room
   Who = Mrs. Martinez (patient)
   How = Unknown, was not witnessed.
   Date/time: 7/2; 1000. Found on floor in day room lying on left side, moaning and holding left leg, crying out with any movement. Stated, "I fell. My leg hurts." Supervisor immediately notified paramedics, and HCP notified. BP [blood pressure] 150/84, P [pulse] 100, R [respirations] 20. Left leg shorter than right. Remained with patient and instructed not to move until paramedics arrived. Blankets applied and pillow under head. Taken to Memorial Hospital by ambulance at 1025. I. Smith, LPN
2. Skin and heel condition monitoring for pressure points; neurovascular checks on left leg. Weight is hanging freely.

Mr. Schnell

1. Possible priority nursing diagnoses include the following:
   - *Acute Pain* related to injury and immobility
   - *Risk for Constipation* related to opioids and immobility
   - *Risk for Impaired Skin Integrity* related to extended recovery time
   - *Social Isolation* related to hospitalization
   - *Decreased Diversional Activity Engagement* related to extended need for bedrest
2. Nursing interventions may include the following:
   - Monitor pain level; administer analgesics as ordered; check pain relief; check position for comfort; provide backrubs.
   - Ensure Mr. Schnell's diet includes fiber and adequate hydration (1.5 to 2 L/day); give stool softener as ordered; monitor daily bowel movements.
   - Ensure Mr. Schnell does the exercises recommended by occupational and physical therapists; reposition him every 2 to 3 hours; have trapeze bar set up for him to use; use skin assessment tool to determine risk for skin breakdown; check for pressure points and signs and symptoms of skin breakdown.
   - Encourage Mr. Schnell's family and friends to alternate visits; request referral to an occupational therapist to assess his social needs.
   - Encourage him to listen to music; encourage visitors; ensure access to hobbies, videos, books, magazines, and comics.

Mr. Kardos

1. Data collection: Neurovascular check including the six Ps; pain level; vital signs.
2. The need to bivalve the cast with evaluation of the extremity by the HCP to determine if further treatment, such as a fasciotomy, is needed.

Mr. Finn

1. Where is your pain located (one or both knees)?
   - Describe your joint pain.
   - "What is your typical day on the job like?"
   - "Do certain activities increase joint pain?"
   - "When is your pain worse: after activity or after rest?"
   - "How long have you experienced joint pain?"
   - "What relieves the joint pain?"

SUGGESTED ANSWERS TO CHAPTER EXERCISES—cont'd

2. Risk factors include that he is overweight, is in late middle age, and has a physically demanding job causing wear and tear.
3. Patient-centered care interventions include pain management, education on weight loss, restoring and maintaining functional ability (e.g., bending ability for work).
4. HCP, occupational therapist, pharmacist, physical therapist, registered nurse.

Mrs. Harris

1. Ask what the nature of her pain is, whether it is worse after activity or rest, and whether she experiences joint stiffness and, if so, when. Follow the **WHAT'S UP?** method of pain data collection.
2. Explain to Mrs. Harris how to balance rest with exercise; to consider use of ice for very hot, swollen joints and heat to decrease stiffness.
3. Observe for joint deformities and indicators of secondary osteoporosis (bone loss).

Mrs. Adam

Unit analysis method:

$$\frac{500 \text{ mg}}{} \times \frac{5 \text{ mL}}{375 \text{ mg}} = 6.7 \text{ mL}$$

Additional Resources

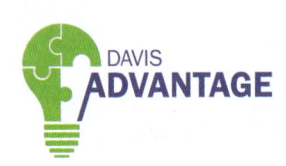

Go to Davis Advantage to complete your learning: strengthen understanding, apply your knowledge, and prepare for the Next Gen NCLEX®.

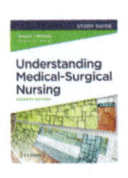

A Study Guide is also available.

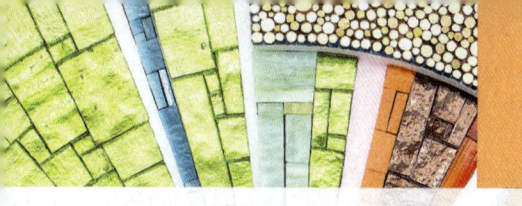

UNIT THIRTEEN Understanding the Neurologic System

CHAPTER 47
Neurologic System Function, Data Collection, and Therapeutic Measures

Heather Thorton, Linda K. Cook, Janice L. Bradford

KEY TERMS

anisocoria (an-ih-suh-KOR-ee-ah)
aphasia (ah-FAY-zhee-ah)
contractures (kon-TRAK-churs)
decerebrate (dee-SER-eh-brayt)
decorticate (dee-KOR-tih-kayt)
dysarthria (dis-AR-three-ah)
dysphagia (dis-FAY-jee-ah)
electroencephalogram (ee-LEK-troh-en-SEF-uh-loh-gram)
myelogram (MY-eh-loh-gram)
nystagmus (nih-STAG-mus)
paresis (puh-REE-sis)
paresthesia (PAR-es-THEE-zhee-ah)
subarachnoid (SUB-uh-RAK-noyd)

CHAPTER CONCEPTS

Cognition
Neurologic regulation

LEARNING OUTCOMES

1. Describe the normal structures and functions of the nervous system.
2. Identify the effects of aging on the nervous system.
3. List data to collect when caring for a patient with a disorder of the nervous system.
4. Identify tests used to diagnose disorders of the nervous system.
5. Plan nursing care for patients undergoing diagnostic tests for disorders of the nervous system.
6. Describe common therapeutic measures for patients with disorders of the nervous system.

NORMAL NEUROLOGIC SYSTEM ANATOMY AND PHYSIOLOGY

The nervous system has two divisions: the central nervous system (CNS), which consists of the brain and spinal cord, and the peripheral nervous system (PNS), which includes the nerves of the autonomic nervous system (ANS). Electrical impulses are transmitted through the nervous system to permit sensory, motor, and integrative activity. Actions are either automatic by reflex or a result of gathering, organizing, and processing data.

Nerve Tissue

Nerve tissue consists of neurons and support cells called neuroglia. Neurons are diverse, including unipolar, bipolar, and multipolar anatomy. Most common is the multipolar neuron with multiple dendrites and a singular axon (Fig. 47.1).

Myelination of axons increases their conduction speed. The level of myelination correlates to the necessity of speed. For example, neurons involved in protective reflexes are heavily myelinated, whereas processing neurons of the CNS lack myelin.

Neuroglial cells include oligodendrocytes, which produce myelin; microglia, which perform phagocytosis; astrocytes, which contribute to the blood-brain barrier; and ependyma, which are involved in production of cerebrospinal fluid (CSF).

Types of Neurons

Functional classification of neurons considers their position and direction of signal: a neuron is a sensory neuron (afferent), a motor neuron

The **cell body** (also called the **soma**) is the control center of the neuron and contains the nucleus.

Dendrites, which look like the bare branches of a tree, receive signals from other neurons and conduct the information to the cell body. Some neurons have only one dendrite; others have thousands.

The **axon**, which carries nerve signals away from the body, is longer than the dendrites and contains few branches. Neurons have only one axon; however, the length of the fiber can range from a few millimeters to as much as a meter.

The axons of many (but not all) neurons are encased in a **myelin sheath**. Consisting mostly of lipid, myelin acts to insulate the axon. In the peripheral nervous system, Schwann cells form the myelin sheath. In the CNS, oligodendrocytes assume this role.

Gaps in the myelin sheath, called **neurofibral nodes** (previously called **nodes of Ranvier**), occur at evenly spaced intervals.

The end of the axon branches extensively, with each axon terminal ending in a **synaptic knob**. Within the synaptic knobs are vesicles containing a neurotransmitter.

Nucleus

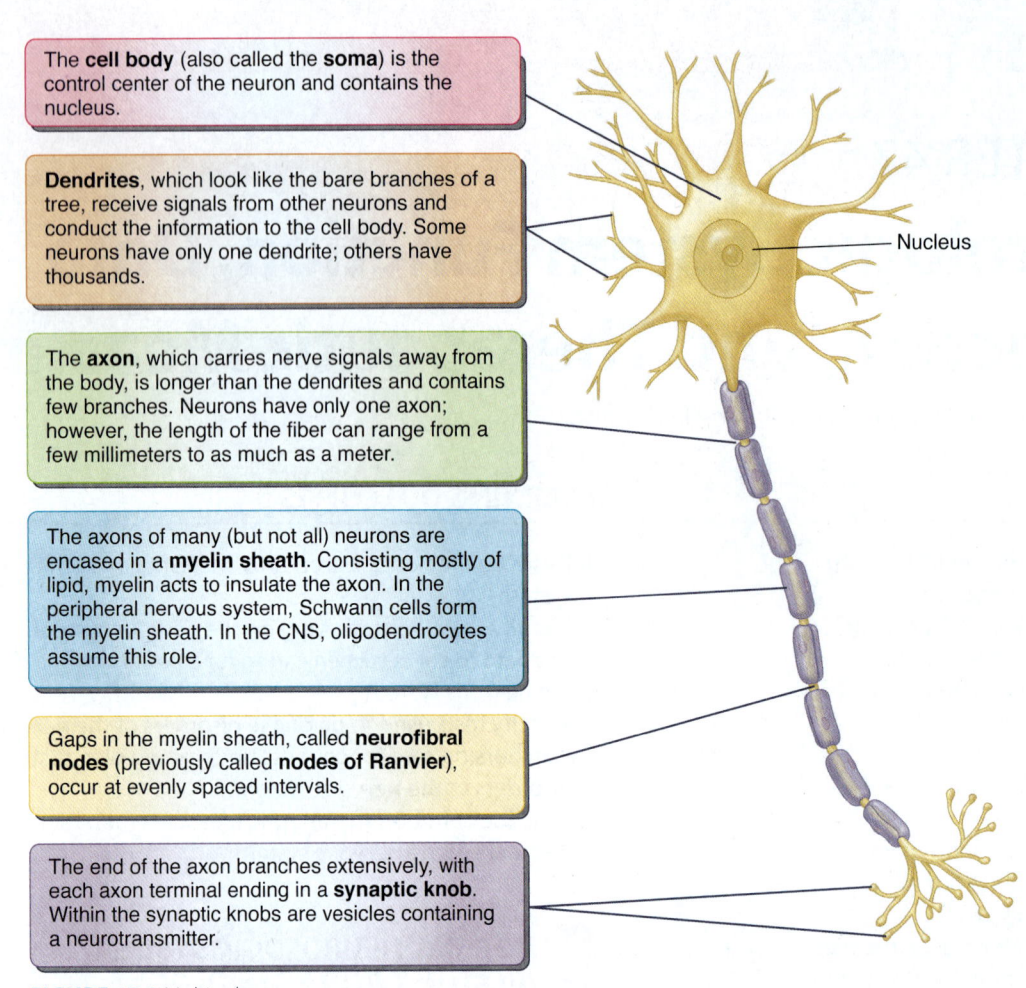

FIGURE 47.1 Multipolar neuron structure.

(efferent), or an interneuron (between the afferent and efferent neurons; Fig. 47.2). Receptors are specialized to detect external or internal changes and then generate electrical impulses. Sensory neurons from receptors in the skin, skeletal muscles, and joints are called *somatic*. Sensory neurons from receptors in internal organs are called *visceral sensory neurons*. Motor neurons that innervate skeletal muscle are called *somatic*. Motor neurons that innervate smooth muscle, cardiac muscle, and glands are called *visceral*.

LEARNING TIP
To remember the difference between *afferent* and *efferent*, try these clues:
- **A**fferent: A is for affect, or sense.
- **E**fferent: E is for effect (action).

Or, think of the alphabet—**A** before **E**: You have to feel or sense (afferent) a stimulus before you can take action (efferent).

Nerve Impulses
A nerve impulse, also called an *action potential*, is a change in the electrical signal of a neuron; the change is caused by the movement of ions across the neuron cell membrane. A neuron at rest is polarized with a positive charge outside the membrane and a relatively negative charge inside the membrane. A threshold stimulus causes a reversal in charge (action potential). A wave of depolarization travels the length of the neuron as a positive feedback loop. Repolarization occurs immediately after, restoring the positive charge outside and the negative charge inside. After a *refractory period* (the brief time after being stimulated when a nerve cannot react to another stimulus), the neuron is polarized again and ready to respond to another stimulus. A myelinated neuron is capable of transmitting hundreds of impulses per second and at speeds of more than 100 meters per second.

Synapses
Neurons typically work in a circuit. When the axon of a neuron must transmit an impulse to the dendrite or cell body of another neuron, the impulse has to cross a small gap called a *synapse*. An electrical impulse is incapable of crossing this microscopic space, so when an impulse reaches the synapse, impulse transmission becomes chemical.

At chemical synapses, impulse transmission is one-way because the neurotransmitter is released only by the presynaptic neuron; the impulse cannot go backward. This is important

FIGURE 47.2 Neurons: sensory, interneurons, motor.

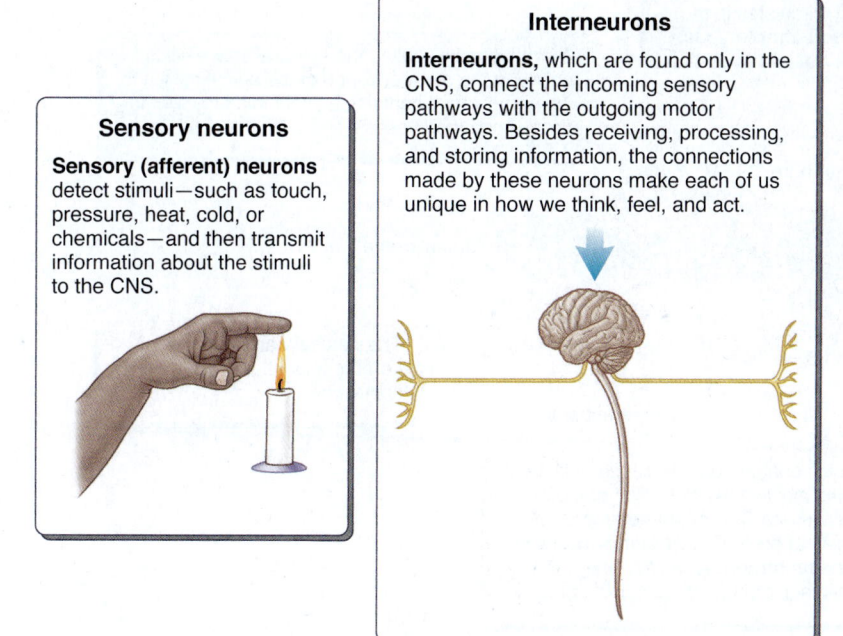

Sensory neurons
Sensory (afferent) neurons detect stimuli—such as touch, pressure, heat, cold, or chemicals—and then transmit information about the stimuli to the CNS.

Interneurons
Interneurons, which are found only in the CNS, connect the incoming sensory pathways with the outgoing motor pathways. Besides receiving, processing, and storing information, the connections made by these neurons make each of us unique in how we think, feel, and act.

Motor neurons
Motor (efferent) neurons relay messages from the brain (which the brain emits in response to stimuli) to the muscle or gland cells.

for the normal activity of functional neurons. The relative complexity of synapses also makes them a potential target for the actions of medications. For example, some antidepressants block the reuptake (reabsorption) of serotonin, a neurotransmitter, back into the proximal nerve endings, increasing the mood-elevating serotonin levels in the synapse.

Nerves and Nerve Tracts

A nerve (whether cranial, spinal, or peripheral) is a group of axons with blood vessels, wrapped in connective tissue. Most nerves are mixed, containing both sensory and motor neurons, but some are not; the optic nerve for vision is sensory only, and autonomic nerves are purely motor.

A nerve tract is a group of thickly myelinated neurons within the CNS; such tracts within white matter appear white due to the myelin sheaths. A nerve tract within the spinal cord carries sensory or motor impulses; those within the brain have sensory, motor, or integrative functions.

Spinal Cord

The spinal cord transmits impulses to and from the brain. It is the integrating center for spinal cord reflexes. The spinal cord is within the vertebral canal formed by the vertebrae of the skeleton. It extends from the foramen magnum of the occipital bone to the intervertebral disc between the first and second lumbar vertebrae. The spinal nerves emerge from the intervertebral foramina.

In cross section, the spinal cord is oval-shaped; internally, it has an H-shaped mass of gray matter surrounded by white matter (Fig. 47.3). Each spinal nerve attaches to the cord by two roots: dorsal and ventral. Meninges (three concentric, external layers of connective tissue) and circulating CSF offer further protection to the spinal cord.

Spinal Nerves

The 31 pairs of spinal nerves are named according to their respective vertebrae: 8 cervical pairs, 12 thoracic, 5 lumbar, 5 sacral, and 1 coccygeal (Fig. 47.4). These nerves are often referred to by letter and number: the second cervical nerve is C2, the tenth thoracic is T10, and so on.

Spinal Cord Reflexes

A reflex is a fast, involuntary, automatic, and predictable response to a stimulus. A spinal cord reflex uses a neural circuit, independent of the brain, called a *spinal reflex arc*. Sensory input triggers motor output.

The somatic spinal cord reflexes include stretch and flexor reflexes (Fig. 47.5). In a stretch reflex, a stretched muscle automatically contracts (e.g., the familiar patellar reflex). All skeletal muscles have such a reflex to keep the body upright without requiring conscious processing as gravity exerts its constant force on the body. Stretch reflexes also prevent potential injury from overstretching a muscle.

Flexor reflexes may also be called *withdrawal* reflexes: the stimulus is painful trauma to tissue, and the response is to pull away from it. Again, this occurs without conscious thought; the brain is not directly involved.

The clinical testing of spinal cord reflexes provides a way to determine the functioning of their reflex arcs. For example, if the patellar reflex is absent, the problem might be in the quadriceps femoris muscle, the femoral nerve, or the spinal cord itself. If the reflex is present, it indicates that all parts of the reflex arc are functioning normally.

UNIT THIRTEEN Understanding the Neurologic System

White matter appears white because of its abundance of myelin. It contains bundles of axons (called **tracts**) that carry impulses from one part of the nervous system to another.

CSF circulates in the **subarachnoid space.**

A small space—called the epidural space—lies between the outer covering of the spinal cord and the vertebrae; it contains a cushioning layer of fat as well as blood vessels and connective tissue.

Posterior horn
Anterior horn
Spinal nerve
Vertebral body

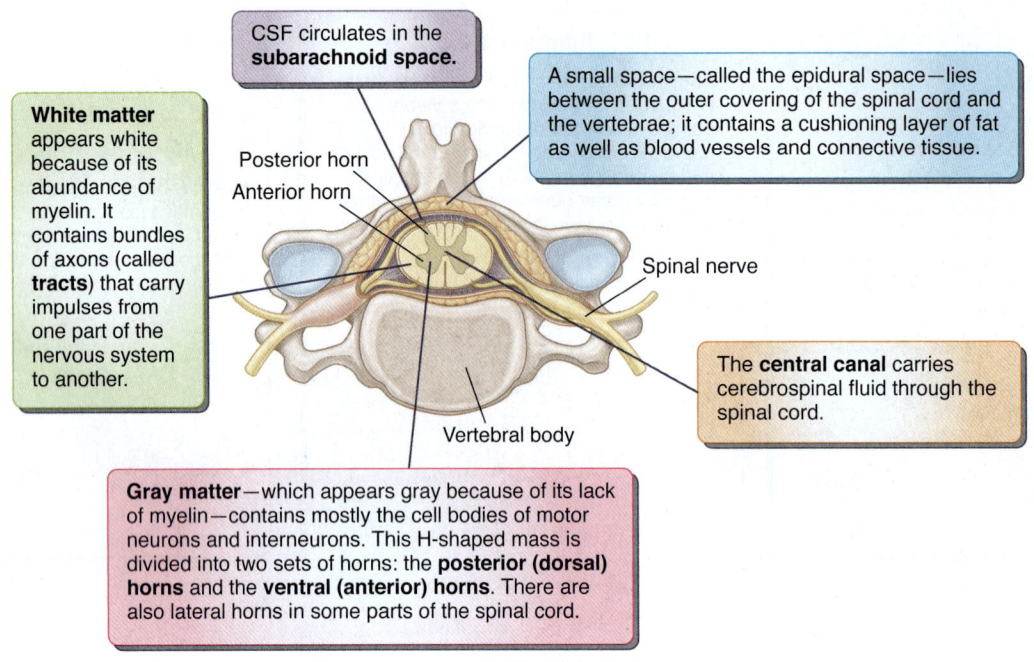

The **central canal** carries cerebrospinal fluid through the spinal cord.

Gray matter—which appears gray because of its lack of myelin—contains mostly the cell bodies of motor neurons and interneurons. This H-shaped mass is divided into two sets of horns: the **posterior (dorsal) horns** and the **ventral (anterior) horns**. There are also lateral horns in some parts of the spinal cord.

FIGURE 47.3 Spinal cord—internal anatomy, cross section, superior view.

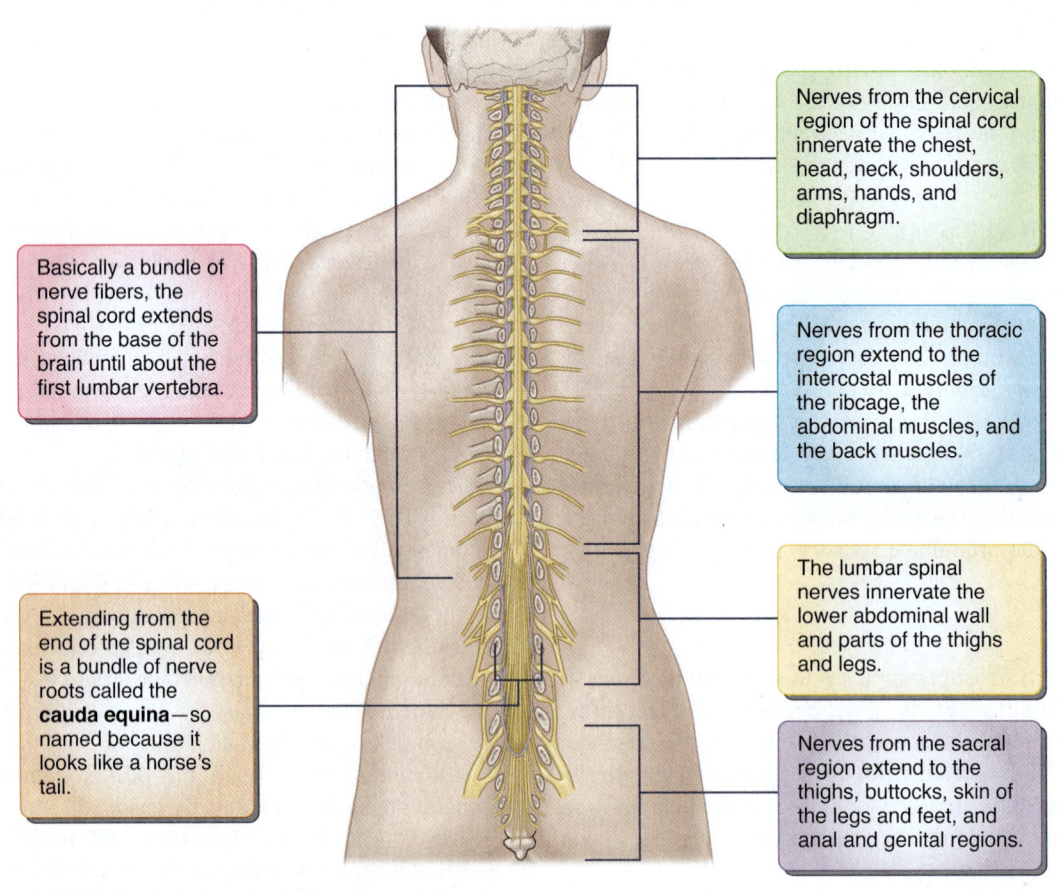

Nerves from the cervical region of the spinal cord innervate the chest, head, neck, shoulders, arms, hands, and diaphragm.

Basically a bundle of nerve fibers, the spinal cord extends from the base of the brain until about the first lumbar vertebra.

Nerves from the thoracic region extend to the intercostal muscles of the ribcage, the abdominal muscles, and the back muscles.

The lumbar spinal nerves innervate the lower abdominal wall and parts of the thighs and legs.

Extending from the end of the spinal cord is a bundle of nerve roots called the **cauda equina**—so named because it looks like a horse's tail.

Nerves from the sacral region extend to the thighs, buttocks, skin of the legs and feet, and anal and genital regions.

FIGURE 47.4 Spinal cord—full length, posterior view.

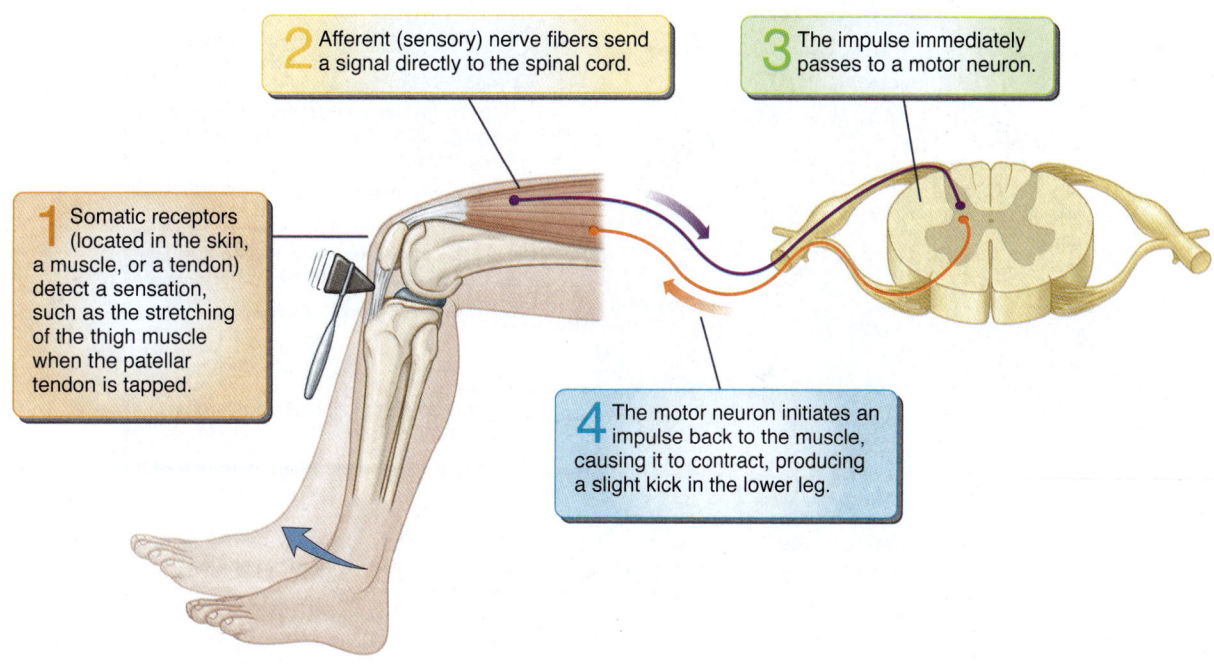

FIGURE 47.5 Somatic spinal reflex.

1. Somatic receptors (located in the skin, a muscle, or a tendon) detect a sensation, such as the stretching of the thigh muscle when the patellar tendon is tapped.
2. Afferent (sensory) nerve fibers send a signal directly to the spinal cord.
3. The impulse immediately passes to a motor neuron.
4. The motor neuron initiates an impulse back to the muscle, causing it to contract, producing a slight kick in the lower leg.

Brain

The brain consists of many parts that function as an integrated whole. The four principal areas are the cerebrum, diencephalon (thalamus and hypothalamus), brainstem (midbrain, pons, and medulla oblongata), and cerebellum (Fig. 47.6).

Meninges

The meninges are the three layers of connective tissue that cover the CNS. Where they enclose the brain, they are referred to as *cranial meninges*.

Ventricles and Cerebrospinal Fluid

The ventricles are four cavities within the brain: two lateral ventricles are located within the cerebral hemispheres, the third ventricle lays midline within the thalamus, and the fourth ventricle is midline between the brainstem and cerebellum. CSF is formed from capillaries of the choroid plexus within and circulates through the four ventricles. Circulation of CSF moves inferiorly within the CNS, into the **subarachnoid** space, and ultimately superiorly to drain into the dural venous sinuses. CSF permits the exchange of nutrients and wastes between the blood and CNS neurons. It also acts as a cushion or shock absorber for the CNS. The pressure and constituents of CSF may be determined by means of a lumbar puncture (spinal tap) and may be helpful in the diagnosis of diseases such as meningitis.

Brainstem: Midbrain, Pons, and Medulla Oblongata

Primarily a reflex center, the midbrain regulates visual reflexes (coordinated movement of the eyes), auditory reflexes (turning the ear toward a sound), and righting reflexes that keep the head upright and contribute to balance. Within the pons are two respiratory centers that work with those in the medulla oblongata to produce a normal breathing rhythm. The medulla oblongata lies just superior to the spinal cord. It regulates the most vital life functions.

Cerebellum

The cerebellum is posterior to the brainstem. The functions of the cerebellum include the involuntary aspects of voluntary movement: coordination, appropriate direction and endpoint of movements, and maintenance of posture and balance. For balance maintenance, the cerebellum uses input from vision, proprioceptors, and equilibrium receptors in the inner ear to detect movement and changes in position.

Diencephalon: Thalamus and Hypothalamus

Deep beneath the cerebral hemispheres, the diencephalon consists primarily of the thalamus and hypothalamus. Above the brainstem, the thalamus acts as a gateway for nearly every sensation traveling to the cerebral cortex. The thalamus filters sensory input, permitting the cerebrum to concentrate on more important sensations with less distraction. The hypothalamus suspends the pituitary gland from a stalk called the infundibulum; they are anatomically and physiologically connected.

Cerebrum

The two cerebral hemispheres form the largest part of the human brain. These right and left hemispheres are connected

• WORD • BUILDING •

subarachnoid: sub—below + arachnoid—middle layer of the meninges

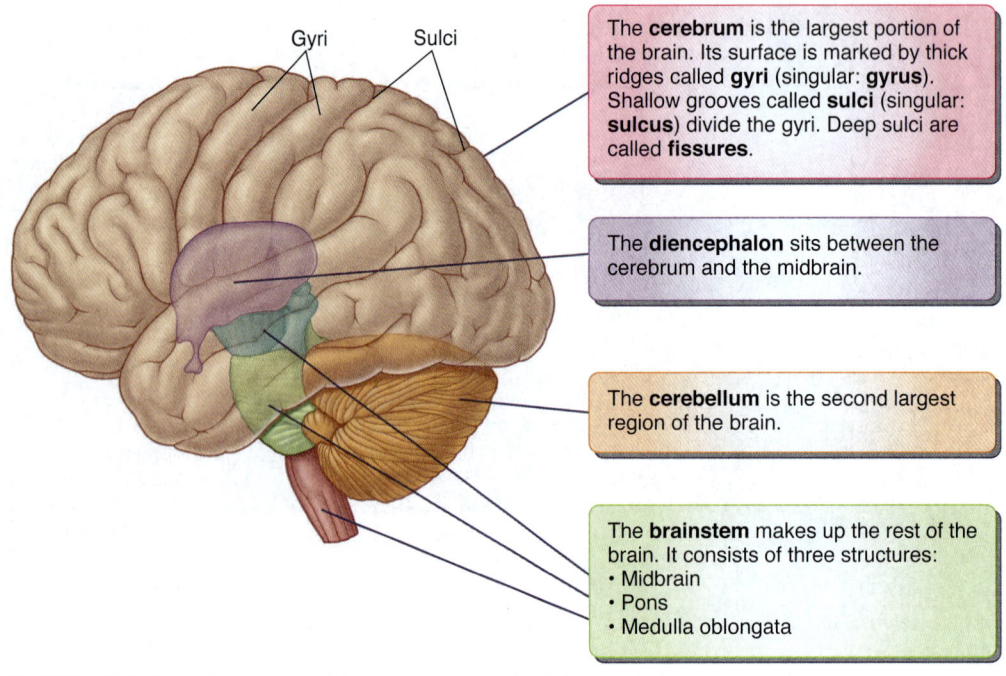

FIGURE 47.6 General structures of the brain—external, left lateral view.

- The **cerebrum** is the largest portion of the brain. Its surface is marked by thick ridges called **gyri** (singular: **gyrus**). Shallow grooves called **sulci** (singular: **sulcus**) divide the gyri. Deep sulci are called **fissures**.
- The **diencephalon** sits between the cerebrum and the midbrain.
- The **cerebellum** is the second largest region of the brain.
- The **brainstem** makes up the rest of the brain. It consists of three structures:
  - Midbrain
  - Pons
  - Medulla oblongata

primarily by the corpus callosum, a band of about 300 million nerve fibers. The cerebral cortex is folded extensively into convolutions (or gyri) that create more surface area for neurons. The deep grooves between the folds are called *fissures*; shallow grooves are called *sulci*. The cerebral cortex is divided into lobes, whose functions have been extensively mapped (Fig. 47.7).

Collectively, the cerebral cortex has areas that enable learning, memory, and thought. It helps form our personalities with complex behaviors that require integration of several cerebral and lower brain areas.

Deep within the white matter of the cerebral hemispheres are masses of gray matter called the *basal nuclei* (*ganglia*). Their functions are concerned with certain subconscious aspects of voluntary movement: regulation of muscle tone, inhibiting tremor, and use of accessory movements such as arm swinging when walking.

LEARNING TIP
The cranial nerves are easier to remember when a mnemonic device is used:

On	Olfactory
Old	Optic
Olympus's	Oculomotor
Towering	Trochlear
Top	Trigeminal
A	Abducens
Finn	Facial
Very	Vestibulocochlear
Graciously	Glossopharyngeal
Viewed	Vagal
A	Accessory
Hop	Hypoglossal

Cranial Nerves

The 12 pairs of cranial nerves emerge from the brainstem except for pair one, which originates from the temporal lobe, and pair two, which originates from the occipital lobe. Some are purely sensory nerves, but others are mixed nerves. The impulses for sight, smell, hearing, taste, equilibrium, and somatic senses of supplied areas are carried by cranial nerves to their respective sensory areas in the brain. Other cranial nerves carry motor impulses to muscles of the face, neck, shoulders, and tongue or to glands. Cranial nerves III, VII, IX, and X contain axons of the somatic and autonomic nervous systems. Table 47.1 summarizes functions of the cranial nerves.

Autonomic Nervous System

The ANS motor output provides dual innervation to effectors—that is, smooth muscle, cardiac muscle, and glands that produce the response (effect). These two divisions (sympathetic and parasympathetic) function in opposition to one other. Their activity is integrated by the hypothalamus. Table 47.2 summarizes both ANS divisions.

Sympathetic Division

The cell bodies of the sympathetic preganglionic neurons are thoracolumbar (in the thoracic and lumbar segments of the spinal cord; Fig. 47.8). The sympathetic division is dominant in stressful situations such as fear, anger, anxiety,

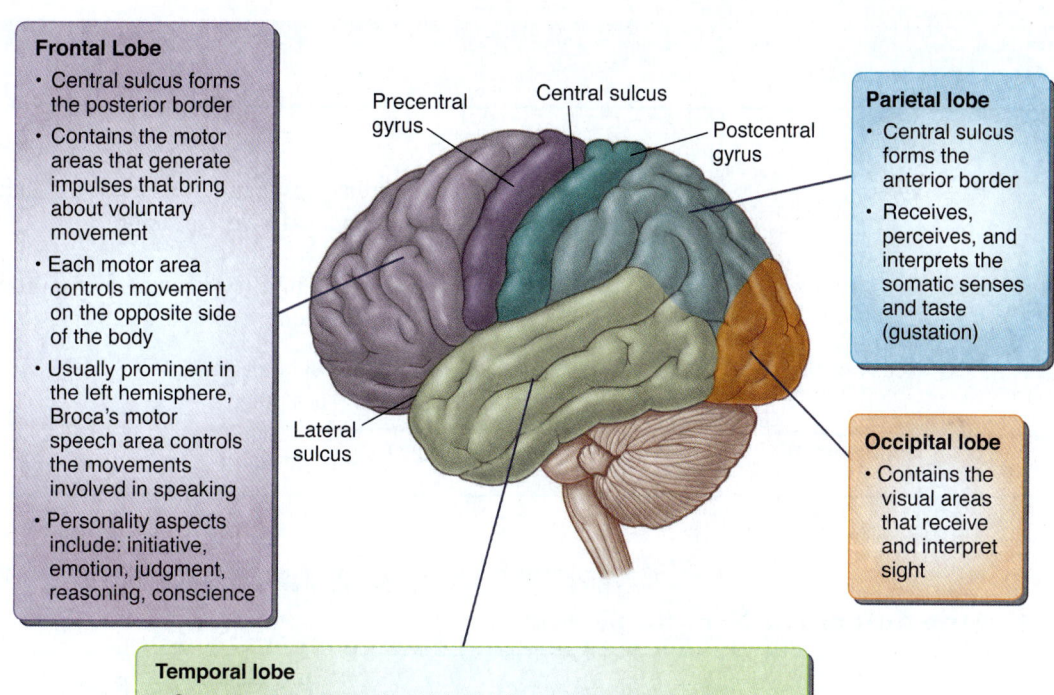

Chapter 47 Neurologic System Function, Data Collection, and Therapeutic Measures

Frontal Lobe
- Central sulcus forms the posterior border
- Contains the motor areas that generate impulses that bring about voluntary movement
- Each motor area controls movement on the opposite side of the body
- Usually prominent in the left hemisphere, Broca's motor speech area controls the movements involved in speaking
- Personality aspects include: initiative, emotion, judgment, reasoning, conscience

Parietal lobe
- Central sulcus forms the anterior border
- Receives, perceives, and interprets the somatic senses and taste (gustation)

Occipital lobe
- Contains the visual areas that receive and interpret sight

Temporal lobe
- Separated from the parietal lobe by the lateral sulcus
- Contains sensory areas for hearing and olfaction (smell)
- Visual recognition
- Also in the temporal and parietal lobes, usually only on the left side, is Wernicke's area where comprehension of speech occurs.

FIGURE 47.7 Cerebrum—lobes, left lateral view.

Table 47.1
Cranial Nerves

Number	Name	Function
I	Olfactory	Sense of smell
II	Optic	Sense of sight
III	Oculomotor	Movement of eyeball Constriction of pupil for bright light or near vision
IV	Trochlear	Movement of eyeball
V	Trigeminal	Sensation in face, scalp, and teeth Contraction of chewing muscles
VI	Abducens	Movement of eyeball
VII	Facial	Sense of taste Contraction of facial muscles Secretion of saliva
VIII	Vestibulocochlear	Sense of hearing Sense of equilibrium
IX	Glossopharyngeal	Sense of taste Secretion of saliva Sensory input for cardiac, respiratory, and blood pressure reflexes Contraction of pharynx, swallowing

Continued

Table 47.1
Cranial Nerves—cont'd

Number	Name	Function
X	Vagus	Sensory input in cardiac, respiratory, and blood pressure reflexes Sensory and motor input to larynx (speaking) Decreased heart rate Contraction of alimentary tube (swallowing, peristalsis) Increased digestive secretions
XI	Accessory	Contraction of neck and shoulder muscles Motor input to larynx (speaking)
XII	Hypoglossal	Movement of the tongue

Table 47.2
Functions of the Autonomic Nervous System

Organ	Sympathetic Response	Parasympathetic Response
Heart (cardiac muscle)	Increase rate	Decrease rate (to normal)
Bronchioles (smooth muscle)	Dilate	Constrict (to normal)
Iris (smooth muscle)	Dilate pupil	Constrict pupil (to normal)
Salivary glands	Decrease secretion	Increase secretion (to normal)
Stomach and intestines (smooth muscle)	Decrease peristalsis	Increase peristalsis for normal digestion
Stomach and intestines (glands)	Decrease secretion	Increase secretion for normal digestion
Internal anal sphincter	Contract to prevent defecation	Relax to permit defection
Urinary bladder (smooth muscle)	Relax to prevent urination	Contract for normal urination
Internal urethral sphincter	Contract to prevent urination	Relax to permit urination
Liver	Change glycogen to glucose	None
Sweat glands	Increase secretion	None
Blood vessels in skin and viscera (smooth muscle)	Constrict	None
Blood vessels in skeletal muscle (smooth muscle)	Dilate	None
Adrenal glands	Increase secretion of epinephrine and norepinephrine	None

excitement, and exercise. The responses prepare the body for physical activity, whether it is actually needed. Heart rate increases, vasodilation in skeletal muscles increases oxygen and glucose supply, bronchioles dilate to take in more oxygen, and the liver converts glycogen to glucose to provide energy. The neurotransmitters of the sympathetic division are acetylcholine and norepinephrine. Acetylcholine is released by sympathetic preganglionic neurons; its inactivator is acetylcholinesterase. Norepinephrine is released by most sympathetic postganglionic neurons at the synapses with the effector cells; its inactivator is catechol O-methyltransferase (COMT) or monoamine oxidase (MAO).

Chapter 47 Neurologic System Function, Data Collection, and Therapeutic Measures

Sympathetic preganglionic neurons begin within the spinal cord.

From the cell bodies, myelinated fibers reach to sympathetic ganglia, most of which exist in chains along both sides of the spinal cord (even though the illustration here depicts the ganglia only along one side). Because the ganglia lie close to the spinal cord, the preganglionic neurons are short.

Not all preganglionic neurons synapse in the first ganglion they encounter. Some travel up or down the chain to synapse with other ganglia at different levels. Others pass through the first ganglion to synapse with another ganglion a short distance away.

Unmyelinated postganglionic fibers leave the ganglia and extend to the target organs. Postganglionic fibers tend to be long.

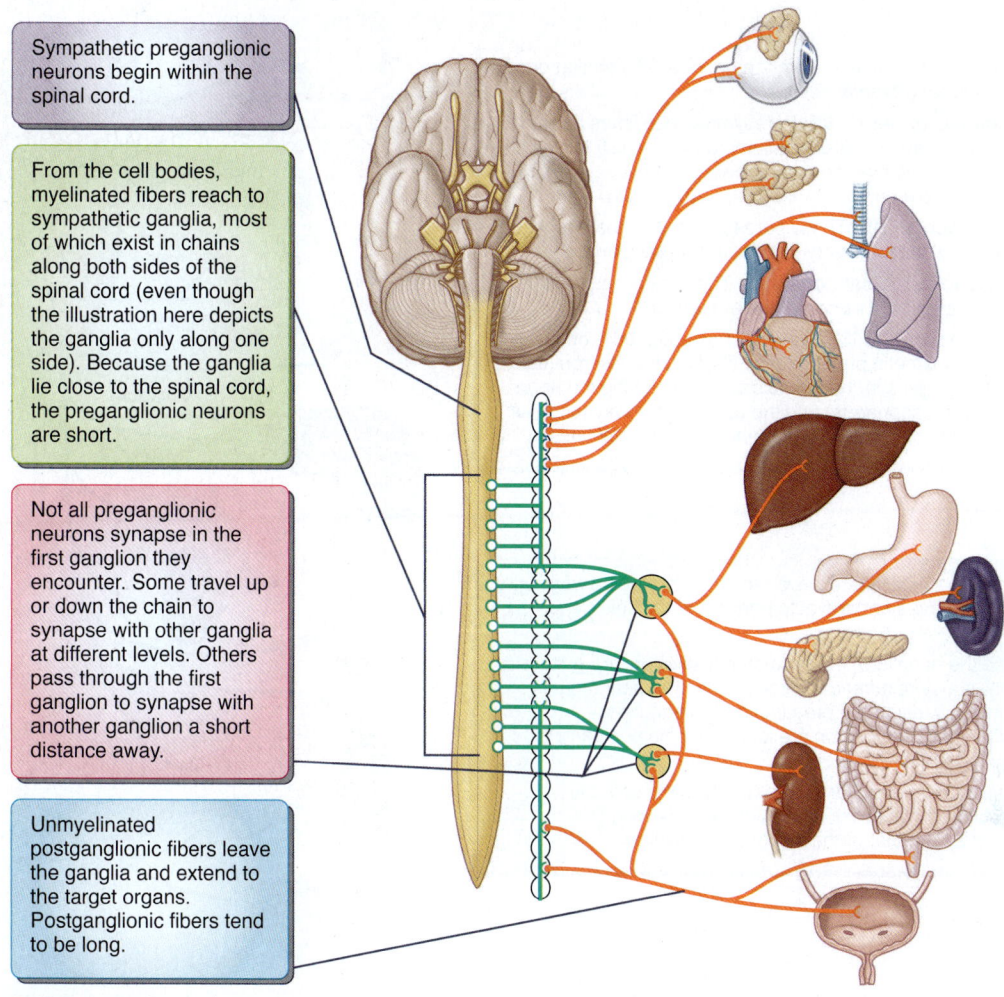

FIGURE 47.8 Sympathetic nervous system.

Parasympathetic Division

Cell bodies of the parasympathetic preganglionic neurons are craniosacral—they exist in the brainstem and sacral segments of the spinal cord (Fig. 47.9). The parasympathetic division dominates during relaxed, stress-free situations to promote normal functioning of several organ systems. Digestion proceeds normally, with increased secretions and peristalsis; defecation and urination may occur; and the heart beats at a normal resting rate (see Table 47.2). Acetylcholine is the neurotransmitter at all parasympathetic synapses, both preganglionic and postganglionic; it is inactivated by acetylcholinesterase.

CRITICAL THINKING & CLINICAL JUDGMENT

Mrs. Stevens received albuterol treatments for her chronic obstructive pulmonary disease (COPD) exacerbation. The medication opened her airways effectively, but after her treatment, she reports that her heart is racing.

Critical Thinking (The Why)
1. What part of the parasympathetic nervous system do you think this medication affects?

Clinical Judgment (The Do)
2. What should you do?

Suggested answers are at the end of the chapter.

PRACTICE ANALYSIS TIP
Linking NCLEX-PN® to Practice
The LPN/LVN provides care that meets the needs of adult clients ages 65 and over.

Aging and the Nervous System

With age, the brain loses neurons. However, this loss represents only a small percentage of the total and is not the usual cause of mental impairment in older adults. Far more common causes of mental changes include depression, malnutrition, infection, hypotension, and side effects of medications. Some forgetfulness and decreased problem-solving ability can be expected. Figure 47.10 presents a concept map showing the effects of the aging process on the neurologic system.

Parasympathetic fibers leave the brainstem by joining one of the following cranial nerves:
- **Oculomotor nerve (III):** Parasympathetic fibers carried in this nerve innervate the ciliary muscle, which thickens the lens of the eye, and the pupillary constrictor, which constricts the pupil.
- **Facial nerve (VII):** These parasympathetic fibers regulate the tear glands, salivary glands, and nasal glands.
- **Glossopharyngeal nerve (IX):** The parasympathetic fibers carried in this nerve trigger salivation.
- **Vagus nerve (X):** This nerve carries about 90% of all parasympathetic preganglionic fibers. It travels from the brain to organs in the thoracic cavity (including the heart, lung, and esophagus) and the abdominal cavity (such as the stomach, liver, kidneys, pancreas, and intestines).

Parasympathetic fibers leave the sacral region by way of pelvic nerves and travel to portions of the colon and bladder.

Unlike the ganglia of the sympathetic division, the ganglia of the parasympathetic division reside in or near the target organ. As a result, the preganglionic fibers of the parasympathetic division are long while the postganglionic fibers are short.

Because the ganglia are more widely dispersed, the parasympathetic division produces a more localized response than that of the sympathetic division.

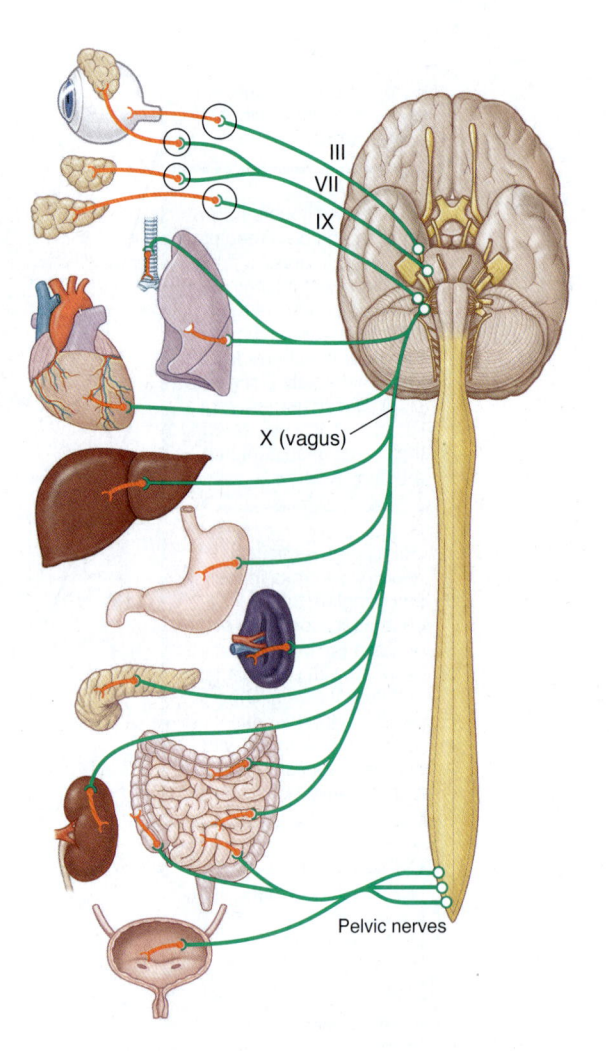

FIGURE 47.9 Parasympathetic nervous system.

NEUROLOGIC SYSTEM DATA COLLECTION

The focus of data collection is to establish the present function of the patient's neurologic system and detect changes from previous observations. A complete neurologic assessment, intended to determine the existence of neurologic disease, is performed by a health-care provider (HCP). Baseline neurologic data collection should be performed on every patient admission (Box 47.1). The data collected provides valuable information about the current functioning of the patient's neurologic system, as well as baseline data for later comparison. This is especially important if the patient has chronic neurologic deficits on admission.

Consider a patient admitted for surgery who had a previous stroke resulting in **paresis** (weakness or partial paralysis) of the right arm. Complete preoperative neurologic data collection would document that the right arm is weaker than the left. If during the postoperative course you find that both arms are equal in strength (i.e., both arms have become equally weak), you would notify the HCP so the patient could be evaluated related to the acute weakness of the left arm.

LEARNING TIP

Sympathetic—S is for STRESS RESPONSE. The sympathetic response is referred to as the *fight-or-flight response*. When thinking of the sympathetic nervous system, imagine getting away from a lion. You need dilated pupils to see the path better, copious production of sweat to lose heat through evaporation, increased rate and force of heart contraction to ensure that enough blood gets to the extremities so you can run faster, dilated bronchioles to get more oxygen to your muscles, decreased digestion to avoid wasting energy, decreased urine output so you will not have to stop, and increased mental alertness so you are always aware of the lion's location.

Parasympathetic—P is for PEACEFUL. The parasympathetic nervous system brings the body back to balance and rest. It is sometimes called the *rest-and-digest response*. Think, "There is no longer a lion. Now my body can go back to normal and start digesting and urinating again!"

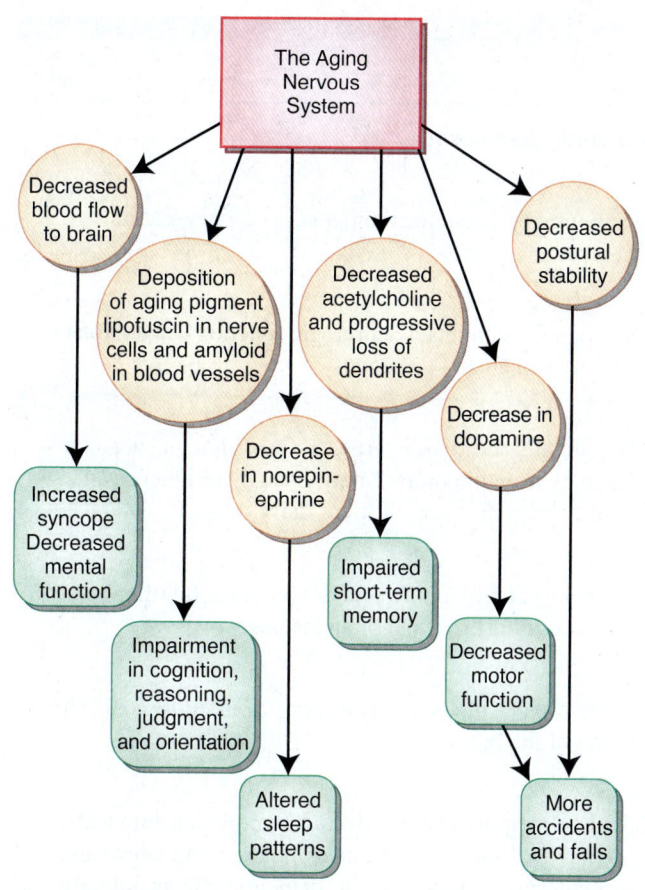

Chapter 47 Neurologic System Function, Data Collection, and Therapeutic Measures

FIGURE 47.10 Aging and the neurologic system.

The results of the baseline data collection are invaluable in planning and implementing safe care. For example, a patient who has a history of seizures needs a safe environment and careful monitoring, and all staff members who interact with such patients should be aware of how to respond to a seizure. Patients with **dysphagia** (difficulty swallowing) may need restrictions on the types of food or fluids they can have. This information must be consistently communicated to all staff involved in the patient's care.

> **PRACTICE ANALYSIS TIP**
> **Linking NCLEX-PN® to Practice**
> The LPN/LVN uses precautions to prevent injury and/or complications associated with a procedure or diagnosis.

> **CUE RECOGNITION 47.1**
> You are caring for a patient after a stroke. You enter his room and find him lying flat in bed and choking on saliva. What should you do?
> *Suggested answers are at the end of the chapter.*

The frequency of neurologic checks depends on the patient's admitting diagnosis, presence of any chronic neurologic disorders, and current functioning of the patient's neurologic system. Orders for neurologic checks vary from every 15 minutes for an acutely ill or injured patient, to every 8 hours for a patient who is close to discharge, to every 24 hours for a resident in long-term care. It is always appropriate to monitor a patient more often than ordered, based on observed changes in the patient's condition, and communicate the findings of those checks to the HCP. Rapid detection and intervention may mean the difference between chronic dysfunction and recovery or even between life and death for the patient.

> **Box 47.1**
> **Basic Neurologic Data Collection**
> - Determine history of neurologic problems.
> - Determine level of consciousness (patient's response to verbal or tactile stimulation) and orientation.
> - Obtain vital signs (specifically blood pressure, pulse, and respirations).
> - Check pupillary response to light.
> - Check strength and equality of hand grip and movement of extremities.
> - Determine ability to sense touch or pain in extremities.

> **BE SAFE!**
> **AVOID FAILURE TO RECOGNIZE!** Use the mnemonic BE FAST to recognize and respond rapidly to a possible stroke (Toral, 2021).
> **B**alance loss
> **E**yesight changes
> **F**ace drooping
> **A**rm weakness
> **S**peech difficulty
> **T**ime (acute onset of symptoms and also the importance of rapid response in stroke management)

Health History

To understand the patient's neurologic status, ask about past and current diagnoses and symptoms, use of prescription and over-the-counter medications, use of recreational drugs, past surgeries, treatments, and risk factors such as family history, diet, exercise, sedentary lifestyle, caffeine intake, and recent stressors. Review of symptoms, as with other body systems, includes asking the **WHAT'S UP?** questions.

Obtain a history of the patient's general health, and then focus on any neurologic symptoms. Symptoms of neurologic disorders vary in type, location, and intensity. It is important to remember that some neurologic disorders can affect the patient's ability to think, remember, speak, or interpret stimuli. It may be necessary to question significant others about duration and severity of symptoms. Table 47.3

• WORD • BUILDING •
dysphagia: dys—difficult + phagia—eating

Table 47.3
Data Collection Related to Mental Status

Questions to Ask During the Health History	Rationale/Significance
Mental Status What is your name? What is the month? Year? Where are you now?	Disorientation is often an initial sign of a neurologic disorder.
Intellectual Function Subtract 7 from 100, then 7 from that answer, and so on (serial 7s).	Most people with intact neurologic function can complete serial 7s in about 90 seconds.
Thought Content What would you do if you smelled smoke? Where would you put milk?	The patient's ability to interpret information and act appropriately is an important safety issue that influences their ability to perform activities of daily living.
Perception Show the patient a pencil and pen and ask what each is.	Agnosia (inability to interpret or recognize familiar objects) can occur in stroke and brain lesions.
Language Ability Read the following sentence: ____.	Different types of aphasia can result from injury to different parts of the brain.
Memory Repeat these four or five words: ____. Repeat them again in 5 minutes.	Impaired memory can be affected by both delirium and dementia. Delirium can cause impaired immediate and short-term memory, whereas dementia affects not only immediate and short-term memory but also the ability to learn new information. It also may be related to stroke.
Pain On a scale of 0 to 10, with 0 as no pain and 10 as the worst you have ever had, what is your pain level?	Pain perception may be altered or impaired by spinal injury, medications, alcohol, stress, and level of consciousness. Some spinal injuries may be critical, but the patient will not report pain.

presents sample questions to ask if the patient has a change in mental status.

In addition to questioning the patient, the nurse observes the patient during the health history. Is the patient shifting positions and exhibiting signs of discomfort? Is the patient able to move about freely? Is the patient able to carry on a coherent conversation?

Physical Examination

The physical examination begins immediately upon meeting the patient and includes evaluating the patient's mental and physical status. The neurologic system is examined using inspection, palpation, and percussion (with a reflex hammer). When conducting the mental status and cognitive portions of the examination, be aware that fatigue, illness, or medications can alter findings. When interpreting neurologic findings, be sure to consider the patient's age, any sensory deficits, educational background, and culture.

Level of Consciousness

Level of consciousness (LOC) exists along a continuum from full wakefulness, alertness, and cooperation to unresponsiveness and/or coma. A fully conscious patient responds to questions spontaneously. As consciousness becomes impaired, a patient may show irritability, a shortened attention span, or an inability to cooperate. LOC should be the first thing checked during a neurologic examination because the information obtained can be used to modify the remainder of the examination if necessary. In addition to neurological disease, consider that a decrease in LOC can be caused by problems such as hypoxia, hypoglycemia, medications, or intoxication.

GLASGOW COMA SCALE. Many health-care institutions use the Glasgow Coma Scale (GCS), an international tool to assess LOC and document findings (Table 47.4). The GCS is used to evaluate patients who have a potential for

Table 47.4
Glasgow Coma Scale

Assessment	Findings	Score
Eye opening	Spontaneous	4
	To verbal stimulus	3
	To painful stimulus	2
	No response	1
Verbal response	Normal conversation	5
	Confused conversation	4
	Inappropriate words	3
	Incomprehensible sounds	2
	No response	1
Motor response	Obeys commands	6
	Localizes pain	5
	Withdraws from pain*	4
	Abnormal flexion	3
	Abnormal extension	2
	No response	1

Note: This scale is for adults only. Criteria specific to children should be used for pediatric cases.
*To elicit pain, place pressure on a nailbed or on the trapezius muscle. Be sure to apply the stimulus long enough to elicit a response.

rapid deterioration in consciousness. When determining LOC, consider the patient's physical ability to respond, considering trauma, medical condition, and medications. For example, a patient who cannot open their eyes because of facial trauma may still have an intact neurologic system.

Motor response is scored in the GCS based on following commands, responding to pain, or displaying abnormal postures. Abnormal postures include decorticate and decerebrate. In **decorticate**, or flexion, posturing, the patient's arms are flexed at the elbow, hands are raised toward the chest, and legs are extended (Fig. 47.11A). This posture indicates significant impairment of cerebral functioning. In **decerebrate**, or extension, posturing, both arms and legs are extended, and arms are internally rotated (Fig. 47.11B). This abnormal posturing indicates damage in the brainstem area.

The total possible score on the GCS ranges from 3 to 15. A score of less than 7 indicates a comatose patient and a score of 15 indicates the patient is fully alert and oriented. When used to score the effects of a head injury, a score of 13 or 14 indicates mild head injury, 9 to 12 indicates moderate injury, and any score of 8 or below indicates severe head injury. For all categories of the GCS, the type of painful stimuli required to elicit a response should be documented. Deterioration in the patient's condition (i.e., a lowering of the GCS score) should be reported to the HCP promptly.

> **Evidence-Based Practice**
>
> **Clinical Question**
> Can technology be used to collect important neurological data during a pandemic?
>
> **Evidence**
> During the COVID-19 pandemic, researchers associated with the Cleveland Clinic found that virtual video calls and smartphone applications could be used to characterize important aspects of Parkinson disease (Alberts et al, 2021). Researchers found that both motor (bradykinesia, functional mobility, etc.) and nonmotor (information processing, attention, and memory) signs and symptoms could be objectively monitored with the assistance of technology.
>
> **Implications for Nursing Practice**
> Make sure you are aware of the available technologies that can be used to gather neurological data when patients are not able to travel to clinics or other appointments.
>
> *Reference:* Alberts, J. L., Miller Koop, M., McGinley, M. P., Penko, A. L., Fernandez, H. H., Shook, S., Bermel, R. A., Machado, A., & Rosenfeldt, A. B. (2021). Use of smartphone technology to gather Parkinson's disease neurological vital signs during the COVID-19 pandemic. *Parkinson's Disease, 2021.* https://doi.org/10.1155/2021/5534282

FOUR SCORE SCALE. The Full Outline of UnResponsiveness (FOUR) Score Coma Scale is a newer tool that has been introduced into many critical care and emergency department areas. Research indicates that it is at least as effective as or more so than the GCS. A major benefit of using the FOUR score scale is that no evaluation of verbal response is necessary, a problem when using the GCS with intubated patients. The FOUR score scale uses four categories: eye response, motor movement, reflexes, and breathing pattern. A maximum of four points can be earned in each of the four areas. The terms *decorticate* and *decerebrate* are not used when assessing the motor response to prevent confusion. The brainstem is evaluated using both pupillary and corneal reflexes along with the cough reflex. Once each component is evaluated and assigned a numerical value, the components are totaled. In general, the lower the FOUR score scale is, the worse the neurological status and poorer prognosis. Conversely, the higher the score, the better the prognosis will be (Fig. 47.12).

Mental Status
Mental status can be affected not only by the aging process but by a variety of neurologic disorders and injuries. A traumatic brain injury (TBI) can result in memory impairment, delayed amnesia, affective (mood) disorders, and dementia. To assess for cognitive impairment, the Mini-Mental State Examination

• WORD • BUILDING •
decorticate: de—down + corticate—cerebral cortex
decerebrate: de—down + cerebrate—cerebrum

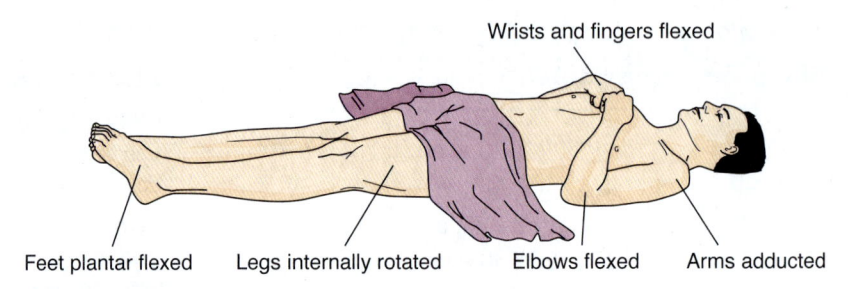

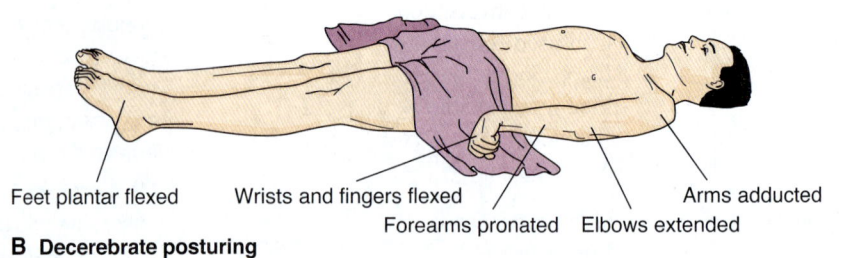

UNIT THIRTEEN Understanding the Neurologic System

A Decorticate posturing
- Wrists and fingers flexed
- Feet plantar flexed
- Legs internally rotated
- Elbows flexed
- Arms adducted

B Decerebrate posturing
- Feet plantar flexed
- Wrists and fingers flexed
- Forearms pronated
- Elbows extended
- Arms adducted

FIGURE 47.11 Abnormal posturing. (A) Decorticate posturing. (B) Decerebrate posturing.

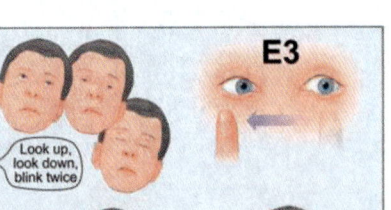

Eye response
- 4 = eyelids open or opened, tracking, or blinking to command
- 3 = eyelids open but not tracking
- 2 = eyelids closed but open to loud voice
- 1 = eyelids closed but open to pain
- 0 = eyelids remain closed with pain

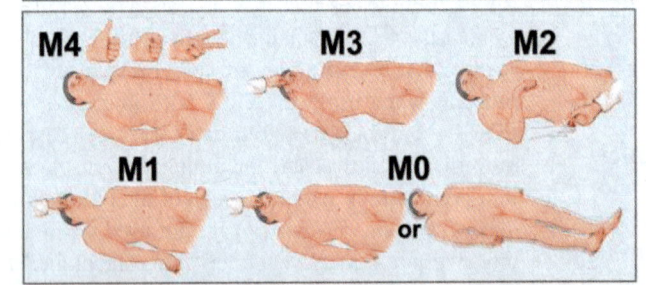

Motor response
- 4 = thumbs-up, fist, or peace sign
- 3 = localizing to pain
- 2 = flexion response to pain
- 1 = extension response to pain
- 0 = no response to pain or generalized myoclonus status

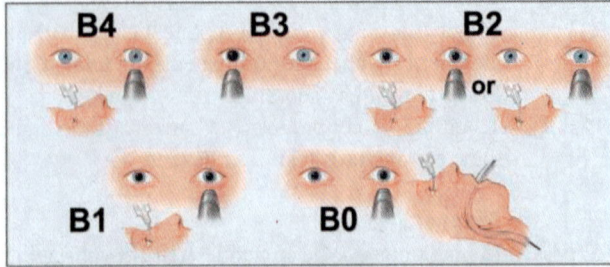

Brainstem reflexes
- 4 = pupil and corneal reflexes present
- 3 = one pupil wide and fixed
- 2 = pupil or corneal reflexes absent
- 1 = pupil and corneal reflexes absent
- 0 = absent pupil, corneal, and cough reflexes

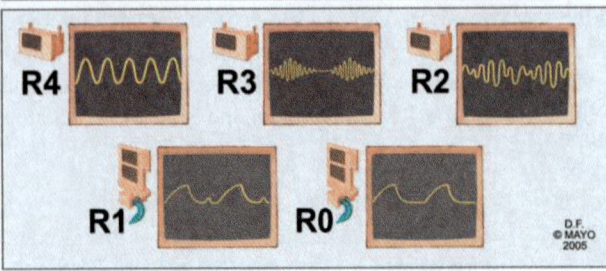

Respiration
- 4 = not intubated, regular breathing pattern
- 3 = not intubated, Cheyne-Stokes breathing pattern
- 2 = not intubated, irregular breathing
- 1 = breathes above ventilator rate
- 0 = breathes at ventilator rate or apnea

FIGURE 47.12 FOUR Score Coma Scale.

(MMSE) or Confusion Assessment Method (CAM) can be used. The MMSE is an assessment tool that tests orientation, registration, attention and calculation, recall, and language. Your clinical site should have an example of the MMSE.

Specialized versions of the CAM scale are available. The basic CAM uses the following criteria to help diagnose delirium (Rieck et al, 2020):

- Acute onset and fluctuating course
- Inattention
- Disorganized thinking
- Altered LOC

Find more about CAM at https://www.nccih.nih.gov.

Change in mental status should be taken seriously, especially when the patient takes multiple medicines or has recently changed medicines. A primary cause of delirium and acute states of confusion is adverse effects from medications. Other causes of acute delirium include vision or hearing impairment, infection, pain, electrolyte or kidney or liver disorders, sleep deprivation, or being in an unfamiliar environment.

> **LEARNING TIP**
> Acute confusion is called *delirium* and often stems from a medical cause or condition (such as a urinary tract infection) in the elderly. It is typically reversible and should be evaluated immediately. Dementia is not reversible and is associated with chronic confusion.

Determining cognitive function includes evaluating the patient's thinking capacity. It is important to determine attention span, ability to concentrate, judgment, memory, orientation, perception, problem-solving ability, and motor function.

Nurses can learn about mental capacity and emotional state by simply interacting with the patient. Behavior, mood, hygiene, grooming, and choice of dress reveal pertinent information about mental status. Mental status examinations can be performed to determine cognitive function, thought processes, and perceptions by observing the patient's verbal and nonverbal responses to questions and specific requests. See Table 47.3 for some ways to collect data in these areas.

> **CUE RECOGNITION 47.2**
> The patient enters the examination room dressed in several heavy layers of clothing during the warm summer months. What do you do?
>
> *Suggested answers are at the end of the chapter.*

Orientation refers to the patient's ability to comprehend themselves in relation to person, location/place, and time. The patient's understanding of the current situation may also be evaluated. A patient who is fully oriented is often referred to as "oriented times three." Typical questions include *What is your name? Where are you? What day is it?* (Keep in mind that we all forget the date from time to time!) You can also ask whether the person knows what season it is (spring, fall, etc.). A resident of a long-term care facility who says they are "at home" may consider the facility home and is not necessarily disoriented. Be sure questions are appropriate to the patient's age, culture, living conditions, lifestyle, and medical condition. If the patient is unable to speak because of a stroke (expressive **aphasia**) or intubation, do not rule out the possibility that the patient is oriented. Give expressively aphasic patients yes-or-no questions such as *Are you in a grocery store? Are you in a bowling alley? Are you in a hospital?* Patients may be able to answer with a shake of the head, eye blinks, or hand squeezes as instructed.

Examination of the Eyes

Examination of pupils is an important part of data collection for the neurological system and cranial nerve evaluation. Size of the pupils at rest is documented in millimeters (Fig. 47.13). If the patient's pupils are unusually large or small, determine whether they have received medications that can affect pupil size. If the pupils are unequal in size (**anisocoria**), without a correlating diagnosis or symptoms, ask patient or significant others whether the person normally has unequal pupils. Anisocoria may be congenital or caused by cataract surgery. Development of unequal pupils in a patient who previously had equal pupils is an emergency and should be reported to HCP immediately. Any deviation from normal round shape of pupils is documented.

The next step is to check pupillary response to light. In a darkened room, a light source (such as a flashlight) is directed at the pupil from the lateral aspect of the eye. This allows the examiner to see the direct and consensual responses to the light. A consensual response means that when one pupil is exposed to direct light, the other pupil also constricts. Absence of a consensual response may indicate a pathological condition in the optic chiasm. Typically, the speed of the reaction to light is described as brisk, sluggish, or absent. Differences in the speed or size of constriction between the two pupils should be reported to the HCP.

Accommodation is the process of visual focusing from far to near. To evaluate accommodation, have the patient focus on an object at a distant point and then refocus on the object at a near point. Pupils should constrict and eyes should converge with the adjustment to the near object. Upon completion of data collection of the pupils, document your findings. PERRLA is a common acronym to note that *p*upils are *e*qual, *r*ound, and *r*eactive to *l*ight and *a*ccommodation. (If accommodation is not performed, do not include the A.)

Next, evaluate for range of motion and for smoothness and coordination of movements. Eyes that move in the same direction in a coordinated manner have a *conjugate* gaze.

• WORD • BUILDING •
aphasia: a—absence + phasia—speech
anisocoria: aniso—unequal + coria—pupil

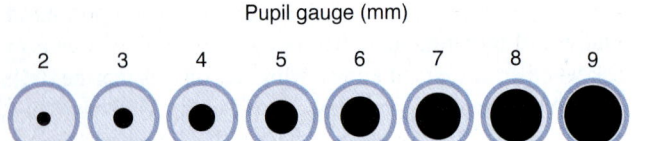

FIGURE 47.13 Documenting pupil size.

A disconjugate gaze is movement of the eyes in different directions. Some patients may be unable to move one or both eyes in a specific direction; this is called *ophthalmoplegia*, often documented as "limited extraocular movements." Always document what the limitation is (e.g., "Patient is unable to look laterally with left eye"). This observation allows colleagues to compare findings and recognize changes.

> **PRACTICE ANALYSIS TIP**
> **Linking NCLEX-PN® to Practice**
> The LPN/LVN performs focused data collection based on client condition (e.g., neurological checks, circulatory checks).

Nystagmus is involuntary movement of the eyes and varies in the speed of the movement and direction. Horizontal nystagmus is the most common. Common causes of nystagmus are phenytoin (Dilantin) toxicity and injury to the brainstem.

Examination of Muscle Function

Examine muscle groups systematically in the upper extremities and then lower extremities, comparing right to left. Compare muscle groups for symmetry of size and strength. Keep in mind the patient's age and general physical condition when evaluating muscle strength. (You would not expect the same amount of strength from a 75-year-old woman as from a 20-year-old man, for example.) If the patient has chronic neurologic deficits, ask whether data collected at this time is different from their usual level of function.

Many HCPs use a 5-point scale to document muscle strength. A score of 5 describes a patient who can move the extremity against gravity and against the resistance of the examiner, displaying normal muscle strength. If the examiner can provide more resistance than the patient can overcome with active movement, the score is 4. If the patient can move the extremity only against gravity but not resistance, the score is 3. If gravity must be eliminated by having the examiner support the extremity to allow the patient to move it, the score is 2. A score of 1 is given if there is no active movement of the extremity but a minimum muscular contraction can be palpated. If the examiner is unable to detect any muscular function, a score of 0 is given.

To test the deltoid muscles, ask the patient to raise their arms at the shoulder. Have the patient resist as you push down on the upper arms. The biceps are tested by having the patient flex the arm at the elbow and bring the palm toward the face, and then resist as you attempt to straighten the arm by pulling on the forearm. With the arm similarly flexed, ask the patient to straighten the arm while you resist the movement.

Hand grasps are tested by having the patient squeeze your fingers. Remember to cross your index and middle fingers to prevent the patient from hurting your fingers. If the patient does not release the grasp when told to, it is a reflex grasp, not a response to command. A reflex palmar grasp may indicate a pathological condition of the frontal lobe.

Check for arm drift by asking the patient to hold both arms straight in front with the palms upward while keeping the eyes closed. A downward drift of the arm or rotation so that the palm is down indicates impairment of the opposite side of the brain. If a pathological condition is present, arm drift may be apparent before differences in muscle strength can be detected.

Checking for leg muscle strength begins with the iliopsoas muscle. Place your hand on the patient's thigh and ask the patient to raise the leg, flexing at the hip. Hip adductors are tested by having the patient bring their legs together against your hands. The hip abductors and gluteus medius and minimus are tested by having the patient move the legs apart against resistance. Hip extension by the gluteus maximus is tested by placing the hand under the thigh and having the patient push down with the leg. The quadriceps femoris extends the knee and is tested by having the patient attempt to straighten the leg at the knee. Hamstrings, responsible for knee flexion, are evaluated by having the patient attempt to keep the heel of the foot against the bed or chair rung. Dorsiflexion is tested by having the patient pull the toes toward the head against resistance. Plantar flexion is tested by having the patient push against the examiner's hand with the ball of the foot.

The Babinski reflex is tested by firmly stroking the sole of the foot. Normal response is flexion of the great toe. If the great toe extends and the other toes fan out, neurologic dysfunction should be suspected if the patient is older than 6 months. Deep tendon reflexes are not usually part of a routine data collection by the nurse. The patient's gait should be evaluated to detect any neurologic dysfunction and to determine ability to ambulate safely. Patients who stagger, weave, or bump into objects may need assistance with walking.

> **BE SAFE!**
> **BE VIGILANT!** If you find that your patient has an unsteady gait, place them on fall precautions based on facility policy. Fall precautions help ensure that procedures are followed to keep the patient safe.

The Romberg test is performed by having the patient stand with feet together and eyes closed. A negative Romberg test means that the patient experiences minimal swaying for up to 20 seconds. A patient who sways or leans to one side is said to have a positive Romberg test, which may be seen in cerebellar dysfunction.

> **BE SAFE!**
> **BE VIGILANT!** A positive Romberg test is common in older adults. Be sure to protect the patient with a positive result from falls. A gait belt may be helpful when assisting the patient with ambulation.

Examination of Cranial Nerves

The cranial nerves are usually not examined in depth during routine bedside neurologic data collection. Testing requires a patient who is able to cooperate with the examiner. Table 47.5 provides testing techniques for collecting data on a patient's cranial nerve function.

Summary of Examination Findings

In all cases, the findings of the neurologic examination should be correlated with the remainder of the physical examination findings. A decreased LOC coupled with a decreased oxygen saturation on pulse oximetry points to hypoxia as a cause. Correlation of vital signs with neurologic signs is particularly important. Bradycardia, increasing systolic blood pressure with widening pulse pressure, and irregular respirations, commonly called the *Cushing triad*, are late indications of increasing intracranial pressure. These findings, in conjunction with a unilateral dilated pupil, may indicate impending herniation of the brain (discussed further in Chapter 48).

DIAGNOSTIC TESTS FOR THE NEUROLOGIC SYSTEM

Laboratory Tests

Specific diagnostic blood tests do not exist for neurologic disorders. However, depending on the history and physical examination, the HCP may include laboratory tests to look for underlying causes of symptoms. Possible tests include thyroid hormone levels, vitamin B_{12}, complete blood count (CBC), electrolytes, creatine kinase (CK) and isoenzymes, venereal disease research lab (VDRL) test (for syphilis), liver function, and renal function. Measurement of erythrocyte sedimentation rate (ESR) and white blood cell (WBC) count may indicate an infection, such as meningitis. Hormone levels, such as prolactin or cortisol, may indicate dysfunction of the pituitary gland related to a brain tumor. Anticholinesterase testing and antibody titers are useful in diagnosing myasthenia gravis. A blood test using an immuno-infrared sensor has been developed to detect amyloid beta misfolding in the blood of those who are at increased risk for the development of Alzheimer disease (Möllers, 2021).

Lumbar Puncture

CSF may be obtained via lumbar puncture and evaluated for glucose and protein levels, presence of bacteria and WBCs, levels of immunoglobulin, antibodies, and culture and sensitivity. See Appendix A for nursing care of a patient undergoing lumbar puncture.

Table 47.5
Data Collection Related to Cranial Nerve Function

Nerve	Test
Olfactory nerve	Ask patient to identify common scents, such as cinnamon and coffee.
Optic nerve	Ask patient to read something or tell how many fingers you are holding up.
Oculomotor nerve	Check pupils for reaction to light and accommodation.
Oculomotor, trochlear, and abducens nerves	Ask patient to follow your finger while moving it in front of their eyes in the positions of a clock: 1, 3, 5, 7, 9, and 11 o'clock.
Trigeminal nerve	Ask patient to identify touch on different parts of the face with eyes closed.
Facial nerve	Ask patient to frown, smile, and wrinkle forehead; check for symmetry.
Vestibulocochlear nerve	Have patient identify a whisper close to each ear. Observe gait for balance.
Glossopharyngeal and vagus nerves	Watch for uvula and palate to rise when patient says "ahh." Touch back of throat with cotton-tipped applicator to elicit gag reflex.
Spinal accessory nerve	Ask patient to turn head and shrug the shoulders against resistance.
Hypoglossal nerve	Ask patient to stick out tongue and move it from side to side.

> **PRACTICE ANALYSIS TIP**
> Linking NCLEX-PN® to Practice
> The LPN/LVN assists with the performance of a diagnostic or invasive procedure.

> **NURSING CARE TIP**
> The idea of a needle being introduced into the spinal canal frightens many people. Give simple, clear directions; help the patient maintain their position; and provide emotional support throughout the procedure.

X-Ray Examination

Spinal x-ray (radiograph) examinations determine the status of individual vertebrae and their relationship to one another. If the patient experiences pain with certain movements, they may be asked to flex and extend the area of the spine being examined while the radiographs are taken. This allows detection of abnormal movement of the vertebrae. Skull radiographs may be taken to detect skull fractures or foreign bodies. No special nursing care is required.

Computed Tomography

A computed tomography (CT) scan is used to diagnose neurologic disorders of the brain or spine. A CT scan can detect hemorrhage, altered ventricle size, cerebral atrophy, tumors, skull fractures, and abscesses. A CT scan is used when magnetic resonance imaging (MRI) is contraindicated because of metal aneurysm clips or other metal implants.

The scan may be performed with or without radiopaque contrast material to enhance the clarity of the images. Contrast material is most common if a tumor is suspected or following surgery in the area to be scanned. CT scans are common in emergency evaluations because they can be done quickly, an important consideration if the patient is mechanically ventilated or has unstable vital signs.

Nursing Care

During a CT scan, the patient must lie still on a movable table. Noncontrast scans take about 10 minutes; contrast scans take 20 to 30 minutes. Patients receiving dye should be warned that they may feel a sensation of warmth following the injection; warmth in the groin area might make them feel as though they have been incontinent of urine. Nausea, diaphoresis, itching, or difficulty breathing can indicate allergy to the dye and should be reported immediately to the HCP. Sedation may be required for patients who are agitated, disoriented, or anxious. Patients should be evaluated for a history of kidney disease, diabetes, and certain medications prior to diagnostic procedures including contrast. Patients who are in pain may need pain medication before the examination. See Appendix A for nursing care of a patient undergoing a CT scan.

Magnetic Resonance Imaging

MRI is used to diagnose degenerative diseases such as multiple sclerosis, arteriovenous malformations, small tumors, hemorrhages, and cerebral and spinal cord edema. An MRI of the mediastinal cavity determines whether the thymus gland is enlarged to facilitate diagnosis of myasthenia gravis. It is a longer procedure that may be difficult for unstable, disoriented, or mechanically ventilated patients. As with CT scan, MRI can be done with or without contrast material. Some facilities can perform magnetic resonance angiograms (MRAs). This test allows visualization of blood vessels and assessment of blood flow without being as invasive as a traditional angiogram. See Appendix A for nursing care of a patient undergoing MRI.

Angiogram

In an angiogram, dye is injected and an x-ray is taken that provides information about the structure of specific vessels as well as overall circulation to an area. See Appendix A for nursing care of a patient undergoing an angiogram.

Myelogram

A **myelogram** is an x-ray examination of the spinal canal and its contents after injection of contrast material. Compression of nerve roots, herniation of intravertebral discs, and blockage of CSF circulation can all be detected by myelogram. See Appendix A for nursing care of a patient undergoing a myelogram.

Electroencephalogram

Electrodes are placed on the scalp to record brain activity during an **electroencephalogram** (EEG). Analysis of the tracing can identify areas of abnormality, such as a seizure focus or areas of slowed activity. See Appendix A for nursing care of a patient undergoing an EEG.

THERAPEUTIC MEASURES FOR THE NEUROLOGIC SYSTEM

Moving and Positioning

Patients who have pain may need help changing positions and ambulating. Use of heat, cold, or analgesics may allow the patient to be more independent in mobility.

If the patient has sensory loss, make sure no part of the body is inadvertently compressed (e.g., a hand caught under a hip or scrotum compressed between the legs). Pressure injuries are a primary concern with the patient who cannot move independently. Collaborate with the physical therapist to determine positioning techniques that maximize the potential for recovery while decreasing the risk for injury and complications.

• WORD • BUILDING •

myelogram: myelo—referring to the spinal cord + gram—picture
electroencephalogram: electro—electrical activity + encephalo—referring to the brain + gram—picture

Patients with paresis, paralysis, or **paresthesia** (abnormal sensation such as burning or tingling) may partially or completely depend on moving and body positioning. Take care to maintain the body in functional positions when making routine position changes. This means keeping the trunk, extremities, hands, and feet in usable positions. For example, hands can be splinted to keep the thumb and fingers opposed, or high-top tennis shoes can be used to keep the feet in an appropriate position for standing or walking.

Contractures and foot drop are complications that are often associated with neurologic disorders. Contractures are permanent muscle contractions with fibrosis of connective tissue that occur from lack of use of a muscle or muscle group. They cause permanent deformities and prevent normal functioning of the affected part. Foot drop occurs when the feet are not supported in a functional position and become contracted in a position of plantar flexion (Fig. 47.14). Use high-top tennis shoes and splints to help prevent foot drop. Splints are commonly used to prevent contractures of the upper and lower extremities and to keep the affected parts in a functional position. If splints are used, the patient must be evaluated for and protected from discomfort and skin breakdown at the splint site.

Mobilization should begin as soon as a patient is medically stable. Initially, this may involve the use of a lift device if the patient is unable to bear weight. Transfer of the patient to a bedside chair or use of ambulation aids may require a multidisciplinary approach. Be careful to recognize any physical or cognitive deficits that might affect safety and adjust the environment to protect the patient. Communicate safety concerns to assistive personnel who interact with the patient.

Activities of Daily Living

The effects of neurologic disorders on activities of daily living (ADLs) can range from an inconvenience to complete dependence. Patients may have trouble bending over to put on their shoes and socks, lifting a full cooking pot, or caring for an infant. A patient with quadriplegia may be completely unable to perform ADLs but can be taught to direct their own personal care. Encourage patients to use strategies they learned in occupational or physical therapy.

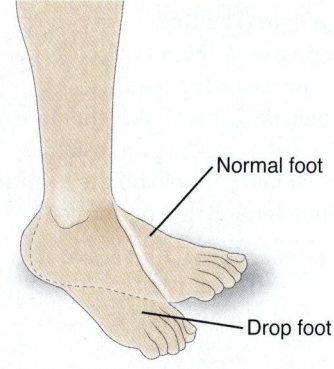

FIGURE 47.14 Contractures, foot drop.

When collecting ADL data on a hospitalized patient, discuss strategies the patient normally uses at home to accomplish ADLs. Every attempt should be made to enable the patient to continue to use these strategies, particularly if the patient is admitted to a long-term care facility. Patients who have intact cognitive function should be included in care planning and encouraged to work collaboratively with caregivers. If strategies the patient uses during ADLs must be changed (e.g., if the patient's transfer technique is unsafe), be sure to explain the rationale for the changes to the patient and significant others. If patients have impaired cognitive function, try to maintain a specific routine that is as close to their normal environment as possible. Normalizing routines may help patients adapt to a change in environment and maximize their ability to function.

Communication

Communication problems associated with neurologic disorders have a variety of causes. Some neurologic disorders cause difficulty speaking (**dysarthria**). Dysfunction of the lips, tongue, or jaw makes speech difficult or impossible to understand. When dysarthric individuals know what they want to say but cannot be understood, they can become very frustrated. This frustration is compounded if the patients are treated as if they have cognitive deficits merely because they have difficulty communicating.

Patients who have had a stroke can experience different types of aphasia. *Expressive aphasia* is difficulty in verbally communicating or inability to verbally communicate with others. The patient may be able to speak in sentences but inappropriately substitutes words, such as "The sky is dish." Word-finding difficulty is another type of expressive aphasia. These patients may tell you, "I want a . . ." and then be unable to complete the sentence. In severe cases of aphasia, the patient may make sounds that resemble words or may only utter sounds. For individuals with no intelligible speech or word-finding difficulty, a picture board with commonly used items may facilitate communication. (See an example of a picture board in Chapter 49.) Keep in mind that patients with expressive aphasia may answer yes or no to all questions regardless of correct answer. For this reason, a nurse should never ask a patient, "Are you Mrs. Gonzalez?" An aphasic patient may say yes even if that is not her name. Instead, ask the patient to state her name. Always check the identification band.

For patients who substitute words, simply correct the substitution and continue the conversation. Patients with expressive aphasia are often aware of and frustrated by their difficulty communicating. Give them time to try to express themselves. If you cannot understand, offer possibilities based on the situation. If the patient is sitting in the chair, ask whether they want to go back to bed or use the bathroom. If the patient is restless, ask if they are in pain.

• WORD • BUILDING •

paresthesia: para—beside + asthesia—sensations
dysarthria: dys—dysfunctional + arthria—movement of the joints used in speech

Some patients use the same word in response to all questions, and for a few patients, that word is a profanity. This is very difficult for their family, particularly if a patient did not normally use profanity in the past. Make it clear to the family that you understand that this behavior is part of the patient's illness.

Receptive aphasia affects the ability to understand spoken language. Again, severity of the aphasia varies. Some patients may understand simple directions such as "sit down" or "squeeze my fingers." In other cases, the nurse may need to pantomime the desired action, such as showing the patient pills and then mimicking taking the pills and drinking water.

> **BE SAFE!**
> **BE VIGILANT!** If the patient has receptive aphasia, assume they cannot understand or follow safety instructions, such as "Do not stand up until I get back." Even going around the corner to get water can give a patient enough time to try to stand up, putting them at risk for a subsequent fall.

Nutrition

Alterations in ability to maintain adequate nutritional intake can have many causes. LOC may be depressed enough that the patient does not recognize hunger or thirst. Decreased LOC or cranial nerve dysfunction may impair the patient's ability to swallow safely. Severe weakness may limit ability to take in enough food to meet the body's requirements. These conditions are often compounded by the increased metabolic rate that accompanies neurologic injury or illness.

If there is question of the patient's ability to swallow, a swallowing evaluation should be performed by a speech therapist. Some institutions use a radiological examination to evaluate the ability to swallow. A small amount of barium is added to food or fluid, and fluoroscopy is used while the patient swallows to allow visualization of the path of the food or fluid. Patients with swallowing difficulty (dysphagia) may have better success with foods or thick liquids than with thin fluids. Liquids may be thickened with special agents to allow easier swallowing. All patients should be positioned as upright as possible while eating or drinking. Patients who have difficulty swallowing should be monitored during eating and not left alone.

If weakness or fatigue is the cause of decreased nutritional intake, several modifications are possible. Serving small portions of food more frequently can increase intake. Using high-protein, high-calorie foods and supplements increases the nutritional content of small amounts of foods.

For patients who cannot swallow or who cannot swallow enough food, enteral (tube) feedings may be needed. If enteral feedings are anticipated for a short duration, a nasogastric tube may be used. Disadvantages of nasogastric tubes include impaired nasal skin integrity and risk of aspiration. The risk of aspiration in neurologically impaired patients who have cognitive impairments is increased, as they may pull out the nasogastric tube due to lack of understanding of its purpose. If long-term enteral feedings are anticipated, a gastrostomy tube may be placed directly through the abdominal wall into the stomach. This feeding method has the advantage of reducing the risks of aspiration and eliminating nasal skin breakdown.

Family

When working with patients who have a neurologic deficit, whether acute or chronic and whether in the hospital, in a long-term care facility, or at home, the family should be included in care and rehabilitation. Depending on the patient's diagnosis and prognosis, the family will need support from staff. It is rewarding to see the patient who has had an accident recover with rehabilitation, but it is also rewarding to promote quality of life for the patient with Alzheimer disease and their family. Communication with the family regarding patient improvements and information about the illness is important. Include the family in the patient's care, such as bathing, feeding, and grooming. Suggest that the family participate in physical, occupational, and speech therapy sessions. Education is of vital importance, especially if the patient is going to be discharged home. Direct the patient and family to support groups and case managers for information regarding financial assistance and community resources during rehabilitation.

> ## CRITICAL THINKING & CLINICAL JUDGMENT
>
> **Mr. Thompson** is a 78-year-old man admitted with heart problems. As you enter his room with his afternoon medications, you find Mr. Thompson confused. He thinks he is at home and that the year is 1968, and he does not understand who you are or why you are there. He recognizes his wife, who is at his bedside, and he knows his own name.
>
> **Critical Thinking (The Why)**
>
> 1. What may be contributing to the confusion?
>
> **Clinical Judgement (The Do)**
>
> 2. What additional data should you collect and what tool(s) can be used to obtain the data?
> 3. What are some important interventions to implement based on Mr. Thompson's current status?
> 4. With whom should you collaborate to ensure follow-up testing or interventions are performed?
>
> *Suggested answers are at the end of the chapter.*

Key Points

- The nervous system has two divisions: the central nervous system, which consists of the brain and spinal cord, and the peripheral nervous system, which includes the nerves of the ANS. A nerve (cranial, spinal, or peripheral) is a group of axons with blood vessels, wrapped in connective tissue containing both sensory and motor neurons.
- There are 31 pairs of spinal nerves and 12 pairs of cranial nerves.
- The cranial nerves are responsible for impulses for sight, smell, hearing, taste, equilibrium, and somatic senses and impulses that innervate the muscles of the face, neck, shoulder and tongue as well as glands.
- The ANS motor output provides dual innervation to effectors; that is, smooth muscle, cardiac muscle, and glands that produce the response. These two divisions (sympathetic [fight-or-flight] and parasympathetic [rest and digest]) function in opposition to one other.
- Be careful about attributing mental impairment to aging. More common causes of mental changes include depression, malnutrition, infection, hypotension, and side effects of medications. Past and current diagnoses and symptoms, use of prescription and over-the-counter medications, use of recreational drugs, past surgeries, treatments, and risk factors such as family history, diet, exercise, sedentary lifestyle, caffeine intake, and recent stressors should be included in the neuro data collection.
- If the patient has cognitive deficits, question the family to get a baseline of the patient's prior level of functioning. LOC exists along a continuum from fully awake, alert, and cooperative to unresponsiveness to any form of external stimuli. Non-neurological sources of decreased LOC include problems such as hypoxia, hypoglycemia, and medications. PERRLA is a commonly used acronym to note that *p*upils are *e*qual, *r*ound, and *r*eactive to *l*ight and *a*ccommodation.
- Possible blood tests for neurological disorders include thyroid hormone levels, vitamin B_{12}, complete blood count, electrolytes, creatine kinase and isoenzymes, VDRL test, liver function, and renal function. In addition, the ESR and WBC count are done to look for an infection, such as meningitis.
- CSF may be obtained via lumbar puncture and evaluated for glucose and protein levels, presence of bacteria and WBCs, levels of immunoglobulin, antibodies, and culture and sensitivity.
- Additional diagnostic tests for the neurologic system include x-rays, computed tomography scan, magnetic resonance imaging, myelogram, and electroencephalogram.
- Patients with sensory impairments need special care to prevent pressure injuries. They may not be able to indicate areas of pressure or pain. Interventions to prevent contractures include splints, positioning, and range of motion. Interventions to help prevent foot drop include splints and high-top sneakers.
- Patients who have intact cognitive function as well as their families should be included in care planning and encouraged to work collaboratively with caregivers. If patients have impaired cognitive function, try to maintain a specific routine that is as close to their normal environment as possible.
- Patients with neurologic deficits may have communication problems, including dysarthria, expressive aphasia, and receptive aphasia.
- Neurological conditions can cause alterations in the ability to maintain an adequate nutritional intake. In addition, these conditions are often compounded by the increased metabolic rate that accompanies neurologic injury or illness.

SUGGESTED ANSWERS TO CHAPTER EXERCISES

Cue Recognition
47.1: Elevate the head of the bed and implement aspiration precautions.
47.2: Collect more data related to mental status and document the findings objectively (also include the patient's perspective of the clothing choice).

Critical Thinking & Clinical Judgment
Mrs. Stevens
1. Albuterol is an adrenergic agonist (sometimes called a *sympathomimetic*), which is given to stimulate the sympathetic nervous system, resulting in open airways in patients with respiratory disease. However, it can also stimulate the cardiac system and cause a rapid heart rate and increased blood pressure.
2. Be sure to monitor vital signs in patients receiving medications that affect the autonomic nervous system.

Mr. Thompson
1. Some possible explanations to explore include hypoxemia, stroke, worsening heart problems causing inadequate flow of blood to the brain, hypoglycemia, or acute confusion (delirium) related to a sudden transition from home to an unfamiliar environment. Use clear and easy-to-understand explanations when discussing the information with Mr. Thompson's family. Tell Mr. Thompson's wife that the HCP will be notified and will determine the cause and whether any follow-up tests or treatments are indicated.

SUGGESTED ANSWERS TO CHAPTER EXERCISES—cont'd

2. The nurse should ask Mrs. Thompson whether this has ever happened before, check his medical history for any disorders that may contribute to neurologic dysfunction, do a quick neurologic examination to determine whether any additional deficits exist, check vital signs and pulse oximetry if available, and notify the HCP immediately if the symptoms are a new finding. The CAM tool will assist the nurse to collect patient data.

3. Acute confusion and/or delirium impacts patient safety. Mr. Thompson should be monitored for fall risk, and fall precautions should be implemented as indicated. Frequent reorientation and use of clear and simple instructions are important, at least until Mr. Thompson returns to his baseline neurological function.

4. If an acute change in mental status is noted, contact the HCP for evaluation. Involve a respiratory therapist, electrocardiogram technician, or others based on assessed needs and orders from the HCP.

Additional Resources

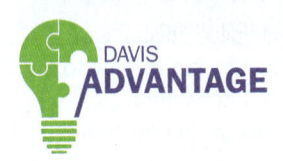

Go to Davis Advantage to complete your learning: strengthen understanding, apply your knowledge, and prepare for the Next Gen NCLEX®.

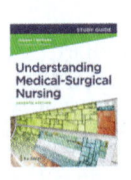

A Study Guide is also available.

CHAPTER 48
Nursing Care of Patients With Central Nervous System Disorders

Lynette P. Harvey, Deborah L. Weaver

KEY TERMS

akinesia (AH-kin-EE-zhee-ah)
ataxia (ah-TAK-see-ah)
bradykinesia (BRAY-dee-kin-EE-zhee-ah)
contralateral (KON-truh-LAT-er-uhl)
craniectomy (KRAY-nee-EK-tuh-mee)
cranioplasty (KRAY-nee-oh-plas-tee)
craniotomy (KRAY-nee-AH-toh-mee)
delirium (dih-LEER-ee-um)
dementia (dih-MENT-sha)
dysreflexia (DIS-re-FLEK-see-ah)
encephalitis (en-SEF-uh-LYE-tis)
encephalopathy (en-SEF-uh-LAHP-ah-thee)
hemiparesis (hem-ee-puh-REE-sis)
hydrocephalus (HY-droh-SEF-uh-luhs)
ipsilateral (IP-sih-LAT-er-uhl)
laminectomy (LAM-ih-NEK-toh-mee)
meningitis (MEN-in-JY-tis)
neurodegenerative (new-roh-de-JEN-er-uh-tiv)
nuchal rigidity (NEW-kuhl ri-JID-ih-tee)
paraparesis (PAR-ah-puh-REE-sis)
paraplegia (PAR-ah-PLEE-jee-ah)
photophobia (FOH-tuh-FOH-bee-ah)
postictal (pohs-TIK-tuhl)
prodromal (proh-DROH-muhl)
quadriparesis (KWA-drih-puh-REE-sis)
quadriplegia (KWA-drih-PLEE-jee-ah)
sciatica (sye-AT-ik-ah)
turbid (TER-bid)

CHAPTER CONCEPTS

Cellular regulation
Cognition
Infection
Mobility
Perfusion
Sexuality

LEARNING OUTCOMES

1. Explain causes, risk factors, and pathophysiology of central nervous system infections, including meningitis and encephalitis.
2. Plan nursing interventions for a patient with a central nervous system infection.
3. Differentiate between the various types of headaches.
4. Identify teaching to be provided for a patient experiencing headaches.
5. List the causes and types of seizures.
6. Describe appropriate interventions for an individual experiencing a seizure.
7. Recognize symptoms in a patient who is developing increased intracranial pressure.
8. Identify nursing interventions that can help prevent increased intracranial pressure.
9. Explain the causes, risk factors, and pathophysiology of injuries to the brain and spinal cord.
10. Plan nursing care for a patient with an injury to the brain or spinal cord.
11. Explain causes, risk factors, and pathophysiology associated with neurodegenerative disorders such as Parkinson, Huntington, and Alzheimer diseases.
12. Plan nursing care for a patient with a neurodegenerative disorder.
13. Plan nursing interventions for the patient with dementia.

Disorders of the central nervous system (CNS) include problems originating in the brain and spinal cord. Because the CNS is the control center for the entire body, disorders in this system can cause symptoms in any part of the body, including pain, confusion, paralysis, and coma. This chapter presents nursing care of patients with these disorders. Care of patients with cerebrovascular disorders is covered in Chapter 49.

CENTRAL NERVOUS SYSTEM INFECTIONS

Infectious agents can enter the CNS via a variety of routes (Table 48.1). Anything that depresses the patient's immune system, such as steroid administration, chemotherapy, radiation therapy, or malnutrition, can make the patient more vulnerable to infection.

Table 48.1
Routes of Entry for Central Nervous System Infections

Route of Entry	Examples
Bloodstream	Insect bite Otitis media
Direct extension	Fracture of frontal or facial bones
Cerebrospinal fluid	Dural tear Poor sterile technique during procedure
Nose or mouth	Meningococcus meningitis
In utero	Contamination of amniotic fluid Rubella Vaginal infection

Table 48.2
Cranial Nerves Affected by Meningitis

Cranial Nerve Affected	Manifestation
III, IV, VI	Ocular palsies Unequal and sluggishly reactive pupils
VII	Facial weakness
VIII	Deafness and vertigo

Meningitis

Pathophysiology and Etiology

Meningitis is an inflammation of the meninges that surround the brain and spinal cord, caused by either bacterial or viral infection. Any microorganism that enters the body can result in meningitis. Bacterial meningitis is a serious infection spread by direct contact with discharge from the respiratory tract of an infected person. Viral meningitis, also called *aseptic meningitis*, is more common and rarely serious. It usually presents with flu-like symptoms, and patients recover in 1 to 2 weeks.

The most common bacteria that cause meningitis are *Neisseria meningitidis, Streptococcus pneumoniae,* Group B *Streptococcus,* and *Haemophilus influenzae* type b (Hib). With current immunization standards in the United States, Hib has decreased in recent years. Bacterial infection generally begins in another area, such as the upper respiratory tract, then enters the blood and invades the CNS, which inflames the meninges and increases intracranial pressure (ICP). Vessel occlusion and necrosis of areas in the brain can occur. Cranial nerve function can be transiently or permanently affected by meningitis (Table 48.2).

Prevention

Vaccines are available against some pathogens. Hib vaccinations begin during infancy. A vaccine against *S. pneumoniae* is recommended for people ages 65 and older and those who have a chronic medical condition. Currently, the Centers for Disease Control and Prevention (CDC, 2019) recommends two doses of meningococcal vaccine (MCV4) for adolescents, one at age 11 or 12 and a booster at age 16. Other groups at increased risk who should be vaccinated are college freshmen living in dormitories, U.S. military recruits, anyone in communal living, anyone with compromised immunity, laboratory personnel, and those traveling to areas of the world where meningococcal disease is common.

Prophylactic treatment is recommended for those who have had significant exposure to anyone infected with meningitis. To destroy the organism from the nasopharynx, antimicrobials such as rifampin (Rifadin), quinolones, or sulfonamides are used.

Signs and Symptoms

The most common symptom of meningitis is a severe headache, caused by tension on blood vessels and irritation of the pain-sensitive dura mater. Other symptoms include a stiff neck, change in level of consciousness, **photophobia** (light sensitivity), and nausea. The patient with meningococcal meningitis may present with petechiae on the skin and mucous membranes.

Nuchal rigidity (pain and stiffness when the neck is moved) is caused by spasm of the extensor muscles of the neck. Positive Kernig and Brudzinski signs are often seen in patients suffering from meningitis. Both signs are caused by inflammation of the meninges and spinal nerve roots. To elicit the Kernig sign, the examiner flexes the patient's hip to 90 degrees and tries to extend the patient's knee. The sign is positive if the patient experiences pain and spasm of the hamstring. The Brudzinski sign is positive when flexion of the patient's neck causes the hips and knees to flex (Fig. 48.1). Nausea and vomiting associated with meningitis are caused by irritation of brain tissue and by increased ICP.

> **LEARNING TIP**
> Kernig starts with a **K**; you test for Kernig sign by bending the **K**nee.
> Brudzinski starts with **B**; you test for Brudzinski sign by lifting the **B**ack of the head.

• WORD • BUILDING •

meningitis: mening—membranous covering of the brain + itis—inflammation
photophobia: photo—light + phobia—fear or intolerance

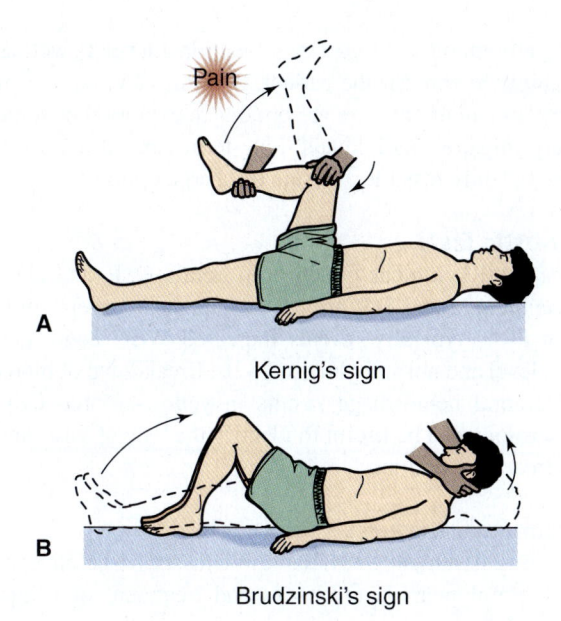

FIGURE 48.1 (A) Kernig sign. (B) Brudzinski sign.

Encephalopathy refers to the mental status changes seen in patients with meningitis, manifested as short attention span, poor memory, disorientation, difficulty following commands, and a tendency to misinterpret environmental stimuli. Late signs include lethargy and seizures.

Complications
Resolution of meningitis depends on how quickly and effectively the disease is treated. Viral meningitis usually has no lasting effects; however, bacterial meningitis can be fatal. Cranial nerve damage can leave a patient blind or deaf. Seizures can continue even after the acute phase of the illness has passed. Cognitive deficits ranging from memory impairment to profound learning disabilities can occur.

Diagnostic Tests
A lumbar puncture is the most informative diagnostic test for a patient with suspected meningitis (see Chapter 47). Viral meningitis is characterized by clear cerebrospinal fluid (CSF) with normal glucose level and normal or slightly increased protein level. No bacteria are seen, but the white blood cell (WBC) count is usually increased. In contrast, the CSF of an individual with bacterial meningitis is **turbid**, or cloudy, because of the elevated number of WBCs. Bacteria are identified by Gram stain and culture, and a sensitivity test is done to identify the most effective antibiotic. The bacteria use the glucose normally found in CSF, thereby lowering the glucose level. The amount of protein in the CSF is elevated. Magnetic resonance imaging (MRI) or computed tomography (CT) scan can be done to evaluate for complications.

Therapeutic Measures
Antibiotics such as vancomycin and cephalosporins are administered for bacterial meningitis. It is important to note the sensitivity report when it is complete to confirm that the antibiotic in use is the best choice. Symptom management is the same for viral or bacterial meningitis. Antipyretics such as acetaminophen are used to control fever; a cooling blanket also can be used. Care should be taken to avoid cooling the patient too much because shivering increases the metabolic demand for oxygen and glucose. Analgesics are given to lessen head and neck pain. Corticosteroids and anti-inflammatory agents are given to decrease cerebral swelling. Nausea and vomiting are controlled with antiemetic medications. The patient with meningococcal meningitis should be placed in droplet isolation for at least the first 24 hours of medication administration to prevent transmission to others.

Patients can become agitated. A quiet, dark environment lessens the stimulation of a patient who has a headache or photophobia and who is agitated, disoriented, or at risk for seizures. An important aspect of nursing care focuses on keeping patients from harming themselves. It is very upsetting to families to see a loved one acting agitated or disoriented. Therefore, it is important to teach the family about symptoms and treatment goals for the patient (Table 48.3).

Encephalitis
Pathophysiology
Encephalitis is an inflammation of brain tissue. Nerve cell damage, edema, and necrosis cause neurologic findings in the areas of the brain affected. Brain hemorrhage can occur in some types of encephalitis. Increased ICP can lead to herniation of the brain (discussed later in this chapter).

Etiology
Viruses are the most common cause of encephalitis. They can be related to time of year or geographic location. Some viruses, such as West Nile virus, are carried by ticks or mosquitoes. Others are systemic viral infections, such as infectious mononucleosis or mumps, which spread to the brain.

Herpes simplex virus (HSV) is the most common non-insect-borne virus to cause encephalitis. Most individuals harbor HSV type 1 in a dormant state. This virus is responsible for sores on the oral mucous membranes, commonly called *cold sores*. Communicable diseases, fever, and emotional stress may cause the virus to become active, but the exact mechanism is not known.

Signs and Symptoms
As with many viruses, symptoms of headache, general malaise, nausea, vomiting, and fever develop over several days. Additional symptoms include nuchal rigidity, confusion, decreased level of consciousness (LOC), seizures, photophobia, **ataxia** (lack of muscle coordination), abnormal sleep patterns, and tremors. The patient may have **hemiparesis** (weakness on one side of the body).

• WORD • BUILDING •

encephalopathy: encephalo—brain + pathy—illness
encephalitis: encephalo—brain + itis—inflammation
hemiparesis: hemi—one side + paresis—partial paralysis

Table 48.3
Meningitis Summary

Signs and Symptoms	Nuchal rigidity Positive Kernig and Brudzinski signs Fever Photophobia Petechial rash on skin and mucous membranes Encephalopathy *No appetite or thirst* *Severe headache*
Diagnostic Tests	Lumbar puncture with cerebrospinal fluid, analysis, culture and sensitivity (C&S) Complete blood count (CBC) C&S nose and throat
Therapeutic Measures	Antimicrobials (if bacterial) Seizure precautions Antipyretics Pain management Reduction of environmental stimuli Education
Complications	Seizures Increased intracranial pressure Hearing loss Vision impairment Cognitive defects
Priority Nursing Diagnoses	*Hyperthermia* *Risk for Acute Confusion* *Self-Care Deficit (Dressing/Feeding/Toileting)* *Acute* or *Chronic Pain* *Risk for Injury* *Impaired Physical Mobility*

The patient with herpes encephalitis develops edema and necrosis (sometimes associated with hemorrhage), most commonly in the temporal lobes. This significant cerebral edema causes increased ICP and can lead to herniation of the brain. A delay in treatment of encephalitis or no treatment can result in death or permanent disability.

Complications
Patients who have had encephalitis can be left with cognitive disabilities and personality changes. Ongoing seizures, motor deficits, and blindness can occur. Changes in cognition and personality are particularly stressful for family members. The patient's behavioral control is a major factor in determining discharge plans. You can assist family members to realistically monitor the patient's functional level as well as their ability to care for the patient. In-home care, outpatient therapy, and adult day care are options to explore. For some severely impaired individuals, long-term care in a facility may be the only feasible and safe discharge option.

Diagnostic Tests
CT scan, MRI, lumbar puncture to obtain CSF, and electroencephalogram (EEG) are used to diagnose encephalitis. CSF analysis typically reveals increased WBC count and protein level and normal glucose levels. Breakdown of blood after cerebral hemorrhage results in yellow-colored CSF. Viral serology can be useful to identify the type of virus and guide treatment options.

Therapeutic Measures
No specific treatment is available for insect-borne encephalitis. Careful neurologic checks and treatment of symptoms can help prevent complications and improve survival. Anticonvulsants, antipyretics, and analgesics are administered to reduce seizures, fever, and headache. Corticosteroids decrease cerebral swelling from inflammation. Sedatives may be given for irritability. Antiviral medications such as acyclovir (Zovirax) may be used, especially for HSV.

> **CUE RECOGNITION 48.1**
>
> You are caring for a patient with encephalitis and notice that their SpO_2 decreases from 94% to 85% after you suction their oral airway. What should you do?
>
> *Suggested answers are at the end of the chapter.*

Nursing Process for the Patient With a Central Nervous System Infection
See "Nursing Process for the Patient With a Communicable or Inflammatory Neurologic Disorder" later in this chapter.

INCREASED INTRACRANIAL PRESSURE

Pathophysiology and Etiology
The skull is a rigid compartment containing three components: brain, blood, and CSF. ICP is the pressure exerted inside the cranial cavity by these components. Normal ICP is 0 to 15 mm Hg. ICP fluctuates with normal physiological changes, such as arterial pulsations, changes in position, and increases in intrathoracic pressure (e.g., coughing or sneezing).

If an increase in one component is not accompanied by a decrease in one or both of the other components, the result is increased ICP (Fig. 48.2). Any patient with a pathological intracranial condition is at risk for increased ICP. Common causes of increased ICP include brain trauma, intracranial hemorrhage, and brain tumors. Prompt detection of changes in neurologic status indicating increased ICP allows intervention aimed at preventing permanent brain damage.

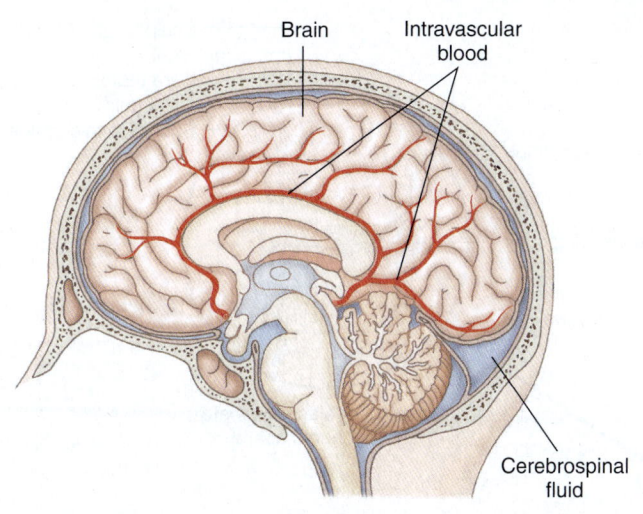

FIGURE 48.2 Any increase in brain tissue, blood, or cerebrospinal fluid can increase intracranial pressure.

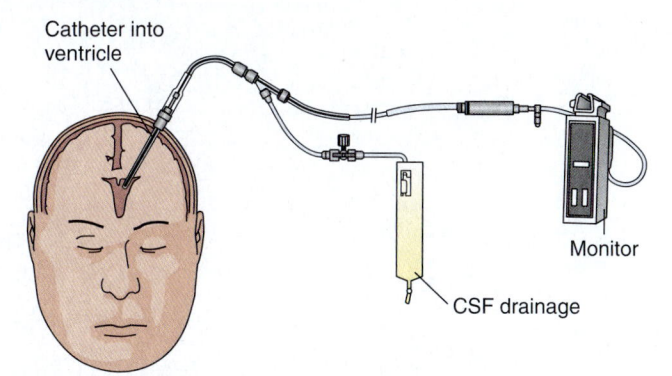

FIGURE 48.3 Ventricular drain. A catheter into the ventricle allows intracranial pressure monitoring and cerebrospinal fluid (CSF) drainage.

The consequences of increased ICP depend on the degree of elevation and speed with which ICP increases. Patients with slow-growing tumors can have significantly increased ICP before they develop symptoms. Conversely, patients with a subarachnoid hemorrhage can sustain a sudden sharp increase in ICP.

The normal body has several methods of compensating for increased ICP. CSF can be shunted into the spinal subarachnoid space. Hyperventilation can trigger constriction of cerebral blood vessels, decreasing the amount of blood within the cranial vault. These compensatory mechanisms are temporary and are not particularly effective for sudden or severe ICP increase.

Signs and Symptoms

Initial symptoms of increased ICP include restlessness, irritability, and decreased LOC because cerebral cortex function is impaired. If not intubated, the patient can hyperventilate, causing vasoconstriction as the body attempts to compensate. As the pressure increases, the oculomotor nerve can be compressed on the side of the impairment. Compression of the outermost fibers of the oculomotor nerve results in diminished reactivity and dilation of the pupil. As the fibers become increasingly compressed, the pupil stops reacting to light. If the compression continues and the brain tissue exerts pressure on the opposite side of the brain from the injury, both pupils become fixed and dilated.

Vital sign changes are a late indication of increasing ICP. The Cushing triad is a classic late sign of increased ICP. It is characterized by bradycardia, decreased respirations, and arterial hypertension (increasing systolic blood pressure while diastolic blood pressure remains the same), resulting in widening pulse pressure. By the time these symptoms appear, the ICP is significantly increased, and interventions may not be successful.

Monitoring

ICP monitoring allows early detection of changes in the pressure on the brain before changes in symptoms are seen. The most common method of monitoring ICP in adults is by placing a catheter in a ventricle of the brain, the cerebral parenchyma, or the subdural or subarachnoid space. This can be done at the bedside or in an operating room. Each of these methods requires anesthetizing the scalp and drilling a hole, called a *burr hole*, into the skull.

Placement of a catheter into one of the lateral ventricles is referred to as *external ventricular drainage* (Fig. 48.3). This method allows for pressure monitoring as well as drainage of CSF to reduce ICP. Disadvantages to this method include difficulty in locating the ventricle for insertion of the catheter and clotting of the catheter by blood in the CSF.

To allow communication with the subarachnoid space, a subarachnoid bolt can be tightly screwed into the burr hole after dura has been punctured (Fig. 48.4). The advantage of a subarachnoid bolt is ease of placement. Disadvantages include occlusion of the sensor portion of the bolt with brain tissue and inability to drain CSF. An intraparenchymal monitor is placed directly into brain tissue. Some physicians believe this type of monitor most accurately reflects the actual situation within the skull. These monitors cannot be used to drain CSF and can become occluded by brain tissue.

Patients with ICP monitors are cared for in an intensive care unit (ICU) and require aggressive nursing care to prevent complications. These patients are often mechanically ventilated and are generally pharmacologically paralyzed and sedated. In addition to meeting the patient's physiological needs and preventing complications, the nurse provides important education and emotional support for family members.

Nursing Process for the Patient With a Communicable or Inflammatory Neurologic Disorder

Data Collection

Collaborate with the registered nurse (RN) to obtain a complete history from the patient, if feasible, and from family members. Pay particular attention to exposure to risk factors. The physical examination must include all body systems because neurologic impairment affects the entire person. Following the initial examination, serial neurologic checks remain important to detect and report

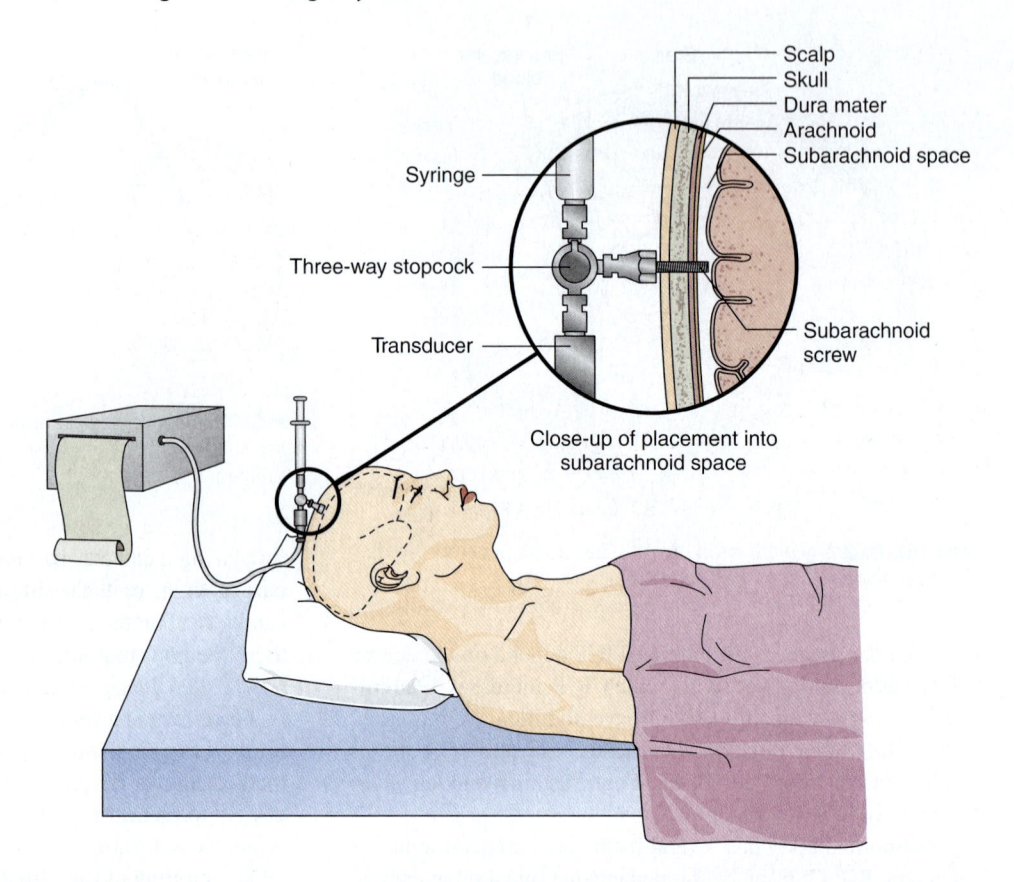

FIGURE 48.4 Subarachnoid bolt monitor.

changes promptly. You can assist with monitoring pupil response, LOC, and vital signs for signs of increased ICP (Box 48.1). Monitor headache on a pain scale or the Pain Assessment in Advanced Dementia (PAINAD) scale if necessary. The Glasgow Coma Scale or the FOUR Score Coma Scale, presented in Chapter 47, are valuable tools to use to monitor LOC.

Nursing Care for the Patient With Communicable or Inflammatory Neurological Disorders

Antipyretics, tepid sponge baths, or cooling blankets may be used to control fever. Determine patient's ability to perform activities of daily living (ADL), and allow them extra time to do so at their own pace. Allow family to assist when appropriate. Manage pain with medications and/or comfort measures and control nausea and vomiting. Maintain seizure precautions if needed (Box 48.2), and report any changes in LOC to the RN or health-care provider (HCP). See Table 48.4 for nursing care of the patient with increased ICP, and refer to Table 48.3 for a summary of care for patients with meningitis.

Box 48.1

Signs and Symptoms of Increased Intracranial Pressure

- Vomiting
- Headache
- Dilated pupil on affected side
- Hemiparesis or hemiplegia
- Decorticate then decerebrate posturing
- Decreasing level of consciousness
- Increasing systolic blood pressure
- Increasing then decreasing pulse rate
- Rising temperature

Box 48.2

Interventions for Seizures

Seizure Precautions
- Pad side rails of hospital bed with commercial pads or bath blankets folded over and pinned in place.
- Keep call light within reach.
- Assist patient when ambulating.
- Keep suction and oral airway at bedside.

Nursing Care During a Seizure
- Stay with patient.
- Do not restrain patient.
- Protect from injury (move nearby objects).
- Loosen tight clothing.
- Turn to side when able to prevent occlusion of airway or aspiration.
- Suction if needed.
- Monitor vital signs when able.
- Be prepared to assist with breathing if necessary.

Patient Education

The nature and focus of teaching depend on the patient's LOC and cognitive status. When appropriate, include both the patient and family members in the education process. If the patient is not able to participate, family members become the focus of teaching.

CRITICAL THINKING & CLINICAL JUDGMENT

Mr. Chung is an 18-year-old college student. He comes to the emergency department with a headache, stiff neck, and fever. When collecting data, you notice a petechial rash on his legs and torso. The HCP diagnoses meningococcal meningitis.

Critical Thinking (The Why)
1. Why would you need to be mindful of certain infection control practices?
2. Why would Mr. Chung be at risk for impaired comfort?
3. What concerns do you have about how Mr. Chung contracted his illness?

Clinical Judgment (The Do)
4. What tests will likely be performed?
5. What patient education should be planned for Mr. Chung?

Suggested answers are at the end of the chapter.

HEADACHES

Headache is a common symptom of neurologic disorders. However, most headaches are transient events and do not indicate a serious pathological condition. If headaches are recurrent, persistent, or increasing in severity, the patient should undergo a neurologic evaluation. This section addresses the most common types of headaches.

Types of Headaches

Headaches are divided into three major types: (1) primary, (2) secondary, and (3) cranial neuralgias, central and primary facial pain, and other headaches. Primary headaches are discussed in this section. Secondary headaches are caused by trauma, infection, or other disorders. Cranial neuralgias and facial pain are discussed in Chapter 50. For more information, visit the International Headache Society at www.ichd-3.org.

Migraine Headaches

Migraine headaches are a neurologic disorder involving brain chemicals and neurologic pathways. Current research suggests that a trigger stimulates a release of chemicals that cause an inflammatory response and overstimulation of the trigeminal nerve, resulting in pain. A migraine may or may not involve an aura, such as vision changes or tingling, that precedes an attack. The tendency to develop migraine

Table 48.4
Measures to Prevent Increased Intracranial Pressure

Preventive Measures	Rationale
Keep head of bed elevated 30 degrees unless contraindicated.	Head elevation reduces intracranial pressure (ICP) in some patients.
Avoid flexing the neck; keep head and neck in midline position.	Neck flexion can obstruct venous outflow.
Administer antiemetics and antitussives as necessary to prevent vomiting and cough.	Coughing and vomiting can increase ICP.
Administer stool softeners.	Straining for bowel movement can increase ICP.
Minimize suctioning. If absolutely necessary, oxygenate first and limit suction passes to one or two.	Suctioning can increase ICP.
Avoid hip flexion.	Hip flexion can increase intra-abdominal and thoracic pressure, which can increase ICP.
Prevent unnecessary noise and startling the patient.	Noxious stimuli can increase ICP in some patients.
Space care activities to provide rest between each disturbance.	Clustering care activities can increase ICP.

headaches is often hereditary. When one or both parents experience migraines, children are more likely to experience them as well. Migraines frequently begin in childhood or adolescence and are more common in women. Common migraine triggers include stress, hormones (menses-related), not eating, changes in barometric pressure, sleep disturbances, odors, neck pain, bright light, and alcohol.

There are two major types of migraine: migraine with aura and migraine without aura. Four phases are generally associated with migraine headaches: prodromal, aura, headache, and resolution. The pre-headache (**prodromal**) phase can include symptoms such as irritability, sleepiness, or food cravings. The aura stage might include visual disturbances, difficulty speaking, and/or numbness or tingling. The headache that follows is often accompanied by nausea and sometimes vomiting; it can last for hours to days. Commonly used descriptors of migraine pain include *throbbing, boring, vise-like,* and *pounding*. The pain is usually on one side of the head. Noise and light tend to worsen the headache, leading patients to find a dark, quiet environment. The final stage, resolution, might be accompanied by sluggishness or confusion.

Treatment of migraine may be prophylactic or directed at an acute episode. Prophylactic treatment is usually reserved for patients experiencing one or more migraine headaches per week. Patients who experience 15 or more days a month with a migraine headache may be treated with botulinum toxin (Botox). Small doses of Botox are injected into specific areas of the head and neck around pain fibers that stimulate release of the inflammatory chemicals. It may take up to three treatments for relief. Treatments are repeated every 3 months.

Lifestyle changes can help prevent migraines such as routine mealtimes, good sleep habits, daily exercise, and avoidance of triggers. Dietary restrictions can be helpful if triggering foods or beverages can be identified.

Several types of medications are available to treat acute migraine headaches. NSAIDs such as naproxen (Naprosyn, Aleve) may be tried first. Ergot (Cafergot), a vasoconstrictor, is effective only if taken before the vessel walls become edematous, usually within 30 to 60 minutes of headache onset. Triptans, such as sumatriptan (Imitrex) and zolmitriptan (Zomig), work at the serotonin receptor sites and have a vasoconstricting action. Treximet combines naproxen and sumatriptan. Lasmiditan, dihydroergotamine, and calcitonin gene-related peptide (CGRP) antagonists are also used. Opioids are habit-forming and are used only as a last resort. The potentially additive effects of multiple medication regimens require careful monitoring.

Tension or Muscle Contraction Headaches

Persistent contraction of the scalp and facial, cervical, and upper thoracic muscles can cause tension headaches. A cycle of muscle tension, muscle tenderness, and further muscle tension is established and may or may not be associated with vasodilation of cerebral arteries. Tension headaches can be associated with premenstrual syndrome or psychosocial stressors such as anxiety, emotional distress, or depression. Symptoms typically develop gradually. Radiation of pain to the crown of the head and base of the skull, varying in location and intensity, is common. *Pressure, aching, steady,* and *tight* are some words patients use to describe tension headaches.

Care must be taken to thoroughly rule out physical causes before attributing the headache to psychosocial origins. Symptom management may include the use of relaxation techniques, yoga/stretching exercises, massage of the affected muscles, rest, localized heat application, nonopioid analgesics, and appropriate counseling.

Cluster Headaches

Vascular disturbance, stress, anxiety, and emotional distress are all proposed causes of cluster headaches. As indicated by the name, these headaches tend to occur in clusters during a time span of several days to weeks. Months or even years can pass between episodes. Alcohol consumption may worsen the episodes.

The patient may state that the headache begins suddenly, typically at the same time of night. *Throbbing* and *excruciating* are often the adjectives used by the patient to describe the pain. The headache tends to be unilateral, affecting the nose, eye, and forehead. A bloodshot, teary appearance of the affected eye is common.

Because of the brief nature of cluster headaches, treatment is difficult. A quiet, dark environment and cold compresses can lessen the intensity of the pain. NSAIDs or tricyclic antidepressants may be prescribed.

Diagnosis of Headaches

Most headaches are diagnosed on the basis of the patient's history and symptoms. MRI, CT scan, skull x-ray, arteriogram, EEG, cranial nerve testing, and lumbar puncture to test CSF may be done to rule out other causes for the headaches.

Nursing Process for the Patient With a Headache

Data Collection

The **WHAT'S UP?** mnemonic is particularly useful in helping the patient provide useful information regarding the headache:

- **W**—Where is the pain? Does it remain in one place or radiate to other areas of the head? Does the headache consistently start in one place?
- **H**—How does the headache feel? Is it throbbing, steady, dull, or bandlike, or does it have other qualities?
- **A**—Aggravating or alleviating factors should be determined. These may include red wine, caffeine, chocolate, and foods containing nitrates or monosodium glutamate (MSG). Other factors include stages of the menstrual cycle, emotional stress, and tension. Alleviating factors might include lying down in a dark room, cold compresses, or medications.

• WORD • BUILDING •

prodromal: pro—before + dromos—running

- **T**—Timing can help with diagnosis. When does it typically occur? How long does it last?
- **S**—Ask the patient to rate the severity on a scale of 0 to 10. Is the severity consistent, or does it vary from headache to headache?
- **U**—Ask about other useful data. For example, are there associated symptoms, such as nausea, vomiting, or bloodshot eyes?
- **P**—Determine the patient's perception of the headache. Does it interfere with the patient's life? If so, how? Has the patient had a previous evaluation of headaches?

Nursing Diagnoses, Planning, and Implementation

Acute Pain related to physiological mechanisms of headache as evidenced by the patient's pain rating

EXPECTED OUTCOME: The headache will be prevented or controlled as evidenced by the patient statement of no pain or acceptable pain rating.

- Assist the patient to identify and reduce or eliminate aggravating factors. Have the patient keep a headache diary for a time, recording the time of day the headache occurs, foods eaten or other aggravating factors, description of the pain, identification of associated symptoms such as nausea or visual disturbances, and other factors related to headache symptoms. *Identification of triggers can help the patient lessen the frequency and intensity of attacks.*
- Encourage the patient to use alleviating techniques such as warm or cold compresses, biofeedback, or stress reduction. *This helps the patient participate in the treatment of the headache and provides a sense of control over their illness.*
- Teach the patient to use relaxation exercises or simple stretching exercises. *These relaxation exercises may be helpful for tension headaches.*
- Provide a dark room and rest *to reduce stimulation during a migraine headache.*
- Teach the patient about medications, appropriate dosage, expected action, side effects, and consequences of misuse. *The patient will need to understand medication administration for appropriate use at home.*

Evaluation

If interventions have been effective, the patient will understand self-care to prevent and treat headaches and will report a reduction in headache pain and occurrences.

SEIZURE DISORDERS

A seizure can be a symptom of epilepsy or other neurologic disorders such as a brain tumor or meningitis. Epilepsy is a chronic neurologic disorder characterized by recurrent seizure activity.

Pathophysiology

The normal stability of the neuron cell membrane is impaired in individuals with seizures. This instability allows for abnormal electrical discharges to occur, causing the characteristic symptoms seen during a seizure.

Seizures can be classified as partial or generalized. Partial seizures begin on one side of the cerebral cortex. In some cases, the electrical discharge spreads to the other hemisphere, and the seizure becomes generalized. Generalized seizures are characterized by involvement of both cerebral hemispheres.

Etiology

Epilepsy can be acquired or idiopathic (unknown cause). Causes of acquired epilepsy include traumatic brain injury and anoxic events. No cause has been identified for idiopathic epilepsy. The most common time for idiopathic epilepsy to begin is before age 20. New-onset seizures after this age are most commonly caused by an underlying neurologic disorder. As the population ages, more older adults are having first-time seizure as a result of bleeding or bruising in the brain related to a fall. Multiple medications in the elder population and untreated hypertension can increase the risk of falls as well as brain injury after a fall.

Signs and Symptoms

Symptoms of seizure activity correlate with the area of the brain where the seizure begins. Some patients experience an aura or sensation that warns that a seizure is about to occur. An aura can be a visual distortion, a noxious odor, or an unusual sound. Patients who experience an aura may have enough time to sit or lie down before the seizure starts, minimizing the risk of injury.

Partial Seizures

Repetitive, purposeless behaviors, called *automatisms*, are the classic symptom of partial seizures. The patient appears to be in a dreamlike state while picking at clothing, chewing, or smacking lips. Patients may be labeled as mentally ill, particularly if automatisms include unacceptable social behaviors such as spitting or fondling themselves. Patients are not aware of behavior or that it is inappropriate. If the patient does not lose consciousness, the seizure is labeled as simple partial and usually lasts less than 1 minute. Older terms for simple partial seizures include *Jacksonian* and *focal motor*. If consciousness is lost, it is called a *complex partial* seizure or *psychomotor* seizure; it can last from 2 to 15 minutes.

Partial seizures arising from the parietal lobe can cause paresthesias on the side of the body opposite the seizure focus. Visual disturbances are seen if the seizure originates in the occipital lobe. Involvement of the motor cortex results in involuntary movements of the opposite side of the body. Typically, movements begin in the arm and hand and can spread to the leg and face.

The **postictal** period is the recovery period after a seizure. Following a partial seizure, the postictal phase may be no more than a few minutes of disorientation.

Generalized Seizures

Generalized seizures affect the entire brain. Two types of generalized seizures are absence seizures and tonic-clonic seizures. Absence seizures, sometimes called *petit mal* seizures, occur most often in children. They are manifested by a period of staring that lasts several seconds.

Tonic-clonic seizures are what most people envision when they think of seizures; they are sometimes called *grand mal* seizures or *convulsions*. Tonic-clonic seizures follow a typical progression. Aura and loss of consciousness may or may not occur. The tonic phase, lasting 30 to 60 seconds, is characterized by rigidity, causing the patient to fall if not lying down. The pupils are fixed and dilated, the hands and jaws are clenched, and the patient may temporarily stop breathing. The clonic phase is signaled by contraction and relaxation of all muscles in a jerky, rhythmic fashion. The extremities can move forcefully, causing injury if the patient strikes furniture or walls. The patient is often incontinent. Biting the lips or tongue can cause bleeding.

The postictal period is usually longer after a tonic-clonic seizure. Patients may sleep deeply for 30 minutes to several hours. Following deep sleep, patients may report headache, confusion, and fatigue. Patients may realize that they had a seizure but not remember the event itself.

Diagnostic Tests

Some diagnostic tests include CT, MRI, PET, and single-photon emission computerized tomography (SPECT) imaging. The most useful test for evaluating seizures is an EEG. An EEG can determine where in the brain the seizures start, the frequency and duration of seizures, and the presence of subclinical (asymptomatic) seizures. Sleep deprivation and flashing light stimulation may be used to evaluate the seizure threshold. See Appendix A for more information on EEGs.

Therapeutic Measures

If an underlying cause for the seizure is identified, treatment focuses on correcting the cause. If no cause is found or seizures continue despite treatment of concurrent disorders, treatment focuses on stopping or preventing seizure activity.

Numerous anticonvulsant medications are available (Table 48.5). Typically, the patient is started on one medication, and the dosage is increased until therapeutic levels are attained or side effects become troublesome. If seizures are not controlled on a single medication, another medication is added. Many anticonvulsants require periodic blood tests to monitor serum levels as well as kidney and liver function. Most of these medications can cause drowsiness, so teach the patient to avoid driving or operating machinery until the effects of the medication are known. Driving is also contraindicated until seizures are under control.

If a patient must discontinue an anticonvulsant, it should be tapered slowly according to manufacturer directions. Stopping abruptly can result in status epilepticus, discussed later. If seizures continue despite anticonvulsant therapy, surgical intervention may be considered.

Seizure alert dogs are specially trained canines that have innate ability, through the sense of smell, to detect an oncoming seizure in their humans before they occur. Not only can seizure alert dogs assist in potentially saving human lives, but they provide needed comfort and reassurance, allowing patients to feel more comfortable when out in public (Epilepsy Foundation, 2020).

Surgical Management

The success of surgical intervention for epilepsy depends on identification of an epileptic focus within nonvital brain tissue. The surgeon attempts to resect the area affected to prevent spread of seizure activity. In some cases, seizures can be cured, but in others, the goal is to reduce the frequency or severity of the seizures. If no focus is identified or if it is in a vital area such as the motor cortex or speech center, surgery is not feasible.

The preoperative assessment for epilepsy surgery is an extensive multistage process. Thorough data collection and teaching are essential. To adequately identify seizure foci, the patient is weaned off anticonvulsant therapy. Increasing the frequency of seizures with weaning is anxiety provoking for patients and family members.

Emergency Care

Emergency care is required when a seizure occurs. The prime objective is to prevent injury during a seizure. It is important to stay with the patient during the seizure activity. Side rails, if used, should be padded to prevent injury if the patient strikes extremities against them. If the patient falls to the floor, move furniture out of the way. Maintain a patent airway, and, if possible, turn the patient on their side to prevent aspiration if vomiting occurs. Do not force an airway or anything else into the patient's mouth once the seizure has begun. Do not restrain the individual because doing so can also increase the risk of injury (see "Patient Perspective: Mrs. Rowley"). Observe and document the patient's behavior during the seizure (e.g., which part of the body was first involved, progression of the seizure, length of time the seizure lasted). After the seizure, check the patient for breathing, suction the oral pharynx if necessary, and, in rare cases, initiate rescue breathing or cardiopulmonary resuscitation (CPR) as indicated.

• WORD • BUILDING •

postictal: post—after + ictal—seizure

Table 48.5
Anticonvulsant Medications

Medication Class/Action

Anticonvulsants—Preventive Agents

Suppress abnormal discharge of neurons and suppress spread of seizure activity from focus to other parts of brain.

Examples	*Nursing Implications*
carbamazepine (Tegretol)	Monitor complete blood count (CBC). Therapeutic level is 6–12 mcg/mL. Do not crush sustained-release (SR) forms.
lacosamide (Vimpat)	Injectable form available. May increase risk of suicidal ideation.
ezogabine (Potiga)	May cause retinal abnormalities. Vision examination necessary at baseline and every 6 months. Monitor for urinary retention.
gabapentin (Neurontin)	Use with opioids may increase the risk of respiratory depression.
levetiracetam (Keppra)	May need reduced dose for older adults. Check white blood cell, red blood cell, and liver function tests.
lamotrigine (Lamictal)	Discontinue therapy and notify health-care provider if rash appears. Monitor blood levels.
topiramate (Topamax)	May cause drowsiness
phenytoin (Dilantin)	Regular dental care essential. Therapeutic level is 10–20 mcg/mL. Binds to tube feedings; hold tube feeding 1 hr before and 2 hr after dose.
phenobarbital (Luminal)	Monitor vital signs. Therapeutic level is 15–40 mcg/mL.
valproic acid (Depakote)	Therapeutic level is 50–100 mcg/mL. Do not crush SR form.

Benzodiazepines—Emergency Agents

Potentiate gamma-amino butyric acid (GABA), an inhibitory neurotransmitter in the central nervous system.

Examples	*Nursing Implications*
lorazepam (Ativan) diazepam (Valium, Diastat)	Given to stop a seizure that has not resolved within 5 minutes. Given via intramuscular or intravenous push route by emergency personnel. Diastat may be given rectally at home.

Patient Perspective

Mrs. Rowley

I have had seizures for 35 years and, as a result of falling during seizures, have experienced cuts, bruises, and a broken bone. I usually have an aura that lets me know a seizure is about to occur. This is helpful if I can get myself to a safe place to prevent falling or being injured.

When a patient is having a seizure, you can best help by using padding such as pillows or blankets for protection, talking calmly, and using gentle touch to prevent injury.

You should not sit on or hold down someone during a seizure. I have had the frightening experience of waking up with a nurse sitting on me and holding down my arms. After you have protected the patient, let the person come out of the seizure naturally. When the seizure is over, I usually want to sleep because seizures are exhausting.

Status Epilepticus

Status epilepticus is characterized by at least 30 minutes of repetitive seizure activity without a return to consciousness. This medical emergency requires prompt intervention to prevent irreversible neurologic damage. Abruptly stopping anticonvulsant therapy is the usual cause of status epilepticus.

Seizure activity precipitates a significant increase in the brain's need for glucose and oxygen. This metabolic demand is even greater during status epilepticus. Irreversible neuronal damage can occur if cerebral metabolic needs cannot be fulfilled. Adequate oxygenation must be maintained, if necessary, by intubating and mechanically ventilating the patient. These patients are also at significant risk for aspiration. Therefore, it is important that the nurse assist in airway maintenance and suction as needed to prevent hypoxia and aspiration pneumonia.

IV diazepam (Valium) or lorazepam (Ativan) is administered to stop active seizures. Diazepam can also be given rectally. Because both medications can cause respiratory depression, careful airway management is required. After obtaining serum medication levels, anticonvulsant therapy is adjusted to achieve therapeutic levels.

If seizures remain resistant to treatment, a barbiturate coma may be induced with IV pentobarbital. The last line of treatment for status epilepticus is general anesthesia or pharmacological paralysis. Both therapies require intubation, mechanical ventilation, and management in an ICU setting. Continuous EEG monitoring is used to verify that seizures have stopped. A patient treated with neuromuscular blockade medications can be seizing without visible manifestations. For more information on seizures, visit the Epilepsy Foundation at www.efa.org.

Psychosocial Effects

Finances can be a major concern to patients with seizure disorders. Some patients with epilepsy experience hiring discrimination or may not qualify for some jobs in which safety is a concern. Remind patients that falsifying information on job applications may be grounds for dismissal. Health insurance coverage issues can create financial hardships for patients on long-term medications. Most patients whose seizures are controlled can work and lead productive lives. A social worker can help explore options for financial assistance if needed.

Patients with poorly controlled seizures should not operate motor vehicles. Many in the United States consider a driver's license a sign of adulthood and independence, and patients who cannot drive can experience lowered self-esteem. Job opportunities may be limited for patients who depend on public transportation. Encourage the patient to obtain a state identification card to use in place of a driver's license for identification.

Patients may limit interpersonal relationships out of fear of having a seizure. The involuntary movements, sounds, and possible incontinence that occur with seizures are embarrassing to patients and can be frightening to others. Role-playing may help the patient determine when and how to confide in others.

> **BE SAFE!**
> **BE VIGILANT!** Never place anything in a patient's mouth during a tonic-clonic seizure; remove objects that could injure patient.

Nursing Process for the Patient With Seizures

Data Collection

Perform a general neurologic examination of the patient with a history of seizures. Determine the type of seizure manifestations and type of aura, if any. Determine the patient's knowledge of the disease and its treatment. It is important to find out whether the patient has the resources to purchase prescribed anticonvulsant medications and whether the medication regimen is adhered to. Medication levels can help determine degree of adherence to therapy.

Nursing Diagnoses, Planning, and Implementation

Risk for Injury related to seizure activity

EXPECTED OUTCOME: The patient will remain free from injury.

- Instruct the patient with generalized seizures to recognize an aura and to get to safety (e.g., lying down away from furniture or other objects) if it occurs. *This helps prevent injury during involuntary movements.*
- Institute seizure precautions for the patient admitted to a health-care institution. Box 48.2 lists precautions and interventions *to prevent injury.*
- Encourage all patients to wear medical alert jewelry or other identification *to alert others to the presence of seizure disorder.*
- Assist patients to identify conditions that trigger seizures. Hypoglycemia, hypoxia, and hyponatremia are all potential triggers of hypersensitive neurons. Teach the patient the importance of a consistent schedule of eating and sleeping. *The patient may be able to prevent seizures by avoidance of triggers.*

Ineffective Health Management related to complex regimen and possible lack of resources

EXPECTED OUTCOME: The patient will follow medication regimen as evidenced by therapeutic medication levels and controlled seizure activity.

- Determine the patient's ability to obtain and pay for medication. *Stopping a medication suddenly can result in status epilepticus.*

- Refer the patient to a case manager or social worker, if needed, *to assist with obtaining resources for medications.*
- Teach the patient about medication action, dose, side effects, schedule, and importance of not stopping treatment suddenly. *Patients with seizures can have several medications to take several times each day. Patients who understand their regimens are more likely to comply.*
- Teach the patient about the importance of regular blood tests if required. *Therapeutic blood levels help prevent seizures (too low) and toxicity (too high).*

> **Risk for Situational lowered self-esteem related to negative perception of self-worth due to perception of disease**
>
> **EXPECTED OUTCOME:** The patient will identify feelings associated with negative self-esteem and explore methods and activities to accept changed lifestyles to express a positive self-appraisal.

- Determine patient's situation that is related to poor self-esteem. *Verbalizing their issues can help patient to begin to accept their situation.*
- Analyze anticipated public reaction to condition. *Role-play potential scenarios and encourage patient not to conceal problem, which may actually increase their risk of injury or negative response when seizure occurs.*
- Explore attitudes of close friends or significant others. *Unfavorable expectations of support can affect patient's self-esteem. Refer patient and/or family to support group (Epilepsy Foundation of America, www.epilepsy.com).*

> **PRACTICE ANALYSIS TIP**
> Linking NCLEX-PN® to Practice
> The LPN/LVN will promote positive self-esteem of client.

Evaluation
Successful care of a patient with epilepsy results in a decrease in seizures to the lowest possible frequency. Patient verbalization of understanding needed lifestyle changes is another indication of success. Patients should be able to state measures to prevent injury if a seizure should occur and should verbalize understanding of all medications and their administration schedules. Therapeutic medication levels can be measured to evaluate adherence to the medication regimen.

TRAUMATIC BRAIN INJURY

Traumatic brain injury (TBI) is a major cause of death and disability in adults. Young men make up a large proportion of brain injury victims.

Pathophysiology
TBI is a complex phenomenon with results ranging from no detectable effect to a persistent vegetative state. Trauma can result in hemorrhage, contusion or laceration of the brain, and damage at the cellular level. In addition to the primary insult, the brain injury can be compounded by cerebral edema, hyperemia, or hydrocephalus.

Etiology
Motor vehicle collisions account for the largest percentage of TBIs. Falls, sports-related injuries, and violence are also common causes of TBI.

The brain is susceptible to various types of injury that can be classified in several ways. The term *closed head injury* or *nonpenetrating injury* is used when there has been rapid back-and-forth movement of the brain that causes bruising and tearing of brain tissues and vessels, but the skull is intact. An *open head injury* or *penetrating injury* refers to a break in the skull. *Acceleration injury* results from a moving object hitting a stationary head. An example of this type of injury is a patient who is hit in the head with a baseball bat. A *deceleration injury* occurs when the head is in motion and strikes a stationary surface. This type of injury is seen in patients who trip and fall, hitting their head on furniture or the floor.

A combination *acceleration-deceleration injury* occurs when the stationary head is hit by a mobile object and the head strikes a stationary surface. A soccer player who sustains a blow to the head and hits the ground with their head can sustain an acceleration-deceleration injury.

Rotational injuries have the potential to cause shearing damage to the brain as well as lacerations and contusions. Rotational injuries can be caused by a direct blow to the head or can occur during a motor vehicle collision in which the vehicle is struck from the side. Twisting of the brainstem can damage the reticular activating system, causing loss of consciousness. Movement of the brain within the skull can result in bruising or tearing of brain tissue where it meets the inside of the skull.

Types of Brain Injury and Signs and Symptoms
Concussion
Cerebral concussion is considered a mild brain injury. Loss of consciousness may occur for 5 minutes or less. Concussion is characterized by headache, dizziness, and/or nausea and vomiting. The patient may describe amnesia of events before or after the trauma. On clinical examination, there is no skull or dura injury and no abnormality detected on CT scan or MRI.

Contusion
Cerebral contusion is characterized by bruising of brain tissue, possibly accompanied by hemorrhage. There can be multiple areas of contusion, depending on the causative

mechanism. Severe contusions can result in diffuse axonal injury. The symptoms of a cerebral contusion depend on the area of the brain involved.

Brainstem contusions affect LOC. Decreased LOC can be transient or permanent. Respirations, pupil reaction, eye movement, and motor response to stimuli can also be affected. The autonomic nervous system can be affected by edema or by hypothalamic injury, causing rapid heart rate and respiratory rate, fever, and diaphoresis.

Hematoma

SUBDURAL HEMATOMA. Subdural hematomas are classified as acute or chronic depending on the time between injury and onset of symptoms. Acute subdural hematoma is characterized by appearance of symptoms within 24 hours following injury. The bleeding is typically venous in nature and accumulates between the dura and arachnoid membranes (Fig. 48.5). About 24% of patients who sustain a severe brain injury develop an acute subdural hematoma. Damage to brain tissue can cause an altered LOC. Therefore, it can be difficult to recognize a subdural hematoma on the basis of clinical examination alone. As the subdural hematoma increases in size, the patient may exhibit one-sided paralysis of extraocular movement, extremity weakness, or dilation of the pupil. LOC can deteriorate further as ICP increases.

Older adults and people with alcoholism are particularly prone to chronic subdural hematomas. Atrophy of the brain, common in these populations, stretches the veins between the brain and dura. A seemingly minor fall or blow to the head can cause stretched veins to rupture and bleed. Often, there are no other injuries associated with the trauma. Because a chronic subdural hematoma can develop weeks to months after the injury, the patient may not remember an injury occurring.

The patient with a chronic subdural hematoma may be forgetful, lethargic, or irritable or may report a headache. If the hematoma persists or increases in size, the patient can develop hemiparesis and pupillary changes. The patient or family members may not associate the symptoms with a previous injury and, therefore, may delay seeking medical care.

EPIDURAL HEMATOMA. About 10% of patients with severe brain injuries develop epidural hematomas. Blood collects between the dura mater and skull. The blood is usually arterial in nature and often associated with skull fracture (see Fig. 48.5). Arterial bleeding can cause the hematoma to become large very quickly. Patients with epidural hematoma typically exhibit a progressive course of symptoms. The patient loses consciousness directly after the injury, then regains consciousness and is coherent for a brief period. The patient then develops a dilated pupil and paralyzed extraocular muscles on the side of the hematoma and becomes less responsive. With no intervention, the patient becomes unresponsive. Seizures or hemiparesis can occur. Once the patient has symptoms, deterioration can be rapid. Airway management and control of ICP must be instituted immediately, or the patient will die.

Diagnostic Tests

A CT scan is usually the first imaging test performed on a patient with a TBI. It is faster and more accessible than MRI. This is particularly important for unstable patients or those with multiple injuries. It is easier to identify skull fractures on a CT scan than on MRI. MRI can be used later to identify damage to the brain tissue.

Neuropsychological testing by a trained specialist can be useful in assessing a patient's cognitive function. This assessment helps direct rehabilitation placement, discharge planning, and return to work or school. Neuropsychological testing identifies problems with memory, judgment, learning, and comprehension. Patients may be able to learn compensation strategies based on results.

Therapeutic Measures

Surgical Management

Surgical treatment of hematomas is discussed under intracranial surgery later in this chapter.

Medical Management

Medical management of TBI involves control of ICP and support of body functions. Patients with brain injuries can be partially or completely dependent on assistance with respiration, nutrition, elimination, movement, and skin integrity.

A variety of techniques are used to control ICP in patients with moderate or severe brain injury. The first step is to insert an ICP monitor to allow measurement of the ICP. Refer to the section on increased ICP earlier in this chapter for further information.

If ICP remains elevated despite drainage of CSF, the next step is use of an osmotic diuretic. The most common medication is IV mannitol (Osmitrol). Mannitol uses osmosis to pull fluid from the brain into the intravascular space and

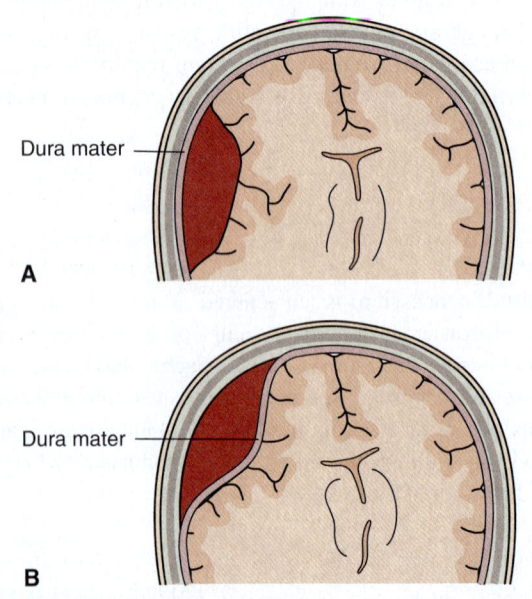

FIGURE 48.5 (A) A subdural hematoma is usually venous and forms between the dura and the arachnoid membranes. (B) An epidural hematoma is usually from an arterial bleed and forms between the dura mater and the skull.

eliminate it via the renal system. Serum osmolarity and electrolytes must be carefully monitored when mannitol is being administered. Some patients experience a rebound increase in ICP after the mannitol wears off.

Mechanical hyperventilation may be used if the patient is still experiencing increased ICP. Hyperventilation is effective in lowering ICP because it causes cerebral vasoconstriction. Vasoconstriction allows less blood into the cranium, thereby lowering ICP. Research has demonstrated, however, that aggressive hyperventilation, particularly within the first 24 hours after injury, can induce ischemia in the already compromised brain. Therefore, hyperventilation is now reserved for increased ICP that does not respond to other treatments.

High-dose barbiturate therapy may be used to induce a therapeutic coma, which reduces the metabolic needs of the brain during the acute phase following injury. Patients in therapeutic coma are completely dependent for all their needs and care. They must be mechanically ventilated and cared for in an ICU setting. Vasopressors may be required to maintain blood pressure, and the patient's temperature should be kept as normal as possible.

Complications
Brain Herniation
If interventions to control ICP are unsuccessful, the patient can experience uncontrolled edema or herniation of brain tissue (Fig. 48.6). Herniation is displacement of brain tissue out of its normal anatomical location. This prevents function of the herniated tissue and places pressure on other vital structures, most commonly the brainstem. Herniation usually results in brain death.

Patients who experience brain death may be suitable organ donor candidates. For some families, the opportunity to donate their loved one's organs provides a sense of purpose in death.

Diabetes Insipidus
Edema or direct injury that affects the posterior portion of the pituitary gland or hypothalamus can result in inadequate release of antidiuretic hormone, causing diabetes insipidus. This results in polyuria and, if the patient is awake, polydipsia. Fluid replacement and IV vasopressin are used to maintain fluid and electrolyte balance. See Chapter 39 for more on diabetes insipidus.

Acute Hydrocephalus
Cerebral edema can interfere with CSF circulation, causing **hydrocephalus.** Initial treatment uses an external ventricular drain, followed by a ventriculoperitoneal shunt if necessary. A shunt drains excess CSF into the peritoneum, where it is reabsorbed into circulation and excreted.

Labile Vital Signs
Direct trauma to or pressure on the brainstem can cause fluctuations in blood pressure, cardiac rhythm, or respiratory pattern. Treatment is aimed at control of ICP.

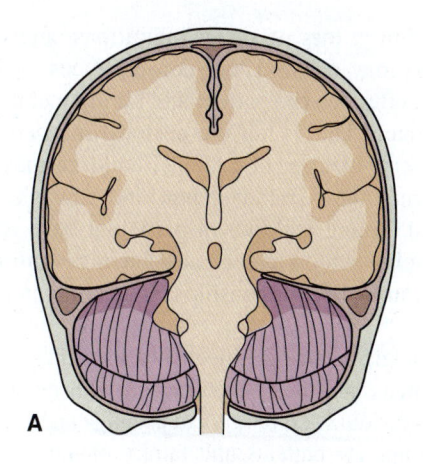

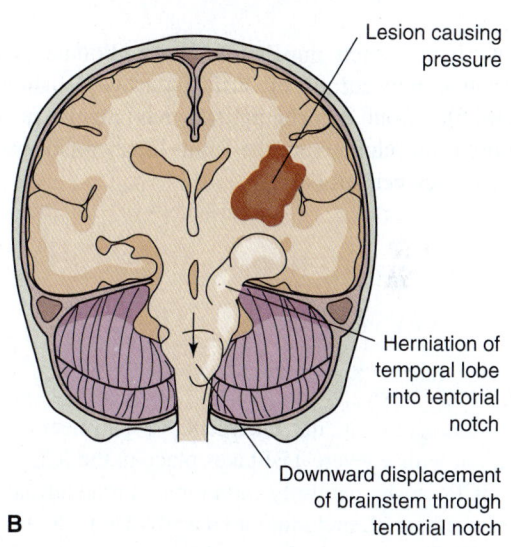

FIGURE 48.6 Herniation of the brain. (A) Normal brain. (B) Herniation of brain tissue into tentorial notch.

Post-Traumatic Stress Disorder
Patients who sustain a concussion can experience ongoing, somewhat vague symptoms. They may report headache, fatigue, difficulty concentrating, depression, or memory impairment. Symptoms can be severe enough to interfere with work, school, and interpersonal relationships. Neuropsychological testing can provide objective evidence of cognitive dysfunction and establish the need for cognitive rehabilitation for post-traumatic stress disorder, or PTSD (see Chapter 57 for more about PTSD). Symptoms can take 3 to 12 months to resolve.

Cognitive and Personality Changes
Alterations in personality and cognition may be the most difficult long-term complication for patients and family members. The patient can have significant short-term memory impairment, which limits their ability to learn new information and can interfere with function at work or school. Impaired judgment can make the patient a safety risk to self or others. It also affects social functioning.

• WORD • BUILDING •

hydrocephalus: hydro—water + cephalus—head

Emotional lability, loss of social inhibitions, and personality changes may occur. These consequences of TBI have a profound effect on the patient and family members. Spouses may state, "This is not the person I married." If behavior is violent, bizarre, or profane, children may be unwilling to bring their friends home and can become socially isolated. Young children in particular have difficulty understanding why a parent is behaving so differently. Disintegration of relationships is not uncommon following TBI.

Neuropsychological testing objectively identifies problems. These deficits can then be addressed with cognitive rehabilitation. Individual and family counseling can be helpful. Support groups for patients and family members may also help.

Motor and speech impairment are additional possible long-term complications of TBI. Intensive rehabilitation provides the best opportunity for maximizing recovery. For more information, visit the Brain Injury Association of America at www.biausa.org.

Nursing Process for the Patient With Traumatic Brain Injury

Acute care is presented here.

Data Collection

After stabilization in the emergency department, care of the patient with a severe TBI takes place in the ICU setting, where ICP can be carefully monitored. Frequent data collection is essential, including a Glasgow Coma Scale score or the FOUR Score (see Chapter 47), pupil responses, muscle strength, and vital signs. Review Box 48.1 for additional signs of increased ICP for which to monitor. Once the patient is stabilized, neurologic damage is assessed. Identification of deficits guides nursing care. Determination of discharge needs should begin as soon as possible. The patient may require extensive rehabilitation, and early referral can speed transfer to an appropriate setting.

Nursing Diagnoses, Planning, and Implementation

Risk for Ineffective Cerebral Tissue Perfusion related to increased ICP

EXPECTED OUTCOME: Changes in cerebral tissue perfusion will be prevented or recognized and reported promptly.

- Monitor vital signs for widening pulse pressure or irregular respirations. *These are signs of increased ICP and should be reported promptly.*
- Monitor Glasgow Coma Scale or FOUR Score Coma Scale and report worsening status promptly. *Decreasing LOC can indicate increased ICP and may necessitate emergency intervention.*
- Implement measures *to prevent increased ICP*. See Table 48.3 for preventive measures and rationale.

Ineffective Airway Clearance related to reduced cough reflex and decreased LOC as evidenced by adventitious lung sounds and dropping SpO_2

EXPECTED OUTCOME: The patient will maintain a clear airway as evidenced by clear breath sounds and SpO_2 of 90% or above.

- Monitor airway and breath sounds. *If the patient has excess secretions and is unable to cough effectively, oropharyngeal suctioning may be necessary.*
- Limit suction passes to one or two at a time for a maximum of 5 to 10 seconds each time. *Suctioning can increase ICP.*
- Keep head of bed elevated 20 to 30 degrees *to reduce risk of aspirating oral secretions and reduce ICP.*
- Turn the patient frequently *to help mobilize secretions and prevent other complications of immobility.*

Ineffective Breathing Pattern related to pressure on respiratory center

EXPECTED OUTCOME: The patient will maintain oxygen saturation (SpO_2) of 90% or above.

- Monitor respiratory rate and depth, arterial blood gases (ABGs), and SpO_2 and report changes. *If respiratory status is deteriorating, mechanical ventilation may be necessary.*
- Elevate head of bed 20 to 30 degrees, but no higher, *to allow chest expansion and ease work of breathing.*
- Administer oxygen as ordered and needed *to prevent hypoxia. Hypoxia promotes brain death.*

Evaluation

The plan of care has been successful if the patient shows no unexpected worsening of neurologic function and injuries and complications are prevented. The patient's airway should be clear, and SpO_2 level should be 90% or above. The patient is kept comfortable, and self-care needs are met.

Rehabilitation

Once the patient is stabilized, evaluation for discharge to a rehabilitation facility is completed. The patient must be able to physically tolerate the rehabilitation program, in which they will be taught to function as independently as possible. The family must be prepared for changes in the patient's ability to function and possible changes in personality. It can take months to years before the patient reaches their maximum potential. In some cases of severe brain damage or continued comatose state, rehabilitation is not feasible, and the patient is discharged to home or a long-term facility for custodial care (Table 48.6).

Table 48.6
Traumatic Brain Injury Summary

Signs and Symptoms	Loss or decrease in level of consciousness (LOC), depending on severity and type of injury Loss of memory before or after the injury Increased intracranial pressure Headache, dizziness Nausea and vomiting Unequal pupils Tachycardia, tachypnea Diaphoresis Hemiparesis
Diagnostic Tests	Computed tomography (CT) scan, magnetic resonance imaging (MRI) Skull x-rays Routine laboratory tests (hemoglobin, electrolytes, coagulation studies, type and crossmatch) Neuropsychological testing
Therapeutic Measures	Control intracranial pressure Surgical management of hematoma Maintain respiratory function Maintain diet/nutrition Maintain skin integrity Prevent complications Education
Complications	Increased intracranial pressure Diabetes insipidus Acute hydrocephalus Post-traumatic syndrome Cognitive and personality changes
Priority Nursing Diagnoses	*Risk for Ineffective Cerebral Tissue Perfusion* *Ineffective Airway Clearance* *Ineffective Breathing Pattern*

CRITICAL THINKING & CLINICAL JUDGMENT

Mr. Evans is a 24-year-old white male who was involved in a motor vehicle collision. His blood alcohol level was 0.24. Mr. Evans has no preexisting medical problems. Emergency medical services personnel report that Mr. Evans was unconscious on their arrival at the scene and then became alert and combative. A CT scan shows a left-sided epidural hematoma. Mr. Evans is admitted to your unit for observation.

Critical Thinking (The Why)
1. Mr. Evans experiences a rapid decrease in consciousness. What do you suspect is happening? What other symptoms might you see?

Clinical Judgement (The Do)
2. What emergency preparations should you have ready?
3. What psychosocial data should you collect?
4. What other members of the health-care team should be consulted?
5. You talk with Mr. Evans's girlfriend, who tells you that in addition to his drinking, he has also developed an addiction to Percocet. What additional steps should you take?

Suggested answers are at the end of the chapter.

BRAIN TUMORS

Brain tumors are neoplastic growths of the brain or meninges. Brain tumors can be characterized by vague symptoms such as headache or visual changes or by focal neurologic deficits such as hemiparesis or seizures.

Pathophysiology and Etiology

Brain tumors cause symptoms by either compressing or infiltrating brain tissue. Tumors can arise from CNS cells or can metastasize from other locations in the body. Primary brain tumors rarely metastasize; however, if they do, it is to the spine.

There is no established cause for primary brain tumors. It is unclear what causes the cells to begin reproducing in an uncontrolled fashion. Risk factors include age (45 and older), exposure to radiation or industrial chemicals, and family history. Whites are more likely to be diagnosed with a brain tumor than are other racial or ethnic groups.

Brain tumors can be classified in several ways. The traditional distinction of benign and malignant is less helpful when classifying brain tumors than when classifying other cancers. A benign tumor in the brainstem can be fatal, whereas a malignant tumor in the frontal lobe may not be. Location of the tumor can be just as important a factor in outcome as the cell type.

Primary tumors are those arising from cells of the CNS. Intra-axial tumors are those that arise from the glial cells within the cerebrum, cerebellum, or brainstem. These tumors infiltrate and invade brain tissue. Extra-axial tumors arise from the skull, meninges, pituitary gland, or cranial nerves; they place pressure on the brain.

Most brain tumors are secondary; they have metastasized from a primary malignancy somewhere else in the body (Fig. 48.7). These tumors commonly spread via the arterial system. If untreated, they cause increased ICP, which can cause the patient's death rather than the primary malignancy.

Signs and Symptoms

The symptoms of a brain tumor are directly related to the location of the tumor in the brain and to the rate of growth. Slow-growing types of tumors such as meningiomas (a tumor arising from the meninges; Fig. 48.8) can get to be quite large before causing symptoms. Conversely, glioblastoma multiforme or metastatic tumors can abruptly cause seizures or hemiparesis. Other types of tumors include oligodendroglioma, astrocytoma, and acoustic neuroma. The suffix *-oma* refers to tumor. The prefix denotes the type of cell from which the tumor arises.

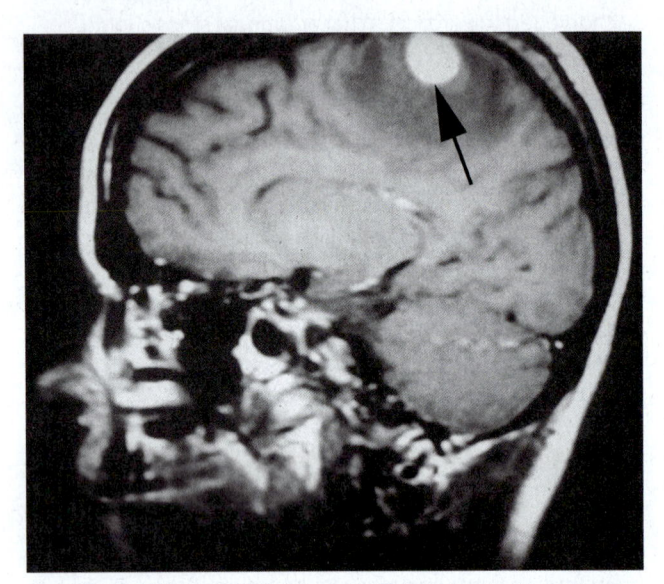

FIGURE 48.7 Metastatic brain tumor. This patient's primary cancer was in the lung.

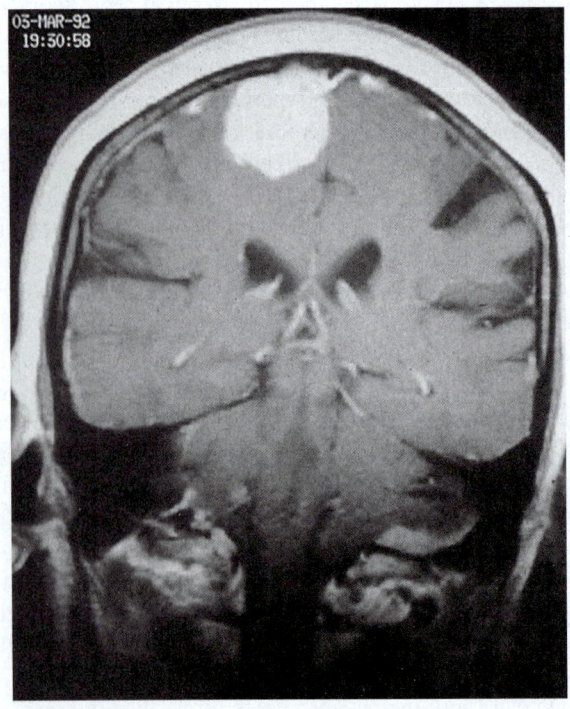

FIGURE 48.8 Meningioma.

The most common early symptom of a brain tumor is fatigue. Other symptoms can include seizures, motor and sensory deficits, nausea and vomiting, headaches, personality changes, confusion, and speech and vision disturbances. If the pituitary gland is involved, additional symptoms related to changes in hormone secretion occur, such as abnormal growth or fluid volume imbalances.

Diagnostic Tests

MRI gives the clearest images of a brain tumor. If the tumor appears to be highly vascular or near major blood vessels, an angiogram may be performed. It is now possible to do a magnetic resonance angiogram (MRA), which involves IV administration of contrast material and is much less invasive than a traditional angiogram. If the tumor is in the region of the pituitary gland, serum hormone levels are evaluated. Biopsy may be done during surgical removal of the tumor or using needle aspiration. Additional tests may be carried out to find a primary cancer site.

Therapeutic Measures

Surgery

Surgical treatment involves removal of the tumor or as much of the tumor as possible. Care of the patient undergoing intracranial surgery is discussed later in this chapter.

Medical Treatment

Medical treatment is aimed at controlling symptoms. Patients who have a seizure are placed on anticonvulsants. If significant cerebral edema is noted on MRI or the patient is suffering from headaches or other symptoms, a steroid such as dexamethasone (Decadron) may be prescribed to lessen edema and reduce symptoms. Typically, patients do not require narcotics for pain relief.

Radiation Therapy

External beam radiation therapy is standard treatment for many patients with a brain tumor. The therapy is typically given 5 days a week for 6 weeks. Some clinicians use a hyperfractionated schedule in which the patient has therapy twice a day for less time per treatment session. Brachytherapy is a means of delivering radiation therapy directly to the tumor. Small catheters are implanted in the tumor, then tiny radioactive particles are inserted into the catheters. The treatment typically takes 3 to 5 days. During this time, the patient is confined to a private room. Interaction with visitors and staff is kept to a minimum to reduce exposure to radioactivity. This therapy is not appropriate for confused individuals because they may not be able to cooperate with restrictions.

Stereotactic radiosurgery is a technique that uses small amounts of radiation directed at the tumor from different angles. A metal frame is affixed to the patient's skull, and the tumor is visualized within the framework on a CT scan or MRI. A computer plan is generated to direct the radiation.

Because multiple small sources are used, the normal brain tissue receives very little radiation, while the majority of the radiation accumulates in the tumor.

Chemotherapy

The blood-brain barrier is a protective mechanism that prevents injurious substances from reaching brain tissue. Unfortunately, it also effectively prevents most chemotherapy agents from reaching the brain. To penetrate the blood-brain barrier, large doses of chemotherapy may be required and may not be well tolerated by other body systems. New treatments are under investigation. Chemotherapy substances may be placed in the cavity left by surgical resection. Other treatments disrupt the blood-brain barrier with mannitol (an osmotic diuretic) and then deliver intra-arterial chemotherapy under general anesthesia. Targeted medication therapy uses a medication such as bevacizumab (Avastin), which stops formation of new blood vessels that support the tumor. Gene therapy is also being used to kill malignant cells.

Complementary and Alternative Therapies

The rate of success for treatment of brain tumors is lower than for treatment of other neoplasms. Patients may be drawn to nontraditional therapies both as potential cures and treatment of symptoms. Encourage patients to look at each option in a rational manner. Some questions they should ask themselves include the following:

- Will this interfere with any of my other treatments or medications?
- What is the cost?
- What are the side effects?
- Is there any objective information (research) available in scholarly journals?
- What does my physician think of this?

Additional information on evaluation of complementary and alternative therapies is found in Chapter 5.

Acute and Long-Term Complications

It is difficult to distinguish between symptoms of a brain tumor and complications of treatment. Seizures, headaches, memory impairment, cognitive changes, and ataxia can be symptoms of the tumor or result from surgery or radiation therapy. Patients can experience hemiparesis or aphasia following surgery. If the tumor continues to grow despite treatment, the patient will experience further decline in function. Gradually, the patient becomes more lethargic and unresponsive. Once the patient becomes comatose, death can occur within a matter of days, particularly if artificial nutrition and hydration are not administered.

Nursing Process for the Patient With a Brain Tumor

Nursing care of the patient with a brain tumor is similar to that for the patient with a brain injury because both experience neurologic deficits.

INTRACRANIAL SURGERY

The primary purpose of intracranial surgery is to remove a mass lesion. These types of lesions include hematomas, tumors, arteriovenous malformations, and, occasionally, contused brain tissue. Other indications for surgery include elevation of a depressed skull fracture, removal of a foreign body, debridement of a wound, or resection of a seizure focus. The term **craniotomy** refers to any surgical opening in the skull. A burr hole is an opening into the cranium made with a drill. **Craniectomy** is the term used to describe removal of part of the cranial bone. **Cranioplasty** refers to repair of bone or use of a prosthesis to replace bone following surgery.

The goal of intracranial tumor surgery is gross total resection (removal) of the tumor. This involves removal of all visible tumor, called *debulking*. Even with the use of an operative microscope, viable tumor cells can be left behind that can cause recurrence. If the entire tumor cannot be removed, the surgeon debulks as much as possible. Radiation can be more effective once the tumor is smaller. In some cases, it is unfeasible to attempt more than a biopsy of the tumor. Location of the tumor or the patient's age or medical condition may not allow the patient to tolerate a full craniotomy. A biopsy may be done under local or general anesthesia, depending on the patient's condition. The goal is to obtain tissue that allows pathological diagnosis of the tumor, which guides further treatment.

Intracranial surgery is usually performed under general anesthesia. Occasionally, a procedure requires that the patient be awake and cooperative.

Preoperative Care

Preoperative care of the patient undergoing intracranial surgery is similar to care of patients having other surgeries (see Chapter 12). The patient undergoes a laboratory workup and anesthesia evaluation. If the patient has cognitive impairments, a family member must be available to provide information and sign consents. A thorough baseline neurologic check should be documented.

Patient education is important preoperatively. The extent of education depends on the patient's ability to absorb new information, influenced by the disease process, cognitive functioning, anxiety, and education level. Family members are involved as needed. Information about the disease process and surgery is provided by the surgeon. The nurse can play an important role in reinforcing and clarifying the information presented.

• WORD • BUILDING •

craniotomy: crani—skull + otomy—incision
craniectomy: crani—skull + ectomy—excision, removal
cranioplasty: crani—skull + plasty—to form

Surgery can last 2 hours for a biopsy to 12 hours or longer for more involved procedures. Anxiety is also a significant concern before surgery. The patient is anticipating serious surgery as well as an unknown outcome. A preoperative visit to the ICU may help prevent anxiety postoperatively. Family members should be accompanied on this visit by a knowledgeable nurse who can explain what they are seeing. Allow time for the patient and family members to express fears and ask questions. Honest and accurate information should be provided.

Family members should be prepared for how the patient will look after surgery. Patients and family members should expect that some or all the patient's hair will be shaved off. Some people prefer to have all their hair shaved rather than just part. The patient should be prepared to see the face swollen after surgery, particularly around the eyes; the periorbital region may be bruised. Many patients wish to wear a scarf or scrub cap after the dressing is removed.

Nursing Process for the Postoperative Care of the Patient Having Intracranial Surgery

Acute care of the postoperative patient is presented here. Also see earlier in this chapter.

Data Collection

After intracranial surgery, the patient will receive care in the ICU. Plan to assist the RN with frequent neurologic assessments in addition to routine postoperative monitoring. Depending on the HCP, patients can be monitored every 15 minutes up to every hour as needed. Many patients undergo a CT scan within the first 24 hours following surgery to assess cerebral edema. Once the patient is awake and alert, plan to determine the patient's response to changes in body image and knowledge base related to care that will be required following discharge.

Nursing Diagnoses, Planning, and Implementation

The primary goal after intracranial surgery is complication prevention. Once the patient is stabilized, goals can change to longer-term outcomes such as acceptance of changes in body image and understanding of self-care following discharge. If the patient has severe deficits following surgery, rehabilitation or long-term care may be necessary. Consultation with a social worker can help with planning for this transition. Priority nursing diagnoses are discussed next.

Risk for Ineffective Cerebral Tissue Perfusion related to edema of the operative site

EXPECTED OUTCOME: The patient will have adequate cerebral tissue perfusion as evidenced by stable or improving neurologic checks.

- Monitor neurologic status as ordered. Report changes promptly. *Deteriorating status can signify increased ICP.*
- Implement measures *to prevent increased ICP.* See Table 48.3 for preventive measures and rationales.
- Position the patient with the head of the bed at 30 degrees or higher, unless ordered otherwise, *to promote venous drainage and minimize increases in ICP.* However, patients who have had a chronic subdural hematoma removed must remain flat. Patients can turn from side to side or lie on their back but should not lie on the operative side.
- Implement seizure precautions *because the patient is at risk for seizures due to cerebral edema.*
- Use caution to protect the many monitoring systems being used. The patient may have an intracranial monitor in place following surgery *to monitor ICP.* Some patients may also have central venous pressure catheters or pulmonary artery catheters *to monitor fluid status.* Urinary catheters are used during the immediate postoperative period *to accurately monitor fluid balance.*
- Monitor dressings for drainage. *Drainage that is blood-tinged in the center with a yellowish ring around it can be CSF leakage. A suspected CSF leak should be reported to the RN or HCP immediately.*

Risk for Infection related to surgical procedure

EXPECTED OUTCOME: The patient will remain free from infection as evidenced by temperature and WBC count within normal limits and incision sites clean and dry.

- Monitor patient for rise in temperature, purulence at incision site, and increase in WBC count. *These are signs of infection and should be reported immediately.*
- Use strict aseptic technique for care of the incision, dressing, and monitoring equipment sites *to reduce risk of infection.*
- Use appropriate hand hygiene *to reduce risk of transmitting infection.*

Disturbed Body Image related to changes in appearance or function as evidenced by patient statement of disturbance or unwillingness to observe changes

EXPECTED OUTCOME: The patient will display an open attitude toward change in appearance, as evidenced by willingness to look in mirror and/or be seen by others.

- Offer a turban, scarf, or hat if the patient desires *to help conceal a shaved head.*
- Portray an accepting attitude toward the patient. *Patients are likely aware of nurses' nonverbal behavior.*
- Allow the patient to express their feelings if desired. *Talking may help the patient work through feelings, but it should not be forced.*

Deficient Knowledge related to change in treatment regimen after surgery as evidenced by patient statement

EXPECTED OUTCOME: The patient and family members will verbalize correct information for follow-up care at home. They will state they have the resources to manage care effectively.

- Teach the patient and family members home management, including medication regimen, wound care, and ordered activity restrictions, including driving. Have the patient and family members verbalize the signs of infection or other possible complications to report. *The patient and family members will assume responsibility for care after discharge unless the patient is being transferred to another facility.*
- Teach the patient and family members seizure precautions and the importance of taking anticonvulsants as ordered. *The patient may be on anticonvulsants to prevent seizures after surgery. If seizure-free for 1 year, the HCP may discontinue anticonvulsants.*
- Consult a social worker or case manager for resources if needed. *The patient may need discharge planning if transfer to another facility is planned. If discharge home is expected, the patient and family members will benefit from a home health-care nurse follow-up. Assistance with obtaining medications can also be provided if necessary.*

Evaluation

Interventions have been effective if the patient's neurologic status is stable and infection and other complications have been prevented. The patient may begin to show evidence of acceptance of changes in body image, although this may not happen until after discharge from the hospital. The patient or family members should be able to demonstrate appropriate follow-up care.

SPINAL DISORDERS

Herniated Discs

Herniated intravertebral discs are a common health problem characterized by pain and paresthesias that follow a radicular (nerve path) pattern. It is not uncommon for patients to have more than one herniated disc or to have herniated discs in different areas of the spine.

Pathophysiology

When the disc between two vertebrae herniates, it moves out of its normal anatomical position. In most cases, the annulus fibrosus, the tough outer ring of the disc, tears. This allows escape of the nucleus pulposus, the soft inner portion of the disc. Displacement of the disc compresses one or more nerve roots, causing the characteristic symptoms (Fig. 48.9).

Etiology

In some cases, a specific event, such as a fall, lifting a heavy object, or a motor vehicle collision, causes a herniated disc. In other instances, the patient cannot identify a triggering incident.

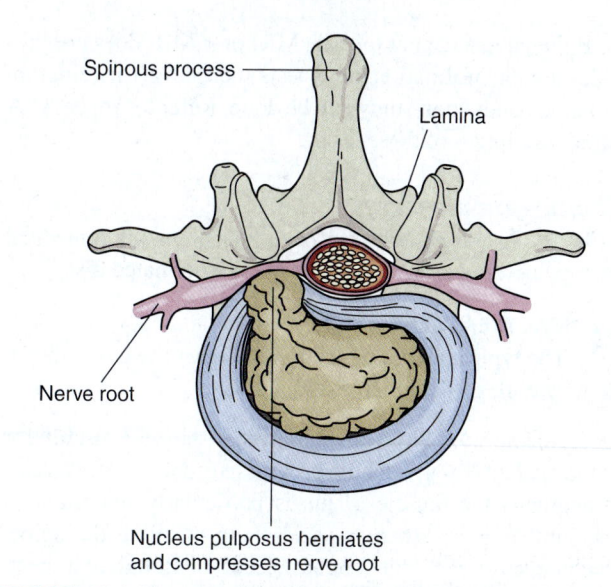

FIGURE 48.9 A herniated disc places pressure on a spinal nerve root.

Signs and Symptoms

Cervical disc herniation causes pain and muscle spasm in the neck. The patient may have decreased range of motion (ROM) secondary to pain. Hand and arm pain is unilateral (one-sided) and follows the distribution of the spinal nerve root. Patients often report numbness or tingling in the extremity. Asymmetrical weakness and atrophy of specific muscle groups may be detected. The severity of the pain or paresthesia does not correlate directly with the severity of the nerve compression. However, weakness and atrophy are indicators of significant nerve compression.

Thoracic herniated discs are not common. This portion of the spine is the least mobile; therefore, less stress is exerted on the discs. Patients with herniated thoracic discs may report pain in the back. It is uncommon to detect muscular weakness.

A herniated lumbar disc is typically characterized by low back pain, pain radiating down one leg, paresthesias, and weakness. Often the sciatic nerve is affected, thus the term **sciatica**. The patient may limp on the affected leg or may have difficulty walking on the heels or toes. Muscle spasm is often present. Pain and muscle spasm can limit the patient's ROM. Depending on the disc affected, the deep tendon reflex of the knee or ankle may be decreased or absent. A severely herniated L5–S1 disc can affect bowel or bladder continence. This is an emergency and should be reported immediately. Use the **WHAT'S UP?** mnemonic to ask about symptoms of herniated discs.

Diagnostic Tests

MRI will detect herniation of a disc and compression or abnormality of the spinal cord. If the patient has previously had surgery in the area of the suspected herniation, the MRI is done with and without contrast to differentiate between scar tissue and a herniated disc.

If the patient cannot tolerate MRI or if MRI does not provide enough information, other tests such as a CT myelogram or nerve conduction study can be done. Refer to Appendix A for a description of these tests.

Therapeutic Measures

Most HCPs and patients prefer to try conservative medical therapy before performing surgery for a herniated disc.

MEDICAL TREATMENT

Rest. The typical recommendation is a day or two of bedrest, then careful, gradual increase in activity.

Physical Therapy. Physical therapy can be very useful for some patients. A gradually progressive course of exercise strengthens the muscles. This is particularly important in the lumbar area, where muscles help stabilize the spine. Techniques such as ultrasound, electrical stimulation, heat, ice, and deep massage can decrease pain and muscle spasm and allow for increased ROM. Instructions in proper body mechanics and strategies for avoiding reinjury are important components of physical therapy.

Traction. Cervical traction is a noninvasive technique sometimes used by physical therapists for patients with herniated cervical discs. The patient's head is placed in a halter-like device. A series of ropes and pulleys connects the halter to a weight that gently pulls the head away from the shoulders. This traction slightly separates the vertebral bodies, allowing the disc to return to its proper position. If it effectively relieves the patient's pain, cervical traction can be done at home as needed. Traction is discontinued immediately if it increases the patient's pain. Lumbar traction is not particularly effective because the lumbar paraspinal muscles are large and strong. The amount of traction needed to overcome the muscular resistance can cause injury.

Medication. Muscle relaxants are often prescribed as a short-term therapy for patients experiencing muscle spasms. These medications decrease pain by decreasing the spasm, helping the patient increase ROM and activity. Muscle spasm is actually a protective mechanism. Muscles tighten and become painful, causing the patient to limit movement. This lessens the chance that the disc will be further injured. However, chronic spasm can cause muscle tearing and scarring. Patients should be warned that drowsiness is a common side effect of muscle relaxants. They should be cautioned against driving or operating machinery until they determine how well they tolerate the medication. Diazepam (Valium) is an effective muscle relaxant but has a strong potential for addiction, so is usually used only if muscle spasm cannot be treated with other medications.

Inflammation of the nerve root is caused by compression and irritation from the herniated disc. NSAIDs can be effective in reducing this inflammation, but there is no way to predict response to a given medication. It may be necessary for the patient to try several NSAIDs before an effective one is found. Because several of these medications are now available without prescription, the patient should be cautioned not to use a nonprescription NSAID at the same time as a prescription NSAID. Patients should be instructed to report any stomach upset to the HCP because NSAIDs can cause gastric bleeding. Occasionally, oral steroids are used on a short-term basis for patients with severe inflammation that does not respond to other treatments. A rapidly tapering dose of steroid over 1 week is often prescribed. Steroids can also cause gastric upset as well as elevated serum glucose levels. Instruct patients with diabetes to monitor glucose levels closely and to consult their HCP if the levels are outside their normal parameters.

Epidural injections may be tried for patients who have no relief with more conservative measures. A mixture of medications, typically a steroid, a long-acting anesthetic, and a long-acting pain reliever, is injected into the epidural space. The anesthetic provides immediate relief, while the steroid reduces swelling for a longer-lasting effect. If relief is obtained, the injection can be repeated every 3 to 4 months. Experts suggest that patients receive a maximum of around four steroid injections per year, because the injectable steroid medicine can weaken nearby joints and ligaments if used excessively (Chou, 2020).

The use of opioid pain medication is a subject of concern in treating patients with herniated discs. Opioids generally are appropriate for short-term treatment of acute pain. However, if treatment is not effective, the pain can become chronic. In that case, the HCP and patient must discuss the potential complications of long-term opioid use, such as constipation, tolerance, and dependence. A referral to a pain clinic for alternative strategies may be appropriate. Alternatives to long-term use of opioids include topical lidocaine patches or NSAID patches as well as the use of agents for neuropathic pain, such as gabapentin (Neurontin) or pregabalin (Lyrica).

Complementary and Alternative Therapy. A transcutaneous electrical nerve stimulator (commonly called a TENS unit) is a noninvasive pain-relief technique. Small electrodes are placed on the skin around the area of the pain. The device then transmits a low-voltage electrical current through the skin. The patient feels a tingling or buzzing sensation that can help block the pain impulses. A physical therapist or pain specialist teaches the patient where to place the electrodes and how to operate the unit. The patient decides when to use it and at what settings. This allows the patient to actively participate in care and have some control over the pain level.

SURGICAL MANAGEMENT.
Surgeries are less common today than in the past because conservative measures are now effective for most patients. If surgery is indicated, several options are available. A **laminectomy** removes one of the laminae, the flat pieces of bone on each side of a vertebra, to relieve pressure or gain access for removal of a herniated

• WORD • BUILDING •

laminectomy: lamin—posterior portion of the vertebra + ectomy—excision, removal

disc. A *discectomy* removes the entire disc. A spinal fusion uses a bone graft to fuse two vertebrae together if the area is unstable. Surgery can be done through a microscope for less scarring and faster recovery. Most patients are discharged within 24 hours of surgery.

A discectomy is generally done for a herniated cervical disc. This can be accomplished via an anterior or posterior approach. Most surgeons replace the disc with bone or another material to prevent collapse of the disc space and create spinal fusion. If bone is used, it may be harvested from the patient's iliac crest or donated from a cadaver. Mobility of the spine is lost in the area of a fusion. Spinal fusions may also be done to correct instability of the spine from other causes, such as scoliosis or degenerative disorders.

A posterior approach is used for a herniated lumbar disc. Typically, the vertical incision is 1 to 2 inches long. It is necessary to pull some muscle away from the bone, which accounts for some of the postoperative pain that patients experience. A laminectomy is done, and the herniated portion of the disc is resected. The remainder of the disc continues to provide a cushion between the intravertebral bodies. The surgeon removes any free fragments and any disc material that appears unstable.

Percutaneous discectomy involves insertion of a large needle into the disc under local anesthesia to aspirate herniated disc material. This technique is not used for severely herniated discs. Laser disc surgery may be used to disintegrate the herniated tissue. Laparoscopic techniques may also be used.

An artificial disc may be used in select patients. It is made of two plastic discs designed to slide so that mobility is not impaired as with spinal fusion. The artificial disc is attached to the vertebra above and below after the damaged disc is removed. This alternative to spinal fusion has been effective for those with single-disc problems. Minimally invasive spinal surgery techniques are becoming more prevalent, as they have a faster recovery time for the patient.

Surgical Complications. As with any surgery, intraoperative hemorrhage is possible, although it is not common in disc surgery. If a postoperative hemorrhage occurs in a patient who has had an anterior cervical discectomy, the airway can become occluded. Monitor the patient for bleeding from the incision and respiratory distress.

If the nerve root is severed during surgery, the patient experiences loss of motor and sensory functions in that nerve's distribution area. This can result in decreased use of the extremity. If the nerve root is damaged or excessive scarring occurs, the patient can experience pain, weakness, or paresthesias. Physical therapy and NSAIDs may effectively improve function and reduce pain.

Lumbar discs can reherniate. This can occur anywhere from 1 week to several years after the initial surgery. If the reherniation occurs within a few weeks to months after the first surgery, the patient usually undergoes a microdiscectomy. Reherniation of a cervical disc does not occur because the entire disc is removed.

Fusion of the cervical spine results in loss of movement at that motion segment, placing increased stress on the discs above and below the fusion. This raises the risk of another herniated disc. Risk is even higher when the patient already has other degenerated discs. Instruct the patient to maintain an exercise program and frequently move the spine through ROM exercises.

Spinal Stenosis

Spinal stenosis is a condition in which the spinal canal compresses the spinal cord (Fig. 48.10). Arthritis is a major cause of spinal stenosis. The facet joints of the spine become inflamed and enlarged, narrowing the diameter of the spinal canal and compressing the spinal cord. Patients may report pain and weakness. Compression of the cervical portion of the spinal cord can result in hyperreflexia and weakness of the arms and hands.

A laminectomy may be done to relieve pressure on the spinal cord. The size of the incision depends on the number of vertebrae involved. Patients requiring laminectomy to relieve spinal cord pressure are often older and may have concurrent illnesses. They may require inpatient rehabilitation before returning home.

Nursing Process for the Patient Having Spinal Surgery

Preoperative Care

In addition to routine teaching, instruct the patient in how to logroll following surgery. This procedure involves keeping the body in alignment and rolling as a unit, without twisting the spine, to prevent injury to the operative site.

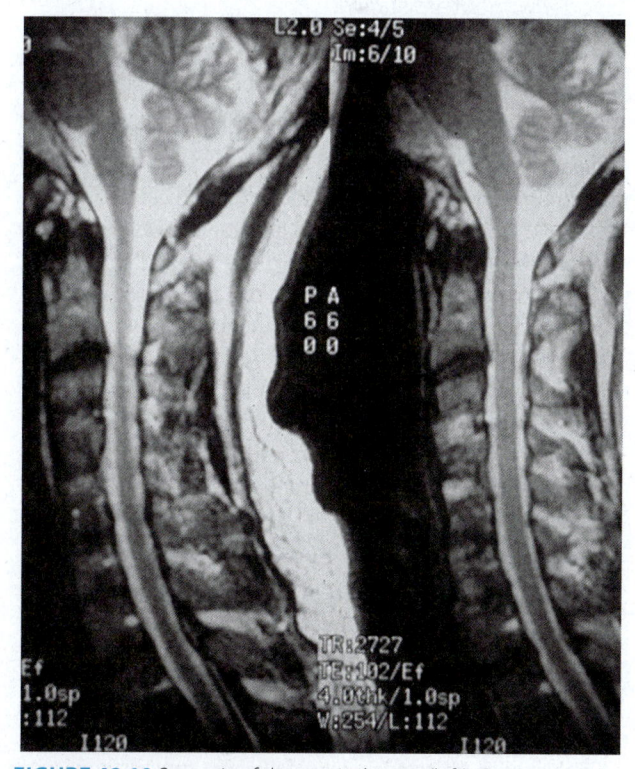

FIGURE 48.10 Stenosis of the cervical spine (left). Compare with normal spinal column (right).

Postoperative Care

DATA COLLECTION. In addition to routine postoperative data collection, monitor extremities for changes in circulation, movement, and sensation. Monitor color, warmth, and presence of pulses in the extremities. Observe movement by asking the patient to move the extremities. Check sensation by gently touching the patient's extremity and asking if feeling is present. Report any changes immediately to the HCP because changes can indicate nerve or circulatory damage.

Monitor pain frequently. The pain that necessitated surgery should be relieved, but the patient may have muscular and incisional pain. Reassure the patient that pain will gradually subside. Monitor surgical dressing and drain (if present) for CSF drainage or bleeding. Any sign of CSF drainage or significant bleeding should be reported to the HCP immediately. If bone was taken from a separate donor site, this site must also be monitored. Intake and output are measured to ensure that the patient is able to void. Notify the HCP if the patient has difficulty voiding.

NURSING DIAGNOSES, PLANNING, AND IMPLEMENTATION. Goals of nursing are to keep the patient safe and free from injury or complications and free from pain. Gradual return to normal physical activity is expected. Possible postoperative diagnoses are discussed next. (A discussion of postoperative pain can be found in Chapter 10.)

Impaired Urinary Elimination related to effects of surgery

EXPECTED OUTCOME: The patient will be able to empty bladder without assistance.

- Monitor urine output for retention. *Patients may have difficulty voiding following lumbar surgery because of anesthesia, immobility, or occasionally because of nerve damage related to surgery.*
- If activity orders allow, assist the patient to get up to urinate (men may need to stand to urinate). *This may help the patient urinate.*
- If the patient is unable to void, try running warm water over the perineum or having the patient take a warm bath or shower. *This may stimulate voiding.*
- If difficulty urinating continues, contact the HCP for an order for intermittent catheterization until the problem resolves. *Urine retention that is not resolved can lead to bladder rupture. Intermittent catheterization is a safe way to empty the bladder.*

Impaired Physical Mobility related to neuromuscular impairment

EXPECTED OUTCOME: The patient will be able to ambulate and prevent complications of immobility after surgery.

- Observe mobility of affected extremities following surgery. *A reduction in expected mobility following surgery indicates nerve damage in surgery and should be reported immediately.*
- Assist the patient to logroll to get out of bed and ambulate on the first postoperative day, as ordered. If spinal fusion has been done, the fused area of the spine will be immobile. *Early mobilization after surgery helps prevent complications.*
- Apply a soft cervical collar to the patient with a cervical laminectomy as ordered *for neck support.*

EVALUATION. The patient is expected to be free of complications and pain, be able to urinate, be able to move all extremities, and return gradually to pre-illness activity level.

SPINAL CORD INJURIES

Injuries to the spinal cord affect people of all ages but take their greatest toll on young people. Spinal cord injuries are characterized by a decrease or loss of sensory and motor functions below the level of the injury.

Pathophysiology

The spinal cord is made up of nerve fibers that allow communication between the brain and the rest of the body. Damage to the spinal cord results in interference with this communication process. Damage may be caused by bruising, tearing, cutting, edema, or bleeding into the cord. The damage can be caused by external forces or by fragments of fractured bone.

Etiology and Types

The causes of spinal cord injury are similar to those of TBI. It is not uncommon for a patient to have both a spinal cord injury and TBI. Motor vehicle collisions are the most common causes of spinal cord injury in the United States. Other causes of injury include falls and acts of violence (World Health Organization, 2021). Assaults can cause cord injury if a knife or bullet penetrates the spinal cord. Diving into shallow water is a common cause of cervical cord injury.

Spinal cord injuries can be classified by location or degree of damage to the cord. A complete spinal cord injury means the patient has no motor or sensory function below the level of the injury. With an incomplete lesion, some function remains. This does not necessarily mean that the remaining function will be useful to the patient. Some patients find that having areas where sensation is intact may be more painful than useful.

The cervical and lumbar portions of the spine are injured more often than the thoracic or sacral segments because the cervical and lumbar areas are the most mobile portions of the spine.

Signs and Symptoms
Cervical Injuries

Signs and symptoms depend on the level at which the cord is damaged (Fig. 48.11). Cervical cord injuries can affect all four extremities, causing paralysis and paresthesias,

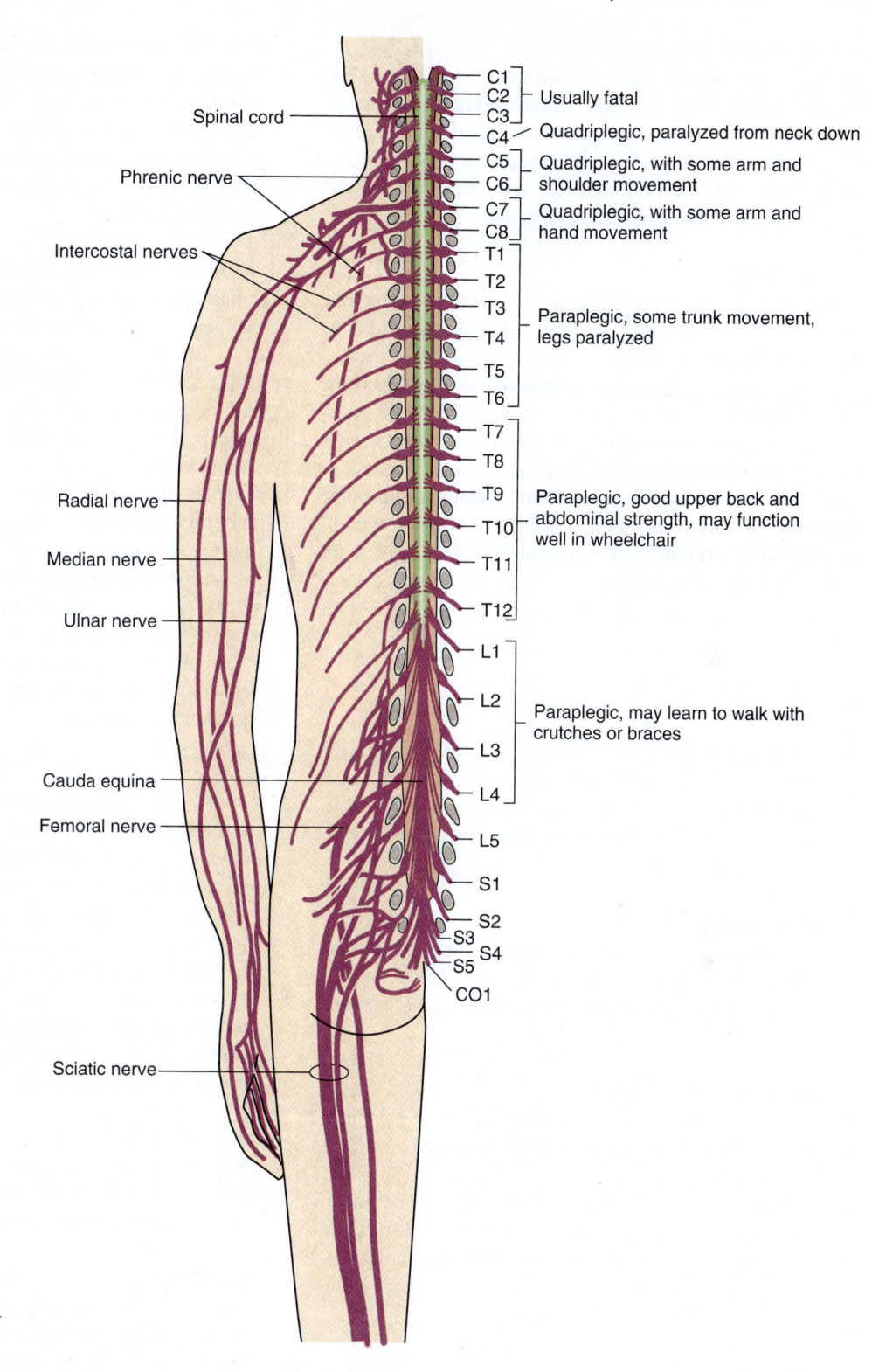

FIGURE 48.11 Spinal cord injury—quadriplegia versus paraplegia.

impaired respiration, and loss of bowel and bladder control. Paralysis of all four extremities is called **quadriplegia**; weakness of all extremities is called **quadriparesis**. If the injury is at C3 or above, the injury is usually fatal because muscles used for breathing are paralyzed. An injury at the fourth or fifth cervical vertebra affects breathing and may necessitate some type of ventilatory support. Such patients typically need long-term assistance with ADLs.

• **WORD • BUILDING** •

quadriplegia: quad—four + plegia—paralysis
quadriparesis: quad—four + paresis—partial paralysis

Thoracic and Lumbar Injuries

Thoracic and lumbar injuries affect the legs, bowel, and bladder. Paralysis of the legs is called **paraplegia;** weakness of the legs is called **paraparesis.** Sacral injuries affect bowel and bladder continence and may affect foot function. Individuals with thoracic, lumbar, and sacral injuries can usually learn to perform ADLs independently.

Spinal Shock

Spinal cord injury has a profound effect on the autonomic nervous system. Immediately after injury, the cord below the injury stops functioning completely. This causes a disruption of sympathetic nervous system function, resulting in vasodilation, hypotension, and bradycardia, called *neurogenic shock* or *spinal shock*. Dilation of the blood vessels allows more blood flow just beneath the skin. This blood cools and is circulated throughout the body, causing hypothermia. The patient is unable to maintain control of body temperature. In addition, all reflexes below the level of the injury are lost, and retention of urine and feces occurs. Spinal shock can last from a week to many weeks in some patients.

Complications
Infection

Impaired respiratory effort, decreased cough, mechanical ventilation, and immobility all predispose a patient with a spinal cord injury to pneumonia. Urinary catheterization, whether indwelling or intermittent, places patients at risk for urinary tract infection.

Deep Vein Thrombosis

Lack of movement in legs inhibits normal blood circulation. Compression stockings, sequential compression devices, and anticoagulant medications may reduce risk of deep vein thrombosis.

Orthostatic Hypotension

Most patients with spinal cord injuries no longer have muscular function in their legs to promote venous return to the heart. They also have impaired vasoconstriction. This leads to pooling of the blood in the legs when the patient moves from a supine to a sitting position. If the movement is sudden, the patient can become dizzy or lightheaded. Gradual elevation of the head, use of elastic stockings, and a reclining wheelchair help lessen this response.

Skin Breakdown

Patients or their caregivers must be diligent about relieving pressure on the skin by position changes and cushioning of bony prominences. It is important to realize that the patient may not be able to feel pain and, therefore, may not ask for position changes. Development of pressure injuries can lead to infection and loss of skin, muscle, or bone. Treatment of pressure injuries is time consuming and expensive and can interfere with work or school.

Renal Complications

Urinary tract infections are an ongoing concern for patients with spinal cord injuries. Caregivers as well as the patient need to be taught to observe the color, clarity, and odor of urine and report changes promptly. Both urinary reflux and untreated urinary tract infections can cause permanent damage to the kidneys.

Depression and Substance Abuse

Patients with spinal cord injury have a higher-than-average incidence of depression and substance abuse (Bombardier et al, 2021). Both factors can interfere with the patient's ability for self-care. Individual or family counseling may be helpful. Some rehabilitation centers have support groups for patients with spinal cord injuries.

Autonomic Dysreflexia

This life-threatening complication occurs in patients with injuries above the T6 level. The spinal cord injury impairs the normal equilibrium between the sympathetic and parasympathetic divisions of the autonomic nervous system. If a noxious stimulus below the spinal cord injury causes activation of the sympathetic system, it will continue unchecked because the parasympathetic responses cannot descend past the spinal cord injury.

The most common cause of autonomic **dysreflexia** is bladder distention. Other causes include bowel impaction, urinary tract infection, ingrown toenails, pressure injuries, pain, and labor in a pregnant woman. Stimulation of the sympathetic nervous system results in cool, pale skin, gooseflesh, and vasoconstriction below the level of the injury. Blood pressure can rise as high as 300 mm Hg systolic. The parasympathetic response results in vasodilation, causing flushing and diaphoresis above the lesion and bradycardia as low as 30 beats per minute. The patient reports a pounding headache and nasal congestion secondary to the dilated blood vessels.

Care of the patient with autonomic dysreflexia is discussed later in this section.

Diagnostic Tests

Plain radiographs are done to identify fractures or displacement of vertebrae. A CT scan is also useful for identifying fractures. MRI can demonstrate lesions within the cord.

Therapeutic Measures

Patients with spinal cord injuries typically are brought to the emergency department. They should be kept immobilized until they are assessed by an HCP. If injury to the spinal cord is detected, the patient needs to remain immobilized.

• WORD • BUILDING •

paraplegia: para—beside + plegia—paralysis
paraparesis: para—beside + paresis—partial paralysis
dysreflexia: dys—abnormal + reflexia—reflex activity

Emergency Management

Emergency management involves careful monitoring of vital signs and airway as well as keeping the patient immobilized. Intubation and mechanical ventilation may be necessary, especially with cervical spine injuries. IV normal saline may be used for fluid replacement and to provide an access site for medication administration. The physician does not rely on fluid administration alone to correct hypotension. It is possible to administer enough fluid to cause pulmonary edema and not correct hypotension. Vasoactive medications may be required. Use of various medications to reduce the extent of injury, including IV steroids, is routine. Emergency medical services (EMS) personnel often start treatment before arrival at the emergency department.

Respiratory Management

Patients with injuries above C4–C5 have some degree of respiratory impairment. The patient may require a tracheostomy and continuous mechanical ventilation or require a ventilator only at night or when fatigued. Some patients are able to breathe by using a phrenic nerve stimulator. This device, similar to a pacemaker, artificially stimulates the phrenic nerve, causing the diaphragm to contract. These patients use a mechanical ventilator at night to lessen the stress on the phrenic nerve and remove the risk of the system failing while the patient is asleep.

Patients can be breathing independently when they first arrive in the emergency department and then experience respiratory compromise as the spinal cord becomes edematous. Edema can compress the spinal cord above the lesion, leading to symptoms at a higher level. This deterioration is usually temporary. Fatigue of the accessory muscles can also cause respiratory compromise. The intercostal muscles are not normally of major importance in respiration. However, if the diaphragm is paralyzed, the intercostal muscles become very important. As these muscles fatigue, the patient's breathing becomes shallow and rapid. Elective intubation and mechanical ventilation protect the patient from expending huge amounts of energy trying to breathe. Feeling their breathing becoming more labored is terrifying, and patients need to be reassured that it is probably a temporary setback. As the edema recedes and the accessory muscles become stronger, the patient may be weaned from the ventilator.

Gastrointestinal Management

Absence of bowel sounds is a common finding on examination. Oral or enteral feedings are not started until bowel function resumes. The metabolic needs of the patient are influenced by the work of breathing and the extent of other injuries. If oral or enteral feedings are not possible, parenteral nutrition begins.

Genitourinary Management

An indwelling urinary catheter is placed to prevent bladder distention and protect skin integrity until spinal shock resolves. Once it is determined what degree of hand function the patient will have, a bladder management program is devised.

Immobilization

The cervical spine can be immobilized with skeletal traction such as Crutchfield or Gardner-Wells tongs (Fig. 48.12). Some patients have a halo brace, a device that attaches to the skull with four small pins. The skull ring attaches to a rigid plastic vest by four poles (Fig. 48.13). This device keeps the head and neck immobile while fusion and healing take place. The advantage over traction is that the patient is not confined to bed.

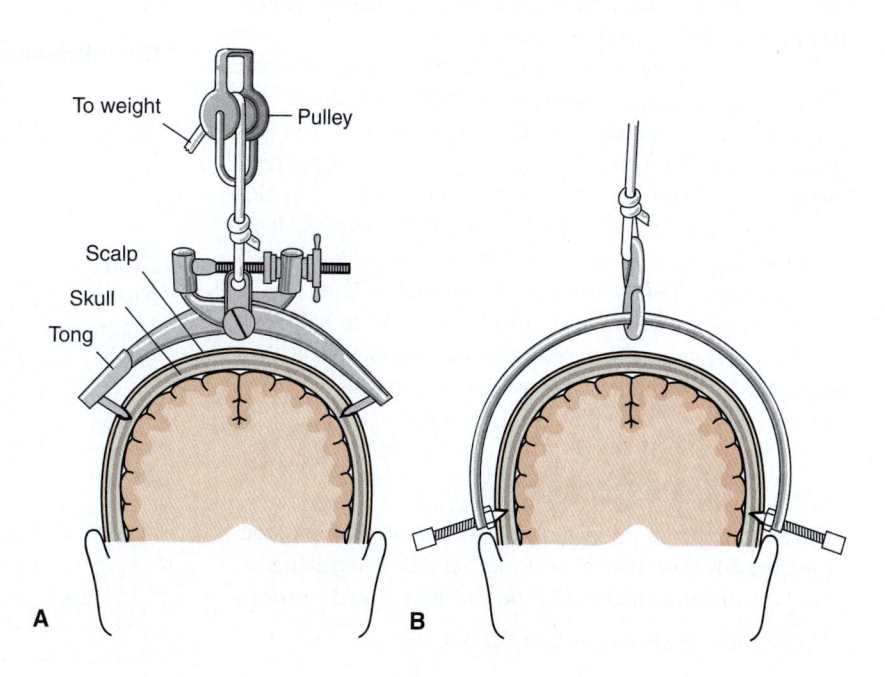

FIGURE 48.12 Skeletal traction for cervical injuries. (A) Crutchfield tongs. (B) Gardner-Wells tongs.

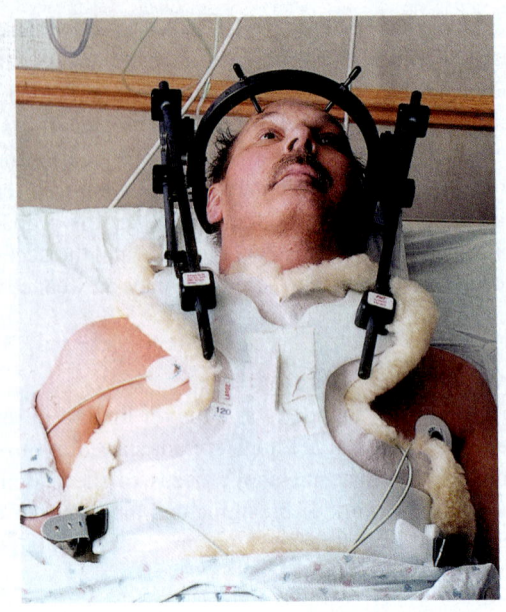

FIGURE 48.13 Halo brace.

Nursing Process for the Patient With a Spinal Cord Injury

Patients with spinal cord injury need ongoing evaluation of all body systems. Frequent neurologic and respiratory checks are essential. Early identification of the patient's support systems can help with discharge and rehabilitation planning. Initial goals for the patient include maintenance of safety and prevention of complications. Long-term goals include rehabilitation and maximizing remaining function.

See "Nursing Care Plan for the Patient With a Spinal Cord Injury," "Gerontological Issues," and Table 48.7.

Table 48.7
Spinal Cord Injury Summary

Signs and Symptoms	Paralysis and paresthesias (depending on level of the lesion) Loss of reflex activity below the level of the lesion Spinal shock initially Risk for autonomic dysreflexia (injuries above sixth thoracic vertebra)
Diagnostic Tests	Radiograph Computed tomography (CT) scan Magnetic resonance imaging (MRI)
Therapeutic Measures	Immobilization Maintenance of airway and respiratory status Bowel and bladder training Nutrition/diet Activity/rehabilitation Prevention of dysreflexia Prevention of skin breakdown Sexual counseling Education
Complications	Infection Deep vein thrombosis Paralysis Orthostatic hypotension Pressure injuries Depression
Priority Nursing Diagnoses	*Impaired Gas Exchange* *Ineffective Airway Clearance* *Risk for Autonomic Dysreflexia* *Reflex Urinary Incontinence* *Constipation* *Impaired Physical Mobility* *Self-Care Deficit (Dressing/Feeding/Toileting/Bathing)* *Risk for Impaired Skin Integrity* *Ineffective Role Performance* *Risk for Sexual Dysfunction* *Anxiety*

PRACTICE ANALYSIS TIP
Linking NCLEX-PN® to Practice
The LPN/LVN will provide care to an immobilized client based on need.

Surgical Management

The goal of surgery following spinal cord injury is to stabilize the bony elements of the spine and relieve pressure on the spinal cord. Surgery may or may not improve functional outcome. Stabilization of the spine allows for earlier patient mobilization, decreasing risk of complications from immobility and speeding the transition to a rehabilitation setting. Patients who have been in cervical traction before surgery may be placed in a halo brace postoperatively.

Unstable thoracic and lumbar fractures may also be treated with surgical implantation of rods to stabilize the spine. It is more difficult to stabilize these areas in the postoperative recovery period. Patients may wear a supportive corset, a rigid brace, or occasionally a body cast to supplement the support provided by the internal fixation devices. For more information, visit the Spinal Cord Injury Model System Information Network at www.spinalcord.uab.edu.

Research is being conducted with stem cells to help with nerve regeneration. Stem cells can be harvested and then processed in a laboratory before reinjection into the body. The goal is improvement in mobility and/or sensation.

CUE RECOGNITION 48.2
You are caring for a patient who is a quadriplegic. Her blood pressure is higher than normal, and her indwelling catheter has had no output in the last 3 hours. What should you do?

Suggested answers are at the end of the chapter.

Gerontological Issues

Aging With Spinal Cord Injury

Individuals aging with a spinal cord injury have an increased risk for developing complications in the following areas:
- Blood pressure control
- Abnormalities in carbohydrate and lipid metabolism related to immobilization
- Cardiovascular disease
- Respiratory complications
- Osteoporosis
- Bladder infections
- Skin injuries
- Chronic pain

PRACTICE ANALYSIS TIP
Linking NCLEX-PN® to Practice
The LPN/LVN will evaluate client oxygen saturation.

Nursing Care Plan for the Patient With a Spinal Cord Injury

See also "Nursing Diagnosis: Ineffective Airway Clearance related to ineffective cough and secretion retention" in Chapter 12 and "Self-Care Deficit (Dressing/Feeding/Toileting/Bathing)" related to reduced mobility later in the chapter.

Nursing Diagnosis: *Risk for Autonomic Dysreflexia* related to stimuli below level of injury
Expected Outcomes: The patient will not demonstrate signs of autonomic dysreflexia as evidenced by stable vital signs. If dysreflexia occurs, it is recognized and corrected promptly.
Evaluation of Outcomes: Is patient free of signs, or are signs recognized and promptly treated?

Intervention	Rationale	Evaluation
Monitor for signs of autonomic dysreflexia (e.g., sudden high blood pressure, bradycardia, headache, pale skin below the injury, gooseflesh). Remember that patients with spinal cord injury are typically hypotensive, so even mild hypertension can represent a dramatic increase from baseline blood pressure.	Autonomic dysreflexia must be recognized quickly to remove cause and prevent complications such as seizures, intracerebral hemorrhage, or death.	Are signs of autonomic dysreflexia present?
If you suspect autonomic dysreflexia, immediately take patient's blood pressure and continue to monitor it every 5 minutes.	Blood pressure must be continually monitored until it is under control, to prevent complications.	Is blood pressure higher than normal for patient? Are emergency interventions warranted?
Place patient in high-Fowler position. Remove elastic stockings or any other garment that could prevent blood from pooling in the periphery.	High-Fowler position uses the effect of orthostasis to control blood pressure. Allowing blood to pool in the periphery can help reduce blood pressure.	Does position change reduce blood pressure?
Evaluate the indwelling catheter for patency. If it is not patent or a catheter is not in place and the bladder is full, obtain order to insert catheter immediately. Monitor blood pressure during catheterization.	A full bladder can be the cause of the stimuli causing the autonomic dysreflexia.	Is catheter patent? Is bladder full? Does emptying bladder resolve autonomic dysreflexia?
Perform a rectal examination to determine whether an impaction is present. Apply anesthetic ointment to the rectum before disimpaction. Have another nurse monitor blood pressure and stop disimpaction if the blood pressure increases.	Fecal impaction can be the stimulus causing the autonomic dysreflexia. Anesthetic is used because further rectal stimulation can exacerbate symptoms.	Is impaction present? Does removal resolve autonomic dysreflexia?

(nursing care plan continues on page 980)

Nursing Care Plan for the Patient With a Spinal Cord Injury—cont'd

Intervention	Rationale	Evaluation
If bowel or bladder distention is not present, examine the patient for other causative mechanisms. If a cause cannot be identified or removal of the cause does not relieve hypertension, notify HCP immediately.	If the cause cannot be found and removed, an antihypertensive agent may be ordered.	Are other causes identifiable? Is an antihypertensive agent ordered?
If hypertension is treated with medication, continue to carefully monitor blood pressure.	Blood pressure can decrease rapidly once the cause of the autonomic dysreflexia is corrected.	Is blood pressure stabilized?
Once the acute episode is past, work with patient and family members to devise a plan to prevent reoccurrence. Teach patient how to direct caregivers in treating autonomic dysreflexia.	Episodes of autonomic dysreflexia can recur, and most can be prevented.	Do patient and caregivers verbalize understanding of how to prevent and treat future episodes of autonomic dysreflexia?

Nursing Diagnosis: Reflex Urinary Incontinence related to spinal cord damage and no sensation to void as evidenced by inability to control flow of urine
Expected Outcomes: The patient's skin will be dry and free of urine; urine elimination will be controlled.
Evaluation of Outcomes: Is the patient clean and dry at all times?

Intervention	Rationale	Evaluation
Determine patient's ability to control urination.	If patient has some control, a bladder training program may be effective.	Is patient able to sense need to urinate? Is any degree of control present?
Implement a bladder training program, using set times for voiding.	Following a voiding schedule can help reduce incontinence.	Is patient able to avoid incontinence with regular voiding?
Use bladder ultrasound to scan bladder for residual urine.	Incomplete voiding can increase risk for urinary tract infection.	Is patient effectively emptying bladder?
Teach the patient or caregiver self-catheterization as ordered, if bladder training is not effective.	Intermittent self-catheterization is associated with fewer complications than an indwelling catheter.	Is patient able to perform self-catheterization correctly?
Monitor appearance of urine, temperature, and white blood cell (WBC) count.	Cloudy urine with an increase in temperature and WBC count indicates urinary tract infection.	Is urine clear and temperature and WBC count within normal limits?
Consult with HCP regarding indwelling Foley catheter if patient is not a candidate for intermittent self-catheterization.	An indwelling catheter can increase risk for infection but may be necessary as a last resort for some patients.	Is Foley catheter necessary? Are signs of infection avoided?

Nursing Diagnosis: Constipation related to immobility and nerve damage as evidenced by passage of hard, dry, or infrequent stools
Expected Outcome: The patient will return to preinjury bowel pattern.
Evaluation of Outcome: Does the patient pass soft stool at regular intervals?

Intervention	Rationale	Evaluation
Determine previous and current bowel pattern and continence.	Decreased or absent sphincter tone, inability to detect the need to defecate, and immobility put patient at risk for incontinence and constipation.	What was previous pattern? How can it be maintained for the patient?

Nursing Care Plan for the Patient With a Spinal Cord Injury—cont'd

Intervention	Rationale	Evaluation
Monitor bowel sounds and abdominal distention.	These are indicators of bowel function.	Are bowel sounds present? Is abdomen soft?
Institute a bowel management program as soon as oral feedings are resumed. Include a suppository on a scheduled daily or every-other-day basis as ordered.	A management program including stool softeners and routine suppository use can help to restore regular defecation.	Does management program keep bowel movements soft and regular and maintain continence?
If possible, have patient sit on a toilet or bedside commode to move bowels.	Sitting allows gravity to help evacuate the bowel.	Does sitting help patient move bowels?
Provide a high-fiber diet with adequate fluid intake.	Fiber and fluids help keep stool soft.	Is patient receiving adequate fiber and fluids?

Nursing Diagnosis: *Impaired Physical Mobility* related to hemorrhage, ischemia, and edema of cord as evidenced by paresis or paralysis
Expected Outcomes: The patient will maintain maximum mobility and be free from complications of immobility.
Evaluation of Outcomes: Is the patient kept mobile without contractures? Is skin intact? Can the patient complete activities of daily living (ADLs) with assistance?

Intervention	Rationale	Evaluation
Determine patient's ability to move independently.	Data collection should guide interventions.	What can patient do independently?
Determine patient's ability to feel pressure and pain.	If patient is unable to feel pain or pressure, it will be even more important to monitor skin and prevent prolonged pressure.	Can patient feel pressure and pain?
Reposition every 2 hours, using supportive devices.	Unrelieved pressure on the skin, especially bony prominences, will result in ischemia and necrosis.	Is skin intact without redness?
Change positions slowly; have patient sit at side of bed before standing (if able) or getting up to a chair.	Patients with cervical spine injuries or patients remaining immobile for long periods are prone to orthostatic hypotension.	Does patient become dizzy when getting up?
Instruct assistive personnel to not grasp the bars when transferring a patient in halo traction.	Grasping the bars can cause harm to the patient or the device.	Do all staff transfer the patient correctly?
Perform active or passive range-of-motion (ROM) exercises at least once every 8 hours. If patient has arm mobility, teach them to participate in as many ROM exercises as possible.	ROM exercises maintain mobility and prevent contractures.	Is patient able to perform ROM exercises with minimal difficulty?
Teach patient importance of repositioning self at least every 2 hours.	Patients with some mobility can learn to reposition themselves; this helps prevent total dependence on caregivers.	Does patient demonstrate correct repositioning every 2 hours?
Teach patient to direct own care if unable to reposition independently.	This allows patient some control over their situation.	Does patient direct own care and prevent complications of immobility?

(nursing care plan continues on page 982)

Nursing Care Plan for the Patient With a Spinal Cord Injury—cont'd

Nursing Diagnosis: *Risk for Impaired Skin* Integrity related to immobility and possible paresthesias
Expected Outcome: The patient's skin will remain intact without redness or breakdown.
Evaluation of Outcome: Is the patient's skin intact?

Intervention	Rationale	Evaluation
Monitor skin frequently. When permitted by the HCP, turn patient frequently and check bony prominences for redness.	The patient who does not have sensation is at increased risk of developing pressure injuries.	Is patient turned and repositioned at least every 2 hours? Is skin intact?
Start preventive measures in the emergency department by being sure to remove anything between patient and the backboard.	Patients have developed pressure injuries from lying on keys or other objects in their pockets.	Are skin surfaces protected from pressure?
Use a pressure-reducing mattress.	Specialty mattresses or beds can reduce pressure but do not reduce need to turn patient.	Is patient on an appropriate mattress?
If on a self-turning bed, make sure patient is not sliding as the bed turns. Avoid pulling and friction on skin when repositioning patient in bed.	Sliding can cause friction and shearing damage to the skin.	Is friction damage to skin avoided?
Ensure that patient's extremities do not get caught in side rails or wheelchair spokes.	Patient may not be aware this is happening, and a pressure injury can result.	Are all patient's body parts accounted for and safe?
If patient is in skeletal traction or a halo brace, check pin sites frequently. Keep sites clean and dry and report any sign of infection.	Skin sites are at risk for infection and breakdown.	Are pin sites clean and dry?
Monitor temperature of bath water (no more than 102°F [38.9°C]).	Patient may not be able to feel burning if water is too hot.	Are burns prevented?

Nursing Diagnosis: *Ineffective Role Performance* related to effects of injury
Expected Outcome: The patient will identify new ways to carry out essential roles.
Evaluation of Outcome: Is the patient able to identify ways to carry out roles?

Intervention	Rationale	Evaluation
Allow patient to verbalize concerns about their roles if desired.	This can help to clarify potential role problems for the patient and begin the process of developing a plan.	Is patient able to identify roles they have filled in the past that will be difficult to carry out due to injury?
Help patient and family members to identify resources.	Interpersonal relationships can be significantly stressed by spinal cord injury. Friends, family members, and members of patient's faith can provide emotional and physical help.	Does patient have adequate support systems in place to provide help?
Consult a social worker to help the patient gain access to appropriate physical and financial assistance.	Loss of income can be temporary or permanent and can add to burden of spinal cord injury. Not all insurance policies cover the extensive inpatient rehabilitation needed by patients with spinal cord injuries. Adaptive equipment is expensive and may not be covered by insurance.	Is patient able to access appropriate financial assistance if needed?

Nursing Care Plan for the Patient With a Spinal Cord Injury—cont'd

Intervention	Rationale	Rationale
Provide information about area support groups.	Individuals who have been through similar experiences can provide support and information for the patient and family.	Is patient willing to contact support groups?

Nursing Diagnosis: *Risk for Sexual Dysfunction* related to autonomic nervous system dysfunction
Expected Outcome: The patient will state they have an acceptable means for sexual expression.
Evaluation of Outcome: Does the patient state satisfaction with sexual function?

Intervention	Rationale	Rationale
If a male patient has an erection during a bath or catheterization, discontinue the procedure and continue later if possible. Maintain a matter-of-fact attitude.	Male patients with quadriplegia may develop an erection during any penile stimulation.	Is patient's dignity maintained during personal care?
Allow patient to voice concerns about sexual function if desired.	Male patients with paraplegia can have difficulty achieving and maintaining an erection.	Is patient able to voice concerns? Is a consult with a urologist or other specialist needed?
Encourage patient and patient's partner to explore alternative methods of sexual expression.	Closeness and touching may be a satisfying alternative.	Is patient able to discuss alternative methods with their partner?
If a male patient wishes to have children, encourage a consult with a fertility specialist or urologist.	Men with spinal cord injuries may not ejaculate in normal manner. A specialist can provide some help for conception if desired.	Is patient given information about conception if desired?

PRACTICE ANALYSIS TIP
Linking NCLEX-PN® to Practice
The LPN/LVN will participate in staff education (e.g., in-services, continued competency).

NEURODEGENERATIVE AND NEUROCOGNITIVE DISORDERS

Neurodegenerative is a term that can apply to any nervous system disorder that causes degeneration, or wasting, of the neurons in the nervous system. The disorders discussed in this section are some of the most common neurodegenerative disorders. *Neurocognitive* is the term to describe acquired neurologic disorders that cause cognitive decline. Management of chronic conditions does not focus on the short-term stay in the hospital because of an exacerbation of the disease process but rather on the long-term goal of helping the patient and family cope with the disease process and maintain the patient's independence for as long as possible. Nursing care involves providing information on management of the illness, prevention and treatment of complications, and referrals to support groups or case managers. As patients decline, there will come a time when family members can no longer care for their loved one in their homes and must consider care in a long-term care facility.

Dementia

Dementia is not a disease but rather a symptom of other neurocognitive disorders. According to the National Institute of Neurological Disorders and Stroke (2019), patients who have dementia have "significantly impaired intellectual functioning that interferes with normal activities and relationships. They also lose their ability to solve problems and maintain emotional control, and they may experience personality changes and behavioral problems, such as agitation, delusions, and hallucinations. While memory loss is a common symptom of dementia, memory loss by itself does not mean that a person has dementia."

Some patients have mild mental status changes that do not interfere significantly with day-to-day functioning. This is sometimes referred to as mild cognitive impairment (MCI). However, patients with MCI are more likely to develop Alzheimer disease than those without MCI.

Etiology and Pathophysiology
There are many causes of dementia, including Parkinson, Huntington, and Alzheimer diseases, which are discussed later in this chapter. Multiple "mini-strokes" (multi-infarct

• **WORD** • **BUILDING** •
neurodegenerative: neuro—nervous system + degenerative—deteriorating
dementia: de—down or from + mentia—the mind

> **Box 48.3**
>
> **Medications That Can Cause Confusion**
> - Anticholinergic agents (atropine [Atropen], some antihistamines)
> - Analgesics (meperidine [Demerol], morphine)
> - Histamine type 2 (H2) receptor antagonists (cimetidine [Tagamet], ranitidine [Zantac])
> - Central nervous system depressants (sleeping pills, tranquilizers, antianxiety agents, alcohol)
> - Steroids (cortisone, prednisone)
>
> For a complete list, check out the Beers Criteria for Potentially Inappropriate Medication Use in Older Adults (https://www.guidelinecentral.com/guideline/340784/).

dementia or vascular dementia) are another common cause. Chronic alcoholism, neurologic infections, head injuries, and many medications (Box 48.3) also can cause changes in mental status, leading to dementia. Although aging is associated with more frequent dementia diagnoses, dementia is not a normal part of aging. In general, thinking is affected by changes in the brain that result from reduced blood flow or from structural changes related to disease states.

Much research has been done to determine factors related to dementia and its prevention. Some studies indicate that patients who have more education, have higher socioeconomic status, and engage in stimulating intellectual and leisure activities are less likely to develop dementia. Some experts believe these individuals develop a sort of cognitive reserve that keeps them functioning at a high level, even when changes in their brains on autopsy indicate dementia. People with less education, fewer leisure activities, and less intellectual stimulation are more likely to develop symptoms of Alzheimer disease.

Signs and Symptoms

Have you ever forgotten something important? Most people have occasional memory lapses, but they do not typically have dementia. In patients with dementia, recent memories are usually affected first. Patients may have difficulty recalling whether they ate breakfast or may accuse a family member of not calling when they called just a few hours earlier. This same patient, however, may easily recall an event or a phone number from childhood.

As patients become more forgetful, they may ask the same questions repeatedly. They can get lost driving or walking in a familiar neighborhood. They can become disoriented to time and be unaware of the year. Patients might say Eisenhower is president, for example, because they remember that as true when they were young. As the disease progresses, they may not recognize where they are and, eventually, can lose recognition of even their own family members.

Later in the course of the dementia, remote memory can be lost. Patients can forget how to perform simple tasks, such as doing the dishes or making a phone call. They may wander and become lost. Safety is a significant issue with a wandering patient; patients have been found wandering in their nightclothes in the middle of a road, unaware of what they are doing. Patients can develop aphasia and become unable to communicate their needs or follow simple instructions. This can become frustrating to both the family and nursing caregivers. Behavioral problems may necessitate admission to a long-term care facility. In very late stages, the patient becomes totally dependent on caregivers.

Diagnostic Tests

Diagnosis of dementia is twofold. First, dementia must be identified; then the focus moves to finding the cause of the mental status change. Early diagnosis is essential, because some causes of MCI may be reversible, and early treatment may delay progression. Neuropsychological testing can determine the degree of memory, personality, and behavior change. The patient should also be tested for depression, which can cause mental status changes but is often easily treated. A review of medications by a knowledgeable nurse, HCP, or pharmacist may reveal a medication that is contributing to the mental changes. MRI, CT scan, positron emission tomography (PET) scan, and blood tests help diagnose underlying causes.

Therapeutic Measures

Medical interventions depend on the cause of the dementia. Table 48.8 lists medications that can be used to delay progression of Alzheimer-related dementia. If medical treatment cannot alter the course of the disease, the focus will shift to delaying progression of symptoms and maintaining patient safety. Excellent nursing care becomes essential for both the patient and family at this point. An important aspect of care in early dementia is determination of the patient's wishes while the patient is still able to make decisions and express desires. Some difficult decisions relate to the patient's continued ability to drive and live alone. Other decisions related to resuscitation, guardianship, and powers of attorney for health care and finances are essential to discuss. For more information on dementia, refer to www.dementiasociety.org.

Nursing Process for the Patient With Dementia

See "Nursing Care Plan for the Patient With Dementia."

Nursing Care Plan for the Patient With Dementia

Nursing Diagnosis: *Risk for Injury* related to impaired memory, thought processes, and judgment
Expected Outcome: The patient will remain free from injury.
Evaluation of Outcome: Is the patient safe and free from injury? Is environment safe?

Intervention	Rationale	Evaluation
Monitor patient's ability to maintain safety.	*As dementia worsens, the patient's needs will change.*	Is patient able to make decisions and negotiate the environment safely?
Keep environment simple and familiar; label doors and objects. Keep patient in familiar environment as long as possible.	*Change can result in confusion; even a minor change in furniture arrangement can result in falls.*	Is patient able to remain in the home with minimum confusion and without injury?
Remove harmful objects (e.g., scissors, matches); store medicines in a locked cabinet; remove knobs from stoves.	*Impaired judgment can make safety a major concern for patients who live at home.*	Is the environment safe for the patient?
Make sure patient has eyeglasses and hearing aids if necessary.	*Impaired sensory perception can increase confusion and risk for falls.*	Is patient able to see and hear effectively?
Use nightlights; remove throw rugs; use safety gates on stairs.	*These can reduce the risk for falls.*	Is environment set up to reduce risk for falling?
Have identification bracelet on patient and identification tags sewn into clothes; put locks on doors to prevent patient from leaving.	*Patients can wander, making them prone to injury.*	Is wandering confined to a monitored area? Is environment set up to allow movement within a safe area?
Provide daily walks or exercise.	*Exercise can decrease wandering.*	Does exercise reduce wandering?

Nursing Diagnosis: *Chronic Confusion* related to dementia
Expected Outcome: The patient will function at optimal cognitive level.
Evaluation of Outcome: Is the patient maintaining optimum cognitive function?

Intervention	Rationale	Evaluation
Monitor changes in thought processes.	*As cognitive function declines, care plan will need to be revised.*	Is patient able to correctly identify objects, remember tasks, speak clearly, and identify person, place, and time?
Provide a box of safe, familiar items, such as empty thread spools or pretty handkerchiefs.	*Patients often rummage through drawers, closets, or boxes. Patients may not recognize difference between their own possessions and others'. Keeping them occupied with a box of safe items may decrease their need to look for things.*	Does a box of items keep patient occupied and content?
Place calendars, clocks, personal items, and seasonal decorations in patient's environment.	*These provide orientation to the present.*	Can patient identify the season or year?
If patient hallucinates or has delusions, do not attempt to correct. Focus instead on the feelings related to the hallucinations, such as "Do you feel frightened?"	*Having feelings validated can help develop trust while not validating the hallucination.*	Does patient respond to refocusing on feelings?
Reduce stressors such as fatigue, overstimulation, or pain.	*Stress may increase dysfunctional behaviors.*	Are stressors eliminated as much as possible? Is patient's behavior calm?

(nursing care plan continues on page 986)

Nursing Care Plan for the Patient With Dementia—cont'd

Intervention	Rationale	Evaluation
Maintain patient's usual routines as much as possible.	*Familiar routines of activities, sleeping, and eating are more comfortable for patients. Change can be stressful.*	Are routines organized around patient rather than the staff?
Communicate clearly. Make eye contact, speak slowly and directly to the patient, and use nonverbal gestures. Use a tone of voice conveying respect and sincerity.	*Unclear communication can increase confusion and stress. Tone of voice plays a role in the ability of the patient to cooperate.*	Do all staff members communicate clearly and respectfully with the patient?
Involve family in care planning and implementation.	*The family knows the patient's preferences and routines best.*	Does family presence help patient stay calm and function at optimum level?
Provide video or audiotapes of patient's family members.	*Familiar sounds and pictures can reduce agitation when family is not present.*	Do video or audiotapes help calm the patient?

Nursing Diagnosis: *Risk for Caregiver Role Strain* related to demands of caring for patient with declining mental status while balancing other demands
Expected Outcomes: The caregiver will have the support needed to safely manage care of the patient. The caregiver will be able to identify when the patient is too difficult to care for and requires more structured care.
Evaluation of Outcomes: Is the caregiver managing demands of caring for the patient? Is the patient safe? Is additional support or a change in environment for the patient indicated?

Intervention	Rationale	Evaluation
Allow caregiver to verbalize concerns related to burden of caring for patient.	*Identification of caregiver concerns and challenges can help the nurse plan appropriate support.*	Does caregiver share concerns? What are caregiver's current support systems?
Observe for signs of depression or stress in the caregiver.	*A stressed or depressed caregiver may have difficulty providing safe care for the patient.*	Are signs of stress present? Does patient care appear to be suffering?
Encourage caregiver to identify family and friends who can provide support. If involved in a local church or religious organization, encourage caregiver to make their needs known.	*There are often resources in the family or community that can be accessed without cost and can help if they know the need exists.*	Can caregiver identify potential resources to contact?
Refer for assistance with caregiving and/or day care utilizing Alzheimer support groups and resources.	*Formal support systems in the community may be available to help relieve some of the caregiver's burden.*	Is caregiver able to obtain support and take some time for himself or herself?
Encourage caregiver to use support systems identified to allow time to care for self; encourage them to take care of own health needs and enjoy regular respite time	*If the caregiver becomes ill due to the stress of caregiving, they will no longer be able to assist the patient.*	Does caregiver maintain own physical and emotional health?
Allow caregiver to grieve over losses, those in the patient as well as loss of control over their own life.	*As the disease progresses, the patient gradually loses awareness of the neurologic deterioration. Occasional lucid moments can be very difficult for patient and caregiver as they realize what has been lost.*	Is the caregiver able to identify feelings of grief, anger, or sorrow?
Discuss progression of the disease process and the possibility of transferring patient to a long-term care facility.	*The caregiver may feel guilt over not being able to care for the patient and may need permission to consider placement at long-term care facility.*	Is caregiver able to identify when home care is too demanding and choose an alternative arrangement?

Table 48.8
Medications Used to Treat Alzheimer-Related Dementia

Medication Class/Action

Cholinesterase Inhibitors

Inhibit cholinesterase, to improve function of acetylcholine in the central nervous system. May improve cognitive function but will not alter course of disease.

Examples	*Nursing Implications*
donepezil (Aricept) tacrine (Cognex) rivastigmine (Exelon) galantamine (Reminyl)	Must be taken regularly; patient may need reminders to take, or family member may need to assist. Monitor for weight loss and report to health-care provider.

N-Methyl-D-Aspartate (NMDA) Antagonist

Reduces binding of glutamate, an excitatory neurotransmitter.

Examples	*Nursing Implications*
memantine (Namenda, Namenda XR, Axura)	Teach patient and family that improvements may take months.

> **PRACTICE ANALYSIS TIP**
> **Linking NCLEX-PN® to Practice**
> The LPN/LVN will assist in the care of the cognitively impaired client.

Delirium

Whereas dementia is chronic and progressive, **delirium** is a mental disturbance that is temporary. It can have either a rapid or gradual onset. Delirium is a medical emergency and should be diagnosed and treated promptly. Delirium is characterized by disorganized thinking and difficulty staying focused. It is seen most in older adults experiencing stress or illness. Patients who are severely ill or who have a history of hypertension, alcoholism, or preexisting dementia are at greatest risk. In many cases, response to medications is the cause (see Box 48.3). The disturbance can also be anything that stresses the person's body, such as pain, oxygen deficiency, urinary catheters, fluid and electrolyte imbalances, a change in environment, or nutritional deficiency. Often, the most effective nursing intervention is to have a family member present to assist with orientation and reassurance. It is beneficial to have continuity in nursing personnel when possible.

> **Nutrition Notes**
> **Nutrition Issues in Dementia**
> The World Health Organization (WHO, 2019) estimates that 50 million people have dementia worldwide, and that figure is expected to triple by 2050. However, some studies have shown a decrease in the prevalence of dementia, which is thought to be related to increased cardiac health (American Speech-Language-Hearing Association, 2020). Poor nutrition may increase behavior symptoms and cause weight loss (Alzheimer's Association, 2020). Brain atrophy, changes in the sense of smell, and high levels of pro-inflammatory cytokines negatively impact appetite and eating behaviors. Problems frequently seen in early- to late-stage dementia patients include difficulty with shopping for groceries and preparing meals, eating regularly, recognizing foods, remembering how to eat and drink independently, and wandering and pacing, which burns excessive calories. Dysphagia is also concerning (Vranešić Bender & Krznarić, 2020).
>
> Patients should be monitored for weight loss, dehydration, and nutrient deficiencies. However, supplements should not be given without evidence of deficiencies. Mealtimes should be routine and in a quiet area with supervision or assistance provided by the same individual whenever possible. Changes in food textures may be necessary with diagnosed dysphagia to prevent malnutrition. Oral liquid supplements may be required to improve nutritional status, as tolerated by patient, but feeding tubes are not recommended (Vranešić Bender & Krznarić, 2020).
>
> *References*
> Alzheimer's Association. (2020). Food and eating. https://www.alz.org/help-support/caregiving/daily-care/food-eating
> American Speech-Language-Hearing Association. (2020). Dementia. https://www.asha.org/practice-portal/clinical-topics/dementia/#collapse_1
> Vranešić Bender, D., & Krznarić, Ž. (2020). Nutritional issues and considerations in the elderly: An update. *Croatian Medical Journal 61*(2), 180–183. https://doi.org/10.3325/cmj.2020.61.180
> World Health Organization. (2019). Dementia. https://www.who.int/news-room/fact-sheets/detail/dementia

> **PRACTICE ANALYSIS TIP**
> **Linking NCLEX-PN® to Practice**
> The LPN/LVN will promote a therapeutic environment.

> **NURSING CARE TIP**
> Patients with delirium or dementia must be kept safe, and interventions are similar for both. One important difference, however, is in how you respond to confusion. If a patient is experiencing delirium, reorient them to the present time and situation. If a patient with dementia is chronically confused, however, reorientation may not be effective. In this case, validate their feelings. An example would be comforting a patient who is calling for a long-lost parent rather than reminding the patient the mother has been gone for 30 years.
>
> It is essential that delirium is not mistaken for dementia. If an older adult is hospitalized and exhibits new-onset confusion, consider that it might be delirium. Correcting electrolyte levels, controlling pain, changing medications, or administering oxygen can be helpful in reversing delirium. See "Nursing Care Plan for the Patient With Dementia" for nursing interventions.

> **Implications for Nursing Practice**
> The HELP program uses nursing staff with the addition of volunteers to provide the following interventions:
>
> 1. Core interventions: Orientation, therapeutic activities, sleep enhancement, early mobilization, visual protocol, hearing protocol, fluid replacement/constipation, feeding assistance
> 2. Additional interventions as needed: Aspiration prevention, infection control, constipation management, pain management, and hypoxia management
> 3. Geriatric nursing assessment and other interventions: Delirium protocol, dementia protocol, screen medications for psychoactive issues, discharge needs assessment
>
> *Reference:* Hsheih, T. T., Yang, T., Gartaganis, S. L., Yue, J., & Inouye, S. K. (2018). Hospital elder life program: Systematic review and meta-analysis of effectiveness. *American Journal of Geriatric Psychiatry 26*(10), 1015–1033. https://doi.org/10.1016/j.jagp.2018.06.007

Parkinson Disease

Parkinson disease is a chronic degenerative movement disorder that arises in the basal ganglia in the cerebrum. Parkinson disease has typically been considered a disease of older adults; however, there are many people with young-onset Parkinson disease. An example is Michael J. Fox (actor and founder of the Michael J. Fox Foundation for Parkinson's Research), who was diagnosed at age 30. The disease is characterized by tremors, changes in posture and gait, rigidity, and slowness of movements. Approximately 60,000 new cases of Parkinson disease are diagnosed each year in the United States; it ranks 14th in causes of death according to the CDC, with prediction that by 2020 the number of cases of Parkinson will increase to 930,000 (Parkinson's Foundation, 2020).

> **Evidence-Based Practice**
>
> **Clinical Question**
> What is the best way to prevent delirium in hospitalized older adults?
>
> **Evidence**
> Delirium is a growing concern for older adults in the hospitalized setting, with occurrence rates as high as 50% among this demographic. It is associated with higher morbidity and mortality rates, longer hospitalizations, and more expensive treatments. Hsheih et al (2018) conducted a systematic literature review of 44 peer-reviewed articles to examine the effectiveness of Hospital Elder Life Program (HELP) to target delirium risk factors and identify the most effective nonpharmacological nursing care interventions to prevent or care for delirium in older adults in the hospital.

Pathophysiology

The substantia nigra is a group of cells located within the basal ganglia, situated deep in the brain. These cells are responsible for the production of dopamine, an inhibitory neurotransmitter. Dopamine facilitates the transmission of impulses from one neuron to another. Parkinson disease is caused by destruction of the cells of the substantia nigra, resulting in decreased dopamine production. Loss of dopamine function results in impairment of semiautomatic movements. Parkinson disease is sometimes called an extrapyramidal disorder because it affects the extrapyramidal tracts in the spinal cord that contain motor neurons.

Acetylcholine, an excitatory neurotransmitter, is secreted normally in individuals with Parkinson disease. The normal balance of acetylcholine and dopamine is interrupted in these patients, causing a relative excess of acetylcholine. This results in the tremor, muscle rigidity, and **akinesia** (loss of muscle movement) characteristics of Parkinson disease.

Etiology

The etiology of Parkinson disease is unknown. It was first described in 1817 by London surgeon James Parkinson. Although scientists now know that the symptoms are caused by death of dopamine-producing cells in the substantia nigra, they do not know what causes the cells to die. There may be a genetic component, especially in younger patients. Certain environmental toxins can also play a role. Parkinson-like symptoms, referred to as *parkinsonism*, can be associated with use of certain medications, such as phenothiazines. Parkinsonism was also linked to an outbreak of encephalitis in the 1920s.

• WORD • BUILDING •
akinesia: a—not + kinesia—movement

Signs and Symptoms

The onset of symptoms in patients with Parkinson disease is usually gradual and subtle. A substantial percentage of the dopamine-producing cells are nonfunctional before the patient becomes symptomatic. Symptoms may be mistakenly attributed to aging or fatigue. In retrospect, patients and their family members often identify a long period in which symptoms were present but not identified as symptoms of Parkinson disease.

The primary symptoms of Parkinson disease are muscular rigidity, **bradykinesia** (slow movement) or akinesia, changes in posture, and tremors. The brain is no longer able to direct the muscles to perform in the usual manner. This lack of communication can profoundly impact the patient's ability to ambulate safely, perform ADLs and job functions, or enjoy leisure activities. The symptoms may also have a significant negative impact on the patient's self-esteem.

The patient may have difficulty initiating movement; this can be particularly apparent when the patient tries to start walking, rise from a sitting position, or begin dressing. Because considerable effort is required to move the rigid muscles, the patient performs voluntary movements very slowly. At times, the patient can experience freezing of gait and be unable to initiate ambulation or negotiate a turn during ambulation.

The extensor muscles are more affected by Parkinson disease than are the flexor muscles. This impaired function of the extensor muscles results in the stooped posture typical of patients with Parkinson disease (Fig. 48.14). Flexion of the hips, knees, and neck shifts the center of gravity forward. The gait is characterized by short, shuffling steps that may increase in speed once the patient finally starts walking. Once in motion, the patient may have difficulty stopping. The patient maintains a broad base when making turns to try to compensate for imbalance. These changes place patients at high risk for falls. Slow movements and stiff muscles make it much harder for patients to catch themselves or to relax muscles to minimize injury if a fall occurs.

Tremors typically begin in the hand and then progress to the **ipsilateral** foot. In most patients, the tremor then moves to the **contralateral** side. Many patients identify one side of the body as more affected by the tremor than the other. Tremor of the hand has been described as a pill-rolling tremor; the thumb typically moves back and forth across the fingers as if the patient is rolling a pill. Tremors typically lessen or disappear during movement and are more noticeable when the extremity is at rest or when trying to hold an object still (called a *resting tremor*). The tremors disappear when the patient is asleep. Inability to hold an object still can make simple acts such as drinking a glass of water or reading a book nearly impossible. The signs and symptoms of Parkinson disease tend to increase in severity when the patient becomes fatigued. Another type of tremor, a benign familial (or essential) tremor, can sometimes be mistaken for Parkinson disease. Table 48.9 details differentiation of these tremors. Treatment is different for each.

The secondary symptoms of Parkinson disease include generalized weakness, muscle fatigue and cramping, and difficulty with fine motor activities. This fine motor dysfunction can make it difficult for the patient to button a shirt or tie shoes. Handwriting typically deteriorates as the disease progresses. A soft, monotone voice and masklike facial expression can make the patient appear lacking in emotional responses. It may be necessary to ask patients about their emotional status and help them develop ways to express emotions. The blink response is diminished, so the patient and significant others must be educated about eye care to prevent corneal abrasions.

Dysfunction of the autonomic system can cause diaphoresis, constipation, orthostatic hypotension, drooling, dysphagia, seborrhea, and frequent urination. Patients who experience seborrhea and diaphoresis need frequent attention to personal hygiene. Drooling and dysphagia can make the patient reluctant to appear in public. Slowness in initiating walking, balance problems, and frequent urination place the patient at risk for urinary incontinence, which can also increase the patient's reluctance to leave home.

Late in the disease, mental function may become slowed, and the patient may develop dementia. This is compounded by the side effects of many anti-Parkinson medications. Death is usually from complications of immobility.

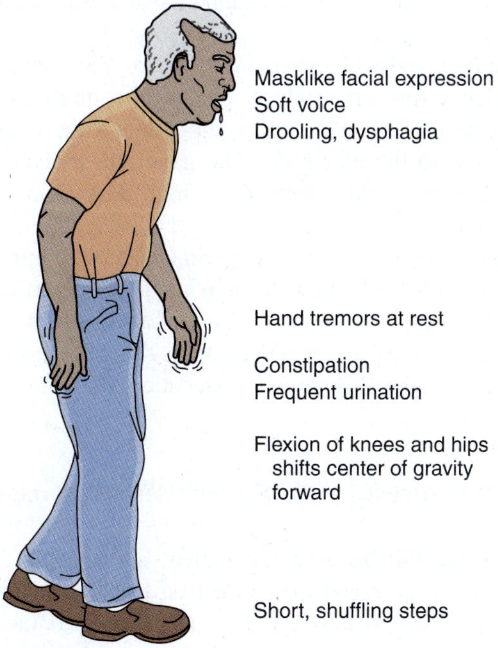

FIGURE 48.14 Manifestations of Parkinson disease.

Labels: Masklike facial expression; Soft voice; Drooling, dysphagia; Hand tremors at rest; Constipation; Frequent urination; Flexion of knees and hips shifts center of gravity forward; Short, shuffling steps

• WORD • BUILDING •

bradykinesia: brady—slow + kinesia—movement
ipsilateral: ipsi—same + lateral—side
contralateral: contra—opposite + lateral—side

Table 48.9
Symptoms of Parkinson Disease Tremor vs. Essential Tremor

Disease	Parkinson Tremor	Benign Familial (Essential) Tremor
Resting tremor	Yes	No
Intention tremor (with movement)	No	Yes
Pill-rolling tremor	Yes	No
Head/voice tremor	No	Yes
Relieved with beta-blocking medication (propranolol)	No	Yes
Relieved with anti-Parkinson medications	Yes	No

Complications

The most typical acute complications of Parkinson disease are related to the patient's difficulties with mobility and balance. Patients are prone to falls, which result in injuries ranging from bruises or fractures to head or spinal cord injuries. Constipation is common because of decreased activity, diminished ability to take in food and fluids, and side effects of anticholinergic medications. Patients are encouraged to increase fiber and fluid in their diets. If constipation is not alleviated by dietary modifications, the patient may need stool softeners.

Muscular rigidity and bradykinesia contribute to joint immobility, which decreases patients' ability to ambulate and care for themselves. Position changes can be painful for patients. Turning sheet and adequate personnel are necessary when turning a patient in bed to prevent stress on the joints. Tremors interfere with ADLs, consume immense amounts of energy, and can prevent the patient from working or performing leisure activities. Swallowing can become so impaired that enteral (tube) feeding is required. Depression is a common complication at any stage of Parkinson disease and may compromise communication, ability to learn, and performance of ADLs. Patients may require counseling or antidepressants.

Diagnostic Tests

No specific tests are used to diagnose Parkinson disease. The diagnosis is based on the history given by the patient and a thorough physical examination. MRI and PET scans may be done to rule out alternative causes of the patient's symptoms.

Therapeutic Measures

There is no cure for Parkinson disease. Treatment aims at controlling symptoms and maximizing the patient's function. Medications used to control symptoms are listed in Table 48.10.

Many patients with Parkinson disease experience fluctuations in motor function related to medication therapy, referred to as the *on-off phenomenon*. Patients may have a decreased response to levodopa, particularly as the dose wears off. As the disease progresses, patients may notice that "off periods" become less predictable and occur more rapidly. The patient may have a delayed or absent response to the next dose of levodopa, resulting in the patient being stuck in the off stage and being significantly disabled for that period. Fluctuations in motor function can be accompanied by other symptoms, such as pain, diaphoresis, anxiety attacks, hallucinations, or mood swings, that increase the disability associated with the episodes (Table 48.10).

Patients taking maximum doses of medication for Parkinson disease symptoms may benefit from a "medication holiday." During a medication holiday, patients are taken off all medications for a time and then restarted on lower doses. Hospitalization may be necessary during this time to maintain patient safety.

Surgical Treatments

Pallidotomy may be an option for patients when rigidity, tremor, and bradykinesia are uncontrollable with medical management. During this stereotactic procedure, a destructive lesion is created in the basal ganglia. The surgery is performed on only one side of the brain. The patient remains awake during the surgery to make sure that the lesion is placed in the appropriate location. These patients need a great deal of education and support before and during the surgery.

Another surgical treatment is deep-brain stimulation in which a tiny electrode is placed into brain tissue. A generator is implanted under the skin on the chest and connected to the electrode. The generator delivers electrical pulses to the electrode, which may help control symptoms.

Some researchers have experimented with implanting stem cells into the brain to develop into dopamine-producing cells; research into gene therapies is also ongoing. These therapies are only experimental at this time. For more information, visit the Parkinson's Foundation Web site at www.parkinson.org.

Nursing Process for the Patient With Parkinson Disease

DATA COLLECTION. Ask the patient about symptoms of Parkinson disease and their effect on level of functioning. Observe ability to move, walk, and perform ADLs safely.

Table 48.10 Medications Used to Treat Parkinson Disease

Medication Class/Action

Dopamine Agonists

Convert into dopamine in the brain.

Examples	Nursing Implications
levodopa (L-dopa) levodopa/carbidopa combination (Sinemet): Carbidopa prevents peripheral breakdown of levodopa so more is available in the central nervous system (CNS).	Teach: Take food shortly after (not before or with) each dose to prevent gastric irritation. May discolor urine and sweat. Take around the clock to control symptoms.

Dopamine Agonists

Stimulate dopamine receptors in the brain.

Examples	Nursing Implications
pramipexole (Mirapex) ropinirole (Requip)	Giving with meals may reduce nausea. Caution about drowsiness and sleep attacks (falling asleep during activities that require alertness, including driving).

Monoamine Oxidase B (MAO-B) Inhibitor

Blocks metabolism of central dopamine, increasing dopamine in CNS.

Examples	Nursing Implications
selegiline (Eldepryl, Zelapar) rasagiline (Azilect)	Can slow progression of Parkinson disease. Administer daily at noon to prevent insomnia. Can cause dangerous interaction with meperidine (Demerol), alcohol, and CNS depressants.

Catechol-O-Methyltransferase (COMT) Inhibitor

Blocks the enzyme COMT to prevent breakdown of levodopa, prolonging levodopa action. For use with levodopa/carbidopa combination (Sinemet).

Examples	Nursing Implications
entacapone (Comtan) carbidopa/levodopa/entacapone combination (Stalevo)	Report elevated temperature, muscular rigidity, altered level of consciousness, and elevated creatine phosphokinase (CKP).

Note: With all anti–Parkinson disease agents, teach patient to check with physician before taking over-the-counter medications, especially cold preparations. Teach patient to rise slowly to prevent orthostasis.

Determine risk for injury related to immobility or falls. Monitor nutritional status and condition of skin. Identify presence of confusion and side effects of medications. Psychosocial data collection includes the patient's and caregiver's responses to the disease, coping strategies, and support systems.

NURSING DIAGNOSES, PLANNING, AND IMPLEMENTATION. The patient with Parkinson disease is at risk for many problems. Priority diagnoses are addressed next. If confusion is present, also see "Nursing Care Plan for the Patient With Dementia" earlier in this chapter.

Impaired Physical Mobility related to muscle stiffness and tremor

EXPECTED OUTCOME: The patient will maintain optimal mobility and ability to ambulate as long as possible.

- Assist the patient to plan daily activities based on anticipated response to medications. *Certain times of day may be less troublesome than others.*
- Consult with physical and occupational therapists to provide assistive devices *to help maintain mobility and provide diversional activities.*

- Provide assistance with ROM exercises *to maintain flexibility of muscles.*
- Teach patients who have difficulty initiating walking to pick up one foot as though attempting to step over something to take the first step. It may also help to take several steps in place before starting to walk. *This may help overcome freezing of gait.*

Self-Care Deficit (Dressing/Feeding/Toileting/Bathing) related to reduced mobility

EXPECTED OUTCOME: The patient's self-care needs will be met as evidenced by patient statement.

- Encourage the patient to participate in ADLs as much as possible. *This helps the patient maintain independence and self-esteem.*
- Consult an occupational therapist *to assist with devices and strategies for maintaining independence.*
- Instruct the patient or family to provide clothing without buttons and supply shoes with adherent fasteners rather than shoelaces *to help maintain independence.*
- Assist the patient and family to make decisions about long-term care. Consult a social worker as needed for assistance. *As the patient ages, so do the family members who are providing care. The point may be reached at which the caregiver is no longer able to meet the increasing needs of the patient. The decision to place the patient in a skilled nursing facility is extremely difficult and emotional.*

Risk for Injury related to reduced mobility and balance

EXPECTED OUTCOME: The patient will remain safe and without injury.

- If the patient is in the hospital or long-term care facility, keep the call light within reach at all times. Remind the patient to request assistance with ambulation. Consider having a sitter, or someone to stay with the patient. *The patient is at risk for injury from falls related to problems with mobility.*
- Maintain bed in the low position, with side rails raised if appropriate (side rails may be prohibited in some institutions). *Maintaining the bed in a low position reduces the risk for injury or fall when getting out of bed. Side rails can increase the risk for injury and must be used carefully.*
- Use an alarm system on the bed and chair that alerts the staff that the patient is getting up *so that staff can assist the patient to get up and ambulate.*
- Avoid use of restraints. *Restraints can increase the risk for injury.*
- Keep environment free from clutter, throw rugs, or items *that can cause a patient to trip.*
- Provide walkers and other assistive devices *to provide support and prevent falls.*

EVALUATION. The care of the patient with Parkinson disease has been successful if the patient remains as mobile and independent as possible. Self-care needs should be met by the patient or others, and the patient should remain safe from injury.

CRITICAL THINKING

Ms. Simpson, 47 years old, has had Parkinson disease for the past 5 years, and the symptoms are becoming progressively worse. She is now admitted for a urinary tract infection.

1. What problems do you foresee when caring for Ms. Simpson?
2. Why do you need to implement safety measures?
3. Ms. Simpson is receiving IV fluids of 5% dextrose in 0.45% saline, 1,000 mL over 12 hours. The RN on duty is accountable for her IV, but as you are bathing her you notice that the bag is nearly full and it has been hanging for 4 hours. How many milliliters should still be in her IV bag after 4 hours?
4. What members of the health-care team should you collaborate with in providing Ms. Simpson's care?

Suggested answers are at the end of the chapter.

Huntington Disease

Huntington disease is a progressive, hereditary, degenerative, incurable neurologic disorder. It was first described in 1872 by George Huntington, a general practitioner in New York. Many cases around the world can be traced to specific individuals.

Pathophysiology and Etiology

Huntington disease (also known as Huntington chorea) is inherited in an autosomal dominant manner, which means that each offspring of an affected parent has a 50% chance of inheriting the disorder. A mutation in a specific gene has been identified; however, the cause of the mutation is not known. A protein called *rhes* may be responsible for the activation of a mutant protein that causes destruction of the cells in the corpus striatum. Destruction also occurs in the caudate nucleus and other deep nuclei of the brain and in portions of the cerebral cortex. This degeneration results in progressive loss of normal movement and intellect. The rate of disease progression varies from person to person.

Signs and Symptoms

Signs usually begin in middle age and develop slowly, becoming progressively more apparent. Cognitive signs can be noticed before movement problems. Patients who are unaware of a hereditary risk for Huntington disease may be incorrectly diagnosed as mentally ill.

The patient can display personality changes and inappropriate behavior. The patient may be euphoric or irritable and can rapidly alternate between moods. Paranoia is common, and behavior can become violent as dementia worsens. The patient eventually becomes incontinent and totally dependent on others for care. Coping with these symptoms is difficult for family and friends as well as professional caregivers. The disease progression and associated symptoms are particularly devastating for offspring, who may not know whether they inherited the disease.

Physical symptoms develop slowly. Huntington disease is characterized by involuntary, irregular, jerky, dancelike (choreiform) movements. Initially, these symptoms take the form of mild fidgeting and facial grimacing, starting in the arms, face, and neck and progressively involving the remainder of the body. Patients display hesitant speech, eye blinking, irregular trunk movements, abnormal tilt of the head, and constant motion (Fig. 48.15). The gait is wide, and the patient may appear to be dancing. Emotional upset, stress, or trying to perform a voluntary task can significantly increase the severity and rate of the abnormal movements; the movements typically diminish or disappear during sleep. Dysphagia can significantly impair the patient's nutritional status.

Depression and suicide are common in the earlier stages of the disease when the patient still has the cognitive ability to carry out a suicidal act. As the disease progresses, the patient becomes increasingly more dependent. Aspiration resulting in respiratory failure is the primary cause of death. Life span following diagnosis is about 10 to 30 years.

Diagnostic Tests

Huntington disease is typically diagnosed based on clinical examination and family history. MRI or CT scan may be helpful. Genetic testing is available for prenatal use and to determine whether an individual has Huntington disease before symptoms arise. This is important because Huntington disease does not become symptomatic until patients are in their 30s or 40s, when they may already have children who could be affected (see "Patient Perspective: Betty").

Therapeutic Measures

Because there is no cure, treatment of Huntington disease focuses on minimizing symptoms and preventing complications. Antipsychotic, antidepressant, and antichoreic medications may be used to treat both the involuntary movements and behavioral outbursts. Tetrabenazine (Xenazine) may reduce involuntary movements by increasing dopamine in the brain.

Physical and occupational therapy can keep the patient mobile and independent for as long as possible. Research on the benefits of transplanting stem cells into the brains of patients with Huntington disease is ongoing but remains experimental.

Patient Perspective

Betty

I was born the second of six children. My mom was diagnosed with Huntington chorea (an old name for Huntington disease) after she had all of us. My brother was diagnosed with Huntington disease at the age of 60. He started out with terrible mood swings and a bad temper, eventually developing movement problems including pronounced facial and tongue movements.

By the time we knew the disease had affected our family, many of us had children and grandchildren of our own. My kids wanted me to be tested. It is a hereditary disease, and you have a 50/50 chance of having it if a parent has it. If I had Huntington disease, then my kids would have a 50/50 chance of having it. If I tested negative, then they and their children would not be at risk.

I was very nervous and afraid of being tested. When I went for the initial visit at the University of Michigan, they observed my movements, how I walked and talked, and my facial movements. They made me go to a psychologist to see whether I could handle the results if they did the blood test that would tell for sure. I understand the suicide rate is kind of high for people with Huntington. After talking for an hour and a half, they decided I could handle the results.

At my next visit, they just drew blood, which was sent out for testing. I had to return to the university 6 weeks later for the results. When I went back, I was a nervous wreck. A friend went with me. When the technician came in, she said the doctor would be with me soon. I immediately had bad thoughts. Then when the technician and doctor came back, they were both smiling and had tears in their eyes—I had tested negative. My friend, the doctor, the technician, and I all hugged and cried.

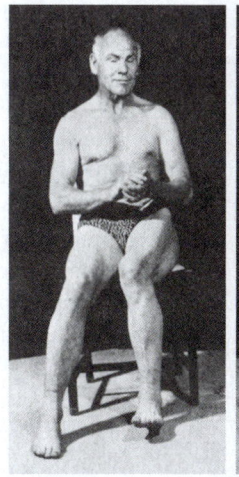

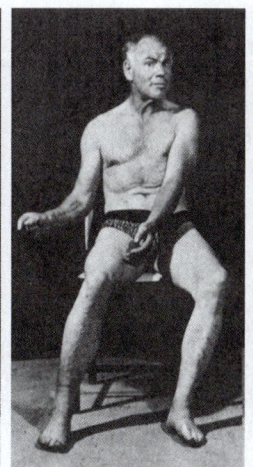

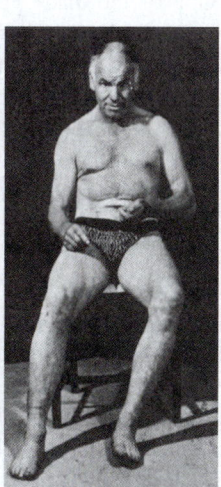

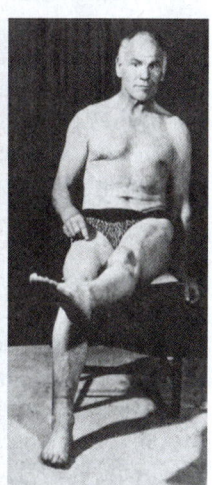

FIGURE 48.15 A 47-year-old patient with Huntington disease. Note constant fidgety movement.

> It is a very hard disease to live with, whether you or another family member has it. My brother has it very bad. Out of my five siblings, four have it for sure, and we think the fifth has it because of mood swings we have observed.
>
> I am the only one of the six who tested clear. I felt very guilty at first that they all had it and I didn't. I'm starting to get over that, but when I see one of them having a bad time with talking, or temper, or movement, the guilt starts to kick in again.

Nursing Care

Patients with Huntington disease typically receive care on an outpatient basis. When a patient with Huntington disease is admitted to an inpatient facility, it is important to obtain as much information as possible about that person's response to medication, daily routine, and emotional and cognitive functioning from the caregivers. For example, knowing a certain patient is afraid of bathtubs but willingly takes showers can prevent unnecessary struggles and outbursts. Providing objects from home can make the new environment seem less threatening. The caregivers may relate that the patient has better cognitive function at a particular time of day. As dementia progresses, the patient responds less to attempts at reasoning. Giving directions in a calm but firm tone may help them cooperate with activities. The environment should be modified to keep the patient safe. Keep in mind that forceful, involuntary movements of patient's extremities can happen at any time and should not be misinterpreted as an attempt to harm caregivers.

Difficulty swallowing typically begins toward the middle of the disease course. Patients exhibit trouble swallowing liquids in particular. At this stage, it may still be possible to teach the patient to hold the chin down to the chest while swallowing, which lessens the chance of aspiration. Have patients sit straight upright while eating. Thickening agents can be added to liquids to help prevent aspiration. Adaptive devices can prolong the patient's ability to eat independently. Soft foods that are easily manipulated in the mouth are most suitable. Patients may have difficulty taking in adequate calories to maintain a normal body weight, even if a caregiver assists with feeding them. One of the many ethical issues faced by these patients and their family members is whether artificial feeding should be used and, if so, for how long. Patients and their family members should be encouraged to discuss end-of-life decisions early in the disease.

For more information, see "Nursing Care Plan for the Patient With Dementia" earlier in chapter.

Alzheimer Disease

Alzheimer disease (also called *dementia of the Alzheimer type [DAT]*) is the most common type of dementia. Dementia is a progressive loss of mental functioning that interferes with memory, ability to think clearly and learn, and eventually ability to function (see discussion of dementia earlier in this chapter).

Alois Alzheimer, a German neurologist, first described the disease in 1907. He described pathological changes, now referred to as *neurofibrillary tangles* and *neuritic plaques*, that he discovered while performing an autopsy on a patient with dementia. Alzheimer disease is a progressively degenerative disease that is inevitably fatal. Alzheimer disease is more common in women than men. Incidence doubles for every 5 years a person lives beyond age 65.

Etiology and Pathophysiology

Many etiologies have been theorized for Alzheimer disease, including viral or bacterial infection and autoimmune dysfunction. Markers associated with Alzheimer disease can be found on several chromosomes. Chromosome 21 in particular has been associated with Alzheimer and is also the location of the genetic abnormality responsible for Down syndrome. Patients older than age 40 who have Down syndrome usually develop Alzheimer disease. The correlation between the two disorders is still being studied. Lifestyle factors that increase risk of Alzheimer disease include hypertension, hypercholesterolemia, and poorly controlled diabetes.

Although the exact cause of Alzheimer disease is unknown, associated structural changes have been well documented. An abnormality exists within the protein of the cell membrane of a neuron. As the axon terminals and dendrite branches disintegrate, they collect in neuritic plaques. Inside the normal brain is a precise arrangement of filaments and tubules responsible for cell integrity. Individuals with Alzheimer disease develop neurofibrillary tangles instead of the normal orderly arrangement. Instead of remaining a small area of abnormality, these neuritic plaques and neurofibrillary tangles spread via axons to other areas of the brain. In addition, patients tend to have a deficiency of acetylcholine in the cerebral cortex. Remember that acetylcholine is a neurotransmitter important for nervous system function.

Advancement of neurofibrillary tangles and neuritic plaques typically affects the hippocampus first, resulting in short-term memory dysfunction. As tangles and plaques spread to the temporal lobe, memory impairment becomes more severe. At this point, the patient may seek assistance from the health-care system. Personality changes and incontinence are inevitable results of Alzheimer disease. These symptoms can be attributed to the spread of plaques and tangles to the frontal lobes of the brain.

It is believed that the younger the patient at the time of onset, the faster the neurofibrillary tangles and neuritic plaques spread. Younger patients tend to deteriorate faster, require complete care earlier, and have a shorter life span.

One area of the brain left relatively untouched by Alzheimer disease is the subcortical area. This structure is responsible for our subconscious urge to survive. The needs for basic requirements such as shelter, food and water, security, and reproduction are controlled by the subcortical area, as are emotional responses to situations. The patient with Alzheimer disease may experience hunger but no longer know how to meet that basic need. Left to their own devices, these individuals would starve.

Signs and Symptoms

The signs and symptoms of Alzheimer disease are typically categorized in three stages.

STAGE 1. This early stage lasts from 2 to 4 years and is characterized by increasing forgetfulness. At this stage, the patient may attempt to cope by using lists and reminders. Interest in day-to-day activities, acquaintances, and surroundings tends to diminish. The patient is reluctant to take on tasks because of uncertainty in how to perform them. If the patient is still working, their performance deteriorates and can result in being terminated from the job.

STAGE 2. The second stage is the longest in duration, lasting 2 to 12 years. Progressive cognitive deterioration causes difficulty doing simple calculations or answering questions. Patients may become irritable, particularly when asked to perform a task that they know they should be able to perform but cannot. It may help the patient to break down the task into manageable steps. Depression is common. Aphasia and the resulting inability to make themselves understood can exacerbate patients' irritability. It is during the middle stage, as cognitive function significantly deteriorates, that the patient may become more physically active. The normal sleep–wake cycle is disrupted, and the patient tends to wander aimlessly, particularly at night. The patient may become lost in familiar surroundings, which compounds the anxiety that typically develops during this stage. Hallucinations and seizures can occur. Management of day-to-day activities, such as feeding a pet or paying bills, becomes overwhelming. Personal hygiene deteriorates, as does appropriate social behavior. Patients may make up stories to cover for deficits, saying that possessions they misplaced were stolen. Some patients hoard food or money.

STAGE 3. The third stage of Alzheimer disease is characterized by progression to complete dependency. The patient loses the ability to converse or control bowel or bladder function. If the patient is still mobile, constant supervision is required to protect from wandering and avoid injury. Emotional control and ability to recognize loved ones are lost. This lack of recognition is particularly devastating for family members. Eventually, the patient is unable to move independently, swallow, or express needs. Death usually occurs from complications of immobility.

The duration of the final stage of Alzheimer disease, characterized by complete dependence, depends in part on the physical stamina and general health of the individual. The healthier the patient, the longer the body will continue to function. Another factor is the decisions that have been made regarding artificial feeding and respiratory support. Few family members or HCPs advocate intubation and mechanical ventilation for patients with Alzheimer disease. The issue of enteral feedings, however, is an emotional one with few easy answers. The use of enteral feedings can prolong the patient's life, despite the absence of cognitive functioning. As with patients suffering from Huntington disease, every effort should be made to determine the patient's wishes before cognitive impairment makes that impossible.

Some experts recognize seven stages of Alzheimer disease. Individuals are evaluated using the Global Deterioration Scale for Assessment of Primary Degenerative Dementia (GDS), which presents a more detailed description of each stage. Predementia (stages 1 through 3) is characterized with no impairment to MCI. In stages 4 and 5, patients have significant memory loss and confusion. In stage 5, the person cannot survive without assistance with ADLs. The final stages (6 and 7) are associated with loss of verbal and basic psychomotor skills, and the brain no longer has control over the body.

Table 48.11 provides a comparison of the symptoms of Parkinson, Huntington, and Alzheimer diseases.

Diagnostic Tests

Alzheimer disease is diagnosed primarily on the basis of clinical examination, history, and elimination of other possible causes of symptoms. MRI can reveal the classic neurofibrillary tangles and neuritic plaques. PET and SPECT scans show areas of neuronal inactivity. Genetic testing and brain imaging can help predict the risk of Alzheimer disease. New blood tests that can predict risk are also being developed.

Table 48.11
Comparisons of Parkinson, Huntington, and Alzheimer Diseases

Symptom	Parkinson	Huntington	Alzheimer
Tremors	Present	Absent	Absent
Bradykinesia/akinesia	Present	Absent	Absent
Muscle rigidity	Present	Absent	Absent
Memory dysfunction	Late	Late	Early
Cognitive dysfunction	Late	Present	Early
Inability to perform activities of daily living	Progressive	Progressive	Progressive
Involuntary movements	Absent	Present	Absent
Depression	Present	Present	Present

Therapeutic Measures

There is no known cure for Alzheimer disease. Treatment has traditionally focused on minimizing the effects of the disease and maintaining independence as long as possible. Acetylcholinesterase (AChE) inhibitors such as donepezil (Aricept) or rivastigmine (Exelon) are thought to inhibit the breakdown of the neurotransmitter acetylcholine (see Table 48.8). Increased levels of acetylcholine in the brain allow better functioning of the remaining neurons. They appear to be most effective for those patients who exhibit mild to moderate symptoms of Alzheimer disease. It can take some time to notice any effects of the medications. Use of AChE inhibitors diminishes the amount of medical care and social service interventions required and delays admission to skilled nursing facilities. This delay in institutionalization can result in significant positive impact on quality of life and financial savings for the patient and family.

Another class of medications, NMDA (*N*-methyl-D-aspartate) antagonists, can prevent overexcitation of NMDA receptors in the brain and allow more normal function. Memantine (Namenda, Axura) is the only medication currently available in this class. These medications can be given at any stage of Alzheimer disease and, like AChE inhibitors, simply slow the patient's decline. The Food and Drug Administration (FDA) recently granted accelerated approval (further testing is needed) for a new medication for Alzheimer Disease. Aducanumab (Aduhelm) targets beta-amyloid plaques in the brain and may reduce cognitive decline.

Antidepressants, antipsychotics, and antianxiety medications can be used as a last resort to control symptoms of depression and behavioral disturbances, but they do not treat the dementia. Patients should be carefully monitored for medication interactions and side effects. For more information, visit the Alzheimer's Association Web site at www.alz.org.

Nursing Process for the Patient With Alzheimer Disease

See the earlier discussion of dementia as well as "Nursing Care Plan for the Patient With Dementia" earlier in this chapter.

CRITICAL THINKING & CLINICAL JUDGMENT

Mrs. Johnson has just become a resident at a long-term care facility. She is diagnosed with Alzheimer disease and is in stage 2 with some signs of stage 3 disease. When you check on her during the evening, you find her walking around her room, talking to herself.

Critical Thinking (The Why)
1. What other signs and symptoms should you check Mrs. Johnson for?

Clinical Judgment (The Do)
2. What nursing interventions should you take to address her behavior?

Suggested answers are at the end of the chapter.

Home Health Hints

Dementia
- Teach caregivers how to handle difficult behavior.
- Try to accommodate rather than change behaviors.
- Changing our response to behaviors often results in a change in the patient's behavior. Try to stay calm.
- Behaviors usually have a purpose and result from the patient not being able to tell us what they need or want—for example, they may be in pain, hungry, or bored.
- Try to disrupt the behavior pattern by using distraction or removing triggers.
- As disease progresses, what has worked in the past may not continue to work, so be flexible.
- Try not to take behavior personally. The patient with dementia is not acting intentionally.
- Keep the patient who wanders safe by covering doorknobs with a piece of cloth or installing a door alarm.
- Take a break. Seek family or friends who can provide a break or community resources for respite.
- Pet therapy, aromatherapy, exercise, and massage or touch have been shown to have positive effects.
- Observe the patient during bathing, grooming, or dressing to check motor function and coordination.
- Teach the caregiver to provide shoes with Velcro closures to promote independence.
- Teach the caregiver and patient to use chairs with armrests so the patient can rise from the chair more easily.
- Teach the caregiver to make a clip-on clothing protector with suspender clips attached to a piece of elastic. A clean napkin or washcloth can be attached for each meal.

Key Points

- Meningitis is an inflammation of the meninges that surround the brain and spinal cord. It can be caused by either bacterial or viral infection. Bacterial meningitis is a serious infection that is spread by direct contact with discharge from the respiratory tract of an infected person. Viral meningitis, also called *aseptic meningitis*, is more common and rarely serious. It usually presents with flu-like symptoms, and patients recover in 1 to 2 weeks.
- Encephalopathy refers to the mental status changes seen in patients with meningitis. These are manifested as short attention span, poor memory, disorientation, difficulty

following commands, and a tendency to misinterpret environmental stimuli. Late signs of meningitis include lethargy and seizures.
- A quiet, dark environment lessens the stimulation of a patient who has a headache or photophobia and who is agitated, disoriented, or at risk for seizures. An important aspect of nursing care focuses on keeping patients from harming themselves.
- Encephalitis is an inflammation of brain tissue. Nerve cell damage, edema, and necrosis cause neurologic findings in the specific areas of the brain affected.
- The patient with herpes encephalitis develops edema and necrosis (sometimes associated with hemorrhage), most commonly in the temporal lobes. This significant cerebral edema causes increased ICP and can lead to herniation of the brain.
- Common causes of increased ICP include brain trauma, intracranial hemorrhage, and brain tumors. Prompt detection of changes in neurologic status indicating increased ICP allows intervention aimed at preventing permanent brain damage.
- Initial symptoms of increased ICP include restlessness, irritability, and decreased LOC because cerebral cortex function is impaired.
- Vital sign changes are a late indication of increasing ICP. The Cushing triad includes bradycardia, irregular respirations, and arterial hypertension (increasing systolic blood pressure while diastolic blood pressure remains the same), resulting in widening pulse pressure. By the time these symptoms appear, the ICP is significantly increased, and interventions may not be successful.
- Headaches are divided into three major types: primary; secondary; and cranial neuralgias, central and primary facial pain, and other headaches. One common type of primary headache is migraine. There are two major types of migraine: migraine with aura and migraine without aura. Other primary headaches are tension and cluster headaches.
- A seizure can be a symptom of epilepsy or other neurologic disorders such as a brain tumor or meningitis. Epilepsy is a chronic neurologic disorder characterized by recurrent seizure activity.
- Seizures can be classified as partial or generalized. Partial seizures begin on one side of the cerebral cortex. In some cases, the electrical discharge spreads to the other hemisphere and the seizure becomes generalized. Generalized seizures are characterized by involvement of both cerebral hemispheres.
- Epilepsy can be acquired or idiopathic (unknown cause). Causes of acquired epilepsy include traumatic brain injury and anoxic events. No cause has been identified for idiopathic epilepsy. The most common time for idiopathic epilepsy to begin is before age 20. New-onset seizures after this age are most commonly caused by an underlying neurologic disorder.
- Repetitive, purposeless behaviors, called *automatisms*, are the classic symptom of partial seizures.
- Generalized seizures affect the entire brain. Two types of generalized seizures are absence seizures and tonic-clonic seizures. Absence seizures, sometimes referred to as petit mal seizures, occur most often in children. They are manifested by a period of staring that lasts several seconds.
- Tonic-clonic seizures are what most people envision when they think of seizures. They are sometimes called *grand mal seizures* or *convulsions*.
- The postictal period is the recovery period after a seizure. Following a partial seizure, the postictal phase may be no more than a few minutes of disorientation. It is usually longer after a tonic-clonic seizure. Patients may sleep deeply for 30 minutes to several hours. Following this deep sleep, patients may report headache, confusion, and fatigue.
- Emergency care is required for seizures. The prime objective is to prevent injury during a seizure. A patient should never be left alone during active seizure activity. Side rails, if used, should be padded to prevent injury if the patient strikes their extremities against them. If the patient falls to the floor, move furniture out of the way. Maintain a patent airway, and, if possible, turn the patient on their side to prevent aspiration if vomiting occurs.
- TBI is a complex phenomenon with results ranging from no detectable effect to a persistent vegetative state. Trauma can result in hemorrhage, contusion or laceration of the brain, and damage at the cellular level. In addition to the primary insult, the brain injury can be compounded by cerebral edema, hyperemia, or hydrocephalus.
- Cerebral concussion is considered a mild brain injury. If there is loss of consciousness, it is for 5 minutes or less. Concussion is characterized by headache, dizziness, or nausea and vomiting. The patient may describe amnesia of events before or after the trauma.
- Cerebral contusion is characterized by bruising of brain tissue, possibly accompanied by hemorrhage. There can be multiple areas of contusion depending on causative mechanism.
- Subdural hematomas are classified as acute or chronic based on the time interval between injury and onset of symptoms. Acute subdural hematoma is characterized by appearance of symptoms within 24 hours following injury. As the subdural hematoma increases in size, the patient may exhibit one-sided paralysis of extraocular movement, extremity weakness, or dilation of the pupil. LOC can deteriorate further as ICP increases.
- Patients with epidural hematoma typically exhibit a progressive course of symptoms. The patient loses consciousness directly after the injury; they then regain consciousness and are coherent for a brief period. The patient then becomes less responsive. If there is no intervention, the patient becomes unresponsive. Once the patient has symptoms, deterioration can be rapid. Airway management and control of ICP must be instituted immediately, or the patient will die.
- If interventions to control ICP are unsuccessful, the patient can experience uncontrolled edema or herniation of brain tissue. Herniation is displacement of brain tissue out of its normal anatomical location. This displacement prevents function of the herniated tissue and places pressure on other vital structures, most commonly the brainstem. Herniation usually results in brain death.

- Brain tumors are neoplastic growths of the brain or meninges. Brain tumors can be characterized by vague symptoms, such as headache or visual changes, or by focal neurologic deficits, such as hemiparesis or seizures.
- The most common early symptom of a brain tumor is fatigue. Other symptoms can include seizures, motor and sensory deficits, nausea and vomiting, headaches, personality changes, confusion, and speech and vision disturbances.
- Therapeutic measures for brain tumors include surgery, radiation, and chemotherapy.
- Spinal disorders include herniated intervertebral discs and spinal stenosis. Both of these conditions may be treated with spinal surgery if other treatments are not effective.
- Injuries to the spinal cord affect people of all ages but take their greatest toll on young people. Spinal cord injuries are characterized by a decrease or loss of sensory and motor functions below the level of the injury.
- Spinal cord injuries can be classified by location or by degree of damage to the cord. A complete spinal cord injury means that there is no motor or sensory function below the level of the injury. With an incomplete lesion, some function remains. This does not necessarily mean that the remaining function will be useful to the patient. Some patients find that having areas where sensation is intact may be more painful than useful.
- Cervical cord injuries can affect all four extremities, causing paralysis and paresthesias, impaired respiration, and loss of bowel and bladder control. Paralysis of all four extremities is called *quadriplegia*; weakness of all extremities is called *quadriparesis*.
- Thoracic and lumbar injuries affect the legs, bowel, and bladder. Paralysis of the legs is called *paraplegia*; weakness of the legs is called *paraparesis*. Sacral injuries affect bowel and bladder continence and may affect foot function.
- Spinal cord injury has a profound effect on the ANS. Immediately after injury, the cord below the injury stops functioning completely. This causes a disruption of sympathetic nervous system function, resulting in vasodilation, hypotension, and bradycardia, called *neurogenic shock* or *spinal shock*.
- Autonomic dysreflexia is a life-threatening complication that occurs in patients with injuries above the T6 level. The spinal cord injury impairs the normal equilibrium between the sympathetic and parasympathetic divisions of the ANS.
- Causes of autonomic dysreflexia include a full bladder, bowel impaction, urinary tract infection, ingrown toenails, pressure injuries, pain, and labor in a pregnant woman. Stimulation of the sympathetic nervous system results in cool, pale skin; gooseflesh; and vasoconstriction below the level of the injury. Blood pressure can rise as high as 300 mm Hg systolic. The parasympathetic response results in vasodilation, causing flushing and diaphoresis above the lesion, and bradycardia as low as 30 beats per minute. The patient reports a pounding headache and nasal congestion secondary to the dilated blood vessels.
- Dementia is not a disease but rather a symptom of a number of neurocognitive disorders. Some patients can have mild mental status changes that do not interfere significantly with day-to-day functioning. This is sometimes referred to as *mild cognitive impairment*. However, patients with MCI are more likely to go on to develop Alzheimer disease than those without MCI.
- Delirium is a mental disturbance that is temporary. It can have either a rapid or gradual onset. Delirium is considered to be a medical emergency and should be diagnosed and treated promptly. Delirium is characterized by disorganized thinking and difficulty staying focused.
- Parkinson disease is a chronic degenerative movement disorder that arises in the basal ganglia in the cerebrum. Dopamine facilitates the transmission of impulses from one neuron to another. Parkinson disease is caused by destruction of the cells of the substantia nigra, resulting in decreased dopamine production. Loss of dopamine function results in impairment of semiautomatic movements
- Huntington disease (also known as *Huntington chorea*) is a progressive, hereditary, degenerative, incurable neurologic disorder that causes uncontrolled movements through the body.
- Alzheimer disease (also called *dementia of the Alzheimer type*) is the most common type of dementia and is a progressively degenerative disease that is inevitably fatal.
- The signs and symptoms of Alzheimer disease are typically broken down into three stages. The first stage lasts from 2 to 4 years and is characterized by increasing forgetfulness. The second stage is the longest in duration, lasting 2 to 12 years. Progressive cognitive deterioration causes difficulty doing simple calculations or answering questions.
- The third stage of Alzheimer disease is characterized by progression to complete dependency. The patient loses the ability to converse or control bowel or bladder function. If the patient is still mobile, constant supervision is required to protect from wandering and avoid injury. Emotional control and ability to recognize loved ones are lost.

SUGGESTED ANSWERS TO CHAPTER EXERCISES

Cue Recognition
48.1: Limit suctioning. If you must suction, oxygenate first and limit passes to 1 or 2.
48.2: Check the catheter for patency/full bladder, noting if emptying the bladder decreases the blood pressure and autonomic dysreflexia.

Critical Thinking & Clinical Judgment
Mr. Chung
1. Because meningococcal meningitis is contagious, he should be placed in droplet isolation. Personal protective equipment, such as gloves, gowns, and masks, should be used. Explain the need for these practices to Mr. Chung and his visitors.

2. Patients with meningitis usually present with head and neck pain with possible nausea and vomiting from increased ICP. Comfort measures include tepid baths; a quiet, dark environment; and minimal stimulation. Administer acetaminophen and analgesics as ordered.
3. The health-care service at his college should be notified of his diagnosis. Close contacts may require prophylactic treatment. If Mr. Chung lives at home rather than at college, his family members should be advised to see their HCP and begin prophylactic treatment.
4. Be prepared to assist with a lumbar puncture.
5. You should use short, simple sentences because he may be very anxious or disoriented. Involve his family. Further education can be provided when he is feeling better.

Mr. Evans
1. Mr. Evans's hematoma may be increasing in size. You might expect to see impaired speech, right-sided weakness, and a rapid decrease in consciousness if Mr. Evans's hematoma is enlarged.
2. Intubation equipment, mannitol, and IV access should be ready. He should be given nothing by mouth (NPO), and the results of laboratory tests should be ready in the event of emergency surgery. The location of Mr. Evans's next of kin must be known.
3. Who are Mr. Evans's support people? Was this drinking episode an isolated incident or a chronic problem that should be addressed if he is discharged safely?
4. Health-care team members needed for Mr. Evans depend on the extent of his injury. They may include a social worker; physical, occupational, and speech therapists; neuropsychologist; dietitian; and possibly neurological/neurosurgical consult.
5. Because of Mr. Evan's narcotic addiction, special care should be taken when addressing his pain and analgesia medications. After initial medical treatment, his addiction issues should be addressed to assist with his chemical dependency.

Ms. Simpson
1. Urinary tract infection is often accompanied by urinary urgency. Ms. Simpson may have difficulty getting to the bathroom quickly and safely.
2. Parkinson patients are at risk for injury due to reduced mobility. All measures should be taken to reduce falls and injury. Keep a bedside commode nearby if the bathroom is not close. Assist Ms. Simpson to the bathroom or commode at regular intervals to prevent urgency. Remind her to ask for help if she needs to get up. Make sure that her call light is within reach.
3. $\dfrac{1{,}000 \text{ mL} \mid 4 \text{ hours}}{12 \text{ hours}} = 333 \text{ mL}$
4. After 4 hours, 1,000 mL − 333 mL = 667 mL should remain in the bag. Because it is still nearly full, the RN should be notified.
5. Occupational, physical, and speech therapy may be involved in Ms. Simpson's care. Speech therapy can help with swallowing problems. Work with nursing assistants to be sure she is mobilized and protected from falls and that swallowing problems are addressed.

Mrs. Johnson
1. Being admitted to a new and unfamiliar facility can increase confusion. Signs of stage 2 Alzheimer disease include memory loss, wandering at night, sleeplessness, irritability, loss of way in familiar surroundings, losing possessions and searching for them, and neglect of personal hygiene. During stage 3 of the disease, the patient will lose weight, recognize hunger but be unable to eat, be unable to communicate verbally or in writing, lose ability to recognize family, become incontinent of urine and feces, and eventually lose ability to stand and walk.
2. Address Mrs. Johnson by her name and ask her what she needs. Reorient her to where she is and assure her that she is safe and being cared for.

Additional Resources

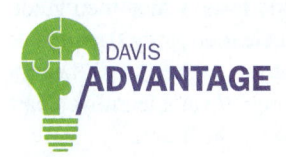

Go to Davis Advantage to complete your learning: strengthen understanding, apply your knowledge, and prepare for the Next Gen NCLEX®.

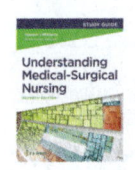

A Study Guide is also available.

CHAPTER 49
Nursing Care of Patients With Cerebrovascular Disorders

Sara E. Wilk, Linda K. Cook

KEY TERMS

aphasia (ah-FAY-zhee-ah)
ataxia (ah-TAK-see-ah)
diplopia (dip-LOH-pee-ah)
dysarthria (dis-AR-three-ah)
dysphasia (dis-FAY-zhee-ah)
embolic (em-BOL-ik)
embolism (EM-buh-lizm)
endarterectomy (end-AR-tur-EK-tuh-mee)
hemiplegia (HEM-ee-PLEE-jee-ah)
hemorrhagic (hem-uh-RAH-jik)
intracerebral (IN-trah-sur-EE-brul)
ischemic (ih-SKEE-mik)
penumbra (puh-NUM-brah)
thrombolytic (throm-buh-LIT-ik)
thrombosis (throm-BOH-sis)
thrombotic (throm-BOT-ik)

CHAPTER CONCEPTS

Collaboration
Caring
Mobility
Perfusion
Self-care

LEARNING OUTCOMES

1. Describe causes, risk factors, and pathophysiology of transient ischemic attack, ischemic stroke, and hemorrhagic stroke.
2. Identify emergency interventions for transient ischemic attack, ischemic stroke, and hemorrhagic stroke.
3. Plan therapeutic measures for transient ischemic attack, ischemic stroke, and hemorrhagic stroke.
4. Identify outcomes that can be expected for a stroke victim.
5. Plan nursing care for a patient with a cerebrovascular disorder.

Cerebrovascular disorders occur when the supply of blood and oxygen to brain cells is inadequate, allowing brain tissue to die and causing a stroke. The most common cerebrovascular disorders include transient ischemic attack, ischemic stroke, and hemorrhagic stroke.

TRANSIENT ISCHEMIC ATTACK

A transient ischemic attack (TIA) is a temporary blockage of blood to the brain that causes a transient (brief) neurologic impairment. The episode typically lasts minutes to hours, and the patient recovers completely. The risk factors, causes, and symptoms of a TIA are identical to those of a stroke. Indeed, if the blockage that causes a TIA does not reverse, an area of the brain is permanently damaged, and the event is a stroke. About 15% of all strokes are preceded by a TIA (American Heart Association/American Stroke Association [AHA/ASA], 2021b). Urgent evaluation of a TIA is essential to decrease the risk of stroke.

Treatment of a TIA focuses on preventing a full stroke. The cause of the TIA may be discovered with diagnostic tests, which then guide treatment. However, the TIA may not have a clear etiology. Treatment, therefore, is mostly centered on minimizing the patient's risk factors for a stroke. Check out the interactive site https://watchlearnlive.heart.org/ to see the effects of a TIA on blood flow to the brain.

STROKE

A stroke (also called *cerebrovascular accident*, or CVA) is caused by the disruption of blood flow to the brain, resulting in death of brain cells. In most cases, permanent disability results. About 795,000 people of all ages are affected each year (Centers for Disease Control and Prevention [CDC], 2020), and risk for stroke increases with age. Because of their increased longevity, 55,000 more women than men have strokes each year (National Stroke Association, 2020). Stroke is the fifth leading cause of death and the leading cause of disability in the United States with 147,810 deaths in 2018 from stroke (AHA/ASA, 2021a). Blacks, Hispanic Americans, and American Indian/Alaska Natives are at higher risk than Asian Americans and Whites (National Heart, Lung, and Blood Institute, 2019). People with lower levels of education, lower socioeconomic status, and those living in the southeastern United States also have an elevated stroke risk.

Pathophysiology

Cerebral function depends on oxygen and glucose delivery to neurons in the brain. The brain cannot store oxygen or glucose, so it relies on a constant supply of these nutrients. Without this supply, brain tissue dies. When a stroke occurs, brain cells begin dying immediately. An area of brain tissue called the **penumbra** surrounds the damaged area. It contains brain cells that are "stunned" and can be revived if the brain is reperfused quickly. However, the brain cells will die if the blood supply is not restored.

The vessel or vessels involved determine the area of the brain affected and symptoms. The duration of ischemia determines whether symptoms are transient or permanent. TIA symptoms generally resolve within 24 hours; however, a TIA can be a warning of an impending stroke.

Etiology

Strokes are classified as either ischemic or hemorrhagic. Ischemic strokes are more common, accounting for about 87% of all strokes (AHA/ASA, 2021b). Hemorrhagic strokes account for the remaining 13%. Find out more about the types of strokes, including helpful videos at www.nih.gov.

Ischemic Stroke

Ischemic stroke occurs when the blood supply to the brain is blocked or significantly slowed. There are two major types: thrombotic or embolic (Fig. 49.1).

THROMBOTIC STROKE. **Thrombotic** strokes occur when occlusion builds up in an artery until it significantly decreases or stops blood flow to the brain. Thrombotic strokes most often occur in the internal or common carotid arteries.

EMBOLIC STROKE. An **embolic** stroke is typically caused by a blood clot that is created somewhere in the body, often within the heart. It then travels through the arteries until it becomes trapped in a smaller vessel, preventing the passage of blood. Typically, the **embolism** will travel and become lodged in the middle, anterior, or posterior cerebral arteries.

RISK FACTORS. Risk factors for ischemic stroke are classified as modifiable or nonmodifiable (Box 49.1). Nonmodifiable risk factors are those that cannot be altered, such as age or gender. Modifiable risk factors are those that can be changed with treatment, such as high blood pressure. Women have additional risks due to hormone changes in pregnancy and menopause. Find out more about a woman's risk of stroke at https://www.goredforwomen.org/en.

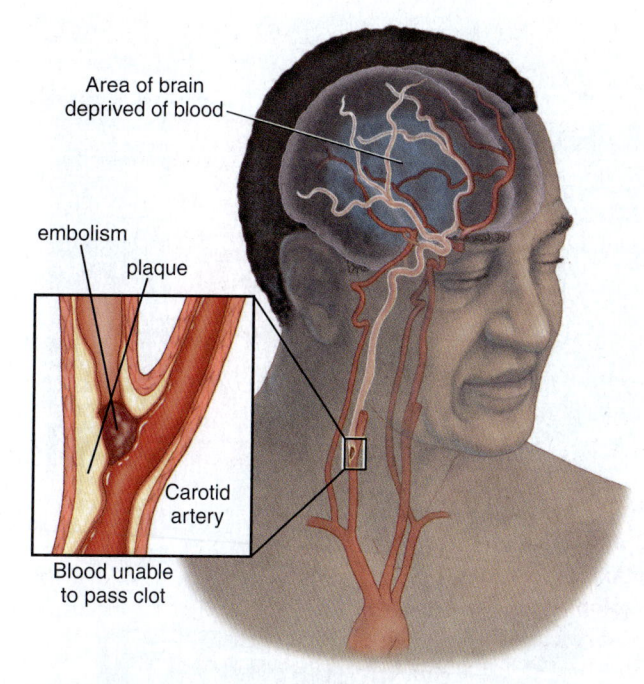

FIGURE 49.1 Embolism and thrombosis.

Box 49.1
Modifiable Risk Factors for Stroke

Men and Women
- Cigarette smoking
- High blood pressure
- Diabetes mellitus
- Cardiovascular disease
- High total cholesterol
- Low high-density lipoprotein (HDL) cholesterol
- Dyslipidemia
- Atrial fibrillation
- Asymptomatic carotid stenosis
- Sickle cell disease
- Obesity
- Excessive alcohol intake
- Poor diet (e.g., high sodium, high fat, low potassium)
- Physical inactivity

Women
- Pregnancy
- Oral contraceptives
- Hormone replacement therapy
- High triglycerides
- History of migraines
- Thick waist

• WORD • BUILDING •

ischemic: isch—to hold back + emia—blood + ic—relating to
thrombotic: thrombus—clot + ic—relating to
embolic: embolism—to throw (as in clot or other debris) + ic—relating to
embolism: embol—to throw + ism—condition

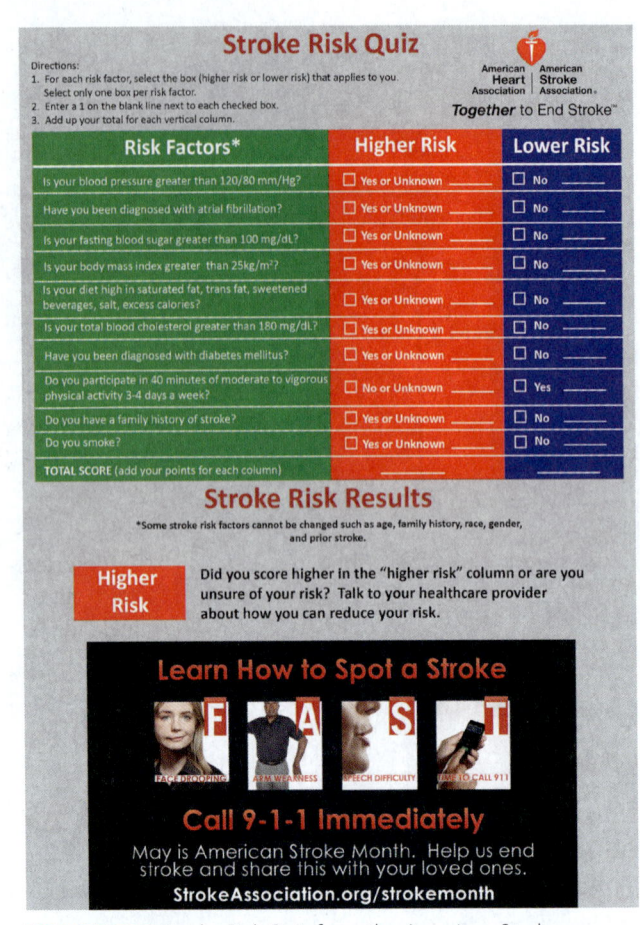

FIGURE 49.2 Stroke Risk Quiz from the American Stroke Association (located at https://www.stroke.org/stroke-risk-scorecard-2018). Reprinted with permission ©2018 American Heart Association, Inc.

Children with sickle cell disease, cardiac anomaly, and hyperlipidemia are also at risk for stroke. Minimizing or eliminating modifiable risk factors can significantly lower risk of a stroke. The Stroke Risk Scorecard from the National Stroke Association (Fig. 49.2) can help determine your risk for stroke.

> **NURSING CARE TIP**
> Copy or print the Stroke Risk from Figure 49.2 and keep it in your pocket for patient teaching opportunities.

Hemorrhagic Stroke

Hemorrhagic strokes are caused by the rupture of a cerebral blood vessel that allows blood to escape the blood vessel, accumulating and compressing the surrounding brain tissue. It can be further classified into two major types: subarachnoid hemorrhage and intracerebral hemorrhage.

SUBARACHNOID HEMORRHAGE. A *subarachnoid* hemorrhage is a stroke that occurs on the surface of the brain, most often the result of a ruptured cerebral aneurysm (covered later in this chapter). Strokes caused by subarachnoid hemorrhage usually are serious and require surgery to correct. They are often fatal.

INTRACEREBRAL HEMORRHAGE. An **intracerebral** hemorrhage is a stroke that occurs in the deeper tissues of the brain, usually caused by uncontrolled hypertension. Patients can experience multiple undetected intracerebral hemorrhages, with minimal deficits noted. However, damage eventually accumulates, and the patient will develop major deficits. Maintaining blood pressure below 130/80 mm Hg should be the goal. We discuss care of patients who have hemorrhagic stroke later in this chapter.

Warning Signs of Stroke

Patients and family members should be taught to recognize signs and symptoms and how to activate emergency medical services (EMS) if these signs occur. Evidence shows that beginning treatment within 1 hour of symptom onset can minimize or avoid permanent loss of function. The acronym FAST, which stands for **F**ace, **A**rms, **S**peech, and **T**ime (see Fig. 49.2), can be used to teach emergency triage nurses, first responders, nonlicensed personnel, and community members to recognize a stroke and respond quickly. Time is extremely important to preserve brain cells. Quick access to the EMS is of particular importance. EMS can focus on delivering a suspected stroke patient to a stroke center for rapid assessment and care.

In addition to FAST, the following five signs or symptoms recognized by the AHA and ASA (2021c) require immediate EMS activation:

- Sudden numbness or weakness of face, arm, or leg, especially on one side of the body
- Sudden confusion or trouble speaking or understanding
- Sudden trouble seeing in one or both eyes
- Sudden trouble walking, dizziness, loss of balance, or coordination
- Sudden severe headache with no known cause

Women may have other unique symptoms, such as sudden onset of the following:

- Nausea
- Facial and limb pain
- Sudden behavioral changes
- Hallucinations
- General weakness
- Chest pain
- Shortness of breath
- Hiccups
- Palpitations

• WORD • BUILDING •

hemorrhagic: hemorrhage—blood loss + ic—relating to
intracerebral: intra—within + cerebral—cerebrum

> **NURSING CARE TIP**
> When reinforcing teaching for a stroke victim and family, repetition is very important. Besides the anxiety and stress they may be feeling, the patient's ability to process information can be altered by the stroke.

> **BE SAFE!**
> **BE VIGILANT!** Before giving a patient with a suspected stroke anything to eat or drink, including medications, the patient should pass a swallow (dysphagia) screening test to prevent possible aspiration. Evaluate the patient's facial features; if there is any apparent weakness or asymmetry, stop and do not give the patient anything by mouth. If no weakness is evident, have the patient swallow about 30 mL of water. If the patient coughs, has difficulty swallowing, or has a wet or gurgly voice afterward, keep the patient NPO (nothing by mouth) until evaluated and cleared by a physician or speech and language pathologist.

Acute Signs and Symptoms

Most patients with stroke symptoms present with sudden or rapidly evolving symptoms. Symptoms are varied and depend on the area of the brain affected (Table 49.1). Common symptoms include visual disturbances, language disturbances, weakness or paralysis on one side of the body, and difficulty swallowing (dysphagia). Signs and symptoms are generally the same for both ischemic and hemorrhagic stroke. Patients may have drowsiness and a severe headache, often described as "the worst headache of my life."

Language Disturbances

Difficulty with language is commonly associated with TIA and stroke. **Aphasia** refers to the absence of language; **dysphasia** refers to difficulty with speech and is not as severe as aphasia. With dysphasia, the patient may experience trouble selecting the correct words, use incomprehensible or nonsense speech, have trouble understanding others' speech, and have trouble writing or reading. Aphasia can be *expressive*, in which the patient knows what he wants to say but cannot speak or make sense, or *receptive*, which is an inability to understand spoken and/or written words. When both expressive and receptive aphasia are present, it is called *global aphasia*. Slurred or indistinct speech because of a motor problem (lack of coordination) is referred to as **dysarthria**. Speech impairment often causes delay in treatment and emphasizes the importance of observation of symptoms by others.

Motor Disturbances

Motor disturbances include paralysis, weakness, and numbness. Sometimes, the first evidence of paralysis or weakness is clumsiness or a feeling of heaviness in a limb. The onset is sudden and typically involves one side of the body (the side opposite the damaged area of the brain). Deficits can appear on both sides of the body if the patient has had a brainstem or vertebrobasilar stroke.

Most commonly, paralysis or weakness affect the arm and face together. Some patients present with complete hemiparesis, with one entire side of the body flaccid. **Ataxia** may be present, which is poor balance or a stumbling, staggering gait. This can be related to damage to the cerebellum or to poor coordination due to weakness or paralysis. If the swallowing muscles are affected, the patient will have trouble swallowing (dysphagia).

Visual Disturbances

Visual field disturbances are also a common symptom of a stroke. The vision loss is painless and can involve loss of all or part of the vision in one eye. Patients often describe the change as a curtain dropping, as fog, or as a gray-out or blackout of vision. The involved eye is on the same side as the diseased artery. Potential visual field abnormalities are shown in Figure 49.3. When checking the patient's vision, stop talking and keep moving across the room. If the patient's eyes do not follow you, there is a good chance he or she has a deficit in that visual field.

Diagnostic Tests

On arrival at the emergency department (ED), a computed tomography (CT) scan will be performed immediately to identify whether symptoms are caused by a hemorrhagic stroke so that the health-care provider (HCP) can determine the appropriate course of treatment. Ischemic stroke changes are not visible on a CT until several days after the event. Interventions for hemorrhagic strokes are different than for ischemic strokes. Care for hemorrhagic strokes is discussed later in this chapter.

After the CT scan, patients may have an electrocardiogram (ECG) to determine whether atrial fibrillation is present. An echocardiogram may be done to determine the presence of other heart disease that increases the risk of thrombus formation. Other tests performed in the ED may include complete blood count (CBC), blood glucose level, metabolic panel, blood typing, prothrombin time (PT), international normalized ratio (INR), and serum pregnancy, if indicated. Stools and emesis may be checked for blood if indicated. The patient will be placed on a cardiac monitor and pulse oximeter. The ED nurse will complete a dysphagia screen before the patient consumes any food or fluids.

Use of the National Institutes of Health Stroke Scale (NIHSS; Fig. 49.4) is recommended to determine the

• WORD • BUILDING •
aphasia: a—absent + phasia—speech
dysphasia: dys—difficult + phasia—speech
dysarthria: dys—difficult + arthria – joint or articulation

Table 49.1
Clinical Manifestations of the Most Common Stroke Symptoms

Left Middle Cerebral Artery Syndrome	Right Middle Cerebral Artery Syndrome	Basilar Artery Syndrome
Weakness of the right face, arm, and leg (arm weakness greater than leg weakness). Decrease in sensation on the right side of the body. Right homonymous hemianopsia (loss of vision in the right temporal field of vision and left nasal field of vision, requiring patients to scan an area in order to visualize objects on their right side). Dysphasia—in most patients, the language center of the brain is located in the left hemisphere. Language deficits may involve the motor speech area (Broca area) and cause patients to have difficulty expressing thoughts and to make errors in speech that they are able to detect. Injury or ischemia to the sensory speech area (Wernicke area) results in an inability to process speech input in the brain, causing patients to make errors in speech of which they are unaware. Inattention or neglect of the right side.	Weakness of the left face, arm, and leg (arm weakness greater than leg weakness). Decrease in sensation on the left side of the body. Left homonymous hemianopsia (loss of vision in the left temporal field of vision and right nasal field of vision, requiring patients to scan an area in order to visualize objects on their right side). Inattention to or neglect of the left side.	Dizziness. Ataxia. Tinnitus. Nausea and vomiting. Weakness on one side of the body that may be ipsilateral to the side of ischemia or injury or contralateral. Decrease in sensation on one side of the body that may be ipsilateral to the side of ischemia or injury or contralateral. Difficulty in the articulation of speech. Difficulty with swallowing and managing oral secretions.

Source: Hoffman, J., & Sullivan, N. (2020) *Medical-surgical nursing: Making connections to practice*, 2nd edition. Philadelphia, PA: F.A. Davis.

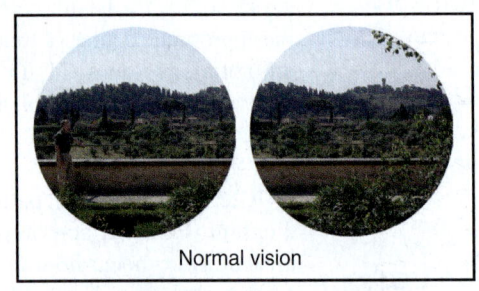

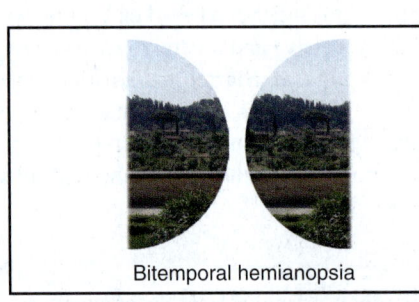

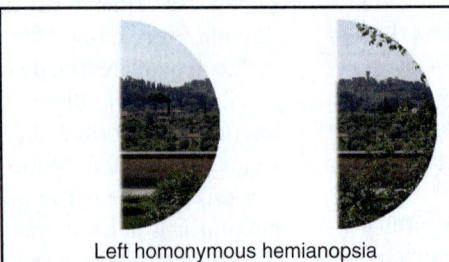

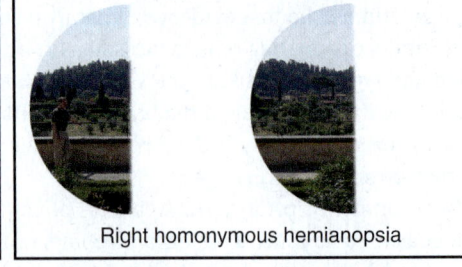

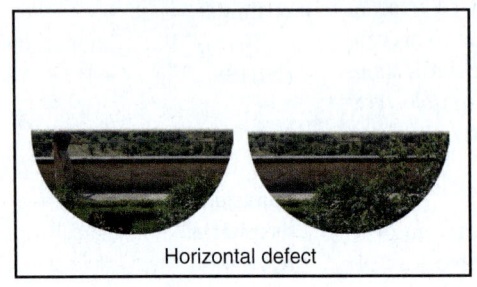

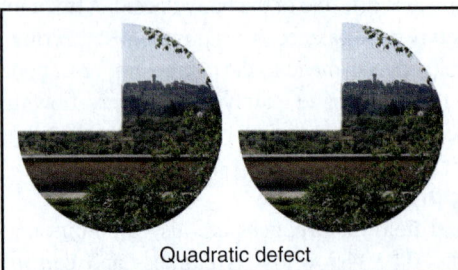

FIGURE 49.3 Visual deficits in stroke.

- Normal vision
- Bitemporal hemianopsia
- Left homonymous hemianopsia
- Right homonymous hemianopsia
- Horizontal defect
- Quadratic defect

Category	Scale Definition	Score
1a. Level of Consciousness (Alert, drowsy, etc.)	0 = Alert 1 = Drowsy 2 = Stuporous 3 = Coma	
1b. LOC Questions (Month, age)	0 = Answers both correctly 1 = Answers one correctly 2 = Incorrect	
1c. LOC Commands (Open/close eyes, make fist/let go)	0 = Obeys both correctly 1 = Obeys one correctly 2 = Incorrect	
2. Best Gaze (Eyes open—patient follows examiner's finger or face)	0 = Normal 1 = Partial gaze palsy 2 = Forced deviation	
3. Visual Fields (Introduce visual stimulus/threat to pt's visual field quadrants)	0 = No visual loss 1 = Partial Hemianopia 2 = Complete Hemianopia 3 = Bilateral Hemianopia (Blind)	
4. Facial Paresis (Show teeth, raise eyebrows and squeeze eyes shut)	0 = Normal 1 = Minor 2 = Partial 3 = Complete	
5a. Motor Arm—Left **5b. Motor Arm—Right** (Elevate arm to 90° if patient is sitting, 45° if supine)	0 = No drift 1 = Drift 2 = Can't resist gravity 3 = No effort against gravity 4 = No movement X = Untestable (Joint fusion or limb amp)	Left Right
6a. Motor Leg—Left **6b. Motor Leg—Right** (Elevate leg to 30° with patient supine)	0 = No drift 1 = Drift 2 = Can't resist gravity 3 = No effort against gravity 4 = No movement X = Untestable (Joint fusion or limb amp)	Left Right
7. Limb Ataxia (Finger-nose, heel down shin)	0 = No ataxia 1 = Present in one limb 2 = Present in two limbs	
8. Sensory (Pin prick to face, arm, trunk, and leg—compare side to side)	0 = Normal 1 = Partial loss 2 = Severe loss	
9. Best Language (Name item, describe a picture and read sentences)	0 = No aphasia 1 = Mild to moderate aphasia 2 = Severe aphasia 3 = Mute	
10. Dysarthria (Evaluate speech clarity by patient repeating listed words)	0 = Normal articulation 1 = Mild to moderate slurring of words 2 = Near to unintelligable or worse 3 = Intubated or other physical barrier	
11. Extinction and Inattention (Use information from prior testing to identify neglect or double simultaneous stimuli testing)	0 = No neglect 1 = Partial neglect 2 = Complete neglect	
	Total Score	

FIGURE 49.4 National Institutes of Health Stroke Scale.

patient's neurologic deficit level (found at https://www.ninds.nih.gov/sites/default/files/NIH_Stroke_Scale.pdf). This 11-point scale determines the severity of a stroke. Nurses can be specially trained and certified to use it. Find out more about the NIHSS at www.nihstrokescale.org.

Once the patient is stabilized, additional tests can be done. Carotid Doppler testing uses ultrasound to detect stenosis of the carotid arteries. Carotid angiography can be done to further determine degree of blockage and help guide treatment.

Therapeutic Measures

Initial emergency care is supportive while test results are pending. ABCs (**A**irway, **B**reathing, and **C**irculation) are monitored. Oxygen is administered to maintain oxygen saturation at or above 94% and the patient's level of consciousness (LOC) is reduced. Vital signs and heart rhythm are monitored. A temperature greater than 99.6°F (37.5°C) is treated because hyperthermia is associated with poorer patient outcomes. When test results verify whether the stroke is hemorrhagic or ischemic, therapeutic interventions are begun.

Some hospitals have a stroke team that evaluates all patients who arrive at the hospital within 2 hours of symptom onset. The stroke team will assess the patient within the first 15 minutes of arrival. Lab tests, ECG, and CT scans will be done, with results back within 45 minutes after assessment. The HCP will make a decision about thrombolytic therapy within 1 hour of arrival.

If the patient is hyperglycemic, blood glucose should be lowered to 140 to 180 mg/dL. According to the AHA/ASA 2018 guidelines, hyperglycemia during the first 24 hours following ischemic stroke is associated with worse outcomes (Powers et al, 2018). If IV fluids are needed, only solutions without glucose are used, such as normal saline solution.

Patients suffering from a stroke can develop increased intracranial pressure (ICP), which further adds to brain damage. Stroke patients are also at risk for repeated strokes. Careful serial neurologic checks and vital signs are needed to promptly detect and report changes.

> **PRACTICE ANALYSIS TIP**
> **Linking NCLEX-PN® to Practice**
> The LPN/LVN participates in client data collection.

Some patients with ischemic stroke may be candidates for **thrombolytic** therapy. This "clotbuster" medication (alteplase [tissue plasminogen activator; tPA]) can lyse (break down) a thrombus (clot), potentially completely reversing stroke symptoms. tPA works best when administered within 4.5 hours of symptom onset, so it is only an option if the patient arrives at the ED quickly after symptoms begin. Some patients awaken after a night's sleep to discover they have had a stroke; their symptom onset is considered the time they went to bed, so they are not candidates for thrombolytic therapy.

Thrombolytic agents can lyse a thrombus by causing conversion of plasminogen to plasmin. Plasmin is the enzyme that causes thrombi to break down. Patients treated effectively with tPA may be able to leave the hospital within 1 or 2 days with no residual effects from the stroke. Thrombolytics are associated with a significant risk of hemorrhage, so all risk of bleeding must be ruled out before these drugs will be considered. They are used very cautiously. If a patient is experiencing an ischemic stroke involving a large blood vessel of the brain, a stent-retrieval device might be used to remove any remnants of the thrombus after the tPA is used (AHA/ASA, 2021d). The device is inserted through the groin and advanced to the affected cerebral vessel.

> **LEARNING TIP**
> Remember: Time lost is brain lost. This means the faster the patient with a stroke receives treatment, the more brain (and brain function) that can be saved. Reminding your patients to recognize the signs and symptoms of a stroke and encouraging them to call 911 if needed could mean the difference between leading a normal life and total disability. **Act FAST!**

Pharmacological Management

Blood pressure control is vital for the stroke patient. Because of the lack of perfusion to certain areas of the brain, the body's response is to increase the systolic blood pressure to force blood into the affected areas. If the patient will receive tPA, blood pressure must be maintained below 185/110 mm Hg to reduce risk of bleeding (Powers et al, 2018). Beta blockers (labetalol) or calcium channel blockers (nicardipine) are often used because they have fast-acting effects and can be given via IV. Table 49.2 lists medications commonly used for cerebrovascular disorders.

If tPA is not given, the HCP may allow the blood pressure to remain high for a period of time to help salvage brain tissue, depending on the source of the stroke and location of the thrombus. This "permissive hypertension" helps blood travel through collateral blood vessels in the brain to reach the affected area. Antihypertensive agents should be given if the systolic pressure exceeds 220 mm Hg or the diastolic pressure exceeds 120 mm Hg (Powers et al, 2018).

• WORD • BUILDING •
thrombolytic: thromb—clot + lytic—causing breakdown

Table 49.2 Medications Used in Cerebrovascular Disorders

Medication Class/Action

Thrombolytic Agents

Dissolve existing clots.

Examples	Nursing Implications
alteplase (tissue plasminogen activator [tPA]; Activase)	Must be administered within 3 to 4.5 hours of symptom onset. Monitor for bleeding.

Antiplatelet Agents

Prevent formation of clots.

Examples	Nursing Implications
aspirin clopidogrel (Plavix) aspirin/dipyridamole (Aggrenox)	Monitor patient for bruising, change in level of consciousness, and prolonged bleeding time.

Anticoagulant Agents

Prolong time to form clots; prevent new clots.

Examples	Nursing Implications
warfarin (Coumadin) heparin	Monitor patient for bruising, change in level of consciousness, and prolonged bleeding time. For warfarin (Coumadin), monitor international normalized ratio (INR) frequently until therapeutic, and then monthly.

Cholesterol-Lowering Agents

Reduce cholesterol level.

Examples	Nursing Implications
simvastatin (Zocor) pravastatin (Pravachol) atorvastatin (Lipitor) lovastatin (Mevacor)	Patient should notify health-care provider if muscle pain or weakness occur.

CUE RECOGNITION 49.1

You are caring for a patient in the extended care facility (ECF) where you work. The patient has a history of cardiovascular disease and is now experiencing trouble talking and weakness on the right side of his body. What do you do?

Suggested answers are at the end of the chapter.

Postemergent Care

After emergent treatment, medical management focuses on controlling the cause of TIA or stroke. The results of the diagnostic tests help the HCP determine the course of treatment. If the patient has residual physical deficits, the HCP will order physical, occupational, and speech therapy consultations to evaluate the patient's functional status and make recommendations for further treatment and rehabilitation.

AHA/ASA guidelines recommend that patients who have a minor stroke receive dual antiplatelet therapy with aspirin and clopidogrel (Plavix) within 24 hours of symptom onset (Powers et al, 2018). Decreasing platelet aggregation lessens the risk of another stroke. The patient in atrial fibrillation may also receive an anticoagulant to prevent thrombus development.

Cholesterol-lowering medication, preferably a statin, will be ordered for patients who have a low-density lipoprotein (LDL) cholesterol level greater than 70 mg/dL. Statins also help minimize the development of atherosclerotic plaques. In addition, they may have a neuroprotective effect and may further decrease risk of a stroke.

Deep vein **thrombosis** (DVT) is of concern when caring for patients who have had a stroke. Decrease in movement, confinement to a hospital bed, and hypercoagulable state all increase risk. Not only can DVTs cause severe pain and complications in the affected leg, but the thrombus can dislodge and travel to the lungs, causing a pulmonary embolism. Prevention involves anticoagulant medication or nondrug treatments such as sequential compression devices.

Stroke patients are at risk for respiratory complications for several reasons, such as an increase in ICP, decreased LOC, and possibly impaired swallowing ability that increase risk for aspiration. Patients should be orally suctioned as needed to keep the airway clear. A patient who vomits should be turned to the side to reduce the risk of aspiration. Oral feedings should be started carefully and progressed slowly. Feedings should begin only after the patient is alert and the ability to swallow safely has been determined by an appropriate swallowing evaluation.

Surgery

Patients with warning signs of stroke or patients who have been stabilized after a stroke may be candidates for surgery. In patients with significant carotid artery occlusion, a carotid **endarterectomy** may be performed. This procedure involves a small incision in the neck and surgical removal of the occlusion from the artery.

Alternatively, a patient who is at high risk for complications with a carotid endarterectomy may have a carotid stent placed. It is placed during a carotid angiogram procedure. A catheter is advanced to the carotid artery, where a balloon is inflated to open the artery by pushing on the plaque. Then a stent (a tiny metal or polymer-based tube) is expanded inside the artery to keep it open and allow better blood flow to the brain. A risk from either procedure is an ischemic stroke.

> ### CRITICAL THINKING & CLINICAL JUDGMENT
>
> **Mr. Jankowski,** 56 years old, has been admitted to your orthopedic unit after knee surgery. While listening to his lungs at the start of the shift, you notice his lung sounds are diminished. You ask whether he is a smoker and learn he has smoked for 40 years. You realize that his smoking history, postoperative status, and reduced mobility all place Mr. Jankowski at risk for DVT and stroke.
>
> **Critical Thinking (The Why)**
> 1. What further data should you collect?
>
> **Clinical Judgment? (The Do)**
> 2. What preventive measures can you provide?
> 3. What resources can you provide to support smoking cessation?
> 4. What other interdisciplinary team members should you collaborate with regarding the respiratory data you have collected?
>
> *Suggested answers are at the end of the chapter.*

Prevention of Stroke

The incidence of stroke can be lessened by reducing controllable risk factors (see Box 49.1). Managing hypertension, cholesterol level, weight, and diabetes can help patients prevent strokes. Smoking cessation is essential. Emboli may be prevented with anticoagulants in people at high risk due to atrial fibrillation. Aspirin or other antiplatelet agents help prevent abnormal clotting.

Educate all patients about new treatments for stroke and the potential for reversal of symptoms with the use of thrombolytic agents. Patients must be taught about risk factors for a stroke, warning signs, and the importance of immediate EMS transport if symptoms occur.

Long-Term Effects of Stroke

Impaired Motor Function and Sensation

Paresthesias and paralysis are common long-term effects of strokes that were not treated with a thrombolytic agent. The side of the body opposite the side of the cerebral infarct (contralateral side) is affected because nerve fibers cross over as they pass from the brain to the spinal cord (Fig. 49.5). Paralysis on one side of the body is called **hemiplegia** (Fig. 49.6). The affected limbs may be weak or totally paralyzed (flaccid). The arm or leg may be weaker, depending on the artery affected. These patients are particularly prone to

Left-side infarct
Right-sided weakness or paralysis
Aphasia (in left–brain-dominant clients)
Depression related to disability common

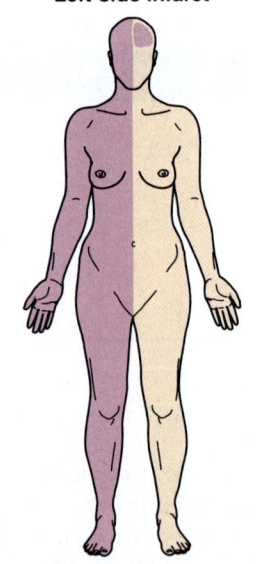

Right-side infarct
Left-sided weakness or paralysis
Impaired judgment/safety risk
Unilateral neglect more common
Indifferent to disability

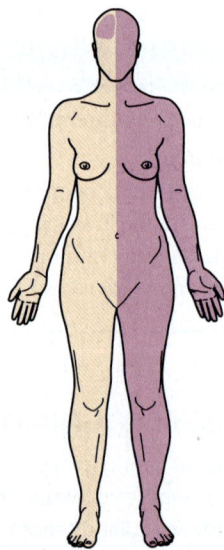

FIGURE 49.5 The side opposite the infarct is affected by a stroke.

• WORD • BUILDING •
thrombosis: thromb—clot + osis—condition
endarterectomy: endo—inside + arter—artery + ectomy—surgical removal of
hemiplegia: hemi—one side + plegia—paralysis

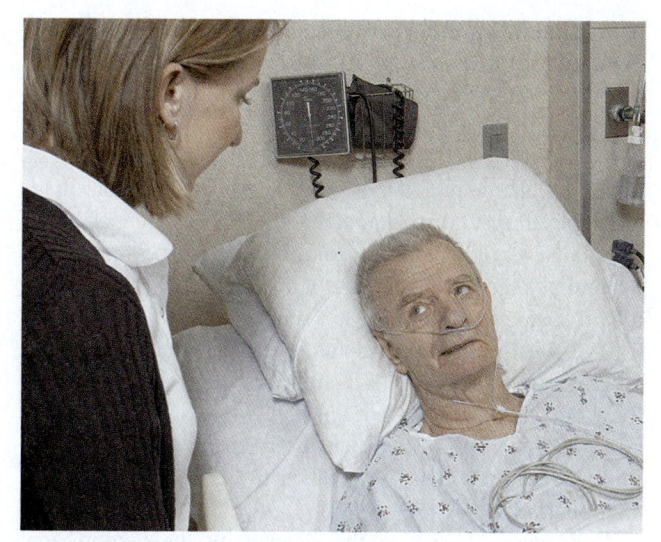

FIGURE 49.6 Hemiplegia: Note the left-sided weakness in this man's smile as result of a stroke.

contractures, which cause permanent immobility of a muscle or joint from fibrosis of connective tissue. Adaptation or assistance with activities of daily living (ADLs) is required.

Patients should be mobilized within 24 hours, if possible, to prevent complications of immobility. Physical and occupational therapy are provided to maximize functioning and to progress the patient toward a return to baseline functioning.

Motor involvement also often affects swallowing and control of urination and bowel function. Sensation changes may prevent awareness of pressure, temperature, or injuries on the affected side. Patients must be taught to be aware of these changes and protect the involved limbs.

Aphasia

If a stroke affects the temporal lobe region, especially on the dominant side, the speech center will likely be affected. Aphasia can be expressive, receptive, or global, as described earlier. Patients may be able to say words but unable to form coherent speech, such as the patient who picks up a fork but calls it a comb. If a patient does not understand, avoid the temptation to speak louder. Remember that it is not the patient's hearing that is affected. Be patient and understanding as the patient tries to communicate. Speech therapy can help the patient relearn to communicate. See the "Nursing Process for the Patient With a Cerebrovascular Disorder" section for interventions for the aphasic patient.

Pseudobulbar Affect

Pseudobulbar affect (PBA) can manifest as emotional lability or instability. Patients may move rapidly from profound sadness to an almost euphoric state and back again. Laughing or crying may have no relationship to the patient's situation at any given moment. Families can be upset by this behavior because they do not understand why a once-happy person is now crying all the time or why the patient laughs inappropriately. You can help by explaining that these responses probably do not reflect how the patient is feeling but are caused by the stroke damage. Dextromethorphan/quinidine (Nuedexta) can reduce these symptoms.

Impaired Judgment

All patients who have had a stroke, particularly those with right-sided lesions, present a high safety risk. Patients may have poor understanding of their limitations and believe that they can perform the same tasks they did before the stroke. Those with left-sided lesions are more likely to hesitate even to try performing ADLs. These generalizations may be the opposite if the individual is left-handed. Precautions must be taken to protect the patient from injury.

If the frontal lobes are involved, learned social behaviors may be lost. The patient may undress in public, use profanity, or make inappropriate sexual advances. These behaviors are extremely difficult for family members. Education and emotional support for significant others are essential. Allowing them to talk about their frustration and anger may facilitate coping. Distracting the patient from inappropriate behavior may help. The patient should not be reprimanded or punished because they do not have the ability to control the behaviors.

Unilateral Neglect

The phenomenon of unilateral neglect is seen predominantly in patients who have right hemisphere infarcts. It has been estimated to affect up to 50% of all patients who have had a stroke (Chen et al, 2015). These patients do not acknowledge the left side of their environment and may not even be aware of their own body on the affected side. Safety is a primary consideration. Essential items such as the call light and telephone should be placed on the patient's right side. Position the bed so the patient's right side is toward the door. Treatment should focus on providing stimuli to all senses on the patient's affected side and prompting the patient to focus on the left side. This involves teaching the patient to purposefully check where the left limbs are positioned and look for safety risks. The patient can learn to turn their head and scan the environment. Patients may also need reminders to accomplish simple tasks, such as turning their plates during meals to recognize the food on the left side of the plate.

Other Long-Term Effects

The stroke patient may experience other complications after the acute phase of the stroke has passed. These include pneumonia, DVT, pulmonary embolism, pressure injuries, malnutrition, and depression. For the homeward-bound patient, education for the patient and family regarding prevention and recognition of these complications will assist the patient in a successful recovery. If a patient needs to receive rehabilitation in a skilled nursing facility, prevention of these issues will be a part of the care plan at the facility. For more information, visit the American Stroke Association at www.strokeassociation.org.

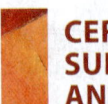

CEREBRAL ANEURYSM, SUBARACHNOID HEMORRHAGE, AND INTRACRANIAL HEMORRHAGE

A cerebral aneurysm is a weakness in the wall of a cerebral artery. It may be congenital, traumatic, or the result of disease. A ruptured aneurysm often causes subarachnoid hemorrhage. It is unknown what causes formation or rupture of congenital aneurysms. Unruptured aneurysms are typically asymptomatic. The exception is a very large aneurysm, which can cause symptoms similar to a brain tumor. Aneurysms can affect children and young, otherwise healthy adults.

Pathophysiology and Etiology

Aneurysms can occur in any of the cerebral arteries, although most occur in the circle of Willis. The most common site is at the bifurcation of an artery. It is theorized that increased turbulence at the bifurcation can cause an outpouching of a congenitally weak arterial wall.

Subarachnoid hemorrhage is the collection of blood beneath the arachnoid mater following aneurysm rupture. Rupture of an arteriovenous malformation or head trauma may also result in subarachnoid hemorrhage (Fig. 49.7). The presence of blood outside the blood vessels is very irritating to brain tissue. It is believed that irritation from blood breakdown is the major cause of vasospasm, a common complication of subarachnoid hemorrhage.

It is unclear what causes an aneurysm to rupture. Some people develop a subarachnoid hemorrhage while performing the Valsalva maneuver, engaging in sexual activity, or physically exerting themselves. For others, the aneurysm ruptures during a quiet, inactive period. If the aneurysm rupture is associated with a particular activity, the patient may be frightened of engaging in that activity again. This may negatively affect the patient's interpersonal relationships if the associated activity was sexual in nature. The patient's partner may feel guilty or responsible for the hemorrhage. Education, emotional support, and confidentiality are essential to help both the patient and significant other.

Signs and Symptoms

Some patients experience a small hemorrhage before diagnosis of subarachnoid hemorrhage. This leakage of blood may cause a mild headache, vomiting, or disorientation. The symptoms may be attributed to a flu-like syndrome. Patients may dismiss symptoms and not seek care.

The most common presentation of rupture of an aneurysm is sudden onset of a severe headache, often reported as the worst of the patient's life. Patients may hold their heads and moan or cry in pain. Sensitivity to light is a common finding that may cause reluctance to cooperate with pupil examinations.

LOC varies based on the severity of the hemorrhage. Patients may be alert and coherent, lose consciousness immediately, or gradually become less responsive. The decreased LOC is caused by increased ICP and impairment of cerebral blood flow. Patients may experience generalized seizures.

Blood in the subarachnoid space causes meningeal irritation. The patient may exhibit nuchal rigidity. The most commonly affected cranial nerves are III and VI. Irritation to these nerves is manifested as an enlarged pupil or abnormal gaze. Motor dysfunction may involve one or both limbs on the side opposite the hemorrhage.

Diagnostic Tests

Because of the severe nature of the symptoms, patients with subarachnoid hemorrhage almost always come to the ED rather than seeking care from a primary HCP. A CT scan or MRI is done to identify and locate a hemorrhage. Precise diagnosis of an aneurysm requires a cerebral angiogram. The contrast material fills the aneurysm if one exists. For a patient with a severe headache facing a life-threatening illness, this test can be frightening. If the patient's neurologic status does not allow cooperation, sedation may be required before and during the examination.

> **PRACTICE ANALYSIS TIP**
> **Linking NCLEX-PN® to Practice**
> The LPN/LVN assists with the performance of a diagnostic or invasive procedure.

Therapeutic Measures

Patients with subarachnoid hemorrhage are cared for in an intensive care unit (ICU). They typically have an arterial line and a central venous pressure monitoring catheter. Blood pressure is carefully monitored because high pressures increase the risk of re-rupture of the aneurysm and low pressures can be associated with ischemia. Values outside parameters identified by the HCP are reported. Typically,

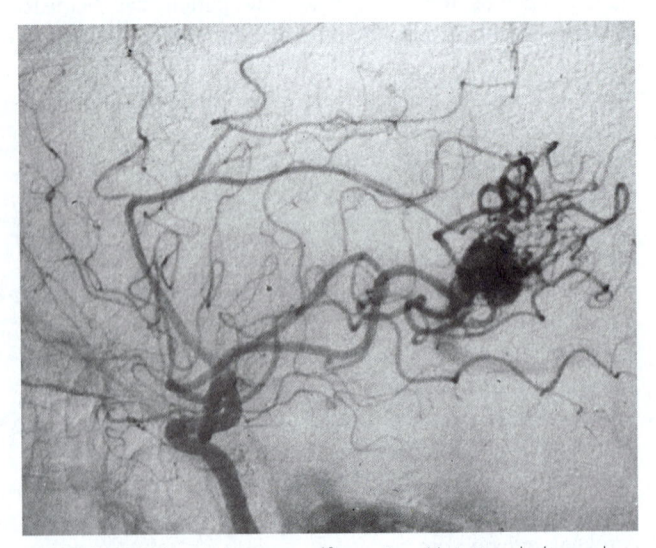

FIGURE 49.7 Arteriovenous malformation. Note tangled vessels.

systolic blood pressure is kept between 120 and 160 mm Hg. Vasoactive drugs may be required to maintain blood pressure within prescribed parameters.

There is no cure for subarachnoid hemorrhage. Treatment consists of correcting the cause of the hemorrhage if possible. Preventing or managing complications and providing supportive care are important aspects of nursing care.

Surgical Management

Definitive treatment involves performing a craniotomy and exposing the aneurysm. If the aneurysm has a neck (berry aneurysm), it is identified and clamped with a metal clip (Fig. 49.8). An aneurysm without a neck may be wrapped with a sterile plastic or muslin wrap. This provides stability to the aneurysm walls, lessening the chance of rupture. In some situations, it is possible to clamp the artery on either side of the aneurysm, removing that portion of the vessel, and the aneurysm, from the circulation. After the removal, ends are reconnected to maintain blood flow.

Nonsurgical Management

Nonsurgical intervention may be provided for aneurysms that are inoperable because of size, configuration, or the patient's medical status. A foreign material such as a metallic or polymer-based coil may be introduced into the aneurysm. A thrombus develops around the foreign body and, if the treatment is successful, occludes the aneurysm. The goal is to fill the aneurysm enough to prevent blood flowing into it, without causing rupture.

Complications
Rebleeding
Recurrent rupture of a cerebral aneurysm carries significant morbidity and mortality rates. Patients are at risk for rebleeding until the aneurysm is surgically repaired. If the aneurysm is wrapped or embolized, risk is much lower than if the aneurysm is left untreated.

Hydrocephalus
Blood in the ventricular system interferes with the circulation and reabsorption of cerebrospinal fluid (CSF), and hydrocephalus can develop. Early in the course of subarachnoid hemorrhage, an external ventricular drain may be used to treat hydrocephalus.

Some patients with subarachnoid hemorrhage require placement of a ventriculoperitoneal shunt to treat hydrocephalus (Fig. 49.9). This procedure involves placement of a catheter into a ventricle in the brain. The catheter is connected to a valve that regulates the rate of CSF drainage. Another catheter connects to the valve and is passed down to the peritoneal cavity. The CSF drains out of the peritoneal catheter and is absorbed into the peritoneal cavity.

Vasospasm
Vasospasm is responsible for most long-term complications of subarachnoid hemorrhage. Vasospasm causes a blood vessel's diameter to narrow. Although it typically begins in the vessel, giving rise to the aneurysm, it may spread to other vessels. This explains why the ischemia or infarct caused by vasospasm can be so widespread and devastating.

The long-term complications of subarachnoid hemorrhage are similar to those of stroke.

Rehabilitation
If the patient can tolerate intensive therapy, discharge from the hospital to a rehabilitation center may occur. Rehabilitation

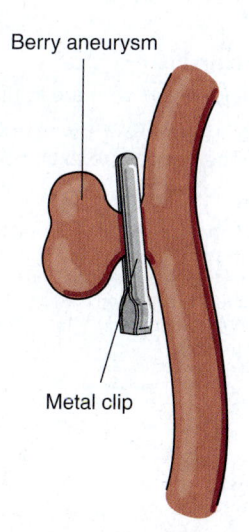

FIGURE 49.8 Surgical management of aneurysms.

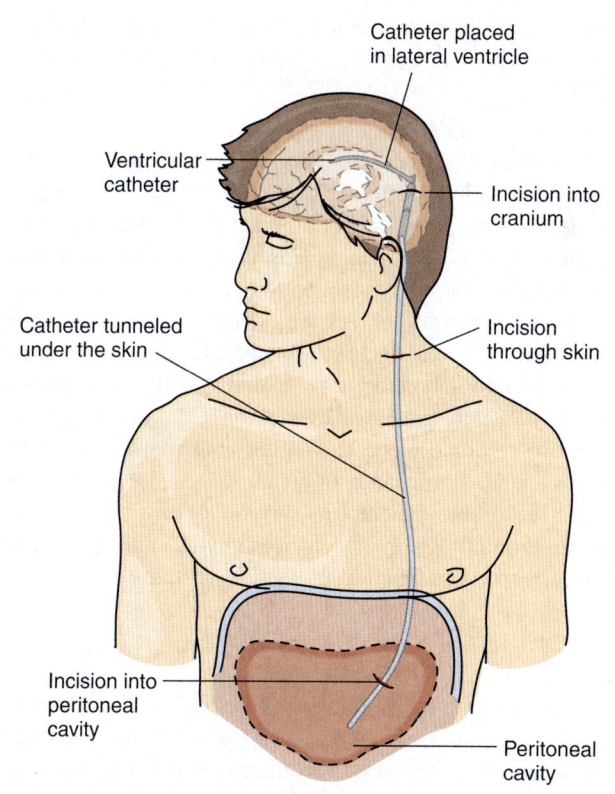

FIGURE 49.9 A ventriculoperitoneal shunt drains cerebrospinal fluid into the peritoneal cavity.

and long-term care are similar whether the patient has had an aneurysm, intracerebral bleed, or an ischemic stroke.

CRITICAL THINKING & CLINICAL JUDGMENT

Mrs. Washington is a 68-year-old Black woman and retired office worker who is admitted to your unit after a right-sided intracerebral hemorrhage. Her daughter states that Mrs. Washington has taken antihypertensive medication for the past 20 years. However, she states that her mother has been forgetful lately and that there are five more pills in the medicine bottle than expected. On admission, Mrs. Washington is oriented only to person and has hemiparesis.

Critical Thinking (The Why)
1. What may have precipitated Mrs. Washington's stroke?
2. On which side do you expect Mrs. Washington's extremities to be affected?

Clinical Judgment (The Do)
3. List two safety concerns and strategies to promote patient safety.
4. List at least two educational needs for Mrs. Washington and her daughter.
5. What health-care team members are important in the interdisciplinary team caring for Mrs. Washington? What is the role of nursing on this team?

Suggested answers are at the end of the chapter.

NURSING PROCESS FOR THE PATIENT WITH A CEREBROVASCULAR DISORDER

Data Collection
Observe the patient for signs of decreased cerebral tissue perfusion. These include decreased LOC, irritability or restlessness, dizziness, syncope, blurred or dimmed vision, **diplopia** (double vision), change in visual fields, unequal pupils or a sluggish or absent pupillary reaction to light, paresthesias, motor weakness, paralysis, or seizures. Recheck frequently and report any change or decline. Monitor vital signs and oxygen levels. Monitor laboratory tests, including CBC, lipid profile, and INR/PT if the patient takes warfarin (Coumadin). Perform a routine respiratory check. Monitor lung sounds for adventitious sounds or a change in breath sounds. Document pain level. Make sure patient can swallow before offering oral intake. Promptly report any changes in vital signs, laboratory values, respiratory function, or neurologic status.

Nursing Diagnoses, Planning, and Implementation
See "Nursing Care Plan for the Patient With Stroke" for nursing diagnoses during acute care. Possible postacute nursing diagnoses are listed next with outcomes and interventions. See also "Caregiver Role Strain" in Chapter 11.

Impaired Physical Mobility related to decreased motor function

EXPECTED OUTCOME: The patient will maintain physical mobility as evidenced by maximum physical mobility within limitations of deficits. The patient will not experience complications related to immobility.

- Consult physical and occupational therapists *to assess the patient's abilities and make specific recommendations related to mobility.*
- Discuss use of constraint therapy with physical and occupational therapists. *Constraint therapy forces the use of the affected limbs by restraining the unaffected side.*
- Maintain the patient in correct body alignment *to prevent contractures and promote comfort.*
- Support affected extremities with pillows *to prevent dislocation injuries and promote comfort.*
- Perform range-of-motion exercises as prescribed by the physical therapist *to prevent contractures and atrophy.*
- Follow physical/occupational therapy recommendations for being up in chair or ambulation. *Prolonged bedrest is associated with complications and poor outcomes.*
- If the patient is unable to get out of bed, turn and reposition at least every 2 hours *to prevent skin, respiratory, and musculoskeletal complications.*

Evidence-Based Practice

Clinical Question
How does exposure to air pollution affect stroke risk?

Evidence
A meta-analysis of 68 studies, with a total of 23 million participants, found that air pollution was associated with an increase in stroke hospital admissions, increased stroke incidence, and increased stroke mortality (Niu et al, 2021).

Implications for Nursing Practice
Nurses should advise those who are at risk for strokes due to other factors (e.g., smoking, hypertension and diabetes) to limit their exposure to air pollution whenever possible.

Reference: Niu, Z., Liu, F., Yu, H., Wu, S., & Xiang, H. (2021). Association between exposure to ambient air pollution and hospital admission, incidence, and mortality of stroke: An updated systematic review and meta-analysis of more than 23 million participants. *Environmental Health and Preventive Medicine, 26*(15). https://doi.org/10.1186/s12199-021-00937-1

• WORD • BUILDING •
diplopia: diplo—double + opia—sight

Imbalanced Nutrition: Less Than Body Requirements related to impaired swallowing and motor deficits

EXPECTED OUTCOME: The patient will maintain adequate nutrition without aspiration as evidenced by stable weight at appropriate level for height and no signs of aspiration.

- Keep patient NPO (nothing by mouth) until swallowing can be evaluated *to prevent aspiration.*
- Perform dysphagia screening. *This quick assessment can identify problems before a complete evaluation can be done:*
  - Observe for facial weakness or inability to completely close mouth.
  - Ask patient to stick out tongue and move it side to side.
  - Observe for drooling.
- If swallowing appears to be intact, have the patient swallow a sip of water from a cup before offering other foods or fluids. Observe for coughing, choking, or noisy lung sounds. *These are signs of difficulty swallowing.*
- Request speech pathologist evaluation if indicated *to diagnose specific swallowing problems and make recommendations.*
- Implement measures to prevent aspiration. *Aspiration can lead to pneumonia, which will greatly complicate the patient's recovery.*
- Stay with the patient during meals.
- Ensure that the patient is fully alert before feeding.
- Place the patient in high-Fowler position or chair for meals.
- Avoid use of straws.
- Use a thickening agent if swallowing study recommends.
- Place food on unaffected side of mouth.
- Remind the patient to swallow twice after each bite.
- Check the patient's mouth for pocketing of food.
- Have suction equipment available.
- Notify HCP if patient is unable to take in adequate oral calories. *A feeding tube may be needed if the patient cannot take in enough calories to maintain nutrition. Advance directives should be consulted before a feeding tube is placed.*
- Assist with insertion and care of feeding tube if needed. *If the patient cannot swallow effectively, a feeding tube may be needed to maintain nutrition.*

See "Nutrition Notes" and Chapter 47 for additional interventions.

Nursing Care Plan for the Patient With Stroke

Nursing Diagnosis: *Risk for Ineffective Cerebral Tissue Perfusion* related to interruption of blood supply
Expected Outcomes: The patient will experience improved cerebral tissue perfusion as evidenced by absence of or reduction in dizziness, syncope, and visual disturbances; improved level of consciousness; pupils equal and reactive to light; and improved motor and sensory function.
Evaluation of Outcomes: Are the patient's symptoms of ineffective perfusion improving?

Intervention	Rationale	Evaluation
Monitor neurologic status at least every 30 minutes initially and then every 4 hours or as ordered. Report changes.	A change in status could indicate decreased perfusion.	Is there a change in neurologic status since the previous documented data?
Monitor vital signs every 30 minutes initially and then every 4 hours or as ordered.	High or low blood pressure can lead to decreased tissue perfusion and recurrent stroke. Temperature above 99.6°F (37.5°C) can worsen ischemic injury to brain tissue.	Are vital signs within normal limits? Are changes reported?
Monitor oxygen saturation and administer oxygen as ordered for peripheral oxygen saturation (SpO_2) less than 92%.	Hypoxemia can increase brain damage.	Is SpO_2 92% or greater?
Monitor blood glucose as ordered and report value greater than 140 mg/dL.	Elevated glucose is associated with worsening of infarct and hemorrhage.	Is glucose level greater than 140 mg/dL? Was HCP notified?
Keep head of bed elevated 20 to 30 degrees. Keep neck in neutral position.	This facilitates venous return and reduces risk of cerebral edema.	Is head of bed elevated? Is neck in neutral position?
Monitor medication for therapeutic and nontherapeutic effects. Monitor coagulation studies if appropriate.	Anticoagulant therapy must be closely monitored to make sure it is at a therapeutic level and not increasing risk for bleeding.	Are coagulation studies within normal or therapeutic ranges? Are signs of bleeding present?

(nursing care plan continues on page 1014)

Nursing Care Plan for the Patient With Stroke—cont'd

Nursing Diagnosis: *Ineffective Airway Clearance* related to stasis of secretions associated with decreased mobility and poor cough effort and airway obstruction resulting from tongue falling back in throat
Expected Outcome: The patient will maintain an open airway as evidenced by respirations quiet and unlabored, 12 to 20 per minute, with SpO_2 greater than 92%.
Evaluation of Outcome: Are respirations quiet, 12 to 20 per minute, with SpO_2 greater than 92%?

Intervention	Rationale	Evaluation
Monitor lung sounds, cough, and respirations.	*Monitoring provides the basis for intervention.*	Are lung sounds clear? Is cough effective? Are respirations quiet and easy?
Position the patient to maintain an open airway.	*Side lying may keep tongue from obstructing airway.*	Is patient positioned to keep airway clear?
Consult with registered nurse or HCP about an oral airway if airway is not clear.	*An oral airway will keep tongue from obstructing airway if needed.*	Is an airway indicated?
Encourage patient to deep breathe and cough if able.	*Coughing and deep breathing will help clear secretions from airway and prevent atelectasis.*	Is patient able to deep breathe and cough? Is cough effective?
If cough is ineffective, suction as needed.	*Suctioning may be needed if patient is unable to swallow secretions or cough effectively.*	Is suctioning indicated? Is airway clear after suctioning?

Nursing Diagnosis: *Risk for Injury* related to seizure, repeat stroke, or hemorrhage secondary to thrombolytic therapy
Expected Outcome: The patient will remain free from injury.
Evaluation of Outcome: Is the patient free from injury? Are problems recognized and reported quickly?

Intervention	Rationale	Evaluation
Monitor neurologic status frequently and report changes promptly.	*Prompt recognition of a repeat stroke is essential.*	Are neurologic checks within normal limits? Are changes reported promptly?
Monitor for signs of hemorrhage for 24 to 36 hours following thrombolytic therapy.	*Hemorrhage is the most common side effect of thrombolytic therapy.*	Are signs of hemorrhage present? Are they reported promptly?
Administer anticonvulsant agent as ordered.	*Patient is at increased risk for seizures following a stroke.*	Is patient seizure free?
Implement seizure precautions (see Chapter 48).	*Precautions help protect patient in event of a seizure.*	Are precautions in place and patient protected? Is patient assisted with mobility?
Assist with transfers and ambulation.	*Patient is at risk for falls because of motor and sensory deficits and impaired judgment.*	Is patient able to call for help when needed?

Nutrition Notes

Feeding Patients With Swallowing Disorders

Swallowing disorders (dysphagia) may occur when an individual suffers from nervous system disorders such as stroke. When dysphagia is suspected, a speech pathologist is consulted to perform comprehensive tests of an individual's ability to swallow foods and liquids. The International Dysphagia Diet Standardization Initiative (2019) recommends a diet prescription that includes the appropriate texture of foods (e.g., regular, easy to chew, soft and bite sized, minced and moist, pureed, and liquidized) and consistency of liquids (e.g., thin, slightly, mildly, moderately, and extremely thick). Recommendations for body and head positioning while eating are also made by the speech pathologist.

Commercially prepared thickeners are designed to provide the appropriate thickness in liquids. The standardized "recipe" must be closely followed by a nurse or family member who has been properly trained and has demonstrated competence. Home recipes (e.g., using instant potato flakes or gelatin) can make foods easier to swallow (American Cancer Society, 2020).

References:
American Cancer Society. (2020). Swallowing problems. https://www.cancer.org/treatment/treatments-and-side-effects/physical-side-effects/eating-problems/swallowing-problems.html
International Dysphagia Diet Standardization Initiative. (2019). The IDDSI framework. https://iddsi.org/framework

Disturbed Sensory Perception related to central nervous system damage

EXPECTED OUTCOME: The patient will adapt to sensory-perceptual deficits as evidenced by avoidance of injury to affected areas.

- Assist the occupational therapist to assess for visual and/or spatial deficits and decreased sensory perception (heat and cold, position of body parts, pressure). *Identification of specific deficits is the first step in creating a plan of care.*
- Reinforce to the patient to scan the environment *to compensate for a visual deficit.*
- Implement plans for skin integrity and mobility *to protect patient from complications related to sensory deficits.*

Risk for Impaired Skin Integrity (irritation or breakdown) related to immobility and incontinence

EXPECTED OUTCOME: The patient's skin integrity will be maintained as evidenced by absence of redness or breakdown.

- Examine the skin often for redness or breakdown, especially around bony prominences, dependent areas, and perineum. *Any signs of breakdown must be treated immediately to prevent further damage.*
- Thoroughly cleanse and dry the perineal area after each episode of incontinence. *Urine and feces can be very irritating to the skin.*
- If incontinence is unavoidable, use a barrier cream such as zinc oxide *to protect skin.*
- Turn and position the patient at least every 2 hours or more often if the patient experiences breakdown. *Pressure impairs circulation and increases risk of breakdown.*
- Use a lift sheet to move the patient in bed *to avoid damage from friction and shear.*
- Consider the use of a pressure-reducing mattress if the patient cannot be out of bed for long periods. *This helps reduce pressure but does not eliminate the need to reposition the patient every 2 hours.*
- If breakdown occurs, contact the HCP or wound care specialist *to obtain treatment recommendations.*

Incontinence (Bowel or Overflow Urinary or Functional Urinary) related to loss of voluntary control of elimination

EXPECTED OUTCOME: Episodes of incontinence are avoided, or, if unavoidable, they will be cleaned up quickly and skin complications avoided.

- Monitor for incontinence of bowel or bladder *so patient can be cleaned promptly and skin protected.*
- Determine usual pattern of urinary and bowel elimination. *Keeping the patient on their regular prehospitalization pattern may help prevent incontinence.*
- Provide assistance with toileting according to the patient's usual schedule. *The patient who is unable to get up unaided may wait too long for help or try to get up alone and be injured.*
- Respond quickly to requests for assistance with toileting *to avoid accidental incontinence.*

Self-Care Deficit (Bathing, Dressing, Feeding, Toileting) related to impaired motor function, spatial-perceptual alterations, and fear of injury

EXPECTED OUTCOME: Self-care will be accomplished as evidenced by the patient's ADL needs being met and the patient becoming increasingly independent.

- Determine the patient's ability to perform ADLs. *Good baseline data will guide development of a care plan.*
- Work with the patient to create a plan for meeting daily physical needs. *The patient will be more likely to participate in a plan if they participated in creating it.*
- Encourage the highest level of independence possible and facilitate the patient's ability to do ADLs. *Providing too much assistance can promote dependence and further loss of mobility.*
- Place objects within reach and within visual field.
- Place food/fluids within the patient's visual field.
- Encourage use of assistive devices.
- Assist the patient with learning to use the nondominant side of body. *If the dominant side is affected, the patient may have to use the nondominant side.*
- Provide positive feedback *to help reduce discouragement with slow progress.*
- Provide education for family members and significant others regarding the patient's deficits and recovery plan. *The family can assist the patient with mobility if they understand what needs to be done.*

Impaired Verbal Communication (dysarthria) related to loss of motor function of the muscles of speech articulation or aphasia or dysphasia related to ischemia of the dominant hemisphere

EXPECTED OUTCOME: Communication needs will be met as evidenced by the patient communicating needs and desires effectively and by avoidance of frustration.

- Listen for difficulties in verbal communication (difficulty speaking, articulating or incorrect ordering of words, inability to find or name words and objects). *Good baseline data will guide planning of care.*
- Consult a speech pathologist for assistance in determining types of aphasia or dysphasia and need for follow-up treatment. *A speech pathologist is*

specially trained to diagnose and treat communication problems and can work with nursing staff to develop a plan of care.
- Implement measures to facilitate communication. *These measures help ensure the patient has their immediate needs met while learning to adapt to communication impairment:*
  - Answer call light in person rather than over an intercom.
  - Monitor needs frequently.
  - Listen carefully, avoid interrupting the patient, and allow ample time for communication.
  - When the patient is tired, ask questions that require short answers.
  - Provide appropriate aids to communication (picture board, magic slate, pencil and paper; Fig. 49.10).
- Provide education to family members and significant others regarding communication problems and interventions *so they can communicate with patient and participate in care.*
- If the patient is unable to communicate, do not assume they cannot hear and understand. Make every effort to speak to the patient and to keep conversation appropriate within the patient's range of hearing. *The patient may understand exactly what is being said, even if they are unable to respond.*
- Contact the HCP if impairment increases. *This may be a sign of stroke extension.*

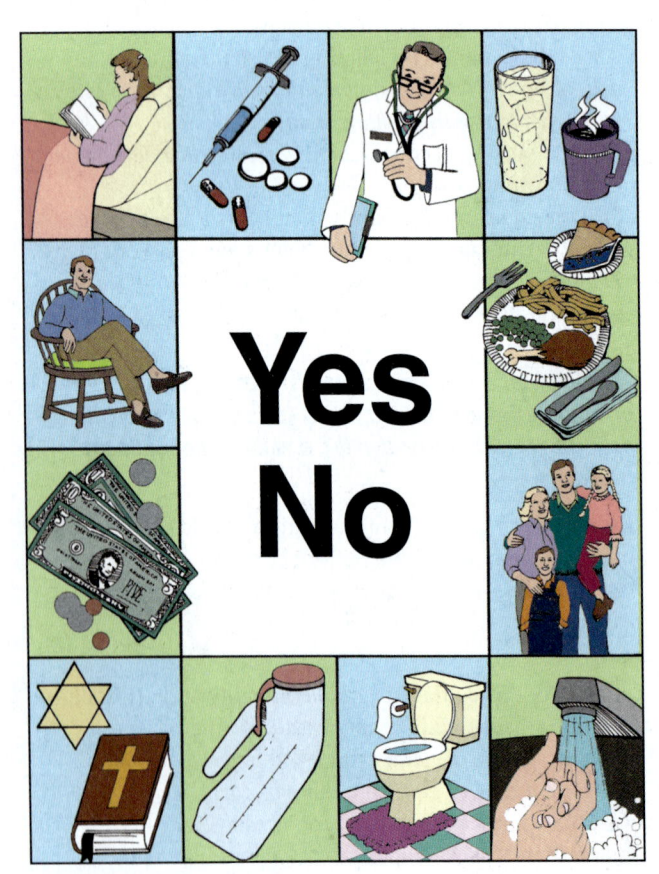

FIGURE 49.10 Picture board.

Acute or Chronic Confusion related to cerebral ischemia

EXPECTED OUTCOME: The patient's thought processes will be as clear as possible within limitations of brain damage as evidenced by responses appropriate to situation; the patient's safety will be maintained, and the patient will feel calm and safe.

- Observe the patient for thought process impairment such as shortened attention span, impaired memory, confusion, slowed or quick and impulsive responses, and aggressive and/or inappropriate responses. *Disturbed thinking can be manifested in a variety of ways. See Chapter 48 for interventions for patients with disturbed thought processes.*

Risk for Falls related to changes in mobility, sensation, or confusion

EXPECTED OUTCOME: The patient will remain safe and free from falls.

- Perform a fall risk assessment according to agency policy *to identify patients at risk.*
- Instruct the patient and family to call for help before the patient gets up *so staff can assist.*
- Keep call light and other essential items within the patient's reach *to prevent falls while trying to access needed items.*
- Provide frequent toileting. *Patients often fall while getting up to use the toilet.*
- Avoid restraints if at all possible. *Restraints are associated with injuries.*

Deficient Knowledge related to diagnosis and treatment

EXPECTED OUTCOME: The patient and family will have the necessary knowledge to make decisions and assist with care.

- Explain what has happened to the patient. Explain tests, procedures, and care activities. *The patient and family members are likely to be very frightened about what is happening. Providing correct information about what a stroke is, tests and procedures, and rationale for care activities helps reduce anxiety.*
- Present information in small amounts and as simply as possible. *The patient may have difficulty managing large amounts of information while acutely ill or if confusion is present.*
- Orient the patient and family to the ICU or other setting and the constant monitoring provided. *This can help reduce anxiety and reassure the patient and family that the patient is receiving competent care.*
- If the patient is to be discharged to home, make sure information is provided related to medications, treatments, and follow-up care. *The patient and family need to know how to provide appropriate care at home.*

- Evaluate the need for home health-care nursing, physical therapy, and occupational therapy, and request appropriate referrals. *The patient will likely need continued therapy after discharge to regain as much function as possible.*

Evaluation

If interventions have been effective, the patient will not experience increased deficits due to decreased perfusion of brain cells. The patient will recover as much physical ability as possible and adjust to remaining deficits to meet self-care needs. Basic needs, including safety, elimination, nutrition, and skin integrity, will be met by the patient or caregiver. The patient will be able to communicate effectively and have needs and desires understood. Caregivers will identify support systems available to help. Table 49.3 provides a summary on stroke.

> **PRACTICE ANALYSIS TIP**
> **Linking NCLEX-PN® to Practice**
> The LPN/LVN collects baseline physical data (e.g., skin integrity, height, weight).

> **Home Health Hints**
> - Referrals to physical, occupational, and speech therapies are often appropriate for patients during rehabilitation. Therapists can make recommendations for assistive devices that can promote the patient's independence. A home health-care aid, homemaker, and respite worker may be needed during the early stages of rehabilitation, especially if the caregiver is an elderly spouse.
> - The home health-care nurse can help the patient progress toward their goals by encouraging compliance with home exercise programs and offering frequent praise for all achievements.
> - Teach the patient and caregiver to keep the home environment free of clutter to prevent falls.
> - Teach the patient and caregiver that a portable phone and other frequently used items can be kept in a bag attached to the patient's walker. In the event of a fall, a portable phone can be used to call for help if the patient is unable to afford a medical alert button.
> - Teach caregivers and patients that a pureed diet can be made at home using a food processor. Baby food can also be purchased to meet swallowing guidelines.
> - Teach patients to wear clothes that are easy to get on and off and shoes with Velcro.
> - Teach patients and caregivers that a bedside commode cover can be kept up for easy access, with patches of Velcro attached to the seat and the frame.

Table 49.3 Stroke Summary

Signs and Symptoms	Dizziness Syncope Visual disturbances Irritability, restlessness, confusion Decreased level of consciousness Unequal pupils Paresthesias Motor weakness Paralysis Seizures Difficulty swallowing, understanding language, speaking
Diagnostic Tests	Computed tomography scan, magnetic resonance imaging (MRI) Electrocardiogram Carotid Doppler Echocardiogram Cerebral angiogram Laboratory: International normalized ratio/prothrombin time, metabolic panel, glucose, complete blood count, partial thromboplastin time, anti-Xa assay, serum pregnancy (if appropriate), oxygen saturation
Therapeutic Measures	Oxygen for peripheral oxygen saturation (SpO_2) less than 92% Antiplatelet, anticoagulant, or thrombolytic medication Physical, occupational, or speech therapy Carotid endarterectomy or stent Knee-high antiembolism stockings
Complications	Stroke evolves, causing more deficits, aspiration pneumonia, skin breakdown, urinary tract infection, malnutrition
Priority Nursing Diagnoses	*Risk for Ineffective Cerebral Tissue Perfusion* *Ineffective Airway Clearance* *Risk for Injury*

Key Points

- A TIA is a temporary blockage of blood to the brain that causes a transient neurologic impairment. The episode typically lasts minutes to hours, and the patient recovers completely.
- If the blockage that causes a TIA does not reverse, an area of the brain is permanently damaged, and the event is a stroke. Treatment of a TIA is focused on preventing a full stroke.
- A stroke, or CVA, is caused by disruption of blood flow to the brain, resulting in the death of brain cells. In most cases, permanent disability results.
- Strokes are classified as either ischemic or hemorrhagic. Ischemic strokes are more common. Ischemic stroke occurs when the blood supply to the brain is blocked or significantly slowed. There are two major types of ischemic strokes: thrombotic or embolic.
- Thrombotic strokes occur when an occlusion builds up in an artery until it significantly decreases or stops blood flow to the brain. An embolic stroke is typically caused by a blood clot that is created somewhere in the body, that then travels through the arteries of the brain until it becomes trapped in a smaller vessel, preventing the passage of blood.
- Hemorrhagic strokes are caused by the rupture of a cerebral blood vessel that allows blood to escape into brain tissue and not travel beyond the point of the rupture. It can be further classified into two major types: subarachnoid hemorrhage and intracerebral hemorrhage.
- The acronym FAST, which stands for **F**ace, **A**rms, **S**peech, and **T**ime, can be used to teach people to recognize a stroke and respond quickly. Time is extremely important to preserve brain cells. Quick access to the emergency medical services is of particular importance.
- Most patients with stroke symptoms present with sudden or rapidly evolving symptoms. Symptoms are varied and depend on the area of the brain affected. Common symptoms include visual disturbances, language disturbances, weakness or paralysis on one side of the body, and difficulty swallowing (dysphagia).
- Diagnostic tests for patients with cerebrovascular disorders include CT scan of the brain; ECG to detect atrial fibrillation; blood work that includes CBC, PT, and INR; and a carotid Doppler ultrasound.
- Initial emergency care is supportive while test results are pending. ABCs (**A**irway, **B**reathing, and **C**irculation) are monitored. Oxygen is administered to maintain oxygen saturation at or above 94%, and the patient's LOC is reduced. Vital signs and heart rhythm are monitored. When test results verify whether the stroke is hemorrhagic or ischemic, therapeutic interventions are begun.
- Some patients with ischemic stroke may be candidates for thrombolytic therapy. This is a "clotbuster" medication (alteplase; tPA]) that can break down a clot and potentially completely reverse stroke symptoms.
- Blood pressure control is vital for the stroke patient. Because of the lack of perfusion to certain areas of the brain, the body's response is to increase the systolic blood pressure to force blood into the affected areas.
- Other therapeutic measures include medications to decrease the risk of clots, usually aspirin and Plavix, as well as statins to decrease cholesterol levels.
- Patients who have had a stroke are at risk for developing DVT and should be checked for signs and symptoms of a DVT. They are also at risk for respiratory complications, especially aspiration.
- Paresthesias and paralysis are common long-term effects of strokes that were not treated with a thrombolytic agent. The side of the body opposite the side of the cerebral infarct is affected because nerve fibers cross over as they pass from the brain to the spinal cord. Paralysis on one side of the body is called hemiplegia. The affected limbs may be weak or totally paralyzed (flaccid).
- Pseudobulbar affect can manifest as emotional lability, or instability, and is a common consequence of stroke. Patients may move rapidly from profound sadness to an almost euphoric state and back again. Laughing or crying may have no relationship to the patient's situation at any given moment. These responses probably do not reflect how the patient is feeling but rather are caused by the stroke damage.
- The phenomenon of unilateral neglect is seen predominantly in patients who have right hemisphere infarcts. These patients do not acknowledge the left side of their environment and may not even be aware of their own body on the affected side. Safety is a primary consideration.
- A cerebral aneurysm is a weakness in the wall of a cerebral artery. It may be congenital, traumatic, or the result of disease. If the aneurysm ruptures, the result is often a subarachnoid hemorrhage.
- Subarachnoid hemorrhage is the collection of blood beneath the arachnoid mater following aneurysm rupture. Rupture of an arteriovenous malformation or head trauma may also result in subarachnoid hemorrhage.
- The most common presentation of rupture of an aneurysm is sudden onset of a severe headache. Typically, a patient will state, "I have never had a headache this bad in my life."
- Patients with subarachnoid hemorrhage are cared for in an ICU setting. They typically have an arterial line and a central venous pressure monitoring catheter. Blood pressure is carefully monitored because high pressures increase the risk of re-rupture of the aneurysm and low pressures can be associated with ischemia.
- Blood in the ventricular system interferes with the circulation and reabsorption of cerebrospinal fluid, and hydrocephalus can develop. Early in the course of subarachnoid hemorrhage, an external ventricular drain may be used to treat hydrocephalus.

- When caring for a patient with a cerebrovascular disorder, observe for signs and symptoms of decreased cerebral tissue perfusion. These include decreased LOC, irritability or restlessness, dizziness, syncope, blurred or dimmed vision, diplopia, change in visual fields, unequal pupils or a sluggish or absent pupillary reaction to light, paresthesias, motor weakness, paralysis, or seizures. Recheck frequently and report any change or decline.

- If interventions have been effective, the patient will not experience increased deficits due to decreased perfusion of brain cells. The patient will recover as much physical ability as possible and adjust to remaining deficits to meet self-care needs. Basic needs, including safety, elimination, nutrition, and skin integrity, will be met by the patient or caregiver.

SUGGESTED ANSWERS TO CHAPTER EXERCISES

Cue Recognition
49.1: Activate the EMS system.

Critical Thinking & Clinical Judgment

Mr. Jankowski
1. Ask Mr. Jankowski about other risk factors for stroke, such as dietary and alcohol habits. Check chart for history of diabetes, hypertension, or heart disease. Check weight and cholesterol levels if drawn. Educate him about risk factors for stroke and how they can be modified. Use the Stroke Risk Quiz and remind him about the FAST acronym (see Fig. 49.2). As a nurse, you will be in a position to recognize risks and help patients modify risk factors for many problems before they occur.
2. Discuss use of an anticoagulant agent or sequential compression device with the RN or HCP.
3. Provide written or audiovisual information on stroke prevention and smoking cessation. Ask the HCP about use of a nicotine patch or other medication for smoking cessation, if Mr. Jankowski is willing.
4. Involve a dietitian for dietary counseling if indicated. Consult the smoking cessation coordinator at your agency if one is on staff or help Mr. Jankowski get connected to a Quit line or support group if he verbalizes interest in smoking cessation.

Mrs. Washington
1. Uncontrolled hypertension, in the presence of a preexisting aneurysm, might have precipitated Mrs. Washington's stroke.
2. Her left extremities will be affected.
3. Mrs. Washington is disoriented. Her room should be as close as possible to the nurse's station. Reorient her to her surroundings and condition frequently. Keep side rails up when Mrs. Washington is alone. Mrs. Washington also has hemiparesis. Obtain a bedside commode because she will probably not be able to walk to the bathroom. Place the call light and telephone on her right side. Assist Mrs. Washington with positioning to prevent injury to her affected limbs.
4. If Mrs. Washington will be going back to her home, you should reinforce to her and her daughter about the relationship of uncontrolled hypertension to intracranial hemorrhage; options for inpatient, outpatient, and in-home therapy; and memory strategies to prevent missed medication doses (e.g., weekly pill box, keeping medications with breakfast food, or an alarm clock or watch).
5. The HCP directs the medical care, but often it is the nurse (typically an RN) who oversees the multidisciplinary team and ensures that everything is being done as ordered. Other important team members include the case manager or discharge planner; dietitian, physical, occupational, and speech therapists; as well as pastoral care if the patient desires.

Additional Resources

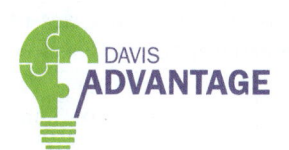

Go to Davis Advantage to complete your learning: strengthen understanding, apply your knowledge, and prepare for the Next Gen NCLEX®.

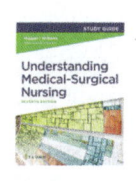

A Study Guide is also available.

CHAPTER 50
Nursing Care of Patients With Peripheral Nervous System Disorders

Jennifer A. Otmanowski, Deborah L. Weaver

KEY TERMS

amyotrophic (ay-MY-oh-TROH-fik)
anticholinesterase (AN-tee-KOH-lin-ESS-ter-ays)
atrophy (AH-troh-fee)
demyelination (dee-MY-uh-lin-AY-shun)
fasciculation (fah-SIK-yoo-LAY-shun)
neuralgia (new-RAL-jee-ah)
neuropathies (new-ROP-uh-thees)
plasmapheresis (PLAZ-mah-fer-EE-sis)
ptosis (TOH-sis)
remyelination (ree-MY-uh-lin-AY-shun)
sclerosis (skleh-ROH-sis)

CHAPTER CONCEPTS

Mobility
Perfusion
Sensory perception
Self-care
Nutrition
Oxygenation

LEARNING OUTCOMES

1. Identify disorders that are caused by disruption of the peripheral nervous system.
2. Explain the pathophysiology, major signs and symptoms, and complications of selected peripheral nervous system disorders.
3. Identify therapeutic measures used for selected peripheral nervous system disorders.
4. List common nursing diagnoses associated with peripheral nervous system disorders.
5. Plan prioritized nursing interventions for patients with peripheral nervous system disorders.
6. Evaluate the effectiveness of nursing care.

The peripheral nervous system (PNS) consists of all nervous system structures outside the central nervous system (CNS). A variety of disorders affect the PNS. Some of these disorders become chronic and cause degeneration of body systems, while others are temporary. Two common types of PNS disorders are discussed in this chapter. The first type is neuromuscular disorders, which can include motor or sensory disorders or both. The second is cranial nerve disorders. Both present a challenge to the nurse caring for the patient and family.

NEUROMUSCULAR DISORDERS

Neuromuscular disorders are chronic and degenerative. They involve a disruption of impulse transmission between neurons and the muscles they stimulate, resulting in muscle weakness. If the muscles of the respiratory system are affected, deadly complications can develop, including pneumonia and respiratory failure. Common neuromuscular disorders include multiple sclerosis, myasthenia gravis, amyotrophic lateral sclerosis, and Guillain-Barré syndrome.

Multiple Sclerosis
Pathophysiology
Multiple sclerosis (MS) is a chronic progressive degenerative disease that affects the myelin sheath of the neurons in the CNS. Myelin is responsible for the smooth transmission of nerve impulses. In MS, the myelin sheath begins to break down (Fig. 50.1) as a result of activation of the body's immune system. The affected nerves become inflamed

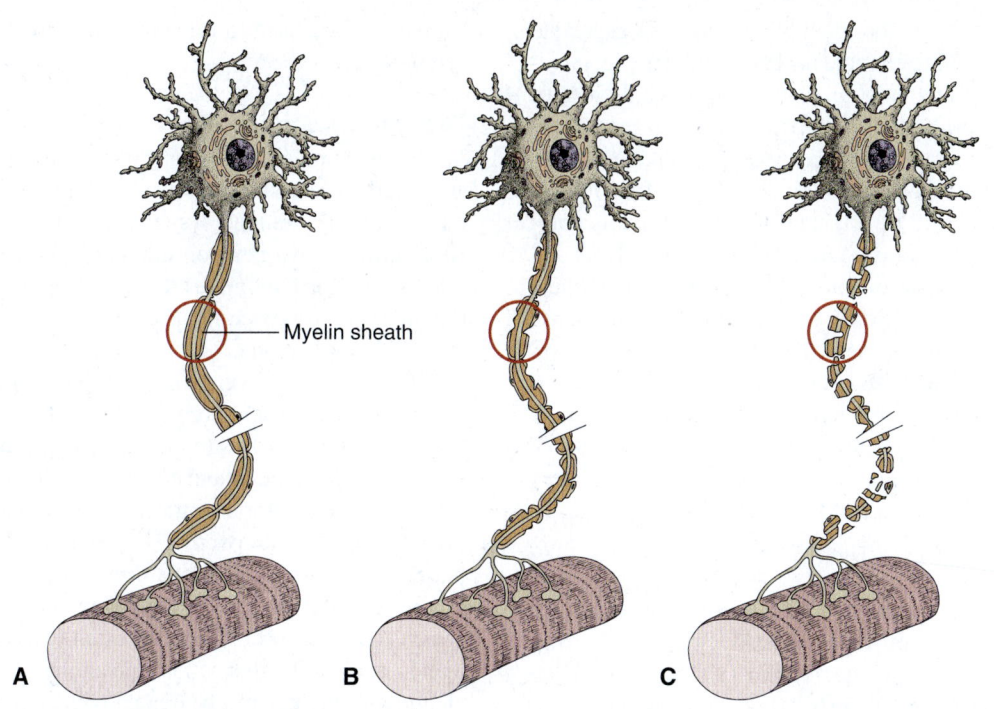

FIGURE 50.1 The myelin sheath breaks down in multiple sclerosis, interrupting transmission of nerve impulses. (A) Normal myelin sheath. (B) Myelin beginning to break down. (C) Total myelin disruption.

and edematous, which interrupts impulses to the muscles. As the disease progresses, **sclerosis**, or scar tissue, damages the nerves. Nerve impulses can become completely blocked, causing permanent loss of muscle function in that area of the body.

Etiology

The cause of MS is not really understood. Damage to the myelin sheath is thought to be from an autoimmune process, but the disease can be related to viral infections, heredity, and other unknown factors. Some research indicates that there is an inherited susceptibility to MS but that development of the disease is triggered by environmental factors (Pytel et al, 2017). The disease usually starts between ages 20 and 50. Women are two to three times more likely than men to develop MS and are more likely to have relapses (National Multiple Sclerosis Society, 2020a). Smokers and those with vitamin D deficiency have a higher risk of MS.

The course of the disease is unpredictable. Symptoms have many variations depending on which nerves are affected. MS is categorized based on the progression of the disease: relapsing-remitting (RRMS), secondary progressive (SPMS), and primary progressive (PPMS). With RRMS, patients experience relapses with increased symptoms that usually resolve. These patients can develop SPMS type in which symptoms do not completely resolve after relapse. When patients have PPMS type, they do not have relapses; neurological function continues to worsen throughout the course of the disease (National Multiple Sclerosis Society, 2020b).

Signs and Symptoms

Symptoms of MS vary greatly among patients. Patients may present with muscle weakness, tingling sensations, numbness, or visual disturbances, usually in one eye at a time. Symptoms may begin slowly over weeks to months or start suddenly and dramatically. MS affects many body systems (Box 50.1).

Box 50.1

Problems Associated With Multiple Sclerosis

- Weakness/paralysis of limbs, trunk, or head
- Diplopia (double vision)
- Slurred speech
- Spasticity of muscles
- Numbness and tingling
- Patchy blindness (scotomas)
- Blurred vision
- Vertigo
- Tinnitus
- Impaired hearing
- Nystagmus
- Ataxia
- Dysarthria
- Dysphagia
- Constipation
- Spastic (uninhibited) bladder
- Flaccid (hypotonic) bladder
- Sexual dysfunction
- Anger, depression, or euphoria

Many factors can trigger the onset of symptoms or aggravate the condition, including extreme heat and cold, fatigue, infection, and physical and emotional stress. Hormonal changes after pregnancy can also cause symptom onset or exacerbation.

Periods of exacerbation and remission lead patients with MS to be uncertain about when the disease will flare up and what body system will be affected. Intense fatigue is common, so immobility can become a problem. Accidents and falls can occur because of muscle weakness or numbness of the trunk and limbs. Some people with MS experience symptoms such as muscle spasticity, bowel or bladder dysfunction, or paralysis. Difficulty with concentration or forgetfulness can also be problematic. Pneumonia can occur from immobility and from weakness of the diaphragm and intercostal muscles. Death, often resulting from respiratory infection, typically occurs 20 to 35 years after diagnosis.

Diagnostic Tests

Diagnosis is based on the patient's history and signs and symptoms. Analysis of cerebrospinal fluid (CSF) may show an increase in immunoglobulin G (IgG) antibodies. Magnetic resonance imaging (MRI) of the brain and spinal cord can detect demyelination. Evoked potential tests may be done to determine slow transmission of nerve impulses. Blood tests are used to rule out other diseases with similar symptoms.

Therapeutic Measures

MS has no cure, although early treatment can delay progression of the disease. Some drugs slow disease progression by modifying the immune system, such as interferon therapy (Betaseron or Avonex) or immunoglobulins (ocrelizumab [Ocrevus]). Teriflunomide (Aubagio) and dimethyl fumarate (Tecfidera) can reduce relapses. Each of these medications has serious side effects.

Other drugs are given to control symptoms. Steroids such as adrenocorticotropic hormone (ACTH, which triggers the body to make its own steroids) and prednisone are given to decrease inflammation and edema of the neurons, which can relieve some symptoms. Anticonvulsants such as carbamazepine (Tegretol) or duloxetine (Cymbalta) help relieve neuropathic pain. The medications diazepam (Valium), baclofen (Lioresal), and tizanidine (Zanaflex) help control muscle spasms. Bladder problems are treated with parasympathetic agents such as bethanechol (Urecholine) and oxybutynin (Ditropan). Fatigue can be treated with antidepressants or an antiviral agent such as amantadine (Symmetrel). Table 50.1 reviews additional medications used to treat PNS disorders.

Table 50.1
Medications Used to Treat Peripheral Nervous System Disorders

Medication Class/Action

Cholinesterase Inhibitors

Increase acetylcholine at synapses.

Examples	**Nursing Implications**
neostigmine (Prostigmin)	Atropine is an antidote.
pyridostigmine (Mestinon)	

Glucocorticoids

Reduce inflammation.

Examples	**Nursing Implications**
prednisone	Provide calcium supplement.
prednisolone	Monitor fluid balance.
methylprednisolone (Solu-Medrol)	May need to treat high blood sugar levels with insulin while on medication.
	Teach:
	Avoid crowds and others with infections.

Immunosuppressants

Suppress immunity and antibody formation.

Examples	**Nursing Implications**
azathioprine (Imuran)	Monitor blood counts.
cyclophosphamide (Cytoxan)	Protect from bleeding and infection.
	Administer with meals to reduce nausea.

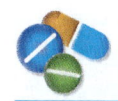

Table 50.1 Medications Used to Treat Peripheral Nervous System Disorders—cont'd

Antispasmodics/Muscle Relaxants

Relax muscles and reduce pain.

Examples	Nursing Implications
dantrolene (Dantrium)	Monitor patient for respiratory depression.
baclofen (Lioresal)	Teach:
tizanidine (Zanaflex)	Avoid operating machinery or driving until effects are known.
benzodiazepines such as diazepam (Valium)	

Anticonvulsants

Treat nerve pain.

Examples	Nursing Implications
phenytoin (Dilantin)	Monitor for fall risk.
carbamazepine (Tegretol)	Monitor complete blood counts.
gabapentin (Neurontin)	Teach:
duloxetine (Cymbalta)	Maintain good oral hygiene with soft bristle brush, floss, and gum massage (phenytoin).

Glutamate Antagonist

Delays progression of amyotrophic lateral sclerosis (ALS).

Examples	Nursing Implications
riluzole (Rilutek)	Monitor for respiratory depression.
ocrelizumab (Ocrevus); also used for multiple sclerosis (MS)	Give on empty stomach.
	Monitor liver function laboratory values.
	Teach:
	Rest.
	Avoid large quantities of caffeine.
	Avoid charcoal-broiled foods.

Disease Modifying Agents

Reduce relapses in relapsing-remitting MS.

Examples	Nursing Implications
alemtuzumab (Lemtrada)	Monitor complete blood count and signs of infection.
glatiramer acetate (Copaxone); also used for ALS	Health-care provider may recommend delaying vaccines.
dimethyl fumarate (Tecfidera)	Other implications based on individual drug action.
fingolimod (Gilenya)	Teach:
teriflunomide (Aubagio)	Avoid others who are ill.
natalizumab (Tysabri)	Do not use if pregnant.

Acute exacerbations are typically treated with high doses of steroids or with ACTH. For those who suffer sudden severe attacks or do not respond to high doses of steroids, plasma exchange, or **plasmapheresis**, may be used to remove antibodies from the blood that are attacking the myelin (Box 50.2).

Rehabilitation after acute exacerbation includes physical, speech, and occupational therapies. Physical therapy can help with strength, coordination, and balance. An occupational therapist can help the patient and family adapt the home environment to the patient's special needs. Assistive devices such as braces, canes, wheelchairs, and splints allow the patient increased mobility and independence. Patients who develop speech difficulties benefit from speech therapy. Exercise also can be beneficial (see "Evidence-Based Practice").

• WORD • BUILDING •

plasmapheresis: plasma—liquid of blood + pheresis—removal

Box 50.2

Plasmapheresis

Plasmapheresis, also known as *plasma exchange therapy*, is a procedure that removes the plasma component from whole blood and replaces it with fresh plasma. The goal is to remove antibodies through plasma exchange, suppressing the immune response and inflammation.

Preprocedure Nursing Care

- Verify that the patient understands the procedure and what to expect, including what the machine looks like (similar to but smaller than a dialysis machine), the need for arterial and venous access sites, and the length of the procedure (2 to 5 hours).
- HCP may order medications held until after the procedure. Some patients may require premedication, especially if they have experienced complications in the past.
- Collect baseline vital signs and weight.
- Review complete blood cell count (CBC), platelet count, and clotting studies.
- Check blood type and crossmatch for replacement blood products.

Postprocedure Nursing Care

- Observe the patient for signs of hypovolemia, such as dizziness and hypotension.
- Apply pressure dressings to the access sites.
- Monitor the patient for infection and bruits at the access site.
- Monitor electrolytes and signs of electrolyte loss. Report imbalances and administer replacement electrolytes as ordered.
- Compare preprocedure and postprocedure laboratory data, such as CBC, platelet count, and clotting times.

Evidence-Based Practice

Clinical Question
Do patients with MS benefit from exercise?

Evidence
The National Multiple Sclerosis Society gathered experts in the field of MS to make recommendations for exercise for patients who have MS. The Society determined that exercise is safe for patients with MS and offers many physical and psychological benefits. It notes that health-care providers should encourage their MS patients to participate in physical activity and exercise (Kalb et al, 2020).

Implications for Nursing Practice
Routinely ask patients about their participation in physical activity.
Offer information (handouts, community resources) regarding physical activity.
Provide encouragement and help with goal setting.

Reference: Kalb, R., Brown, T. R., Coote, S., Costello, K., Dalgas, U., Garmon, E., Glesser, B., Halper, J., Karpatkin, H., Keller, J., Ng, J. V., Pilutti, L. A., Rohrig, A., Asch, P. V., Zackowski, A., & Moti, R. W. (2020). Exercise and lifestyle physical activity recommendations for people with multiple sclerosis throughout the disease course. *Multiple Sclerosis Journal, 26*(12). https://doi.org/10.1177/1352458520915629

Nursing Care

See "Nursing Care Plan for the Patient With a Progressive Neuromuscular Disorder." In addition to reviewing routine care, instruct the patient to avoid factors that can exacerbate symptoms. These triggers include stressful situations, extreme

---

Nursing Care Plan for the Patient With a Progressive Neuromuscular Disorder

Nursing Diagnosis: Ineffective Airway Clearance related to respiratory muscle weakness, and impaired cough and gag reflexes
Expected Outcomes: The patient will maintain a patent airway as evidenced by clear lung sounds and freedom from signs and symptoms of respiratory distress.
Evaluation of Outcomes: Is the patient's airway patent, and are lung sounds clear? Is the patient free of signs and symptoms of respiratory distress?

Intervention	Rationale	Evaluation
Monitor respiratory rate and depth, breath sounds, oxygen saturation (SpO$_2$), and arterial blood gases (as ordered). Report deterioration.	*Increasing respiratory distress indicates progressing muscle weakness that may require mechanical ventilation or end-of-life decisions.*	Is patient's respiratory rate status stable, or is intervention indicated?
Evaluate cough, swallow, and gag reflexes frequently. Notify HCP if absent.	*Impaired reflexes place patient at risk for aspiration and possible pneumonia.*	Is patient able to cough effectively? Is gag reflex intact?
Observe patient for breathlessness while speaking.	*Inability to speak without breathlessness indicates declining respiratory function.*	Is patient able to finish sentences without needing to take a breath?
Encourage patient to cough and deep breathe every 2 hours.	*Effective coughing helps keep airway clear.*	Does patient have the strength to cough effectively?

Nursing Care Plan for the Patient With a Progressive Neuromuscular Disorder—cont'd

Intervention	Rationale	Evaluation
Elevate head of bed.	The Fowler position improves lung expansion, decreases work of breathing, improves cough efforts, and decreases risk for aspiration.	Does elevation of head of bed help relieve dyspnea and prevent aspiration?
Suction secretions as needed, noting color and amount of secretions.	Muscle weakness can result in inability to clear airway.	Does patient require suctioning to clear airway? What color are secretions?

Nursing Diagnosis: *Impaired Physical Mobility* related to muscle weakness
Expected Outcomes: The patient will maintain optimum mobility and activity level, identify measures to help maintain mobility, and perform exercises that help promote mobility.
Evaluation of Outcomes: Is optimal activity level maintained? Can the patient identify measures that will help maintain mobility? Does the patient perform exercises that help maintain mobility?

Intervention	Rationale	Evaluation
Determine pre-illness and current level of mobility.	Assessment guides care planning.	What was patient able to do prior to illness or exacerbation?
Identify factors that affect ability to be mobile and active.	Some factors that interfere with mobility can be modified.	Are interfering factors modified effectively?
Encourage patient to perform self-care to maximum ability.	Promotes sense of control and independence for patient.	Does patient perform self-care activities? Is assistance required?
Consult physical therapist to provide safe transferring and exercise recommendations.	Exercise can improve strength and mobility.	Does patient follow exercise recommendations? Is mobility maintained?
Consult physical therapist or occupational therapist to provide assistive devices (e.g., canes, braces, walker, wheelchair) for walking, transferring, and other activities.	Assistive devices decrease fatigue and promote independence, comfort, and safety.	Does patient use assistive devices safely during activities? Do they help keep patient active?
Reposition frequently if patient is immobile.	Prevents skin breakdown and stasis of pulmonary secretions.	Is skin intact?
Provide active/passive range-of-motion exercises if needed on a regular basis.	Prevents contractures and disuse atrophy.	Does patient have any contractures or atrophy?
Plan activities with a balance of frequent rest periods.	Rest decreases fatigue.	Is fatigue controlled?

Nursing Diagnosis: *Impaired Verbal Communication* related to impaired respiratory and muscle function
Expected Outcome: The patient will be able to communicate needs.
Evaluation of Outcome: Does patient indicate that needs are met with minimal frustration?

Intervention	Rationale	Evaluation
Determine ability to speak and communicate.	Assessment is essential to planning appropriate communication interventions.	Can patient speak and communicate needs?
Request referral for speech therapy if indicated.	Speech therapist can help with speech clarity or recommend appropriate alternative communication techniques.	Is referral completed if indicated?
Observe for nonverbal signs of pain or distress, such as restlessness, agitation, and grimacing.	Patient may not be able to tell you if in pain or distress.	Are signs of pain or distress present? Are they attended to?

(nursing care plan continues on page 1026)

Nursing Care Plan for the Patient With a Progressive Neuromuscular Disorder—cont'd

Intervention	Rationale	Evaluation
Use a picture board or paper and pencil. Ask questions that require a yes or no answer.	*These do not require patient to speak to communicate.*	Do alternative methods help patient communicate needs?
Use an unhurried, calm, and caring approach while providing care.	*This will help decrease anxiety and provide emotional support to patient and family.*	Do patient and family appear anxious? Does calm approach help?
Explain all procedures.	*Patient can still hear and needs to know what is happening.*	Does patient indicate understanding?

temperature changes, infection, and illness. Rest, exercise, and a balanced diet are important self-care steps to control symptoms. Any infection, especially respiratory, should be reported immediately to the health-care provider (HCP). Two excellent sources of information on MS are the National Multiple Sclerosis Society at www.nationalmssociety.org and the Multiple Sclerosis Foundation at www.msfocus.org.

> **PRACTICE ANALYSIS TIP**
> Linking NCLEX-PN® to Practice
> The LPN/LVN assures availability and safe functioning of client care equipment.

> **PRACTICE ANALYSIS TIP**
> Linking NCLEX-PN® to Practice
> The LPN/LVN uses transfer assistive devices (e.g., gait/transfer belt, slide board, mechanical lift).

Myasthenia Gravis
Pathophysiology
Myasthenia gravis (MG) means "grave muscle weakness," or weakness of voluntary or skeletal muscles of the body. MG is a chronic disease of the neuromuscular junction (Fig. 50.2). Normally, a neuron releases the chemical neurotransmitter acetylcholine (ACh) at the neuromuscular junction. Receptors on muscle tissue take up ACh, resulting in contraction. In MG, the body's immune system is activated, producing antibodies that attack and destroy ACh receptors at the neuromuscular junction. ACh cannot stimulate muscle contraction because the number of ACh receptors has been reduced, which causes loss of voluntary muscle strength.

Etiology
MG is a chronic autoimmune process. No specific cause has been found, but certain viruses may initiate the autoimmune process. Genetic susceptibility may also play a role.

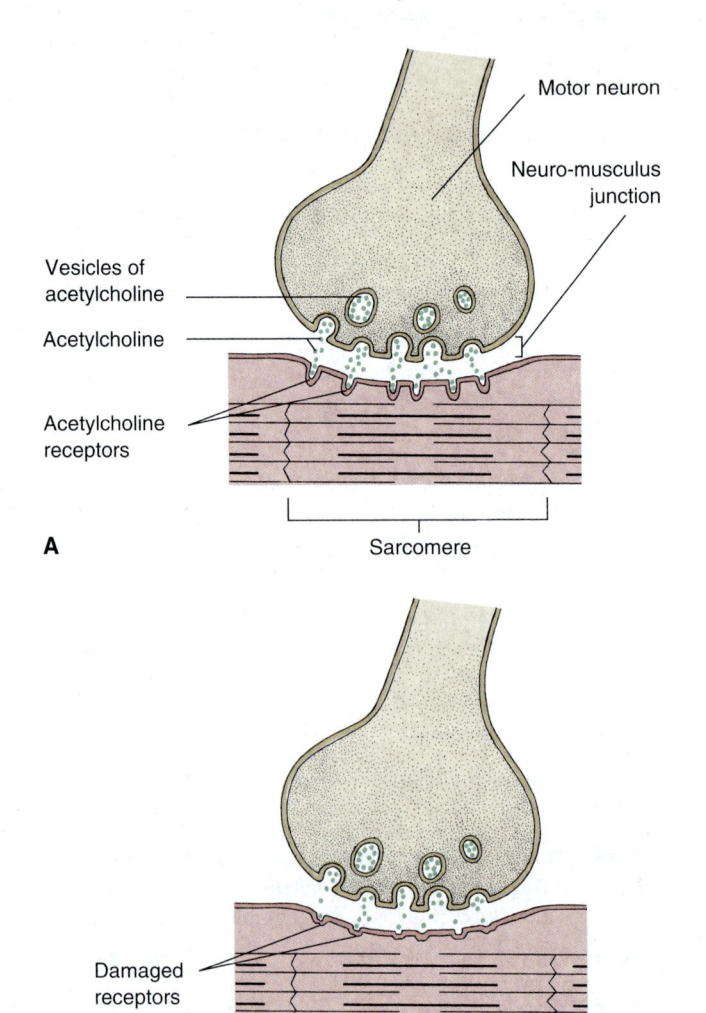

FIGURE 50.2 Myasthenia gravis. (A) Normal neuromuscular junction. (B) Note damaged acetylcholine receptor sites in myasthenia gravis.

Disorders of the thymus gland are often associated with MG. All ethnic groups and both genders can develop this disease. Peak age of onset in women is ages 20 to 30. Men are affected more often after age 60. MG occurs more often in women than in men.

Signs and Symptoms

MG results in progressive extreme muscle weakness. The classic sign of MG is increased muscle weakness during activity and improvement in muscle strength after rest. Muscles are strongest in the morning when the person is rested. Activities affected by MG include eye and eyelid movements, chewing, swallowing, speaking, and breathing as well as skeletal muscle function. Patients often present with drooping of the eyelids (**ptosis**). Facial expressions become masklike. After long conversations, the patient's voice may fade. Falls occur because of weakness of the arm and leg muscles. Patients with MG, like those with MS, experience periods of exacerbation and remission of symptoms. Exacerbations can be caused by emotional or physical stress such as menses, illness, trauma, extremes in temperature, pregnancy, electrolyte imbalance, surgery, and drugs that block action at the neuromuscular junction.

Complications

Major complications associated with MG result from weakness of muscles that assist with swallowing and breathing. Aspiration, respiratory infections, and respiratory failure are the leading causes of death. Sudden onset of muscle weakness in patients with MG resulting from undermedication is called a *myasthenic crisis*. Overmedication with **anticholinesterase** drugs causes a *cholinergic crisis*. The first sign of a cholinergic crisis is weakness of the facial muscles, including the tongue, that may impact the patient's ability to talk or swallow (Table 50.2). Both myasthenic crisis and cholinergic crisis require immediate medical attention.

Table 50.2
Comparison of Myasthenic Crisis and Cholinergic Crisis

	Myasthenic Crisis	Cholinergic Crisis
Cause	Too little medication	Too much medication
Signs and Symptoms	Ptosis Difficulty swallowing Difficulty speaking Dyspnea Weakness	Salivation Lacrimation Urinary incontinence Diarrhea Gastrointestinal cramping Emesis Increased bronchial secretions Sweating Miosis (constriction of pupils) Bradycardia Increasing muscle weakness Dyspnea

> **LEARNING TIP**
> Symptoms of cholinergic crisis can be remembered with the acronym **SLUDGE**, which stands for **s**alivation, **l**acrimation, **u**rination, **d**iarrhea, **g**astrointestinal (GI) cramping, and **e**mesis. A severe crisis has been described as "liquid pouring out of every body orifice."

Diagnostic Tests

Diagnosis of MG is based on history of symptoms and physical examination of the patient. A simple test involves the patient looking upward for 2 to 3 minutes. Increased ptosis occurs if MG is present. After a brief rest, the eyelids can be opened without difficulty. Another test is done by injecting edrophonium (Tensilon), an anticholinesterase drug, intravenously. If muscle strength improves dramatically (e.g., the patient can suddenly open the eyes wide), MG is diagnosed. However, improvement is only temporary. An increased number of anti-ACh receptor antibodies in the blood are present in 90% of patients with MG. Electromyography (EMG) may be done to rule out other conditions. Pulmonary function tests may be done to predict potential myasthenic crisis leading to respiratory failure.

Therapeutic Measures

No cure is currently available for MG. Treatment is aimed at controlling symptoms. Removal of the thymus gland (thymectomy) can decrease production of ACh receptor antibodies and decrease symptoms in most patients. Medications used to treat MG include the anticholinesterase drugs neostigmine (Prostigmin) and pyridostigmine (Mestinon). These drugs improve MG symptoms by destroying the acetylcholinesterase that breaks down ACh. Remember that ACh causes muscles to contract. If ACh is allowed more time to attach to remaining muscle tissue receptors, the muscle contracts and strength is increased. Steroids such as prednisone and immunosuppressants are used to suppress the body's immune response. The monoclonal antibody rituximab (Rituxan) is an IV-administered medication used in some cases of MG; it works by affecting the immune system. Plasmapheresis can be used to remove antibodies from the patient's blood. IV immunoglobulin (IVIg) helps restore normal immune function.

Nursing Process for the Patient With Myasthenia Gravis

DATA COLLECTION. Determine the patient's baseline muscle strength. Ask how much activity is tolerated before fatigue and muscle weakness occur. Identify the patient's support systems and determine whether the patient's needs

• **WORD • BUILDING** •

anticholinesterase: anti—against + cholinesterase—chemical that breaks down acetylcholine

are being met. Determine the knowledge base of the patient and family. Check respiratory function and swallowing ability.

NURSING DIAGNOSES, PLANNING, AND IMPLEMENTATION.

Activity Intolerance related to muscle weakness

EXPECTED OUTCOME: The patient will improve activity tolerance as evidenced by the ability to carry out necessary activities.

- Schedule anticholinesterase drugs so that peak action occurs when increased muscle strength is needed *so that the patient has strength for activities such as meals and physical therapy.*
- Reinforce the scheduling of activities such as grocery shopping and other errands at times when medication is at peak action *so that muscle strength is adequate for the activity.*
- Be aware of symptoms and treatment of myasthenic and cholinergic crises *so that quick intervention can be carried out to prevent worsening symptoms.*
- Reinforce symptoms of crisis conditions to patients and family members *because both crises constitute medical emergencies and require immediate intervention* (see Table 50.2).
- Reinforce methods to conserve energy, such as sitting down to do grooming and housekeeping activities whenever possible. *This helps the patient conserve energy to manage activities of daily living (ADLs).*
- Remind the patient to rest between activities *to allow time for muscle strength to be restored.*
- Reinforce the importance of avoiding people with infections and exposure to cold *to minimize risk for respiratory infections, which can exacerbate symptoms and increase risk for ineffective airway clearance.*
- Instruct the patient to eat nutritious, well-balanced meals *to maintain strength and resistance to infections, which can exacerbate symptoms.*
- Remind the patient to use only medications that are prescribed by the HCP. If multiple providers are used, all medications should be checked with the HCP who is treating the MG. *Many medications can exacerbate muscle weakness or interfere with medications used to treat MG* (Box 50.3).
- Provide information about support groups *that can provide encouragement and assistance to patients and their families.*

EVALUATION. If the plan of care has been effective, the patient's activity and self-care needs will be met, either by the patient or by other support individuals.

Also see "Nursing Care Plan for the Patient With a Progressive Neuromuscular Disorder" earlier in this chapter. More information can be found at the Myasthenia Gravis Foundation of America Web site at www.myasthenia.org.

Box 50.3
Medications That Can Exacerbate Symptoms of Myasthenia Gravis

- Antibiotics (some)
- Alpha interferon
- Anticholinergic agents
- Beta blockers
- Botulinum toxin
- Calcium channel blockers
- Chloroquine
- Lithium
- Magnesium
- Neuromuscular blocking agents (such as those used during surgery)
- Penicillamine
- Prednisone
- Procainamide
- Quinidine

CRITICAL THINKING & CLINICAL JUDGMENT

Alba is referred to a neurologist because of muscle weakness.

Critical Thinking (The Why)
1. What history can differentiate between multiple sclerosis (MS) and myasthenia gravis (MG)?
2. What physical examination can be done to differentiate between MS and MG?

Clinical Judgment (The Do)
3. The neurologist prepares to do an edrophonium (Tensilon) test and asks you to prepare 2 mg of Tensilon for IV injection. It is supplied as 10 mg per milliliter. How much should you draw up?
4. In preparing for a case management meeting for a patient with a neuromuscular disease, which health-care team members should be invited?
5. Alba is eventually diagnosed with MG. In her next visit to your clinic, Alba reports an exacerbation with increased weakness and swallowing difficulty. While reconciling her medications, you notice she was started on a beta blocker, metoprolol, for hypertension by her primary physician. What should you do?

Suggested answers are at the end of the chapter.

PRACTICE ANALYSIS TIP
Linking NCLEX-PN® to Practice
The LPN/LVN will:

1. Evaluate the appropriateness of HCP order for client.
2. Reconcile and maintain medication list or medication administration record (e.g., prescribed medications, herbal supplements, over-the-counter medications).

Amyotrophic Lateral Sclerosis

Pathophysiology and Etiology

Amyotrophic lateral sclerosis (ALS; also called *Lou Gehrig disease*) is a progressive, degenerative condition that affects motor neurons responsible for the control of voluntary muscles. In the brain and spinal cord, upper and lower motor neurons begin to degenerate and form scar tissue or die, blocking transmission of nerve impulses. Without stimulation, muscles **atrophy**, and muscle strength and coordination decrease. As the disease progresses, more muscle groups, including muscles controlling breathing and swallowing, become involved. The heart and GI tract are controlled involuntarily and are not affected by ALS. The ability to think and reason is also unaffected.

ALS can occur at any age but usually does not appear until adulthood. The cause of ALS is unknown but likely has a genetic component. Smoking and other toxins appear to increase risk.

Signs and Symptoms

Symptoms are vague early in the course of ALS. Primary symptoms include progressive muscle weakness and decreased coordination, which can begin in the arms, legs, or muscles of speech and swallowing. Atrophy of muscles and **fasciculation** (twitching) also occur. Muscle spasms can cause pain. Difficulty with chewing and swallowing places the patient at risk for choking and aspiration as the disease progresses. Inappropriate emotional outbursts of laughing and crying can occur. Speech becomes increasingly difficult. Bladder and bowel functions remain intact, yet problems such as constipation and urinary urgency, hesitancy, or frequency can occur.

Late in the disease, communication becomes limited to moving and blinking the eyes in response to questions. Pulmonary function becomes severely compromised to the point of requiring mechanical ventilator assistance if the patient chooses. Other complications can include extreme malnutrition, falls, pulmonary emboli, and heart failure. ALS eventually leads to death from respiratory complications such as atelectasis, respiratory failure, and pneumonia.

Diagnostic Tests

Diagnosis is made on the basis of clinical symptoms. Additional tests such as CSF analysis, electroencephalogram (EEG), nerve biopsy, nerve conduction velocity (NCV), or EMG may be done to rule out other conditions. Blood enzymes can be increased as a result of muscle atrophy.

Therapeutic Measures

ALS has no cure; treatments are palliative in nature. Goals of treatment are aimed at maintaining function for as long as possible and emotionally supporting the patient and family. Glycopyrrolate (Robinul) may be administered to decrease saliva production. Carbamazepine or phenytoin may be used for muscle cramps. Baclofen may be used for spasms. Riluzole (Rilutek) slows the progression of the disease and can prolong life by 3 to 4 months. Edaravone (Radicava) reduces the glutamate in the body, which damages the motor nerves, slowing decline in function.

Nonpharmacological measures such as physical therapy, massage, position changes, and diversional activities can help control pain. Enteral feedings via a surgically placed gastrostomy tube help provide adequate nutrition. Prevention of infections, such as pneumonia and urinary tract infection (UTI), is vital. Meticulous skin care minimizes the incidence of pressure injuries. Physical, occupational, and speech therapies allow the patient to maximize function for as long as possible. Therapy can also decrease the occurrence of complications such as aspiration, falls, and contractures. As the disease progresses, mechanical ventilation may be needed. Patients may choose supportive hospice care instead of life-prolonging mechanical ventilation.

Patients with speech problems may benefit from use of alternative communication. A variety of systems are available; most involve laptop computers that patients use to type words or symbols to generate speech. Support groups and counseling provide emotional support for the patient and family.

Nursing Care

See "Nursing Care Plan for the Patient With a Progressive Neuromuscular Disorder" earlier in this chapter.

PATIENT EDUCATION. Reinforce information given by the HCP to the patient and family about ALS and its prognosis. Support groups can provide emotional support as the patient and family deal with the likely reality of untimely death. Assistive devices and exercises help prevent complications. Patients should avoid exposure to persons with infections because an infection can be deadly to a patient with a debilitating disease. Request a consultation with a palliative care specialist or other resource personnel to help the patient and family develop an advance directive.

> **NURSING CARE TIP**
>
> When planning care, remember that a person with amyotrophic lateral sclerosis has an intact mind; it is the body that is deteriorating.

> **CUE RECOGNITION 50.1**
>
> You are answering the triage phone at the neurology office when a patient with MC calls with a report of increasing weakness with changes in speech and swallowing. What do you do?
>
> *Suggested answers are at the end of the chapter.*

• WORD • BUILDING •

amyotrophic: a—without + myo—muscle + trophy—nourishment + ic—related to

atrophy: a—without + trophy—nourishment

> **CRITICAL THINKING &
> CLINICAL JUDGMENT**
>
> **Mr. Miller** has been having difficulty swallowing. He is diagnosed with ALS.
>
> **Critical Thinking (The Why)**
> 1. What are the priority nursing diagnoses for Mr. Miller?
>
> **Clinical Judgment (The Do)**
> 2. What actions can the nurse take to support the patient and his family in coping with ALS?
> 3. What health-care team members should be consulted for his care?
>
> *Suggested answers are at the end of the chapter.*

Guillain-Barré Syndrome

Pathophysiology

Guillain-Barré syndrome (GBS) is a rare neuromuscular disease affecting only 1 in every 100,000 persons. Both men and women in the United States are affected equally. Onset is usually between 30 and 50 years of age. GBS is an inflammatory disorder characterized by abrupt onset of symmetrical paresis (weakness) that progresses to paralysis. The myelin sheath of the spinal and cranial nerves is destroyed by a diffuse inflammatory reaction. The peripheral nerves are infiltrated by lymphocytes, which leads to edema and inflammation. Segmental **demyelination** causes atrophy of the axons, resulting in slowed or blocked nerve conduction. Typically, demyelination begins in the most distal nerves and ascends in a symmetrical fashion. **Remyelination** is a much slower process. It occurs in a descending pattern and is accompanied by a resolution of symptoms.

There are four recognized variants of GBS; only the most common type, ascending GBS, is addressed in this chapter. It is characterized by progressive weakness and numbness that begins in the legs and ascends body. Numbness tends to be mild, but muscle weakness usually progresses to paralysis. The paralysis can ascend all the way to cranial nerves or stop between the legs and head. Deep tendon reflexes are either depressed or absent. Respiratory failure requiring mechanical ventilation happens in 17% to 30% of patients with GBS (Garg, 2017).

Etiology

GBS is believed to result from an autoimmune response to a viral infection or certain vaccines, although the exact cause is unknown. Usually, the viral illness affects the respiratory or GI system and occurs within 2 weeks before onset of neurologic symptoms. The most common organism with GBS is *Campylobacter jejuni*, a common cause of gastroenteritis.

Signs and Symptoms

GBS is divided into three stages.

STAGE 1: ONSET OF SYMPTOMS. The first stage starts with the onset of symptoms and lasts until the progression of symptoms stops. This stage can last from 24 hours to 3 weeks. It is characterized by abrupt and rapid onset of muscle weakness and paralysis, with little or no muscle atrophy. Patients with ascending GBS may gradually notice a reduced ability to take deep breaths or have conversations and may feel short of breath. These patients are terrified that they will not be able to breathe and may require intubation and artificial ventilation.

The autonomic nervous system is often affected by GBS. Patients can experience unstable blood pressure, cardiac arrhythmias, urine retention, or paralytic ileus. Patient reports of discomfort range from annoying numbness and cramping to severe pain. The discomfort is exacerbated by the patient's inability to move voluntarily.

STAGE 2: PLATEAU. The second stage is the plateau stage, when symptoms are most severe but progression has stopped. It can last from 2 to 14 days. Patients may become discouraged if no improvement is evident.

STAGE 3: RECOVERY. Axonal regeneration and remyelination occur during the third stage, recovery. This stage lasts from 6 to 24 months, and symptoms slowly improve. Most patients with GBS recover in a few months to a year. A few patients experience chronic disability.

Complications

Complications can include respiratory failure, infection, and depression. It is important to discuss the possible need for intubation early in the patient's illness. The decision to intubate in GBS is different from other PNS disorders because GBS patients are expected to recover. It is important to be vigilant in monitoring pulse oximetry, respiratory rate and depth, and dyspnea to predict the need for intervention and maintain the patient's safety.

Patients with GBS are prone to pneumonia and UTIs. Maintaining infection control practices and maximizing the patient's nutritional status help decrease the likelihood of infection. Immobility leads to problems such as skin breakdown, pulmonary embolus, deep vein thrombosis, and muscle atrophy. Patients with GBS have little time to adjust to their illness and deterioration; they often fear they will not recover function. Calm, supportive reassurance is important.

Diagnostic Tests

A lumbar puncture is performed to obtain CSF. The CSF analysis shows a normal cell count with an elevated protein level. EMG and NCV tests are done to evaluate nerve function. Pulmonary function testing helps confirm impending respiratory problems.

• WORD • BUILDING •

demyelination: de—down or from + myelin—sheath surrounding neurons + ation—process

remyelination: re—repeat + myelin—sheath surrounding neurons + ation—process

Therapeutic Measures
During the initial stages, patients are partially or completely dependent for all needs. They are often frightened and anxious. Oxygen and mechanical ventilation may be required. Plasma exchange may be used to remove the patient's plasma and replace it with fresh plasma. This procedure is thought to lessen the body's immune response. Immunoglobulin therapy may help reduce the severity of the disease. Supportive interventions include anticoagulants to prevent deep vein thrombosis and analgesics for pain. Intensive rehabilitation helps the patient regain function during the recovery phase.

Nursing Care for the Patient With Guillain-Barré Syndrome
See "Nursing Care Plan for the Patient With a Progressive Neuromuscular Disorder" earlier in this chapter. Check the patient's vital signs, arterial blood gases (ABGs), and oxygen saturation (SpO_2) to monitor respiratory status. Monitor gag, corneal, and swallowing reflexes to determine whether safety measures are needed to prevent aspiration or injury to the eyes. Be prepared to reinforce teaching provided to the patient and family about the disease and treatment. Table 50.3 summarizes and compares MS, MG, ALS, and GBS.

Postpolio Syndrome
Pathophysiology and Etiology
Postpolio syndrome affects survivors of polio 20 to 40 years after they have recovered from infection caused by the poliomyelitis virus. Up to 40% of patients who had polio develop postpolio syndrome.

Signs and Symptoms
Postpolio syndrome involves further weakening of the muscles that were affected with the first poliovirus infection. Symptoms range from fatigue to progressive muscle weakness and atrophy. Sleeping problems, joint pain, scoliosis, and respiratory compromise can occur. Some people suffer great debilitation; others have fewer problems.

Diagnostic Tests
Diagnosis is made on the basis of history and by ruling out other disorders.

Therapeutic Measures
No interventions have been found to be effective at this time. Physical therapy can help the patient increase exercise tolerance. An occupational therapist can help the patient with assistive devices to conserve energy.

Restless Legs Syndrome
Restless legs syndrome (RLS) is an uncomfortable sensation in the legs, causing the sufferer to constantly feel the need to move the legs. It typically occurs at rest or at night.

Pathophysiology and Etiology
RLS is believed to be related to imbalance of dopamine and serotonin in the brain and may have a hereditary component. Some medications can aggravate RLS. Patients with chronic medical conditions such as kidney failure, iron deficiency, diabetes, Parkinson disease, and peripheral neuropathy may develop RLS. Symptoms of RLS can improve as these medications are discontinued and illnesses are treated.

Signs and Symptoms
Patients often complain of unpleasant sensations such as creeping, crawling, throbbing, pulling, or pins and needles in the legs. Symptoms occur as the person is resting and often increase in severity during sleep. Moving the legs temporarily relieves symptoms.

RLS can interfere with falling and staying asleep, resulting in daytime fatigue and exhaustion. The resulting sleep deprivation can impact work performance and ADLs.

Both men and women and all ages are affected by RLS. The incidence in women is twice as high as in men. People often fail to report symptoms to their HCP, as they believe their symptoms will not be taken seriously or treated.

Diagnostic Tests
No specific tests exist to diagnose RLS. Diagnosis is based on the patient's report of symptoms. The HCP will order a blood test for iron deficiency and may test to rule out other disorders. Patients should be asked about their medication history, whether family members have similar symptoms, and whether they experience daytime sleepiness.

Therapeutic Measures
Treatment of RLS is aimed at improving symptoms. Encourage patients to eliminate caffeine and establish routine sleep and exercise habits. Use of heat and cold therapies, leg massages, and warm baths may also help reduce symptoms. A vibrating pad (Relaxis) is approved by the Food and Drug Administration and has helped some RLS sufferers.

Medications such as pramipexole (Mirapex), ropinirole (Requip), and rotigotine (Neupro) may be ordered for moderate to severe RLS to increase serum dopamine levels. Opioids, anticonvulsants, and benzodiazepines may be prescribed when other therapies are ineffective.

Nursing Care
Nursing care targets patient education about lifestyle changes and medications to control symptoms. Conduct a thorough sleep history if the patient complains of insomnia. A sleep specialist can be consulted for additional help.

CRANIAL NERVE DISORDERS

Cranial nerves are the peripheral nerves of the brain. There are 12 pairs of cranial nerves that innervate areas including the head, neck, and special sensory structures (see Chapter 48). Cranial nerve problems are classified as peripheral **neuropathies.** Disorders can affect the sensory, motor, or both branches of a single nerve. Causes of cranial nerve

• WORD • BUILDING •

neuropathies: neuro—nerve + pathies—disease

Table 50.3
Summary of Peripheral Nervous System Disorders

	Multiple Sclerosis	Myasthenia Gravis	Amyotrophic Lateral Sclerosis	Guillain-Barré Syndrome
Signs and Symptoms	Muscle weakness Muscle paralysis Visual disturbances Fatigue	Progressive severe weakness of voluntary muscles Muscles regain strength with rest Masklike face	Progressive muscle weakness Decreased coordination Muscle twitching Muscle spasms Pain Emotional outbursts Difficulty with speech	Three stages: 1. Ascending paralysis 2. Plateau 3. Descending resolution Pain, cramping, or numbness
Diagnosis	CSF analysis MRI gMS Dx (blood test)	Ptosis test Tensilon test EMG	CSF analysis EEG Nerve biopsy NCV	CSF EMG NCV
Therapeutic Measures	Interferon therapy Steroids Immunosuppressants Plasmapheresis Anticonvulsants Antiviral agents Muscle relaxants Physical therapy Speech therapy	Plasmapheresis Thymectomy Anticholinesterase agents Steroids	Antispasmodics/quinine Riluzole (Rilutek) Physical therapy Massage Muscle relaxants Diversional activities Enteral feeding Alternative communications devices	Plasmapheresis Ventilation support Physical therapy
Complications	Falls Muscle spasms Bowel and bladder problems; risk for UTI Forgetfulness Extreme fatigue	Aspiration Respiratory infections Respiratory failure Myasthenic crisis or cholinergic crisis	Communication problems Risk for aspiration Pain Respiratory failure	Respiratory infection Respiratory failure Depression Fatigue UTI Complications of immobility
Priority Nursing Diagnoses	*Ineffective Airway Clearance* *Impaired Physical Mobility* *Imbalanced Nutrition: Less Than Body Requirements* *Impaired Verbal Communication*			

CSF = cerebrospinal fluid; EEG = electroencephalogram; EMG = electromyography; MRI = magnetic resonance imaging; NCV = nerve conduction velocity; UTI = urinary tract infection.

---

disorders include tumors, infections, inflammation, trauma, and unknown causes. Two common cranial nerve problems are trigeminal neuralgia (tic douloureux) and Bell palsy.

Trigeminal Neuralgia
Pathophysiology and Etiology
Trigeminal **neuralgia** (TN), sometimes called *tic douloureux*, involves the fifth cranial (trigeminal) nerve. This nerve has three branches that include both sensory and motor functions. The branches innervate areas of the face, including the forehead, nose, cheek, gums, and jaw. TN affects only the sensory portion of the nerve. Irritation or chronic compression of the nerve is suspected to cause symptoms. This condition is more common in women and usually begins about age 50 to 60.

• WORD • BUILDING •
neuralgia: neur—nerve + algia—pain

Signs and Symptoms

TN causes recurring episodes of intense pain, described as sudden, jabbing, burning, or knifelike. Episodes of pain begin and end suddenly, lasting a few seconds to minutes. Attacks occur in clusters from a few times a year to up to hundreds of times daily. Pain is felt in the skin on one side of the face. A slight touch, cold breeze, talking, or chewing can trigger attacks of pain. The areas of the face where pain occurs are referred to as *trigger zones*. Areas affected include the lips, upper or lower gums, cheeks, forehead, or side of the nose (Fig. 50.3). Sleep provides a period of relief from the pain. Therefore, persons with TN may sleep most of the time to avoid painful attacks. They also may refrain from activities such as talking, face washing, teeth brushing, shaving, and eating to prevent pain. Frequent blinking and tearing of the eye on the affected side also occur.

Diagnostic Tests

Diagnosis is generally made by MRI combined with a history of symptoms and direct observation of an attack.

Therapeutic Measures

Initial management includes carbamazepine (Tegretol) or oxcarbazepine (Oxtellar XR) to reduce transmission of painful nerve impulses. Commonly administered analgesics and opioids are typically not effective in managing the sharp, intense pain.

If medications are ineffective, microvascular decompression may be done to relieve compression on the nerve. Other methods such as radiation, injection, or heat may be used to destroy the sensory portion of the trigeminal nerve. These interventions leave the patient with varying degrees of numbness and are supported by only limited evidence. Complementary and alternative therapies such as botulinum toxin (Botox) injection, acupuncture, electrical stimulation, and nutritional therapy have also been used with varying success.

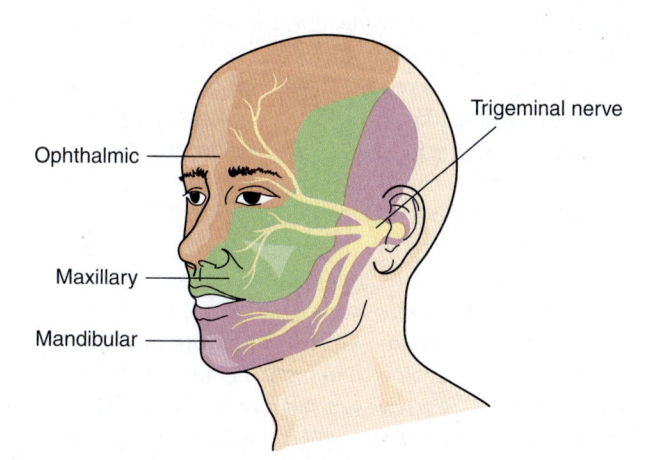

FIGURE 50.3 Areas innervated by the three main branches of the trigeminal nerve (cranial nerve V) are affected in trigeminal neuralgia.

The patient will need to learn to protect anesthetized areas of the face after nerve procedures. If corneal sensation is lost, goggles and sunglasses should be used as needed to protect the affected eye. An eye patch may be needed at night to prevent injury during sleep. Artificial tears may also be needed to prevent corneal damage.

Bell Palsy

Pathophysiology and Etiology

In Bell palsy, the facial nerve (cranial nerve VII) becomes inflamed and edematous, interrupting nerve impulses. This condition is thought to arise from nerve trauma from a viral infection such as herpes simplex (most common), herpes zoster, influenza B, or Epstein-Barr. Loss of motor control typically occurs on one side of the face; bilateral facial palsy occurs rarely. Contracture of facial muscles can occur if recovery is slow. Men and women are affected equally. Bell palsy is more common in women in the third trimester of pregnancy, people with immune disorders such as HIV, and people with diabetes. It occurs in all ages, including children.

Signs and Symptoms

Onset of symptoms may be sudden or progress over a 2- to 5-day period. Pain behind the ear may precede the onset of facial paralysis. Other vague initial symptoms are dry eye or tingling around the lips with progression to the more recognizable symptoms of Bell palsy. The patient may be unable to close the eyelid, wrinkle the forehead, smile, raise the eyebrow, or close the lips effectively. The mouth is pulled toward the unaffected side (Fig. 50.4). Drooling of saliva occurs, and the affected eye has constant tearing. Sense of taste is lost over the anterior two-thirds of the tongue. Speech difficulties occur. Most patients recover completely within 6 months (see "Patient Perspective").

> **PRACTICE ANALYSIS TIP**
> **Linking NCLEX-PN® to Practice**
> The LPN/LVN assists in the care of a client experiencing sensory/perceptual alterations.

Diagnostic Tests

History of the onset of symptoms is used to diagnose Bell palsy. Observation of the patient confirms the diagnosis. EMG may be done. The possibility of a stroke must be ruled out.

Therapeutic Measures

Prevention of complications is the goal of treatment. Prednisone may be given over 7 to 10 days to decrease inflammation. Antiviral agents such as acyclovir (Zovirax) may be used in combination with prednisone in severe cases. Eye drops to provide artificial tears and eye protection are needed if the eyelid does not completely close. Analgesics

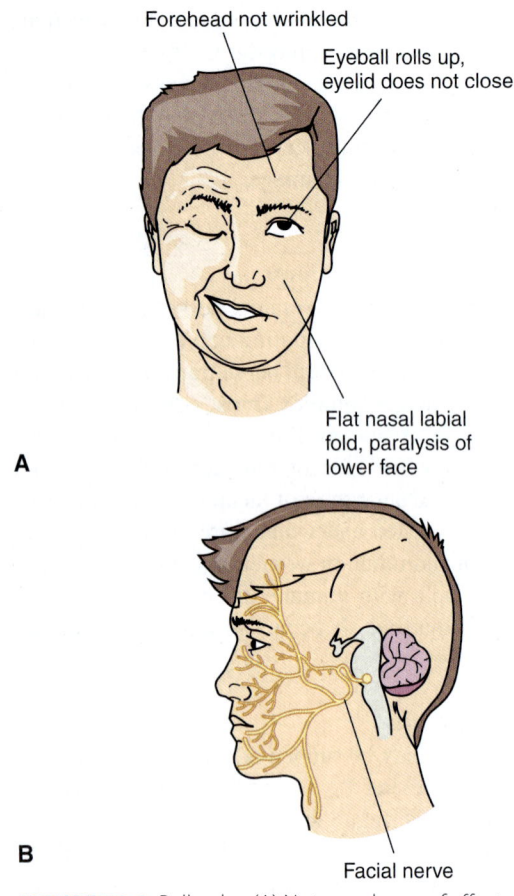

FIGURE 50.4 Bell palsy. (A) Note weakness of affected side of face. (B) Distribution of facial nerve.

are given for pain control. Moist heat and gentle massage to the face and ear can ease pain. A facial sling can be used to aid in eating and support of facial muscles.

> **BE SAFE!**
> **AVOID FAILURE TO RECOGNIZE!** You can prevent aspiration by recognizing neurological patients at risk for aspiration and initiating appropriate preventive interventions. Patients at risk may cough or sneeze during meals, have uncoordinated or delayed swallowing, pocket food, or have a wet-sounding voice after meals. Collaborate with HCP and speech therapy.

Nursing Process for the Patient With a Cranial Nerve Disorder

Data Collection

Monitor pain using the **WHAT'S UP?** format, being sure to include factors that trigger pain. Are sensory or motor problems associated with the pain? Determine the effect of the disorder on the patient's life, including nutritional status, general and oral hygiene, behavior, and emotional state. Carefully document all findings.

Patient Perspective
Angela

I woke up that Thursday morning with the same intense pain in my forehead that I had been experiencing for the past week. When I rolled out of bed, I realized that I didn't have morning breath (or so I thought). Knowing that I had not brushed my teeth yet, I did so and noticed that I could not taste the toothpaste. The fruit cup I ate for lunch tasted like bleach. I chomped on each bite, then carefully attempted to swallow. It was like I had been injected with several shots of Novocain. My throat felt like it had closed, and each swallow took a concentrated effort. Over the course of eating my fruit, I managed to bite my tongue three times.

I was 35 weeks pregnant and on strict bedrest due to pregnancy-induced hypertension and severe edema (which later spiraled into toxemia). We attributed the numbness in my mouth to the edema. I had already swollen up like a balloon and had experienced intense numbness in my extremities since the 12th week of pregnancy. As the afternoon progressed, I grew more and more concerned. I knew something was not quite right. By 5:30 that evening, I had lost control of the entire left side of my face. I called my obstetrician, and she said to get to the emergency department (ED) because I was either having a stroke or had developed Bell palsy. The doctor at the ED confirmed that I had Bell palsy and prescribed valacyclovir (Valtrex) and prednisone to treat it.

The symptoms I experienced were severe pain in my forehead, not being able to breathe out of the left side of my nose, and difficulty chewing, swallowing, and saying most consonants. I completely lost the ability to smile, blink, close my eye, raise my eyebrow, or use a straw or blow. My eyesight in the left eye blurred, and I could not go out at night due to the intense pain behind my eye triggered by headlights and having to use eye drops every 5 to 20 minutes.

I delivered my baby 2 weeks after being diagnosed with Bell palsy. During labor, I continuously asked for my eye drops, and the pain in my head was so fierce that it overshadowed the contractions.

After delivery, I was desperate for my face to be "fixed." I tried everything that anyone suggested—herbal supplements, chiropractic medicine, facial massage, laser treatments, facial exercise, shock treatments, a neurologist consultation, and physical therapy. The only thing that has worked for me is time (and lots of it)!

For the first 15 weeks after being diagnosed, I wanted to hide from the world. However, here it is, 7 months later, and I have come to terms with it. I am constantly aware of it, though I have regained a tremendous amount of the muscle control. I still have not shared a "real smile" with my daughter and do not blink my left eye. Covering my mouth when I smile or laugh so others do not see has become almost like a reflex now.

Chapter 50 Nursing Care of Patients With Peripheral Nervous System Disorders

Nursing Diagnoses, Planning, and Implementation

Acute Pain related to inflammation or compression of the nerve

EXPECTED OUTCOME: The patient will state pain is controlled at an acceptable level.

- Administer medications as needed for pain. Anticonvulsant and antidepressant agents used to treat neuropathic pain must be given routinely to prevent pain. *Medications prevent or decrease pain and increase comfort.*
- Discuss and implement alternative and complementary pain relief measures *to complement medications and increase the patient's control over pain.*
- Plan hygiene activities when pain relief is at its peak *to decrease discomfort with activities.*
- Provide alternative communication methods (e.g., paper and pencil, dry erase board, communication board, visual pain scale). *The patient may not be able to speak clearly or may not want to speak due to pain.*
- Remind patient to chew on the opposite side of the face *to avoid triggering pain and injury.*
- Encourage use of an electric razor rather than blades *to prevent injury to numb areas.*
- Provide measures for trigeminal neuralgia *to reduce pain triggers:*
  - Provide soft cloths for facial hygiene using lukewarm water.
  - Avoid touching the patient's face.
  - Provide a soft bristle toothbrush for oral care.
  - Protect the face from cold or wind.
- Provide measures for Bell palsy *to reduce pain and prevent muscle atrophy:*
  - Provide warm, moist compresses as needed.
  - Massage face.
  - Assist with facial exercises as prescribed by physical therapy.
  - Provide a facial sling.

Imbalanced Nutrition: Less Than Body Requirements related to fear of triggering pain as evidenced by poor intake and weight loss

EXPECTED OUTCOME: The patient will maintain sufficient nutrition as evidenced by stable weight.

- Weigh patient twice weekly and record *to monitor weight loss or gain.*
- Provide small, frequent meals *to promote nutrition without increasing pain.*
- Provide soft, easy-to-chew foods at lukewarm temperature *to prevent triggering pain.*
- Provide a high-protein and high-calorie diet. *Protein and calories are needed for cellular repair.*
- Avoid hot or cold foods and drinks. *Temperature extremes can trigger pain. If foods are associated with pain, the patient may avoid them.*
- Encourage oral hygiene after each meal and at bedtime *to prevent gum and tooth disease as triggers for pain.*
- Insert an enteral feeding tube as ordered into the nostril on the unaffected side if nutrition is severely impaired *to provide means for nutrient intake while avoiding painful nerve areas.*

Risk for Injury to Eyes related to inability to blink (Bell palsy)

EXPECTED OUTCOME: The patient's cornea will remain intact and without injury.

- Administer eye drops or eye ointment as ordered by the HCP *to protect the eye.*
- The patient should use a patch over the affected eye *to protect the eye.*
- Advise the patient to wear glasses or goggles, especially when outside or in areas with particles in the air, *to protect the eyes.*

Evaluation

Nursing care has been successful if the patient reports that pain is controlled, nutrition is maintained with no inappropriate weight loss, and the eyes are intact and without injury.

> **LEARNING TIP**
> Remember: Trigeminal neuralgia (cranial nerve V) is a sensory disorder; Bell palsy (cranial nerve VII) is a motor disorder.

Key Points

- PNS disorders can be acute or chronic. Two common types of PNS disorders are neuromuscular disorders (motor or sensory) and cranial nerve disorders.
- MS is a chronic progressive degenerative disease where the myelin sheath begins to break down due to the activation of the immune system. MS patients experience a variety of symptoms, including muscle weakness, tingling sensations, numbness, or visual disturbances, usually in one eye at a time. Symptoms may begin slowly over weeks to months or start suddenly and dramatically.
- Periods of exacerbation and remission lead patients with MS to be uncertain about when the disease will flare up and what body system will be affected.
- MG is a chronic autoimmune process that causes weakness of the voluntary or skeletal muscles.

- MG results in progressive extreme muscle weakness. The classic sign of MG is increased muscle weakness during activity and improvement in muscle strength after rest. Muscles are strongest in the morning when the person is rested. Activities affected by MG include eye and eyelid movements, chewing, swallowing, speaking, and breathing, as well as skeletal muscle function.
- ALS, also called *Lou Gehrig disease*, is a progressive, degenerative condition that affects motor neurons, blocking transmission of nerve impulses.
- As the ALS progresses, more muscle groups, including muscles controlling breathing and swallowing, become involved.
- ALS symptoms begin in the arms, legs, or muscles of speech and swallowing. Atrophy of muscles and fasciculation also occur. Late in the disease, the patient may only be able to communicate with eye blinking. ALS eventually leads to death from respiratory complications such as atelectasis, respiratory failure, and pneumonia.
- GBS is an inflammatory disorder caused by an autoimmune response to a viral infection and on rare occasions after certain vaccines. Symmetrical paresis and paralysis usually begin in lower extremities and can progress to respiratory involvement.
- Postpolio syndrome affects survivors of polio and involves progressive weakness and muscle atrophy.
- RLS is an uncomfortable sensation in the legs, causing the sufferer to constantly feel the need to move the legs especially at night.
- Cranial nerve disorders include trigeminal neuralgia and Bell palsy. TN, sometimes called *tic douloureux*, occurs when the fifth cranial nerve (trigeminal) becomes irritated. TN affects only the sensory portion of the nerve. It causes intense recurring episodes of pain described as sudden, jabbing, burning, or knifelike on one side of the face. Episodes may happen frequently or intermittently.
- In Bell palsy, the facial nerve (cranial nerve VII) becomes inflamed and edematous, causing interruption of nerve impulses. Bell palsy can often be traced back to a viral infection such as Epstein-Barr, herpes simplex, or herpes zoster. Loss of motor control typically occurs on one side of the face. The patient with Bell palsy may be unable to close the eyelid, wrinkle the forehead, smile, raise the eyebrow, or close the lips effectively. The eyes should be protected from injury. Patients can have drooling, eye tearing, speech difficulty and loss of taste. Most patients recover completely within 6 months.

SUGGESTED ANSWERS TO CHAPTER EXERCISES

Cue Recognition
50.1: Follow the office protocol for securing emergency assistance for this patient.

Critical Thinking & Clinical Judgment
Alba
1. Muscle weakness caused by MG improves with rest, unlike that caused by MS.
2. Have Alba look up for 2 to 3 minutes. If ptosis occurs, have her close her eyes for several minutes. If she can open her eyelids and look up, MG is likely. Of course, diagnosis will be done by a neurologist.
3. $\dfrac{2 \text{ mg}}{10 \text{ mg}} \times 1 \text{ mL} = 0.2 \text{ mL}$
4. The team may include a nurse, occupational therapist, physical therapist, neurologist, pharmacist, dietitian, and primary HCP for other health issues.
5. Notify the neurologist that the patient is taking metoprolol, a medication that can cause exacerbations. See Table 50.3 for other medications that may cause exacerbations in patients with MG. Alba will most likely need to be hospitalized for this exacerbation due to the potential effects on her respiratory system.

Mr. Miller
1. Priority nursing diagnoses include *Ineffective Airway Clearance* and *Risk for Aspiration related to muscle weakness*. If a patient's respiratory system is compromised by a disease, nursing care should be focused on maintaining pulmonary function to preserve life.
2. Providing compassionate care to the patient and providing information about the disease and its prognosis to the patient and family establish an honest and supportive relationship. Support groups provide resources and emotional support.
3. The team may include a registered nurse, respiratory therapist, speech pathologist, neurologist, and dietitian. In addition, find out who at your institution helps patients make end-of-life decisions. A palliative care specialist or social worker can help the patient and family work through some difficult decisions and develop an advance directive.

Additional Resources

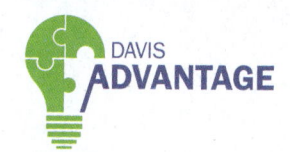

Go to Davis Advantage to complete your learning: strengthen understanding, apply your knowledge, and prepare for the Next Gen NCLEX®.

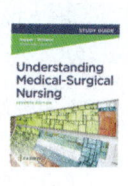

A Study Guide is also available.

UNIT FOURTEEN Understanding the Sensory System

CHAPTER 51
Sensory System Function, Data Collection, and Therapeutic Measures: Vision and Hearing

Lazette V. Nowicki, Janice L. Bradford

KEY TERMS

accommodation (ah-KOM-uh-DAY-shun)
arcus senilis (AR-kuss seh-NIL-iss)
cochlear implant (KOK-lee-ur IM-plant)
consensual response (kon-SEN-shoo-uhl ree-SPONS)
electroretinography (ee-LEK-troh-RET-in-AH-gruh-fee)
esotropia (ESS-oh-TROH-pee-ah)
exotropia (EKS-oh-TROH-pee-ah)
hearing aid (HEER-ing AYD)
hypotropia (HY-poh-TROH-pee-ah)
nystagmus (nye-STAG-mus)
ophthalmologist (AHF-thal-MAW-luh-jist)
ophthalmoscope (ahf-THAL-muh-skohp)
optician (op-TISH-uhn)
optometrist (op-TOM-uh-trist)
otalgia (oh-TAL-jee-ah)
otorrhea (OH-toh-REE-ah)
ototoxic (OH-toh-TOK-sik)
ptosis (TOH-sis)
Rinne test (RIN-eh test)
Romberg test (RAHM-berg test)
Snellen chart (SNEL-en chart)
tropia (TROH-pee-ah)
Weber test (VAY-ber test)

CHAPTER CONCEPTS

Safety
Sensory perception
Teaching and learning

LEARNING OUTCOMES

1. Describe the normal anatomy of the sensory system.
2. Explain the normal function of the sensory system.
3. List data to collect when caring for a patient with a disorder of the sensory system.
4. Identify diagnostic tests commonly performed to diagnose disorders of the sensory system.
5. Plan nursing care for patients undergoing diagnostic tests for sensory disorders.
6. Describe therapeutic measures for patients with disorders of the sensory system.

It is difficult to imagine experiencing inability to see or hear the world around us. Nurses assist patients in maintaining or coping with deficits in these primary senses.

VISION

Normal Anatomy and Physiology of the Eye
External Structures
Several structures protect the eye from desiccation (extreme dryness) and debris (Figs. 51.1 and 51.2).

Structure of the Eyeball
Most of the eyeball is within the orbit, the bony socket that protects the eye from trauma. The six extrinsic muscles that move the eyeball are attached to the orbit and to the outer surface of the eyeball. Four rectus muscles move the eyeball side to side or up and down. Two oblique muscles rotate the eye. The cranial nerves that innervate these muscles are the oculomotor, trochlear, and abducens (third, fourth, and sixth cranial nerves, respectively). Actions of the six extrinsic eye muscles allow voluntary control of movement. They are also innervated by the autonomic nervous system to perform convergence, alignment of the visual axis of each eye on the same field of view.

The wall of the eyeball has three layers: the outer fibrous tunic (sclera and cornea), the middle vascular tunic (choroid, ciliary body that suspends the lens, and iris), and the inner nervous tunic (retina; Fig. 51.3). The lens divides the interior of the eye into two main cavities: anterior cavity and posterior cavity. Anterior to the lens is the ring-shaped curtain called the iris. The iris divides the anterior cavity into two chambers: anterior chamber and posterior chamber (Fig. 51.4).

Chapter 51   Sensory System Function, Data Collection, and Therapeutic Measures: Vision and Hearing   1039

Eyebrow: Perhaps the most significant role of the eyebrows is to enhance facial expressions, aiding in nonverbal communication. They also help keep perspiration out of the eye and shield the eye from glare.

Eyelashes: These hairs along the edges of the eyelids help keep debris out of the eye. Touching the eyelashes stimulates the blink reflex.

Eyelids (palpebrae): Formed primarily by the orbicularis oculi muscle covered with skin, the eyelids protect the eye from foreign bodies and block light when closed to allow for sleeping. Periodic blinking also helps moisten the eyes with tears and wash out debris.

Conjunctiva: The conjunctiva is a transparent mucous membrane that lines the inner surface of the eyelid and covers the anterior surface of the eyeball (except for the cornea). It secretes a thin mucous film to help keep the eyeball moist. It is very vascular, which becomes apparent when eyes are "bloodshot," a result of dilated vessels in the conjunctiva.

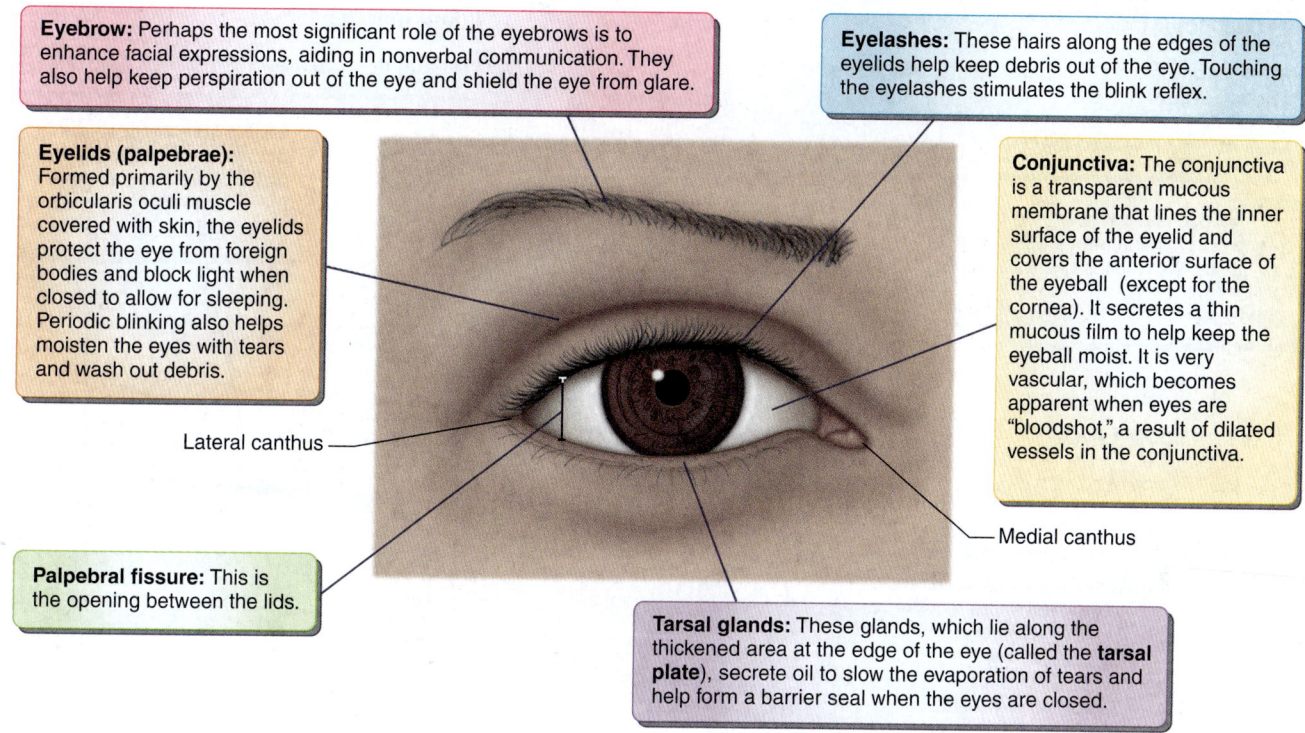

Lateral canthus

Medial canthus

Palpebral fissure: This is the opening between the lids.

Tarsal glands: These glands, which lie along the thickened area at the edge of the eye (called the **tarsal plate**), secrete oil to slow the evaporation of tears and help form a barrier seal when the eyes are closed.

FIGURE 51.1 Accessory structures of the eye.

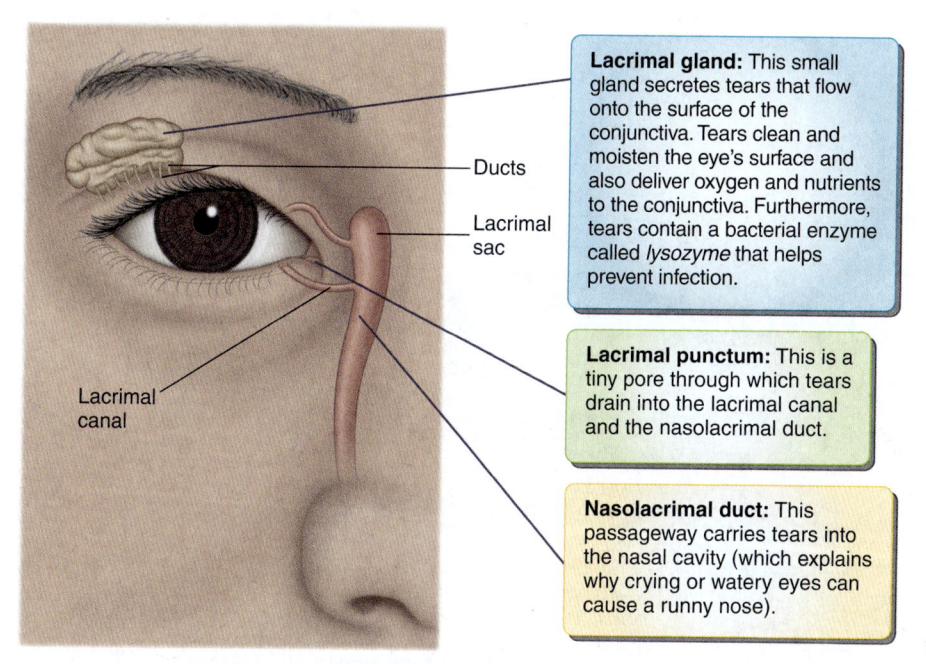

Ducts

Lacrimal sac

Lacrimal gland: This small gland secretes tears that flow onto the surface of the conjunctiva. Tears clean and moisten the eye's surface and also deliver oxygen and nutrients to the conjunctiva. Furthermore, tears contain a bacterial enzyme called *lysozyme* that helps prevent infection.

Lacrimal canal

Lacrimal punctum: This is a tiny pore through which tears drain into the lacrimal canal and the nasolacrimal duct.

Nasolacrimal duct: This passageway carries tears into the nasal cavity (which explains why crying or watery eyes can cause a runny nose).

FIGURE 51.2 Lacrimal apparatus.

The retina lines the posterior two-thirds of the eyeball and contains the photoreceptors (rods and cones). Rods detect the presence of light while cones respond to photons (the basic particle of light) of differing wavelengths. The fovea centralis is a small depression in the macula lutea of the posterior retina. It is directly behind the center of the lens and contains only cones. The fovea centralis, therefore, is the area of most acute color vision. Rods are proportionately more abundant toward the periphery of the retina, so night vision is best at the sides of the visual field.

Neurons called *ganglion cells* transmit the impulses generated by the rods and cones. These neurons all converge at the optic disc and pass through the wall of the eyeball as the optic nerve. The optic disc may also be called the *blind spot* because no rods or cones are present.

Fibrous Outer Layer

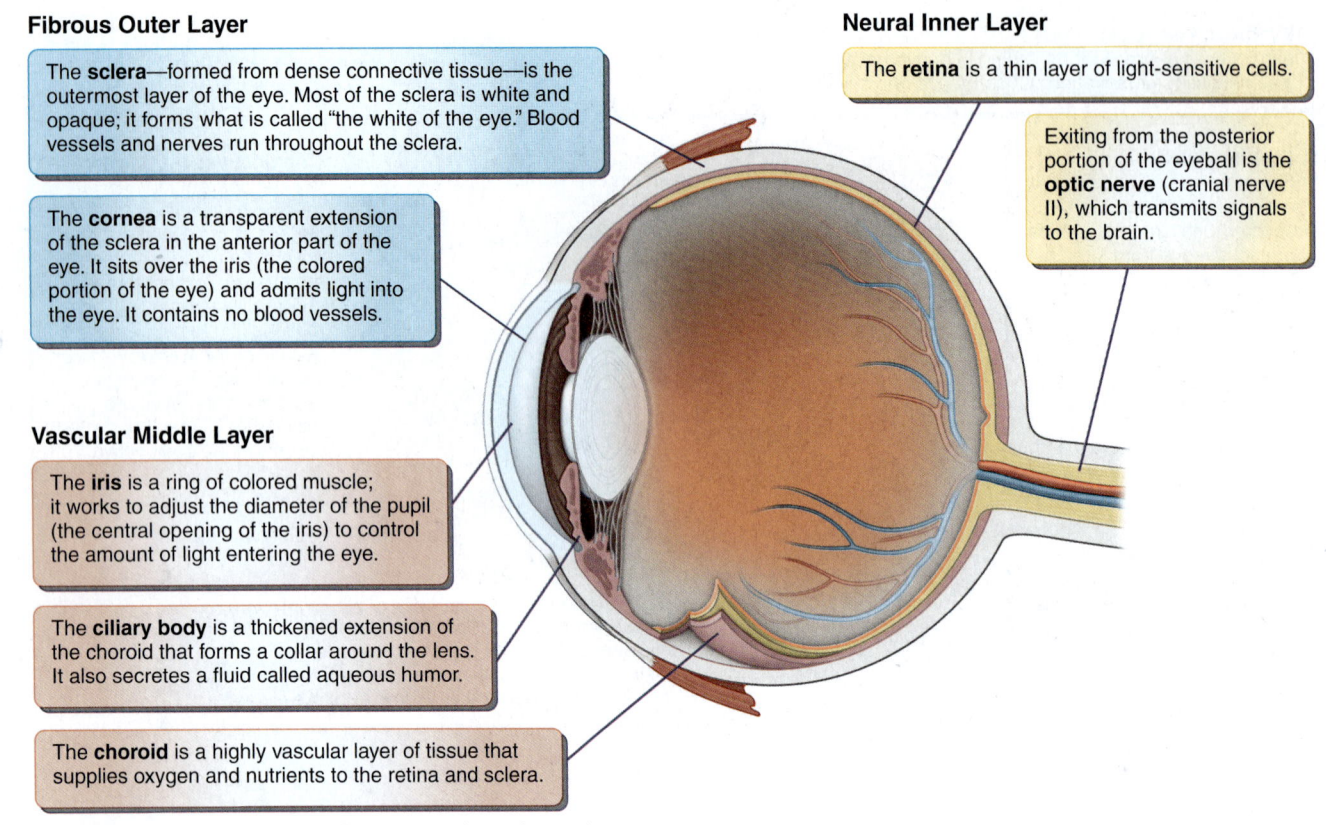

The **sclera**—formed from dense connective tissue—is the outermost layer of the eye. Most of the sclera is white and opaque; it forms what is called "the white of the eye." Blood vessels and nerves run throughout the sclera.

The **cornea** is a transparent extension of the sclera in the anterior part of the eye. It sits over the iris (the colored portion of the eye) and admits light into the eye. It contains no blood vessels.

Vascular Middle Layer

The **iris** is a ring of colored muscle; it works to adjust the diameter of the pupil (the central opening of the iris) to control the amount of light entering the eye.

The **ciliary body** is a thickened extension of the choroid that forms a collar around the lens. It also secretes a fluid called aqueous humor.

The **choroid** is a highly vascular layer of tissue that supplies oxygen and nutrients to the retina and sclera.

Neural Inner Layer

The **retina** is a thin layer of light-sensitive cells.

Exiting from the posterior portion of the eyeball is the **optic nerve** (cranial nerve II), which transmits signals to the brain.

FIGURE 51.3 Eye tissue layers—fibrous, vascular, and neural.

The space between the lens and the cornea is the **anterior cavity**. This cavity is further divided into an *anterior chamber* (anterior to the iris) and a *posterior chamber* (posterior to the iris but anterior to the lens). A clear, watery fluid called **aqueous humor** fills the anterior cavity.

The **lens** is a transparent disc of tissue just behind the pupil, between the anterior and posterior cavities. The lens changes shape for near and far vision.

The **posterior cavity** is the larger cavity lying posterior to the lens. It is filled with a jelly-like substance called **vitreous humor**. This semi-solid material helps keep the eyeball from collapsing.

- Anterior chamber
- Scleral venous sinus
- Posterior chamber

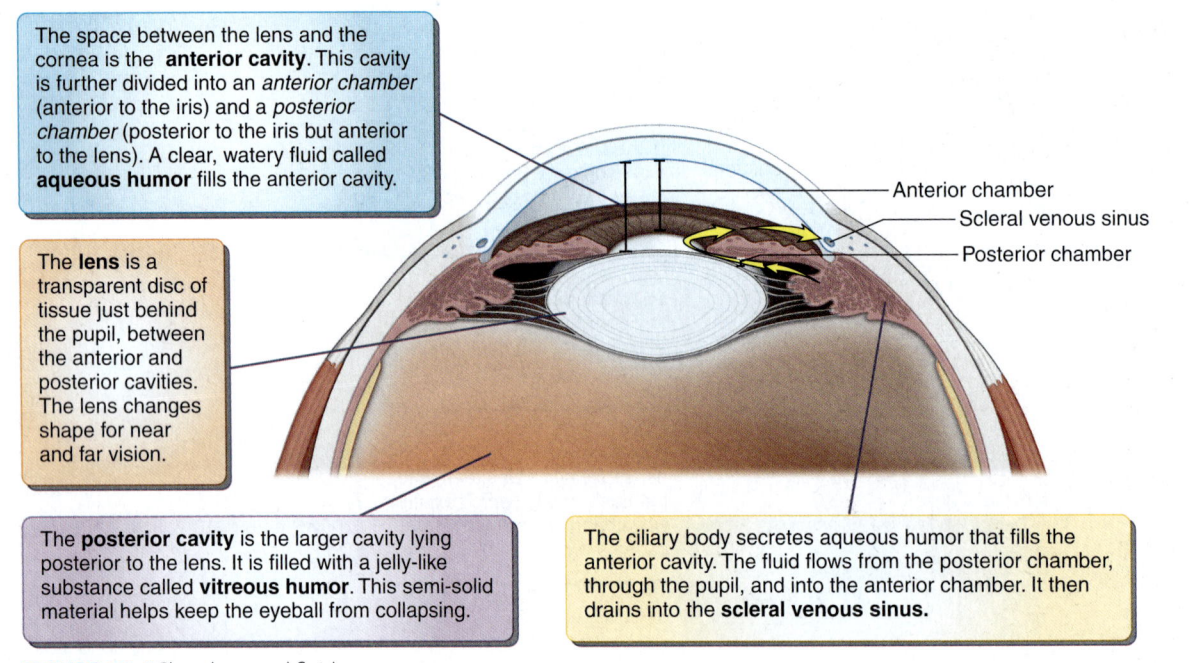

The ciliary body secretes aqueous humor that fills the anterior cavity. The fluid flows from the posterior chamber, through the pupil, and into the anterior chamber. It then drains into the **scleral venous sinus.**

FIGURE 51.4 Chambers and fluids.

Physiology of Vision

Vision involves the focusing of light rays on the retina and the transmission of the subsequent nerve impulses to the visual areas of the cerebral cortex. The refractive structures of the eye are, in order, the cornea, aqueous humor, lens, and vitreous humor. The lens is the only adjustable part of this focusing system. When the eye shifts focus to a nearby object, accommodation of the lens occurs (Fig. 51.5). Also, the pupil constricts in near vision to force photons through the thickness of the lens (Fig. 51.6). Accommodation and pupil constriction increase the number of photons that strike the fovea centralis.

Lens thins
Ciliary muscle relaxed

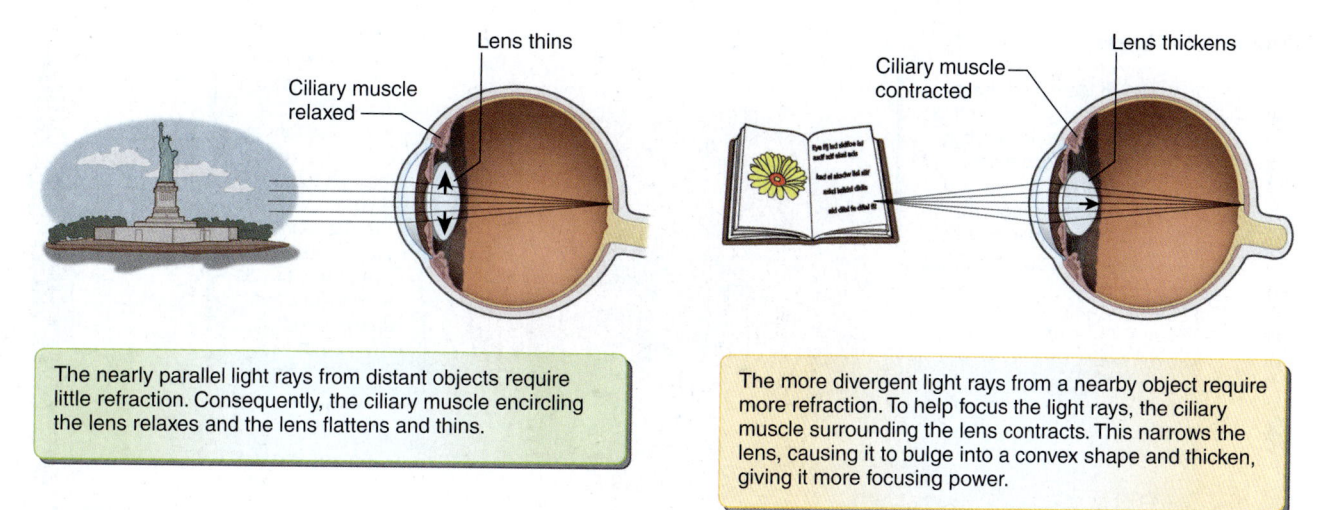

The nearly parallel light rays from distant objects require little refraction. Consequently, the ciliary muscle encircling the lens relaxes and the lens flattens and thins.

Lens thickens
Ciliary muscle contracted

The more divergent light rays from a nearby object require more refraction. To help focus the light rays, the ciliary muscle surrounding the lens contracts. This narrows the lens, causing it to bulge into a convex shape and thicken, giving it more focusing power.

FIGURE 51.5 Accommodation of the lens.

Pupil

Pupillary constrictor muscles

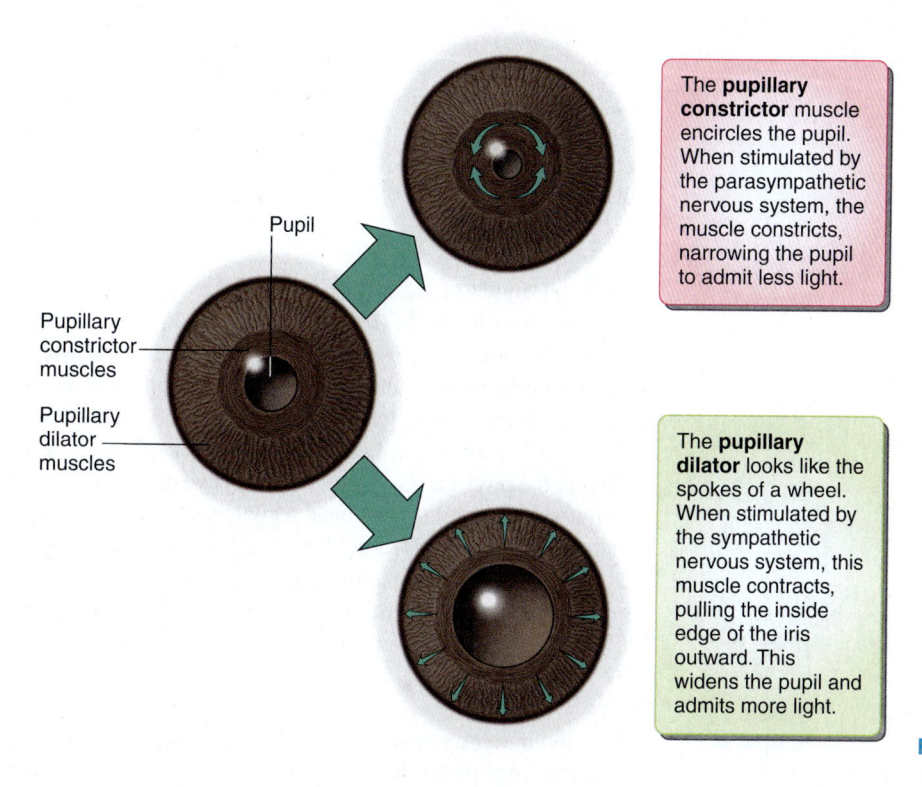

Pupillary dilator muscles

The **pupillary constrictor** muscle encircles the pupil. When stimulated by the parasympathetic nervous system, the muscle constricts, narrowing the pupil to admit less light.

The **pupillary dilator** looks like the spokes of a wheel. When stimulated by the sympathetic nervous system, this muscle contracts, pulling the inside edge of the iris outward. This widens the pupil and admits more light.

FIGURE 51.6 Constriction of the pupil.

When photons strike the retina, they stimulate chemical reactions in the rods and cones. Resultant changes generate a nerve impulse for transmission. Rods generate an action potential in dim light but only allow shades of gray vision. The cones are specialized to respond to a portion of the visible light spectrum; there are red-absorbing, blue-absorbing, and green-absorbing cones. Combinations of these cone types allow color interpretation (Fig. 51.7).

Refraction inverts the image onto the photoreceptors in the retina. Impulses from the rods and cones are transmitted to the ganglion neurons, which converge at the optic disc and become the optic nerve. The optic nerves from both eyes converge at the optic chiasma just in front of the pituitary gland. Here, the medial fibers of each optic nerve cross to the other side. This crossing permits each visual area to receive impulses from both eyes, which is important for binocular (two eyes) vision. The visual areas are in the occipital lobes of the cerebral cortex, where the upside-down retinal images are righted and the slightly different pictures from the two eyes are integrated into one image. This integration results in binocular vision, which also provides depth perception.

Aging and the Eye

The most common changes in the aging eye are those in the lens (Fig. 51.8), which may become partially or totally opaque. The lens loses its elasticity with age; most people

Rods
- Are located at the periphery of the retina
- Are active in dim light
- Are responsible for night vision
- Cannot distinguish colors from each other

Nucleus

Cones
- Are concentrated in the center of the retina (but are also scattered throughout the retina)
- Are active in bright light
- Are primarily responsible for sharp vision
- Are responsible for color vision

Nucleus

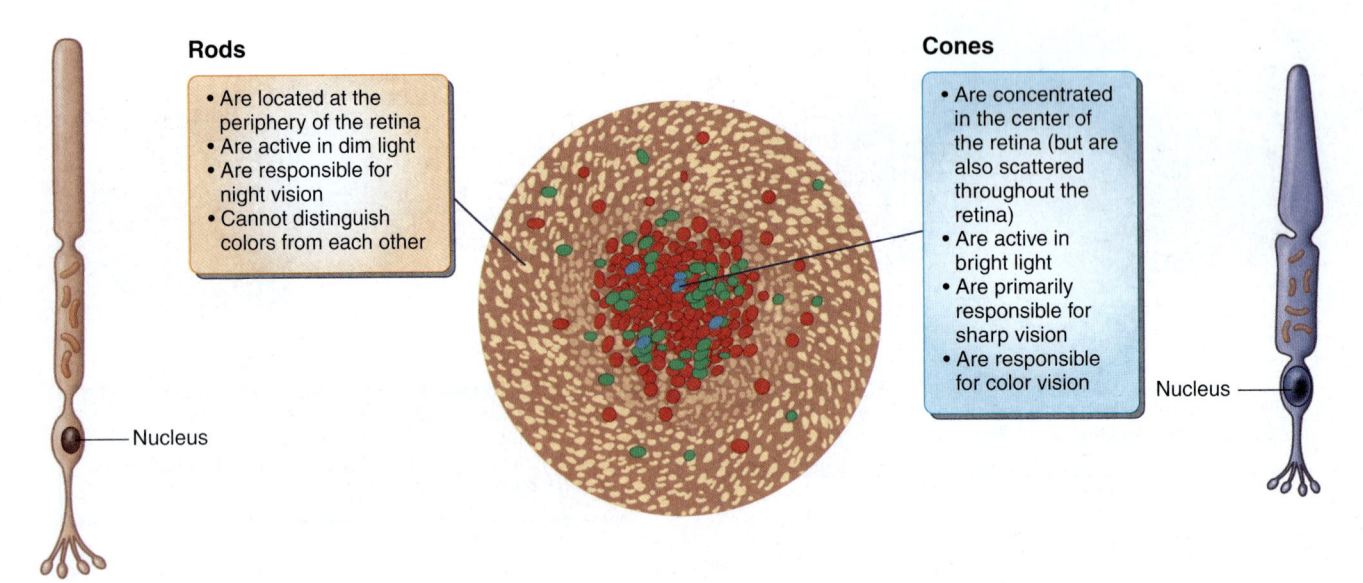

FIGURE 51.7 Action of photoreceptors.

FIGURE 51.8 Aging and the sensory system.

become farsighted and need corrective lenses for near vision by about age 40. Peripheral vision may decline. Depth perception decreases and glare intensifies, both of which can affect safety. Color vision fades with lesser discrimination of blue, green, and violet colors. Red, yellow, and orange colors are seen best.

Sensory System Data Collection of the Eye and Visual Status

Data collection of the eye begins with a subjective health history and objective observation, testing, and physical examination. Licensed practical nurses/licensed vocational nurses (LPN/LVNs) assist the health-care provider (HCP) in conducting the physical examination. Many eye diseases have no symptoms, so adults must have a comprehensive eye examination. Goals from Healthy People 2030 are to increase the percentage of adults having comprehensive eye examinations in the last 2 years to a target of 61.1 % of the population (Office of Disease Prevention and Health Promotion, 2020a).

Health History

Ask about family history that can affect vision, including diabetes, hypertension, glaucoma, cataracts, and blindness. Eye disorders and diseases can be genetically transmitted. Patients are asked about general health status and disorders such as diabetes, hypertension, cancer, thyroid disorders, or rheumatoid arthritis. A medication review checks for eye side effects. The patient is asked about eye symptoms or changes in visual acuity (Table 51.1).

Physical Examination

VISUAL ACUITY. Visual acuity is measured in several ways (Table 51.2). It often begins with the use of a **Snellen chart** or an E chart to measure distance acuity. A handheld visual acuity chart (Rosenbaum card) measures near acuity. The Snellen chart has lines of letters labeled for visual acuity that range in size from the largest letters at the top to the smallest

Table 51.1
Subjective Data Collection for the Eye

Questions to Ask During the Health History	Rationale
Family History	
Do you have any family members with a history of diabetes? Hypertension? Cataracts? Glaucoma? Blindness? Diabetes mellitus? Do any family members wear glasses or contact lenses? Is their vision corrected with the lens?	Many eye disorders are genetically transmitted.
Health History	
What health problems do you currently have? How are they treated? What health problems or trauma to your eyes have you had in the past?	Some metabolic disorders are precursors to eye disorders, such as diabetes and hypertension.
What medications do you take?	Look for ocular effects of systemic medications.
How often do you have eye examinations? When was the last time you had an eye examination? Do you wear protective eyewear (e.g., sunglasses, safety goggles) and hats in the sun?	Identify preventive practices and need for further teaching.
Visual Acuity	
Do you wear glasses or contact lenses? Have you had any changes in vision, such as difficulty seeing distances or up close, sensitivity to light, or difficulty seeing at night? Do you have double vision? Do you have clouded vision? Do you see halos around lights? Does it look like you are looking through a veil or web? Is there pain? Itching? Tearing? Burning? Dryness? Do you have headaches? If so, what are the precipitating events?	Any of these signs and symptoms could indicate visual disorders/disturbances.

at the bottom (Fig. 51.9). For the Snellen or E chart test, people stand 20 feet from the chart. They cover one eye and read aloud a line of letters. The lowest line (smallest letters) on the chart that the patient can read accurately designates the visual acuity of that eye. The E chart is used for people with literacy issues. The patient indicates the direction of the E-shaped figure. The handheld visual acuity chart is held by the patient 14 inches from the eyes to read the letters. The LogMAR chart was created to provide better visual acuity measurement than the other visual acuity charts. Similar to the Snellen chart, it measures distance acuity.

Normal vision is defined as 20/20. This means the patient can see at 20 feet what the normal eye clearly sees at 20 feet. Moderate low vision is defined as 20/70 through 20/160. Legal blindness in the United States occurs at 20/200 in the best eye with the best possible correction. Most people defined as blind still have some sight. The LogMAR rates 20/20 vision as 0.00, low vision as 0.5 through 1.3, and higher than 1.3 as legal blindness.

The vision acuity test is done on each eye separately and then both eyes together. A documentation example of low vision acuity findings is: "oculus dexter (OD) [right eye] 20/70, oculus sinister (OS) [left eye] 20/70, oculus uterque (OU) [both eyes] 20/70." This example means the patient must be 20 feet from an object to see what a patient with normal vision would see from 70 feet away. The test is done with and without the patient's corrective lenses, if applicable. When corrective lenses are used, documentation reflects this as "OD 20/70 without correction, OD 20/20 with correction."

VISUAL FIELDS. Peripheral vision is the distance the eye sees objects up, down, right, and left while looking straight ahead. The confrontation visual field test is a basic, quick test, named because the HCP faces the patient 2 feet away. Then, the HCP compares their own normal ability to see peripheral objects with the patient's ability to see these objects. The patient covers one eye and stares at the HCP. The HCP covers their own corresponding eye (e.g., if the

Table 51.2
Objective Data Collection for the Eye

Abnormal Findings	Possible Causes
Visual Acuity	
Hyperopia, myopia, presbyopia blurred or cloudy vision	Refractive error, opacity, or disorder of pathway.
Visual Fields	
Peripheral field loss	Retinopathy, macular degeneration, or glaucoma.
Muscle Balance and Eye Movement	
Nystagmus Inability to move in all six fields	Cranial nerve impairment, inner ear conditions, stroke or diseases of the central nervous system.
Asymmetry of corneal light reflex	Muscle weakness such as with a lazy eye
Drifting eye with cover test	Muscle weakness.
Pupillary Reflexes	
Dilated, fixed, or constricted pupils Absence of constriction or convergence	Medications, recreational drug use, brain or eye injury.
External Structures	
Ptosis Opaque whitening of outer rim of cornea Corneal opaqueness	Nerve dysfunction Arcus senilis Cataract, trauma

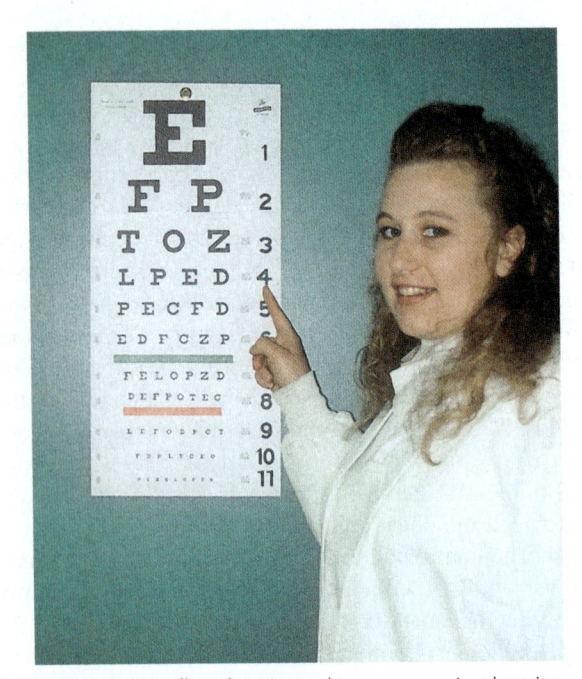

FIGURE 51.9 A Snellen chart is used to measure visual acuity.

patient's right eye is covered, the HCP's left eye is covered). The HCP extends their arm to the side and moves their fingers back into the visual field from three directions: superior, inferior, and temporal (middle). The patient indicates when the fingers are seen. The patient has full visual fields if the patient and HCP see the fingers at the same place for both eyes. Perimetry is computerized testing that maps one's peripheral vision. It gives more accurate results and tracks vision changes over time.

MUSCLE BALANCE AND EYE MOVEMENT. To test extraocular muscle balance and cranial nerve function, the patient and HCP face each other. The patient looks straight ahead. The HCP moves their finger in the six cardinal fields of gaze, returning to the point of origin between each field of gaze (Fig. 51.10). The patient follows the HCP's finger without moving the head. The purpose is to see if the patient's eyes can follow the HCP's finger in all fields of gaze without **nystagmus**, an involuntary, cyclical, rapid movement of the eyes.

The corneal light reflex test checks muscle balance, conducted by shining a penlight toward the cornea while the patient stares at an object straight ahead. The light reflection

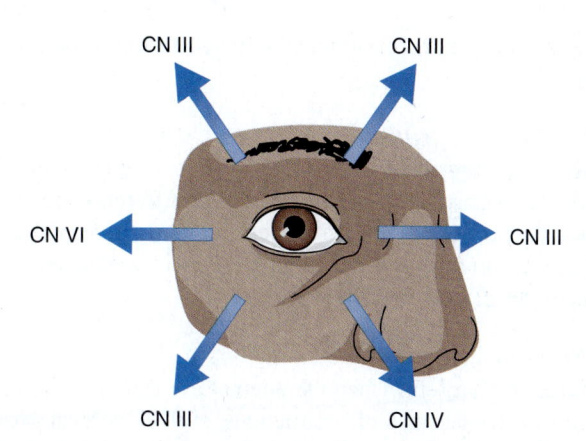

FIGURE 51.10 Six cardinal fields of gaze.

should be at exactly the same place on both pupils. If eyes lack symmetry, muscle weakness could be present.

The cover test is used along with an abnormal corneal light reflex test to evaluate eye muscle balance. Deviation of the eye away from the visual axis is known as **tropia**. Deviation toward the nose is **esotropia**. Movement laterally is **exotropia**. Downward deviation is **hypotropia**.

PUPILLARY REFLEXES. When observed, the pupils should be round, symmetrical, and reactive to light. To test pupillary response to light, both consensual and direct examinations should be completed. A slightly darkened room works best. The patient looks straight ahead, and the size of the pupil is noted. A penlight is shone toward the pupil from the side of the eye. Movement of the pupil is observed. The pupil should quickly constrict. The size of the pupil is noted when it constricts, known as direct response.

To conduct a consensual pupil examination, observe the eye just tested for reaction while shining the penlight into the other eye. The observed pupil should constrict. This is known as **consensual response**. Repeat the procedure for the opposite eye.

The HCP proceeds to test for **accommodation**, or the ability of the pupil to respond to near and far distances. The patient is told to look at an object far away. The size and shape of the pupils are observed. The HCP continues to observe pupils as the patient focuses on a near object (the HCP's penlight or finger) about 5 inches from the patient's face. Normally, the patient's eyes turn inward and the pupils constrict. These responses—convergence and constriction— are called *accommodation* (see "Gerontological Issues: Age-Related Changes in Vision"). HCPs use the acronym PERRLA to indicate pupils equal, round, reactive to light, and accommodation. If accommodation is not tested along with the other tests, the acronym used is PERRL.

INSPECTION AND PALPATION OF EXTERNAL STRUCTURES. Extraocular structures are inspected and presence of eyebrows, symmetry, hair texture, size, and extension of the brow are noted. The HCP first inspects and palpates the orbital area for edema, lesions, puffiness, and tenderness.

> **Gerontological Issues**
>
> **Age-Related Changes in Vision**
> Older adults commonly have vision changes such as the following:
> - Presbyopia, an inability to focus up close because of decreased elasticity in the ocular lens
> - Narrowing of the visual field and more difficulty with peripheral vision
> - Decreased pupil size and responsiveness to light
> - Difficulty with vision in dimly lit areas or at night (requires more light to see adequately)
> - Increased opacity of the lens, which causes sensitivity to glare, blurred vision, and interference with night vision
> - Yellowing of the lens, which reduces ability to differentiate low-tone colors of blues, greens, and violets (yellow, orange, and red hues are more clearly visible)
> - Distorted depth perception and difficulty correctly judging the height of curbs and steps
> - Decreased lacrimal secretions
>
> Because visual accommodation decreases with aging, older adults have an increased risk of falling. An older person has difficulty making a visual adjustment when moving from a well-lit room into the evening darkness, for example, or when stepping out of a dark area into the sunlight. The increased time needed to accommodate to near and far and to dark and light is often the reason that older adults do not drive at night.
>
> One of the most effective ways to improve vision for older adults is to ensure that their eyeglasses are cleaned daily and as needed.

Then, eyelids are inspected for symmetry, presence of eyelashes, eyelash position, tremors, flakiness, redness, and swelling. The patient is asked to open and close the eyelids. When open, the eyelid should cover the iris margin but not the pupil. The distance between the upper and lower eyelid, the palpebral fissure, is inspected and should be equal in both eyes. If the palpebral fissure is nonsymmetrical, observe for **ptosis**, drooping of the eyelid common in stroke patients. Next, the medial canthus of the lower lid is gently palpated and observed for exudate. The eyelids are palpated for nodules. The eye is palpated for firmness over the closed eyelid.

External eyes are inspected for color and symmetry of the irises, clarity of the cornea, and depth and clarity of the anterior chamber. Shining a light obliquely across the cornea shows the clearness of the cornea, which should be transparent without cloudiness. In individuals older than 40, bilateral

• WORD • BUILDING •

esotropia: eso—inward + tropia—movement of the eye
exotropia: exo—out + tropia—movement of the eye

opaque whitening of the outer rim of the cornea known as **arcus senilis** may occur. It is caused from lipid deposits and is considered normal. It does not affect vision.

INTERNAL EYE EXAMINATION. Examination of the internal eye is done by an HCP. A dark room allows the pupil to dilate. Anticholinergic mydriatic eye drops that cause dilation may be used but are not always necessary. An **ophthalmoscope** is a handheld instrument with a light source. It magnifies the internal structures of the eye. For the examination, the patient is asked to hold the head still while looking at a distant object. They are informed that the bright light could be uncomfortable. The HCP can examine the internal eye using a stationary device called a *slit-lamp microscope*. For this examination, the patient is seated and rests the chin on a support while a microscope and a bright light source are directed into the eye.

Estimation of intraocular pressure is measured by using one of several types of tonometers. The procedure may be performed using anesthetic drops. Readings above the normal range of 10 to 21 mm Hg may indicate glaucoma.

> **CUE RECOGNITION 51.1**
>
> You are caring for an older adult patient who stumbles when he gets up to use the bathroom at night. He states he has difficulty seeing at night. Upon examination of his eye and lens, you observe opacity. What action do you take?
>
> *Suggested answers are at the end of the chapter.*

Diagnostic Eye Tests

Exudate Culture
If exudate from any part of the eye or surrounding structure is present, an eye culture may be ordered. Results of the culture guide anti-infective treatment.

Digital Imaging
Digital imaging is a newer way of viewing most of the retina without the use of dilating eye drops. The instrument takes a digital picture of the retina in 2 seconds. Digital imaging assists in early detection of eye disease. A permanent photographic reference for the retina is obtained.

Optical Coherence Tomography
Optical coherence tomography takes a picture of the retina. Light beams are shone into the eye at various angles. The amount of interference is measured, creating a detailed image of retinal depth.

Fluorescein and Indocyanine Green Angiography
Angiography with dye is a test using special cameras to find leaking or damaged blood vessels in retinal or deeper choroidal circulation. The patient is asked about prior dye reactions, then the pupil is dilated with intravenously injected dye that travels to the eye's circulation, making its blood vessels visible. Fluorescein is used for diabetic retinopathy and retinal vascular disease. Indocyanine green is used for the wet form of macular degeneration when blood is present.

Electroretinography
Electroretinography is used to diagnose diseases of the rods and cones. The procedure evaluates differences in electrical potential between the cornea and retina in response to light wavelengths and intensity. The test is conducted with electrodes placed directly on the eye.

Ultrasonography
Ultrasound is useful when the internal eye cannot be visualized directly because of obstructions, such as corneal opacities or bloody vitreous. The eye is numbed with anesthetic drops. A transducer probe is placed on the eye to perform the ultrasound.

Imaging Tests
X-ray films show bone structure and tumors. Computed tomography (CT) scan and magnetic resonance imaging (MRI) visualize ocular structures and abnormalities of the eye and surrounding tissues.

Therapeutic Measures for the Eye and Vision

Nurses have an important role in screening and educating people about care for healthy eyes and the prevention of disease and helping them cope with visual deficits. See Box 52.1 in Chapter 52 for methods to interact with people with visual impairments. To learn about promoting vision health, visit www.lighthouseguild.org. For blindness resources, visit the American Foundation for the Blind at www.afb.org or the National Federation of the Blind at www.nfb.org.

Eye Examinations
The American Optometric Association (2021) guidelines suggest eye examinations for people ages 18 to 64 every 2 years. For those younger than 64 at risk for eye disease, eye examinations should be done every 1 to 2 years or as directed by the HCP. Those 65 and older should have annual or as-directed eye examinations.

Eye care providers include the ophthalmologist and optometrist. An **ophthalmologist** is a physician who specializes in diagnosing and treating eye diseases. An **optometrist** (doctor of optometry) specializes in eye examinations to identify visual defects, diagnose problems, prescribe corrective lenses or other treatments, and refer for medical treatment. An **optician** is trained to grind and fit lenses prescribed by an ophthalmologist or optometrist.

Eye Hygiene
It is important to keep debris out of the eyes to prevent scratching of the eye's delicate surfaces. When a foreign object gets into the eye, such as dirt or an eyelash, teach people not to rub the eye. Tears can wash out the object by pulling the upper eyelid down over the eye briefly. When wiping the eyes, wipe from the inner canthus to the outer canthus.

Nutrition for Eye Health

Adequate nutrition is important for eye health (see "Nutrition Notes"). Inadequate vitamin intake can result in corneal damage and night blindness from a lack of vitamin A. Optic neuritis can result from a vitamin B deficiency.

> **Nutrition Notes**
>
> **Nutrition and Eye Disease**
> Antioxidants, including anthocyanins, carotenoids, flavonoids, and vitamins, can reduce age-related eye disorders (ARED) (Khoo et al, 2019). Antioxidants such as flavonoids aid in prevention of eye-related diseases through anti-inflammatory properties. According to the National Eye Institute (2020), research has found supplements containing vitamins and minerals may reduce the risk of developing advanced age-related macular degeneration (AMD). The study found beta carotene in the original formula may increase the risk of lung cancer in individuals who smoke. The National Eye Institute suggests there is no benefit from supplemented omega-3 fatty acids or increased zinc. The National Eye Institute continues with ongoing research and recommended formulation of supplements for AMD.

Eye Safety and Prevention of Injury

Many people in the United States suffer eye injuries each year, usually from common activities such as microwave cooking, lawn care, shooting rubber bands, and BB gun use. Most of these injuries could be prevented with education and use of safety measures (Table 51.3).

Eye Irrigation

If it is necessary to irrigate foreign bodies or chemical substances from the eye, prepare the patient by explaining the procedure. (See the "Irrigating the Eye and Ear" procedure in your resources on Davis Advantage.)

Guide Dogs for the Blind and Visually Impaired

Guide dogs are trained to lead blind and visually impaired people around obstacles. While dogs are working, they should not be approached, touched, or fed without their owner's permission. Most dogs do not like to be petted or patted on the head, so ask the owner the dog's petting preference (often the chest, back, and near the tail) if permission is given to touch the dog.

Medication Administration

Most eye medications are applied as drops, ointments, or irrigations (see Chapter 52). The nurse must know the normal dosage and strength, desired action, side effects, and contraindications of the medication for safe administration. The steps for application of eye medications ("Administering Eye and Ear Medications") can be found under "Procedures" on Davis Advantage. Systemic adverse reactions from eye medications can occur.

Table 51.3 Eye Safety and Injury Prevention

To Protect From:	Use These Eye Safety Measures
Foreign objects	Always wear safety goggles when working with tools or yard equipment.
Chemical splashes	Use splash shields around body fluids or chemicals. Close eyes to avoid getting hairspray in them.
Corneal lens abrasions/infections from contact lenses	Follow manufacturer's or eye care professional's directions for length of use and cleaning procedures. Do not wear contact lenses too long.
Ultraviolet light (UV)	Wear UV-protective sunglasses at all ages. Wear a hat to shield sun. Wear sunglasses with side shields after administration of mydriatics.
Visual deficits	Update prescription of glasses yearly. Wear glasses that fit properly, are clean, and are free of scratches.
Computer vision syndrome (digital eye strain)	Position the center of the computer screen 4 to 5 inches below eye level and the screen 20 to 28 inches from the eyes. Avoid glare on the computer screen. Blink frequently to prevent dry eyes. Rest eyes: Every 20 minutes, look 20 feet away for 20 seconds. Take a break every 2 hours for 15 minutes.
Eye injury from sports	Wear protective eyewear with polycarbonate lenses, facemasks, or helmets while participating in sports.

PUNCTAL OCCLUSION. After eye drop administration, eyelids should be closed for 2 minutes without blinking, about the time it takes for absorption of the medication into the eye. At this same time, the puncta (tear duct) on the eyelid of the eye in which medication was administered should have pressure applied to it by either the nurse, wearing gloves, or the patient (see Fig. 51.2). The index finger is placed on the corner of the eye. Pressure is applied against the bone along the nose (not into the eye). This allows the eye drop to remain in the eye longer for greater effect. It also reduces systemic absorption and side effects. Some eye medications have serious cardiac or respiratory effects. Reinforce patient teaching on proper instillation of eye medications.

> **NURSING CARE TIP**
> Teach patients to refrigerate eyedrops, if not contraindicated, for 15 to 30 minutes before instillation to help them feel whether the drops go into the eye or miss and fall onto the face.

EYE PATCHING. After treating an injured or infected eye, the HCP may order the eye to be patched. Apply ointment or drops if ordered and ask the patient to keep the eyelid shut. Place a disposable cotton gauze eye patch over the eye socket depression. Eye patching protects the eye from further damage by keeping the lids closed. Sometimes an additional metal shield is placed over the soft pads to protect the eye from external injury. The patch is taped in place, and the patient is instructed to rest the eyes. Suggest quiet activities, such as listening to music or an audio book. Watching television or reading is not recommended because the patched eye will follow the movement of the unpatched eye.

HEARING

Normal Anatomy and Physiology of the Ear

The ear consists of three areas: the outer ear, the middle ear, and the inner ear. The inner ear contains the receptors for the senses of hearing and equilibrium.

Outer Ear
The outer ear consists of the auricle and the auditory canal (Fig. 51.11).

Middle Ear
The middle ear is an air-filled cavity in the temporal bone (see Fig. 51.11). Vibrations of the tympanic membrane caused by sound are transmitted through the three auditory bones (ossicles). The stapes then transmits vibrations to the fluid-filled inner ear at the oval window.

Inner Ear
The inner ear is a cavity in the temporal bone called the bony labyrinth, lined with membranes called the *membranous labyrinth*. The fluid between bone and membrane is called *perilymph*, and fluid within the membrane is called *endolymph*. The structures of the bony labyrinth include the semicircular canals, vestibule, and cochlea (Fig. 51.12).

The process of hearing involves transmission of vibrations and the generation of nerve impulses. When sound waves enter the auditory canal, vibrations are transmitted by the tympanic membrane, malleus, incus, stapes, oval window of the inner ear, perilymph and endolymph within the cochlea, and hair cells of the organ of Corti. When the hair cells bend, they generate impulses that are carried by the eighth cranial nerve to the brain. The auditory areas, for both hearing and interpretation, are in the temporal lobes of the cerebral cortex.

The inner ear also has receptors for equilibrium. Dynamic equilibrium receptors are within the semicircular canals, whereas static equilibrium receptors are within the vestibule (Fig. 51.13). Within the utricle and saccule of the vestibule, the hair cells bend in response to gravity on the otoliths as the position of the head changes. The impulses generated are carried by the vestibular branch of the eighth cranial nerve to the cerebellum, medulla, and pons. The cerebellum sends this information continuously to the cerebral motor cortex. The cerebellum and brainstem use this information to maintain equilibrium at a subconscious level; the cerebrum interprets the conscious awareness of the position of the head.

When the head moves, movement of the endolymph bends the cupula within the ampulla. The bending of the hair cells at its base generates impulses carried by the vestibular branch of the eighth cranial nerve to the cerebellum and brainstem. Then impulses are sent to the cerebral cortex and interpreted as directional acceleration or deceleration; this information is used to maintain equilibrium during movement.

> ### Gerontological Issues
>
> **Age-Related Changes in Hearing**
> Presbycusis is an age-related change in which progressive hearing loss is caused by loss of hair cells and decreased blood supplying the ear. This results in the loss of hearing high-pitched sounds (pitch = cycles per second; loudness = decibels). Because the ability to hear pitch, rather than volume, is lost, it is not helpful to talk louder to a patient with this type of hearing loss. In fact, talking louder can make it more difficult to discriminate sounds. Loss of high-pitched hearing causes the older adult to hear distracting background noises more clearly than conversation.
>
> It is important to know what helps a person hear best. Deafness or decreased hearing acuity is one of the main reasons that older adults withdraw from social activities. Older adults who have a hearing loss may need adaptive equipment in their home for safety. Using a hearing aid may increase hearing for those who do not have nerve damage deafness. The use of flashing lights instead of buzzers or alarms increases the safety of an older adult who is not able to hear a smoke detector or fire alarm.

Chapter 51 Sensory System Function, Data Collection, and Therapeutic Measures: Vision and Hearing

Outer Ear

The **auricle (pinna)** is the visible part of the ear. Shaped by cartilage (except for the lobule), this part of the ear funnels sound into the auditory canal.

The lined **auditory canal** leads through the temporal bone to the eardrum. (The opening of the bony tunnel to the outside of the body is called the **external acoustic meatus**.) Glands lining the canal produce secretions that mix with dead skin cells to form cerumen (ear wax). Cerumen waterproofs the canal and also traps dirt and bacteria. The cerumen usually dries and then, propelled by jaw movements during eating and talking, works its way out of the ear.

Ossicles:
Malleus
Incus
Stapes
Semicircular canals
Vestibular nerve
Cochlear nerve
Cochlea
Round window
Eustachian tube

Outer ear | Middle ear | Inner ear

Middle Ear

Auditory ossicles: The three smallest bones in the body connect the eardrum to the inner ear; they are named for their shape:
- **Malleus** (hammer)
- **Incus** (anvil)
- **Stapes** (stirrup)

The stapes fits within the **oval window** of the vestibule, which is where the inner ear begins.

Tympanic membrane (or eardrum): This membranous structure separates the outer ear from the middle ear; it vibrates freely in response to sound waves.

Oval window

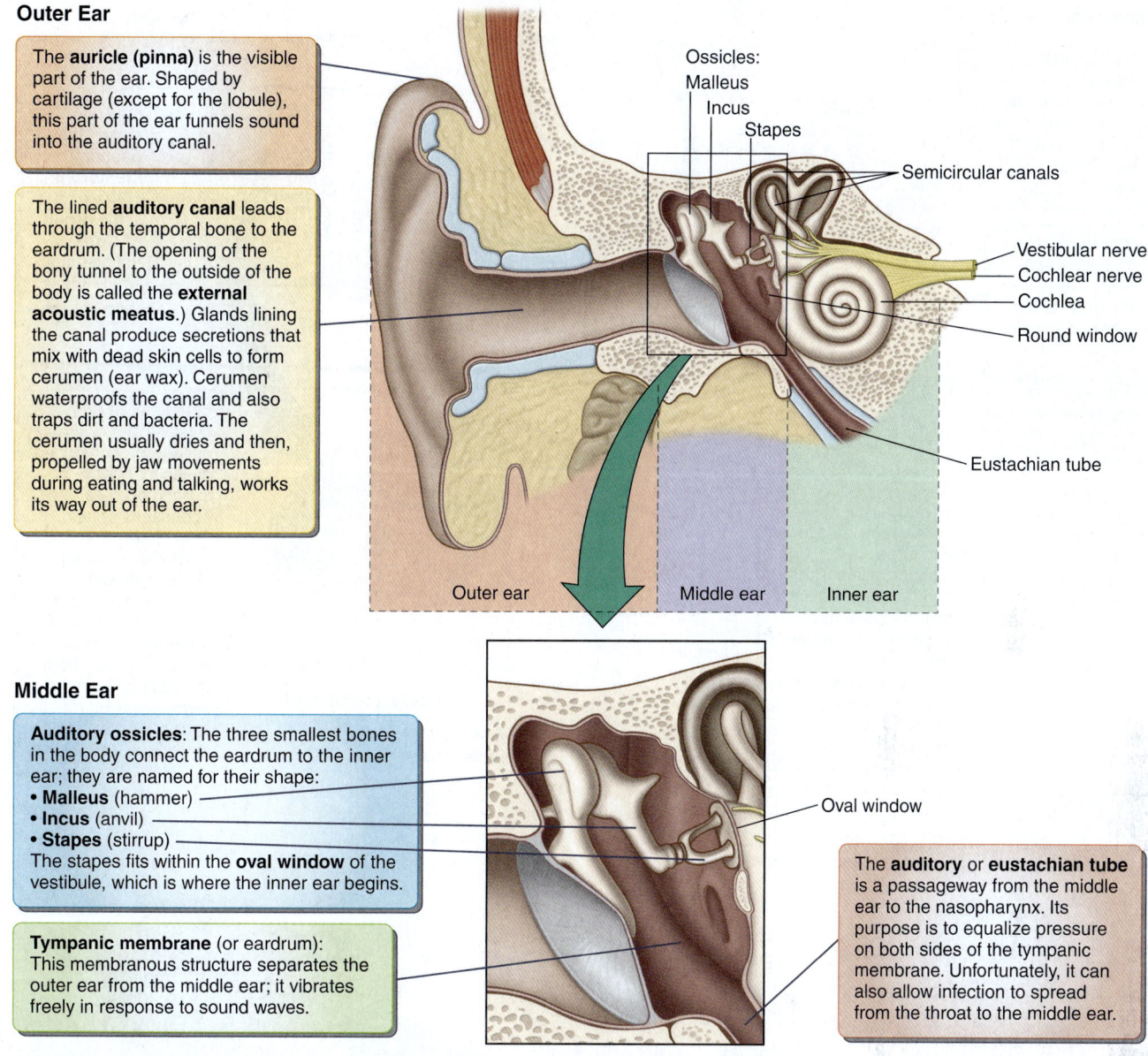

The **auditory** or **eustachian tube** is a passageway from the middle ear to the nasopharynx. Its purpose is to equalize pressure on both sides of the tympanic membrane. Unfortunately, it can also allow infection to spread from the throat to the middle ear.

FIGURE 51.11 Outer and middle ear.

Aging and the Ear

In the ear, cumulative damage to the hair cells in the organ of Corti usually becomes apparent sometime after age of 60 (see Fig. 51.8). Damaged hair cells cannot be replaced. Ability to hear high frequencies is usually lost first (presbycusis), whereas hearing may still be adequate for lower-pitched ranges. The high-pitched sounds *f, s, k,* and *sh* are common losses. Also, it becomes more difficult to filter out background noises, so loud environments make it difficult to hear conversations (see "Gerontological Issues: Age-Related Changes in Hearing").

Sensory System Data Collection of the Ear and Hearing Status

A quiet environment is helpful for collecting accurate hearing data. Document the patient's behavior, as it may provide information related to a hearing loss.

Health History

Patient's self-appraisal of their hearing or related symptoms and family observations are obtained during the health history (Table 51.4). Data collection regarding symptoms includes asking **WHAT'S UP?** questions (see Chapter 1). Symptoms related to the ear may include decreased hearing or loss of hearing, **otorrhea** (discharge), **otalgia** (ear pain), itching, fullness, tinnitus (ringing, buzzing, or roaring in the ears), or vertigo (dizziness). Note exposure to medications that are potentially **ototoxic**, such as certain antibiotics or diuretics (see Chapter 52).

• WORD • BUILDING •

otorrhea: oto—related to the ear + rrhea—to flow
otalgia: ot—related to the ear + algia—signifying pain
ototoxic: oto—related to the ear + toxic—poison

1050 UNIT FOURTEEN Understanding the Sensory System

Inner Ear

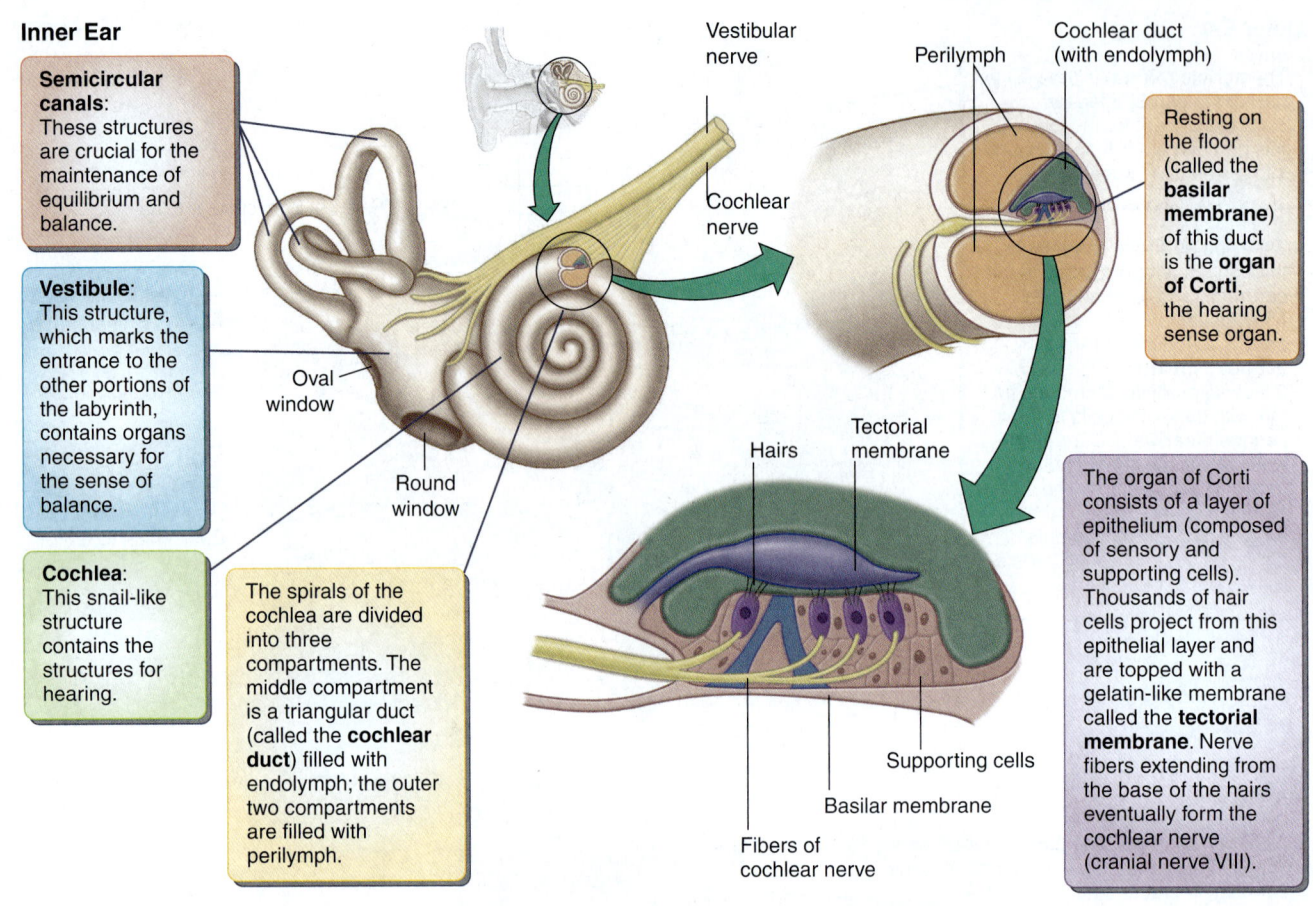

Semicircular canals: These structures are crucial for the maintenance of equilibrium and balance.

Vestibule: This structure, which marks the entrance to the other portions of the labyrinth, contains organs necessary for the sense of balance.

Cochlea: This snail-like structure contains the structures for hearing.

The spirals of the cochlea are divided into three compartments. The middle compartment is a triangular duct (called the **cochlear duct**) filled with endolymph; the outer two compartments are filled with perilymph.

Labels: Vestibular nerve, Cochlear nerve, Oval window, Round window, Perilymph, Cochlear duct (with endolymph), Hairs, Tectorial membrane, Supporting cells, Basilar membrane, Fibers of cochlear nerve

Resting on the floor (called the **basilar membrane**) of this duct is the **organ of Corti**, the hearing sense organ.

The organ of Corti consists of a layer of epithelium (composed of sensory and supporting cells). Thousands of hair cells project from this epithelial layer and are topped with a gelatin-like membrane called the **tectorial membrane**. Nerve fibers extending from the base of the hairs eventually form the cochlear nerve (cranial nerve VIII).

FIGURE 51.12 Inner ear.

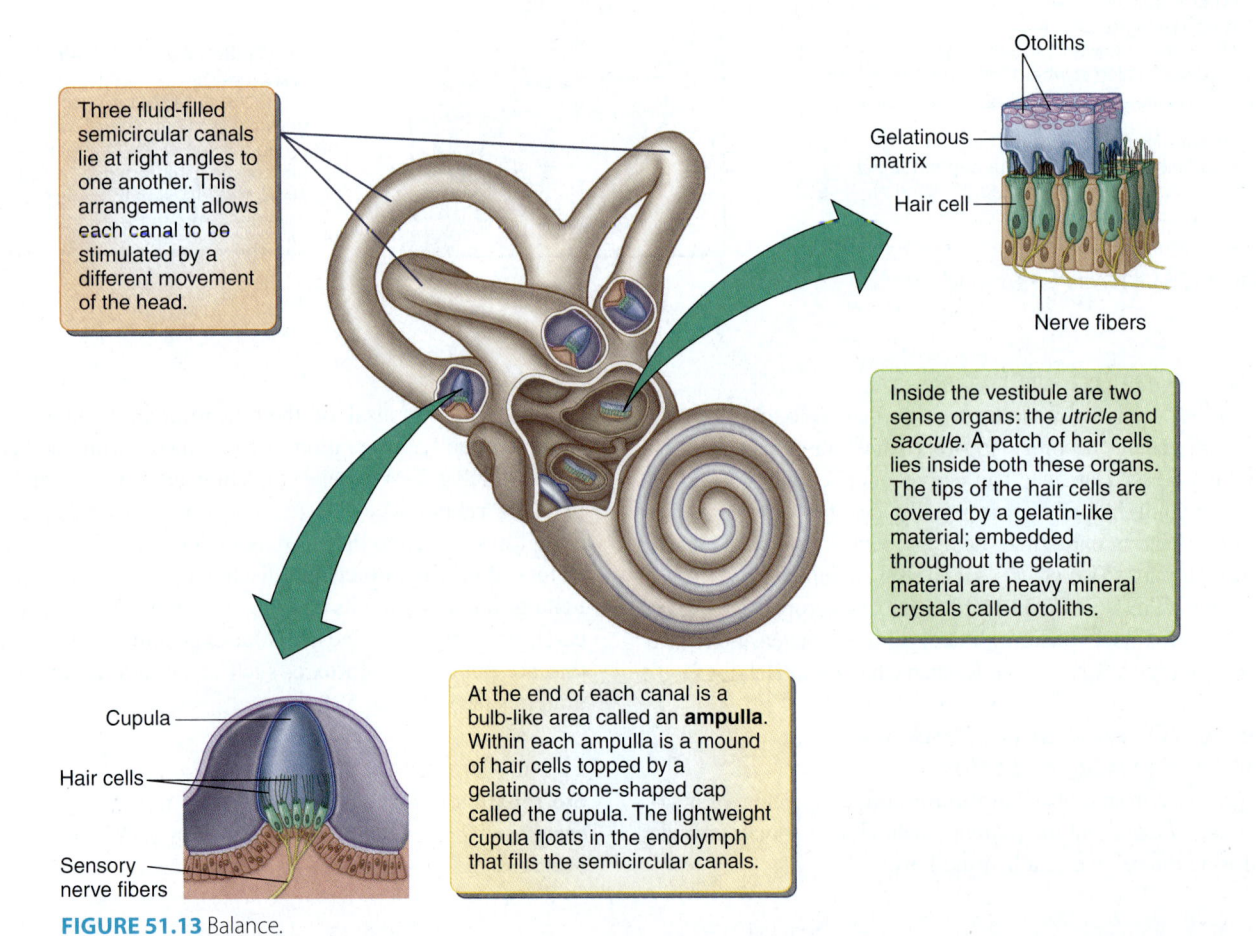

Three fluid-filled semicircular canals lie at right angles to one another. This arrangement allows each canal to be stimulated by a different movement of the head.

Labels: Otoliths, Gelatinous matrix, Hair cell, Nerve fibers, Cupula, Hair cells, Sensory nerve fibers

Inside the vestibule are two sense organs: the *utricle* and *saccule*. A patch of hair cells lies inside both these organs. The tips of the hair cells are covered by a gelatin-like material; embedded throughout the gelatin material are heavy mineral crystals called otoliths.

At the end of each canal is a bulb-like area called an **ampulla**. Within each ampulla is a mound of hair cells topped by a gelatinous cone-shaped cap called the cupula. The lightweight cupula floats in the endolymph that fills the semicircular canals.

FIGURE 51.13 Balance.

Table 51.4
Subjective Data Collection for the Ear

Questions to Ask During the Health History	Rationale
Family History	
Has any family member had any hearing problems or loss? Has any family member had Ménière disease?	Some ear diseases may be genetic.
Health History	
What childhood illnesses have you had?	Mumps, measles, or scarlet fever can affect hearing.
What current diseases do you have? Hospitalizations?	Diseases and their treatments can affect hearing.
What is your sodium intake? How much alcohol do you drink?	Sodium and alcohol intake can affect amount of endolymph in the inner ear, affecting hearing.
What medications do you take?	Many medications are ototoxic and can cause hearing loss.
What are your swimming habits?	Swimming can cause swimmer's ear.
Have you had any injuries or surgeries to the ear?	Recent trauma or surgeries can affect hearing.
Do you have any allergies? Have you had a recent or past upper respiratory or ear infection?	Allergies can cause nasal congestion, leading to middle ear congestion and/or infection.
Do you have otorrhea, otalgia, itching, fullness, tinnitus, or vertigo? Have you had any falls related to vertigo? Any restrictions in walking or driving due to vertigo? Do you have a fever, nausea, or vomiting?	These symptoms can indicate outer, middle, or inner ear infections; ototoxicity; or other ear diseases. Falls and mobility issues are safety concerns when considering care.
Have you been exposed to pressure changes such as with flying or diving?	Barotrauma may occur due to pressure changes.
Hearing Impairment	
Have you noticed any hearing loss, either gradually or suddenly? Do you have difficulty understanding certain words or entire conversations? Do you have difficulty hearing when there is a lot of background noise? Do you hear better with one ear than the other? Do you wear a hearing aid or other assistive device? If so, what is the device and for which ear is it used?	Patient may have hearing loss in one or both ears.
Have your friends or family commented on your decreased hearing? How does your hearing loss affect your daily life? Do you feel frustrated or embarrassed because of your hearing loss? How do your friends and family react to your hearing loss?	Others may notice hearing loss signs in patient. Hearing loss can cause social isolation.
Are you exposed to loud noises (e.g., current/past job, transportation, machinery, or music)?	Loud noises can cause damage to the ear, leading to hearing loss over time.
Self-Care Behaviors	
Have you had your hearing checked? If so, when? How do you clean your ears? How do you protect your ears from loud noises?	Provides information about patient's ear self-care and health.

> **CUE RECOGNITION 51.2**
>
> While completing admission data collection on a resident patient, she asks you to repeat questions several times. She also answers your questions in a very loud tone. What action do you take?
>
> *Suggested answers are at the end of the chapter.*

Physical Examination

Physical examination of the ear begins by observing the patient's behavior (Box 51.1). Note how the patient communicates and observe how they talk. Note slurred speech. Examination of the ear includes inspection, palpation, testing of auditory acuity, balance testing, and otoscopic examination by the HCP (Table 51.5). Document all findings.

INSPECTION AND PALPATION OF THE EXTERNAL EAR. Inspection of the external ear begins with the auricle and the ear canal. A small bump on the inside of the helix (the upper external ear margin), Darwin's tubercle, is normal. The ear canal should be inspected before obtaining an infrared ear temperature because the presence of excess cerumen can alter the accuracy of the reading. To inspect the external ear canal, tip the adult patient's head toward the opposite side of the ear. Use a penlight or otoscope to inspect the canal.

Next, the auricles and mastoid process are palpated. The mastoid process (bony prominence located behind the earlobe) should be smooth and hard, not tender or swollen.

AUDITORY ACUITY TESTING. Three assessment tests evaluate auditory function. The whisper voice test identifies hearing function in each ear. Ask the patient to occlude one ear with a finger and push on the tragus to mask sound. Stand 1 to 2 feet away on the opposite side, behind the patient's field of vision, to prevent lip reading. Whisper two-syllable words toward the unoccluded ear, varying each whisper in volume. Ask the patient to restate the whispered words. Repeat the process on the other ear. Ask the patient if hearing was better in one ear than in the other ear. Normally, the patient should hear a soft whisper equally well in both ears. Findings of better hearing in one ear than the other or an inability to hear a soft whisper can indicate hearing impairment.

A second acuity test is the **Rinne test**, performed with a tuning fork to differentiate between conductive and sensorineural hearing loss. To perform the test, strike the tuning fork and place it on the patient's mastoid process (Fig. 51.14). Verify that the patient can hear the tuning fork, then instruct them to tell you immediately when they no longer hear the sound. Then, place the vibrating tuning fork 2 inches in front of the ear. Again, ask the patient whether they hear the tuning fork and to indicate when the sound stops. Normally, air conduction (AC) is heard for twice as long as bone conduction (BC). Normal findings are when the patient reports hearing the tuning fork when placed in front of the ear (AC) after it is no longer heard on the mastoid process (BC). Normal results are recorded as "AC greater than BC." The test is repeated on the other ear. Abnormal findings can indicate conduction or sensorineural problems (Table 51.6).

The **Weber test** is a third test to determine hearing acuity, also performed using a tuning fork. Place the vibrating tuning fork on the center of the patient's forehead or head (Fig. 51.15). Verify that the patient can hear the tuning fork. If the patient says yes, ask if they hear the sound better in the left ear, better in the right ear, or the same in both ears. It is important to give the patient these three choices. Normally, the patient hears the sound the same in both ears (see Table 51.6). Ensuring a patient can hear is important during care to ensure clear communication. Healthy People 2030 has set a goal to increase the percentage of adults ages 20 to 69 who have their hearing assessed from 21.8% to 24.4% of the population (Office of Disease Prevention and Health Promotion, 2020b).

BALANCE TESTING. When the patient reports dizziness, nystagmus, or problems with equilibrium, simple tests can evaluate vestibular function. Plan for patient safety before testing. The first test is simply to observe the patient's gait by having them walk away from the HCP and then walk back. Note balance, posture, and movement of arms and legs. The patient should be able to walk in an upright position with no difficulties in balance or movement.

Romberg test (falling test) is another simple test of vestibular function. If a fall appears likely, be prepared to support the patient during the test to prevent injury. Instruct the patient to stand with feet together, first with eyes open and then with eyes closed. Normally, the patient has no difficulty maintaining a standing position with only minimal swaying. If the patient has difficulty maintaining balance or loses balance (a positive Romberg test), the patient may have an inner ear problem.

> **Box 51.1**
>
> ### Behaviors Indicating Hearing Loss
>
> Adults with hearing loss may show any or all the following behaviors:
> - Turns up volume on the television or radio.
> - Frequently asks, "What did you say?"
> - Leans forward or turns head to one side during conversations to hear better.
> - Cups hand around ear during conversation.
> - Says people are talking softly or mumbling.
> - Speaks in an unusually loud or quiet voice.
> - Answers questions inappropriately or not at all.
> - Has difficulty hearing high-frequency consonants.
> - Avoids group activities.
> - Shows loss of sense of humor.
> - Has strained or serious look on face during conversations.
> - Appears to ignore people or does not participate.
> - Is irritable or sensitive in interpersonal relations.
> - Reports ringing, buzzing, or roaring noise in ears.

Table 51.5
Objective Data Collection for the Ear

Abnormal Findings	Possible Causes
Inspection and Palpation of the External Ear	
Asymmetrical size and placement	Congenital deformities.
Breaks in the skin, discharge, inflammation, or growths.	Infections, poorly fitting hearing aid, skin cancer, or trauma.
Excessive cerumen or drainage, irregular color, consistency, and odor.	Infection or trauma. Excessive cerumen can alter hearing and cause inaccurate tympanic temperature readings.
Note for presence of lesions, tophi, or masses during palpation. No foreign bodies should be seen.	Tophi (deposits of uric acid crystals in external ear margin) occur in gout. A mass could indicate cancer.
Tenderness of auricle when palpated or odor from ear.	Tenderness and odor can indicate infection.
Auditory Acuity Testing	
Abnormal Rinne and Weber tests (see Table 51.6).	Abnormal results can indicate conductive, sensorineural, mixed, or neural hearing loss.
Balance Testing	
Difficulty sitting and/or walking as well as increased swaying or falling with Romberg test may be due to balance difficulties.	Inner ear infection or disorder.
Otoscopic Examination	
Ear canal may be reddened and swollen; drainage may be present; excessive cerumen or foreign object may be present.	This could be caused by infection, improper care, or excessive cerumen production.
Internal otoscope examination is completed by experienced practitioner and eardrum may be dull, bulging, retracted, or reddened.	Middle ear infection or blockage.
Other	
Does the patient watch the practitioner's mouth or lean toward the practitioner?	Behaviors may indicate hearing loss and the patient's effort to compensate.

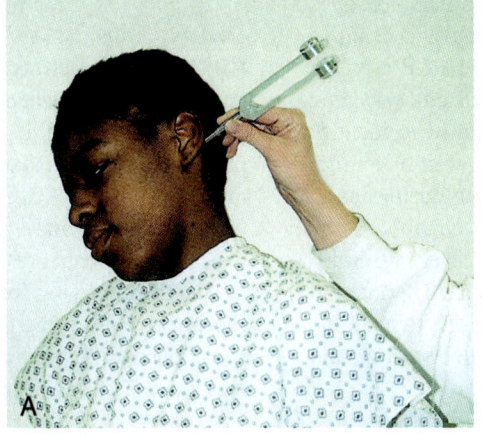

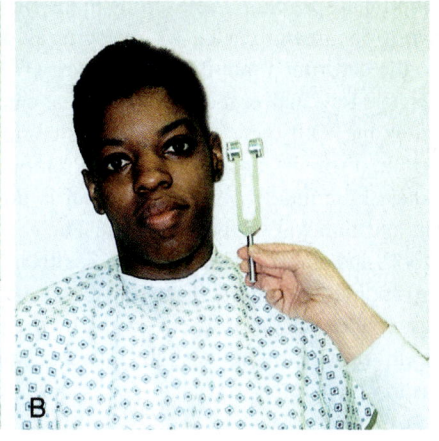

FIGURE 51.14 Rinne test. (A) Bone conduction. (B) Air conduction.

Table 51.6
Auditory Acuity Tuning Fork Tests

Test	Normal Hearing Results	Conductive	Sensorineural Hearing Loss
Rinne test	Air conduction heard twice as long as bone conduction	Bone conduction heard longer than air conduction in affected ear	Air conduction heard longer than bone conduction in affected ear (but may be less than 2:1 ratio)
Weber test	Tone heard in center of the head; no lateralization	Sound heard louder in affected ear	Sound heard louder in better ear

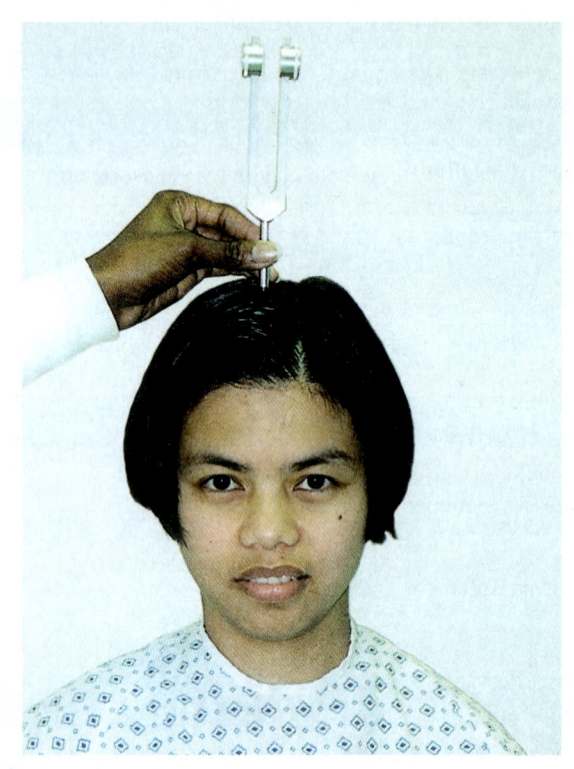

FIGURE 51.15 Weber test.

OTOSCOPIC EXAMINATION. An otoscope is an instrument consisting of a handle, a light source, a magnifying lens, and an optional speculum for inserting in the ear. Some otoscopes have a pneumatic device for injecting air into the canal to test the eardrum's mobility and integrity. The HCP uses the otoscope to visualize the external ear, ear canal, and tympanic membrane. Otoscopic examination is completed to identify specific disorders or infections or to remove wax or foreign bodies. Examination of the ear canal is done during insertion and removal of the speculum. The ear canal should be smooth and empty with no redness, scaliness, swelling, drainage, nodules, foreign objects, or excessive wax. The internal otoscopic examination is conducted by the HCP to examine the eardrum. It should be slightly conical, shiny, smooth, and a pearly gray color.

Evidence-Based Practice
Clinical Question
Does age and hearing loss affect balance and listening?

Evidence
An experimental study examined older adults (OA) and older adults with age-related hearing loss (ARHL) and found both had more difficulty with cognitive and balance activities than did young adults (YA). Twenty-nine YA, 26 OA, and 32 ARHL completed dual cognitive and balance tasks in both quiet and noisy environments. The results demonstrated that YA were able to dual task and were able to flexibly distribute their attention between auditory and balance tasks. The OA and ARHL groups had negative effects with increased noise. The ARHL group focused more on balance than on the cognitive tasks in noisy environments.

Implications for Nursing Practice
Noise negatively impacted task prioritization. Understanding that noisy distractions can impact balance in OA and ARHL populations could help reduce the risk of falls.

Reference: Bruce, H., Aponte, D., St-Onge, N., Phillips, N., Gagne, J., & Li, K. (2019). The effects of age and hearing loss on dual-task balance and listening. *Journals of Gerontology Series B, 74*(2), 275–283. https://doi.org/10.1093/geronb/gbx047

Diagnostic Tests for the Ear and Hearing
Audiometric Testing
An audiologist uses audiometric testing as a screening tool to determine type and degree of hearing loss. The audiometer produces a stimulus that consists of a musical tone, pure tone, or speech. To test AC, the patient sits in a soundproof booth, wears earphones, and signals the audiologist when and if a tone is heard. Each ear is tested separately. The patient is exposed to sounds of varying frequency or pitch (hertz) and intensity (decibels). By varying the levels of the sound, a hearing level is established (Table 51.7). Earphone testing can be used to measure AC, level of speech hearing, and understanding of

speech. For BC testing, a vibrator is placed on the mastoid process, and the earphones are removed. Testing proceeds as with AC.

A patient with normal hearing should have the same AC as BC hearing levels. Differences in AC and BC hearing can provide information about the location and type of hearing loss.

Tympanometry

Tympanometry tests the movement of the tympanic membrane (ear drum) and evaluates middle ear function. The test is not done if the ear canal is obstructed or the ear drum is perforated. The tympanometer probe applies varying amounts of pressure to vibrate the tympanic membrane. The results are graphed on a tympanogram. The patient is informed that the tympanometry may cause transient vertigo. The patient is asked to report any nausea or dizziness felt during the test.

Caloric Test

The caloric test is used by the HCP to test the function of the eighth cranial nerve and assess vestibular reflexes of the inner ear that control balance. The test is not done if the ear canal is obstructed or the ear drum is perforated. The test is performed first on one ear and then the other. Warm (112°F [44.5°C]) or cold (86°F [30°C]) water is instilled into the ear canal. Expected eye movements and nystagmus are noted. Dizziness may also be felt. No nystagmus is seen if the patient has a disease of the labyrinth, such as Ménière disease.

Electronystagmogram

The electronystagmogram is used to diagnose causes of unilateral hearing loss of unknown origin, vertigo, or ringing in the ears. The test is contraindicated in patients with pacemakers. It is similar to the caloric test. Usually tranquilizers, alcohol, stimulants, and antivertigo agents are avoided for 1 to 5 days before the test. The patient should also avoid tobacco and caffeine on the day of the test. The patient may experience nausea, vertigo, or weakness following the test.

Computed Tomography Scan

A CT scan is used to visualize the temporal and mastoid bones, the middle and inner ears, and the eustachian tube.

Magnetic Resonance Imaging

MRI examines membranous organs, nerve, and blood vessels of the temporal bone for disease.

Laboratory Tests

CULTURE. Culture of drainage from the ear canal or a surgical incision is important to diagnose and treat acute infections with the appropriate anti-infective agent. Often with chronic infections, the culture is less helpful because gram-negative bacilli cover up the original pathogen. Drainage from the external ear is collected using a culture swab kit and taken to the laboratory immediately.

PATHOLOGY EXAMINATION. Pathology examination of tissue obtained during surgery is completed to rule out a malignancy and identify any unusual problems. A cholesteatoma (cyst of epithelial cells and cholesterol found in the middle ear) is identified by a pathology examination.

Table 51.7 Common Noise Levels

Human hearing threshold	0–25 decibels (dB)
Quiet room	30–40 dB
Conversational speech	60 dB
Heavy traffic	70 dB
Alarm clock	80 dB
Vacuum cleaner	80 dB
Unsafe noise levels begin	**90 dB**
Circular saw	100 dB
Rock music	120 dB
Jet planes	120–130 dB
Pain threshold	**130 dB**
Firearms	140 dB

CRITICAL THINKING & CLINICAL JUDGMENT

Mr. Frank is at his HCP's office when his wife expresses concern about his changing behavior during the past 6 months. She says that Mr. Frank no longer enjoys talking to neighbors or visiting with friends and seems irritable. He has also lost his sense of humor and does not always answer her questions appropriately.

Critical Thinking (The Why)
1. What do you think is occurring with Mr. Frank?
2. What would be the expected findings of data collection tests?

Clinical Judgment (The Do)
3. What examination techniques or tests do you use to gather data related to Mr. Frank's signs and symptoms?
4. Which other members of the health-care team do you collaborate with for Mr. Frank's care?
5. What teaching for these symptoms and their effect on Mr. Frank's lifestyle do you reinforce?
6. What safety issues do you address with Mr. Frank?

Suggested answers are at the end of the chapter.

Therapeutic Measures for the Ear and Hearing

Medications

The most common medications to treat ear disorders include anti-infectives, anti-inflammatories, antihistamines, decongestants, cerumenolytics, and diuretics. Anti-infectives can be administered systemically or as a topical solution. Ear medications are usually given as drops (see "Administering Eye and Ear Medications" under "Procedures" on Davis Advantage). Anti-inflammatories, antihistamines, and decongestants are used with acute infections to reduce nasal and middle ear congestion. Cerumenolytics are used to soften cerumen and remove it from the ear canal. Diuretics are used with some inner ear disorders to reduce pressure caused by fluids.

Ear Health Maintenance

Safe routine cleaning and ear care should be taught to all patients to prevent eardrum injury (Fig. 51.16). All patients can benefit from ear and hearing protection education, found in Table 51.8.

Assistive Hearing Devices

Hearing aids are instruments that amplify sound (see Chapter 52). Certain hearing aids are designed to amplify sounds and attenuate certain portions of the sound signal.

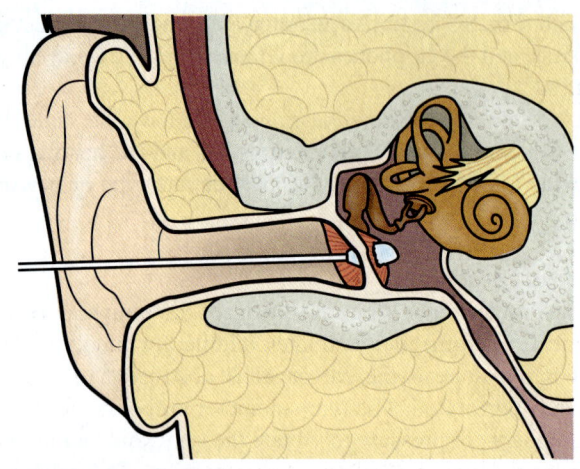

FIGURE 51.16 Ear drum perforation. Avoid putting things into the ear canal for cleaning to prevent injury.

A small battery serves as the energy source. Digital hearing aids contain computers that convert sound waves into numerical codes before amplifying. This provides clearer and crisper sound that is programmable to each person's hearing loss. Digital hearing aids are more expensive than analog hearing aids (which convert sound waves into electrical signals for amplifying). Technology for assistive devices

Table 51.8
Prevention of Ear Problems

Patient Education	Rationale
Caring for the External Ear	
Wash external ear with soap and water only.	Keeps external ear clean.
Do not routinely remove wax from the ear canal.	Wax serves as a protective mechanism to lubricate and trap foreign material. The ear is generally self-cleaning. Wax is normally removed through talking, eating, and showering.
Preventing Ear Trauma	
Avoid inserting any objects or solutions into the ear. Avoid swimming in polluted areas.	Prevents traumatizing the ear and tympanic membrane or exposing the ear to infection.
Avoid flying when the ear or upper respiratory system is congested.	Prevents barotrauma due to pressure changes.
Preventing Damage from Noise Pollution	
Avoid exposure to excessive occupational noise levels. Avoid other causes of excessive noise such as use of firearms and high-intensity music.	Normal speech is 60 decibels (dB). Above 80 dB is uncomfortable. If there is ringing in the ear, damage may be occurring. Occupational noise is the primary cause of hearing loss.
Use protective earplugs or earmuffs if exposure to loud noise cannot be avoided.	Hearing loss can occur due to exposure to loud noises. Protects ears from hearing loss by decreasing exposure to loud noises.

Chapter 51 Sensory System Function, Data Collection, and Therapeutic Measures: Vision and Hearing

Table 51.8
Prevention of Ear Problems—cont'd

Patient Education	Rationale
Instruct adults to have hearing checked every 2 to 3 years.	Degenerative changes occur in the ear with aging.
Early Detection of Hearing Loss	
Monitor for side effects of ototoxic drugs. Instruct patient to report dizziness, decreased hearing acuity, or tinnitus.	Prevents side effects of medications from causing hearing loss.
Caution older patients who use aspirin that it is ototoxic and can cause tinnitus.	Older patients may have hearing loss and not be able to hear the tinnitus.
Instruct patient to report acute symptoms of ear pain, swelling, drainage, or plugged feeling.	Many medical problems can be prevented with prompt treatment.
Instruct patient to blow nose with both nostrils open during upper respiratory infections (colds).	Prevents infected secretions from moving up the eustachian tubes into the middle ear.

using Bluetooth and smartphones with amplification apps is available. Several types of hearing aids are commonly used today (see www.fda.gov/medical-devices/hearing-aids/types-hearing-aids):

- The in-the-ear aid fits into the ear.
- The behind-the-ear aid rests behind the ear and connects to the earmold in the ear canal by plastic tubing (see Fig. 52.6 in Chapter 52).
- The canal aid fits into the ear canal and is nearly unseen.

To care for a hearing aid, ensure it is turned off and the battery is removed when not in use. This reduces battery expense for the patient, who may be on a fixed income. When turning the hearing aid on, the volume should be turned up just until it squeals, then turned down until the patient indicates it is at the best level for hearing. Hearing aids can be water-resistant but should be removed before showering or swimming. Newer electronic hearing aids should not be cleaned with soap and water and must be protected from humidity and perspiration. Hearing aids can be cleaned daily with a soft dry cloth. Some hearing aids have a wax guard in place to protect the electronics. Ear wax should be removed daily from the hearing aid to ensure proper functioning. A soft brush or cotton-tipped swab can also be used to clean the small tip that fits into the ear.

Other types of assistive hearing devices are middle ear implants and cochlear implants. The middle ear implant (visit http://www.medel.com/us) is for those with a sensorineural hearing loss. It provides sound perception by enhancing the normal middle ear hearing function. A **cochlear implant** has a microelectronic processor to convert sound into electrical signals, a transmission system to relay signals to the implanted parts, and a long, slender electrode placed in the cochlea to deliver the electrical stimuli directly to the fiber of the auditory nerve. A person who has profound deafness with complete hearing loss may benefit from this technology.

SAFETY PRODUCTS. Products such as visual-alarm smoke detectors (flashing light) or alarms that vibrate the bed to alert a person with a hearing impairment of a fire are available.

Hearing Service Dogs
Hearing service dogs are trained to respond to sounds that a person who is hearing impaired or cannot hear. Examples include a crying baby, smoke alarm, or oven timer.

Key Points

- Several structures protect the eye from debris and desiccation: the bony orbit, the muscles that move the eye, and the three layers of the eyeball.
- Vision involves the focusing of light rays on the retina and the transmission of the subsequent nerve impulses to the visual areas of the cerebral cortex.
- The most common changes in the aging eye are those in the lens. With age, the lens may become partially or totally opaque, and it loses its elasticity. Most people become farsighted as they age and by 40 years begin to need corrective lenses.
- Visual acuity is often measured using a Snellen chart or an E chart to measure distance acuity and a handheld visual acuity chart (a Rosenbaum card) to measure near acuity.
- When observed, the pupils should be round, symmetrical, and reactive to light.

- Testing for accommodation checks ability of the pupil to respond to near and far distances.
- Diagnostic tests of the eye include exudate culture, digital imagery, optical coherence tomography, fluorescein and indocyanine green angiography, electroretinography, ultrasound, and x-rays.
- Nurses have an important role in screening and educating people about care for healthy eyes and the prevention of disease.
- During eye drop administration, the puncta (tear ducts) on the eyelids should have pressure applied by either the nurse, wearing gloves, or the patient with a tissue, for 1 to 5 minutes depending on the type of medication to avoid systemic effects such as cardiovascular effects.
- The ear consists of three areas: the outer ear, the middle ear, and the inner ear. The inner ear contains the receptors for the senses of hearing and equilibrium.
- The outer ear consists of the auricle and the auditory canal. The middle ear is an air-filled cavity in the temporal bone. Vibrations of the tympanic membrane caused by sound are transmitted through three auditory bones (ossicles). The inner ear is a cavity in the temporal bone called the bony labyrinth, lined with membranes called the membranous labyrinth. Structures of the bony labyrinth include semicircular canals, vestibule, and cochlea.
- In the ear, cumulative damage to the hair cells in the organ of Corti usually becomes apparent sometime after the age of 60. Damaged hair cells cannot be replaced.
- Ability to hear high frequencies is usually lost first (presbycusis), whereas hearing may still be adequate for lower-pitched ranges.
- Physical examination of the ear begins by observing how the patient communicates. Note slurred speech. Examination of the ear includes inspection, palpation, testing of auditory acuity, balance testing, and otoscopic examination by the HCP.
- Auditory function is evaluated with three assessment tests: Rinne, Weber, and whisper tests.
- When the patient reports dizziness, nystagmus, or problems with equilibrium, simple tests can be performed to evaluate vestibular function observe how the patient walks and perform a Romberg test.
- Diagnostic tests for ears and hearing include audiometric testing, tympanometry, caloric test, electronystagmogram, CT scan, MRI, and laboratory tests done on ear drainage or tissue.
- Hearing aids are instruments that amplify sound. Certain hearing aids may be designed to amplify sounds and attenuate certain portions of the sound signal. Digital hearing aids provide clearer and crisper sound that is programmable to each person's hearing loss.
- Other types of assistive hearing devices are middle ear implants and cochlear implants. The middle ear implant is for those with a sensorineural hearing loss. It provides sound perception by enhancing the normal middle ear hearing function.

SUGGESTED ANSWERS TO CHAPTER EXERCISES

Cue Recognition

51.1: Make the environment safe. Place call light by patient and ask him to call for assistance, provide adequate night lighting for the patient, clear the pathway to the bathroom, and make ambulatory aids accessible if any are used. Discuss data collection findings with the HCP.

51.2: You suspect your patient has some hearing loss. You can ask if she has any known hearing loss. You can also use a quick screening app for hearing to check your patient's hearing at World Health Organization at https://www.who.int/health-topics/hearing-loss/hearwho. You could assist with a whisper, Rinne, and Weber tests to detect hearing loss. During data collection, you can speak clearly, face your patient, and speak in lower tones.

Critical Thinking & Clinical Judgment

Mr. Frank
1. He is likely exhibiting behaviors of hearing loss.
2. For inspection of ear, cerumen impaction may be found. For a whisper voice test, the whisper is not heard in the affected ear. For a Rinne test, bone conduction is heard longer than air conduction in the affected ear. For a Weber test, sound is heard louder in the affected ear.
3. Ear inspection, a whisper voice test, a Rinne test, and a Weber test might be performed.
4. An audiologist.
5. Explaining to Mr. and Mrs. Frank symptoms of hearing loss will help them understand Mr. Frank's behaviors. Explore with them the effects of these symptoms on daily life so they can develop plans for coping with the hearing loss until an intervention is implemented.
6. Mr. Frank may not hear telephones or alarms such as smoke or carbon monoxide detectors, so alternatives such as visual alarms could be considered. If he drives, he may not hear car horns or emergency vehicles, which he should be aware of so he can compensate.

Additional Resources

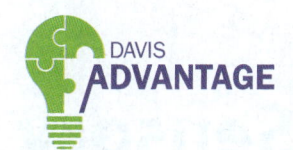

Go to Davis Advantage to complete your learning: strengthen understanding, apply your knowledge, and prepare for the Next Gen NCLEX®.

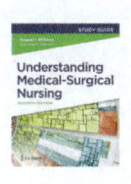

A Study Guide is also available.

CHAPTER 52
Nursing Care of Patients With Sensory Disorders: Vision and Hearing

Lazette V. Nowicki

KEY TERMS

astigmatism (uh-STIG-mah-TIZM)
blepharitis (BLEF-uh-RY-tis)
blindness (BLYND-ness)
carbuncle (KAR-bun-kul)
cataract (KAT-uh-rakt)
chalazion (kah-LAY-zee-on)
conductive hearing loss (kon-DUK-tiv HEER-ing LOSS)
conjunctivitis (kon-JUNK-ti-VY-tis)
enucleation (ee-NEW-klee-AY-shun)
external otitis (eks-TER-nuhl oh-TY-tis)
furuncle (FYOOR-un-kul)
glaucoma (glaw-KOH-mah)
hordeolum (hor-DEE-oh-lum)
hyperopia (HY-per-OH-pee-ah)
macula (MAK-yoo-la)
Ménière disease (ma-NEAR di-ZEEZ)
miotics (my-AH-tiks)
myopia (my-OH-pee-ah)
myringoplasty (mir-IN-goh-PLAS-tee)
myringotomy (MIR-in-GOT-uh-mee)
otosclerosis (OH-toh-skle-ROH-sis)
photophobia (FOH-toh-FOH-bee-ah)
presbycusis (PREZ-by-KYOO-sis)
presbyopia (PREZ-by-OH-pee-ah)
retinopathy (ret-i-NAH-puh-thee)
sensorineural (SEN-suh-ree-NEW-ruhl)
stapedectomy (stay-puh-DEK-tuh-mee)

CHAPTER CONCEPTS

Safety
Sensory perception
Teaching and learning

LEARNING OUTCOMES

1. Explain the pathophysiology of each disorder of the sensory system.
2. Define blindness and the refractive errors of vision.
3. Explain the etiologies, signs, and symptoms of each sensory disorder.
4. Assist with planning nursing care for patients undergoing tests for sensory disorders.
5. Identify therapeutic measures for each sensory disorder.
6. Identify medications contraindicated for patients with acute angle-closure glaucoma.
7. List three ototoxic drugs.
8. List data to collect when caring for patients with disorders of the sensory system.
9. Assist with planning nursing care for patients with disorders of the eye or ear.
10. Assist with planning nursing care interventions for the patient with a hearing impairment.

VISION DISORDERS

Early detection of visual problems can lessen their impact on a person's life. Nurses play an important role in assisting patients with visual problems (Table 52.1).

Infections and Inflammation

Eye infections can result from bacteria or viruses. Bacteria include *Staphylococcus* and *Streptococcus*. Viruses include herpes simplex virus, cytomegalovirus, and human adenovirus. Inflammation can be caused by allergies to environmental substances; irritation from chemicals found in perfumes, makeup, sprays, or plants; or mechanical irritation such as with sunburn.

Conjunctivitis

Conjunctivitis is inflammation of the conjunctiva, caused by either a virus or bacteria. Viral conjunctivitis occurs more often than bacterial conjunctivitis. It is highly contagious. The virus is usually transmitted

• WORD • BUILDING •
conjunctivitis: conjunctive—joining membrane + itis—inflammation

Table 52.1
Eye Disorder Summary

Signs and Symptoms	Pain Redness, secretions, itchiness Sensation of pressure in eyes Visual disturbances
Diagnostic Tests	Visual acuity Amsler grid (identifies visual field disturbances) Ophthalmoscopic examination of internal and external eye Slit-lamp examination (identifies abnormalities on cornea and sclera) Tonometry (identifies intraocular pressure)
Therapeutic Measures	Medications to reduce intraocular pressure, treat infections, anesthetize the eye Surgery
Complications	Worsening vision or loss of vision Acute pain
Priority Nursing Diagnoses	*Anxiety* *Deficient Knowledge* *Risk for Injury*

via contaminated eye secretions on a hand that then touches or rubs an eye, infecting it. The virus is hardy and may live on dry surfaces for 2 weeks or more. Viral conjunctivitis lasts 2 to 4 weeks. Bacterial conjunctivitis (commonly called *pinkeye*) is usually due to staphylococcal or streptococcal bacteria and is also highly contagious. Conjunctivitis can also be caused by the organisms *Haemophilus influenzae*, *Chlamydia trachomatis*, and *Neisseria gonorrhoeae*. Trachoma, a form of conjunctivitis caused by a viral strain of *Chlamydia trachomatis*, is the most common preventable cause of blindness worldwide. Conjunctivitis is commonly transmitted among children and then to family members. Signs and symptoms include conjunctival redness and crusting exudate on the lids and in the corners of the eyes. Itching, pain, and excessive tearing also occur.

> **BE SAFE!**
> **TAKE ACTION!** Conjunctivitis is highly contagious. If a patient has conjunctivitis, use contact precautions to prevent spreading the organism to other people.

Viral conjunctivitis treatment includes eye washes or eye irrigations to cleanse the conjunctiva. This relieves the inflammation and pain. Bacterial conjunctivitis is treated with antibiotic eye drops or ointments (Table 52.2). Adults generally prefer eye drops because they do not impair vision. Ointments are used when the eye is resting (at night). Hand hygiene prevents the spread of conjunctivitis. To prevent transmitting the infection to others, persons with conjunctivitis should not share handkerchiefs, tissues, towels, cosmetics, linens, or eating utensils.

Blepharitis

Blepharitis is a chronic inflammatory process affecting the edges of the eyelids. Causes may include bacterial colonization (usually *Staphylococcus*), parasitic infestation (mites), seborrhea (dandruff), rosacea (a chronic skin disease usually affecting middle-aged and older adults), irritants (cosmetics, smoke, contact lens/contact lens solutions), medications (retinoids or chemotherapeutic agents), or abnormalities of the tarsal glands (also called the *meibomian glands*) and their lipid secretions. Posterior blepharitis is more common, and the tarsal glands become blocked, which promotes bacterial growth. Anterior blepharitis, less common, is characterized by inflammation at the base of the eyelashes. Symptoms usually affect both eyes, and the patient may have red, swollen, or itchy eyelids along with a gritty or burning sensation, pink eyes, excessive tearing, crusting of eyelashes in the morning, flaking of eyelid skin, light sensitivity, and blurred vision. Dry eye disease is a frequent complication.

Treatment requires commitment to long-term daily cleansing and good hygiene. Each eyelid is cleansed with cotton-tipped swabs or a clean cloth (one for each eye) dipped in diluted baby shampoo or warm water. Eyelids chronically infected with *Staphylococcus* may thicken and lose eyelashes. Anterior blepharitis is managed with an antibiotic ointment (e.g., bacitracin [Bactrim], erythromycin [E-Mycin]) applied to the eyelid edges at bedtime for 2 weeks. Posterior blepharitis is treated with azithromycin 1% ophthalmic solution (AzaSite) with one drop twice a day for 10 to 14 days. *Domodex* mites are treated with oral ivermectin or topical tea tree oil.

Keratoconjunctivitis Sicca (Dry Eye Disease)

Dry eye results from inadequate lubrication of the eye due to reduced tear production and/or excessive evaporation. Risk increases after age 50. Most patients have chronic symptoms such as dryness, irritation, redness, light sensitivity, excessive tearing (but the eye is actually dry), and blurred vision. Treatment includes frequent blinking, smoking cessation, minimizing air conditioning or heating, reducing screen time, taking eye breaks (closed with blinking), using warm compresses for tarsal gland swelling, requesting prescription medications that are nondrying, and using over-the-counter artificial tears or prescribed eye drops such as cyclosporine (Restasis) or lifitegrast (Xiidra). Less common treatments are topical glucocorticoids, punctal plugs, autologous serum tears (serum from patients own blood formulated into eye drops), tear stimulation medications, and scleral contact lenses. A newer treatment uses intense pulsed light therapy to treat tarsal (meibomian) gland dysfunction and stimulate the natural flow of oil into the tears.

Table 52.2
Ophthalmic Medications

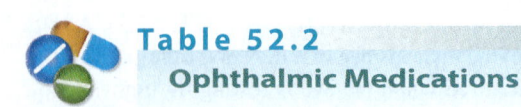

Medication Class/Action

Diagnostic Aids

Fluorescein Sodium
Used for staining of eye; lesions of foreign objects pick up bright yellow-orange stain.

Examples	*Nursing Implications*
fluorescein (AK-Fluor)	Irrigate stain from eye with caution as stain is colorfast.

Topical Anesthetics
Provide local anesthesia to area, making examination painless. Also used to reduce pain of injury.

Examples	*Nursing Implications*
tetracaine (Pontocaine)	Teaching: Keep eyelid closed to keep eye moist as blink reflex is temporarily lost.

Antiangiogenetics

Inhibits growth of new blood vessels and slows progression of wet age-related macular degeneration.

Examples	*Nursing Implications*
pegaptanib (Macugen)	Monitor for 1 week after administration to detect infection.

Eye Allergy Symptom Relief
Relieves red, itchy eyes caused by allergies.

Examples	*Nursing Implications*
nedocromil (Alocril) azelastine (Astelin) naphazoline (Naphcon) olopatadine (Patanol)	Caution patient not to wear soft contact lenses while eyes are red.

Anti-infectives

Antibiotics
Treat bacterial eye infections.

Examples	*Nursing Implications*
ciprofloxacin (Ciloxan) gatifloxacin (Zymar) polymyxin B and trimethoprim ophthalmic (Polytrim) tobramycin (Tobrex) sulfacetamide (Bleph-10, Isopto Cetamide, Sodium Sulamyd)	Follow instructions for instillation.

Antivirals
Treat viral eye infections.

Examples	*Nursing Implications*
trifluridine (Viroptic)	Follow administration instructions.

Antifungals
Treat fungal eye infections.

Examples	*Nursing Implications*
natamycin (Natacyn)	Follow instructions for instillation.

Table 52.2 Ophthalmic Medications—cont'd

Medication Class/Action

Anti-Inflammatories

Steroidal
Reduce inflammation of conjunctiva, cornea, or eyelids due to infection, edema, allergic reaction, cataract surgery, or burns.

Examples	Nursing Implications
dexamethasone (Decadron) tobramycin and dexamethasone (TobraDex)	Follow instructions for instillation.

Nonsteroidal
Reduce ocular inflammation and pain after cataract surgery, usually within 2 days.

Examples	Nursing Implications
ketorolac (Acular) bromfenac (Xibrom)	Follow instructions for instillation.

Lubricants

Moisten eyes in healthy and ill persons.

Examples	Nursing Implications
artificial tears (Lacri-Lube, Tears Plus)	Explain that ointment distorts vision.

Miotics

Lower intraocular pressure by stimulating papillary and ciliary sphincter muscles.

Examples	Nursing Implications
pilocarpine (Pilocar) physostigmine (Isopto Eserine)	Pupil will be smaller than normal with little or no reaction to light.

Beta-Adrenergic Blockers

Reduce intraocular pressure by reducing aqueous humor formation and increasing its outflow.

Examples	Nursing Implications
timolol (Timoptic) betaxolol (Betoptic)	Monitor for bradycardia, heart block, or wheezing.

Mydriatics

Dilate pupils for examination or surgical procedures.

Examples	Nursing Implications
atropine (Isopto Atropine)	Dilated pupils cannot protect eye from bright light, so dark glasses are needed until medication effects wear off.

Cycloplegics

Paralyze muscles of accommodation for examination or surgical procedures.

Examples	Nursing Implications
cyclopentolate (Cyclogyl)	Contraindicated in patients with glaucoma as it increases intraocular pressure.

Hordeolum and Chalazion

Another type of eyelid infection is a **hordeolum**. An external hordeolum (also known as a *sty*) is a small staphylococcal abscess in the sebaceous gland at the base of the eyelash (either the glands of Zeis or glands of Moll). A sty is a small, raised, reddened area. Use of cosmetics around the eyes may contribute to hordeolum formation. A second type of abscess is a **chalazion** (internal hordeolum). It may form in the connective tissue of the eyelids, specifically in the tarsal glands. A chalazion is larger than a sty. While a sty may be tender, a chalazion often puts pressure on the cornea, causing discomfort. Hordeola usually heal on their own within a few days. They require no treatment. Chalazions may require surgical incision and drainage if they do not drain on their own. If either type of abscess persists, administration of oral antibiotics may be prescribed. Warm compresses applied for 5 to 15 minutes, three to five times a day, may increase comfort and aid healing.

Evidence-Based Practice

Clinical Question
Is widespread use of face masks associated with increased incidence of chalazion?

Evidence
A retrospective study of multicenters of two West Coast institutions compared the number of patients with chalazion in June through August 2020 to the same interval in 2016, 2017, 2018, and 2019. A significant increase in chalazion was shown during the widespread use of masks during the COVID-19 pandemic.

Implications for Nursing Practice
While patients and staff are wearing face masks, their breath is entering the periocular region. Measures that help prevent chalazion formation when wearing masks include use of antiseptic mouthwash containing hydrogen peroxide, alcohol, or povidone iodine; good hand hygiene; avoidance of touching the face; avoidance of excessive mask adjustment; and use of adhesive tape over one's mask on the bridge of the nose to minimize upward direction of air toward the eye.

Reference: Silkiss, R., Paap, M., & Ugradar, S. (2021). Increased incidence of chalazion associated with face mask wear during the COVID-19 pandemic. *American Journal of Ophthalmology Case Reports, 22*, 1–4. https://doi.org/10.1016/j.ajoc.2021.101032

Keratitis

PATHOPHYSIOLOGY AND ETIOLOGY. Keratitis is inflammation of the cornea. It may be acute or chronic, superficial or deep. The depth of keratitis is determined by the affected layers of the cornea. Keratitis may be associated with bacterial conjunctivitis, a viral infection such as herpes simplex, a corneal ulcer, or diseases such as tuberculosis and syphilis. People who have dry eyes or decreased corneal sensation, are immunosuppressed, or wear contact lens or practice poor eye hygiene are at increased risk.

SIGNS AND SYMPTOMS. The cornea has many pain receptors. Any inflammation of the cornea is painful. Pain increases with movement of the lid over the cornea. Other signs and symptoms of keratitis include redness, decreased or blurred vision, **photophobia** (eye sensitivity to light), feeling that something is in the eye, and tearing. In advanced cases, the cornea may appear opaque (cloudy).

DIAGNOSTIC TESTS. Assessment of keratitis or corneal ulcer is done with a slit lamp or a handheld light. The cornea is examined by shining the light source obliquely (diagonally) across the cornea. This shows opacity in the cornea. Fluorescein stain may be used to outline the area of involvement. When the stained area is viewed with a blue light, disruption in the corneal surface shows up clear. If the patient has pain from blepharospasm, a topical ophthalmic anesthetic such as proparacaine can be administered.

THERAPEUTIC MEASURES. Therapeutic measures may include topical antibiotics, topical corticosteroids, topical interferons, antiviral medications for herpes simplex, cycloplegic agents (to keep the iris and ciliary body at rest), and warm compresses. Corneal transplant may be needed for severe damage. The eye may be patched to decrease the amount of eyelid movement over the cornea during healing.

COMPLICATIONS. Corneal infections are usually serious and often threaten eyesight. Corneal tissue may become thin and susceptible to perforation. Untreated keratitis can cause permanent scarring of the cornea, resulting in permanent loss of vision.

Nursing Process for the Patient With Infection and Inflammation of the Eye

DATA COLLECTION. Table 52.3 reviews subjective data. Objective data collection includes the condition of the conjunctiva, eyelids, and eyelashes; the presence of exudate, tearing, any visible abscess on the palpebral border, or a palpable abscess in the eyelid; opacity of the cornea; and visual acuity testing comparing unaffected and affected eyes.

NURSING DIAGNOSES, PLANNING, AND IMPLEMENTATION.

> *Acute Pain related to inflammation or infection of the eye or surrounding tissues*
>
> **EXPECTED OUTCOME:** The patient's pain will be decreased or absent as evidenced by lower rating on a pain scale.

- Identify presence and level of the patient's pain. *Use of dark glasses, rubbing the eye, squinting, and avoiding light may be indicators of pain that can be observed.*
- Administer eye medications as ordered *to relieve eye pain.*

• WORD • BUILDING •
photophobia: photo—light + phobia—fear of

Table 52.3
Subjective Data Collection for Eye Inflammation, Eye Infection, or Visual Impairment

W: Where is it?	What part of the eye or visual field is affected? What characteristics can be seen? Blurry? Hazy? Dark? Halos around lights?	
H: How does it feel?	Pressure? Itchy? Irritated? No pain? Painful? Headaches? How does visual impairment make the patient feel? Fearful? Anxious? Depressed? Helpless? Hopeless? Accepting?	
A: Aggravating and alleviating factors	Is there photosensitivity? Is vision better at a distance or close up? Is it worse when blinking? Reading? Watching television? Only at night?	
T: Timing	Was there exposure to a pathogen? Previous infection or irritation? Was onset sudden? When did the symptoms start? How long have symptoms persisted? Do they come and go? Is visual impairment progressively getting worse?	
S: Severity	Does pain or visual impairment affect the patient's activities of daily living? If so, how severely? Does the patient need assistance to cook, dress, bathe, read mail, pay bills, access health care, obtain transportation, maintain household, or shop?	
U: Useful data for associated symptoms	What is typical eye hygiene? Is the patient infected with lice? Immunosuppressed? Do other members of the family or peer group have infection symptoms? Is there exudate? Are the eyelids stuck together on awakening? Does the patient wear contact lenses, soft contact lenses overnight, or disposable contact lenses? Does the patient have dry eyes? Is the patient infected with tuberculosis, syphilis, or HIV? Does the patient have diabetes, hypertension, a family history of retinitis pigmentosa, a history of eye infection, or eye trauma? Has the patient recently traveled out of the country?	
P: Perception of the problem by the patient	What does the patient think is wrong? How severe does the patient think visual impairment is?	

- Apply warm or cool packs as ordered *to assist in soothing the eye.*
- Patch affected eye as ordered to help reduce pain *by decreasing the movement of the eye across the eyelid.*

Risk for Injury related to visual impairment

EXPECTED OUTCOME: The patient remains free of injury.

- Identify and plan interventions for visual impairments *to promote safety.*
- Advise the patient with one eye patched not to drive *to prevent injury because depth perception is altered.*
- Reinforce teaching to use caution when ambulating and reaching for things *to prevent injury because inflamed eyes often do not focus well and may have exudate, tearing, or ointment present, which can interfere with vision.*

Deficient Knowledge related to eye disease, preventive measures, and treatment from lack of previous experience

EXPECTED OUTCOME: The patient will be able to explain the eye disease, preventive measures, and treatment. The patient will demonstrate correct application of eye medications.

- Reinforce teaching about eye disease, preventive measures, care of the affected eye, and medication administration *for understanding and adherence to therapeutic plan.*
- Observe the patient administering eye medications after reinforcing teaching *to evaluate understanding.*
- Reinforce teaching the patient and their family how *to prevent spreading infection, including hand hygiene, if it is contagious.*
- Reinforce teaching about contact lens hygiene *to prevent reinfection of the eye.*
- Reinforce teaching to not wear contact lenses or use eye makeup when the eye or surrounding structure is inflamed *to prevent irritation.*

EVALUATION. The plan of care has been successful if pain is reduced to an acceptable rating, vision improves or returns to pre-illness levels, injury does not occur as a result of visual impairment, and infection does not occur as a result of poor eye hygiene or contact lenses. The patient explains eye disease, preventive measures, and treatment accurately, and prescribed treatment is stated or demonstrated correctly (e.g., administering eye medications).

Refractive Errors
Pathophysiology and Etiology

Refraction is the bending of light rays as they enter the eye. *Emmetropia* is normal vision. It means that the light rays are bent to focus images precisely on the macula of the retina.

Ametropia describes any refractive error. When an image is not clearly focused on the retina, a refractive error is present. Ametropia occurs when parallel light rays entering the eye are not refracted (bent) to focus precisely on the retina. Refractive errors account for the largest number of impairments in vision. There are four common ametropic disorders: hyperopia, myopia, astigmatism, and presbyopia.

HYPEROPIA. **Hyperopia** (farsightedness) is caused when the globe or eyeball is too short from the front to the back, causing the light rays to focus beyond the retina. People who are hyperopic see faraway images more clearly than nearby images. Hyperopia is corrected with convex lenses (Fig. 52.1).

MYOPIA. **Myopia** (nearsightedness) is caused by light rays focusing in front of the retina. The eyeball is elongated. The light rays do not reach the retina. Distance vision is blurred. Items close are clear. Myopia is corrected with concave lenses (see Fig. 52.1).

> **LEARNING TIP**
> To remember the type of vision a person has, use this saying: *You are what you say*. For example, if you say you are farsighted, it means that you have clear vision of faraway images but difficulty seeing images that are nearer. If you say you are nearsighted, it means that you have clear vision of images that are near but difficulty seeing images that are farther away.

ASTIGMATISM. **Astigmatism** results from unequal curvatures in the shape of the cornea. When parallel light rays enter the eye, the irregular cornea causes the light rays to be refracted to focus on two different points. This results in either myopic or hyperopic astigmatism. The person with astigmatism has blurred vision with distortion. Corneal irregularities can be caused by injury, inflammation, corneal surgery, or an inherited autosomal dominant trait.

PRESBYOPIA. **Presbyopia** is an age-related condition in which the eye's lens gradually loses its elasticity. This makes it difficult for the lens to change shape, reducing its ability to focus light onto the retina to see close objects. This condition differs from the other errors of refraction that relate to the shape of the eyeball. People often compensate for presbyopia by holding objects farther away. It occurs at about age 40. There is no way to stop the lens from becoming more rigid. Reports of eyestrain and mild frontal headache occur. Treatment includes contact lenses, eyeglasses, or surgery. Vuity (pilocarpine HCL ophthalmic solution 1.25%) is the first FDA-approved eye drop that constricts the pupils to improve presbyopia.

Signs and Symptoms
Difficulty reading or seeing objects is reported with errors of refraction. The eyestrain that occurs as one strains to improve visual acuity often causes a headache.

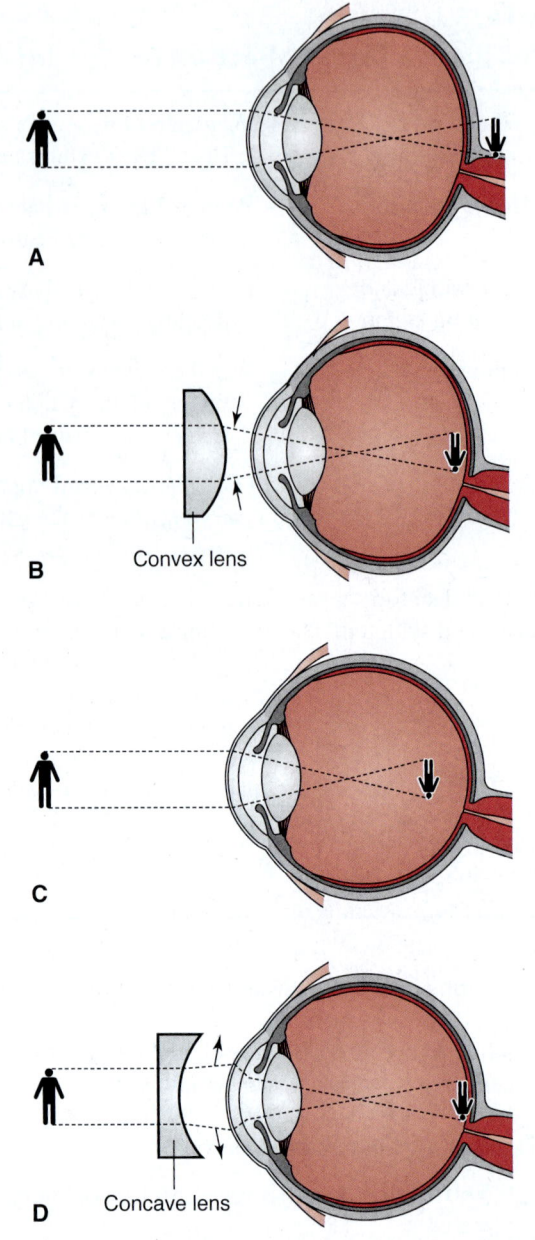

FIGURE 52.1 Refractive disorders. (A) Hyperopia (farsightedness). The eyeball is too short, causing the image to focus beyond the retina. (B) Corrected hyperopia. (C) Myopia (nearsightedness). A long eyeball causes the image to focus in front of the retina. (D) Corrected myopia.

Diagnostic Tests
A refractive error can be estimated by use of a Snellen chart. A retinoscopic examination definitively identifies the refractive error. Before this examination, a cycloplegic medication is often instilled (see Table 52.2). A cycloplegic medication dilates the pupil. It temporarily paralyzes the ciliary muscle to prevent accommodation. The internal and external eye are examined. Trial lenses via retinoscope are used to identify

• WORD • BUILDING •

presbyopia: presby—old man + opia—concerning vision

the type of lens to correct the refractive error in each eye. With a cycloplegic agent, blurred vision might be present. Sunglasses should be worn until the agent wears off. In addition, the patient should be instructed that driving and reading might not be possible until the effect of the cycloplegic medication is gone.

Therapeutic Measures
Refractive errors are commonly treated with either eyeglasses or contact lenses. The corrective lenses bend the parallel light rays so that they converge on the macular portion of the retina. Laser-assisted in situ keratomileusis (LASIK) and photorefractive keratectomy (PRK) are surgical procedures that correct refractive errors. With LASIK and PRK, laser energy makes the cornea flatter to correct myopia, or more cone shaped with hyperopia. Small incision lenticule extraction (SMILE) provides correction of refractive error with a much smaller incision than LASIK. For patients ages 21 to 45 years, an implantable collamer lens is an option that does not remove eye tissue but works with the patient's lens to correct refractive errors. Intrastromal corneal rings can be implanted in the eye to flatten a Bulging cornea to correct vision.

Blindness
Pathophysiology and Etiology
Blindness is complete or almost complete absence of sight. Blindness in adults is caused by various factors that impair nerve transmission of light images or by damage to the optic nerve or brain, such as cataracts, glaucoma, diabetes, hypertension, and trauma. Blindness may be permanent or transient, complete or partial. It may occur only in darkness (night blindness).

Signs and Symptoms
Total vision loss may be reported. In other cases, vision may be described as blurred, distorted, or absent in specific areas of the visual field. Vision may be reported as blurry or hazy with corneal visual problems, cataracts, diabetic retinopathy, or refractive errors. Objects may appear dark or absent in the peripheral field with glaucoma or retinitis pigmentosa (rare inherited degeneration of the pigmented layer of the retina). The center of the visual field may appear dark for individuals with diabetic retinopathy or macular degeneration (Fig. 52.2). Half the visual field may be impaired in patients with hemianopia, which results from a defect in the optic pathways in the brain and occurs with stroke.

Diagnostic Tests
Diagnostic tests include a visual field examination, tonometry, and slit-lamp microscope examination. Retinal angiography follows blood flow through the retinal vessels to detect vascular changes. Ultrasonography may be used to visualize changes in the posterior eye that cannot be directly examined because of other pathological conditions. These conditions include a cloudy cornea, a bloody vitreous, or an opaque lens. The IDx-DR is a newer device that takes pictures of the

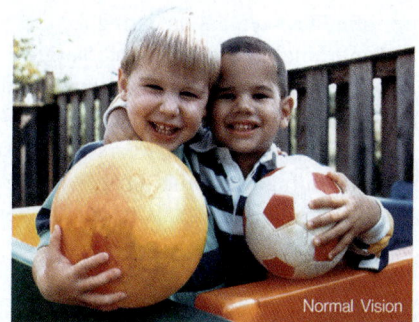

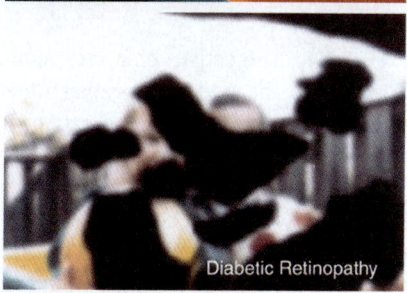

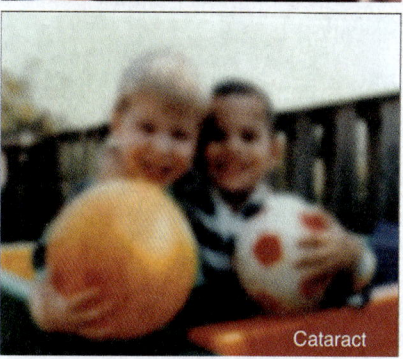

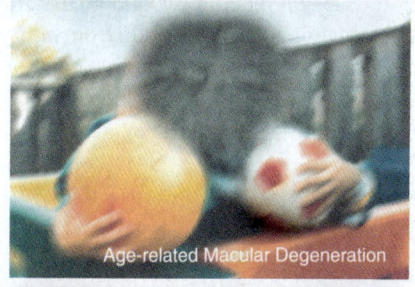

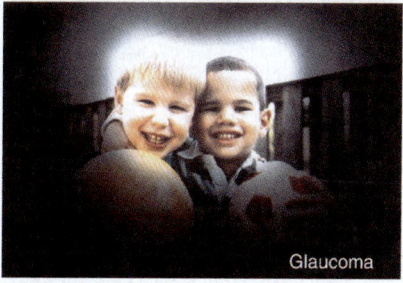

FIGURE 52.2 Visual field abnormalities. (A) Normal vision. (B) Diabetic retinopathy. (C) Cataracts. (D) Macular degeneration. (E) Advanced glaucoma.

fundus for early detection of diabetic retinopathy and macular edema. This exam can be done in the health-care provider's office and referrals can be made to eye specialists sooner.

Therapeutic Measures

Treatment for blindness centers on caring for the underlying condition and may include medications, surgical intervention, corrective eyewear, and referral to supportive services. For retinal disorders, a device called the *Argus II* may be implanted into the eye. The patient wears special sunglasses with a video camera that transmits images to the Argus II. This retinal prosthetic sends signals to healthy retinal cells that send the signals to the brain.

Nursing Process for the Patient With Visual Impairment

DATA COLLECTION. Subjective data are collected (see Table 52.3). Observe the patient to gather objective data. Do they squint or rub the eyes? Is the patient using compensatory measures (e.g., magnifying glass, sitting close to the television, using large-print reading materials, avoiding reading, using eyeglasses)? Psychosocial data are important. Blind people may be withdrawn or socially isolated. They can have low self-esteem, poor coping mechanisms, or poor interpersonal skills.

NURSING DIAGNOSES, PLANNING, AND IMPLEMENTATION. Nursing care begins by understanding how to interact with a patient who is visually impaired (Box 52.1). The patient's level of independence is included in planning care. Patients with minimal visual impairment or who have attended rehabilitation may be able to function independently. Patients who have recently become visually impaired may be completely dependent. They will need to learn ways of coping to become independent.

Planning focuses on meeting several goals. They include self-care needs, keeping the patient safe from injury, and supporting the grieving process. Inform the patient of agencies, services, and devices that promote independence. Families must be included in planning. They need to understand and be supportive of the self-image and role performance changes that can occur.

Self-Care Deficit (Bathing, Dressing, Feeding) related to impaired vision

EXPECTED OUTCOME: The patient will demonstrate ability to perform activities of daily living (ADLs), with assistance if necessary.

- Observe patient's performance of ADLs to *determine patient's ability to adequately dress and feed self.*
- Assist with grooming and dressing (such as pre-matching coordinated clothing or laying coordinated clothing out for patient to dress) as required. *Ensures patient's grooming and dressing needs are met.*
- Provide assistance with preparing food and feeding as required; for severe vision loss, use the face of a clock for referencing location of foods on a plate. *Ensures patient's feeding needs are met.*

Risk for Injury related to visual impairment

EXPECTED OUTCOME: The patient remains free of injury.

- Provide for optimal care of assistive appliances such as eyeglasses, including maintenance of proper prescription, fit, and cleaning. *Improperly fitting or dirty eyeglasses may impair vision even further. Older adults should have their eyeglass prescription checked yearly.*
- Structure environment to compensate for visual loss by adding color and contrast (e.g., chairs and carpeting in contrasting colors, bright tape or paint on stairs, medicine bottles color-coded with colored dot stickers). *Makes the environment easier to visualize and interpret, and assists in depth perception and identifying medications.*

Box 52.1

Interacting With a Patient Who Has a Visual Impairment

- Identify yourself when entering a room and at each contact with the patient.
- Use a normal tone of voice and do not yell, as this is not a hearing impairment.
- Speak directly to the patient, not through a companion.
- If the patient has a seeing eye dog, do not play with the dog, pet it, or feed it without consulting the patient—the dog is working! Make sure the patient's dog is near the bed, on a mat provided especially for the dog, preferably on the side of the bed that is less likely to be used by staff. Instruct staff and visitors about the seeing eye dog.
- When orienting the patient to the hospital room, explain the location of items they may need, such as the water pitcher, call light, bed controls, urinal, and tissues. Attempt to keep these items in the same place at all times.
- Ask the patient what their needs are; do not assume the patient needs help with everything.
- Explain procedures before beginning them. Speak to the patient before touching them.
- Explain activity occurring in the room or within the patient's auditory range.
- At mealtime, explain the location of items on the tray by comparing their position to the numbers on a clock if doing so is agreeable to the patient (e.g., milk at 2:00, peas at 7:00).
- When seating the patient, place the patient's hand on the arm of the chair.
- When walking with the patient, allow them to grasp an arm and walk a half step behind. Be aware of obstacles on either side when walking.
- Tell the patient when you leave the area so they do not continue conversation in empty room.

- Introduce other assistive devices such as handheld magnifying glasses, tableside magnifiers, television magnifiers, large-print items, talking watches, and phones, alarm clocks, and calculators with large numbers. *Patients may not be aware of assistive devices that could help them adapt to vision loss during activities such as watching television or reading letters and magazines. Allows patient to rely on hearing rather than vision.*

> **Deficit Knowledge related to new onset of impaired vision.**
>
> **EXPECTED OUTCOME:** The patient will understand resources that will allow maintenance of independence.

- Refer to an ophthalmologist, occupational therapist, or resources from such organizations as American Foundation for the Blind or Prevent Blindness. *Specialized clinicians can provide detailed examination and treatment. Specialized resource groups assist people in coping with vision loss and maximizing abilities.*

EVALUATION. The outcomes for a patient with a visual impairment are met if the patient demonstrates the ability to complete ADLs with increasing independence, remains free of injury, and demonstrates the ability to contact agencies and services for those with visual impairments.

Diabetic Retinopathy
Pathophysiology and Etiology
Retinopathy is a disorder in which vascular changes occur in the retinal blood vessels, most commonly with diabetes. Pathological changes in diabetic retinopathy are related to excess glucose, changes in retinal capillary walls, formation of microaneurysms, and constriction of retinal blood vessels. Nonproliferarative and proliferative are two forms of diabetic retinopathy.

Nonproliferative retinopathy results from microaneurysms on the retinal capillary walls, occluded vessels, or hard exudates. Microaneurysms may leak blood into the central retina or macula. Leakage may cause edema. The patient may notice a decrease in color discrimination and visual acuity.

Proliferative retinopathy is characterized by the formation of new blood vessels. They grow into the retinal and optic disc area to increase the blood supply to the retina. The newly formed blood vessels are fragile and abnormal, and they often leak blood into the vitreous and retina. In addition, the newer vessels may grow into the vitreous, causing a traction effect that pulls the vitreous away from the retina, then pulls the retina away from the choroid. This condition is called retinal detachment (discussed later).

Signs and Symptoms
Central visual acuity or color vision may decrease due to macular edema (see Fig. 52.2). Many patients with diabetic retinopathy have no symptoms until the proliferative stage when vision is lost. Visual loss at the last stage usually cannot be restored. If people with diabetes have changes in visual acuity or color discrimination, they should immediately contact their health-care provider (HCP).

Complications
Early treatment for diabetic retinopathy is very successful in preventing further visual loss. However, existing visual loss cannot be reversed. Therefore, it is essential for patients with diabetes to have a comprehensive eye examination through dilated pupils at least once each year. Careful control of diabetes and hypertension during the first 5 years after diagnosis is vital. It can delay onset of diabetic retinopathy. Healthy People 2030 has an objective to increase the number of annual eye examinations performed for adults over 18 years old who have been diagnosed with diabetes (Office of Disease Prevention and Health Promotion, 2020).

Diagnostic Tests
Diabetic retinopathy can only be diagnosed with examination of the internal eye. First, the pupil is dilated with a cycloplegic agent. Then an ophthalmoscope is used to view the internal eye. Retinoangiography may also be used to enhance the examination. In the initial stages, vessels may appear swollen and tortuous (twisted).

Therapeutic Measures
Treatment of diabetic retinopathy is to stop the leakage of blood and fluid into the vitreous and retina. Surgical or pharmacologic methods can be used. The leaking microaneurysm can be sealed with a laser. Lasers can also shrink abnormal blood vessels. If blood has already leaked into the vitreous, a vitrectomy is performed to drain vitreous humor out of the eye chamber. It is replaced with saline or silicon oil (oil often removed months later). The replacement fluid is necessary to support the structures of the eyeball until healing can occur. Use of intravitreal corticosteroids is beneficial.

Nursing Process for the Patient With Diabetic Retinopathy
DATA COLLECTION. Risk factors for diabetic retinopathy are identified. The patient may not have symptoms to report.

NURSING DIAGNOSIS, PLANNING, AND IMPLEMENTATION. The planning phase of the nursing process for diabetic retinopathy focuses on prevention of visual loss with early detection and treatment. If the patient has entered the final stage and is already visually impaired, the "Nursing Process for the Patient With Visual Impairment" is used.

> **Ineffective Health Self-Management**
>
> **EXPECTED OUTCOME:** The patient will state ability to manage therapeutic regimen.

• WORD • BUILDING •
retinopathy: retino—having to do with the retina + pathy—illness, disease, or suffering

- Determine whether the patient with a visual impairment who is diabetic can monitor blood glucose and draw up and administer the correct amount of insulin. *Specialty devices are available that can be preset to draw up the correct amounts of insulin. Family members may have to assist the patient. Controlling blood sugar levels helps prevent complications.*
- Reinforce teaching to control blood pressure with lifestyle changes and medications *to help prevent complications.*
- Reinforce teaching the patient the importance of yearly comprehensive eye examinations *to detect visual changes for treatment.*

EVALUATION. The patient goal is met if the patient is able to manage the therapeutic regimen.

Retinal Detachment
Pathophysiology and Etiology
Retinal detachment is a separation of the retina from the choroid layer beneath it (see Fig. 51.3). This allows fluid to enter the space between the layers. Retinal detachment has three possible causes: a hole or tear in the retina that allows fluid to flow between the two layers; fibrous tissue in the vitreous humor that contracts and pulls the retina away from its normal position; or fluid or exudate accumulation in the subretinal space that separates the retinal layers.

Signs and Symptoms
Patients experiencing a retinal detachment report a sudden change in vision. Initially, as the retina is pulled, patients report seeing flashing lights and then floaters. The flashing lights are caused by vitreous traction on the retina. Floaters are caused by bleeding into the vitreous fluid. When the retina detaches, patients often describe it as "looking through a veil" or "cobwebs" and finally "like a curtain being lowered over the field of vision," with darkness resulting. There is no pain. The retina does not contain sensory nerves. The patient typically has a loss of visual acuity in the affected eye. There is loss of peripheral vision.

Diagnostic Tests
Indirect ophthalmoscopy allows the examiner to visualize the retina. It may be pale, opaque, and in folds with retinal detachment. The type of detachment is diagnosed. If lesions are present in the eye, the slit-lamp examination magnifies them. Ultrasound can also be used to detect retinal detachment or retinal breaks.

Therapeutic Measures
Emergency medical treatment must be sought to protect vision. The amount of vision restored varies depending on the affected area. One or more procedures are performed to treat retinal tears or detachment. They include lasers, cryopexy, pneumatic retinopexy, or scleral buckling.

LASER SURGERY. Laser surgery focuses a laser beam at the torn area of the retina, causing a controlled burn. This forms scars around the tear and reattaches the retina to surrounding tissue.

CRYOPEXY. Cryopexy is the placement of a supercooled probe on the sclera over the affected area. The probe freezes and scars the tear or hole, a principle similar to the laser procedure.

PNEUMATIC RETINOPEXY. Pneumatic retinopexy, done in the HCP's office, is time-consuming for the patient. It involves injecting air or gas into the eye chamber to hold the retina in place. The patient must be extremely compliant with the treatment regimen. They must recline for about 16 hours before the procedure so the retina can fall back toward the choroid. Because air rises, the patient must maintain a prone position that keeps the air bubble against the detached area for up to 8 hours a day for 3 weeks.

SCLERAL BUCKLING. Scleral buckling is a surgical procedure for retinal detachment. A silicon buckle under a thin band of silicon around the sclera is tightened to create an indentation that brings the choroid in contact with the retina. Cryosurgery or laser surgery is usually used to permanently adhere the retina and choroid layers together. Vitrectomy is often done as well.

Complications
With any retinal procedure, there is risk of increased intraocular pressure (IOP), retinal tears, and recurrent retinal detachment.

Nursing Process for the Patient With Retinal Detachment
DATA COLLECTION. Subjective data include patient observation of the loss of peripheral vision, changes in visual acuity, and the presence of floaters, flashing lights, cobwebs, or veil-like visual impairments. The patient should not report pain. Objective data include the patient's visual acuity, visual fields, ability to perform ADLs, and level of anxiety.

NURSING DIAGNOSES, PLANNING, IMPLEMENTATION, AND EVALUATION. See "Nursing Process for the Patient Having Eye Surgery" later in this chapter.

> **CLINICAL JUDGMENT**
>
> **Mr. Samuel**, your neighbor, is working in the yard when a branch strikes his right eye. When you go to check on him, he reports seeing flashes of light and then, a short time later, a dark shadow over his right eye.
>
> 1. What do you have Mr. Samuel do?
> 2. After having a scleral buckling procedure, Mr. Samuel reports nausea. What action should the nurse take?
> 3. Ondansetron (Zofran) 4 mg intramuscular is ordered. Ondansetron 2 mg/mL in 2 mL/vial is available. How many milliliters will the nurse give?
>
> *Suggested answers are at the end of the chapter.*

> **BE SAFE!**
> **Avoid Failure to Recognize and Communicate**
> - Severe eye pain, decreased vision, halos lights, and headache could indicate angle-closure glaucoma, which is an ophthalmic emergency and should be reported immediately.
> - Report immediately to the HCP any sudden changes in a patient's vision such as flashing lights, floaters, "cobwebs," or "curtain lowered over field of vision," which could indicate serious problems such as a detached retina.

Glaucoma

Glaucoma is a group of diseases that damage the optic nerve. All but one type cause increased pressure within the eye that damages the optic nerve. The optic nerve transmits visual information from the eye to the brain. The damage to this nerve is silent, progressive, and irreversible. Loss of peripheral vision occurs, followed by reduced central vision and eventually blindness (see Fig. 52.2). Normal tension glaucoma with optic nerve damage can also occur. It is a form of primary open-angle glaucoma. Glaucoma has no cure. Treatment plans must be followed to prevent any further vision loss and blindness.

Pathophysiology

There are different types of glaucoma generally categorized by the anterior chamber: open-angle glaucoma (OAG) and angle-closure glaucoma (ACG). The most common form of glaucoma is primary open-angle glaucoma (POAG). ACG is also known as narrow-angle glaucoma. Both OAG and ACG can be divided into primary and secondary. Secondary glaucoma may result from infections, tumors, or injuries. Congenital or infantile glaucoma can occur in infants or up to age 2 to 3 years.

POAG occurs when the drainage system of the eye, the trabecular meshwork and scleral venous sinus, degenerates and blocks the flow of aqueous humor and/or there is an increased aqueous production. ACG occurs in people who have an anatomically narrowed angle at the junction where the iris meets the cornea. When nearby eye structures such as the iris protrude into the anterior chamber, the angle is occluded, blocking the flow of aqueous fluid. ACG is considered a medical emergency and results in partial or total blindness if not treated.

Etiology and Prevention

Incidences of POAG increase in those age 40 and older (age 40 for African Americans [Glaucoma Research Foundation, 2017] and age 50 for European Americans), in people with diabetes, and in those with a family history of glaucoma. POAG occurs four to five times more in African Americans than in European Americans. The incidence of ACG is highest among Asians, women over age 45, and people who are nearsighted. Those in high-risk groups or over age 60 should have yearly eye examinations.

Signs and Symptoms

POAG usually develops bilaterally. The onset is usually gradual and painless. The patient may have no noticeable symptoms. After some time, peripheral vision gradually decreases. Central vision is not usually affected until late in the disease.

ACG is an ophthalmic emergency. It typically has a unilateral, rapid onset. The patient may report severe pain over the affected eye, decreased vision, halos around lights, headache, and nausea and vomiting. Eye redness and a cloudy cornea may occur. Increased IOP can cause nausea and vomiting.

Diagnostic Tests

Measuring IOP and identifying optic nerve damage and visual loss diagnose glaucoma. Tonometry detects increased IOP (normal is 12 to 20 mm Hg), present in about 50% of glaucoma cases. In ACG, IOP may exceed 50 mm Hg. The GDx Access, a laser device, detects nerve damage long before the patient has symptoms. A visual field examination checks for peripheral vision loss. Corneal thickness is measured, as it can affect IOP. With gonioscopy, a special lens is used to look at the angle where the iris meets the cornea to identify POAG or ACG.

Therapeutic Measures

Treatment for POAG focuses on decreasing IOP by opening the aqueous flow. Medications and laser therapy are considered first-line therapy. Cholinergic agents (**miotics**) such as physostigmine (Isopto Eserine) or pilocarpine (Pilocar) are given to constrict the pupil, which pulls the iris away from the drainage canal. This allows the aqueous fluid to flow freely. Beta blockers such as timolol (Timoptic) and betaxolol (Betoptic) may be given to slow the production of aqueous fluid, which helps decrease IOP. Steroid eye drops may be ordered to reduce inflammation. The patient having an acute attack of ACG is also given these types of medications, as well as analgesics, and placed on bedrest.

Patients with glaucoma need lifelong monitoring of IOP. With no symptoms, adherence to medication treatment is often an issue. Other factors that cause nonadherence are the patient's age, inability to afford medication, and not understanding the seriousness of the disease. Patients should carry medical alert identification and medications for their glaucoma to help prevent administration of medications in emergency situations that are contraindicated for ACG. The implanted EYEMATE system remotely tracks eye pressure in patients with glaucoma. HCP's can then adjust glaucoma eye drop doses remotely.

Many categories of medications are contraindicated with POAG and ACG regardless of route and can cause blockage of the eye's drainage system. They include glucocorticoids (topical, ocular, oral, or inhaled), systemic sympathomimetics (ephedrine, pseudoephedrine-containing medications, decongestants, tricyclic antidepressants, antipsychotics, and selective serotonin uptake inhibitors), and anticholinergics. Before a medication is given, the nurse must determine that it is not contraindicated in POAG and ACG in order to prevent serious complications.

> **LEARNING TIP**
> Mydriatic medications are contraindicated in ACG. They can cause an acute episode of increased intraocular pressure by dilating the pupil and pushing the iris back. This blocks the outflow of aqueous humor.
> Miotic medications constrict the pupil. They can be given to patients with ACG.
> To remember the pupillary action of mydriatic medications and miotic medications so that the appropriate medication is given and contraindicated ones are never given, think of the following:
> - **D** = **d**ilate = my**d**riatic = **d**o not give.
> - No D = constricts = miotic = okay to give.

Surgical Management

Laser trabeculoplasty is often used first for POAG. A narrow laser beam opens drainage in the trabecular meshwork to allow aqueous humor to flow freely. Selective laser trabeculoplasty uses low-level laser that affects selected pigmented tissue in the eye to improve drainage of aqueous humor through the trabecular meshwork (Fig. 52.3). Surgical therapy (trabeculectomy) can be used for patients who have not responded to laser therapy or medication or have severe visual loss at baseline. Surgery creates an area where the aqueous humor can flow freely or reduce aqueous humor production, preventing increased IOP. Traditional trabeculectomy removes part of the trabecular meshwork. Glaucoma drainage devices (shunts) carry aqueous humor away. For ACG, laser peripheral iridotomy or surgical iridectomy is performed. Laser iridotomy creates a small hole on the edge of the iris so aqueous fluid can flow out of the area. Prophylactic laser iridotomy may be performed on the other eye to prevent ACG.

Nursing Process for the Patient With Glaucoma

DATA COLLECTION. The patient should be monitored for pain, loss of central and peripheral vision, understanding of disease and adherence to treatment regimen, and ability to conduct ADLs.

NURSING DIAGNOSES, PLANNING, AND IMPLEMENTATION. The goal of nursing care for the patient with glaucoma is to prevent further visual loss and promote comfort if the patient is experiencing pain with acute glaucoma. See "Nursing Process for the Patient With Visual Impairment" earlier in this chapter and "Nursing Process for the Patient Having Eye Surgery" later in this chapter for additional nursing diagnoses.

Acute Pain related to increased intraocular pressure

EXPECTED OUTCOME: The patient will report that pain is relieved.

- Give analgesics as needed for ACG glaucoma *to relieve pain.*

Risk for Injury related to decreased vision

EXPECTED OUTCOME: The patient will not be injured as a result of visual impairment.

- Refer the patient to support services that *provide adaptive visual devices.*
- Reinforce teaching to the patient and their family to keep walking areas clutter free and not to rearrange furniture without patient's knowledge *to prevent falls or injury.*

Deficient Knowledge related to medical regimen and disease process due to no prior experience

EXPECTED OUTCOME: The patient will demonstrate correct instillation of eye medications and be able to verbalize understanding of condition and treatment.

- If needed, use large-print labels or audiotaped directions *if the patient is unable to see the label on the eye drop bottle.*
- If needed, place large, multicolored dot stickers on medication bottles and on corresponding instruction cards *for patients with multiple medications.*
- Reinforce teaching the patient the need for regular eye examinations through dilated pupils *to monitor disease and detect complications.*
- Reinforce teaching the patient how to administer medications with a return demonstration *to ensure that eye drops are administered properly.*
- Reinforce teaching the patient to rest their hand on the forehead *if the patient has trouble keeping the hand steady when administering eye drops.*

EVALUATION. Interventions are successful if the patient maintains an acceptable level of comfort, has no further loss of vision, and can care for self with assistance. Also, the patient does not suffer injury as a result of the visual impairment, demonstrates correct instillation of eye medications, and can verbalize understanding of condition and treatment.

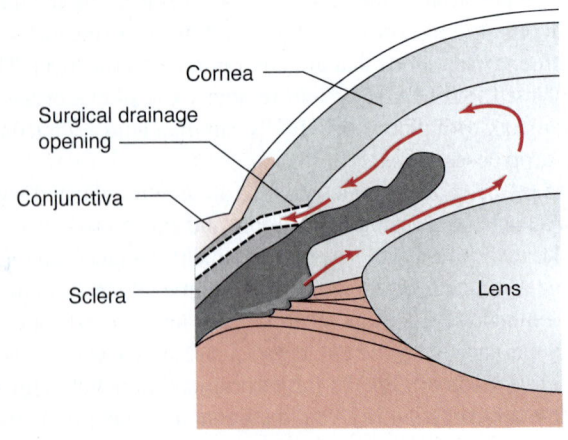

FIGURE 52.3 Flow of aqueous humor after trabeculoplasty (*arrows*).

Cataracts

Pathophysiology and Etiology
A **cataract** is an opacity in the lens of the eye that may cause a loss of visual acuity (see Fig. 52.2). Vision is diminished because the light rays are unable to reach the retina through the clouded lens. Factors that contribute to cataract development include age, ultraviolet (UV) radiation (sunlight), diabetes, smoking, steroids, nutritional deficiencies, alcohol consumption, intraocular infections, trauma, and congenital defects.

Signs and Symptoms
Cataracts are painless. Symptoms of cataract formation may include loss of vision, difficulty with night vision, reading fine print or seeing in bright light, increased sensitivity to glare such as when driving at night, and myopic shift (increase in nearsightedness).

Diagnostic Tests
Cataracts are diagnosed with an eye examination. Visual acuity is tested for near and far vision. The direct ophthalmoscope and slit-lamp microscope are used to examine the lens, which appears opaque, and other internal structures.

Surgical Management
When cataracts begin to interfere with daily living and quality of life, intraocular lens implant surgery is recommended. One eye is treated at a time. Outpatient laser (with a LenSx laser) or no-stitch cataract surgery to remove the cloudy lens is performed. Implantable lenses come in various types. They are inserted after lens removal. Some lenses reduce the need for eyeglasses. Postoperative activity restrictions vary among surgeons, but heavy lifting and strenuous activity may be restricted. Patients should avoid swimming until directed to by the surgeon. Complications are rare.

Nursing Process for the Patient With Cataracts
DATA COLLECTION. The patient is monitored for visual deficits to assist care planning. Knowledge needs about the disease, treatment, and postoperative care are identified.

NURSING DIAGNOSES, PLANNING, IMPLEMENTATION, AND EVALUATION. Preoperative and postoperative nursing care is the primary nursing responsibility for the patient with cataracts, as discussed next.

Nursing Process for the Patient Having Eye Surgery
DATA COLLECTION. Subjective data to collect include type of visual impairment, which eye is affected, presence of pain, and anxiety. Objective data may include visual acuity with and without corrective lenses and peripheral field measurements. Eye tearing, redness, or swelling is noted.

NURSING DIAGNOSES, PLANNING, AND IMPLEMENTATION.

> **Risk for Injury related to altered visual acuity**
>
> **EXPECTED OUTCOME:** The patient will remain free of injury.

- Ambulate with assistance and use clearly marked stairs *to prevent injury*.

> **Deficient Knowledge related to preoperative and postoperative eye care**
>
> **EXPECTED OUTCOME:** The patient will verbalize preoperative and postoperative care directions.

- Reinforce teaching the patient about disease process, preoperative and postoperative care, and how to administer eye medications as instructed *to increase patient knowledge*.
- Reinforce teaching the patient to seek medical care for sudden or worsening pain, watery or bloody discharge, or sudden loss of vision *because these are signs of hemorrhage or problems*.

> **Anxiety related to visual alteration and surgery**
>
> **EXPECTED OUTCOME:** The patient will report reduced anxiety.

- Give the patient the opportunity to discuss their feelings about vision loss or surgery *to reduce anxiety*.

EVALUATION. The patient goals have been met if the patient is free of injury, verbalizes preoperative and postoperative directions, and reports reduced anxiety.

> **CUE RECOGNITION 52.1**
>
> You are assisting with a new admission at a skilled nursing facility. The resident reports that he has had diabetes for 20 years and has not had an eye examination in 5 years. What action do you take?
>
> *Suggested answers are at the end of the chapter.*

Macular Degeneration

Pathophysiology and Etiology
Age-related macular degeneration (AMD) is the leading cause of permanent impairment of close-up vision or reading in U.S. residents ages 65 and older (Centers for Disease Control and Prevention [CDC], 2020). It involves deterioration and scarring within the **macula**, the area on the retina where light rays converge for the sharp, central vision needed to read and see small objects (Fig. 52.4). The macula is also responsible for color vision.

There are two types of AMD: dry (atrophic) and wet (exudative). In dry AMD, which accounts for 70% to 90% of cases, photoreceptors in the macula fail and are not replaced because of age (CDC, 2020). In the wet form, retinal tissue degenerates, allowing vitreous fluid or blood into the subretinal space. New fragile blood vessels form (angiogenesis). This compromises the macular tissue, causing subretinal edema. Eventually, fibrous scar tissue forms, severely limiting central vision.

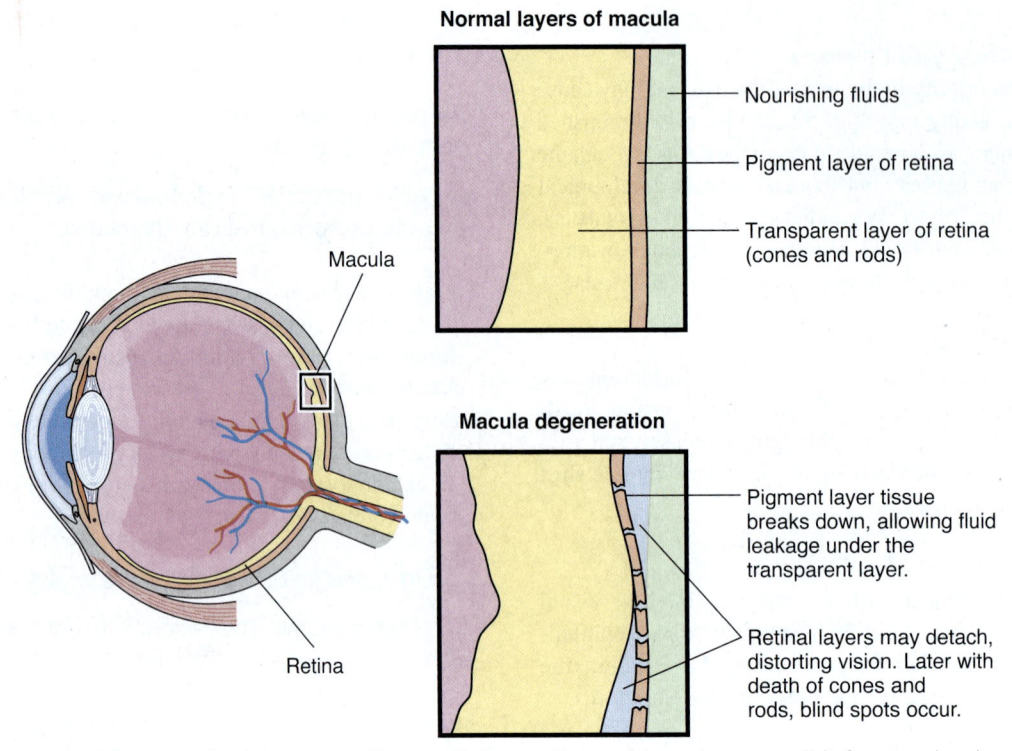

FIGURE 52.4 Macular degeneration. The macula is a small area of the retina responsible for central and color vision.

People at higher risk of developing AMD include White individuals as well as those older than 60 with a family history of macular degeneration, who have diabetes, who smoke, and who are frequently exposed to UV light.

> **NURSING CARE TIP**
> Most damaging exposure to UV light occurs before age 18. It is important for everyone of all ages to use adequate UV protective sunglasses.

Prevention
A healthy lifestyle is important. A nutritious diet high in carotenoids, lutein, zeaxanthin, and zinc has been associated with decreased risk of AMD. A Mediterranean diet including dark green leafy vegetables (e.g., kale, collard greens, lettuce, spinach) and orange- and yellow-colored fruits and vegetables (e.g., peppers, corn) is helpful. Measuring macula pigment optical density is an important screening tool. Physical activity has a protective effect against AMD. Smoking increases the risk of developing AMD. Hypertension should be monitored and controlled.

Signs and Symptoms
Early AMD is often asymptomatic. Dry AMD is characterized by slow, progressive loss of central and near vision (see Fig. 52.2). People usually have the condition in both eyes in varying degrees. Vision loss is often noticed as difficulty with reading or driving. Wet AMD has the same loss of central and near vision, but onset is sudden and causes more severe vision loss. Vision loss can occur in one or both eyes, described as blurred vision, distortion of straight lines, and a dark or empty spot in central area of vision. Some patients have decreased ability to distinguish colors.

Diagnostic Tests
Visual acuity for near and far vision and an examination of the internal eye structures with an ophthalmoscope is done. The examiner uses an Amsler grid (Fig. 52.5) to detect central vision distortion. A color vision test evaluates color differentiation. Patients are given an Amsler grid to look at regularly to monitor vision changes. If any grid lines look crooked or disappear, the patient should contact the HCP. (See "How to Use Amsler Grid" under "Patient Teaching Guidelines" in your resources on Davis Advantage.) Digital imaging, an optical coherence tomography retinal scan (similar to a computed tomography [CT] scan), or IV fluorescein (dye) angiography are used to evaluate blood vessel leakage or abnormalities in the eye.

Therapeutic Measures
Unfortunately, no treatment exists for dry AMD. Prevention is important when possible. Most patients with dry AMD do not lose peripheral vision or become totally blind and instead are legally blind (less than 20/200 vision with correction). Low-vision telescopic glasses can enhance remaining vision. A telescope implant is available for those with

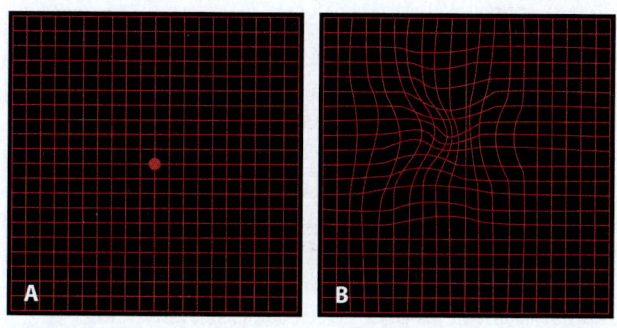

FIGURE 52.5 An Amsler grid is used for self-assessment to identify central vision blind spots or distortions. (A) Normal Amsler grid. The red on black grid was developed to increase better accuracy with the test. (B) Abnormal Amsler grid with distortion and small area of central vision loss.

end-stage AMD. It is placed in only one eye after the eye's natural lens is removed to help restore central vision. Visit www.centrasight.com for more information.

Wet AMD is treated with intermittent injection into the eye of an antiangiogenesis medication (e.g., ranibizumab [Lucentis] or aflibercept [Eylea]). Medications that are antiangiogenetic prevent formation of fragile blood vessels that can leak and bleed. Older treatment options are less common because of the availability of antiangiogenesis medications. They include laser photocoagulation that seals the leaking blood vessels or photodynamic therapy. With either type of AMD, patients must adapt to significant visual loss. (See "Nursing Care Plan for the Patient With Visual Impairment" earlier in this chapter.)

Nursing Process for the Patient With Macular Degeneration

See "Nursing Process for the Patient With Visual Impairment" earlier in this chapter.

Trauma

Eye emergencies and trauma must be immediately treated. Examples include foreign bodies, chemical burns, UV exposure, direct heat sources, abrasions, lacerations from dragging something across the eye, and penetrating wounds. Penetrating wounds are the most serious eye injury. They increase the risk for infection and blindness.

Signs and Symptoms

Foreign bodies produce pain when the eyeball or eyelid moves. The eye tears excessively to irrigate the noxious substance out of the eye. Injuries that irritate or penetrate layers of the cornea result in mild to severe pain. With corneal abrasions, pain may be delayed for several hours. Other symptoms with abrasions, lacerations, and foreign bodies include conjunctival redness, photosensitivity, decreased visual acuity, erythema, and pruritus. Acute pain and burning are characteristic symptoms of a burn to the eye. Penetrating wound symptoms depend on the area of the eye and the extent of the damage.

Diagnostic Tests

Visual acuity is tested. It is important to establish baseline acuity to evaluate effectiveness of treatment. Many patients resist acuity testing because of discomfort. Testing includes examination by slit-lamp microscope and direct ophthalmoscope. Fluorescein staining is used to evaluate abrasions.

Therapeutic Measures

Foreign bodies are treated with a normal saline flush. This irrigates the object out of the eye or to a point where it can be removed with a swab. Topical antibiotic ointment is prescribed to prevent infection. Chemical burns must be treated immediately with a 15- to 20-minute irrigation at an eye wash station or with sterile solution at a medical facility. Topical antibiotic ointments are prescribed. Burns from heat or UV radiation are not irrigated.

Abrasions and lacerations are cleansed with normal saline. Then they are treated with anti-infective ointments or drops.

An eye specialist treats penetrating wounds. After the injury, both eyes should be covered to prevent ocular movement. Any protruding object should be stabilized but not removed until the HCP can assess the patient.

Complications

If the eye cannot be saved with medical treatment, surgical removal may be needed. This procedure is called **enucleation** (entire eyeball removal).

Nursing Care for the Patient With Eye Trauma

FOREIGN BODIES. The eye is inspected for foreign bodies, which may be visible on the eyeball. Assist the HCP, who will evert the eyelid to examine the surface and irrigate the eye.

BURNS. Identification of the type of burn is done because treatment options vary. Immediate irrigation of the eyes is performed once it has been established that a chemical burn has taken place, unless contraindicated for the chemical. Medication and eye patching are applied as indicated.

ABRASIONS AND LACERATIONS. The eye is examined for visible lacerations and then cleansed, medicated, and patched as indicated.

PENETRATING WOUNDS. The patient is kept calm and relaxed to minimize eye movement and increased IOP. If a protruding object is present, the object is stabilized with tape or other supports.

HEARING DISORDERS

Hearing Loss

Hearing loss is a common disability in the United States, with 5.9% of the population reporting hearing disability.

• WORD • BUILDING •

enucleation: e—removed from + nuclear—center

Hearing disability is more common in older adults and in men (Okoro et al, 2018). It can be acquired or congenital and ranges from difficulty understanding words or hearing certain sounds to total deafness (Table 52.4). Hearing loss can affect communication, social activities, and work activities and diminish quality of life. Nurses have a responsibility to communicate with patients with hearing impairments and provide needed information regarding health care.

Conductive Hearing Loss

Conductive hearing loss, a mechanical problem, is interference with conduction of sound impulses to the inner ear through the external auditory canal, eardrum, or middle ear. The inner ear is not involved in pure conductive hearing loss. Causes of conductive hearing loss include cerumen, foreign bodies, infection, perforation of the tympanic membrane, trauma, fluid in the middle ear, cysts, tumors, cholesteatoma, and otosclerosis. Many causes, such as infection, foreign bodies, and impacted cerumen, can be corrected. Hearing devices may improve hearing for conditions resulting in conductive hearing loss that cannot be corrected, such as scarred tympanic membrane or otosclerosis.

Sensorineural Hearing Loss

Sensory hearing loss originates in the cochlea and involves the hair cells and nerve endings. Neural hearing loss originates in the nerve or brainstem. **Sensorineural** hearing loss results from hereditary hearing loss, congenital viral infections or malformations, or disease or trauma to the sensory or neural components of the inner ear. Causes of nerve deafness include complications of infections (such as measles, mumps, and meningitis), ototoxic medications (Table 52.5), trauma, noise, neuromas, arteriosclerosis, and aging.

Presbycusis is hearing loss caused by the aging process, resulting from degeneration of the organ of Corti. This degeneration often begins after age 50. The person develops an inability to decipher high-frequency sounds (consonants s, z, t, f, and g) that interferes with the ability to understand what is said, especially in noisy environments. The older adult commonly has more difficulty understanding higher-pitched female voices than lower-pitched male voices.

Other Types of Hearing Loss

Mixed hearing loss occurs when an individual has both conductive and sensorineural hearing loss, caused by a combination of any of the disorders previously discussed. Central hearing loss occurs when the central nervous system cannot interpret normal auditory signals. This condition is associated with disorders such as cerebrovascular accidents and tumors. Functional hearing loss has no organic cause or lesion that can be found. Also called *psychogenic hearing loss*, it is triggered by emotional stress.

Therapeutic Measures

The goal of medical management is to improve the patient's hearing. The source of the hearing impairment should be identified and addressed. With any permanent hearing

Table 52.4
Hearing Loss Summary

Signs and Symptoms	Difficulty understanding words or certain sounds Total deafness Ringing, buzzing, or roaring noise Changes in social and work activities, turning up volume on the television, asking, "What did you say?" Reports that people are talking softly Speaks in a quiet or loud voice and answers questions inappropriately Avoids group activities, loss of sense of humor, appears aloof
Diagnostic Tests	Rinne and Weber tests Audiometric testing
Therapeutic Measures	Cerumenolytics Anti-infectives Anti-inflammatories Assistive devices (e.g., hearing aids, implantable middle ear hearing devices, cochlear implants)
Complications	Safety issues Withdrawal from social activities and relationships
Priority Nursing Diagnoses	*Impaired Verbal Communication* *Impaired Social Interaction* *Deficient Knowledge*

Table 52.5
Ototoxic Medications

Aminoglycoside antibiotics	amikacin (Amikin) gentamicin (Garamycin) neomycin streptomycin tobramycin (Tobrex)
Other antibiotics	erythromycin (E-Mycin) minocycline (Minocin) vancomycin (Vancocin)
Diuretics	bumetanide (Bumex) furosemide (Lasix) hydrochlorothiazide (Hydrocot)
Other drugs	cisplatin (Platinol) methotrexate (Rheumatrex) salicylate (Bayer, Ecotrin)

loss, use of a hearing aid should be considered (Fig. 52.6; see Chapter 51). Surgical intervention may be available if hearing aids do not work. Implantable middle ear hearing aids can improve sound perception for patients with moderate to severe sensorineural hearing loss. Cochlear implants can restore up to half of the patient's hearing (Fig. 52.7). Visit www.nidcd.nih.gov/health/cochlear-implants for more information.

Nursing Process for the Patient With Hearing Impairment

DATA COLLECTION. Nursing care includes identifying patients at risk for hearing impairment (Table 52.6). Patients who have renal or hepatic disease, use ototoxic medications, or have previously used ototoxic medications are at risk for hearing impairment. If the patient uses ototoxic medications, gather data for tinnitus, sensorineural hearing loss, and vestibular dysfunction, which could indicate ototoxicity. Medications should be discontinued if signs of ototoxicity are present. Monitor for vertigo, horizontal nystagmus (fast side-to-side eye movements), nausea, vomiting, and spinning or rocking sensation while still. When collecting data for the patient with hearing impairment, include family members. They can often report what the patient cannot hear.

Objective data collection should start with a normal conversation with the patient. Observe the patient for difficulty understanding the conversation or questions. Clarity of the patient's speech is determined. Physical examination

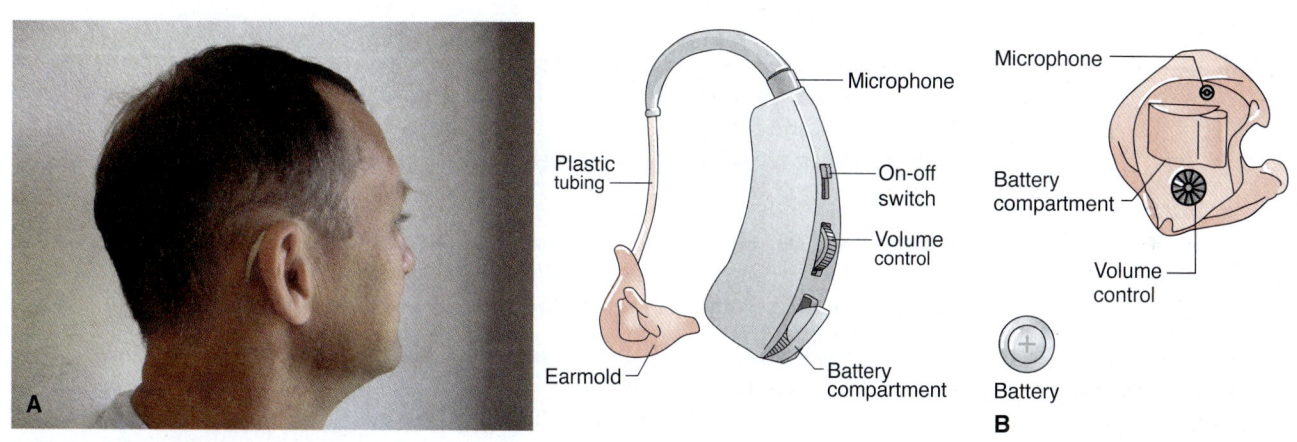

FIGURE 52.6 Hearing aids. (A) Behind-the-ear hearing aid. (B) In-the-ear hearing aid.

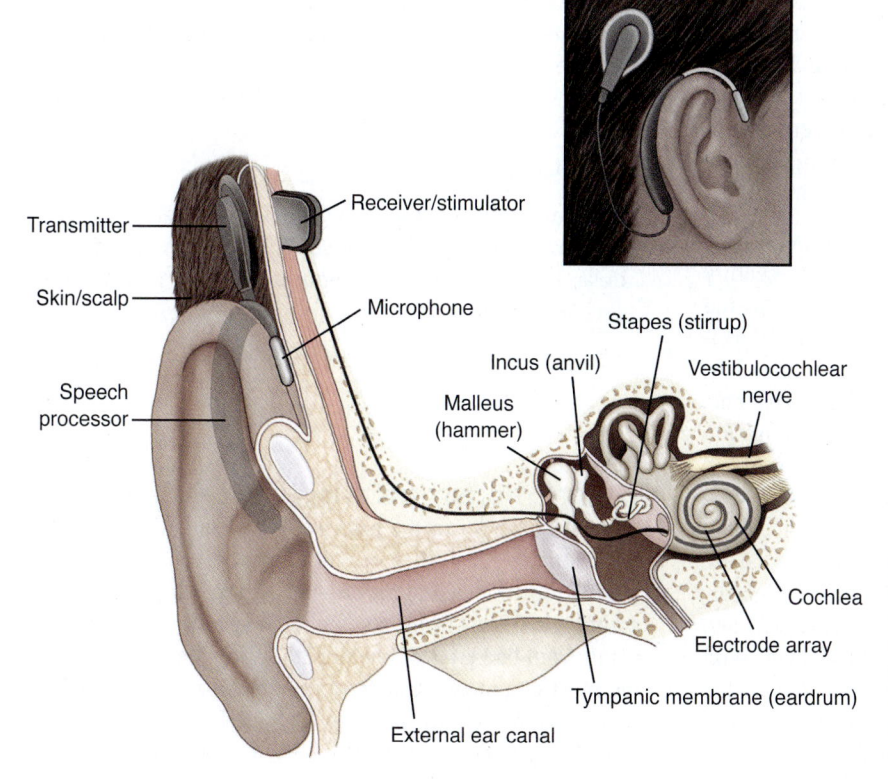

FIGURE 52.7 Cochlear implant. A cochlear implant is an electronic device that uses a speech processor that fits behind the ear. It captures sound signals and sends them to a receiver implanted under the skin. The message is transmitted to the cochlea, which stimulates the auditory nerve, and the brain interprets the signals as sound.

Table 52.6
Subjective Data Collection for Hearing Disorders

W: Where is it?	Are both ears affected? Is one side worse than the other?
H: How does it feel?	Are certain words unclear or entire conversations? Are high-frequency sounds (consonants *s, t, z, f, g*, and female voices) unclear or difficult to understand? Is any pain associated with the hearing loss? Any tinnitus or vertigo?
A: Aggravating and alleviating factors	Is hearing worse in large groups or when there is a lot of background noise? Is hearing improved in a quiet environment or when speaking only to an individual? Is it easier to understand someone when seeing the person's lips move? Does the patient own or use any assistive hearing devices? Are they effective? What type is used?
T: Timing	When did the hearing loss start? Was it gradual or sudden? Is the hearing loss associated with any illness or traumatic event? Is it associated with any recent flying? Any history of ototoxic drug use?
S: Severity	Does it cause communication impairment? How much? Does it affect activities of daily living? Does it affect or limit usual social activities? Have family or friends commented on decreased hearing? Does the patient avoid communication or social activities because of difficulty hearing? Is the patient having difficulties hearing telephone voices, radio, television, or movies?
U: Useful data for associated symptoms	Is there any fever, nausea, vomiting, or dizziness? Is there any history of occupational or environmental exposure to loud noises? What are the usual ear self-care habits? Any history of impacted cerumen? Has the patient ever had cerumen removed from ears?
P: Perception of the problem by the patient	What does the patient feel is wrong? Does the patient think that he or she has a hearing problem? How does the patient feel about hearing assistive devices? How does the patient perceive the hearing loss, and how is it influencing the patient's life?

includes the whisper voice, Rinne, and Weber tests (see Chapter 51). Test results estimate conductive or sensorineural hearing loss. Data help determine whether an external, middle, or inner ear problem is the underlying cause. The HCP may examine the ear canal for impacted cerumen or a tympanic membrane problem. Assistive hearing devices should be noted and inspected for proper functioning.

NURSING DIAGNOSES, PLANNING, AND IMPLEMENTATION. Planning focuses on helping the patient optimize hearing while promoting communication and adjustment to impaired hearing (Box 52.2 and Box 52.3). During the COVID-19 pandemic, social distancing and face masks added to the challenge of clear communication with hearing impaired patients (National Institute on Deafness and Other Communication Disorders [NIDCD], 2021). Tips for communication when wearing a face covering can be found on the NIDCD Web site (www.nidcd.nih.gov/about/nidcd-director-message/cloth-face-coverings-and-distancing-pose-communication-challenges-many). Nursing management for the patient with hearing impairment focuses on enhancing communication and quality of life (see "Nursing Care Plan for the Patient With Hearing Impairment"). Families should be included in discussions about therapeutic hearing devices, enhancing communication, and limiting patient social isolation.

EVALUATION. The patient's goals are met if the patient communicates effectively, engages in usual social activities, uses assistive hearing device, copes with emotional reaction to hearing impairment, and demonstrates care of a hearing aid.

CUE RECOGNITION 52.2

You are caring for a resident who has been taking furosemide (Lasix) for several years. The HCP increased the dose, and now your patient reports very loud ringing in the ears. What do you do?

Suggested answers are at the end of the chapter.

External Ear
Infections

PATHOPHYSIOLOGY AND ETIOLOGY. Infection is the most common disorder of the external ear. **External otitis** is the infection that most often occurs. Exposure to moisture, contamination, or local trauma provides an ideal environment for pathological growth in the external ear. External otitis may result from bacterial or fungal pathogens. Staphylococci are the most common causative organism. *Pneumocystis* infections may be seen in patients who have HIV. Bacterial or fungal external otitis that occurs when water is left in the ear

Box 52.2
Communicating With a Patient Who Has a Hearing Impairment

- Do not avoid conversation with a person who has hearing loss.
- Obtain the patient's attention before beginning to speak.
- If the listener uses a hearing device, ensure that it is operational and in place before beginning to communicate. Give the person time to adjust hearing device before speaking.
- Ensure an optimal environment by reducing background noises (e.g., turn off television and radio, close the door, or move to a quieter area).
- When wearing a mask is necessary, use a transparent mask so that your mouth and facial expression can be viewed.
- Face the person being spoken to and maintain eye contact.
- Do not smile, chew gum, or cover your mouth when talking.
- Avoid standing in the glare of bright sunlight or other bright lights.
- Speak clearly at a normal rate and volume near the good ear. Do not shout or overarticulate.
- If the listener has difficulty with high-pitched sounds, lower the pitch of your voice.
- Encourage nonverbal communication, such as touch or gestures, as appropriate.
- Inform the listener of topics to be discussed and when a change of topic occurs. Stick to a topic for a while and avoid quick shifts.
- Use short sentences and check for understanding. If the listener does not understand after the message is repeated, rephrase the message.
- Allow extra time for the listener to respond, and do not rush the listener.
- Use written communication if the person is unable to communicate verbally.
- Use active listening with attentive body posture, pleasant facial expressions, and a calm, unhurried manner.

Box 52.3
Care of Hearing Aids

Explain to the patient the following regarding care of hearing aids:

- Apply hair or medicinal sprays before inserting hearing aid to protect the hearing aid.
- Insert hearing aid over a soft surface to prevent damage if the hearing aid is dropped.
- Turn hearing aid on and increase volume once it is inserted.
- Check battery or lower the volume if sound is not clear or is intermittent. Buzzing noise may indicate that the battery door is not completely closed.
- Minimize whistling noise by ensuring that the volume is not too high, the aid fits securely, and the aid is free from earwax.
- Remove hearing aid before showering or bathing. Do not immerse it in water.
- Clean the hearing aid's body daily with a dry, soft cloth. Clean earmold with small brush or toothpick to keep free of earwax.
- Turn the hearing aid volume down and then off when not in use to conserve battery.

See "Care of Hearing Aids" under "Patient Teaching Guidelines" in your resources on Davis Advantage.

---

and washes away protective earwax is known as swimmer's ear. External otitis occurs more often in the summer months but can be seen year-round in patients who swim indoors.

A localized infection called ear canal **furuncle** (abscess) results when a hair follicle becomes infected. A **carbuncle** forms when several hair follicles are involved in forming the abscess. Most furuncles and carbuncles erupt and drain spontaneously.

Otomycosis is an infection caused by fungal growth. It is typically seen after topical corticosteroid or antibiotic use. Otomycosis occurs more often in hot weather.

An infection of the auricle is called perichondritis. It can result in necrosis of ear cartilage.

SIGNS AND SYMPTOMS. The most common sign of infection of the external ear is pain (Table 52.7). An early indication of infection is pain with gentle pulling on the pinna (outer ear). The patient may also experience pain when moving the jaw or when the otoscope is inserted into the ear canal. Pruritus (itching) is a common symptom that can be an early sign of infection. Signs of inflammation are present on the external ear. The ear canal may become swollen or occluded. As a result, hearing may be diminished. Redness, swelling, and drainage can be observed during otoscopic examination. If drainage is present, it usually starts out clear and becomes purulent as the disease progresses. The patient may also be febrile.

DIAGNOSTIC TESTS. A complete blood cell count with elevated white blood cell counts and discharge cultures helps diagnose infections. Culture and sensitivity tests isolate the specific infective organism and determine which antibiotics would be most effective to treat the infection. The Rinne and Weber tests can indicate conductive hearing impairment.

Impacted Cerumen

PATHOPHYSIOLOGY AND ETIOLOGY. Normally, the ear is self-cleaning. However, cerumen (wax) may become impacted, blocking the ear canal. Factors that contribute to impaction include large amounts of hair in the ear canal, exposure to dusty or dirty areas, improper ear cleaning, aging (because cerumen is drier as secretions decrease from shrinking ceruminous glands and keratin continues to collect), use of hearing aids, obstruction of the ear canal due to disease, narrowing of the ear canal, and bony growths secondary to an osteophyte or osteoma.

Nursing Care Plan for the Patient With Hearing Impairment

Nursing Diagnosis: *Impaired Verbal Communication* related to impaired hearing
Expected Outcome: The patient will use effective communication techniques.
Evaluation of Outcome: Is the patient able to communicate effectively to have needs met and reduce social isolation?

Intervention	Rationale	Evaluation
Inspect ear canals for mechanical obstruction. If cerumen is found, request order for cerumenolytic, if not contraindicated. If canal is clear, continue gathering data by using a tuning fork, loud ticking clock, or verbal cues to determine auditory ability at various distances.	Hearing loss may result from buildup of cerumen in the auditory canal. Determination of hearing ability assists in developing interventions appropriate to patient's hearing level.	Is ear canal free of mechanical obstruction? Is patient able to hear verbal input? If not, how severe is the impairment?
Enhance hearing by giving auditory cues in quiet surroundings.	The presence of background noise, such as television, radio, or large numbers of people, makes hearing more difficult.	Are auditory cues being delivered in an environment free of extraneous background noises?
Enhance understanding of auditory cues in a well-lit area but not in front of a window (which may cause glare). Get patient's attention before speaking; face patient, speak slowly, add hand gestures, and adjust voice pitch lower without shouting.	Hearing is enhanced when additional cues assist patient in understanding the message. Use of hand gestures to point, lip-reading, facial expression, and lower pitch all assist communication.	Are auditory cues being understood by patient? Are instructions given in a step-by-step format with written cues?
Provide for optimal care of assistive appliances such as hearing aids by making sure cerumen has been cleaned from the device, batteries are charged, and appliance is placed correctly in ear.	Appliances that are not functioning properly will not assist patient in hearing.	Is patient's hearing aid placed correctly? Is cerumen blocking sound conduction? Do batteries work?
Introduce assistive devices such as hearing amplifiers, telephone amplifiers, telephones with extra-loud bells, written communication, devices such as smoke detectors with visual indicators, and sign language.	Patients may not be aware of assistive devices that could help them adapt to hearing loss and continue previous activities, such as talking on the telephone or listening to television.	Is patient aware of assistive devices that will allow them to continue to verbally communicate with others? Is patient able to use the devices to compensate for auditory impairment?
Refer to specialized clinician such as an audiologist or occupational therapist or to specialized resources from such groups as the National Association of the Deaf or American Speech-Language-Hearing Association.	Specialized clinicians can provide detailed examination and treatment. Specialized resource groups have networks in place to help patients cope with loss and maximize abilities.	Does patient know whom to call for detailed examination and treatment? Does patient know that specialized clinicians and resource groups help with hearing impairment? Does patient know how to access specialists?

SIGNS AND SYMPTOMS. The patient may experience hearing loss, a full feeling, ear pain, or a blocked ear if cerumen has become impacted (see Table 52.7). Otoscopic examination reveals cerumen blocking part or all of the ear canal.

DIAGNOSTIC TESTS. Audiometric testing reveals conductive hearing loss in the affected ear. Hearing acuity can be decreased by 45 decibels because of impacted cerumen. Whisper voice, Rinne, and Weber tests also indicate conductive hearing loss.

Masses

PATHOPHYSIOLOGY AND ETIOLOGY. Benign masses of the external ear are usually cysts from sebaceous glands. Other benign masses are lipomas, warts, keloids, and infectious polyps. Aural polyps can occur in the external or middle ear

Table 52.7
Ear Disorders Summary

Signs and Symptoms	*External ear:* Pain, pruritus, swelling, redness, drainage, lacerations, contusion, hematomas, abrasion, blistering, hearing loss, foreign body *Middle ear:* Fever, earache, feeling of fullness in affected ear, nausea, vomiting, mastoid tenderness, redness and bulging of the tympanic membrane, hearing loss, vertigo, disorientation *Inner ear:* Vertigo, tinnitus, hearing loss, pain, fever, nausea, vomiting, headache, fullness in the ears
Diagnostic Tests	Complete blood count (CBC) Audiometric, Rinne, Weber, and whisper voice tests Ear drainage culture Imaging studies
Therapeutic Measures	Cerumenolytics to remove earwax Anti-infectives, anti-inflammatories, analgesics *External ear:* Debridement, surgical repair, application of protective covering for trauma *Middle ear:* Myringotomy, myringoplasty, stapedectomy *Inner ear:* Antibiotics, surgical removal of tumor, lifestyle changes, labyrinthectomy, diuretics, antihistamines, vasodilators, and antiemetics
Complications	*External ear:* Spread of infection to other parts of the ear, disfigurement, loss of hearing, scarring *Middle ear:* Perforation of tympanic membrane, cholesteatoma, tympanosclerosis, mastoiditis, permanent hearing loss *Inner ear:* Loss of hearing
Priority Nursing Diagnoses	Acute Pain Risk for Injury Deficient Knowledge

SIGNS AND SYMPTOMS. Changes in skin appearance can occur with benign or malignant masses. Usually, masses cause conductive or sensorineural hearing loss. Pain may occur, typically described as deep and radiating inward on the affected side. Ear drainage may be present. As the condition progresses, facial paralysis may occur. Otoscopic examination provides visualization of the mass.

DIAGNOSTIC TESTS. A biopsy may be obtained to determine whether the mass is benign or malignant. Imaging studies are also used to diagnose tumors. Audiometric studies reveal any hearing impairment.

Trauma
PATHOPHYSIOLOGY AND ETIOLOGY. Injuries to the external ear are commonly caused by a blow to the head, automobile accidents, burns, foreign bodies lodged in the ear canal, or cold temperatures. Cotton ball pieces and insects are the most common foreign bodies found in adult ears.

SIGNS AND SYMPTOMS. Lacerations, contusions, hematomas, abrasions, erythema, and blistering are seen with thermal or physical trauma. Repeated trauma to the ear can cause swelling, known as cauliflower ear. This is more common among boxers, rugby players, martial artists, and wrestlers. Conductive hearing loss can occur if the ear canal is partially or totally blocked. Patients who have contusions or hematomas commonly report numbness, pain, and paresthesia of the auricle. Symptoms associated with foreign bodies include decreased hearing, itching, pain, and infection. Care is taken during otoscopic examination not to push the foreign body farther into the ear canal.

DIAGNOSTIC TESTS. Imaging studies may be needed to determine the extent of the trauma. Audiometric, whisper voice, Rinne, and Weber tests may demonstrate conductive hearing loss.

Complications of External Ear Disorders
Untreated infections can spread, causing cellulitis, abscesses, middle ear infection, and septicemia. Metastasis occurs if malignant tumors are not treated. Infection, trauma, and malignant tumors may cause temporary or permanent hearing loss, disfigurement, discoloration, and scarring.

Therapeutic Measures for External Ear Disorders
For external ear infections, topical antibiotics are given. Systemic antibiotics are used for severe infections that are localized or have spread to surrounding tissues. Analgesics are used to control pain. Topical or systemic steroids may be used to treat inflammation. The ear is thoroughly cleaned before starting topical treatment. If the external ear canal has drainage or is swollen shut, a wick may be inserted to aid in removing drainage or to administering medication into the ear canal. If the patient is asymptomatic, cerumen removal is not recommended. In symptomatic patients, cerumen may be removed with cerumenolytics, or trained clinicians can remove

and may perforate the tympanic membrane. Actinic keratosis is a precancerous lesion found on the auricle. It may be seen in older adults. Malignant tumors such as basal cell carcinoma on the pinna and squamous cell in the ear canal may develop and can spread.

cerumen manually or with gentle irrigation (Fig. 52.8). (See "Irrigating the Eye and Ear" under "Procedures" in your resources on Davis Advantage.) Irrigation is not used if the patient has a history of perforated tympanic membrane or other contraindications. Debridement, surgical repair, or application of a protective covering may be done when trauma occurs to the external ear. Surgical management consists of incision and drainage of abscesses. Excision of cysts or cutaneous carcinomas may also be required.

> **PRACTICE ANALYSIS TIP**
> Linking NCLEX-PN® to Practice
> The LPN/LVN will perform irrigation (e.g., ear and eye).

Nursing Process for the Patient With External Ear Disorders

DATA COLLECTION. Subjective data obtained in a patient history include reports of pain, fullness, previous cerumen impaction, itching, or hearing loss. Onset, duration, and severity of symptoms are also part of the data. Additional data include patient's occupation, previous ear problems, hearing aid use, and typical ear hygiene. Observation for objective data includes redness, swelling, drainage, furuncles, carbuncles, lesions, abrasions, lacerations, growths, cerumen, scaliness, or crusting. The patient may report pain when the ear is palpated. Basic hearing acuity tests are conducted to evaluate hearing loss (see Chapter 51).

NURSING DIAGNOSES, PLANNING, AND IMPLEMENTATION.

Acute Pain related to inflammation or trauma

EXPECTED OUTCOME: The patient's pain will be relieved as evidenced by a lower rating on a pain scale within 30 minutes of report of pain.

- Monitor pain using a pain scale, and determine optimum analgesic schedule with the patient *to maximize pain control*.
- Implement nonpharmacological methods, such as relaxation, massage, music, guided imagery, or distraction techniques *to relieve pain*.
- Apply heat as ordered to the area *to promote comfort*.
- Offer liquid or soft foods *to relieve pain when chewing*.

Risk for Injury related to self-cleaning of external ear

EXPECTED OUTCOME: The patient will explain or demonstrate prescribed treatment.

- Explain ear care (Box 52.4) *to prevent injury*.
- Reinforce teaching the patient the treatment regimen *to ensure completion of treatment*.

Deficient Knowledge related to lack of information on preventive ear care

EXPECTED OUTCOME: The patient will explain or demonstrate procedures to maintain wellness of the external ear.

- Explain the procedure before removal of cerumen *to decrease anxiety*.
- If a wick is inserted into the ear canal, explain to the patient that it is used *to monitor for drainage, report excessive drainage to HCP, and wick medicine into the ear canal*.
- Reinforce teaching the patient how to use topical antibiotics, oral antibiotics, and/or anti-inflammatory medications *to promote healing*.
- Reinforce teaching the patient how to complete the prescribed treatment and maintain ear health (see Box 52.4). Include keeping the ear clean and dry and use of earplugs or cotton with petroleum jelly *to avoid getting water in the ears during an infection*.

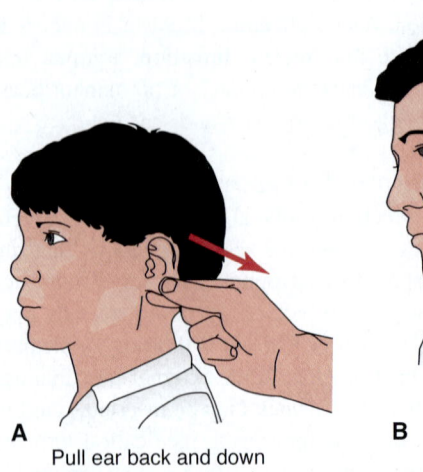

A Pull ear back and down to straighten ear canal in a child

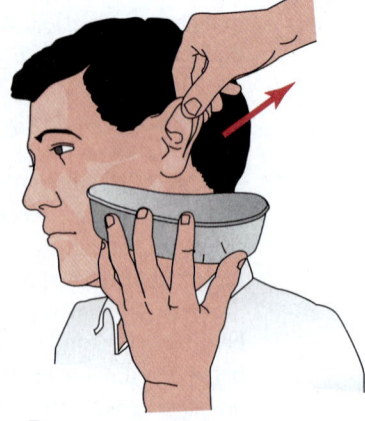

B Pull ear up and back to straighten ear canal in an adult

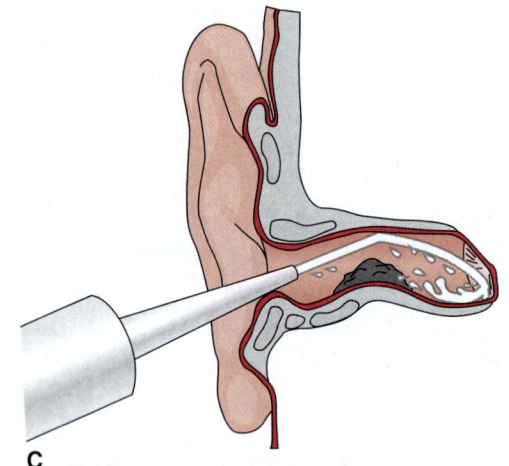

C Irrigation – Fluid is aimed off top of ear canal wall behind impacted cerumen

FIGURE 52.8 Ear irrigation. (A) Child. (B) Adult. (C) Irrigation.

Box 52.4

Ear Care

1. Cleanse the external ear with a wet washcloth. Gently cleanse the helix.
2. The ear has an effective self-cleaning system that continually moves protective earwax outward to prevent buildup. Cleaning attempts, particularly with swabs, can cause a wax impaction. Never insert anything into the ear canal, including cotton-tipped swabs, hair pins, matchsticks, safety pins, toothpicks, paper clips, or fingers. The thin skin of the ear canal is very fragile and can become abraded and then infected from being touched with these objects.
3. A person with a history of ear infections, perforated tympanic membrane, or swimmer's ear should prevent moisture from entering the ear canal and should avoid swimming in contaminated water. Moisture or water in the ear canal can be prevented by using earplugs.
4. For frequent swimming, use swim earplugs (custom or over-the-counter), an ear conditioner to prevent ear dryness, and an ear dryer after swimming.
5. Do not try home remedies for ear care without consulting a health-care provider.
6. A person with an upper respiratory infection should gently blow the nose with both nares open to prevent microbes from being forced into the eustachian tubes.

See "Ear Care" under "Patient Teaching Guidelines" in your resources on Davis Advantage.

EVALUATION. The outcomes for the patient are met if the patient indicates pain is relieved as evidenced by a lower rating on a pain scale, hearing improves or returns to pre-illness level, the patient states or demonstrates prescribed treatment (e.g., administering ear drops or ointments), and the patient explains or demonstrates measures to maintain wellness of the external ear.

Middle Ear, Tympanic Membrane, and Mastoid Disorders

Infections

PATHOPHYSIOLOGY AND ETIOLOGY. The most common disease of the middle ear, *otitis media* is a general term for inflammation of the middle ear, mastoid, and eustachian tube. Inflammation of the nasopharynx causes most cases of otitis media. As inflammation occurs, the nasopharyngeal mucosa becomes edematous, producing discharge. When fluid, pus, or air builds up in the middle ear, the eustachian tube becomes blocked. This impairs middle ear ventilation.

With various types of otitis media, inflammation can occur alone, with infective drainage, or with noninfective drainage. The first type is otitis media without effusion, an inflammation of the middle ear mucosa without drainage. The second type occurs with a bacterial infection of the middle ear mucosa, called *acute* otitis media. The infected fluid becomes trapped in the middle ear. If the infection continues longer than 3 months, *chronic* otitis media results. The third type is *otitis media with effusion.* Other names include *serous otitis media, nonsuppurative otitis media,* and *glue ear.* With this type of otitis media, noninfective fluid accumulates within the middle ear.

SIGNS AND SYMPTOMS. Acute otitis media commonly follows an upper respiratory infection or exacerbation of seasonal allergic rhinitis. Fever, earache, and feeling of fullness in the affected ear are common symptoms (see Table 52.7). As purulent drainage forms, pain and conductive hearing loss occur. Nausea and vomiting may be present. Purulent drainage may be evident in the external ear canal if the tympanic membrane ruptures. Otoscopic examination reveals a reddened, bulging tympanic membrane, and reduced tympanic membrane mobility when pneumatic pressure is applied.

Symptoms of otitis media with effusion may go undetected in adults because there are no signs of infection. The patient may report fullness, bubbling, or crackling and may have slight conductive hearing loss, report allergies, or breathe through the mouth. Otoscopic examination can reveal a bulging tympanic membrane. The eardrum is not reddened.

COMPLICATIONS. Buildup of fluid and pressure in the middle ear can cause a spontaneous perforation of the tympanic membrane with acute or chronic infection. The patient usually experiences pain before the rupture and relief after the rupture. The fluid in the middle ear moves through the perforation into the ear canal. This relieves pressure and pain. A tympanic membrane perforation causes hearing loss. The location and size of the perforation determine its extent. Damage to ossicles can occur with perforation.

Repeated infections in the middle ear or mastoid can cause a cholesteatoma, an epithelial cyst-like sac that fills with debris such as degenerated skin and sebaceous material. The cholesteatoma can be located on either side of the tympanic membrane. Damage can affect the middle ear structures as a result of pressure necrosis. The cholesteatoma causes conductive hearing loss. As the disease progresses, facial paralysis and vertigo may occur.

Tympanosclerosis is another complication of repeated middle ear infections that consists of deposits of collagen and calcium on the tympanic membrane. The condition can slowly progress to the area around the middle ear ossicles. These deposits appear as chalky white plaques on the tympanic membrane and contribute to conductive hearing loss.

Mastoiditis can occur if acute otitis media is not treated. The infection spreads to the mastoid area, causing pain. The use of antibiotics has resulted in acute mastoiditis becoming relatively uncommon. Chronic mastoiditis is still seen with repeated middle ear infections.

DIAGNOSTIC TESTS. An elevated white blood cell count may be seen. Cultures on ear drainage identify the specific infective organism. Conductive hearing loss is usually present on audiometric studies and Rinne, Weber, and whisper voice tests. Imaging studies may be done to diagnose infection.

THERAPEUTIC MEASURES. Bacterial infections are treated with topical and systemic antibiotics. Topical antibiotics may contain steroids to help with inflammation. Oral analgesics are given to control pain.

A modified Politzer ear device can equalize pressure in the middle ear and aid fluid drainage. The device, marketed as the EarPopper (www.earpopper.com), emits a stream of air into the nasal cavity to gently open the eustachian tubes and relieve negative pressure. This allows pressure to equalize and fluid to drain.

Surgical intervention includes several techniques. Paracentesis may be performed with a needle and syringe. The tympanic membrane is punctured with the needle, and fluid drained from the middle ear. A **myringotomy** may also be performed with an incision in the tympanic membrane. Fluid drains out or is suctioned out of the middle ear. Another technique is laser-assisted myringotomy, which vaporizes a hole in the tympanic membrane. Various types of transtympanic tubes may be inserted to keep the incision open. With the transtympanic tube keeping the incision in the tympanic membrane open, pressure is equalized. Further fluid formation and buildup is prevented. The transtympanic tubes are left in place until the infection is cured. Most tubes spontaneously extrude in 3 to 12 months. They rarely have to be removed.

Reconstructive repair of a perforated tympanic membrane is called a **myringoplasty**. One technique involves placing Gelfoam over the perforation. A graft from the temporal muscle behind the ear or tissue from the external ear is then placed over the perforation and Gelfoam. The Gelfoam is absorbed, and the graft repairs the perforation.

A mastoidectomy involves incision, drainage, and surgical removal of the mastoid process if the infection has spread to the mastoid area.

Otosclerosis

PATHOPHYSIOLOGY AND ETIOLOGY. **Otosclerosis**, hardening of the ear, results from formation of new bone along the stapes. With the new bone growth, the stapes becomes immobile, causing conductive hearing loss. The formation of new bone growth begins in adolescence or early adulthood and progresses slowly. Hearing loss is apparent after age 40 and steadily increases with age. Otosclerosis is more common in women than in men. The disease usually affects both ears. Although the exact cause is unknown, most patients have a family history of otosclerosis, so it likely has a hereditary component.

SIGNS AND SYMPTOMS. The primary symptom of otosclerosis is progressive hearing loss. The patient usually experiences bilateral conductive hearing loss, particularly with soft, low tones. Medical treatment is sought when the hearing loss interferes with the ability to take part in conversations. The patient may experience tinnitus. Otoscopic examination reveals a pinkish-orange tympanic membrane because of vascular and bony changes in the middle ear.

DIAGNOSTIC TESTS. Audiometric testing indicates the type and extent of the hearing loss. Imaging studies indicate the location and extent of excessive bone growth. The whisper voice test and normal conversation show decreased hearing. The patient hears best with bone conduction in the Rinne test, whereas lateralization to the most affected ear occurs with the Weber test.

THERAPEUTIC MEASURES. Otosclerosis has no cure. However, hearing aids may improve patient hearing. Reconstruction of necrotic ossicles may restore some hearing. Various methods are used to reposition and replace some or all of the ossicles. Unfortunately, surgeries are not always successful over time. Ossiculoplasty is the reconstruction of the ossicles. Prostheses made of plastic, ceramic, or human bone are used to partially or completely replace the necrotic ossicles.

Stapedectomy is the treatment of choice for otosclerosis. Either part or all of the stapes is removed and replaced with a prosthesis placed between the incus and the oval window. Advances in surgical treatment include use of lasers for improved visualization, less trauma, and greater surgical precision. The goal is to restore vibration from the tympanic membrane to the oval window and allow sound transmission. Many patients experience improved hearing immediately; others do not have improvement until swelling subsides. Complications of ossiculoplasty and stapedectomy include extrusion of the prosthesis, infection, hearing loss, dizziness, and facial nerve damage.

NURSING CARE. Initially, the patient may be on bedrest for several hours, then asked to ambulate to determine tolerance. When the patient is in bed, instruct them to lie on the side of the unaffected ear or the back during the first week. The cotton ball placed in the ear during surgery may be changed as needed with drainage. Occasionally, the patient may

> ## CLINICAL JUDGMENT
>
> **Mrs. Springhorn** is an 83-year-old woman who is scheduled to be discharged from the hospital after a stapedectomy. She lives alone at home and is able to care for herself.
>
> 1. What will you do to communicate with Mrs. Springhorn to ensure that she understands the discharge instructions?
> 2. What teaching methods do you reinforce to enhance communication?
> 3. What ear care instructions do you address with Mrs. Springhorn?
> 4. What teaching do you reinforce for Mrs. Springhorn to monitor for postoperative complications?
> 5. Which other members of the health-care team do you collaborate with for Mrs. Springhorn?
>
> *Suggested answers are at the end of the chapter.*

• **WORD • BUILDING** •

myringoplasty: myringo—tympanic membrane + plasty—surgical repair
otosclerosis: oto—ear + sclerosis—hardening
stapedectomy: stape(s)—stirrup + ectomy—excision of

experience nausea or dizziness. Antiemetics can be used to prevent vomiting. The patient's safety should be ensured if dizziness occurs. Oral analgesics are given for pain. To prevent dislodgment or damage to the prosthesis, patients are instructed to sneeze with the mouth open, and not to blow their nose, sniff, fly in an airplane, scuba dive, exercise, lift heavy objects, or use ear plugs for several weeks. Showering and hair washing may be allowed 2 days after surgery with a Vaseline-covered cotton ball in the ear. If the patient develops a cold, the HCP should be contacted.

Trauma

PATHOPHYSIOLOGY AND ETIOLOGY. Trauma, such as a blasting force, a blunt injury to the side of the head, or sudden changes in atmospheric pressure, can perforate the tympanic membrane and fracture the middle ear ossicles. Blasts cause injury from direct pressure on the ear. Blunt injury to the head can cause temporal skull fractures and trauma to the middle and inner ear. Barotrauma caused by sudden changes in atmospheric pressure in the ears can occur during scuba diving and airplane take-offs and landings. Pressure changes can occur during normal atmospheric conditions such as nose blowing, heavy lifting, and sneezing. During rapid pressure changes, the eustachian tube does not ventilate because of occlusion or dysfunction. Negative pressure develops in the middle ear and can cause the tympanic membrane to rupture or damage to the middle and inner ear.

SIGNS AND SYMPTOMS. Pain and hearing loss are the most common symptoms of trauma. Other symptoms of barotrauma include fullness of the ears, vertigo, nausea, disorientation, edema of the affected area, and hemorrhage in the external or middle ear. In severe cases of barotrauma when scuba diving, symptoms can cause drowning or cerebral air embolism from an overly rapid ascent. Otoscopic examination may reveal a retracted, reddened, and edematous tympanic membrane.

DIAGNOSTIC TESTS. Audiometric studies are completed to determine the hearing loss. Imaging studies may be done to determine the extent of middle and inner ear damage. Conductive or sensorineural hearing loss may be evident, depending on the extent and location of the damage.

Nursing Process for the Patient With Middle Ear, Tympanic Membrane, and Mastoid Disorders

DATA COLLECTION. Table 52.8 reviews subjective data that should be collected. The external ear should be inspected and palpated to obtain objective data. Pain with palpation is indicative of external ear problems, not middle ear problems. Pain over the mastoid area can indicate a mastoid problem. The middle ear and mastoid cavity cannot be visualized directly. The tympanic membrane is the only middle ear structure that can be directly visualized with an otoscope. Objective data also includes vital signs, noting any elevation in temperature. Any drainage from the ear should be noted and described. Hearing acuity is screened with the whisper voice, Rinne, and Weber tests.

NURSING DIAGNOSES, PLANNING, AND IMPLEMENTATION.

Risk for Infection related to pressure necrosis or surgical procedure

EXPECTED OUTCOME: The patient will have no signs of infection (i.e., no drainage from ear, no tenderness over mastoid, negative culture, afebrile).

- Reinforce teaching the patient not to blow their nose by pinching off nares *to prevent spread of upper respiratory infections up the eustachian tube.*
- Reinforce teaching the patient not to insert anything into the ear canal *to prevent ear damage* (see Box 52.4).
- Reinforce teaching the patient how to correctly remove cerumen from ear *to prevent infection or damage.*

Acute Pain related to fluid accumulation, inflammation, or infection

EXPECTED OUTCOME: The patient will indicate pain is decreased or absent as evidenced by a lower rating on a pain scale.

- Monitor pain using a pain scale, and determine optimum analgesic schedule with the patient *to maximize pain control.*
- Use nonpharmacological measures such as heat, distraction, and relaxation techniques *for pain reduction.*
- Reinforce teaching the patient how to administer ear drops or ear ointment *to help resolve infection and decrease pain.* See "Administering Eye and Ear Medications" under "Procedures" in your resources on Davis Advantage.
- Reinforce teaching the patient to take all prescribed antibiotics, even after symptoms are relieved, *to ensure that the infection is completely resolved.*

Deficient Knowledge related to no prior experience with a middle ear disorder

EXPECTED OUTCOME: The patient will state an understanding of methods for preventing problems in the middle ear, tympanic membrane, and mastoid process or impending surgery.

- Include the patient's family in teaching sessions *to enhance learning and assist with retention of information.*
- Reinforce teaching the patient to avoid trauma to the ear, loud noise exposure, and environmental or occupational conditions *to prevent damage to the ear.*
- Reinforce teaching the patient to yawn or perform jaw-thrust maneuver (opening mouth wide and moving jaw) *to equalize ear pressure, which helps maintain ear health.*
- Reinforce teaching patient methods of effective communication *to compensate for hearing loss* (see "Nursing Care Plan for the Patient With Hearing Impairment" earlier in chapter).

Table 52.8
Subjective Data Collection for Middle Ear, Tympanic Membrane, Mastoid, or Inner Ear Disorders

W: Where is it?	Are both ears affected? Is it deep within the head?
H: How does it feel?	Is there pressure? Drainage? Fullness? Vertigo? Tinnitus? Is it painful? If so, is it sharp, dull, continuous, intermittent, throbbing, localized? No pain?
A: Aggravating and alleviating factors	Are there any allergies? Is it worse with change of position or movement? Is there relief with heat or drainage? Is there relief with analgesics or other medications?
T: Timing	When did it start? Was it a sudden onset? How long have symptoms persisted? Has there been any recent upper respiratory infection, airline travel, scuba diving, trauma, or weight lifting?
S: Severity	Does it cause hearing impairment? How much? Does it affect activities of daily living, nutritional intake, work?
U: Useful data for associated symptoms	Is there fever, headache, drainage from the ear canal, nausea, vomiting, dizziness? Is there a family history of otosclerosis? Any previous ear problems or ear surgeries?
P: Perception of the problem by the patient	What do you think is wrong? Has the problem occurred before? If so, what was the same and what was different?

- Reinforce teaching preoperative and postoperative instructions and provide written instructions *to promote patient understanding* (Box 52.5).
- Reinforce teaching the patient how to avoid getting water in the ear postoperatively *to prevent moisture from reaching surgical site.*

EVALUATION. Goals for the patient are met if there is no ear drainage or pain over mastoid and if the patient has negative culture and remains afebrile. Also, the patient states that no pain is present or pain is decreased, verbalizes care of ears and methods to prevent further infection, describes signs requiring medical attention, and verbalizes the rationale and outcome for any upcoming surgery as well as preoperative and postoperative instructions.

Inner Ear
Labyrinthitis

PATHOPHYSIOLOGY AND ETIOLOGY. Labyrinthitis (also known as vestibular neuritis) is inflammation or infection of the inner ear by viral or bacterial pathogens. The bacterium or virus enters the inner ear from the middle ear, meninges, or bloodstream. Serous labyrinthitis is acute labyrinthitis that sometimes follows drug intoxication or overindulgence in alcohol. It can also be caused by an allergy. Diffuse suppurative labyrinthitis occurs when acute or chronic otitis media spreads into the inner ear or after middle ear or mastoid surgery. Destruction of soft tissue structures from infection can cause permanent hearing loss.

SIGNS AND SYMPTOMS. Vertigo, tinnitus, and sensorineural hearing loss are the most common symptoms. Vertigo, or dizziness, occurs when vestibular structures are involved. Tinnitus, or ringing in the ear, occurs when the infection is in the cochlea. Sensorineural hearing loss can be caused by infections in the cochlea or vestibular structures. Nystagmus on the affected side may occur. Other signs and symptoms include pain, fever, ataxia, nausea, vomiting, and beginning nerve deafness.

DIAGNOSTIC TESTS. Complete blood count (CBC) is done to diagnose infection. Hearing evaluation by an audiologist may reveal mild to complete hearing loss. Rinne and Weber tests indicate conductive or sensorineural hearing loss.

THERAPEUTIC MEASURES. Antibiotics are used to treat bacterial inner ear infections. Viral infections usually run their course in about 1 week and can be treated with glucocorticoids. Mild sedation may help the patient relax. Although no specific medicine relieves dizziness, antihistamines can be used if they prove helpful on an individual basis. Antiemetics may be used for nausea and vomiting. Patients may be placed on bedrest.

NURSING CARE. Nursing management includes helping the patient manage symptoms and self-care. Educate the patient about safety issues while on bedrest and sedatives to prevent falls and injury. The patient should avoid turning the head quickly to help alleviate vertigo. The patient is assisted to cope with anxiety that may occur because of the frustration surrounding hearing loss or loss of work.

Neoplastic Disorders
PATHOPHYSIOLOGY AND ETIOLOGY. Inner ear tumors can be benign or malignant. Acoustic neuroma, affecting the eighth cranial nerve, is the most common benign tumor. It is slow-growing and can occur at any age, typically developing unilaterally. As it spreads, it compresses the nerve and adjacent structures.

Box 52.5
Preoperative and Postoperative Nursing Interventions for the Patient Having Ear Surgery

Preoperative Care

For the patient undergoing ear surgery, the nurse collects data, determines the patient knowledge base, notes the patient's mental readiness, and obtains baseline physiological data.

- Ask about the type of surgery and anesthesia that will be used.
- Help alleviate the patient's fear by encouraging the patient to ask questions. Ensure that all questions are answered before surgery by the appropriate person.
- Explain types of pain control, packing or dressings to expect, and postoperative restrictions that may be ordered.
- Obtain and document baseline vital signs.
- Ensure that the informed operative consent is signed.
- Document the patient's current medications.
- Leave hearing devices for interactions in place until surgery.

Postoperative Care

Postoperatively, the nurse is responsible for monitoring the patient's physiological status and discharge teaching.

- Monitor vital signs.
- Explain that an occlusive dressing may decrease hearing.
- Instruct patients with ear tubes to avoid getting water in the ear and to use a shower cap or earplugs as ordered.
- Instruct the patient to seek medical care if excessive bleeding or drainage occurs. If a cotton plug is to be left in place, instruct the patient to change it daily and as needed.
- Instruct patient to sneeze with mouth open and avoid blowing the nose.
- Explain ordered activity restrictions such as flying and heavy lifting.
- Explain use of pain medication and to take antibiotics as ordered.
- Instruct the patient to call the HCP's office for a follow-up appointment.

See "Post-op Ear Care Surgery" under "Patient Teaching Guidelines" in your resources on Davis Advantage.

Malignant tumors arising from the inner ear are rare. Squamous and basal carcinomas arise from the epidermal lining of the inner ear.

SIGNS AND SYMPTOMS. Early symptoms of acoustic neuroma include progressive unilateral sensorineural hearing loss of high-pitched sounds, unilateral tinnitus, and intermittent vertigo. Headache, pain, and balance disorders may be present. Symptoms progress as the tumor spreads to other structures. Acoustic neuromas generally grow slowly, but some tumors grow quickly. The symptoms vary depending on the area of the ear that is involved.

DIAGNOSTIC TESTS. Neurologic, audiometric, and vestibular testing are used to diagnose neuroma. Auditory brainstem evoked response and electronystagmography are completed. A CT scan and magnetic resonance imaging (MRI) are used to determine the size and location of the tumor.

THERAPEUTIC MEASURES. Preferred method of treatment involves surgical removal of the tumor. If labyrinth is destroyed, permanent hearing loss results. Steroids and radiation may decrease size of the tumor, including inoperable tumors. Small tumors can be observed for growth and treated if necessary.

NURSING CARE. Nursing care focuses on preparing the patient for surgery and adjusting to the diagnosis and the resulting hearing loss (see Box 52.5).

> **BE SAFE!**
> **TAKE ACTION!** Provide fall precautions for any patient's report of vertigo or dizziness in order to prevent falls and patient injury.

Ménière Disease

PATHOPHYSIOLOGY AND ETIOLOGY. Ménière disease is a balance disorder. This disease causes dilation of the membranous labyrinth resulting from a disturbance in the fluid physiology of the endolymphatic system. Its exact etiology is unknown but may stem from hypersecretion, hypoabsorption, deficit membrane permeability, allergies, viral infection, hormonal imbalance, or mental stress. The disease usually develops between ages 40 and 60. The symptoms range from vague to severe and debilitating.

SIGNS AND SYMPTOMS. A triad of symptoms of vertigo, hearing loss, and tinnitus characterizes Ménière disease. Recurring episodes of the incapacitating triad of symptoms along with nausea and vomiting occur. Attacks may happen suddenly or the patient may experience warning signs such as headache or fullness in the ears. During an acute episode, the patient experiences vertigo for 20 minutes to 24 hours. Vertigo is usually accompanied by nausea and vomiting, followed by dizziness and unsteadiness. The patient is uncoordinated and displays gait changes. Hearing loss is often described as a fluctuating fullness in the ears. Tinnitus is present. Irritability, depression, and withdrawal are common. Vital signs usually remain normal. It takes several weeks for symptoms to resolve, and hearing loss in the affected ear remains. The patient then enters a stage of remission until the next attack. The acute episodes occur two to three times yearly. Eventually the patient has complete remission with some degree of permanent hearing loss.

DIAGNOSTIC TESTS. Audiometric studies identify the type and magnitude of the hearing loss. Neurologic testing and radiographic studies rule out other pathological conditions. A caloric stimulation test checks for damage to the acoustic nerve (involved in hearing and balance). The test is normal if nystagmus (fast side-to-side eye movements) occurs.

THERAPEUTIC MEASURES. Medical treatment consists of prophylactic treatment between attacks and symptomatic treatment for acute attacks. A salt-restricted diet, diuretics, antihistamines, and vasodilators are used during prophylactic treatment. The patient should avoid alcohol, caffeine, and tobacco use. Medication for vertigo (meclizine [Antivert], tranquilizers, glucocorticoids, and vagal blockers may be needed during acute attacks. The patient may be placed on bedrest during acute attacks. The goals of medical treatment are to preserve hearing and to reduce symptoms.

Surgical treatment is used only when medical management has failed. When involvement is unilateral, a labyrinthectomy can be performed. This causes complete loss of hearing in that ear. Another surgical intervention establishes a shunt from the inner ear to the subarachnoid space. This procedure helps drain the fluid and prevent future hearing loss. Another treatment is intratympanic gentamicin (Garamycin) injection, which is usually done in the HCP's office. This treatment can cause hearing loss.

NURSING CARE. Nursing management focuses on managing symptoms and providing safety during acute attacks. Because of the unpredictability of Ménière disease, nursing care focuses on emotional support for the patient during remission periods. Provide emotional support and resources to help the patient cope with the unpredictable nature of the disease and its physical impairments.

Nursing Process for the Patient With Inner Ear Disorders

DATA COLLECTION. Subjective data are collected (see Table 52.8). Objective data are collected through examination of gross hearing; the whisper voice, Rinne, and Weber tests; a physical examination; and laboratory data. The nurse should gather data and note any nutritional deficiencies, including dehydration, weight loss, or weight gain. An unsteady gait or temperature are also noted.

NURSING DIAGNOSES, PLANNING, AND IMPLEMENTATION. Planning focuses on helping the patient maintain a normal lifestyle, remain free of injuries, cope with the illness or hearing loss, and maintain adequate nutrition and hydration.

Anxiety related to unpredictability of sudden and severe acute attacks

EXPECTED OUTCOME: The patient will state that anxiety is decreased.

- Encourage the patient to express concerns about hearing loss and the unpredictability of acute attacks *to identify causes of anxiety.*
- Monitor for signs of anxiety such as fidgeting, restlessness, apprehension, shakiness, and increased heart rate *to determine whether anxiety is present.*
- Explore with the patient techniques that have and have not worked in the past *to determine which techniques to use to reduce anxiety.*
- Use a calm reassuring approach *to help install confidence.*
- Provide a quiet environment and diversional activities *to calm the patient.*
- Provide information regarding diagnosis and treatment *to promote understanding and reduce anxiety.*

Risk for Injury related to impaired equilibrium

EXPECTED OUTCOME: Patient will not be injured from falling due to alterations in equilibrium.

- Institute fall precautions *to help prevent injury.*
- Ensure that the environment is safe and free of obstacles (e.g., throw rugs, electrical cords in walkways, poor lighting) *to prevent falls.*
- Monitor for signs of headache or fullness in the ears *to detect an oncoming attack.*
- Reinforce teaching the patient to avoid sudden movement of the head during periods of vertigo *to prevent increasing symptoms.*
- Reinforce teaching the patient on correct dosage and administration of medications *to help ensure resolution of symptoms.*
- Reinforce teaching the patient to avoid use of alcohol, caffeine, and tobacco *to decrease disruptions of equilibrium.*
- Reinforce teaching the patient to call for assistance when ambulating or remain on bedrest if indicated until symptoms are relieved *to minimize risk of falling and injury.*

Imbalanced Nutrition: Less Than Body Requirements related to nausea and vomiting

EXPECTED OUTCOME: The patient will experience adequate nutrition and hydration with relief of nausea and vomiting.

- Monitor for signs of nausea, vomiting, and inadequate hydration *to determine baseline information.*
- Medicate as ordered *to relieve symptoms and prevent episodes of nausea and vomiting.*
- Institute a salt-restricted diet, if ordered, and instruct the patient on low- and high-sodium foods *to reduce fluid retention.*
- Reinforce teaching the patient to use deep breathing, voluntary swallowing, and eating slowly *to suppress the vomiting reflex.*

EVALUATION. Goals for the patient have been met if signs of anxiety are decreased and if the patient remains free from injury and maintains weight within normal range with no signs of dehydration.

CLINICAL JUDGMENT

Mrs. Belmont is a 48-year-old woman diagnosed with Ménière disease. She is currently in a state of remission. She states that she is fearful that the next attack will occur during her daughter's upcoming wedding.

1. What data do you collect about Mrs. Belmont's attacks?
2. What instructions do you provide to Mrs. Belmont to use during her attacks?
3. What will you do to address Mrs. Belmont's fears about future attacks?

Suggested answers are at the end of the chapter.

Key Points

- Conjunctivitis (pink eye) is inflammation of the conjunctiva by a virus or bacteria and is highly contagious.
- Blepharitis is chronic inflammation of the eyelid edges. The cause may include staphylococcal infection, seborrhea (dandruff), rosacea, or abnormalities of the tarsal glands.
- Dry eye results from inadequate lubrication due to reduced quality or amount of tears.
- An external hordeolum, or sty, is a small staphylococcal abscess in the sebaceous gland at the base of the eyelash. Chalazion is another type of abscess that forms in the tarsal glands and is larger than a stye.
- Keratitis is inflammation of the cornea. Corneal infections are usually serious. Corneal tissue may become thin and susceptible to perforation. This can result in permanent loss of vision.
- Hyperopia (farsightedness) is caused by light rays focusing behind the retina. People who are hyperopic see far away images more clearly than images that are close.
- Myopia (nearsightedness) is caused by light rays focusing in front of the retina. Distance vision is blurred. Items that are close are clear.
- Astigmatism results from unequal curvatures in the shape of the cornea. The person with astigmatism has blurred vision with distortion.
- Presbyopia is an age-related condition in which the eye's lens gradually loses its elasticity. The lens is less able to focus light onto the retina to see close objects.
- Blindness is the complete or almost complete absence of the sense of sight.
- Retinopathy is a disorder in which vascular changes occur in the retinal blood vessels. It is most common in persons with diabetes.
- Retinal detachment is a separation of the retina from the choroid layer that is beneath it. Emergency medical treatment must be sought to help protect vision.
- Glaucoma is a group of diseases that damage the optic nerve. The damage to it is silent, progressive, and irreversible. Loss of peripheral vision occurs, which is then followed by reduced central vision and eventually blindness. Patients with glaucoma need lifelong monitoring of IOP.
- A cataract is an opacity in the lens of the eye that may cause a loss of visual acuity. Intraocular lens implant surgery is used to correct cataracts.
- AMD involves deterioration and scarring within the macula leading to permanent vision loss.
- Injuries to the eye include foreign bodies, chemical burns, UV exposure, direct heat sources, abrasions, lacerations from dragging something across the eye, and penetrating wounds.
- Nursing diagnoses for patient with visual impairment include *Self-care Deficit* related to impaired vision, *Risk for Injury* related to impaired vision, and *Deficient Knowledge* related to new onset of impaired vision.
- Conductive hearing loss is a mechanical problem that interferes with conduction of sound.
- Sensory hearing loss originates in the cochlea and involves the hair cells and nerve endings. Neural hearing loss originates in the nerve or brainstem. Sensorineural hearing loss results from disease or trauma to the sensory or neural components of the inner ear.
- External otitis may be caused by bacterial or fungal pathogens.
- Benign masses of the external ear are usually cysts resulting from sebaceous glands.
- Injuries to the external ear are commonly caused by a blow to the head, automobile accidents, burns, foreign bodies lodged in the ear canal, or cold temperatures. Cotton ball pieces and insects are the most common foreign bodies found in adult ears.
- Otitis media is a general term for inflammation of the middle ear, mastoid, and eustachian tube. Buildup of fluid, pus, or air in the middle ear blocks the eustachian tube. This can lead to perforation of the tympanic membrane and hearing loss.
- Mastoiditis can occur if acute otitis media is not treated and spreads to the mastoid area.
- A myringotomy is an incision made in the tympanic membrane to drain fluid out of the middle ear. Various types of transtympanic tubes may be inserted which equalize pressure so that fluid formation and buildup is prevented.
- Otosclerosis, or hardening of the ear, results from the formation of new bone along the stapes. This makes the stapes immobile and causes conductive hearing loss. Stapedectomy is the treatment of choice.
- Trauma, such as a blasting force, a blunt head injury, or sudden changes in atmospheric pressure, can cause the tympanic membrane to perforate and middle ear ossicles to fracture.
- Acoustic neuroma, a tumor of the eighth cranial nerve, is the most common benign tumor.
- Ménière disease is a balance disorder with a triad of symptoms of vertigo, hearing loss, and tinnitus. Its cause is unknown. It is characterized by episodic bouts of symptoms and remission.
- Nursing diagnosis for patients with hearing impairment include *Impaired Verbal Communication* related to impaired hearing.

SUGGESTED ANSWERS TO CHAPTER EXERCISES

Cue Recognition
52.1: Gather data about his ability to see and make the environment safe. Discuss with HCP the need for the patient to have an eye examination and referral to optometrist or ophthalmologist. Patients with diabetes are at risk for developing diabetic retinopathy and cataracts and should have annual eye examinations.

52.2: Hold the Lasix and contact the HCP. Lasix is ototoxic, and the increased dose could be causing the ringing in the resident's ears. Ototoxicity can result in loss of hearing.

Critical Thinking & Clinical Judgment
Mr. Samuel
1. You should have Mr. Samuel seek immediate assistance, patch both eyes, and have someone take him to receive medical treatment immediately.
2. The nurse should ensure that an antiemetic is ordered postoperatively on the patient's return to the unit. When Mr. Samuel reports nausea, the antiemetic should be given *promptly*.
3. The nurse should recognize that the concentration is 2 mg/1 mL, and the volume of the vial is 2 mL. The concentration is what is required to calculate the dose:

$$\frac{4 \text{ mg}}{} \cdot \frac{1 \text{ mL}}{2 \text{ mg}} = 2 \text{ mL}$$

Mrs. Springhorn
1. Gain her attention, face her and stand in her visual field, avoid glare, speak clearly, inform her of topics to be discussed, check for understanding, allow extra time for more explanation, reduce background noises, use nonverbal communication, and do not cover your mouth when talking.
2. Use active listening. Use written communication to enhance spoken words. Use demonstration and return demonstration. Allow questions. Do not hurry. Provide information in short segments. Determine understanding at each session.
3. Place the operative ear upward or lie on back when in bed. Sneeze with the mouth open. Do not blow nose, sniff, fly in an airplane, or lift heavy objects. Exercise as instructed. Shower and wash hair as instructed. If a cold develops, call the HCP. If dizzy, be careful when standing up.
4. Reinforce teaching that complications could include extrusion of the prosthesis, infection, hearing loss, dizziness, and facial nerve damage and to report these to the surgeon immediately.
5. Discuss care with the discharge planner and possibly have a home health aide assist at home.

Mrs. Belmont
1. You should ask Mrs. Belmont about specific signs she may have had before previous attacks, such as headache or fullness in the ears. You should also ask her specifically what symptoms she has during attacks. Common symptoms include the triad of vertigo, hearing loss, and tinnitus. She may also have nausea, vomiting, and unsteady gait.
2. Encourage her to ensure safety to prevent falling. Discuss treatment that Mrs. Belmont has used with previous attacks. Ask her which treatments helped. Recommend taking ordered medications such as tranquilizers and vagal blockers; maintaining adequate fluid and nutritional intake; ambulating with assistance; limiting salt in her diet; and avoiding alcohol, caffeine, and tobacco use.
3. Provide emotional support. Discuss methods to help her cope with the disease, such as counseling and relaxation techniques. Discuss with Mrs. Belmont prophylactic treatment, such as a salt-restricted diet, diuretics, antihistamines, and vasodilators.

Additional Resources

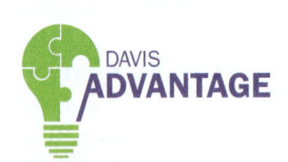

Go to Davis Advantage to complete your learning: strengthen understanding, apply your knowledge, and prepare for the Next Gen NCLEX®.

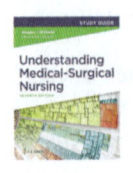

A Study Guide is also available.

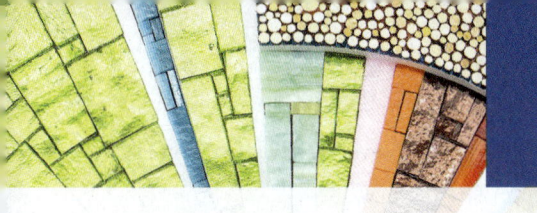

UNIT FIFTEEN Understanding the Integumentary System

CHAPTER 53
Integumentary System Function, Data Collection, and Therapeutic Measures

Rita Bolek Trofino, Janice L. Bradford

KEY TERMS

alopecia (AH-low-PEE-she-ah)
ecchymosis (EK-ih-MOH-sis)
erythema (AIR-ih-THEE-mah)
petechiae (peh-TEE-kee-eye)
turgor (TUR-gur)

CHAPTER CONCEPT

Tissue integrity

LEARNING OUTCOMES

1. Explain normal structures and functions of the integumentary system.
2. Identify the effects of aging on the integumentary system.
3. List data to collect when caring for a patient with an integumentary system disorder.
4. Identify laboratory and diagnostic tests commonly used to diagnose integumentary disorders.
5. Describe therapeutic measures that are used for patients with integumentary disorders.

NORMAL INTEGUMENTARY SYSTEM ANATOMY AND PHYSIOLOGY

The skin, its accessory structures, and the subcutaneous tissue form the integumentary system, the covering of the body that separates the living internal environment from the external environment. The skin itself is considered an organ and consists of two layers: the outer epidermis and the inner dermis (Fig. 53.1).

Epidermis, Dermis, and Hypodermis

The epidermis has up to five epithelial layers. The innermost epidermal layer is called the *stratum germinativum*. This is where mitosis occurs to produce new epidermal cells. The rate of mitosis is fairly constant but increases from chronic abrasion to the skin, as in callus formation. The new cells, keratinocytes, produce the protein keratin and a water-repelling sealant. As they are pushed to the surface of the skin, they die and become the *stratum corneum*, the outermost epidermal layer. These cells resist abrasion and water entry and exit.

The stratum corneum consists of many layers of dead, keratinized cells. An unbroken stratum corneum is an effective barrier against pathogens and most chemicals, although even microscopic breaks can permit their entry. As dead cells are worn off the surface of the skin (which contributes to the removal of pathogens), they are continuously replaced by cells from beneath. Loss of large portions of the stratum corneum (and deeper), as with extensive third-degree burns, greatly increases the risk for infection and dehydration.

Melanocytes are cells in the lower epidermis that produce the protein melanin. The amount of melanin is a genetic characteristic that gives color to skin and hair. When skin is exposed to ultraviolet (UV)

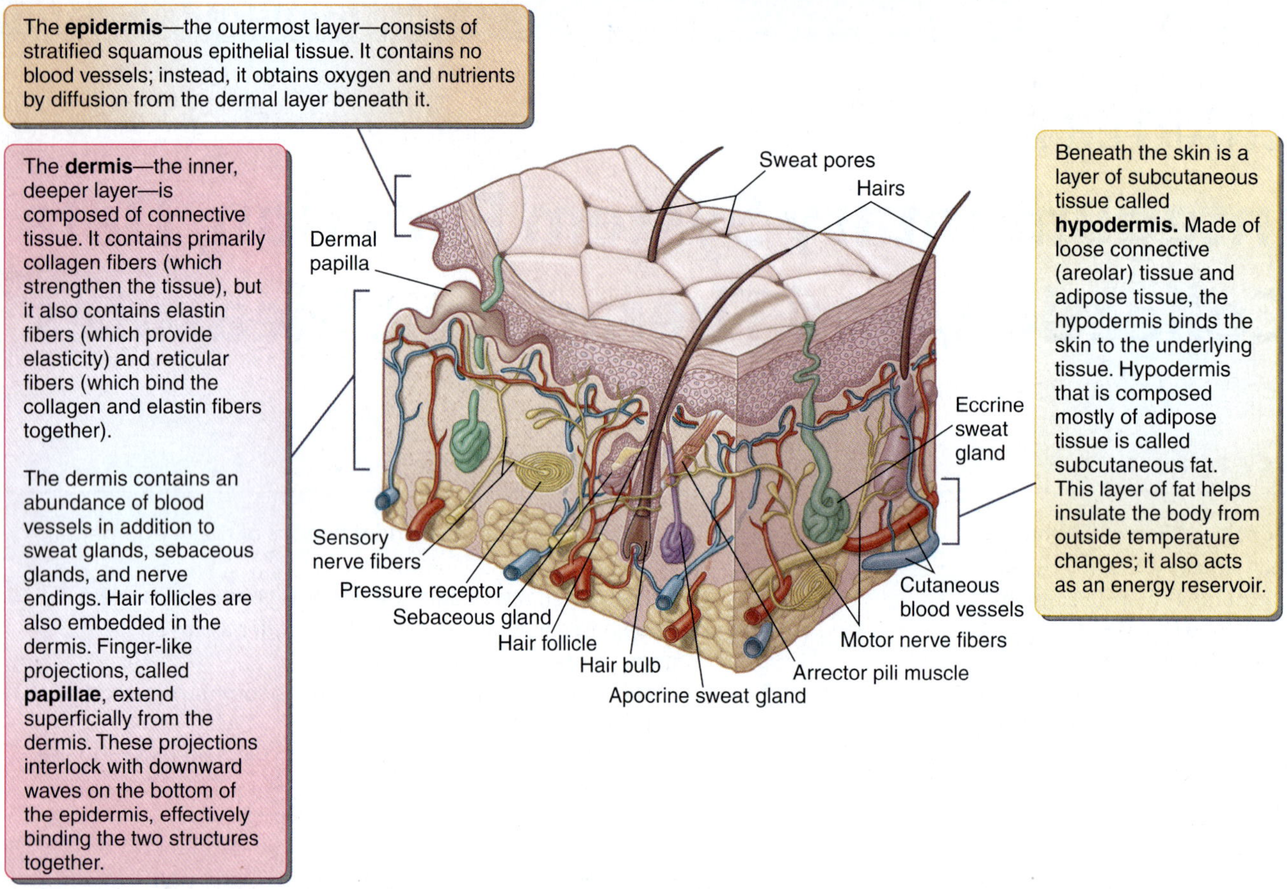

The epidermis—the outermost layer—consists of stratified squamous epithelial tissue. It contains no blood vessels; instead, it obtains oxygen and nutrients by diffusion from the dermal layer beneath it.

The dermis—the inner, deeper layer—is composed of connective tissue. It contains primarily collagen fibers (which strengthen the tissue), but it also contains elastin fibers (which provide elasticity) and reticular fibers (which bind the collagen and elastin fibers together).

The dermis contains an abundance of blood vessels in addition to sweat glands, sebaceous glands, and nerve endings. Hair follicles are also embedded in the dermis. Finger-like projections, called **papillae**, extend superficially from the dermis. These projections interlock with downward waves on the bottom of the epidermis, effectively binding the two structures together.

Beneath the skin is a layer of subcutaneous tissue called **hypodermis**. Made of loose connective (areolar) tissue and adipose tissue, the hypodermis binds the skin to the underlying tissue. Hypodermis that is composed mostly of adipose tissue is called subcutaneous fat. This layer of fat helps insulate the body from outside temperature changes; it also acts as an energy reservoir.

FIGURE 53.1 Structure of the skin.

rays from the sun or artificial lighting, production of melanin is incorporated into the epidermal cells, darkening them. Melanin is a pigment barrier to prevent further exposure of living cells in the stratum germinativum to UV rays. UV rays are mutagenic, or capable of damaging the DNA in cells and causing mutations that can result in malignancy.

Also in the epidermis are intraepidermal macrophages (Langerhans cells), a type of macrophage that presents foreign antigens to immune cells. This is the first step in the destruction of pathogens that penetrate the epidermis.

Extensive collagen fibers in the dermis give the skin its strength as an organ. Elasticity results from these elastic fibers, allowing stretched skin to return to its proper position.

The hypodermis (also known as the *subcutaneous layer*) consists of areolar and adipose tissue. This subcutaneous adipose tissue cushions, insulates, and stores energy as triglyceride. The subcutaneous tissue contains abundant leukocytes that destroy pathogens that enter through broken skin.

Hair
Human hair with significant function includes the eyelashes and eyebrows, which keep dust and sweat out of the eyes, and nostril hair, which filters air entering the nasal cavities. Hair on the head provides thermal insulation (Fig. 53.2).

Nails
Nail roots are found at the ends of the fingers and toes. Nail growth is similar to hair growth. Mitosis in the nail root is a continuous process to produce new, keratinized cells. As these cells die, they form the visible nail. Nails protect the ends of the digits from mechanical injury and are useful for picking up small objects.

Receptors
Sensory receptors for the cutaneous senses reside in the dermis. Receptors for heat, cold, and pain are free nerve endings; encapsulated nerve endings are specific for touch and pressure. The sensitivity of an area of skin is determined by the density of receptors present.

Glands
Cutaneous exocrine glands lie within the dermis and secrete to the surface of the skin through ducts. These include sudoriferous glands (both eccrine and apocrine), sebaceous (oil) glands (Fig. 53.3), ceruminous glands (cerumen), and ciliary glands (tears).

Water lost to eccrine gland secretion, at minimum, is about 500 mL per day through insensible perspiration. Excessive loss can rise to a liter per day in extreme heat or during vigorous exercise. Such dehydration and electrolyte loss must be replaced to avoid imbalances.

Chapter 53   Integumentary System Function, Data Collection, and Therapeutic Measures

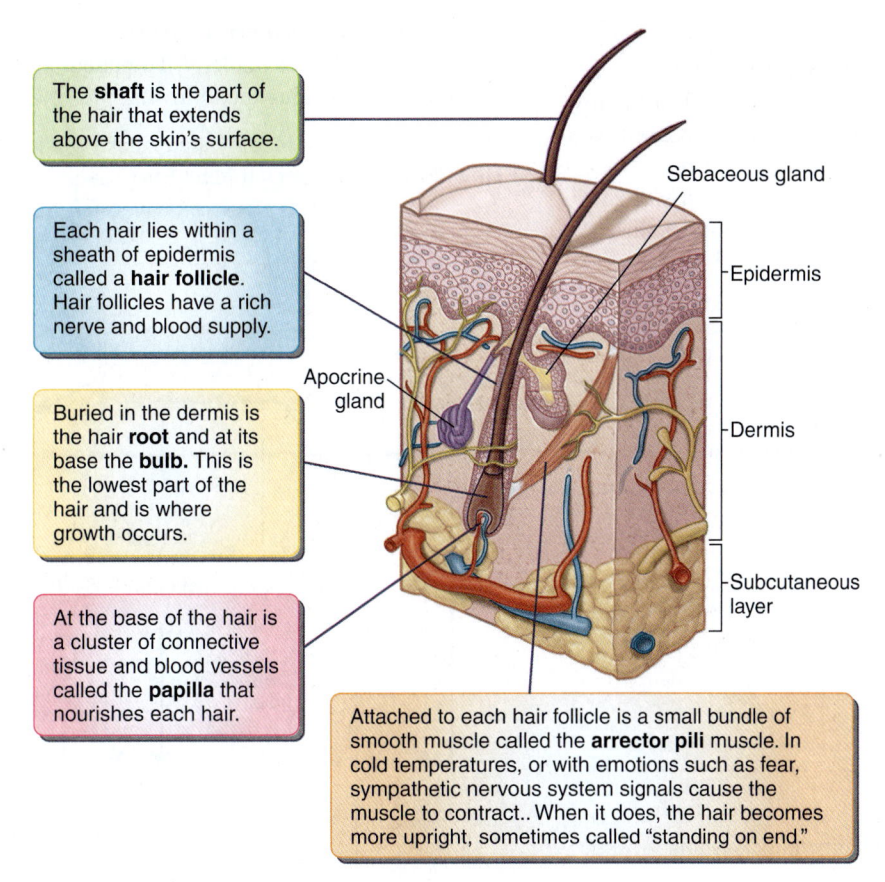

The shaft is the part of the hair that extends above the skin's surface.

Each hair lies within a sheath of epidermis called a **hair follicle**. Hair follicles have a rich nerve and blood supply.

Buried in the dermis is the hair **root** and at its base the **bulb**. This is the lowest part of the hair and is where growth occurs.

At the base of the hair is a cluster of connective tissue and blood vessels called the **papilla** that nourishes each hair.

Attached to each hair follicle is a small bundle of smooth muscle called the **arrector pili** muscle. In cold temperatures, or with emotions such as fear, sympathetic nervous system signals cause the muscle to contract.. When it does, the hair becomes more upright, sometimes called "standing on end."

FIGURE 53.2 Hair.

Eccrine glands
- Contain a duct that leads from a secretory portion (consisting of a twisted coil in the dermis), through the dermis and epidermis, and onto the skin's surface
- Are widespread throughout the body, but are especially abundant on the palms, soles, forehead, and upper torso
- Produce a transparent, watery fluid called sweat, which contains potassium, ammonia, lactic acid, uric acid, and other wastes
- Sweat plays a chief role in helping the body maintain a constant core temperature and also helps the body eliminate wastes.

Apocrine glands
- Contain a duct that leads to a hair follicle (as opposed to opening onto the skin's surface)
- Are located mainly in the axillary and anogenital (groin) regions
- Are scent glands that respond to stress and sexual stimulation
- Begin to function at puberty
- Sweat produced by these glands does not have a strong odor unless it accumulates on the skin; when this occurs, bacteria begin to degrade substances in the sweat, resulting in body odor.

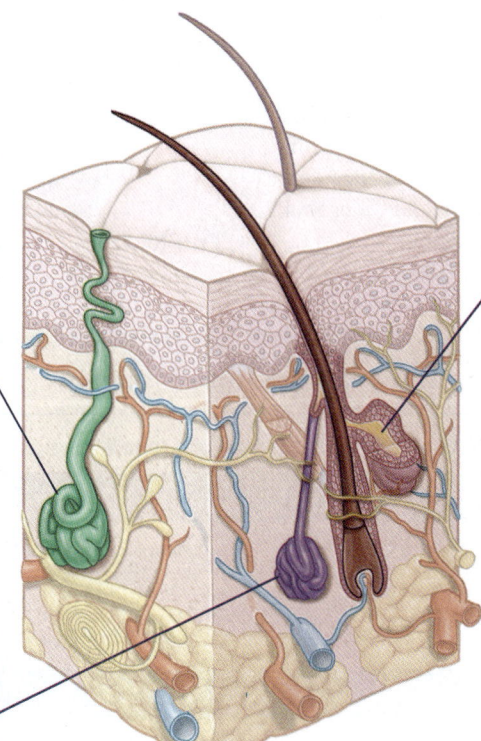

Sebaceous glands
Sebaceous glands, which open into a hair follicle, secrete an oily substance called sebum. Sebum helps keep the skin and hair from drying out and becoming brittle. Sebum has a mild antibacterial and antifungal effect. Under the influence of sex hormones, sebum production increases during adolescence. When excess sebum accumulates in the gland ducts, pimples and blackheads can form. (When the accumulated sebum is exposed to air, it darkens, forming a blackhead. A pustule results if the area becomes infected by bacteria.)

FIGURE 53.3 Glands.

Blood Vessels

Blood vessels in the dermis serve the usual function of tissue nourishment, but the arterioles are also involved in maintaining body temperature. Blood carries heat produced by active organs and distributes it throughout the body. In a warm environment, dilation of blood vessels in the dermis increases blood flow and loss of heat to air. Constriction of blood vessels in a cold environment decreases blood flow to the skin and conserves body heat.

Stressful situations also cause vasoconstriction in the dermis, which allows blood to circulate to more vital organs, such as the heart, liver, brain, or muscles.

Other functions of the skin are the formation of vitamin D from cholesterol when the skin is exposed to the UV rays of the sun and the excretion of small amounts of ammonia, urea, and sodium chloride in sweat.

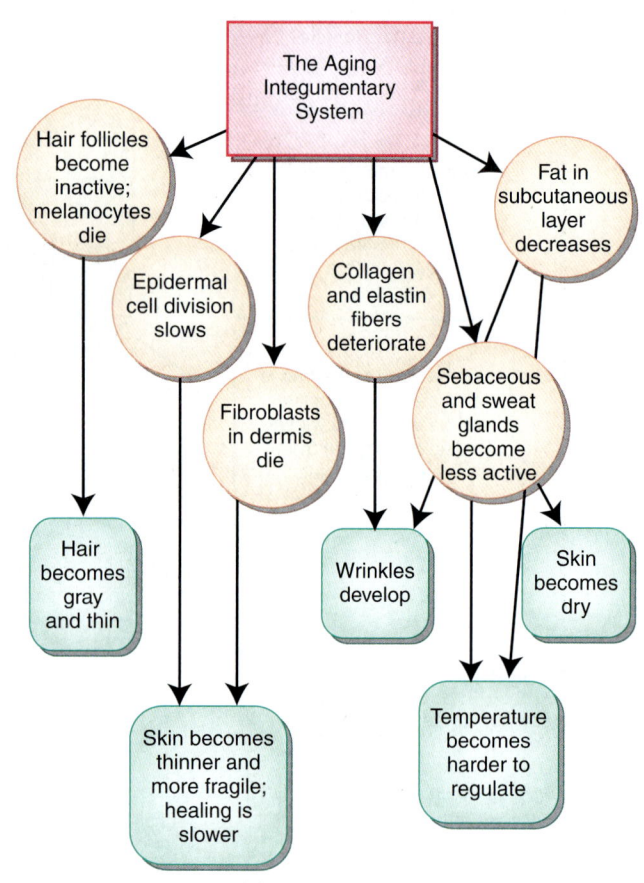

Aging and the Integumentary System

The effects of age on the integumentary system are often quite visible. Figure 53.4 summarizes the effects of aging.

INTEGUMENTARY SYSTEM DATA COLLECTION

Health History

Many factors influence the integumentary system. A skin problem may be a patient's only problem or be a manifestation of an underlying systemic condition or psychological stress. Most important, the skin can visibly communicate a patient's health. Therefore, good data collection can help determine whether a problem is a skin disease or a sign of a more systemic disorder. Repeat data collection is recommended with any change in condition or every shift in an acute care setting. Table 53.1 provides examples of general questions that can be asked of the patient to gather information.

If further data collection is needed, *WHAT'S UP?* questioning can be used. For example, if the patient has a rash, you can respond by pursuing the following information:

- **W**here is it? Is that the only area where you have a rash?
- **H**ow does it feel? Does it itch? Burn? Hurt? Sting?

FIGURE 53.4 Aging and the integumentary system.

Table 53.1
Subjective Data Collection for the Integumentary System

Questions to Ask During the Health History	Rationale
History	
Do you or anyone in your family have a history of dryness, rashes, itching, skin disease, psoriasis, eczema, dermatitis, asthma, hay fever, hives, or allergies?	These conditions may be hereditary.
Risk Factors	
Have you noticed any changes in your skin, such as a sore that does not heal, rashes, lumps, or a change in an existing mole?	Sores that do not heal, moles that change color, or lumps may indicate cancer. Slow healing can also be associated with diabetes. Brown staining of the skin in the lower legs is associated with venous stasis.

Table 53.1
Subjective Data Collection for the Integumentary System—cont'd

Questions to Ask During the Health History	Rationale
Have you had any recent trauma to your skin?	A break in skin integrity can lead to infection.
Do you tend to sunburn easily? Do you use sunblock? Do you go to tanning salons or use a sun lamp?	Repeat sunburns and tanning are a risk factor for skin cancer.
Hair	
Do you wear a wig or hairpiece?	Adequate examination of the scalp requires permission for removal of a wig or hairpiece.
Have you noticed a change in hair growth or hair loss?	Hair loss can result from systemic illness or treatment or sometimes from infections or hair care products.
Nails	
Have you experienced recent trauma to or changes in your nails? Do you wear artificial nails?	Nail changes may be caused by circulatory problems. Artificial nails may mask changes.
Medications	
What medications do you take every day (prescription and over the counter)?	The patient may be taking medication for a skin disorder. Many medications cause skin reactions, from hives and photosensitivity to serious inflammatory conditions.
What medications did you take most recently? When did you take your last dose?	This might help pinpoint the cause of a new reaction.
Exposures	
What is your occupation?	Occupational exposures can lead to skin problems.
How often do you bathe or shower?	Frequent bathing can cause dry skin.
What kind of soap do you use?	Some soap may cause allergic reactions.
What recreational activities do you participate in?	Skin disorders can be caused by gym equipment that was not cleaned properly. Poison ivy may result from being in wooded areas.
Have you or any members of your immediate family or your coworkers had recent skin problems?	Some skin disorders are contagious.
Have you traveled recently?	This could help pinpoint causes of suspicious skin changes.
Is there anything in your current environment, at home or work, that may cause skin problems (e.g., animals, plants, chemicals, infections, new carpeting, new soaps or detergents)?	Various environmental factors cause contact dermatitis; some chemicals can cause skin disorders.
Does anything that touches your skin cause a rash?	This may help pinpoint causes of contact dermatitis.

- **A**ggravating and alleviating factors. Does scratching aggravate it? Does anything else aggravate it, such as soaps and detergents? What relieves it? How have you treated it in the past?
- **T**iming. How long have you had this problem? Does it recur?
- **S**everity. How bad is the discomfort on a scale of 0 to 10, with 0 being comfortable and 10 being unable to touch the area?
- **U**seful other data. Do you have other symptoms besides the rash? Are any other members of your family experiencing this rash? Is there a family history of this type of rash?
- **P**atient's perception. What do you think is causing your rash?

Physical Examination

Examination of skin involves not only the entire skin area, but also hair, nails, scalp, and mucous membranes. The main techniques used in physical examination of the skin are inspection and palpation. Make sure the patient is undressed but adequately draped in a well-lit and warm environment. Use a handheld magnifying glass or penlight to see small details and light the area being inspected. Use a ruler to measure any skin conditions as necessary.

Normally, skin is intact, abrasion-free, smooth, dry, well-hydrated, and warm. Skin **turgor** (tension) is firm and elastic. Skin surface is flexible and soft. Color ranges from light to ruddy pink or olive in light-skinned patients and light brown to deep brown in dark-skinned patients.

Be aware of normal developmental changes when performing an examination. The skin of the neonate is very thin and friable (easily broken). During adolescence, skin becomes thicker, with active sebaceous, eccrine, and apocrine glands. Body hair changes during adolescence as a result of hormonal influences. In older patients, skin loses some of its elasticity and moisture. Activity of sebaceous and sweat glands decreases. The older patient's skin is thinner, more fragile, and more wrinkled. Very obese and very thin people may be more susceptible to skin irritation.

Inspection

Inspect each area of the skin for color, moisture, lesions/intactness, edema, vascular lesions, turgor, and cleanliness. This examination should be done in an orderly sequence, such as hair, scalp, buccal mucosa, nails, and then the general skin surface from head to toe.

COLOR. Skin color can be influenced by many factors, including temperature, oxygenation, blood flow, exposure to UV rays, and positioning. Because skin color can differ genetically from very light to very dark, collecting data can be difficult for the novice practitioner.

In general, healthy patients have an even skin tone that matches their genetic background. Light-skinned patients may have pink or yellow to olive undertones. Patients with naturally dark skin may have a reddish undertone, with pinkish buccal mucosa, tongue, nails, and lips.

Commonly noted alterations include pallor, **erythema** (redness), jaundice, cyanosis, and brown coloring. Pallor is paleness or a decrease in color, caused by vasoconstriction, decreased blood flow, or decreased hemoglobin levels from anemia. Pallor is best noted on the face, conjunctivae, nailbeds, and lips. If a dark-skinned patient is pale, the mucous membranes have an ash-gray color, lips and nailbeds appear paler than usual, and the skin appears yellow-brown to ash gray.

Erythema, red discoloration, can result from vasodilation or increased blood flow to the skin from fever or inflammation. Erythema is best noted on the face or in an area of trauma. Erythema presents in dark-skinned patients as a purplish-gray color.

Jaundice, a yellow-orange discoloration, can result from liver disease. Although skin is affected by jaundice, the best place to inspect for jaundice is in the sclera of the eye.

Cyanosis, or bluish discoloration, can indicate a cardiac, pulmonary, or perfusion problem. The best places to inspect for cyanosis are the lips, nailbeds, conjunctivae, and palms. People of Mediterranean descent normally have a bluish tone to their lips; this is not cyanosis. Cyanosis in a dark-skinned patient presents as a gray cast to the skin. Nailbeds, palms, and soles may have a blue cast.

A brown color in an otherwise light-skinned patient may be caused by increased melanin production. This can indicate chronic exposure to sunlight or pregnancy. It is best seen on areas exposed to the sun; changes in pregnancy can be seen on the face, areolae, and nipples. A brownish color may result from chronic peripheral vascular disease, especially on the lower legs.

MOISTURE/DRYNESS. Skin moistness provides clues to the patient's level of hydration. Observe skin for dryness, moisture, scales, and flakes. Moisture may be found in skinfold areas. Skin is normally smooth and dry. Flaking and scaling can indicate dry skin or an inflammatory disorder.

LESIONS. A lesion is any change or injury to tissue. Observation of skin lesions helps determine the cause of a skin disorder. Lesions are described as primary or secondary. Primary lesions are the initial reaction to a disease process. Secondary lesions are changes that take place in the primary lesion because of trauma, scratching, infection, or various stages of a disease. Lesions are further described according to type and appearance (Fig. 53.5).

When collecting data and documenting about skin lesions, note the colors of the lesion and its size (usually in centimeters), location, distribution, and configuration. Configuration refers to the pattern of the lesions (Fig. 53.6). Also note any exudate, including amount, color, and odor, and accompanying symptoms. Gently stretching skin over the affected area makes lesions stand out more for better visualization.

EDEMA. Edema occurs because of excess fluid in the tissues. It can cause the skin to become stretched, dry, and shiny. Examine and document the location, distribution, and color

PRIMARY LESIONS

Macule:
Flat, nonpalpable change in skin color, with different sizes, shapes, color; usually smaller than 1 cm (e.g., rubella, scarlet fever, freckles)

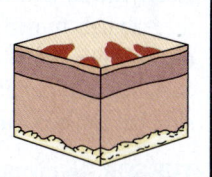

Papule:
Palpable solid raised lesion that is less than 1 cm in diameter due to superficial thickening in the epidermis (e.g., ringworm, wart, mole)

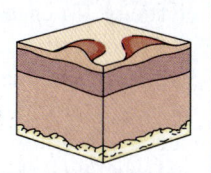

Nodule:
Solid elevated lesion that is larger and deeper than a papule (e.g., fibroma, intradermal nevi)

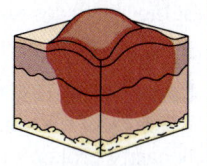

Vesicle:
A small, blisterlike raised area of the skin that contains serous fluid, up to 1 cm in diameter (e.g., poison ivy, shingles, chickenpox)

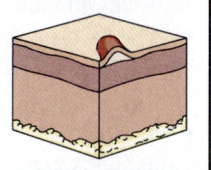

Bulla:
A fluid-filled vesicle or blister larger than 1 cm (e.g., burns, contact dermatitis)

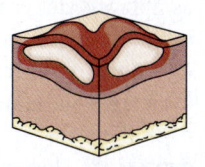

Pustule:
Small elevation of skin or vesicle or bulla that contains lymph or pus (e.g., impetigo, scabies, acne)

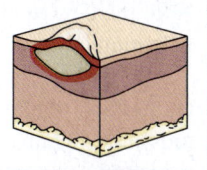

Wheal:
Round, transient elevation of the skin caused by dermal edema and surrounding capillary dilatation; white in center and red in periphery (e.g., hives, insect bites)

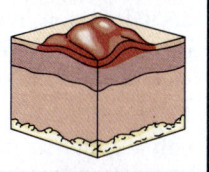

Plaque:
A patch or solid, raised lesion on the skin or mucous membrane that is greater than 1 cm in diameter (e.g., psoriasis)

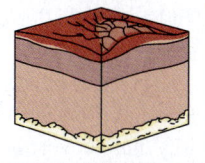

Cyst:
A closed sac or pouch which consists of semisolid, solid, or liquid material (e.g., sebaceous cyst)

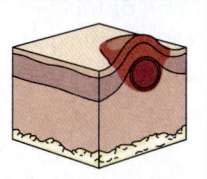

SECONDARY LESIONS

Scale:
Dry exfoliation of dead epidermis that may develop as a result of inflammatory changes (e.g., very dry skin, cradle cap, psoriasis)

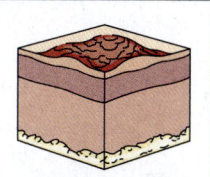

Crust:
A scab formed by dry serum, pus, or blood (e.g., infected dermatitis, impetigo)

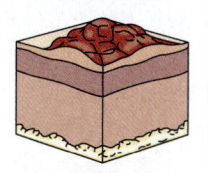

Excoriation:
Traumatized abrasions of the epidermis or linear scratch marks (e.g., scabies, dermatitis, burns)

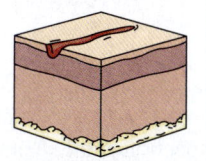

Fissure:
A slit or cracklike sore that extends into dermis, usually due to continuous inflammation and drying (e.g., athlete's foot, anal fissure)

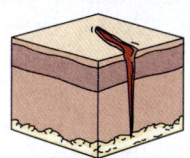

Ulcer:
An open sore or lesion that extends to the dermis (e.g., pressure sores)

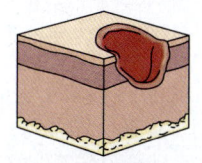

Lichenification:
Thickening and hardening of skin from continued irritation such as from intense scratching

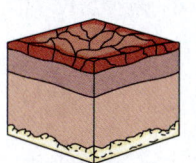

Scar:
A mark left in the skin due to fibrotic changes following healing of a wound or surgical incision

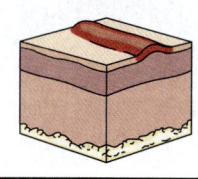

FIGURE 53.5 Description of skin lesions.

Discrete
Individual lesions are separate and distinct.

Grouped
Lesions are clustered together.

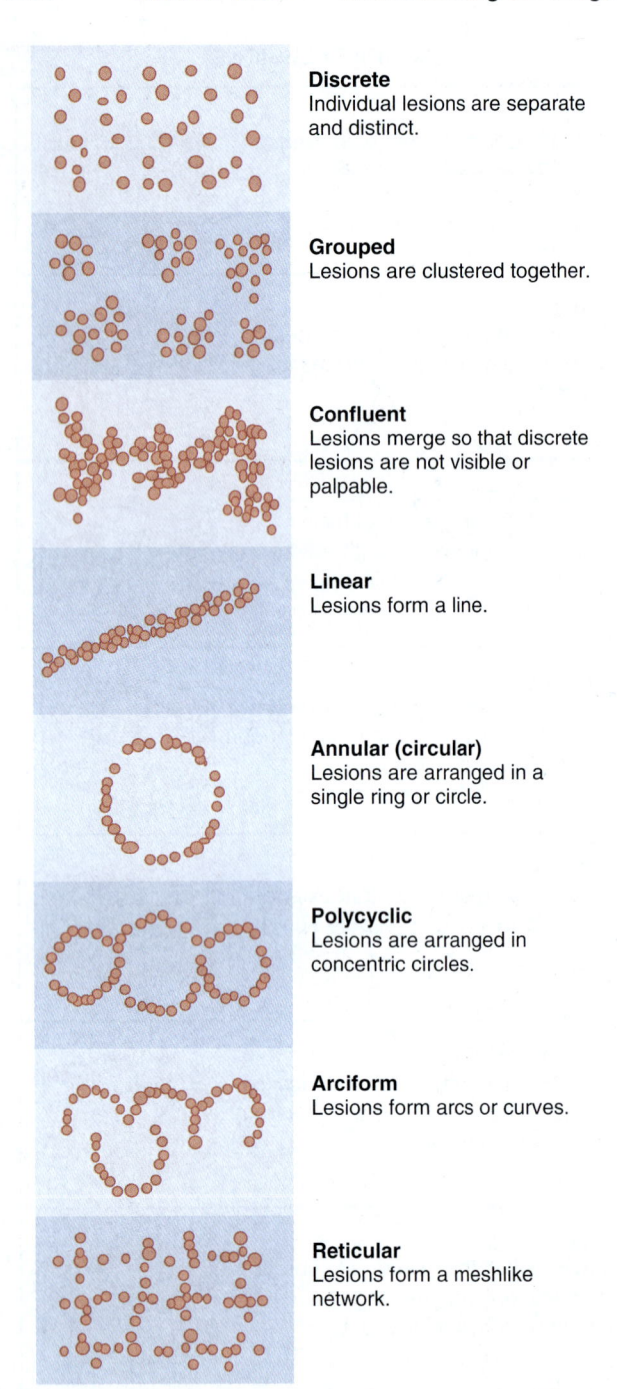

Confluent
Lesions merge so that discrete lesions are not visible or palpable.

Linear
Lesions form a line.

Annular (circular)
Lesions are arranged in a single ring or circle.

Polycyclic
Lesions are arranged in concentric circles.

Arciform
Lesions form arcs or curves.

Reticular
Lesions form a meshlike network.

FIGURE 53.6 To determine configuration, observe the relationship of the lesions to each other. Then characterize the configuration by choosing one of the patterns illustrated in the chart.

---

and petechiae (see Fig. 28.1 and Fig. 28.2 in Chapter 28). **Ecchymosis** is a bruise that changes color from blue-black to greenish brown or yellow over time. **Petechiae** are reddish-purple spots smaller than 0.5 mm in diameter. In the dark-skinned patient, petechiae are usually not visible on the skin but can be visualized in the conjunctivae and oral mucosa.

TURGOR. Skin turgor is a measure of the amount of skin elasticity. To check for turgor, pinch the skin on the back of the forearm or over the sternum between the thumb and forefinger and then release. Normally, skin lifts easily and quickly returns to its normal state. Poor skin turgor is indicated by "tenting" of the skin, with gradual return to its normal state. Poor skin turgor can indicate dehydration. Normal aging produces some loss of skin elasticity; the preferred place to check skin turgor in older adults is over the sternum.

GENERAL INTEGRITY AND CLEANLINESS. Examine the integrity of the skin. Older adults have thin, fragile skin that is easily broken or torn. Be sure to check between toes and skinfolds and under a pendulous abdomen or breasts. Check over bony prominences for signs of pressure. Note general cleanliness and odors.

Palpation

Palpation is used with inspection. Wear gloves for palpation as appropriate, especially if a lesion is moist or draining or infection is suspected. Use the dorsum (back) of the hand to palpate temperature because this part is most sensitive to changes in temperature. Use fingertips to gently palpate over the skin to determine size, contour (flat, raised, or depressed), and consistency (soft or indurated) of lesions. Note the degree of pain or discomfort associated with light palpation of lesions.

If edema is suspected, palpate those areas to check for tenderness, mobility, and consistency. Press the edematous area (against bone, if possible) with your thumb for 5 seconds and release. When pressure from fingers leaves an indentation, it is called *pitting edema*. For edema in an extremity, measure and record circumference in centimeters, and monitor it for increase or decrease in size.

Inspect and/or palpate the hair over the entire body for color, quantity, thickness, and texture. Note any areas of **alopecia** (hair loss). Determine any recent changes in color and growth pattern. Note cleanliness, redness, scaling, flakes, and tenderness.

Terminal hair is on the scalp, eyebrows, axillae, and pubic areas and on the face and chest of men. Vellus hair is soft, tiny hair covering the body. Normally, body hair has uniform distribution. Loss of hair on the extremities can indicate impaired circulation. Note male or female pubic hair distribution. Scalp hair can normally be thick, thin, coarse,

---

of edematous areas. If edema is unilateral, compare it with the opposite side of the body. Measure edematous extremities to track changes over time. Dependent edema occurs in the part of the body that is at the lowest point, typically the feet and ankles, or in the sacrum if the patient is lying down.

VASCULAR CHANGES. Two common abnormal vascular changes result from bleeding under the skin: ecchymosis

• **WORD** • **BUILDING** •

ecchymosis: ec—out + cchymos—juice + is—condition

smooth, shiny, curly, or straight. Loss of scalp hair may indicate thyroid or other health issues. Describe scalp hair distribution and cleanliness.

Nails can reflect general health. Examine fingers and nails for color, shape, texture, thickness, and abnormalities. Normally, nails appear pink, smooth, hard, and slightly convex (160-degree angle), with a firm base. Older adults' nails may have a yellowish-gray color, thickening, and ridges. Brown or black pigmentation between the nail and nail base is normal in dark-skinned patients. Abnormal findings include clubbing, which may indicate hypoxia, and spoon nails (concave nails, also called *koilonychia*), which can be associated with anemia. Thick nails may indicate fungal infection. Palpate for nail consistency, and observe for redness, swelling, or tenderness around the nail area. Table 53.2 describes other nail abnormalities.

Describe abnormal skin conditions in detail. Include findings such as color of lesion, pain, swelling, redness, location, size, drainage (including amount, color, and odor), and eruption patterns. If equipment is available, an excellent way to supplement documentation is by photographing the area; serial photographs can be mounted in the chart to document healing progression. "Gerontological Issues" describes data collection and care specific to older adults.

> **NURSING CARE TIP**
> When scraping scales for culture, position the patient so that the skin lesion is vertical. Place the slide against the skin below the lesion. Be sure to wear gloves when collecting specimens and perform hand hygiene before and after.

Table 53.2
Abnormalities of the Nails

Physical Examination Finding	Description	Possible Causes
Beau lines	Transverse depressions in the nails	Systemic illnesses or nail injury
Splinter hemorrhages	Red or brown streaks in the nailbed	Minor trauma, subacute bacterial endocarditis, or trichinosis
Paronychia	Inflammation of the skin at the base of the nail	Local infection or trauma

Gerontological Issues

Care of Older Patients' Feet

Many older people are unable to bend down or bring the feet up high enough to see or care for them. Take time to examine and take special care of your older patients' feet. General guidelines for inspection include the following:

- Inspect feet for redness or pressure injuries over bony prominences.
- Inspect feet for dryness or cracking.
- Inspect between toes for cracking, wounds, or excess moisture.
- Inspect and palpate for calluses.
- Inspect toenails for thickening.
- Palpate dorsalis pedis and posterior tibial pulses for circulatory status.
- Check patient's sensation using a wisp of cotton, monofilament, or light touch.

Actions to promote healthy feet include the following:

- Soak the patient's feet briefly in warm water and wash using a gentle soap. Test the water to be sure it is not too warm, especially for the patient with reduced sensation.
- Thoroughly dry the feet, including between the toes. Water left to evaporate can cause drying, cracking, and fungal infection.
- Use a pumice stone to help remove dry dead skin over heels or calluses. Work gently, rubbing the stone in one direction only and removing only a small amount of dead skin at one time. Only use a pumice stone on a patient with diabetes mellitus under direction of a podiatrist.
- Use a cream or lotion that does not contain alcohol to moisturize the feet. *Do not* apply between toes. Apply it with gentle massage while moving the patient's feet through range-of-motion exercises. To prevent falls, never apply lotion before the patient steps into the tub or shower.
- Use gauze or a commercially made pad to decrease pressure and friction in areas between toes that cross or other areas where breakdown is likely.
- Encourage the patient to wear cotton or dry weave socks that keep feet dry from perspiration.
- Encourage the patient to wear comfortable leather shoes or hard-soled slippers to avoid injury to the feet and prevent falls. Patients with diabetes should be encouraged to wear closed-toe shoes.
- Take extra care to monitor and care for feet in patients with diabetes because of their increased risk for injury and slow healing (Chapter 40).

DIAGNOSTIC TESTS FOR THE INTEGUMENTARY SYSTEM

Laboratory Tests
Cultures
Skin cultures determine the presence of fungi, bacteria, and viruses. When a fungal infection is suspected, use a gloved hand to gently scrape scales from the lesion into a Petri dish or other indicated container. The specimen is treated with a 10% potassium hydroxide solution to make fungi more prominent. It can remain at room temperature until sent to the laboratory.

If a viral culture is ordered, the fluid is expressed (gently squeezed) from an intact vesicle, collected with a sterile cotton swab, and placed in a special viral culture tube. If the lesion has crusts, they are removed or punctured before swabbing. The viral culture tube must be kept in ice and sent to the laboratory as soon as possible.

Bacterial cultures may be collected with a sterile swab or wound culture kit. Box 53.1 gives specific instructions.

Skin Biopsy
A skin biopsy is indicated for deeper infections, suspicious lesions, or evaluation of current treatment. A biopsy is an excision of a small piece of tissue for microscopic examination. Three common types of skin biopsies are punch, shave, and incisional.

A punch biopsy uses a small, round cutting instrument called a punch to cut a cylinder-shaped plug of tissue for a full-thickness specimen. A shave biopsy removes just the area that has risen above the rest of the skin. An incisional biopsy uses a scalpel to make a deep incision and almost always requires sutures for closure.

For all biopsies, explain the procedure, assist in preparing a sterile field, calm and comfort the patient during the procedure, and assist in dressing the site after the procedure. The most uncomfortable part of the procedure is usually injection of a local anesthetic. Explaining the procedure and calming the patient can reduce the trauma of the procedure.

Other Diagnostic Tests
Wood Light Examination
A Wood light examination involves the use of UV rays to detect fluorescent materials in the skin and hair present in certain diseases such as tinea capitis (ringworm). This examination is performed with a handheld black light (Wood light) in a darkened room.

Skin Testing
Patch and scratch tests are performed for suspected allergic contact dermatitis. These are usually done by a dermatologist on uninvolved skin, such as the upper back or arms. Any hair in the area must be shaved.

For a scratch test, skin is superficially scratched or pricked with an allergen for an immediate reaction. If a reaction such as a wheal occurs, the test is positive for that allergen. Resuscitation equipment should be in the immediate vicinity in case of severe allergic (anaphylactic) reaction.

For a patch test, allergens are applied under occlusive tape patches; a delayed hypersensitivity reaction develops in 48 to 96 hours. The skin should be free of oils to promote patch adhesion, so cleanse the area first with alcohol. The test site must remain dry and free from moisture. The patch is removed in 2 days. Any reaction is noted, with a final reading in 2 to 5 days.

CUE RECOGNITION 53.1

You are working in an allergy clinic. Twenty minutes after administration of a series of scratch tests, a patient complains of severe itching and says she can't seem to catch her breath. What do you do?

Suggested answers are at the end of the chapter.

THERAPEUTIC MEASURES FOR THE INTEGUMENTARY SYSTEM

Open Wet Dressings
Wet compresses may be ordered for acute, weeping, crusted, inflamed, or ulcerated lesions. Wet dressings decrease inflammation, cleanse and dry wounds, and promote drainage of infected areas. They may be ordered either sterile or clean depending on infection risk. Solutions commonly consist of room temperature to cool tap water or normal saline solution, aluminum acetate solution (Burow solution), or magnesium sulfate. The dressing is saturated with the solution before it is applied, usually every 3 to 4 hours for 15 to 30 minutes.

Wet dressings should not be prescribed for more than 72 hours because skin may become too dry or macerated. Cool compresses should be reapplied every 5 to 10 minutes as they become warm from body heat. If warm compresses are used, monitor the skin closely to prevent burns.

Box 53.1

Steps in Culturing a Wound

1. Use sterile saline to remove excess drainage and debris from the wound. Purulent material may have different bacteria than those causing the infection.
2. Using a sterile calcium alginate swab in a rotating motion, swab wound and wound edges 10 times in a diagonal pattern across the entire surface of the wound.
3. Do not swab over eschar or slough.
4. Place swab in culture tube, label, and send to laboratory.

PRACTICE ANALYSIS TIP
Linking NCLEX-PN® to Practice
Use measures to maintain or improve client skin integrity.

> **NURSING CARE TIP**
> To prevent chilling, no more than one-third of the body should be treated with a wet dressing at one time. Keep the patient warm during wet dressing treatment.

Balneotherapy

Balneotherapy (therapeutic bath) is useful in applying medications to large areas of the skin as well as for debridement (removing old crusts), removing old medications, and relieving itching and inflammation. Water temperature should be kept at a comfortable level, and hot water avoided. The bath should last for 15 to 30 minutes, while maintaining warmth. Fill the tub halfway. Keep the room warm to minimize chilling. Advise patient to wear loose clothing after bath.

Water and saline solution are used for weeping, oozing, and erythematous lesions. Colloidal baths (such as oatmeal or Aveeno) are used for widely distributed skin lesions, drying, and relief of itching. Medicated tar baths, such as Balnetar, are used for chronic eczema and psoriasis. Loose skin crusts can be removed after the bath. The room should be well ventilated because tars are volatile.

To increase hydration after the bath, a lubricating agent is applied to damp skin if prescribed. Bath oils, such as Alpha Keri or Lubath, are used for lubrication and to relieve itching.

> **BE SAFE!**
> **BE VIGILANT!** A nonslip bathmat should be used in treatment baths, as some treatments may make the tub slippery.

Topical Medications

Many types of topical medications are used to treat skin conditions, including lotions, ointments and creams, powders, gels, pastes, and intralesional therapy. Systemic medications may be given for more serious conditions.

Lotions tend to cool the skin through water evaporation. They may have a protective effect and be antipruritic (anti-itch). Lotions may be applied with cotton, gauze, gloves, or a soft brush.

Ointments and creams have a varied base (greasy, nongreasy, or penetrating), depending on the drug applied. These medications can protect the skin, provide lubrication, and prevent water loss. They are used for localized or chronic skin conditions. Ointments and creams cause some reduction in blood flow to the skin. They are applied with a gloved hand or wooden tongue depressor.

Powders usually have a zinc oxide, talc, or cornstarch base. They are used to absorb moisture and reduce friction. Antifungal powders may be used in skinfolds. Powders are usually supplied with a shaker top. They should be shaken onto a gauze pad or gloved hand away from the patient's face, then applied by gently patting or rubbing onto the affected area. Avoid use of powders in patients with respiratory disease or tracheostomies.

> **NURSING CARE TIP**
> Avoid applying too much powder in skinfold areas, as this can cause dermatitis and fungal infection. Shake powder gently to avoid possible inhalation by the nurse or the patient.

Gels, or semisolid emulsions, become liquid with topical application. They are usually greaseless and do not stain. Many topical steroids are prescribed in this manner.

Pastes are semisolid substances comprising ointments and powders. They are used for inflammatory disorders. Mineral oil can facilitate removal of pastes.

Topical corticosteroids reduce or relieve pain and itching by decreasing inflammation. Steroids should be used sparingly according to package directions. Overuse of topical corticosteroids can cause thinning of the skin. Some clinicians use steroid inhalers (usually used for patients with asthma) to apply a fine mist of medication to affected areas.

Intralesional therapy may be used for anti-inflammatory action. This procedure uses a sterile suspension of a corticosteroid injected just below the lesion with a tuberculin syringe. Local atrophy may occur if the injection is made into subcutaneous tissue. Common conditions that are treated with this therapy include psoriasis and keloids.

> **CLINICAL JUDGMENT**
>
> **Mr. Evans** comes to the doctor's office with atrophic skin (thin, shiny, and pink with visible vessels) at the area of psoriasis where he is applying his corticosteroid ointment. He says that he has been applying a thick layer of ointment four times a day.
>
> 1. What should you advise Mr. Evans about his treatment?
> 2. What complications can occur if he continues to use too much ointment?
> 3. What should you include when you document his skin condition?
>
> *Suggested answers are at the end of the chapter.*

Dressings

Dressings may be used to enhance absorption of topical medications, promote retention of moisture, protect from infection, prevent evaporation of medication, and reduce pain and itching. Occlusive dressings (for sealing a wound) are commonly used for skin disorders. For an occlusive dressing, an airtight plastic film is applied directly over the topical agent. Corticosteroids are also available in a special plastic surgical tape that can be cut to size. See "Nursing Care Plan for the Patient With an Occlusive Dressing."

Nursing Care Plan for the Patient With an Occlusive Dressing

Nursing Diagnosis: *Impaired Skin Integrity* related to open lesions
Expected Outcome: The patient will experience improved skin integrity as evidenced by reduction in size of lesion.
Evaluation of Outcome: Is there a decrease in wound size?

Intervention	Rationale	Evaluation
Inspect areas of lesions for changes in size, color, swelling, dead skin, and drainage three times a day or as ordered.	*Areas of redness, swelling, pain, and drainage may indicate infection.*	Are lesions free of redness, swelling, pain, and drainage?
Cleanse wound as prescribed. Lightly pat dry.	*Cleansing helps provide a healthy granulation area for healing.*	Is wound clean and free of debris, crusts, and exudate?
Apply prescribed topical agent to moist skin as ordered. Apply sparingly or as directed.	*Depends on agent and reason prescribed.*	Does area exhibit signs that treatment is effective (e.g., decrease in size and number of lesions, free from infection, less itching)?
Cut plastic film to size and apply. Cover with an appropriate dressing to seal edges.	*Film enhances absorption of medication and helps retain moisture.*	Is the topical agent adherent to the skin?
Remove dressing for 12 of 24 hours.	*Continued use may cause skin atrophy, folliculitis, erythema, and systemic absorption of medication.*	Are there signs of healthy granulation tissue? Is skin pink? Are there fewer open areas? Is dressing removed for at least 12 hours every 24 hours?

Nursing Diagnosis: *Disturbed Body Image* related to presence of lesions or wound
Expected Outcomes: The patient will verbalize acceptance of condition. The patient will be willing to participate in care of lesion or wound.
Evaluation of Outcomes: Does the patient verbalize acceptance of condition? Does the patient participate in care of lesions?

Intervention	Rationale	Evaluation
Determine the patient's feelings regarding condition.	*Data collection provides a baseline for care. If patient denies condition, he or she may not comply with care.*	Does patient state willingness to follow care instructions?
Care for patient with an accepting attitude.	*Patient will be aware of nurse's response to the appearance of the skin.*	Does patient appear comfortable allowing nurse to provide care for lesion or wound?
Allow opportunities for patient to verbalize concerns about condition.	*Verbalization allows patient to begin to accept changes and problem solve.*	Does patient verbalize feelings appropriately?
Provide referrals to support groups and counselors as appropriate.	*Patient may benefit from talking to others with similar condition or to another professional for objective evaluation.*	Is patient receptive to appropriate referrals?
Assist patient in concealing lesion or wound in a safe and appropriate manner.	*Long sleeves and long pants may help conceal and protect lesions and prevent further skin damage.*	Is patient able to conceal lesions if desired?

> **PRACTICE ANALYSIS TIP**
> Linking NCLEX-PN® to Practice
> Perform wound care and/or dressing change.

Proper application of a plastic wrap dressing includes washing the area, lightly patting it dry, applying the medication to moist skin, covering the medicated area with plastic wrap, and covering with a dressing to seal the edges. Wet dressings and ointments should be applied only to affected areas, not to healthy intact skin, because this can cause maceration of good skin. Plastic wrap dressings should be used for no more than 12 hours a day.

> **NURSING CARE TIP**
> Continued use of occlusive dressings can cause skin atrophy, folliculitis, maceration, erythema, and systemic absorption of the medication. To prevent some of these complications, the dressing is removed for at least 12 of every 24 hours.

Hydrocolloid dressings (e.g., DuoDERM, Tegaderm) can help protect areas exposed to pressure and treat pressure injuries in early stages. Gels, pastes, and granules can fill in deep wounds to promote granulation and aid healing. See Chapter 54 for dressings used specifically for pressure injuries. A skin tear (superficial flap of skin exposing underlying dermis) should be covered with a nonadherent dressing such as Xeroform and wrapped with gauze. Table 53.3 summarizes various types of wound dressings.

Table 53.3
Common Dressings

Dressing Type/Examples	Description	When Used
Alginates: ALGICELL Kaltostat Melgisorb SeaSorb Tegagen	Derived from brown seaweed; conform to the shape of the wound.	When packed into wound, absorb exudate and form a soft gel to maintain moist environment for wound healing.
Antimicrobial dressings: Acticoat Aquacel Ag IODOSORB Kerlix AMD SilvaSorb Gel Tegaderm Ag Mesh	Topical dressings derived from such agents as silver, iodine, and polyhexamethylene biguanide.	Intended for use in draining, nonhealing wounds that have bacterial contamination, such as burns, surgical wounds, diabetic ulcers, pressure injuries, and leg ulcers.
Collagen dressings: CellerateRX Gel Fibracol Plus Collagen Stimulin	Collagen is the most abundant protein in the body; its fibers are found in connective tissues, skin, bone, ligaments, and cartilage.	To stimulate new tissue development.
Promogran matrix: Prisma Ag	Oxidized regenerated cellulose and collagen. Binds metalloproteases, which protect growth factors.	For diabetic foot ulcers, venous leg ulcers, and surgical wounds.
Composite dressings: Alldress Covaderm 3M Medipore CombiDERM Stratasorb	Combine two or more distinct products into a single dressing.	May absorb exudate and also cover a wound, for example.
Hydrocolloid dressings: AQUACEL DuoDERM Tegaderm Absorbent Comfeel Plus Exuderm PrimaCol Ultec	Occlusive or semiocclusive dressings made of pectin, gelatin, and carboxymethylcellulose.	Used when a moist environment is needed that allows clean wounds to granulate; provides autolytic debriding.

Continued

Table 53.3
Common Dressings—cont'd

Dressing Type/Examples	Description	When Used
Hydrogels: DuoDERM Gel SAF-Gel Amerigel AquaSite CarraDres SilvaSorb Aquasorb FlexiGel Hypergel	Water- or glycerine-based amorphous gels, impregnated gauzes, or sheet dressings.	Used when a moist healing environment is needed to promote granulation and epithelialization and facilitate autolytic debridement.
Impregnated gauze: Mesalt Xeroform Xeroflo Adaptic Curity Non-adherent Dermagran Vaseline Petrolatum Gauze Iodoform Packing AMD Gauze	Woven or nonwoven material impregnated by the manufacturer with substances such as iodinated agents, petrolatum, zinc, bismuth tribromophenate, chlorhexidine gluconate, crystalline sodium chloride, or aqueous saline.	Used for a variety of conditions, depending on the agent added to the dressing.
Transparent films: Bioclusive Plus Tegaderm CarraFilm OpSite Mefilm Polyskin II DermaView Suresite	Adhesive semipermeable polyurethane membrane dressings that are waterproof and impermeable to bacteria and contaminants yet permit water vapor to cross the barrier.	Used when a moist healing environment is needed, promoting formulation of granulation tissue and autolysis of necrotic tissue.
Wound fillers: FlexiGel Strands Iodosorb Gel Iodoflex Pads	Sterile products that absorb exudate and conform to the shape of the wound bed.	Used when wound has exudate and would benefit from debriding.

Other items commonly used with topical treatments for skin conditions include gauze or cotton cloth held in place with:

- Small, stretchable tubular material (e.g., Surgitube) for fingers, toes, and extremities
- Disposable polyethylene gloves sealed at the wrist for hands
- Cotton socks or plastic bags for feet
- Disposable adult briefs or cotton adult briefs for the groin and perineal areas
- Cotton cloth held in place with dress shields for the axillae
- Cotton or light flannel pajamas for the trunk
- A shower cap for the scalp
- A facemask made from gauze and stretchable dressings with holes cut out for eyes, nose, mouth, and ears

The HCP or a wound care specialist should specify the type of dressing and materials needed.

Key Points

- The skin, accessory structures, and subcutaneous tissue form the integumentary system, the covering of the body that separates the internal environment from the external environment.
- The skin itself is an organ that has two layers: the outer epidermis and the inner dermis.
- The epidermis has up to five epithelial layers. The innermost layer, called the *stratum germinativum*, is where mitosis occurs to produce new epidermal cells.
- As these cells are eventually pushed to the surface of the skin, they die and become the *stratum corneum*, the outermost epidermal layer.
- The hypodermis, or subcutaneous layer, consists of areolar and adipose tissue. This subcutaneous adipose tissue cushions, insulates, and stores energy as triglyceride.
- Human hair includes eyelashes and eyebrows, which keep dust and sweat out of the eyes, and nostril hair, which filters air entering the nostrils. Head hair provides thermal insulation.
- Nail roots are found at the ends of the fingers and toes. Mitosis in the nail root continuously produces new cells. As these cells die, they form the visible nail.
- Cutaneous exocrine glands within the dermis secrete to the surface of the skin through ducts. These include sudoriferous glands (both eccrine and apocrine), sebaceous glands, ceruminous glands, and ciliary glands that make tears.
- Blood vessels in the dermis serve the function of tissue nourishment; arterioles also help maintain body temperature.
- A skin problem may be the patient's primary problem or a manifestation of stress or another health problem. A thorough skin inspection can help determine a patient's health status.
- Normal skin is intact, with no abrasions, smooth, dry, hydrated, and warm.
- Inspect each area for color, moisture, intactness/lesions, edema, vascular lesions, turgor, and cleanliness. Examination should take an orderly sequence, such as hair, scalp, buccal mucosa, nails, and then the general skin surface from head to toe.
- A lesion is any change or injury to tissue. Inspection of skin lesions helps determine the cause of a skin disorder.
- Edema occurs because of excess fluid in the tissues. It can cause skin to become stretched, dry, and shiny.
- Two common abnormal vascular changes result from bleeding under the skin: petechiae and ecchymosis.
- Diagnostic tests for skin disorders include skin cultures, skin biopsy, Wood light examination, and skin testing for allergies.
- Wet compresses may be ordered for acute, weeping, crusted, inflamed, or ulcerated lesions. These dressings decrease inflammation, cleanse and dry a wound, and promote drainage of infected areas.
- Balneotherapy (therapeutic bath) is used to apply medications to large areas of the skin, debride the wound, remove old medication, and reduce inflammation and itching.
- Many types of topical medications are used to treat skin conditions, such as lotions, ointments and creams, powders, gels, pastes, and intralesional therapy.
- Dressings enhance absorption of topical medications, promote retention of moisture, prevent evaporation of medication, and reduce pain and itching. Occlusive dressings (for sealing a wound) are commonly used for skin disorders.
- Hydrocolloid dressings can protect areas exposed to pressure and treat early pressure injuries.

SUGGESTED ANSWERS TO CHAPTER EXERCISES

Cue Recognition

53.1: Follow clinic policy to activate an emergency response. Sit the patient up and start oxygen. Make sure resuscitation equipment with epinephrine is in the room.

Critical Thinking & Clinical Judgment

Mr. Evans

1. Advise Mr. Evans to apply the ointment in a thin layer and usually only twice daily (as ordered). He may be sensitive or allergic to the medication. Most likely, he is applying too much, too often.
2. Too much ointment will cause further skin damage. Continued thinning puts Mr. Evans at risk for injury, and injury puts him at risk for infection.
3. Note the size (usually in centimeters), location, color, distribution, and configuration of lesions. Describe exactly what you see, avoiding judgments about what you think it is. Document any instruction you provided related to how his medication should be applied.

Additional Resources

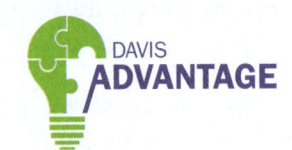

Go to Davis Advantage to complete your learning: strengthen understanding, apply your knowledge, and prepare for the Next Gen NCLEX®.

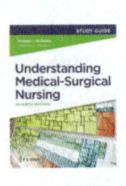

A Study Guide is also available.

CHAPTER 54
Nursing Care of Patients With Skin Disorders

Rita Bolek Trofino

KEY TERMS

cellulitis (sell-yoo-LYE-tis)
comedo (KOH-meh-doh)
dermatitis (DER-mah-TYE-tis)
dermatomycosis (DER-mah-toh-my-KOH-sis)
eschar (ESS-kar)
lichenified (lye-KEN-i-fyde)
onychomycosis (ON-ih-koh-my-KOH-sis)
pediculosis (peh-DIK-yoo-LOH-sis)
pruritus (proo-RY-tus)
psoriasis (suh-RY-ah-sis)
purulent (PURE-you-lent)
pyoderma (PYE-oh-DER-mah)
seborrhea (SEB-uh-REE-ah)

CHAPTER CONCEPTS

Mobility
Nutrition
Tissue integrity

LEARNING OUTCOMES

1. Explain the pathophysiology of each of the skin disorders listed in this chapter.
2. Describe the etiologies, signs, and symptoms of each of the skin disorders.
3. Describe current therapeutic measures that are used for each of the skin disorders.
4. List data to collect when caring for patients with disorders of the integumentary system.
5. Recognize the role of the nurse in preventing pressure injuries.
6. Plan nursing care for patients with each of the skin disorders.
7. Explain how to know whether your nursing interventions have been effective.

Skin disorders cover a wide array of diseases and conditions; they can be generalized, localized, acute, chronic, or traumatic. This chapter covers common skin disorders nurses may encounter.

PRESSURE INJURIES

Pathophysiology and Etiology

Patients often refer to pressure injuries with old terms such as *bedsores*, *decubitus ulcers*, or *pressure ulcers*. Essentially, a pressure injury is a lesion caused by prolonged pressure against the skin. Pressure injuries result from tissue anoxia and begin to develop within minutes to hours of unrelieved pressure on the skin. A primary cause of pressure injuries is spending long periods in one position, causing the weight of the body to compress the capillaries against a bed or chair, especially over bony prominences. Other causes include pressure from a tight splint or cast, traction, or another device. Patients who are immobile, have decreased circulation, or have impaired sensory perception or neurologic function are at risk for pressure injuries.

Mechanical forces (e.g., pressure, friction, and shear) cause pressure injuries to form. The pressure level that closes capillaries in healthy people is 25 to 32 mm Hg. When pressure applied to the skin exceeds pressure in the capillary bed, blood supply to the tissues is decreased, impairing cellular metabolism, eventually causing tissue ischemia. This reduction in blood flow causes the skin to *blanch* (lose color). The longer the pressure lasts, the greater the risk of skin breakdown and the development of a pressure injury.

Friction is created when the skin surface rubs over a stationary surface. *Shearing* occurs when the patient slides down in bed when the head of the bed is raised or when they are pulled or repositioned but not lifted off the sheets. With shearing, the skin and subcutaneous tissue remain stationary while fat, muscle, and bone shift in the direction of body movement. As a result, damage occurs deep within the tissues.

Any patient experiencing prolonged pressure is at risk for a pressure injury. Older patients have increased risk because of normal aging changes of the skin. Thin patients are at greatest risk because they have little padding when pressure is present. Obesity also is a contributing factor because adipose tissue is poorly vascularized and is therefore more likely to develop ischemic changes. Impaired peripheral circulation also makes the skin more susceptible to ischemic damage. See Chapter 24 for more information on problems caused by poor circulation.

Prevention

Use a Validated Assessment Tool

Use an assessment tool such as the Braden Scale for Predicting Pressure Sore Risk to monitor patients for physical condition, mental status, activity, mobility, and incontinence to determine the risk for pressure injuries. Advanced age, low diastolic blood pressure, elevated body temperature, and inadequate intake of protein are risk factors associated with the development of pressure injuries. Table 54.1 shows the Braden instrument.

> **BE SAFE!**
> **BE VIGILANT!** The National Quality Forum lists pressure injury as a *Serious Reportable Event*. Medicare and many private insurers will not pay for treatment of any stage 3, stage 4, or unstageable pressure ulcers acquired after admission/presentation to a health-care facility (https://psnet.ahrq.gov/primer/never-events). Therefore, it is essential to (1) do a careful skin examination and document with photographs all pressure injuries on admission; and (2) be vigilant with care to prevent development or worsening of pressure injuries.

CLEANSE THE SKIN. Gently cleanse the skin daily with tepid water and mild soap to prevent drying. To reduce friction, pat skin dry rather than rubbing. After bathing, prevent dryness by lubricating skin with moisturizers. Thoroughly dry skin-to-skin surfaces, such as under the breasts, in the groin and abdominal folds, and between the toes, to prevent prolonged exposure to moisture.

PREVENT DAMAGE FROM INCONTINENCE. If the patient is incontinent, clean the skin promptly with tepid water and mild soap, pat dry, and apply a moisture barrier to prevent breakdown.

AVOID MASSAGING AFFECTED AREAS. Avoid massaging bony prominences or reddened skin areas. Blood vessels are damaged by massage when ischemia is present or when they lie over a bone.

> **BE SAFE!**
> **AVOID FAILURE TO COMMUNICATE!** You can help prevent damage to capillary beds by advising nursing personnel and family members to avoid massaging reddened areas and to discontinue use of donut-shaped pillows for pressure relief.

MAINTAIN MOBILITY. A mobility program specific to each patient must be developed. Maintain the highest possible level of mobility, as follows:

- Teach patients to shift weight every 15 minutes, if possible, when lying or sitting.
- Provide frequent active or passive range-of-motion exercises and turn patient according to a written repositioning schedule. If patients are on bedrest, turn and reposition them at least every 2 hours, preferably more often because ischemia development can begin rapidly in the presence of pressure.
- When positioning patients on their side, place them at a 30-degree angle or less, not directly on the trochanter, because this area is especially sensitive to pressure and can quickly break down. Patients placed on the trochanter usually become restless and squirm around.
- If the patient is seated in a chair, repositioning every hour is important.

REDUCE PRESSURE, FRICTION, AND SHEAR DAMAGE. Avoid elevating the head of the bed more than 30 degrees to reduce pressure on the coccyx as well as friction and shear damage from sliding down in the bed. Use a sheet to lift and move patients. Provide a bed trapeze to help patients to move themselves.

ELEVATE HEELS AND AVOID PRESSURE ON CALVES. Elevate the patient's heels off the bed with pillows placed lengthwise under the calf or with heel elevators. Take care so pillows do not apply pressure to the calves.

PROTECT BONY PROMINENCES FROM PRESSURE. Be sure to protect the patient's elbows, sacrum, scapulae, ears, and occipital area from pressure.

PREVENT ISCHEMIA. Avoid the use of donut-shaped cushions. They create a circle of pressure that cuts off the circulation to the surrounding tissue, promoting ischemia rather than preventing it.

PROTECT SKIN CONTACT SURFACES. Pad skin contact surfaces, especially bony prominences, so they do not press against each other. For example, place a small pillow between the knees when the patient is in a side-lying position.

Table 54.1
Braden Scale for Predicting Pressure Sore Risk

Patient's Name:
Evaluator's Name:
Date of Assessment:

SENSORY PERCEPTION Ability to respond meaningfully to pressure-related discomfort	**1. Completely Limited** Unresponsive (does not moan, flinch, or grasp) to painful stimuli, due to diminished level of consciousness or sedation. OR Limited ability to feel pain over most of body.	**2. Very Limited** Responds only to painful stimuli. Cannot communicate discomfort except by moaning or restlessness. OR Has a sensory impairment which limits the ability to feel pain or discomfort over 1/2 of body.	**3. Slightly Limited** Responds to verbal commands, but cannot always communicate discomfort or the need to be turned. OR Has some sensory impairment which limits ability to feel pain or discomfort in 1 or 2 extremities.	**4. No Impairment** Responds to verbal commands. Has no sensory deficit which would limit ability to feel or voice pain or discomfort.
MOISTURE Degree to which skin is exposed to moisture	**1. Constantly Moist** Skin is kept moist almost constantly by perspiration, urine, etc. Dampness is detected every time patient is moved or turned.	**2. Very Moist** Skin is often, but not always, moist. Linen must be changed at least once a shift.	**3. Occasionally Moist** Skin is occasionally moist, requiring an extra linen change approximately once a day.	**4. Rarely Moist** Skin is usually dry. Linen requires changing only at routine intervals.
ACTIVITY Degree of physical activity	**1. Bedfast** Confined to bed.	**2. Chairfast** Ability to walk severely limited or nonexistent. Cannot bear own weight and/or must be assisted into chair or wheelchair.	**3. Walks Occasionally** Walks occasionally during day, but for very short distances, with or without assistance. Spends majority of each shift in bed or chair.	**4. Walks Frequently** Walks outside room at least twice a day and inside room at least once every 2 hours during waking hours.
MOBILITY Ability to change and control body position	**1. Completely Immobile** Does not make even slight changes in body or extremity position without assistance.	**2. Very Limited** Makes occasional slight changes in body or extremity position but cannot make frequent or significant changes independently.	**3. Slightly Limited** Makes frequent though slight changes in body or extremity position independently.	**4. No Limitation** Makes major and frequent changes in position without assistance.

Continued

Table 54.1
Braden Scale for Predicting Pressure Sore Risk—cont'd

NUTRITION Usual food intake pattern	**1. Very Poor** Never eats a complete meal. Rarely eats more than 1/3 of any food offered. Eats two servings or less of protein (meat or dairy products) per day. Takes fluids poorly. Does not take a liquid dietary supplement. OR Is NPO and/or maintained on clear liquids or IVs for more than 5 days.	**2. Probably Inadequate** Rarely eats a complete meal and generally eats only about 1/2 of any food offered. Protein intake includes only 3 servings of meat or dairy products per day. Occasionally will take a dietary supplement. OR Receives less than optimum amount of liquid diet or tube feeding.	**3. Adequate** Eats over half of most meals. Eats a total of 4 servings of protein (meat, dairy products) per day. Occasionally will refuse a meal but will usually take a supplement when offered. OR Is on a tube feeding or TPN regimen, which probably meets most of nutritional needs.	**4. Excellent** Eats most of every meal. Never refuses a meal. Usually eats a total of 4 or more servings of meat and dairy products. Occasionally eats between meals. Does not require supplementation.
FRICTION AND SHEAR	**1. Problem** Requires moderate to maximum assistance in moving. Complete lifting without sliding against sheets is impossible. Frequently slides down in bed or chair, requiring frequent repositioning with maximum assistance. Spasticity, contractures, or agitation leads to almost constant friction.	**2. Potential Problem** Moves feebly or requires minimum assistance. During a move skin probably slides to some extent against sheets, chair, restraints, or other devices. Maintains relatively good position in chair or bed most of the time but occasionally slides down.	**3. No Apparent Problem** Moves in bed and in chair independently and has sufficient muscle strength to lift up completely during move. Maintains good position in bed or chair.	

© Copyright Barbara Braden and Nancy Bergstrom, 1988. Reprinted with permission.
Note. NPO = nothing by mouth; TPN = total parenteral nutrition.

Total Score

INTERVENTIONS FOR SPECIFIC RISK LEVEL AT RISK (15–18)*
FREQUENT TURNING
MAXIMAL REMOBILIZATION
PROTECT HEELS
MANAGE MOISTURE, NUTRITION, AND FRICTION AND SHEAR
PRESSURE-REDUCTION SUPPORT SURFACE IF BED- OR CHAIRBOUND

*If other major risk factors are present (advanced age, fever, poor dietary intake of protein, diastolic pressure below 60 mm Hg, hemodynamic instability), advance to next level of risk.

SPECIFIC CONDITION MANAGEMENT
MANAGE MOISTURE
USE COMMERCIAL MOISTURE BARRIER
USE ABSORBANT PADS OR DIAPERS THAT WICK & HOLD MOISTURE
ADDRESS CAUSE IF POSSIBLE
OFFER BEDPAN/URINAL AND GLASS OF WATER IN CONJUNCTION WITH TURNING SCHEDULES

Table 54.1
Braden Scale for Predicting Pressure Sore Risk—cont'd

MODERATE RISK (13–14)* TURNING SCHEDULE USE FOAM WEDGES FOR 30° LATERAL POSITIONING PRESSURE-REDUCTION SUPPORT SURFACE MAXIMAL REMOBILIZATION PROTECT HEELS MANAGE MOISTURE, NUTRITION, AND FRICTION AND SHEAR *If other major risk factors present, advance to next level of risk.	**MANAGE NUTRITION** INCREASE PROTEIN INTAKE INCREASE CALORIE INTAKE TO SPARE PROTEINS SUPPLEMENT WITH MULTIVITAMIN (SHOULD HAVE VITAMINS A, C, & E) ACT QUICKLY TO ALLEVIATE DEFICITS CONSULT DIETITIAN
HIGH RISK (10–12) INCREASE FREQUENCY OF TURNING SUPPLEMENT WITH SMALL SHIFTS PRESSURE-REDUCTION SUPPORT SURFACE USE FOAM WEDGES FOR 30° LATERAL POSITIONING MAXIMAL REMOBILIZATION PROTECT HEELS MANAGE MOISTURE, NUTRITION, AND FRICTION AND SHEAR	**MANAGE FRICTION AND SHEAR** ELEVATE HOB NO MORE THAN 30° USE TRAPEZE WHEN INDICATED USE LIFT SHEET TO MOVE PATIENT PROTECT ELBOWS & HEELS IF BEING EXPOSED TO FRICTION
VERY HIGH RISK (9 or below)* ALL OF THE ABOVE USE PRESSURE-RELIEVING SURFACE IF PATIENT HAS INTRACTABLE PAIN OR SEVERE PAIN EXACERBATED BY TURNING OR ADDITIONAL RISK FACTORS *Low-air-loss beds do not substitute for turning schedules.	**OTHER GENERAL CARE ISSUES** NO MASSAGE OF REDDENED BONY PROMINENCES NO DONUT TYPE DEVICES MAINTAIN GOOD HYDRATION AVOID DRYING THE SKIN

© Barbara Braden, 2001.

USE PRESSURE-REDISTRIBUTING MATTRESSES AND CUSHIONS. Provide an appropriate mattress and chair cushion to redistribute pressure for immobile patients.

PREVENT MALNUTRITION AND DEHYDRATION. Prevent malnutrition and dehydration by ensuring an adequate intake of protein, calories, and fluid. Provide 2,500 mL of fluid each day if not contraindicated by other medical problems. Consult a dietitian if necessary.

"Gerontological Issues" summarizes additional preventive measures. See also "Evidence-Based Practice."

Gerontological Issues

Interventions to Prevent Skin Breakdown

- Avoid use of soap and water on dry skin areas. Use a moisture barrier cream or ointment on dry skin before bathing to protect the skin from the drying effects of water.
- Regularly wash (and dry thoroughly) between toes.
- Toilet patient often, and institute a bowel program to prevent incontinence.
- Use perineal cleansing products to cleanse urine and feces residue from the perineum and anal area. These products are specially designed to break down and facilitate the complete removal of urine and feces without irritating the skin.
- Use moisturizing creams that have no alcohol or perfume, which can irritate the skin.
- Avoid pressure, especially over bony areas, by assisting the older adult to change positions on a regular schedule.
- Remind the patient to change position or shift weight frequently while sitting in a chair to avoid prolonged pressure.
- Examine skin for red areas. If redness occurs, positioning schedule should be more frequent.

- Keep fingernails short to avoid scratching.
- Use pillows and pads to help maintain alignment with position changes. Use specialized mattresses and chair cushions designed to decrease pressure. Keep the patient's heels off the bed with pillows under the calves for support and to prevent pressure.
- Encourage the older adult to be out of bed and active throughout the day. Remember to examine skin and reposition frequently even when out of bed because areas of pressure occur whether the patient is in or out of bed.
- Provide a high-protein, vitamin-rich diet if not contraindicated.
- Monitor for dehydration and encourage fluids if not contraindicated.
- Make sure bed linens are kept dry and unwrinkled.

Signs and Symptoms

A developing pressure injury usually begins with a reddened area, often over a bony prominence, that does not blanch with pressure. You learned to check for capillary refill by pressing on a fingertip and watching it turn white (blanch), then red again. If redness returns within 3 seconds, then capillary refill is considered adequate. A pressure injury stays red and does not blanch. If pressure is not relieved and healing does not occur, it can progress to an open, ulcerated area. In a dark-skinned patient, blanching may be difficult to see. Observe for changes in skin color rather than blanching. Stages of pressure injuries are discussed in the section on data collection.

The most common sites for pressure injuries are the sacrum, heels, elbows, lateral malleoli, greater trochanters, ischial tuberosities, base of the skull, scapulae, and ears. Most patients experience pain. A pain report requires continual monitoring, documentation, and treatment.

> **LEARNING TIP**
> Pressure injuries may be described according to a three-color system:
> - *Black* wounds indicate tissue necrosis.
> - *Yellow* wounds have slough, which is a layer of dead tissue. It is usually yellow, creamy, or tan in color. It may have exudate and may be infected.
> - *Red* wounds are pink or red. These are in the healing stage.
>
> These are guidelines. Collaborate with the registered nurse (RN) to do a complete assessment to determine actual cause of color changes.

A wound may contain a mixture of black, yellow, and red colors. Necrotic (black) wounds are the worst because they contain dead tissue. Beefy red wounds are desired because they are healing wounds. It is important to treat the worst color present first, or healing will be delayed. For example, if a wound is both yellow and black, dead tissue must be removed before infection can be effectively treated. This is a helpful system for patients and families to describe wounds to the home health-care nurse, as colors are easily recognized and understood by most people.

Complications

Wound infection is a common complication. New pressure injuries can also appear, or the injury can progress to a deeper wound. Some wounds take a prolonged time to heal or may never heal.

Diagnostic Tests

All open pressure injuries are colonized with bacteria. This means that bacteria are present, but the wound is not necessarily infected. In most cases, adequate cleansing and debridement prevent bacterial colonization from advancing to clinical infection. Culture and sensitivity tests may identify the causative organism in suspected infection sites. (See Chapter 53 for instructions to obtain a culture.) Results need to be interpreted to distinguish between true wound infection and bacterial colonization. If the wound is healing by secondary intention, it becomes colonized by bacterial flora from the skin and from the environment. If, however, the wound is extensive, bacterial growth may exceed the defenses of the local tissue, and a true wound infection will result.

If the wound does not show signs of healing or an ischemic wound is suspected, noninvasive (e.g., Doppler studies) or invasive (e.g., arteriogram) arterial blood supply studies are recommended. Biopsies may be performed for large, extensive unhealing wounds to ensure cancer is not a complicating factor.

Therapeutic Measures

Treatment varies according to the size, depth, and stage of the pressure injury; the special needs of the patient; and health-care provider (HCP) preference. All pressure must be removed from the affected area for healing to occur. Cleanliness must be maintained. Basic treatment includes debridement, cleansing, and dressing of the wound to provide a moist and healing environment.

Debridement

Debridement is the removal of dead or nonviable tissue from a wound to help clean the wound and facilitate formation of granulation tissue. It may be done with or without surgery. Nonsurgical debridement includes mechanical, enzymatic, and autolytic methods. Surgical debridement is used only if the patient has sepsis or cellulitis or to remove extensive eschar. **Eschar** is a black or brown hard scab or dry crust,

• WORD • BUILDING •
eschar: eschara—scab

or thick, black, leatherlike tissue that forms from necrotic tissue. It may hide the true depth of the wound and must be removed for the wound to heal.

MECHANICAL DEBRIDEMENT. Scissors and forceps can be used for mechanical debridement to selectively remove nonviable tissue. Dextranomer beads, another method of mechanical debridement, can be sprinkled over the wound to absorb exudate and products of tissue breakdown as well as surface bacteria. Whirlpool baths and wet-to-dry saline gauze dressings may be used for mechanical debridement. For wet-to-dry dressings, wet gauze is placed directly on the wound (avoiding surrounding healthy tissue) and allowed to dry completely. The drying process causes the gauze to adhere to the wound; when it is pulled off, tissue is pulled off with it. This results in nonselective debridement because viable tissue may also be removed. These methods are painful, so the patient should be premedicated for pain and monitored carefully.

ENZYMATIC DEBRIDEMENT. Enzymatic debridement involves application of a topical enzyme debriding agent. Most debriding agents are proteolytic enzymes that selectively digest necrotic tissue. Carefully apply them according to package directions, only to the wound, and avoiding contact with healthy tissue.

AUTOLYTIC DEBRIDEMENT. Autolytic debridement is use of a synthetic dressing or moisture-retentive dressing over the injury. The eschar self-digests via the action of enzymes present in the fluid environment of the wound. This method is not used for infected wounds, because the infection would worsen.

SURGICAL DEBRIDEMENT. Surgical debridement involves removal of devitalized tissue, slough, or thick, adherent eschar with a scalpel, scissors, or other sharp instrument. *Slough* is loose, yellow to tan stringy necrotic tissue. Slough, like eschar, can be tightly adhered to the wound bed.

Depending on the amount of dead tissue, surgical debridement may be performed in the operating room, a treatment room, or the patient's room. Following surgical debridement, grafting may be required to close the wound if it is a full-thickness injury, if there is loss of joint function, or for cosmetic purposes. For procedures without anesthesia, premedicate the patient for pain. Continually monitor for pain during the procedure, especially in case of a donor site for grafting.

Wound Cleansing

A pressure injury should be thoroughly cleansed using a handheld showerhead or irrigating system with a pressure between 4 and 15 pounds per square inch (psi). A 30 mL syringe with an 18-gauge needle works well. Pressure less than 4 psi does not adequately cleanse the wound, and pressure greater than 15 psi may damage tissue. If an irrigating system is used, 250 mL of normal saline solution (sometimes tap water for home care) should be used to thoroughly cleanse the wound. If the wound is red, gentle irrigation with a needleless 30 to 60 mL syringe can prevent trauma and bleeding. If the wound has been diagnosed as being infected, flushing with a 30 to 60 mL syringe and an 18-gauge needle provides the pressure to remove bacteria.

> **LEARNING TIP**
> Dilution is the solution to wound pollution!

ONCE THE WOUND HAS BEEN CLEANSED AND DEBRIDED, APPLY A DRESSING. Wounds heal more rapidly in a moist environment, with minimal bacterial colonization and a healing temperature—optimally about 98.6°F (37°C). Cooler temperatures can impede healing. A healing temperature is reached approximately 12 hours after the wound is covered with an occlusive dressing. If a dressing is frequently removed, the wound may not reach its healing temperature, and healing may be impaired. When possible, the dressing should be left in place for extended periods. Draining wounds may require frequent dressing changes.

> **LEARNING TIP**
> The epidermis "skates" on moisture, so wounds must be kept moist to heal.

Wound Dressings

Dressings vary according to size, location, depth, stage of injury, and preference of the HCP. Common dressing materials for pressure injuries include hydrogel dressings, polyurethane films, hydrocolloid wafers, biological dressings, alginates, and cotton gauze. See Chapter 53 for more information on dressing types. An appropriate dressing promotes an optimum healing environment. Hypoallergenic tape should be used to secure dressings if necessary. Skin protectants may be applied to protect unaffected tissue from topical agents. In all cases, pressure should be kept off the wound. No treatment will be effective if pressure continues to damage the tissue.

> **PRACTICE ANALYSIS TIP**
> Linking NCLEX-PN® to Practice
> The LPN/LVN will provide care for client drainage device (e.g., chest tube, wound drain).

Negative Pressure Wound Therapy

Negative pressure wound therapy (NPWT) can effectively heal large open pressure injuries (Fig. 54.1). In NPWT, a wound is packed loosely with a sterile sponge and covered with an occlusive dressing. A vacuum source is placed in the wound and gentle negative pressure applied. The negative

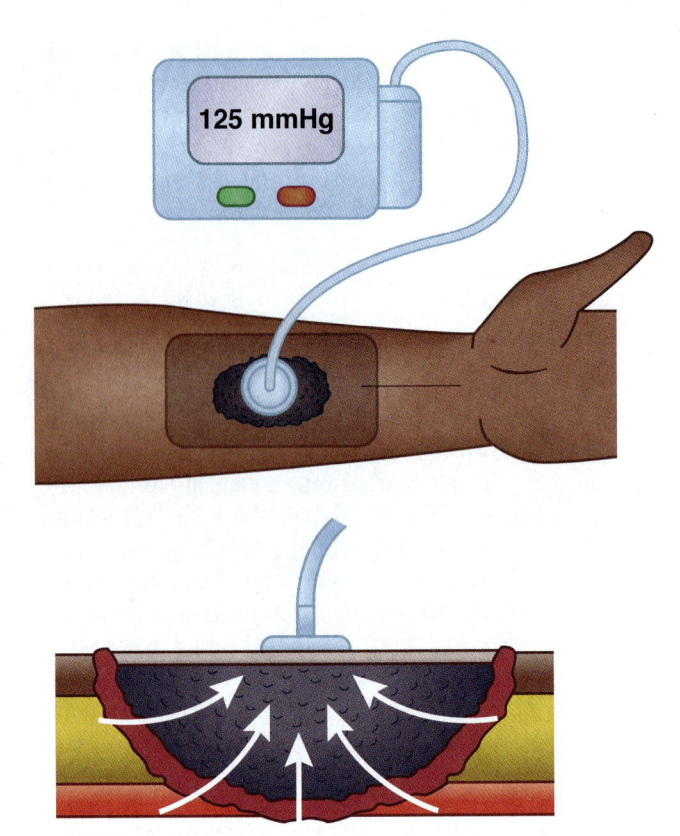

FIGURE 54.1 Negative pressure wound therapy.

pressure removes excess drainage and infectious material, reducing pressure on delicate new tissue. With small vessels decompressed, circulation increases, accelerating healing. NPWT also maintains a moist environment for optimal healing. Evidence strongly supports NPWT for nonischemic diabetic foot pressure injuries. It is also effective for other deep wounds. Risks of NPWT include bleeding in at-risk patients such as those on anticoagulant therapy.

> **BE SAFE!**
> **AVOID FAILURE TO RESCUE!** Be very cautious when using a continuous NPWT device with any patient who is on anticoagulant therapy. NPWT can increase risk of bleeding.

Other Therapies
Much research is ongoing in the field of wound healing. Some success has been shown with electrical stimulation, ultrasound, platelet-derived growth factor application, silver-based products, hyperbaric oxygen therapy, and ozone-oxygen treatments.

Evidence-Based Practice

Clinical Question
What are best practices for preventing and caring for pressure injuries on the heels?

Evidence
The National Pressure Injury Advisory Panel performed a systematic review of research relating to pressure injuries in collaboration with 14 wound organizations from 12 countries. Best practices include the following:

1. Check perfusion status of the heels and feet when collecting data.
2. For patients at risk of heel pressure injury or those with stage 1 or 2 injuries, elevate the heels using a specially designed device or a pillow along the length of the calf that avoids pressure on the Achilles tendon and the popliteal vein. Ensure that there is no pressure under the heel.
3. For stage 3 or 4 injury, use a specially designed device to offload all pressure from the heel.
4. Use a prophylactic dressing in addition to other measures to prevent heel pressure injury.

Implications for Nursing Practice
Monitoring heels should be a routine part of skin care for all patients with impaired mobility. Reducing pressure and protecting heels are easy and low-cost measures that can save patients much pain and misery.

Reference: European Pressure Ulcer Advisory Panel, National Pressure Injury Advisory Panel and Pan Pacific Pressure Injury Alliance. (2019). *Prevention and Treatment of Pressure Ulcers/Injuries: Quick Reference Guide.* Emily Haesler (Ed.). PUAP/NPIAP/PPPIA. https://international guideline.com/static/pdfs/Quick_Reference_Guide-10Mar2019.pdf

Nursing Process for the Patient With a Pressure Injury

Data Collection
Collaborate with the RN to evaluate status of the pressure injury along with underlying causes and barriers to healing. Monitor risk factors for impaired healing, such as prolonged immobility, incontinence, and inadequate nutrition and hydration. Also monitor intact skin to prevent development of new pressure injuries.

Use a disposable measuring guide or ruler to measure the diameter of the injury in centimeters. Imagine a clock superimposed over the wound, with 12 o'clock at the head and 6 o'clock at the feet. Measure in centimeters from 12 to 6 o'clock and from 9 to 3 o'clock. Depth can be measured with a cotton-tipped applicator. Also, gently probe a cotton-tipped applicator under the skin edges to detect tunneling and measure lateral tissue destruction.

Several staging systems are available for pressure injuries based on the depth of tissue destroyed. Most systems stage wounds from stage 1 to stage 4. Additional stages may include deep tissue injury and an unstageable injury (Table 54.2). An unstageable pressure injury typically must be debrided to allow healing. One exception to debridement is stable, dry, intact eschar on the heels or ischemic limb (National Pressure Ulcer Advisory Panel, 2016). In this instance, eschar serves as the body's natural (biological) cover and should not be removed.

Table 54.2
Pressure Injury Stages

Stage 1: The skin is still intact, but the area is red and does not blanch when pressed. There may also be warmth, hardness, and discoloration of the skin.

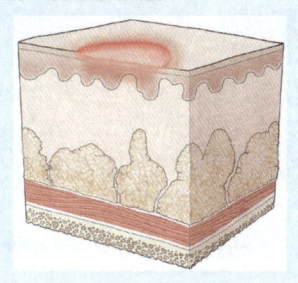

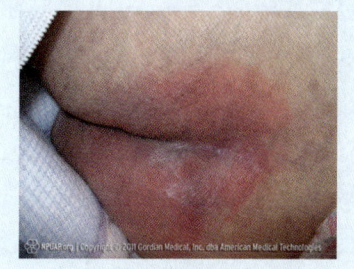

Stage 2: Partial-thickness skin loss with exposed dermis. The wound bed is pink or red and moist; it may appear as an intact or ruptured blister. Skin loss may result from shearing.

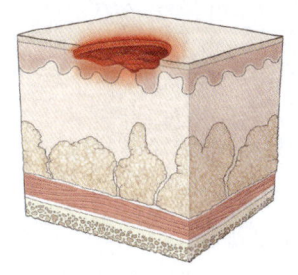

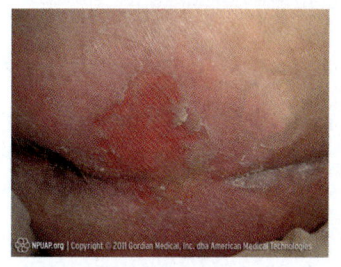

Stage 3: Full-thickness skin loss with visible fat showing. Granulation, slough, and/or eschar may be seen. Undermining and tunneling may occur.

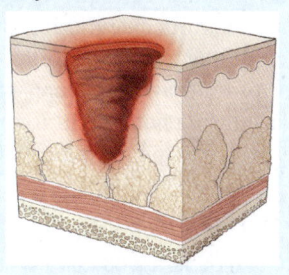

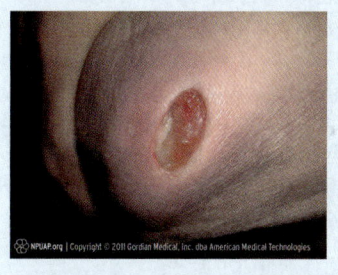

Stage 4: Full-thickness skin loss with exposed muscle, bone, and/or tendons. Slough or eschar may be present.

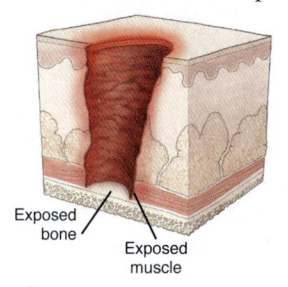

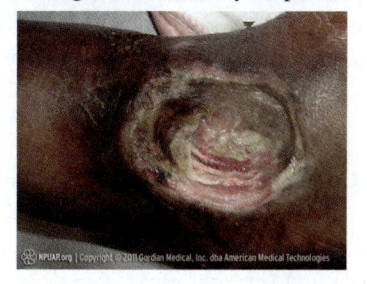

Continued

Table 54.2
Pressure Injury Stages—cont'd

Unstageable: Full-thickness skin and tissue loss is hidden by slough or eschar so that the depth cannot be evaluated. A stage 3 or stage 4 pressure injury may be revealed once the wound bed is debrided.

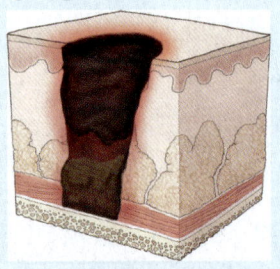

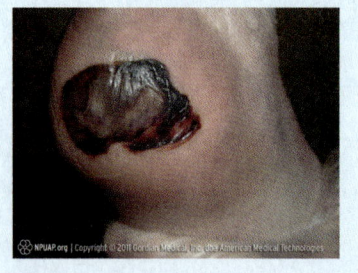

Deep Tissue Injury: Intact or nonintact skin area with persistent, nonblanchable, dark red-maroon-purple discoloration or epidermal separation revealing a dark wound bed or blood-filled blister.

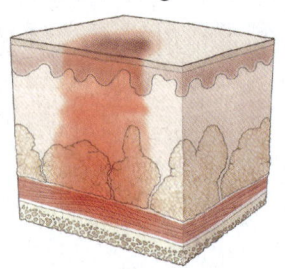

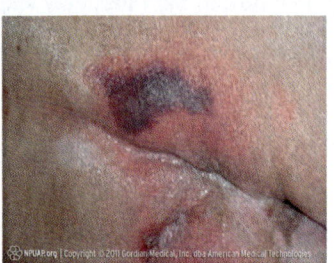

Observe wound exudate. Two common types are serosanguineous and purulent. *Serosanguineous* exudate is amber fluid consisting of serum and blood. **Purulent** fluid contains pus. It varies in color and odor depending on which bacteria are present. Creamy yellow pus may indicate *Staphylococcus*. Beige pus that has a fishy odor may suggest *Proteus*. Green-blue pus with a fruity odor may indicate *Pseudomonas*. Brown pus with a fecal odor may suggest *Bacteroides*. The wound must be cultured to accurately identify bacteria.

Gently palpate the wound with a gloved hand to determine the texture of granulations. Granulation tissue has a budding appearance from the development of tiny new capillaries. If the granulations are healthy, they have a slightly spongy texture.

Document all findings carefully in the medical record so all health-care team members can monitor the progress of healing. Take photographs if possible. Many institutions have specific forms for drawing pictures of the locations and sizes of wounds and for photographs to monitor the healing process. Follow policy at the institution where you work.

CUE RECOGNITION 54.1

You are caring for a patient who has a synthetic dressing, and you see that exudate is causing the adhesive seal to leak. What should you do?

Suggested answers are at the end of the chapter.

Nursing Care Plan for the Patient With a Pressure Injury

In addition to the nursing diagnoses that follow, be sure to manage the patient's pain, especially prior to dressing changes.

Nursing Diagnosis: *Impaired Skin Integrity* related to pressure on skin surface, reduced circulation, or immobility
Expected Outcomes: The patient's skin integrity will improve as evidenced by a decrease in wound size and depth, and no development of additional pressure injuries.
Evaluation of Outcomes: Is there a decrease in wound size? Are there new pressure injuries?

Intervention	Rationale	Evaluation
Monitor status of pressure injury according to stage, color, exudate, texture, size, and depth.	*Appropriate care is based on data.*	What stage is pressure injury? Is it improving or worsening?

• WORD • BUILDING •
purulent: purulentus—pus

Nursing Care Plan for the Patient With a Pressure Injury—cont'd

Intervention	Rationale	Evaluation
Determine and remove cause of pressure (e.g., immobility, friction, shearing).	*This allows for correction and prevents further trauma.*	What is the cause of the pressure injury? Is cause removed?
Cleanse wound gently with warm water; rinse; pat dry gently with gauze. Do not rub the area.	*Cleansing reduces number of bacteria. Drying prevents maceration of skin. Gentle handling prevents further trauma.*	Is wound clean and dry?
Debride or assist with debridement of wound as prescribed.	*Debridement removes drainage and wound debris and permits granulation of tissue.*	Does wound look clean and free of debris? Is granulation tissue present?
Apply topical agents and/or dress wound as prescribed. Make sure dressing stays intact with movement and edges do not roll, causing more pressure.	*Dressings protect underlying wound and help promote healing.*	Is dressing applied appropriately?
Position patient off the pressure injury; reposition at least every 2 hours.	*Prevents further pressure and trauma on the injured area.*	Is patient positioned off the pressure injury?
If the pressure injury is on the leg, provide for frequent rest periods with leg elevated; if immobile, reposition every 2 hours.	*Elevation promotes circulation; repositioning prevents further tissue breakdown.*	Is leg elevated? Is patient repositioned every 2 hours?

Nursing Diagnosis: *Risk for Infection* related to open wound
Expected Outcomes: The patient will not experience wound infection or systemic sepsis as evidenced by clean wound bed and temperature and white blood cell count within normal limits.
Evaluation of Outcomes: Is the patient free from symptoms of local and systemic infection?

Intervention	Rationale	Evaluation
Examine wound at every dressing change. Check for areas of tenderness, swelling, redness, heat, and drainage. Report changes.	*Allows for early recognition of infection and response to treatment.*	Are signs of infection present? Are they reported promptly?
Monitor temperature at least every 12 hours.	*Elevated body temperature is a sign of infection.*	Is patient afebrile?
Provide meticulous wound care using sterile technique (see *Impaired Skin Integrity*).	*Helps decrease the level of contamination and prevent infection.*	Is wound showing signs of healing without purulent drainage?
Use thorough hand hygiene technique.	*Prevents cross-contamination.*	Does nurse take proper precautions?

NURSING CARE TIP
Many institutions now have nurses who are specially trained in wound care. Consult one of these nurses for expert wound assessment and treatment recommendations.

CLINICAL JUDGMENT
Mr. Russ is an 84-year-old man admitted from home to the medical-surgical unit after a fall that fractured his femur. He has a history of type 2 diabetes. He had an open reduction and internal fixation of his femur and is now in a brace.

He is 6 feet tall and weighs 160 pounds. His appetite is poor; his wife states he has lost 15 lb in the past 3 months. He is sometimes urine incontinent.

1. How can you be vigilant in identifying risks and preventing skin breakdown in Mr. Russ?
2. What other members of the health-care team can you collaborate with when planning care for Mr. Russ?

Suggested answers are at the end of the chapter.

CUE RECOGNITION 54.2

Your patient yesterday had a blanchable reddened area on his coccyx. Today the area is nonblanchable. What do you do?

Suggested answers are at the end of the chapter.

INFLAMMATORY SKIN DISORDERS

Dermatitis

Pathophysiology and Etiology

Dermatitis is inflammation of the skin characterized by itching, redness, and skin lesions with varying borders and distribution patterns. There are three common types of dermatitis: contact dermatitis, atopic dermatitis, and seborrheic dermatitis. Contact dermatitis is caused by exposure to an allergen or irritant such as soap, perfume, or poison ivy. Atopic dermatitis tends to be hereditary and is associated with allergies, asthma, and hay fever. Seborrheic dermatitis occurs most often on the scalp, usually in individuals with oily skin. All types tend to be chronic and respond well to treatment but are prone to recur. Table 54.3 lists common types of dermatitis.

Table 54.3
Common Types of Dermatitis

Type	Description
Contact	Acute or chronic condition; caused by contact with irritant or allergen
• Irritant contact	Caused by direct contact with an irritating substance, such as soap, detergent, strong medication, astringent, cosmetic, or industrial chemical
• Allergic contact	From contact with an allergen, such as perfume, tanning lotion, medication, hair dye, poison ivy, poison oak; contact results in cell-mediated immune response
Atopic	Chronic inherited condition; may be associated with respiratory allergies or asthma; can vary between bright red macules, papules, oozing, and **lichenified** or hyperpigmented areas
Seborrheic	Chronic, inflammatory disease usually accompanied by scaling, itching, and inflammation; **seborrhea** is excessive production of sebaceous secretions; found in areas with abundant sebaceous glands (e.g., scalp, face, axilla, groin) and where there are folds of skin; can appear as dry, moist, or greasy scales, yellow or pink-yellow crusts, redness, and dry flakiness; can be associated with emotional stress; genetic predisposition may exist

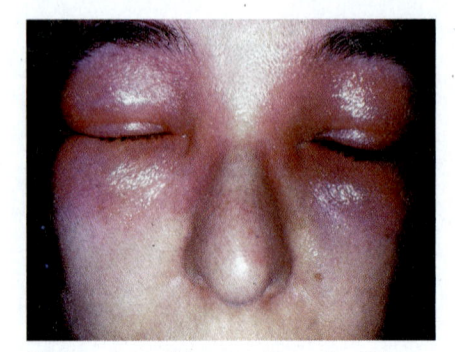

Contact dermatitis caused by nail polish.

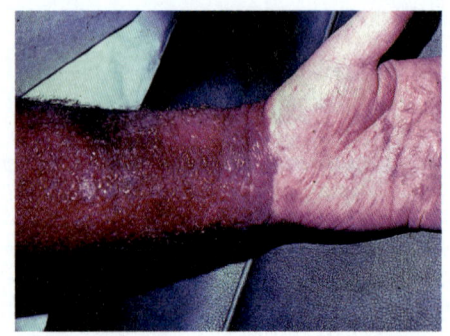

Contact dermatitis caused by topical anesthetic.

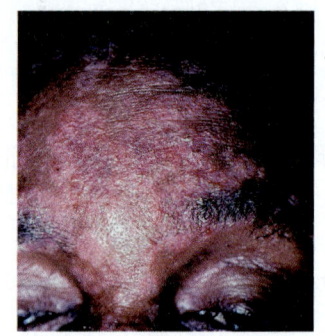

Seborrheic dermatitis.

• WORD • BUILDING •

dermatitis: derma—skin + itis—inflammation
lichenified: leichen—scaly growth + facere—to make
seborrhea: sebum—tallow + rhoia—flow

Prevention

The patient should prevent irritation to the skin by avoiding irritants, allergens, and excessive heat and dryness and by controlling perspiration. Baths should be short, in tepid water. Deodorant soaps should be avoided; mild superfatted soaps are recommended instead. Dry skin can be lubricated with creams, oils, or ointments as appropriate. Itching and scratching should be prevented as much as possible.

Signs and Symptoms

Itching and rashes or lesions are the main clinical manifestations of dermatitis. Lesions vary depending on the type and location of dermatitis. Rashes and lesions may present as dry and flaky scales, yellow crusts, redness, fissures, macules, papules, and vesicles. (These are described in Chapter 53.) Scratching can make any of these lesions worse and increase infection risk.

> **NURSING CARE TIP**
> Itching and scratching can occur during sleep, causing a rash to worsen. Have the patient wear cotton gloves at night to prevent scratching.

Complications

Lesion or rash worsens with continued irritation, exposure to offending agents, or scratching. Skin infections are common due to the many open areas and breaks in the skin. They may also occur due to the patient's reluctance to properly wash the affected area because of pain from the lesions. Some infections can become systemic.

Diagnostic Tests

Diagnosis is usually based on history, symptoms, and clinical findings. If infection is suspected, cultures of the lesions may be ordered to identify the infecting agent.

Therapeutic Measures

Treatment varies according to symptoms. Basic treatment aims to control itching, alleviate discomfort and pain, decrease inflammation, control or prevent crust formation and oozing, prevent infection, prevent further damage to the skin, and heal the lesions as much as possible.

Patients can receive some relief from itching, or **pruritus**, and discomfort with antihistamines, analgesics, and antipruritic medications as ordered. Colloidal oatmeal preparations added to baths may also help.

> **BE SAFE!**
> **AVOID FAILURE TO RESCUE!** Monitor older adults on antihistamines that have sedating effects. These medications may pose an increased risk for confusion and falls.

Steroids such as hydrocortisone or methylprednisolone may be used to suppress inflammation. They can be administered as topical, intralesional, or systemic agents. The specific type used depends on the type of lesion, body area involved, and extent of the lesion. Topical administration is preferred as systemic steroids can cause serious side effects, including adrenal suppression.

Tub baths and wet dressings help control oozing and prevent further crust formation; they also loosen exudates, scales, and other wound debris, providing a clean area for topical application of medication. Protect skin by lightly patting dry, avoiding friction, and avoiding hot water. Advise the patient to use a sunscreen agent when outdoors.

Nursing Process for the Patient With Dermatitis

DATA COLLECTION. Use the **WHAT'S UP?** format to evaluate the rash, as described in Chapter 53. Also refer to Chapter 53, Table 53.1, for specific questions to ask. Observe the rash or lesions for character, distribution, description, tenderness, signs of scratching, and other associated problems.

> **NURSING CARE TIP**
> Teledermatology (telederm) is increasingly used by patients to access high-quality dermatologic care. Secure HIPAA-compliant confidential apps allow the HCP to visualize and assess various dermatologic conditions in the privacy of the patient's home.

NURSING DIAGNOSES, PLANNING, AND IMPLEMENTATION.

> *Impaired Skin Integrity related to rash, lesions, and scratching*
>
> **EXPECTED OUTCOME:** The patient's skin integrity will improve as evidenced by reduction in lesions and absence of signs or symptoms of infection.

- Monitor skin condition regularly *to determine whether treatment is working.*
- Cleanse the area as ordered by the HCP, taking care not to irritate the skin further, *to keep area clean and prevent infection.*
- Provide cool moist compresses, dressings, or tepid tub baths *to help relieve inflammation and itching, debride lesions, and soften crusts and scales.*
- Pat the skin dry rather than rubbing *to prevent further trauma.*
- Apply topical agents to clean skin as ordered *to help suppress inflammation and itching.*
- Provide skin care at bedtime *to help promote comfortable sleep.* Many antihistamines also have a sedative effect.

• WORD • BUILDING •

pruritus: prur—itch + itis—condition

- Encourage patient to eat a high-protein diet *to promote healing and replace lost protein*. If lesions are generalized, protein can be lost through oozing of serum. Confirm appropriateness of high-protein diet with HCP.
- Encourage use of gloves or mitts, especially at night, *to help prevent scratching*.
- Advise the patient to keep fingernails short *to prevent scratching*.
- Inform the patient that applying slight pressure with a clean cloth *may help relieve itching*.
- Encourage use of a humidifier in the home *to help maintain hydration of skin and control itching during dry weather, especially in winter*.
- Teach the patient how to manage the condition at home. *Most skin conditions are cared for by the patient or family*.
- Teach relaxation exercises *to help the patient cope with distressing symptoms*.

> **Disturbed Body Image related to visible rash or lesions**
>
> **EXPECTED OUTCOME:** The patient will have improved body image as evidenced by a statement of acceptance of the condition and ability to socialize with others.

- Allow patients to verbalize concerns if they wish to do so. Talking about concerns may help the patient to begin *to work through feelings about body image* but should not be forced.
- Refer to support group, if available, *to receive support from others in similar circumstances*.
- Display an accepting attitude while caring for skin lesions. *The patient will be quick to pick up your reaction to the lesions, especially if it is negative*.
- Encourage the patient to participate in skin care *to allow more control over the situation*.
- Encourage the patient to wear long sleeves or other appropriate covering if the patient desires *to make the lesions less noticeable*.

> **NURSING CARE TIP**
>
> Advise patients that when applying topical medications, more is not better!

EVALUATION. If medical and nursing care have been effective, lesions will be controlled or in remission, the patient will state that itching and discomfort are controlled, the patient can socialize without undue difficulty, and the patient will be able to describe and demonstrate self-care measures.

Psoriasis
Pathophysiology and Etiology
Psoriasis is a chronic inflammatory skin disorder in which the epidermal cells proliferate abnormally fast. Usually, epidermal cells take about 27 days to shed. With psoriasis, the cells shed every 4 to 5 days. The abnormal keratin forms loosely adherent scales with dermal inflammation.

The exact cause is not known; however, it is autoimmune in nature, with T cells attacking healthy skin cells, increasing skin cell, T-cell, and white cell production. Many patients have a family history of psoriasis. The average age at onset is 27 years, although it can begin at any age. The condition can be severe if the onset is in childhood.

Psoriasis is characterized by exacerbations and remissions. Many factors influence the suppression and outbreak of lesions and vary among individuals. Sun and humidity may suppress lesions. Aggravating factors include streptococcal pharyngitis, stress, hormone changes, cold weather, skin trauma, smoking, alcohol, and certain drugs (e.g., antimalarial agents, lithium, beta blockers).

Prevention
Because the exact etiology is not known, measures to prevent exacerbation of symptoms are specific to patient circumstances. General preventive measures include avoiding upper respiratory infections, especially streptococcal infections; coping with emotional stress; avoiding skin trauma, including sunburns; and avoiding medications that can precipitate a flare-up.

Signs and Symptoms
Signs and symptoms vary by patient and the type of psoriasis. Lesions are red papules that join to form plaques with distinct borders (Fig. 54.2). Silvery scales develop on untreated lesions. Areas most often affected are the elbows and knees, scalp, umbilicus, and genitals. Other signs and symptoms include nail involvement, involvement in the gluteal fold (called *intergluteal pinking*), itching, and dry or brittle hair.

Complications
Because of the nature of the disease with lesions and itching, secondary infections can occur. Psoriatic arthritis can develop, with nail changes and destructive arthritis of large joints, the spine, and interphalangeal joints. If the psoriasis becomes severe and widespread, fever, chills, increased cardiac output, and benign lymphadenopathy can result.

Diagnostic Tests
Testing depends on severity of psoriasis. Usually, diagnosis is based on physical assessment. Skin biopsy or other diagnostic tests may be performed to rule out concurrent disease or secondary infection.

• WORD • BUILDING •

psoriasis: psor—itch + iasis—inflammation

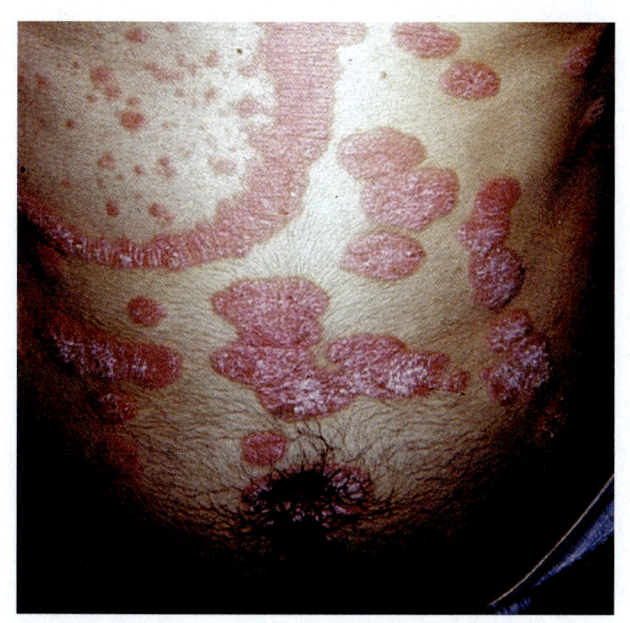

FIGURE 54.2 Psoriasis. Note bright red scaly plaque with silvery scales.

Therapeutic Measures

Treatment varies according to the type and extent of the disease as well as patient preference. Basic treatment strives to decrease rapid epidermal proliferation, inflammation, and itching and scaling. The patient may be instructed to bathe daily in a tub and remove scales with a soft brush.

A variety of topical and systemic agents are used to treat psoriasis. Topical corticosteroids may be used to reduce inflammation. Occlusive dressings enhance penetration of medications (see Chapter 53). Salicylic acid can loosen or remove scales. Synthetic vitamin D cream slows proliferation of skin cells. Fish oil supplements reduce inflammation in some patients.

Tar preparations may be prescribed along with corticosteroids. The tar acts as an antimitotic, slowing the epidermal cell division. Occlusive dressings are not used with tars. Anthralin is a substance extracted from coal tar that suppresses mitotic activity. Anthralin may be mixed with salicylic acid in a stiff paste. The patient must be closely observed because anthralin is a strong irritant and can cause chemical burns. It is usually applied for no longer than 2 hours. Both coal tar and anthralin are commonly used in combination with ultraviolet (UV) light. They are usually administered in inpatient settings or specialized outpatient clinics.

Topical preparations for the scalp are used in shampoo form. Reinforce the need to read package instructions; preparations generally need to be left in the hair for a period of time to work.

UV light may be designated as UVB (shorter wavelength) or UVA (longer wavelength). UVA is from an artificial source, such as special mercury vapor lamps. The amount of exposure depends on the patient's condition, pigmentation, and susceptibility to burning. The patient must wear eye guards during treatments. Oral psoralen tablets (a photosensitizing agent) followed by exposure to UVA is called PUVA therapy. PUVA therapy temporarily inhibits DNA synthesis, which is antimitotic. Because psoralen is a photosensitizing agent, the patient must wear dark glasses not only during the treatment period but also for the entire day after a treatment. Possible side effects include increased skin carcinomas, premature skin aging, and actinic keratosis (premalignant lesions of the skin). The patient should be observed closely for redness, tenderness, edema, and eye changes. Initial and follow-up eye examinations, skin biopsies, urinalysis, and blood tests may be ordered.

Retinoids are oral agents such as acitretin (Soriatane) that promote skin cell differentiation and inhibit malignancies from forming in the skin. They may be used with UV therapy.

Antimetabolites, usually used for cancer chemotherapy, are reserved for the most severe cases. Methotrexate is the most common agent. Because of its hepatotoxicity, it is contraindicated in patients with liver disease, alcoholism, renal disease, and bone marrow suppression. Other systemic agents, such as cyclosporine and etanercept (Enbrel), work by altering the immune system.

Nursing Care

Nursing care for the patient with psoriasis is the same as nursing care for the patient with dermatitis. Collaborate with the RN to teach the patient to use prescribed medications and how to identify and avoid triggers. Explain that drinking alcohol can interfere with some treatments. Consult with the HCP about recommending small amounts of sunlight to help improve skin lesions.

CLINICAL JUDGMENT

Mrs. Long arrives at the health-care clinic stating that the shampoo prescribed for her scalp psoriasis is not working. She says that she washes her hair thoroughly with the medicated shampoo and then rinses completely. She wants to know why her scalp shows no signs of improvement.

1. What additional information should you collect?
2. What can you advise her?

Suggested answers are at the end of the chapter.

INFECTIOUS SKIN DISORDERS

A variety of infections can affect the skin. The most common disorders are discussed in this section. Table 54.4 provides a summary of additional skin infections.

Herpes Simplex

Pathophysiology and Etiology

Herpes simplex virus (HSV) infection is a common viral infection that tends to recur repeatedly. There are two types

Table 54.4
Infectious Skin Disorders

Type	Description	Complications	Treatment/Nursing Care
Impetigo Contagiosa 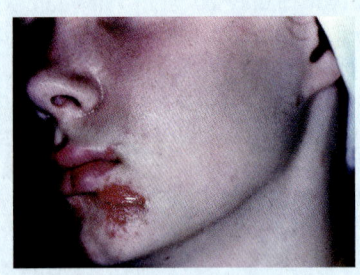 Impetigo on the face	Common contagious, infectious, inflammatory skin disorder usually caused by *Streptococcus* or *Staphylococcus aureus*; sources of infection include swimming pools, pets, dirty fingernails, beauty and barber shops, and contaminated clothing, towels, and sheets; may occur secondary to scrapes, cuts, insect bites, burns, dermatitis, poison ivy. Rash appears as oozing, thin-roofed vesicle that rapidly grows and develops a honey-colored crust; crusts are easily removed, and new crusts appear; lesions heal in 1 to 2 weeks if allowed to dry. Rash is contagious until all lesions are healed.	Glomerulonephritis may occur up to 6–7 weeks after infection. Lesions may spread. Lesions may persist if not permitted to dry. Secondary **pyoderma**, or acute inflammatory purulent dermatitis, can occur if lesions are unresponsive to treatment.	Administer systemic antibiotics as prescribed. Apply topical antibiotics after crust removal. Wash gently with a mild soap or soak with warm, moist compresses to aid in removal of crusts and debris, and to provide a clean bed for topical therapy. Keep fingernails short and clean and use gloves or hand mitts as necessary to prevent scratching. Teach proper disposal or washing of any material that comes in contact with lesions.
Furuncles and Carbuncles 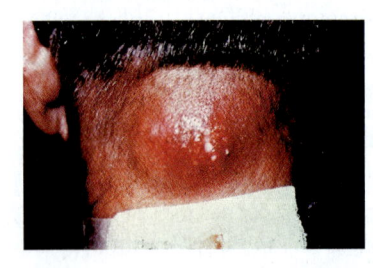	Furuncle: Small, tender boil that occurs deep in one or more hair follicles and spreads to surrounding dermis; usually caused by *Staphylococcus*; usually on body areas prone to excessive perspiration, friction, and irritation (e.g., buttocks, axillae); can recur; eventually comes to a soft yellow, black, or white head with localized pain and surrounding cellulitis; lymphadenopathy may be present. Carbuncle: Abscess of skin and subcutaneous tissue; deeper than a furuncle; usually caused by *Staphylococcus*; usually appears where skin is thick, fibrous, and inelastic (e.g., back of neck, upper back, and buttocks); associated symptoms may include fever, pain, leukocytosis, and prostration.	Furuncles may progress to more severe carbuncles. Carbuncles may progress to infection of bloodstream. Further spread of infection can occur to self and others.	Administer antibiotics as ordered. Prevent trauma; avoid squeezing or irritation. Cleanse surrounding skin with antibacterial soap, followed by application of antibacterial ointment. Surgical incision and drainage may be performed. Cover draining lesions with dressings. Follow standard precautions to prevent cross-contamination. Cover mattress and pillows with plastic and wipe daily with a disinfectant. Wash all linens, towels, and clothing after each use. Properly discard razor blades after each use.

• **WORD** • **BUILDING** •

pyoderma: pyo—pus + derma—skin

of herpes simplex: HSV-1, caused by type 1 virus, which occurs above the waist and causes a fever blister or cold sore (Fig. 54.3), and HSV-2, caused by type 2 virus, which occurs below the waist and causes genital herpes. Chapter 44 covers genital herpes.

Primary infection occurs through direct contact, respiratory droplet, or fluid exposure from another infected person. Following initial infection, the virus lies dormant in nerve ganglia near the spinal column, where the immune system cannot destroy it. The patient is asymptomatic.

Recurrence of symptomatic infection can happen spontaneously or be triggered by stressors such as fever, sunburn, illness, menses, fatigue, or injury. The secondary lesion may appear isolated or as groups of small vesicles or pustules on an erythematous base. Crusts eventually form, and lesions heal in one to four weeks without treatment. The lesions are contagious for 2 to 4 days before dry crusts form.

Prevention
Avoidance of contact with a known infected lesion during the blistering phase can prevent primary lesions. Patients should also be taught to avoid sharing contaminated items such as toothbrushes, lipsticks, and drinking glasses. This disease can recur spontaneously. Avoidance of stressors may delay a recurrence. The use of sunscreens, especially on the lips, may be helpful.

Signs and Symptoms
Some patients have a prodromal phase of burning or tingling at the site for a few hours before eruption. The area becomes erythematous and swollen. Vesicles and pustules erupt in 1 to 2 days. There may be redness with no blistering. Lesions can burn, itch, and cause pain. Attacks vary in frequency but diminish with age. Each outbreak is contagious until scabs form.

Complications
If HSV is present in the vagina at childbirth, the newborn may be infected (meningoencephalitis or a panvisceral infection may occur). If the person touches the affected area and rubs the eyes, eyes can become severely infected. Secondary bacterial infection of lesions can occur. Rarely, herpes encephalitis can occur, which is deadly if not treated promptly.

Diagnostic Tests
Cultures of the lesions provide a definitive diagnosis. Most lesions are diagnosed on the basis of history, signs, and symptoms.

Therapeutic Measures
There is no complete cure for HSV. Recurrences will happen. Topical acyclovir (Zovirax) ointment is the drug of choice for primary lesions, to suppress the multiplication of vesicles. Docosanol (Abreva) is an over-the-counter topical antiviral agent that may be effective. Oral antivirals (acyclovir, famciclovir, or valacyclovir) may be recommended for severe or frequent attacks (i.e., six or more attacks per year) or for patients who are immunosuppressed. Various lotions, creams, and ointments may be prescribed to accelerate drying and healing of lesions (e.g., camphor, phenol, alcohol). Antibiotics may be indicated for secondary infections.

Herpes Zoster (Shingles)
Pathophysiology
Herpes zoster, or shingles, is an acute inflammatory and infectious disorder that produces a painful eruption of bright red edematous vesicles along the distribution of nerves from one or more posterior ganglia. This eruption follows the course of the cutaneous sensory nerve and is almost always unilateral (one sided; Fig. 54.4).

Etiology
Herpes zoster is caused by the varicella zoster virus, the virus that causes chickenpox. After a case of chickenpox, the virus remains dormant in nerve tissue near the brain and spinal cord. Herpes zoster is a reactivation of this latent varicella virus. Eruption usually occurs posteriorly and progresses anteriorly and peripherally along the dermatome. The total duration of the outbreak can vary from 10 days to 5 weeks.

Shingles occurs most commonly in older adults or in those who have a diminished resistance, such as the patient with AIDS, on immunosuppressant agents, or with a malignancy or injury to the spine or a cranial nerve.

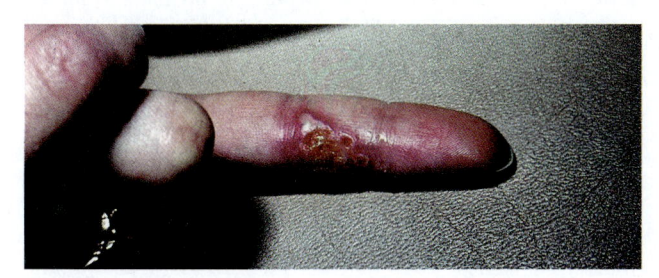

FIGURE 54.3 Herpes simplex.

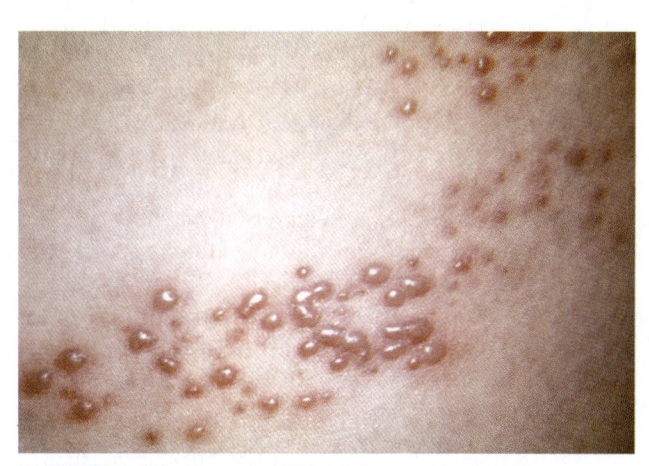

FIGURE 54.4 Herpes zoster (shingles).

Prevention

Avoidance of persons with herpes zoster during the contagious phase (a few days before eruption until vesicles dry or scab) is the best prevention. Varicella vaccine (Varivax) in children and adults who have not had chickenpox can reduce risk of varicella infection. Zostavax is a vaccine that many people received to prevent shingles before 2017 when Shingrix was developed. Shingrix is recommended for all adults older than 50. It reduces the risk of shingles outbreak and reduces severity if an outbreak does occur.

Signs and Symptoms

In addition to vesicles and plaques, there may be irritation, itching, fever, malaise, and, depending on the location of lesions, visceral involvement. Lesions may be very painful; the incidence of pain increases with age.

Complications

Postherpetic neuralgia, persistent dermatomal pain, and hyperesthesia (very sensitive skin) are common in older adults and can last for weeks to months after the lesions have healed. The incidence and severity of these complications increase with age.

Ophthalmic herpes zoster affects the fifth cranial nerve. Consultation with an ophthalmologist is essential because this complication can affect eyesight. Other complications can occur with facial and acoustic nerve involvement, including hearing loss, tinnitus, facial paralysis, and vertigo. Full-thickness skin necrosis and scarring can occur if lesions do not heal properly; systemic infection can occur from scratching, causing the virus to enter the bloodstream.

Diagnostic Tests

Diagnosis is usually confirmed by history and physical examination of the patient and associated signs and symptoms. Cultures may be ordered if secondary bacterial infections are suspected.

Therapeutic Measures

Treatment aims to control the outbreak, reduce pain and discomfort, and prevent complications. Mild cases may heal without medication. Antiviral agents such as acyclovir are used for more severe cases. They are most effective if started within 72 hours of the onset of the rash. Analgesics may be prescribed for pain and discomfort. Anticonvulsants (e.g., gabapentin [Neurontin]) or antidepressants (e.g., amitriptyline [Elavil]) may be effective for neuropathic pain.

Use of corticosteroids is controversial, but they may help reduce discomfort and improve quality of life when used with antiviral agents. Topical steroids should not be applied if a secondary infection is present because they suppress the immune system. Antihistamines can be administered to control itching. Antibiotics are prescribed for secondary bacterial infections.

In addition to medications, cool compresses or baths may help with pain and itching. Topical agents containing lidocaine may also be helpful.

Fungal Infections
Pathophysiology and Etiology

Dermatomycosis, a fungal infection of the skin, occurs with impairment of skin integrity in a warm, moist environment. This infection is transmitted through direct contact with infected humans, animals, or objects. *Tinea* is the term to describe fungal skin infections; the name used after tinea indicates the body area affected. For example, tinea capitis is a fungal infection of the scalp, and tinea pedis is athlete's foot. The term *candidiasis* is used when *Candida* is the infecting organism. Common fungal infections and treatments are described in Table 54.5.

Cellulitis
Pathophysiology and Etiology

Cellulitis is inflammation of the skin and subcutaneous tissue resulting from infection, usually with *Staphylococcus* or *Streptococcus* bacteria. Methicillin-resistant *Staphylococcus aureus* (MRSA) is a common cause that is resistant to many antibiotics. Cellulitis can occur because of skin trauma or a secondary bacterial infection of an open wound, such as a pressure injury. It also may be unrelated to skin trauma. It most often affects extremities, especially the lower legs.

Prevention

Good hygiene and prevention of cross-contamination are important. If an open wound is present, preventing infection and promoting healing are critical.

Signs and Symptoms

The initial sign of cellulitis is a localized area of inflammation that may become more generalized if not treated promptly. Common clinical manifestations include warmth, redness, localized edema, pain, tenderness, fever, and lymphadenopathy. The infection can worsen rapidly and become systemic if not treated effectively.

Diagnostic Tests

Culture and sensitivity testing of pustules or drainage is necessary to identify the infecting organism. Blood cultures may also be indicated to rule out bacteremia.

Therapeutic Measures

Topical and systemic antibiotics are prescribed according to culture and sensitivity test results. High-risk patients are hospitalized for IV antibiotics. Debridement of nonviable tissue is necessary if an open wound is present. Systemic antibiotics are indicated if fever and lymphadenopathy are present.

Elevation of the extremity can reduce pain and swelling. Monitor vital signs and report hypotension and tachycardia as such changes can indicate systemic infection. Measure the extremity daily and document to monitor progress.

• WORD • BUILDING •

cellulitis: cellu—cell + itis—inflammation

Table 54.5
Fungal Infections

Type	Description	Treatment/Nursing Care
Tinea Pedis (Athlete's Foot) 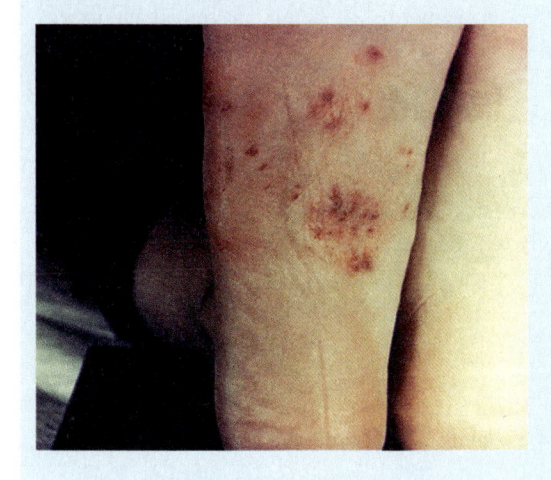	Common fungal infection, most frequently seen in those with warm, diaphoretic feet; occlusive shoes; or friction/trauma to the feet. Four types: Interdigital (between the toes), chronic hyperkeratotic (chronic plantar erythema and scaling), inflammatory/vesicular (vesicles on plantar surface), and ulcerative (vesicular lesions and ulcers between toes and on plantar surface).	Administer topical antifungal agents as ordered; may be oral in more severe or unresponsive cases. Apply topical agents in a thin layer; treat for time specified, even after apparent clearing. Wet dressings or vinegar soaks may be ordered to dry blisters. Reinforce prevention measures: Keep feet dry; dry carefully between toes; apply foot powder and wear cotton socks to absorb perspiration; if weather permits, use perforated shoes or sandals; avoid plastic or rubber-soled shoes; wear water shoes in public showers and near swimming pools.
Tinea Capitis (Ringworm of Scalp) 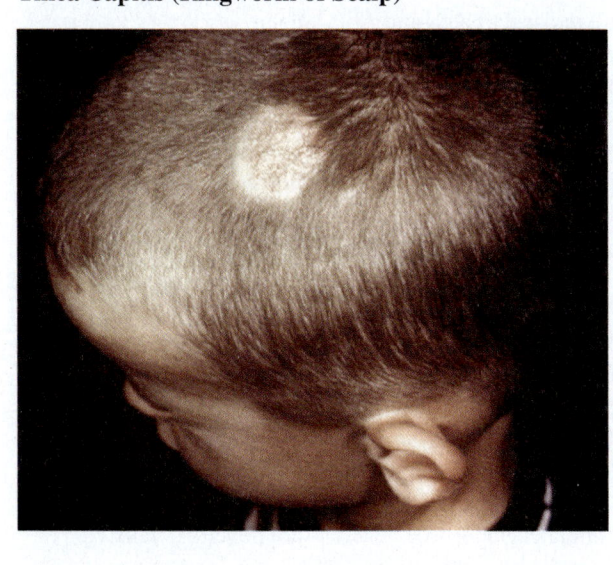	Contagious fungal infection of the scalp; commonly causes hair loss in children. Appears as scattered round, red, scaly patches; small papules or pustules may be evident at edges of patches; hair is brittle at site, breaks off, and temporary areas of baldness result; mild itching, tenderness, and pain may be present. Kerion is a severe inflammation of the scalp with resulting alopecia that sometimes occurs with tinea capitis.	Administer systemic antifungals as prescribed; relapse rate is high with topical agents. Oral corticosteroids are indicated for kerion inflammation to help prevent alopecia. Instruct family on contagious aspect of disease and need to monitor family members. Teach prevention measures: Never share combs, brushes, pillowcases, or headgear.

Continued

Table 54.5
Fungal Infections—cont'd

Type	Description	Treatment/Nursing Care
Tinea Corporis (Tinea Circinata, Ringworm of Body) 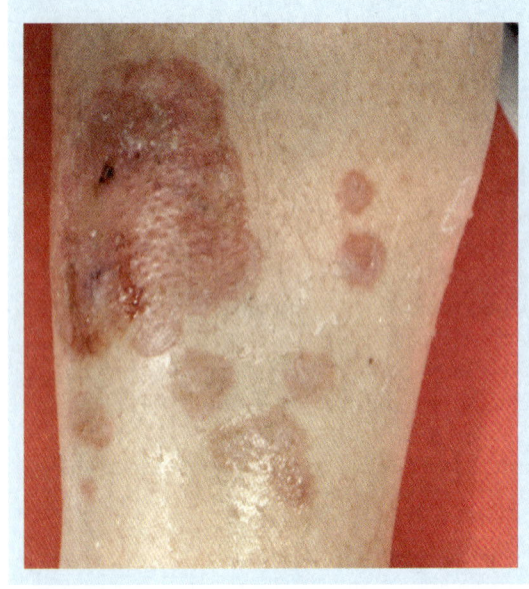	Fungal infection of the body that appears as an erythematous macule; progresses to rings of vesicles or scale with a clear center that appears alone or in clusters; usually occurs on exposed areas of body; can be moderately to intensely itchy.	Administer topical or systemic antifungal agents as prescribed. Infected pet is common source of infection. Reinforce prevention measures: avoid heat, moisture, and friction; keep skin areas, especially folds, dry; use clean towel and washcloth daily; wear cotton clothing, especially on hot, humid days.
Tinea Cruris (Ringworm of Groin, Jock Itch) 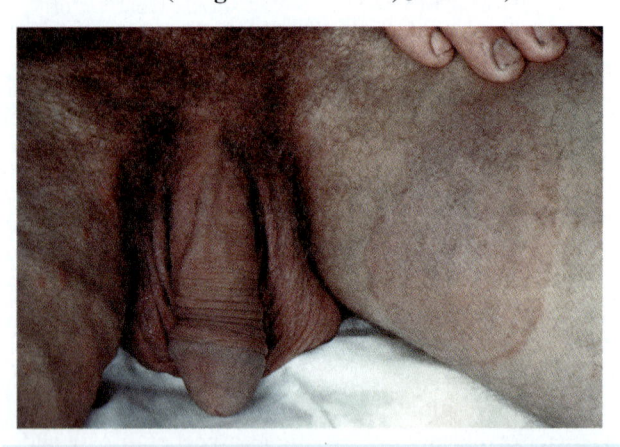	Infection of groin, inner thighs, and buttocks area; may occur with tinea pedis; often in obese people who participate in athletics. Lesion first appears as a small red scaly patch and then progresses to a sharply demarcated plaque with elevated scaly or vesicular borders; itching can range from minimal to severe.	Topical antifungals are prescribed; apply in a thin layer to rash and a few centimeters beyond border. Unresponsive cases may require oral antifungal agent. Teach patient prevention measures: Bathe daily and change to clean underwear. Avoid tight clothing. Do not share personal items. Treat tinea pedis to prevent spread.
Tinea Unguium (Ringworm of Nails, Onychomycosis) 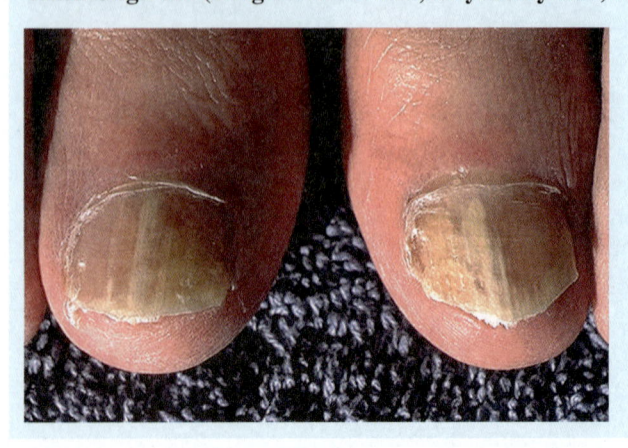	Chronic fungal infection of nails, usually the toenails; a lifelong disease. There is yellow thickening of nail plate; it is friable and lusterless. Eventually crumbly debris accumulates under free edge of the nail and causes nail plate to become separated; over time, the nail may become thickened, painful, and destroyed.	Systemic antifungals are rarely given for toenail involvement but may be prescribed for fingernail involvement. Topical antifungals are usually ineffective because they do not penetrate nails. Nail may have to be surgically removed (nail avulsion). Keep nails neatly trimmed and buffed flat; gently scrape out any nail debris.

• WORD • BUILDING •

onychomycosis: onycho—fingernail or toenail + myco—fungus + osis—condition

Table 54.5
Fungal Infections—cont'd

Type	Description	Treatment/Nursing Care
Candidiasis/Thrush 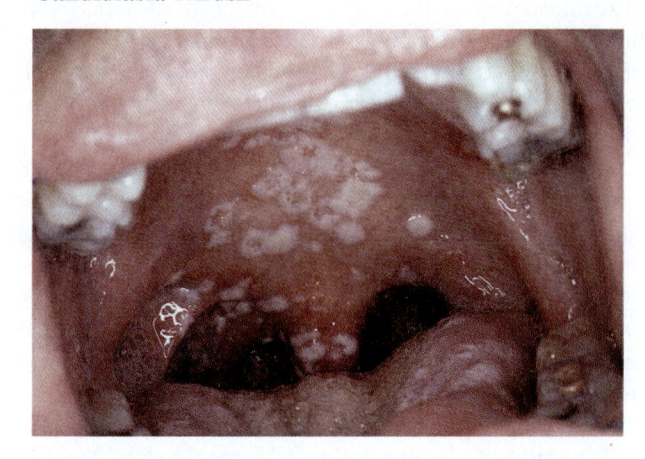	Oral candidiasis is called *thrush*. Infection of skin or mucous membranes with *Candida*. Grows in warm moist areas such as under breasts, in groin, vagina, or oral mucous membranes. Appears as white patches in mouth, white vaginal discharge, or red irritated areas in skinfolds. May occur because of antibiotic therapy because normal flora that usually keep *Candida* in check are destroyed, or with corticosteroid therapy.	Administer oral or topical antifungal agents as ordered. Examples include nystatin "swish and swallow" or lozenges for oral thrush, nystatin powder or ointment for skin infection, or vaginal suppositories or creams. Teach patient to keep skin clean and dry, especially in skinfold areas. Treatment is important to prevent systemic infection.

Outlining the affected area with a marker can also help monitor progress but may be difficult if the borders are not clear.

Acne Vulgaris
Pathophysiology, Etiology, and Signs and Symptoms

Acne vulgaris is a common skin disorder of the sebaceous glands and their hair follicles that usually occurs on the face, chest, upper back, and shoulders. The most common cause is hormonal changes during puberty. The initial lesions are called comedones (singular: **comedo**). Closed comedones, or whiteheads, are small white papules with tiny follicular openings. These may eventually become open comedones, or blackheads. The color is not caused by dirt but by lipids and melanin pigment. Scarring occurs because of significant skin inflammation; picking can worsen inflammation and lead to further scarring. The resulting inflammation can lead to papules, pustules, nodules (Fig. 54.5), cysts, or abscesses.

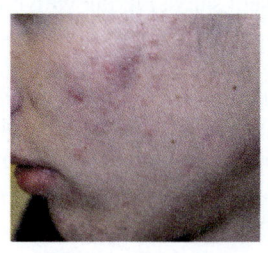

FIGURE 54.5 Acne vulgaris.

Therapeutic Measures

Medical treatment helps control lesions and prevent new lesions. Effective topical agents include benzoyl peroxide, an antibacterial agent that may help prevent pore plugging; antibiotics (e.g., erythromycin, tetracycline) to kill bacteria in follicles; vitamin A acid (Retin-A, tretinoin) to loosen pore plugs and prevent occurrence of new comedones; and acids such as salicylic or azelaic, which open pores; azelaic acid also reduces bacteria. Topical agents may be used alone or in combination. It may take 3 to 6 weeks before improvement is seen.

Systemic antibiotics (long-term and low-dose) and isotretinoin (Accutane) are usually reserved for severe cases of acne. The patient must be closely monitored for side effects. Estrogen therapy (oral contraceptives) may be prescribed for young women; however, risks often outweigh the benefits. Women should know that some antibiotics reduce effectiveness of oral contraceptives.

Nursing Process for the Patient With a Skin Infection
Data Collection

Subjective data collection regarding a skin infection can begin with the **WHAT'S UP?** Acronym:

- **W**here is the skin infection located?
- **H**ow does it feel? Does it itch, burn, or hurt?
- What **A**ggravates or **A**lleviates the symptoms?
- **T**iming: How long has it been present?
- How **S**evere is it?

- Useful other data: Is there swelling, drainage, or fever?
- Patient's Perception: What does the patient think caused the infection?

Collection of objective data includes observing the affected area and describing the infection in terms of type and configuration of lesions, color, size, and presence of drainage. Also observe for swelling and check for elevated temperature. If the patient has cellulitis of an extremity, be sure the provider is aware. Measure and document circumference of the extremity daily and as needed. Determine the patient's understanding of cause of infection and infection control measures.

NURSING DIAGNOSES, PLANNING, AND IMPLEMENTATION.

Risk for Infection (worsening infection or spread to other areas)

EXPECTED OUTCOME: The infected area will not spread to other areas on the patient or to other individuals.

- Monitor and document size and location of infected area daily and as needed *to identify improvement or new spread of infection.*
- Monitor temperature every 8 hours and prn. *An increasing temperature can indicate worsening or systemic infection.*
- Monitor for signs and symptoms of systemic spread of infection, such as hypotension, tachycardia, and increasing temperature. Systemic infection must be reported and treated promptly *to prevent complications, including sepsis.*
- Use standard precautions, including careful hand hygiene, when providing patient care *to prevent transmission to yourself or to others.*
- Implement appropriate isolation precautions for the patient with a contagious infection. Contact precautions are usually sufficient, although airborne precautions may be necessary if immunocompromised individuals are present. *Isolation reduces spread of infection.*
- Instruct the patient on wound care, appropriate hand hygiene, and disposal of soiled dressings. The patient must follow precautions *to protect self and others.*
- Instruct the patient on use of prescribed anti-infective agents, including the importance of taking it exactly as directed *to prevent development of a resistant infection.*
- For the patient with acne, advise keeping hands away from the face and avoiding touching or squeezing pimples. Keep hair clean and off the face. These measures help *to prevent spread, secondary infection, and scarring.*

See Chapter 10 for interventions for pain.

Evaluation

If interventions have been effective, the skin lesions will improve and will not spread to new areas or to others. The patient will state that pain is manageable.

PARASITIC SKIN DISORDERS

Pediculosis

Pathophysiology and Etiology

Pediculosis is a lice infestation. There are three basic types: pediculosis capitis (head lice), pediculosis corporis (body lice), and pediculosis pubis (pubic, or crab, lice). Generally, the lice bite the skin and feed on human blood, leaving their eggs and excrement, which can cause intense itching. The lice are oval and are approximately 2 mm in length.

In pediculosis capitis, the female louse lays eggs (nits) close to the scalp, where they become firmly attached to hair shafts. The most common areas of infestation are the back of the scalp and behind the ears. The nits are about 1 to 5 mm in length and appear silvery white and glistening. Transmission is by direct contact or contact with infested objects, such as combs, brushes, wigs, hats, and bedding. It is most common in children and in people with long hair.

Pediculosis corporis is caused by body lice that lay eggs in the seams of clothing and then pierce the skin. Areas of the skin usually involved are the neck, trunk, and thighs.

Pediculosis pubis is caused by pubic, or crab, lice. It is generally localized in the genital region but can also be seen on hairs of the chest, axillae, beard, and eyelashes. Lice are about 2 mm in length and have a crablike appearance. It is chiefly transmitted through sexual contact and sometimes by infested bed linens.

Prevention

Prevention involves avoidance of contact with infected persons and objects. Brushes, combs, hats, and other personal items should not be shared. Good personal hygiene and routine clothes washing are other preventive measures; however, even someone with meticulous hygiene can develop an infestation after contact with the organism.

Signs and Symptoms

Pediculosis capitis may not itch or may cause intense itching and scratching, especially at the back of the head. Nits may be noticeably attached to hair. A papular rash may be seen.

Pediculosis corporis may appear as tiny hemorrhagic points. Excoriations may be noted on the back, shoulders, abdomen, and extremities. It may also cause intense itching.

Pediculosis pubis results in mild to severe itching, especially at night. Black or reddish-brown dots (lice excreta) may be noted at the base of hairs or in underclothing. Gray-blue macules may be noted on the trunk, thighs, and axillae; this results from insect saliva mixing with bilirubin.

Complications

Secondary bacterial infections can occur with pediculosis capitis, resulting in impetigo, furuncles, pustules, crusts, and matted hair. Complications include secondary infection and hyperpigmentation. Most important, body lice may be vectors for rickettsial or other systemic disease. Complications with pediculosis pubis include dermatitis and coexistence of other sexually transmitted infections.

Diagnostic Tests
Diagnosis is made through history and physical examination. The patient may also be tested for other sexually transmitted infections if pediculosis pubis is present.

Therapeutic Measures
Medical treatment is aimed at killing the parasites and mechanically removing nits. Over-the-counter pediculicides containing pyrethrins or permethrin are the most commonly recommended compounds. These agents should kill the lice and nits, although some lice develop pesticide resistance and require mechanical removal. Permethrin (Nix) remains active for about a week, killing adult lice immediately and nits when they hatch days later. Pyrethrins (RID, A-200 Pyrinate) must be reapplied in 1 week to kill newly hatched lice. Prescription treatments include benzyl alcohol lotion (Ulesfia), ivermectin lotion (Sklice), malathion lotion (Ovide), and spinosad (Natroba). Physostigmine ophthalmic ointment can be applied to affected eyebrows and eyelashes. Other medications should not be applied to eyebrows or eyelashes.

If initial treatment is not effective, lindane may be prescribed. This controversial, highly toxic topical medication is only used if other treatments have failed. Complications are treated, as appropriate, with antipruritics, topical corticosteroids, and systemic antibiotics.

Patient Education
Reassure the patient and family that head lice can happen to anyone and that it is not a sign of uncleanliness. Lice infestations are treated on an outpatient basis, so patient education is important. Package instructions should be followed for correct usage of all medications.

Instruct the patient to bathe with soap and water and disinfect combs and brushes in hot, medicated soapy water. A fine-toothed comb dipped in vinegar can be used to remove nits from hairy areas. Nits can be removed from eyebrows and eyelashes with a cotton-tipped applicator after treatment. Clothing, linens, and towels should be laundered in hot water and detergent; unwashable clothing should be dry-cleaned or sealed in a plastic bag for 10 days. Treatment should start immediately to prevent rapid spread. Family members and close contacts (sexual contacts with pediculosis pubis) should be examined for infestation and change into clean clothing.

Shampoos and lotions kill nits but do not remove them. To loosen nits from the scalp, hair may be soaked in equal parts vinegar and water, then covered with a shower cap for 15 minutes. Then comb hair with a fine-toothed comb and thoroughly rinse or shampoo to mechanically remove the nits. Infested children should avoid direct contact with other children. However, children may be able to stay in class because by the time of diagnosis, the infestation has often been present for a month or more.

> **NURSING CARE TIP**
> Some lice-infested items cannot be dry-cleaned or washed, such as mattresses and upholstered furniture. Advise patients to thoroughly vacuum upholstered furniture. The lice die in 3 to 4 days without human contact.

Scabies
Pathophysiology and Etiology
Scabies is a contagious skin disease caused by the mite *Sarcoptes scabiei*. It results from intimate or prolonged skin contact or prolonged contact with infected clothing, bedding, or animals (e.g., dogs, cats, other small animals). The parasite burrows into the superficial layer of the skin (Fig. 54.6). Burrows appear as short, wavy, brownish black lines. The patient is asymptomatic while the organism multiplies, but it is most contagious at this time. Symptoms do not occur until almost 4 weeks after the time of contact.

Prevention
All persons (and animals) in intimate contact with an infected patient should be treated at the same time to eliminate the mites. Mites survive less than 24 hours without human contact. Bed linens, clothes, and towels should be washed in hot water and dried at high heat, but furnishings need not be cleaned. Clean clothing and linens should be applied.

Signs and Symptoms
Major complaints are itching and rash. Itching can be intense, especially at night. It begins about 1 month after infestation and may persist for days to weeks after treatment. The rash appears as small, scattered erythematous papules, concentrated in finger webs, axillae, wrist folds, umbilicus, groin, and genitals. Crusts and scales may be present. Male patients may have excoriated papules on the penis and groin area.

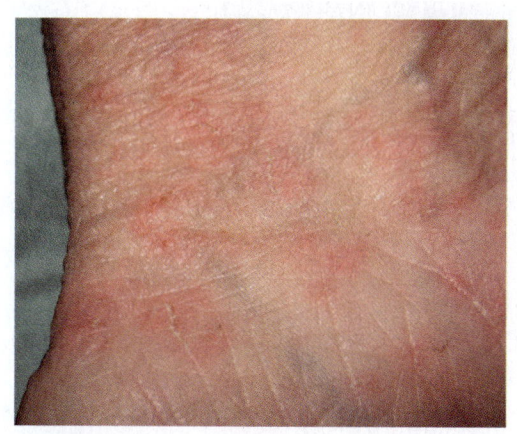

FIGURE 54.6 Scabies.

Complications

Hypersensitivity reactions to the mite can result in crusted lesions, vesicles, pustules, excoriations, and bacterial superinfections.

Diagnostic Tests

Diagnosis is confirmed by a superficial shaving of a lesion and microscopic evaluation for adult mites, eggs, or feces.

Therapeutic Measures

Topical scabicides (e.g., permethrin [Elimite], crotamiton [Crotan]) are used for chemical disinfection. Package instructions should be followed for each medication. Antipruritics may be prescribed for itching.

Patient Education

A warm soapy bath or shower removes scales and skin debris. Advise the patient to apply topical medication as ordered, follow medication directions, treat family members and close contacts simultaneously to eliminate mites, wear clean clothing, and use clean linens. Remind the patient that itching may continue for up to 2 weeks after treatment until the allergic reaction subsides. (Dead mites remain in the epidermis until exfoliated.)

> **NURSING CARE TIP**
> Animals infested with scabies should be treated by a veterinarian to avoid infecting humans.

SKIN LESIONS

Skin lesions can be either benign (noncancerous) or malignant. Benign lesions are described in Table 54.6. Malignant lesions are discussed next. Also see "Cultural Considerations."

Cultural Considerations

- People who have dark skin have a tendency toward an overgrowth of connective tissue components that protect against infection and repair after injury. Keloid formation is one example of this overgrowth.
- Black individuals and others who have tightly coiled hair may find that after shaving, the hairs curls back on itself and penetrates the skin. This can cause pustules and small keloids. Depilatories or electric razors can help prevent nicking the skin, another cause of keloids.
- Persons with dark skin have an increased incidence of birthmarks and congenital melanocytosis (also called *Mongolian spots*) compared with light-skinned people. Congenital melanocytosis may disappear over time. The nurse must be cautious not to mistake these spots for bruising, which can indicate injury or abuse.
- For people with very light skin, prolonged exposure to the sun may increase incidence of skin cancer. Teach patients to protect themselves from sun exposure to reduce risk of skin cancer. Nevi (freckles and skin discolorations) are more common in light-skinned individuals but occur across all racial and ethnic groups.

Table 54.6
Benign Skin Lesions

Type	Description	Treatment
Cyst 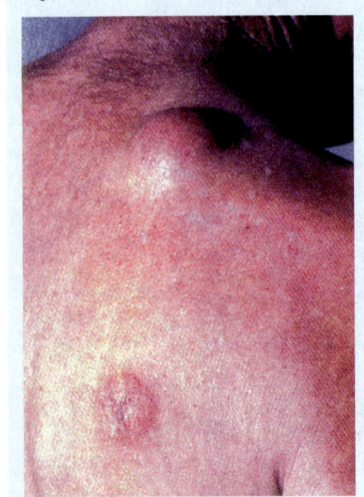 Epidermoid cyst.	A saclike growth with a defined wall that may contain liquid, semifluid, or solid material. An epidermoid cyst is the most common type of cyst. It results from proliferation of epidermal cells in the dermis. Rarely, it is associated with carcinoma development.	Not all cysts need to be treated. Treatments include intralesional steroid therapy and antibiotics, if indicated. If excision is done, the entire cyst wall is removed to prevent recurrence.

Table 54.6
Benign Skin Lesions—cont'd

Type	Description	Treatment
Seborrheic Keratosis 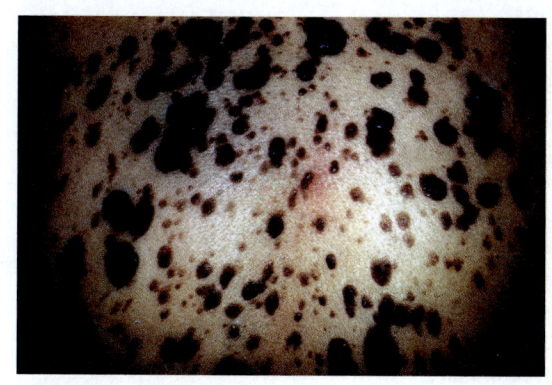 Seborrheic keratosis.	A benign skin lesion with pigmented light tan to dark brown patches. The plaques or papules have a "stuck-on" appearance caused by the proliferation of epidermal cells and keratin piled on the skin surface. Cause is unknown, but it tends to occur in middle-aged to older patients, most commonly on the trunk, scalp, face, and extremities.	Treatment is cosmetic only, or if lesion becomes irritated from friction. Topical agents may be used to reduce lesion size or height. Liquid nitrogen cryotherapy or light curettage may be performed if necessary for removal.
Keloid 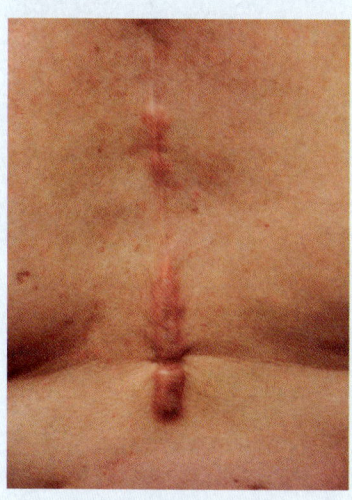 Keloid.	A benign growth of fibrous tissue (scar formation) at the site of trauma or surgical incision; occurs in various sizes. Growth of tissue is out of proportion to what is needed for normal healing. The lesion extends beyond the original injury and occurs mainly in middle-aged and older adult patients and darker-skinned patients.	Treatment varies and is not always successful; a larger scar may ensue. Some treatment options include compression therapy, corticosteroid injections into lesions, excision, and laser therapy.
Pigmented Nevus (Mole) 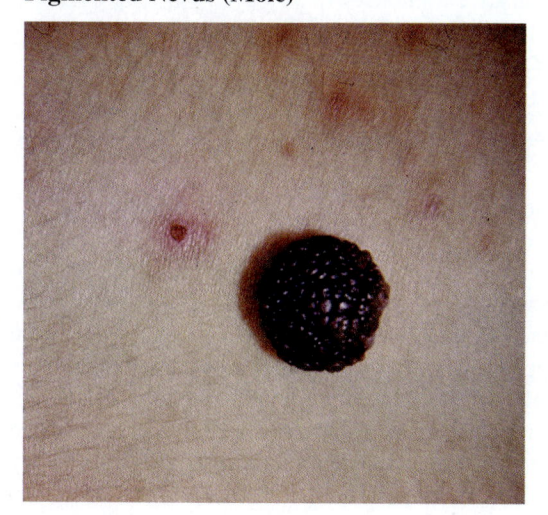 Dermal mole.	A benign, flesh-colored to dark brown macule or papule located randomly over the entire skin surface of the body. Can be inherited or acquired and occurs mostly in light-skinned patients. Usually begin to appear between 1 and 4 years of age, increasing in number into adulthood. Some contain a few hairs. There are many variations. Rate of transformation to a malignant melanoma is higher in congenital moles and larger lesions. Clinical signs of melanoma include change in color or size; inflammation of surrounding skin; irregular or spreading borders; variegated colors, especially a bluish pigmentation; bleeding; and oozing, crusting, and itching. Usually, nevi larger than 1 cm should be carefully examined.	Treatment is indicated for risk of melanoma, unsightly nevi (cosmetic), repeated irritation (rubbing from belt, bra), trauma, large moles, and patient report of a change in the mole. Surgical removal can include excision (preferred) or surgical shave. All excised moles should be sent for histological examination.

Continued

Table 54.6
Benign Skin Lesions—cont'd

Type	Description	Treatment
Wart 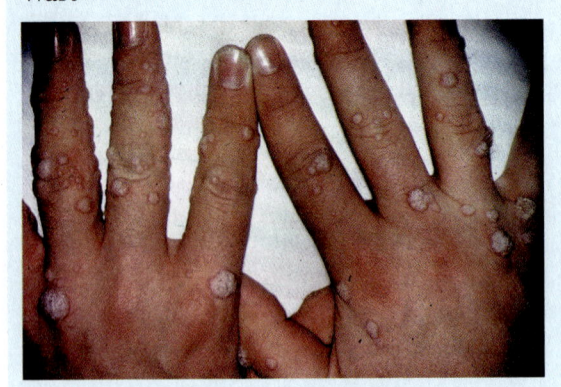 Warts.	Small, common, benign growth of the skin resulting from the hypertrophy of the papillae and epidermis; caused by a virus. Common warts, often seen on hands and fingers, appear as raised, flesh-colored papules that have a rough surface. May crack, fissure, bleed, and be painful to lateral pinching and direct, firm pressure. Plantar warts occur on the sole of the foot. They may appear granular, pitted, or protuberant, with a callous of surrounding normal skin. Incubation period can be weeks to months. Virus spread by direct contact.	Patient should be cautioned not to spread lesions by picking or biting them. Treatment is indicated for symptomatic warts and for cosmetic purposes. General treatments include keratolytic agents (e.g., salicylic acid plasters) to soften and reduce keratin; cryotherapy (liquid nitrogen); and light electrodesiccation and curettage (requires local anesthesia).
Hemangioma (Angioma)	Benign vascular tumor of dilated blood vessels that can have varied clinical manifestations Nevus flammeus involves mature capillaries on the face and neck. It is a congenital neoplasm that appears as a pink-red to bluish purple macular patch. Port-wine stains or port-wine angiomas appear as violet-red macular patches, usually singular lesions, growing proportionately as the child grows. Lesions can persist indefinitely. Cherry hemangiomas are commonly seen in older adults. They appear as small round papules that can vary in color from red to purple.	Nevus flammeus is usually treated for cosmetic reasons. Port-wine stains, if large enough, may be treated surgically or with pulse-dye laser therapy. Cosmetics to camouflage the affected area are also available. Treatment for cherry hemangiomas is usually not prescribed, except for cosmetic purposes.

Malignant Skin Lesions
Pathophysiology and Etiology

The most common type of cancer in the United States is skin cancer, which includes basal cell carcinoma, squamous cell carcinoma, and malignant melanoma. Most cases of skin cancer are preventable. The major cause of skin malignancies is overexposure to ultraviolet rays, most commonly sunlight. Other risk factors include light skin and blue eyes, multiple moles, family history, history of x-ray therapy, exposure to certain chemical agents (e.g., arsenic, coal tar), burn scars, and immunosuppressive therapy.

Basal cell carcinoma arises from the basal cell layer of the epidermis. It is the most common type of skin cancer. This tumor is mainly seen on sun-exposed areas of the body, appearing as a small pearly or translucent papule with a rolled and waxy edge, depressed center, telangiectasia (lesion formed by dilation of vessels), crusting, and ulceration (Fig. 54.7). Metastasis is rare, although it may be locally invasive.

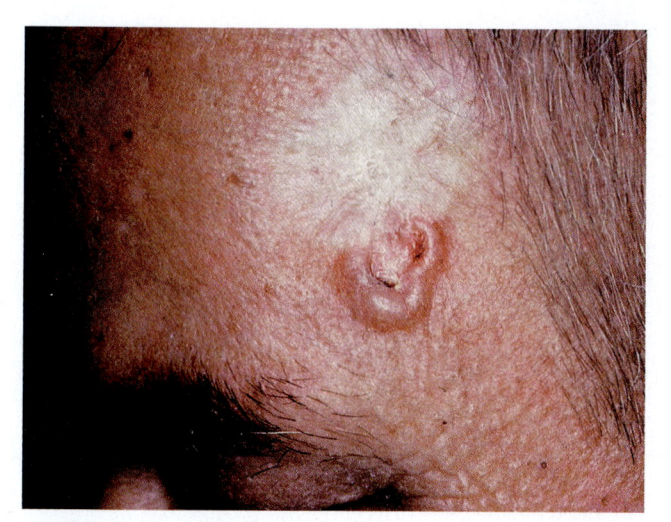

FIGURE 54.7 Basal cell carcinoma.

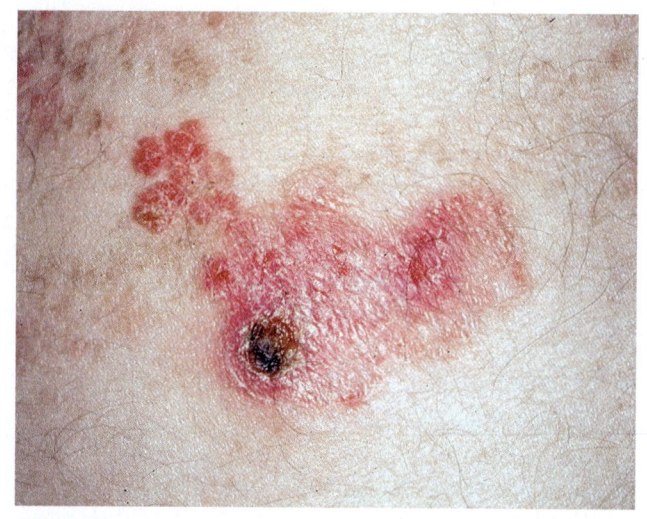

FIGURE 54.8 Squamous cell carcinoma. Surface is fragile and bleeds easily.

Squamous cell carcinoma arises from the epidermis. It can occur on sun-exposed areas of the skin and mucous membranes, mainly seen on the lower lip, neck, tongue, head, and dorsal surfaces of the hands. The lesion appears as a single, crusted, scaled, eroded papule, nodule, or plaque (Fig. 54.8). A neglected lesion appears more rough, scaly, and dark-colored. The lesion is fragile and prone to oozing and bleeding. Untreated squamous cell carcinoma can metastasize to distant areas of the body.

Malignant melanoma, as the name implies, is a malignant growth of pigment cells (melanocytes; Fig. 54.9). It is highly metastatic, with a higher mortality rate than basal or squamous cell carcinomas. It can occur anywhere on the body; about half of cases arise from preexisting nevi, or moles. There are three general types: lentigo maligna, superficial spreading, and nodular.

Lentigo maligna melanoma appears as a slow-growing dark macule on exposed skin surfaces (especially the face) of older adults. The lesion has irregular borders and brown, tan, and black coloring. Prognosis is good if treated early.

Superficial spreading melanoma is the most common melanoma. It can occur anywhere on the body and is usually seen in middle-aged persons. The lesion appears as a slightly elevated plaque with an irregular border. Color varies in combinations of black, brown, and pink. The fragile surface may bleed or ooze. Eventually the plaque develops into a nodule. The cure rate is excellent in the plaque phase; prognosis is poor in the nodular phase.

Nodular melanoma occurs suddenly as a spherical papule or nodule on the skin or in a mole. Coloration is blue-black, blue-gray, or reddish blue that may have a rim of inflammation. The lesion is fragile and bleeds easily. Metastasis occurs rapidly. This type of melanoma has the least favorable prognosis. Early diagnosis and treatment are important.

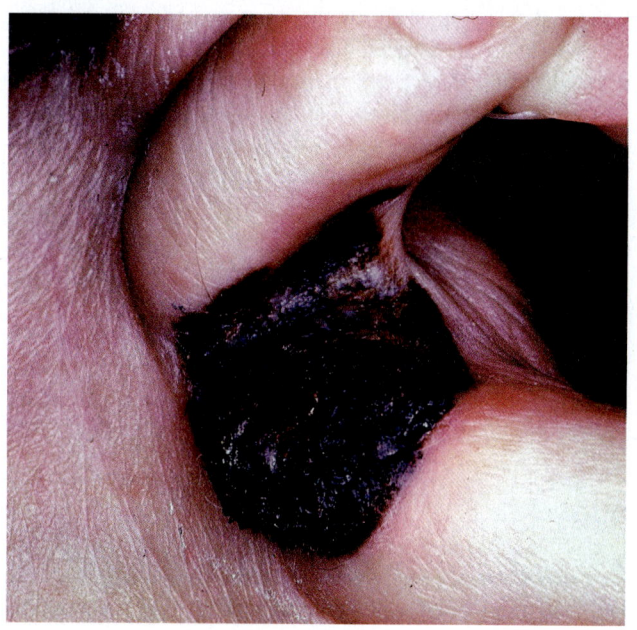

FIGURE 54.9 Malignant melanoma.

NURSING CARE TIP
To help patients find melanomas as early as possible, encourage them to examine their skin regularly and report any lesions that fit this profile:
- Asymmetrical shape
- Irregular or poorly defined border
- Variable color
- Diameter larger than that of a pencil eraser
- Changing appearance

Prevention

Risk of most types of skin cancer can be reduced by limiting or avoiding direct exposure to UV rays (e.g., sun, tanning booths). If exposure to the sun is necessary, it should be avoided during the time of its highest intensity (between 1000 and 1600). The patient should use a protective sunscreen with sun protection factor (SPF) of 30 or more and wear sun-protective clothing such as hats and long sleeves. The patient should seek medical advice if a mole or lesion changes in color, size, shape, sensation, or character.

Diagnostic Tests

A definitive diagnosis is made by biopsy. Other tests may be performed on the basis of the results of the pathological examination.

Therapeutic Measures

Medical treatment depends on type, thickness, and location of the lesion; stage of the disease; and age and general health of the patient. Generally, lesions are surgically excised with a 1 to 2 cm margin to make sure no cancer cells remain. Lymph nodes may also be removed. *Mohs surgery* is a technique in which the surgeon removes layers of cancerous skin, which is then examined under a microscope; additional layers are removed until no cancerous cells remain.

Grafting may be necessary for closure or repair. Chemotherapy may be used if metastasis is present. Radiation therapy may be used as adjunct treatment or recommended for patients with a deeply invasive tumor or those who are poor surgical risks. Other therapies include cryosurgery or curettage and electrodesiccation.

Nursing Care

Perform a complete skin examination. Document size, location, color, surface characteristics, pain, discomfort, itching, and bleeding. Note when the patient first discovered the lesion.

Nursing care of the patient with cancer is covered in Chapter 11. Specific nursing care related to cryosurgery includes preparing the patient for the procedure. Explain that minor discomfort can be expected. The patient may experience swelling, local tenderness, and hemorrhagic blister formation 1 to 2 days after the procedure. After the procedure, the area is cleansed as ordered and prescribed ointments are applied.

Specific nursing care for curettage and electrodesiccation includes preparing the patient for the procedure. After local anesthesia, a dermal curette is used to scrape away the lesion, followed by electrodesiccation of the remaining wound; the wound heals by secondary intention, usually with minimal scarring. After the procedure, the wound is cleansed and dressed as prescribed.

DERMATOLOGICAL SURGERY

Plastic or reconstructive surgery is performed to correct defects, scars, and malformations and to restore function or prevent further loss of function. This type of surgery is usually an elective procedure; it may be prescribed by the HCP or requested by the patient to improve body image. Common types of plastic surgical procedures are listed in Table 54.7. Care of the surgical patient is covered in Chapter 12.

Home Health Hints

- Measure wounds weekly with a disposable centimeter measuring guide.
- SurgiNet or a similar stretchy cover can be used to cover dressings for patients with tape sensitivities or fragile skin. They are also good for additional support to prevent a dressing from falling off.
- Ask the HCP for an order for a surgical stockinette for patients with edema who cannot tolerate or apply compression stockings but need gentle compression to promote wound healing.
- A special pressure-reducing mattress and hospital bed may be necessary for patients with pressure injuries.
- Reinforce dietary measures to promote healing, including adequate protein intake. Good sources of protein include lean meats, nuts, and eggs.
- Advise patients and caregivers to prevent pressure injuries by keeping skin well lubricated with unscented lotions, changing position at least every 2 hours, and changing briefs when damp. Teach patients in wheelchairs to use armrests to shift their weight every 15 minutes.
- Unless the patient or caregiver has been instructed on how to perform the dressing change and has performed a return demonstration, inform them to contact the home health-care agency if the dressing becomes soiled or falls off.
- Inform patients that they can wear a cast shoe over a dressing on the foot. This will help protect the dressing and provide additional support for the patient while ambulating.

Table 54.7
Common Plastic Surgical Procedures

Operation	Description	Purpose	Possible Complications	Postoperative Nursing Care Considerations
Rhinoplasty (Nose)	Removal of excessive nasal cartilage, tissue, or bone; reshaping of nose	Correct congenital or acquired septal defects; improve cosmetic shape of nose	Hemorrhage, hematoma; temporary ecchymosis and edema; infection, septal perforation	Monitor dressing and packing for bright-red bleeding; monitor vital signs and level of consciousness; maintain semi-Fowler position to minimize edema.
Blepharoplasty (Eyelid)	Incisions on upper and lower lids with excision of fat and skin and primary closure	Removal of bags under eyes and wrinkles and bulges	Corneal injury; hematoma; ectropion; rarely visual loss and wound infection	Administer antibiotic ointment as ordered; maintain eye dressings; maintain semi-Fowler position to minimize edema.
Rhytidoplasty (Facelift)	Incision anterior to ear with removal of excessive skin and tissue; the subcutaneous tissue and fascia are folded and stretched	Removal of excessive wrinkling or sagging skin	Hemorrhage; hematoma; ecchymosis, and edema (temporary); wound infection; facial nerve damage	Surgical improvement lasts from 5 to 10 years; apply antibiotic ointment to suture line; maintain semi-Fowler position to minimize edema.
Otoplasty (Ear)	Incision of ear for correction of defect	Correct congenital defects; correct deformities; improve cosmetic shape of ear	Hemorrhage; hematoma; edema; wound infection	Maintain ear dressing for about 1 week; protect ear at times of sleep for about 3 weeks.

Key Points

- A pressure injury caused by prolonged pressure against the skin. It is caused by spending long periods in one position, causing the weight of the body to compress capillaries. Mechanical forces lead to the formation of pressure injuries.
- Use an assessment tool such as the Braden Scale for Predicting Pressure Sore Risk to determine risk for pressure injuries based on physical condition, mental status, activity, mobility, and incontinence.
- Avoid massaging bony prominences or reddened skin, which can damage blood vessels.
- If patients are on bedrest, turn and reposition them at least every 2 hours.
- Pad skin contact surfaces, especially bony prominences, to shield them from each other.
- Provide an appropriate pressure-relieving or pressure-reducing mattress and chair cushion for immobile patients.
- Wound infection is common. Some wounds take a long time to heal or never heal.
- Basic treatment for a pressure injury includes debridement, cleansing, and dressing.

- Commonly used dressing materials include hydrogel dressings, polyurethane films, hydrocolloid wafers, biological dressings, alginates, and cotton gauze.
- Negative pressure wound therapy may be effective for healing large open pressure injuries.
- Most staging systems categorize pressure injuries from stage 1 to stage 4.
- Dermatitis is inflammation of the skin. It is characterized by itching, redness, and skin lesions, with varying borders and distribution patterns. Three common types include contact dermatitis, atopic dermatitis, and seborrheic dermatitis.
- Psoriasis is a chronic inflammatory skin disorder in which epidermal cells proliferate abnormally fast. The abnormal keratin forms loosely adherent scales with dermal inflammation.
- HSV infection is a common viral infection that recurs and has no cure. There are two types of herpes simplex: that caused by type 1 virus (HSV-1), which occurs above the waist and causes a fever blister or cold sore, and that caused by type 2 virus (HSV-2), which occurs below the waist and causes genital herpes.
- Herpes zoster, or shingles, is an acute inflammatory and infectious disorder that produces a painful vesicular eruption of bright red edematous plaques.
- Postherpetic neuralgia, persistent dermatomal pain, and hyperesthesia are common in older adults and can last for weeks to months after the lesions have healed.
- Ophthalmic herpes zoster affects the fifth cranial nerve and can be a serious complication. Consultation with an ophthalmologist is essential.
- Dermatomycosis is a fungal infection of the skin that occurs through direct contact with infected humans, animals, or objects. *Tinea* is the term used to describe fungal skin infections. The name used after tinea indicates the body area affected.
- Cellulitis is inflammation of the skin and subcutaneous tissue resulting from infection, usually with *Staphylococcus* or *Streptococcus* bacteria.
- Pediculosis is an infestation by lice. Generally, the lice bite the skin and feed on human blood, leaving their eggs and excrement, which can cause intense itching.
- Scabies is a contagious skin disease caused by the mite *Sarcoptes scabiei*. The parasite burrows into the superficial layer of the skin.
- Skin lesions can be benign (noncancerous) or malignant. The most common type of cancer in the United States is skin cancer.
- Malignant melanoma is a malignant growth of pigment cells. It is highly metastatic, with a higher mortality rate than basal or squamous cell carcinomas.
- Risk of skin cancer can be reduced by limiting or avoiding direct exposure to UV rays.
- Plastic or reconstructive surgery is performed to correct defects, scars, and malformations and to restore function or prevent further loss of function.

SUGGESTED ANSWERS TO CHAPTER EXERCISES

Cue Recognition
54.1: Change the dressing.
54.2: Realize that early tissue damage indicates stage I pressure injury and treat accordingly.

Critical Thinking & Clinical Judgment
Mr. Russ
1. You can do the following:
   - Perform a Braden Scale assessment. A specialty pressure-relieving bed may be appropriate for Mr. Russ.
   - Change Mr. Russ's position at least every 2 hours if not more frequently. Keep his heels off of the bed at all times by propping them on pillows.
   - Request a dietary consult because the body cannot meet the increased healing demands if there is an albumin deficiency. Mr. Russ may need increased protein (contraindicated in kidney failure). He may also need fats, carbohydrates, vitamins, and minerals for wound healing. A dietitian can help determine the amounts of calories and types of foods for the best prevention and/or healing.
   - If Mr. Russ is able to sit up in a chair, provide a chair cushion to prevent skin breakdown and have him shift his weight every 15 minutes.
   - Mr. Russ is wearing a brace, so examine the underlying tissue for pressure areas. Braces and splints must be padded to avoid skin breakdown.
   - Involve HCP, dietitian, wound nurse, RN, physical therapist, and nursing assistant. The nursing assistant is one of the most important members of this team because they are often responsible for bathing and turning patients. Ask to be called to examine Mr. Russ's skin during bathing and teach the assistant warning signs to report.

Mrs. Long
1. Ask how long she is leaving the shampoo in her hair. For medicated scalp shampoos to work properly, they must remain on the scalp for several minutes.
2. Advise Mrs. Long to read the package instructions carefully for each product because they vary from product to product.

Additional Resources

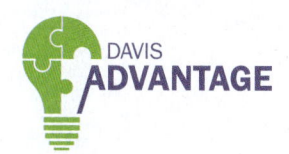

Go to Davis Advantage to complete your learning: strengthen understanding, apply your knowledge, and prepare for the Next Gen NCLEX®.

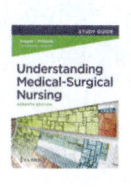

A Study Guide is also available.

CHAPTER 55
Nursing Care of Patients With Burns

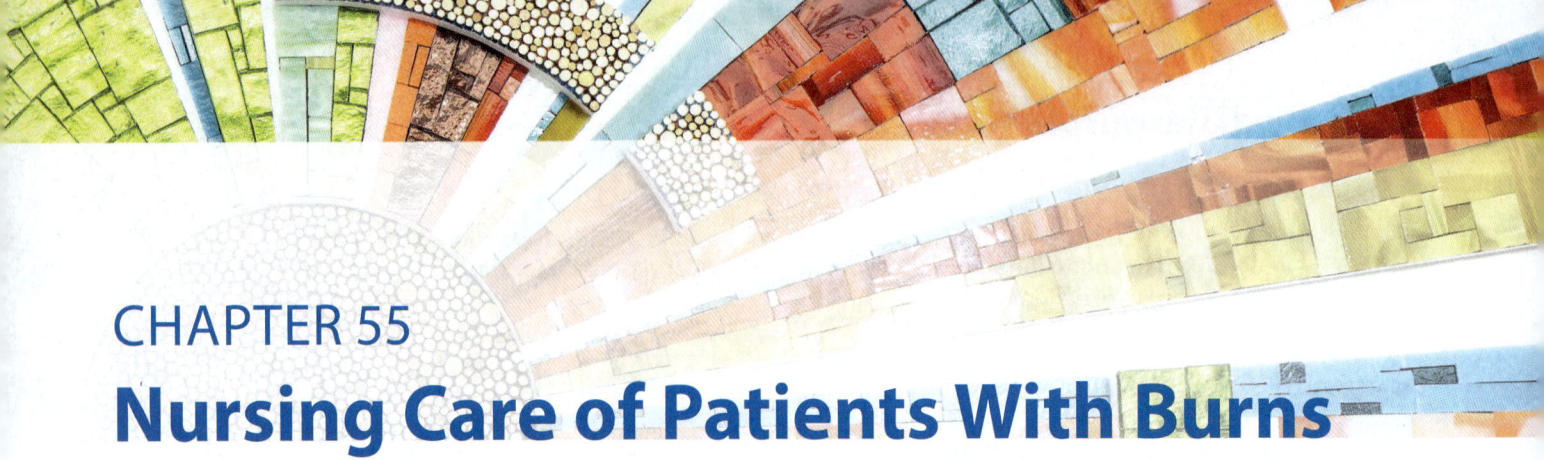

Rita Bolek Trofino

KEY TERMS

autograft (AW-toh-graft)
epithelialization (ep-ih-THEEL-ee-al-eye-ZAY-shun)
escharotomy (es-kar-AHT-oh-mee)
hemochromogen (HEEM-oh-KROH-moh-jen)

CHAPTER CONCEPTS

Comfort
Fluid and electrolytes
Self
Tissue integrity

LEARNING OUTCOMES

1. Explain the pathophysiology of burns.
2. Describe current therapeutic measures used for burns.
3. List data to collect when caring for patients with burns.
4. Plan nursing care for patients with burns.
5. Explain how you will know whether your nursing interventions have been effective.

Many people are hospitalized each year for burns. Burns affect not only the skin but also every major body system. Smoke inhalation and wound infections complicate care for burn patients.

PATHOPHYSIOLOGY AND SIGNS AND SYMPTOMS

Burns are wounds caused by an energy transfer from a heat source to the body, heating the tissue enough to cause damage. Locally, heat denatures cellular protein and interrupts blood supply. The three zones of tissue damage that occur with burns are described in Figure 55.1.

The amount of skin damage is related to (1) temperature of the burning agent, (2) agent that caused the burn, (3) duration of exposure, (4) conductivity of tissue, and (5) thickness of involved dermal structures. Alterations in normal skin function from a major burn injury include loss of protective functions, impaired ability to regulate temperature, increased infection risk, sensory function changes, fluid loss, impaired skin regeneration, and impaired secretory and excretory functions. A burn over 45% of the body is considered a major burn injury.

Systemic Responses
Alterations in functional capacity of the skin from a burn affect virtually all major body systems.

Fluid Balance
Following a major burn, damaged cells release inflammatory mediators. The resulting inflammation causes increased capillary permeability, which leads to leakage of plasma and proteins into the tissue. This results in blisters and edema with a loss of intravascular volume. Water loss by evaporation through the burned tissue can be 4 to 15 times the normal amount. Increased metabolism leads to further water loss through the respiratory system.

maintained until wound closure. Hypermetabolism is further compromised by associated injuries, surgical interventions, and the stress response. Severe catabolism begins early. It is associated with a negative nitrogen balance, weight loss, and decreased wound healing. Elevated catecholamine (epinephrine, norepinephrine) levels are triggered by the stress response. This, along with elevated glucagon levels, can stimulate hyperglycemia.

Gastrointestinal Problems
Some gastrointestinal problems that can develop with a major burn include gastric dilation, peptic ulcers, and paralytic ileus. Most of these problems occur in response to fluid shifting, dehydration, opioid analgesics, immobility, depressed gastric motility, and the stress response.

Renal Function
Acute renal insufficiency can occur because of hypovolemia and decreased cardiac output. Fluid loss and inadequate fluid replacement can lead to decreased renal blood flow and glomerular filtration rate. Extensive burns can cause destruction of muscle, creating myoglobin casts that block renal tubules and lead to renal failure.

Pulmonary Effects
Pulmonary effects are mostly related to smoke inhalation. However, hyperventilation may occur with any moderate to major burn injury, usually proportional to the severity of the burn. Oxygen consumption increases because of the hypermetabolic state, fear, anxiety, and pain.

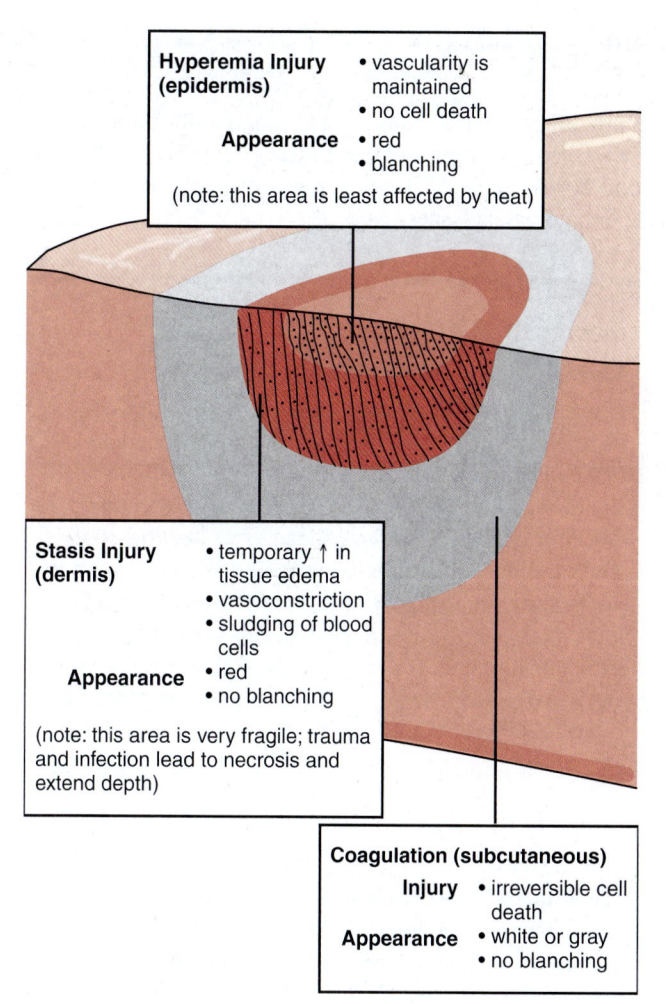

FIGURE 55.1 Three zones of tissue damage.

Cardiac Function
A major burn is followed by an initial decrease in cardiac output. This is further compromised by the loss of circulating plasma volume. Severe hematologic changes resulting from tissue damage and vascular changes occur in patients with major burns. Plasma moves into the interstitial space because of increased capillary permeability. In the first 48 hours after a burn, fluid shifts lead to hypovolemia and, if untreated, hypovolemic shock. Loss of intravascular fluid causes a relative increase in hematocrit, and red blood cells are destroyed. The intense heat decreases platelet function and half-life. Leukocyte and platelet aggregation may progress to thrombosis.

Loss of Thermoregulation
The skin is the largest organ of the body and the first line of defense for the body. It helps protect from infection and trauma and assists with temperature regulation. Patients with major burns are at high risk for heat loss and hypothermia. In full-thickness burns, the sweat glands are destroyed, which also affects thermoregulation.

Metabolic Changes
Burn patients have very high metabolic demands. A high metabolic rate proportional to the severity of the burn is usually

> **BE SAFE!**
> **BE VIGILANT!** It is not uncommon to administer massive volumes of IV fluids to severe burn patients. They must receive close hemodynamic monitoring to avoid fluid overload.

Immune Function
With the skin destroyed, the body loses its first line of defense against infection. Major burns also depress immunoglobulin (Ig)A, IgG, and IgM.

> **BE SAFE!**
> **BE VIGILANT!** You must be vigilant in monitoring for and protecting from infection, which represents a real and life-threatening risk to severely burned patients.

> **PRACTICE ANALYSIS TIP**
> **Linking NCLEX-PN® to Practice**
> The LPN/LVN will apply principles of infection control (e.g., aseptic technique, isolation, sterile technique, universal/standard precautions).

Evaluation of Burn Injuries

The severity of a burn injury is determined by the depth of tissue destruction (Table 55.1 and Fig. 55.2), percentage of body surface area injured, cause of the burn, age of the patient, related injuries, medical history (e.g., heart disease, diabetes), and location of the burn wound.

The size of a burn wound is estimated on the basis of parts of the body affected. A quick and common method is the Rule of Nines. This method divides the body into segments with areas of either 9% or multiples of 9% of the total body surface, with the perineum counted as 1% (Fig. 55.3). This formula is easy to use but not as accurate when assessing children. A more accurate method uses a table with a relative anatomical scale or diagram that estimates total burned area by ages and by smaller anatomical areas of the body. The practitioner will overestimate the size of a severe electrical burn injury. Damage to internal organs and tissues will not be evident on the skin, and symptoms may worsen over time.

> **NURSING CARE TIP**
> For a quick estimation of percentage of burn injury on an adult patient, the palm of your hand is about 1%.

> **CLINICAL JUDGMENT**
> **Mr. Weinberg** is admitted to the hospital with superficial and deep partial-thickness burns. His wife asks how long it will take for the burns to heal. What should you tell her? (See Table 55.1.)
> Suggested answers are at the end of the chapter.

ETIOLOGY

Burn injuries have many causes, commonly flames; contact burns; scalding; and chemical, electrical, and radiation burns. Table 55.2 summarizes these causes; see also "Gerontological Issues."

> **Gerontological Issues**
>
> **Burn Injury and the Older Adult**
> Older adults face the threat of serious complications or death in a fire as a result of several factors. Older adults have thinner skin, and many suffer from comorbidities such as diabetes and hypertension. These chronic conditions can increase recovery time and lead to a longer hospital stay. Prevention measures for older adults should consider vision and hearing impairments as well as limited mobility. Individuals must be able to evacuate in case of a fire and seek help if a burn injury occurs. Nurses should target prevention measures toward the most common activities that can lead to fire or burn injury: smoking and cooking.

> **BE SAFE!**
> **BE VIGILANT!** Most burns are preventable. Prevention should focus on all areas, including electrical safety, fire safety, cooking safety, and scald prevention, especially in very young children and older adults.

Table 55.1
Classification of Burn Depth

Classification	Formerly	Areas Involved	Appearance	Sensitivity	Healing Time
Partial thickness (superficial)	First to second degree	Epidermis, Papillae of dermis	Bright red to pink, Blanches to touch, Serum-filled blisters, Glistening, moist	Sensitive to air, temperature, and touch	7–10 days
Partial thickness (deep)	Second degree	Epidermis, half to seven-eighths of dermis	Blisters may be present, Pink to light red to white, Soft and pliable, Blanching present	Pressure may be painful because of exposed nerve endings	14–21 days; may need grafting to decrease scarring
Full thickness	Third to fourth degree	Epidermis, Dermis, Tissue, Muscle, Bone	Snowy white, gray, or brown, Texture is firm and leathery, Inelastic	No pain because nerve endings are destroyed, unless surrounded by areas of partial-thickness burns	Grafting necessary to complete healing

Hermans, M. H. E. An introduction to burn care. *Advances in Skin and Wound Care, 32*(1), 9–18. https://doi.org/10.1097/01.ASW.0000549711.42146.32

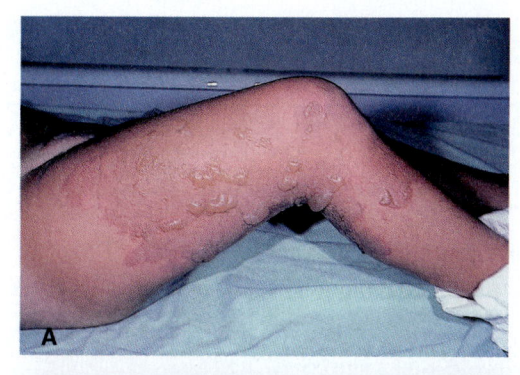

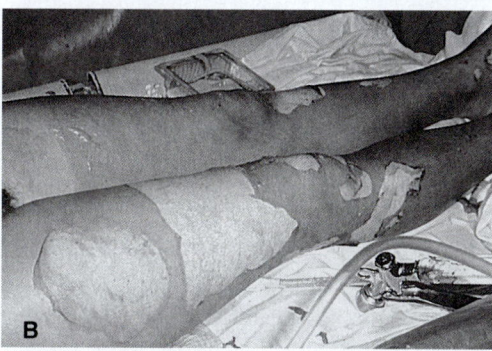

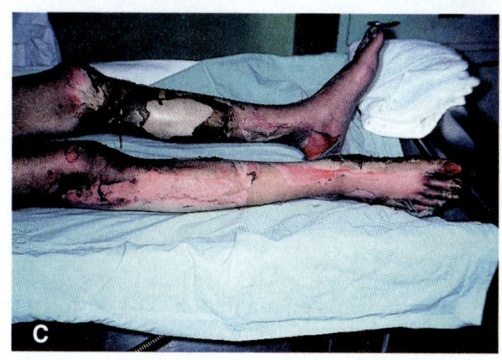

Chapter 55 Nursing Care of Patients With Burns   1141

FIGURE 55.2 (A and B) Partial-thickness burns. (C) Full-thickness burn.

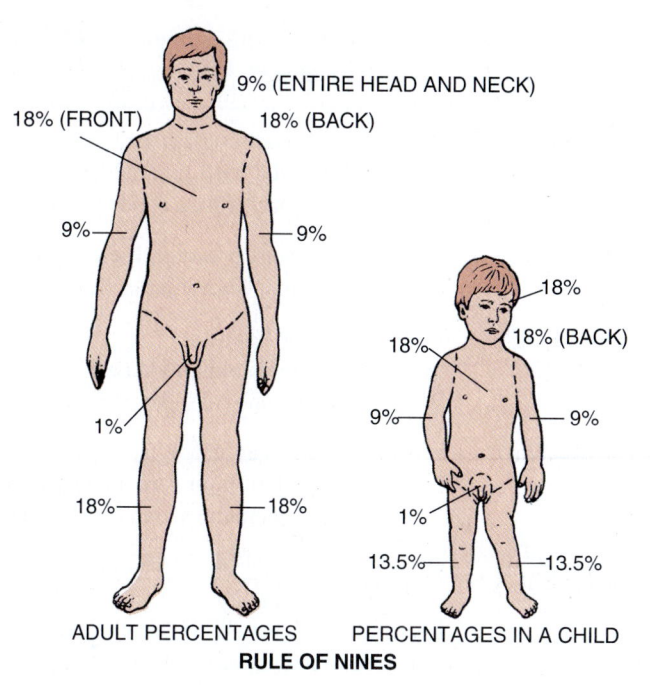

FIGURE 55.3 Estimation of extent of burn injury.

RULE OF NINES

ADULT PERCENTAGES:
- 9% (ENTIRE HEAD AND NECK)
- 18% (FRONT)
- 18% (BACK)
- 9%, 9%
- 1%
- 18%, 18%

PERCENTAGES IN A CHILD:
- 18%
- 18% (BACK)
- 9%, 9%
- 1%
- 13.5%, 13.5%

> **BE SAFE!**
> **BE VIGILANT!** Advise patients to keep the temperature of their hot water heater at 120°F or just below the medium setting—a safe bathing temperature—and to check water temperature before entering a bath or shower.

COMPLICATIONS

A major complication with a flame burn in an enclosed space is inhalation injury, a significant cause of morbidity and mortality associated with burn injuries. Treatment of inhalation injury takes precedence over other injuries. (Remember your ABCs? Airway always comes first.) Infection is another common complication with a major burn. Incidence of infection increases with the size of the burn wound because the skin is the first line of defense against microorganisms.

Neurovascular compromise can also occur with a major burn. Eschar formation creates pressure and contributes to decreasing blood flow to areas distal to the burned area. Other systemic complications were reviewed in the "Systemic Responses" section earlier in this chapter.

DIAGNOSTIC TESTS

Burns are diagnosed by physical assessment. Various diagnostic tests are performed for systemic reactions, infection, and other complications. Common laboratory tests include complete blood count (CBC) and differential, blood urea nitrogen (BUN), serum glucose and electrolytes, serum protein and albumin levels, urinalysis, urine cultures, and clotting studies. If an inhalation injury is suspected, arterial blood gases, bronchoscopy, and carboxyhemoglobin levels are tested. X-rays, electrocardiogram, and wound cultures are completed if indicated.

CLINICAL JUDGMENT

Mrs. Rivera is admitted to the emergency department after sustaining injuries from a house fire. Both arms and hands are burned, she has a right leg fracture and a possible neck fracture, her lips are swollen, her face is sooty, and she is spitting up grayish-blackish sputum.

1. What is your priority concern with these injuries?
2. An IV line with normal saline is ordered at 1 L over 6 hours. How many milliliters per hour should be set on the controller?
3. Approximately what percentage of her body is burned?
4. What members of the health-care team will collaborate on Mrs. Rivera's care?

Suggested answers are at the end of the chapter.

Table 55.2
Common Causes of Burns

Flame	House fire is a common cause. Usually associated with an inhalation injury. Flash injury occurs from a sudden ignition or explosion.
Contact	Hot tar, hot metals, or hot grease can produce a full-thickness injury on contact. E-cigarette-related burn injuries due to battery explosion and liquid ignition.
Scald	A burn from hot liquid. More common in children younger than age 5 and adults older than age 65. With an immersion scald, there are usually no splash marks; usually involves lower regions of body.
Chemical	Usually occurs in an industrial setting. Extent and depth of injury are directly proportional to concentration and quantity of agent, duration of contact, and chemical activity and penetrability of agent.
Electrical	One of the most serious types of burn injury; can be full thickness with possible loss of limbs; can cause internal injuries. Entry wound is usually ischemic, charred, and depressed. Exit wound may have an explosive appearance. Extent of injury depends on voltage, resistance of body, type of current, amperage, pathway of current, and duration of contact. Bones offer greatest resistance to the current, resulting in great damage. Tissue fluid, blood, and nerves offer least resistance; therefore, the current travels this path.
Radiation	Can occur in an industrial setting, as a result of treatment of disease, or from ultraviolet light (sun or tanning salons). Severity depends on type of radiation, duration of exposure, depth of penetration, distance from source, and absorbed dose.

Table 55.3
Stages of Burn Care

Stage	Duration
I: Emergent	From onset of injury to completion of fluid resuscitation
II: Acute	From start of diuresis to near completion of wound closure
III: Rehabilitation	From wound closure to return of optimal level of physical and psychosocial function

THERAPEUTIC MEASURES

Therapeutic interventions vary according to the severity of the burn and the stage the patient is in. Treatment is managed across three overlapping stages (Table 55.3).

Emergent Stage

At the time of injury, the burning process must be stopped. Clothes are immediately removed. The wound is cooled with tepid water. The patient is covered with clean sheets to decrease shivering and contamination. The burn wound is a lower priority than the ABCs (airway, breathing, circulation) of trauma resuscitation. Emergency rescuers at the scene will stabilize the victim by establishing an airway, ensuring oxygenation, inserting an IV line, and stabilizing fractures, hemorrhage, and spinal and other injuries. Inhalation injury is suspected if the patient sustained a burn from a fire in an enclosed space or was exposed to smoldering materials, if the face and neck are burned, if there are vocal changes, or if the patient is coughing up carbon particles. If a pulmonary injury is present, humidified oxygen is administered. IV fluids are given to prevent and treat hypovolemic shock. The patient is treated for pain with IV opioid analgesics.

An accurate history of the injury is obtained to determine severity, potential complications, and associated trauma. The patient's medical history is also obtained. Admission

> **NURSING CARE TIP**
> If the patient is unable to communicate effectively, interview all involved witnesses to determine the cause of the injury as well as past and current medical history and medications the patient is taking. Getting a full description of the cause of the injury may lead to the detection of other injuries that may not be readily visible.

to the facility and burn care treatment are explained to the patient and family.

Acute Stage

If the patient is in a facility with a special burn unit, multidisciplinary care from a burn team is provided during the acute stage. Management goals include wound closure with no infection, minimum scarring, maximum function, maintenance of comfort as much as possible, adequate nutritional support, and maintenance of fluid, electrolyte, and acid-base balance. The patient continues to be medicated for pain as needed, especially before painful treatments. Patient-controlled analgesia (PCA) is very effective. Nutritional support may be maintained via nasogastric enteral feeding (see "Nutrition Notes").

> **PRACTICE ANALYSIS TIP**
> **Linking NCLEX-PN® to Practice**
> Provide nonpharmacological measures for pain relief (e.g., imagery, massage, repositioning).

> **Nutrition Notes**
>
> **Burns**
> The goals of nutritional support in burned patients are to (1) meet metabolic needs, (2) promote wound healing, (3) promote resistance to infection, and (4) reduce protein loss.
>
> Early (within 4 to 6 hours of injury) use of nasogastric enteral feeding has been shown to reduce the incidence of mortality and infectious morbidity. Indirect calorimetry (IC) should be utilized to determine calorie needs, and needs should be reevaluated more than once per week. If IC is unavailable, calorie needs should be individualized per each patient. Complete assessment of the individual is required to determine nutritional needs. Needs vary greatly due to total body surface area of the burn, age, weight, nutritional status, and disease state. Refer to a registered dietitian for complete quality care.
>
> When oral intake is possible, but intake is inadequate, supplemental enteral feeding is the preferred route. Parenteral nutrition poses an infection risk and is reserved for use in those for whom enteral feeding is not feasible or calorie and protein needs are not met enterally.
>
> *Reference:* Natarajan, M. (2019). Recent concepts in nutritional therapy in critically ill burn patients. *International Journal of Nutrition, Pharmacology, Neurological Diseases, 9*(1), 4–36. https://doi.org/10.4103/ijnpnd.ijnpnd_58_18

The wound is cleansed and debrided daily to promote healing, prevent infection, and provide a clean bed for grafting. Wound cleansing is achieved by showering (using a shower trolley or shower chair) and bedside care.

Debridement, or removal of nonviable tissue (eschar), can be done mechanically, surgically, with chemicals, or with a combination of these methods. Mechanical debridement can involve the use of scissors and forceps to manually excise loose, nonviable tissue or the use of wet-to-moist or wet-to-dry fine-mesh gauze dressings (see Chapter 54). Chemical debridement involves the use of a proteolytic enzymatic agent that digests necrotic tissue. Surgical debridement is the excision of full-thickness and deep partial-thickness burns followed by a skin graft.

If the patient has a circumferential burn (one that surrounds an extremity or area), an increase in tissue pressure secondary to tissue edema occurs. The burn then acts like a tourniquet, impeding arterial and venous flow and impairing distal pulses. Common sites for these burns are the extremities, trunk, and chest. If this occurs on the chest and trunk, respiratory insufficiency can occur as a result of restricted chest expansion. An **escharotomy** may be immediately needed to relieve pressure. An escharotomy is a linear excision through the eschar to the superficial fat that allows for expansion of the skin and return of blood flow or chest expansion (Fig. 55.4).

> **CUE RECOGNITION 55.1**
> You are caring for a patient with circumferential burns to his right leg. You cannot find his right popliteal pulse. What should you do?
>
> *Suggested answers are at the end of the chapter.*

> **NURSING CARE TIP**
> Remember to provide adequate padding of the bed before an escharotomy because this procedure can be accompanied by copious amounts of drainage. Provide for appropriate disposal of the drainage. Premedicate for pain prior to the procedure. For an extremity escharotomy, monitor the patient for return of distal pulses.

After the area is cleaned, the burn dressing and topical treatment are prescribed. The type of dressing and topical agent are chosen depending on the area involved, the extent and depth of injury, and health-care provider (HCP) preference. Common topical agents are listed in Table 55.4.

Dressings may be open, closed, biological, synthetic, or a combination. The open method is the use of a topical agent without any dressing. The closed method involves the use of an occlusive dressing over the wound. General principles for dressings include the following:

1. Limit the bulk of the dressing to facilitate range of motion.
2. Never wrap skin-to-skin surfaces (e.g., wrap fingers or toes separately; place a donut gauze dressing around the ear).
3. Base dressings on the size of wounds, absorption, protection, and type of debridement.
4. Wrap extremities from distal to proximal to promote venous return.
5. Do not wrap dressings too tightly. Check peripheral pulses often.
6. Elevate affected extremities.

• WORD • BUILDING •

escharotomy: eschara—scab + otomy—incision

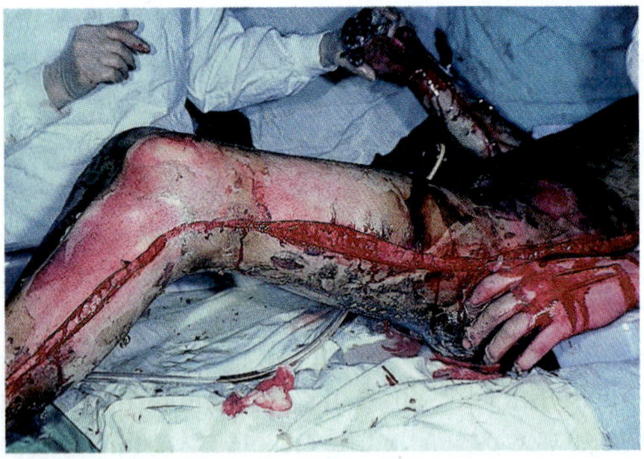

FIGURE 55.4 Escharotomy.

Table 55.4
Common Topical Broad-Spectrum Antibiotic Agents

Examples	Nursing Implications
silver sulfadiazine 1% cream (Silvadene)	Intermediate penetration of eschar. Butter on in thick layer. Cover with light dressings once or twice a day.
mafenide acetate (Sulfamylon)	Premedicate for pain. Butter on. Open exposure method. Apply three to four times daily. Keeps eschar soft for easier debridement.
silver nitrate solution 0.5%	Poor penetration of eschar. Ineffective on established wound infections. Apply with wet dressings and change twice daily. Soak every 2 hours.
bacitracin (Baciguent)	Poor penetration of eschar. Butter on. Reapply every 4 to 6 hours.
gentamicin (Garamycin)	Painful on application. Apply gently three to four times daily.
mupirocin (Bactroban)	May cause burning, itching, and pain on application. Apply three times daily.
neomycin/ bacitracin/ polymyxin (Neosporin)	Apply one to three times daily.

The term *biological dressing* refers to a dressing that uses tissue from living or deceased humans (cadaver skin) or deceased animals (e.g., pigskin). It also refers to cellular dressings that may use animal tissue, human tissue, or synthetics. Biological dressings help with wound healing and stimulate **epithelialization**. These dressings may be used as donor site dressings, to manage a partial-thickness burn, or to cover a clean, excised wound before autografting. Some cellular wound dressings have varied layers that form a matrix onto which the patient's own cells migrate over a few weeks to form a new dermis. A very thin layer of the person's own skin is then grafted onto this new dermis.

Synthetic dressings are used in the management of partial-thickness burns and donor sites. Synthetic dressings are more readily available, less costly, and easier to store than biological dressings. They are made from a variety of materials and come in many sizes and shapes. Most of these dressings contain no antimicrobial agents.

Biological and synthetic dressings are used as temporary wound coverings over clean partial- and full-thickness injuries. They act as skin substitutes to help maintain the wound surface until healing occurs, a donor site becomes available, or the wound is ready for autografting.

> **PRACTICE ANALYSIS TIP**
> Linking NCLEX-PN® to Practice
> The LPN/LVN will perform wound care and/or dressing change.

> **CUE RECOGNITION 55.2**
> You are caring for a burn patient who has a synthetic dressing over his burn wound. You notice exudate that is leaking out of the adhesive seal. What should you do?
> *Suggested answers are at the end of the chapter.*

Skin Grafts
AUTOGRAFT. An **autograft** is a skin graft from the patient's unburned skin placed on the clean, excised burn. Two common types of autografts are the split-thickness skin graft (STSG), which includes the epidermis and part of the dermis, and the full-thickness skin graft (FTSG), which includes the epidermis and entire dermal layer.

Split-Thickness Skin Graft. An STSG (0.006 to 0.016 inch or 0.15 to 0.41 mm) may be applied as a sheet graft or a meshed graft. A sheet graft is used for cosmetic effect on the face, neck, upper chest, breast, or hand. It is placed on the area as a full sheet. A meshed graft is passed through a "mesher" that produces tiny splits in the skin, similar to a fishnet, with openings

• WORD • BUILDING •
epithelialization: epi—over + thele—nipple + ization—condition
autograft: auto—self + graft—tissue transplant

in the shape of diamonds (Fig. 55.5). This permits the skin to expand one and a half to nine times its original size. The meshing allows for coverage of a large burn area with a small piece of skin by stretching it and securing it with sutures or staples. A mesh graft is especially useful when a patient's burns are extensive, resulting in few available donor sites. Graft "take," or vascularization, is complete in about 3 to 5 days.

Full-Thickness Skin Graft. An FTSG (0.035 to 0.040 inch or 0.9 to 1.02 mm) can be a sheet graft or pedicle flap. These grafts are used over areas of muscle mass, soft tissue loss, hands, feet, and eyelids. They are not used for extensive wounds because donor sites usually require STSG for closure or closure from the wound edges. A pedicle graft or flap is a skin flap and subcutaneous tissue still attached at one corner by a "pedicle" to a blood supply (artery and vein); it is attached to an adjacent area in need of grafting. Once the distal part of the graft takes, it remains in place and the flap is divided, with the remainder returning to the original site. Pedicle flaps are not as popular as free skin flaps because they require multiple surgeries and take longer for the graft site and donor site to heal. Table 55.5 provides a comparison of split-thickness and full-thickness skin grafts.

Donor sites are considered partial-thickness wounds. They usually heal in 10 to 14 days depending on thickness, method of grafting, and the general health of the patient. Treatment for the donor site varies with the patient, area of the body, and HCP preference. Considerations for care include promoting comfort and preventing trauma and infection. Use of semiocclusive, transparent dressings (e.g., OpSite, Biobrane, Tegaderm) provides a moist healing environment and is associated with reduced risk of infection. The donor site is very painful. Appropriate pain medications are provided, along with nonpharmacologic measures (e.g., back rubs or distraction).

With any type of graft, the patient must keep the graft site immobilized until the graft takes to prevent movement or slippage of the grafted skin. Dressings may be bulky to assist in immobilization. These dressings must not be disturbed. The involved area requires frequent circulatory checks, including observation of color, warmth, sensation, pulses, and capillary refill. Any involved extremities must be elevated to maintain circulation. A graft has been successful if there is good adherence of the graft to the wound with no evidence of necrosis or infection.

Rehabilitation Stage

The therapy started during the acute phase continues in the rehabilitation phase. There is wound closure with a goal to return the patient to an optimum level of physical and psychosocial function. This may take months to years to accomplish, depending on the extent of the injury. Reconstructive surgeries may be ongoing for many years.

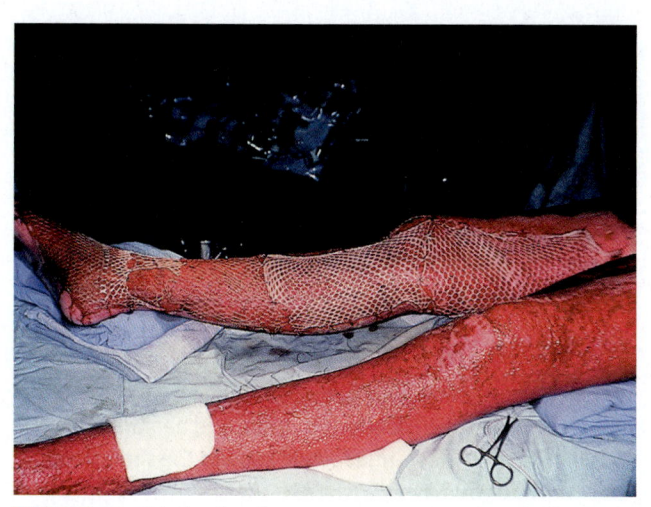

FIGURE 55.5 Meshed graft.

Table 55.5
Comparison of Split-Thickness and Full-Thickness Skin Grafts

	Split-Thickness Skin Graft	*Full-Thickness Skin Graft*
Layers	Epidermis Partial layer of dermis	Epidermis Entire dermal layer
Advantages	Donor site may be reused. Healing of donor site is more rapid; results in a good "take."	Allows more elasticity over joints. Can reconstruct cosmetic defects. Soft, pliable. Gives full appearance. Provides good color match. Less hyperpigmentation. May allow hair growth.
Disadvantages	Prone to chronic breakdown. Likely to hypertrophy. More likely to contract.	Donor site takes longer to heal. Requires split-thickness skin graft to heal or closure from wound edges.

Braza, M. E., and Fahrenkopf, M. P. (2020). Split-thickness skin grafts. [Updated 2020 Jul 31]. In *StatPearls* [Internet]. Treasure Island, FL: StatPearls Publishing. https://www.ncbi.nlm.nih.gov/books/NBK551561

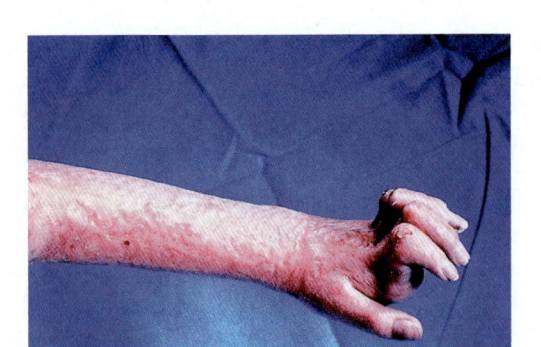

FIGURE 55.6 Burn deformity: contracture.

Two things to keep in mind when caring for the patient with a major burn are (1) the most comfortable position (flexion) is the position of contracture, and (2) the burn wound will shorten until it meets an opposing force. Have you ever seen a contracture? They are uncomfortable and debilitating. To avoid contractures (Fig. 55.6), a specific exercise program starts 24 to 48 hours after injury, along with use of splinting devices to maintain proper positioning and stretching. Hypertrophic scarring, or a proliferation of scar tissue, can be minimized or prevented with a pressure garment (Fig. 55.7).

As the burn heals, itching may occur and be intense at times. It is important to control itching as scratching can impair healing and increase risk of infection (see "Evidence-Based Practice").

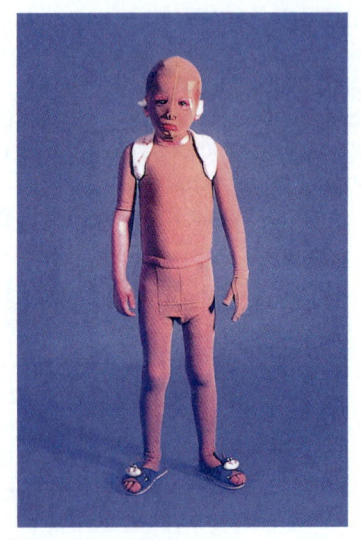

FIGURE 55.7 Full-body pressure garment.

the patient, burn location (e.g., face, hands) and changes in body image, recovery from injury, cause of the injury (especially if related to negligence or a deliberate act), and ability to continue at the preburn level of normal daily activities. The patient may experience disruption of role function and general health and coping ability. Treatment involves the patient and family members. Referrals to support groups, counselors, and psychiatrists are important during this stage.

Evidence-Based Practice

Clinical Question
What nursing interventions are helpful for treating itching in a healing burn?

Evidence
Itching (pruritis) can interfere with activities of daily living. Treatment of itching can include pharmacological and nonpharmacological approaches. Pharmacological treatments include medications such as antihistamines, gabapentin, and topical anesthetics. Treatments that can be carried out by nurses include using pressure, colloidal oatmeal baths, moisturizers, and massage therapy. Check with the HCP before use.

Implications for Nursing Practice
Postburn itching affects about 80% to 100% of burn patients. Asking about postburn itching should be a part of routine care. Pruritus can cause discomfort and distress. Determine the intensity and impact of itching on a 0 to 10 scale and advocate for appropriate orders.

Reference: Chung, B. Y., Kim, H. B., Jung, M. J., Kang, S. Y., Kwak, I. S., Park, C. W., & Kim, H. O. (2020). Post-burn pruritus. *International Journal of Molecular Sciences, 21*(11), 3880. https://doi.org/10.3390/ijms21113880

CRITICAL THINKING

Mrs. Potter is recovering from partial-thickness burns and skin grafts. She mentions that she and her family have planned a much-needed vacation to the shore. What concerns do you have?

Suggested answers are at end of the chapter.

NURSING CARE TIP
Use caution with heating pads, water temperature, and electrical equipment when working with your patients. Burns are considered Never Events because they can be prevented, and thus hospitals will not be paid by Medicare for treating burns acquired during hospitalization.

NURSING PROCESS FOR A PATIENT WITH A BURN INJURY

Data Collection
A major burn is painful and frightening for the patient and the family. Obtain information from the patient, family, and rescuers.

General information to collect for all burns (in addition to normally collected data, such as medical history, allergies, and current medications) includes extent, depth, type, and

Psychosocial Effects of Burn Injury
A burn affects the patient's psychosocial status in many ways. The magnitude of these effects varies with the age of

location of the burn; burn agent; duration of contact with the burning agent; severity and location of pain; and associated injuries. Determine immediate first aid treatment provided at the scene. Obtain psychosocial information, including other people injured, additional losses (e.g., home, pets), whether the patient was at fault, and how this injury affects the patient's role function.

If the injury occurred in an enclosed space with flames or smoldering materials, suspect an inhalation injury. If an electrical injury has occurred, ask about voltage, duration of contact, host susceptibility (wet or dry skin), entry and exit sites, and associated falls. The outward appearance of a severe electrical burn may be deceiving. Damage to internal organs and tissues might not be evident at first. With injury to bones, damage will manifest from the inside out. With chemical burns, determine the type of agent and duration of exposure.

Nursing Diagnoses, Planning, Implementation, and Evaluation

See "Nursing Care Plan for the Patient With a Major Burn Injury" and Table 55.6. Priority nursing diagnoses are presented here. Additional diagnoses such as *Body Image Disturbance* become important during the rehabilitation stage. For more information on burns, go to the American Burn Association Web site at www.ameriburn.org.

Nursing Care Plan for the Patient With a Major Burn Injury

Nursing Diagnosis: *Impaired Gas Exchange* related to upper airway edema, carbon monoxide (CO) poisoning, and edema of alveolar capillary membranes, as evidenced by abnormal arterial blood gases (ABGs) and elevated CO level
Expected Outcomes: The patient's gas exchange will be improved as evidenced by patent airway, CO level less than 10%, clear lung sounds, partial pressure of oxygen (PaO_2) 80 to 100 mm Hg, partial pressure of carbon dioxide ($PaCO_2$) 35 to 45 mm Hg, oxygen saturation (SpO_2) 95%, responsiveness, and awareness.
Evaluation of Outcomes: Are oxygenation levels improved? Do the lungs sound clear on auscultation? Is the patient aware of their surroundings? Are signs of respiratory distress absent (e.g., retractions, nasal flaring, use of accessory muscles)?

Intervention	Rationale	Evaluation
Monitor respiratory status; auscultate breath sounds every 15 minutes or as needed. Note any adventitious breath sounds. Observe for chest excursion. Monitor ability to cough.	*Regular monitoring detects changes in pulmonary function for planning care.*	What is patient's respiratory status? Are any adventitious lung sounds noted? Has a change occurred?
Monitor ABGs and SpO_2 and CO levels.	*Helps guide oxygen therapy.*	Is oxygenation adequate?
Monitor for nasal flaring, retractions, wheezing, and stridor.	*Stridor may signal upper airway involvement. Nasal flaring, retractions, and wheezing may indicate lower airway involvement.*	Does patient exhibit signs of upper or lower airway involvement?
Administer humidified 100% oxygen via tight-fitting facemask as ordered.	*Provides oxygen for adequate gas exchange.*	Is oxygen administered appropriately? Are ABGs improving?
Elevate head of bed (if no cervical spine injuries or no history of multiple trauma).	*Decreases swelling of face and neck. Increases ability to expand lungs.*	Is head of bed elevated? Is there any change in facial or neck swelling?
Provide appropriate pulmonary care: turn, cough, deep breathe every 2 to 4 hours.	*Mobilizes secretions and promotes lung expansion.*	Is patient receiving vigorous pulmonary care? Is it affecting outcomes?
Provide incentive spirometer every 2 to 4 hours.	*Promotes lung expansion to prevent atelectasis and mobilize secretions.*	Is patient able to take deep breaths? Are lungs clear?
Suction frequently as needed/ordered.	*Keeps airways free of secretions.*	Is suctioning effective? Are lungs clear?

(nursing care plan continues on page 1148)

Nursing Care Plan for the Patient With a Major Burn Injury—cont'd

Intervention	Rationale	Evaluation
Obtain sputum cultures as ordered. Note amount, color, and consistency of pulmonary secretions.	Carbonaceous sputum indicates smoke inhalation injury. Infection changes color, amount, and consistency of sputum. Culture and sensitivity (C&S) assists in selection of appropriate antibiotic.	Is patient coughing up any sputum? Has character of sputum been reported and documented?
Administer bronchodilators and antibiotics as prescribed.	Bronchodilators decrease bronchospasms and edema. Antibiotics fight infection.	Are medications effective?

Nursing Diagnosis: *Impaired Skin Integrity* related to thermal injury as evidenced by presence of burn lesions
Expected Outcomes: The patient's skin integrity will be improved as evidenced by the stopping of burning process and healing of burned areas with no infection present.
Evaluation of Outcomes: Did burning process stop? Is burned area healing and free from infection?

Intervention	Rationale	Evaluation
Obtain history of burning agent.	Provides information related to depth, duration of contact, and resistance of tissues. If fire scenario, consider possible inhalation injury.	What caused this thermal injury? How long was patient in contact with agent?
Assist with assessment of burning process. If heat is felt on wound, cool with tepid tap water or sterile water, while keeping patient from chilling.	Depth of injury increases with length of exposure to burning agent.	Is heat felt over wounds? Has burn process been effectively stopped?
Remove clothing and jewelry.	These items can retain heat and thermal agent, thereby increasing depth of injury. Jewelry can be constrictive when edema develops.	Are clothing and jewelry removed and constriction avoided?
Do not apply ice.	Ice causes vasoconstriction, further increasing skin damage. Ice also causes a decrease in core body temperature, which may promote shock.	Is burning stopped without the use of ice?
Cover patient with clean sheet or blanket.	Prevents excessive heat loss. Decreases pain from air exposure. Protects patient from environmental contamination.	Is patient covered and protected?
For all chemical burns, initiate immediate copious tepid water lavage for 20 minutes along with simultaneous removal of contaminated clothing. Do not neutralize chemical because this takes too much time and resulting reaction may generate heat and cause further skin injury.	Dilution and removal of chemical agent halts burning process. Lavage dissipates heat.	Has lavage been initiated?
Brush off dry chemicals before lavage.	Prevents further burn damage due to reaction of dry chemical with water.	Are dry chemicals removed?
Use heavy rubber gloves or thick gauze for removal of clothing.	Protects health-care workers from injury.	Do health-care workers remain safe?

Nursing Care Plan for the Patient With a Major Burn Injury—cont'd

Intervention	Rationale	Evaluation
Cleanse wound at bedside or via showering.	*Promotes healing and helps decrease infection.*	Is burn wound clean and free of wound debris?
Assist registered nurse (RN) or HCP to assess the burn area for extent (percentage) and depth (thickness) of injury.	*Provides basis for triage of care. Important for calculating resuscitation fluid therapy.*	What is the estimation of percentage of burn injury? What is depth of injury?
Assist RN or HCP with debriding wound via surgical, chemical, or mechanical means. Apply topical agent as prescribed.	*Promotes healing and healthy granulation bed. Most agents prevent infection and promote healing.*	Is eschar present? Is wound free of wound debris? Is agent applied as directed?
Apply dressing as prescribed.	*Dressing types vary and are influenced by area, extent, and depth of injury as well as by topical agent used. Dressing protects burn area and promotes healing.*	Is dressing applied appropriately?
Do not wrap skin surface to skin surface (e.g., wrap fingers and toes separately; donut bandage around ears).	*Wrapping separately prevents webbing and contractures.*	Are skin surfaces separated? Are webbing and contractures avoided?
Limit bulk of dressings.	*Mobility is enhanced with less bulky dressing.*	Is patient's mobility maximized?
Wrap extremities from distal to proximal.	*Circulation is increased when extremities are wrapped distal to proximal.*	Is wrapping done correctly? Is edema of distal extremity avoided?

Nursing Diagnosis: Acute Pain related to burns or graft donor sites as evidenced by patient's rating on appropriate pain scale, restlessness, and sleeplessness
Expected Outcomes: The patient will experience pain control as evidenced by pain rating acceptable to patient and nonverbal cues, such as less restlessness and ability to rest or sleep.
Evaluation of Outcomes: Does the patient verbalize pain control? How many hours of rest/sleep does the patient get in 24 hours? Does the patient state they feel rested?

Intervention	Rationale	Evaluation
Collect data related to pain using **WHAT'S UP?** mnemonic. Rate pain on appropriate pain scale.	*Provides baseline to monitor response to therapy.*	Is patient's individual response to pain documented?
Observe for varied responses to acute pain: increase in blood pressure, pulse, and respirations; increased restlessness and irritability; increased muscle tension; facial grimaces; guarding.	*Responses to pain are variable. These parameters change in response to pain.*	What are patient's responses to pain? Do responses change with treatment?
Acknowledge presence of pain. Explain causes of pain.	*Encourages trust and understanding.*	Is patient more trusting of the nurse and the treatments?
Administer opioids as ordered. Use patient-controlled analgesia (PCA) as appropriate.	*Opioids are needed for severe burn pain. PCA allows patient more control.*	Is patient being medicated for pain appropriately?

(nursing care plan continues on page 1150)

Nursing Care Plan for the Patient With a Major Burn Injury—cont'd

Intervention	Rationale	Evaluation
Offer diversional activities (e.g., music, TV, books, games, relaxation techniques).	Helps patient focus on something other than pain.	Does patient use diversional activities? Do they help?
Position patient for comfort in good body alignment.	Increases comfort.	Is patient positioned as comfortably as possible?
Elevate burned extremities.	Elevation decreases edema and pain.	Are extremities elevated? Is pain reduced?
Maintain comfortable environment (e.g., bed cradle, comfortable environmental temperature of 86–91.4°F [30–33°C], quiet environment).	Pressure from bed linens may cause discomfort; with loss of integument, body cannot self-regulate temperature.	Does patient verbalize comfort of environment?

Nursing Diagnosis: *Deficient Fluid Volume* related to evaporative losses from wound, capillary leak, and decreased fluid intake as evidenced by urine output less than 30 to 50 mL per hour, hypotension, tachycardia, and weight loss
Expected Outcomes: The (adult) patient will maintain adequate circulating volume as evidenced by urine output of 30 to 50 mL/hr, blood pressure within normal limits, heart rate between 60 and 100 beats per minute, and stabilized body weight.
Evaluation of Outcomes: Is urine output maintained at least at 30 to 50 mL/hr? Are blood pressure and heart rate within normal limits? Is the patient's weight stable?

Intervention	Rationale	Evaluation
Obtain admission weight and monitor weight daily.	Helps measure fluid loss or gain.	Is patient's weight documented? Is it stable?
Record intake and output (I&O) hourly during emergent/acute stages.	Serves as guide for fluid loss and replacement.	Is urine output adequate?
Examine for signs and symptoms of hypovolemia (e.g., hypotension, tachycardia, tachypnea, extreme thirst, restlessness, disorientation).	Fluid volume loss is multifocal (e.g., through increased capillary permeability, insensible loss).	Does patient exhibit any signs or symptoms of hypovolemia?
Monitor electrolytes and complete blood count (CBC) and report abnormal results to HCP.	Serves as guide for electrolyte replacement and blood product replacement.	What are patient's laboratory values? Are abnormal results reported?
Administer or monitor IV fluids as ordered via large-bore IV catheter.	Fluid replacement begins immediately to prevent hypovolemia. Large vessels are needed for rapid delivery of fluids.	Is patient's fluid replacement adequate? Is catheter patent?
Insert indwelling urinary catheter.	Accurate urine output measurement is essential for fluid replacement calculation.	Is catheter patent and output recorded?
Monitor urine for amount, specific gravity, and **hemochromogen**.	Specific gravity helps predict volume replacement. Hemochromogen can cause renal tubular damage.	What are patient's urine values?

• WORD • BUILDING •
hemochromogen: hemo—blood + chromo—color + gen—producing

Nursing Care Plan for the Patient With a Major Burn Injury—cont'd

Intervention	Rationale	Evaluation
Administer osmotic diuretics as ordered; monitor response to therapy.	*Decreased urine output can be caused by decreased renal flow (due to myoglobin in urine).*	What is urine output? Has it changed due to therapy?
Monitor gastrointestinal function for absent bowel sounds. Maintain nasogastric tube as ordered.	*Splanchnic constriction due to hypovolemia can cause a paralytic ileus.*	Are patient's bowel sounds within normal limits? Is nasogastric tube patent?

Nursing Diagnosis: *Impaired Physical Mobility* related to burn healing, pain, and contractures
Expected Outcomes: The patient will maintain adequate physical mobility as evidenced by ability to ambulate, move in bed, and tolerate activity.
Evaluation of Outcomes: Is the patient able to sit? Is the patient able to get out of bed? Is the patient able to walk with or without assistance?

Intervention	Rationale	Evaluation
Encourage ambulation as able.	*Helps prevent atelectasis and pneumonia.*	Is patient optimally mobilized?
Perform active and passive range of motion exercises on affected areas.	*Prevents contractures and hypertrophic scarring.*	Do affected areas remain mobile?
Provide support above and below affected joints. Apply splints and functional devices as ordered.	*Maintains functional position of extremities.*	Are immobilized joints in a functional position?
For lower extremity burns, apply bandages and elastic bandages before patient is in upright position.	*Promotes venous return and minimizes edema formation.*	Does patient tolerate being upright? Is edema minimized?

Nursing Diagnosis: *Ineffective Peripheral Tissue Perfusion* related to circumferential burns, blood loss, and decreased cardiac output as evidenced by weak pulses, cool extremities, limited movement, and sensation
Expected Outcomes: The patient will maintain adequate tissue perfusion as evidenced by presence of peripheral pulses, minimal edema, intact sensation and motion, and warm extremities.
Evaluation of Outcomes: Are peripheral pulses present? Are extremities warm, with adequate sensation, movement, and circulation? Is edema decreased?

Intervention	Rationale	Evaluation
Monitor pulses on burned extremities every 15 minutes until stable, then every hour.	*If pulses diminish, an escharotomy may be indicated.*	Are pulses present and documented?
Use Doppler ultrasound as needed to detect weak pulses. Check capillary refill, sensation, color, swelling, and movement.	*Monitors peripheral perfusion.*	Is the extremity warm, with adequate color, sensation, movement, and capillary refill?
Monitor for numbness, tingling, and increased pain in burned extremity.	*Can be indicative of increased pressure from edema.*	Does patient report numbness, tingling, or pain?
Measure circumference of burned extremities.	*Monitors edema formation.*	Is there evidence of edema? Is it getting better or worse?
Report changes in data findings promptly.	*Emergency intervention may be indicated.*	Does patient require an emergency intervention?

(nursing care plan continues on page 1152)

Nursing Care Plan for the Patient With a Major Burn Injury—cont'd

Intervention	Rationale	Evaluation
Elevate burned extremity above level of the heart.	Enhances venous return and decreases edema formation.	Are all burned extremities elevated above heart level? Is edema decreasing?
Apply burn dressing loosely	Prevents constriction and allows for expansion as edema forms.	Is dressing limiting circulation?
Assist with muscle compartment pressure measurement.	Helps determine need for escharotomy (if pressure exceeds 25 mm Hg).	What is patient's pressure?
Assist with escharotomy as needed.	If indicated, removal of eschar allows for edema expansion and permits peripheral perfusion.	Does patient require an escharotomy? Is edema relieved?

Nursing Diagnosis: *Risk for Infection*
Expected Outcome: The patient will not develop a wound infection or sepsis.
Evaluation of Outcome: Is there healthy granulation tissue on unhealed areas with no evidence of infection? Are donor sites free of infection? Have skin grafts taken? Is there absence of clinical manifestation of infection (e.g., temperature 98.6°F [37°C], normal white blood cell count)?

Intervention	Rationale	Evaluation
Use sterile technique with wound care.	The unhealed burn wound is an excellent culture medium for bacterial growth.	Is sterile technique used for all wound care?
Maintain protective isolation with careful hand hygiene.	Prevents spread of bacteria from patient to patient or nurse to patient.	Do all persons in contact with patient maintain proper precautions?
Administer immunosupportive medications as prescribed (tetanus and gamma globulin).	Immunoglobulins are depressed at time of severe burn injury.	Have medications been administered if indicated?
Perform wound care as prescribed, which may include the following: inspect and debride wounds daily; culture wound three times a week or at sign of infection; shave hair at least 1 inch around burn areas if necessary (excluding eyebrows); inspect invasive line sites for inflammation (especially if line is through a burn area).	Provides quick identification of bacterial wound invasion and decreases incidence of infection. Presence of hair increases medium for bacterial growth.	What does wound look like? Is it debrided? What are culture results? Does hair present a risk for infection?
Continually monitor for and report signs and symptoms of sepsis (e.g., temperature elevation, change in sensorium, changes in vital signs and bowel sounds, decreased output, positive blood and wound cultures).	The burn patient is at risk for sepsis until wound is healed.	Does patient exhibit any signs or symptoms of sepsis?
Administer systemic antibiotics and topical agents as prescribed.	Antibiotics prevent or treat infection.	Does patient require systemic antibiotics? Are topical agents applied appropriately? Is wound healing?

Table 55.6
Burn Summary

Signs and Symptoms	Pain Superficial partial-thickness burn: pink to red skin, blisters Deep partial-thickness burn: pink to light red or white skin, blisters, blanching Full-thickness burn: white, gray, or brown color; firm and leathery
Diagnostic Tests	Wound cultures Complete blood count (CBC), blood urea nitrogen (BUN), glucose, electrolytes, urine studies
Therapeutic Measures	IV fluid replacement Antibiotic/antimicrobial agents Analgesics
Complications	Shock Wound infection
Priority Nursing Diagnoses	*Impaired Gas Exchange* *Impaired Skin Integrity* *Deficient Fluid Volume* *Acute Pain* related to burns or graft donor sites *Impaired Physical Mobility* *Ineffective Peripheral Tissue Perfusion* *Risk for Infection*

Key Points

- Burns are wounds caused by an energy transfer that heats tissue enough to cause damage. Alterations resulting from a major burn injury include loss of protective functions, impaired ability to regulate temperature, increased risk of infection, changes in sensory function, loss of fluids, impaired skin regeneration, and impaired secretory and excretory functions.
- Fluid is lost after a major burn causing blisters and edema, with a loss of intravascular volume. Water loss occurs by evaporation through the burned tissue and increased metabolism.
- A burn is followed by an initial decrease in cardiac output and loss of circulating plasma volume. Severe hematologic changes occur in patients with major burns.
- Some gastrointestinal problems that can develop with a major burn include gastric dilation, peptic ulcers, and paralytic ileus.
- Fluid loss and inadequate fluid replacement can lead to decreased renal blood flow and glomerular filtration rate. Extensive burns can cause destruction of muscle, creating myoglobin casts that can block renal tubules and lead to renal failure.
- Pulmonary effects are mostly related to smoke inhalation. However, hyperventilation may occur with any moderate to major burn injury, usually proportional to burn severity.
- With skin destroyed, the body loses its first line of defense against infection. Major burns also depress immunoglobulin (Ig)A, IgG, and IgM.
- The severity of a burn injury is determined by the depth of tissue destruction, percentage of body surface area injured, cause of the burn, age of the patient, related injuries, medical history (e.g., heart disease, diabetes), and location of the burn wound.
- The size of a burn wound is estimated on the basis of parts of the body affected. A quick and common method is the Rule of Nines, which divides the body into segments with areas of 9% or multiples of 9%.
- The most common causes include flames; contact burns; scalding; and chemical, electrical, and radiation burns.
- Inhalation injury is a major cause of morbidity and mortality associated with burn injuries caused by flames.
- Burns are diagnosed by physical assessment. Various diagnostic tests are performed for systemic reactions, infection, and other complications. These include blood work, x-rays, electrocardiogram, and wound cultures.
- At the time of the injury, after burning has stopped, the wound itself is a lower priority than the ABCs (airway, breathing, circulation) of trauma resuscitation.
- In the acute stage, the wound is cleansed and debrided daily to promote healing, prevent infection, and provide a clean bed for grafting.
- An escharotomy may be immediately needed to relieve pressure. This linear excision through the eschar to the superficial fat allows for expansion of the skin and return of blood flow or chest expansion.

- After the area is cleaned, the burn dressing and topical treatment are chosen depending on the area involved, the extent and depth of injury, and HCP preference.
- Dressings may be open, closed, biological, synthetic, or a combination of methods
- Skin grafting may be done to close the wound. An autograft is a graft from the patient's unburned skin (donor site) that is placed on the clean, excised burn.
- The two common types of autografts are STSG, which includes the epidermis and part of the dermis, and FTSG, which includes the epidermis and entire dermal layer.
- Donor sites are considered partial-thickness wounds. They usually heal in 10 to 14 days, but this depends on the thickness and method of grafting and the general health of the patient.
- The involved area requires frequent circulatory checks, including observation of color, warmth, sensation, pulses, and capillary refill.
- A graft has been successful if there is good adherence of the graft to the wound with no evidence of necrosis or infection.
- A burn affects the patient's psychosocial status related to the age of the patient, location of the burn (e.g., face, hands) and changes in body image, recovery from injury, cause of the injury (especially if related to negligence or a deliberate act), and ability to continue at the preburn level of normal daily activities.
- General information to collect for burns includes extent, depth, type, and location of the burn; burn agent; duration of contact with the burning agent; severity and location of pain; and associated injuries. Determine the immediate first aid treatment provided at the scene.
- The priority nursing diagnoses for patients with burns include *Impaired Gas Exchange, Impaired Skin Integrity, Deficient Fluid Volume, Acute Pain, Ineffective Peripheral Tissue Perfusion*, and *Risk for Infection*.
- Treatment involves the patient and family members. Referrals to support groups, counselors, and psychiatrists are important during the rehabilitation stage.

SUGGESTED ANSWERS TO CHAPTER EXERCISES

Cue Recognition
55.1: Check with a Doppler ultrasound.
55.2: Change the dressing as allowed/ordered.

Critical Thinking & Clinical Judgment
Mr. Weinberg
Superficial partial-thickness burns usually heal in 7 to 10 days. Deep partial-thickness burns may take up to 3 weeks. These estimated healing times depend on the location of the injury, the health of the patient, and whether he remains infection free.

Mrs. Rivera
1. Mrs. Rivera has an inhalation injury. This takes precedence over the burn and other injuries.
2. $\dfrac{1 \text{ L}}{6 \text{ hr}} \times \dfrac{1{,}000 \text{ mL}}{1 \text{ L}} = 167 \text{ mL/hr}$
3. Approximately 18%.
4. Burn care requires a true interdisciplinary approach. She has a major burn, so the burn nurse will collaborate with a burn physician, plastic surgeon, pulmonary physician, orthopedic surgeon, physician assistant or nurse practitioner, physical therapist, occupational therapist, and dietitian.

Mrs. Potter
Burned and graft areas will be sensitive to sunlight for up to 1 year. These areas should be covered, and she must use sunscreen anytime she is out in the sun. Her HCP should offer guidance as to whether any exposure is safe and, if so, what type of sunscreen agent is recommended. In addition, if any areas are not completely healed, she will be at risk for infection.

Additional Resources

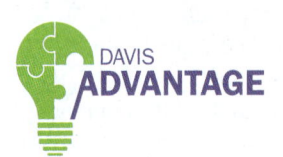

Go to Davis Advantage to complete your learning: strengthen understanding, apply your knowledge, and prepare for the Next Gen NCLEX®.

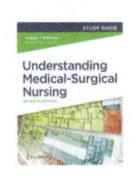

A Study Guide is also available.

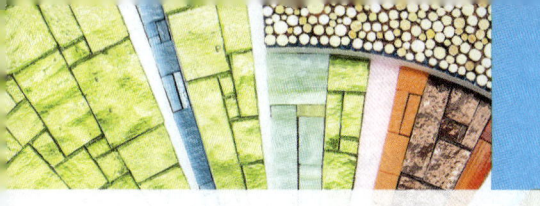

UNIT SIXTEEN Understanding Mental Health Care

CHAPTER 56
Mental Health Function, Data Collection, and Therapeutic Measures

Marina Martinez-Kratz

KEY TERMS

adaptation (a-dap-TAY-shun)
affect (AF-ekt)
anxiety (ang-ZY-uh-tee)
cognitive (KOG-nih-tiv)
coping (KOH-ping)
electroconvulsive therapy
  (ee-LEK-troh kun-VUL-siv THER-uh-pee)
imagery (IM-ij-ree)
insight (IN-site)
mental health (MEN-tuhl HELTH)
mental illness (MEN-tuhl ILL-ness)
milieu (meel-YOO)
psychoanalysis (SY-koh-uh-NAL-ih-sis)
psychopharmacology
  (SY-koh-FAR-mah-KAH-luh-jee)
psychotherapy (SY-koh-THER-uh-pee)
stress (STRESS)
stressor (STRESS-ur)

CHAPTER CONCEPTS

Cognition
Communication
Mood and affect
Stress and coping

LEARNING OUTCOMES

1. Define mental health and mental illness.
2. Describe the components of a mental health status assessment.
3. Describe the *Diagnostic and Statistical Manual of Mental Disorders* (5th ed.; *DSM-5*) as a tool to diagnose mental illness.
4. Identify common ego defense mechanisms.
5. Describe characteristics of a therapeutic milieu.
6. Explain how psychoanalysis, behavior management, cognitive behavioral therapy, counseling, group therapy, electroconvulsive therapy, and relaxation therapy are carried out.
7. Describe the role of the licensed practical nurse/licensed vocational nurse (LPN/LVN) in mental health nursing.

REVIEW OF NEUROLOGIC ANATOMY AND PHYSIOLOGY

When studying mental illnesses, it is important to review and understand the anatomy and physiology of the brain and central nervous system (CNS). The brain is involved in many functions, including thinking, decision making, speaking, emotion, memory, motor and sensory activity, and the basic functions of temperature regulation and breathing. Refer to Chapter 47 to review the nerves, structure of neurons, synapses, neurotransmitters, and the autonomic nervous system as well as the structure and function of the brain. Table 56.1 presents the hypothesized roles of CNS neurotransmitters in mental illness.

MENTAL HEALTH AND MENTAL ILLNESS

Opinions within the mental health community differ as to definitions of mental health and mental illness. **Mental health** has been defined in many ways. These definitions include the ability to do the following:

- Be flexible.
- Take responsibility for one's own actions.
- Form close relationships.
- Make appropriate judgments.
- Solve problems.
- Cope with daily **stress**.
- Have a positive sense of self.

1155

Table 56.1
Neurotransmitters in the Central Nervous System

Location/Function	Possible Implications for Mental Health
Cholinergics	
Acetylcholine Autonomic nervous system (ANS): Sympathetic and parasympathetic presynaptic nerve terminals, parasympathetic postsynaptic nerve terminals Central nervous system (CNS): Cerebral cortex, hippocampus, limbic structures, basal ganglia *Functions:* Sleep, arousal, pain perception, movement, memory	*Decreased levels:* Alzheimer disease, Huntington disease, Parkinson disease *Increased levels:* Depression
Monoamines	
Norepinephrine ANS: Sympathetic postsynaptic nerve terminals CNS: Thalamus, hypothalamus, limbic system, hippocampus, cerebellum, cerebral cortex *Functions:* Mood, cognition, perception, locomotion, cardiovascular functioning, sleep and arousal	*Decreased levels:* Depression *Increased levels:* Mania, anxiety states, schizophrenia
Dopamine Frontal cortex, limbic system, basal ganglia, thalamus, posterior pituitary, spinal cord *Functions:* Movement and coordination, emotions, voluntary judgment, release of prolactin	*Decreased levels:* Parkinson disease, depression *Increased levels:* Mania, schizophrenia
Serotonin Hypothalamus, thalamus, limbic system, cerebral cortex, cerebellum, spinal cord *Functions:* Sleep and arousal, libido, appetite, mood, aggression, pain perception, coordination, judgment	*Decreased levels:* Depression *Increased levels:* Anxiety states
Histamine Hypothalamus	*Decreased levels:* Depression
Amino Acids	
Gamma-Aminobutyric Acid (GABA) Hypothalamus, hippocampus, cortex, cerebellum, basal ganglia, spinal cord, retina *Functions:* Slowdown of body activity	*Decreased levels:* Huntington disease, anxiety disorders, schizophrenia, various forms of epilepsy
Glycine Spinal cord, brainstem *Functions:* Recurrent inhibition of motor neurons	*Toxic levels:* Glycine encephalopathy; decreased levels are correlated with spastic motor movement
Glutamate and Aspartate Pyramidal cells of the cortex, cerebellum, and primary sensory afferent systems; hippocampus, thalamus, hypothalamus, spinal cord *Functions:* Relay of sensory information and in the regulation of various motor and spinal reflexes	*Increased levels:* Huntington disease, temporal lobe epilepsy, spinal cerebellar degeneration

Table 56.1
Neurotransmitters in the Central Nervous System—cont'd

Location/Function	Possible Implications for Mental Health
Neuropeptides	
Endorphins and Enkephalins Hypothalamus, thalamus, limbic structures, midbrain, brainstem; enkephalins are also found in the gastrointestinal tract *Functions:* Modulation of pain and reduced peristalsis (enkephalins)	Modulation of dopamine activity by opioid peptides may indicate some link to the symptoms of schizophrenia
Substance P Hypothalamus, limbic structures, midbrain, brainstem, thalamus, basal ganglia, spinal cord; also found in gastrointestinal tract and salivary glands *Function:* Regulation of pain	*Decreased levels:* Huntington disease and Alzheimer disease *Increased levels:* Depression
Somatostatin Cerebral cortex, hippocampus, thalamus, basal ganglia, brain stem, spinal cord *Function:* Inhibits release of norepinephrine; stimulates release of serotonin, dopamine, acetylcholine	*Decreased levels:* Alzheimer disease *Increased levels:* Huntington disease

Source: Morgan, K. I., & Townsend, M. C. (2020). *Davis Advantage for essentials of psychiatric mental health nursing* (8th ed.). Philadelphia, PA: F.A. Davis.

Mental illness can be defined as experiencing the following:

- Impaired ability to think
- Impaired ability to feel
- Impaired ability to make sound judgments
- Impaired ability to adapt
- Difficulty in **coping** or inability to cope with reality
- Difficulty in forming or inability to form strong personal relationships

It is important to remember that mental health and mental illness exist on a continuum. It is natural for emotions to ebb and flow from day to day in response to the degree of stress experienced. People who remain mentally healthy can cope with and keep their stress in perspective. Others are not able to do so and over time may develop physical or emotional illnesses because of present and past life stresses.

Etiologies

The line between mental illness and other brain or neurologic disorders is being blurred as we learn more about how the brain functions. As scientists study the brains of people who have mental illnesses, they conclude that mental illness is caused by a variety of biological, genetic, and environmental factors. Changes in the brain's structure, chemistry, and function are associated with expressions of mental illness. However, it is important to note that while mental illnesses can be categorized as brain diseases, not all brain diseases are mental illnesses.

Explanations of mental illness in this unit include concepts from the psychological and the psychobiological (or biological) theories. When pertinent, other theories (e.g., behavioral, environmental) are presented. Most mental illnesses have no identifiable cause. Some etiological theories have stronger positive correlations to illnesses than others. When appropriate, this unit gives the most current or most widely accepted view of an etiology.

Social and Cultural Environments

Many behavioral health professionals believe that social and cultural environments greatly influence the way people develop and process life experiences. It is part of the nurse's role to learn about traits that are common among cultures and traits that differ. It is essential to recognize that each person is a unique individual while understanding broad cultural customs and beliefs.

Spirituality and Religion

Spirituality and religion are extremely important to some patients and unimportant to others. A person's success in recuperating from physical or emotional illness may be deeply tied to spiritual beliefs. It is necessary to be comfortable talking to the patient about spiritual needs while taking care not to impose personal values on the patient. If you are not comfortable in these situations, you should offer to call the spiritual or religious leader of the patient's choice.

For more information about mental health and illness, visit the Web sites of the National Institute of Mental Health at www.nimh.nih.gov, the American Psychological Association at www.apa.org, the American Psychiatric Nurses Association at www.apna.org, and the International Society of Psychiatric-Mental Health Nurses at www.ispn-psych.org.

NURSING DATA COLLECTION RELATED TO MENTAL HEALTH

During the assessment/data collection phase of the nursing process, a mental status examination is performed. This series of questions, activities, and observations evaluates the following eight areas:

- Appearance and behavior
- Level of awareness and reality orientation
- Thinking/content of thought
- Memory
- Speech and ability to communicate
- Mood and **affect**
- Judgment
- Perception

Many tools of varying names, lengths, and formats are used to evaluate mental capabilities. Table 56.2 is a sample mental status examination.

After data have been collected, the LPN/LVN collaborates with the registered nurse (RN) to develop nursing diagnoses (Box 56.1).

DIAGNOSTIC TESTS

Physicians use diagnostic criteria to diagnose mental illness. It is important to rule out physical illness as a cause of symptoms. A health-care provider (HCP) may refer a patient to a psychiatrist or another mental health professional for further testing and diagnosis.

The diagnostic tool used most widely by psychiatrists and other mental health professionals is the *Diagnostic and Statistical Manual of Mental Disorders*, fifth edition, or *DSM-5* (American Psychiatric Association, 2013). *DSM-5*, a complex diagnostic tool, groups illnesses into categories of clinical disorders. Although as an LPN/LVN you are not responsible for completing the assessment or making a diagnosis, you can contribute valuable information to the diagnostic process.

Batteries of psychological tests can be administered and interpreted by psychiatrists, psychologists, social workers, or advanced practice nurses. Age, hand tremors, vision, language barriers, educational background, and HCP interpretation can influence the results of these tests.

Some disorders can mimic mental health disorders, so the following diagnostic tests may be performed to either confirm or rule out a diagnosis of a mental illness:

- Laboratory tests can rule out problems such as electrolyte imbalances, hypothyroidism, infections, dehydration, drug toxicity, or pregnancy.
- Computed tomography (CT) scans or magnetic resonance imaging (MRI) can rule out tumors, lesions, or other physical problems.
- Positron emission tomography (PET) scans can identify how brain areas are functioning by showing chemical activity or metabolism.

COPING AND EGO DEFENSE MECHANISMS

"Oh, just learn to cope with it." "Get a grip." "Don't make a mountain out of a molehill." Most people have heard or given these phrases as advice at some point. But what do they mean? What is coping? Coping is the way one adapts psychologically, physically, and behaviorally to a **stressor**. People have different ways of coping with stressors. Culture, religion, individual belief systems, experience, and personal choice influence responses to stress. It is not the value of a behavior that we determine as nurses; it is the desired outcome that is important. What is an effective coping skill? Is it healthy? Does it work? How do we as nurses observe and measure it?

Effective Coping Skills

Effective coping skills offer healthy choices for dealing with stressors. Individuals might use humor, prayer, exercise, or problem-solving. Effective coping skills are conscious mechanisms. Hospitalization is stressful for patients and families. Many things are unknown and unfamiliar. The patient may not understand the illness or implications of the treatment plan. It is common for patients to use coping mechanisms during hospitalization. The process of effective coping is sometimes called **adaptation**. Allowing the patient to practice new coping techniques will give them confidence and decrease the stress that can accompany change.

Often, mild **anxiety** can be positive. A little anxiety can make people more alert and ready to respond. The *fight-or-flight mechanism* can help one adapt to (or escape from) a dangerous situation. However, too much anxiety can cloud consciousness and interfere with the ability to make appropriate choices or recall new adaptive tools that have been learned. Helpful nursing roles include actively listening to the patient's thoughts and feelings about the stressor, assisting with identifying precipitating factors and patterns to stress, encouraging the patient to problem-solve, and helping develop alternative solutions to a problem.

CLINICAL JUDGMENT

Mr. Joseph is noted wailing loudly and continuously after the death of his wife. It is disturbing the other patients on the hospital wing. One of the nurses comments, "He is a real nut case. Get him out of here." What is an appropriate response to this nurse? To the husband? How would you document his behavior?

Suggested answers are at the end of the chapter.

Chapter 56 Mental Health Function, Data Collection, and Therapeutic Measures 1159

Table 56.2
Sample Mental Status Examination

Type of Examination	Normal Parameters	Alterations From Normal
Appearance and Behavior		
Observations about dress, hygiene, posture, and appearance and about the patient's actions and reactions to health-care personnel.	Clean, combed hair. Clothing intact and appropriate to weather or situation. Teeth/dentures in good repair. Posture erect. Cooperates with health-care personnel.	Displays either unusual apathy or concern about appearance. Displays uncooperative, hostile, or suspicious behaviors toward health-care personnel.
Subjective and objective assessment of patient's degree of alertness (wakefulness) and degree of patient's knowledge of self.	Awareness is measured on a continuum that ranges from unconscious to manic. "Normal alertness" is the desired behavior. Facilities may provide a standard format for this assessment, but observations can be documented as well if the patient is not able to stay awake for even short intervals or if the patient is overly active and has difficulty staying in one place. Orientation is assessed by asking questions relating to person, place, and time, such as "Who is this sitting next to you?" or "Where are you right now?"	Outcome is not considered within accepted normal limits if the patient is difficult to arouse and keep awake or if the patient has difficulty feeling calm. Abnormal results of orientation are the patient's inability to correctly answer orientation questions or inability to answer commonly known questions, such as "Who is the president?"
Thinking/Content of Thought		
Subjective assessment of what the patient is thinking and the process the patient uses in his or her thinking.	Formal testing may be done by a psychologist or psychiatrist to determine patient's general thought content and pattern. Nurses may contribute to the assessment of thought by documenting statements the patient makes regarding daily care and routines.	Abnormal behaviors include flight of ideas, loose associations, phobias, delusions, and obsessions.
Memory		
Subjective assessment of the mind's ability to recall recent and remote (long-term) information. Speech and ability to communicate are also assessed	*Recent memory:* Recall of events immediately past or within 2 weeks before the assessment, such as news. One technique is to ask the patient what they had for breakfast that day or what they did yesterday afternoon. *Remote memory:* Recall of events of the past beyond 2 weeks before assessment. Patients may be asked where they were born, where they went to grade school, etc.	Inability to accurately perform recent or remote (long-term) recall exercises within parameters. May indicate symptom of delirium or dementia.

Continued

Table 56.2
Sample Mental Status Examination—cont'd

Type of Examination	Normal Parameters	Alterations From Normal
Speech and Ability to Communicate		
Objective and subjective assessment of how the patient uses verbal and nonverbal communication. Stuttering, repetition of words, and words that the patient makes up (neologisms) are also assessed.	Patient can coherently produce words appropriate to age, education, and life experience. Rate of speech reflects other psychomotor activity (e.g., faster if the patient is agitated). Volume is not too soft or too loud. Speech is fluid and appropriate.	Limited speech production. Rate of speech is inconsistent with other psychomotor activity. Volume is not appropriate to situation (speaks louder or softer than appropriate). Presence of stuttering, word repetition, or neologisms may indicate physical or psychological illness.
Mood and Affect		
Objective and subjective assessment of the patient's stated feelings and emotions. Affect measures the outward expression of those feelings.	Mood is the stated emotional condition of the patient and should reflect situations as they occur. Facial expression and body language (affect) should match (be congruent with) the stated mood. Affect should change to fluctuate with the changes in mood.	Mood and affect do not match (e.g., facial expression does not appear sad while the patient is expressing sad feelings).
Judgment		
Subjective assessment of a patient's ability to make appropriate decisions about their situation or to understand concepts.	When given a proverb or situation to solve, such as "You can't teach an old dog new tricks," the patient should be able to give an acceptable interpretation, such as "Old habits are hard to break" or "It is hard to learn something new."	Patient cannot interpret the sayings or complete problem-solving questions appropriately. The patient might answer very literally, "Dogs can't learn anything when they get old."
Perception		
Assessment of the way a person experiences reality. Observation of the patient's statements about their environment and the behaviors expressed in association with those statements. Assessment of the patient's insight into their condition.	All five senses are monitored for the patient's perception of reality. Perceptions of environment are accurate. Insight into condition is appropriate.	Hallucinations (false sensory perceptions) may occur with schizophrenia. Illusions are misperceptions of reality. The patient is unable to state understanding of the origin of the illness; associated behaviors are inappropriate. Many people with schizophrenia or mania have poor insight because of impairment of prefrontal cortex functioning during psychosis.

Box 56.1
Nursing Diagnoses Commonly Used to Address Mental Health Problems

Anxiety (mild to panic)
Body Image, Disturbed
Chronic Sorrow
Communication, Impaired Verbal
Communication, Readiness for Enhanced
Community Health, Deficient
Compromised Human Dignity, Risk for
Coping, Compromised Family
Coping, Defensive
Coping, Disabled Family
Coping, Ineffective
Decision-Making, Readiness for Enhanced
Decisional Conflict
Decreased Diversional Activity Engagement
Denial, Ineffective
Family Processes, Dysfunctional
Family Processes, Interrupted
Fear
Grieving
Grieving, Complicated
Grieving, Risk for Complicated
Health Behavior, Risk-Prone
Hope, Readiness for Enhanced
Hopelessness
Impaired Resilience
Impaired Resilience, Risk for
Impulse Control, Ineffective
Injury, Risk for
Labile Emotional Control
Loneliness, Risk for
Mood Regulation, Impaired
Moral Distress
Personal Identity, Disturbed
Post-trauma Syndrome, Risk for
Power, Readiness for Enhanced
Powerlessness
Powerlessness, Risk for
Rape-Trauma Syndrome
Relationship, Ineffective
Relationship, Risk for Ineffective
Religiosity, Impaired
Religiosity, Readiness for Enhanced
Religiosity, Risk for Impaired
Relocation Stress Syndrome, Risk for
Resilience, Readiness for Enhanced
Role Performance, Ineffective
Self-Care Deficit (Bathing, Dressing, Feeding, or Toileting)
Self-Esteem, Chronic Low
Self-Esteem, Risk for Low (Chronic or Situational)
Self-Mutilation
Sexual Dysfunction
Sleep Pattern, Disturbed
Social Interaction, Impaired
Social Isolation
Spiritual Well-Being, Readiness for Enhanced
Stress Overload
Suicidal Behavior, Risk for
Violence, Risk for (Self-Directed or Other-Directed)

Ineffective Coping Skills

Sometimes coping behaviors are ineffective. When conscious techniques are not successful, people may unconsciously fall into habits that give the illusion of coping. These habits, called *ego defense mechanisms*, act as mental pressure valves. Their purpose is to reduce or eliminate anxiety. They give the impression that they are helping alleviate the stress. Sometimes ego defense mechanisms can be helpful. When they are overused or are the only means used to deal with anxiety, however, they can become ineffective and unhealthy. People are not born with coping behaviors; the behaviors are learned as responses to stress. Often, they develop by age 10. They may appear conscious, but they are for the most part unconscious mechanisms. Some commonly used ego defense mechanisms are listed in Table 56.3.

CRITICAL THINKING & CLINICAL JUDGMENT

Mrs. Beison, a 44-year-old mother of three teenagers, is diagnosed with breast cancer. She is refusing treatment because she does not believe she has cancer. She says if anything is wrong, her vitamins will take care of it.

Critical Thinking (The Why)
1. What ego defense mechanism is Mrs. Beison using? Is it effective or ineffective? Why?

Clinical Judgment (The Do)
2. How can you help? Are there other health-care professionals who could assist?

Suggested answers are at the end of the chapter.

CUE RECOGNITION 56.1

You are caring for a patient with an alcohol use disorder. Whenever you attempt to discuss the patent's alcohol use, he states, "I don't have a drinking problem. I can quit any time I want." What ego defense mechanism is the patient showing overuse of?

Suggested answers are at the end of the chapter.

THERAPEUTIC MEASURES

People who experience alterations in mental health have special treatment needs. When emotional health is threatened, many daily activities can be altered as well. **Cognitive** ability (the ability to think rationally and to process thoughts) can be impaired. Emotional responses can be decreased or even absent in some conditions. This can be extremely frightening and lead to a worsening of the mental disorder or even development of another disorder. This section provides an overview of selected therapies to help patients deal with alterations in mental health.

Therapeutic Communication

Many people take communication for granted. In the mental health setting, communication is a tool to relate therapeutically with patients. It is important to be intentional about the

Table 56.3
Ego Defense Mechanisms

Mechanism	Description	Examples
Denial	Usually the first defense learned and used. Unconscious refusal to see reality; not conscious lying.	The alcoholic states, "I can quit any time I want to."
Repression (stuffing)	An unconscious "burying" or "forgetting" mechanism. Excludes or withholds from consciousness events or situations that are unbearable.	A step deeper than "denial." A patient may "forget" about an appointment they do not want to keep.
Rationalization	Using a logical-sounding excuse to cover up true thoughts and feelings. The most frequently used defense mechanism.	"I made a medication error because the doctor's orders were confusing." "I failed the test because the teacher wasn't clear about what would be on it."
Compensation	Making up for something perceived as an inadequacy by developing some other desirable trait.	The small boy who wants to be a basketball center instead becomes an honor roll student. The physically unattractive person who wants to model instead becomes a famous designer.
Reaction formation (overcompensation)	Similar to compensation, except the person usually develops the exact opposite trait.	The small boy who wants to be a basketball center becomes a political voice to decrease the emphasis on sports in the elementary grades. The physically unattractive person who wants to be a model speaks out for eliminating beauty pageants.
Regression	Emotionally returning to an earlier time in life when the patient experienced far less stress. Commonly seen in patients while hospitalized.	Children who are toilet trained begin to wet the bed after the birth of a younger sibling. Adults who have a "temper tantrum."
Projection	Ascribing one's own unacceptable qualities or feelings to someone else. May lead to scapegoating.	A patient might state, "My sister is so jealous of me," when actually the patient is jealous of her sister. An anxious patient may say to the nurse, "Why do I make you so nervous?"
Displacement (transference)	"Kick-the-dog syndrome," or transferring anger and hostility to another person or object that is perceived to be less powerful than oneself.	Parent loses job without notice and then goes home and verbally abuses spouse, who unjustly punishes child, who slaps the dog.
Restitution (undoing)	Make amends for a behavior one thinks is unacceptable. Makes an attempt at reducing guilt.	A person gives a treat to a child who is being punished for a wrongdoing. The person who sees someone lose a wallet with a large amount of cash does not return the wallet but puts extra in the collection plate at the next church service.
Conversion reaction	Anxiety is channeled into physical symptoms. Often, the symptoms disappear soon after the threat is over.	Nausea develops the night before a major exam, causing the person to miss the exam. Nausea may disappear soon after the scheduled test is finished.
Avoidance	Unconsciously staying away from events or situations that might cause feelings of aggression or anxiety.	"I can't go to the class reunion tonight. I'm just so tired, I have to sleep."

messages we communicate to patients. Therapeutic communication is accomplished through deliberate use of verbal and nonverbal techniques. Other considerations when communicating are the patient's values, attitudes, beliefs, culture, religion, social status, gender, and age or developmental level.

Verbal therapeutic communication techniques can facilitate an interpersonal interaction. For instance, if you ask a patient to explain something to you in more detail, you are using the verbal therapeutic communication technique of *exploring*. Verbal communication is also influenced by the tone, pitch, speed, and volume of speech. Some commonly used therapeutic communication techniques are listed in Table 56.4.

Components of *nonverbal communication* include physical appearance, dress, body movement and posture, touch, facial expression, and eye contact. It is believed that most communication takes place nonverbally, so while you are saying one thing to a patient, your body language could be saying something else. Silence is useful, as it gives both the nurse and the patient a chance to collect their thoughts and organize what they are going to say.

Table 56.4
Verbal Therapeutic Communication Techniques

Technique	Description	Examples
Encouraging descriptions of perceptions	Asking the patient what they are seeing or hearing	"Tell me what the voices are saying to you."
Encouraging comparison	Asking the patient to compare similarities or differences	"How is this medication working for you compared to the last time you used it?"
Exploring	Looking deeper into a subject, idea, or experience	"Tell me more about the last time you were depressed."
Focusing	Concentrating on a single idea or event	"Tell me more about how your divorce made you feel."
Formulating a plan of action	Assisting the patient to come up with a plan to cope with stress	"When this happens in the future, how could you handle it more constructively?"
Giving broad openings	Allowing the patient to steer the interaction	"What would you like to work on today?"
Giving recognition	Acknowledging or showing awareness	"I see you went to your therapy group today."
Making observations	Verbalizing what is observed	"I noticed you seemed upset after your visit."
Offering self	Extending one's presence	"I am available to talk whenever you would like."
Offering general leads	Giving the patient encouragement to continue	"I see. . . ." "Go on. . . ."
Placing event in time or sequence	Clarification of events in time	"Was this before or after your first hospitalization?"
Presenting reality	Defining reality in simple terms	"The voices may seem real to you, but they are a symptom of your illness."
Restating	Repeating the main idea of what the patient has verbalized	"It sounds as if you are feeling frustrated."
Reflecting	Statements, questions, or feelings are stated back to the patient	"What do you think you should do?"
Seeking clarification	Searching for understanding of what was said	"Tell me if this is what you meant when you said. . . ."
Verbalizing the implied	Putting into words what the patient has implied or said indirectly	"You must be feeling very sad right now."

Table 56.5
Communication Blocks

Mechanism	Description	Examples to Avoid
Agreeing/disagreeing	Implies that the patient's ideas or feelings are somehow right or wrong	"That is right on target. I agree 100%."
Asking "why" questions	Implies that the patient knows the reason for their behavior and feelings	"Why were you feeling so angry?"
Changing the subject	Takes control of the conversation away from the patient	Patient: "I am feeling so hopeless." Nurse: "Did you go to group therapy today?"
Giving advice	Implies that the nurse knows what is best	"I think you should. . . ."
Giving approval or disapproval	Passes judgment on the patient's ideas or opinions	"That sounds like a bad idea."
Giving false reassurance	Devalues the patient's feelings	"Everything will be all right."
Self-focusing behavior	Focuses on nurse's own feelings at the expense of the patient's	"That happened to me once. Let me tell you about it."
Double-bind messages	When the nonverbal message doesn't match the verbal message	"I'm listening," as the nurse fidgets in her chair, doesn't make eye contact, and then coughs.

Barriers to effective communication are called *communication blocks*. A nurse who tells a patient, "Don't worry, everything will be all right," has given false reassurance. This communicates to the patient that their concerns are not taken seriously. Common communication blocks are listed in Table 56.5.

Milieu

One area over which you can have some control is the therapeutic environment. In the mental health setting, this environment is called the **milieu** or therapeutic milieu. It is believed that environment influences behavior. Milieu therapy is the systematic management of the social environment as a treatment modality.

A therapeutic milieu provides containment, support, structure, involvement, and validation during the patient's stay. The goals of milieu therapy are resocialization, ego development, and prevention of regression. Resocialization occurs when patients help govern the running of the mental health unit and attend regular meetings to set rules and assign tasks. Ego development is fostered with structured activities that are provided to assist the patient to learn coping and social skills. Regression is discouraged when patients help with washing dishes or other small jobs that foster independence. Common milieu interventions include role modeling, positive reinforcement, a schedule of events, consistent expectations and rules for behavior, and unit meetings. Milieu therapy is difficult in this era of managed care because of shorter hospital stays.

Psychopharmacology

Psychopharmacology is the use of medications to treat psychological disorders. Since the introduction of the phenothiazine class of drugs in the 1950s, the number of medications for treating mental health disorders has increased greatly, with newer medications having fewer side effects. The reason for using medications is twofold: First, the medications manage the symptoms, helping the patient feel more comfortable emotionally. Second, the patient is generally more receptive and able to focus on other types of therapy if medications are effective. More information on psychoactive drugs is provided in Chapter 57.

Psychotherapy

Psychotherapy is the form of treatment chosen by the psychologist, psychiatrist, social worker, or advanced practice mental health nurse. Goals of psychotherapy include the following:

- Reducing the patient's emotional discomfort.
- Increasing the level of the patient's social functioning.
- Increasing the ability of the patient to behave or perform in a manner appropriate to the situation.

Several specific types of psychotherapy are described next.

• WORD • BUILDING •

psychopharmacology: psycho—soul or mind + pharmaco—drug or medicine + ology—study of
psychotherapy: psycho—soul or mind + therapy—treatment

Psychodynamic Therapy

Psychodynamic therapy is based on **psychoanalysis**. It consists of clarifying the meaning of events, feelings, and behavior, thereby gaining **insight**. Psychoanalysis was developed from Sigmund Freud's psychoanalytic theory. Freud believed that anxiety was the primary motivation for behavior and that all behavior had meaning. The role of the patient is to provide the therapist with clues to the unconscious source of problems and to try to develop insights into behavior. The role of the therapist is to uncover these unconscious experiences and interpret their meanings to the patient. Some believe that psychodynamic therapy will lose popularity as we gain a better understanding of the role of the brain, neurotransmitters, and genetics in mental health.

Behavior Management

Behavior management (also called *behavior modification*) is a treatment method that stems from the studies of behavioral theorists such as B. F. Skinner and Ivan Pavlov. It is a common treatment modality used in extended care facilities, with children and adolescents, and with individuals who have a low level of cognitive functioning.

According to behavior management theory, all behavior is learned; therefore, it can be unlearned. The belief is that behavior can be shaped by either positive or negative reinforcement. *Positive reinforcement* is the act of rewarding the patient with something pleasant when the desired behavior has been performed. For instance, if a patient has a habit of using foul language to fulfill needs, the desired behavior change might be to go to a staff member and ask appropriately for what they need. If this patient loves to be outside but is not allowed out except at supervised times, a suitable positive reinforcement might be to allow 15 more minutes outdoors when desired behavior is exhibited.

Negative reinforcement is the act of responding to the undesired behavior by taking away a privilege or adding a responsibility. Negative reinforcement can be misinterpreted as punishment. Parents who ground their children for unacceptable behavior are using negative reinforcement; requiring the child to perform extra household tasks for a stated period is reinforcing the fact that the behavior has consequences. The child may not repeat the undesired behavior after negative reinforcement has been used.

It is necessary to avoid violating the Patient's Bill of Rights when performing behavior management with patients. A signed consent from the patient is advised when using this form of therapy. The patient must understand the consequences of the behavior to be changed and the purpose for the chosen consequence. If the person is incapable of understanding the situation or unable to remember the consequences, behavior management will be ineffective.

Cognitive Behavioral Therapy

Jean Piaget and Aaron T. Beck are cognitive theorists who have greatly contributed to modern cognitive behavioral therapy. Cognitive behavioral therapists believe that people experience mental illness due to cognitive distortions about their situations. Cognitive behavioral therapy stresses ways of rethinking situations. The therapist confronts the patient with certain distortions of thinking and helps the patient to work out ways of thinking differently. This type of treatment is used frequently for affective or mood disorders.

Feeling sad about an unpleasant experience (such as the death of a loved one) is acceptable and normal. However, long-term depression about the death is an extreme emotion and considered unhealthy. In this situation, therapy may help the patient see the death as a sad loss and begin to move forward. Behavioral techniques are also often used with phobias or panic disorders, in which fear may interfere with reasoning.

Cognitive behavioral therapy is gaining in popularity because it is usually shorter than other types of therapy and therefore less costly to the patient. Patients are given "homework" specific to their needs; they practice their assignments between sessions. Cognitive behavioral therapy in combination with medications can provide effective treatment for depression.

Counseling

Counseling is the provision of help or guidance by an HCP. The profession of counseling is licensed and regulated differently by state and sometimes also by municipality. Nurses prepared at an LPN/LVN level or at an RN level, in some areas and with special advanced education, can practice some forms of counseling.

You may be asked or expected to accompany patients to counseling sessions or facilitate a group discussion. Remember, these are confidential sessions even if they are group-oriented. Patients are there to work; others are there by invitation for specific reasons.

Group Therapy

Therapy groups are formed for many reasons; they can be ongoing or short-term depending on the needs of the patients or type of disorder. Group therapy is a cost-effective means of treatment. For example, Alcoholics Anonymous (AA) and similar 12-step, self-help groups are well-established, ongoing groups formed to treat a specific problem. Family counseling sessions may occur with individual therapists with a specialty in the problem area for that family. Marriage counseling may be done in a group with other couples. Often, peer counselors are used.

Therapists and counselors are tools, or facilitators, in the therapeutic process. Patients must take the suggestions given by the therapist, try them, and see what works for them. You can help by reinforcing the work patients do to stay mentally healthy and develop effective life skills.

• WORD • BUILDING •

psychoanalysis: psycho—soul or mind + analysis—dissolving

> **PRACTICE ANALYSIS TIP**
> **Linking NCLEX-PN® to Practice**
> The LPN/VN will:
> - Use therapeutic communication techniques with client.
> - Reinforce education to caregivers/family on ways to manage client with behavioral disorders.
> - Assist client to cope/adapt to stressful events and changes in health status.
> - Promote a therapeutic environment.
> - Incorporate behavioral management techniques when caring for a client.
> - Identify client use of effective and ineffective coping mechanisms.
> - Collect data regarding client psychosocial functioning.
> - Collect data on client potential for violence to self and others.
> - Participate in client group session.

Electroconvulsive Therapy

Electroconvulsive therapy (ECT) is a form of treatment for severely depressed patients who have not responded to psychotropic medications. ECT passes an electric current through the brain to produce a tonic-clonic (grand mal) seizure. Most mental health professionals believe ECT stimulates an increase in circulating levels of the neurotransmitters serotonin, norepinephrine, and dopamine in the brain. Essentially, ECT affects neurotransmitter activity much like antidepressant medications do. ECT may be frightening to patients; it is important for the nurse to provide education and information to the patient and family. Many changes have been made in this form of therapy since the 1940s, and ECT is currently a safe and effective treatment for resistant depression.

Procedure

ECT often takes place in the recovery room of an operating suite with ready access to emergency equipment. Informed consent must be obtained by the HCP. About 30 minutes before the procedure, the patient is given medication to dry secretions and counteract stimulation of the vagus nerve, which can cause bradycardia and syncope. Patients are given short-acting anesthetic before treatment and a smooth muscle relaxant to minimize injury. Before giving the muscle relaxant, a blood pressure cuff is placed on one of the patient's lower limbs and inflated to ensure that seizure activity can be visually monitored in this limb. Blood pressure and pulse are carefully monitored before and after treatment. The patient is oxygenated with pure oxygen during and after the seizure until spontaneous respirations return. During treatment, an electrical stimulus is delivered to the brain via unilateral or bilateral electrodes. The amount of electrical energy used is individualized to the patient. The seizure must last at least 30 seconds for efficacy. Seizure activity is monitored with an electroencephalogram (EEG) and movement in the cuffed limb.

Side Effects

Side effects of ECT can be unpleasant but are usually temporary. The patient may feel confused and forgetful immediately after the treatment from both the ECT and the medication that was used before the treatment. If the seizure was severe, the patient may have some muscle soreness and report a headache.

ECT is not used indiscriminately. It is used when other therapies have not been helpful and is usually reserved for treatment-resistant depression (see "Patient Perspective").

> **Patient Perspective**
>
> **Ethel**
>
> My mom is 83 years old and has had a total of 35 electroconvulsive therapy (ECT) treatments for severe depression in her lifetime. If you met her, you'd never know; you'd find her delightful. She's a sweet, little, plump German lady with a big heart. I am a nurse, and when I tell fellow nurses about my mom, they often ask me why I didn't get her on antidepressants. I want to scream, "How dumb do you think I am?!" Of course, Mom is on antidepressants. But at intervals they don't work, and she sinks into severe depression. My choice then is to help her have ECT or let her stay depressed and miserable and put her in a nursing home. And she would soon die, because when she is depressed, she refuses to move, doesn't sleep, and is horribly miserable.
>
> The first time my mom was scheduled for ECT, one of the nurses in our local community hospital told her to refuse it, that no one should have to go through that. It was a cruel thing to do. My mom doesn't do well in counseling; she doesn't believe in it. In her mind, you don't talk about your "dirty linen." My mom was in an abusive relationship with my father for 47 years, and she hid all the problems away and doesn't talk about them to this day. I'm so grateful to have my mom doing okay and grateful that ECT treatments exist. With ECT, my mother is doing well and enjoying life. Without treatment, she would be gone. Please understand that there are times when ECT treatments are the best thing for severely depressed people, when other treatments have been ineffective.

Nursing Care

The patient should receive nothing by mouth (NPO) for at least 4 hours before a treatment. Remind the patient to empty his or her bladder and to remove dentures, contact lenses, hair pins, and other items on the body. Following ECT, carefully monitor vital signs and document the patient's subjective and objective responses to the treatment. Stay with the patient until he or she is oriented and able to care for him or herself. Withhold oral medications and food until the gag reflex returns. Ensure that the patient is kept safe after ECT therapy.

CUE RECOGNITION 56.2

Your patient is scheduled for ECT in 1 hour. You find she just had a candy bar and a soda. What do you do?

Suggested answers are at the end of the chapter.

Relaxation Therapy

A variety of relaxation techniques can be taught to help patients manage responses to stress. Relaxation exercises such as deep, rhythmic breathing increase oxygenation and provide distraction from stressors. Breathing exercises may be coupled with progressive muscle relaxation exercises. For this technique, patients are taught to start at the head and neck and systematically tense and then relax muscle groups as they progress toward the lower extremities. Soft music may enhance the patient's ability to fully relax.

Guided **imagery** is the use of the imagination to promote relaxation. For this technique, the patient is assisted to imagine a pleasurable experience from their past, such as lying on a beach or soaking in a warm bath. Use of all senses is encouraged: for a beach image, the patient might see a beach, feel the warm sun, smell salt air, and hear waves crashing against the shore. The patient might also be taught to visualize being successful in a problem situation.

Relaxation techniques may be used individually, but they are often used in combination with each other or with other therapies for maximum effect. See Chapter 5 for more information on relaxation and imagery.

Home Health Hints

- Observe for indications that the patient is at risk of falls, especially if the patient is experiencing orthostatic hypotension from medications.
- Reconcile medications at each visit, checking for missed doses, compliance, and new or discontinued medications.
- Ask depressed patients about suicide ideations at every visit. Report to RN or HCP if needed.

BE SAFE!

BE VIGILANT! During home visits, watch for signs of potential violence such as shouting, verbal abuse, or drug or alcohol misuse, and always have a clear path to an exit in the event the agitation escalates.

Key Points

- Mental health has been defined in many ways and encompasses the ability to be flexible, take responsibility for own actions, form close relationships, make appropriate judgments, solve problems, cope with daily stress, and have a positive sense of self.
- Mental illness can be defined as impaired ability to think, feel, make sound judgments, or adapt, as well as difficulty coping with reality and difficulty forming strong personal relationships.
- Changes in brain structure, chemistry, and function are associated with mental illness.
- Although mental illnesses can be categorized as brain diseases, not all brain diseases are mental illnesses.
- Collecting data from a patient with mental illness includes a mental status examination. This series of questions, activities, and observations evaluates eight areas: appearance and behavior, level of awareness and reality orientation, thinking/content of thought, memory, speech and ability to communicate, mood and affect, judgment, and perception.
- The diagnostic tool used most widely by psychiatrists and other mental health professionals is the *DSM-5*, which groups illnesses into categories of clinical disorders. It is a complex diagnostic tool.
- Some disorders mimic mental health disorders, so the following diagnostic tests may be performed to confirm or rule out a diagnosis of a mental illness: laboratory tests, CT scans, MRI, and PET scans.
- Effective coping skills offer healthy choices for dealing with stressors. Individuals might use humor, prayer, exercise, or problem-solving, for example. Effective coping skills are also conscious mechanisms.
- Sometimes coping behaviors are ineffective. When conscious techniques are not successful, people may unconsciously fall into habits that give the illusion of coping.
- When these ego defense mechanisms are overused or used alone for anxiety, they can become ineffective and unhealthy.
- People who experience alterations in their mental health have special treatment needs. Cognitive ability can be impaired. Emotional responses can be decreased or even absent in some conditions.
- Therapeutic communication is accomplished through the deliberate use of verbal and nonverbal techniques. Other areas to consider are the patient's personal values, attitudes, beliefs, culture, religion, social status, gender, and age or developmental level.
- Components of *nonverbal communication* include physical appearance, dress, body movement and posture, touch, facial expression, and eye contact.
- In the mental health setting, the therapeutic environment is called the *milieu* or *therapeutic milieu*. It is believed that environment influences behavior.

- Psychotherapy is the form of treatment chosen by the psychologist, psychiatrist, social worker, or advanced practice mental health nurse.
- Psychodynamic therapy is based on psychoanalysis. It consists of clarifying the meaning of events, feelings, and behavior, thereby gaining insight into them.
- According to behavior management theory, all behavior is learned and can be unlearned with positive or negative reinforcement.
- Cognitive behavioral therapists believe that people experience mental illness due to cognitive distortions about their situations. Cognitive behavioral therapy stresses ways of rethinking situations. The therapist confronts the patient with certain distortions of thinking and then helps the patient to work out ways of thinking about them differently.
- Group therapy is a cost-effective means of providing treatment.
- ECT is used for severely depressed patients who have not responded to psychotropic medications. Mental health professionals believe ECT affects neurotransmitter activity much like antidepressant medications.
- Relaxation techniques can help patients manage their responses to stress. Relaxation exercises such as deep, rhythmic breathing can increase oxygenation and provide distraction from stressors.

SUGGESTED ANSWERS TO CHAPTER EXERCISES

Cue Recognition

56.1: The patient is displaying denial.

56.2: Notify the provider, who will likely cancel the procedure.

Critical Thinking & Clinical Judgment

Mr. Joseph

Different people cope in different ways. This may be a healthy way to cope in this grieving husband's culture. Gently guide him to a room where he can express his emotions without disturbing others. Ask if he would like you to contact someone to come help support him. Document objectively: "Patient's husband weeping loudly; guided to consultation room for privacy." As an LPN/LVN, your best course of action may be to report the RN's comment objectively to your supervisor.

Mrs. Beison

1. Mrs. Beison is overusing the ego defense mechanism denial to cope with her cancer diagnosis. Although at times denial can be an effective coping mechanism, if Mrs. Beison continues to deny her disease and refuse treatment, her life will be in danger.
2. You can help Mrs. Beison verbalize her fears about cancer and cancer treatment, and provide accurate information to help her make wise choices. If needed, a psychiatric evaluation can be requested. If she is found to be mentally competent, then her wishes must be respected.

Additional Resources

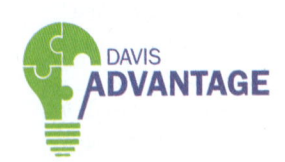

Go to Davis Advantage to complete your learning: strengthen understanding, apply your knowledge, and prepare for the Next Gen NCLEX®.

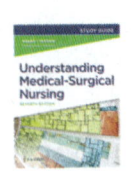

A Study Guide is also available.

CHAPTER 57
Nursing Care of Patients With Mental Health Disorders

Marina Martinez-Kratz

KEY TERMS

abuse (uh-BYOOS)
addiction (ah-DIK-shun)
alogia (ah-LOH-jee-uh)
anhedonia (AN-heh-DOH-nee-uh)
anorexia nervosa (AN-uh-REK-see-ah nur-VOH-sah)
avolition (A-voh-LISH-un)
bipolar (bye-POH-lur)
bulimia nervosa (buh-LEE-mee-ah ner-VOH-sah)
codependence (KOH-dee-PEN-dense)
compulsion (kum-PUHL-shun)
delirium tremens (dee-LEER-ee-um TREE-menz)
delusions (dee-LOO-zhuns)
dependence (dee-PEN-dense)
displacement (dis-PLACE-ment)
dysfunctional (dis-FUNK-shun-uhl)
eustress (YOO-stress)
hallucinations (hah-LOO-sih-NAY-shuns)
illusions (ih-LOO-zhuns)
mania (MAY-nee-ah)
obsession (ob-SESH-un)
phobia (FOH-bee-ah)
tolerance (TALL-er-ense)
withdrawal (with-DRAW-ul)

CHAPTER CONCEPTS

Addiction
Behaviors
Cognition
Communication
Family
Mood and affect
Self
Stress and coping

LEARNING OUTCOMES

1. Identify etiological theories for common mental health disorders.
2. Describe signs and symptoms of common mental health disorders.
3. Describe therapeutic management for each of the disorders.
4. Identify actions, side effects, and nursing considerations for selected classifications of psychoactive medications.
5. Plan nursing interventions for patients with mental health disorders.
6. Discuss the role of the licensed practical nurse/licensed vocational nurse (LPN/LVN) in the care of patients with mental health disorders.

As we saw in Chapter 56, people with mental health problems may experience impaired ability to think, feel, make sound judgments, adapt to changes, cope with stressors, and form strong relationships with others. This chapter covers some of the more common mental health disorders you will see in medical, surgical, and extended care settings. Patients with mental health disorders may need modified care planning to help them manage both mental and physiological illnesses.

ANXIETY DISORDERS, OBSESSIVE-COMPULSIVE AND RELATED DISORDERS, AND TRAUMA- AND STRESSOR-RELATED DISORDERS

Anxiety Disorders

Do you ever experience stress? How does it make you feel? Is it possible to live a completely stress-free existence? Stress is everywhere in our society. It produces anxiety and is most often associated with negative situations. However, the good things that happen to us, such as a marriage or a job promotion, also produce stress. The stress from positive experiences is called **eustress**. Eustress can produce just as much anxiety as negative stressors. A *stressor* is any person or situation that produces an anxiety response. Stress and stressors are different for each person; therefore, it is important to ask patients what their personal stress producers are.

• WORD • BUILDING •
eustress: eu—normal or good + stress

Anxiety is the uncomfortable feeling of dread in response to extreme or prolonged periods of stress. It is commonly ranked as mild, moderate, severe, or panic. It is believed that mild anxiety is a normal part of being human that helps us develop new ways of coping with stress.

Anxiety may also be influenced by one's culture. For example, it may be acceptable for some groups to acknowledge and discuss stress, while other cultures may believe that discussing personal problems is inappropriate. Understanding how cultural beliefs influence behaviors can be complicated and can make assessment challenging. The nurse should approach behavioral data collection by documenting observed behaviors and voiced patient and family concerns, ensuring that documentation is judgment-free and sticks to the facts.

Anxiety is usually called either *free-floating anxiety* or *signal anxiety*. Free-floating anxiety is described as a general feeling of impending doom. The person cannot pinpoint the cause but might say something like, "I just know something bad is going to happen if I go on vacation." Signal anxiety is an uncomfortable response to a known stressor ("Finals are only a week away, and I've got nausea again"). Both types of anxiety are involved in various anxiety disorders.

Etiological Theories

Psychoanalytical theorists believe that anxiety is a conflict between the *id* (the "all for me" part of the personality) and the *superego* (the conscience), which is repressed in early development but emerges again in adulthood.

Biological theorists view anxiety differently. One biological theory points to the sympathoadrenal (fight-or-flight) responses to stress to explain signs and symptoms of anxiety. This theory notes that blood vessels constrict because epinephrine and norepinephrine have been released, causing blood pressure to rise. Another biological theory implicates a lack of the neurotransmitter gamma-aminobutyric acid (GABA) in anxiety. GABA is an inhibitory neurotransmitter that prevents postsynaptic excitation.

If the body adapts to the stress, hormone levels adjust and body functions return to a homeostatic state. If the body does not adapt to the stress, the immune system is challenged and risk for physical illness increases.

You may observe psychological responses to physical illness. It is important to recognize the relationship between physical and emotional responses to stress. Some examples of medical conditions that occur because of the body's response to stress are shown in Table 57.1.

Diagnosis

Because so many symptoms are associated with anxiety disorders, it is important for patients to have a complete physical examination before an anxiety disorder is diagnosed. Some medical disorders, such as hyperthyroidism, can mimic anxiety; hypothyroidism can mimic depression.

Types of Anxiety

SPECIFIC PHOBIA. Specific **phobias** are the most common anxiety disorder. There are more than 700 documented phobias. Specific phobias are defined as irrational fears of distinct objects or situations, such as snakes, bridges, or flying. The person is very aware of the fear, and even the fact that it is irrational, but cannot gain control over the stressor. Therefore, the fear continues.

The psychoanalytic view implies that it really is not the object that is the source of fear but that the fear results from defense mechanism called **displacement**. For example, the person with a phobia of snakes may have seen a frightening movie in which someone died from a snakebite. The object of the phobia would be a symbol for the underlying cause, such as fear of dying.

SOCIAL ANXIETY DISORDER (SOCIAL PHOBIA). Social anxiety disorder is a social phobia characterized by a persistent fear of behaving or performing in a way that will be embarrassing or humiliating. Examples include public speaking, eating in front of others, or using public restrooms. The fear is disproportionate to the situation.

PANIC DISORDER. Panic is a state of extreme fear that cannot be controlled; it may be referred to as a *panic attack*. Panic episodes are recurrent and occur unpredictably. Patients may present at the emergency department because they believe they are having a heart attack or other significant physical illness. Patients must exhibit several episodes within a specified time frame to be given the diagnosis of panic disorder. Some of the symptoms associated with panic disorder include the following:

- Fear (usually of dying, losing control of oneself, or "going crazy")
- Feelings of impending doom
- Dissociation (feeling that it is happening to someone else or not happening at all)
- Nausea
- Diaphoresis
- Chest pain
- Palpitations
- Shaking

GENERALIZED ANXIETY DISORDER. In generalized anxiety disorder (GAD), the anxiety itself (also referred to as *excessive worry* or *severe stress*) is the expressed symptom. Patients with GAD worry about everything. Symptoms that may be present in GAD include the following:

- Restlessness or feeling "on edge"
- Shaking
- Palpitations
- Dry mouth
- Nausea and/or vomiting
- Being easily frightened
- Hot flashes
- Chills
- Muscle aches
- Hypervigilance (excessive attention to stimuli)
- Polyuria
- Difficulty swallowing

Nursing care of patients with anxiety is discussed after "Trauma- and Stressor-Related Disorders."

Table 57.1 Responses to Stress

Stress-Related Medical Condition	Pathophysiology	Outcome of Stress on the Body
Lowered immunity	Stress interferes with effectiveness of antibodies Possibly related to interactions among the hypothalamus, pituitary gland, adrenal glands, and immune system	Increased susceptibility to colds and other viruses and illnesses
Burnout	Stress- or work-related emotional exhaustion and depression	Emotional detachment
Migraine, cluster, and tension headaches	Tightening of skeletal muscles Dilating of cranial arteries	Nausea, vomiting, tight feeling in or around head and shoulders, tinnitus, inability to tolerate light, weakness of a limb
Hypertension	Role of stress not positively known Thought to contribute to hypertension by negatively interacting with kidneys, autonomic nervous system, and endocrine system	Resistance to blood flow through the cardiovascular system, causing pressure on the arteries Can lead to stroke, heart attack, and kidney failure
Coronary artery disease	Not fully understood Stress may be associated with behavioral factors such as overeating, physical inactivity, and obesity.	Hypertension, hypercholesterolemia, atherosclerosis, diabetes
Cancer	Stress lowers the immune response.	Lowered immunity may allow for overcolonization of opportunistic cancer cells.
Asthma	Autonomic (parasympathetic) nervous system stimulates mucus, increases blood flow, and constricts airways. May be associated with other stress-related conditions such as allergy and viral infection	Wheezing, coughing, dyspnea, apprehension May lead to respiratory infections, respiratory failure, or pneumothorax

Obsessive-Compulsive and Related Disorders

The *Diagnostic and Statistical Manual of Mental Disorders, Fifth Edition*, or *DSM-5* (American Psychiatric Association, 2013), groups obsessive-compulsive and related disorders in a distinct category separate from the anxiety disorders. Disorders in this category have common features such as obsessive preoccupation and repetitive behaviors and include obsessive-compulsive disorder, body dysmorphic disorder, and trichotillomania (hair-pulling disorder) as well as two new disorders: hoarding disorder and excoriation (skin-picking) disorder.

Obsessive-Compulsive Disorder

Obsessive-compulsive disorder (OCD) occurs in 2% to 3% of the adult population in the United States. It is the fourth-most common psychiatric diagnosis. It consists of two parts: the **obsession** (repetitive thought, urge, or images) and the **compulsion** (an excessive or unrealistic repetitive act that the individual feels driven to perform in response to the obsession). An example of OCD is the need to check that doors are locked numerous times before one can sleep or leave the house. This need may prevent the person from sleeping or leaving the house at all. Some individuals wash hands compulsively to the point of having raw and bleeding hands. Behaviors become ritualistic, and the person cannot stop the thought or the action. Performing the action (such as checking the locks or hand washing) is the mechanism that reduces anxiety. Although the nurse should not interfere with repetitive acts, OCD patients can be helped by therapeutic interventions such as cognitive behavioral therapy or medications such as fluoxetine (Prozac). Nursing care of patients with OCD is discussed after "Trauma- and Stressor-Related Disorders."

Trauma- and Stressor-Related Disorders

The *DSM-5* groups trauma- and stressor-related disorders. Patients diagnosed have been exposed to a traumatic or stressful event, such as war or natural disaster, and experience specific symptoms. Disorders in this category are posttraumatic stress disorder (PTSD), reactive attachment disorder, disinhibited social engagement disorder, acute stress disorder, and adjustment disorders.

Posttraumatic Stress Disorder

PTSD develops in response to some unexpected emotional or physical trauma with a *real threat of death or harm* in which the patient was helpless. People who have fought in wars, been raped, survived violence or natural disaster, or survived severe illness (such as COVID-19) are some who are susceptible to suffering from PTSD.

An associated condition is *survivor guilt* expressed by those who have survived a tragedy. A survivor of an airline crash may say, "Why me? Why did I make it? I should have died too!" This is especially true if a loved one died in the tragedy.

Symptoms may appear immediately or not until years later. A key symptom of PTSD is *flashbacks* in which the person relives the traumatic event as if it were happening that moment. Sounds and smells associated with the trauma may trigger the flashback.

Signs and symptoms of PTSD include the following:

- Flashbacks or dissociative reactions
- Recurrent intrusive memories of the traumatic event
- Recurrent intrusive dreams/nightmares related to the traumatic event
- Intense psychological distress at exposure to internal or external cues that resemble an aspect of the traumatic event
- Marked physical reaction to internal or external cues that resemble an aspect of the traumatic event
- Persistent avoidance of stimuli associated with the traumatic event
- Social withdrawal
- Feelings of low self-esteem
- Changes in relationships with significant others
- Difficulty forming new relationships
- Hypervigilance
- Irritability and outbursts of anger seemingly for no obvious reason
- Depression
- Chemical dependency

Therapeutic Measures for Patients With Anxiety, Obsessive-Compulsive, or Trauma-Related Disorders

Treatment for these disorders is individualized and may include one or more of the following: medications (psychopharmacology), individual psychotherapy, group therapy, systematic desensitization, hypnosis, imagery, relaxation exercises, and biofeedback.

Psychopharmacology may involve benzodiazepines, an antianxiety classification of medications. Benzodiazepines are used for short-term treatment because of the strong potential for dependency. Individuals who need long-term therapy for anxiety or have chemical dependency tendencies may be treated with buspirone (BuSpar), selective serotonin reuptake inhibitors (SSRIs), the sedating antihistamine hydroxyzine hydrochloride (Atarax) or hydroxyzine pamoate (Vistaril), or the antihypertensive agent clonidine (Catapres). Table 57.2 provides a review of medications.

In *systematic desensitization*, the patient is exposed gradually (rating the fear on a scale from 1 to 10) to the object that causes anxiety. *Hypnosis* places the patient in a subconscious state and helps them recall and subsequently deal with events that may be producing anxiety. A meta-analysis showed that hypnosis was more effective in reducing anxiety when combined with other psychological interventions than as a stand-alone treatment (Valentine et al, 2019). Additional therapies are discussed in Chapter 56.

Nursing Process for the Patient With an Anxiety, Obsessive-Compulsive, or Trauma-Related Disorder

Data Collection

Observe the patient's anxiety level and level of functioning. Ask about triggers of anxiety and coping mechanisms that have been successful or unsuccessful in the past. Stay alert for physical symptoms such as changes in vital signs, diaphoresis, or tremor. Ask about suicidal thoughts and observe for suicidal behavior. It is important to identify anxiety and intervene at lower levels before escalation to severe or panic anxiety levels (Table 57.3).

Nursing Diagnoses, Planning, and Implementation

> **Anxiety related to response to stressors**
>
> **EXPECTED OUTCOME:** The patient will verbalize that anxiety is controlled. The patient will identify triggers and patterns for anxiety and demonstrate techniques to control anxiety. Physical signs of anxiety, such as tremors or changes in vital signs, will be absent.

- Assist the patient to identify triggers of and patterns to anxiety. *Recognition of patterns can help guide care and allow the patient to initiate measures to stop anxiety from progressing.*
- Maintain a calm milieu and manner. *A chaotic environment can increase the patient's anxiety. Anxiety is contagious and may be transmitted from staff to patient.*
- Maintain open communication. Encourage the patient to verbalize thoughts and feelings. Observe nonverbal communication. *Honesty in dealing with patients helps them learn to trust others and enhances their self-esteem.*

Table 57.2
Medications Used for Alterations in Mental Health

Medication Class/Action

Typical Antipsychotics

Block mainly D_2 dopamine receptors (used less often because of serious extrapyramidal side effects).

Examples	*Nursing Implications*
chlorpromazine (Thorazine) haloperidol (Haldol) fluphenazine (Prolixin) trifluoperazine (Stelazine)	For short-term use because of side effects. Monitor for extrapyramidal side effects. Have patient rise slowly to counter orthostatic hypotension. Offer ice chips, gum, or hard candy for dry mouth. Monitor urinary and bowel elimination. Do not use/take with alcohol or other central nervous system (CNS) depressants. *Teach:* Use sunscreen when outside.

Atypical Antipsychotics

Block multiple dopamine and serotonin receptors.

Examples	*Nursing Implications*
asenapine (Saphris) clozapine (Clozaril) lurasidone (Latuda) risperidone (Risperdal, Risperdol Consta) olanzapine (Zyprexa) quetiapine (Seroquel, Seroquel XR) ziprasidone (Geodon) aripiprazole (Abilify, Abilify Maintena) paliperidone (Invega, Invega Sustenna)	Monitor complete blood count for clozapine. Monitor for weight gain. Monitor glucose level for onset of type 2 diabetes. Use gloves when administering risperidone. Long-acting injections are administered weekly to monthly to improve patient compliance. *Teach:* Take lurasidone with food. Sublingual forms can dissolve in hands; make sure hands are dry and take immediately. Do not eat or drink for 10 minutes.

Antidepressants

Selective Serotonin Reuptake Inhibitor (SSRIs)
Block the reuptake of serotonin at the presynaptic receptor.

Examples	*Nursing Implications*
fluoxetine (Prozac) sertraline (Zoloft) paroxetine (Paxil) escitalopram (Lexapro) citalopram (Celexa) fluvoxamine (Luvox) trazodone (Desyrel)	Allow time for side effects to subside. Do not administer after 1500 to keep excitation from affecting sleep. *Teach:* Takes 6–8 weeks for therapeutic effects to occur. Do not stop drug abruptly. Do not take with other serotonin-type medications including St. John's wort and S-adenosyl-L-methionine (SAMe).

Continued

Table 57.2
Medications Used for Alterations in Mental Health—cont'd

Medication Class/Action

Tricyclic Antidepressants
Partially block the reuptake of serotonin and norepinephrine at the presynaptic receptor; used infrequently because of side effects.

Examples	*Nursing Implications*
amitriptyline (Elavil) nortriptyline (Pamelor) imipramine (Tofranil)	Decreases effects of antihypertensives. Lowers seizure threshold. Will affect oral contraceptives. *Teach:* Takes 6–8 weeks for therapeutic effects to occur. Do not stop drug abruptly. Overdose can cause fatal arrhythmias.

Selective Serotonin Norepinephrine Reuptake Inhibitors (SNRIs)
Block the reuptake of serotonin and norepinephrine.

Examples	*Nursing Implications*
venlafaxine (Effexor, Effexor XR) duloxetine (Cymbalta) desvenlafaxine (Pristiq)	Monitor blood pressure for systolic hypertension. *Teach:* Do not take with other serotonin-type medications, including St. John's wort and SAMe. Do not stop drug abruptly.

Tetracyclic Antidepressants
Block multiple serotonin and histamine receptors; adreno receptor antagonist.

Examples	*Nursing Implications*
mirtazapine (Remeron) maprotiline (Ludiomil)	Administer at bedtime to counteract sedating effects. *Teach:* Do not take with alcohol or other CNS depressants.

Norepinephrine-Dopamine Reuptake Inhibitor (NDRI)
Inhibits reuptake of norepinephrine and dopamine.

Examples	*Nursing Implications*
bupropion (Wellbutrin, Zyban)	May be prescribed for smoking cessation.

Antianxiety Agents

Benzodiazepines
Potentiate effects of gamma-aminobutyric acid (GABA), which causes a calming effect.

Examples	*Nursing Implications*
alprazolam (Xanax) diazepam (Valium) lorazepam (Ativan) clonazepam (Klonopin)	For short-term use only; can be addictive. Use cautiously in older adults. Do not use in pregnant patients. *Teach:* Do not operate heavy machinery. Do not stop drug abruptly.

BuSpar
Action is unknown.

Examples	*Nursing Implications*
buspirone (BuSpar)	Non–habit-forming with little sedating effect. *Teach:* Takes 3–6 weeks for drug to work.

Table 57.2
Medications Used for Alterations in Mental Health—cont'd

Medication Class/Action

Anticonvulsant Mood Stabilizers

Antikindling effect; affect GABA receptors.

Examples	*Nursing Implications*
carbamazepine (Tegretol)	Loading dose may be ordered for acute mania.
lamotrigine (Lamictal)	Monitor for bleeding.
valproic acid (Depakote)	Use cautiously in older adults and in patients with liver or renal disease.
	Do not use in pregnant or breastfeeding patients.
	Teach:
	Use sunscreen.
	Report any signs of rash immediately.

Antimanic Agent

Lithium
Decreases postsynaptic receptor sensitivity.

Example	*Nursing Implications*
lithium carbonate (Eskalith)	Narrow therapeutic range increases risk of toxicity.
	Monitor blood levels.
	Do not use in cardiac or renal disease.
	Do not use with diuretics.
	Do not use in pregnant patients.
	Check interactions with other medications.

Antiparkinsonian Agents
Restore the natural balance of acetylcholine and dopamine in the CNS to manage extrapyramidal side effects.

Examples	*Nursing Implications*
benztropine (Cogentin)	Caution in patients with hypersensitivity, glaucoma, or history of urine retention.
trihexyphenidyl (Artane)	
diphenhydramine (Benadryl)	

Table 57.3
Anxiety Summary

Signs and Symptoms	*Phobia:* Irrational fear of object or situation
	Panic disorder: Extreme fear, feelings of impending doom, palpitations
	Generalized anxiety disorder: Worry, restlessness, palpitations
Diagnosis	History of symptoms; physical causes for symptoms must be ruled out first
Therapeutic Measures	Antianxiety medication
	Selective serotonin reuptake inhibitors
	Systematic desensitization
	Psychotherapy
	Relaxation exercises
Primary Nursing Diagnosis	*Anxiety*

- Encourage patient to use positive self-talk, such as, "I can do this. Anxiety can't kill me." *This helps patient replace negative anxious thoughts with positive statements to reduce anxiety.*
- Report and document any changes in behavior, such as positive or negative alterations in the way a patient responds to the nursing staff, the treatment plan, or other people and situations. *Any change can be significant to the patient's care.*
- Encourage activities but avoid placing the patient in a competitive situation. *Activities that are enjoyable and nonstressful provide diversion and give staff members an opportunity to provide positive feedback about the progress the patient is making. Competitive situations can produce anxiety.*
- Encourage problem-solving and assist to develop alternative solutions. Help the patient to identify what has worked in the past. *This can help the patient focus on strategies that were effective in the past and eliminate those that are ineffective.*
- Stay with a patient during acute severe or panic levels of anxiety. *Feelings of being abandoned can increase anxiety. The nurse's presence provides a feeling of safety for the patient.*
- Implement suicide precautions if indicated. *The patient may need to be protected from self-harm until treatment is effective.*
- Consider your own level of anxiety. *An anxious nurse may make the patient more anxious.*

Evaluation

The patient will be able to implement strategies to control anxiety, recognize triggers of anxiety, and state they feel less anxious. Physical signs, such as tremors or changes in vital signs, will be improved.

> **CLINICAL JUDGMENT**
>
> **Tommy** has come to the clinic with numerous cracks on his hands. They are bleeding and very sore. Tommy tells you that he has to wash his hands all the time. His mother says he washes for 2 to 3 hours at a time, and he will not stop when she tells him to. The doctor has diagnosed Tommy with obsessive-compulsive disorder and has explained the illness to Tommy and his mother. When the doctor leaves the room, Tommy's mother begins to cry. "What did he just say? What am I supposed to do? What did I do wrong that Tommy got this illness?"
>
> How can you respond therapeutically? What team member would you use as a resource?
>
> *Suggested answers are at the end of the chapter.*

MOOD DISORDERS

Mood disorders (also called *affective disorders*) are disorders in which the major symptom is extreme changes or instability in mood (emotions) and affect (the outward expression of the mood). Moods involving both highs and lows are bipolar disorders; low moods without highs are depressive disorders. Mood disorders are diagnosed when symptoms interfere with normal daily functioning. People of all ages and ethnic and socioeconomic groups develop mood disorders.

Etiological Theories

Psychoanalytic theory explains that people who have suffered loss are at risk for developing depression. Depression is also associated with unresolved anger and has been described as "anger turned inward." In other words, people who cannot or do not deal appropriately with anger may turn these feelings within and become depressed.

Cognitive theorists believe the ways people perceive events and situations may lead to depression. Instead of being disappointed in oneself for failing an exam, people with tendencies toward depression may exaggerate the emotion and turn the situation into something much deeper, such as thoughts of "I'm stupid" or "I'll never get anywhere."

Biological theories offer genetic links and neurotransmitter dysfunctions as two etiologies. Serotonin, norepinephrine, and dopamine influence mood. If these neurotransmitters are elevated, mood is elevated; if they are low, mood is low. Some biological theorists also believe that there is a connection between these neurotransmitters and female hormones.

Differential Diagnosis

Symptoms of depression may occur in conjunction with those of other disorders, such as schizophrenia or drug side effects or overuse. Heart failure, nutritional deficiencies, drug toxicity, thyroid disease, fluid and electrolyte imbalances, infections, and diabetes can be associated with depression. Physical causes for symptoms must be ruled out before a diagnosis of depression can be made. A common assessment scale used by many providers is the Patient Health Questionnaire (PHQ-9). You can access it for use at https://patient.info/doctor/patient-health-questionnaire-phq-9.

Types of Mood Disorders

Major (Unipolar) Depression

Major depression is an episodic condition. Its symptoms interfere with the person's usual social or occupational functioning. Depressed people may be described as viewing the world through "gray-tinted glasses." The *DSM-5* specifies that symptoms of major depression include either depressed mood or **anhedonia** (loss of pleasure in things that are usually pleasurable) along with at least five of the following symptoms:

- Significant weight loss or gain—more than 5% in a month
- Increase or decrease in appetite
- Sleep pattern disturbances—insomnia or hypersomnia
- Increased fatigue or loss of energy
- Increased agitation or psychomotor retardation

• WORD • BUILDING •

anhedonia: an—not + hedonia—pleasure

- Decreased ability to think, remember, or concentrate
- Feelings of guilt or hopelessness
- Indecisiveness
- Suicidal ideation

Bipolar Disorder

About 4.4 percent of people in the United States eventually develop **bipolar** disorder (National Institute of Mental Health [NIMH], 2021). Formerly called *manic depressive illness*, bipolar disorder is a mood disorder in which patients experience the mood states of **mania** (extreme elation or agitation) and extreme depression. Bipolar depression is more severe than major depression. Affected people stay depressed longer, relapse more often, display more depressive symptoms, have more delusions and hallucinations, commit suicide more often, require more hospitalizations, and overall experience more disability.

Affected people can cycle slowly (over weeks, months, or even years), or they can be "rapid cyclers" who change moods several times in an hour. Research indicates that individuals with bipolar disorder may not experience periods of normal mood alternating with periods of abnormal mood as previously believed. Instead, some bipolar illness is characterized by frequent mood lability, with both manic and depressive symptoms, that are sometimes milder and sometimes more severe (Chakrabarty et al, 2020).

Common signs of major depression were covered in the preceding section. Common signs of mania include the following:

- Excessive high (euphoric) moods lasting at least 1 week
- Increased energy, activity, and restlessness
- Decreased need for sleep
- Grandiosity (unrealistic belief in one's abilities or powers)
- Extreme irritability and distractibility
- Uncharacteristically poor judgment
- Pressured and rapid speech
- Flight of ideas or subjective experience that one's thoughts are racing
- Increase in goal-directed behavior
- Excessive involvement in pleasurable activities that have a high potential for unpleasant consequences, such as sex, substance abuse, or shopping sprees
- Obnoxious, provocative, or intrusive behavior

Therapeutic Measures for Patients With Mood Disorders

Most people with major depression respond to treatment. Bipolar disorder is more difficult to treat. Some common medical treatments for *all* mood disorders include the following:

- Antidepressant medications
- Mood stabilizers
- Psychotherapy
- Electroconvulsive therapy (ECT)

Lithium was once the drug of choice for bipolar disorder. This antimanic medication has a very narrow therapeutic range, so toxic drug levels can easily develop. Blood must be drawn regularly to assess for serum lithium levels in the therapeutic range. It is infrequently used today.

Mood stabilizers, such as the anticonvulsants valproic acid (Depakote) and lamotrigine (Lamictal), are now more common than lithium to treat bipolar disorder. Atypical antipsychotics are also commonly used with a mood stabilizer when the patient is in an acute manic state. Antidepressant agents, if used, should be monitored carefully because they can trigger a manic episode. See Table 57.2 for a summary of medications. Also see "Nutrition Notes."

Psychotherapy for the patient and family may be helpful for any type of mood disorder. It can help the patient understand the illness and learn problem-solving and other adaptive coping behaviors. For young children, play therapy is the most common and effective form of therapy. ECT is an option for individuals with rapid-cycling bipolar disorder or major depression that is not responsive to conventional treatment.

Nutrition Notes

Food-Drug Interactions in Patients Taking Lithium

Lithium carbonate (Eskalith), used to treat bipolar disorder, is absorbed, distributed, and excreted alongside sodium. Fluctuations in sodium and caffeine intake may affect lithium metabolism and should remain consistent while a patient is being treated with lithium:

- Decreased sodium and caffeine or caffeine intake with decreased fluid intake may lead to retention of lithium and overmedication.
- Increased sodium or caffeine intake from food or medications and increased fluid intake may hasten excretion of lithium, resulting in worsening signs and symptoms of mania.

Reference: National Alliance on Mental Illness. (2019). Lithium. https://nami.org/About-Mental-Illness/Treatments/Mental-Health-Medications/Types-of-Medication/Lithium

---

BE SAFE!

BE VIGILANT! When collecting data from your patient, ask about herbal supplements and over-the-counter (OTC) medications they use in addition to prescription medications. Many people take St. John's wort, an OTC herbal supplement, for depression. Although it may be effective for some people with mild depression, it can interact with many prescribed medications that influence serotonin levels. If combined with prescription serotonin-type antidepressants, it can cause serotonin syndrome, an excess of serotonin resulting in agitation, confusion, diarrhea, muscle spasms, and even death (Bartlett, 2017).

CLINICAL JUDGMENT

Mr. Zenz is the director of nursing at an extended care facility. His usual behavior is rather sullen, and he comes across as quiet or sad to various members of the staff. His management style at the facility is to let people do their jobs; he rarely interferes unless staff let him know of a problem. Recently, however, staff members have noticed a change in Mr. Zenz. He spends more time interacting with staff and residents. He moves quickly, speaks loudly, and has set unrealistic goals for the staff. He frequently says he has called the owner of the facility to tell him of his new ideas. He says he has not slept in several days, and he feels terrific. He has changed his wardrobe and has begun pointing out specific performance issues to staff. He jokes with staff. Staff members are made aware that he has bipolar disorder and has quit taking his medications. His wife has asked for the staff's help. Remember: He is your boss.

How do you respond to Mrs. Zenz? How do you approach Mr. Zenz?

Suggested answers are at the end of the chapter.

Nursing Process for the Patient With a Mood Disorder

See "Nursing Care Plan for the Patient With Depression." Also see Table 57.4.

Nursing Care Plan for the Patient With Depression

Nursing Diagnosis: *Ineffective Coping*
Expected Outcomes: The patient will cope effectively as evidenced by verbalizing the ability to cope and asking for help when needed and by demonstrating new effective coping strategies.
Evaluation of Outcomes: Does the patient exhibit increased ability to problem-solve and cope with stressors?

Intervention	Rationale	Evaluation
Use therapeutic communication techniques to allow patient to verbalize feelings.	Verbalization of feelings in a supportive environment can assist patient to work through issues.	Does patient verbalize feelings to nursing staff?
Assist patient to describe stressors and identify their existing coping skills and knowledge.	Providing validation of actual stress and available coping resources and strategies aids in positive adaptation to stress.	Is patient able to identify stressors? Does patient have some effective coping skills on which to draw?
Help patient set realistic goals.	Achievement of small steps toward a goal can help the patient feel empowered.	Does patient set realistic goals?
Encourage patient to make choices and participate in care.	Active involvement in care increases the possibility of positive adjustment.	Is patient actively involved in care?

Nursing Diagnosis: *Powerlessness*
Expected Outcomes: The patient will have reduced feelings of powerlessness as evidenced by verbal expression of having control over life, situation, or care and by participation in care or decision making when opportunities are provided.
Evaluation of Outcomes: Does the patient identify feelings of powerlessness? Does the patient identify factors that are controllable and actively participate in care?

Intervention	Rationale	Evaluation
Assist the patient to identify factors contributing to powerlessness.	Correct identification of actual or perceived problems is essential to providing appropriate support.	Is patient able to identify factors contributing to powerlessness?
Help patient to identify factors that are or are not under their control.	Identifying factors within patient's control encourages patient to take some control over the situation.	Is patient able to identify what is controllable and what is not controllable in their life?
Allow ventilation of powerless feelings.	Sharing feelings in groups can lead to the realization that similar feelings are experienced by others and reduce feelings of powerlessness.	Is patient sharing feelings with nursing staff and in therapeutic groups?
Encourage patient to actively participate in care with goal-directed activities.	Goal-directed behavior increases self-efficacy and empowerment.	Does patient set realistic goals daily and achieve them daily?

Nursing Care Plan for the Patient With Depression—cont'd

Nursing Diagnosis: *Risk for Suicidal Behavior*
Expected Outcome: The patient will not cause self-harm.
Evaluation of Outcome: Did the patient remain free from self-harm during hospitalization? Does the patient have ongoing support following discharge?

Intervention	Rationale	Evaluation
Ask patient directly about suicidal ideations each shift.	*Ongoing assessment of suicidal risk is essential to patient safety.*	Is patient verbalizing warning signs of suicide?
Create a safe environment for patient.	*Patient safety is a nursing priority.*	Are means of harming self kept from patient?
Initiate suicide precautions according to agency protocol.	*Patient must be protected until risk is reduced.*	Is increased surveillance of patient implemented and communicated to all staff?
Encourage patient to seek out nursing staff when experiencing suicidal thoughts.	*Active listening and therapeutic communication by staff provide patient with empathy and alternatives to acting on suicidal thoughts.*	Does patient seek out nursing staff when experiencing suicidal thoughts?

Healthy People 2030 (Office of Disease Prevention and Health Promotion, 2020) has an objective to reduce suicides from 14.2 to 12.8 suicides per 100,000 population by 2030.

SCHIZOPHRENIA

Schizophrenia is becoming more widely viewed as a group of illnesses rather than a single condition. The term *schizophrenia* (which means "split mind") was first used by a Swiss psychiatrist, Eugene Bleuler (1911). Schizophrenia is a serious disorder of thought and association characterized by inability to distinguish between what is real and what is not as well as by hallucinations, delusions, and limited socialization. People who have schizophrenia may not be able to differentiate between "theirs" and what is "everybody else's" in relation to social functioning. Poor self-esteem may be present. It is difficult for them to focus on one topic for any length of time. Schizophrenia is not the same as dissociative identity disorder (once called *multiple personality disorder*). Schizophrenia often begins during adolescence or young adulthood. It develops over time, and symptoms may go unnoticed for a time before diagnosis.

There are four phases of schizophrenia:

1. *Schizoid personality*. Those in this phase are perceived as being indifferent, cold, and aloof. They are often described as loners and don't seem to enjoy close relationships with others. In adolescence, these behaviors may be dismissed as normal for age. Not all individuals with schizoid personality develop schizophrenia.
2. *Prodromal phase*. Affected people continue to socially withdraw and begin to show peculiar or eccentric behavior. Role functioning is impaired, personal hygiene is neglected, and disturbances are evident in communication, ideation, and perception.
3. *Schizophrenia*. This is the third, active phase of the disorder. Psychotic symptoms are prominent and include delusions, hallucinations, and impairment in work, social relations, and self-care.
4. *Residual phase*. Symptoms are like the prodromal phase, with flat affect and impairment in role functioning.

Table 57.4 Depression Summary

Signs and Symptoms	*Unipolar (major):* Depressed mood, weight changes, anhedonia, sleep disturbance, social withdrawal *Bipolar:* Signs and symptoms of depression cycling with euphoria, delusions, hallucinations
Diagnosis	History; physiological causes must be ruled out
Therapeutic Measures	Antidepressant medication, mood stabilizers (anticonvulsants), psychotherapy, electroconvulsive therapy
Primary Nursing Diagnoses	*Ineffective Coping* *Powerlessness* *Risk for Suicide*

> **PRACTICE ANALYSIS TIP**
> **Linking NCLEX-PN® to Practice**
> The LPN/LVN will assist in the care of a client experiencing sensory/perceptual alterations.

Evidence-Based Practice

Clinical Question
How do young people living with mental illness view their lives and manage their health?

Evidence
A systematic review of qualitative literature included 54 research papers and 304 study findings. They were combined into nine categories and four synthesis statements (Woodgate et al, 2017). Young people living with mental illness expressed the need for a different way of being, felt challenged to get through difficult times, and yearned for acceptance. There are numerous barriers for accessing help.

Implications for Nursing Practice
Young people living with mental illness need continuous support and plans of care with multiple coping strategies, using a collaborative interdisciplinary approach. Decreasing barriers to accessing help as well as offering a therapeutic approach when interacting with this population is important.

References: National Institute of Mental Health. (2021). Bipolar disorder. https://www.nimh.nih.gov/health/statistics/bipolar-disorder

Woodgate, R. L., Sigurdson, C., Demczuk, L., Tennent, P., Wallis, B., & Werner, P. (2017). The meanings young people assign to living with mental illness and their experiences managing their health and lives: A systematic review of qualitative evidence. *JBI Database of Systematic Reviews and Implementation Reports, 15*(2), 276–401. https://doi.org/10.11124/JBISRIR-2016003283

Positive and Negative Symptoms

Positive symptoms of schizophrenia are those that reflect an "excess" or distortion of normal functioning. Patients are usually hospitalized for exacerbation of positive symptoms, which include hallucinations, delusions, disorganized thinking, and disorganized behavior. **Delusions** are fixed, false beliefs that cannot be changed by logic or factual proof. Patients may exhibit delusions of grandeur, persecution, or guilt. **Hallucinations** are false sensory perceptions. They can affect any of the five senses; auditory and visual delusions are most common. For example, a person might see a person no one else sees or hear voices that no one else hears. In contrast, **illusions** are mistaken perceptions of reality. For example, a person may see a glowing sunset and think the horizon is on fire. Both typical and atypical antipsychotic medications work well to manage the positive symptoms of schizophrenia.

Negative symptoms of schizophrenia represent loss of normal functioning. They include affective blunting or flattening, **alogia, avolition,** apathy, anhedonia, and social isolation. These are often the most debilitating symptoms of schizophrenia because they keep the individual from living a normal life. Negative symptoms respond to atypical antipsychotic medications but not the typical antipsychotic agents.

Pathophysiology and Etiology

Schizophrenia is widely believed to result from a combination of neurobiological and environmental factors. Psychological factors as are no longer considered a valid cause because most researchers and clinicians consider schizophrenia a brain disease.

The role of genetics in schizophrenia (neurobiological or nature theory) has been examined in twin studies, family studies, and adoption studies for many years. A study done on 31,524 sets of Danish twins found a 79% rate of genetic contribution. In fraternal twins alone, the percentage drops dramatically (Hilker et al, 2018).

Other studies have examined brain structure and the relationship between neurotransmitters and schizophrenia. Patients with a diagnosis of schizophrenia typically have elevated dopamine levels or a brain that overreacts to the amount of dopamine present. Glutamate is an excitatory neurotransmitter that also appears to be related to schizophrenia. The glutamate theory proposes that there is an excess of glutamate of the brain (Uno & Coyle, 2019). The brains of patients with a diagnosis of schizophrenia show a significant loss of gray matter, enlarged ventricles, and diminished prefrontal cortex functioning. Today, schizophrenia is primarily thought of as a series of brain disorders characterized by brain abnormalities and neurotransmitter dysfunction.

Environmental factors that increase risk of schizophrenia include central nervous system damage during childbirth, some infections, and substance abuse.

Symptoms

Patients with paranoid symptoms tend to exhibit unusual suspicions and fears. The person may also be hostile and aggressive or have delusions of persecution or grandeur. Those with persecutory delusions may state that they feel tormented or followed by people. Patients often integrate people around them into their delusions. They may feel that nursing staff, relatives, or announcers on the radio or television are trying to harm them. In delusions of grandeur, patients might state that they are God or are on the phone with the president of the United States.

Hallucinations often accompany delusions and can affect any of the five senses. The most common hallucinations are auditory, followed by visual. Patients diagnosed with

• **WORD** • **BUILDING** •

alogia: a—not + logia—(able to) speak
avolition: a—not + volition—energy or initiative to do something

schizophrenia talk about hearing voices. These voices are frightening and derogatory to the patient and trigger many of the actions performed by people with paranoid schizophrenia. Patients experience increased fear, anxiety, and suicidal ideation as a result of the voices. You may see or hear patients who seem to argue with themselves but are actually arguing with the voices. Describing the voices is difficult, but imagine that you are in a room with six televisions on different stations at the same time. This example comes close to what some patients have described.

Therapeutic Measures

Medications, social skills training, and individual and family psychotherapy are indicated for patients with schizophrenia. Prescribed classifications of medications may include the typical and atypical antipsychotics, which block dopamine action in the brain. There are different dopamine tracts in the brain. Typical antipsychotics have a greater effect on the D_2 dopamine receptors of the motor function tract, resulting in extrapyramidal side effects such as parkinsonism (see Table 57.2). Anticholinergic medications such as benztropine (Cogentin) or trihexyphenidyl (Artane) combat the extrapyramidal side effects of the typical antipsychotic by helping return balance among dopamine, acetylcholine, and other neurotransmitters. Newer, atypical antipsychotic medications such as lurasidone (Latuda) and risperidone (Risperdal) have fewer extrapyramidal side effects but have other side effects. Atypical antipsychotics are effective in treating both the positive and negative symptoms of schizophrenia.

Psychotherapy can include individual, group, and family therapy (Table 57.5). ECT is used in some severe cases; it is not usually used until other methods of therapy have been exhausted. Referral of the patient and family to organizations such as the National Alliance on Mental Illness (www.nami.org) provides helpful education and support. Table 57.6 provides suggestions for responding to patients experiencing hallucinations.

Nursing Process for the Patient With Schizophrenia

Data Collection

Observe the patient with schizophrenia for positive and negative symptoms, including hallucinations, delusions, and illusions. Observe interactions with others. Monitor the patient for response to medications, including side effects. Determine the person's ability to function and manage activities of daily living (ADLs).

Nursing Diagnoses, Planning, and Implementation

Social Isolation related to inability to trust and delusional thinking

EXPECTED OUTCOME: The patient will willingly attend milieu activities and initiate interactions with staff and peers.

Table 57.5
Schizophrenia Summary

Signs and Symptoms	Disorganized speech and behavior Ineffective thinking and decision making Trouble functioning at school and work; self-care deficits *Positive symptoms:* Hallucinations, delusions *Negative symptoms:* Apathy, flat affect, anhedonia
Diagnosis	History Psychiatric evaluation DSM-5 criteria
Therapeutic Measures	Antipsychotic medications Anticholinergic agents to control side effects Psychotherapy Family education Social skills training and therapy
Primary Nursing Diagnosis	*Social Isolation*

- Establish a therapeutic rapport with the patient. *This will help the patient learn to interact with others.*
- Convey acceptance and unconditional positive regard for the patient. *An accepting attitude may facilitate trust and increase feelings of self-worth.*
- Assure the patient of their safety. *An isolative patient may be fearful of the other patients or staff members.*
- Offer to accompany patient to milieu activities. *An isolative patient may be more likely to be present in the milieu if accompanied by a supportive individual.*
- Acknowledge the patient's efforts to interact and attend activities. *Positive reinforcement may encourage the patient's attempts at interaction.*

Evaluation

If interventions have been effective, the patient will participate in therapy and interact with other staff and patients.

CLINICAL JUDGMENT

Anne is a young woman receiving chemotherapy on your oncology unit. While preparing to invite her to a movie in the day room, you observe her standing in the corner of her room, trembling. You ask her what's wrong, and she responds that she's talking to the woman in the wall. Your first instinct is to giggle, but you ask her, "What woman?"

Table 57.6
Suggested Interventions for Patients With Schizophrenia Who Are Hallucinating

Suggested Action	Rationale
"Mr. R., I don't see any snakes. It is time for lunch. I will walk to the dining room with you."	Lets the patient know you heard him, but brings him immediately into the reality of time of day and the need to go to the dining room.
"I see a crack in the wall, Mr. R. It is harmless; you are safe. Susan is here to take you down to occupational therapy now."	This is in response to a probable illusion. It lets the patient know that you see something. It validates his fear, but it tells him what you see and then moves him into the here and now.
"I know that your thoughts seem very real to you, Ms. C., but they do not seem logical to me. I would like for you to come to your room and get dressed now, please."	Again, you are validating the patient's concern without exploring and focusing on the delusion.
"Ms. C., it appears to me that you are listening to someone. Are you hearing voices other than mine?"	This method validates your impression of what you see. This is as far as you will go into exploring what she may be hearing.
"Thank you, Ms. C. I want to help you focus away from the other voices. I am real; they are not. Please come with me to the reading room."	Responds to her in the present and reinforces her response to you. Attempts to redirect her thinking.

She tells you that you wouldn't understand and says, "You helped put her there, and you told me that it is my job to be sure she can't get out." You report this to the charge nurse, who calls the physician. Tests are run, and it is determined that Anne is not experiencing side effects from the chemotherapy. Further workup delivers the diagnosis of schizophrenia for Anne.

1. What therapeutic responses are appropriate for this situation? How will you get Anne to the movie or to participate in other care activities?
2. What special needs might Anne now experience relating to her chemotherapy, if any?
3. What actions can team members take to promote trust with Anne?

Suggested answers are at the end of the chapter.

PERSONALITY DISORDERS

How many times have you heard, "She has such a good personality"? What determines an individual's personality? Personality is composed of enduring patterns or traits that determine how someone perceives, relates to, and thinks about the environment and self. Personality develops as the person adjusts to physical, emotional, social, and spiritual environments. Personality traits or patterns are reflected in how individuals cope with feelings and impulses, see themselves and others, respond to their surroundings, and find meaning in relationships.

Etiology
The causes of personality disorders are unknown. Genetic and family environmental factors as well as neurobiological and other social factors are thought to play a role.

Diagnosis
Personality disorders are diagnosed when personality patterns or traits are inflexible, enduring, pervasive, and maladaptive and cause significant functional impairment or subjective distress. In the United States, 9.1% of the population has been diagnosed with a personality disorder (NIMH, 2017).

Personality disorders are characterized by the following:

- *Behavioral manifestations:* Dysfunctional patterns of daily behavior and impulse control
- *Affective manifestations:* Inappropriate range, intensity, mood lability, and emotional response
- *Cognitive manifestations:* Inaccurate interpretation of self, others, and events
- *Sociocultural manifestations:* Ineffective interpersonal functioning

Patients with personality disorders exhibit common problem behaviors that create difficulty in daily living. *Manipulation* is a control behavior that uses and exploits others for personal gain. *Narcissism* is self-centered behavior in which the individual feels entitled to special favors or feels justified in not obeying authority and rules. *Impulsive behavior* creates difficulties for those patients who act without considering the consequences of their own behavior.

The *DSM-5* lists 10 personality disorders that are organized into three diagnostic clusters: Cluster A: Odd and Eccentric, Cluster B: Dramatic and Erratic, and Cluster C: Anxious and Fearful. This text covers two of the more common personality disorders in Cluster B: borderline personality disorder (BPD) and antisocial personality disorder (ASPD).

Borderline Personality Disorder

Individuals with BPD display a pattern of instability of interpersonal relationships, self-image, and affect with marked impulsivity. The personality pattern is present by early adulthood and occurs across a variety of situations. Other symptoms may include intense fear of abandonment, anger and irritability, chronic feelings of emptiness, and transient paranoia or dissociative symptoms. Patients with BPD often engage in idealization and devaluation of others, alternating between high positive regard and great disappointment. This defense mechanism is called *splitting*. Self-mutilation and recurrent suicidal behavior, gestures, and threats are common.

Antisocial Personality Disorder

ASPD is characterized by a pervasive pattern of disregard for and violation of the rights of others. It begins in childhood or early adolescence and continues into adulthood. Individuals with ASPD have a lack of empathy and/or remorse for their actions. They fail to conform to social norms, often leading to legal problems or criminal behavior. Behavior can be impulsive and aggressive, with a reckless disregard for the safety of self or others. Deceitfulness and consistent irresponsibility are common.

Therapeutic Measures

Psychotherapy

Psychotherapy is the primary treatment for personality disorders. Using insight and knowledge gained in psychotherapy, patients can learn healthy ways to manage their illness. Types of psychotherapy to treat personality disorders include cognitive behavioral therapy and psychoeducation. *Cognitive behavioral therapy* helps patients identify unhealthy, negative beliefs and behaviors and replace them with healthy, positive ones. *Dialectical behavior therapy* is a type of cognitive behavioral therapy that teaches skills to tolerate stress, regulate emotions, and improve relationships with others. *Psychodynamic psychotherapy* focuses on increasing the patient's awareness of unconscious thoughts and behaviors, developing new insights and motivations, and resolving conflicts. Psychoeducation teaches the patient and family members about their illness, including treatments, coping strategies, and problem-solving skills.

No medications are specifically approved to treat personality disorders. However, several types of psychiatric medications may help with various common symptoms. Antidepressant medications are used to treat depressed mood, anger, impulsivity, irritability, or hopelessness. Mood-stabilizing medications are used to help even out mood swings or reduce irritability, impulsivity, and aggression. Antianxiety medications can address anxiety, agitation, or insomnia. Antipsychotic medications can help with paranoia, aggression, anger, and impulsiveness.

Nursing Process for the Patient With a Personality Disorder

Data Collection

A priority nursing action is determining the presence of suicidal or homicidal ideation. Mood and affect might be described as depressed, angry, or labile. Mood can indicate a higher risk for self-injury. Observe for paranoia, manipulative behaviors, and impulsiveness as well as history of violence. It will also be necessary to obtain a medical history, psychiatric history, developmental history, and information about sociocultural background.

Nursing Diagnosis, Planning, and Implementation

Risk for Other-Directed Violence related to impulsivity, impaired judgment, and disregard for the rights of others

EXPECTED OUTCOME: The patient will not harm self or others. The patient will discuss feelings with staff instead of acting on them. The patient will verbalize adaptive coping strategies for use when hostile or suicidal feelings occur.

- Monitor the patient's behavior frequently. *Close monitoring is required so that intervention can occur if required to ensure safety.*
- Remove all dangerous objects from the patient's environment (e.g., sharp items, belts, ties, straps, breakable items, smoking materials). *Safety is a nursing priority.*
- Redirect violent behavior by means of physical outlets for the patient's anxiety (e.g., exercise machines, walking). *Physical activity can be an effective way of relieving tension and stress.*
- Maintain a calm attitude toward the patient. *Anxiety is contagious and can be transmitted from staff members to patient.*
- Encourage appropriate verbal expression of emotions. *Verbalization of feelings in a nonthreatening environment may assist the patient to develop insight into the situation.*

Evaluation

The patient will be able to discuss anger with staff, engage in physical activity to cope with tension, and act responsive to calm interaction. The patient and others are safe from harm, and environmental safety has been maintained.

AUTISM SPECTRUM DISORDERS

Autism spectrum disorders (ASDs) are lifelong neurodevelopmental disabilities that are typically recognized during the second year of life. ASD prevalence is believed to occur in up to 2% of the U.S. population and occurs four times more in males than in females.

Etiology

ASDs are characterized by abnormal brain development and function. Although specific causes are unknown, an ASD likely has multiple etiologies, including genetic factors. A range of studies has found that in 10% to 37% of cases, the child has an associated medical condition such as maternal rubella or other genetic syndromes. Current research is also showing that the frontal lobe and amygdala appear to have abnormal growth patterns in patients with ASDs. Several studies show that the amygdala, which controls emotions, undergoes disproportionate enlargement in ASDs (Xu et al, 2020). A large Swedish study showed that genetic factors account for 83% of autism diagnoses (Sandin et al, 2017). These may include advanced parental age, low birth weight, and fetal exposure to valproate, an anticonvulsant.

Signs and Symptoms

An ASD is characterized by (1) deficits in social communication and social interaction and (2) restricted and repetitive behaviors (RRBs), interests, and activities. Patients with ASDs tend to have communication deficits such as responding inappropriately in conversations, misreading nonverbal cues, or having difficulty building friendships appropriate to their age. They may desire friendship and interaction with others, but inability to understand the emotions, motivations, and perspectives makes relationships difficult. In addition, patients who have ASDs may be overly dependent on routines, highly sensitive to changes in their environment, or intensely focused on inappropriate items.

Therapeutic Measures

Early intervention can greatly improve a child's development and help children from birth to 3 years learn important skills. Interventions include therapy to help the child talk, walk, and interact with others.

Various treatments address deficits in communication, social interaction, and behaviors. Applied behavior analysis (ABA) has become widely accepted among health-care professionals and is used in many schools and treatment clinics. ABA encourages positive behaviors and discourages negative behaviors to improve a variety of skills.

Occupational therapy teaches skills that help the patient with ADLs such as dressing, eating, bathing, and relating to people. Sensory integration therapy helps the patient cope with sensory information, including sights, sounds, and smells. Sensory integration therapy may help a patient who cannot tolerate certain sounds or physical touch. Speech therapy helps improve the patient's communication skills either verbally or by using sign language, gestures, or picture boards. The Picture Exchange Communication System uses picture symbols to teach communication skills.

Medications do not cure for ASDs or address its key symptoms. Some medications can help people with ASDs function better by managing high energy levels, inability to focus, depression, or seizures. The U.S. Food and Drug Administration has approved the use of the antipsychotic medications risperidone (Risperdal) and aripiprazole (Abilify) to treat patients with ASDs who exhibit behavioral problems such as tantrums, aggression, or self-injurious behaviors. Referral of the patient and family to organizations such as Autism Speaks (www.autismspeaks.org/family-services/resource-guide) can provide helpful education and support.

Nursing Process for the Patient With an Autism Spectrum Disorder

Data Collection

Collect data related to developmental spurts or lags or loss of previously acquired skills. Observe the caregiver-patient relationship for bonding, anxiety, tension, and difficult fit. Discuss the patient's social, communication, and behavioral strengths and limitations with the caregiver. Observe the patient's communication style and verbal and nonverbal skills. Determine risk of injury to self and others and be alert for the potential for abuse.

Nursing Diagnosis, Planning, and Implementation

Impaired Social Interaction related to neurological alterations

EXPECTED OUTCOME: The patient will interact appropriately and develop a trusting relationship with at least one staff member. The patient will function appropriately in the inpatient milieu.

- Assign consistent staff to the patient. *This is essential to the development of trust.*
- Provide positive reinforcement for the patient's voluntary interactions with others. *Positive reinforcement enhances self-esteem and encourages repetition of desirable behaviors.*
- Provide direct feedback about the patient's interactions with others in a nonjudgmental manner. *Direct feedback from a trusted individual may help to alter behaviors in a positive manner.*
- Help the patient learn how to respond more appropriately in interactions with others. Practice new skills through role-play. *Practicing skills in role-play facilitates use in real situations.*
- Give positive feedback when eye contact is used. *Positive reinforcement enhances self-esteem and encourages repetition of desirable behaviors.*

Evaluation

If the plan has been successful, the patient will establish trust with at least one staff member, engage in voluntary interaction with others, be responsive to feedback regarding interactions, be responsive to role-plays, and make eye contact.

EATING DISORDERS

Anorexia Nervosa

Anorexia nervosa is an eating disorder recognized by the American Psychiatric Association. It most commonly occurs in females between ages 13 and 18. Males account for less than 10% of those with anorexia nervosa. Depression and anxiety often are also present. Anorexia nervosa is thought to be multifactorial in origin. Patients may have a phobia about weight gain, fear losing control, and mistrust others.

> **PRACTICE ANALYSIS TIP**
> Linking NCLEX-PN® to Practice
> The LPN/LVN will monitor and provide for client nutritional needs.

Signs and Symptoms

DSM-5 criteria for anorexia nervosa include restriction of energy intake, intense fear of gaining weight, and disturbance in the way one's body weight or shape is experienced. The *DSM-5* further specifies whether the disorder is a restricting type (dieting, fasting) or binge-eating/purging type (self-induced vomiting; misuse of laxatives, diuretics, or enemas). Severity of the disorder is determined by current body mass index. As the disease progresses, additional symptoms appear, including electrolyte imbalance, cardiac arrhythmias, constipation, dry skin, lanugo (downy hair covering body), bradycardia, hypothermia, hypotension, muscle wasting, and facial puffiness. Often, patients with anorexia nervosa deny the existence of any problem. They may develop bizarre food rituals and sometimes weigh themselves several times a day.

Complications

Chronic poor nutrition takes its toll on the body. Complications from starvation occur as the body tries to conserve energy. Pulse and blood pressure fall. Heart and kidney failure are a risk. Osteoporosis and muscle loss occur. Vitamin and electrolyte imbalances result. Diabetes may develop.

Therapeutic Measures

Treating this disorder is complex and requires a multidisciplinary approach. Patients often do not see the need for medical intervention. They do not usually seek help on their own and often resist treatment. When treatment is sought, often through a concerned person's urgings, a medical and psychological workup is necessary. Nutritional status is also evaluated to determine urgency of intervention. Establishing a trusting relationship, which can be difficult, is a key element in initiating treatment. Early treatment results in a better prognosis.

The priority is restoration of nutritional health. A significant number of anorexia nervosa patients eventually die of starvation and complications. Hospitalization and refeeding are indicated for those who are underweight with severe weight loss, life-threatening electrolyte imbalances, and arrhythmias or other symptoms. Nutrition is supplied by IV infusions containing electrolytes. Oral food supplements may also be given. Restoring normal weight is a long, slow process. Gains may be small, with setbacks along the way. Praise and rewards for small achievements in weight gains (not food intake) are positive reinforcements that aid recovery. Programs that treat eating disorders are often set up on a reward system, with privileges being increased as progress occurs.

The patient's distorted self-image and need for control are underlying causes of the disorder that must be addressed in conjunction with the nutritional aspect. Psychotherapy and behavior modification that includes participation of the patient's family members are used to treat anorexia nervosa. Restoration of control and development of a healthy self-image are the main focuses of therapy. Educating the patient on normal body weight, symptoms of the illness, effects on the body, and methods to feel more control can be helpful. Individual or group therapy is often used. The Maudsley approach is an evidence-based treatment for adolescents with anorexia nervosa (Dalle Grave et al, 2019). During treatment, a support system is vital to success. Visit www.nationaleatingdisorders.org for resources for patients and families.

Bulimia Nervosa

Bulimia nervosa criteria is identified by the *DSM-5* as recurrent episodes of binge eating and inappropriate compensatory behaviors (purges) to avoid weight gain. Behaviors can include self-induced vomiting, misuse of laxatives or diuretics, fasting, or excessive exercise. Binging and purging both occur at least once a week for 3 months or more and do not occur exclusively during episodes of anorexia nervosa. The individual's self-evaluation is unduly influenced by body shape and weight. Severity is specified by the number of purges per week. Individuals with bulimia nervosa are often within a normal weight range.

Signs and Symptoms

Patients with bulimia nervosa exhibit many of the same signs and symptoms as patients with anorexia nervosa, with a few exceptions. Bulimic patients often have enamel erosion of the front teeth and staining caused by the acid content of the emesis. They also spend a great deal of time locked in the bathroom vomiting, especially after meals. Their knuckles may be calloused or have small cuts from self-induced vomiting. They may have a chipmunk appearance from enlarged parotid glands secondary to self-induced vomiting. Electrolyte imbalances occur from dehydration. Loss of potassium and sodium may result in arrhythmias, heart failure, and death. As electrolyte imbalance worsens, metabolic alkalosis develops because of the loss of gastric acid in the stomach contents. Signs of metabolic alkalosis include hypokalemia and hypocalcemia. Laxative use results in irregular bowel movements.

Therapeutic Measures

Treatment for bulimia nervosa is essentially the same as for the patient with anorexia nervosa.

Nursing Process for the Patient With an Eating Disorder

Caring for patients with eating disorders is challenging. Gaining the patient's genuine cooperation by using therapeutic communication and setting realistic, mutual goals are important for establishing trust and preventing relapse. To work with patients with an eating disorder, a therapeutic relationship must be developed to facilitate effective interactions. Empathy, acceptance of the patient, trust, warmth, and unconditional positive regard are important.

Data Collection

Data are collected related to inadequate nutrition. Note changes in weight (15% or more below expected weight), poor skin turgor, poor muscle tone, lanugo, amenorrhea, electrolyte imbalances, swollen parotid glands, and hypothermia. Data collection findings may also include a normal weight, enamel erosion of front teeth, and metabolic alkalosis for the patient with bulimia. Note abnormal diagnostic studies such as anemia, electrolyte imbalances, altered endocrine studies, and electrocardiogram changes.

Nursing Diagnoses, Planning, and Implementation

Imbalanced Nutrition: Less Than Body Requirements related to inadequate food intake and/or inappropriate compensatory behaviors

EXPECTED OUTCOME: The patient will establish a dietary pattern and gain weight toward desired individual weight range.

- Monitor patient's weight *to determine baseline* and monitor patient's progress *toward goal.*
- Monitor vital signs and laboratory studies *to detect changes in cardiac function related to electrolyte imbalances.*
- Promote a consistent approach *to enhance acceptance by the patient and to build trust.*
- Promote a pleasant eating environment and record intake *to enhance patient intake.*
- Provide six small meals and snacks *to prevent gastric dilation.*

Disturbed Body Image related to psychosocial or cognitive/perceptual changes

EXPECTED OUTCOME: The patient will verbalize satisfaction with body appearance.

- Identify and document the patient's verbal and nonverbal responses to own body *to provide baseline understanding of the patient's perceptions of body image.*
- Listen to the patient and acknowledge reality of concerns regarding treatment and progress *to establish therapeutic relationship.*
- Monitor frequency of negative statements about self *to determine whether interventions are helping the patient.*
- Assist with referrals to social services or counseling *to help the patient overcome psychosocial issues.*
- Provide care in a nonjudgmental manner *to maintain the patient's dignity.*
- Use positive praise when the patient verbalizes positive comments about own body. *Praise reinforces the behavior and increases likelihood of repeating the desired behavior.*
- Encourage the patient to verbalize consequences of an eating disorder that have influenced self-concept *to help the patient realize the negative impact of the eating disorder.*

Evaluation

The patient's goals are met if they gain weight toward expected weight goal, verbalize satisfaction with body appearance, and increase the number of positive statements about own appearance.

SUBSTANCE USE DISORDERS

Substance (alcohol and drug) use disorders are serious conditions. People start using alcohol and drugs for many reasons, often to feel accepted by a peer group or to feel comfortable and reduce anxiety in a social situation. People mistake the temporary high as a stimulant. In reality, alcohol is a depressant. Any chemical can be potentially dangerous.

> **PRACTICE ANALYSIS TIP**
>
> **Linking NCLEX-PN® to Practice**
> The LPN/LVN will:
>
> - Provide information for prevention of high-risk behaviors (e.g., substance abuse, sexual practices, smoking cessation).
> - Identify signs and symptoms of substance abuse, chemical dependency, withdrawal, or toxicity.

It is important to understand the following terms and their definitions:

- **Addiction:** Repeated compulsive use of a substance that continues despite negative consequences (physical, social, legal).
- **Tolerance:** A condition in which increased amounts of a substance are needed over time to achieve the same effect as that previously obtained with smaller doses.
- Physical **withdrawal** syndrome: A physiological response to the abrupt stopping or reduction of a substance used (usually) for a long time. Withdrawal symptoms are specific to the substance used.

Substance use disorders are conditions in which the patient does the following:

- Takes more of the substance or takes it over a longer period of time than intended (**abuse**)
- Has a persistent desire to or unsuccessful efforts to cut down or control use
- Experiences strong craving for the substance
- Is unable to fulfill major role obligations at home, work, or school
- Needs more of the substance and at more frequent intervals to achieve the same "high," or desired effect of the substance (tolerance)
- Spends significant time obtaining the substance
- Gives up important social or professional functions to use the substance
- Has tried at least once to quit but still obsesses about the substance
- Experiences difficulty with job, family, or social activities because of use or withdrawal symptoms
- Uses the substance regardless of the problems it causes
- Experiences the substance-specific withdrawal syndrome
- Uses the substance to avoid withdrawal symptoms

Nurses need to be informed about substance use disorders for several reasons. First, many patients on medical-surgical units have substance use–related disorders. The disorder affects their healing and the effect of their medications. Second, as part of the human experience, you have a significant chance of having a close personal or family relationship with someone who has a substance use disorder. Third, perhaps most important, you are part of a profession whose members are statistically high users and abusers of drugs and alcohol. Ten percent of nurses will abuse drugs or alcohol at some point during their careers (American Addiction Centers, 2019). If you note signs of impairment in a colleague, you ethically must report the behaviors to your supervisor.

> **PRACTICE ANALYSIS TIP**
> **Linking NCLEX-PN® to Practice**
> The LPN/LVN will respond to the unsafe practice of a health-care provider (e.g., intervene, report).

Substance use disorders are not a one-person illness; they affect personal and professional relationships with people who are associated with the user. The relationships in a family or work environment with a substance abuser are often **dysfunctional**. Dishonesty and inability to discuss the situation are strong components of the disease. People who live or work in the dysfunctional group typically begin to cover up for the substance user's behaviors and lack of responsibility. Family members or friends may take sides, be dishonest with each other, and erode the bond within that group. Eventually, their actions lead to **codependence**, which can be as serious as the substance use. Codependent members of a group begin to lose their own sense of identity and purpose and exist solely for the abuser. Their actions take away the opportunity for the user to take responsibility for their own actions. This is called *enabling*.

Denial is a common ego defense mechanism used by people who are substance abusers. The person who is dependent on a substance often uses statements such as "I can quit anytime I want to" or "I just need a little bump to loosen me up."

Sometimes patients who are actively using drugs or alcohol when admitted to an inpatient setting or who are cut off from substances abruptly experience physiological withdrawal. Withdrawal from alcohol specifically can progress to a condition called **delirium tremens** (DTs). DTs develop when alcohol intake is significantly reduced and neurotransmitters previously suppressed by alcohol are no longer suppressed. Their rebound causes a phenomenon known as brain hyperexcitability, which leads to visual hallucinations, tremors, and possibly tonic-clonic seizures. Elevated blood pressure and pulse and cardiac arrhythmias also may occur. Symptoms of withdrawal begin within 4 to 12 hours after the patient has stopped drinking and will peak in 24 to 48 hours. Hospitalization is needed to maintain the patient's safety.

Types of Substance Use Disorders
Alcohol Use Disorders

Alcohol use disorders are present in all walks of life, at all economic levels, and in both genders. Sometimes a fine line exists between a social drinker and a person who has an abuse condition. One factor used to make that differentiation is the degree of need or compulsion to drink. There is a high incidence of alcohol use and abuse among older adults, teenagers, and even younger children. Alcoholism either directly or indirectly decreases a person's life expectancy by an average of 10 to 12 years.

Patients with alcohol use disorders may experience the following:

- Binges usually lasting 2 days or more
- Blackouts (unable to recall what happened during a period of drinking)
- Vomiting and dehydration
- Disorientation
- Increased vulnerability to infections, accidents, and other injuries

Other Substance Use Disorders

Many substances other than alcohol can be addictive. Caffeine and nicotine are two that are readily available. Coffee, tea, soda, and cigarettes are everywhere in our society and very addicting. Many experts believe the single-most difficult addiction to overcome is to nicotine.

• WORD • BUILDING •

dysfunctional: dys—bad or difficult + functional—performance

Illegal substances such as cannabis (in some states), heroin, cocaine, crack, phencyclidine (more commonly known as PCP), and prescription medications for pain and mental health treatment are also potentially addictive. The United States is in the midst of an opioid epidemic that includes everything from prescription medications to heroin (National Institute on Drug Abuse, 2021). Deaths from heroin and prescription opioid overdoses are occurring in record numbers. Methamphetamine (meth) abuse is a major problem affecting families and society. Inhalants such as lighter fluid, paint, paint thinners, and gasoline also can be used to get high; in the United States, these substances are used mainly by teenagers. The term for their use is *huffing*. These are highly neurotoxic substances, potentially lethal, and usually available in the house or garage.

The signs and symptoms of drug abuse and dependence can be similar to those of alcohol abuse. Additional signs of drug abuse include the following:

- Red, watery eyes
- Runny nose
- Hostile behavior
- Paranoia
- Needle tracks on arms or legs

Etiological Theories

Why do some people develop substance use disorders and others do not? Is it the substance or the person? Some theorists believe in the existence of an addictive personality that may explain addictions to food, sex, and gambling as well as alcohol, drugs, and other dependencies. Psychoanalytical theorists believe that people who develop substance use disorders are people who failed to successfully pass through the "oral" stage of development.

Biological theories include numerous studies that imply some sort of genetic metabolic disorder. Many studies were done on twins born to an alcoholic parent or parents and separated from the parents shortly after birth. The number of twins who were born of alcoholic parents but raised by nonalcoholic adoptive or foster parents and yet developed alcohol use disorder was consistently elevated.

Cognitive behavioral theorists suggest the way in which a person perceives being high may influence the act of becoming high. It can be an innocent beginning: obtaining relief from valid prescription medications can, according to cognitive theory, leave people perceiving that the drugs offer a miracle cure. It becomes appealing to want that kind of relief again; soon a pattern is formed, and other substances may be added.

Differential Diagnosis

A patient with a substance use disorder may be admitted to the hospital for medical problems associated with substance use (e.g., dehydration, liver failure) or unrelated problems (e.g., cancer, diabetes). Nursing data collection, unexplained tolerance to pain medication, or symptoms of withdrawal may lead you or the physician to pursue the possibility of substance dependency. Laboratory tests can rule out physiological problems. Blood levels of alcohol or drugs can also be measured. A patient who is uncommonly anxious for early discharge should also be further assessed.

> **BE SAFE!**
> **BE VIGILANT!** Careful data collection on admission to a facility can uncover addiction issues. Intervention at this early point prior to onset of withdrawal symptoms can keep the patient safe from harm and more comfortable.

Therapeutic Measures

Treatment for and recovery from a substance use disorder is a slow process. With few exceptions, a person who has a substance use disorder and who is recovering cannot ever use that substance again or they will risk the chance of returning to previous patterns of use. Some treatment options are described next. Several forms of treatment may be used together.

SUPPORT GROUPS. Support groups are a common and effective treatment for substance use disorder. For alcoholism, the most famous is Alcoholics Anonymous (AA), a 12-step program that offers support through others who have stopped drinking. For more information, visit www.aa.org. Another program for women dealing with alcoholism is Women for Sobriety (www.womenforsobriety.org). For those who abuse drugs, Narcotics Anonymous (NA; www.na.org) is a well-known support group.

COGNITIVE BEHAVIORAL THERAPY. Cognitive behavioral therapy is used as an adjunct for control of substance abuse. Cognitive behavioral therapists believe that with homework and practice, a person can learn to think differently about the event that led to the substance abuse. When the person changes the belief system about the activating event, they can practice more positive thoughts and behaviors.

PSYCHOTHERAPY. Psychotherapy provides one-to-one therapy. Because substance use affects an entire family, family or group therapy is important in reinstating honest communication. A commitment to stop the substance abuse is required. Therapy will help with only some of the issues resulting from substance abuse.

SCREENING, BRIEF INTERVENTION, AND REFERRAL TO TREATMENT. The three-part Screening, Brief Intervention, and Referral to Treatment (SBIRT) is an evidence-based practice to identify, reduce, and prevent health problems related to use, abuse, and dependence on alcohol and illicit drugs (McManama O'Brien et al, 2019). This approach combines screening with brief behavioral counseling interventions. SBIRT is like other preventive health screening measures in that it provides an effective way to identify patients who are at risk for substance use. In addition, it offers an appropriate intervention.

MEDICATIONS. In the United States, aversion and anticraving medications to treat alcohol use disorders have been approved. If a comorbid anxiety or depressive disorder accompanies the alcohol abuse, other medications may be prescribed. Antidepressant or nonaddictive antianxiety drugs are most often prescribed.

The aversion medication disulfiram (Antabuse) is sometimes prescribed as a deterrent to alcohol use. Disulfiram should never be administered without the patient's full informed consent. If a patient taking disulfiram ingests alcohol, a severe reaction causes chest pain, nausea, vomiting, confusion, and other symptoms. Those taking disulfiram also can be adversely affected if they use products that contain alcohol, such as cologne, mouthwash, aftershave, or cough syrup. The effects of disulfiram last 2 to 3 weeks after the last dose.

The medication acamprosate (Campral) is thought to work by restoring GABA-glutamate equilibrium. Acamprosate may help combat cravings and is specifically indicated for maintenance of abstinence from alcohol in patients who have stopped drinking. Naltrexone (ReVia) may reduce the desire to drink. Naltrexone helps patients remain abstinent and can interfere with the tendency to want to drink more after relapsing with a single drink.

Use of benzodiazepines such as diazepam (Valium) and lorazepam (Ativan) can help prevent symptoms of DTs during acute withdrawal by neurotransmitter action but are not used long term because of risk for **dependence**.

To treat abuse of opioids, a combination of the drugs buprenorphine and naloxone (Suboxone) relieves withdrawal symptoms and opioid cravings. It works by binding with the same receptor sites as opioids. If Suboxone is taken correctly, the individual will feel drug-free without cravings or withdrawal symptoms.

Methadone acts as a sort of "step down" for people addicted to certain opioid drugs. It can be legally prescribed and dispensed. Methadone is also potentially addicting, and its critics believe it is only a substitute for heroin. It is typically given once a day. Psychotherapy is also provided for patients in methadone programs.

HOSPITALIZATION. Therapy may range from inpatient hospitalization to halfway houses to eventual independence, usually with attendance at AA or NA meetings. Hospitalization may be necessary during the acute withdrawal stage. It is common for patients to seek treatment multiple times. This should not be interpreted as a weakness in the patient or the treatment program. It is only a sign that the person is learning more about the disorder and the need to help themselves. People with all kinds of chronic diseases experience relapse at times.

Nursing Process for the Patient With Substance Use Disorders

Nursing care for people who have drug use disorders is essentially the same as for those who have alcohol use disorders. It is important to remember that nurses and physicians cannot "fix" the patient who uses substances. The desire to not use a substance must come from the person who is using it. Table 57.7 provides a substance use summary.

Table 57.7 Substance Abuse Summary

Signs and Symptoms	Inability to fulfill obligations at work, school, or home
	Recurrent legal or interpersonal problems
	Continued use despite social and interpersonal problems
	Participation in hazardous situations while impaired
Diagnosis	History
	Liver function studies
	Serum drug or alcohol levels
	Evaluate for other coexisting disorders (bipolar disorder)
Therapeutic Measures	12-step programs
	Cognitive behavioral therapy
	Psychotherapy
	SBIRT
	For alcohol use: Disulfiram (Antabuse), acamprosate (Campral), naltrexone (ReVia)
	For opioid use: Buprenorphine and naloxone (Suboxone), methadone
	Benzodiazepines for acute withdrawal
Primary Nursing Diagnoses	*Ineffective Coping*
	Ineffective Denial

CUE RECOGNITION 57.1

You are caring for a patient who had emergency surgery for appendicitis. You enter his room to check his vital signs and level of pain. His blood pressure and pulse are elevated, and he is diaphoretic and anxious. What do you do?

Suggested answers are at the end of the chapter.

Data Collection

For patients suspected of alcohol use disorder, a common screening tool to determine whether a patient has a drinking problem is the CAGE questionnaire (Ewing, 1984):

- Have you ever felt you should **C**ut down on your drinking?
- Have people **A**nnoyed you by criticizing your drinking?
- Have you ever felt bad or **G**uilty about your drinking?
- Have you ever had a drink first thing in the morning (as an "**E**ye opener") to steady your nerves or get rid of a hangover?

A yes answer to two or more questions suggests a drinking problem. Some organizations also use the CAGE questionnaire to screen for substance abuse, although it has not been validated for use in substance use disorders.

Alcohol also can have many physiological effects. See Chapter 32 for assessment of patients with liver disorders.

Nursing Diagnoses, Planning, and Implementation

Ineffective Coping related to lack of effective coping mechanisms as evidenced by abuse of a substance

EXPECTED OUTCOME: The patient will accept responsibility for their behavior, verbalize acceptance of the relationship between substance abuse and personal problems, and identify effects of the substance on the body.

- Help the patient to identify recent behavior while under the influence of the substance. *Patients need to see the relationship between their substance abuse and personal problems.*
- Expect sobriety. *This establishes sobriety as the norm.*
- Teach about the physical impact of drugs and alcohol on the body. *Many patients lack accurate information about the effects of substance abuse on the body.*
- Be honest and be aware of your own thoughts and feelings about addictions. *Effective communication is essential for a therapeutic relationship.*
- Provide group support such as a 12-step program. *Peer support is an effective treatment that is often more acceptable to patients than other treatments.*
- Confront the patient immediately if projection, rationalization, or denial behaviors are noted. *Projection, rationalization, and denial are ego defense mechanisms that discourage the patient from accepting responsibility for behavior.*
- Use positive reinforcement. *Positive reinforcement for successes is important when helping a person with an addiction. Every step is a big one in this field; every step taken is a new one.*
- Provide a safe environment. *Patients who are chemically addicted may become suicidal or display other bizarre behavior, especially during withdrawal. A patient under the influence of alcohol or another chemical may have poor impulse control or judgment. Maintaining a safe milieu and calm demeanor will help the patient through this difficult time.*
- Remain alert to the possibility that the patient may be using a substance even in the hospital. Report and document all findings and behaviors that may be potential safety hazards for the patient. *Being hospitalized does not guarantee that a patient has no access to the chemical or way of using it in your presence. Unfortunately, family members or friends sometimes smuggle in drugs or alcohol to patients.*
- Practice "tough love." "Doing for" patients may be tempting, but it is not in the patient's best interest most of the time. *Tough love encourages patients to be responsible for their own healing.*

Evaluation

Does the patient verbalize acceptance of responsibility for own behavior? Does the patient understand the relationship between personal problems and substance abuse? Does the patient understand the effects of substance abuse on the body?

For additional information, visit the Web sites of the National Institute on Alcohol Abuse and Alcoholism (www.niaaa.nih.gov) and the National Institute on Drug Abuse (www.drugabuse.gov).

CRITICAL THINKING

Maria, a 17-year-old student, is behaving oddly. She has always been rather loud and even has been referred to as "obnoxious" by several of her peers. As the school nurse, you have observed her sitting alone, as if waiting for someone, but when you approach, she barely greets you and then moves away. What are your concerns about Maria? What are some of the possibilities that might be affecting her? How can you approach her more effectively the next time you see her?

Suggested answers are at the end of the chapter.

MENTAL ILLNESS AND THE OLDER ADULT

It is not uncommon for older adults to be admitted to the hospital with a tentative diagnosis of "change in mental status." It is important to distinguish between physical and mental disorders in these cases. Some neurocognitive disorders that affect older adults' mental status are as follows:

- *Major neurocognitive disorder* is an impairment of mental functioning that interferes with daily activities and relationships. Causes of major neurocognitive disorder may include Alzheimer disease, Lewy body dementia, vascular disease, Huntington disease, and HIV.
- *Delirium* is an acute change in mental status needing immediate evaluation and treatment. This is often due to a physiological condition such as an infection. It typically can be reversed if recognized and the underlying cause removed. Read more about dementia and delirium in Chapter 48.
- *Pseudodementia* is a condition in which the patient appears to have a major neurocognitive disorder but is really experiencing depression. Treating the depression can help reverse the mental status changes.
- *Depression* in older adults should not be viewed as a normal part of aging; it should be diagnosed and treated. Older adults may be dealing with physical and mental decline, loss of function, isolation, and loss of a spouse and friends. Depression may be expressed through bodily symptoms such as pain. If not evaluated and treated, depression can lead to suicide (see "Gerontological Issues"). Review Chapter 15, "Nursing Care of Older Adult Patients."

Older adults often need assistance to develop or enhance skills required to cope with life events. Self-care and personal independence in care choices can be encouraged.

Gerontological Issues

Suicide and the Older Adult

Older adults have higher suicide rates than younger adults, with those over 85 years old having the highest risk (American Foundation for Suicide Prevention, 2021). Comments by any older adult referring to hopelessness or desire to die must be explored to identify suicide risk. Comments such as "I am useless. I can't do anything anymore" should be taken seriously. If an older adult is thought to be depressed, the Geriatric Depression Scale (GDS) can be used to assess further risk (Greenberg, 2020; Yesavage, 1983).

To adequately determine suicide potential, ask questions that establish whether the older adult has done the following:

- Thought about ending their life
- Attempted to end their life in the past
- Developed a plan to end their life
- Has started to give away personal possessions as gifts
- Set the plan into action (i.e., bought a gun, has a full bottle of pills in the bedside table)

Any older adult who has a plan to end their life and the ability or resources to do so must be immediately referred for psychological evaluation. Never leave a person with suicidal thoughts alone.

If necessary, crisis intervention for a suicidal older adult should include the following:

- Remove any items that the older adult could use to inflict an injury or end their life, such as razors, jewelry with pins or sharp points, and mirrors.
- Arrange reliable direct supervision and observation, considering personnel and family resources. Often, hospital admission is the most appropriate intervention for a person at high risk for suicide.
- Help the older adult talk about the crisis or life event that has devastated their desire to live. For example, encourage reminiscence about the patient's spouse or allow the person to express the frustration of being unable to physically meet the daily demands of life.
- Collaborate with a mental health worker to develop a "do no harm" or suicide contract with the older adult. Outline a short-term, structured plan to keep the older adult safe. Focus on decreasing social isolation by requiring personal social contacts. These could include staying at a daughter's home for a weekend, going to the senior center for lunch, calling a specific person who is willing and wants to listen to feelings and concerns, exercising, taking a walk outside, or volunteering at a nursing home, hospital, or school.

References: American Foundation for Suicide Prevention. (2021). Suicide statistics. https://afsp.org/suicide-statistics
Greenberg, S. A. (2020). The Geriatric Depression Scale. *Try This: Best Practices in Nursing Care to Older Adults*, 4, 1–2. https://hign.org/consultgeri/try-this-series/geriatric-depression-scale-gds
Yesavage, J. A., Brink, T. L., Rose, T. L., Lum, O., Huang, V., Adey, M. B., & Leirer, V. O. (1983). Development and validation of a geriatric depression screening scale: A preliminary report. *Journal of Psychiatric Research, 17*(1), 37–49. https://doi.org/10.1016/0022-3956(82)90033-4

Home Health Hints

- Observe family members for evidence of caregiver role strain.
- Connect patients and families with pharmacies that will deliver medications to the home. Some pharmacies offer prefilled dose packs.
- Maintain communication with and act as a liaison between the psychiatrist and primary care provider as needed.
- Assist patient and family to identify resources such as support groups and respite care.
- Teach patients about their illness and medications and how to manage their symptoms.
- Focus on the patient's strengths. How can the patient assist in their own recovery?

Key Points

- Anxiety is the feeling of dread that occurs in response to stress. It can be mild, moderate, severe, or panic.
- Specific phobias, the most common anxiety disorder, are defined as irrational fears of distinct objects or situations, such as snakes, bridges, or flying. The person is aware of the irrational fear but cannot control it.
- Social anxiety disorder is characterized by a fear of embarrassing oneself in a public setting.
- Panic is a state of extreme uncontrollable and unpredictable fear. A person may have panic disorder if they have several panic attacks in a short time frame.
- In GAD, anxiety itself is the main symptom.
- OCD consists of both the obsession (repetitive thought, urge, or images) and the compulsion (an excessive or unrealistic repetitive act).
- Patients with OCD can be helped by therapeutic interventions such as cognitive-behavioral therapy or medications such as fluoxetine (Prozac).
- PTSD develops in response to some unexpected emotional or physical trauma in which the person was helpless.

- A key symptom of PTSD is *flashbacks* in which the person relives the traumatic event, often triggered by sounds or smells.
- Mood disorders (also called *affective disorders*) cause extreme changes or instability in mood and affect. Moods involving both highs and lows are bipolar disorders; low moods without any highs are described as depressive disorders.
- Major depression is an episodic condition that interferes with social or occupational functioning.
- Bipolar disorder is a mood disorder that causes states of mania and extreme depression. Bipolar depression is more severe than major depression.
- Schizophrenia is a serious disorder of thought and association that causes hallucinations, delusions, and limited socialization as well as inability to discern reality.
- Patients are usually hospitalized for exacerbation of positive symptoms, which include hallucinations, delusions, disorganized thinking, and disorganized behavior.
- Patients with paranoid symptoms tend to exhibit unusual suspicions and fears. The person may also be hostile and aggressive or have delusions of persecution or grandeur.
- Data collection for schizophrenia includes observing for positive and negative symptoms, including hallucinations, delusions, and illusions.
- Personality disorders include personality patterns or traits that are inflexible, enduring, pervasive, and maladaptive, and cause significant functional impairment or subjective distress.
- Patients with personality disorders exhibit behaviors that create problems in daily living. *Manipulation* is a control behavior that uses and exploits others for personal gain. *Narcissism* is self-centered behavior in which the individual feels entitled to special favors or feels justified in not obeying authority and rules. *Impulsive behavior* creates difficulties for those patients who act without considering the consequences of their own behavior.
- Individuals with borderline personality disorder display a pattern of instability of interpersonal relationships, self-image, and affect. There is marked impulsivity.
- ASPD is characterized by a pervasive pattern of disregard for and violation of the rights of others. Individuals with ASPD have a lack of empathy and/or remorse for their actions.
- Psychotherapy is the primary way to treat personality disorders. Patients can learn healthy ways to manage their illness.
- A priority nursing action for patients with mood disorders is determination of suicidal or homicidal ideation. Mood and affect might be identified as depressed, angry, or labile.
- An ASD is characterized by deficits in social communication and social interaction, as well as restricted and repetitive behaviors, interests, and activities.
- Patients with ASDs tend to have communication deficits, such as responding inappropriately in conversations, misreading nonverbal cues, or having difficulty building friendships appropriate to their age.
- Anorexia nervosa signs and symptoms include restriction of energy intake, an intense fear of gaining weight, and a disturbance in the way one's body weight or shape is experienced.
- The *DSM-5* further specifies if the eating disorder is a restricting type (dieting, fasting) or binge-eating/purging type (self-induced vomiting; misuse of laxatives, diuretics, or enemas).
- Bulimia nervosa criteria is identified by the *DSM-5* as recurrent episodes of binge eating and recurrent inappropriate compensatory behaviors (purges) to avoid weight gain. Behaviors include self-induced vomiting, misuse of laxatives or diuretics, fasting, or excessive exercise.
- Substance use disorders affect personal and professional relationships with people who are associated with the user. The term *dysfunctional* refers to unhealthy relationships in a family or work environment with a substance abuser.
- Alcohol use disorders are present in all walks of life, economic levels, and genders.
- Patients with alcohol use disorders may experience binges usually lasting 2 days or more, blackouts, vomiting and dehydration, disorientation, and increased vulnerability to infections, accidents, and other injuries.
- The signs and symptoms of drug abuse and dependence can be similar to those of alcohol abuse. Additional signs of drug abuse include red, watery eyes; runny nose; hostile behavior; paranoia; and needle tracks on arms or legs.
- Therapy for substance abuse may range from inpatient hospitalization to halfway houses to eventual independence, usually with attendance at Alcoholics Anonymous or Narcotics Anonymous meetings. Hospitalization may be necessary during the acute withdrawal stage. It is common for patients to seek treatment multiple times.
- For patients suspected of alcohol use disorder, a common screening tool to determine whether a patient has a drinking problem is the CAGE questionnaire.
- It is not uncommon for older adults to be admitted to the hospital with a tentative diagnosis of "change in mental status." It is important to distinguish between physical and mental disorders in these circumstances.
- Older adults often need assistance to develop or enhance skills required to cope with life events. Self-care and personal independence in care choices can be encouraged.

Chapter 57 Nursing Care of Patients With Mental Health Disorders

SUGGESTED ANSWERS TO CHAPTER EXERCISES

Cue Recognition
57.1: Consult with the RN to assess for alcohol withdrawal.

Critical Thinking & Clinical Judgment

Tommy
You can reassure Tommy's mother that his OCD is not her fault. Tell her that Tommy can learn to control his illness with medications and therapy. The family must be part of the therapy for both Tommy's and the family's sake. Positive communication between Tommy and his family is encouraged. Tommy's mother can also be encouraged to attend a support group herself. Suggest to Tommy's mother that she meet with a counselor or behavioral therapist to learn more about the causes and treatment of the disorder.

Mr. Zenz
It is important to be supportive of Mrs. Zenz while maintaining her husband's confidentiality and privacy. Encouraging Mrs. Zenz to talk to Mr. Zenz's HCP is appropriate. Empathic statements such as "It must be confusing and difficult to watch your husband change moods so quickly" are good tools to use. It may be a bit more challenging to approach him directly. Ask if you can speak frankly and share specific observations (e.g., "The residents appear frightened when you approach them quickly and speak loudly"). This may help him reflect. Chances are, however, in a manic stage, Mr. Zenz will not hear your concern. Advise his wife to speak with the next person in the chain of command, or you can report specific behaviors that are becoming problematic.

Anne
1. Appropriate communication skills include being positive, reassuring, and not reinforcing the hallucinations. "I don't see or hear a woman, Anne. It is time for the movie. I'd like you to come with me for a while at least" is an example of an appropriate verbal interaction. Reinforcing expectations is also appropriate; you might say, "Anne, part of your care plan includes attending one unit activity each day. This is the last opportunity for you to meet your care plan objective for today."
2. At all times, nurses need to be aware of drug interactions. Anne will most likely be medicated for her schizophrenia, and those medications can interact unfavorably with her chemotherapy. If she is receiving oral medications, it may be necessary to check her mouth to ensure she is swallowing them.
3. Work with team members to provide a therapeutic and low stimulus environment for Anne. Good nursing data collection skills are essential.

Maria
Several things may explain Maria's behavior, including depression, drug use, schizophrenia, or an eating disorder. Next time you see Maria, you might try constructively confronting her behavior by saying something like "Maria, you used to be much more outgoing. We always were friendly, and now you leave when I'm near. That change in you concerns me. I'm here if you want to talk." Or "Maria, I noticed your behavior is changing. You are loud one moment and very quiet the next. That is unusual for you. What's happening?"

Additional Resources

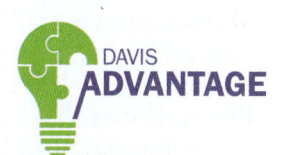

DAVIS ADVANTAGE Go to Davis Advantage to complete your learning: strengthen understanding, apply your knowledge, and prepare for the Next Gen NCLEX®.

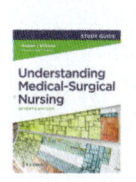

A Study Guide is also available.

APPENDIX A
Diagnostic Tests

This appendix is intended to be a quick reference only. Please check a diagnostic test reference manual for comprehensive information.

GENERAL CONSIDERATIONS FOR ALL TESTS

- Ensure that an informed consent form is signed before any invasive procedure.
- Check orders for need to withhold food or fluids before test.
- Preparation if contrast media will be used *to prevent reaction or nephrotoxicity*: (1) Check for and report allergies to contrast media (which may be reported as an iodine allergy); (2) report low glomerular filtration rate (GFR) or elevated creatinine/blood urea nitrogen (BUN) levels *because contrast media is nephrotoxic and excreted by the kidneys*; (3) consider patient risk factors for contrast-induced nephropathy (renal disease, diabetes, hypertension, chemotherapy) and discuss with health-care provider (HCP). *Prophylaxis orders such as providing IV hydration or prophylactic premedication such as acetylcysteine (Mucomyst) may be indicated*; (4) if patient is taking metformin, hold it as ordered before the test (typically 1 or 2 days) and then for 48 hours as ordered after the test until renal function is determined to be normal *to reduce risk for lactic acidosis if acute renal failure develops due to the contrast media*; (5) teach that the patient may experience a feeling of warmth or experience a salty or metallic taste when contrast media is injected; (6) encourage increased fluids after test *to promote excretion of contrast media*.
- Reinforce patient education for test.

Test or Procedure	Description	Reasons Done	Preprocedure Nursing Considerations	Postprocedure Nursing Considerations
Angiography • abdominal • adrenal • carotid • coronary • pulmonary • renal	Contrast media is injected through a catheter, usually via femoral artery or vein, and then radiographs are taken at intervals to view vasculature.	To view patency and distribution of blood vessels.	See General Considerations for precare for contrast media. Report history of bleeding/clotting disorders. Medications that interfere with clotting are stopped about 1 week before examination. Ensure patent IV is in place.	See General Considerations for postcare for contrast media. Monitor vital signs and circulatory status as ordered. Maintain pressure on insertion site as ordered. Report bleeding or hematoma formation.
Biopsy	Removal of tissue for microscopic examination. May be done with needle, punch, incision, or endoscopically.	To diagnose cancerous or other lesions.	Premedicate for pain relief.	Monitor vital signs and biopsy site as ordered.

Test or Procedure	Description	Reasons Done	Preprocedure Nursing Considerations	Postprocedure Nursing Considerations
Computed axial tomography (CAT), computed tomography (CT)	Multiple x-ray beams provide three-dimensional cross-section visualization of internal structures. Contrast media may be used.	To visualize abnormal structures or masses.	Ask if claustrophobic (depending on scanner); patient could be in scanner for up to 1 hour. Premedicate anxious or claustrophobic patients as ordered. See General Considerations for precare for contrast media.	See General Considerations for postcare for contrast media.
Electrocardiography (ECG, EKG)	Electrodes provide a graphic display of the electrical current during the cardiac cycle.	To evaluate electrical function of the heart; diagnose arrhythmias.	Explain test to patient.	None specific.
Electroencephalography (EEG)	Electrodes on scalp evaluate electrical activity of the brain.	To evaluate brain activity, lesions, and seizures.	Ensure patient's hair is clean and dry. Check orders for medications such as sedatives or stimulants that may need to be weaned or withheld before test.	Wash adhesive from hair before it hardens and becomes difficult to remove. Oil or witch hazel may make removal easier. Instruct patient about resuming medications as ordered.
Endoscopy • bronchoscopy • colonoscopy • colposcopy • gastroscopy • sigmoidoscopy	A flexible fiber-optic tube and camera are inserted into a body cavity to observe structures.	To observe for abnormalities, remove polyps, obtain biopsy specimens, suction secretions, coagulate bleeding sites, and more.	Check orders for preparation such as NPO (nothing by mouth), laxatives, and enemas. Premedicate as ordered.	Check for swallow and gag reflexes after upper endoscopy before offering food or fluids.
Lumbar puncture (spinal tap)	A small needle is used to withdraw cerebrospinal fluid for examination. The needle is typically inserted between the L3–4 or L4–5 vertebrae.	To diagnose infection, central nervous system (CNS) disease, or cancers. Sometimes used to inject medication.	Premedicate as ordered. Assist patient to sit leaning forward or lay curled up on side according to HCP preference. Be prepared to assist with procedure.	Label specimens and take to laboratory. Monitor site. Implement activity restrictions if ordered. Encourage fluids.

Continued

Test or Procedure	Description	Reasons Done	Preprocedure Nursing Considerations	Postprocedure Nursing Considerations
Magnetic resonance imaging (MRI)	Magnetic field and radiofrequency energy are used to obtain a detailed image of tissues. Contrast media may be used.	To visualize structural abnormalities in organs and tissues.	Ask patient about any metals in the body, including metallic foreign bodies, tattoos with metal-based inks, or cardiac or orthopedic implants and their designation as MR safe (no hazard), MR conditional (able to carefully use MRI), or MR unsafe (unacceptable risk). Metals can interact with the powerful magnets and be contraindications with MRI. Remove all jewelry. Ask if claustrophobic; patient will be in scanner for up to 1 hour. Consider open MRI availability. If needed, request order for sedative or analgesic to be given 1 hour before test. Explain that patient must lie still in an enclosed area for prolonged period and to expect loud knocking sounds during test. See General Considerations for precare for contrast media.	See General Considerations for postcare for contrast media.
Myelography	Contrast media is injected into cerebrospinal space following lumbar puncture. Radiographs are then taken to outline the vertebrae.	Identifies spinal column abnormalities.	Same as lumbar puncture.	Maintain bedrest with head elevated less than 30 degrees. Monitor for seizures. See General Considerations for postcare for contrast media.

Test or Procedure	Description	Reasons Done	Preprocedure Nursing Considerations	Postprocedure Nursing Considerations
Nuclear scan • heart • lungs • CNS • thyroid • bone • other	Radioactive substances are administered (orally, inhaled, or IV), and then a special scanner observes where the substance is distributed.	To show both structure and function abnormalities.	Check HCP orders for preparation, which may differ for each scan type. Explain that the amount of radioactive material is very small, and no special precautions are needed.	Encourage hydration to promote excretion of radioactive material.
Radiograph (x-ray)	X-ray beams identify internal structures, especially high-density structures such as bone. Contrast media may be used with some tests.	To identify differences in tissue densities. Can help diagnose a variety of structural or other disorders.	Have patient remove jewelry from area to be x-rayed. For bowel prep, laxatives or enemas may be ordered before some gastrointestinal x-rays.	If barium has been used as contrast media to outline the bowel, administer laxative as ordered and increase fluid intake to help evacuate barium before it hardens. See General Considerations for postcare for contrast media.
Ultrasonography • endoscopic ultrasound • transesophageal echocardiogram • transrectal ultrasound • transvaginal	High-frequency sound waves are passed through soft tissues to outline tissues and masses. Gel is used on skin and transducer to improve conduction of sound waves.	To identify alterations in soft tissues and organs.	Check orders for preparation if ultrasound will be done endoscopically.	None specific.

APPENDIX B
Normal Adult Reference Common Laboratory Values

BLOOD, PLASMA, OR SERUM VALUES

Reference Range		
Determination	Conventional	SI
Albumin	3.7–5.1 g/dL	37–51 g/L
Aldolase	Less than 8.1 units/L	
Ammonia	10–80 mcg/dL	5.87–47 micromol/L
Amylase	100–300 units/L	
B-type natriuretic peptide (BNP)	Less than 100 pg/mL	Less than 100 ng/L
Pro-BNP (N-Terminal)	Age 0–74: Less than 125 pg/mL	Age 0–74: Less than 125 ng/L
	Age 75 and older: Less than 449 pg/mL	Age 75 and older: Less than 449 ng/mL
Bilirubin, Total	Less than 1.2 mg/dL	Less than 21 micromol/L
Blood Gases, Arterial		
O_2 Saturation	95–99%	
PCO_2	35–45 mm Hg	4.7–6 kPa
Blood Gas Value (pH)	7.35–7.45	7.35–7.45
PO_2	80–95 mm Hg	10.6–12.6 kPa
Calcium, Total	8.2–9.6 mg/dL	2.1–2.4 mmol/L
Carbon dioxide, plasma or serum (venous)	23–29 mEq/L	23–29 mmol/L
Chloride, Blood	97–107 mEq/L	97–107 mmol/L
Cholesterol, Total and Fractions		
Cholesterol, Total	Less than 200 mg/dL	Less than 5.2 mmol/L
Low-density lipoprotein (LDLC)	Less than 100 mg/dL	Less than 2.59 mmol/L
High-density lipoprotein (HDLC)	Greater than 60 mg/dL	Greater than 1.55 mmol/L
Creatine kinase (CK)	Male: 50–204 units/L	
	Female: 36–160 units/L	

Reference Range		
Determination	*Conventional*	*SI*
CK isoenzymes		
CK-BB	Absent	
CK-MB	0%–4%	
CK-MM	96%–100%	
CK-MB by immunoassay	0–5 ng/mL	
Creatinine		
Male	0.6–1.21 mg/dL	54–107 micromol/L
Female	0.5–1.11 mg/dL	45–98 micromol/L
D-Dimer	0–0.5 mcg/mL FEU (FEU = Fibrinogen Equivalent Units)	0–2.7 nmol/L
Erythrocyte sedimentation rate (ESR) (Westergren method)		
Male	*Under age 50:* Less than 15 mm/hr	
	Over age 50: Less than 20 mm/hr	
Female	*Under age 50:* Less than 25 mm/hr	
	Over age 50: Less than 30 mm/hr	
Glucose, Fasting	Less than 100 mg/dL	Less than 5.6 mmol/L
Iron		
Male	65–175 mcg/dL	11.6–31.3 micromol/L
Female	50–170 mcg/dL	9–30.4 micromol/L
Iron-binding capacity	250–450 mcg/dL	45–81 micromol/L
Lactate dehydrogenase	90–176 units/L	
Lipase	0–60 units/L	
Magnesium, Blood	1.6–2.2 mg/dL	0.66–0.91 mmol/L
Myoglobin		
Male	28–72 ng/mL	1.6–4.1 nmol/L
Female	25–58 ng/mL	1.4–3.3 nmol/L
Osmolality, Serum	275–295 mOsm/kg	275–295 mmol/kg
Phosphatase (alkaline)		
Male	35–142 units/L	
Female	25–125 units/L	
Phosphorus, Blood	2.5–4.5 mg/dL	0.8–1.4 mmol/L
Potassium, Blood	3.5–5.3 mEq/L	3.5–5.3 mmol/L
Protein, Total	6–8 g/dL	60–80 g/L

Continued

Reference Range		
Determination	*Conventional*	*SI*
Sodium, Blood	135–145 mEq/L	135–145 mmol/L
Transaminase, alanine aminotransferase (ALT)		
Male	19–36 units/L	19–36 units/L
Female	24–36 units/L	24–36 units/L
Transaminase, aspartate aminotransferase (AST)		
Male	20–40 units/L	0.34–0.68 microkat/L
Female	15–30 units/L	0.26–0.51 microkat/L
Triglycerides	Less than 150 mg/dL	Less than 1.7 mmol/L
Troponin I	Less than 0.03 ng/mL	Less than 0.03 mcg/L
Troponin T		
Male	Less than or equal to 15 ng/L	Less than or equal to 15 mcg/L
Female	Less than or equal to 10 ng/L	Less than or equal to 10 mcg/L
Urea Nitrogen, Blood (BUN)	8–21 mg/dL	2.9–7.5 mmol/L
Uric Acid, Blood		
Male	4–8 mg/dL	0.24–0.47 mmol/L
Female	2.5–7 mg/dL	0.15–0.41 mmol/L

URINALYSIS REFERENCE VALUES

Dipstick	
pH	4.5–8
Protein	Negative
Glucose	Negative
Ketones	Negative
Hemoglobin	Negative
Bilirubin	Negative
Urobilinogen	Up to 1 mg/dL
Nitrite	Negative
Leukocyte esterase	Negative
Specific gravity	1.005–1.03

Microscopic Examination	
Red blood cells (RBCs)	Less than 5/hpf
White blood cells (WBCs)	Less than 5/hpf
Renal cells	None seen
Transitional cells	None seen
Squamous cells	Rare; usually no clinical significance
Casts	Rare hyaline; otherwise, none seen
Crystals in acid urine	Uric acid, calcium oxalate, amorphous urates
Crystals in alkaline urine	Triple phosphate, calcium phosphate, ammonium biurate, calcium carbonate, amorphous phosphates
Bacteria, yeast, parasites	None seen

HEMATOLOGIC VALUES

Determination	Conventional	SI
Coagulation Screening Tests		
Bleeding time (template)	2.5–10 minutes	
Prothrombin time (PT)	10–13 seconds	
International normalized ratio (INR)	0.9–1.1 for patients not receiving anticoagulation therapy 2–3 for patients receiving conventional anticoagulation therapy with warfarin 2.5–3.5 for patients receiving intensive anticoagulation therapy with warfarin	
Partial Thromboplastin Time, activated (aPTT)	25–35 seconds	
Complete Blood Count (CBC)		
Hematocrit		
Male	42–52	0.42–0.52
Female	36–48	0.36–0.48
Hemoglobin		
Male	14–17.3 g/dL	140–173 mmol/L
Female	11.7–15.5 g/dL	117–155 mmol/L
Platelet count	150–450 × 10^3/microL	150–450 × 10^9/L
Red Blood Cell (Erythrocyte) Count		
Male	4.51–6.01 × 10^6/microL	4.51–6.01 × 10^{12}/L
Female	4.01–5.51 × 10^6/microL	4.01–5.51 × 10^{12}/L

Red Blood Cell (RBC) Indices

	Mean Corpuscular Volume (fl)	Mean Corpuscular Hemoglobin (pg/cell)	Mean Corpuscular Hemoglobin Concentration (g/dL)	RBC Distribution Width Index
Male	77–97	26–34	32–36	11.6–14.8
Female	78–98	26–34	32–36	11.6–14.8

White Blood Cell (WBC) Count and Differential

Conventional Units WBC × 10^3/microL	Neutrophils Total (Absolute and %)	Lymphocytes Bands (Absolute and %)	Monocytes Segments (Absolute and %)	Basophils (Absolute and %)	Eosinophils (Absolute and %)
4.5–11.1	2.7–6.5	1.5–3.7	0.2–0.4	0.05–0.5	0–0.1
	40%–75%	12%–44%	4%–9%	0%–5.5%	0%–1%

THERAPEUTIC DRUG LEVELS

Reference Range

Determination	Conventional	SI
Carbamazepine	4–12 mcg/mL	16.9–50.8 micromol/L
Digoxin	0.5–2 ng/mL	0.6–2.6 nmol/L
Ethanol	None detected	None detected
Lithium	0.6–1.2 mEq/L	0.6–1.2 mmol/L
Phenobarbital	15–40 mcg/mL	64.6–172.4 micromol/L
Phenytoin (Dilantin)	10–20 mcg/mL	40–79 micromol/L
Salicylate, anti-inflammatory	10–30 mg/dL	0.7–2.2 mmol/L

MISCELLANEOUS VALUES

Determination	Conventional	SI
Carcinoembryonic antigen (CEA)		
Smoker	Less than 5 ng/mL	Less than 5 mcg/L
Nonsmoker	Less than 2.5 ng/mL	Less than 2.5 mcg/L
Gastrin	Less than 100 pg/mL	Less than 48.1 pmol/L
Immunological tests		
Alpha-1-antitrypsin (a-1)	126–226 mg/dL	1.26–2.26 g/L
Antinuclear antibodies (ANA)	Titer of 1:40 or less	
Anti-DNA	*Negative:* Less than 5 IU *Indeterminate:* 5–9 IU *Positive:* 9 IU	

Reference range values may differ from one institution to another. hpf × high-power field; SI × International System of Units.

Source: Data from Van Leeuwen, A. M., & Bladh, M. L. (2021). *Davis's comprehensive handbook of laboratory and diagnostic tests with nursing implications* (9th ed.). Philadelphia, PA: F.A. Davis.

Glossary

ablation: Removal of part, pathway, or function by surgery, chemical electrocautery, or radio-frequency.

abrasion: A scraping away of skin or mucous membrane as a result of injury or by mechanical means.

abuse: Misuse; excessive or improper use. May refer to substances or individuals.

accommodation: A reflex action of the eye for focusing.

acidosis: An actual or relative increase in the acidity of blood caused by an accumulation of acid or a loss of base.

acquired immunodeficiency syndrome (AIDS): Suppression or deficiency of the cellular immune response, acquired by exposure to human immunodeficiency virus (HIV).

active immunity: Acquired immunity attributable to the presence of antibodies or of immune lymphoid cells formed in response to antigenic stimulus.

activities of daily living (ADLs): Activities and behaviors that are performed in the care and maintenance of self (e.g., bathing, dressing, eating).

acupuncture: Alternative or complementary technique using needles inserted at specific points to create analgesia or treat certain conditions.

acute coronary syndromes: Group of conditions, including unstable angina, non-Q-wave myocardial infarction, and ST segment elevation myocardial infarction, caused by a lack of oxygen to the heart muscle.

acute pulmonary hypertension: An excessive buildup of pressure in the pulmonary arteries caused by sudden obstruction of the pulmonary artery.

adaptation: Adjustment to changes in internal or external conditions or circumstances; coping.

addiction: Psychological dependence characterized by drug seeking and craving for an opioid or other substance for effects other than the intended purpose of the substance.

adjunct: An addition to the principal procedure or course of therapy.

adjuvant: Something that assists something else, such as a second form of treatment added to treat a disease.

administrative law: Establishes the licensing authority of the state to create, license, and regulate the practice of nursing.

adnexa: Appendages or accessory organs.

advance medical directive: A set of documents (living will and durable medical power of attorney) that explain a person's end-of-life wishes and direct care when the patient is no longer able to do so.

adventitious: Abnormal or extra; often refers to extra breath sounds, such as wheezes or crackles.

advocate: Someone who makes sure a person's wishes are adhered to; someone who represents the best interests of the patient.

aerobic: Living only in the presence of oxygen.

affect: Emotional tone.

afterload: The forces impeding the blood flow out of the heart (vascular pressure, aortic compliance, blood mass, and viscosity).

agenesis: Failure of an organ or part to develop or grow.

agonist: A substance that causes a response. Typically refers to an opioid that binds to opioid receptors in the central nervous system to relieve pain.

akinesia: Absence or loss of the power of voluntary movement.

alkalosis: An actual or relative decrease in the acidity of blood caused by loss of acid or accumulation of base.

allograft: Transplanted organ, tissue, or cells from one individual to another of the same species who is not genetically identical. Donors can be living (related or unrelated) or cadaveric.

allopathic: Method of treating disease with remedies that produce effects different from those caused by the disease.

alopecia: The loss of hair from the body and the scalp.

alternative modality: Refers to a therapy used *instead* of a conventional modality. An example is using acupuncture instead of analgesics for pain.

amenorrhea: The absence or suppression of menstruation. Amenorrhea is normal before puberty, after menopause, and during pregnancy and lactation.

amputation: The removal of a limb or other appendage or outgrowth of the body.

anaerobic: Able to live without oxygen. Often refers to bacteria.

analgesic: A drug that relieves pain.

anaphylactic shock: Systemic reaction that produces life-threatening changes in the circulation and bronchioles.

anaphylaxis: A sudden severe allergic reaction to an allergen.

anastomose: To surgically connect two parts.

anemia: A condition in which there is reduced delivery of oxygen to the tissues as a result of reduced numbers of red cells or hemoglobin.

anergic: Related to the diminished ability of the immune system to react to an antigen.

anesthesia: Controlled temporary medical treatment creating a lack of awareness, feeling, sensation, and the ability to feel pain; used during surgery, procedures, and tests.

anesthesiologist: A physician who specializes in anesthesiology.

aneurysm: A sac formed by the localized dilation of the wall of an artery, a vein, or the heart.

angina pectoris: Severe pain and pressure in the chest caused by insufficient supply of blood and oxygenation to the heart.

angioedema: A localized edematous reaction of the deep dermis or subcutaneous or submucosal tissues appearing as giant wheals.

anion: Electrolyte that carries a negative electrical charge.

anisocoria: Inequality in size of the pupils of the eyes.

ankylosing spondylitis: Inflammatory autoimmune disease of the spine causing stiffness and pain with eventual fusing of some of the vertebrae; a type of arthritis of the spine.

annuloplasty: Repair of a cardiac valve.

anorexia: Absence or loss of appetite for food. Seen in depression, with illness, and as a side effect of some medications.

anorexia nervosa: Refusal to maintain body weight at or above a minimal normal weight for age and height.

antagonist: Medication used to counteract the effects of another substance, usually an opioid (e.g., naloxone).

anteflexion: The abnormal bending forward of part of an organ.

anteversion: A tipping forward of an organ as a whole, without bending.

anthrax: A disease caused by the spore-forming bacterium *Bacillus anthracis* that has three clinical forms in humans: inhalational, cutaneous, and gastrointestinal.

antibody: An immunoglobulin molecule having a specific amino acid sequence that gives it the ability to adhere to and interact only with the specific antigen that induced its synthesis.

anticholinesterase: A substance that breaks down acetylcholinesterase.

antidiuretic: Lessening urine excretion.

antigens: Protein markers on the surface of cells that identify the type of cell.

antitussive: An agent that prevents or relieves cough.

anuria: Complete suppression of urine formation by the kidney.

anxiety: The uncomfortable feeling of apprehension or dread that occurs in response to a known or unknown threat.

aphasia: Defect or loss of the power of expression by speech, writing, or signs, or of comprehension of spoken or written language, caused by disease or injury of the brain centers, such as stroke syndrome.

aphthous stomatitis: Small, white, painful ulcers (also known as canker sores) that appear on the inner cheeks, lips, gums, tongue, palate, and pharynx.

apnea: Absence of breathing.

appendicitis: Inflammation of the vermiform appendix.

arcus senilis: A benign white or gray opaque ring in the corneal margin of the eye.

arrhythmia: Irregular rhythm, especially heartbeat.

arteriosclerosis: Term applied to a number of pathological conditions in which there is gradual thickening, hardening, and loss of elasticity of the walls of the arteries.

arthritis: Inflammation of a joint.

arthrocentesis: Puncture of a joint space with a needle to remove fluid accumulated in the joint.

arthrogram: X-ray examination, with air or a contrast medium injected, of a synovial joint, often the knee or shoulder.

arthroplasty: Surgery to reshape, reconstruct, or replace a diseased or damaged joint.

arthroscopy: Examination of the interior of a joint with an arthroscope.

articular: Pertaining to a joint.

artificial feeding: Feeding via a tube into the stomach or intestine when a person is unable to take oral nutrition.

artificial hydration: Administration of water via IV or gastric tube when a person is unable to take oral fluids.

ascites: Abnormal accumulation of fluid in the peritoneal cavity.

asepsis: A condition free from germs, infection, and any form of life.

aseptic: Free of pathogenic organisms; asepsis.

asphyxia: A condition in which there is a deficiency of oxygen in the blood and an increase in carbon dioxide in the blood and tissues.

aspiration: Accidental drawing in of foreign substances into the trachea and lungs during inspiration. Removal of fluid or tissue from the body, such as an aspiration biopsy.

assessment: An appraisal or evaluation of a patient's condition.

asterixis: Hand-flapping tremor and involuntary movements of tongue and feet; may be present in hepatic encephalopathy.

astigmatism: An error of refraction in which a ray of light is not sharply focused on the retina but is spread over a more or less diffuse area.

ataxia: Failure of muscular coordination; irregularity of muscular action.

atelectasis: Collapsed or airless condition of the lung or portion of lung, caused by obstruction or hypoventilation.

atheroma: Fatty deterioration or thickening of the walls of the larger arteries occurring in atherosclerosis.

atherosclerosis: A form of arteriosclerosis characterized by accumulation of plaque, blood, and blood products lining the wall of the artery, causing partial or complete blockage of an artery.

atrial depolarization: Electrical activation of the atria.

atrial systole: Contraction of the atria.

atrioventricular (AV) node: Located in lower right atrium; receives an impulse from the sinoatrial (SA) node and relays it to the ventricles.

atrophy: Without nourishment; wasting.

atypical: Deviating from normal.

augmentation: The act or process of increasing in size, quantity, degree, or severity.

auscultation: Process of listening for sounds within the body, usually of the internal organs of the chest (heart, lungs) or abdomen (stomach, intestines).

autograft: A graft of tissue from one part of an individual's body to another part of the same individual's body.

autoimmune disease: Produced when the body's normal tolerance of the antigens on its own cells is disrupted.

Ayurvedic: An ancient Hindu system of medicine that improves health by harmonizing mind and body.

azotemia: An increase in nitrogenous bodies in the blood, especially urea, as measured by the serum blood urea nitrogen (BUN) level.

bacteria: One-celled organisms that can reproduce but need a host for food and supportive environment. Bacteria can be harmless, normal flora, or disease-producing pathogens.

balanitis: Inflammation of the skin covering the glans penis.

bariatric: Branch of medicine that deals with the prevention, control, and treatment of obesity.

basal cell secretion test: Part of a gastric analysis; measures the amount of gastric acid produced in 1 hour.

behavior management: Treatment method that uses positive and negative reinforcement to alter behavior.

belief: Something accepted as true. Does not have to be proven.

beneficence: Actions taken and treatments provided are to benefit a person and promote welfare.

benign: Not progressive; for example, a tumor that is not cancerous.

beta-hemolytic streptococci: Gram-positive bacteria that, when grown on blood-agar plates, completely hemolyze the blood and produce a clear zone around the bacteria colony. Group A beta-hemolytic streptococci cause disease in humans.

bigeminy: Occurring every second beat, as in bigeminal premature ventricular contractions.

bimanual: With both hands.

biofeedback: A form of therapy that uses sensors to monitor the status of an autonomic body function such as heart rate, blood pressure, respiratory rate, or muscle tension.

bioprosthesis: Prosthesis consisting of an animal part or containing animal tissue (e.g., porcine heart valve).

biopsy: A sample of tissue removed for examination.

bioterrorism: Biological agent use or threat of use with a pathological organism for terrorist purposes.

bipolar: Having two poles or pertaining to both poles. Bipolar disorder is characterized by episodes of manic and depressive behavior.

blanch: To lose color.

blebs: Irregularly shaped fluid-filled elevations of the skin, such as a blister. May also occur in lung tissue; if a lung bleb ruptures, pneumothorax will occur.

blepharitis: Inflammation of the glands and lash follicles along the margin of the eyelids.

blindness: Lack or loss of ability to see.

bolus: A dose of IV medication injected all at once.

botulism: A paralytic illness caused by a potent neurotoxin produced by *Clostridium botulinum,* an anaerobic, spore-forming bacterium.

bradycardia: A slow heartbeat characterized by a pulse rate below 60 beats per minute.

bradykinesia: Abnormal slowness of movement; sluggishness.

breakthrough pain: Pain that occurs while medicated with long-acting analgesics.

bronchiectasis: Chronic dilation of a bronchus or bronchi, usually associated with secondary infection and excessive sputum production.

bronchitis: Inflammation of the mucous membrane of the bronchial airways; may be viral or bacterial.

bronchodilator: A drug that expands the bronchial tubes by relaxing bronchial smooth muscle.

bronchospasm: Spasm of the bronchial smooth muscle resulting in narrowing of the airways; associated with asthma and bronchitis.

bruit: A humming heard when auscultating a blood vessel that is caused by turbulent blood flow through the vessel.

bulimia nervosa: Recurrent episodes of binge eating and self-induced vomiting.
bulla: Large blisters or skin lesions filled with fluid. Bullae in lung tissue are filled with air. Often occurs in chronic obstructive lung disease.
bundle of His: A bundle of fibers of the impulse-conducting system of the heart. Originates in the atrioventricular (AV) node.
bursae: A small fluid-filled sac or saclike cavity situated in tissues such as joints where friction would otherwise occur.
calculi: An abnormal concentration, usually composed of mineral salts, occurring within the body, chiefly in the hollow organs or their passages. Also called *stones,* as in kidney stones and gallstones.
cancer: A general name for more than 100 diseases in which abnormal cells grow out of control; a malignant tumor.
cannula: A flexible tube that can be inserted into the body and guided by a stiff, pointed rod. For example, an IV cannula is guided by a metal needle.
capillary permeability: The ability of substances to diffuse through capillary walls into tissue spaces.
capillary refill: The amount of time required for color to return to the nailbed after having been compressed, normally 3 seconds or less. Indicator of peripheral circulation.
caput medusae: Dilated veins around the umbilicus, associated with cirrhosis of the liver.
carbuncle: A necrotizing infection of skin and subcutaneous tissue composed of a cluster of boils.
carcinoembryonic antigens (CEA): A class of antigens normally present in fetal cells; CEA level is elevated in many cancers and is measured to guide cancer treatment.
carcinogen: Specific agent known to promote the cancer process.
cardiac output: A measure of the pumping ability of the heart; amount of blood pumped by the heart per minute.
cardiac tamponade: The life-threatening compression of the heart by the fluid accumulating in the pericardial sac surrounding the heart.
cardiogenic shock: Occurs when the heart muscle is unhealthy and contractility is impaired.
cardiomegaly: Enlargement of the heart.
cardiomyopathy: A group of diseases that affect the myocardium's (heart muscle's) structure or function.
cardioplegia: Arrest of myocardial contraction, as by use of chemical compounds or cold temperatures in cardiac surgery.
cardioversion: An elective procedure in which a synchronized shock is delivered to attempt to restore the heart to a normal sinus rhythm.
cataract: Opacity of the lens of the eye.
cation: Electrolyte that carries a positive electrical charge.
ceiling effect: The dose of medication at which the maximum therapeutic effect is achieved. Increasing the dose beyond the therapeutic dose will not result in increased relief and may result in undesirable side effects.
cell-mediated immunity: Production of lymphocytes by thymus in response to antigen exposure.
cellulitis: Spreading bacterial infection of the skin and subcutaneous tissues.
cerebrovascular: Pertaining to the blood vessels of the cerebrum or brain.
cervicitis: Inflammation of the cervix.
chalazion: A small eyelid mass resulting from chronic inflammation of a meibomian gland.
chancre: A hard, syphilitic primary ulcer, the first sign of syphilis, appearing approximately 2 to 3 weeks after infection.
chemotherapy: The treatment of disease with medication; often refers to cancer therapy.
chiropractic: Treatment modality that uses manual adjustment of the vertebral column and extremities to remove interference with nerve function.
cholecystitis: Inflammation of the gallbladder.
choledocholithiasis: Gallstones in the common bile duct.
choledochoscopy: An endoscopic test of the gallbladder and common bile duct.
cholelithiasis: Gallstones in the gallbladder.
chorea: A nervous system condition marked by involuntary muscular twitching of the limbs or facial muscles.
chronic illness: An illness that is long lasting or recurring and usually interferes with a person's ability to perform activities of daily living.
circumcise: Surgical removal of the foreskin covering the head of the penis.
cirrhosis: Chronic disease of the liver, associated with fat infiltration and development of fibrotic tissue.
civil law: Provides the rules by which individuals seek to protect their personal and property rights.
claudication: Severe pain in the calf muscle from inadequate blood supply.
clinical judgment: The outcome of critical thinking and decision making; the action that results from critical thinking.
Clostridioides difficile: A gram-positive bacterium that can overgrow when normal gut microbiota has been destroyed, as with antibiotic therapy, causing a life-threatening infection.
clubbing: A condition in which the ends of the fingers and toes appear bulbous and shiny, most often the result of lung disease.
cochlear implant: A device consisting of a microphone, signal processor, external transmitter, and implanted receiver to aid hearing.
codependence: A situation in which the significant others in a family group begin to lose their own sense of identity and purpose and exist solely for another.
cognitive: The ability to think rationally and to process thoughts.
colectomy: Excision of the colon or a portion of it.
colic: Spasm of a hollow organ or duct, causing pain.
colitis: Inflammation of the colon.
collateral circulation: Small branches off of larger blood vessels that will increase in size and capacity next to a main blood vessel that is obstructed.
colonization: The presence of pathogenic microbes in the body, without development of a symptomatic infection.
colonoscopy: Examination of the upper portion of the rectum with a colonoscope.
colostomy: An artificial opening (stoma) created in the large intestine and brought to the surface of the abdomen for evacuating the bowels.
colporrhaphy: Surgical repair of the vagina.
colposcopy: Examination of the vulva, vagina, and cervix by means of a magnifying lens and a bright light.
comedone: Skin lesion that occurs in acne vulgaris (closed form: whitehead; open form: blackhead).
commissurotomy: Surgical incision of any commissure, as in cardiac valves to increase the size of the orifice.
complementary modality: Refers to a therapy used *in addition* to a conventional modality. For example, a nurse might suggest guided imagery or relaxation techniques for pain control in addition to prescribed drug therapy.
compliance: The ability to alter size or shape in response to an outside force; the ability of the lungs to distend.
compulsion: A recurrent, unwanted, and distressing urge to perform an act.
conductive hearing loss: Impaired transmission of sound waves through the external ear canal to the bones of the middle ear.
condylomata acuminata: Warts in the genital region caused by the human papillomavirus (HPV); a contagious sexually transmitted infection.
condylomatous: Pertaining to a condyloma.
confidentiality: Maintaining privacy of patient information. The patient and their care can be discussed only in the professional setting.
congestive heart failure: Buildup of fluid in either the lungs (left-sided heart

failure) or systemically (right-sided heart failure) that results from impaired cardiac pumping function.

conization: The removal of a cone of tissue, as in partial excision of the cervix uteri.

conjunctivitis: Inflammation of the conjunctiva of the eye.

consensual response: Reaction of both pupils when one eye is exposed to greater intensity of light than the other.

constipation: A condition of sluggish or difficult bowel action/evacuation.

contraceptive: Any process, device, or method that prevents conception.

contractures: Abnormal accumulations of fibrosis connective tissue in skin, muscle, or joint capsule that prevent normal mobility at that site.

contralateral: Originating in or affecting the opposite side of the body.

conversion disorder: An illness that emerges from overuse of the conversion reaction defense mechanism, in which there is impaired physical functioning that appears to be neurologic, but no organic disease can be identified.

coping: The process of contending with the stresses of daily life in an effort to overcome or work through them.

cor pulmonale: Hypertrophy or failure of the right ventricle from disorders of the chest wall, lungs, and pulmonary vessels, as with increased pulmonary pressure caused by chronic obstructive pulmonary disease (COPD).

coronary artery disease: Narrowing of the coronary arteries sufficient to prevent adequate blood supply to the myocardium.

coronavirus disease: Disease caused by the severe acute respiratory syndrome coronavirus 2 *(SARS-CoV-2)* that was first identified in 2019.

craniectomy: Excision of a segment of the skull.

cranioplasty: Any plastic repair operation on the skull.

craniotomy: Any incision through the cranium.

crepitation: A crackling sound such as that heard in the chest with lung inflammation or with grating of the ends of a fractured bone.

crepitus: *See* crepitation.

criminal law: Regulates behaviors for citizens within a country.

critical thinking: Use of knowledge and skills to make the best decisions possible in patient care situations.

cryotherapy: The therapeutic use of cold.

cryptorchidism: A birth condition in which one or both of the testicles has or have not descended into the scrotum.

culdocentesis: The procedure for obtaining material from the posterior vaginal cul-de-sac by aspiration or surgical incision through the vaginal wall, performed for therapeutic or diagnostic reasons.

culdoscopy: Direct visual examination of the female viscera through an endoscope introduced into the pelvic cavity through the posterior vaginal fornix.

culdotomy: Incision or needle puncture of the cul-de-sac of Douglas through the vagina.

cultural awareness: Being aware of history and ancestry and having an appreciation of and attention to the crafts, arts, music, foods, and clothing of various cultures.

cultural competence: Having an awareness of one's own culture and not letting it have an undue influence over another person's culture. Having the knowledge and skills about a culture that are required to provide care.

cultural diversity: Representing two or more cultures; the differences among cultures. Presence of various ethnicities within society.

cultural sensitivity: Being aware of and sensitive to cultural differences. Avoiding behavior or language that may be offensive to another person's cultural beliefs.

culture: The socially transmitted behavior patterns, beliefs, values, customs, arts, and all other characteristics of people that guide their worldview.

curet: A loop, ring, or spoon-shaped instrument, attached to a handle and having sharp or blunt edges; used to scrape tissue from a surface.

customs: The usual ways of acting in a given circumstance or something that an individual or group does out of habit. For example, many people in the United States eat turkey on Thanksgiving.

cyanosis: Slightly bluish, grayish, or dark purple discoloration of the skin caused by the presence of abnormal amounts of reduced hemoglobin in the blood.

cystic: Pertaining to cysts or the urinary bladder.

cystitis: Inflammation of the urinary bladder.

cystocele: A bladder hernia that protrudes into the vagina.

cystoscopy: A diagnostic procedure using an instrument (cystoscope) via the urethra to view the bladder.

cytomegalovirus: Species-specific herpesvirus; usually harmless to those with functional immune systems. May cause fatal pneumonia in those who are immunocompromised. Affects retina and may cause blindness in those with acquired immunodeficiency syndrome (AIDS).

cytotoxic: Destructive to cells.

debridement: The removal of foreign material and contaminated and devitalized tissues from or adjacent to a traumatic or infected area until surrounding healthy tissue is exposed.

decerebrate: Abnormal extension posture indicating brainstem damage.

decorticate: Abnormal flexion posture indicating cerebral damage.

defibrillation: Use of an electrical device that applies countershock to the heart through electrodes placed on the chest wall to stop fibrillation of the heart.

degeneration: Deterioration.

dehiscence: A splitting open (i.e., rupture) of an incision.

dehydration: A condition resulting from excessive loss of body fluid that occurs when fluid output exceeds intake.

delirium: Acute, reversible state of disorientation and confusion with difficulty focusing attention, inability to sleep, and hyperactivity due to an underlying cause.

delirium tremens: An acute alcohol withdrawal syndrome marked by acute, transient disturbance of consciousness.

delusions: False beliefs that are firmly maintained despite incontrovertible proof to the contrary.

dementia: A broad term that refers to cognitive deficit, including memory impairment.

demyelination: Loss of myelin from neurons.

deontology: The study of moral obligations and commitments, including medical ethics.

dependence: A state of reliance on something. Psychological craving for a drug that may or may not be accompanied by a physiological need.

depression: A mental disorder marked by altered mood and loss of interest in daily activities.

dermatitis: Inflammation of the skin.

dermatomycosis: A fungal infection of the skin.

dermoid: Resembling the skin.

developmental stage: An age-defined period with specific psychological tasks that need to be accomplished to maintain ego as proposed by Erik Erikson, a psychoanalyst.

diabetes mellitus: A chronic disease characterized by impaired production or use of insulin and high blood glucose levels.

diaphysis: Long bone shaft.

diarrhea: Passage of fluid or unformed stools.

diastolic blood pressure: The amount of pressure exerted on the wall of the arteries when the ventricles are at rest. The bottom number of a blood pressure measurement.

diffusion: The tendency of molecules of a substance (gaseous, liquid, or solid) to move from a region of high concentration to one of lower concentration.

dilation and curettage: A surgical procedure that expands the cervical canal of the uterus (dilation) so that the surface

lining of the uterine wall can be scraped (curettage).
diplopia: Double vision.
displacement: Transference of emotion from the original idea with which it was associated to a different idea, allowing the patient to avoid acknowledging the original source.
disseminated intravascular coagulation: A pathological form of coagulation that is diffuse (widespread) rather than localized, as would be the case in normal coagulation. Clotting factors are consumed to such an extent that generalized bleeding may occur.
distributive shock: Excessive dilation of the venules and arterioles, leading to decreased distribution of blood, resulting in shock.
diverticulitis: Inflammation of a diverticulum (a sac or pouch in the walls of a canal or organ, usually the colon), especially inflammation involving diverticula of the colon.
diverticulosis: The presence of diverticula in the absence of inflammation.
do not resuscitate (DNR): An order not to do cardiopulmonary resuscitation (CPR) at the end of life.
dormant: Condition of greatly reduced metabolic activity permitting long-term survival and possible reactivation of bacterial endospores, protozoan cysts, larval stages of worm parasites, and viruses.
Dressler syndrome: Postmyocardial infarction syndrome; pericarditis.
durable power of attorney: Person legally designated to speak for a patient when the patient is no longer able to speak for themself.
dysarthria: Imperfect articulation of speech caused by disturbances of muscular control resulting from central or peripheral nervous system damage.
dysfunctional: Family or work environment that does not function effectively, sometimes because of problems of members.
dysmenorrhea: Pain in association with menstruation.
dyspareunia: Occurrence of pain in the labia, vagina, or pelvis during or after sexual intercourse.
dysphagia: Inability to swallow or difficulty swallowing.
dysplasia: Abnormal development of tissue.
dyspnea: Subjective sense of labored breathing that occurs because of insufficient oxygenation.
dysreflexia: State in which an individual with a spinal cord injury at or above T6 experiences an uninhibited sympathetic response to a noxious stimulus.
dysrhythmia: Another name for arrhythmia.

dysuria: Difficult or painful urination.
ecchymoses: A bruise of varying size, the color of which may be blue-black, changing to greenish yellow or yellow with time.
ectasia: Replacement of normal tissue with fibrous tissue.
ectopic: Out of normal position. For example, ectopic hormones are secreted from sites other than the gland where they would normally be found.
edema: Collection of excess fluid in body tissues.
ejaculation: The release of semen from the male urethra.
electrocardiogram (ECG): A recording of the electrical activity of the heart.
electrocautery: Cauterization using platinum wires heated to red or white heat by an electric current, either direct or alternating.
electrocoagulated: Coagulation of tissue by means of a high-frequency electric current.
electroconvulsive therapy (ECT): A type of somatic therapy in which an electric current is used to produce convulsions to treat such conditions as depression.
electroencephalogram: A record produced by electroencephalography; tracing of the electrical impulses of the brain.
electrolytes: Substances that when dissolved in water can conduct electricity, such as potassium or sodium.
electroretinography: Measurement of the electrical response of the retina to light stimulation.
elopement: Leaving a facility unsupervised when unable to protect oneself.
emboli: Solid, liquid, or gaseous masses of undissolved matter traveling with the fluid current in a blood or lymphatic vessel.
embolism: Foreign substance or blood clot that travels through the circulatory system until it obstructs a vessel.
emphysema: Distention of interstitial tissue by gas or air; chronic pulmonary disease marked by terminal bronchiole and alveolar destruction and air trapping.
empyema: Pus in a body cavity, especially the pleural space.
encephalitis: Inflammation of the brain.
encephalopathy: Dysfunction of the brain.
endarterectomy: Excision of thickened atheromatous areas of the innermost coat of an artery.
endogenous: Produced or originating from within a cell or organism.
endometritis: Inflammation of the endometrium of the uterus.
endorphins: Naturally occurring opioids in the body, many times more potent than analgesic medications.
endoscope: A device consisting of a tube and optical system for observing the inside of a hollow organ or cavity. Can be flexible or rigid.
endothelium: A single layer of squamous epithelium cells that line the blood vessels, heart, and lymphatic vessels; it is very smooth to prevent abnormal clotting.
enkephalins: One type of endorphin.
enteral nutrition: Feeding using the gastrointestinal tract, including an oral diet or a tube feeding.
enteritis: Inflammation of the intestines, particularly of the mucosa and submucosa of the small intestine.
enucleation: Removal of an organ or other mass intact from its supporting tissues, as of the eyeball from the orbit.
epidemic: A widespread occurrence of disease in a large number of people.
epidemiological: The study of the distribution and determinants of health-related states and events in populations and the application of this study to the control of health problems.
epididymitis: Inflammation or infection of the epididymis.
epidural: Situated on or outside the dura mater.
epinephrine: A hormone secreted by the adrenal medulla in response to stimulation of the sympathetic nervous system.
epiphyses: Ends of long bone.
epispadias: A congenital male defect in which the opening of the urethra is on the dorsum of the penis, instead of the tip.
epistaxis: Nosebleed.
epithelialization: The growth of skin over a wound.
equianalgesic: Drug doses having equal pain-killing effect. The same degree of pain relief may require different doses of different medications or different routes.
erectile dysfunction: Inability to have an erection sufficient for sexual intercourse.
erection: Enlargement and hardening of the penis caused by engorgement of blood.
erythema: Diffuse redness over the skin.
eschar: Hard scab or dry crust that results from necrotic tissue.
escharotomy: Removal of a slough or scab formed on the skin and underlying tissue of severely burned skin.
esophagogastroduodenoscopy: An endoscopic procedure that allows the physician to view the esophagus, stomach, and duodenum.
esophagoscopy: Examination of the esophagus using an endoscope.
esotropia: Strabismus in which there is deviation of the visual axis of one eye toward that of the other eye, resulting in diplopia. Also called *cross-eyed*.
essential hypertension: Chronic elevation of blood pressure resulting from an unknown cause.

ethical: Describes behavior guided by a system of moral principles or standards.
ethics: Branch of philosophy that answers questions about morality such as good and bad or right and wrong.
ethnic: Pertaining to a religious, racial, national, or cultural group. For example, individuals may identify with the Jewish, Catholic, or Islamic religions.
ethnocentrism: The tendency to think that one's own ways of thinking, believing, and acting are the only right ways. People who are different are seen as strange or bizarre. An example is one who believes that one's own religious beliefs are the only right beliefs and other religions are wrong.
eustress: Stress from positive experiences.
euthyroid: Normal thyroid function.
evaluation: The judgment of something, such as evaluation of outcomes in the nursing process.
evisceration: Extrusion of viscera outside the body, especially through a surgical excision.
exacerbation: Aggravation of symptoms.
exertional dyspnea: Subjective sense of labored breathing that occurs because of insufficient oxygenation due to activity.
exophthalmos: Abnormal protrusion of the eyeball.
exotropia: Abnormal turning outward of one or both eyes; divergent strabismus.
expectorant: Agent that promotes removal of pulmonary secretions.
expectorate: The process of coughing up materials from the air passageways leading to the lungs.
external otitis: Inflammation of the external ear.
extracardiac: Outside the heart.
extracellular: Outside the cell.
extracorporeal shock-wave lithotripsy (ESWL): Noninvasive treatment using shock waves to break up gallstones or kidney stones.
extravasation: The escape of fluids into surrounding tissue.
extrinsic factors: External variables.
exudate: Accumulated fluid in a cavity; oozing of pus or serum; often the result of inflammation.
fasciculation: Twitching.
fasciotomy: Incision of fascia.
fetor hepaticus: Foul breath associated with liver disease.
fibrocystic: Consisting of fibrocysts, which are fibrous tumors that have undergone cystic degeneration or accumulated fluid.
fidelity: Obligation to be faithful to commitments made to self and others.
filtration: The process of removing particles from a solution by allowing the liquid portion to pass through a membrane or other partial barrier, such as in the kidneys.

fissure: A narrow slit or cleft, especially one of the deeper or more constant furrows separating the gyri of the brain; a crack-like skin wound.
fistula: Any abnormal, tubelike passage within body tissue, usually between two internal organs, or leading from an internal organ to the body surface.
flaccid: Weak, lax, soft muscles.
flail chest: Condition of the chest wall caused by two or more fractures on each affected rib resulting in a segment of rib that is not attached on either end; the flail portion moves paradoxically in with inspiration and out with expiration.
fluoroscope: A device consisting of a fluorescent screen suitably mounted, either separately or in conjunction with an x-ray tube, by means of which the shadows of objects interposed between the tube and the screen are made visible.
fluoroscopy: The use of a fluoroscope for medical diagnosis or for testing various materials by roentgen rays.
full-thickness burn: Burn involving epidermis, dermis, tissue, muscle, and bone.
fungi: A general term for a group of eukaryotic organisms (e.g., mushrooms, yeasts, molds).
furuncle: An acute circumscribed inflammation of the subcutaneous layers of the skin or of a gland or hair follicle.
gastrectomy: Any surgery that involves partial or total removal of the stomach.
gastric acid stimulation test: A test that measures the amount of gastric acid for 1 hour after subcutaneous injection of a drug that stimulates gastric acid secretion.
gastric analysis: A test performed to measure secretions of hydrochloric acid and pepsin in the stomach.
gastric lavage: Washing out of the stomach.
gastritis: Acute: Inflammation of the stomach mucosa (heartburn or indigestion). Chronic: Recurring gastritis classified as type A (asymptomatic) or type B (symptomatic).
gastroduodenostomy: Excision of the pylorus of the stomach with anastomosis of the upper portion of the stomach to the duodenum.
gastroepiploic: Pertaining to the stomach and greater omentum.
gastrojejunostomy: Subtotal excision of the stomach with closure of the proximal end of the duodenum and side-to-side anastomosis of the jejunum to the remaining portion of the stomach.
gastroparesis: Paralysis of the stomach, resulting in poor emptying.
gastroplasty: Surgery to decrease the size of the stomach to treat morbid obesity.
gastroscopy: Examination of the stomach and abdominal cavity by use of a gastroscope.

gastrostomy: Surgical creation of a gastric fistula through the abdominal wall.
gavage: Feeding with a stomach tube or with a tube passed through the nares, pharynx, and esophagus into the stomach. The food is in liquid or semiliquid form at room temperature.
glaucoma: A group of eye diseases characterized by increased intraocular pressure.
glomerulonephritis: A form of nephritis in which the lesions involve primarily the glomeruli.
glossitis: Inflammation of the tongue.
glycosuria: Abnormal amount of glucose in the urine, often associated with diabetes mellitus.
goitrogens: Foods or medications that cause a goiter.
gout: A common group of arthritic disorders marked by deposition of monosodium urate crystals in joints and other tissues.
gravida: Number of times a woman has been pregnant.
gummas: A soft granulomatous tumor of the tissues characteristic of the tertiary stage of syphilis.
gynecomastia: Excessive breast tissue on a male.
hallucinations: False perceptions having no relation to reality and not accounted for by any exterior stimuli.
hand hygiene: Cleansing of the hands with hand washing or an alcohol-based hand sanitizer solution as defined by the Centers for Disease Control and Prevention.
health literacy: Degree to which a person has the capacity to obtain, process, and understand basic health information and services to make the best-informed health decisions.
hearing aid: An instrument to amplify sounds for those with hearing loss.
heatstroke: An acute and dangerous reaction to heat exposure, characterized by high body temperature, usually higher than 105°F (40.5°C).
Helicobacter pylori: Bacterium that can cause a peptic ulcer.
hemarthrosis: Bleeding into a joint.
hematochezia: Blood in the feces.
hematoma: A localized collection of extravasated blood, usually clotted, in an organ, space, or tissue.
hematuria: Blood in the urine.
hemiparesis: Weakness affecting one side of the body.
hemipelvectomy: The surgical removal of half of the pelvis and the leg.
hemiplegia: Paralysis of only one side of the body.
hemodialysis: A method for replacing the filtering function of the kidneys by circulating a person's blood through tubes made of semipermeable membranes.

hemolysis: The destruction of the membrane of red blood cells with the liberation of hemoglobin, which diffuses into the surrounding fluid.
hemophilia: A hereditary blood disease marked by greatly prolonged coagulation time, with consequent failure of the blood to clot and abnormal bleeding.
hemoptysis: Coughing up of blood from the respiratory tract.
hemorrhoids: A mass of dilated, tortuous veins in the anorectum involving the venous plexuses of that area.
hemothorax: Blood in the pleural space; may be associated with trauma, tuberculosis, or pneumonia.
hepatitis: Inflammation of the liver, most often caused by a virus.
hepatomegaly: Enlargement of the liver.
hepatorenal syndrome: Severe kidney failure in patients with liver disease.
hepatosplenomegaly: Enlargement of the liver and spleen.
herd immunity: Occurs when a significant portion of the community becomes immune to a specific disease through infection or vaccination.
hernia: The protrusion or projection of an organ or a part of an organ through the wall of the cavity that normally contains it.
herpetic: Pertaining to herpes.
heterograft: Graft from one species to another species (animal to man). Another name for xenograft.
hiatal hernia: A condition in which part of the stomach protrudes through and above the diaphragm.
high-density lipoprotein (HDL): Plasma lipids bound to albumin consisting of lipoproteins. It has been found that those with high levels of HDL have less chance of having coronary artery disease.
histamine: A substance produced in the body that increases gastric secretion, increases capillary permeability, and contracts the bronchial smooth muscle. Plays a role in allergic reaction.
holistic: The view that people and other organisms function as complete units that cannot be reduced to the sum of their parts. In health care, holistic care encompasses the person's body, mind, and spirit along with the environment and society in which the person lives.
homeopathy: System of medicine based on the theory that "like cures like" and uses tiny doses of a substance that create the symptoms of disease.
homeostasis: Maintaining a constant balance, especially whenever a change occurs.
homograft: Graft from a donor of the same species as the recipient.
hopelessness: Subjective state in which a person sees limited or unavailable alternatives.
hordeolum: A sty; bacterial infection of the gland(s) at the base of the eyelashes.
hospice: A service provided to patients and their families in the last 6 months of life to manage symptoms and provide emotional support.
host: The organism from which a parasite obtains its nourishment.
human immunodeficiency virus (HIV): A retrovirus that causes acquired immunodeficiency syndrome (AIDS).
human trafficking: The act of recruiting, harboring, transporting, providing, or obtaining a person for labor or as a sex worker though the use of force, fraud, or coercion.
humoral: Pertaining to body fluids or substances contained in them.
hydrocele: A collection of fluid in the scrotal sack.
hydrocephalus: A condition caused by enlargement of the cranium caused by abnormal accumulation of cerebrospinal fluid within the cerebral ventricular system.
hydronephrosis: Abnormal dilation of kidneys caused by obstruction of urine flow.
hydrostatic: Pertaining to the pressure of liquids in equilibrium and to the pressure exerted by liquids.
hyperalgesia: Increased sensitivity to pain; extreme response to pain.
hypercalcemia: An excessive amount of calcium in the blood.
hyperglycemia: Excess glucose in the blood.
hyperkalemia: An excessive amount of potassium in the blood.
hyperlipidemia: Excessive quantity of fat in the blood.
hypermagnesemia: Excess magnesium in the blood.
hypernatremia: Excess sodium in the blood.
hyperopia: Farsightedness.
hyperplasia: Excessive increase in the number of normal cells.
hypertension: Abnormally elevated blood pressure.
hypertensive emergency: Systolic blood pressure above 180 mm Hg and diastolic blood pressure above 120 mm Hg.
hypertensive urgency: Occurs when blood pressure is as elevated as in a hypertensive emergency but without progression of target-organ dysfunction.
hypertonic: Exerts greater osmotic pressure than blood.
hypertrophy: An increase in the size of an organ or structure, or of the body, owing to tissue growth rather than tumor formation.
hyperuricemia: An excess of uric acid or urates in the blood.
hyperventilation: Increased ventilation that results in a lowered carbon dioxide (CO_2) level (hypocapnia).
hypervolemia: An abnormal increase in the volume of circulating blood.
hypocalcemia: Reduced amount of calcium in the blood.
hypoglycemia: Below-normal amount of glucose in the blood.
hypokalemia: Reduced amount of potassium in the blood.
hypomagnesemia: Reduced amount of magnesium in the blood.
hyponatremia: Reduced amount of sodium in the blood.
hypoperfusion: Low blood flow that occurs when the circulatory system cannot deliver adequate oxygenated blood to the organs and tissues, as in shock.
hypophysectomy: Surgical removal of the pituitary gland.
hypoplasia: Underdevelopment of a tissue organ or body.
hypospadias: A congenital male defect in which the opening of the urethra is on the underside of the penis, instead of the tip.
hypotension: Blood pressure below 90 mm Hg systolic.
hypothermia: Body temperature below 95°F (35°C).
hypotonic: Pertaining to defective muscular tone or tension; having a lower concentration of solute than intracellular or extracellular fluid.
hypotropia: Downward deviation of the eye away from the visual axis.
hypovolemia: The most common form of dehydration resulting from the loss of fluid from the body; results in decreased blood volume.
hypovolemic: Low volume of blood in the circulatory system.
hypovolemic shock: Shock that occurs when blood or plasma is lost in such quantities that the remaining blood cannot fill the circulatory system despite constriction of the blood vessels.
hypoxemia: Deficient oxygenation of the blood.
hypoxia: Diminished availability of oxygen to the body tissues.
hysterectomy: Surgical removal of the uterus through the abdominal wall or vagina.
hysterosalpingogram: Radiograph of the uterus and fallopian tubes.
hysteroscopy: Endoscopic direct visual examination of the canal of the uterine cervix and the cavity of the uterus.
hysterotomy: Incision of the uterus.
icterus: Yellowing of the skin and the sclera of the eye.
ileostomy: An artificial opening (stoma) created in the small intestine (ileum) and brought to the surface of the abdomen for the purpose of evacuating feces.
illness: The state of being sick.
illusions: Mistaken perceptions of reality.

imagery: The use of the imagination to promote relaxation.
immune (or idiopathic) thrombocytopenic purpura: A disorder in which the immune system destroys platelets, resulting in slowed blood clotting and bleeding risk.
immunocompromised: Having an immune system that is not capable of reacting to a pathogen or tissue damage.
immunosenescence: Aging of the immune system.
impaction: A dry, hard mass of feces that cannot be pushed out of the rectum or colon.
imperforate: Without an opening.
in situ: Localized, not invading surrounding tissue.
in vitro fertilization: Fertilization in a test tube.
incontinence: Loss of control such as with urine or stool. *See* urinary incontinence.
induction: The process or act of causing to occur, as in anesthesia induction.
induration: Area of hardened tissue.
infective endocarditis: Inflammation of the heart lining caused by microorganisms.
infiltration: The accumulation of an external substance (such as IV fluids) within tissues.
informatics: The study of digital information and information systems.
inspection: Use of observation skills to systematically gather data that can be seen.
insufficiency: The condition of being inadequate for a given purpose, such as heart valves that do not close properly.
insufflation: Inflation of the abdomen during laparoscopic or endoscopic procedures to enhance visualization of structures.
intermittent claudication: Pain in the calf of a lower extremity, usually brought on by activity or exercise, that ceases with rest caused by arterial occlusive disease.
international normalized ratio: The World Health Organization's standard for reporting the prothrombin time assay test when the thromboplastin reagent developed by the first International Reference Preparation is used.
interstitial: Between tissues.
intervention: One or more actions taken in order to modify an effect.
intracellular: Located within a blood cell.
intracranial: Within the cranium or skull.
intraoperative: Occurring during a surgical procedure.
intravascular: Located within the blood vessels.
intravenous: Within or into a vein.
intrinsic factors: Internal variables.
intussusception: The slipping of one part of an intestine into another adjacent to it.

ipsilateral: On the same side; affecting the same side of the body.
ischemia: Condition of inadequate blood supply.
isoelectric line: The period when an electrical tracing is at zero and is neither positive nor negative.
isolated systolic hypertension: The systolic pressure is 160 mm Hg or more, but the diastolic pressure is lower than 95 mm Hg.
isotonic: A fluid that has the same osmolarity as the blood.
jaundice: Yellowing of the skin and the sclera of the eye.
Kaposi sarcoma: A vascular malignancy that is often first apparent in the skin or mucous membranes but may involve the viscera.
ketoacidosis: A condition in which fat breakdown produces ketones, which cause an acidic state in the body; may be associated with weight loss or diabetes mellitus.
Kussmaul respirations: Term describing deep respirations of an individual with ketoacidosis.
laceration: A wound or irregular tear of the flesh.
lactic acid: By-product of anaerobic metabolism.
laminectomy: The excision of a vertebral posterior arch, usually to remove a lesion or herniated disc.
laparoscopy: Exploration of the abdomen with an endoscope.
laparotomy: Surgical opening of the abdomen; an abdominal operation.
laryngeal edema: Sudden swelling of the larynx occurring with severe allergic reactions.
laryngectomy: Surgical removal of the larynx.
laryngitis: Inflammation of the larynx.
laser ablation: Therapeutic destruction of a growth or part of a growth by laser treatment.
lavage: Washing out of a cavity.
law: The further formalization of moral considerations.
leadership: The process of socially influencing others to obtain their assistance and support to accomplish a common task.
leiomyoma: A myoma consisting principally of smooth muscle tissue.
leukemia: A malignancy of the blood-forming cells in the bone marrow.
leukocytosis: An increase in the number of leukocytes in the blood, generally caused by the presence of infection.
leukopenia: Abnormal decrease of white blood cells, usually below 5,000/mm^3.
liability: The level of responsibility that society places on individuals for their actions.
libido: Sexual drive, conscious or unconscious.

lichenified: Thickened or hardened from continued irritation.
limitation of liability: Steps that health-care professionals can take to limit their liability.
living will: A document instructing health-care workers about a patient's preferences when the patient is no longer able to communicate. Implementation of living wills varies by state.
lobectomy: Surgical removal of a lobe of any organ or gland.
low-density lipoprotein (LDL): A lipoprotein that transports cholesterol and triglycerides from the liver to peripheral tissues.
lower gastrointestinal (GI) series: The use of barium sulfate as an enema to facilitate x-ray and fluoroscopic examination of the colon.
lymphadenopathy: Any disorder of the lymph nodes.
lymphangitis: Inflammation of lymphatic channels or vessels.
lymphedema: An abnormal accumulation of tissue fluid (potential lymph) in the interstitial space.
lymphocytes: Cells present in the blood and lymphatic tissue that provide the main means of immunity for the body; white blood cells.
lymphoma: A usually malignant lymphoid neoplasm.
macrodrop: A large drop (typically 15–20 drops per mL). In IV therapy, may refer to an administration device used to deliver large drops of IV solution.
macular degeneration: Age-related breakdown of the macular area of the retina of the eye.
maleficence: Committing harm or evil.
malignant: Growing, resisting treatment; used to describe a tumor of cancerous cells.
malingerer: Someone who pretends to be in pain or be ill.
malpractice: A breach of duty arising out of the relationship that exists between the patient and the health-care worker.
mammography: Use of radiography to study breast tissue.
mammoplasty: Plastic surgery of the breast.
mania: Mood disturbance characterized by excessive energy and elevated mood.
marsupialization: Process of raising the borders of an evacuated tumor sac to the edges of the abdominal wound and stitching them there to form a pouch that easily drains.
mastalgia: Pain in the breast.
mastectomy: Excision of the breast.
mastitis: Inflammation of the breast.
mastopexy: Correction of a pendulous breast by surgical fixation and plastic surgery.

mediastinum: A septum or cavity between two principal portions of an organ.
megacolon: Extremely dilated colon.
melena: Black, tarry feces caused by action of intestinal secretions on free blood.
menarche: The initial menstrual period, normally occurring between the ninth and 17th year of life.
Ménière disease: A recurrent and usually progressive group of symptoms including progressive deafness, ringing in the ears, dizziness, and a sensation of fullness or pressure in the ears.
meningitis: Inflammation of the membranes of the spinal cord and brain.
menopause: The period that marks the permanent cessation of menstrual activity, usually occurring between the ages of 35 and 58.
mental health: State of being adjusted to life; able to be flexible, successful, maintain close relationships, solve problems, make appropriate judgments, and cope with daily stresses.
mental illness: Any illness that affects the mind or behavior.
metastasis: Movement of bacteria or body cells (especially cancer cells) from one part of the body to another.
microbiota: Microorganisms inhabiting a bodily organ or part such as the gut or skin.
microdrop: A small drop (60 drops per mL). In IV therapy, may refer to an administration device used to deliver small drops of IV solution.
milieu: Environment.
miotic: An agent that causes the pupil to contract.
moral distress: Distress experienced when the right thing to do cannot be carried out because of institutional constraints.
morbidity: State of being diseased.
mortality: Condition of being mortal; number of deaths in a population.
mucolytic: Agent that liquefies sputum.
mucopurulent cervicitis: Inflammation of the cervix producing mucus and purulent discharge.
mucositis: Inflammation of a mucous membrane.
multifocal: Many foci (areas) or sites.
murmur: An abnormal sound heard on auscultation of the heart and adjacent large blood vessels.
myalgia: Muscle pain or tenderness.
myectomy: Surgical removal of a hypertrophied muscle.
myelogram: The film produced by radiography of the spinal cord after injection of a contrast medium into the subarachnoid space.
myocardial infarction: Death of myocardial cells as a result of oxygen deprivation due to an obstruction of the blood supply. Commonly referred to as a heart attack.
myocarditis: The inflammatory process that causes nodules to form in the myocardial tissue; the nodules become scar tissue over time. Inflammation of the heart muscle.
myocardium: Heart muscle.
myomectomy: Removal of a portion of muscle or muscular tissue.
myopia: The error of refraction in which rays of light entering the eye parallel to the optic axis are brought to a focus in front of the retina; nearsightedness.
myringoplasty: Surgical reconstruction of the tympanic membrane.
myringotomy: Incision of the tympanic membrane, usually performed to relieve pressure and allow for drainage of either serous or purulent fluid in the middle ear behind the tympanic membrane.
myxedema: Condition resulting from hypofunction of the thyroid gland.
nasoseptoplasty: Surgical correction of the nasal septum.
naturopathy: System of medicine that uses natural therapies such as nutrition, herbs, hydrotherapy, counseling, physical medicine, and homeopathy.
negligence: An unintentional tort.
neoplasm: New abnormal tissue growth, as in a tumor.
nephrectomy: Surgical removal of a kidney.
nephrogenic: Caused by the kidneys.
nephrolithotomy: Incision of a kidney for removal of kidney stones.
nephropathy: Any disease of the kidney.
nephrosclerosis: Hardening of the kidney associated with hypertension and disease of the renal arterioles.
nephrostomy: Creation of a permanent opening into the renal pelvis.
nephrotoxin: A toxin having a specific destructive effect on kidney tissue.
neuralgia: Nerve pain.
neurogenic: Originating in the nervous system.
neuropathic: Resulting from peripheral nerve injury.
neuropathy: A general term denoting functional disturbances and pathological changes in the peripheral nervous system.
neutrophils: Type of white blood cells including granulocytes (neutrophils, eosinophils, and basophils), monocytes, and lymphocytes (T cells and B cells).
nociception: The body's normal reaction to noxious stimuli, such as tissue damage, with the release of pain-producing substances.
nociceptive: Pain sensitive.
nocturia: Excessive urination at night.
nodal or junctional rhythm: A cardiac rhythm with its origin at the atrioventricular (AV) node.
nonmaleficence: The requirement that health-care providers do no harm to their patients, either intentionally or unintentionally.
norepinephrine: A hormone produced by the adrenal medulla, similar in chemical and pharmacological properties to epinephrine, but chiefly a vasoconstrictor with little effect on cardiac output.
normoglycemia: Normal blood glucose.
nosocomial infection: Infection acquired in a health-care agency.
nuchal rigidity: Rigidity of the nape, or back, of the neck.
numeracy: Ability to understand and use numbers in everyday life.
nursing diagnosis: A standardized label placed on a patient's problem to make it understandable to all nurses.
nursing process: An orderly, logical approach to administering nursing care so that the patient's needs for such care are met comprehensively and effectively.
nystagmus: Involuntary, cyclical, rapid movement of the eyes in response to vertical, horizontal, or rotary movement.
obesity: Abnormal amount of fat on the body ranging from 20% to 30% above average weight for age, sex, and height.
objective data: Factual data obtained through physical examination and diagnostic tests; objective data are observable or knowable through the five senses.
obsession: Repetitive thought, urge, or emotion.
obstipation: Intractable constipation.
obstructive shock: Shock caused by indirect pump failure.
occult blood: Blood not seen by the naked eye.
oliguria: Diminished urination.
oncology: The study of cancer and cancer treatment.
oncovirus: Viruses linked to cancer in humans.
onychomycosis: Disease of the nails caused by fungus.
oophorectomy: Surgical removal of the ovaries.
ophthalmia neonatorum: Conjunctivitis in the newborn resulting from exposure to infectious or chemical agents.
ophthalmologist: A physician who specializes in the treatment of disorders of the eye.
ophthalmoscope: An instrument used for examining the interior of the eye, especially the retina.
opioid: A narcotic drug with morphine-like effects. True opioids are derived from opium.
optician: One who specializes in filling prescriptions for corrective lenses for eyeglasses and contact lenses.
optometrist: A doctor of optometry who diagnoses and treats conditions and diseases of the eye per state laws.

orchiectomy: Removal of one or both testicles; a treatment for prostate cancer.

orchitis: Inflammation of a testis.

orgasm: Pleasurable physical release sensation related to physical, sexual, and psychological stimulation.

orientation: The ability to comprehend and to adjust oneself in an environment with regard to time, location, and identity of persons.

orthopnea: Labored breathing that occurs when lying flat; relieved when sitting up; associated with left ventricular heart failure.

osmolality: Osmotic concentration; ionic concentration of the dissolved substances per unit of solvent.

osmolarity: Concentration of the substances in body fluids.

osmosis: The passage of solvent through a semipermeable membrane that separates solutions of different concentrations.

osteoblast: Produce bone matrix during growth and replace matrix during normal remodeling or in repair of fractures.

osteoclast: Resorb bone matrix when more calcium is needed in the blood or during repair.

osteomyelitis: Inflammation of bone, especially the marrow, caused by a pathogenic organism.

osteopathic: System of medicine emphasizing the interrelationship of the body's nerves, muscles, bones, and organs; involves treating the whole person.

osteoporosis: A condition in which there is a reduction in the mass of bone per unit volume.

osteosarcoma: A malignant sarcoma of a bone.

otalgia: Pain in the ear.

otorrhea: Inflammation of the ear with purulent discharge.

otosclerosis: A condition characterized by chronic, progressive deafness, especially for low tones.

ototoxic: Having a detrimental effect on the eighth cranial nerve or the organs of hearing.

pain: An unpleasant sensory and emotional experience associated with actual or potential tissue damage, or described in terms of such damage. Pain is whatever the patient says it is whenever the patient says it occurs.

palliation: The relief of symptoms without the intent to cure disease.

palpation: Use of the fingers or hands to feel something.

pancreatectomy: Removal of all or part of the pancreas.

pancreatitis: Inflammation of the pancreas.

pancytopenia: Abnormal depression of all of the cellular elements of the blood.

pandemic: The occurrence of a disease affecting large numbers of people that spreads across more than one continent or around the world.

panhysterectomy: Excision of the entire uterus and cervix.

panmyelosis: Increased level of all bone marrow components, red blood cells, white blood cells, and platelets.

para: Number of deliveries a woman has had from pregnancies after 20 weeks' gestation.

paradoxical respiration: Chest movement on respiration that is opposite to that expected.

paranoia: Behavior that is marked by delusions of persecution or delusional jealousy.

paraparesis: Partial paralysis of the lower extremities.

paraphimosis: Uncircumcised foreskin that has swollen and stuck behind the head of the penis.

paraplegia: Paralysis of the lower body, including both legs, resulting from a spinal cord lesion.

parenteral: A medication delivery route that is "beside" rather than in the intestine, such as intramuscular, IV, or subcutaneous.

parenteral nutrition: Nutrition by IV route, either centrally or peripherally.

paresis: Weakness; incomplete paralysis.

paresthesia: A heightened sensation, such as burning, prickling, or tingling.

paroxysmal nocturnal dyspnea: Sudden attacks of shortness of breath that usually occur during sleep. Person wakes gasping for breath and sits up to relieve symptoms; associated with left ventricular heart failure.

partial-thickness burn: Burn in which the epithelializing elements remain intact.

passive immunity: Reinforcement of the immune system with immune serum for such conditions as tetanus, diphtheria, and venomous snake bite.

paternalism: A unilateral and sometimes unreasonable decision by health-care providers that implies they know what is best, regardless of the patient's wishes.

pathogen: A microorganism or substance capable of producing a disease.

pathological fracture: Fracture resulting from weakening of the bone structure by pathological processes such as neoplasia or osteomalacia.

patient-controlled analgesia (PCA): An apparatus that delivers an IV analgesic to relieve pain, which is controlled by the patient.

pedicle: The stem that attaches a new growth.

pediculosis: Infestation with lice.

pemphigus: Acute or chronic serious skin disease characterized by the appearance of bullae (blisters) of various sizes on normal skin and mucous membranes.

penumbra: An area of brain tissue surrounding damage from a stroke that may be revived if the brain is reperfused quickly.

peptic ulcer disease: A condition in which the lining of the esophagus, stomach, or duodenum is eroded.

perception: A unique impression of events by an individual. These impressions are strongly influenced by personality, cultural orientation, attitudes, and life experiences.

percussion: A tapping technique used by physicians and advanced practice nurses to determine the consistency of underlying tissues.

percutaneous: Through the skin; may refer to an injection, a medication application, or a biopsy.

perfusion: Supplying an organ or tissue with blood.

pericardial effusion: A buildup of fluid in the pericardial space.

pericardial friction rub: Friction sound heard over the fourth left intercostal space near the sternum; a classic sign of pericarditis.

pericardial tamponade: Compression of the heart by an abnormal filling of the pericardial sac with blood.

pericardiectomy: Excision of part or all of the pericardium.

pericardiocentesis: Surgical perforation of the pericardium.

pericardiotomy: Incision of the pericardium.

pericarditis: Inflammation of the pericardium (two thin layers of a saclike membrane surrounding the heart).

perimenopausal: The phase before the onset of menopause, during which the cycle of a woman with regular menses changes, perhaps abruptly, to a pattern of irregular cycles and increased periods of amenorrhea.

perinatal: Concerning the period beginning after the 28th week of pregnancy and ending 28 days after birth.

perioperative: Occurring in the period immediately before, during, and after surgery.

periosteum: Connective tissue covering all outer bone surfaces except at joints that protects, is involved in bone growth and repair, and participates in the blood supply of bone.

peripheral arterial disease: Disease of the peripheral arteries that interferes with adequate flow of blood.

peripheral vascular resistance: Opposition to blood flow through the vessels.

peristalsis: Progressive, wavelike movement that occurs involuntarily in hollow tubes of the body such as the alimentary (digestive) canal; causes contents of tube to be moved onward.

peristomal: Area around a stoma.
peritoneal dialysis: The employment of the peritoneum surrounding the abdominal cavity as a dialyzing membrane for the purpose of removing waste products or toxins accumulated as a result of renal failure.
peritonitis: Inflammation of the peritoneum.
personal protective equipment: Items worn to protect oneself and one's patients from direct transmission of organisms (including gloves, surgical masks, goggles, gowns, and shoe booties) based on the task to be performed and the type of isolation precautions in use.
petechiae: Small, purplish, hemorrhagic spots on the skin that appear in certain illnesses and bleeding disorders.
phagocytosis: Ingestion and digestion of bacteria and particles by phagocytes, cells that have the ability to ingest and destroy particulate substances such as bacteria, protozoa, and cell debris.
pharyngitis: Inflammation of the mucous membranes and lymph tissues of the pharynx, usually caused by infection.
pheochromocytoma: Rare tumor of the adrenal system that secretes catecholamines.
phimosis: Uncircumcised foreskin that cannot be moved down from the head of the penis.
phlebitis: Inflammation of a vein; may be due to irritating IV fluids or thrombosis.
phlebotomy: Entry into a vein for the removal or withdrawal of blood.
phobia: A persistent, irrational, intense fear of a specific object, activity, or situation.
photophobia: Abnormal visual intolerance to light.
physical dependence: A pharmacological phenomenon characterized by signs and symptoms of withdrawal when medication is withdrawn.
phytoestrogens: Naturally occurring plant sterols that have an estrogen-like effect.
pinocytosis: Reabsorption of small proteins from renal filtrate by attachment to the membranes of the tubule cells and then engulfment and digestion.
plague: A severe febrile illness caused by the gram-negative coccobacillus *Yersinia pestis* that is usually transmitted by the bite of an infectious flea.
plaque: A deposit of fatty material on the lining of an artery.
plasmapheresis: Removal of blood to separate cells from plasma.
pleurodesis: Creation of adhesions between the parietal and visceral pleura to treat recurrent pneumothorax.
pneumocystis pneumonia (PCP): An acute pneumonia caused by the fungus *Pneumocystis jiroveci*.
pneumonectomy: Surgical removal of all or part of a lung.
pneumonia: Pulmonary inflammation usually due to infection with bacteria, viruses, or other pathogens.
pneumonitis: Pulmonary inflammation due to causes other than infection.
pneumothorax: Air in the pleural space.
poikilothermy: The absence of sufficient arterial blood flow, causing the extremity to become the temperature of the environment.
point of maximum impulse (PMI): The area of the chest where the greatest force can be felt with the palm of the hand when the heart contracts or beats. Usually at the fourth to fifth intercostal space in the midclavicular line.
polycythemia: Excessive red cells in the blood.
polydipsia: Excessive thirst.
polyneuropathy: A disease involving multiple nerves.
polyphagia: Excessive eating.
polyuria: Excessive urination.
portal hypertension: Persistent blood pressure elevation in the portal circulation of the abdomen.
postcoital: After sexual intercourse.
postictal: Occurring after a sudden attack, such as an epileptic seizure.
postmortem care: Care after death.
postoperative: Following a surgical operation.
postprandial: After a meal.
powerlessness: Perceived lack of control over a situation.
prehabilitation: Preoperative functional, physical, and lifestyle preparation to promote the best possible surgical and recovery outcome.
preload: End-diastolic stretch of cardiac muscle fibers; equals end-diastolic volume.
preoperative: Preceding an operation.
preprandial: Before a meal.
presbycusis: Progressive, bilaterally symmetrical perceptive hearing loss occurring with age; usually occurs after age 50 and is caused by structural changes in the organs of hearing.
presbyopia: Diminution of accommodation of the lens of the eye occurring normally with aging, and usually resulting in hyperopia, or farsightedness.
pressure injury: An open sore or lesion of the skin that develops because of prolonged pressure against an area.
priapism: Erection that lasts too long.
primary hypertension: Abnormally elevated blood pressure of unknown cause. Also called *essential hypertension*.
probiotics: Supplements of live bacteria or yeast that assist the body's naturally occurring gut microbiota. Often recommended after antibiotic therapy to reestablish the normal microbiota.
proctitis: Inflammation of the rectum and anus.
proctosigmoidoscopy: Visual examination of the rectum and sigmoid colon by use of a sigmoidoscope.
prodrome: A symptom indicating the onset of a disease or event, such as a seizure.
prostaglandins: Chemical neurotransmitters usually associated with pain at the site of an injury.
prostatectomy: Removal of the prostate gland.
prostatitis: Inflammation or infection of the prostate gland.
protozoa: Single-celled parasitic organisms that can move and live mainly in the soil.
pruritus: Severe itching.
pseudoaddiction: Syndrome in which behaviors similar to addiction appear as a result of inadequate pain control and patient fear of not receiving adequate pain medications and pain relief.
psoriasis: Chronic inflammatory skin disorder in which epidermal cells proliferate abnormally fast.
psychoanalysis: Form of therapy based on the theories of Sigmund Freud regarding the dynamics of the unconscious.
psychogenic: Of mental origin.
psychological dependence: Obsession of obtaining drugs for use other than medicinal; addiction.
psychopharmacology: The study of the action of drugs on psychological functions and mental states.
psychosomatic: Having bodily symptoms of psychological, emotional, or mental origin; illness traceable to an emotional cause.
psychotherapy: A method of treating disease (especially mental illness) by mental rather than pharmacological means.
ptosis: Drooping of eyelid.
puerperal: Concerning the puerperium, or period of 42 days after childbirth.
pulmonary edema: Severe fluid congestion in the alveoli of the lungs; life threatening. Usually a result of heart failure or pneumonia.
pulse deficit: A condition in which the number of pulse beats counted at the radial artery is less than those counted in the same period of time at the apical heart rate.
purpura: Hemorrhage into the skin, mucous membranes, internal organs, and other tissues.
purulent: Fluid that contains pus.
pyelogram: A diagnostic procedure involving x-ray of the kidneys; may be done after injection of a dye into the bloodstream or directly into the kidneys.
pyelonephritis: Inflammation of the kidney and renal pelvis.

pyoderma: Any acute, inflammatory, purulent bacterial dermatitis.
QSEN project: Quality and Safety Education for Nurses project; focuses on nursing education that promotes the continual improvement of quality and safety in patient care.
quadrigeminy: PVC occurs every fourth beat (three normal beats and then a PVC).
quadriparesis: Weakness involving all four limbs caused by spinal cord injury.
quadriplegia: Paralysis of all four limbs caused by spinal cord injury.
radiation therapy: Cancer treatment with ionizing radiation.
range of motion (ROM): The range of movement of a body joint.
Raynaud disease: A primary or idiopathic vasospastic disorder characterized by bilateral and symmetrical pallor and cyanosis of the fingers and toes.
reality orientation: A process to orient a person to facts such as names, dates, and time, through the use of verbal and nonverbal repeating messages.
rectocele: Protrusion or herniation of the posterior vaginal wall with the anterior wall of the rectum through the vagina.
red blood cells: Erythrocytes; circulating blood cells that contain hemoglobin and carry oxygen to tissues.
regurgitation: A backward flowing, as in the backflow of blood through a defective heart valve.
reminiscence therapy: Use of life reflection with a therapist to resolve conflicts or bring closure to life events.
remyelination: Replacement of myelin on neurons.
replantation: The replacement of an organ or other structure, such as a digit, limb, or tooth, to the site from which it was previously lost or removed.
reservoir: A person, animal, arthropod, plant, soil, or substance in which an infectious agent normally lives and multiplies, on which it depends for survival.
resorption: To absorb again, as in removal of bone tissue by absorption.
respiratory excursion: Downward movement of the diaphragm with inspiration.
respite care: Short-term, intermittent care for the chronically ill; provides rest for the family members or caregivers from the stress of sustained caregiving.
respondeat superior: An institution that employs a worker may be liable for the acts or omissions of its employees.
retinopathy: Disease of the retina of the eye.
retroflexion: A bending or flexing backward.
retrograde: Moving backward; degenerating from a better to a worse state.
retrograde cholangiopancreatography: An endoscopic procedure that permits the physician to visualize the liver, gallbladder, and pancreas using an endoscope, dye, and x-ray examinations.
retroversion: A turning, or a state of being turned back; the tipping of an entire organ.
rhabdomyolysis: Rapid skeletal muscle tissue breakdown that releases damaged cell contents, such as myoglobin, into the bloodstream, which are harmful to the kidneys and can lead to kidney damage.
rheumatic carditis: Serious complication of rheumatic fever in which all layers of the heart become inflamed.
rheumatic fever: A hypersensitivity reaction to antigens of group A beta-hemolytic streptococci.
rhinitis: Inflammation of the nasal mucosa, usually associated with congestion, itching, sneezing, and nasal discharge.
rhinoplasty: Plastic surgery of the nose.
rickettsia: A genus of bacteria of the tribe rickettsiae that multiply only in host cells.
Rinne test: A test of hearing done with tuning forks.
Romberg test: A test to determine if a person has the ability to maintain body balance when the eyes are shut and the feet are close together.
Roux-en-Y: For gastric bypass surgery, a small stomach pouch the size of a thumb is created with staples, then a Y-shaped section of the small intestine is attached to the pouch to allow food to bypass the lower stomach and duodenum.
rule of nines: A formula for estimating percentage of body surface area, particularly helpful in judging the percentage of skin that has been burned.
sacral radiculopathy: Pathology of sacral nerve roots.
salpingectomy: Surgical removal of the fallopian tubes.
salpingitis: Inflammation of a fallopian tube.
salpingoscopy: Endoscopic visualization of the fallopian tubes.
scleroderma: A chronic manifestation of progressive systemic sclerosis in which the skin is taut, firm, and edematous, limiting movement.
sclerosis: A hardening or induration of an organ or tissue, especially from excessive growth of fibrous tissue.
seborrhea: Disease of the sebaceous glands marked by increase in the amount and often alteration of the quality of sebaceous secretions.
secondary hypertension: High blood pressure that is a symptom of a specific cause, such as a kidney abnormality.
semipermeable: Partly permeable; said of a membrane that will allow fluids but not a dissolved substance to pass through it.
sensorineural: Hearing loss caused by impairment of a sensory nerve.
sensory deprivation: No or minimal stimulation of the senses that creates the potential for maladaptive coping.
sensory overload: Excessive stimulation of the senses that creates the potential for maladaptive coping.
sepsis: Systematic infection caused by microorganisms in the bloodstream.
serologic: Study of substances present in blood serum.
sanguineous: Bloody.
serosanguineous: Fluid consisting of serum and blood.
serous: Watery fluid resembling serum.
serotonin: A chemical neurotransmitter important in sleep/wake cycles. Reduced serotonin levels are associated with depression.
shock: A clinical syndrome in which the peripheral blood flow is inadequate to return sufficient blood to the heart for normal function, particularly transport of oxygen to all organs and tissues.
sinoatrial (SA) node: Node at the junction of the superior vena cava and right atrium, regarded as the starting point of the heartbeat.
sinusitis: Inflammation of the sinuses; may be due to viral or bacterial infection, or to allergies.
Snellen chart: A chart imprinted with lines of black letters graduating in size from smallest on the bottom to largest on top; used for testing visual acuity.
somatoform: Denoting psychogenic symptoms resembling those of physical disease; psychosomatic.
spider angioma: Thin reddish-purple vein lines close to the skin surface.
spirituality: Sense of connectedness with all of life and the universe.
splenectomy: Excision of the spleen.
splenomegaly: Enlargement of the spleen.
standard precautions: Guidelines recommended by the Centers for Disease Control and Prevention to reduce the risk of the spread of infection.
stapedectomy: Excision of the stapes to improve hearing, especially in cases of otosclerosis.
Staphylococcus: A genus of gram-positive bacteria; they are constantly present on the skin and in the upper respiratory tract and are the most common cause of localized suppurating infections.
status asthmaticus: Prolonged period of unrelieved asthma symptoms.
steatorrhea: Fat in the stools; may be associated with pancreatic disease.
stenosis: The constriction or narrowing of a passage or orifice, such as a cardiac valve.

stent: Any mold or device used to hold tissue in place or to provide a support, graft, or anastomosis while healing is taking place.

stereotype: An opinion or belief about an individual or group that may not be true.

sternotomy: The operation of cutting through the sternum.

stoma: A mouth, small opening, or pore.

stomatitis: Inflammation of the mouth.

stress: The physical (gravity, mechanical, pathogenic, injury) and psychological (fear, anxiety, crisis, joy) forces that are experienced by individuals.

stressor: Any person or situation that produces an anxiety response.

striae: A line or band of elevated or depressed tissue; may differ in color or texture from surrounding tissue.

subarachnoid: Below or under the arachnoid membrane and the pia mater of the covering of the brain and spinal cord.

subdural: Beneath the dura mater.

subjective data: Information that is provided verbally by the patient.

suffering: A state of severe distress associated with events that threaten the intactness of the person. Emotional pain associated with real or potential tissue damage.

summons: A notice of suit, issued by a court.

suprapubic: Bone of the groin (or region) located above the pubic arch.

surgeon: A medical practitioner who specializes in surgery.

synarthrosis: Immovably fixed joint between bones connected by fibrous tissue (sutures of the skull).

synovitis: Inflammation of the synovial membrane that may be the result of an aseptic wound, a subcutaneous injury, irritation, or exposure to cold and dampness.

systolic blood pressure: Maximal pressure exerted on the arteries during contraction of the left ventricle of the heart. The top number of a blood pressure measurement.

tachycardia: An abnormal rapidity of heart action, usually defined as a heart rate greater than 100 beats per minute in adults.

tachydysrhythmia: An abnormal heart rhythm with rate greater than 100 beats per minute in an adult.

tachypnea: Abnormally rapid respiratory rate.

tamponade: Compression of a part.

telenursing: Delivering nursing care from a distance with the use of telecommunications.

tension pneumothorax: Abnormal accumulation of air with buildup of pressure in the pleural space; life-threatening.

teratoma: A congenital tumor containing one or more of the three primary embryonic germ layers.

terminal illness: An illness that will probably cause death in 6 months or less.

tetanus: A highly fatal disease caused by the bacillus *Clostridium tetani* and characterized by muscle spasm and convulsions.

tetany: Muscle spasms, numbness, and tingling caused by changes in pH and low serum calcium.

therapeutic privilege: Limitation for veracity used by health-care providers when telling patients the truth would cause them greater harm.

thoracentesis: Insertion of a large-bore needle into the pleural space to remove air or fluid.

thoracotomy: Surgical incision into the chest wall.

thrill: Palpation of a vibration on the surface of the skin. Can be caused by turbulent blood flow through a blood vessel (as with a fistula or graft) or cardiac abnormalities.

thrombi: Blood clots.

thrombocytopenia: Abnormal decrease in the number of blood platelets.

thrombolytic: Agent that dissolves or splits up a thrombus, an aggregation of blood factors.

thrombophlebitis: The formation of a clot and inflammation within a vein.

thrombosis: Formation, development, or presence of a thrombus, an aggregation of blood factors.

tidaling: Rise and fall; may refer to water in water-seal chamber of a chest drainage system.

titration: Adjustment of medication up or down to meet patient needs.

tolerance: The response of the body to medication that requires increased medication administration to achieve the same effect. Often refers to opioids.

torts: Lawsuits involving civil wrongs.

toxemia: Spread of the poisonous products of bacteria throughout the body.

tracheostomy: A surgical opening in the neck into the trachea to provide an airway when the trachea is obstructed.

tracheotomy: An opening in the neck into the trachea.

traditions: Practices and customs handed down through the generations, often by word of mouth.

transcellular: Across cell membranes.

transdermal: Entering through the dermis, or skin, as in administration of a drug applied to the skin in ointment or patch form.

transillumination: The passage of strong light through a body structure to permit inspection of an observer on the opposite side.

transjugular intrahepatic portosystemic shunt (TIPS): Shunt that sidetracks venous blood around the liver to the vena cava for treatment of ascites.

transmyocardial: Across all layers of the heart.

trauma: Physical injury caused by an external force.

trauma-informed care: Special care based on knowing trauma survivors' personal experiences (such as those of abuse, Holocaust survivors, veterans, or victims of large-scale disasters) to avoid triggers that could cause re-traumatization.

Trendelenburg position: A position in which the patient's head is low and the body and legs are on an elevated and inclined plane. Also called *Trendelenburg's position*.

triage: The assignment of degrees of urgency to wounds or illnesses to decide the order of treatment of patients or casualties.

trichinosis: A disease caused by the roundworm *Trichinella spiralis*, which is spread by eating raw or undercooked meat from pigs or wild animals that contains *Trichinella* larvae.

trigeminy: Occurring every third beat, as in trigeminal premature ventricular contractions.

tropia: A manifest deviation of an eye from the normal position when both eyes are open and uncovered.

tumor: An abnormal growth of cells or tissues; tumors may be benign or malignant.

turbid: Cloudy.

turgor: The resistance of the skin to being grasped between the fingers. Dehydration causes poor skin turgor.

unifocal: Coming or originating from one site or focus.

upper gastrointestinal (GI) series: X-ray and fluoroscopic examinations of the stomach and duodenum after the ingestion of a contrast medium.

uremia: An excess in the blood of urea, creatinine, and other nitrogenous end products of protein and amino acid metabolism.

urethritis: Inflammation of the urethra.

urethroplasty: Plastic repair of the urethra.

urinary incontinence: Inability to control urine excretion, creating accidental urinary leakage.

urodynamic: The study of the holding or storage of urine in the bladder, the facility with which it empties, and the rate of movement of urine out of the bladder during urination.

urosepsis: Sepsis resulting from urinary tract infection.

urticaria: Hives signifying an allergic reaction.

utilitarian: Consequences or outcomes of a dilemma are the most important element.

vaginitis: Inflammation of the vagina.

vaginosis: Infection of the vagina.
values: Ideals or concepts that give meaning to an individual's life.
valvotomy: Cutting through a valve.
valvuloplasty: Plastic or restorative surgery on a valve, especially a cardiac valve.
varices: Dilated veins.
varicocele: Varicose veins of the scrotum; can lead to infertility.
varicose veins: Swollen, distended, and knotted veins, usually in the subcutaneous tissue of the leg.
vasculitis: Inflammation of a vessel.
vasectomy: Surgically cutting and sealing the vas deferens to prevent sperm from getting outside the body. Used as a birth control method for men.
vector: Living organism that transmits disease.
venous stasis ulcers: Poorly healing ulcers that result from inadequate venous drainage.
ventricular diastole: The period of relaxation of the two ventricles.
ventricular escape rhythm: The naturally occurring rhythm of the ventricles when the rest of the cardiac conduction system fails.
ventricular repolarization: Reestablishment of the polarized state of the muscle after contraction.
ventricular systole: The contraction of the two ventricles.
ventricular tachycardia: A series of at least three beats arising from a ventricular focus at a rate greater than 100 beats per minute.
veracity: Truthfulness.
verrucous: Wartlike, with raised portions.
vesicant: Agent that causes blistering of tissue. Some chemotherapy agents are vesicants.
vesicular: Pertaining to vesicles or small blisters.
virulence: The power of an organism to cause disease.
virus: The smallest organism identified by use of electron microscopy; intracellular parasites that may cause disease.
viscosity: Thickness, as of the blood.
vulvovaginitis: Inflammation of the vulva and vagina.
volvulus: A twisting of the bowel on itself, causing obstruction.
Weber test: A test for unilateral deafness.
white blood cells: Leukocytes; the body's primary defense against infection.
withdrawal: Symptoms caused by cessation of administration of a drug, especially a narcotic or alcohol, to which the individual has become either physiologically or psychologically addicted.
worldview: The way individuals look on the world to form values and beliefs about life and the world around them.
xenograft: Graft from one species to another species (animal to man).
xerostomia: Dry mouth caused by reduction in secretions.

Photo & Illustration Credits

Chapter 1
Fig 1.1: NCSBN. Copyright © 2019 National Council of State Boards of Nursing, Inc. (NCSBN®). All rights reserved.

Chapter 2
Fig 2.1: From Ackley, B. J., Ladwig, G. B., Swan, B. A., & Tucker, S. J. (2008). *Evidence-based nursing care guidelines: Medical-surgical interventions.* Philadelphia: Elsevier, with permission.

Chapter 8
Fig 8.2: From Hoffman, J. J., and Sullivan, N. J. (2021). *Davis Advantage for medical-surgical nursing: Making connections to practice.* (2nd ed.). Philadelphia: FA Davis.

Chapter 10
Fig 10.3: From the International Association for the Study of Pain, with permission.
Fig 10.4: From Warden, V., Hurley, A. C., & Volicer, L. (2003). Development and psychometric evaluation of the Pain Assessment in Advanced Dementia (PAINAD) Scale. *Journal of the American Medical Directors Association, 4*(1), 9–15. Developed and tested by clinicians and researchers at the New England Geriatric Research Education and Clinical Center, a Department of Veterans Affairs center of excellence with divisions at EN Rogers Memorial Veterans Hospital, Bedford, MA, and VA Boston Health System. www.amda.com
Fig 10.5: From the Purdue Frederick Company, Norwalk, CT.

Chapter 11
Figs 11.7 & 11.10: Photo courtesy of Dinesh Patel, MD, Medical Oncology, Internal Medicine, Zanesville, OH.
Fig 11.8: Data from the American Cancer Society. (2020). *Cancer facts and figures 2020.* Atlanta, GA. From https://www.cancer.org/content/dam/cancer-org/research/cancer-facts-and-statistics/annual-cancer-facts-and-figures/2020/cancer-facts-and-figures-2020.pdf
Fig 11.11: Photo courtesy of National Cancer Institute (NCI).

Chapter 15
Fig 15.2: Courtesy of Desin, LLC.

Chapter 17
Fig 17.1: Copyright 1999. Robert Wood Johnson Foundation. Used with permission from the Robert Wood Johnson Foundation. (From Emanuel, L. L., von Gunten, C. F., & Ferris, F. D. (Eds.). (1999). *The Education for Physicians on End-of-Life Care [EPEC] curriculum.* Chicago: The EPEC Project. Copyright Robert Wood Johnson Foundation.)

Chapter 20
Fig 20.1: Modified from United States Department of Health and Human Services. (2021). The HIV life cycle. https://hivinfo.nih.gov/understanding-hiv/fact-sheets/hiv-life-cycle

Chapter 25
Figs 25.10, 25.11, 25.12, 25.13, 25.15, 25.16, 25.17, 25.18: Modified from Jones, S. A. (2008). *ECG success: Exercises in ECG interpretation.* Philadelphia: F.A. Davis.

Chapter 28
Fig 28.4: Courtesy of Sandoz Pharmaceutical Corp., East Hanover, NJ.
Fig 28.6: From Huether, S. E., & McCance, K. L. (1996). *Understanding pathophysiology.* St. Louis, MO: Mosby, p. 548, with permission.
Figs 28.7: Courtesy of Paul A. Volberding, MD, University of California, San Francisco.

Chapter 29
Fig 29.22: Courtesy of Axcan Scandipharm, Birmingham, AL.
Fig 29.23: Courtesy of Deknatel Snowden Pencer, Inc., Tucker, GA.
Fig 29.26: Courtesy of Passy-Muir, Inc., Irvine, CA.

Chapter 30
Fig 30.1: Courtesy of ArthroCare, Inc., Austin, TX.
Figs 30.2AB: Courtesy of Philips Respironics, Murrysville, PA.
Fig 30.4A: Courtesy of UltraVoice Ltd., Newtown Square, PA.
Fig 30.4B: Courtesy of InHealth Technologies, Carpinteria, CA.

Chapter 31
Fig 31.6: From U.S. Department of Health & Human Services, *Get on a path to a healthier you (quitting).* Retrieved from https://betobaccofree.hhs.gov/gallery/quit.html
Fig 31.13: From the National Cancer Institute, June 1998.

Chapter 32
Figs 32.6AB: Courtesy Dr. Russell Tobe.

Chapter 35
Fig 35.1: From the Centers for Disease Control and Prevention/Dr. Thomas F. Sellers; Emory University, 1963.

Chapter 39
Fig 39.2AB: From Chanson, P., & Salenave, S. (2008). Acromegaly. *Orphanet Journal of Rare Disease, 3*(17). Published online June 25, 2008, PMCID. © 2008 Chanson and Salenave, licensee BioMed Central Ltd.
Fig 39.5: Courtesy of the CDC Public Health Image Library (PHIL), #15470.

Chapter 40
Fig 40.5: Courtesy of Medtronic MiniMed, Inc.
Fig 40.6: Courtesy of Roche Diabetes Care, Inc.

Chapter 41
Fig 41.9: From National Cancer Institute, created by Rhoda Baer (Photographer).

Chapter 47
Fig 47.12: From Wijdicks, E. F. M., Bamlet, W. R., Marmatton, B. V., Manno, E. M., & McClelland, R. L. (2005). Validation of a new coma scale: The FOUR Score. *Annals of Neurology, 58*(4), 585–593. https://doi.org/10.1002/ana.20611. Figure 1 and Table 1. Used with permission. © Mayo, 2005.

Chapter 48
Fig 48.15: From Spillane, J. D. (1968). *An atlas of clinical neurology.* New York: Oxford University Press, p. 219, with permission.

Chapter 49
Fig 49.2: From the National Stroke Association, © 2015. Reprinted by permission of National Stroke Association. Please visit www.stroke.org for stroke education resources.
Fig 49.4: Modified from National Institutes of Health, National Institute of Neurological Disorders and Stroke. Stroke Scale. https://www.stroke.nih.gov/documents/NIH_Stroke_Scale_508C.pdf

Chapter 52
Fig 52.2: From National Eye Institute, National Institutes of Health. https://medialibrary.nei.nih.gov

Chapter 54
Fig 54.4: Courtesy of CDC/ K.L. Herrmann.
Fig 54.6: Courtesy of Dr. Loretta Fiorillo.
UNFigs 54.2, 54.4, 54.6, 54.8, 54.10, 54.12: National Pressure Ulcer Advisory Panel Copyright. Reprinted with permission of the copyright holder, Gordian Medical, Inc. dba American Medical Technologies.
UNFigs 54.18, 54.19: Courtesy of CDC.
UNFigs 54.20, 54.21: Courtesy of CDC/Dr. Lucille K. Georg.
UNFig 54.22: Courtesy of CDC/Dr. Edwin P. Ewing, Jr.
UNFig 54.23: Courtesy of CDC/Sol Silverman, Jr., DDS.

INDEX

Note: Page numbers followed by f refer to figures; page numbers followed by t refer to tables; page numbers followed by b refer to boxes; **medication entries are in boldfaced type**.

A

Abdomen assessment, 581–583, 582f
   in secondary survey, 194t
Abdominal aortic aneurysm (AAA), 396–397, 396f
Abdominal hernias, 633–634, 633f
Abdominal trauma, 196
   deficient fluid volume and, 198
Abducens nerve, 935t
Ablation, catheter, 413, 414
ABO blood types, 451, 452t
Abortion, 837–839
Abrasions, 194
   eye, 1075
Abscesses
   anorectal, 638
   in Crohn disease, 626
Absence seizures, 960
Absorption disorders, 634–635, 635t
Abuse
   mandatory reporting of, 26
   recognizing elder, 195, 243
Acceleration-deceleration injury, 963
Accessory nerve, 936t
Accommodation, visual, 943
Acetaminophen, 123, 124t
   acute liver failure and, 656, 656b
   preoperative, 173t
Acetylcholine (ACh), 887, 936, 1156t
Acid-base balance, 65
   chronic kidney disease (CKD) and, 713
   control of, 65
   respiration and, 490, 492
Acid-base imbalances, 65, 66f, 66t
Acidic agents, 874t
Acidosis, 66t, 490
   in shock, 106
Acne vulgaris, 1127, 1127f
Acquired immunodeficiency syndrome (AIDS). *See* HIV/AIDS
Acquired von Willebrand syndrome, 471
Acromegaly, 744, 744f
Action potential, 930
Activated partial thromboplastin time (aPTT), 458t
Active immunity, 266
Active listening, 5–6
Active transport, 51
Activities of daily living (ADLs), 214, 215
   after stroke, 1009
   assistive devices for, 224, 224f
   contractures and, 22f, 223
   long-term care services, 236–237
   osteoporosis and, 911, 919
   therapeutic measures for neurologic system, 947
Activity. *See also* Exercise
   after myocardial infarction (MI), 389
   chronic heart failure (HF) and, 432, 438
   in long-term care facilities, 238

Acupressure, 43f
Acupuncture, 42, 43f
Acute bronchitis, 533–534
Acute care, 235–236
Acute care for elders (ACE) units, 236
Acute compartment syndrome, 906–907, 907f
Acute coronary syndrome (ACS)
   myocardial infarction (MI) (*see* Myocardial infarction)
   silent ischemia, 384
   sudden cardiac death, 384
Acute gastritis, 607
Acute heart failure (HF), 385t, 428–429, 428t
Acute hydrocephalus, 965
Acute kidney injury (AKI), 708–710, 710t
Acute liver failure, 655–656, 656b, 660–661
Acute lymphocytic leukemia (ALL), 475
Acute pain, 119
Acute pancreatitis, 662–664, 665–666
Acute poststreptococcal glomerulonephritis, 707
Acute pulmonary hypertension, 111
Acute respiratory distress syndrome (ARDS), 562–563
Acute respiratory failure, 562
Adaptation, 1158
Addiction, 122. *See also* Alcohol use disorders; Substance use disorders
Addison disease, 757–758
Adenocarcinoma, 564
Adenoiditis, 525
Adenosine SPECT-CT thallium imaging, 333t
Adenosine triphosphate (ATP), 51
Adherence, 306
Adipose tissue, 725f
Adjunct agents, anesthesia, 176
Adjustable gastric banding, 601, 602f
Adjuvants, 123, 124–125t, 127
Administrative laws, 28
Adrenal cortex, 727, 733t
Adrenalectomy, 760–761
Adrenal glands, 724f, 725f, 727, 728f
Adrenal glands disorders
   adrenocortical insufficiency/Addison disease, 757–758
   Cushing syndrome, 758–760, 758t, 759f
   medications for, 762t
   pheochromocytoma, 756–757
Adrenal medulla, 727, 732t
Adrenergic bronchodilators, 550t
Adrenocortical insufficiency (AI), 757–758
Adrenocorticotropic hormone (ACTH), 724, 725f, 727, 731t
Adult day-care service, 237t
Adult foster care service, 237t
Advance directives, 167, 248
Adventitious breath sounds, 495, 498t
Advocate, nurse as patient's, 252
Aerobic bacteria, 85
Affective disorders, 1176–1179

Afterload, 426
Agenesis, 828
Age-related macular degeneration (AMD), 1067, 1067f, 1073–1075, 1074f, 1075f
Aging. *See also* Gerontological issues; Older adults
   cancer risk and, 146
   cardiovascular system and, 323, 323f
   cultural diversity and, 37
   defined, 222–223
   developmental stage, 213–215, 214f
   diverticulosis and diverticulitis and, 624
   ear and, 1049, 1054
   endocrine system and, 728, 733f
   eye and, 1041–1042, 1042f
   gastrointestinal, hepatobiliary and pancreatic systems and, 576–577, 577f
   hematologic and lymphatic systems and, 453, 454f
   hypertension and, 344
   hyperthermia and, 202
   immune system and, 213, 268, 268f
   integumentary system and, 225, 1094, 1094f
   mental health and, 1190–1191
   musculoskeletal system and, 887, 890f
   nervous system and, 937, 939f
   physiological changes with, 223–229, 224f
   reproductive system and, 227–228, 795, 796f
   respiratory system and, 492f
   spinal cord injuries and, 979
   surgery and, 166
   urinary system and, 678–679, 679f
   urinary tract infection (UTI) and, 696
   vision and hearing loss with, 215, 228–229
AIDS wasting syndrome, 302, 304, 305t
Airway assessment, in primary survey, 192–193, 193f
Alcoholics Anonymous (AA), 1165
Alcohol use
   acute pancreatitis and, 662–663
   cancer and, 145
   chronic pancreatitis and, 664
   malignant breast disorders and, 816
   surgery and, 167
Alcohol use disorders, 1187
   subdural hematomas and, 964
Aldosterone, 727
Aldosterone antagonists, 435
Aldosterone receptor antagonists, 348t
Alkaline phosphatase (ALP), 890, 893t
Alkalosis, 66t, 490
Allergen immunotherapy, 275
Allergic rhinitis, 278–279
Allergies, 176, 269, 271. *See also* Asthma
   therapeutic measures for, 275
Allograft, 361
Allopathic/Western medicine, 42
Alogia, 1180
Alopecia, 155, 1098–1099

Alpha-1 blockers, 347t
Alpha-adrenergic agents, 112t
Alpha-adrenergic antagonists, 850t
Alpha-glucosidase inhibitors (AGIs), 775t
Alpha-reductase inhibitors, 850t
Altered mental status in chronic heart failure (HF), 431
Alveoli, 491f
Alzheimer disease, 994–996, 995t
Ambulatory surgery discharge, 189
Amebicides, 874t
Amenorrhea, 823t, 825
    lactational, 837
American Cancer Society (ACS), 142
American Indian medicine, 43
American Society for Parenteral and Enteral Nutrition, 69
Ametropia, 1066
Amino acid metabolism, 575
Amino acids, 1156t
Aminoglycosides, 98t
    hearing loss due to, 1076t
Amphotericin B, 100t
Amputation, 194–195, 924–926
Amyotrophic lateral sclerosis (ALS), 1029–1030, 1032t
Anabolic (bone-forming) medications, 912
Anaerobic bacteria, 85
Anal fissures, 638
Analgesia
    balanced approach to, 127
    fears related to, 166
    patient-controlled analgesia (PCA), 71–72, 128
    procedural sedation and, 177
    scheduling options for, 127
Analgesics, 123
    medication administration routes, 128, 129–130t
    for osteoarthritis (OA), 916
    preoperative, 173t
    urinary, 698t
Anaphylactic shock, 108, 109t, 194, 266
Anaphylaxis, 194, 279, 280t
    after blood administration, 460
    due to insect stings or bites, 203
Anemia, 462–465
    aplastic, 465–466, 466f
    in chronic heart failure (HF), 431
    chronic kidney disease (CKD) and, 713–714
    defined, 462
    nutrition and, 463
    pernicious, 288
    sickle cell, 467–470, 468f, 469f
Anesthesia
    fears related to, 166
    general, 176
    local or regional, 176–177, 177f
Anesthesiologists, 167
Aneurysms, 396–397, 396f, 397t
Angina pectoris, 380–381
    medications for, 382–383t
Angioedema, 280–281
Angiography, 331t, 333t, 336, 336f, 946
Angioma, 1132t
Angioplasty, 399
Angiotensin-converting enzyme (ACE) inhibitors, 347t, 432, 433t
Angiotensin II receptor blockers (ARB), 348t, 433t, 435

Angiotensin receptor neprilysin inhibitors (ARNIs), 433t, 435
Angular cheilosis, 604b
Anhedonia, 1176, 1180
Animal-assisted activities (AAA), 46, 46f
Animal-assisted therapy (AAT), 46
Anions, 57
Anisocoria, 943
Ankle-brachial index, 394
Ankylosing spondylitis, 293–294
Annuloplasty, 361
Anorectal abscess, 638
Anorectal problems, 637–638
Anorexia, 154, 598
Anorexia nervosa, 1185
Anterior pituitary gland, 723–724, 725f, 731t
Anthrax, 205, 205f, 206t
Antiangiogenetics, 1062t
Antianxiety agents, 1174t
Antiarrhythmics, 410t
Antibiotic-associated diarrhea (AAD), 101
Antibiotic prophylaxis, 604b
Antibiotic-resistant infections, 97
Antibiotics, 97–99t
    for burns, 1144t
    for Crohn disease, 627
    hearing loss due to, 1076t
    for irritations and inflammations of the vagina and vulva, 828t
    ophthalmic, 1062t
    preoperative, 173t
    for sexually transmitted infections (STIs), 873–874t
    for urinary tract infection (UTI), 698t
Antibodies, 88, 264, 265f, 265t
    HIV/AIDS, 305
    monoclonal, 275
    responses by, 265–266, 267f
Anticholinergics
    for arrhythmias, 410t
    for chronic obstructive pulmonary disease (COPD), 550t
    in end-of-life care, 259t
Anticholinesterases, 1027
Anticoagulants
    for arrhythmias, 410t
    for myocardial infarction (MI), 388t
    for pulmonary embolism (PE), 558
    for stroke, 1007t
    for venous thromboembolism (VTE) disease, 372, 372–373t
Anticonvulsant mood stabilizers, 1175t, 1177
Anticonvulsants, 125t
    for multiple sclerosis (MS), 1023t
    for seizure disorders, 960, 961t
Antidepressants, 1173–1174t, 1177
Antidiuretic hormone (ADH), 51, 726f, 731t
    imbalances of, 740–743, 741t, 742b
    medications for, 761t
Antiembolism devices, 337–338
Antiemetics
    for pancreatic and gallbladder disorders, 665t
    preoperative, 173t
Antifungals, 100t
    for irritations and inflammations of the vagina and vulva, 828t
    ophthalmic, 1062t

Antigens, 88, 264
    HIV/AIDS, 305
    serum sickness and, 284
Antihistamines
    for hemolytic transfusion reactions, 284t
    for shock, 113t
Anti-inflammatory agents, 113t
    ophthalmic, 1063t
Anti-inflammatory synthetic corticosteroid, 628t
Anti-ischemic agents, 383t
Antimalarials, 292t
    for osteoarthritis (OA), 918t
Antimanic agents, 1175t
Antimicrobial resistance (AMR), 879
Antimitotic agents, 874t
Antiparkinsonian agents, 1175t
Antiplatelets
    for coronary artery disease (CAD), 382t, 383
    for myocardial infarction (MI), 388t
    for stroke, 1007t
Antiprotozoals
    for irritations and inflammations of the vagina and vulva, 828t
    for sexually transmitted infections (STIs), 874t
Antipruritics, 279
Antipsychotics, 1173t
Antipyretics
    preoperative, 173t
    for serum sickness, 284
Antiresorptive medications, 911–912
Antiretroviral (ARV) therapy, 297, 306–309, 307–308t
    CD4 T-lymphocyte count and, 306
    pre-exposure prophylaxis, 301
Antisecretory agents, 610t
Antisocial personality disorder (ASPD), 1183
Antispasmodics, 1023t
Antitussive agents, 549
Antivirals, 100t
    for hepatitis, 653
    ophthalmic, 1062t
    for respiratory viruses, 526
    for sexually transmitted infections (STIs), 874t
Anxiety, 166
Anxiety disorders, 1169–1170
    diagnosis, 1170
    etiological theories of, 1170
    mild, 1158
    nursing process, 1172, 1176
    summary, 1175t
    therapeutic measures for, 1172
    types of, 1170
Anxiolytics
    to increase comfort at end of life, 259t
    preoperative, 173t
Aortic regurgitation, 356t, 358–359
Aortic stenosis, 355–356t, 358
Aphasia, 943, 947–948, 1003, 1009
Aphthous stomatitis, 603
Aplastic anemia, 465–466, 466f
Apnea, 494
Apocrine glands, 1092, 1093f
Appendicitis, 623, 624f
Arcus senilis, 1046
Arrhythmias. *See* Cardiac arrhythmias
Arterial blood gases (ABGs), 495, 498t
    acid-base balance and, 65, 66t

Arterial pressure points, 198f
Arterial stiffness index, 334
Arterial thrombosis and embolism, 393–394
Arteries, heart, 320, 322f
Arthritis, 900
　osteoarthritis (OA), 914–919, 914f, 915f, 917–918t
　rheumatoid arthritis (RA), 914t
Arthrocentesis, 890, 895t
Arthrography, invasive, 894t
Arthroplasty, 921
Arthroscopy, 891–892, 895t
Artificial feeding and hydration, 250
Ascites, 657, 659, 659f
Asepsis, 93, 93b
Aseptic technique, 174–175
ASKMME! (Ask, Search, thinK, Measure, Make it happen, and Evaluate), 11
Aspartate, 1156t
Asphyxia, 204
Aspiration, 198
　in older patients, 226
Aspiration pneumonia, 538
Aspirin, 552
Aspirin-exacerbated respiratory disease (AERD), 520
Assault and battery, 195
Assessment tools, pain, 131–132, 132f, 133f, 134f
Assistive hearing devices, 1056–1057
Assistive personnel (AP), 13, 17
Asterixis, 657–658
Asthma, 550–554
　complications, 552, 554t
　diagnostic tests, 552, 554t
　etiology, 551
　pathophysiology, 551
　prevention, 551
　signs and symptoms, 551–552, 554t
　therapeutic measures, 552–554, 552f, 553f, 554t
　triggers, 551
Astigmatism, 1066
Astrocytes, 929
Asystole, 418, 418f
Ataxia, 1003
Atelectasis, 167, 169
　due to lung cancer, 565
　due to pneumonia, 539
　due to pulmonary fibrosis, 545
Atherosclerosis, 323, 323f
　diagnostic tests, 378
　etiology of, 378
　pathophysiology, 377–378
　risk factors for, 378–379t
　therapeutic measures, 379
Atlas vertebrae, 885
Atopic dermatitis, 279
Atrial depolarization, 405
Atrial fibrillation (AF), 413–414, 414f
Atrial flutter, 413, 413f
Atrial natriuretic hormone, 319
Atrioventricular (AV) node, 319, 320f
　arrhythmias originating in, 412–415, 412–415f
Atrophic vaginitis, 827t
Atrophy, muscle, 1029
Atypical antipsychotics, 1173t

Audiometric testing, 1054–1055, 1055t
Auditory acuity testing, 1052, 1054t
Augmentation, breast, 821, 821f
Aura, 959
Auscultation, 329–330, 329f
　abdominal, 582
　endocrine system, 729
　respiratory system, 495, 497f
Autism spectrum disorders (ADSs), 1183–1184
Autoclaves, 93
Autocratic (authoritarian) leadership, 18
Autogenic drainage, 501
Autograft, 361, 1144
Autoimmune disorders, 288–294, 288t. See also Immune disorders
　ankylosing spondylitis, 293–294
　Crohn disease, 626–627, 626f, 627f
　gastritis, 607
　Hashimoto thyroiditis, 289
　idiopathic autoimmune hemolytic anemia, 288–289
　pernicious anemia, 288
　rheumatic fever, 354
　systemic lupus erythematosus (SLE), 289–293, 289b, 290b, 291t, 292–293t, 292f
Autolytic debridement, 1113
Automatic external defibrillators (AEDs), 249, 421, 421f
Autonomic dysreflexia, 975
Autonomic nervous system (ANS), 934–937
　function of, 936t
　parasympathetic division, 937, 938, 938f
　sympathetic division, 934, 936, 937f, 938
Autonomic nervous system agents, 112t
Autonomy, 3, 21, 22, 24
Avascular necrosis, 921
Avian influenza, 527
Avolition, 1180
Avulsions, 194, 902t, 903f
Axons, 929, 930f
Ayurvedic medicine, 42
Azotemia, 713

B

Bacillus Calmette-Guérin (BCG) Live vaccine, 149, 541
Bacteria, 83–85, 85t
　cancer risk factor, 144–145
Bacterial infections
　conjunctivitis, 1060–1061
　external ear, 1078–1079
　pneumonia, 538
　tuberculosis (TB), 540–543
　vaginosis, 827t
Bactericidal antibiotics, 97–99t
Balance and ear, 1048, 1050f
　aging and, 1054
　Ménière disease and, 1087–1088
　testing of, 1052
Balanced electrolyte solutions, 74
Balneotherapy, 1101
Bariatric surgery, 600–602, 602f
Barium enema, 588–589, 588f
Barium swallow, 588
Barrel chest, 494
Barrier contraceptive methods, 835–836, 835–836f
Barrier methods for safer sex, 881t

Bartholin cysts, 840–841
Bartholin's glands, 793f
Basal cell carcinoma, 1132, 1133f
Basal nuclei, 934
Basilar artery syndrome, 1004t
Basophils, 450t, 451
B cells, 264, 451, 453
　humoral immunity, 265, 267f
Beau lines, nails, 1099t
Behavior management, 1165
Bell palsy, 1033–1034, 1034f
Beneficence, 21, 22
Benign breast disorders, 816
Benign prostatic hyperplasia (BPH), 795
　diagnostic tests, 852
　etiology of, 852
　pathophysiology, 852
　signs and symptoms, 852
　surgical treatment of, 853–857, 853f, 854f, 857f
Benign skin lesions, 1130–1132t
Benign tumors, 142
　bone, 912
　breast, 816
Benzodiazepines, 125t, 961t, 1174t
Beta-adrenergic blockers, 1063t
Beta blockers
　for angina pectoris, 382t, 383
　for arrhythmias, 410t
　for chronic heart failure (HF), 433t, 435
　for hypertension, 346–347t
　for myocardial infarction (MI), 389t
　for shock, 112t
Beta-lactam antibiotics, 698t
Bigeminy, 415
Biguanide, 775t
Bile, 575, 576f
Bile acid dissolution agents, 665t
Bile acid sequestrants, 665t
Bilevel continuous positive airway pressure (BiPAP), 193
Biliopancreatic diversion with duodenal switch, 601, 602f
Bilirubin, 453, 575–576, 576f, 582
Bimanual palpation, 803, 806t
Biofeedback, 45
　for pain, 128
Biological response modifiers, 917t
Biological variations, 36
Biologic response modifiers, 628t
Bioprosthesis, 361
Biopsy, 149–150
　bone marrow, 457
　bone or muscle, 892–893, 895t
　breast, 800–801
　endocrine system, 737
　immune system, 274t
　lymph node, 457
　masses of external ear, 1081
　for oral cancer, 603
　percutaneous liver, 590–591
　renal, 689
　skin, 1100, 1134
Bioterrorism agents, 205, 205f, 206–208t
Bipolar disorder, 1177
Bird flu, 527
Bisphosphonates, 911
Blebs, 547

Index

Bleeding. *See also* Hemorrhagic disorders
   fractures and, 906
   gastric, 611–612, 612t
   hemophilia and, 473–475
   interventions to prevent, 467b
   intracerebral stroke, 1002
   lower gastrointestinal, 638
   related to trauma, 197, 198, 198f, 368
   total hip replacement and, 922–923
Bleeding time, 458t
Blepharitis, 1061
Blepharoplasty, 1135t
Blindness, 1067–1069, 1067f, 1068b
   guide dogs for people with, 1047
Blind spot, 1039
Blom-Singer voice prosthesis, 528
Blood
   ABO types, 451, 452t
   administration of, 458–459, 458t
   cell formation, 448, 449f
   cell values and disorders, 450t
   clotting of, 451, 453f
   components of, 448, 449f
   diagnostic tests of, 456
   gas transport in, 489–490
   general functions of, 448
   monitoring of, 459–460
   normal pH of, 450
   osmolarity of, 51
   plasma, 448, 451
   platelets, 450t, 451
   red blood cells (RBCs), 450t, 451, 452f
   Rh factor, 451
   warmed, 459
   washed or leukocyte-depleted, 459
   white blood cells (WBCs), 88, 263, 450t, 451
Blood glucose levels, 727–728, 730f, 732t, 766, 766f. *See also* Diabetes mellitus
   self-monitoring of, 776, 776f
Blood pressure, 321–322, 322f. *See also* Hypertension
   data collection on, 325–326, 327b
   measurement and categories of, 342–343, 343t
   orthostatic, 325–326, 326b
Blood products, 458–459, 458t
Blood tests. *See* Serological tests
Blood transfusion, 458–460, 458t
   HIV/AIDS transmission by, 302
Blood urea nitrogen (BUN) level, 53, 55
Blood vessels
   capillaries, 320–321, 322f
   heart, 320–321, 322f
   renal, 676
   skin, 1094
Blunting or flattening in schizophrenia, 1180
Blunt trauma, 194
Boards of nursing, 26
Body temperature
   at end of life, 253
   hyperthermia and, 201–202, 202b
   hypothermia and, 174, 200–201, 200t
   plasma and, 450
Bone and soft tissue disorders, 899–913. *See also* Musculoskeletal and connective tissue disorders
   bone cancer, 912–913
   bursitis, 900
   carpal tunnel syndrome, 900
   dislocations, 900
   fractures (*see* Fractures)
   osteomyelitis, 906, 909–910, 910f
   osteoporosis, 801, 910–912
   Paget disease, 912
   rotator cuff injury, 900
   sprains, 900
   strains, 899
Bone density, 223–224
   DEXA scans of, 801, 893
   systemic lupus erythematosus (SLE) and, 290
Bone health assessment, 801
Bone marrow biopsy, 457
Bones
   aging and, 22f, 223–224
   biopsy of, 892–893, 895t
   injuries to, 196, 198, 224
   rib fractures, 560–561
   skeletal structure of, 885, 886f
   synovial joints, 885, 888f
   tissue and growth of, 885
Bone-seeking cancers, 912
Borderline personality disorder (BPD), 1183
Botulism, 207t
Bouchard nodes, 915
Braden Skin Scale, 16, 1108, 1109–1111t
Bradycardia, 409, 410f
Bradykinesia, 989, 990
Brain, 933–934
   brainstem, 933, 934f
   cerebellum, 933, 934f
   cerebrum, 933–934, 934f, 935f
   diencephalon, 933, 934f
   effects of shock on, 106
   head trauma and, 195, 196b
   herniation, 965, 965f
   meninges, 933
   neurotransmitters of, 1156–1157t
   traumatic brain injury (TBI), 963–967, 964–965f, 967t
   tumors of, 967–969, 968f
   ventricles and cerebrospinal fluid (CSF), 933
Brainstem, 933, 934f
   contusions of, 964
Brain tumors, 967–969, 968f
BRCA1 and BRCA2 genes, 800, 801, 816–817
Breakthrough pain, 126
Breast augmentation, 821, 821f
Breast cancer. *See* Malignant breast disorders
Breast disorders
   benign, 816
   malignant, 816–821, 819t, 820t
Breast examination, 796, 798–799, 800f, 817
Breastfeeding, 837
Breast modification surgeries, 821–822, 821–822f
Breast reduction, 821, 821f
Breasts
   diagnostic tests of, 799–801, 800f
   mammary glands, 724, 725f, 726f, 791, 793f
Breast self-examination (BSE)
   female, 798–799, 800f, 806t, 817
   male, 811
Breathing
   assessment of, in primary survey, 193
   changes at end of life, 253
   Cheyne-Stokes, 431
   deep, 167, 169
   exercises for, 501
   major trauma and, 197
   mechanism of, 487–489
   positioning for, 501–502, 502f
   respiration rate and ease and, 328
Bronchial tree, 487, 489f
Bronchiectasis, 534, 534f
Bronchitis
   acute, 533–534
   chronic, 546, 546f
Bronchodilators, 534, 540, 550t, 554
Bronchoscopy, 499
Bronchospasm, 551, 552
Brudzinski sign, 952, 953f
Bruit, 328
Buddhist persons, 361
Buerger disease, 395
Bulbourethral glands, 792, 794, 795f
Bulimia nervosa, 1185–1186
Bullae, 547, 1097f
Bundle of His, 318, 320f
Burns, 199–200, 1138–1154
   acute stage, 1143–1145
   causes of, 1140, 1142t
   diagnostic tests, 1141
   emergent stage, 1142–1143
   evaluation of injuries, 1140, 1140t, 1141f
   eye, 1075
   nursing process for, 1146–1152
   pathophysiology and signs and symptoms, 1138–1140, 1139f, 1140t, 1141f
   psychosocial effects of, 1146
   rehabilitation stage, 1145–1146, 1146f
   skin grafts for, 1144–1145, 1145f
   summary of, 1153t
   systemic responses to, 1138–1139
   therapeutic measures, 1142–1146, 1142t, 1144–1145t, 1144–1146f
   three zones of tissue damage, 1139f
Bursae, 885
Bursitis, 900
BuSpar, 1174t

C

CAGE questionnaire, 1189–1190
Calcitonin, 726f, 732t
   osteoporosis and, 911
Calcium
   bone growth and, 885
   imbalances in, 62–64, 62f, 63f, 63t
   intake of, 801, 802t
   laboratory tests for, 890, 893t
   osteoporosis and, 911, 912
Calcium channel blockers (CCB)
   for arrhythmias, 411t
   for coronary artery disease (CAD), 382t, 383
   for hypertension, 348t
Caloric test, 1055
Cancer, 140–163
   anatomy and physiology of normal cells and, 140–142, 141f
   benign tumors, 142, 144t
   bladder, 702–705
   bone, 912–913
   cervical, 147–148, 841–842, 842f
   classification of, 146–147, 147t
   colorectal, 639–640t, 639–641, 641f
   defined, 142
   diagnosis of, 149–150, 150t

early detection and prevention, 147–149, 148f
endometrial, 842
esophageal, 603–604
gastric, 612–613, 613f, 613t
HIV/AIDS and, 304
Hodgkin lymphoma, 480–481
home health care, 161
hospice care and, 161, 162f
inner ear, 1086–1087
kidney, 705
larynx, 527–531, 528f, 528t, 529f
liver, 662
lung, 148, 563–566, 564f, 565t, 566f
metastasis of, 147, 147f, 150–151, 151t
mortality rates, 147
multiple myeloma, 478–480, 479f
nursing process for, 156–161
oncological emergencies, 162
oncology and, 142
oral, 603, 605f
ovarian, 842
pancreas, 667–668, 668f
pathophysiology and etiology, 142–144
penis, 860
prostate, 858–859
research on new therapies for, 156
resources, 143b
risk factors, 144–146
skin, 1132–1134, 1133f
staging and grading, 150–151, 151t
survivorship and, 161
testicular, 861
thyroid gland, 752–753
treatment for, 151–156
vulvar, 841
Candida albicans, 304, 305t
Candidiasis, 827t, 1124, 1127t
Canker sores, 603
Cannabidiol (CBD), 47
Cannabis, 47
Cannula, 69
Capillaries, 320–321, 322f
Capillary fragility test, 458t
Capillary refill, 113, 328
Capnography, 499
Capsule endoscopy, 589
Caput medusae, 581
Carbapenems, 97t
Carbohydrate counting, 772t
Carbohydrate metabolism, 575
Carbuncles, 1122t
Carcinogens, 144
Carcinomas, 146
Cardiac arrhythmias, 106, 404–424
  automatic external defibrillators (AEDs) for, 421, 421f
  cardiac conduction system and, 404
  cardiac pacemakers for, 418–420, 419f
  cardioversion for, 413, 420
  cardioverter defibrillators for, 421
  as complication of myocardial infarction (MI), 385t
  components of cardiac cycle and, 405–407, 405–407f
  defibrillation for, 420, 420f
  electrocardiogram (ECG) and, 404–405, 405f
  home health care, 422

interpretation of cardiac rhythms and, 405f, 407–408, 407f, 407t, 408f
  normal sinus rhythm (NSR) and, 409
  nursing process for, 421–422
  originating in the atria, 412–415, 412–415f
  originating in the sinoatrial node, 409, 410–411t, 410f, 411–412, 411f
  ventricular arrhythmias, 415–418, 416f, 418f
Cardiac biomarkers, 330–331t, 334
Cardiac catheterization, 333t, 336–337
Cardiac computed tomography scan, 331t
Cardiac conduction pathway, 318, 320f
Cardiac cycle, 318, 320f, 404
  normal sinus rhythm (NSR), 318, 320f, 409
  PR interval, 405, 405f, 408
  P wave, 405, 405f, 407f, 408
  QRS complex, 406, 406f
  QRS interval, 406, 406f, 408
  QT interval, 405f, 406, 408
  ST segment, 407, 407f
  T wave, 406, 406f
  U wave, 406, 407f
Cardiac disorders, inflammatory and infectious
  cardiac trauma, 368
  cardiomyopathy, 368–370, 369f, 369t, 370b
  infective endocarditis (IE), 362–366, 363f, 364f, 364t, 365t
  myocarditis, 367–368
  pericarditis, 366–367, 366t, 367f
Cardiac glycosides, 411t, 434t, 435
Cardiac magnetic resonance imaging (MRI), 331t, 335
Cardiac output, 105–106, 319
  blood pressure and, 342
  heart failure (HF) and compensatory mechanisms to maintain, 427–428
Cardiac pacemakers, 318, 320f, 418–420, 419f
  sudden death risk with, 436
Cardiac rehabilitation, 391
  QRS interval, 408
Cardiac resynchronization therapy, 436
Cardiac rhythms, interpretation of, 407t
  heart rate, 408, 408f
  PR interval, 408
  P waves, 407f, 408
  QT interval, 408
  regularity of, 407–408, 407f
Cardiac surgery, 338–340, 339f
Cardiac tamponade, 196, 367
Cardiac transplantation, 441–445, 442f
Cardiac trauma, 368
Cardiac troponin I or T, 330t, 334
Cardiac valve repairs, 361–362
Cardiac valvular disorders, 353–376
  aortic regurgitation, 356t, 358–359
  aortic stenosis, 355–356, 358
  heart valves and, 353–354, 354f
  mitral regurgitation, 355t, 357–358
  mitral stenosis, 355t, 356–357, 357f
  mitral valve prolapse, 354, 355t, 356
  nursing process for, 359–361, 359t
  rheumatic fever, 354
  valve repairs for, 361–362
Cardiogenic shock, 108, 109t, 194
  as complication of myocardial infarction (MI), 385t
Cardiomegaly, 370
Cardiomyopathy, 368–370, 369f, 369t, 370b

Cardiopulmonary bypass, 339, 339f
Cardiopulmonary resuscitation (CPR), 249
  bystander, 417
Cardiovascular diseases and disorders, 323
  acute coronary syndrome (ACS), 384–393, 385–386t, 385f, 387–388f, 387b, 388–389t, 390f
  atherosclerosis, 377–379, 378–379t, 378f
  atypical symptoms of, 323
  cardiomyopathy, 368–370, 369f, 369t, 370b
  coronary artery disease (CAD), 378–379t, 379–384, 381f, 382–383t
  HIV/AIDS and, 313
  infective endocarditis (IE), 362–366, 363f, 364f, 364t, 365t
  inflammatory and infectious, 362–370
  myocardial infarction (MI) (*see* Myocardial infarction)
  myocarditis, 367–368
  pericarditis, 366–367, 366t, 367f
  peripheral vascular disease (PVD), 393–400, 396f, 397t, 399f
  valvular disorders, 353–376
  venous thromboembolism (VTE) disease, 370–374
Cardiovascular system, 317–341
  aging and, 225, 323, 323f
  blood pressure, 321–322, 322f
  blood vessels, 320–321, 322f
  burns and, 1139
  data collection, 323–330, 324–326t, 327b, 328–329f
  diagnostic tests, 330–333t, 330–337, 336f
  heart, 317–319, 318–320f
  invasive studies, 333t, 336–337, 336f
  laboratory tests, 330–331t, 334
  noninvasive studies, 331–332t, 334–336
  normal anatomy and physiology, 317–323, 318–323f
  postoperative, 179
  renin-angiotensin-aldosterone system, 106, 322, 322f
  surgery of, 338–340, 339f
  therapeutic measures, 337–340
  trauma and, 198
Cardioversion, 413, 420
Carpal tunnel syndrome, 900
Casts, 903, 905f
  extremity care after removal of, 909b
Cataracts, 1067, 1067f, 1073
Catechol-O-methyltransferase (COMT) inhibitor, 991t
Cather-associated UTI, 96
Cations, 57
CD4 T-lymphocyte count, 306
Cecostomy, 643t
Ceiling effect, 123
Celiac disease, 634–635
Cell body, 930f
Cell-mediated immunity, 264–265, 266f
Cells
  genetic code and protein synthesis in, 142, 143f
  malignant, 142, 144t
  mitosis, 142, 143f
  mutations of, 142
  nucleus, 140, 141f
  schematic of, 141f
  structure of, 140
  tissues and, 142

Cellular changes due to sexually transmitted infections (STIs), 871
Cellular chemokine receptor type 5 (CCR5) antagonists, 308t
Cellulitis, 1124, 1127
Centers for Disease Control (CDC), 93
Centers for Medicare & Medicaid Services (CMS)
  hospital-acquired conditions (HACs), 16
  long-term care facilities and, 238, 239t
Central-acting alpha-2 agonists, 347t
Central nervous system (CNS)
  assessment of, in primary survey, 193
  HIV-associated neurocognitive disorder and, 304
  musculoskeletal system and, 886–887
  neurotransmitters, 1156–1157t
Central nervous system (CNS) disorders, 951–999
  brain tumors, 967–969, 968f
  headaches, 957–959
  increased intracranial pressure (ICP), 954–957, 955f, 956b, 956f, 957t
  infections, 951–954, 952t, 953f, 954t
  intracranial surgery for, 969–971
  neurodegenerative and neurocognitive disorders, 983–996, 984b, 987t, 989f, 990t, 991t, 993f, 995t
  seizure disorders, 956b, 959–963, 961t
  spinal cord injuries, 195–196, 196f, 197, 197t, 974–983
  spinal disorders, 971–974, 971f, 973f
  traumatic brain injury (TBI), 963–967, 964–965f, 967t
Central venous access devices (CVAD), 74, 76, 79–80, 79f
Cephalosporins, 98t
  for sexually transmitted infections (STIs), 873t
Cerebellum, 933, 934f
Cerebral aneurysm, 1010–1012, 1010f, 1011f
  rehabilitation after, 1011–1012
Cerebral edema, 197–198
Cerebral tissue perfusion
  related to cerebral edema, 197–198
  related to severe anoxia, 204
Cerebrospinal fluid (CSF), 933
Cerebrovascular accident (CVA). See Stroke
Cerebrovascular disorders, 1000–1019
  cerebral aneurysm, subarachnoid hemorrhage, and intracranial hemorrhage, 1010–1012, 1010f, 1011f
  home health care, 1017
  nursing process, 1012–1017, 1016f
  stroke, 1000–1009, 1001–1002f, 1001b, 1004–1005f, 1004t, 1007t, 1008–1009f
  transient ischemic attack (TIA), 1000
Cerebrum, 933–934, 935f
Certified nurse midwives (CNMs), 17
Certified nursing assistants (CNAs), 17
Certified registered nurse anesthetists (CRNAs), 17
Cerumen, impacted, 1079–1080
Cervical cancer, 841–842, 842f
  screening for, 147–148
Cervical caps, 835–836, 836f, 881t
Cervical cord injuries, 974–975, 975f
Chalazion, 1064
Chancre, 875, 876f

Changes, health-care delivery, 15
Chemical pneumonia, 538
Chemical restraints, 239
Chemicals as cancer risk, 145
Chemoreceptors, 490
Chemotherapy, 153–156, 154f, 155f, 155t
  bone cancer, 913
  brain tumors, 969
  leukemia, 476
  lung cancer, 565
  malignant breast disorders, 817
Chernobyl nuclear disaster, 752
Chest assessment in secondary survey, 194t
Chest drainage, 506–508, 507b, 507f
Chest pain in chronic heart failure (HF), 429
Chest physiotherapy (CPT), 504, 505f, 534
Chest trauma, 196–198
  flail chest, 196, 561
  pneumothorax, 559–560, 560f
  rib fractures, 560–561
Chest x-ray, 331t, 334, 499
  for pleural effusion, 544
  for pneumonia, 539, 540f
  for pulmonary fibrosis, 545
  for tuberculosis (TB), 542
Cheyne-Stokes respiration, 431
Chiropractic medicine, 42
Chlamydia, 145, 804, 871
  antibiotics for, 873t
  testing for, 804
Cholecystitis, 668–672, 670t, 671f, 672t
Choledocholithiasis, 668–672, 670t, 671f, 672t
Cholelithiasis, 668–672, 670t, 671f, 672t
Cholesterol absorption inhibitors, 380t
Cholesterol-lowering agents, 380t
  for coronary artery disease (CAD), 383, 383t
  for myocardial infarction (MI), 389t
  for stroke, 1007t
Cholesterol tests, 331t, 334
Cholinergics, 1156t
Cholinesterase inhibitors, 1022t
  for dementia, 987t
Chorea, 354
Choroid, 1038, 1040f
Chronic airflow limitation, 545–550, 546f, 547t, 548–549f, 550t
Chronic bronchitis, 546, 546f
Chronic Disease Self-Management Program (CDSMP), 215
Chronic gastritis, 607
Chronic glomerulonephritis, 707
Chronic heart failure (HF)
  complications of, 430t, 431
  diagnostic tests, 430t, 431–432
  home health care, 441
  nursing process for, 437–438t, 437–441, 440b
  signs and symptoms, 429, 430t, 431
  therapeutic measures, 430t, 432–437, 433–435t, 436–437f, 438–440
Chronic illness, 211–221
  changing roles and, 218
  coping with impact of, 216–220, 218b
  defined, 215
  definitions of health, wellness, and, 211
  effects of, 216
  family and caregivers of patients with, 218, 218b
  finances and, 219–220

  gerontological influence, 215–216
  health promotion and, 220
  home health care, 219
  hope and, 217
  incidence of, 215
  nurse's role in supporting and promoting, 212
  nursing care for, 220
  powerlessness and hopelessness in, 214, 216, 217f
  respite care and, 219
  sexuality and, 217–218
  surgery and, 166
  types of, 215, 215t
Chronic kidney disease (CKD), 706–707, 710–711
  effects on body systems, 712t
  kidney transplantation for, 718, 718f
  nursing process for, 718–719
  symptoms of, 711–714, 711t, 713b, 713f
  therapeutic measures, 711t, 714–717, 715–717f, 715b, 717b
Chronic liver disease, 656–662, 657t, 658–660f, 660–661
Chronic lymphocytic leukemia (CLL), 475
Chronic myelogenous leukemia (CML), 475
Chronic obstructive pulmonary disease (COPD), 545–550, 546f, 547t, 548–549f, 550t, 551f
Chronic pain, 119
Chronic pancreatitis, 664, 665t
Chronic renal diseases, 706–707
Chronic sorrow, 216
Chvostek sign, 62, 63f
Chyme, 574
Cilia, 88
Ciliary body, 1038, 1040f
Circuits of circulation, 322–323
Circulatory overload, intravenous (IV) therapy, 78t
Circulatory system
  assessment of, in primary survey, 193
  circuits of circulation, 322–323
  long-term effects of diabetes mellitus on, 780–781
  postoperative, 182–183
Circumcision, 807
Cirrhosis, 656–662, 658–660f
  ascites and, 657, 659, 659f
  clotting defects and, 657
  hepatic encephalopathy and, 657–658
  hepatorenal syndrome and, 658, 659f
  portal hypertension and, 657, 658f
  Wernicke-Korsakoff syndrome and, 658–659
Civil laws, 28
CK3 (CK-MM) isoenzyme, 890, 893t
CK-MB isoenzyme, 330t, 334
Clean technique, 93
Clinical judgment, 2–3
  acute liver failure, chronic liver disease, cirrhosis, 661
  acute pancreatitis, 664
  adolescents and contraceptives, 835
  advance directive, 250
  Alzheimer disease, 996
  amyotrophic lateral sclerosis (ALS), 1030
  anaphylaxis, 279
  ankylosing spondylitis, 294
  aortic stenosis, 358
  asthma, 552

autonomic nervous system (ANS), 937
barium enema, 589
bowel obstruction, 637
breast examination, 799
burns, 200, 1140, 1141
cancer, 160–161
cardiovascular disease, 330
cerebral aneurysm, 1012
cholecystitis, 669
chronic heart failure (HF), 436, 441
chronic kidney disease (CKD), 718
chronic obstructive pulmonary disease (COPD), 557
complementary and alternative modalities, 48
coping skills, 1161
Crohn disease, 631
cultural influences on nursing care, 37–38
cystic fibrosis (CF), 555
dehydration, 54
diabetes mellitus, 770
duodenal ulcer, 611
electrolyte imbalances, 57
embolectomy, 400
end of life care, 254
enteral nutrition (EN), 595
epistaxis, 519
erectile dysfunction, 865
female reproductive system and age, 804
fractures, 905, 907
fractures in older adults, 896
GI bleeding, 579
hearing and aging, 1055
hepatitis, 655
HIV/AIDS, 313
home health care, 241, 244
hypercalcemia, 64
hypertension, 349
infections, 102
infective endocarditis (IE), 365–366
influenza, 527
insulin injections, 774
intravenous (IV) therapy, 75, 76
latex allergy, 271
leukemia, 478
liver biopsy, 591
male reproductive system, 811
Ménière disease, 1088
meningitis, 957
menopause, 825
mental illness, 1158
mitral valve prolapse (MVP), 356
mood disorders, 1178
musculoskeletal system, 890
myasthenia gravis (MG), 1028
myocardial infarction (MI), 391
nephrosclerosis, 707
neurologic system, 948
nursing process and, 3–5, 3f, 4–5t
obsessive-compulsive disorder (OCD), 1176
older adult health concerns, 214, 215, 219, 228
osteoarthritis (OA), 916
pacemakers, 420
pain, 122, 127, 128, 136
pneumonia, 539
postoperative patient, 184
premature ventricular contractions (PVCs), 416
pressure injuries, 1117–1118
psoriasis, 1101, 1121

respite care and, 219
rheumatoid arthritis (RA), 921
schizophrenia, 1181–1182
scleral buckling, 1070
sexually transmitted infections (STIs), 880
shock, 114
stapedectomy, 1084
stroke, 1008
systemic lupus erythematosus (SLE), 293
testicular cancer, 861
tonsillectomy, 525
total hip replacement, 922
tracheostomy, 510
transurethral resection of the prostate (TURP), 857
trauma and, 199
traumatic brain injury (TBI), 967
trichomoniasis, 876
tuberculosis (TB), 543
urinary drainage system, 682
urinary tract infection (UTI), 699
ventricular tachycardia, 417
warfarin, 457
Clinical latency stage, HIV/AIDS, 299
Clinically assisted nutrition and hydration (CANH), 250
Clinical nurse specialists (CNSs), 17
Clitoris, 793f
Closed head injury, 963
Closed pneumothorax, 559
Closed reduction, 902
Closed wounds, 194
Clostridioides difficile, 101
Clostridium tetani, 195
Clotting, 451, 453f
  cirrhosis and defects in, 657
Clubbing, finger, 328, 328f
Cluster headaches, 958
Coaching leadership, 18
Coagulation studies, 456, 458t
Cochlear implant, 1077f
Cochrane Database of Systematic Reviews, 10
Cognition
  aging and, 230
  changes at end of life, 254
  in chronic heart failure (HF), 431
  traumatic brain injury (TBI) and, 965
Cognitive ability, 1161
Cognitive-behavioral interventions for pain, 128
Cognitive behavioral therapy (CBT), 1165
  for substance use disorders, 1188
Coitus interruptus, 837
Colectomy, 627, 640t
Colic, biliary, 669
Collaboration, 2, 7, 17
  evidence-based practice (EBP), 13
Collaborative home health care, 240–241, 240t
Collateral circulation, 379
Colon cancer screening, 148
Colonization, 83
Colonoscopy, 590
Colony-stimulating factors, 155f
Color, skin, 1096
Colorectal cancer, 639–640t, 639–641, 641f
Colostomy, 642–643, 643f, 643t
Colporrhaphy, 829
Colposcopy, 805, 843
Combination agents for HIV/AIDS, 308t

Combined alpha and beta blockers, 347t
Comminuted fractures, 902t, 903f
Commissurotomy, 361
Common cold, 522–523, 523t
Communication
  active listening in, 5–6
  avoiding failures of, 3
  blocks to, 1164, 1164t
  cultural diversity and, 34
  with health-care team, 5–6
  therapeutic, 1161, 1163, 1163t
  therapeutic measures for neurologic system, 947–948
Compact bone, 885
Compassion, 17
Compassion fatigue, 253
Complementary and alternative modalities, 41–49
  American Indian medicine, 43
  animal-assisted therapy and animal-assisted activities, 46, 46f
  Ayurvedic medicine, 42
  benign prostatic hyperplasia (BPH), 853
  brain tumors, 969
  cannabis, 47
  categories and types of, 44t
  chiropractic medicine, 42
  detoxing and cleansing, 46
  difference between, 41
  heat and cold application, 46
  herbal therapy, 44, 45t
  herniated discs, 972
  home health, 48
  homeopathic medicine, 42
  introduction of new systems into traditional Western health care, 42–43
  for malignant breast disorders, 817
  massage therapy, 45
  naturopathic medicine, 43
  osteoarthritis (OA), 916
  osteopathic medicine, 43
  relaxation therapies, 44–45, 46b
  rheumatoid arthritis (RA), 920
  role of license practical nurse/licensed vocational nurse in, 47–48
  safety and effectiveness of, 47, 47b
  Traditional Chinese medicine, 42, 43f
Complement cascade, 265
Complete blood count (CBC)
  HIV/AIDS and, 305–306
  respiratory system and, 495
Complete heart block (CHB), 414–415, 414f
Complications
  abdominal hernias, 633
  absorption disorders, 634
  acute pancreatitis, 663, 663t
  acute respiratory distress syndrome (ARDS), 563
  adrenocortical insufficiency (AI), 757
  allergic rhinitis, 278
  anaphylaxis, 280t
  aneurysms, 397t
  anorexia nervosa, 1185
  aortic stenosis, 358
  appendicitis, 623
  asthma, 552, 554t
  bariatric surgery, 601
  benign prostatic hyperplasia (BPH), 858t
  blood administration, 459–460

Complications (*continued*)
  brain tumors, 969
  breast surgery, 822
  burns, 1141, 1153t
  cardiac transplantation, 443
  cardiomyopathy, 369t
  cerebral aneurysm, 1011, 1011f
  chlamydia, 872t
  cholecystitis, cholelithiasis, choledocholithiasis, 669
  chronic heart failure (HF), 430t, 431
  chronic kidney disease (CKD), 711t
  chronic liver disease and cirrhosis, 657–659, 657t
  chronic obstructive pulmonary disease (COPD), 547
  chronic pancreatitis, 664
  colorectal cancer, 639–640
  condylomata (HPV), 872t
  constipation, 619
  COVID-19, 526
  Crohn disease and ulcerative colitis, 629
  dehydration, 53
  dermatitis, 1119
  diabetes mellitus, 777–782, 777t, 778t, 782f
  diabetic nephropathy, 706
  diabetic retinopathy, 1069
  ear disorders, 1081, 1081t
  encephalitis, 954, 954t
  eye disorders, 1061t
  eye trauma, 1075
  fluid excess, 55
  fractures, 906–908, 907f, 908t
  gastric cancer, 613t
  gastric surgery, 614–615
  gastroesophageal reflux disease (GERD), 605–606, 606t
  glomerulonephritis, 708t
  gonorrhea, 872t
  Guillain-Barré syndrome (GBS), 1030
  hearing loss, 1076t
  heart valve replacement, 362
  hemolytic transfusion reaction, 283t
  hepatitis, 653
  herpes simplex, 872t, 1123
  herpes simplex lesions, 1123
  herpes zoster (shingles), 1123
  HIV/AIDS, 302, 303t, 304, 305t, 310–311b
  hypercalcemia, 64
  hyperkalemia, 61
  hypernatremia, 59
  hypertension, 343t, 345
  hyperthyroidism, 749
  hypocalcemia, 63
  hypokalemia, 60
  hyponatremia, 58
  hypothyroidism, 746
  infective endocarditis (IE), 363, 364t
  keratitis, 1064
  lung cancer, 564–565, 567t
  malignant breast disorders, 820t
  meningitis, 953
  menopause, 825
  middle ear infections, 1083
  mitral regurgitation, 358
  mitral stenosis, 357
  mitral valve prolapse (MVP), 354
  myasthenia gravis (MG), 1027, 1027t
  myocardial infarction (MI), 385t, 386t
  obesity, 599, 600f
  pancreatic cancer, 667
  Parkinson disease, 990
  pediculosis, 1128–1129
  peptic ulcer disease (PUD), 608, 609t
  pericarditis, 366t, 367, 367f
  peritonitis, 624
  pleurisy, 544
  pneumonia, 539, 540t
  pneumothorax, 561t
  pressure injuries, 1112
  prostate cancer, 858
  prostatitis, 849
  psoriasis, 1120
  pulmonary embolism (PE), 558, 559t
  renal calculi, 700, 700t
  respiratory viruses, 526
  scabies, 1130
  shock, 106–107
  spinal cord injuries, 975, 978t
  splenectomy, 483–484
  stroke, 1008–1009, 1008f, 1009f, 1017t
  syphilis, 872t
  systemic lupus erythematosus (SLE), 291t
  testicular cancer, 861
  transplant rejection, 286
  traumatic brain injury (TBI), 965–966, 965f, 967t
  trichomoniasis, 872t
  tuberculosis (TB), 541
  ulcerative colitis, 629
  urinary tract infection (UTI), 696t
  venous thromboembolism (VTE) disease, 373–374, 373t
Compression stockings, 337–338, 372
Computed tomography (CT)
  breast, 800, 806
  chest, 499
  colonography, 589
  ear, 1055
  endocrine system, 737
  musculoskeletal system, 893, 894–895t, 895f
  neurologic system, 946
Computed tomography angiography (CTA), 334–335
Concussion, 963
Condoms, 301–302, 301b, 835, 835f, 881t
Conductive hearing loss, 1076
Condylomata, 872t
Condylomata acuminata, 877–878, 878f
Condylomatous growths, 871
Confidentiality, 22–23
Confusion Assessment Method (CAM), 943
Congenital malformations, female reproductive system, 828–829
Congenital syphilis, 875
Congestive heart failure (HF), 426
Conjunctiva, 1039f
Conjunctivitis, 1060–1061
Connective tissue disorders, 913–921
  gout, 913–914, 913f
  osteoarthritis (OA), 914–919, 914f, 915f, 917–918t
  rheumatoid arthritis (RA), 919–921, 919f, 920f
Constipation, 226–227, 618–620, 619t, 621b
Contact dermatitis, 285–286, 287
Contact inhibition, 143–144
Contact vulvovaginitis, 827t
Continuing care retirement community, 237t
Continuous infusion, 70
Continuous quality improvement (CQI), 19, 19f
Continuous renal replacement therapy (CRRT), 710
Contraceptive implants, 834
Contraceptives, 818t, 833–837, 835–836f
Contractures, 22f, 223, 947, 947f
Contralateral tremor, 989
Contrast-induced acute kidney injury, 688–689, 689f
Controlling in management process, 19
Contusion, brain, 963–964
Coombs' test, 456
Coordinating in management process, 19
Coping
  aging and, 230
  with cardiac transplantation, 444
  with chronic heart failure (HF), 440–441
  defined, 1158
  effective, 1158
  ineffective, 1161, 1162t
Cornea, 1038, 1040f
  keratitis, 1064
Coronary artery bypass graft (CABG), 389–390, 390f
Coronary artery disease (CAD), 377, 378
  angina pectoris, 380–381, 382–383t
  diagnostic tests, 381
  medications for angina pectoris, 382–383t
  risk factors for, 378–379t
  signs and symptoms, 381, 381f
  smoking and, 379
  therapeutic measures, 381
Coronavirus. *See* COVID-19 (coronavirus disease 2019)
Cor pulmonale, 427
Correctional nursing, 236
Corticosteroids, 124t
  for allergic rhinitis, 278
  for atopic dermatitis, 279
  for chronic obstructive pulmonary disease (COPD), 550t
  for Crohn disease and ulcerative colitis, 628t
  for gout, 913
  for hemolytic transfusion reactions, 284t
  for osteoarthritis (OA), 917t
  for rheumatoid arthritis (RA), 920
  for systemic lupus erythematosus (SLE), 293t
Corticotropin-releasing hormone (CRH), 724
Cortisol, 727
Coughing, 167, 169, 499, 501
  in chronic heart failure (HF), 429
  huff, 501
  in older patients, 226
Coumarin, 372t
Counseling, 1165
  on HIV/AIDS, 301
COVID-19 (coronavirus disease 2019), 86, 86f, 87f, 89, 90, 90–91t
  complications of, 526
  diagnostic test for, 526
  difficulties for hearing impaired persons during, 1078

increase in chalazion due to face mask use and, 1064
incubation period of, 526
myocarditis and, 367–368
neurologic data collection using virtual technology during, 941
nursing care for, 527
in older patients, 228
oxygen saturation test and, 499
pneumonia and, 538
prevention, 526
signs and symptoms, 526
transmission of, 525–526
Cowper's glands, 795f
COX-2 inhibitors, 124t
Crackles and wheezes in chronic heart failure (HF), 429
Cranial nerve disorders, 1031–1032
 Bell palsy, 1033–1034, 1034f
 nursing process, 1034–1035
 trigeminal neuralgia (TN), 1032–1033, 1033f
Cranial nerves, 934–937, 935–936t, 938f
 affected by meningitis, 952, 952t
 disorders of, 1031–1035, 1033f, 1034f
 in neurologic system examination, 945, 945t
Cranioplasty, 969
Craniotomy, 969
C-reactive protein (CRP), 378
Creatine kinase (CK), 330t, 334, 890, 893t
Crepitation, 888
Crepitus, 494
Criminal laws, 28
Critical thinking, 1–2
 about evidence, 12–13
 about pain, 122, 126, 127, 128
 ACE inhibitors, 436
 acute liver failure, chronic liver disease, cirrhosis, 661
 acute pancreatitis, 664
 Alzheimer disease, 996
 amyotrophic lateral sclerosis (ALS), 1030
 anaphylaxis, 279
 asthma, 552
 attitudes, 3
 autonomic nervous system (ANS), 937
 barium enema, 589
 bowel obstruction, 637
 breast examination, 799
 burns, 200, 1146
 cancer, 160–161
 cardiac transplantation, 445
 cardiovascular disease, 330
 cerebral aneurysm, 1012
 chest tube, 508
 cholecystitis, 669
 chronic heart failure (HF), 431, 432
 chronic obstructive pulmonary disease (COPD), 557
 complementary and alternative modalities, 48
 coping skills, 1161
 cultural influences on nursing care, 37–38
 cystic fibrosis (CF), 555
 defined, 2
 dehydration, 54
 diabetes mellitus, 770
 disseminated intravascular coagulation (DIC), 472

electrolyte imbalances, 57
end of life care, 254
enteral nutrition (EN), 595
epistaxis, 519
erectile dysfunction, 865
ethical decisions, 26
female reproductive system and age, 804
fractures, 905
fractures in older adults, 890, 896
GI bleeding, 579
growth hormone deficiency, 744
hearing and aging, 1055
Hodgkin lymphoma, 481
home health care, 241
hypercalcemia, 64
hypertension, 345
hypoglycemia, 779
hypothyroidism, 748
infection risk, 96
infective endocarditis (IE), 365–366
influenza, 527
intravenous (IV) therapy, 76
liver biopsy, 591
male reproductive system, 811
Maslow hierarchy of human needs and, 7
meningitis, 957
middle-aged adult health concerns, 213
mitral valve prolapse (MVP), 356
myasthenia gravis (MG), 1028
myocardial infarction (MI), 391
neurologic system, 948
older adult health concerns, 214, 215, 218
pacemakers, 420
Parkinson disease, 992
pneumonia, 539
sexually transmitted infections (STIs), 880
shock, 106, 113–114
stroke, 1008
substance use disorders, 1190
syndrome of inappropriate ADH (SIADH), 742–743
testicular cancer, 861
thyroid-stimulating hormone, 733
tonsillectomy, 525
tracheostomy, 510
transurethral resection of the prostate (TURP), 857
trauma and, 199
traumatic brain injury (TBI), 967
trichomoniasis, 876
tuberculosis (TB), 543
type 2 diabetes foot complications, 782
urinary tract infection (UTI), 699
ventricular tachycardia, 417
vigilance in, 5
warfarin, 457
Crohn disease, 626–627, 626f, 627f, 631
Crust, 1097f
Cryopexy, 1070
Cryptorchidism, 860
Crystalloid solutions, 73–74
Culdocentesis, 843
Culdoscopy, 805, 805f
Culdotomy, 843
Cultural awareness, 32
Cultural competence, 32
Cultural diversity, 34

Cultural groups in the United States, 31
Cultural humility, 32
Cultural influences on nursing care, 31–40
 characteristics of cultural diversity, 34
 concepts related to culture, 32
 concepts related to spirituality, 32–33
Culturally and linguistically appropriate services (CLAS), 38b
Culturally responsive care, 31, 38, 38b
Cultural sensitivity, 32
Cultural values/beliefs/differences, 31, 33–34
 cancer rates, 145
 cardiac valve options and, 361
 characteristics, 32b
 Chernobyl nuclear disaster and cancer, 752
 Crohn disease and ulcerative colitis, 626
 culturally responsive care for, 31, 38, 38b
 culture defined, 32
 Ellis-van Creveld Syndrome, 743
 fasting, 54
 G6PD deficiency, 463
 health-care values, beliefs, and practices, 33–34
 home health care, 39
 nutritional assessment and, 579, 579b
 organ donation, 662, 718
 pain and, 119, 120, 133
 racial and ethnic groups in the United States, 37–38
 respiratory system, 494
 sickle cell anemia, 468
 skin lesions, 1130
 space, 34–37
 type 2 diabetes and, 773
Cushing syndrome, 758–760, 758t, 759f
Customs, 31
Cyanosis, 113, 328, 494
 in chronic heart failure (HF), 431
 in chronic obstructive pulmonary disease (COPD), 547
Cyclic breast discomfort, 816
Cycloplegics, 1063t
Cystadenomas, 840
Cystic fibrosis (CF), 554–555
Cystitis, 697
Cystocele, 829, 830f
Cystourethrography, 811, 812t
Cysts
 reproductive system, 840–841
 skin, 1097f, 1130t
Cytochrome P450 enzymes, 338
Cytology, 150
 Pap smear, 147–148, 803–804
Cytolytic vaginosis, 827t
Cytomegalovirus (CMV), 304, 305t
Cytoprotective agents, 156
Cystoscopy, 701

D

Data collection. *See also* Objective data; Subjective data
 acute liver failure, chronic liver disease, cirrhosis, 660
 adrenocortical insufficiency (AI), 757–758
 anemia, 465
 aneurysms, 397
 autism spectrum disorders (ADSs), 1184

Data collection (*continued*)
  blindness, 1068
  blood pressure, 325–326, 327b
  bone health, 801
  bowel obstruction, 637
  burns, 1146–1147
  cancer, 156
  cardiac arrhythmias, 421
  cardiac transplantation, 443
  cardiac valvular disorders, 359t
  cardiovascular system, 323–330, 324–326t, 327b, 328–329f
  cataracts, 1073
  cerebrovascular disorder, 1012
  chest trauma, 561
  chronic heart failure (HF), 437, 437–438t
  chronic kidney disease (CKD), 718
  colorectal cancer, 640–641
  constipation, 619–620
  coronary artery disease (CAD) and angina, 383
  cranial nerve disorder, 1034
  Cushing syndrome, 760
  dehydration, 53–54
  dermatitis, 1119
  diabetes insipidus, 741
  diabetes mellitus, 783, 783t
  diabetic retinopathy, 1069
  diarrhea, 622
  displacement disorders, 830–831
  ear and hearing status, 1049–1052, 1051t, 1053t
  ear disorders, 1082
  eating disorders, 1186
  endocrine system, 728–729
  erectile dysfunction, 865
  eye infection and inflammation, 1064, 1065t
  female reproductive system, 797–799t, 800f, 802f, 802t, 805f
  fluid excess, 55–56
  fractures, 908
  gallbladder disorder, 671
  gastric bleeding, 612
  gastric surgery, 613–614
  gastroesophageal reflux disease (GERD), 606
  glaucoma, 1072
  from grieving family, 260
  hearing loss, 1077–1078, 1078t
  hematologic and lymphatic systems, 454, 455t
  hemophilia, 474
  hepatitis, 653–654
  HIV/AIDS, 314, 314b
  home health care, 244
  hyperparathyroidism, 756
  hypertension, 349–350, 349f
  hyperthyroidism, 750
  hypoparathyroidism, 755
  hypothermia, 200
  hypothyroidism, 746
  immune system, 268–271, 269t, 270t
  increased intracranial pressure (ICP), 955–956, 956b
  infections, 101–103
  infectious skin disorders, 1127–1128
  infective endocarditis (IE), 364, 365t
  inflammatory bowel disease, 629–630
  inflammatory or infectious gastrointestinal disorder, 625
  inner ear disorders, 1088
  integumentary system, 1094–1099
  intracranial surgery, 970
  intravenous (IV) therapy, 75
  irritable bowel syndrome (IBS), 632
  lung cancer, 565
  lymphangitis, 400
  male reproductive system, 805–812, 808–810t, 811b, 811f, 812t
  mental status, 1158, 1159–1160t
  middle ear, tympanic membrane, and mastoid disorders, 1085, 1086t
  multiple myeloma, 480
  musculoskeletal system, 887–890, 891t, 892t, 893t
  myocardial infarction (MI), 390
  nausea and vomiting, 599
  near-drowning, 204
  neurologic system, 938–945, 939b, 940t, 941t, 942f, 944f, 945t
  obesity, 602
  obstructive disorders, 555
  osteoarthritis (OA), 916
  ostomy, 643–644, 643f
  pain, 131–132, 132f, 133f, 134f
  pancreatic cancer, 668
  pancreatitis, 665
  Parkinson disease, 990–991
  peripheral arterial disorders, 395
  personality disorders, 1183
  poisoning and drug overdose, 203
  postoperative, 178, 179, 182, 183–184, 187–188
  preoperative, 169, 170t
  prostatitis, 849
  pulmonary embolism (PE), 559
  pulse, 327–328
  renal calculi, 701–702
  respiratory failure, 563
  respiratory system, 492, 493t
  restrictive disorders, 545
  retinal detachment, 1070
  rheumatoid arthritis (RA), 920
  schizophrenia, 1181
  seizure disorders, 962
  sensory system, 1042–1046, 1043–1044t, 1044–1045f
  sexually transmitted infections (STIs), 879
  shock, 111
  sickle cell anemia, 470
  spinal surgery, 974
  substance use disorders, 1189–1190
  surgical wound, 187
  syndrome of inappropriate ADH (SIADH), 742
  thoracic surgery, 567
  thyroidectomy, 753
  transgender population, 812–813
  transurethral resection of the prostate (TURP), 857
  trauma, 197
  traumatic brain injury (TBI), 966
  tuberculosis (TB), 543
  type I hypersensitivity disorder, 281
  urinary tract infection (UTI), 697
  venous insufficiency, 398
  venous thromboembolism (VTE) disease, 374
Dawn phenomenon, 777

D-dimer, 495, 558
Death and dying. *See also* End of life
  from acute liver failure, 655–656
  from anaphylactic shock, 108
  from cancer, 147
  care at time of and after, 259–260
  cultural influences on, 37
  good, 247–248
  grief over, 260–261, 260t
  identifying symptoms of impending, 248, 248f
  nurse's experience with, 261
  process of, 253–254
Debridement, 185, 1112–1113
Debulking, 969
Deceleration injury, 963
Decerebrate posturing, 941, 942f
Decision making, ethical, 24–26
Decompression, gastrointestinal, 595
Decorticate posturing, 941, 942f
Deep breathing, 167, 169, 499, 501
Deep vein thrombosis (DVT), 370, 373–374. *See also* Venous thromboembolism (VTE) disease
  fractures and, 906
  spinal cord injuries and, 975
  stroke and, 1008
  total hip replacement and, 923
Defecation posture modification device (DPMD), 620
Defibrillation, 420, 420f
Dehiscence, wound, 185, 187f
Dehydration, 52–54, 52b, 54b, 621
Delayed reaction, 284
Delegation process, 20
Delirium, 230–231, 943, 1190
Delirium tremens (DTs), 1187
Delusions, 1180
Dementia, 230, 943, 983–986
  Alzheimer disease, 994–996, 995t
  diagnostic tests, 984
  HIV/AIDS-associated, 304
  home health care, 996
  long-term care services for, 237–238
  nursing process, 984–986
  pathophysiology and etiology, 983–984, 984b
  signs and symptoms, 984
  therapeutic measures, 984, 987t
Democratic (participative) leadership, 18, 18f
Demyelination, 1030
Dendrites, 930f
Dental care, 602–603, 604b
Dental implants, 604b
Dentures, 604b
Deontology, 24
Depressed fractures, 902t
Depression, 230, 1179t
  major, 1176–1177
  in older adults, 1190
  spinal cord injuries and, 975
Dermatitis, 1118–1120, 1118t
Dermatomycosis, 1124
Dermis, 1091–1092
Dermoid cysts, 841
Descending or sigmoid colostomy, 643t
Desquamation, 152
Detoxing and cleansing, 46
  liver and, 576

Developmental stages, 212–215, 212t
   middle-age, 213
   older adult, 213–215, 214f
   young adult, 212–213
Deviated septum, 520
Dextrose solutions, 73
Diabetes insipidus, 740–741, 741t, 965
Diabetes mellitus, 765–766
   complications of, 777–782, 777t, 778t, 782f
   diagnostic tests, 769, 769f, 769t, 777t
   diet and, 770–771, 771f, 772t
   exercise and, 771–772
   home health care, 785–786
   hypertension and, 344
   injectable hypoglycemic medication for, 774–776, 775–776t
   medication for, 772–773f, 772–776, 774t, 775–776t
   natural remedies for, 776
   oral hypoglycemic medication for, 774
   pancreas transplant in, 777
   pathophysiology and etiology, 766, 766f
   prevention, 770
   self-management education, 783, 785–786
   self-monitoring of blood glucose in, 776, 776f
   signs and symptoms, 768, 777t
   surgery in patients with, 782–783
   therapeutic measures, 770–777, 771–773f, 772t, 774–776t, 776–777f, 777t
   types of, 767–768, 767t
   urine glucose and ketone monitoring in, 776–777, 777f
   weight loss for, 771
Diabetic ketoacidosis (DKA), 779–780
Diabetic nephropathy, 706
Diabetic retinopathy, 1067, 1067f, 1069–1070
Diagnostic and Statistical Manual of Mental Disorders, 5th edition, 1158
Diagnostic tests. *See also* Nursing diagnoses, planning, and implementation
   absorption disorders, 634, 635t
   acromegaly, 744
   acute pancreatitis, 663, 663t
   acute respiratory distress syndrome (ARDS), 563
   acute respiratory failure, 562
   adrenocortical insufficiency (AI), 757
   allergic rhinitis, 278
   Alzheimer disease, 995
   amyotrophic lateral sclerosis (ALS), 1029
   anaphylaxis, 279, 280t
   anemia, 463
   aneurysms, 396, 397t
   angioedema, 281
   ankylosing spondylitis, 294
   aortic regurgitation, 359
   aortic stenosis, 358
   aplastic anemia, 466
   appendicitis, 623
   asthma, 552, 554t
   atherosclerosis, 378, 379t
   atopic dermatitis, 279
   Bell palsy, 1033
   benign prostatic hyperplasia (BPH), 852, 858t
   bladder cancer, 703
   blindness, 1067
   bone cancer, 912–913
   of bones, 801
   brain tumors, 968
   breasts, 799–801, 800f
   bronchiectasis, 534
   burns, 1141, 1153t
   cancer, 147–149, 148f, 149–150, 150t
   cardiomyopathy, 369t, 370
   cardiovascular system, 330–333t, 330–337, 336f
   cataracts, 1073
   cellulitis, 1124
   cerebral aneurysm, 1010
   cervical cancer, 841
   chlamydia, 871, 872t
   cholecystitis, cholelithiasis, choledocholithiasis, 669–670, 672t
   chronic heart failure (HF), 430t, 431–432
   chronic kidney disease (CKD), 711t
   chronic liver disease and cirrhosis, 657t
   chronic obstructive pulmonary disease (COPD), 547–548, 547t
   chronic pancreatitis, 664
   cirrhosis, 659
   colorectal cancer, 639, 639t
   condylomata (HPV), 872t
   constipation, 619, 619t
   contact dermatitis, 285
   coronary artery disease (CAD), 381
   Crohn disease, 626–627, 629t
   Cushing syndrome, 759
   cystic fibrosis (CF), 555
   dehydration, 53
   dementia, 984
   depression, 1179t
   dermatitis, 1119
   diabetes insipidus, 740, 741t
   diabetes mellitus, 769, 769f, 769t, 777t
   diabetic nephropathy, 706
   diabetic retinopathy, 1069
   diarrhea, 622, 622t
   disorders related to development of the genital organs, 828
   displacement disorders, 829, 831t
   disseminated intravascular coagulation (DIC), 472, 472t
   diverticulosis and diverticulitis, 625
   dysmenorrhea, 823
   ear and hearing, 1054–1055, 1055t
   ear disorders, 1081t
   ear trauma, 1081
   encephalitis, 954, 954t
   endocrine system, 729–737, 731–737t
   endometrial cancer, 842
   erectile dysfunction, 863
   esophageal cancer, 603
   external ear infection, 1079
   eye and vision, 1046
   eye disorders, 1061t
   eye trauma, 1075
   female reproductive system, 806t
   fibrocystic breast disease, 816
   fibroid tumors, 839
   fluid excess, 55
   fractures, 902
   gastric cancer, 613t
   gastroesophageal reflux disease (GERD), 605, 606t
   genital parasites, 878
   genital warts, 878
   glaucoma, 1071
   glomerulonephritis, 707–708, 708t
   goiter, 751
   gonorrhea, 872t, 875
   gout, 913
   growth hormone deficiency, 743
   Guillain-Barré syndrome (GBS), 1030
   Hashimoto thyroiditis, 289
   headaches, 958
   hearing loss, 1076t
   hematologic and lymphatic systems, 456–457, 458t
   hemolytic transfusion reaction, 283, 283t
   hemophilia, 474
   hepatitis, 653, 654t
   herniated discs, 971–972
   herpes simplex, 872t, 877
   herpes simplex lesions, 1123
   herpes zoster (shingles), 1124
   hiatal hernia, 605
   HIV/AIDS, 303t, 304–306
   Hodgkin lymphoma, 481
   Huntington disease, 993
   hyperkalemia, 61
   hypernatremia, 59
   hyperparathyroidism, 755
   hyperthyroidism, 749
   hypocalcemia, 63
   hypogammaglobulinemia, 294
   hypokalemia, 60
   hyponatremia, 59
   hypoparathyroidism, 754
   hypothyroidism, 746
   idiopathic autoimmune hemolytic anemia, 288
   immune system, 271, 271–274t
   immune thrombocytopenic purpura (ITP), 473
   impacted cerumen, 1080
   infectious disease, 89
   infective endocarditis (IE), 363, 364t
   inner ear tumors, 1087
   integumentary system, 1100
   irritable bowel syndrome (IBS), 631
   irritations and inflammations of the vagina and vulva, 826
   keratitis, 1064
   kidney cancer, 705
   labyrinthitis, 1086
   laryngeal cancer, 527, 528t
   laryngitis, 525
   leukemia, 475, 476t
   lower gastrointestinal bleeding, 638
   lung cancer, 565, 567t
   macular degeneration, 1074, 1075f
   male infertility, 866
   male reproductive system, 811–812, 812t
   malignant breast disorders, 817, 820t
   masses of external ear, 1081
   Ménière disease, 1087
   meningitis, 953
   menstrual flow and cycle disorders, 823
   mental health, 1158
   middle ear infections, 1083
   middle ear trauma, 1085
   mitral regurgitation, 358
   mitral stenosis, 357

Diagnostic tests (continued)
  mitral valve prolapse (MVP), 354
  mood disorders, 1176
  multiple myeloma, 479
  multiple sclerosis (MS), 1022
  musculoskeletal system, 890–896, 893t, 894–895t
  myasthenia gravis (MG), 1027
  myocardial infarction (MI), 386t, 387
  myocarditis, 368
  non-Hodgkin lymphomas, 482
  oral cancer, 603
  osteoarthritis (OA), 915
  osteomyelitis, 910
  osteoporosis, 911
  otosclerosis, 1084
  ovarian cancer, 842
  pancreatic cancer, 667
  Parkinson disease, 990
  pediculosis, 1129
  pelvic inflammatory disease (PID), 871
  peptic ulcer disease (PUD), 608–609, 609t
  pericarditis, 366–367, 366t
  peripheral arterial disease (PAD), 394
  peritonitis, 624
  pernicious anemia, 288
  personality disorders, 1182–1183
  pharyngitis, 523
  pheochromocytoma, 756
  pleural effusion, 544
  pleurisy, 544
  pneumonia, 539, 540f, 540t
  pneumothorax, 560, 561t
  polycystic ovary syndrome (PCOS), 840
  polycythemia, 471
  postpolio syndrome, 1031
  preoperative, 167, 168t
  pressure injuries, 1112
  prostate cancer, 858
  prostatitis, 849
  psoriasis, 1120
  pulmonary edema, 428, 428t
  pulmonary embolism (PE), 558, 559t
  pulmonary fibrosis, 545
  reactive hypoglycemia, 786
  refractive errors, 1066–1067
  renal calculi, 700–701, 700t
  respiratory system, 495–499, 497f, 498t, 499f
  respiratory viruses, 526
  restless legs syndrome (RLS), 1031
  retinal detachment, 1070
  rheumatoid arthritis (RA), 920
  scabies, 1130
  schizophrenia, 1181t
  seizure disorders, 960
  sickle cell anemia, 468
  sinusitis, 521
  skin cancer, 1134
  sleep apnea, 522
  small-bowel obstruction, 636, 636t
  spinal cord injuries, 975, 978t
  stroke, 1003, 1005f, 1017t
  substance use disorders, 1188, 1189t
  syndrome of inappropriate ADH (SIADH), 741t, 742
  syphilis, 872t, 875–876
  systemic lupus erythematosus (SLE), 290, 291t
  testicular cancer, 861
  thyroid gland cancer, 752
  tonsillitis/adenoiditis, 525
  toxic shock syndrome (TSS), 827
  transplant rejection, 286
  traumatic brain injury (TBI), 964, 967t
  trichomoniasis, 872t, 876
  trigeminal neuralgia (TN), 1033
  tuberculosis (TB), 541–542, 542t
  ulcerative colitis, 629, 629t
  urinary system, 683–688t, 683–689, 689f
  urinary tract infection (UTI), 696t
  urticaria, 280
  venous thromboembolism (VTE) disease, 373t, 374
  viral rhinitis/common cold, 522
  vulvar cancer, 841
Dialysis, 714
  hemodialysis, 710, 714–716, 715–716f, 715b
  peritoneal, 716–717, 717b, 717f
Diaphragmatic breathing, 501
Diaphragms, 835–836, 836f, 881t
Diaphysis, 885
Diarrhea, 620–623, 622t
  antibiotic-associated, 101
Diazepam (Valium), preoperative, 173t
Diencephalon, 933, 934f
Diet. *See* Nutrition and diet factors
Dietary Approaches to Stop Hypertension (DASH), 344, 345, 379
Diethylstilbestrol (DES), 146
Diffusion, 51
Digital imaging of eye, 1046
Digitalis, 440
Digital rectal examination (DRE), 809–810, 812t
Dilated cardiomyopathy, 368
Dilation and curettage (D&C), 823
Dilation and evacuation (D&E), 838
Diplopia, 1012
Dipyridamole SPECT-CT thallium imaging, 333t
Directing in management process, 18
Direct injection/intravenous push, 71
Directly observed therapy (DOT), 541
Direct thrombin inhibitors, 372t
Direct transmission, 86, 86f, 87f
Direct vasodilators, 348t
Disability-associated incontinence, 690
Disability/central nervous system assessment in primary survey, 193
Disaster response, 204–205
  bioterrorism agents, 205, 205f, 206–208t
Discectomy, 973
Discharge
  after total hip replacement, 923
  from hospital-based care to home health care, 241
  PACU, 180, 180b
  postoperative patient, 189
Discoid lupus erythematosus (DLE), 289
Disease modifying agents, 1023t
Disease-modifying antirheumatic drugs (DMARDs), 917t, 920
Dislocations, 900
Displaced fractures, 902t, 903f
Displacement, 1170
Displacement disorders, 829–831, 830f, 831t
Dissecting aneurysms, 396, 396f
Disseminated intravascular coagulation (DIC), 471–472, 472t
Distention, gastric, 614–615
Distraction for pain, 128
Distributive shock, 108–111, 109t, 194
Diuretics, 55, 59
  for chronic heart failure (HF), 434t, 435, 440
  for chronic kidney disease (CKD), 714
  hearing loss due to, 1076t
  for hypertension, 346t
Diverticulosis and diverticulitis, 624–625, 625f, 625t
DNA (deoxyribonucleic acid), 140, 142, 143f
Doctors of nursing practice (DNPs), 17
Documentation
  appropriate, 29
  home health care, 244
Dogs
  guide, 1047
  hearing service, 1057
  seizure alert, 960
Do not resuscitate (DNR) order, 249
Dopamine, 1156t
Dopamine agonists, 991t
Doppler ultrasound, 332t, 336
Double-barrel stoma, 643
Double pneumonia, 538
DPP-4 inhibitor, 775t
Drains, surgical wound, 187
Dressings
  for burns, 1144
  open wet, 1100
  skin, 1101, 1103–1104, 1103–1104t, 1113
  surgical wound, 187
Dressler syndrome, 366
Drowning, 204
Drug-induced lupus erythematosus (DILE), 289
Drug injections, HIV/AIDS transmission by, 302, 311t
Drug use. *See* Substance use disorders
Dry eye disease, 1061
Dual-energy x-ray absorptiometry (DEXA) scan, 801, 893
Ductus deferens, 792
Dumping syndrome, 615
Durable medical power of attorney (DPOA), 248
Dwarfism, 743f
Dysarthria, 947, 1003
Dysmenorrhea, 823–824
Dyspareunia, 828
Dysphagia, 523, 939
Dysphasia, 1003
Dyspnea, 495
  in chronic heart failure (HF), 429
Dysrhythmia, 409

E

Ear. *See also* Hearing
  aging and, 1049, 1054
  data collection on, 1049–1052, 1051t, 1053t
  diagnostic tests, 1054–1055, 1055t
  health maintenance of, 1056, 1056–1057t, 1056t
  irrigation of, 1082, 1082f
  normal anatomy and physiology, 1048, 1049f, 1050f

physical examination of, 1052–1054, 1052b, 1053f, 1054t
therapeutic measures, 1055f, 1056–1057, 1056–1057t
Ear disorders
external, 1078–1083, 1082f, 1083b
inner, 1086–1088, 1087b
middle, 1083–1086, 1086t
summary, 1081t
Eating disorders, 1185–1186
Ebola virus disease, 90, 90–91t
Ecchymosis, 1098
Eccrine glands, 1092, 1093f
Echinocandins, 100t
Echocardiogram, 332t, 335
Economic issues, 16, 17b
Ectopic hormone production and lung cancer, 564–565
Ectopic pregnancy, 838
Eczema, 279
Edema
in chronic heart failure (HF), 431
pitting, of skin, 55, 329, 329f
pulmonary, 385t, 428–429, 428t
skin, 1096, 1098
Ego defense mechanisms, 1161, 1162t
Ehler-Danlos syndrome, 354
Ejaculation, 795, 807
retrograde, 854
Ejaculatory ducts, 792
Ejection fraction, heart, 319
Electrocardiogram (ECG), 332t, 335, 404–405, 405f
interpretation of cardiac rhythms, 405f, 407–408, 407f, 407t, 408f
pacemaker activity, 419, 419f
Electroconvulsive therapy (ECT), 1166
Electroencephalogram (EEG), 946
Electrolarynx, 528
Electrolyte imbalances, 57–64
calcium imbalances, 62–64, 62f, 63f, 63t
chronic kidney disease (CKD) and, 712–713, 713b
extracellular and intracellular electrolytes, 57, 58f
magnesium imbalances, 64
potassium imbalances, 60–62
sodium imbalances, 58–60, 58b
Electrolyte solutions, 74
Electronic infusion devices (EIDs), 73, 73f
Electronystagmogram, 1055
Electrophysiological studies, 333t, 337
Electroretinography, 1046
Elimination problems
constipation, 226–227, 618–620, 619t, 621b
diarrhea, 101, 620–623, 622t
Ellis-van Creveld Syndrome, 743
Elopement, 237
Embolectomy, 399
Emboli, 357
arterial, 393–394
as complication of myocardial infarction (MI), 385t
Embolic stroke, 1001
Embolism, 1001
Emergency management
seizure disorders, 960
spinal cord injuries, 977, 977–978f

Emergent conditions
bioterrorism agents, 205, 205f, 206–208t
burns, 199–200
disaster response, 204–205
fractures, 902, 904b
frostbite, 201
hypertensive emergency, 349
major trauma, 194–199, 196b, 196f, 197t, 198f
near-drowning, 204
oncological emergencies, 162
poisoning and drug overdose, 202–204
primary survey in, 192–193, 193f
psychiatric emergencies, 204
secondary survey in, 193, 194t
shock, 194
stroke, 1002, 1003
triage for, 192, 193f, 205
Emmetropia, 1065
Emotional responses to surgery, 166
Empathy, 17
Emphysema, 546, 548f
surgery for, 549
Empty nest, 213
Empyema, 544
Encephalitis, 953–954
Encephalopathy, 953
Endarterectomy, 399–400, 1008
Ending the HIV Epidemic: A Plan for America (EHE), 300
Endobronchial valve, 549
Endocrine disorders, 739–764
adrenal glands, 756–762, 758t, 759f, 761–762t
causes of, 739, 740t
medications used in, 761–762t
parathyroid gland, 754–756, 755t
pituitary gland, 740–745, 741t, 742b, 743–745f
summary of, 761t
thyroid gland, 227, 745–754, 745t, 747t, 749f, 752f
Endocrine-metabolic system
aging and, 227
Hashimoto thyroiditis, 289
Endocrine pancreas disorders, 765–789
diabetes mellitus, 765–786
reactive hypoglycemia, 786–787
Endocrine system, 723–738
adrenal glands, 724f, 725f, 727, 728f
aging and, 728, 733f
data collection, 728–729
diagnostic tests of, 729–737, 731–737t
hormone tests, 729–730, 731–733t
hypothalamus and pituitary gland, 723–724, 724f, 725f
normal anatomy and physiology, 723–728, 724f
pancreas, 575t, 576, 576f, 724f, 727–728, 729f
parathyroid glands, 724f, 727, 727f
thyroid gland, 724, 724f, 725f, 726f
End of life, 247–262, *See also* Death and dying
advance directives, living wills, and durable medical power of attorney for, 167, 248
artificial feeding and hydration at, 250
cardiopulmonary resuscitation and, 249
choices for, 249–251
chronic obstructive pulmonary disease (COPD) and planning for, 549–550

communicating with parents and their loved ones at, 251–252, 252f
compassion fatigue, 253
cultural influences on, 37
do not resuscitate (DNR) order, 249
dying process at, 253–254
grief over, 260–261, 260t
hospice care at, 250–251, 251t
hospitalization at, 250
identifying symptoms of impending death at, 248, 248f
medications to increase comfort at, 259t
nursing care plan, 254–258
postmortem care, 259–260
Endometrial cancer, 842
Endometriosis, 824, 824f
Endorphins, 122, 1157t
Endoscope, 164
Endoscopic retrograde cholangiopancreatography (ERCP), 589–590
Endoscopy, 150, 589, 589f
female reproductive system, 805, 805f, 806t
gynecological, 843
lower gastrointestinal, 590
Endothelium, 317, 320, 322f
End stoma, 642
Enhanced Recovery After Surgery (ERAS) Society, 166
Enkephalins, 122, 1157t
Enteral nutrition (EN), 592–595, 593–594t
therapeutic measures for neurologic system, 948
Enteritis, 871
Environmental control, 35–36
Environmental gastritis, 607
Environmental/occupational safety and HIV/AIDS, 310t
Enzymatic debridement, 1113
Enzymes, muscle, 890
Eosinophils, 450t, 451
Ependyma, 929
Epidemic, 89
Epidermis, 1091–1092
Epididymis, 792
Epididymitis, 860
Epidural blocks, 176
Epilepsy, 959, 960. *See also* Seizure disorders
Epinephrine, 105–106, 275, 279
Epiphyses, 885
Epispadias, 807
Epistaxis, 518–519, 519f
Epithelialization, 1144
Epstein-Barr virus (EBV), 90–91
cancer risk factor, 144
Equianalgesic doses, 125, 126t
Erectile dysfunction, 862–865, 863t, 864f, 865t
Erection, 807
Erikson, Erik, 212
Erythema, 1096
Erythropoietin, 155f
Eschar, 1112–1113
Escharotomy, 1143, 1144f
Escherichia coli (E. coli), 92
Esophageal cancer, 603–604
Esophageal speech, 528
Esophageal varices, 607, 659
cirrhosis and, 657
Esophagogastroduodenoscopy (EGD), 589

Esophagus, 573, 573f
Esotropia, 1045
Estimated average glucose, 769
Estrogen, 791, 794t
  osteoporosis and, 912
Estrogen antagonists, 818t
Estrogen-progestin contraceptive ring, 834–835
Ethics and values, 20–26
  abortion and, 839
  basic principles of, 21, 22–24
  building blocks of, 22–24
  changing issues in, 20–21
  defined, 20
  dilemmas in, 21, 24–26
  ethical decision making, 24–26
  nursing code of ethics, 21
  nursing obligations, 21
  theories of, 24
  use of, 24
Ethnocentrism, 32
Evaluation of outcomes, 4t
  acute liver failure, chronic liver disease, cirrhosis, 661
  adrenocortical insufficiency (AI), 758
  anemia, 466
  aneurysms, 397
  anxiety, obsessive-compulsive, or trauma-related disorders, 1176
  autism spectrum disorders (ADSs), 1184
  blindness and visual impairment, 1069
  bowel obstruction, 637
  cancer, 160
  cerebrovascular disorder, 1017, 1017t
  chest trauma, 561
  chronic kidney disease (CKD), 719
  colorectal cancer, 641
  constipation, 620, 621b
  coronary artery disease (CAD) and angina, 384
  cranial nerve disorder, 1035
  Cushing syndrome, 760
  dermatitis, 1120
  diabetes insipidus, 741
  diabetes mellitus, 783
  diabetic retinopathy, 1070
  diarrhea, 623
  displacement disorders, 831
  ear disorders, 1083
  eating disorders, 1186
  erectile dysfunction, 865
  eye infection and inflammation, 1065
  fractures, 909
  gallbladder disorder, 672
  gastric bleeding, 612
  gastric surgery, 614
  gastroesophageal reflux disease (GERD), 606
  glaucoma, 1072
  grieving family, 261
  headaches, 959
  hearing loss, 1078
  hemophilia, 475
  hepatitis, 655
  HIV/AIDS, 313
  hyperparathyroidism, 756
  hyperthermia, 202
  hyperthyroidism, 751
  hypoparathyroidism, 755
  hypothermia, 201
  infections, 101–103
  infectious skin disorders, 1128
  infective endocarditis (IE), 364
  inflammatory bowel disease, 630
  inflammatory or infectious gastrointestinal disorder, 626
  inner ear disorders, 1088
  intracranial surgery, 971
  intravenous (IV) therapy, 76
  irritable bowel syndrome (IBS), 633
  laryngectomy, 531
  lung cancer, 566
  lymphangitis, 401
  middle ear, tympanic membrane, and mastoid disorders, 1086
  multiple myeloma, 480
  nausea and vomiting, 599
  near-drowning, 204
  obesity, 602
  obstructive disorders, 557
  osteoarthritis (OA), 919
  ostomy, 646
  pain, 136
  pancreatic cancer, 668
  pancreatitis, 666
  Parkinson disease, 992
  peripheral arterial disorders, 396
  personality disorders, 1183
  poisoning and drug overdose, 203
  postoperative, 179, 188
  preoperative patient, 171
  prostatitis, 852
  renal calculi, 702
  respiratory failure, 563
  restrictive disorders, 545
  rheumatoid arthritis (RA), 921
  schizophrenia, 1181
  seizure disorders, 963
  sickle cell anemia, 470
  spinal surgery, 974
  substance use disorders, 1190
  syndrome of inappropriate ADH (SIADH), 742
  thoracic surgery, 568
  thyroidectomy, 754
  transurethral resection of the prostate (TURP), 857
  trauma, 198
  traumatic brain injury (TBI), 966
  tuberculosis (TB), 543
  type I hypersensitivity disorder, 281
  urinary system diagnostic tests, 689
  urinary tract infection (UTI), 697
  vascular surgery, 400
  venous insufficiency, 398
  venous thromboembolism (VTE) disease, 374
Event recorder, 332t
Evidence
  delirium in hospitalized older adults, 988
  identifying nursing, 10
  levels of, 10t
  neurological data collection during pandemic, 941
Evidence-based practice (EBP), 2, 9–14
  age and hearing loss effects on balance and listening, 1054
  air pollution and stroke risk, 1012
  bystander CPR, 417
  cancer, 158
  cardiac magnetic resonance imaging, 335
  chalazion, 1064
  cholecystectomy, 671
  chronic kidney disease (CKD) and diabetes, 710
  colonoscopy preparation, 590
  common cold prevention, 523
  complementary and alternative modalities, 47
  defecation posture modification devices (DPMD), 620
  defined, 9
  Dietary Approaches to Stop Hypertension (DASH), 345
  eHealth-based interventions in cardiac rehabilitation, 391
  end of life communication, 252
  exercise for glucose control in diabetes mellitus, 787
  family presence during resuscitation, 199
  heart failure (HF), 429
  HIV/AIDS and cardiovascular disease, 313
  hospital readmission after home health care, 243
  hyponatremia, 59
  identifying nursing evidence for, 10
  infection control, 95
  itching in healing burns, 1146
  levels of, 10t
  Mediterranean diet, 227
  microbial growth with nail polish, 175
  multimorbidity resilience, 217
  multiple sclerosis (MS) and exercise, 1024
  oral anticoagulant intervention, 371
  osteoarthritis (OA), 915
  for pain, 130
  polycystic ovary syndrome (PCOS), 840
  pressure injuries, 1114
  process, 10–13, 11f
  quality and safety in, 13–14
  question framework PICO(T), 11b
  reasons for using, 10
  sepsis and septic shock, 110
  smoking cessation, 501
  systemic lupus erythematosus (SLE), 290
  thyroid function and weight, 752–753
  who should provide nursing care based on, 13
  yoga benefits, 540
  young people living with mental illness, 1180
Evidence-informed practice (EIP), 9
Evisceration, wound, 185, 187f
Ewing sarcoma, 912
Excoriation, 1097f
Exercise. See also Activity
  atherosclerosis and, 379
  bone density and, 223–224
  breathing, 501
  cardiac rehabilitation and, 391
  cardiovascular system and, 337
  diabetes mellitus and, 771–772
  in long-term care facilities, 238
  multiple sclerosis (MS) and, 1024
  musculoskeletal system aging and, 887
  osteoarthritis (OA) and, 916
  osteoporosis and, 912
  for pain, 130
  preoperative, 167, 169
  range of motion, 22f, 223
  yoga, 540

Exercise stress echocardiogram, 332t, 336
Exertional dyspnea, 429
Exhalation, 488–489
Exophthalmos, 749, 749f
Exotropia, 1045
Expectorants, 534
Exposure, in primary survey, 193
Expressive aphasia, 947–948, 1003
Extensively drug resistant TB, 541
External ear, 1048, 1049f
    disorders of, 1078–1083, 1082f, 1083b
External fixation, 904, 905f, 906
Extracellular fluid (ECF), 50
Extracorporeal membrane oxygenation (ECMO), 436
Extravasation, 76, 77t
Extremities assessment in secondary survey, 194t
Exudate
    eye, 1046
    throat, 523
Eye. *See also* Vision
    accessory structures of, 1039f
    aging and, 1041–1042, 1042f
    diagnostic tests of, 1046
    examination guidelines for, 1046
    hygiene of, 1046
    internal examination of, 1046
    irrigation of, 1047
    lacrimal apparatus of, 1039f
    long-term effects of diabetes mellitus on, 781
    muscle balance and movement of, 1044–1045, 1045f
    in neurologic system examination, 943–944, 944f
    normal anatomy and physiology, 1038–1041, 1039–1042f
    nutrition for healthy, 1047
    physical examination of, 1042–1043, 1044f, 1044t
    therapeutic measures, 1046–1048, 1047t
    trauma to, 1075
Eye allergy medications, 1062t
Eyeball, structure of, 1038, 1040f
Eyebrow, 1039f
Eyelashes, 1039f
Eyelids, 1039f
    blepharitis of, 1061
Eye patching, 1048

F

Face masks, 1064
Facial nerve, 935t, 938f
    Bell palsy, 1033–1034, 1034f
Factor Xa inhibitors, 373t
Fallopian tubes, 791, 791f, 792f
Falls, 195, 214–215, 912
    prevention, in long-term care facilities, 238–239
Family and caregivers
    communication with patients and, about end of life, 251–252, 252f
    compassion fatigue in, 253
    of patients with chronic illness, 218–219, 218b
    therapeutic measures for neurologic system and, 948
Family history, hypertension, 344
Family organization, 35
Family visitation, PACU, 180
Fasciculation, 1029
Fasciotomy, 907
Fasting blood glucose level, 769, 769f, 769t
Fat embolism syndrome, 907–908, 908t
Fatigue and weakness in chronic heart failure (HF), 429
Fecal microbiota transplantation, 101
Feeding, artificial, 250
    therapeutic measures for neurologic system, 948
Feet, care of older patients', 1099
Female condoms, 881t
Female reproductive system. *See also* Breasts
    data collection, 796–805, 797–799t, 800f, 802f, 802t, 805f
    diagnostic procedures for, 806t
    hormones of, 794t, 801, 806t
    normal anatomy and physiology, 790–791, 791f, 792–793f
    ovarian and menstrual cycles, 791
    pregnancy termination, 837–839
    reproductive life planning, 833–837, 836f
Female reproductive system disorders, 815
    benign, 839–841
    breast disorders, 816–822, 818t, 820t, 821–822f
    displacement disorders, 829–831, 830f, 831t
    fertility disorders, 831–833, 832t
    irritations and inflammations of the vagina and vulva, 825–826, 827t, 828t
    malignant, 841–843, 842f
    menstrual disorders, 822–825, 823t, 824f, 825t
    related to development of the genital organs, 828–829
    surgery for, 843–845
    toxic shock syndrome (TSS), 826–828
    tumors, 839–843, 842f, 843t
Fentanyl (Sublimaze), 126
    preoperative, 173t
Fever after blood administration, 459
Fibrates, 380t
Fibrocystic breast disease, 816
Fibroid tumors, 839
Fidelity, 22
Fight-or-flight mechanism, 938, 1158
Filters, infusion, 73
Filtration, 51
Finances and chronic illness, 219–220
Fissures
    brain, 934
    intestinal, 626
    skin, 1097f
Fistulas, intestinal, 626
5-aminosalicylates, 628t
Flail chest, 196, 561
Flu. *See* Influenza
Fluid balance, 50–52
    burns and, 1138
    control of, 51
    fluid gains and fluid losses, 52
    movement of fluids and electrolytes in the body, 51–52
    normal distribution of total body water, 51f
Fluid excess, 54–57, 55f, 56t, 57t
    monitoring for, 460
Fluid imbalances, 52–57
    dehydration, 52–54, 52b, 54b
    fluid excess, 54–57, 55f, 56t, 57t
Fluid retention in chronic heart failure (HF), 438
Fluid volume decrease
    due to hemorrhage or abdominal organ injury, 198
    due to hyperthermia, 202
Fluorescein and indocyanine green angiography, 1046
Fluoroquinolones, 98t
    for sexually transmitted infections (STIs), 873t
    for urinary tract infection (UTI), 698t
Folk practices, 33
Follicle-stimulating hormone (FSH), 725f, 731t, 791, 794t
Food allergies, 275
Food/water safety and HIV/AIDS, 310t
Foot circles, 169
Foot complications of diabetes mellitus, 781–782, 782f
Foot drop, 947, 947f
Foot neuropathy, 225
Foreign bodies in eye, 1075
Four Score Scale, 941, 942f, 956
Fractures, 196
    complications of, 906–908, 907f, 908t
    diagnostic tests, 902
    emergency treatment, 902, 904b
    etiology and types, 901, 902t, 903f
    management of, 902–906, 904b, 905f
    in older adults, 224, 890, 896
    pathophysiology, 900–901, 901f
    rib, 560–561
    signs and symptoms, 901–902
Frail Elderly Syndrome, 216
Frailty, 216, 223, 223b, 250
Frank-Starling phenomenon, 428
Free-floating anxiety, 1170
Frontal lobe, 935f
Frostbite, 201
Frostnip, 201
Full Outline of UnResponsiveness (FOUR) Score Coma Scale, 941, 942f, 956
Full thickness burns, 1140t, 1141f
Full-thickness skin graft, 1145, 1145t
Fungal infections
    candidiasis, 827t, 1124, 1127t
    external ear, 1078–1079
    skin, 1124, 1125–1126t
Fungal pneumonia, 538
Fungi, 85, 85t
Furosemide (Lasix), 55
Furuncles, 1122t
Fusion inhibitors, 307t
Fusiform aneurysms, 396, 396f

G

Gallbladder
    disorders of, 668–672, 670t, 671f, 672t
    medications for, 576, 576f
Gallium/thallium scans, 895t, 896
Gallstones, 668–672, 670t, 671f, 672t
Gamma-aminobutyric acid (GABA), 1156t
Ganglion cells, 1039
Gas transport in the blood, 489–490
Gastric acid, 88

Gastric bleeding, 611–612, 612t
Gastric bypass, 601
Gastric cancer, 612–613, 613f, 613t
Gastric juice, 574
Gastric surgery, 613–614f, 613–615
Gastritis, 607, 607b, 608t
Gastroduodenostomy, 613
Gastroesophageal reflux disease (GERD), 605–606, 606t
Gastrointestinal, hepatobiliary and pancreatic systems
  aging and, 576–577, 577f
  diagnostic tests of, 583–591
  health history, 577–579, 578–579t, 579b
  home health care, 595–596
  laboratory tests, 583–587t, 583–588
  normal anatomy and physiology, 572–577, 573–574f, 575t, 576–577f
  physical examination, 579–581, 580–581t
  radiographic tests of, 588–589, 588f
  therapeutic measures, 591–595, 591f, 592–594t
Gastrointestinal disorders
  abdominal hernias, 633–634, 633f
  absorption disorders, 634–635, 635t
  anorectal problems, 637–638
  anorexia, 154, 598
  appendicitis, 623, 624f
  bleeding, 638
  colorectal cancer, 639–640t, 639–641, 641f
  constipation, 226–227, 618–620, 619t, 621b
  Crohn disease, 626–627, 626f, 627f, 631
  diarrhea, 101, 620–623, 622t
  diverticulosis and diverticulitis, 624–625, 625f, 625t
  esophageal cancer, 603–604
  esophageal varices, 607
  gastric bleeding, 611–612, 612t
  gastric cancer, 612–613, 613f, 613t
  gastric surgery for, 613–614f, 613–615
  gastritis, 607, 607b, 608t
  gastroesophageal reflux disease (GERD), 605–606, 606t
  hiatal hernia, 604–605, 605f, 606f
  inflammatory and infectious disorders, 623–626, 624f, 625f, 625t
  inflammatory bowel disease, 626–630, 626f, 627f, 628t, 629t, 631
  intestinal obstruction, 635–637, 636f, 636t
  irritable bowel syndrome (IBS), 630–633
  lower, 618–648
  Mallory-Weiss tear (MWT), 606–607
  nausea and vomiting, 598–599
  obesity, 599–602, 600f, 602f
  oral cancer, 603, 605f
  oral health and dental care and, 602–603, 604b
  oral inflammatory disorders, 603
  ostomy and, 629, 642–646, 642f, 643f, 643t, 644t
  peptic ulcer disease (PUD), 608–611, 609t, 610t
  peritonitis, 623–624
  problems of elimination, 618–623, 619t, 621b, 622t
  ulcerative colitis, 626, 626f, 627–629, 628t, 629t
  upper, 598–617

Gastrointestinal system
  aging and, 226–227
  burns and, 1139
  changes at end of life, 253
  chemotherapy effects on, 154
  decompression, 595
  effects of shock on, 106
  infections in, 103
  intubation of, 591–592, 591f, 592t
  postoperative function, 187–188
  spinal cord injuries and, 977
Gastrojejunostomy, 613
Gastroscopy, 589, 589f
Gender
  coronary artery disease (CAD) and, 381
  fall risk and, 224
  multiple sclerosis (MS) and, 1021
  myocardial infarction (MI) and, 386–387
  osteoporosis and, 910
  roles and, 35
  urinary tract infection (UTI) and, 696
General anesthesia, 176
Generalized anxiety disorder (GAD), 1170
Generalized seizures, 960
Genetics, 140, 142
  breast cancer and, 800, 801, 816–817
  cancer and, 145
Genetic testing
  for cancer, 148
  immune system, 271, 274t
Genital parasites, 878
Genital ulcers, 871
Genital warts, 874t, 877–878, 878f
Genitourinary and reproductive system. *See also* Female reproductive system; Male reproductive system; Urinary system
  aging and, 227–228, 795, 796f
  chemotherapy and, 155
  normal anatomy and physiology, 790–795
  reproductive life planning, 833–837, 835–836f
  spinal cord injuries and, 977
  transgender population data collection, 812–813
Genitourinary tract infections, 96, 103
Genotyping, HIV/AIDS, 306
Gerontological issues. *See also* Aging; Older adults
  absence of fever with infection, 87
  antihypertensive therapy, 345
  arrhythmia risk, 412
  burn injury, 1140
  burn prevention, 199
  care of feet, 1099
  chronic illness, 215–216
  cultural influences on, 37
  dehydration, 52, 54b, 621
  diabetes mellitus, 787
  diverticulitis, 624
  falls, 912
  hearing changes, 1048
  HIV/AIDS, 301
  home health care safety, 243
  hypokalemia, 621
  immune system, 268
  injuries caused by falls versus battery or assault, 195
  intravenous (IV) therapy, 75

  medication metabolism, 577
  monitoring for fluid excess, 460
  myocardial infarction (MI), 387
  oral hygiene, 602–603
  osteoporosis, 911
  pain, 132, 183
  postoperative pain, 183
  preoperative, 171
  respiratory infections, 539
  sexually transmitted infections (STIs), 879
  shock, 111
  skin breakdown, 1111–1112
  spinal cord injuries, 979
  suicide, 1191
  technology use for, 224, 224f
  tuberculosis (TB), 541
  vision changes, 1045
Gestational diabetes mellitus (GDM), 768
Gigantism, 743f
Gingival recession, 604b
Gingivitis, 604b
Glands, skin, 1092, 1093f
Glasgow Coma Scale (GCS), 193, 197, 940–941, 941t, 942f, 956
Glaucoma, 1067, 1067f, 1071–1072, 1072f
Global aphasia, 1003
Global Deterioration Scale for Assessment of Primary Degenerative Dementia (GDS), 995
Glomerular filtration, 676, 678f
Glomerulonephritis, 707–708, 708t
Glossopharyngeal nerve, 935t, 938f
Glucagon-like peptide-1 receptor agonists, 775t
Glucocorticoids, 1022t
Glutamate, 1156t
Glutamate antagonists, 1023t
Glycine, 1156t
Glycohemoglobin, 769
Glycopeptides, 98t
Glycoprotein IIb/IIIa inhibitors, 389t
Goiter, 751–752, 752f
Goitrogens, 751
Gold preparations, 918t
Gonorrhea, 872, 872t, 875
  antibiotics for, 873t
Good death, 247–248
Goodpasture syndrome, 707
Gout, 913–914, 913f
Grafts, skin, 1144–1145, 1145f
Gram-negative bacteria, 84, 85t
Gram-positive bacteria, 84, 85t
Granulocyte-colony-stimulating factor (G-CSF), 155f
Graph paper, electrocardiogram, 405, 405f
Gravity drip, 71f, 72–73
Greater vestibular glands, 793f
Green House Project model, 237t, 238
Greenstick fractures, 902t, 903f
Grief
  nursing process for family experiencing, 260–261
  stages of, 260, 260t
Group A streptococci, 354
Group therapy, 1165
Growth hormone (GH), 723, 725f, 731t
  disorders related to imbalance of, 743–744, 743–744f
  medications for, 761t

Growth hormone-inhibiting hormone (GHIH), 723
Growth hormone-releasing hormone (GHRH), 723
Guided imagery, 44, 46b, 1167
Guide dogs, 1047
Guillain-Barré syndrome (GBS), 1030–1031, 1032t
Gummas, 875
Gunshot wounds, 194
Gynecomastia, 807

H

H1N1, 527
Hair, 1092, 1093f
　alopecia, 155, 1098–1099
Hair loss with chemotherapy, 155
Hallucinations, 1180–1181, 1182t
Hand hygiene, 92–93, 92f
Hashimoto thyroiditis, 289
Head
　assessment of, in secondary survey, 194t
　trauma to, 195, 196b
Headaches
　diagnosis, 958
　nursing process, 958–959
　types, 957–958
Health, definition of, 211
Health-care delivery, 15–16
Health-care providers (HCPs), 17
　cultural influences on choice of, 36
　occupational exposure to HIV/AIDS, 302
　oncology and, 142
Health-care team
　in collaborative home health care, 240–241, 240f
　communication with, 5–6
　pain management and, 120–121, 133, 135
　surgical, 175b
Health history, 169
　cardiovascular system, 323, 324–325t
　ear and hearing, 1049
　endocrine system, 728
　female reproductive system, 796, 797–798t
　gastrointestinal, hepatobiliary and pancreatic systems, 577–579, 578–579t
　hematologic and lymphatic systems, 454, 455–456t
　immune system, 269–270
　integumentary system, 1094–1095t, 1094–1096
　male reproductive system, 807
　musculoskeletal system, 887–888
　neurologic system, 939–940, 940t
　respiratory system, 492, 493t
　sensory system, 1042, 1043t
　urinary system, 679, 680–681t
Health Insurance Portability and Accountability Act (HIPAA), 27–28
Health promotion
　cardiovascular system, 337
　chronic illness and, 220
　for middle-aged adults, 213
　for older adults, 214, 231, 232t
　for young adults, 213
Healthy Vegetarian Dietary Pattern, 344
Hearing, 1048–1057. *See also* Ear

　aging and, 1042f, 1054
　behaviors indicating loss of, 1052b
　data collection on, 1049–1052, 1051t, 1053t
　diagnostic tests, 1054–1055, 1055t
　normal anatomy and physiology of the ear, 1048, 1049f
　therapeutic measures, 1056–1057t, 1056–1058
Hearing aids, 1056–1057, 1077f, 1079b
Hearing disorders. *See also* Ear disorders
　communicating with patient who has, 1079b
　hearing aids for, 1056–1057, 1077f, 1079b
　hearing loss, 1048, 1049, 1075–1078, 1076t, 1077f, 1078t
　nursing care for patient with, 1080
Hearing service dogs, 1057
Heart
　blood vessels, 320–321, 322f
　cardiac conduction pathway and cardiac cycle, 318, 320f
　cardiac cycle, 318, 320f, 404, 405–407, 405–407f
　cardiac output, 105–106, 319
　cardiac pacemakers for, 318, 320f, 418–420, 419f
　cardiac structure and function, 317–318, 318f
　cardiomyopathy of, 368–370, 369f, 369t, 370b
　conduction system of, 404
　coronary blood flow in, 318–319, 319f
　effects of shock on, 106, 108
　hormones and, 319
　infective endocarditis (IE) of, 362–366, 363f, 364f, 364t, 365t
　layers of, 362, 363f
　location of, 317
　murmur in, 329, 354
　myocarditis, 367–368
　pericarditis of, 366–367, 366t, 367f
　regulation or heart rate, 319, 321f
　structure of coronary blood vessels and, 317–318, 318f
　trauma to, 368
　valves of, 353–354, 354f
　venous thromboembolism (VTE) disease of, 370–374
Heart failure (HF), 425–447
　cardiac transplantation for, 441–445, 442f
　chronic, 429–441, 430t, 433–435t, 436–437f, 437–438t, 440b
　compensatory mechanisms to maintain cardiac output in, 427–428
　as complication of myocardial infarction (MI), 385t
　congestive, 426
　left-sided, 426, 426t, 427f
　overview of, 425–427, 426t, 427f, 427t
　pathophysiology, 426
　pulmonary edema, 385t, 428–429, 428t
　right-sided, 426–427, 427t, 428f
Heart rate, 319, 321f, 408, 408f
　pulse and, 327–328
Heart valve replacement, 361–362
Heat and cold application, 46
　for osteoarthritis (OA), 916
　for pain, 130
　for rheumatoid arthritis (RA), 920
Heat cramps, 202
Heat exhaustion, 202

Heatstroke, 202
Heberden nodes, 915
Helicobacter pylori (*H. pylori*), 144–145
　gastric cancer and, 612–613
　gastritis and, 607, 608t
　peptic ulcer disease (PUD) and, 608–610, 609t
Helminths, 85
Hemangioma, 1132t
Hemarthrosis, 890
Hematocrit, 53, 55, 450t
Hematologic disorders
　hemorrhagic disorders, 471–475, 472t, 473b
　home health care, 484
　multiple myeloma, 478–480, 479f
　red blood cell disorders, 462–471, 465t, 466f, 467b, 468–469f
　white blood cell disorders, 475–478, 476t
Hematologic system
　aging and, 453, 454f
　chemotherapy effects on, 154, 155f
　diagnostic tests, 456–457, 458t
　normal anatomy and physiology, 448–451, 449f, 450t
　nursing assessment of, 454–455, 455–456t
　therapeutic measures, 458–460, 458t
Hematoma, 76, 77t, 964, 964f
Hemipelvectomy, 924
Hemiplegia, 1008–1009, 1009f
Hemodialysis, 710, 714–716, 715–716f, 715b
Hemodynamic monitoring, 333t, 337
Hemoglobin, 450t, 451
Hemolysis, 451
Hemolytic transfusion reaction, 282–283, 283t, 284t, 459
Hemophilia, 473–475
Hemorrhagic disorders. *See also* Bleeding
　cerebral aneurysm, 1010–1012, 1010f, 1011f
　disseminated intravascular coagulation (DIC), 471–472, 472t
　hemophilia, 473–475
　immune thrombocytopenic purpura (ITP), 472–473, 473b
Hemorrhagic stroke, 1002
Hemorrhoids, 637–638
Hemothorax, 559
Hemovac drains, 187
Heparin, 372t
Hepatic encephalopathy, 657–658, 659–660
Hepatic portal circulation, 575
Hepatitis, 649–655
　complications of, 653
　defined, 649
　diagnostic tests, 653, 654t
　hepatitis A, 649, 650–652t, 652
　hepatitis B, 144, 148–149, 305t, 649, 650–652t, 652, 878
　hepatitis C, 305t, 649, 650–652t, 652, 878
　hepatitis D, 649, 650–652t
　hepatitis E, 649, 650–652t
　home health care, 655
　nursing process for, 653–655
　pathophysiology and etiology of, 649
　prevention, 652
　signs and symptoms, 652–653, 653f
　therapeutic measures, 653, 653b
Hepatomegaly, 427
Hepatorenal syndrome, 658, 659f

Hepatosplenomegaly, 875
Herbal therapy, 44, 45t
   for benign prostatic hyperplasia (BPH), 853
   for erectile dysfunction, 864
Herd immunity, 89
Hernias
   abdominal, 633–634, 633f
   hiatal, 604–605, 605f, 606f
Herniated discs, 971–973, 971f
Herniation, brain, 965, 965f
Herpes simplex virus (HSV), 603, 872t, 876–877, 877f, 1121–1123
   antivirals for, 874t
   encephalitis and, 953–954
   HIV/AIDS-associated, 305t
Herpes zoster (shingles), 228, 1123–1124, 1123f
   HIV/AIDS-associated, 305t
Heterograft, 361
Hiatal hernia, 604–605, 605f, 606f
High-density lipoproteins (HDLs), 378, 379, 380t
High-frequency chest wall oscillation vest, 504
Highly active antiretroviral therapy (HAART), 297
High-sensitive C-reactive protein (hs-CRP), 330t, 334
Hindu persons, 361
Hip replacement, 921–924, 922f, 923b
Histamine, 277, 1156t
HIV/AIDS, 144, 297–316
   clinical latency stage, 299
   complications of, 302, 304, 305t, 310–311b
   counseling on, 301
   development of, 297, 298b
   diagnostic tests, 303t, 304–306
   history and incidence, 299
   home health for, 315
   information resources on, 298t
   mode of transmission, 300–301
   parenteral transmission of, 302
   pathophysiology, 299, 300f
   perinatal transmission of, 302
   pre-exposure prophylaxis (PrEP), 301
   prevention, 300–302, 301b, 308–309
   progression of, 299
   resources for, 315
   sexual transmission of, 301–302, 301b
   signs and symptoms, 302, 303f, 303t
   in special populations, 879
   therapeutic measures, 303t, 305t, 306–314
HIV-associated neurocognitive disorder, 304
Hives, 280
   after blood administration, 459
Hodgkin lymphoma, 480–481, 482t
Holistic belief system, 33
Holistic care, 229
Holistic nursing, 41
Holter monitor, 332t, 335
Home health care
   autonomous nature of, 241
   cancer and, 161
   cardiac arrhythmias, 422
   cardiovascular conditions, 401
   cerebrovascular disorders, 1017
   chronic heart failure (HF), 441
   chronic illness, 219
   collaborative, 240–241, 240f
   complementary and alternative modalities, 48
   cultural influences on, 39
   dementia, 996
   diabetes mellitus and, 785–786
   documentation in, 244
   eligibility for, 240, 240b
   end of life and, 251
   gastrointestinal, hepatobiliary and pancreatic systems, 595–596
   genital warts, 878
   hematologic and lymphatic systems, 484
   hepatitis, 655
   HIV/AIDS and, 315
   hypertension, 350–351
   immune disorders, 295
   infection control in, 243–244
   intravenous (IV) therapy, 80–81
   liability issues in, 242b
   lower respiratory tract disorders, 568
   mental health, 1167, 1191
   musculoskeletal system, 896
   musculoskeletal system disorders, 926
   nursing process in, 244–245
   for older adults, 232–233
   ostomy, 645
   pain, 136
   patient education in, 244
   postoperative, 189
   private-duty nursing, 245
   role of LPN/LVN in, 241–242, 242f
   safety considerations in, 242–243, 243b
   skin care, 1134
   steps in visits in, 242
   telenursing, 245
   transition from hospital-based nursing to, 241
   urinary system, 693
   venous thromboembolism (VTE) disease, 374–375
Homeopathic medicine, 42
Homeostasis, 223
Homocysteine, 330t, 334
Homograft, 361
Hope, 217
Hopelessness, 214, 217f
Hordeolum, 1064
Hormone replacement therapy (HRT)
   for menopause, 824
   osteoporosis and, 912
Hormones
   cancer risk and, 145–146
   effects on kidneys, 678t
   endocrine system, 723–724, 729–730, 731–733t
   female reproductive, 794t, 801, 806t
   heart and, 319
   male reproductive, 794t, 811–812, 812t
Hormone therapy
   for male reproductive disorders, 850–851t, 864
   for malignant breast disorders, 816, 818t
Hospice care, 250–251, 251t
   for cancer, 161, 162f
Hospital-acquired conditions (HACs), 16, 17b
   catheter-associated UTI, 96
   pneumonia, 538
Hospitalization
   at end of life, 250
   for substance use disorders, 1189
Host (infection), 83, 87
Huff coughing, 501
Human immunodeficiency virus (HIV). See HIV/AIDS
Human monoclonal antibody, 293t
Human papillomavirus (HPV), 144, 148, 877–878, 878f
   cervical cancer and, 841–842
   condylomata, 872t
   penis cancer and, 860
   vaccine, 842, 877
Human trafficking, 27, 27b
Humility
   cultural, 32
   intellectual, 3
Humoral immunity, 265, 267f
Huntington disease, 992–994, 993f, 995t
Hydration, artificial, 250
Hydrocele, 807, 860
Hydrocephalus
   acute, 965
   cerebral aneurysm, 1011, 1011f
Hydromorphone hydrochloride (Dilaudid), 173t
Hydronephrosis, 702, 703f, 704f
Hydrostatic pressure, 51
Hyperalgesia, 125
Hypercalcemia, 63–64
   as cancer emergency, 162
Hyperglycemia, 777, 778t
Hyperkalemia, 61–62, 334
   chronic kidney disease (CKD) and, 712–713, 713b
   third-degree atrioventricular block and, 415
   ventricular fibrillation and, 417
Hypermagnesemia, 64
Hypermenorrhea, 823t
Hypernatremia, 59–60
Hyperopia, 1066, 1066f
Hyperosmolar hyperglycemic state (HHS), 780
Hyperparathyroidism, 755–756, 755t
Hyperpolarization-activated cyclic nucleotide-gated (HCN) channel blockers, 434t, 435
Hypersensitivity reactions, 277–287
   type I, 277–281, 278f, 280t
   type II, 281–283, 282f, 283t, 284t
   type III, 283–284, 285f
   type IV, 284–287, 286f, 286t
Hypertension, 342–352. *See also* Blood pressure
   categories of, 342–343, 343t
   complications of, 343t, 345
   diagnosis of, 343
   home health care, 350–351
   hypertensive emergency, 349
   hypertensive urgency, 349
   nursing process for, 349–350, 349f
   portal, 657, 658f
   risk factors for, 344–345
   signs and symptoms, 343, 343t
   social determinants of health (SDOH) and, 343–344
   special considerations, 349
   therapeutic measures, 343t, 345, 346–348t
   types of, 343
Hypertensive emergency, 349
Hypertensive urgency, 349
Hyperthermia, 201–202, 202b
Hyperthyroidism, 227, 747t, 748–751, 749f

Hypertonic solutions, 52, 74
Hypertrophic cardiomyopathy, 368–369
Hypertrophy, 345, 840
Hyperuricemia, 913
Hypervolemia, 54
Hypnosis, 1172
Hypocalcemia, 62–63, 62f, 63f, 63t
Hypodermis, 1091–1092
Hypodermoclysis, 81
Hypogammaglobulinemia, 294–295
Hypoglossal nerve, 936t
Hypoglycemia, 727, 770, 777–779, 778t
  injectable hypoglycemic medication for, 774–776, 775–776t
  oral hypoglycemic medication for, 774
  reactive, 786
Hypokalemia, 60–61, 61b, 334, 621
Hypomagnesemia, 64, 334
  ventricular fibrillation and, 417
Hypomenorrhea, 823t
Hyponatremia, 58–59, 58b
Hypoparathyroidism, 754–755, 755t
Hypophysectomy, 741, 744–745, 745f
Hypoplasia, 828
Hypospadias, 807
Hypotension and spinal cord injuries, 975
Hypothalamus, 723–724, 724f, 725f, 933
Hypothermia, 200–201, 200t
  intraoperative, 174
Hypothyroidism, 227, 745–748, 745t, 747t
Hypotonic solutions, 52, 74
Hypotropia, 1045
Hypovolemia, 52
Hypovolemic shock, 107, 109t, 194
Hypoxia, 451
Hysterectomy, 823, 844–845
Hysterosalpingogram, 804
Hysteroscopy, 805, 843
Hysterotomy, 838–839

I

Identities, 31
Idiopathic autoimmune hemolytic anemia, 288–289
Ileoanal pouch, 629
Ileocolectomy, 640t
Ileostomy, 642, 642f, 643t
Illness, definition of, 211
Immobilization after spinal cord injuries, 977, 977–978f
Immune deficiencies, 294–295
Immune disorders, 277–296
  allergic rhinitis, 278–279
  anaphylaxis, 279, 280t
  angioedema, 280–281
  atopic dermatitis, 279
  autoimmune disorders (*see* Autoimmune disorders)
  contact dermatitis, 287
  hemolytic transfusion reaction, 282–283, 283t, 284t
  home health care, 295
  immune deficiencies, 294–295
  type I hypersensitivity reactions, 277–281, 278f, 280t
  type II hypersensitivity reactions, 281–283, 282f, 283t, 284t
  type III hypersensitivity reactions, 283–284, 285f
  type IV hypersensitivity reactions, 284–287, 286f, 286t
  urticaria, 280
Immune system, 88, 263–276
  aging and, 213, 228, 268, 268f
  antibodies, 88, 264, 265–266, 265f, 265t, 267f
  antigens, 88, 264
  burns and, 1139
  cancer risk and, 146
  data collection on, 268–271, 269t, 270t
  diagnostic tests, 271, 271–274t
  lymphocytes, 263, 264
  microbiota and, 268
  normal anatomy and physiology, 263–265, 264f, 265f, 265t
  therapeutic measures, 275
Immune thrombocytopenic purpura (ITP), 472–473, 473b
Immunity
  defined, 263
  herd, 89
  mechanisms of, 264–265, 266f
  types of, 266
Immunomodulators, 628t
Immunosenescence, 213, 268, 268f
Immunosuppressants, 293t
  for multiple sclerosis (MS), 1022t
  for osteoarthritis (OA), 917t
Immunotherapy, 275
  for allergic rhinitis, 278–279
  for malignant breast disorders, 817
Impacted cerumen, 1079–1080
Impacted fractures, 902t, 903f
Impaction, fecal, 619
Impaired judgment after stroke, 1009
Imperforate, 828
Impetigo contagiosa, 1122t
Implantable cardioverter defibrillators (ICD), 421
  sudden death risk with, 436
Implantable replacement heart, 436
Incentive spirometry, 169, 504, 505f
Incision pain, 169
Increased intracranial pressure (ICP), 195, 196b, 197, 954–957
  monitoring, 955, 955f, 956f
  nursing care, 956–957, 956b, 957t
  pathophysiology and etiology, 954–955, 955f
  signs and symptoms, 955
  traumatic brain injury (TBI) and, 964–965
Incretins, 732t
Indirect transmission, 86–87, 86f, 87f
Induction, anesthesia, 176
Indwelling urinary catheters, 692, 692b
Infection control, 91–92
  anemia and, 467b
  asepsis, 93, 93b
  hand hygiene for, 92–93, 92f
  in health-care agencies, 92–96
  in home health care, 243–244
  ultraviolet environmental disinfection, 93
Infection prevention, 83, 84f
  CDC guidelines for, 93
  genitourinary tract infections, 96
  in long-term care facilities, 240
  respiratory tract infections, 96
  standard precautions and transmission-based precautions, 94–95t, 96
  surgical wound infections, 96
Infections, 83–104
  acute bronchitis, 533–534
  after amputation, 925
  after spinal cord injuries, 975
  anthrax, 205, 205f, 206t
  antibiotic-resistant, 97
  botulism, 207t
  bronchiectasis, 534, 534f
  central nervous system (CNS), 951–954, 952t, 953f, 954t
  control of, 91–96
  diarrhea due to, 620
  due to diabetes mellitus, 781
  external ear, 1078–1079
  eye, 1060–1065, 1062–1063t, 1065t
  fractures and, 906
  Helicobacter pylori (H. pylori), 144–145, 607, 608t
  hepatitis, 649–655, 650–652t, 653b, 653f, 654t
  herpes simplex virus type 1 (HSV-1), 603, 1121–1123
  HIV/AIDS (*see* HIV/AIDS)
  human body's defense mechanisms against, 88–89
  infection process, 83–87, 84f
  infectious disease, 89–91, 90–91t
  infective endocarditis (IE), 362–366, 363f, 364f, 364t, 365t
  laryngitis, 525
  lymphangitis, 400–401
  middle ear, 1083–1084
  nursing process for, 101–103
  opportunistic, with HIV/AIDS, 304, 305t, 310–311b
  overwhelming postsplenectomy infection (OPSI), 483–484
  pharyngitis, 523, 525
  plague, 208t
  pneumonia, 538–540, 540f, 540t
  prostatitis, 849–852, 850–851t
  related to tissue trauma, 198
  respiratory viruses, 525–527
  risk factors for, 88–89
  sexually transmitted (STIs), 804, 869–883
  sinus, 520–521
  skin, 1121–1128, 1122t, 1123f, 1125–1127t, 1127f
  tonsillitis/adenoiditis, 525
  total hip replacement and, 922
  toxic shock syndrome (TSS), 826–828
  tuberculosis (TB), 540–543, 542t
  urinary tract, 96, 228, 695–699, 696t, 698t
  viral rhinitis/common cold, 522–523, 523t
Infections, central nervous system (CNS), 951
  encephalitis, 953–954
  meningitis, 952–953, 952t, 953f, 954t
  routes of entry, 952t
Infectious agents, 83–86, 85t
Infectious disease
  herd immunity, 89
  immunity, 89
  laboratory assessment, 89
  localized, 89
  pandemic, 89

Infectious disease (continued)
  sepsis, 89
  therapeutic measures, 97–100t, 97–101
  types of, 89–91, 90–91t
Infectious mononucleosis (IM), 90–91
Infectious skin disorders
  acne vulgaris, 1127, 1127f
  cellulitis, 1124, 1127
  fungal infections, 1124
  furuncles and carbuncles, 1122t
  herpes simplex, 1121–1123
  herpes zoster (shingles), 1123–1124, 1123f
  impetigo contagiosa, 1122t
Infective endocarditis (IE), 362–366, 363f, 364f, 364t, 365t
Infertility
  female, 831–833, 832t
  male, 811–812, 865–866
Infiltration, 76, 77t
Inflammation
  bursitis, 900
  encephalitis, 953–954
  eye, 1060–1065, 1062–1063t, 1065t
  gallbladder, 668–672, 670t, 671f, 672t
  gout, 913, 913f
  middle ear infections, 1083–1084
  oral, 603
  prostatitis, 849–852, 850–851t
  skin disorders, 1118–1121, 1118t, 1121f
  urinary tract infection (UTI), 696–697
  vagina and vulva, 825–826, 827t, 828t
Inflammatory and infectious cardiac disorders
  cardiac trauma, 368
  cardiomyopathy, 368–370, 369f, 369t, 370b
  infective endocarditis (IE), 362–366, 363f, 364f, 364t, 365t
  myocarditis, 367–368
  pericarditis, 366–367, 366t, 367f
Inflammatory and infectious gastrointestinal disorders
  appendicitis, 623, 624f
  diverticulosis and diverticulitis, 624–625, 625f, 625t
  inflammatory bowel disease (IBD), 626–627f, 626–630, 626f, 628–629t, 631
  lower gastrointestinal disorders, 623–626, 624f, 625f, 625t
  peritonitis, 623–624
Inflammatory bowel disease (IBD), 626–630, 631
  Crohn disease, 626–627, 626f, 627f
  ulcerative colitis, 626, 626f, 627–629, 628t, 629t
Inflammatory exudate, 88
Inflammatory response, 88
Inflammatory skin disorders
  dermatitis, 1118–1120, 1118t
  psoriasis, 1101, 1120–1121, 1121f
Influenza
  diagnostic tests, 526
  HIV/AIDS and, 305t
  incubation period of, 526
  nursing care for, 527
  in older patients, 228
  prevention, 526
  signs and symptoms, 526
  therapeutic measures, 526
  transmission of, 525–526

Informatics
  defined, 15
  evidence-based practice (EBP), 14
Informed consent, 171–172
Infusion Nurses Society, 69
Inhalation, 487–488
Inhalation agents for anesthesia, 176
Inhaled poisons, 203
Inhalers, 504, 504f
Inhibin, 794t
Injectable contraceptive medications, 834
Injectable hypoglycemic medication, 774–776, 775–776t
Injected poisons, 203
Injuries
  abdominal, 196, 198
  assault and battery, 195
  burn (see Burns)
  chest, 196, 197, 198
  ear, 1081
  eye, 1047, 1047t
  fall, 195, 214–215
  fracture, 196, 198, 224
  frostbite, 201
  head, 195
  major trauma, 194
  near-drowning, 204
  neck, 198
  orthopedic, 196
  pressure, 225, 1107–1118, 1109–1111t, 1114f, 1115–1116f
  spinal cord, 195–196, 196f, 197, 197t, 974–983
  stings and bites, 203–204
  traumatic brain injury (TBI), 963–967, 964–965f, 967t
Inner ear, 1048, 1050f
  disorders of, 1086–1088, 1087b
Inotropes, 411t, 434t, 435
Inpatient surgery discharge, 189
Insect stings or bites, 203
Inspection
  abdominal, 581–582
  ear, 1052
  endocrine system, 728–729
  eye area, 1045–1046
  integumentary system, 1096–1098, 1097–1098f
  respiratory system, 494, 494f, 495f, 496t
Inspiration, 487–488
Institute for Safe Medication Practices, 16
Instrumental activities of daily living (IADLs), 214, 215
  long-term care services, 236–237
Insufficiency, valvular, 353
Insufflation, 805
Insulin, 772–773f, 772–774, 774t
  reaction, 777
Integrase inhibitors, 308t
Integrity, 3, 213
Integumentary system, 1091–1106. See also Skin
  aging and, 225, 1094, 1094f
  data collection, 1094–1099
  diagnostic tests, 1100
  disorders of (see Skin disorders)
  normal anatomy and physiology of, 1091–1094, 1092f, 1093f
  therapeutic measures, 1100–1104, 1103–1104t

Intellectual autonomy, 3
Intellectual humility, 3
Intellectual integrity, 3
Intelligent assistive technology (IAT), 224, 224f
Interarticular fractures, 902t, 903f
Interferon, 88
Intermittent claudication, 394
Intermittent infusion, 70–71, 71f
Intermittent pneumatic compression devices, 338
Intermittent urinary catheterization, 692
Internal fixation, 904, 905f
International normalized ratio (INR), 361, 458t
Interneurons, 931f
Interstitial fluid, 51, 51f
Intestinal obstruction, 635–637, 636f, 636t
Intra-aortic balloon pump (IABP), 436, 436f
Intracellular fluid (ICF), 50, 51f
Intracerebral hemorrhage, 1002
Intracranial hemorrhage, 1010–1012, 1010f, 1011f
Intracranial surgery, 969–971
Intragastric balloon, 601
Intraoperative phase, 166t, 174–176, 175b, 175f
  anesthesia, 176–177, 177f
Intrauterine devices, 833
Intravascular fluid, 51, 51f
Intravenous (IV) therapy, 69–82
  anesthesia, 176
  central venous access devices (CVAD), 74, 76, 79–80, 79f
  complications of, 76, 77–78t
  defined, 69
  home, 80–81
  indications for, 70
  intravenous access, 74–75
  methods of infusion, 72–73
  nursing process for patient receiving, 75–76
  parenteral nutrition (PN), 70, 80
  subcutaneous infusion (hypodermoclysis), 81
  types of fluids, 73–74
  types of infusions, 70–72, 71f
  venous thromboembolism (VTE) disease and, 372
Intubation, 510, 510f, 513
  gastrointestinal, 591–592, 591f, 592t
Intussusception, 635, 636f
Invasive tests
  arthrography, 894t
  gastrointestinal, hepatobiliary and pancreatic systems, 586–587t
In vitro fertilization (IVF), 831–832, 833
Ipsilateral foot, 989
Iris, 1038, 1040f
Irrigation
  ear, 1082, 1082f
  eye, 1047
Irritable bowel syndrome (IBS), 630–633
Ischemia
  angina pectoris and, 380
  tissue, 106
Ischemic stroke, 1001–1002, 1001b, 1001f, 1002f
Isoelectric line, ECG, 405
Isotonic solutions, 51–52, 74

J

Jackson-Pratt drains, 187
Jaundice, 581–582
  in hepatitis, 653, 653f

Jewish persons, 361
Joanna Briggs Institute, 10
Johns Hopkins Fall Risk Assessment Tool (JHFRAT), 239
Joint Commission, The, 16, 29
Joints
    aging and, 887
    appendicular skeleton, 887t
    dislocations of, 900
    osteoarthritis (OA) and replacement of, 916
    rheumatoid arthritis (RA) and replacement of, 920
    synovial, 885, 888f
Jugular neck veins, 328
Justice, 21

K

Kegel exercises, 690, 690b, 829, 830, 831
Keloid, 1131t
Keratitis, 1064
Keratoconjunctivitis sicca, 1061
Kernig sign, 952, 953f
Ketone monitoring, 776–777
Kidneys
    acid-base balance and, 676
    acute kidney injury (AKI), 708–710, 710t
    blood chemistry studies, 685–686t
    cancer of, 705
    chronic kidney disease (CKD), 706–707, 710–718, 711–712t, 713b, 713f, 715–717f, 715b
    effects of hormones on, 678t
    effects of shock on, 106
    formation of urine in, 676, 678f
    long-term effects of diabetes mellitus on, 781
    nephrons, 676, 677f
    normal anatomy and physiology, 675–676, 676f
    polycystic kidney disease, 705–706
    pyelonephritis of, 697
    renal calculi, 699–702, 699f, 700t, 701f
    transplantation of, 718, 718f
Knee replacement, 924, 924f
Knowledge base, nursing, 7
Kock pouch, 642, 642f
Kupffer cells, 575
Kussmaul respirations, 780

L

Labia majora, 793f
Labia minora, 793f
Labile vital signs, 965
Laboratory tests
    blood, 456, 458t
    breast, 801
    cancer, 150
    cardiovascular system, 330–331t
    ear, 1055
    endocrine system hormones, 736–737t
    gastrointestinal, hepatobiliary and pancreatic systems, 583–587t, 583–588
    hepatitis, 654t
    male reproductive system, 811
    musculoskeletal system, 890, 893t
    neurologic system, 945
    Pap tests, 147–148, 803–804, 878
    respiratory system, 495
    skin cultures, 1100
    urinary system, 683–686t, 683–687
Labyrinthitis, 1086
Lacerations, 194
    eye, 1075
    lung, 196
Lacrimal apparatus, 1039f
Lacrimal gland, 1039f
Lacrimal punctum, 1039f
Lactational amenorrhea method, 837
Lactic acid, 106
Lactose intolerance, 634–635
Laissez-faire (delegative) leadership, 18
Laminectomy, 972–973
Language disturbances with TIA and stroke, 1003
Laparoscopy, 805, 805f, 806t, 843
Large-bowel obstruction, 636–637
Large intestine, 573f, 574
Laryngectomy, 528–531, 528f, 529f
Laryngitis, 525
Larynx, 487, 488f
    cancer of, 527–531, 528f, 528t, 529f
Laser-assisted in situ keratomileusis (LASIK), 1067
Laser surgery, 164
    for retinal detachment, 1070
Latent TB infection (LTBI), 540, 542–543
Latex allergy, 271
Leadership, 17–18
    and delegation for LPN/LVN, 19–20, 19f
    management functions, 18–19
    in nursing practice, 17–20, 18f, 19f
    styles of, 18, 18f
Leadless pacemakers, 418–419
Left middle cerebral artery syndrome, 1004t
Left-sided heart failure (HF), 426, 426t, 427f, 430t
Left transverse colostomy, 643t
Legal concepts, 26–29
    advanced directives, 167
    Health Insurance Portability and Accountability Act (HIPAA), 27–28
    human trafficking, 27, 27b
    mandatory reporting, 26
    regulation of nursing practice, 26
    required reporting to licensing board, 26
Leg exercises, 169
Leiomyomas, 839
Lens, eye, 1038, 1040f, 1041f
Lesions, skin, 1096, 1097f, 1098f, 1130, 1130–1132t, 1133f
Lesser vestibular glands, 793f
Leukemia, 146–147, 475–478, 476t
Leukocyte-depleted blood, 459
Leukocytes, 88
Leukopenia, 154
Level of consciousness (LOC), 940–941, 941f, 942f
    brainstem contusions and, 964
    cerebral aneurysm and, 1010
    nutrition therapeutic measures for neurologic system, 948
LGBTQ community, sexually transmitted infections (STIs) in, 879
Liability, nursing, 28
    in home health care, 242b
Licensed practical nurses (LPNs), 17
    leadership and delegation for, 19–20, 19f
    patient care settings, 235–246
    role in complementary and alternative modalities, 47–48
    role in home health care, 241–242, 242f
    role in long-term care services, 238
Licensed vocational nurses (LVNs), 17
    leadership and delegation for, 19–20, 19f
    patient care settings, 235–246
    role in complementary and alternative modalities, 47–48
    role in home health care, 241–242, 242f
    role in long-term care services, 238
Licensing board, required reporting to, 26
Lichenification, 1097f
Lifestyle
    adaptation after amputation, 926
    cancer risk and, 145, 148
    cardiovascular system and, 337
    hypertension risk and, 344
    migraines and, 958
    osteoporosis and, 910–911
Lighting in long-term care facilities, 239
Limitation of liability, 28
Lincomycins, 99t
Lipids, 331t, 334
    medications for lowering, 379, 380t
    metabolism of, 575
Lipoproteins, 331t
Listening, active, 5–6
Lithium, 1175t, 1177
Lithotripsy, 701, 701f
Liver
    anatomy of, 573f, 574–575
    effects of shock on, 106
    functions of, 575–576
    percutaneous biopsy of, 590–591
    secretions by, 575t
    transplantation of, 662
Liver disorders, 649–662
    acute liver failure, 655–656, 656b
    cancer, 662
    chronic liver disease and cirrhosis, 656–662, 657t, 658–660f
    hepatitis, 649–655, 650–652t, 653b, 653f, 654t
Liver scans, 589
Liver transplantation, 662
Living wills, 248
Lobectomy, 565, 566, 566f
Local anesthesia, 176–177, 177f
Localized infection, 89
    due to intravenous (IV) therapy, 77t
Long-acting beta agonist (LABA) bronchodilators, 554
Longitudinal fractures, 902t, 903f
Long-term care services, 223, 236–240, 237t
    dementia care, 237–238
    disaster plans for, 205
    infection prevention in, 240
    lighting in, 239
    Medicare and Medicaid participation requirements for, 238, 239t
    patient safety and wellness in, 238–240
    restraints in, 239
    role of LPN/LVN in, 238
    types of, 236–238
Loop diuretics, 55
    for chronic heart failure (HF), 434t
    for hypertension, 346t

Loop stoma, 642–643
Lorazepam (Ativan), 173t
Lou Gehrig disease, 1029–1030
Low-density lipoproteins (LDLs), 378, 379, 380t
Lower esophageal sphincter, 573
Lower gastrointestinal disorders, 618–648
    abdominal hernias, 633–634, 633f
    absorption disorders, 634–635, 635t
    anorectal problems, 637–638
    appendicitis, 623, 624f
    bleeding, 638
    colorectal cancer, 639–640t, 639–641, 641f
    constipation, 226–227, 618–620, 619t, 621b
    Crohn disease, 626–627, 626f, 627f, 631
    diarrhea, 101, 620–623, 622t
    diverticulosis and diverticulitis, 624–625, 625f, 625t
    inflammatory and infectious disorders, 623–626, 624f, 625f, 625t
    inflammatory bowel disease, 626–630, 626f, 627f, 628t, 629t, 631
    intestinal obstruction, 635–637, 636f, 636t
    irritable bowel syndrome (IBS), 630–633
    ostomy and, 629, 642–646, 642f, 643f, 643t, 644t
    peritonitis, 623–624
    problems of elimination, 618–623, 619t, 621b, 622t
    ulcerative colitis, 626, 626f, 627–629, 628t, 629t
Lower gastrointestinal endoscopy, 590
Lower respiratory tract disorders, 533–571
    chest trauma, 559–562, 560f, 561t
    home health care, 568
    infectious disorders, 533–543, 534f, 540f, 540t, 542t
    lung cancer, 563–566, 564f, 565t, 566f
    obstructive disorders, 545–557, 546f, 547t, 548–549f, 550t, 551–553f, 554t
    pulmonary vascular disorders, 557–559, 558f, 559t
    respiratory failure, 562–563
    restrictive disorders, 543–545
    thoracic surgery and, 566–568
Low molecular weight heparin (LMWH), 372, 388t
Lubricants, eye, 1063t
Lumbar injuries, 975
Lumbar puncture, 945
Lumpectomy, 817
Lung cancer
    complications of, 564–565
    diagnostic tests, 565, 567t
    etiology of, 564
    pathophysiology, 563–564, 564f
    prevention, 564
    screening for, 148
    signs and symptoms, 564, 567t
    therapeutic measures, 565, 565t, 566f, 567t
Lungs, 487, 490f
    abnormal sounds in, 498t
    acute respiratory distress syndrome (ARDS), 562–563
    alveoli, 491f
    asthma and, 550–554, 552–553f, 554t
    chronic obstructive pulmonary disease (COPD) of, 545–550, 546f, 547t, 548–549f, 550t
    lacerations of, 196
    respiratory failure, 562
    restrictive disorders of, 543–545
    transplantation of, 567
    upper respiratory tract disorders of, 518–532
Lung volume reduction surgery (LVRS), 549
Luteinizing hormone (LH), 725f, 731t, 791, 794t
Lymph, 452
Lymphangiography, 457
Lymphangitis, 400–401
Lymphatic disorders, 483t
    Hodgkin lymphoma, 480–481, 482t
    home health care, 484
    non-Hodgkin lymphomas, 481–482, 482f, 482t
    splenic disorders, 482–484
Lymphatic system, 263–264, 454f
    aging and, 453, 454f
    components of, 451
    diagnostic tests, 456–457, 458t
    lymphangitis, 400–401
    lymphatic vessels, 452
    lymph nodes and nodules, 264, 264f, 452–453
    normal anatomy and physiology, 451–453, 454f
    nursing assessment of, 454–455, 455–456t
    spleen, 453
    therapeutic measures, 458–460
    thymus, 453
Lymph nodes, 264, 264f, 452–453
    biopsy of, 457
Lymphocytes, 263, 264, 450t
    HIV/AIDS and, 305–306
Lymphomas, 147, 483t
Lymph vessels, 264, 264f, 321
Lysozymes, 88

M

Macrocytic anemia, 463
Macrolides, 99t
    for sexually transmitted infections (STIs), 873t
Macrophages, 88, 451
Macrovascular complications of diabetes mellitus, 780–781
Macular degeneration, 1067, 1067f, 1073–1075, 1074f, 1075f
Macules, 1097f
Magnesium imbalances, 64, 334
Magnetic resonance angiography (MRA), 331t
Magnetic resonance imaging (MRI), 150
    breast, 800, 806t
    cardiac, 331t, 335
    ear, 1055
    endocrine system, 737
    musculoskeletal system, 893, 894–895t, 895, 895f
    neurologic system, 946
Major depression, 1176–1177
Major neurocognitive disorder, 1190
Maleficence, 21
Male genitourinary disorders, 848–868
    benign prostatic hyperplasia (BPH), 795, 852–857, 853f, 854f, 857f, 858t
    infertility, 811–812, 865–866
    penile disorders, 859–860
    prostate disorders, 848–859, 850–851t, 853f, 854f, 857f, 858t
    sexual functioning, 861–866, 862f, 863t, 864f, 865t
    testicular disorders, 860–861
Male reproductive system
    condoms, 301–302, 301b, 835, 835f
    data collection, 805–812, 808–810t, 811b, 811f, 812t
    diagnostic tests of, 811–812, 812t
    hormones of, 794t, 811–812, 812t
    normal anatomy and physiology, 791–792, 794–795, 795f
    sexual functioning, 861–866, 862f, 863t, 864f, 865t
Malignant breast disorders, 145–146, 820t
    diagnostic tests, 817, 820t
    nursing care for, 819–820
    pathophysiology and etiology, 816
    screening for, 147
    staging of, 817
    therapeutic measures, 817, 820t
Malignant cells, 142, 144t
Malignant hyperthermia, 168b
Malignant melanoma, 1132–1133, 1133f
Malignant skin lesions, 145, 145f, 1132–1134, 1133f
Malingerers, 119
Mallory-Weiss tear (MWT), 606–607
Malnutrition
    in chronic heart failure (HF), 431
    in Crohn disease and ulcerative colitis, 629
Malpractice, 28
    insurance against complaints of, 29
Mammary glands, 724, 725f, 726f, 791, 793f
Mammography, 799–800, 800f, 806t
Mammoplasty, 821–822, 821–822f
Management functions, 18–19
Mandatory reporting, 26
    human trafficking, 27, 27b
Mania, 1177
Marsupialization, 841
Masks, oxygen, 503
Maslow's hierarchy of human needs, 6, 6f
Massage therapy, 45
    for pain, 130
Masses, external ear, 1080–1081
Mastectomy, 817
Mastitis, 816
Mastoid disorders, 1085–1086, 1086t
Mastoidectomy, 1084
Mastoiditis, 1083
Mastopexy, 821, 821f
McBurney point, 624f
Mechanical assistive devices for chronic heart failure (HF), 436
Mechanical debridement, 1113
Mechanical infusion devices, 73
Mechanical ventilation, 513–515, 513f, 514t, 515b
    for chronic obstructive pulmonary disease (COPD), 549
Medial canthus, 1039f
Medicaid, 238, 239t
Medical asepsis, 93
Medical office nursing, 236
Medical Orders for Life-Sustaining Treatment (MOLST), 249
Medical Orders for Scope of Treatment (MOST), 249

Medicare, 238, 239t
Medication errors, 16
Medications
   allergic rhinitis, 278
   Alzheimer disease, 996
   angina pectoris, 382–383t
   ankylosing spondylitis, 294
   anticoagulant, 372, 372–373t
   antihypertensive, 345, 346–348t
   antimicrobial resistance (AMR) and, 879
   antiretroviral, 297, 301, 306–309, 307–308t
   anxiety, obsessive-compulsive, or trauma-related disorders, 1172, 1173–1175t
   asthma, 554
   atherosclerosis, 379
   brain tumors, 968
   cardiovascular system, 338
   chemotherapy, 153–156, 154f, 155f, 155t
   cholecystitis, cholelithiasis, choledocholithiasis, 670
   chronic heart failure (HF), 432, 433–435t, 435–436, 440
   chronic kidney disease (CKD), 714
   chronic obstructive pulmonary disease (COPD), 549, 550t
   chronic pancreatitis, 664, 665t
   colorectal cancer, 639
   contraceptive, 834
   Crohn disease, 627, 628t
   dementia, 987t
   diabetes mellitus, 772–773f, 772–776, 774t, 775–776t
   ear disorder, 1056
   endocrine disorders, 761–762t
   erectile dysfunction, 863–864
   fluid excess, 55
   gastritis, 608t
   gastrointestinal, hepatobiliary and pancreatic system, 577, 579
   herniated discs, 972
   hypertension, 345
   immune disorder, 275
   to increase comfort at end of life, 259t
   injectable hypoglycemic, 774–776, 775–776t
   insulin, 772–773f, 772–774, 774t
   irritable bowel syndrome (IBS), 632
   lupus erythematosus triggered by, 289, 289b
   male reproductive organ disorders, 850–851t
   management of, in older adults, 231
   mood disorders, 1177
   multiple sclerosis (MS), 1022–1023, 1022–1023t
   myocardial infarction (MI), 388, 388–389t
   ophthalmic, 1062–1063t
   opioid addiction and, 121–122
   oral hypoglycemic, 774
   osteoarthritis (OA), 916, 917–918t
   osteoporosis, 911
   ototoxic, 1076t
   Parkinson disease, 990, 991t
   peptic ulcer disease (PUD), 610t
   preoperative, 172, 173t
   rheumatoid arthritis (RA), 920
   seizure disorders, 960, 961t
   sexually transmitted infections (STIs), 873–874t
   shock, 112–113t
   sinus bradycardia, 409, 410–411t
   stroke, 1006, 1007t
   systemic lupus erythematosus (SLE), 292–293t
   that can cause confusion, 984b
   that can exacerbate myasthenia gravis (MG), 1028b
   for therapeutic abortion, 838
   thrombolytic, 373t, 387–388
   topical skin, 1101
   for treating infections, 97–100t, 97–101
   for treating substance use disorders, 1188–1189
   ulcerative colitis, 628t
   urinary tract infection (UTI), 698t
Mediterranean-Style Dietary Pattern, 344
Mediterranean-type glucose-6-phosphate dehydrogenase (G6PD) deficiency, 463
Medulla oblongata, 933
Megakaryocytes, 451
Melanin, 1091–1092
Melanocytes, 1091
Menarche, 816
Ménière disease, 1087–1088
Meninges, 933
Meningitis, 952–953, 952t, 953f, 954t
Menometrorrhagia, 823t
Menopause, 795, 824–825
   malignant breast disorders and late, 816
   musculoskeletal system changes after, 887
Menorrhagia, 823t
Menstrual cycle, 791
Menstrual disorders
   dysmenorrhea, 823–824
   endometriosis, 824, 824f
   flow and cycle, 823, 823t
   menopause, 824–825
   premenstrual syndrome and premenstrual dysphoric disorder, 822
   summary of, 825t
Mental health
   cognitive behavioral therapy (CBT) and, 1165
   counseling and, 1165
   defined, 1155
   diagnostic tests, 1158
   electroconvulsive therapy (ECT) and, 1166
   group therapy and, 1165
   home health care, 1167, 1191
   milieu, 1164
   nursing data collection related to, 1158, 1159–1160t
   nursing diagnoses commonly used to address problems with, 1161b
   in older adults, 1190–1191
   psychopharmacology and, 1164
   psychotherapy for, 1164–1165
   relaxation therapy for, 44–45, 46b, 128, 1167
   social and cultural environments and, 1157
   spirituality and religion and, 1157
   therapeutic communication and, 1161, 1163, 1163t
   therapeutic measures, 1161–1167, 1163–1164t
Mental health disorders, 1169–1193
   anxiety disorders, 1169–1170, 1171t
   autism spectrum disorders (ADSs), 1183–1184
   eating disorders, 1185–1186
   medications used for, 1172, 1173–1175t
   mood disorders, 1176–1179
   obsessive-compulsive and related disorders, 1171
   in older adults, 1190–1191
   personality disorders, 1182–1183
   schizophrenia, 1179–1182, 1181t, 1182t
   substance use disorders, 167, 202–204, 1186–1190, 1189t
   trauma- and stressor-related disorders, 1172
Mental illness
   defined, 1157
   diagnostic tests, 1158
   etiologies of, 1157
   social and cultural environments and, 1157
Mental status
   changes at end of life, 254
   data collection on, 939–940, 940t
   physical examination for, 941, 943
Meperidine (Demerol), 126
Metabolic acidosis, 66t
   with compensation, 66t
Metabolic alkalosis, 66t
   with compensation, 66t
Metabolic syndrome, 768
Metabolism, 575
   aging and, 577
   burns and, 1139
Metastasis, cancer, 147, 147f, 150–151, 151t
   lung cancer, 565
Metered-dose inhalers (MDIs), 540, 554
Methicillin-resistant staphylococcus aureus (MRSA), 97
   cellulitis, 1124
Metoclopramide (Reglan), 173t
Microbiota and the immune system, 268
Microcytic anemia, 463
Microglia, 929
Microvascular angina, 381
Microvascular complications of diabetes mellitus, 781
Midazolam (Versed), 173t
Midbrain, 933
Middle-aged adults, 213
Middle ear, 1048, 1049f
   disorders of, 1083–1086, 1086t
Migraine headaches, 957–958
Milieu, 1164
Milk ejection, 724
Minimally invasive surgery, 164
   coronary artery bypass, 340, 390
Mini-Mental State Examination (MMSE), 941, 943
Miotics, 1063t
Mitosis, 142, 143f
Mitral regurgitation, 355t, 357–358
Mitral stenosis, 355t, 356–357, 357f
Mitral valve prolapse (MVP), 354, 355t, 356
Mixed hearing loss, 1076
Mobility
   after amputation, 925
   impaired due to neck injury or bone injury, 198
   neurologic system therapeutic measures, 947
   in Parkinson disease, 989, 989f
   postoperative, 188–189
   prevention of pressure injuries and, 1108
Mode of transmission, infection, 86–87, 86f, 87f
Modulation of pain, 122
Mohs surgery, 1134

Moisture/dryness of skin, 1096
Mole, 1131t
Monoamine oxidase B (MAO-B) inhibitors, 991t
Monoamines, 1156t
Monoclonal antibodies, 275
    for colorectal cancer, 639
    for osteoporosis, 912
    for systemic lupus erythematosus (SLE), 293t
Monocytes, 450t, 451
Mons pubis, 793f
Mood disorders, 1176–1179
Moral distress, 21
Morning hyperglycemia, 777
Morphine sulfate, 173t
Morse Fall Scale, 239
Motor disturbances with stroke, 1003
Motor neurons, 930, 931f
Mouth, 572–573, 573f
Moving and positioning, as therapeutic measure for neurologic system, 946–947
Mucolytic agents, 534
Mucopurulent cervicitis (MPC), 870
Mucous membranes as defense against infections, 88
Multiple-gated acquisition (MUGA) scan, 333t
Multiple myeloma, 478–480, 479f
Multiple sclerosis (MS), 1020–1026, 1032t
    diagnostic tests, 1022
    nursing care, 1024–1026
    pathophysiology, 1020–1021, 1021f
    signs and symptoms, 1021–1022, 1021b
    therapeutic measures, 1022–1023, 1022–1023t, 1024b
Murmur, 329, 354
Muscle contraction headaches, 958
Muscle relaxants, 1023t
Muscles
    aging and, 887
    amyotrophic lateral sclerosis (ALS) and, 1029–1030
    biopsy of, 892–893, 895t
    enzyme tests, 890
    eye, 1044–1045, 1045f
    in neurologic system assessment, 944
    neuromuscular junction, 887, 889f
    respiratory, 491f
    structure and arrangements, 886, 889f
    superficial, 886, 889f
Musculoskeletal and connective tissue disorders, 899–928
    bone and soft tissue disorders, 899–913
    bone cancer, 912–913
    connective tissue disorders, 913–921, 913f, 914t, 915f, 917–918t, 919f, 920f
    fractures, 900–909, 901f, 902t, 903f, 904b, 905f, 907f, 908t
    home health care, 926
    osteomyelitis, 906, 909–910, 910f
    osteoporosis, 910–912
    Paget disease, 912
    surgery for, 921–926, 922f, 923b, 924f
Musculoskeletal system, 884–898
    aging and, 22f, 223–224, 887, 890f
    anatomy and physiology of, 884
    bone tissue and bone growth, 885
    data collection, 887–890, 891f, 892t, 893t
    diagnostic tests, 890–896, 893t, 894–895t

    home health care, 896
    muscle structure and arrangements, 886, 889f
    nervous system and, 886–887
    neuromuscular junction, 887, 889f
    respiratory muscles, 491f
    skeletal structure, 885, 886f
    synovial joints, 885, 888f
    tissues and functions of, 884–886
Muslim persons, 54, 361
Mutations, genetic, 142
Myalgia, 525
Myasthenia gravis (MG), 1026–1028, 1026f, 1027t, 1028b, 1032t
    medications that can exacerbate, 1028b
Mycobacterium avium complex (MAC), 304, 305t
Mycobacterium tuberculosis, 540
Mydriatics, 1063t
Myectomy, 370
Myelin sheath, 930f
    Guillain-Barré syndrome (GBS) and, 1030
    multiple sclerosis (MS) and (*see* Multiple sclerosis)
Myelography, 894t, 895, 946
Myocardial infarction (MI), 378
    complications of, 385t, 386t
    coronary artery bypass graft (CABG) and, 389–390, 390f
    diagnostic tests, 386t, 387
    medications for, 388, 388–389t
    pathophysiology, 384–385, 385f
    signs and symptoms, 386, 386t
    therapeutic measures, 386t, 387–389, 387b, 388–389t, 388f
Myocarditis, 108, 367–368
Myocardium, 106
Myoglobin, 890, 893t
Myopia, 1066, 1066f
Myringoplasty, 1084
Myringotomy, 1084

N

Nadir, 154
Nail polish, 175
Nails, 1092, 1099, 1099t
Naloxone (Narcan), 122, 127, 203
Nasal cannula, 502–503, 502f
Nasal polyps, 520
Nasal samples, 497
Nasogastric tubes, 591–592, 591f, 592t
Nasolacrimal duct, 1039f
National Association of Licensed Practical Nurses, 21
National Center for Complementary and Integrative Health (NCCIH), 41
National Council of State Boards of Nursing, 2
National Institute for Occupational Safety and Health, 69
National Institutes of Health Stroke Scale, 1003, 1005f
National Quality Forum, 16
Natural family planning, 837
Natural killer (NK) cells, 264
Naturopathic medicine, 43
Nausea and vomiting, 598–599
NCLEX-PN, 2, 7
Near-drowning, 204

Nebulized mist treatments (NMT), 503–504, 503f
    for pneumonia, 539, 540
Neck injury, 198
Negative pressure wound therapy (NPWT), 1113–1114, 1114f
Negative reinforcement, 1165
Negligence, 28
Neoplasms, 142, 146
    inner ear, 1086–1087
Neoplastic fractures, 902t
Nephrons, 676, 677f
Nephropathy due to diabetes mellitus, 781
Nephrosclerosis, 707
Nephrotic syndrome, 706–707
Nephrotoxins, 708–709, 710t
Nerve conduction studies, 894t, 896
Nerve injury, 76
Nerve tissue, 929–931, 930f
    cranial nerves, 934, 935–936t, 938f, 945, 945t, 1031–1035, 1033f, 1034f
    impulses, 930
    nerves and nerve tracts, 931
    synapses, 930–931
    types of neurons, 929–930, 931f
Neurodegenerative and neurocognitive disorders, 983–996
    Alzheimer disease, 994–996, 995t
    delirium, 230–231, 943, 987–988, 1190
    dementia, 230, 237–238, 304, 943, 983–986, 984b, 987t
    Huntington disease, 992–994, 993f, 995t
    Parkinson disease, 225, 988–992, 989f, 990t, 991t, 995t
Neurofibral nodes, 930f
Neurogenic shock, 109t, 111, 975
Neuroleptics, 259t
Neurologic system, 929–950
    aging and, 224–225, 939f
    autism spectrum disorders (ADSs), 1183–1184
    chemotherapy and, 156
    data collection, 938–945, 939b, 940t, 941t, 942f, 944f, 945t
    diagnostic tests, 945–946
    normal anatomy and physiology, 929–937, 930–935f, 935–936t, 937–938f, 1155, 1156–1157t
    postoperative, 179–180
    therapeutic measures, 946–948, 947f
Neuromuscular disorders
    amyotrophic lateral sclerosis (ALS), 1029–1030, 1032t
    Guillain-Barré syndrome (GBS), 1030–1031, 1032t
    multiple sclerosis (MS), 1020–1026, 1021b, 1021f, 1024b, 1032t
    myasthenia gravis (MG), 1026–1028, 1026f, 1027t, 1028b, 1032t
    postpolio syndrome, 1031
    restless legs syndrome (RLS), 1031
Neuromuscular junction, 887, 889f
Neurons
    aging and, 937
    structure of, 930f
    types of, 929–930, 931f
Neuropathic pain, 122–123
Neuropathies, 1031
    due to diabetes mellitus, 781

Neurotransmitters, 936, 1156–1157t
  neuromuscular junction, 887
Neurovascular complications
  of fractures, 906
  of total hip replacement, 923
Neurovascular data collection, 893t
Neutropenia, 154
Neutrophils, 265, 450t, 451
Never-events, 16
Niacin, 380t
Nitrates
  for coronary artery disease (CAD), 382t
  for myocardial infarction (MI), 389t
Nitroglycerin, 381, 382t, 383b
Nitroimidazoles, 98t
N-methyl-D-aspartate (NMDA) antagonist, 987t
Nociception, 122
Nocturia, 227
  in chronic heart failure (HF), 431
Nodes of Ranvier, 930f
Nodules, 1097f
Nonalcoholic steatohepatitis (NASH), 656
Noninvasive positive-pressure ventilation (NIPPV), 515–516, 515f
Noninvasive tests, gastrointestinal, hepatobiliary and pancreatic systems, 586t
Nonmaleficence, 22
Nonnucleoside reverse transcriptase inhibitors (NNRTIs), 299, 307t
Nonopioid analgesics, 123, 124t
Nonpenetrating injuries, 368
  to head, 963
Nonpharmacological therapies for pain
  cognitive-behavioral interventions, 128
  physical agents, 130
Non-small cell lung cancer (NSCLC), 563–564, 565
Nonsteroidal anti-inflammatory drugs (NSAIDs)
  asthma exacerbated by, 552
  for bone and soft tissue disorders, 899–900
  for gout, 913
  for osteoarthritis (OA), 916, 918t
  for pain, 123, 124t
  for rheumatoid arthritis (RA), 920
  for systemic lupus erythematosus (SLE), 292t
Nontunneled central catheter, 79
Nonunion modalities with fractures, 906
Nonverbal communication, 1163
Norepinephrine, 105–106, 936, 1156t
Norepinephrine-dopamine reuptake inhibitors (NDRIs), 1174t
Normal cells, anatomy and physiology of, 140–142, 141f
Normal flora, 83
Normal sinus rhythm (NSR), 318, 320f, 409
Nose and nasal cavities, 486, 487t
  deviated septum, 520
  disorders of, 518–522, 519f, 520b, 521f
  epistaxis, 518–519, 519f
  nasal polyps, 520
  nasal samples, 497
  rhinoplasty, 520
  sinusitis, 520–521
  sleep apnea and, 521–522, 521f
  surgery of, 520, 520b

Nuchal rigidity, 952
Nuclear imaging, 150
Nuclear medicine scans, 894t, 896
Nuclear radioisotope imaging, 333t, 336
Nuclear scanning
  hepatobiliary, 589
  thyroid, 737
Nucleoside reverse transcriptase inhibitors (NRTIs), 299, 307t
Nucleus, cell, 140, 141f
Nurse, patient loss and, 261
Nurse practice act, 26
Nurse practitioners (NPs), 17
Nursing applications of complementary and alternative modalities, 47–48
Nursing assessment and strategies
  biological variations and, 36
  choice of health care providers and, 36
  cultural differences in time orientation and, 35
  cultural diversity in social organization and, 35
  death and end-of-life issues, 37
  environmental control and, 35–36
  hematologic and lymphatic systems, 454–455, 455–456t
  personal space and, 34–37
  respiratory system, 492, 493t, 494–495, 494–495f
Nursing care and process
  abdominal hernias, 634
  abortion, 839
  absorption disorders, 635
  acute liver failure, chronic liver disease, cirrhosis, 656, 660–661
  adrenocortical insufficiency (AI), 757–758
  Alzheimer disease, 996
  amyotrophic lateral sclerosis (ALS), 1029
  anemia, 463–464
  aneurysms, 397
  ankylosing spondylitis, 294
  anxiety, obsessive-compulsive, or trauma-related disorders, 1172, 1176
  aplastic anemia, 466, 467b
  asthma, 554
  autism spectrum disorders (ADSs), 1184
  bladder cancer, 705
  blindness, 1068–1069, 1068b
  bone cancer, 913
  bowel obstruction, 637
  brain tumors, 969
  burns, 1146–1152
  cancer, 156–161
  cardiac arrhythmias, 421–422
  cardiac transplantation, 443–444
  cardiac valvular disorders, 359–361, 359t
  cardiomyopathy, 370b
  cataracts, 1073
  central nervous system (CNS) infection, 954
  cerebrovascular disorder, 1012–1017, 1016f
  chest drainage, 507b
  chest trauma, 561
  chronic heart failure (HF), 437–438t, 437–441, 440b
  chronic illness, 220
  chronic kidney disease (CKD), 718–719
  chronic liver disease and cirrhosis, 660–661
  chronic obstructive pulmonary disease (COPD), 550

clinical judgment and, 3–5, 3f, 4–5t
collaboration in, 2, 7
colorectal cancer, 640–641
communicable or inflammatory neurological disorders, 956–957, 956b, 957t
communication with health-care team in, 5–6
computed tomography, 946
constipation, 619–620
contact dermatitis, 286, 287
coronary artery disease (CAD), 383–384
Crohn disease, 627
cultural influences on, 31–40
Cushing syndrome, 760
dehydration, 53–54
dementia, 984–986
dermatitis, 1119–1120
dermoid cysts, 841
deviated septum, 520
diabetes insipidus, 741
diabetes mellitus, 783–785, 783t
diabetic retinopathy, 1069–1070
diarrhea, 622–623
disorders related to development of the genital organs, 829
displacement disorders, 830–831
disseminated intravascular coagulation (DIC), 472
dysmenorrhea, 824
eating disorders, 1186
electroconvulsive therapy (ECT), 1166
end of life care, 254–258
endometriosis, 824
endoscopy, 805
epistaxis, 519
erectile dysfunction, 865
external ear disorders, 1082–1083, 1082f, 1083b
external fixation of lower extremity, 906
eye infection and inflammation, 1064–1065, 1065t
eye trauma, 1075
fertility testing and treatment, 832–833
fluid excess, 55–57, 56t, 57t
fractures, 908–909
gallbladder disorder, 671–672
gastric bleeding, 612
gastric surgery, 613
gastroesophageal reflux disease (GERD), 606
glaucoma, 1072
glomerulonephritis, 708
goiter, 752
gout, 913–914
growth hormone deficiency, 743–744
Guillain-Barré syndrome (GBS), 1031
gynecological cancers, 843
gynecological surgery, 843
Hashimoto thyroiditis, 289
headaches, 958–959
hearing loss, 1077–1078, 1078t
hemodialysis, 715b
hemolytic transfusion reaction, 283
hemophilia, 474–475
hepatitis, 653–655
hiatal hernia, 605
HIV/AIDS, 309–314
Hodgkin lymphoma, 481
home health care, 244–245

Nursing care and process (*continued*)
   Huntington disease, 994
   hyperparathyroidism, 756
   hypertension, 349–350, 349f, 350
   hyperthermia, 202
   hyperthyroidism, 750–751
   hypogammaglobulinemia, 295
   hypoparathyroidism, 755
   hypophysectomy, 744–745, 745f
   hypothermia, 200–201
   hypothyroidism, 746–748
   hysterectomy, 844–845
   idiopathic autoimmune hemolytic anemia, 288–289
   immune thrombocytopenic purpura (ITP), 473, 473b
   increased intracranial pressure (ICP), 955–956, 956b
   infections, 101–103
   infective endocarditis (IE), 364–365
   inflammatory bowel disease, 629–630, 631
   inflammatory or infectious gastrointestinal disorder, 625–626
   inner ear disorders, 1088
   inner ear tumors, 1087
   intracranial surgery, 970–971
   intravenous (IV) therapy, 75–76
   irritable bowel syndrome (IBS), 632–633
   irritations and inflammations of the vagina and vulva, 826
   kidney cancer, 705
   knowledge base in, 7
   labyrinthitis, 1086
   leukemia, 476–478
   lower gastrointestinal bleeding, 638
   lower respiratory infections, 535–537
   lung cancer, 565–566
   lymphangitis, 400–401
   macular degeneration, 1075
   male reproductive system, 812
   malignant breast disorders, 819–820
   mammoplasty, 822
   mastitis, 816
   mechanical ventilation, 514–515, 515b
   Ménière disease, 1088
   menopause, 825
   menstrual flow and cycle disorders, 823
   middle ear, tympanic membrane, and mastoid disorders, 1085–1086, 1086t
   mood disorders, 1178–1179
   multiple myeloma, 480
   multiple sclerosis (MS), 1024–1026
   myasthenia gravis (MG), 1027–1028
   myocardial infarction (MI), 390, 392–393
   myocarditis, 368
   nausea and vomiting, 599
   near-drowning, 204
   non-Hodgkin lymphomas, 482
   noninvasive positive-pressure ventilation (NIPPV), 515–516
   obesity, 602
   obstructive disorders, 555–557
   occlusive dressing, 1102
   oral or esophageal cancer, 604
   osteoarthritis (OA), 916
   osteomyelitis, 910
   osteoporosis, 912
   ostomy, 643–646
   otosclerosis, 1084–1085
   pain, 131–136, 132–135f
   pancreatic cancer, 668
   pancreatitis, 665–666
   Pap smear, 803–804
   Parkinson disease, 990–992
   for patients with pacemakers, 419–420
   patient with hearing impairment, 1080
   peptic ulcer disease (PUD), 610
   pericarditis, 367
   peripheral arterial disorders, 395–396
   pernicious anemia, 288
   personality disorders, 1183
   pneumonia, 540
   pneumothorax, 560
   poisoning and drug overdose, 203
   polycythemia, 471
   for postoperative patients, 181–182
   postoperative phase, 178–189
   premenstrual syndrome and premenstrual dysphoric disorder, 822
   preoperative phase, 169–171, 170t
   pressure injuries, 1114–1118, 1115–1116f
   prioritizing care in, 6–7
   prostatitis, 849, 851–852
   psoriasis, 1121
   pulmonary edema, 429
   pulmonary embolism (PE), 558–559
   radiography, 804–805
   renal calculi, 701–702
   respiratory failure, 563
   respiratory viruses, 527
   restless legs syndrome (RLS), 1031
   restrictive disorders, 545
   retinal detachment, 1070–1071
   rheumatoid arthritis (RA), 920–921
   schizophrenia, 1181
   seizure disorders, 962–963
   sexually transmitted infections (STIs), 879–880
   shock, 111, 113–115, 114t
   sickle cell anemia, 470
   sinusitis, 521
   skin cancer, 1134
   spinal cord injuries, 978, 979–983
   spinal surgery, 973–974
   substance use disorders, 1189–1190
   syndrome of inappropriate ADH (SIADH), 742
   systemic lupus erythematosus (SLE), 290, 292–293
   testicular cancer, 861
   thoracic surgery, 567
   thyroidectomy, 753–754
   thyroid gland cancer, 752–753
   total laryngectomy, 528–531, 529f
   toxic shock syndrome (TSS), 828
   tracheostomy, 511–513
   transplant rejection, 287
   transurethral resection of the prostate (TURP), 855–857
   trauma, 197–199, 197t, 198f
   traumatic brain injury (TBI), 966
   tuberculosis (TB), 543
   type I hypersensitivity disorder, 281
   upper respiratory infections, 524
   urinary incontinence, 690, 691–692
   urinary system diagnostic tests, 689
   urinary tract infection (UTI), 697
   vascular surgery, 399–400
   venous insufficiency, 398
   venous thromboembolism (VTE) disease, 374
Nursing code of ethics, 21
Nursing diagnoses, planning, and implementation, 7. *See also* Diagnostic tests
   acute liver failure, chronic liver disease, cirrhosis, 660–661
   adrenocortical insufficiency (AI), 758
   anemia, 465–466
   aneurysms, 397
   anxiety, obsessive-compulsive, or trauma-related disorders, 1172
   autism spectrum disorders (ADSs), 1184
   blindness, 1068–1069
   bowel obstruction, 637
   burns, 1147–1152
   cancer, 156
   cardiac arrhythmias, 421
   cardiac transplantation, 443–444
   cardiac valvular disorders, 360
   cataracts, 1073
   cerebrovascular disorder, 1012–1017, 1016f
   chest trauma, 561
   chronic heart failure (HF), 438–441, 440b
   chronic kidney disease (CKD), 718–719
   colorectal cancer, 641
   constipation, 620
   coronary artery disease (CAD) and angina, 383–384
   cranial nerve disorder, 1035
   Cushing syndrome, 760
   dermatitis, 1119–1120
   diabetes insipidus, 741
   diabetes mellitus, 783
   diabetic retinopathy, 1069–1070
   diarrhea, 623
   displacement disorders, 831
   ear disorders, 1082, 1083b
   eating disorders, 1186
   erectile dysfunction, 865
   eye infection and inflammation, 1064–1065
   fractures, 908–909
   gallbladder disorder, 671–672
   gastric bleeding, 612
   gastric surgery, 614
   gastroesophageal reflux disease (GERD), 606
   glaucoma, 1072
   grieving family, 260
   headaches, 959
   hearing loss, 1078
   hemophilia, 474
   hepatitis, 654–655
   HIV/AIDS, 309–314
   home health care, 244–245
   hyperparathyroidism, 756
   hypertension, 350
   hyperthermia, 202
   hyperthyroidism, 750
   hypoparathyroidism, 755
   hypothermia, 200–201
   infectious skin disorders, 1128
   infective endocarditis (IE), 364
   inflammatory bowel disease, 630
   inflammatory or infectious gastrointestinal disorder, 625–626

inner ear disorders, 1088
intracranial surgery, 970–971
irritable bowel syndrome (IBS), 632–633
laryngectomy, 529–530
lung cancer, 565–566
middle ear, tympanic membrane, and mastoid disorders, 1085–1086
multiple myeloma, 480
myasthenia gravis (MG), 1028, 1028b
myocardial infarction (MI), 390
nausea and vomiting, 599
near-drowning, 204
obesity, 602
obstructive disorders, 556–557
osteoarthritis (OA), 916, 918–919
ostomy, 644–646
pain, 131–132, 132f, 133f, 134f
pancreatic cancer, 668
pancreatitis, 665–666
Parkinson disease, 991–992
peripheral arterial disorders, 395
personality disorders, 1183
poisoning and drug overdose, 203
postoperative, 178–179, 188–189
preoperative, 170–171
prostatitis, 849
pulmonary embolism (PE), 559
renal calculi, 702
respiratory failure, 563
restrictive disorders, 545
retinal detachment, 1070
rheumatoid arthritis (RA), 920–921
schizophrenia, 1181
seizure disorders, 962–963
sexually transmitted infections (STIs), 879–880
sickle cell anemia, 470
spinal surgery, 974
substance use disorders, 1190
syndrome of inappropriate ADH (SIADH), 742
thoracic surgery, 567–568
thyroidectomy, 753–754
transurethral resection of the prostate (TURP), 857
trauma, 197–198, 198f
traumatic brain injury (TBI), 966
tuberculosis (TB), 543
type I hypersensitivity disorder, 281
urinary system diagnostic tests, 689
urinary tract infection (UTI), 697
vascular surgery, 400
venous insufficiency, 398
venous thromboembolism (VTE) disease, 374
Nursing homes, 237t
Nursing knowledge base, 7
Nursing practice issues, 15–30
   compassion, 17
   economic issues, 16, 17b
   ethics and values, 20–26
   health-care delivery, 15–16
   infectious skin disorders, 1127–1128
   leadership, 17–20, 18f, 19f
   legal concepts, 26–29
   nursing and the health-care team, 17
Nutrition and diet factors
   acute pancreatitis, 663
   anemia, 463

artificial feeding and hydration, 250
atherosclerosis, 379
bariatric surgery and, 600–601
bone density, 223–224
burns and, 1143
calcium and vitamin D recommendations, 801, 802t
cancer care, 159
cancer risk, 145, 148, 149
cardiovascular system and, 337, 338
celiac disease, 634–635
chronic heart failure (HF), 432
chronic kidney disease (CKD), 712–713, 713b, 714
constipation, 621
Crohn disease, 627
delirium, 987
diabetes mellitus, 770–771, 771f, 772t
diarrhea, 622
Dietary Approaches to Stop Hypertension (DASH), 344, 345
eating and drinking changes during end-of-life care, 253
enteral, 592–595, 593–594t
eye health, 1047
fluid excess, 55
food allergies, 275
gallbladder disease, 670
gastric surgery, 615
history taking on, 579
HIV/AIDS, 313
hypertension, 344
hypocalcemia, 63, 63t
hypoglycemia, 779
lithium and, 1177
liver disease, 660
low FODMAP diet, 632
macular degeneration, 1074
myocardial infarction (MI), 389
in older adults, 226
osteoporosis and, 824–825, 911, 912
ostomies, 645
parenteral, 70, 80, 595
postoperative, 188
potassium, 57t
pressure injuries and, 1111
renal calculi, 700
respiratory disease, 556
sodium intake reduction, 57
surgery, 166
therapeutic measures for neurologic system, 948
thyroid function, 751
ulcerative colitis, 629
vitamin K and blood clotting, 361
Nystagmus, 944

O

Obesity, 599–602, 600f, 602f
   malignant breast disorders and, 816
Objective data. *See also* Data collection; Subjective data
   cardiovascular system, 326t
   diabetes mellitus, 783t
   ear, 1053t
   endocrine system, 735t
   eye, 1042–1043, 1044t

female reproductive system, 799t
gastrointestinal, hepatobiliary and pancreatic systems, 580–581t
hematologic and lymphatic systems, 454, 456t
immune system, 270–271, 270t
infective endocarditis (IE), 365t
male reproductive system, 810t
musculoskeletal system, 892t
respiratory system, 496t
urinary system, 681–682t
Oblique fractures, 902t, 903f
Obsessive-compulsive disorder (OCD), 1171
   nursing process, 1172, 1176
   therapeutic measures for, 1172
Obstipation, 619
Obstructive disorders, 545–557
   asthma, 550–554, 552–553f, 554t
   chronic obstructive pulmonary disease/chronic airflow limitation, 545–550, 546f, 547t, 548–549f, 550t
   cystic fibrosis (CF), 554–555
   intestinal obstruction, 635–637, 636f, 636t
Obstructive hypertrophic cardiomyopathy, 369
Obstructive shock, 109t, 111, 194
Obstructive sleep apnea (OSA), 521–522, 521f
Occipital lobe, 935f
Occlusive cardiovascular disorders, 377–403
   acute coronary syndrome (ACS), 384–393, 385–386t, 385f, 387–388f, 387b, 388–389t, 390f
   atherosclerosis, 377–379, 378–379t, 378f
   coronary artery disease (CAD), 378–379t, 379–384, 381f, 382–383t
   lymphatic system, 400–401
   peripheral vascular disease (PVD), 393–400, 396f, 397t, 399f
Occult blood, 583
Occupational exposures and cancer, 145
Oculomotor nerve, 935t, 938f
Older adults. *See also* Aging; Gerontological issues
   cardiovascular system in, 225
   cognitive and psychological changes in, 230–231
   delirium in hospitalized, 988
   developmental stage of, 213–215, 214f
   diabetes mellitus in, 787
   endocrine-metabolic system in, 227
   gastrointestinal system in, 226–227
   genitourinary system in, 227–228
   health promotion for, 214, 231, 232t
   HIV/AIDS in, 301
   home health care of, 232–233
   immune system in, 228
   integumentary system in, 225
   mental health in, 1190–1191
   muscular system in, 223
   nervous system in, 937, 939f
   neurologic system in, 224–225
   perception and attitude of, 222–223
   physiological changes in, 223–229, 224f
   respiratory system in, 225–226
   sensory system in, 215, 228–229
   sexuality in, 229, 229b, 879
   skeletal system in, 22f, 223–224, 887, 890f
Olfactory nerve, 935t
Oligodendrocytes, 929

Oligomenorrhea, 823t
Oliguria, 106
Oncology, 142
Oncoviruses, 144
Ondansetron (Zofran), 173t
Open colectomy, 640t
Open head injury, 963
Open pneumothorax, 559
Open reduction with internal fixation, 904, 905f
Open wet dressings, 1100
Open wounds, 194
Operating room setup, 174–175, 175f
Ophthalmia neonatorum, 875
Ophthalmoplegia, 944
Ophthalmoscope, 1046
Opioid addiction, 121–122
Opioid analgesics, 123
Opioid antagonists, 127
Opioids, 123, 124t, 125–126
    for chronic obstructive pulmonary disease (COPD), 549
    to increase comfort at end of life, 259t
    preoperative, 173t
Optical coherence tomography, 1046
Optic nerve, 935t, 1040f
Oral cancer, 603, 605f
Oral cavity, 572–573, 573f, 581
Oral contraceptives, 834
Oral glucose tolerance test (OGTT), 769
Oral health and dental care, 602–603, 604b
Oral hypoglycemic medication, 774
Oral inflammatory disorders, 603
Oral sections at end of life, 253
Orchitis, 860–861
Organ donation, cultural considerations in, 662, 718
Organelles, 140
Organizing in management process, 18
Orgasm, 807
Orientation, assessment of, 943
Orthopedic trauma, 196
Orthopnea, 429
Orthostatic blood pressure, 325–326, 326b
Orthostatic hypotension and spinal cord injuries, 975
Os coxae, 885
Osler nodes in infective endocarditis (IE), 363, 364f
Osmolarity, 51, 74
Osmosis, 51
Osmotic pressure, 51
Osteoblasts, 885
Osteocytes, 885
Osteomyelitis, 906, 909–910, 910f
Osteons, 885
Osteopathic medicine, 43
Osteoporosis, 801
    diagnostic tests, 911
    fall prevention and, 912
    menopause and, 824–825
    nursing care, 912
    pathophysiology, 910
    prevalence, 910
    prevention, 911
    signs and symptoms, 911
    therapeutic measures, 911–912
    types and risk factors, 910–911

Osteosarcoma, 912
Ostomy, 629, 644t
    ileostomy, 642, 642f
Otitis, external, 1078
Otitis media, 1083–1084
Otomycosis, 1079
Otoplasty, 1135t
Otosclerosis, 1084–1085
Otoscopic examination, 1054
Outcome and Assessment Information Set (OASIS), 244
Outer ear, 1048, 1049f
    disorders of, 1078–1083, 1082f, 1083b
Ovarian cancer, 842
Ovarian cysts, 840
Ovaries, 724f, 725f, 726f, 790, 791f
Overflow incontinence, 690
Overwhelming postsplenectomy infection (OPSI), 483–484
Ovulation, 791
Oxazolidinones, 99t
Oxygen needs
    in chronic heart failure (HF), 438–439
    reducing, 502
Oxygen saturation test, 497–499
Oxygen therapy, 502
    cardiovascular system and, 338
    for chronic heart failure (HF), 432, 440
    chronic obstructive pulmonary disease (COPD), 548–549
    for fluid excess, 55
    high-flow devices, 503
    low-flow devices, 502–503, 502f
    for myocardial infarction (MI), 388
    for pulmonary embolism (PE), 558
    risks of, 503, 503f
    transtracheal catheter, 503, 503f
Oxyhemoglobin, 451, 489–490
Oxytocin, 724, 726f, 731t, 794t

P

Pacemakers, 318, 320f, 418–420, 419f
    sudden death risk with, 436
Paget disease, 912
Pain, 118–139
    acute, 119
    after amputation, 925
    appendicitis, 624f
    biliary colic, 669
    chronic, 119
    in chronic heart failure (HF), 429
    culture and, 119, 120
    definition of, 119
    dysmenorrhea, 823–824
    endometriosis, 824
    external ear infection, 1079
    health-care team management of, 120–121, 133, 135
    home health care, 136
    incision, 169
    medication administration routes for, 128, 129–130t
    multiple myeloma, 479
    myocardial infarction (MI), 386, 386t
    myths and barriers to effective management of, 121
    nonpharmacological therapies for, 128–130

    nursing process for, 131–136, 132–135f
    opioid addiction and, 121–122
    other interventions for, 128–130
    pain puzzle, 118
    placebos and, 128
    postoperative, 179, 183
    referred, 122, 123f
    related to tissue trauma, 197
    risks of uncontrolled, 119
    suffering, 119
    transmission mechanisms of, 122–123, 123f
    treatment options for, 123–130, 124–125t, 126f, 129–130t
Pain Assessment in Advanced Dementia (PAINAD) Scale, 131–132, 133f, 956
Palliation, 151
Palpation, 328–329
    abdominal, 582–583
    breast, 796
    ear, 1052
    endocrine system, 729
    eye area, 1045–1046
    integumentary system, 1098–1099, 1099t
    respiratory system, 494, 497f
Palpebral fissure, 1039f
Pancreas
    as digestive organ, 575t, 576, 576f
    as endocrine organ, 724f, 727–728, 729f, 732t
    transplant of, 777
Pancreas disorders
    cancer, 667–668, 668f
    pancreatitis, 662–668, 665t
Pancreatic supplements, 665t
Pancreatitis
    acute, 662–664, 665–666
    chronic, 664, 665t
    definition of, 662
Pandemic, 89
Panic disorder, 1170
Panmyelosis, 471
Pap tests, 147–148, 803–804, 878
Papules, 1097f
Paralysis
    Guillain-Barré syndrome (GBS) and, 1030
    with stroke, 1003
Paranasal sinuses, 494, 497f
Paraparesis, 975
Paraphimosis, 859–860
Paraplegia, 975
Parasites, genital, 878
Parasitic skin disorders, 1128–1130, 1129f
Parasympathetic nervous system, 937, 938, 938f
Parathyroidectomy, 756
Parathyroid glands, 724f, 727, 727f, 732t
    hyperparathyroidism, 755–756, 755t
    hypoparathyroidism, 754–755, 755t
    ultrasound of, 737
Parenteral nutrition (PN), 70, 80, 595
Parenteral transmission of HIV/AIDS, 302
Paresis, 938
Parietal lobe, 935f
Parkinson disease, 225, 988–992, 995t
    complications, 990
    diagnostic tests, 990
    etiology, 988
    nursing process, 990–992
    pathophysiology, 988

signs and symptoms, 989, 989f, 990t
  surgery, 990
  therapeutic measures, 990, 991t
Paronychia, nails, 1099t
Paroxysmal nocturnal dyspnea, 429
Partial seizures, 959–960
Partial thickness burns, 1140t, 1141f
Passive immunity, 266
Passive transport, 51
Patching, eye, 1048
Patch tests, skin, 1100
Paternalism, 22
Pathogens, 83
  urticaria, 280
Pathological fractures, 902t, 903f
Pathophysiology and etiology
  abdominal hernias, 633, 633f
  absorption disorders, 634
  acne vulgaris, 1127
  acromegaly, 744
  acute kidney injury (AKI), 708–709
  acute pancreatitis, 662–663
  acute respiratory distress syndrome (ARDS), 562
  acute respiratory failure, 562
  adrenocortical insufficiency (AI), 757
  allergic rhinitis, 278
  Alzheimer disease, 994
  amyotrophic lateral sclerosis (ALS), 1029
  anaphylaxis, 279
  anemia, 463
  angioedema, 280
  ankylosing spondylitis, 293–294
  anxiety, 1170
  aortic regurgitation, 358
  aortic stenosis, 358
  aplastic anemia, 465
  appendicitis, 623
  arterial thrombosis and embolism, 393
  asthma, 551
  asystole, 418
  atherosclerosis, 377–378
  atopic dermatitis, 279
  atrial fibrillation (AF), 413
  atrial flutter, 413
  autism spectrum disorders (ADSs), 1184
  Bartholin cysts, 840–841
  Bell palsy, 1033
  benign prostatic hyperplasia (BPH), 852
  bladder cancer, 703
  blindness, 1067
  brain tumors, 967
  bronchiectasis, 534, 534f
  burns, 1138–1140, 1139f, 1140t, 1141f
  cancer, 142–144
  cataracts, 1073
  cellulitis, 1124
  cerebral aneurysm, 1010, 1010f
  cervical cancer, 841
  chlamydia, 871
  cholecystitis, cholelithiasis, choledocholithiasis, 669
  chronic kidney disease (CKD), 711, 711t
  chronic liver disease and cirrhosis, 657
  chronic obstructive pulmonary disease (COPD), 546–547, 546f
  chronic pancreatitis, 664
  colorectal cancer, 639
  constipation, 618–619
  contact dermatitis, 285
  Crohn disease, 626, 626f, 627f
  Cushing syndrome, 758–759
  cyclic breast discomfort, 816
  cystic fibrosis (CF), 554
  cystocele, 829
  dehydration, 52
  dementia, 983–984, 984b
  dermatitis, 1118, 1118t
  dermatomycosis, 1124
  dermoid cysts, 841
  deviated septum, 520
  diabetes insipidus, 740
  diabetes mellitus, 766, 766f
  diabetic ketoacidosis (DKA), 779–780
  diabetic nephropathy, 706
  diabetic retinopathy, 1069
  diarrhea, 620, 622t
  disorders related to development of the genital organs, 828
  displacement disorders, 829
  disseminated intravascular coagulation (DIC), 471–472
  diverticulosis and diverticulitis, 624, 625f
  dysmenorrhea, 823
  encephalitis, 953
  endometrial cancer, 842
  endometriosis, 824
  epistaxis, 518
  erectile dysfunction, 862–863
  esophageal cancer, 603
  external ear infections, 1078–1079
  external ear trauma, 1081
  fibrocystic breast disease, 816
  fibroid tumors, 839
  flail chest, 561
  fluid excess, 54
  fractures, 900–901, 901f
  gastritis, 607
  gastroesophageal reflux disease (GERD), 605
  genital parasites, 878
  glaucoma, 1071
  glomerulonephritis, 707
  goiter, 751
  gonorrhea, 872
  gout, 913, 913f
  growth hormone deficiency, 743
  Guillain-Barré syndrome (GBS), 1030
  Hashimoto thyroiditis, 289
  heart failure (HF), 426
  hemolytic transfusion reaction, 282
  hemophilia, 473
  hepatitis, 649
  herniated discs, 971, 971f
  herpes simplex, 876–877, 1121, 1123f
  herpes zoster (shingles), 1123, 1123f
  hiatal hernia, 604–605
  HIV/AIDS, 299, 300f
  Hodgkin lymphoma, 480
  Huntington disease, 992
  hypercalcemia, 63
  hyperkalemia, 61
  hypernatremia, 59
  hyperosmolar hyperglycemic state (HHS), 780
  hyperparathyroidism, 755
  hyperthyroidism, 748
  hypocalcemia, 62
  hypogammaglobulinemia, 294
  hypokalemia, 60
  hyponatremia, 58
  hypoparathyroidism, 754
  hypothyroidism, 745–746, 745t
  idiopathic autoimmune hemolytic anemia, 288
  immune thrombocytopenic purpura (ITP), 472–473
  impacted cerumen, 1079
  increased intracranial pressure (ICP), 954–955, 955f
  infective endocarditis (IE), 363
  inner ear tumors, 1086–1087
  irritable bowel syndrome (IBS), 630–631
  irritations and inflammations of the vagina and vulva, 825–826
  keratitis, 1064
  labyrinthitis, 1086
  large-bowel obstruction, 636
  laryngeal cancer, 527
  leukemia, 475
  lower gastrointestinal bleeding, 638
  lung cancer, 563–564, 564f
  macular degeneration, 1073–1074, 1074f
  male infertility, 866
  malignant breast disorders, 816
  masses of external ear, 1080–1081
  mastitis, 816
  Ménière disease, 1087
  meningitis, 952, 952t
  menopause, 824
  menstrual flow and cycle disorders, 823, 823t
  middle ear infections, 1083
  middle ear trauma, 1085
  mitral valve prolapse (MVP), 354
  mood disorders, 1176
  multiple myeloma, 478–479, 479f
  multiple sclerosis (MS), 1020–1021, 1021f
  myasthenia gravis (MG), 1026, 1026f
  myocardial infarction (MI), 384–385, 385f
  nasal polyps, 520
  non-Hodgkin lymphomas, 482
  oral cancer, 603
  osteoarthritis (OA), 914–915, 915f
  osteomyelitis, 909, 910f
  osteoporosis, 910
  otosclerosis, 1084
  ovarian cancer, 842
  pancreatic cancer, 667
  Parkinson disease, 988
  pediculosis, 1128
  pelvic inflammatory disease (PID), 870
  peptic ulcer disease (PUD), 608
  pericarditis, 366
  peripheral arterial disease (PAD), 394
  peritonitis, 623–624
  pernicious anemia, 288
  personality disorders, 1182
  pharyngitis, 523
  pheochromocytoma, 756
  pleural effusion, 544
  pleurisy, 543
  pneumonia, 538
  pneumothorax, 559, 560f
  polycystic ovary syndrome (PCOS), 840

Pathophysiology and etiology (continued)
  polycythemia, 470
  postpolio syndrome, 1031
  premature atrial contractions (PACs), 412
  premature ventricular contractions (PVCs), 416
  premenstrual syndrome and premenstrual dysphoric disorder, 822
  pressure injuries, 1107–1108
  prostate cancer, 858
  prostatitis, 849
  psoriasis, 1120
  pulmonary edema, 428
  pulmonary embolism (PE), 557, 558f
  pulmonary fibrosis, 544
  reactive hypoglycemia, 786
  rectocele, 829
  refractive errors, 1065–1066
  renal calculi, 699–700
  reproductive system cysts, 840
  respiratory viruses, 525–526
  restless legs syndrome (RLS), 1031
  retinal detachment, 1070
  rheumatoid arthritis (RA), 919, 919f
  rib fractures, 560–561
  scabies, 1129, 1129f
  schizophrenia, 1180
  seizure disorders, 959
  shock, 105–106
  sickle cell anemia, 467–468, 468f
  sinus bradycardia, 409
  sinusitis, 520–521
  sinus tachycardia, 411
  sleep apnea, 521–522, 521f
  small-bowel obstruction, 635–636
  spinal cord injuries, 974
  stress responses, 1171t
  stroke, 1001–1002, 1001b, 1001f, 1002f
  substance use disorders, 1188
  syndrome of inappropriate ADH (SIADH), 742
  syphilis, 875
  systemic lupus erythematosus (SLE), 289–290, 290b
  testicular cancer, 861
  third-degree atrioventricular block, 415
  thyroid gland cancer, 752
  tonsillitis/adenoiditis, 525
  toxic shock syndrome (TSS), 826
  transplant rejection, 286
  traumatic brain injury (TBI), 963
  trichomoniasis, 876
  trigeminal neuralgia (TN), 1032
  tuberculosis (TB), 540–541
  ulcerative colitis, 627–629
  uterine or cervical polyps, 840
  uterine position disorders, 829
  uterine prolapse, 830
  varicose veins, 397
  venous thromboembolism (VTE) disease, 370–371
  ventricular fibrillation, 417
  ventricular tachycardia, 417
  viral rhinitis/common cold, 522
  vulvar cancer, 841
Patient care settings, 235–246
  acute care, 235–236
  correctional nursing, 236
  fractures, 909b
  home health care, 240–245, 240b, 240f, 242b, 242f, 243b
  long-term care services, 236–240, 237t, 239t
  LPN/LVN employment settings, 235
  medical office nursing, 236
Patient-centered care
  evidence-based practice (EBP), 13
  prioritization in, 6–7
Patient-controlled analgesia (PCA), 71–72, 128
Patient education
  abortion, 839
  acute liver failure, chronic liver disease, cirrhosis, 661
  breast self-examination, 799, 800f
  cardiac valvular disorders, 360–361
  cardiomyopathy, 370b
  chronic heart failure (HF) medications, 440, 440b
  communicable or inflammatory neurological disorders, 957
  dehydration, 54
  diabetes mellitus self-management, 783, 785–786
  displacement disorders, 831
  disseminated intravascular coagulation (DIC), 472
  dysmenorrhea, 824
  endometriosis, 824
  endoscopy, 805
  erectile dysfunction, 865
  fertility testing and treatment, 832–833
  fluid excess, 56
  fractures, 909
  gallbladder disorder, 672
  gynecological surgery, 843
  Hashimoto thyroiditis, 289
  hemolytic transfusion reaction, 283
  HIV/AIDS, 310–311b
  Hodgkin lymphoma, 481
  home health care, 244
  hyperthyroidism, 750
  hypogammaglobulinemia, 295
  hypophysectomy, 745
  hypothyroidism, 748
  immune thrombocytopenic purpura (ITP), 473, 473b
  infective endocarditis (IE), 365
  laryngectomy, 531
  mastitis, 816
  menopause, 825
  myocardial infarction (MI), 390–391
  obstructive disorders, 557
  osteoarthritis (OA), 919
  pain, 136
  pancreatic cancer, 668
  pancreatitis, 666
  pediculosis, 1129
  polycythemia, 471
  premenstrual syndrome and premenstrual dysphoric disorder, 822
  preoperative, 167, 169
  prostate cancer, 859
  rheumatoid arthritis (RA), 921
  scabies, 1130
  sickle cell anemia, 470
  splenectomy, 483
  sterilization, 837
  total hip replacement, 923
Patient Health Questionnaire (PHQ-9), 1176
Patient rights, 28–29
Patient Self-Determination Act, 248
Peak expiratory flow rate (PEFR), 552, 552f, 553f
Pediculosis, 1128–1129
Pelvic examination, 801–803, 802f, 806t
Pelvic inflammatory disease (PID), 870–871
Penetrating injuries, 194
  to abdomen, 196
  to eye, 1075
  to head, 963
  to heart, 368
Penicillin, 97t
  for sexually transmitted infections (STIs), 873t
Penile disorders, 859–860
Penis, 794–795, 795f
Penumbra, 1001
Peptic ulcer disease (PUD), 608–611, 609t, 610t
Perception
  abdominal, 582
  and attitude toward aging, 222–223
  of pain, 122
Percussion
  endocrine system, 729
  respiratory system, 494
Percutaneous balloon valvotomy, 357, 357f
Percutaneous coronary intervention with stenting, 387, 388f
Percutaneous liver biopsy, 590–591
Percutaneous nephrolithotomy, 701
Percutaneous transluminal cardiac angioplasty (PTCA), 387
Perfusion, 425
Perianesthesia care unit (PACU), 177–178, 177f, 178b
  discharge from, 180, 180b
  family visitation in, 180
  nursing process for, 178–180
Pericardial effusion, 367
Pericardial friction rub, 330, 366
Pericardial tamponade, 111
Pericardiectomy, 367
Pericardiocentesis, 367, 367f
Pericarditis, 366–367, 366t, 367f
  as complication of myocardial infarction (MI), 385t
Perichondritis, 1079
Perimenopause, 824
Perinatal transmission of HIV/AIDS, 302
Periosteum, 885
Peripheral arterial disease (PAD), 394–395
Peripherally inserted central catheter (PICC), 79f, 80
Peripheral nervous system disorders, 1020–1037
  cranial nerve disorders, 1031–1035, 1033f, 1034f
  neuromuscular disorders, 1020–1031, 1021b, 1021f, 1024b, 1026f, 1027t, 1028b
  summary, 1032t
Peripheral vascular disease (PVD)
  aneurysms, 396–397, 397t
  arterial thrombosis and embolism, 393–394
  endarterectomy, 399–400
  peripheral arterial disease (PAD), 394–395
  Raynaud disease, 395

thromboangiitis obliterans, 395
varicose veins, 397–398
vascular surgery for, 398–399, 399f
venous insufficiency, 398
Peripheral vascular resistance (PVR), 342, 426
Peristalsis, 573
Peritoneal dialysis, 716–717, 717b, 717f
Peritonitis, 623–624
Permanent pacemakers, 418–419, 419f
Pernicious anemia, 288
Personality changes with traumatic brain injury (TBI), 965–966
Personality disorders, 1182–1183
Personal protective equipment (PPE), 302
Pessary, 829
Petechiae, 454, 1098
abdominal, 582
in infective endocarditis (IE), 363, 364f
Petit mal seizures, 960
Pet-related issues and HIV/AIDS, 311–312t
Peyronie disease, 859
Phagocytosis, 88, 575
Phantom pain, 925
Pharmacists, 17
Pharyngitis, 523, 525
Pharynx, 487, 487f, 573, 573f
Pheochromocytoma, 756–757
PH imbalances, 490
Phimosis, 859–860
Phlebitis, 76, 77t
Phlebotomy, 471
Phobias, specific, 1170
Phosphodiesterase-4 inhibitor, 550t
Phospholipids, 331t, 334
Phosphorus, laboratory tests for, 890, 893t
Physical activity. *See* Exercise
Physical dependence, 121–122
Physical examination
cardiovascular system, 323, 326t
ear, 1052–1054, 1052b, 1053f, 1054t
endocrine system, 728–729
eye, 1042–1043, 1044f, 1044t
gastrointestinal, hepatobiliary and pancreatic systems, 579, 581
hematologic and lymphatic systems, 454, 456t
integumentary system, 1096–1099, 1097–1098f, 1099t
male reproductive system, 807–810
musculoskeletal system, 888
neurologic system, 940–945, 941t, 942f, 944f, 945t
preoperative assessment, 169
respiratory system, 494–495, 494–495f, 497f
urinary system, 679–682, 681–682t
Physical restraints, 239
Physical therapy for herniated discs, 972
Physician Orders for Life-Sustaining Treatment (POLST), 249
Physician Orders for Scope of Treatment (POST), 249
Phytoestrogens, 824
PICO(T), 11b
Piggyback (secondary) intermittent infusion, 70–71, 71f
Pigmented nevus, 1131t
Pineal gland, 724f
Pituitary gland, 723–724, 724f, 725f, 731t

Pituitary gland disorders
related to antidiuretic hormone imbalance, 740–743, 741t, 742b
tumors, 744–745, 745f
Placebos, 128
Plague, 208t
Planning in management process, 18
Plaque
arterial, 344, 378, 378f
skin, 1097f
Plasma, 448, 451
gas transport and, 489–490
multiple myeloma and, 478–480, 479f
Plasmapheresis, 1023, 1024b
Plasma proteins, 575
Platelets, 450t, 451, 453f
Pleural effusion, 544
due to lung cancer, 564
Pleural membranes, 487
Pleurisy, 543–544
Pleurodesis, 560
Pneumatic retinopexy, 1070
Pneumococcal pneumonia, HIV/AIDS-associated, 305t
Pneumocystis pneumonia (PCP), 304, 305t
Pneumonectomy, 565, 566, 566f
Pneumonia, 538–540, 540f, 540t
due to lung cancer, 565
in older patients, 228
Pneumothorax, 559–560, 560f
Poikilothermy, 328
Point of maximum impulse (PMI), 328
Poisoning and drug overdose, 202–204
Polycystic kidney disease, 705–706
Polycystic ovary syndrome (PCOS), 840
Polycythemia, 470–471, 547
Polydipsia, 768
Polymenorrhea, 823t
Polyphagia, 768
Polyps
nasal, 520
uterine or cervical, 840
Polyuria, 768
Pons, 933
Portal hypertension, 657, 658f
Portal of entry, 84f, 87
Portal of exit, 84f, 86
Ports, intravenous (IV) therapy, 80
Positioning
breathing and, 501–502, 502f
chronic heart failure (HF) and, 438
as therapeutic measure for neurologic system, 946–947
Positive feedback loop, 724
Positive reinforcement, 1165
Positron emission tomography (PET), 333t, 336
endocrine system, 737
Post-attachment inhibitors, 308t
Postcoital douching, 837
Posterior pituitary gland, 724, 731t
Postictal period, seizure disorders, 960
Postmortem care, 259–260
Postoperative phase, 166t
abdominal hernia repair, 634
admission to perianesthesia care unit, 177f, 178–180, 178b
adrenalectomy, 761

amputation, 925
bariatric surgery, 601–602
cardiovascular function in, 179
circulatory function in, 182–183
ear surgery, 1087, 1087b
family visitation, 180
gastrointestinal function in, 187–188
home health for, 189
hypophysectomy, 745
intracranial surgery, 970
laryngectomy, 528–531
mobility in, 188–189
neurologic function in, 179–180
nursing process, 178–180
nutrition in, 188
pain in, 179, 183
patient discharge and, 189
respiratory function in, 178–179
spinal surgery, 974
splenectomy, 483
surgical wound care, 185–187, 185f, 186f, 186t, 187f
thoracic surgery, 567
thyroidectomy, 753
total hip replacement, 922
transfer to nursing unit, 180, 180f
urinary function in, 183–184
Postpolio syndrome, 1031
Postprandial hyperinsulinemic hypoglycemia, 615
Post-traumatic stress disorder (PTSD), 1172
concussion and, 965
Potassium
food sources of, 57t
imbalances in, 60–62, 334
Potassium-sparing diuretics, 346t
Powerlessness, 216, 217f
Preadmission surgical patient assessment, 167, 168b, 168t
Prediabetes, 768
Pre-exposure prophylaxis (PrEP), HIV/AIDS, 301
Pregnancy
HIV/AIDS in, 302
termination of, 837–839
Prehabilitation, 166
Preload, 427
Premature atrial contractions (PACs), 412–413, 412f
Premature ventricular contractions (PVCs), 415–418, 416f, 418f
Premenstrual dysphoric disorder (PMDD), 822
Premenstrual syndrome (PMS), 822
Preoperative medications, 172, 173t
Preoperative phase, 166–167, 166t
adrenalectomy, 760–761
amputation, 924–925
ear surgery, 1087, 1087b
factors influencing surgical outcomes, 166–167
hypophysectomy, 744–745
informed consent, 171–172
intracranial surgery, 969–970
medications for, 172, 173t
nursing process for, 169–171, 170t
ostomy, 643
preadmission surgical patient assessment, 167, 168b, 168t

Preoperative phase (continued)
  preoperative teaching, 167, 169
  preparation for surgery, 172
  spinal surgery, 973
  splenectomy, 483
  thoracic surgery, 567
  thyroidectomy, 753
  total hip replacement, 921
  warming, 173–174
Preoperative teaching, 167, 169
Preoperative warming, 173–174
Preparation for surgery, 172
Prepuce, 793f
Presbycusis, 1048, 1049, 1076
Presbyopia, 1066
Present-on-admission (POA) reporting, 16
Pressure injuries, 225
  Braden Skin Scale and, 16, 1108, 1109–1111t
  complications of, 1112
  diagnostic tests, 1112
  nursing process for, 1114–1118, 1115–1116f
  pathophysiology and etiology of, 1107–1108
  prevention of, 1108
  signs and symptoms, 1112
  stages of, 1115–1116f
  therapeutic measures, 1112–1114, 1114f
Prevention
  abdominal hernias, 633
  acute pancreatitis, 663
  acute respiratory distress syndrome (ARDS), 562
  acute respiratory failure, 562
  asthma, 551
  cancer, 147–149, 148f
  cellulitis, 1124
  cervical cancer, 842
  chronic obstructive pulmonary disease (COPD), 547
  coronary artery disease (CAD), 379–380
  dehydration, 52
  dermatitis, 1119
  diabetes mellitus, 770
  diarrhea, 620–621
  ear problems, 1056–1057t
  eye injury, 1047, 1047t
  fluid excess, 55
  glaucoma, 1071
  gout, 913–914
  hepatitis, 652
  herpes simplex lesions, 1123
  herpes zoster (shingles), 1124
  HIV/AIDS, 300–302, 301b, 308–309
  hypercalcemia, 64
  hyperkalemia, 61
  hypernatremia, 59
  hypocalcemia, 62
  hypokalemia, 60
  hyponatremia, 58, 58b
  infective endocarditis (IE), 363
  laryngeal cancer, 527
  lung cancer, 564
  macular degeneration, 1074
  male infertility, 866
  malignant breast disorders, 816–817
  meningitis, 952
  osteoporosis, 911
  pediculosis, 1128
  pneumonia, 538–539
  pressure injuries, 1108
  prostatitis, 849
  psoriasis, 1120
  pulmonary embolism (PE), 557
  renal calculi, 700
  respiratory viruses, 526
  scabies, 1129
  skin cancer, 1134
  stroke, 1008
  testicular cancer, 861
  toxic shock syndrome (TSS), 826–827
  tuberculosis (TB), 541
  venous thromboembolism (VTE) disease, 371–372, 372–373t
  viral rhinitis/common cold, 522–523
Priapism, 859
Primary hypertension, 343
Primary intermittent infusion, 70
Primary survey, emergent conditions, 192–193, 193f
PR interval, 405, 405f, 408
Prions, 85–86
Prioritization of care, 6–7
Privacy, 22
  social media and, 28
Private-duty nursing, 245
Procedural sedation and analgesia, 177
Prochlorperazine (Compazine), 173t
Proctitis, 871
Prodromal phase, schizophrenia, 1179
Progesterone, 791, 794t
Progressive muscle relaxation, 44
Projectile injuries, 194
Prolactin, 725f, 731t, 794t
Promethazine hydrochloride (Phenergan), 173t
Prophylactic antiembolism devices, 372
Prostaglandins, 123
Prostate cancer screening, 148
Prostate disorders, 848
  cancer, 858–859
  prostatitis, 849–852, 850–851t
Prostate gland, 792, 794, 795f
Prostate-specific antigen (PSA), 811
Prostatic acid phosphatase (PAP), 811
Prostatitis, 849–852, 850–851t
Prostheses, limb, 925
Protease inhibitors, 307t
Protected health information (PHI), 27–29
Prothrombin time (PT), 458t
Protozoa, 85, 85t
Pseudoaddiction, 122
Pseudobulbar affect (PBA), 1009
Pseudodementia, 1190
Pseudomonas aeruginosa, 92
Psoriasis, 1101, 1120–1121, 1121f
Psychiatric emergencies, 204
Psychodynamic therapy, 1165
Psychogenic hearing loss, 1076
Psychological dependence, 122
Psychopharmacology, 1164
Psychosocial development. See Developmental stages
Psychosocial effects
  of burn injury, 1146
  of seizure disorders, 962
  of traumatic brain injury (TBI), 965–966
Psychotherapy, 1164–1165, 1181, 1183, 1188
Ptosis, 1027
Pulmonary angiography, 499
Pulmonary edema, 428–429, 428t
  as complication of myocardial infarction (MI), 385t
Pulmonary effects of burns, 1139
Pulmonary embolism (PE), 557–559, 558f, 559t
  versus fat embolism syndrome, 908t
Pulmonary fibrosis, 544–545
Pulmonary function studies, 499, 500t
Pulmonary vascular disorders, 557–559, 558f, 559t
Pulse, 327–328
Pulse deficit, 327
Punctal occlusion, 1047–1048
Puncture wounds, 194
Pupil, 1041f, 1045
Pupillary reflexes, 1045
Pupillary response, 943–944, 944f
Purpura, 454
Pursed-lip breathing, 501
Purulent drainage
  from pressure injuries, 1116
  from surgical wounds, 185
Purulent exudate, 88
Pustule, 1097f
P waves, 405, 405f, 407f, 408
Pyelonephritis, 697
Pyloric obstruction, 615
Pyrimidine synthesis inhibitors, 917t

Q

Qi meridians, 43f
QRS complex, 406, 406f
QRS interval, 406, 406f, 408
QT interval, 405f, 406, 408
Quadrigeminy, 416
Quadriparesis, 975
Quadriplegia, 975
Quality, evidence-based practice (EBP), 13–14
Quality and Safety Education for Nurses (QSEN), 13–14
Quality improvement (QI), 13
  continuous, 19, 19f
Quality of care, 29
QuantiFERON-TB test, 542

R

Racial and ethnic groups
  asthma and, 551
  HIV and, 879
  hypertension and, 344
  malignant breast disorders and, 816
  observing for jaundice in different, 582
  stroke and, 1001
  type 2 diabetes and, 773
  in the United States, 37–38
Radiation as cancer risk, 145
Radiation therapy, 145, 151–152, 153f
  bone cancer, 913
  brain tumors, 968–969
  laryngeal cancer, 528
  leukemia, 476
  malignant breast disorders, 817
Radical prostatectomy, 854, 857, 857f, 859
Radioactive iodine therapy, 749, 751

Radioactive iodine uptake test, 737
Radiography
　endocrine system, 737
　eye area, 1046
　female reproductive system, 804
　fractures, 902
　gastrointestinal, hepatobiliary and pancreatic systems, 588–589, 588f
　musculoskeletal system, 894t, 896
　neurologic system, 946
　osteoporosis, 911
　rheumatoid arthritis (RA), 920
Radioisotopes, 332–333t
Radiology, 150
Random blood glucose, 769
Randomized controlled trials, 10
Range of motion (ROM), 22f, 223
　musculoskeletal system physical examination, 888
Raynaud disease, 395
Reactive hypoglycemia, 786
Rebleeding, cerebral aneurysm, 1011
Receptive aphasia, 948, 1003
Receptors, skin, 1092
Recombinant DNA technology, 275
Reconstruction mammoplasty, 821–822, 821–822f
Rectocele, 829, 830f
Red blood cell (RBC) disorders
　anemia, 462–465, 465t
　aplastic anemia, 465–466, 466f
　polycythemia, 470–471
　sickle cell anemia, 467–470, 468f, 469f
Red blood cells (RBCs), 450t, 451
　breakdown of, 452f
Reduced hemoglobin, 451
Reed-Sternberg cells, 480–481
Referred pain, 122, 123f
Reflexes, spinal cord, 931, 933f
Refractive errors, 1065–1067, 1066f
Refractory period, 930
Regadenoson SPECT-CT thallium imaging, 333t
Regional anesthesia, 176–177, 177f
Registered nurses (RNs), 17
Regulation of nursing practice, 26
Regurgitation, 353
　aortic, 356t, 358–359
　mitral, 355t, 357–358
Rehabilitation
　burns, 1145–1146, 1146f
　cerebral aneurysm, 1011–1012
　multiple sclerosis (MS), 1023
　ostomy, 646
　pulmonary, 549, 551f
　traumatic brain injury (TBI), 966
Relaxation therapies, 44–45, 46b, 128, 1167
　for pain, 128
Religious traditions, 24, 32–33. See also Spirituality
　cardiac valve options and, 361
Reminiscence therapy, 213
Remodeling, airway, 551
Remyelination, 1030
Renal biopsy, 689
Renal calculi, 699–702, 699f, 700t, 701f
Renal filtrate, 676, 678f
Renal system. See Urinary system

Renin-angiotensin-aldosterone system, 106, 322, 322f
Replantation, 924
Reproductive life planning, 833–837, 835–836f
Reproductive system. See Female reproductive system; Genitourinary and reproductive system; Male reproductive system
Required reporting, 26
Research, 9, 12b
Reservoir, infection, 86
Residential care community, 237t
Residual phase, schizophrenia, 1179
Resilience, multimorbidity, 217
Resorption, 885
Respirations, rate and ease of, 328
Respiratory acidosis, 66t, 490
　with compensation, 66t
Respiratory alkalosis, 66t, 490
　with compensation, 66t
Respiratory excursion, 494
Respiratory failure, 562–563
Respiratory system, 486–517. See also Lower respiratory tract disorders; Upper respiratory tract disorders
　acid-based balance and, 490, 492
　aging and, 225–226, 492f
　allergic rhinitis, 278–279
　burns and, 1139
　chemical regulation and respiration, 490
　diagnostic tests of, 495–499, 497f, 498t, 499f
　gas transport in the blood and, 489–490
　larynx, 487, 488f
　lungs and pleural membranes, 487, 490f
　mechanism of breathing, 487–489
　muscles of, 491f
　near-drowning and, 204
　normal anatomy and physiology, 486–492, 487–491f, 487t
　nose and nasal cavities, 486, 487t
　nursing assessment of, 492, 493t, 494–495, 494–495f
　pharynx, 487, 487f
　physical examination of, 494–495, 494–495f, 496t, 497f
　postoperative, 178–179
　protective mechanisms, 486, 487t
　spinal cord injuries and, 977
　sputum culture and sensitivity, 496–497, 499f
　trachea and bronchial tree, 487, 489f
　with trauma, 197
Respiratory system interventions
　autogenic drainage, 501
　breathing exercises, 501
　chest drainage, 506–508, 507b, 507f
　chest physiotherapy (CPT), 504, 505f
　deep breathing and coughing, 499, 501
　high-frequency chest wall oscillation vest, 504
　huff coughing, 501
　incentive spirometry, 504, 505f
　inhalers, 504, 504f
　intubation, 510, 510f, 513
　mechanical ventilation, 513–515, 513f, 514t, 515b
　nebulized mist treatments, 503–504, 503f
　noninvasive positive-pressure ventilation (NIPPV), 515–516, 515f
　oxygen therapy, 502–503, 502–503f

　positioning, 501–502, 502f
　reducing oxygen consumption, 502
　smoking cessation, 499, 500t
　suctioning, 510
　thoracentesis, 505–506
　tracheostomy, 508–509f, 508–510, 511–513
　vibratory positive expiratory pressure device, 505, 505f
Respiratory tract disorders, lower, 533–571
　chest trauma, 559–562, 560f, 561t
　home health care, 568
　infectious disorders, 533–543, 534f, 540f, 540t, 542t
　lung cancer, 563–566, 564f, 565t, 566f
　obstructive disorders, 545–557, 546f, 547t, 548–549f, 550t, 551–553f, 554t
　pulmonary vascular disorders, 557–559, 558f, 559t
　respiratory failure, 562–563
　restrictive disorders, 543–545
　thoracic surgery and, 566–568
Respiratory tract disorders, upper, 518–532
　infectious disorders, 522–527, 523t
　malignant disorders, 527–531, 528f, 528t, 529f
　nose and sinus disorders, 518–522, 519f, 520b, 521f
Respiratory tract infections, 96, 102
Respite care, 219
Respondeat superior, 28
Rest-and-digest response, 938
Restless legs syndrome (RLS), 1031
Restraints in long-term care facilities, 239
Restrictive cardiomyopathy, 369
Restrictive disorders, 543–545
　empyema, 544
　pleural effusion, 544
　pleurisy, 543–544
　pulmonary fibrosis, 544–545
Resuscitation
　do not resuscitate (DNR) order and, 249
　drowning and, 204
　as end-of-life choice, 249
　family presence during, 199
Reticulocytes, 450t, 451
Retina, 1038, 1039, 1040f, 1046
Retinal detachment, 1070–1071
Retinopathy, 781
Retraction of chest wall, 494
Retrograde ejaculation, 854
Rhabdomyolysis, 890, 907
Rheumatic fever, 354
Rheumatoid arthritis (RA), 914t
　diagnostic tests, 920
　etiology, 919
　nursing process for, 920–921
　pathophysiology, 919, 919f
　signs and symptoms, 919–920, 920f
　therapeutic measures, 920
Rh factor, 451
Rhinitis, viral, 522–523, 523t
Rhinophototherapy, 278
Rhinoplasty, 520, 1135t
Rhytidoplasty, 1135t
Rib fractures, 560–561
Ribs, 885
RICE (Rest, Ice, Compression, and Elevation) therapy, 899, 900

Rickettsiae, 85
Right middle cerebral artery syndrome, 1004t
Right-sided heart failure (HF), 426–427, 427t, 428f, 430t
Right transverse colostomy, 643t
Rinne test, 1052, 1053f, 1054t
Robotic-assisted surgery, 166
Robotic devices, 224, 224f
Roles, chronic illness and changing, 218
Romberg test, 944–945, 1052
Rotational injury, 963
Rotator cuff injury, 900
Roux-en-Y gastric bypass, 601, 602f
Rugae, 574
Rule of Nines for burns, 1140, 1141f

S

Saccular aneurysms, 396, 396f
Sacrum vertebrae, 885
Safer sex practices, 301–302, 301b
Safety
   avoiding failure to communicate for, 3
   complementary and alternative modalities, 47, 47b
   ear health, 1056, 1056f
   evidence-based practice (EBP), 13–14
   eye, 1047, 1047t
   home health care, 242–243, 243b
   in long-term care facilities, 238–240
   medication, in older adults, 231
   medication errors, 16
   postoperative dehiscence or evisceration, 185
   radiation therapy, 152, 153f
Salicylates, 124t
Saline lock, 70
Salivary glands, 573, 573f, 575t
Salivation, 573
Salpingoscopy, 805
Sandwich generation, 213
Sarcomas, 146
Scabies, 1129–1130, 1129f
Scales, 1097f
Scar, 1097f, 1131t
Scheduling options for analgesics, 127
Schizoid personality, 1179
Schizophrenia, 1179–1182
   nursing process, 1181
   pathophysiology and etiology, 1180
   positive and negative symptoms, 1180
   symptoms, 1180–1181
   therapeutic measures, 1181, 1181t, 1182t
Sclera, 1038, 1040f
Scleral buckling, 1070
Sclerosis in pneumothorax, 560
Scratch tests, skin, 1100
Screening, Brief Intervention, and Referral to Treatment (SBIRT), 1188
Sebaceous glands, 1092, 1093f
Seborrheic keratosis, 1131t
Secondary diabetes, 768
Secondary hypertension, 343
Secondary survey, emergent conditions, 193, 194t
Sedatives, preoperative, 173t
Segmental resection, 565, 566, 566f
Seizure disorders
   diagnostic tests, 960
   emergency care, 960
   etiology, 959
   increased intracranial pressure and, 956b
   nursing process, 962–963
   pathophysiology, 959
   psychosocial effects, 962
   signs and symptoms, 959–960
   status epilepticus, 962
   surgical management, 960
Selective serotonin norepinephrine reuptake inhibitors (SNRIs), 1174t
Selective serotonin reuptake inhibitors (SSRI), 1173t
Self-Management Resource Center, 215
Self-monitoring for asthma, 552, 552f
Self-monitoring of blood glucose (SMBG), 776, 776f
Semiassisted/assisted living, 237t
Semi-Fowler/high Fowler positioning, 55, 55f
   for chronic heart failure (HF), 438
Seminal vesicles, 792, 794, 795f
Semipermeable membrane, 51
Sensorineural hearing loss, 1076, 1076t
Sensory disorders. *See* Hearing disorders; Vision disorders
Sensory neurons, 930, 931f
Sensory system
   aging and, 215, 228–229, 1041–1042, 1042f, 1045
   data collection on, 1042–1046, 1043–1044t, 1044–1045f
   hearing, 1048–1057
   vision, 1038–1048
Sepsis, 89, 108–109
   peritonitis, 624
   signs and symptoms, 110f
Septal rupture, 385t
Septicemia, intravenous (IV) therapy, 78t
Septic shock, 108–109, 109t
   urosepsis, 697
Septoplasty, 520, 520b
Serious reportable events (SREs), 16
Serological tests
   diabetes mellitus, 769, 769f, 769t
   endocrine system hormones, 729–730, 731–733t
   gastrointestinal, hepatobiliary and pancreatic systems, 584–585t
   HIV/AIDS, 306
   kidney function, 685–686t
   musculoskeletal system, 890, 893t
   preoperative, 168t
   syphilis, 875–876
Serosanguineous drainage, 187
Serotonin, 1156t
Serotonin-norepinephrine reuptake inhibitor, 125t
Serous drainage, 187
Serum sickness, 284
Serum sodium level, 59
Seventh Day Adventists, 361
Severe acute respiratory syndrome (SARS), 527
Sexuality
   aging and, 229, 229b, 879
   barrier methods for safer sex and, 881t
   chronic illness and, 217–218
   HIV/AIDS and, 311t
   myocardial infarction (MI) and, 391
Sexually transmitted infections (STIs), 804, 869–883
   antimicrobial resistance (AMR) and, 879
   barrier methods for safer sex and, 881t
   cellular changes due to, 871
   chlamydia, 145, 804, 871, 872t
   condylomata (HPV), 872t
   disorders and syndromes related to, 870–871
   genital parasites, 878
   genital ulcers due to, 871
   gonorrhea, 872, 872t, 875–876, 876f
   hepatitis B and C, 878
   herpes simplex virus (HSV), 305t, 603, 872t, 874t, 876–877, 877f
   HIV/AIDS, 301–302, 301b
   human papillomavirus (HPV), 144, 148, 841–842, 860, 872t, 877–878, 878f
   medications used to treat, 873–874t
   mucopurulent cervicitis (MPC) due to, 870
   nursing process for, 879–880
   pelvic inflammatory disease (PID) due to, 870–871
   proctitis and enteritis due to, 871
   risk factors for, 870
   syphilis, 306, 872t, 873–874t, 875–876, 876f
   trichomoniasis, 827t, 872t, 874t, 876
   urethritis due to, 870
   vulvovaginitis due to, 870
Shingles, 228, 305t, 1123–1124, 1123f
Shock, 105–117
   anaphylactic, 108, 109t, 194, 266
   cardiogenic, 108
   classification of, 107–111, 109t, 110f
   complications from, 106–107
   distributive, 108–111
   effect on organs and organ systems, 106, 108t
   as emergent condition, 194
   hypovolemic, 107
   metabolic and hemodynamic changes in, 105–106
   pathophysiology, 105–106
   stages of, 107t
   therapeutic measures, 111, 111t, 112–113t
   vital signs in, 197
Shock-wave lithotripsy, 701, 701f
Short-acting beta agonists (SABA), 554
Sickle cell anemia, 467–470, 468f, 469f
Sigmoidoscopy, 590
Signal anxiety, 1170
Signal-averaged ECG, 335
Signs and symptoms
   abdominal hernias, 633
   absorption disorders, 634
   acne vulgaris, 1127, 1127f
   acromegaly, 744, 744f
   acute liver failure, 656
   acute pancreatitis, 663, 663t
   acute respiratory distress syndrome (ARDS), 563
   acute respiratory failure, 562
   adrenocortical insufficiency (AI), 757
   allergic rhinitis, 278
   Alzheimer disease, 994–995
   amyotrophic lateral sclerosis (ALS), 1029
   anaphylaxis, 279, 280t
   anemia, 464, 465t
   aneurysms, 396, 397t

angioedema, 280
ankylosing spondylitis, 294
anorexia nervosa, 1185
anxiety, 1170, 1175t
aortic regurgitation, 359
aortic stenosis, 358
aplastic anemia, 466, 466f
appendicitis, 623
arterial thrombosis and embolism, 393
asthma, 551–552, 554t
asystole, 418
atopic dermatitis, 279
atrial fibrillation (AF), 414
atrial flutter, 413
autism spectrum disorders (ADSs), 1184
Bartholin cysts, 840–841
Bell palsy, 1033, 1034f
benign prostatic hyperplasia (BPH), 852, 858t
bladder cancer, 703
blindness, 1067, 1067f
bone cancer, 912
brain tumors, 968, 968f
bronchiectasis, 534
bulimia nervosa, 1185
burns, 1138–1140, 1139f, 1140t, 1141f, 1153t
cardiomyopathy, 369–370, 369t
cardiovascular disease, 323
cataracts, 1073
cellulitis, 1124
cerebral aneurysm, 1010
cervical cancer, 841
chlamydia, 871, 872t
cholecystitis, cholelithiasis, choledocholithiasis, 669, 670t, 672t
chronic heart failure (HF), 429, 430t, 431
chronic kidney disease (CKD), 711–714, 711t, 713b, 713f
chronic liver disease and cirrhosis, 657, 657t, 658f
chronic obstructive pulmonary disease (COPD), 547, 547t
chronic pancreatitis, 664
colorectal cancer, 639, 639t
condylomata (HPV), 872t
constipation, 619, 619t
contact dermatitis, 285
coronary artery disease (CAD), 381, 381f
Crohn disease, 626, 629t
Cushing syndrome, 759, 759f
cyclic breast discomfort, 816
cystic fibrosis (CF), 554–555
cystocele, 829
dehydration, 53
dementia, 984
depression, 1179t
dermatitis, 1119
dermoid cysts, 841
deviated septum, 520
diabetes insipidus, 740, 741t
diabetes mellitus, 768, 777t
diabetic nephropathy, 706
diabetic retinopathy, 1069
diarrhea, 621, 622t
disorders related to development of the genital organs, 828
displacement disorders, 831t

disseminated intravascular coagulation (DIC), 472
diverticulosis and diverticulitis, 624–625, 625t
dysmenorrhea, 823
ear disorders, 1081t
ear trauma, 1081
encephalitis, 953–954, 954t
endometrial cancer, 842
endometriosis, 824
esophageal cancer, 603
external ear infection, 1079
eye disorders, 1061t
eye trauma, 1075
fibroid tumors, 839
flail chest, 561
fluid excess, 55
fractures, 901–902
gastric bleeding, 611–612, 612t
gastric cancer, 613, 613t
gastritis, 607
gastroesophageal reflux disease (GERD), 605, 606t
genital parasites, 878
genital warts, 877–878, 878f
glaucoma, 1071
glomerulonephritis, 707, 708t
goiter, 751, 752f
gonorrhea, 872, 872t
gout, 913
growth hormone deficiency, 743
Guillain-Barré syndrome (GBS), 1030
Hashimoto thyroiditis, 289
hearing loss, 1076t
hemolytic transfusion reaction, 283t
hemophilia, 473–474
hepatitis, 652–653, 653f
herniated discs, 971
herpes simplex, 872t, 876–877, 877f
herpes simplex lesions, 1123
herpes zoster (shingles), 1124
hiatal hernia, 605
HIV/AIDS, 302, 303f, 303t
Hodgkin lymphoma, 480–481
Huntington disease, 992–993, 993f
hypercalcemia, 64
hyperkalemia, 61
hypernatremia, 59
hyperparathyroidism, 755
hypertension, 343, 343t
hyperthyroidism, 747t, 749, 749f
hypocalcemia, 62, 62f, 63f
hypogammaglobulinemia, 294
hypokalemia, 60
hyponatremia, 58
hypoparathyroidism, 754, 755t
hypothyroidism, 746
idiopathic autoimmune hemolytic anemia, 288
immune thrombocytopenic purpura (ITP), 473
impacted cerumen, 1080
increased intracranial pressure (ICP), 955
infective endocarditis (IE), 363, 364f, 364t
inner ear tumors, 1087
irritable bowel syndrome (IBS), 631
irritations and inflammations of the vagina and vulva, 826
keratitis, 1064
kidney cancer, 705

labyrinthitis, 1086
large-bowel obstruction, 636
laryngeal cancer, 527, 528t
laryngitis, 525
leukemia, 475, 476t
lower gastrointestinal bleeding, 638
lung cancer, 564, 567t
macular degeneration, 1074
male infertility, 866
malignant breast disorders, 816, 820t
masses of external ear, 1081
mastitis, 816
Ménière disease, 1087
meningitis, 952–953, 953f
menopause, 824
middle ear infections, 1083
middle ear trauma, 1085
mitral regurgitation, 357–358
mitral stenosis, 356–357
mitral valve prolapse (MVP), 354
multiple myeloma, 479
multiple sclerosis (MS), 1021–1022, 1021b
myasthenia gravis (MG), 1027
myocardial infarction (MI), 386, 386t
myocarditis, 368
non-Hodgkin lymphomas, 482, 482f
oral cancer, 603
osteoarthritis (OA), 915
osteomyelitis, 909
osteoporosis, 911
otosclerosis, 1084
ovarian cancer, 842
pancreatic cancer, 667
Parkinson disease, 989, 989f, 990t
pediculosis, 1128
pelvic inflammatory disease (PID), 870
peptic ulcer disease (PUD), 608, 609t
pericarditis, 366, 366t
peripheral arterial disease (PAD), 394
peritonitis, 624
pernicious anemia, 288
pharyngitis, 523
pheochromocytoma, 756
pleural effusion, 544
pleurisy, 543
pneumonia, 539, 540t
pneumothorax, 559–560, 561t
polycystic ovary syndrome (PCOS), 840
polycythemia, 471
postpolio syndrome, 1031
premature atrial contractions (PACs), 413
premature ventricular contractions (PVCs), 416
pressure injuries, 1112
prostate cancer, 858
prostatitis, 849
psoriasis, 1120, 1121f
pulmonary edema, 428, 428t
pulmonary embolism (PE), 557, 559t
pulmonary fibrosis, 545
rectocele, 829
refractive errors, 1066
renal calculi, 700, 700t
reproductive system cysts, 840
respiratory viruses, 526
restless legs syndrome (RLS), 1031
retinal detachment, 1070
rheumatoid arthritis (RA), 919–920, 920f

Signs and symptoms (*continued*)
  rib fractures, 560–561
  scabies, 1129
  schizophrenia, 1180–1181, 1181t
  seizure disorders, 959–960
  sepsis, 110f
  shock, 106, 107t
  sickle cell anemia, 468, 469f
  sinus bradycardia, 409
  sinusitis, 521
  sinus tachycardia, 411
  sleep apnea, 522
  small-bowel obstruction, 636, 636t
  spinal cord injuries, 974–976, 975f, 978t
  stroke, 1002–1003, 1004t, 1017t
  substance use disorders, 1189t
  syndrome of inappropriate ADH (SIADH), 741t, 742, 742b
  syphilis, 872t, 875
  systemic lupus erythematosus (SLE), 290, 291t, 292f
  testicular cancer, 861
  third-degree atrioventricular block, 415
  thyroid disorders, 747t
  thyroid gland cancer, 752
  tonsillitis/adenoiditis, 525
  toxic shock syndrome (TSS), 826
  transplant rejection, 286, 286t
  traumatic brain injury (TBI), 963–964, 964f, 967t
  trichomoniasis, 872t, 876
  trigeminal neuralgia (TN), 1033, 1033f
  tuberculosis (TB), 541
  ulcerative colitis, 629, 629t
  urinary tract infection (UTI), 696, 696t
  urticaria, 280
  uterine position disorders, 829
  uterine prolapse, 830
  varicose veins, 397
  venous thromboembolism (VTE) disease, 373, 373t
  ventricular fibrillation, 417
  ventricular tachycardia, 417
  vigilance about, 5
  viral rhinitis/common cold, 522, 523t
  vulvar cancer, 841
Silent ischemia, 384
Single-photon emission computed tomography (SPECT-CT) thallium imaging, 332t
Sinoatrial (SA) node, 318, 320f
  arrhythmias originating in, 409, 410–411t, 410f, 411–412, 411f
Sinus bradycardia, 409, 410f
Sinuses, 494, 497f
  disorders of, 518–522, 519f, 520b, 521f
  sinusitis, 520–521
Sinusitis, 520–521
Sinus tachycardia, 106, 196, 409, 411–412, 411f
Situation-Background-Assessment/Analysis Recommendation (SBAR), 5
Skeletal system. *See also* Musculoskeletal system
  aging and, 22f, 223–224, 887, 890f
  appendicular joints, 887t
  muscles, 886
  structure of, 885–886, 886f, 887f
  synovial joints, 885, 888f
  tissues and function of, 884–885

Skeletal traction, 903–904
Skene's glands, 793f
Skin. *See also* Integumentary system
  aging and, 225, 1094, 1094f
  atopic dermatitis, 279
  blood vessels of, 1094
  Braden Skin Scale, 16, 1108, 1109–1111t
  cancer, 145, 145f, 1132–1134, 1133f
  in chronic heart failure (HF), 431
  color of, 1096
  contact dermatitis, 285–286, 287
  cyanosis of, 328
  as defense mechanism against infections, 88
  diagnostic tests, 1100
  dressings for, 1101, 1103–1104, 1103–1104t, 1113
  frostbite of, 201
  glands of, 1092, 1093f
  grafting of, 1144–1145, 1145f
  moistness of, 1096
  normal anatomy and physiology, 1091–1094, 1092f, 1093f
  physical examination of, 1096–1099, 1097–1098f, 1099t
  plastic or reconstructive surgery, 1134, 1135f
  receptors on, 1092
  spinal cord injuries and breakdown of, 975
  structure of, 1091–1092, 1092f
  testing for immune system, 274t
  tetanus and, 195
  therapeutic measures, 1100–1104, 1103–1104t
  total hip replacement and breakdown of, 922
  turgor, 53, 1098
  ulcers in, 398
  wounds to, 194
Skin disorders, 1107–1137
  burns, 199–200, 1138–1154
  home health care, 1134
  infectious, 1121–1128, 1122t, 1123f, 1125–1127t, 1127f
  inflammatory, 1118–1121, 1118t, 1121f
  lesions, 1096, 1097f, 1098f, 1130, 1130–1132t, 1133f
  parasitic, 1128–1130, 1129f
  pressure injuries, 1107–1118, 1109–1111t, 1114f, 1115–1116f
Skin traction, 903
Skull, 885
Sleep and rest
  aging and, 231
  changes at end of life, 254
  chronic heart failure (HF) and, 438
  pain effects on, 133
Sleep apnea, 521–522, 521f
Sleeve gastrectomy, 601, 602f
Small-bowel obstruction, 635–636, 636f, 636t
Small cell lung cancer (SCLC), 563
Small House model, 237t, 238
Small incision lenticule extraction (SMILE), 1067
Small intestine, 573f, 574, 575t
Smoking
  acute pancreatitis and, 663
  atherosclerosis and, 379
  bladder cancer and, 703
  cancer and, 145, 148
  cardiovascular system and, 337, 379

  cessation of, 499, 500t, 548, 549f
  chronic obstructive pulmonary disease (COPD) and, 546–547
  chronic pancreatitis and, 664
  lung cancer and, 564
  malignant breast disorders and, 816
  pancreatic cancer and, 667
  surgery and, 167
Smooth muscle relaxers, 850t
Snakebites, 203–204
Snellen chart, 1043, 1044f
Social anxiety disorder, 1170
Social determinants of health (SDOH), 343–344
Social isolation in schizophrenia, 1180
Social media, 28
Social organization, 35
Sodium, food sources of, 56t
Sodium chloride solutions, 73–74
Sodium-glucose cotransporter 2 (SGLT2) inhibitors, 435–436, 776t
Sodium imbalances, 58–60, 58b
Sodium intake, 57
  chronic heart failure (HF) and, 432, 440
Sodium-potassium pumps, 51
Solutions
  balanced electrolyte, 74
  crystalloid, 73–74
  osmolarity of, 51–52, 74
Soma, 930f
Somatic pain, 122
Somatostatin, 1157t
Somatotropin, 725f
Somogyi effect, 777
Sonography, 804
Space, personal, 34–37
  time orientation and, 35
Specific phobias, 1170
Speed shock, intravenous (IV) therapy, 78t
Sperm, 792, 794, 795
Spermatozoa, 795
Spermicides, 836–837
Spider angiomas, 582
Spinal blocks, 176
Spinal cord
  ankylosing spondylitis and, 293–294
  compression of, 162
  cross section, 931, 932f
  reflexes, 931, 933f
  spinal nerves, 931, 933f
  trauma to, 195–196, 196f, 197, 197t
  vertebral column and, 885, 887f
Spinal cord injuries, 195–196, 196f, 197, 197t, 974–983
  aging and, 979
  complications, 975
  diagnostic tests, 975
  etiology and types, 974
  nursing care plan, 979–983
  nursing process, 978
  pathophysiology, 974
  signs and symptoms, 974–976, 975f
  surgical management, 978
  therapeutic measures, 975
Spinal disorders, 971–974
  herniated discs, 971–973, 971f
  nursing process for spinal surgery, 973–974
  spinal stenosis, 973, 973f

Spinal shock, 975
Spinal stenosis, 973, 973f
Spiral fractures, 902t, 903f
Spiritual distress, 216
Spirituality, 24, 32–33
　spiritual distress and, 216
　suffering and, 119
Spleen, 453
　disorders of, 482–484
Splenectomy, 275, 483–484
Splenomegaly, 427, 482–483
Splinter hemorrhages, nails, 1099t
Splints, 902–903, 947
Split-thickness skin graft, 1144–1145, 1145f, 1145t
Splitting, 1183
Spongy bone, 885
Sprains, 900
Sputum culture, 496–497, 499f
Squamous cell carcinoma, 1132–1133, 1133f
Stable angina, 380
Standard precautions, 94–95t, 96
Stapedectomy, 1084
Staphylococcus aureus, 92
　cellulitis, 1124
　osteomyelitis and, 909
　preoperative nasal cultures for, 167
　toxic shock syndrome (TSS) and, 826–828
Starling's law, 319
State boards of nursing, 26
Statins, 380t
　for coronary artery disease (CAD), 383, 383t
　for myocardial infarction (MI), 389t
　for stroke, 1007t
Status asthmaticus, 552
Status epilepticus, 962
STEADI (Stopping Elderly Accidents, Deaths & Injuries) initiative, 238
Steatorrhea, 615
Stem cell transplant, 476
Stenosis, 353
　aortic, 355–356t, 358
　mitral, 355t, 356–357, 357f
Stents, 399
Stereotypes, 32
Sterilization, 837
Sternotomy, 339
Sternum, 885
Stomach, 573–574, 573f, 574f, 575t
Stomas, 639, 641f, 642–643, 643f, 643t.
　See also Ostomy
Stomatitis, 154
Stool tests, 583, 583t, 588
　in diarrhea, 622
Strain echocardiogram, 332t
Strains, 899
Stratum germinativum, 1091–1092
Strep throat, 523
Streptococcus
　cellulitis, 1124
Stress fractures, 902t, 903f
Stress incontinence, 690
Stress-induced gastritis, 607
Stressors, 1158
Stress response, 938, 1170, 1171t
Striae, 582
Stroke, 1000–1009
　acute signs and symptoms, 1002–1003, 1004t
　air pollution and risk of, 1012
　diagnostic tests, 1003, 1005f
　etiology of, 1001–1002, 1001b, 1001f, 1002f
　hemorrhagic, 1002
　ischemic, 1001–1002, 1001b, 1001f, 1002f
　long-term effects, 1008–1009, 1008f, 1009f
　pathophysiology, 1001
　prevention, 1008
　summary, 1017t
　therapeutic measures, 1006–1008, 1007t
　warning signs of, 1002
Stroke volume, heart, 319
ST segment, 407, 407f
St. Thomas's Risk Assessment Tool in Falling Elderly Inpatients (STRATIFY), 239
Student nurses, 17
Subarachnoid hemorrhage, 1010–1012, 1010f, 1011f
Subarachnoid space, 933
Subarachnoid stroke, 1002
Subclinical infection, 83
Subcutaneous immunotherapy (SCIT), 275
Subcutaneous infusion, 81
Subdural hematoma, 964, 964f
Subjective data. *See also* Data collection; Objective data
　cardiovascular system, 324–325t
　diabetes mellitus, 783t
　ear, 1051t
　endocrine system, 734t
　eye infection and inflammation, 1065t
　female reproductive system, 797–798t
　hearing loss, 1078t
　hematologic and lymphatic systems, 454, 455t
　immune system, 268–270, 269t
　infective endocarditis (IE), 365t
　integumentary system, 1094–1095t
　male reproductive system, 808–809t
　middle ear, tympanic membrane, and mastoid disorders, 1086t
　musculoskeletal system, 891t
　respiratory system, 492, 493t
　urinary system, 680–681t
Sublingual immunotherapy (SLIT), 275
Substance P, 1157t
Substance use disorders, 1186–1190
　overdose, 202–204
　spinal cord injuries and, 975
　surgery and, 167
　types, 1187–1188
Suctioning, tracheostomy tube, 510
Sudden cardiac death, 384
　pacemakers and, 436
Suffering, 119
Suicide and older adults, 1191
Sulci, 934, 935f
Sulfonamides, 99t
　for urinary tract infection (UTI), 698t
Sulfonylureas, 775t
Summons, 28
Superficial muscles, 886, 889f
Superior vena cava syndrome (SVCS), 162
　due to lung cancer, 564
Support groups for substance use disorders, 1188
Suprapubic urinary catheters, 692
Surface trauma, 194–195

Surgery, 164–191
　abdominal aortic aneurysm (AAA), 397
　abdominal hernias, 634
　adrenalectomy, 760–761
　amputation, 194–195, 924–926
　appendectomy, 623
　atrial fibrillation (AF), 414
　bariatric, 600–602, 602f
　benign prostatic hyperplasia (BPH), 853–857, 853f, 854f, 857f
　bone cancer, 913
　brain tumors, 968
　breast modification, 821–822, 821–822f
　cancer, 151
　cardiac, 338–340, 339f
　cardiac transplantation, 441–445, 442f
　cardiac valve repair, 361–362
　cataracts, 1073
　cerebral aneurysm, 1011, 1011f
　cholecystectomy, 670, 671f
　chronic heart failure (HF), 437
　cochlear implant, 1077f
　colorectal cancer, 639, 640–641, 640t
　coronary artery bypass graft (CABG), 389–390, 390f
　for Crohn disease, 627
　defined, 164
　dermatological, 1134, 1135t
　discharge after, 189
　diverticulosis and diverticulitis, 625
　ear, 1087, 1087b
　endarterectomy, 399–400, 1008
　gastric, 613–614f, 613–615
　glaucoma, 1072, 1072f
　gynecological, 843–845
　hematomas, 964
　hemorrhoids, 638
　herniated discs, 972–973
　hiatal hernia, 605, 606f
　hospital room preparation, 172, 174t
　hypophysectomy, 741, 744–745, 745f
　hysterectomy, 823, 844–845
　intracranial, 969–971
　intraoperative phase, 166t, 174–178, 175b, 175f, 177f
　kidney transplantation, 718, 718f
　for laryngeal cancer, 528–531, 528f, 529f
　liver transplantation, 662
　for lung cancer, 565, 566f
　for malignant breast disorders, 817
　middle ear, 1084
　musculoskeletal, 921–926, 922f, 923b, 924f
　nose, 520, 520b
　oral cancer, 603, 605f
　for osteoarthritis (OA), 916
　pancreatic cancer, 667–668, 668f
　parathyroidectomy, 756
　Parkinson disease, 990
　patient arrival in surgery department, 172–174
　in patients with diabetes mellitus, 782–783
　penile implant, 864, 864f
　postoperative phase, 166t, 178–189, 178b, 180b, 180f, 185–187f, 186t
　preadmission surgical patient assessment, 167
　preoperative phase, 166–167, 166t, 168t, 170t, 173t
　preparation for, 172

Surgery (continued)
　procedure suffixes, 165t
　radical prostatectomy, 854, 857, 857f, 859
　recovery from intestinal, 644t
　for removal of emphysematous lung tissue, 549
　retinal detachment, 1070
　for rheumatoid arthritis (RA), 920
　rhinoplasty, 520
　seizure disorders, 960
　septoplasty, 520
　skin cancer, 1134
　spinal, 972–974
　spinal cord injuries, 978
　splenectomy, 275
　stroke and, 1008
　thoracic, 566–568
　thyroidectomy, 749, 752, 753–754
　tonsillectomy, 525
　total joint replacement (TJR), 921–924, 922f, 923b, 924f
　transfer from, 177–178, 177f
　transfer to surgery department, 172
　transurethral resection of the prostate (TURP), 853–854, 853f, 854f
　types and phases of, 164–174
　ulcerative colitis, 629
　urgency level and purpose, 165t
　vascular, 398–399, 399f
　vasectomy, 861–862, 862f
　wound care after, 185–187, 185f, 186f, 186t, 187f
Surgical asepsis, 93
Surgical debridement, 1113
Surgical team, 175b
Surgical wound infections, 96
Survey process, 29
Survivorship, cancer and, 161
Susceptible host, 87
Swine flu, 527
Sympathetic nervous system, 934, 936, 937f
Sympatholytics, 346–347t
Sympathomimetics, 284t
Symptom data collection, 2b
Synapses, 930–931
Synaptic knob, 930f
Synarthrosis, 885
Syndrome of inappropriate ADH (SIADH), 564–565, 740, 741t, 742–743, 742b
Synovial joints, 885, 888f
Syphilis, 306, 872t, 875–876, 876f
　antibiotics for, 873–874t
Systematic desensitization, 1172
Systematic reviews, 10
Systemic lupus erythematosus (SLE), 289–293, 291t, 292f
　medications associated with triggering, 289b

T

Tachycardia, 106, 196
　automatic external defibrillators (AEDs) for, 421, 421f
　chronic heart failure (HF) and, 429
　defibrillation for, 420, 420f
　sinus, 409, 411–412, 411f
　ventricular, 416–417
Tachypnea, 106, 204
Tai chi, 224

Targeted therapies for malignant breast disorders, 817
Target-organ disease, 345
Tarsal glands, 1039f
T-cell modulators, 918t
T cells, 264, 451, 453
　cell-mediated immunity, 264–265, 266f
Team, health-care
　collaboration among, 2, 7, 13, 17
　communication with, 5–6
Teamwork, evidence-based practice (EBP), 13
Technetium pyrophosphate or technetium-99m (TC-99m) sestamibi imaging, 333t, 336
Technology
　assistive, 224, 224f
　for chronic heart failure (HF), 436–437, 436–437f
　robotic-assisted surgery, 166
　telenursing, 245
Teeth, 572
Telenursing, 245
Temporal lobe, 935f
Temporary pacemakers, 418
Tension headaches, 958
Tension pneumothorax, 111, 559
Tenting, 53
Terminal restlessness at end of life, 254
Testes, 724f, 725f, 792, 795f
Testicular disorders, 860–861
Testicular self-examination (TSE), 810, 811b, 811f, 812t, 861
Testosterone, 794t
Testosterone suppressing/blocking agents, 850t
Tetanus, 195
Tetany, 754
Tetracyclic antidepressants, 1174t
Tetracyclines, 99t
　for sexually transmitted infections (STIs), 873t, 874t
Tetrahydrocannabinol (THC), 47
Thalamus, 933
Theological perspectives, 24
Therapeutic communication, 1161, 1163, 1163t
Therapeutic measures
　abdominal hernias, 633–634
　absorption disorders, 635
　acne vulgaris, 1127
　acromegaly, 744
　acute kidney injury (AKI), 710
　acute liver failure, 656
　acute pancreatitis, 663t, 664
　acute respiratory distress syndrome (ARDS), 563
　acute respiratory failure, 562
　adrenocortical insufficiency (AI), 757
　after cardiac transplantation, 443
　allergic rhinitis, 278–279
　Alzheimer disease, 996
　amyotrophic lateral sclerosis (ALS), 1029
　anaphylaxis, 279, 280t
　anemia, 463
　aneurysms, 397, 397t
　angioedema, 281
　ankylosing spondylitis, 294
　anorexia nervosa, 1185
　anxiety, obsessive-compulsive, or trauma-related disorders, 1172, 1175t
　aortic regurgitation, 359

　aortic stenosis, 358
　aplastic anemia, 466
　appendicitis, 623
　arterial thrombosis and embolism, 394
　asthma, 552–553f, 552–554, 554t
　asystole, 418
　atherosclerosis, 379, 379t
　atopic dermatitis, 279
　atrial fibrillation (AF), 414
　atrial flutter, 413
　autism spectrum disorders (ADSs), 1184
　Bartholin cysts, 841
　Bell palsy, 1033–1034
　benign prostatic hyperplasia (BPH), 853–857, 853f, 854f, 857f, 858t
　bladder cancer, 703–705
　blindness, 1068
　bone cancer, 913
　brain tumors, 968–969
　bronchiectasis, 534
　bulimia nervosa, 1186
　burns, 1142–1146, 1142t, 1144–1145t, 1144–1146f, 1153t
　cancer, 151–156
　cardiomyopathy, 369t, 370
　cardiovascular system, 337–340
　cellulitis, 1124
　cerebral aneurysm, 1010–1011
　cervical cancer, 841–842, 842f
　chlamydia, 871, 872t
　cholecystitis, cholelithiasis, choledocholithiasis, 670–671, 671f, 672t
　chronic heart failure (HF), 430t, 432–437, 433–435t, 436–437f
　chronic kidney disease (CKD), 711t, 714–717, 715–717f, 715b, 717b
　chronic liver disease and cirrhosis, 657t
　chronic obstructive pulmonary disease (COPD), 547t, 548–550, 549f, 550t, 551f
　chronic pancreatitis, 664, 665t
　cirrhosis-associated disorders, 659–660, 659–660f
　colorectal cancer, 639, 639t
　condylomata (HPV), 872t
　constipation, 619, 619t
　contact dermatitis, 285–286
　coronary artery disease (CAD), 381
　Crohn disease, 627, 628t, 629t
　Cushing syndrome, 759–760
　cyclic breast discomfort, 816
　cystic fibrosis (CF), 555
　cystocele, 829
　dehydration, 53
　dementia, 984, 987t
　depression, 1179t
　dermatitis, 1119
　dermoid cysts, 841
　deviated septum, 520
　diabetes insipidus, 740–741, 741t
　diabetes mellitus, 770–777, 771–773f, 772t, 774–776t, 776–777f, 777t
　diabetic ketoacidosis (DKA), 780
　diabetic nephropathy, 706
　diabetic retinopathy, 1069
　diarrhea, 622, 622t
　disorders related to development of the genital organs, 829

displacement disorders, 829, 831t
disseminated intravascular coagulation (DIC), 472
diverticulosis and diverticulitis, 625
dysmenorrhea, 823
ear and hearing, 1055f, 1056–1057, 1056–1057t
ear disorders, 1081–1082, 1081t
encephalitis, 954, 954t
endometrial cancer, 842
endometriosis, 824
epistaxis, 519, 519f
erectile dysfunction, 863–865, 864f
esophageal cancer, 603–604
eye and vision, 1046–1048, 1047t
eye disorders, 1061t
eye trauma, 1075
fertility disorders, 831–832, 866
fibrocystic breast disease, 816
fibroid tumors, 839
flail chest, 561
fluid excess, 55
fractures, 902–906, 904b, 905f
gastric bleeding, 612
gastric cancer, 613, 613f, 613t
gastritis, 607
gastroesophageal reflux disease (GERD), 606, 606t
gastrointestinal, hepatobiliary and pancreatic systems, 591–596, 591f, 592–594t
genital parasites, 878
genital warts, 878
glaucoma, 1071
glomerulonephritis, 708, 708t
goiter, 751–752
gonorrhea, 872t, 875
gout, 913
growth hormone deficiency, 743
Guillain-Barré syndrome (GBS), 1031
Hashimoto thyroiditis, 289
hearing loss, 1076–1077, 1076t, 1077f
hematologic and lymphatic systems, 458–460, 458t
hemolytic transfusion reaction, 283, 283t
hemophilia, 474
hepatitis, 653, 653b
herniated discs, 972
herpes simplex, 872t, 877, 1123
herpes zoster (shingles), 1124
hiatal hernia, 605
HIV/AIDS, 303t, 306–314
Hodgkin lymphoma, 481
Huntington disease, 993
hypercalcemia, 64
hyperkalemia, 61–62
hypernatremia, 60
hyperosmolar hyperglycemic state (HHS), 780
hyperparathyroidism, 755–756
hypertension, 343t, 345
hyperthyroidism, 749–750
hypocalcemia, 63, 63t
hypogammaglobulinemia, 294–295
hypokalemia, 60–61, 61b
hyponatremia, 59
hypoparathyroidism, 754
hypothyroidism, 746
idiopathic autoimmune hemolytic anemia, 288

immune system, 275
immune thrombocytopenic purpura (ITP), 473
infectious diseases, 97–100t, 97–101
infective endocarditis (IE), 363–364, 364t
inner ear tumors, 1087
integumentary system, 1100–1104, 1103–1104t
irritable bowel syndrome (IBS), 631–632
irritations and inflammations of the vagina and vulva, 826
keratitis, 1064
kidney cancer, 705
labyrinthitis, 1086
large-bowel obstruction, 637
laryngeal cancer, 528, 528f, 528t, 529f
laryngitis, 525
leukemia, 476, 476t
lower gastrointestinal bleeding, 638
lung cancer, 565, 565t, 567f
macular degeneration, 1074–1075
malignant breast disorders, 817, 820t
mastitis, 816
Ménière disease, 1087–1088
meningitis, 953
menopause, 824
menstrual flow and cycle disorders, 823
mental health, 1161–1167, 1163–1164t
middle ear infections, 1083–1084
mitral regurgitation, 358
mitral stenosis, 357, 357f
mitral valve prolapse (MVP), 356
mood disorders, 1177
multiple myeloma, 479–480
multiple sclerosis (MS), 1022–1023, 1022–1023t, 1024b
myasthenia gravis (MG), 1027
myocardial infarction (MI), 386t, 387–389, 387b, 388–389t, 388f
myocarditis, 368
nasal polyps, 520
nausea and vomiting, 599
neurologic system, 946–948, 947f
non-Hodgkin lymphomas, 482
obesity, 599
oral cancer, 603, 605f
osteoarthritis (OA), 916, 917–918t
osteomyelitis, 910
otosclerosis, 1084
ovarian cancer, 842
for pain, 123–130, 124–125t, 126t, 129–130t
pancreatic cancer, 667–668, 668f
Parkinson disease, 990, 991t
pediculosis, 1129
pelvic inflammatory disease (PID), 871
peptic ulcer disease (PUD), 609t, 610
pericarditis, 366t, 367
peripheral arterial disease (PAD), 395
peritonitis, 624
pernicious anemia, 288
personality disorders, 1183
pharyngitis, 523
pheochromocytoma, 756–757
pleural effusion, 544
pleurisy, 544
pneumonia, 540, 540t
pneumothorax, 560, 561t
polycystic ovary syndrome (PCOS), 840

polycythemia, 471
postpolio syndrome, 1031
premature atrial contractions (PACs), 413
premature ventricular contractions (PVCs), 416
premenstrual syndrome and premenstrual dysphoric disorder, 822
pressure injuries, 1112–1114, 1114f
prostate cancer, 858–859
prostatitis, 849, 850–851t
psoriasis, 1121
pulmonary edema, 428–429, 428t
pulmonary embolism (PE), 558, 559t
pulmonary fibrosis, 545
reactive hypoglycemia, 786
rectocele, 829
refractive errors, 1067
renal calculi, 700t, 701, 701f
reproductive system cysts, 840
respiratory system, 499–516, 500t, 502–505f, 507–510f, 507b, 513f, 514t, 515b, 515f
respiratory viruses, 526
restless legs syndrome (RLS), 1031
retinal detachment, 1070
rheumatoid arthritis (RA), 920
rib fractures, 561
scabies, 1130
schizophrenia, 1181, 1181t, 1182t
shock, 111, 111t, 112–113t
sickle cell anemia, 469–470
sinus bradycardia, 409, 410–411t
sinusitis, 521
sinus tachycardia, 411–412
skin cancer, 1134
sleep apnea, 522
small-bowel obstruction, 636, 636t
spinal cord injuries, 975, 978t
stroke, 1006–1008, 1007t, 1017t
substance use disorders, 1188–1189, 1189t
syndrome of inappropriate ADH (SIADH), 741t, 742
syphilis, 872t, 876
systemic lupus erythematosus (SLE), 290, 291t
testicular cancer, 861
third-degree atrioventricular block, 415
thyroid gland cancer, 752
tonsillitis/adenoiditis, 525
toxic shock syndrome (TSS), 827
transplant rejection, 286–287
traumatic brain injury (TBI), 964–965, 967t
trichomoniasis, 872t, 876
trigeminal neuralgia (TN), 1033
tuberculosis (TB), 542–543
ulcerative colitis, 628t, 629, 629t
urinary system, 690–693, 690b, 692b, 692f
urinary tract infection (UTI), 696t, 698t
urticaria, 280
uterine or cervical polyps, 840
uterine position disorders, 829
uterine prolapse, 830
varicose veins, 397–398
venous stasis ulcers, 398
venous thromboembolism (VTE) disease, 373t, 374
ventricular fibrillation, 417–418
ventricular tachycardia, 417
viral rhinitis/common cold, 522
vulvar cancer, 841

Thermography, 800, 806t
Thermoregulation
    burns and, 1139
    hyperthermia, 201–202, 202b
    hypothermia, 174, 200–201, 200t
Thiazide and thiazide-like diuretics
    for chronic heart failure (HF), 434t
    for hypertension, 346t
Third-degree atrioventricular block, 414–415, 414f
Third spacing, 52
Thoracentesis, 505–506
Thoracic cage, 885
Thoracic injuries, 976
Thoracic surgery, 566–568
Thoracic vertebrae, 885
Thoracotomy, 566
Thrill, 327
Throat culture, 497
Thrombectomy, 399
Thromboangiitis obliterans, 395
Thrombocytes, 450t
Thrombocytopenia, 154
Thrombolytic agents, 373t, 387–388, 389t
    for stroke, 1006, 1007t
Thrombophlebitis. *See* Venous thromboembolism (VTE) disease
Thrombosis, 77t, 387
    arterial, 393–394
    fractures and, 906
    postoperative, 182–183
    venous (*see* Venous thromboembolism (VTE) disease)
Thrombotic stroke, 1001
Thrombus, 357
Thrush, 604b, 1127t
Thymus, 453, 724f
Thyroidectomy, 749, 752, 753–754
Thyroid gland, 724, 724f, 725f, 726f
    biopsy of, 737
    nuclear scanning of, 737
    serum tests of, 732t
    ultrasound of, 737
Thyroid gland disorders
    goiter, 751–752, 752f
    hyperthyroidism, 227, 747t, 748–751, 749f
    hypothyroidism, 227, 745–748, 745t, 747t
    medications for, 761t
    thyroid cancer, 752–753
Thyroid-stimulating hormone (TSH), 724, 725f, 726f, 731t
Thyrotoxic crisis, 749, 754
Thyroxine, 732t
Tic douloureux, 1032–1033, 1033f
Tilt table test, 336
Time orientation, 35
Tinea, 1124
Tinea capitis, 1125t
Tinea corporis, 1126t
Tinea cruris, 1126t
Tinea pedis, 1125t
Tinea unguium, 1126t
Tissues, 142
T lymphocytes, 88, 451
Tobacco use. *See* Smoking
Tolerance, drug, 121
Tongue, 572–573

Tonic-clonic seizures, 960
Tonicity, 51
Tonsillitis, 525
Tonsils, 452–453
Topical medications for skin, 1101
Torts, 28
Total artificial heart, 436
Total colectomy, 640t
Total hip replacement (THR), 921–924, 922f, 923b
Total incontinence, 690
Total joint replacement (TJR), 921–924, 922f, 923b, 924f
Total knee replacement (TKR), 924, 924f
Total proctocolectomy, 640t
Toxemia, 106
Toxic shock syndrome (TSS), 826–828
Trachea, 487, 489f
Tracheoesophageal puncture (TEP), 528
Tracheostomy, 508–509f, 508–510, 511–513
Traction, 903–904
    for herniated discs, 972
Traditional Chinese medicine, 42, 43f
Traditions, 31
Transcellular fluid, 51, 51f
Transdermal contraceptive patch, 835
Transdermal patches, 126
Transduction of pain, 122
Transesophageal echocardiogram, 332t
Transfer from surgery, 177–178, 177f
Transfer to nursing unit, 180, 180f
Transfer to surgery, 172
Transfusion-associated circulatory overload (TACO), 460
Transfusion-related acute lung injury (TRALI), 460
Transgender population data collection, 812–813
Transient ischemic attack (TIA), 1000, 1003
Transillumination, 807
Transjugular intrahepatic portosystemic shunt (TIPS), 659
Transmission-based precautions, 94–95t, 96
Transmission of pain, 122
Transplantation
    kidney, 718, 718f
    liver, 662
    lung, 567
    pancreas, 777
    rejection of, 286–287, 286t
Transtracheal catheter, 503, 503f
Transurethral resection of the prostate (TURP), 853–854, 853f, 854f
Transverse fractures, 902t, 903f
Trauma
    abdominal, 196, 198
    cardiac, 368
    chest, 196–198, 559–562, 560f, 561t
    external ear, 1081
    eye, 1075
    head, 195, 196b
    infections related to, 198
    major, 194–199
    mechanism of injury in, 194
    middle ear, 1085
    nursing process for, 197–199, 197t, 198f
    orthopedic, 196
    renal system, 705

    spinal, 195–196, 196f, 197, 197t
    surface, 194–195
Trauma- and stressor-related disorders, 1172
    nursing process, 1172, 1176
    therapeutic measures, 1172
Traumatic amputation, 924
Traumatic brain injury (TBI), 963–967
    complications, 965–966, 965f
    diagnostic tests, 964
    nursing process, 966
    pathophysiology, 963
    rehabilitation, 966
    therapeutic measures, 964–965
    types and signs and symptoms, 963–964, 964f
Traumatic pneumothorax, 559
Treatment. *See* Therapeutic measures
Tremors, 225
    in Parkinson disease, 989
Triage, 192, 193f
    disaster response, 205
Triazoles, 100t
Trichomoniasis, 827t, 872t, 876
    amebicides/antiprotozoals for, 874t
Tricyclic antidepressants, 125t, 1174t
Trigeminal nerve, 935t
    trigeminal neuralgia, 1032–1033, 1033f
Trigeminal neuralgia (TN), 1032–1033, 1033f
Trigeminy, 416
Triglycerides, 331t, 334
Triiodothyronine, 732t
Trochlear nerve, 935t
Tropia, 1045
Trousseau sign, 62, 62f
T-SPOT test, 542
Tuberculin skin test, 541–542, 542t
Tuberculosis (TB), 540–543, 542t
    HIV/AIDS-associated, 304, 305t
Tubular reabsorption and secretion, 676, 678f
Tumor necrosis factor inhibitors, 917–918t
Tumor-node-metastasis (TNM) system, 150–151, 151t
Tumors, 142
    benign, 142, 144t
    brain, 967–969, 968f
    female reproductive system, 839–843, 842f, 843t
    inner ear, 1086–1087
    pituitary, 744–745, 745f
    types of, 146–147, 147t
Tunneled catheters, 79, 79f
Turgor, skin, 53, 1098
T waves, 406, 406f
Tympanic membrane, 1085–1086, 1086t
Tympanometry, 1055
Tympanosclerosis, 1083
Type 1 diabetes, 767, 767t
Type 2 diabetes, 767–768, 767t
Type I hypersensitivity reactions, 277–281, 278f, 280t
    allergic rhinitis, 278–279
    anaphylaxis, 279, 280t
    angioedema, 280–281
    atopic dermatitis, 279
    nursing process for, 281
    urticaria, 280
Type II hypersensitivity reactions, 281–283

hemolytic transfusion reaction, 282–283, 283t, 284t
Type III hypersensitivity reactions, 283–284, 285f
   serum sickness, 284
Type IV hypersensitivity reactions, 284–287, 286f
   contact dermatitis, 285–286, 287
   transplant rejection, 286–287, 286t
Typical antipsychotics, 1173t

U

Ulcerative colitis, 626, 626f, 627–629, 628t, 629t
Ulcers, skin, 1097f
Ultrasonography, 150
   endocrine system, 737
   eye, 1046
   female reproductive system, 799–800, 806t
   male reproductive system, 811, 812t
   musculoskeletal system, 894–895t, 896
Ultraviolet environment disinfection, 93
UltraVoice, 528
Unconsciousness at end of life, 254
Undetectable viral load, 306
Unilateral neglect after stroke, 1009
Unlicensed assistive personnel (AP), 13, 17
Upper gastrointestinal disorders, 598–617
   anorexia, 154, 598
   esophageal cancer, 603–604
   esophageal varices, 607
   gastric bleeding, 611–612, 612t
   gastric cancer, 612–613, 613f, 613t
   gastric surgery for, 613–614f, 613–615
   gastritis, 607, 607b, 608t
   gastroesophageal reflux disease (GERD), 605–606, 606t
   hiatal hernia, 604–605, 605f, 606f
   Mallory-Weiss tear (MWT), 606–607
   nausea and vomiting, 598–599
   obesity, 599–602, 600f, 602f
   oral cancer, 603, 605f
   oral health and dental care and, 602–603, 604b
   oral inflammatory disorders, 603
   peptic ulcer disease (PUD), 608–611, 609t, 610t
Upper respiratory tract disorders, 518–532
   infectious disorders, 522–527, 523t
   malignant disorders, 527–531, 528f, 528t, 529f
   nose and sinus disorders, 518–522, 519f, 520b, 521f
Ureteroscopy, 701
Ureters, 677
Urethra, 677, 794–795
Urethral strictures, 699
Urethritis, 696–697
   due to sexually transmitted infections (STIs), 870
Urge incontinence, 690
Uric acid, 890, 893t
   in gout, 913
Urinalysis, 683–684t
Urinary analgesics, 698t
Urinary bladder, 677
   cancer of, 702–705
Urinary catheters, 692, 692b, 702, 703f, 704f
Urinary function, postoperative, 183–184
Urinary incontinence
   bladder cancer and, 704–705
   management of, 690, 690b
   in older adults, 228
   skin injury due to, 1108
Urinary retention, 690, 692f
Urinary system, 675–694. *See also* Genitourinary and reproductive system
   aging and, 678–679, 679f
   burns and, 1139
   characteristics of urine, 677–678
   data collection, 679–682, 680–682t
   diagnostic procedures, 683–688t, 683–689, 689f
   elimination of urine, 677
   formation of urine, 676, 678f
   home health care, 693
   normal anatomy and physiology, 675–679, 676–679f, 678t
   spinal cord injuries and, 975
   therapeutic measures, 690–693, 690b, 692b, 692f
Urinary system disorders, 695–722
   acute kidney injury (AKI), 708–710, 710t
   chronic kidney disease (CKD), 706–707, 710–718, 711–712t, 713b, 713f, 715–717f, 715b
   glomerulonephritis, 707–708, 708t
   polycystic kidney disease, 705–706
   renal system trauma, 705
   renal system tumors, 702–705
   urinary tract infections (UTI), 96, 228, 695–699, 696t, 698t
   urological obstructions, 699–702, 699f, 700t, 701f
Urinary tract infection (UTI), 695–699
   catheter-associated, 96
   in older patients, 228
   risk factors for, 696
   signs and symptoms, 696, 696t
   therapeutic measures, 696t, 698t
   types of, 696–697
Urination reflex, 677
Urine
   characteristics of, 677–678
   elimination of, 677
   formation of, 676, 678f
   hydronephrosis, 702, 703f, 704f
Urine glucose monitoring, 776–777, 777f
Urine studies, 684–685t
Urine tests, 585t
   endocrine system hormones, 733
   preoperative, 168t
Urolithiasis, 699–702, 699f, 700t, 701f
Urological obstructions
   hydronephrosis, 702, 703f, 704f
   renal calculi, 699–702, 699f, 700t, 701f
   urethral strictures, 699
Urosepsis, 697, 852
Urticaria, 280, 459
Uterine position disorders, 829, 830f
Uterine prolapse, 830, 830f
Uterus, 791, 791f, 792f
   hysterectomy, 823, 844–845
Utilitarianism, 24
U waves, 406, 407f

V

Vaccines
   Bacillus Calmette-Guérin (BCG), 149, 541
   cancer prevention and, 148–149
   COVID-19, 526
   HPV (Gardasil), 842, 877
   meningitis, 952
   pneumococcal, 226, 228, 268, 305t, 470, 539, 545, 549, 569
   Shingrix, 228, 268, 1124
   varicella, 1124
Vacuum-assisted closure (VAC), 185
Vagina, 791, 791f, 792f
   irritations and inflammations of, 825–826, 827t, 828t
Vaginitis, 826, 827t
Vaginosis, 826, 827t
Vagus nerve, 936t, 938f
Valves, heart, 353–354, 354f
   rupture, as complication of myocardial infarction (MI), 385t
Valvuloplasty, 357, 357f
Vancomycin-resistant enterococci (VRE), 97
Varicella zoster
   herpes zoster (shingles), 228, 305t, 1123–1124, 1123f
   HIV/AIDS-associated, 305t
Varicocele, 807, 860
Varicose veins, 397–398
Vascular bypass surgery, 399
Vascular grafts, 399
Vascular inflammatory response, 88
Vascular surgery, 398–399, 399f
Vas deferens, 792
Vasectomy, 861–862, 862f
Vasodilators, 435t, 440, 850t
Vaso-occlusive crisis, 468
Vasopressors, 411t
Vasospasm, cerebral aneurysm, 1011
Vasospastic angina, 381
Veins, heart, 320, 322f
   venous thromboembolism (VTE) disease of, 370–374
Veins, varicose, 397–398
Venous air embolism, intravenous (IV) therapy, 78t
Venous insufficiency, 398
Venous spasm, intravenous (IV) therapy, 77t
Venous stasis ulcers, 398
Venous thromboembolism (VTE) disease, 76
   home health care, 374–375
   immobility and, 372
   IV therapy and, 372
   pancreatic cancer and, 667
   pathophysiology and etiology, 370–371, 371t
   prophylactic antiembolism devices and, 372
   prophylactic medications for, 372, 372–373t
   total hip replacement and, 923
Ventilation, 487
   mechanical, 513–515, 513f, 514t, 515b
Ventilation-perfusion scan, 499
Ventilator-associated pneumonia, 538
Ventricles, brain, 933
Ventricular assist devices, 436–437, 437f
Ventricular fibrillation (VF), 417–418, 418f
   automatic external defibrillators (AEDs) for, 421, 421f
   defibrillation for, 420, 420f
Ventricular tachycardia, 416–417
   automatic external defibrillators (AEDs) for, 421, 421f
   defibrillation for, 420, 420f
Veracity, 23
Verbal communication, 1163, 1163t

Vertebrae, 885, 887f
Vertebral column, 885, 887f
  herniated discs, 971–973, 971f
Vesicant medications, 153
Vesicles, 1097f
Vestibule, 793f
Vestibulocochlear nerve, 935t
Vibratory positive expiratory pressure device, 505, 505f
Video-assisted thoracoscopic surgery (VATS), 567
Video games, 224
Vigilance, 5
Viral infections
  conjunctivitis, 1060–1061
  hepatitis, 649–655, 650–652t, 653b, 653f, 654t
  pneumonia, 538
Viral load testing, HIV/AIDS, 306
Viral rhinitis/common cold, 522–523, 523t
Virchow's triad, 371, 371t
Viruses, 85, 85t
  cancer risk factor, 144
  respiratory, 525–527
Visceral pain, 122
Visceral sensory neurons, 930
Viscosity, blood, 342
Vision, 1038–1048. *See also* Eye
  aging and, 1041–1042, 1042f, 1045
  examination guidelines for, 1046
  normal anatomy and physiology of the eye, 1038–1041, 1039–1042f
  physiology of, 1040–1041, 1041f
  testing of, 1042–1044, 1044f, 1044t
  therapeutic measures, 1046–1048, 1047t
Vision disorders
  blindness, 1067–1069, 1067f, 1068b
  cataracts, 1067, 1067f, 1073
  conjunctivitis, 1060–1061
  diabetic retinopathy, 1067, 1067f, 1069–1070
  eye trauma, 1075
  glaucoma, 1067, 1067f, 1071–1072, 1072f
  infections and inflammation, 1060–1065, 1062–1063t, 1065t
  macular degeneration, 1067, 1067f, 1073–1075, 1074f, 1075f
  ophthalmic medications for, 1062–1063t
  refractive errors, 1065–1067, 1066f
  retinal detachment, 1070–1071
  summary, 1061t
Visual acuity, 1043–1044, 1044t
Visual disturbances with stroke, 1003, 1004f
Visual fields, 1043–1044, 1044f
Vital signs
  heart and great vessels trauma and, 198
  in shock, 197
Vitamin A deficiency, 1047
Vitamin B deficiency, 615
  vision and, 1047
Vitamin D, 576
  bone health and, 801, 802t
  for chronic kidney disease (CKD), 714
  osteoporosis and, 911, 912
Vitamin intake
  liver storage of, 576
  red blood cells and, 451
Vitamin K, 361
  deficiency of, in absorption disorders, 634
Volvulus, 635, 636f
Vulva, 791, 791f
  cancer of, 841
  irritations and inflammations of, 825–826, 827t, 828t
Vulvovaginitis, 870

W

Walking pneumonia, 538
Warfarin, 457
Warmed blood, 459
Warming, preoperative, 173–174
Warts, 1132t
Washed blood, 459
Water-pushing pressure, 51
Weakness with stroke, 1003
Wearable cardioverter defibrillator (WCD), 421
Weber test, 1052, 1054f, 1054t
Wedge resection, 565, 566, 566f
Weight loss
  chronic heart failure (HF) and, 432, 440
  diabetes mellitus and, 771
  osteoarthritis (OA) and, 916
  thyroid function and, 752–753
Wellness
  definition of, 211
  in long-term care facilities, 238–240
  nurse's role in supporting and promoting, 212
Wernicke-Korsakoff syndrome, 658–659
West Nile virus, 527
Wheal, 1097f
White blood cells (WBCs), 88, 263, 450t, 451
  disorders of, 475–478, 476t
Wong Baker FACES Pain Scale, 131, 132f
Wood light examination, 1100
Worldview, 32
Wound, ostomy, and continence nurse (WOCN), 643
Wound care, surgical, 185–187, 185f
  dehiscence and evisceration in, 185, 187f
  healing phases and, 186f, 186t
Wounds
  abrasion, 194
  amputation, 194–195
  avulsion, 194
  cleansing of skin, 1113
  closed versus open, 194
  laceration, 194
  puncture, 194
  skin cultures, 1100b
  surgical, 185–187, 185f, 186f, 186t, 187f
  tetanus, 195

X

Xenograft, 361
Xerostomia, 154, 604b
X-rays. *See* Radiography

Y

Yoga, 540
Young adult development stage, 212–213

Z

Zika virus disease, 90–91t, 91

Prefixes, Suffixes, and Combining Forms

a-, an-. Without; away from; not
ab-, abs-. From; away from; absent
abdomin-, abdomino-. Abdomen
-ad. Toward; in the direction of
aden-, adeno-. Gland
adip-, adipo-. Fat
-aemia. Blood
aer-, aero-. Air
-algesia, -algia. Suffering; pain
andro-. Man; male; masculine
angi-, angio-. Blood or lymph vessels
aniso-. Unequal; asymmetrical; dissimilar
ankyl-, ankylo-. Crooked; bent; fusion or growing together of parts
ant-, anti-. Against
ante-. Before
antero-. Anterior; front; before
arteri-, arterio-. Artery
arthr-, arthro-. Joint
-ase. Enzyme
-asis, esis, -iasis, -isis, -sis. Condition; pathological state
aut-, auto-. Self
axo-. Axis; axon
bacteri-, bacterio-. Bacteria; bacterium
bi-, bis-. Two; double; twice
bili-. Bile
bio-. Life
blast-, -blast. Germ; bud; embryonic state of development
blephar-, blepharo-. Eyelid
brady-. Slow
bronch-, bronchi-, broncho-. Airway
cardi-, cardio-. Heart
cat-, cata-, cath-, kat-, kata-. Down; downward; destructive; against; according to
cent-. Hundred
cephal-, cephalo-. Head
cervic-, cervice-. Head; the neck of an organ
chrom-, chromo-. Color
-cide. Causing death
contra-. Against; opposite
crani-, cranio-. Skull; cranium
cry-, cryo-. Cold
cyan-, cyano-. Blue
cyst, cysto-, -cyst. Cyst; urinary bladder
cyt-, cyto-, -cyte. Cell
derm-, derma-, dermato-, dermo-. Skin
di-. Double; twice; two; apart from
dors-, dorsi-, dorso-. Back
-dynia. Pain
dys-. Difficult; bad; painful
ec-, ecto-. Out; on the outside
-ectomy. Excision
ef-, es-, ex-, exo-. Out
electr-, electro-. Electricity
-emesis. Vomiting
-emia. Blood

en-. In; into
end-, endo-. Within
ent-, ento-. Within; inside
enter-, entero-. Intestine
ep-, epi-. Upon; over; at; in addition to; after
erythr-, erythro-. Red
eury-. Broad
ex-. Out; away from; completely
exo-. Out; outside of; without
extra-. Outside of; in addition; beyond
-facient. Causing; making happen
-ferous. Producing
ferri-, ferro-. Iron
fluo-. Flow
fore-. Before; in front of
-form. Form
-fuge. To expel; to drive away; fleeing
gaster-, gastero-, gastr-, gastro-. Stomach
gen-. Producing; forming
-gen, -gene, -genesis, -genetic, -genic. Producing; forming
glosso-. Tongue
gluc-, gluco-, glyc-, glyco-. Sugar; glycerol or similar substance
gyn-, gyne-, gyneco-, gyno-. Woman; female
hem-, hema-, hemato-, hemo-. Blood
hemi-. Half
hepat-, hepato-. Liver
heter-, hetero-. Other; different
histo-. Tissue
homo-. Same; likeness
hydra-, hydro-, hydr-. Water
hyp-, hyph-, hypo-. Less than; below; under
hyper-. Above; excessive; beyond
hyster-, hystero-. Uterus
-ia. Condition, esp. an abnormal state
-iasis. SEE *-asis*
-iatric. Medicine; medical profession; physicians
in-. In; inside; within; intensive action; negative
infra-. Below; under; beneath; inferior to; after
inter-. Between; in the midst
intra-, intro-. Within; in; into
ipsi-. Same
irid-, irido-. Iris
-ism. Condition; theory
iso-. Equal
-itis. Inflammation of
kera-, kerato-. Horny substance; cornea
kolp-, kolpo, colp-, colpo-. Vagina
kypho-. Humped
leuk-, leuko-. White; colorless; rel. to a leukocyte
lip-, lipo-. Fat
-lite, -lith, lith-, litho-. Stone; calculus

-logia, -logy. Science of; study of
lumbo-. Loins
-lysis. 1. Setting free; disintegration; 2. In medicine, reduction of; relief from
macr-, macro-. Large; long
mal-. Ill; bad; poor
med-, medi-, medio-. Middle
mega-, megal-, megalo-. Large; of great size
-megalia, -megaly. Enlargement of a body part
melan-, melano-. Black
mening-, meningo-. Meninges
-meter. Measure
metr-, metra-, metro-. Uterus
micr-, micro-. Small
mon-, mono-. Single; one
muc-, muci-, muco-, myxa-, myxo-. Mucus
multi-. Many; much
musculo-, my-, myo-. Muscle
my-, myo-. SEE *musculo-*
myel-, myelo-. Spinal cord; bone marrow
naso-. Nose
necr-, necro-. Death; necrosis
neo-. New; recent
nephr-, nephra-, nephro-. Kidney
neur-, neuri-, neuro-. Nerve; nervous system
non-. No
normo-. Normal; usual
oculo-. Eye
-ode, -oid. Form; shape; resemblance
-odynia, odyno-. Pain
olig-, oligo-. Few; small
-ology. Science of; study of
-oma. Tumor
onco-. Tumor; swelling; mass
oo-, ovi-, ovo-. Egg; ovum
oophor-, oophoro-, oophoron-. Ovary
ophthalm-, ophthalmo-. Eye
-opia. Vision
optico-, opto-. Eye; vision
orchi-, orchid-, orchido-. Testicle
orth-, ortho-. Straight; correct; normal; in proper order
os-. Mouth; bone
-osis. Condition; status, process; abnormal increase
oste-, osteo-. Bone
ostomosis, -ostomy, -stomosis, -stomy. A created mouth or outlet
ot-, oto-. Ear
-otomy. Cutting
-ous. 1. Possessing; full of; 2. Pertaining to
pan-. All; entire
para-, -para. 1. Prefix: Near; alongside of; departure from normal; 2. Suffix: Bearing offspring